KU-613-969

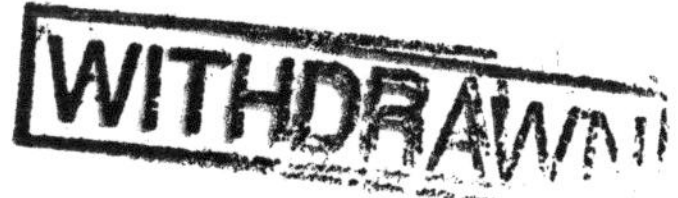
WITHDRAWN

Textbook of

VETERINARY DIAGNOSTIC RADIOLOGY

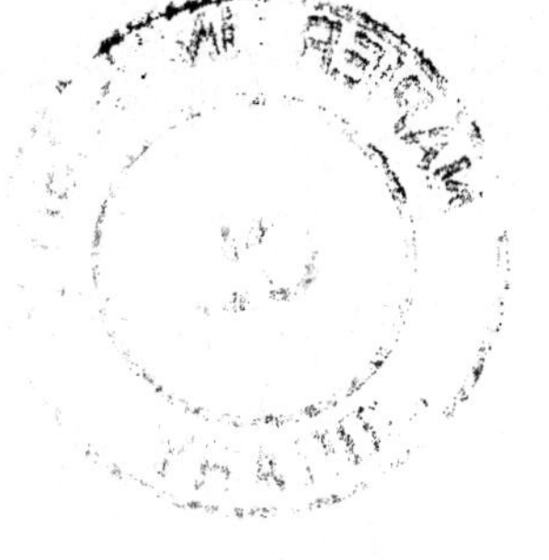

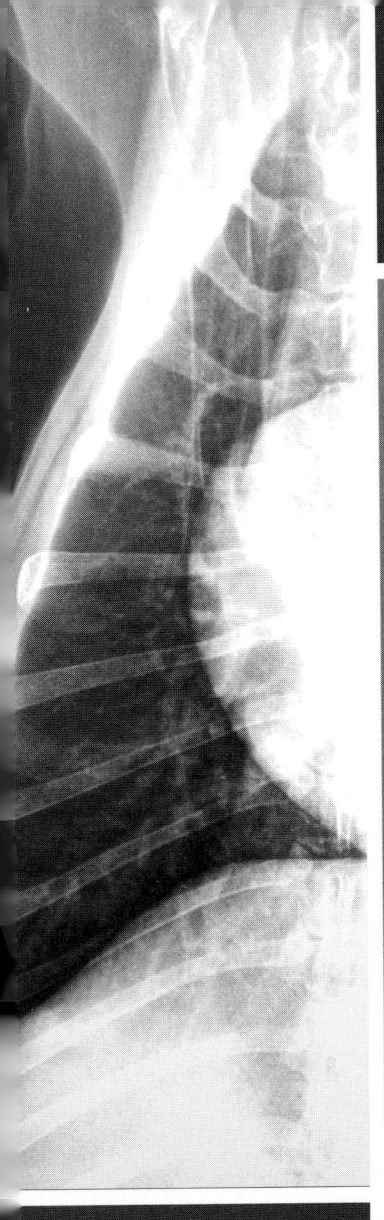

Textbook of

VETERINARY DIAGNOSTIC RADIOLOGY

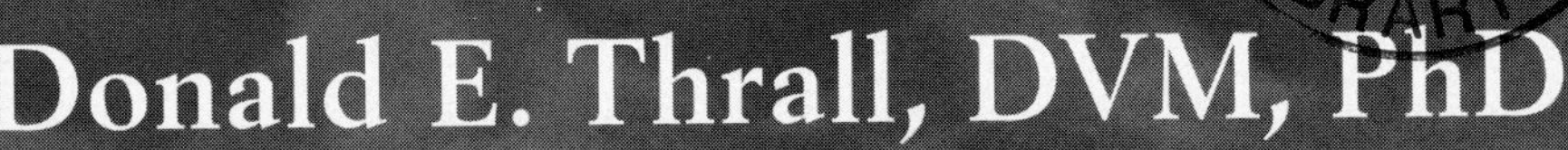

Donald E. Thrall, DVM, PhD
Professor of Radiology
College of Veterinary Medicine
North Carolina State University
Raleigh, North Carolina

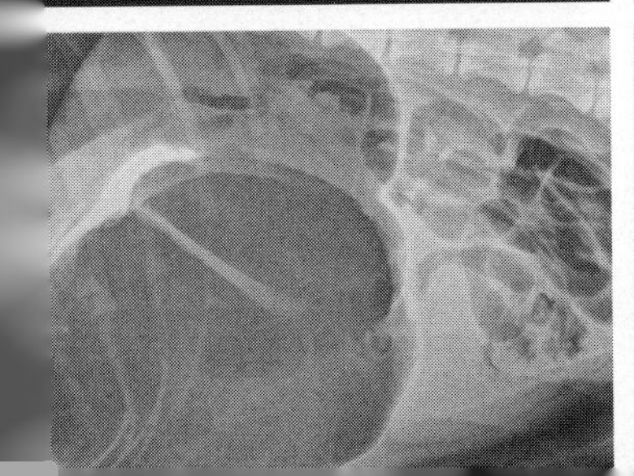

SAUNDERS
ELSEVIER

Fifth Edition

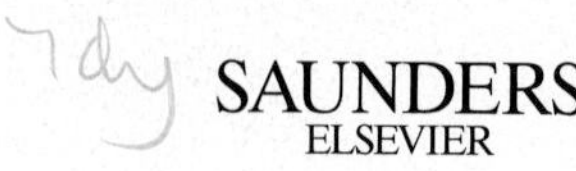

SAUNDERS
ELSEVIER

11830 Westline Industrial Drive
St. Louis, Missouri 63146

TEXTBOOK OF VETERINARY DIAGNOSTIC RADIOLOGY, FIFTH EDITION

ISBN: 978-1-4160-2615-0

Notice

Neither the Publisher nor the Authors assume any responsibility for any loss or injury and/or damage to persons or property arising out of or related to any use of the material contained in this book. It is the responsibility of the treating practitioner, relying on independent expertise and knowledge of the patient, to determine the best treatment and method of application for the patient.

The Publisher

ISBN: 978-1-4160-2615-0

Publishing Director: Linda Duncan
Acquisitions Editor: Anthony Winkel
Developmental Editor: Shelly Stringer
Publishing Services Manager: Patricia Tannian
Project Manager: Claire Kramer
Designer: Andrea Lutes

Printed in the United States of America

Last digit is the print number: 9 8 7 6 5 4 3 2 1

CONTRIBUTORS

Graeme S. Allan, BVSc, MVSc, FACVSc, DACVR, MRCVS
Adjunct Professor
Faculty of Veterinary Science
University of Sydney
Sydney, Australia
Veterinary Imaging Associates
Newtown, Australia

Laura J. Armbrust, DVM, DACVR
Assistant Professor of Radiology
Department of Clinical Sciences
College of Veterinary Medicine
Kansas State University
Manhattan, Kansas

Anne Bahr, DVM, MS, DACVR
Assistant Professor and Chief, Radiology
Department of Large Animal Clinical Sciences
College of Veterinary Medicine
Texas A&M University
College Station, Texas

Robert J. Bahr, BS, DVM, DACVR
Associate Professor
Veterinary Clinical Sciences
Oklahoma State University
Stillwater, Oklahoma

Clifford R. Berry, DVM, DACVR
Adjunct Associate Professor
Department of Small Animal Clinical Sciences
University of Tennessee
Knoxville, Tennessee

Darryl N. Biery, DVM, DACVR
Emeritus Professor of Radiological Sciences
Department of Clinical Sciences
School of Veterinary Medicine
University of Pennsylvania
Philadelphia, Pennsylvania

Lisa G. Britt, DVM, MS, DACVR
Assistant Clinical Professor, Veterinary Radiology
Department of Veterinary Medicine and Surgery
University of Missouri
College of Veterinary Medicine
Columbia, Missouri
Veterinary Medical Teaching Hospital
Columbia, Missouri

Valeria Busoni, DVM, PhD, DECVDI
Service d'Imagerie Médicale
Département des Sciences Cliniques
Faculté de Médecine Vétérinaire–Université de Liége
Liége, Belgium

Wm. Tod Drost, DVM, DACVR
Associate Professor and Head, Radiology Section
Veterinary Clinical Sciences
The Ohio State University
Columbus, Ohio

Sue J. Dyson, MAm, VetMB, PhD, DEO, FRCVS
Head of Clinical Orthopaedics
Centre for Equine Studies
Animal Health Trust
Newmarket
Suffolk, United Kingdom

Stephanie C. Essman, DVM, MS, DACVR
Assistant Professor, Veterinary Radiology
Department of Veterinary Medicine and Surgery
University of Missouri
College of Veterinary Medicine
Columbia, Missouri
Veterinary Medical Teaching Hospital
Columbia, MO, USA

Daniel A. Feeney, DVM, MS, DACVR
Professor of Veterinary Radiology
Department of Veterinary Clinical Sciences
College of Veterinary Medicine
University of Minnesota
St. Paul, Minnesota

Eric A. Ferrell, DVM, DACVR
Radiologist
Affiliated Veterinary Specialists
Maitland, Florida

Lisa J. Forrest, VMD, DACVR
Associate Professor
University of Wisconsin-Madison
School of Veterinary Medicine
Madison, Wisconsin

Paul M. Frank, DVM, DACVR
Assistant Professor of Clinical Radiology
College of Veterinary Medicine
University of Georgia
Athens, Georgia

John P. Graham, MVB, MSc, DVR, MRCVS, DACVR, DECVDI
Affiliated Veterinary Specialists
Maitland, Florida

George A. Henry, DVM, DACVR
Associate Professor
Department of Small Animal Clinical Sciences
College of Veterinary Medicine
University of Tennessee
Knoxville, Tennessee

Gary R. Johnston, DVM, MS, DACVR
Professor of Veterinary Radiology
College of Veterinary Medicine
Western University of Health Sciences
Pomona, California

Stephen K. Kneller, DVM, MS, DACVR
Department of Veterinary Clinical Medicine
College of Veterinary Medicine
University of Illinois
Urbana, Illinois

Christopher R. Lamb, MA, VetMB, DACVR, DECVDI, MRCVS, ILTM
Senior Lecturer in Radiology
Department of Veterinary Clinical Sciences
The Royal Veterinary College
University of London
London, United Kingdom
Head of Radiology Service
Queen Mother Hospital for Animals
The Royal Veterinary College
London, United Kingdom

Martha Moon Larson, DVM, MS, DACVR
Professor of Radiology
Small Animal Clinical Sciences
Virginia-Maryland Regional College of Veterinary Medicine
Blacksburg, Virginia

Jimmy C. Lattimer, DVM, MS, DACVR
Associate Professor, Veterinary Radiology
Department of Veterinary Medicine and Surgery
University of Missouri–Columbia
Columbia, Missouri
Veterinary Medical Teaching Hospital
Columbia, Missouri
Adjust Associate Professor
Department of Nuclear Sciences and Engineering Institute
University of Missouri–Columbia
Columbia, Missouri

Mary B. Mahaffey, DVM, MS, DACVR
Professor Emeritus
Department of Anatomy and Radiology
The University of Georgia
Athens, Georgia
Radiologist
Oconee Veterinary Imaging & Diagnostics
Watkinsville, Georgia

Federica Morandi, DVM, MS, DECVDI, DACVR
Assistant Professor of Radiology
Department of Small Animal Clinical Sciences
College of Veterinary Medicine
The University of Tennessee
Knoxville, Tennessee

Rachel C. Murray, MA, VetMB, MS, PhD, MRCVS, DACVS, DECVS
Head of Orthopaedic Research
Animal Health Trust
Lanwades Park
Kentford
Newmarket, United Kingdom

Stephanie G. Nykamp, DVM, DACVR
Assistant Professor
Clinical Studies
Ontario Veterinary College
University of Guelph
Guelph, Ontario, Canada

Richard D. Park, DVM, PhD, DACVR
Professor
Environmental and Radiological Health Sciences
Colorado State University
Fort Collins, Colorado
Head of Diagnostic Imaging Section
Veterinary Medical Center
Colorado State University
Fort Collins, Colorado

Anthony P. Pease, DVM, MS, DACVR
Assistant Professor of Radiology
Department of Molecular and Biomedical Sciences
College of Veterinary Medicine
North Carolina State University
Raleigh, North Carolina

Robert D. Pechman, Jr., DVM, DACVR
Visiting Professor of Diagnostic Imaging
Veterinary Clinical Sciences
College of Veterinary Medicine
Oklahoma State University
Stillwater, Oklahoma

Rachel E. Pollard, DVM, PhD, DACVR
Assistant Professor of Diagnostic Imaging
University of California
Davis, California

Elizabeth A. Riedesel, DVM, DACVR
Associate Professor
Veterinary Clinical Sciences
Iowa State University
Ames, Iowa

Ian D. Robertson, BVSc, DACVR
Clinical Associate Professor
Department of Molecular and Biomedical Sciences
College of Veterinary Medicine
North Carolina State University
Raleigh, North Carolina

Valerie F. Samii, DVM, DACVR
Associate Professor
Department of Veterinary Clinical Sciences
College of Veterinary Medicine
The Ohio State University
Columbus, Ohio

Tobias Schwarz, DVM, MA, DVR, MRCVS, DACVR, DECVDI
Assistant Professor of Radiology
Department of Surgical Sciences
School of Veterinary Medicine
University of Wisconsin
Madison, Wisconsin

James E. Smallwood, DVM, MS
Alumni Distinguished Professor
Molecular Biomedical Sciences
North Carolina State University
Raleigh, North Carolina

Kathy A. Spaulding, DVM, DACVR
Clinical Professor
Large Animal Clinical Sciences
College of Veterinary Medicine and Bio Med
Texas A&M University
College Station, Texas

Amy S. Tidwell, DVM, DACVR
Associate Professor
Clinical Sciences
School of Veterinary Medicine
Tufts University
New Grafton, Massachusetts

Robert L. Toal, DVM, MS, DACVR
Radiologist, SouthPaws Veterinary Specialists and Emergency Center
Fairfax, Virginia

Russell L. Tucker, DVM, DACVR
Director of Radiology
Associate Professor
Veterinary Clinical Sciences
College of Veterinary Medicine
Washington State University
Pullman, Washington

Barbara J. Watrous, DVM, DACVR
Professor Emeritus
Clinical Sciences
College of Veterinary Medicine
Oregon State University
Corvallis, Oregon

William R. Widmer, DVM, MS, DACVR
Professor of Diagnostic Imaging
Department of Veterinary Clinical Sciences
Purdue University
West Lafayette, Indiana

Erik R. Wisner, DVM, DACVR
Professor and Vice Chair
Department of Surgical and Radiological Sciences
School of Veterinary Medicine
University of California
Davis, California

Robert H. Wrigley, BVSc, MS, DVR, MRCVS, DACVR, DECVDI
Professor of Diagnostic Imaging
Department of Environmental and Radiological Health Sciences
Colorado State University
Fort Collins, Colorado
Head of Ultrasound Section
Veterinary Medical Center Teaching Hospital
Fort Collins, Colorado

PREFACE TO THE FIFTH EDITION

The primary objective of this book is to serve as an instructional aid for students of imaging; this has been the goal since the first edition and I am excited to say that the changes made to this fifth edition go even further in accomplishing this objective. Students at all levels should be able to find material in this edition that helps in the interpretation of both basic and challenging images. Valuable features of prior editions, such as the self-assessment questions and the atlas of normal anatomy, have been retained, but extensive changes have been introduced and new media used. The normal anatomy material has been dispersed throughout the text so that rather than being sequestered in the back of the book, it can be consulted more conveniently.

The interface between the book and the World Wide Web that has been developed for this fifth edition is very exciting. A Web portal will host the self-assessment exercises that students can complete online and thereafter obtain immediate grading. For some chapters, movies are available online that will assist in the explanation of complex physical principles, such as sonographic and magnetic resonance (MR) imaging physics, or dynamic disease processes, such at tracheal collapse and esophageal disorders. For each chapter, a list of key points has been created to emphasize the major points of focus, and this material is also available through the Web portal. Finally, for chapters dealing with specific anatomic areas, one or two case studies will be available for each chapter through the Web portal. Students will be given a history and access to images and asked to formulate an opinion. Once this exercise is complete, the answer can be accessed to determine whether the correct approach or assessment was chosen. I believe these additions raise the utility of this edition to an entirely new level and one that should excite students even more about veterinary imaging.

As in the second, third, and fourth editions, all chapters have been reviewed carefully, making for an extensive, substantive revision. No chapter has escaped in-depth scrutiny, assuring that the latest and most accurate information is included. In the fourth edition four new chapters were introduced that covered the basic aspects of interpretation pertaining to radiographic images of the axial skeleton in small and large animals, the appendicular skeleton in small and large animals, and the thorax and abdomen in small animals. Details of positioning, specific anatomic features of the body part in question, methods of radiographic viewing, and assessment and applications of specialized imaging modalities are some of the topics covered in these introductory chapters. In the fifth edition these chapters have been expanded, with many new illustrations, and form the basis of interpretation that can be applied when assessing the more detailed chapters dealing with specific anatomic areas.

Veterinary imaging is becoming increasingly complex. The digital world is engulfing the specialty. As a result, new chapters on the basic principles of digital imaging and the MR imaging features of brain disease in small animals have been included. Also, the MR and computed tomography (CT) features of diseases outside of the brain have been expanded, and chapters covering the physical principles of ultrasonography and CT and MR imaging have been updated significantly.

The basis of interpretation used in this textbook remains centered on the description of radiographic abnormalities in terms of Roentgen signs—changes in size, shape, location, opacity, number, and margination. I believe that students who have a firm understanding of Roentgen sign description will be less inclined to make errors by jumping immediately to a diagnosis and will instead thoroughly consider radiographic changes in an orderly and efficient manner.

Thanks are extended to all who have used prior editions of this work and to those who have pointed out errors or omissions, thereby allowing this edition to be what I believe is the best one yet. Finally, I think it is impossible for one person to prepare a meaningful, comprehensive textbook of veterinary imaging. I am fortunate to have had so many talented authors take time from their busy schedules to prepare material for this book. Many new authors have contributed to this fifth edition, and many familiar names are again found as contributors. The expertise of this team heightens the quality of the information contained on these pages, and I am honored by their participation.

Donald E. Thrall

CONTENTS

SECTION I Physics and Principles of Interpretation

SECTION II The Axial Skeleton

SECTION III The Appendicular Skeleton

SECTION IV Neck and Thorax

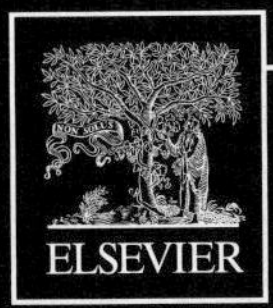

evolve

To access your Student Resources, visit:

http://evolve.elsevier.com/Thrall/vetrad/

Evolve® Student Resources for ***Thrall: Textbook of Veterinary Diagnostic Radiology, 5th Edition*** offers the following features:

Student Resources

- **Case Studies**
  49 in-depth, real-life situations that encourage you to successfully work through challenging cases. Case studies include all relevant data, including pertinent history, clinical signs, and radiographic images for you to make a systematic evaluation and diagnosis.

- **Video/Audio Clips**
  22 video clips and audio files assist in the understanding of complex physical principles (e.g., sonographic and MRI physics) or dynamic disease processes (e.g., tracheal collapse and esophageal disorders).

- **Chapter Quizzes**
  An on-line test bank that contains multiple choice and true/false self-assessment exercises for every chapter.

- **Key Points**
  Bulleted information emphasizes and reinforces the take-home messages in every chapter.

- **Bonus Chapters**
  2 bonus chapters provide still-current and practical information from the fourth edition:
  - Visual Perception and Radiographic Interpretation by Marc Papageorges, DVM, MS, PhD, DACVR
  - Abdominal Masses by Charles R. Root, DVM, MS, DACVR

- **An Atlas of Normal Radiographic Anatomy of the Dog and Horse**
  Compiles all normal radiographic anatomy chapters from the fifth edition into a single atlas in a digital image format:
  - Radiographic Anatomy of the Axial Skeleton
  - Radiographic Anatomy of the Appendicular Skeleton
  - Radiographic Anatomy of the Cardiopulmonary System
  - Radiographic Anatomy of the Abdomen

- **Useful Guidelines for Radiographic Interpretation**
  - A Systematic Checklist for Evaluating Abdominal Radiographs
  - Thoracic Radiographic Paradigm for Interpretation

http://evolve.elsevier.com/Thrall/vetrad/

Textbook of VETERINARY DIAGNOSTIC RADIOLOGY

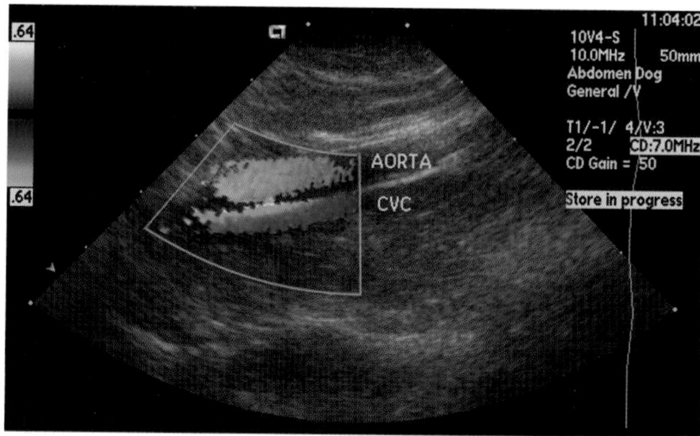

Fig. 3-12 Doppler image of the distal aorta and caudal vena in a dog. The aorta is in the near field and is red. The caudal vena cava is in the far field and is blue. According to the color scale, red represents blood flowing toward the transducer and blue represents blood flowing away from the transducer. The colors are assigned by the ultrasound machine and are related to the direction of blood flow. In other words, arteries will not always be red and veins will not always be blue. Blood flow velocity ranges from 0.64 m/s toward the transducer (red/yellow) to 0.64 m/s away from the transducer (blues). The *black bar* in the middle of the scale represents 0 m/s. Yellow and light blue represent faster velocities in their respective directions.

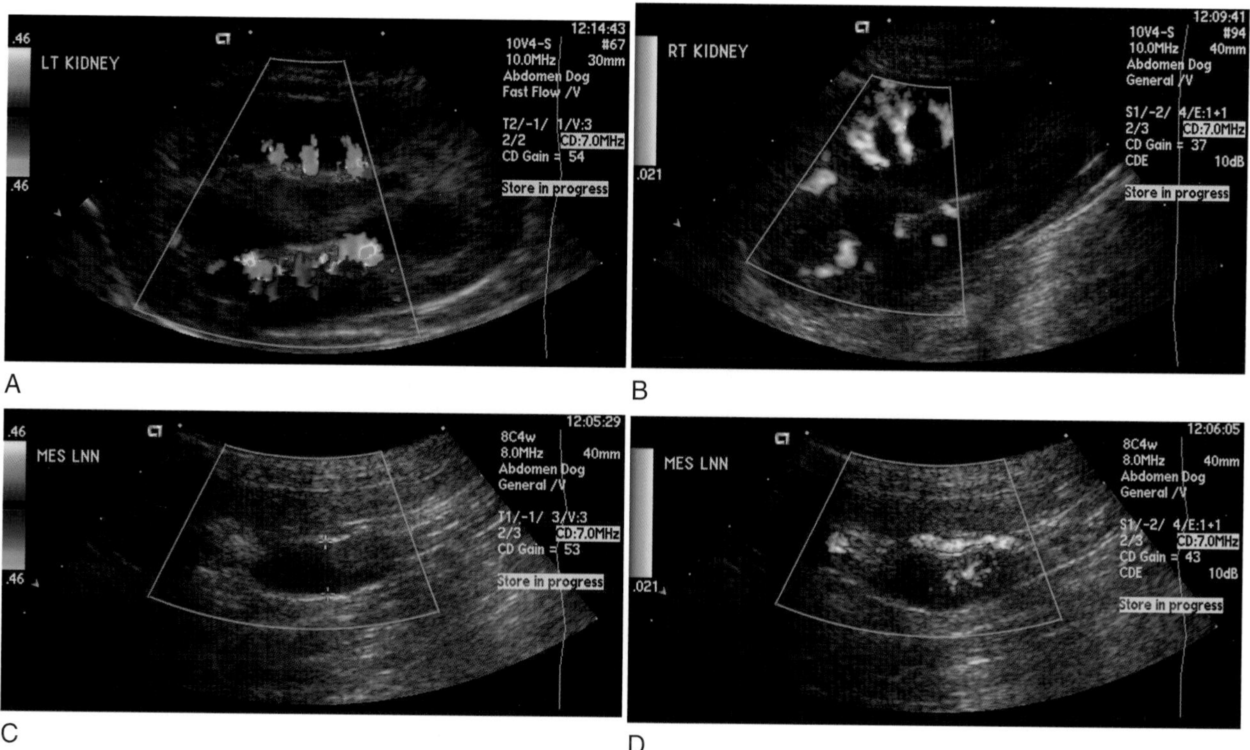

Fig. 3-13 Images of the left kidney in a dog. **A,** Color Doppler image showing blood flow within the kidney. Red hues indicate blood flow toward the transducer and blue hues, away from the transducer. Note the color scale at *left*. **B,** Power Doppler image showing blood flow in the same kidney. Because power Doppler is not direction dependent, only one hue is used (orange in this case). Lower-velocity blood flow can be detected with power Doppler compared with color Doppler. Compared to **A**, blood flow is noted further into the renal cortex by using power Doppler. **C,** Image of a mesenteric lymph node in a dog with color Doppler (note color scale). No blood flow is noted by color Doppler in or around the mesenteric lymph node. **D,** Image of a mesenteric lymph node in a dog with power Doppler active. A blood vessel is noted in the immediate near field to the lymph node and blood flow is noted within the lymph node.

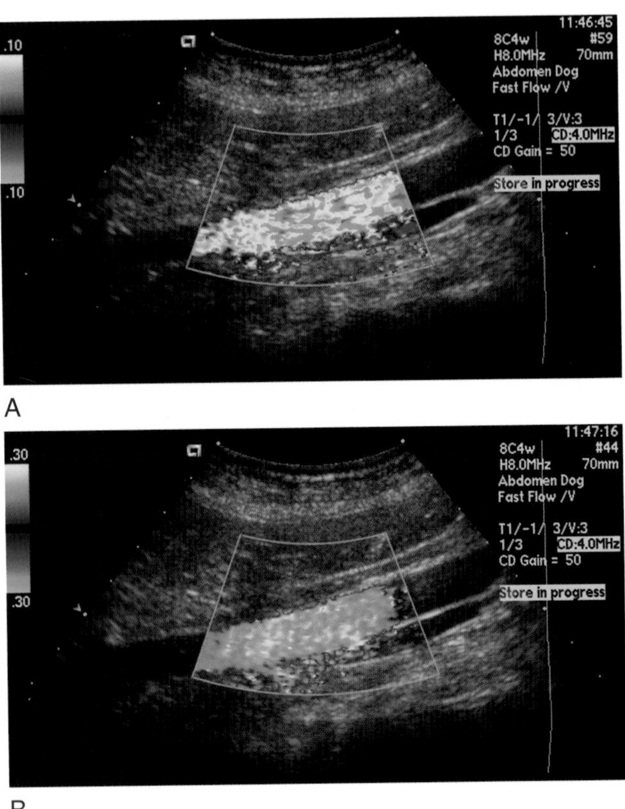

Fig. 3-15 Color Doppler image of the distal aorta in a dog. **A,** Color Doppler aliasing is seen as a mixture of red and blue hues. As the blood flow velocity exceeds 0.10 m/s toward the transducer, the computer changes the color coding from yellow to light blue. **B,** The aliasing was corrected by increasing the velocity scale to 0.30 m/s. Increasing the velocity scale increased PRF. The mixture of red and yellow hues within the aorta represents different velocity of blood flow.

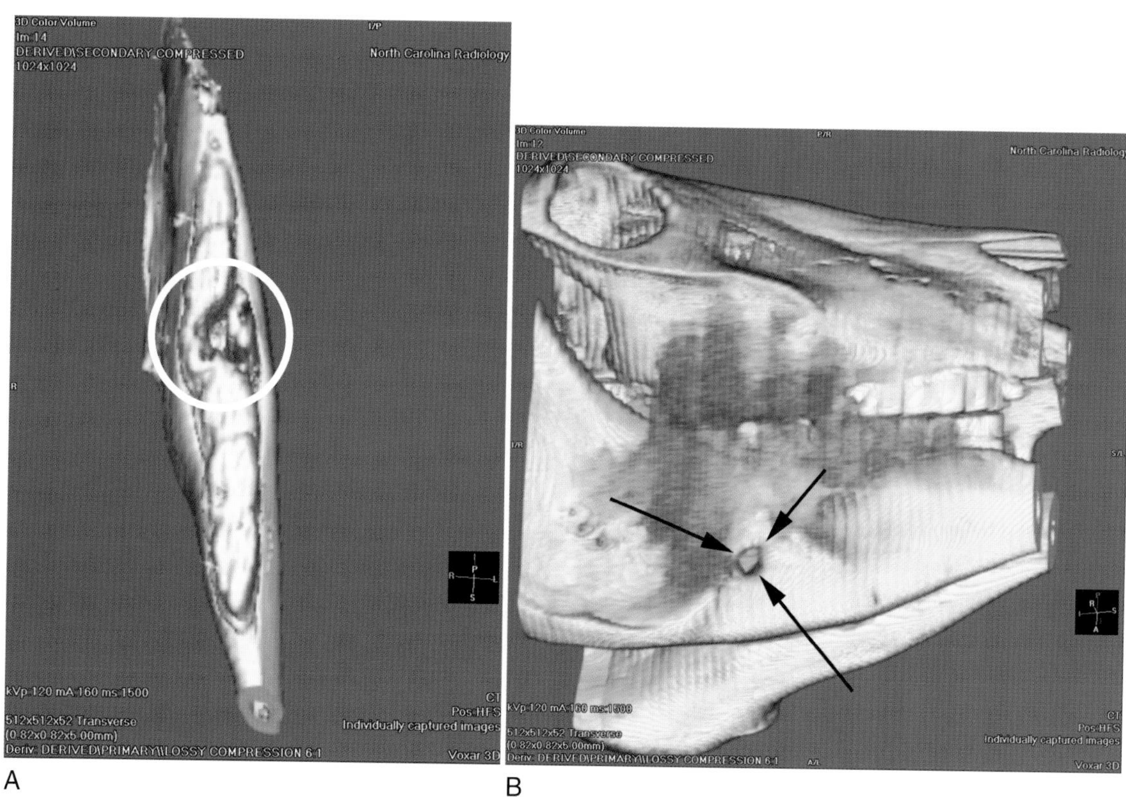

Fig. 10-3 Three dimensional reconstructions of the apical tooth root abscess in Figure 10-2. Note the fracture of the first molar along the sagittal plane (**A**, *circle*) as well as the defect in the mandible (**B**, *arrow*).

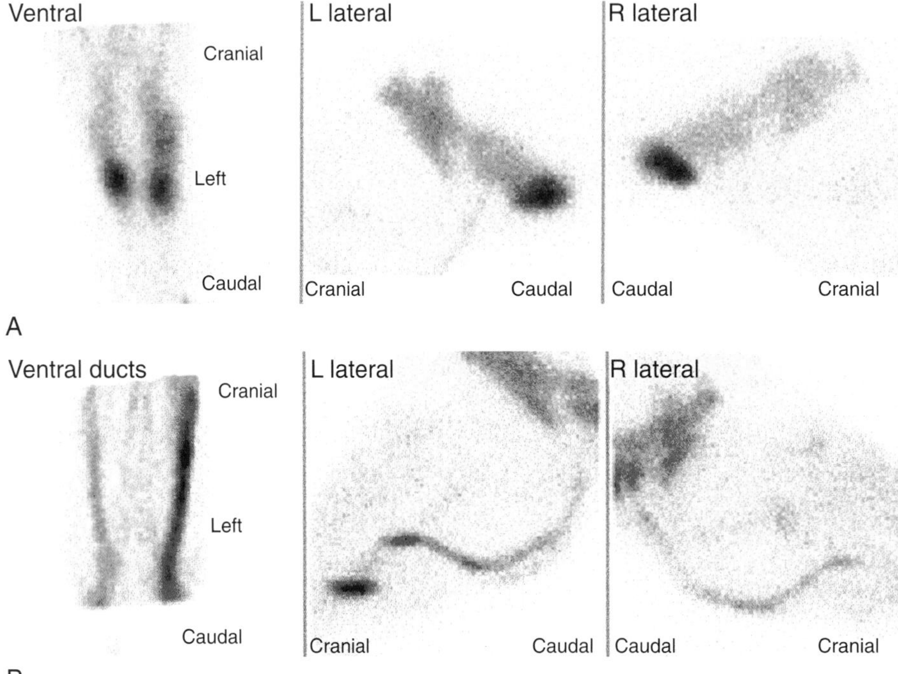

Fig. 10-31 A, Scintigraphic images acquired 20 minutes after 50 mCi of technetium-99m pertechnetate was administered intravenously. The parotid salivary glands are shown, with the right having slightly less activity then the left. **B,** The same horse after being fed a peppermint. Activity is detected within the left parotid salivary duct to a greater degree than the right parotid salivary duct. (Images courtesy of Dr. Nathan Dykes, Cornell University, Ithaca, NY.)

SECTION I

Physics and Principles of Interpretation

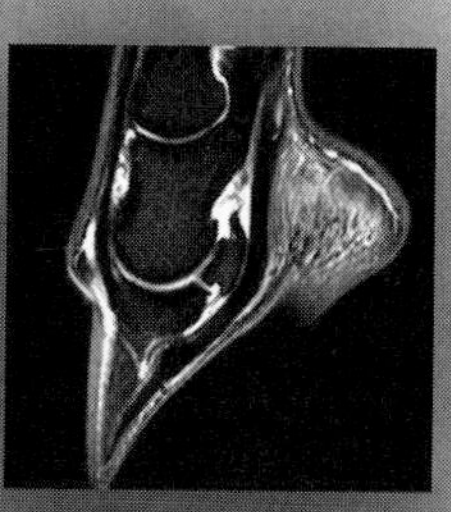
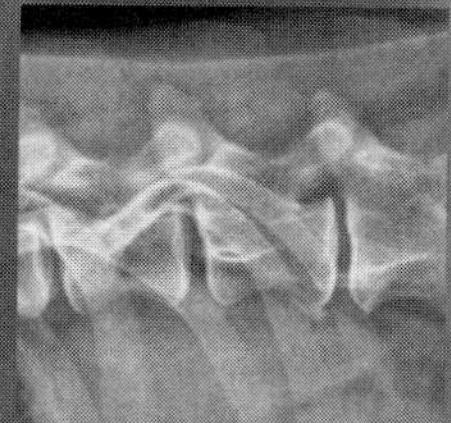
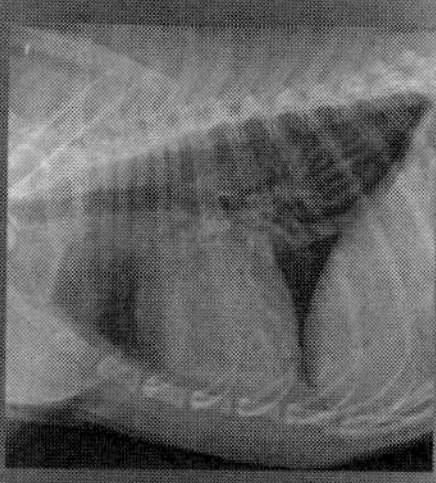
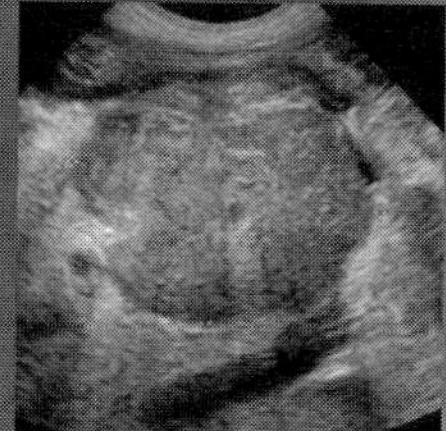
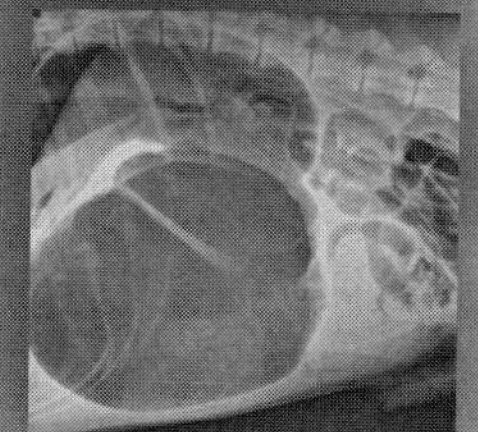

CHAPTER • 1
Physics of Diagnostic Radiology, Radiation Protection, and Darkroom Theory

Donald E. Thrall
William R. Widmer

X-rays were discovered on November 8, 1895, by Wilhelm Conrad Roentgen, a German physicist.[1] These new "rays" were quickly put to use for medical purposes, and many sophisticated medical applications were soon devised. For example, angiography was first described in 1896, only 1 year after the discovery of x-rays. The discovery of x-rays revolutionized the diagnosis and treatment of disease in human beings and animals. In 1901, Roentgen was awarded the first Nobel Prize for Physics in recognition of his discovery.

More than 100 years after their discovery, x-rays remain in widespread use for many aspects of medical imaging. Although x-rays are valuable for medical purposes, the interaction of x-rays with tissue produces ionization, which can produce significant biologic damage. Because x-rays are widely applied yet potentially harmful, their basic principles must be understood.

BASIC PROPERTIES OF X-RAYS

X-rays and gamma rays are types of electromagnetic radiation. The distinction between x-rays and gamma rays is their source; x-rays are produced by electron interactions outside the nucleus, and gamma rays are emitted from unstable nuclei. Other familiar types of electromagnetic radiation include radio waves, radar, microwaves, and visible light (Table 1-1).

Electromagnetic radiation is a combination of electric and magnetic fields that travel together. Electromagnetic radiation can be represented as a "sine wave" model (Fig. 1-1). Sine waves are characterized by two related parameters—frequency and wavelength. The velocity of electromagnetic radiation, which is the speed of light, is the product of the frequency and the wavelength.

$$\text{Velocity (m/sec)} = \text{frequency (per sec)} \times \text{wavelength (m)}$$

All types of electromagnetic radiation travel at the speed of light; thus frequency is inversely proportional to wavelength. The energy of electromagnetic radiation is related to wavelength by the formula:

$$\text{Energy} = \text{Planck's constant} \times \frac{\text{speed of light}}{\text{wavelength}}$$

Energy is therefore also inversely proportional to wavelength.

The energy unit for electromagnetic radiation is the *electron volt* (eV). One electron volt is the energy of an electron accelerated by a potential difference of 1 V. Electromagnetic radiation with energies greater than 15 eV, a very low absolute energy, can produce ionization within cells. X-rays used for diagnosis have energies greater than 1000 times this amount; thus the need to understand their principles and how to use them safely should be clear.

Some physical properties of electromagnetic radiation cannot be adequately explained by theories of wave propagation. The photon, or quantum concept, was developed to explain the apparent particulate behavior of x-rays and gamma rays and how they interact with a target to create an image or cause radiation damage. A photon is a discrete bundle of electromagnetic radiation. Properties of x-rays and gamma rays are given in Box 1-1.

The ionizing property of x-rays and gamma rays renders them hazardous. Ionization occurs when a photon ejects an electron from an atom, thereby creating an ion pair consisting of the negatively charged electron and the positively charged atom (Fig. 1-2). Because DNA is involved in metabolic and clonogenic cell processes, an ionization in DNA may result in *biologic amplification*. In other words, a lesion induced in one cell's DNA can affect progeny cells for future generations. Ionization in DNA can lead to an increased (1) rate of mutation; (2) rate of abortion or fetal abnormalities, if irradiated in utero; (3) susceptibility to disease and shortened life span; (4) risk of cancer; and (5) cataracts.[2] Ionization in cells is exploited in radiation therapy with the intention of killing cancer cells.

RADIATION PROTECTION

A goal in diagnostic radiology is to obtain maximum diagnostic information with minimal exposure of the patient, radiology personnel, and general public. This section reviews radiation protection principles. Because blind adherence to rules cannot substitute for the exercise of sound judgment, these principles may be modified in unusual circumstances on the professional advice of experts with recognized competence in radiation protection.*

Radiation Units

For many years the roentgen, rad, and rem were the units used to quantify radiation exposure, radiation absorption, and equivalent dose, respectively. In 1977 the International System of Units (SI units) was developed in keeping with the trend toward universal adoption of the metric system.[3] Because the roentgen, rad, and rem are not coherent with the SI system, their corresponding SI units are coulomb per kilogram and joule per kilogram, respectively.

*Local, state, and national regulations supersede any recommendations given in this chapter.

Table • 1-1

Wavelength of Common Types of Electromagnetic Radiation

TYPE OF ELECTROMAGNETIC RADIATION	WAVELENGTH (CM)
Radio waves	30,000
Microwaves	10
Visible light	0.0001
X-rays	0.00000001

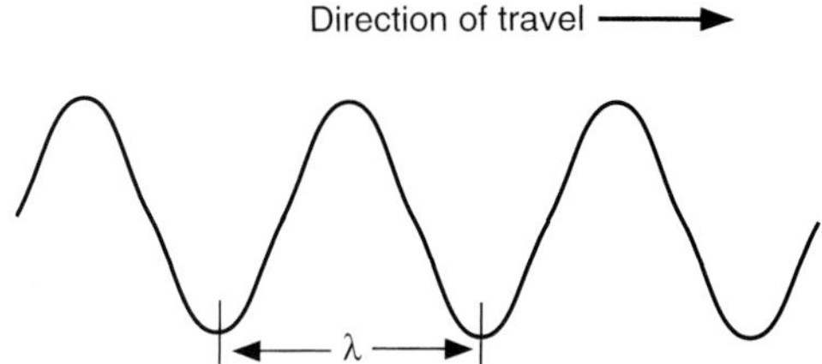
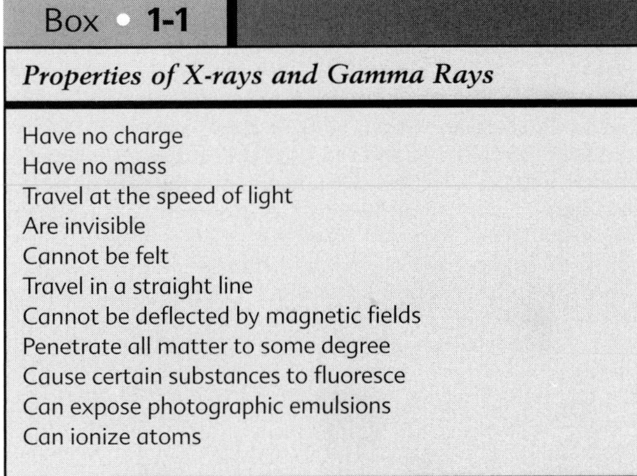

Fig. 1-1 Sine wave model of electromagnetic radiation. The distance between crest or trough separation, λ, is the wave length. Another characteristic of waves is their frequency, f, or the number of waves per unit time. The velocity (c) of a wave is related to wavelength and frequency by the formula, $c = f \times \lambda$. Electromagnetic radiation travels at a constant speed—the speed of light.

Box • 1-1

Properties of X-rays and Gamma Rays

Have no charge
Have no mass
Travel at the speed of light
Are invisible
Cannot be felt
Travel in a straight line
Cannot be deflected by magnetic fields
Penetrate all matter to some degree
Cause certain substances to fluoresce
Can expose photographic emulsions
Can ionize atoms

Given that ionizing radiation has no mass and no charge, it can only be indirectly detected. That is, it cannot be felt, weighed, or detected by its perturbation of an electric field (see Box 1-1). The amount of radiation exposure is commonly quantified by measuring the number of ionizations, in other words, the electric charge, produced by x-rays in air.

Exposure Quantity

Measurement of the amount of radiation striking a subject is often needed. This measurement is based on the number of ion pairs produced in air by the oncoming radiation and is expressed in the SI system as coulombs of charge per kilogram of air (C/kg). The previous word used to describe exposure quantity was the roentgen. One roentgen is equal to the production of 2.58×10^{-4} C/kg in air. No special name has been given to exposure quantity in the SI system, and exposure is quantified only in terms of coulombs per kilogram.

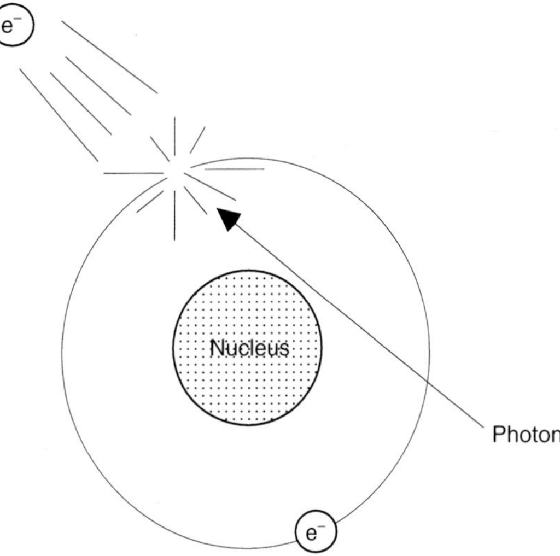

Fig. 1-2 The principle of ionization. A photon ejects an electron from an atom, causing ionization, forming an ion pair: the negatively charged electron and the positively charged atom. After this ionization event, the photon, depending on its energy, may be completely absorbed, or it may interact with other atoms to produce more ionization. The ejected electron can interact with biologic molecules, such as DNA, and produce damage to macromolecules that results in cell death.

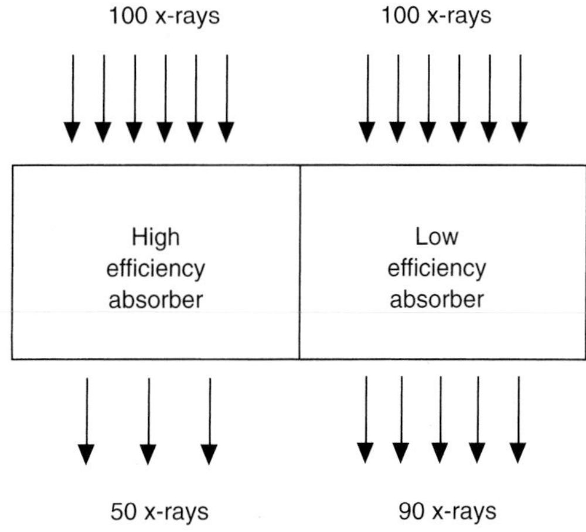

Fig. 1-3 Two materials are exposed to 100 x-rays. Thus the exposure dose, or dose in coulombs per kilogram, is the same for both. However, the efficiency of x-ray absorption is not the same. The absorber on the left absorbs 50% of x-rays, whereas the absorber on the right only absorbs 10%. Therefore the absorbed dose will be higher in the absorber on the left even though the exposure dose is the same. An example of a high-efficiency absorber is bone compared with soft tissues such as fat and muscle.

Absorbed Dose

The efficiency of x-ray absorption in various materials varies considerably. Therefore the radiation "dose" to objects with different absorption efficiencies will not be constant when these objects are exposed to the same quantity of radiation (Fig. 1-3). The SI unit for absorbed dose is the gray (Gy).

The gray is defined as the amount of radiation such that the absorbed energy is 1 joule/kg of tissue. Before SI units were accepted, the unit of absorbed dose was the rad, which is equal to 100 ergs/g. By using appropriate conversion factors, it can be shown that 1 Gy = 100 rad. In soft tissue, exposure to 2.58×10^{-4} C/kg (1 roentgen) amounts to an absorbed dose of approximately 0.9 cGy (0.9 rad). Because bone is a more efficient absorber of x-rays than is soft tissue, exposure to bone of 2.58×10^{-4} C/kg (1 roentgen) results in a bone-absorbed dose of greater than 0.9 cGy. This differential between exposure and absorption in soft tissue versus bone may be as great as a factor of 4 or 5 with low-energy radiation. Differential x-ray absorption among various tissues in the body is the basis of radiographic image formation. As will be discussed later, the differential between exposure dose and absorbed dose is inversely proportional to photon energy.

Dose Equivalent

In living tissue, absorption of the same dose in Gy from different types of radiation may not produce the same biologic effect. For example, damage from particulate radiation, such as alpha particles and neutrons, is greater on a Gy-for-Gy basis than damage from the same dose of x-rays. This is related to differences in "ionization density" for different types of radiation. For example, a high-mass, heavily charged particle, such as an alpha particle (a helium nucleus: two nuclear protons, two nuclear neutrons, no orbital electrons) creates many ionizations that are very close to one another in the tissue compared with a low-mass, lightly charged particle such as an electron. Electrons set in motion by x-rays interacting with tissue (ionization) are the major source of damage resulting from x-ray exposure. Therefore deposition of 1 Gy from alpha particle absorption does more biologic damage than deposition of 1 Gy from x-ray absorption. Damage from different types of radiation may be compared by a weighting factor, which is a numeric factor describing the relative effectiveness of a particular type of radiation to photons. The weighting factor for photons is 1.0; it is greater than 1.0 for charged or particulate types of radiation such as electrons, neutrons, or alpha particles. In the SI system, the unit of dose equivalency is the Sievert (Sv); the Sv is derived from the product of the absorbed dose in Gy and the weighting factor. Before SI units were accepted, the unit of dose equivalency was the rem. The rem was derived from the product of the absorbed dose in rads and the weighting factor. Because 1 Gy = 100 rads, 1 Sv = 100 rem. As a rule of thumb, an absorbed dose of 1 Gy from photons results in an approximately equivalent dose of 1 Sv.

Radiation Safety

The United States Nuclear Regulatory Commission (NRC) is the official source for establishing guidelines for radiation protection. The NRC has indicated that the annual occupational radiation dose to individual adults should be limited to a maximum of 0.05 Sv (5 rem).[4] The NRC has not established an upper limit for cumulative exposure. Previously, the NRC had recommended that cumulative exposure be less than 5 rem/yr × (n minus 18), where *n* is the age of the individual. This recommendation has been overruled in favor of the ALARA (*as low as reasonably achievable*) principle. Although the NRC is the official body regarding exposure limits for ionizing radiation, other groups also make recommendations regarding exposure to ionizing radiation. For example, the National Council on Radiation Protection (NCRP), a governmental scientific group, meets regularly to review recent radiation research and update radiation safety recommendations. According to the NCRP, the objectives of radiation protection are the following:

1. To prevent clinically significant radiation-induced effects by adhering to dose limits that are below the apparent or practical threshold
2. To limit the risk of cancer and heritable effects to a reasonable level in relation to societal needs and values and benefits gained[5]

These objectives can be met through adherence to the principle of ALARA—that is, limiting exposure of radiation workers to a level as low as reasonably achievable—and by applying established dose levels for controlling occupational and general public exposure.[6]

Maximum permissible dose is the maximal amount of absorbed radiation that can be delivered to an individual as a whole-body dose or as a dose to a specific organ and still be considered safe. The term "safe" in this context means that no evidence exists that individuals receiving the maximum dose mentioned will suffer harmful immediate or long-term effects to the body as a whole or to any individual structure or organ. Although the effect of very low doses of radiation is not known with certainty, the fact that any amount of radiation will have some effect on the subject is safe to assume. Thus whenever an individual is exposed to ionizing radiation, some biologic damage may occur, so following the ALARA principle is of paramount importance. An analogy could be made to an individual smoking a cigarette only once a month. No evidence exists that physical damage could result from this frequency of smoking; however, with increasing frequency of smoking, the probability steadily escalates by virtue of its cumulative effect. Unfortunately, no threshold for either cigarette smoking or radiation has been established under which damage will not occur or over which damage will definitely result.

In December 1989, the National Academy of Sciences Committee on the Biological Effects of Ionizing Radiation (BEIR) produced its latest report, which concluded that radiation risks had until then been underestimated. Specifically, it stated that the likelihood of cancer induction after exposure to low radiation doses is three to four times higher than previously thought.[7] Much of their data were derived from studies of survivors of the World War II atomic bomb detonations in Japan. Very few large human exposures to radiation have been documented; however, events such as Hiroshima, Nagasaki, and Chernobyl have provided information on human tolerance to low-level radiation exposure. Also, the Department of Energy has recently released information derived from human radiation exposure experiments that were conducted during the Cold War period of the 1950s and 1960s.

Even though ALARA is the official method of choice for limiting exposure to radiation, recommendations for upper limits of exposure have also been established by the NCRP to guide those involved in radiation work. The NCRP recommends the following[8]:

1. An individual worker's lifetime effective dose should not exceed age in years × 10 mSv (age in years × 1 rem), and no occupational exposure should be permitted until age 18 years. Therefore an individual's lifetime effective dose equivalent in rems should not exceed the value of his or her age in years.
2. The effective dose in any 1 year should not exceed 50 mSv (5 rem).
3. For the general public, radiation exposure (excluding that related to medical use) should not exceed 1 mSv (0.1 rem).
4. Once pregnancy is declared, the monthly limit of exposure to the embryo or fetus should not exceed 0.5 mSv (0.05 rem). Specific controls for occupationally exposed women are no longer recommended until a pregnancy is declared.

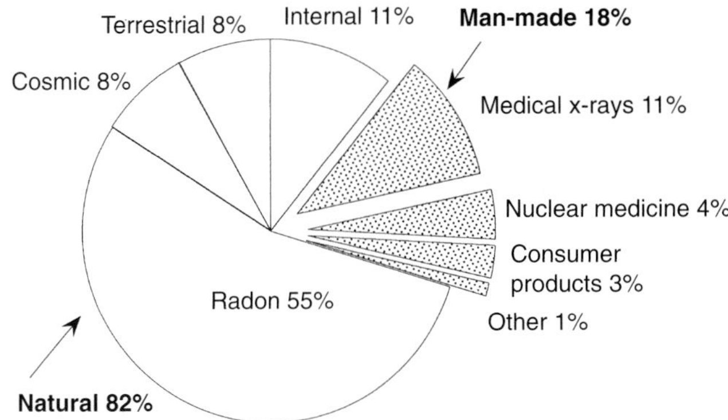

Fig. 1-4 An estimate of sources of exposure dose from ionizing radiation in the United States.

Table • 1-2

Radiation Doses Received from Some Familiar Activities

EVENT	RADIATION DOSE RECEIVED (MSV)
Flight from Los Angeles to Paris	0.05
Thoracic radiograph	0.22
Apollo X astronauts' moon flight	4.8
Whole-mouth dental x-ray	9.1
Exposure to accident at Three Mile Island	11.0
Mammography	15.0
Barium enema	80.0
Heart catheterization	450.0

Doses are whole body in some instances and regional in others.

The difference in opinion between the NRC and the NCRP regarding limits for cumulative exposure can be confusing. The NRC is the agency officially responsible for identifying federal exposure standards. However, the NRC has elected to eliminate any recommendations regarding cumulative exposure limits, probably because of the uncertainty of such predictions. The NCRP, on the other hand, has elected to establish an estimate for acceptable cumulative exposure, which is much more conservative than that previously recommended by the NRC. Regardless, the radiation worker should adhere to the principle of ALARA regarding occupational exposure and use the most conservative of any conflicting recommendations.

In addition to occupational exposure, the population is continually exposed to very low levels of radiation, both natural and manmade. A breakdown of relative exposure of the U.S. public to radiation by various sources was published by the NCRP in 1987 (Fig. 1-4).[9] In brief, the average U.S. citizen receives 3.6 mSv (360 mrem) annually. Of this figure, more than 80% is attributable to the inhalation of radon gas. The relative levels of different sources of exposure may vary on the basis of geographic location. For example, because of the greater altitude, exposure to cosmic radiation is higher in Colorado than in North Carolina, and in Eastern Pennsylvania, household radon exposure is much greater than in most other areas of the United States. Typical radiation doses received from some familiar activities are shown in Table 1-2.

Biologic Principles

X-rays produce ionization in tissue. Because most tissue is 70% water, ionization of water is common and results in the formation of chemically active free radicals. These free radicals account for most radiation damage to DNA. A small fraction of radiation-induced damage in DNA results from direct ionization. DNA changes include base nucleotide damage, DNA strand breakage, and DNA cross-linkage. These effects may be minimal and quickly repaired enzymatically, or they can result in cell lethality. DNA is uniquely sensitive because it is a large target relative to other intracellular structures and possesses little redundancy within any one cell. The principle of biologic amplification as previously described is another reason why DNA damage can have serious consequences.

Depending on the tissue, a given dose of x-rays can have effects varying in magnitude from imperceptible to lethal. For example, a tissue that does not divide, such as muscle, may receive a high dose but exhibit few side effects. Conversely, actively dividing tissues, such as intestinal epithelium and bone marrow, are quite responsive to radiation. This does not mean that nondividing tissue is less sensitive overall, just that damage is less obvious.

Two other tissues, gonadal and fetal, are of crucial importance regarding radiation safety. Irradiation of these tissues at sensitive stages can result in biologic amplification of any damage caused. The younger the fetus or embryo, the greater the potential for damage. Consequences of such damage include embryonic death, congenital malformation, or a growth defect.

Practical Considerations

Radiation workers in veterinary practices must be aware of the risks of radiation. They should be skilled in patient positioning for radiography, machine operation, and image processing techniques so that repeat studies are minimized. Workers should be instructed on the proper use and care of radiation protection devices. Reduction of radiation exposure to an individual from external radiation sources may be achieved by any one or any combination of the following measures:

1. Distance: increasing the distance of the individual from the radiation source
2. Time: reducing the duration of exposure
3. Shielding: use of protective barriers between the individual and the radiation source

In veterinary medicine, shielding and distance are readily controlled. Shielding may be composed of permanent protective barriers and structural shielding such as walls containing lead, concrete, or other materials sufficient to provide the required degree of radiation attenuation. Shielding may also be a protective barrier incorporated into equipment, such as an aluminum filter in the x-ray tube to remove scattered radiation or a collimator to limit the size of the primary x-ray beam. Or shielding may consist of mobile or temporary devices used as the occasion demands, such as movable screens or lead-impregnated aprons or gloves.

Protective aprons and gloves are usually 0.5 mm Pb equivalent, and they must be worn when positioning patients for radiography. Although these devices are heavy and seemingly provide considerable protection, they are designed solely for protecting against scattered radiation and must never be placed in the primary beam. In addition, mishandling of lead aprons and gloves results in damage to the equipment and thus less protection. Protective equipment should be treated with respect; it is used to protect the health of the radiation worker.

Pregnant and potentially pregnant women, and individuals younger than 18 years, must not hold animal patients during radiographic examinations. A radiation protection supervisor (who may also be the user) should be designated for every installation. This supervisor assumes the responsibilities defined below and is in charge of establishing safe working conditions that comply with all pertinent federal, state, and local regulations. Radiation protection supervisors should be familiar with the basic principles of radiation protection to carry out their responsibilities properly, although they may wish to consult appropriate qualified experts for advice.

The following are suggested responsibilities of the radiation protection supervisor:

1. Establish and supervise the implementation of written operating procedures
2. Periodically review procedures to ensure their conformity with local regulations
3. Instruct personnel in proper radiation protection practices
4. Oversee conduction of indicated radiation surveys and keep records of such surveys and tests, including summaries of corrective measures recommended or instituted
5. Routinely observe and periodically test interlock switches and warning signals
6. Ensure that warning signs and signals are properly located
7. Determine the cause of each known or suspected case of excessive abnormal exposure and take steps to prevent its recurrence

Personnel Monitoring

Personnel monitoring is used to check the adequacy of the radiation safety program, disclose improper radiation protection practices, and detect potentially serious radiation exposure situations. A radiation badge is a common personnel monitoring device. A radiation film badge consists of a plastic holder that contains a paper-wrapped piece of photographic film. When struck by ionizing radiation, the film becomes exposed, and the degree of film blackness can be related to the amount of exposure. Radiation badges may contain thermoluminescent dosimeters rather than film. These dosimeters trap electrons energized by oncoming radiation, and the number of trapped electrons can be quantified and related to the amount of exposure. Radiation badges should be analyzed at least quarterly; weekly analysis is preferable.

Personnel monitoring should be performed in controlled areas for each occupationally exposed individual who has a reasonable possibility of receiving a dose exceeding one fourth the applicable maximum permissible dose. A qualified expert should be consulted on establishment and evaluation of the personnel monitoring system. Devices worn for the monitoring of occupational exposure should *not* be worn by the individual when he or she is exposed as a patient for medical or dental examinations. Monitoring devices should be worn on the chest or abdomen, except for special circumstances. When a protective apron is worn, the monitoring device should be worn on the outside of the apron for monitoring the radiation environment but may be worn inside the apron when an estimate of the body exposure is desired.

Basic Radiation Safety Rules for Diagnostic Radiology

1. Only personnel involved in the procedure should be in the room at the time of exposure.
2. Persons younger than 18 years and pregnant women must not be in the room during the examination.
3. Personnel who assist with radiographic examinations should have a rotating duty roster to minimize exposure to any one person.
4. Sandbags, sponges, tape, or other restraining devices should be used for positioning the patient rather than manual restraint.
5. Anesthesia or tranquilization should be used to facilitate patient restraint when possible.
6. No part of the body should be in the primary beam, whether or not protected by gloves or aprons.
7. An x-ray tube, x-ray machine, or cassette should never be handheld during the exposure.
8. Protective aprons should always be worn when positioning an animal.
9. Protective gloves should be worn if hands are placed near the primary beam.
10. Protective glasses should be worn if the work level is heavy. These glasses provide 0.25 mm Pb equivalent protection to the lens.
11. Thyroid shields should be considered. These are "mini-aprons" that are worn around the neck to protect the thyroid gland.
12. Collimate the primary beam so each film has an unexposed border, proving that the primary beam does not exceed the size of the cassette.
13. Use the fastest film screen combination compatible with the production of diagnostic images.
14. All personnel should wear radiation badges outside the lead apron.
15. Plan the procedure carefully and double-check machine settings.

PRODUCTION OF X-RAYS

When high-speed electrons strike metal, x-rays are produced. X-ray tubes provide for acceleration of electrons and their subsequent interaction with a metal target. Electric current is passed through the cathode (filament) of the x-ray tube in much the same way that an electric current is used to heat the filament of a light bulb. The heat allows electrons to "boil" off the surface of the filament into an electron cloud around the filament. The number of electrons in the cloud is directly related to the amount of electric current passing through the filament, which in turn is regulated by the milliamperage (mA) control on the panel of the x-ray machine. Increasing milliamperage is analogous to increasing the wattage of a light bulb. A 100-W bulb has a hotter filament and emits more light rays per unit time than does a 60-W bulb. More current flows through the filament of a 100-W bulb than through a 60-W bulb.

X-rays are produced at the anode (target). Electrons that have been produced at the filament remain stationary; thus a mechanism is needed to make them strike the metallic anode. This is accomplished by applying a voltage differential between the anode and cathode. Electrons are negatively charged. Therefore, if the anode is positive with respect to the filament of the cathode, the electrons will be attracted to the anode (opposite charges attract) and strike it. The energy of x-rays produced is a function of the energy of the electrons striking the anode. Electrons traveling through a larger potential voltage difference will have a higher energy level. The potential voltage difference is adjusted with the kilovoltage peak (kVp) control on the x-ray panel. Increasing kilovoltage peak increases the voltage difference between the anode and cathode; thus electrons are accelerated to higher velocities and have greater energy when striking the anode. This enables the production of high-energy x-rays (Fig. 1-5).

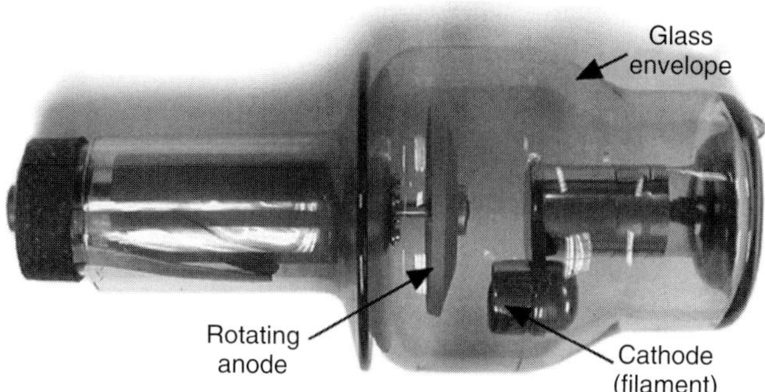

Fig. 1-5 A rotating-anode x-ray tube. The anode rotates at high speed, dissipating heat over a large surface area. Electrons emanate from the cathode. The x-ray tube is encased in a glass envelope from which air has been evacuated; this vacuum prevents electrons from interacting with air molecules on their way to the anode. (Courtesy of Oak Ridge Associated Universities.)

When electrons strike the anode, x-rays are produced by either collisional or radiative interactions.[10] Collisional interactions involve a collision between a high-speed electron and an atom in the anode. The oncoming electron ejects an orbital electron from the anode atom with subsequent release of energy as an x-ray (Fig. 1-6). X-rays produced by this mechanism have specific energies relating to the energy required to eject the target electron from its shell (the binding energy) and are therefore called characteristic x-rays. X-rays created by collisional interactions account for only a small fraction of the total x-rays produced in a diagnostic x-ray tube.

In a radiative interaction (Fig. 1-7), the oncoming high-speed electron passes close to the nucleus of the target atom (attracted by the opposite charge) but an electron is not ejected from the atom. As the oncoming electron slows as it bends around the nucleus, it releases energy in the form of electromagnetic radiation, called bremsstrahlung or "braking radiation." The energy released in the form of bremsstrahlung has a broad spectrum, depending on the amount of energy lost from the electrons as they are deflected to various degrees by the nucleus. Most oncoming electrons have many "braking" interactions with atoms of the target as their kinetic energy is dissipated.

A range (spectrum) of x-ray energies is produced for any given combination of milliamperage and kilovoltage peak. This results because most electrons undergo multiple braking interactions, resulting in production of x-rays with different energy, and a wide range of electron energies arrives at the anode (Fig. 1-8). The maximum x-ray photon energy achievable is one with energy equal to the kilovoltage peak. For this to occur, an electron must be accelerated at maximal velocity (a function of kilovoltage peak) and lose all of its energy in one interaction. The number of x-ray photons in the spectrum with energy equal to the kilovoltage peak is very small (see Fig. 1-8).

The difference between kilovoltage peak and kiloelectron volt* must be understood. The kilovoltage peak refers to the maximum voltage applied to the x-ray tube across the anode-cathode gap. In the United States, electric current is alternating; thus for any given kilovoltage peak setting, the voltage potential difference across the anode-cathode gap fluctuates between positive 110 V and negative 110 V (Fig. 1-9). The term kiloelectron volt (keV) is a unit of energy that describes the energy of either electrons or photons. If the kiloelectron peak is set at 100 (100,000 V maximum differential between the anode and cathode), electrons traveling from anode to cathode have energies equal to or less than 100 keV (100,000 eV). Few electrons achieve energy of 100 keV because of the fluctuating nature of the voltage across the anode-cathode gap; that is the

*An electron volt (eV) is the amount of energy an electron gains as it is accelerated by a potential difference of 1 V. 1 keV = 1000 eV.

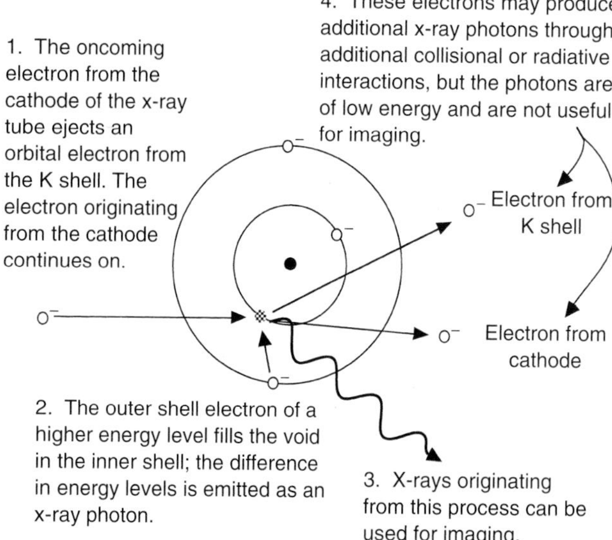

Fig. 1-6 The collision model of x-ray production. An electron from the filament in an x-ray tube is accelerated to high speed through a voltage difference and strikes a target atom. In some collisions, the oncoming electron will eject an orbital electron from the target atom and continue on at a different angle. Atoms with vacancies in electron shells are unstable, and the vacancy is quickly filled by a more peripheral electron or a free electron. When this occurs, energy that was deposited by the original oncoming electron, which resulted in ejection of the target electron, is released in the form of electromagnetic radiation, called a *characteristic* x-ray. In general, electrons in shells near the nucleus are tightly bound and have less kinetic energy than those in peripheral shells.

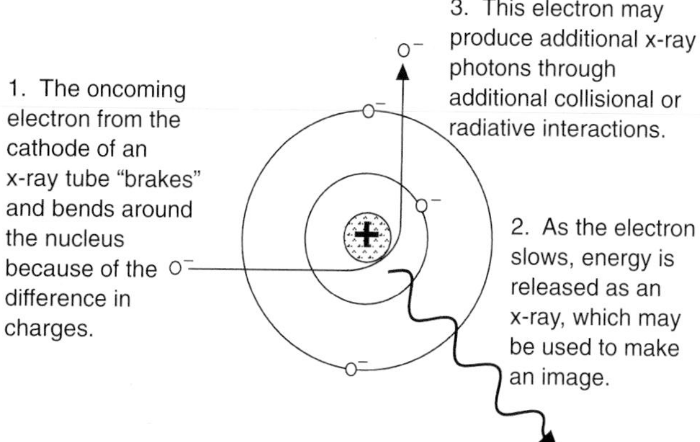

Fig. 1-7 The radiative, or braking, model of x-ray production. An electron from the filament in an x-ray tube is accelerated to high speed through a large potential difference. Because of the difference in charge between the electron (negative) and the nucleus (positive), the electron is deflected as it nears the nucleus. As the deflected electron decelerates, it releases electromagnetic radiation in the form of an x-ray. Because deflected electrons may pass within various distances of the nucleus, braking radiation has a spectrum of energies.

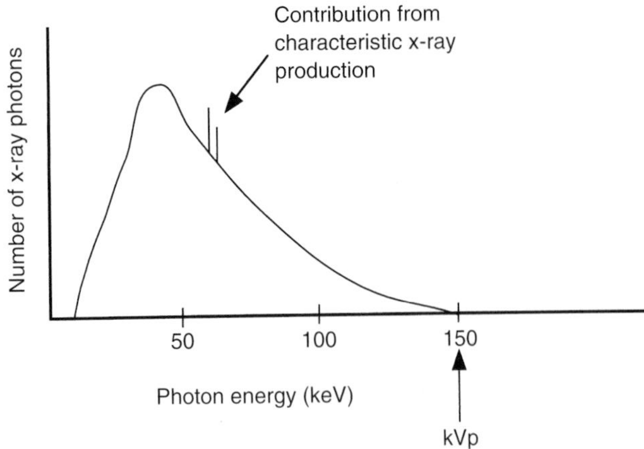

Fig. 1-8 The spectrum of x-ray energy produced by braking and characteristic radiation. The maximum energy x-ray photon achievable is equal to the kilovoltage peak (kVp). For this to occur, an electron must be accelerated at maximal velocity and lose all of its energy in one interaction. As illustrated, the number of x-rays in the spectrum with energy equal to the kilovoltage peak is very small.

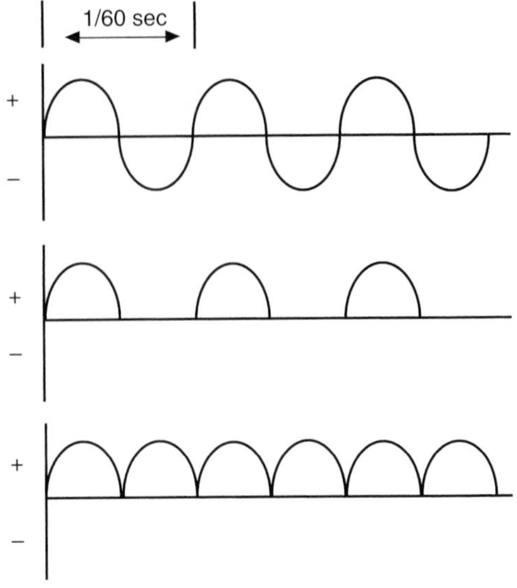

Fig. 1-9 The concept of rectification. The *upper panel* shows the fluctuation typical of alternating current. One complete cycle occurs each 1/60 sec. If this current were used for voltage application in the x-ray tube, the cathode (filament) would be positive in relation to the anode (target) 50% of the time. When the cathode is positive, any free electrons at the anode created by heat buildup would travel to the cathode and damage it. The *middle panel* illustrates the fluctuation obtained when current is not allowed to flow during the negative phase of the cycle. In this instance, electrons will not flow from the anode to the cathode. One disadvantage of this type of current modification is a loss of potentially useful current during the negative phase of the cycle. Methods have been developed to reverse the direction of current flow in half the cycle. The resultant waveform is shown in the *bottom panel*. This is called full-wave rectification and results in one useful pulse of current every $^1/_{120}$ sec.

voltage is at its maximum value for only an instant during each cycle. If a 100-keV electron loses all its energy in one interaction, it produces an x-ray photon with energy of 100 keV. But this is very uncommon. Only a few x-ray photons in the beam will have an energy that is equal to the kilovoltage peak, and it is unusual for an electron to lose all its energy in one interaction (see Fig. 1-8).

A basic discussion of problems relating to the use of alternating current for production of x-rays is necessary. If alternating current (see Fig. 1-9) were used for x-ray production, at times during the current cycle the cathode would be positive in relation to the anode. Any free electrons at the surface of the anode, present because of the high temperature of the anode, would be attracted to the cathode and damage it. To avoid this, alternating current is converted to direct current by a process called *rectification*. An in-depth discussion of rectification is beyond the scope of this text. What must be understood here is that rectification results in the anode always being positive with respect to the cathode. Thus electrons only travel from the cathode to the anode.

Most of the energy (more than 90%) of the electrons striking the anode is converted to heat. Therefore, x-ray tube targets must be constructed of high–melting point substances, such as tungsten. Additionally, as an ancillary heat dissipation mechanism, the anode may rotate to increase the effective surface area struck by the oncoming high-speed electrons. Anode rotation prevents the target from melting or becoming "pitted," as would happen if electrons continually struck the same target region. Targets in x-ray tubes are also typically constructed of a high–atomic number material, such as tungsten, because the efficiency of x-ray production from electron interactions is directly related to atomic number.

The focal spot is the region of the target struck by electrons and is the site of x-ray production. The smaller the focal spot, the better the detail on the radiograph. A practical example of this principle is the sharpness of a shadow cast by a large versus a small light source. A shadow cast by a small light source, assuming the distance from the light to the object is constant, will always be sharper than a shadow cast by a large light source. Therefore having a small focal spot is desirable. Angling the anode is one way to make the focal spot of the x-ray tube appear smaller than it really is while at the same time maintaining a larger area on the anode being struck by electrons to facilitate heat distribution (Fig. 1-10).

Some x-ray machines allow the operator to select the focal spot size. A small focal spot is useful when greater image detail is necessary. One disadvantage of using the small filament is that lower milliamperage values must also be used to prevent the filament from overheating.

As already stated, increasing milliamperage increases the number of x-rays produced. The number of x-rays produced can also be controlled by the length of time the x-ray tube is energized. The timer on the x-ray machine panel controls the length of time current is applied to the cathode and voltage is applied across the anode-cathode gap. X-rays are produced only when a source of electrons and a voltage differential are present across the anode-cathode gap.

The concept of milliampere seconds (mAs) is used to quantify the amount of radiation produced by the x-ray tube and is analogous to leaving a 60-W bulb burning twice as long as a 120-W bulb. In both instances, the total number of light rays emitted would be roughly the same, although the intensity at any one time would be twice as great for the 120-W bulb. A milliampere second is the product of milliamperage (the setting on the control panel) and time, in seconds. A variety of combinations of milliamperage and time can be used to produce the same number of x-rays (Table 1-3).

X-ray generators provide electrical energy to the x-ray tube.[11,12] Components within the generator permit the operator to select kilovoltage peak, milliamperage, and exposure time. X-ray generators also protect the x-ray tube from being damaged by excessive exposure factors. The main components

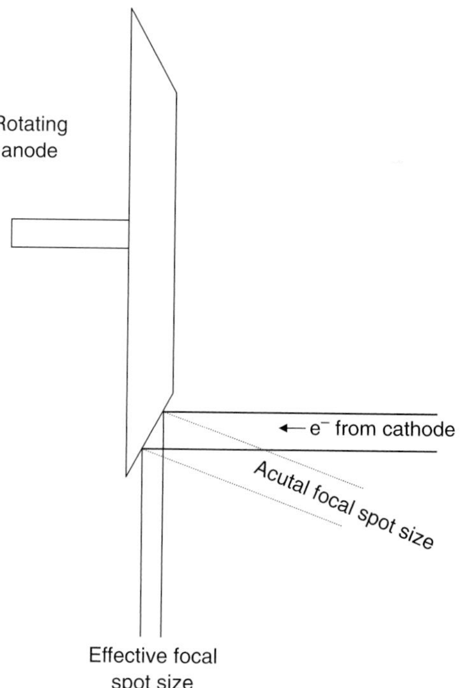

Fig. 1-10 The effective focal spot size principle. By angling the anode, the size of the effective focal spot is decreased, whereas the area on the anode that is struck by electrons remains large and thus facilitates heat distribution.

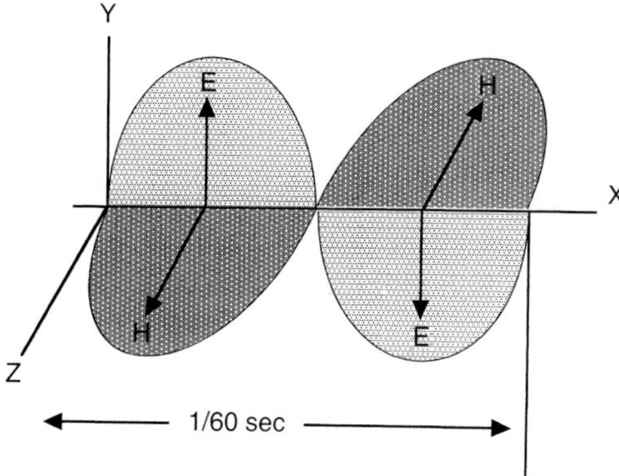

Fig. 1-11 The concept of electromagnetic radiation. Oscillating electric *(E)* and magnetic *(H)* fields move in orthogonal planes. Here the *E* field moves in the *Y* direction and the *H* field moves in the *Z* direction. Time is in the *X* direction.

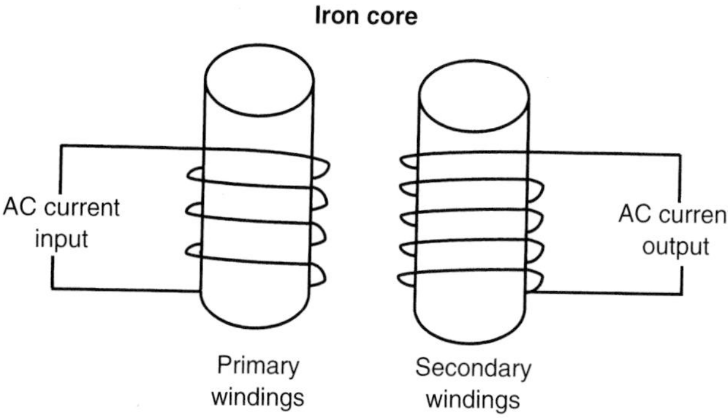

Fig. 1-12 A step-up transformer. The magnetic field in the primary winding induces a current in the secondary winding. Because more turns are present in the secondary windings, the voltage will be increased—here by a factor of 5/4 because the secondary side has five turns and the primary side has four turns. Energy must be conserved, thus amperage will drop proportionately (by a factor of 4/5) on the output side.

Table • 1-3

Constant Milliampere Seconds Can Be Produced by a Variety of Milliamperage and Time Combinations

mA	TIME (SEC)	mAS
50	0.1	5
100	0.05	5
500	0.01	5
1000	0.005	5

of an x-ray generator are the high-voltage circuit (which regulates voltage potential across the anode-cathode gap, e.g., kilovoltage peak), the filament circuit (which regulates filament current in the x-ray tube, e.g., milliamperes), and circuits for automatic exposure control.

X-ray generation requires potential differences of 40,000 to 120,000 V (40 to 120 kVp) in the x-ray tube. Thus transformers are needed to boost the relatively weak input voltage from a standard power source (110 to 120 V) by 500- to 1000-fold. A transformer is a complex device, and only a simplified explanation follows. Transformers convert a given input voltage to a new output voltage. A moving charge such as an electric current produces a magnetic field. The magnetic field oscillates in conjunction with the sinusoidal change in polarity of a 60-Hz electric current (Fig. 1-11). A moving (oscillating) magnetic field generates a flow of electrons (current) in a wire that is capable of conducting electricity. The transformer exploits this phenomenon by using the magnetic field of input current of a primary circuit to induce a current in an adjacent, secondary circuit. The primary and secondary circuits are arranged in parallel opposing coils or windings and are insulated, so no contact is made between them (Fig. 1-12). If the number of windings of each circuit is equal, the transformer will generate identical output current and voltage in the secondary circuit. However, if the secondary circuit has more windings than the primary circuit, the induced current will have a higher voltage. This is because the magnetic field or flux generated by the primary windings interacts with a greater number of secondary windings. The ratio of the number of secondary and primary windings is proportional to the output voltage. Thus, if twice as many secondary as primary windings are present, the output voltage will be twice the input voltage. Such a transformer is called a *step-up transformer.* In x-ray generators, the incoming (line) voltage of the primary circuit of the step-up transformer can be adjusted using the kilovoltage peak selector. This results in selectable output voltage from the secondary circuit that is applied to the x-ray tube. This type of transformer is called an autotransformer.

The generator also houses a low-energy circuit that supplies current to the filament of the x-ray tube. Only a weak

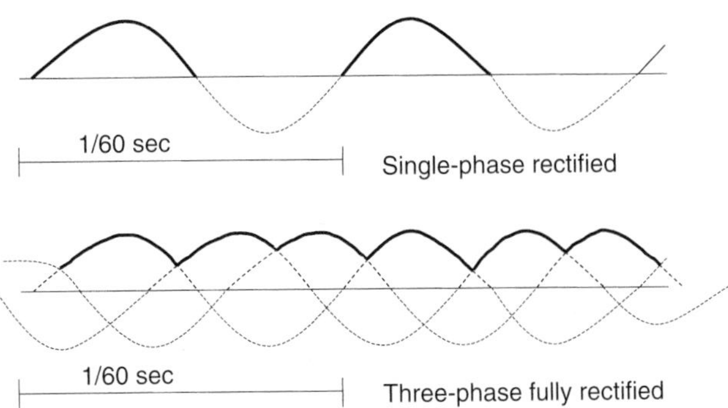

Fig. 1-13 The ripple factor. In single-phase, unrectified x-ray machines, voltage fluctuates from zero to +110 V to zero in $^1/_{120}$ sec, followed by no voltage fluctuation for $^1/_{120}$ sec, then from zero to +110 V to zero in the next $^1/_{120}$ sec, and so forth. By introducing three separate current sources (waves), each out of phase by the same amount of time, the ripple from peak to peak is diminished. Use of three separate current sources is called three-phase technology. The ripple factor is illustrated by the *dark line* connecting the tops of the current cycles. This clearly has been reduced by the three-phase method.

current is needed to heat the tungsten filament of the cathode, and even a standard 110-V, 5 A, 60-Hz current is too strong. Therefore *a step-down tra*nsformer is used to reduce the incoming voltage to approximately 10 V. The step-down transformer has adjustable primary windings, allowing it to function as the milliamperage selector. Overall, the step-down transformer has fewer secondary than primary windings. The milliamperage selector controls the current passing through the filament, and thus the number of electrons available for acceleration to the cathode, where x-rays are produced.

Several types of generators exist, but only three are discussed: single- and three-phase generators and high-frequency generators.[12] Single-phase generators are connected to a single-phase alternating current input line (Fig. 1-13). Single-phase generators are problematic because the polarity of the alternating current reverses every $^1/_{60}$ second. Therefore only half of each cycle is useful for accelerating electrons across the tube (see the previous discussion on rectification). Even with full-wave rectification, the large fluctuation between maximum and minimum voltage, or *ripple factor,* during an exposure (evident in Fig. 1-13) is undesirable. However, with a three-phase alternating current, the ripple factor is significantly reduced because the alternating current arrives in three separate phases regarding time. Three identical lines supply the transformer of a three-phase generator, allowing the three waveforms to be 120 degrees out of phase with each other (see Fig. 1-13). This obviously provides less fluctuation between maximum and minimum voltage, giving a smaller ripple factor. Although this feature of a three-phase generator is desirable, it adds to the complexity of the x-ray machine and increases cost. Advantages of three-phase generators include shorter exposure times and higher kilovoltage peak. Many large, standing x-ray machines use three-phase generators, and portable units have single-phase generators.

High-frequency generators are the current state-of-the-art power source for x-ray tubes. These generators produce extremely high-frequency, high-voltage output that has a near-zero ripple factor. First, incoming three-phase alternating line current is converted into direct current. Next, the current is chopped into a high-frequency square wave current and fed to the primary windings of a step-up transformer. The frequency of the tube current is 500 to 4000 Hz, which produces a low ripple factor. The generator also contains capacitors in the high-voltage circuit that help "hold" the voltage potential constant across the x-ray tube. With additional smoothing, the final waveform across the tube is almost a flat line, or of constant voltage. High-frequency generators are also compact, relatively inexpensive, and easily maintained. Therefore they are the most desired type of x-ray generator and are commonly used in x-ray machines that are manufactured for veterinary practices.

INTERACTION OF RADIATION WITH MATTER

To understand how radiographs are produced by using x-rays, an understanding of how photons interact with matter is necessary. Five possible mechanisms of interaction exist of a photon with matter: (1) coherent scattering, (2) photoelectric effect, (3) Compton scattering, (4) pair production, and (5) photodisintegration. Pair production and photodisintegration have no relevance to diagnostic radiology and are not discussed. A basic description of the coherent, photoelectric, and Compton processes is given; sources for more detailed reading are available.[10]

Coherent Scattering

A photon interacts with an object and changes its direction, but the subject does not absorb the photon and a change in photon energy does not occur. The fraction of x-rays striking a patient that undergoes coherent scattering is small, approximately 5%. Coherent scattering is not useful in the production of the radiograph and is, in fact, disadvantageous because the scattered photons may strike the x-ray film and degrade image quality or they may strike the radiographer, thereby increasing personnel exposure.

Photoelectric Effect

The photoelectric effect is the interaction process that ultimately results in an image being formed. The x-ray striking the patient is totally absorbed (Fig. 1-14) and, therefore, no scattered radiation exists to contend with. The absorption of the x-ray results in less exposure of the film under that particular part of the patient. The absorbed x-ray photon ejects an electron, called a photoelectron, from an inner shell of a tissue atom. The photoelectron may produce multiple ionization events in the tissue and is eventually absorbed in the patient. When the vacancy created by ejection of the photoelectron is filled by a peripheral shell electron, or a free electron, a characteristic x-ray is given off (see Fig. 1-14). This is the same type of characteristic x-ray given off in the target of an x-ray tube when the oncoming electron from the cathode creates a vacancy in a target atom. The energy of characteristic radiation is a function of the atomic number of the atom from which it arises. Thus with a large atomic number atom such as tungsten (the target of the x-ray tube), the characteristic x-ray is actually part, albeit small, of the useful x-ray beam. But in the body the energy of characteristic x-rays is so low that they are absorbed locally and therefore contribute to the absorbed dose in the patient being radiographed, but not to production of the radiographic image. The probability of a photoelectric interaction is directly proportional to the cube of the atomic number (proportional to Z^3) and inversely proportional to the cube of the photon energy (proportional to $1/E^3$). The relation between the photoelectric process and the atomic number of the absorber (the patient) is very important. This relation "magnifies" differences in absorption ability of various tissue types, such as bone versus soft tissue and soft tissue versus fat. If it were not for the atomic number dependence of the photoelectric effect, there would be insufficient differential absorption of x-ray photons between tissues for the resultant image to have any contrast; that is, all tissues would appear of similar opacity on the radiograph and the

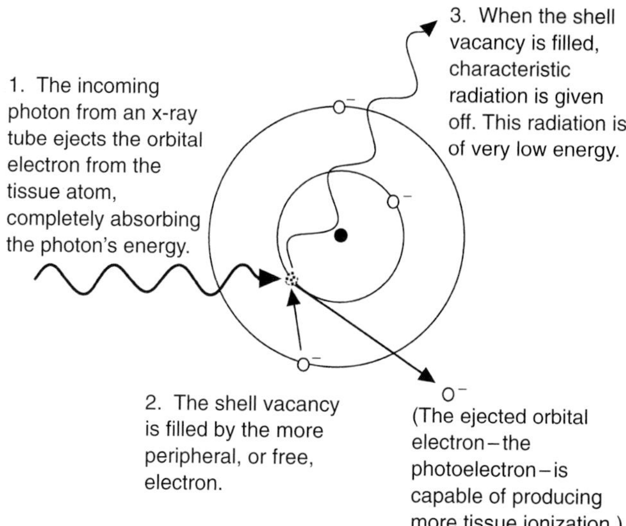

Fig. 1-14 The photoelectric effect. An x-ray from the x-ray tube ejects an electron, usually from an inner shell of a tissue atom. The incoming x-ray is completely absorbed. Electrons in shells near the nucleus are tightly bound and have less kinetic energy than those in peripheral shells. Electrons in the most peripheral shells are essentially "free" because of their weak attraction to the positively charged nucleus. Therefore, as a photoelectron is ejected from the K shell, replacement electrons must give up energy before they can occupy the shell. This energy is released in the form of a photon, called characteristic radiation because shell energy levels are specific to the type of atom. In tissue, the energy of the characteristic radiation is extremely low and is absorbed.

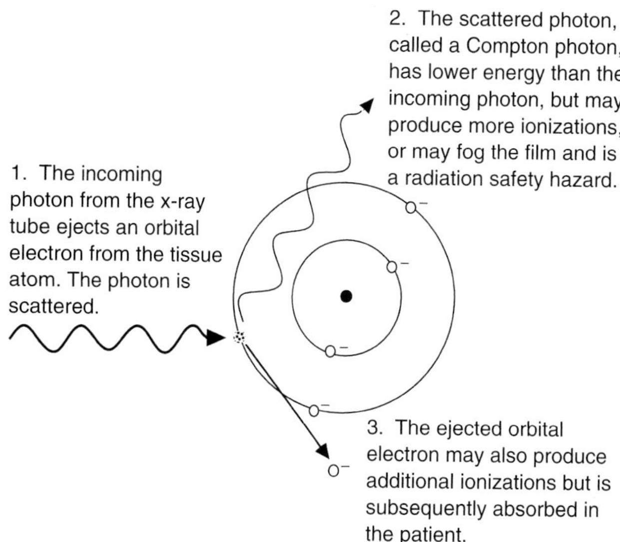

Fig. 1-15 The Compton absorption process. An x-ray produced in the x-ray tube ejects an electron, usually from an outer shell, of a tissue atom. The incoming photon is scattered, not absorbed as in the photoelectric process, but it has lower energy. The ejected electron and scattered photon may continue and produce additional ionizations.

radiograph would be useless. Another advantage of the photoelectric effect is the lack of a scattered photon. Scattered photons are disadvantageous because they result in exposure of the x-ray film (film fog) and personnel. However, patient dose associated with the photoelectric effect is high because the entire incoming photon is absorbed in the patient. The decrease in probability of photoelectric absorption as the energy of the photon beam increases results in a loss of contrast between tissues of various types when very high-energy photons are used for radiography.

Compton Scattering

Almost all scattered radiation that is encountered in diagnostic radiology results from Compton scattering. In the Compton reaction, an incoming x-ray photon interacts with a peripheral shell electron of the patient. The electron is ejected, and the photon is scattered at a different angle; the scattered photon also has lower energy than the original photon (Fig. 1-15). The scattered electron is called either a Compton electron or a recoil electron. The probability of a Compton reaction depends on the total number of electrons in the absorber (patient), which in turn depends on its physical density (grams per cubic centimeter) and number of electrons per gram. The probability of a Compton interaction decreases as photon energy increases. Because most elements contain approximately the same number of electrons per unit mass, the probability of a Compton reaction is independent of atomic number. Such independence is disadvantageous. For example, the atomic number dependence of photoelectric absorption results in great differences in absorption, and thus good tissue contrast, between tissues. With Compton absorption being independent of atomic number, Compton absorption results in poorer image contrast. Thus, if the energy of the x-ray beam is such that Compton absorption predominates, the image will have very little contrast. This is why radiography should use x-ray beams that have an energy in which the photoelectric absorption reaction predominates. The photon scattering that occurs with Compton interactions is also disadvantageous because the scattered photons are radiation safety considerations for bystanders; they also degrade the image by producing fog.

BASIC CONCEPT OF MAKING A RADIOGRAPH

To make a radiograph the patient is placed between the x-ray tube and the x-ray film (Fig. 1-16). The spectrum of energy of x-rays produced by a diagnostic x-ray tube is broad. X-ray photons of very low energy serve no useful purpose because they are absorbed by the patient and make no useful contribution to creation of the image. Therefore filters are routinely placed in the x-ray tube housing to remove low-energy x-rays. Some x-rays passing through the filter are absorbed by the beam-shaping collimator or tube housing and do not strike the patient. The collimator serves to limit the primary beam and prevent nonuseful radiation from leaving the tube housing. This nonuseful radiation would only increase patient dose, degrade image quality because of fogging, and increase the radiation dose to bystanders. In Figure 1-16, three x-rays are seen leaving the collimator. The left one completely penetrates the patient and will be recorded on the x-ray film. Some fraction of the x-rays must penetrate the patient or no information would be recorded on the film. The middle x-ray hits a structure within the patient and is completely absorbed. This is also necessary and emphasizes an important point: radiographs are possible only because of differential absorption of x-rays by the patient. The x-ray on the right hits the patient and is scattered. In this instance, the x-ray will strike a bystander. If the bystander is not wearing a protective apron and gloves, he or she will receive unnecessary radiation dose. If the angle of scatter had been different, the scattered x-ray may have struck the x-ray film, causing film fog.

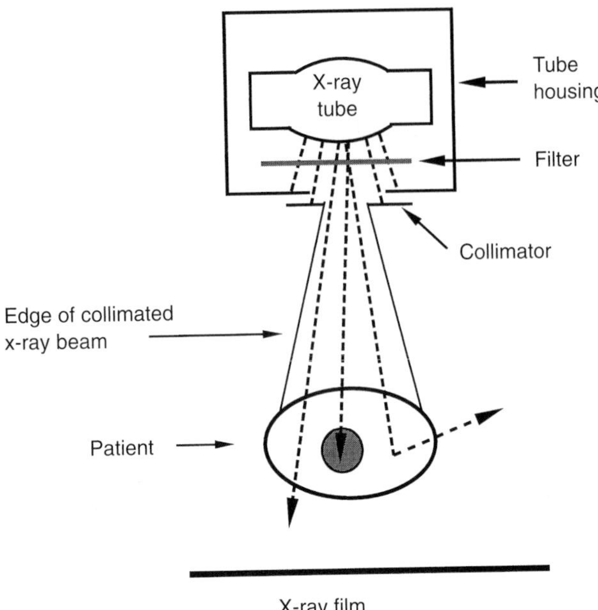

Fig. 1-16 The schematic relation between x-ray tube, patient, and cassette. The fate of three x-ray photons striking the patient is also shown.

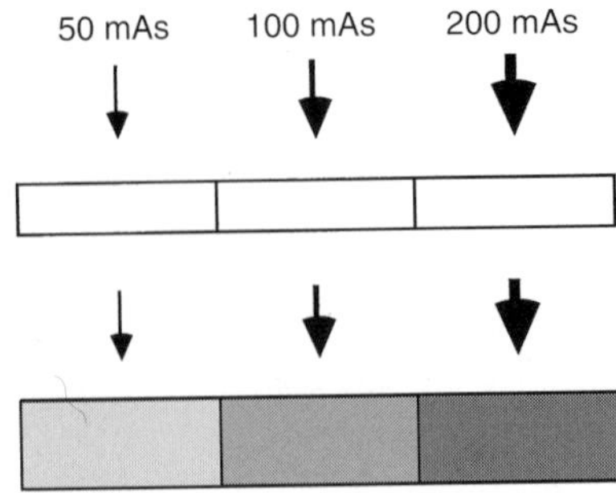

Fig. 1-17 The number of x-rays reaching the film, and therefore film blackness, can be controlled by changing the milliamperage setting on the control panel. Increasing milliampere seconds (mAs), while keeping the kilovoltage peak (kVp) constant, will result in more x-rays striking the patient and thus proportionally more x-rays will pass through the patient or object. Thus as milliamperage is increased, film blackness also increases.

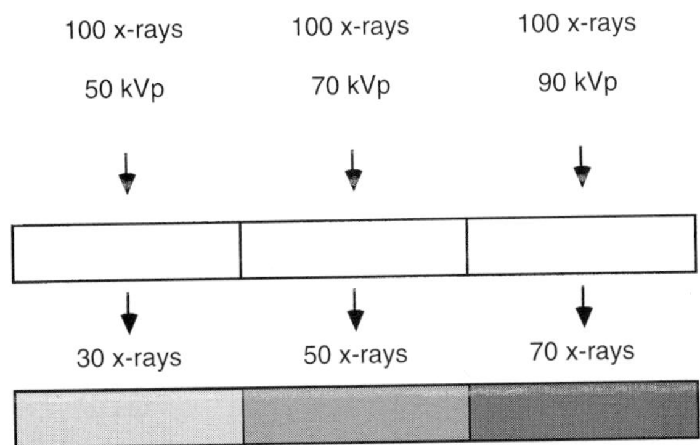

Fig. 1-18 The number of x-rays reaching the film, and therefore film blackness, can be controlled by changing the kilovoltage peak (kVp) setting on the control panel. Increasing kilovoltage peak while keeping milliamperage constant results in x-rays having more energy. As energy increases, the likelihood of penetration without interaction increases. This will result in more x-rays hitting the film and an increase in film blackness.

A radiograph is a visible image of the internal makeup of an object. Some method of recording the image of the patient must occur if it is to be critically assessed. Fortunately, one of the important characteristics of x-rays is their ability to expose photographic emulsions. Therefore x-rays passing through the patient can expose the photographic emulsion in the film in such a manner as to present a picture of the composition of the body. Some important aspects of this process must be understood at this point in the text, although the radiographic image itself is dealt with in greater detail in Chapter 5.

A new method of radiographic image production, that of using x-rays to create a digital image file that can be viewed and manipulated on a computer monitor, is quickly gaining acceptance in veterinary medicine. This technology is discussed in more detail in Chapter 2.

Film Blackness/Opacity

X-ray film is photographic film with a light-sensitive emulsion containing silver halide. After x-rays or visible light, silver halide crystals become sensitized and precipitate during development, forming neutral silver deposits. These neutral silver deposits appear black on processed film. Unexposed crystals are removed during fixation, leaving clear areas on the film. Thus the amount of precipitated silver in any particular part of the film determines how black, gray, or clear that part of the film appears. This film darkening is directly related to the number of x-rays that reach that part of the film from the patient. The degree of film blackness is affected by the number of x-rays striking the film, which in turn is affected by the x-ray machine output (milliampere seconds). When more x-rays are emitted, more reach the film (Fig. 1-17).

Film blackness is also affected by the energy of the x-ray beam (kilovoltage peak). The higher the kilovoltage peak, the higher the x-ray energy, the more x-rays that will penetrate the patient, and the greater the film blackness (Fig. 1-18).

The distance from the x-ray tube to the film also affects film blackness. This distance is referred to as the focal spot/film distance (FFD). As the FFD increases, film blackness decreases because the intensity of x-rays in the x-ray beam (x-rays/unit area) decreases (Fig. 1-19).

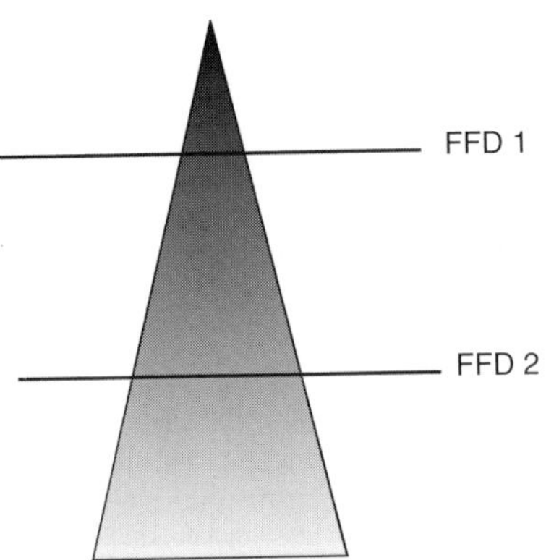

Fig. 1-19 As distance from the x-ray source (anode) increases, the intensity of x-rays in the beam (x-rays/unit area) decreases because of beam divergence. This example shows that as the FFD increases, the film blackness of the resultant radiograph decreases. To obtain film blackness at FFD 2 that is similar to that at FFD 1 in this example, the number of x-rays produced at the anode (milliamperage) would have to be increased.

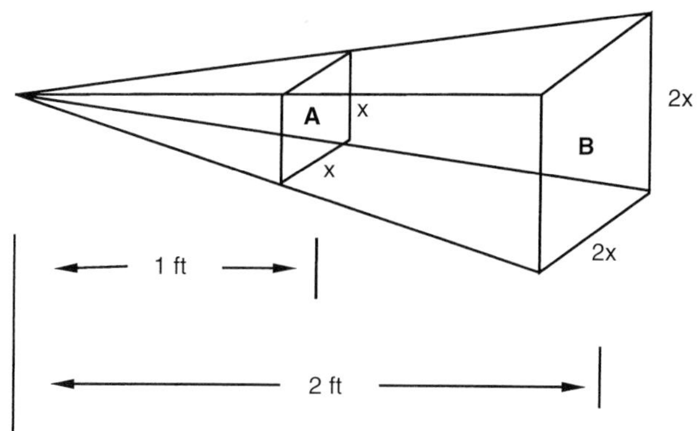

Fig. 1-20 The intensity of an x-ray beam (x-rays/unit area) changes with the square of the distance. At a distance of 1 foot, the diverging x-ray beam covers an area represented by square A with each side of dimension *x*, or an area of (x) times (x) = x^2. At 2 feet, the diverging beam covers a square B in which each side is now twice as long as it was at 1 foot. The area covered by the beam at 2 feet is therefore (2x) times (2x) = $4x^2$, which is four times the area at 1 foot. Because the intensity of the beam originating at the anode is constant, the intensity falling on the small square must spread out over an area that is four times as large by the time it reaches the large square.

The amount of change in intensity of the x-ray beam as a function of distance is described by the inverse square law equation:

$$\frac{I_1}{I_2} = \frac{(d_2)^2}{(d_1)^2}$$

where *I* is intensity in terms of number of x-rays/unit area, *d* is distance, I_1 is intensity at d_1, and I_2 is intensity at d_2. Therefore, as FFD increases, intensity and film blackness decrease; this decrease is a function of the square of the distance, not simply the distance (Fig. 1-20).

As an example, assume that at an FFD of 50 inches, the intensity of the x-ray beam at the level of the film is 100 x-rays/cm^2. What will the intensity be if the FFD is decreased to 25 inches? Intuitively, the intensity must be greater at a shorter distance, but the exact solution can be obtained. I_1 = 100 x-rays/cm^2, d_1 = 50 inches, I_2 = ?, d_2 = 25 inches. Substituting, the equation becomes:

$$\frac{100}{I_2} = \frac{(25)^2}{(50)^2};$$

$$\frac{100}{I_2} = \frac{625}{250};$$

$$\frac{100}{I_2} = 0.25;$$

$$I_2 = 400\text{x-rays/cm}^2$$

Therefore, by decreasing the distance from the x-ray source to the film by a factor of two, the intensity increases not by a factor of two but by a factor of four—that is, the square of the distance change.

The inverse square relation has other practical implications. Suppose an exposure of 100 mAs is needed to make a radiograph of the abdomen with a 40-inch FFD. When another x-ray machine is used, the maximum FFD that can be obtained is 30 inches. What milliamperage must be used to maintain the same radiographic opacity as at a 40-inch FFD? Common sense states that because the distance is shorter, a lower milliamperage must be used. The exact milliamperage value can be calculated from the inverse square principle. The inverse square law equation noted previously cannot be used for this calculation because it relates intensity change as a function of distance. In this example, the same photon intensity should be maintained at the film, which is now 10 inches closer to the x-ray tube. The question is, how much does the milliamperage have to decrease to maintain the same intensity? In this situation, a direct relation exists between the milliamperage needed to maintain the same intensity and distance, so the equation is as follows:

$$\frac{mAs_1}{mAs_2} = \frac{(d_1)^2}{(d_2)^2}$$

and from the above, mAs_1 = 100, mAs_2 = ?, d_1 = 40 inches, d_2 = 30 inches, and the proper expression is:

$$\frac{100}{mAs_2} = \frac{(40)^2}{(30)^2};$$

$$\frac{100}{mAs_2} = \frac{1600}{900};$$

$$\frac{100}{mAs_2} = 1.77;$$

$$mAs_2 = \frac{100}{1.77};$$

$$mAs_2 = 56.25 \text{ mAs}$$

Thus, the new measurement at a 30-inch FFD is 56.25 mAs and is lower than the original value of 100 mAs, which was needed at a 40-inch FFD. In this example, the intensity (x-rays/unit area) at the film will be the same under either circumstance—that is, 100 mAs at 40 inches, or 56.25 mAs at 30 inches.

Therefore FFDs are chosen as a compromise between long values, which preserve radiographic detail, and short values, which require lower milliamperage values. Use of a long FFD to preserve detail cannot be recommended because the large milliamperage values needed to maintain x-ray intensity at the film are potentially harmful to the x-ray tube; to obtain high milliamperage values, longer exposure times are needed, which may result in patient motion, a cause of image unsharpness. FFD values are typically in the range of 40 to 60 inches. Short FFD is often used in large animal applications where minimal space is available and reduced exposure time is needed to limit motion artifact. Thus the above equation has significant practical value because it is needed to determine the proper milliamperage for a shorter FFD.

FACTORS AFFECTING IMAGE DETAIL

Motion

Motion is the biggest enemy of detail in veterinary radiology because any motion will induce image unsharpness. To avoid motion unsharpness, a fast exposure time is used. In some x-ray machines, the timer is capable of millisecond exposures. When exposure times become very short, the milliamperage must be very large; otherwise, the milliamperage will be too low to produce the necessary level of film blackness. Milliampere values up to 1500 can be obtained in some x-ray machines. In private practice, however, choice of milliamperage values is more limited and most machines have maximum values of 300 mAs. This means exposure times must be longer to obtain suitable values, and motion

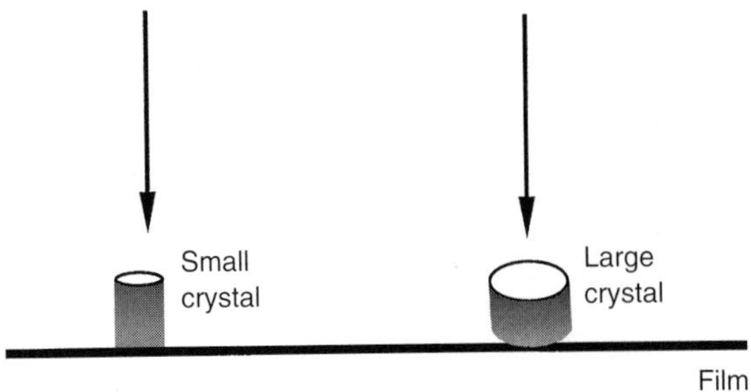

Fig. 1-21 An x-ray carrying information from the patient is about to interact with an x-ray film crystal. On the left (small crystal, slow, or detail film) the information from the patient will be deposited over a smaller area than on the right (large crystal, fast film). Therefore detail will be better on the left, but more radiation will be necessary to make the radiograph because the probability of an x-ray leaving the patient and hitting the crystal will be less with small crystals than with large crystals.

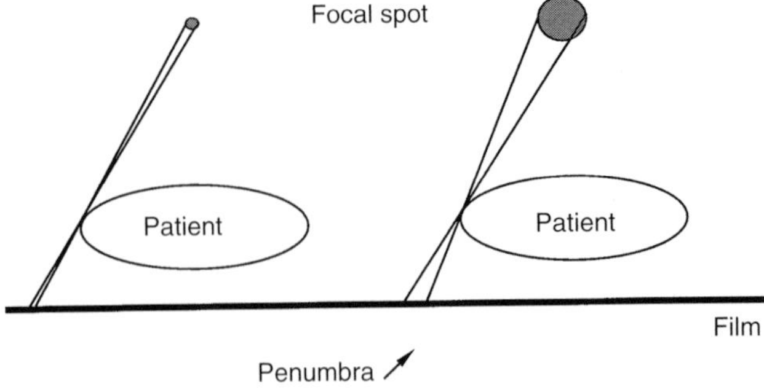

Fig. 1-22 The effect of focal spot size on detail. With large focal spots, the edge unsharpness, or the penumbra, is larger. This contributes to image unsharpness.

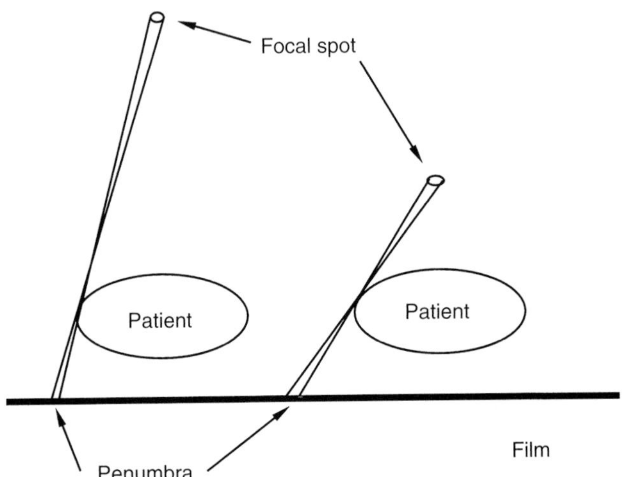

Fig. 1-23 The effect of FFD on detail. At short FFDs, x-rays from either side of the focal spot will create a larger area of edge unsharpness (penumbra) on the film than at long FFDs. At short FFDs, information from the patient is spread out over a larger area of the film (magnification), resulting in loss of detail. This is synonymous with photographic enlargement. As a photograph is enlarged, detail decreases because the information is spread out over a larger area.

becomes more of a problem. Motion can be combated by (1) not using a long FFD (requires more milliamperage and, therefore, longer exposure time), (2) not using detail film, (3) using high-speed screens (rare-earth), and (4) using a grid with a medium grid ratio (e.g., 8 : 1). All these factors are included in the subsequent discussion.

Film Speed

X-ray film is available in a variety of speeds. Film speed is related to the size of the silver halide crystals in the emulsion or to the thickness of the silver halide layer. X-rays (or light from the intensifying screen) are more likely to interact with (hit) a large silver halide crystal or the increased number of silver halide crystals in a thicker crystal layer. Thus degree of film blackness from a constant exposure is greater for films with larger silver halide crystals or thicker crystal layers. Fast films, or high-speed films, have larger silver halide crystals or thicker layers of silver halide crystals. Slow films have smaller crystals or thinner layers of crystals. The detail of the radiographic image is inversely related to the speed of the film. Detail is greater with slow films (small crystals) because the area exposed by each x-ray is smaller, that is, less amplification of information is conferred by each x-ray (Fig. 1-21).

Focal Spot Size

Some x-ray tubes have a large and a small focal spot, both of which are operator selectable. Use of a small focal spot results in improved detail (Fig. 1-22). The disadvantage of using the small focal spot is that lower milliamperage values must be used to prevent the filament from burning out. With the small focal spot, edges of anatomic structures are projected much more sharply than with the large focal spot. This edge unsharpness is called *penumbra*. In practice, small focal spots are not used frequently because of the associated milliamperage limitations.

Focal Spot/Film Distance

Detail is also related to FFD. As previously mentioned, FFD affects detail (Fig. 1-23). The following is known about FFD values: (1) the advantage of keeping FFD long is optimization of detail, (2) the advantage of keeping FFD short is decreased radiographic technique (milliamperage) requirements, and (3) compromise and 40- to 60-inch values are typical.

Object-Film Distance

The distance of the patient from the film also affects detail. This parameter is called object-film distance (OFD) (Fig. 1-24). Changes in OFD affect detail more than do changes in FFD, although both obviously have some effect on detail. Therefore, when a patient is radiographed, the patient should be kept as close to the x-ray film as possible.

Intensifying Screens

In reality, the sensitivity of the film emulsion to x-rays is much lower than its sensitivity to visible light. Therefore converting the x-ray energy into visible light and then using the visible light to expose the film is more convenient. This is possible because of the property of x-rays to cause certain compounds to fluoresce (see Box 1-1). Intensifying screens are used to convert x-rays into visible light. Intensifying screens are composed of layers of phosphorescent crystals that emit light when struck by an x-ray (Fig. 1-25). The phosphorescent crystals of intensifying screens should not be confused with the silver halide crystals in the film emulsion.

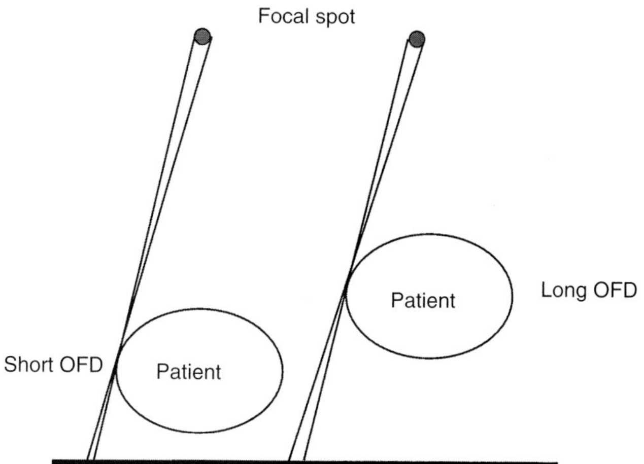

Fig. 1-24 In this example, the film focal distance is the same in both instances. The OFD is different, being long on the right and short on the left. As OFD increases, magnification and edge unsharpness increase, resulting in a decrease in radiographic detail. Note how much larger the image of the object will be on the right compared with the left.

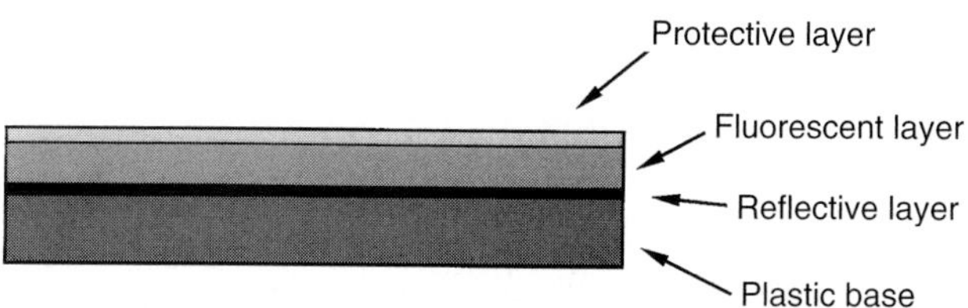

Fig. 1-25 The anatomy of an intensifying screen. Intensifying screens are covered with a protective layer. Beneath this is the phosphorescent layer, which fluoresces (converts x-rays into visible light) when struck by x-rays. A reflective layer lies deep beneath the fluorescent layer, which reflects light back in the direction of the x-ray film. The film contacts the protective layer. The plastic base provides support for the intensifying screen.

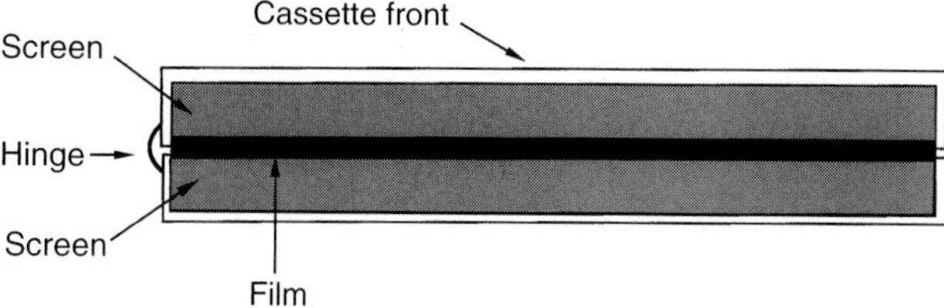

Fig. 1-26 The anatomy of a cassette. X-ray film is placed in a cassette, sandwiched between two intensifying screens. This increases the efficiency of the entire system over that achieved if only one screen were used. Use of two screens decreases detail compared with only one screen, however.

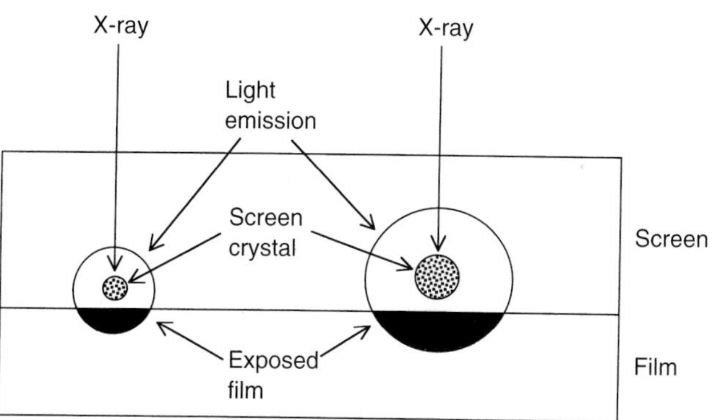

Fig. 1-27 Effect of intensifying screen crystal size on detail. Shown is a screen that contains crystals of two sizes. (This is for illustration purposes only because screens are never constructed with more than one size of phosphorescent crystal.) The crystal on the left is smaller, and that part of the screen will be slower (require more radiation to produce light, because the chance of an x-ray hitting a small crystal is less) than the right side, where the crystals are bigger. An x-ray is shown hitting each crystal. A halo of light is emitted from each crystal. The halo is bigger on the right, resulting in a larger area of x-ray film being exposed. Therefore less detail will be seen on the right because the information being recorded from the patient is spread over a larger area of the film. Screens for optimizing detail, so-called detail screens, have smaller crystals than regular speed screens but require more radiation to produce an acceptable radiograph.

For radiography, x-ray film is sandwiched between two intensifying screens in a cassette (Fig. 1-26). The front of the cassette is a low atomic number, low physical density material that does not absorb a significant portion of the incident x-ray beam. The cassette is constructed in such a manner as to compress the film between the screens to ensure good film-screen contact. If there is not good contact between the film and the screens, light from the screens would diffuse over a larger distance and detail would be degraded.

Both the thickness of the phosphor layer and the size of the crystals in the phosphor layer can be varied (Fig. 1-27). As with x-ray film, an increased chance exists for interaction between an x-ray and the intensifying screen when the phosphor crystals are large or the phosphor layer is thick; but the radiographic detail is decreased with large crystals or thicker phosphor layers because light produced by the screen diffuses over a wider area. In some intensifying screens, particularly those with a thick phosphor layer, a light-absorbing dye is added to the phosphor layer to reduce the amount of diffused light reaching the x-ray film; this leads to increased radiographic detail. These light-reducing dyes also result in more radiation required to produce a satisfactory radiographic image.

Intensifying screens are used because they can convert a few absorbed x-rays into many light rays, thereby decreasing the number of incident x-rays needed to make a radiograph. This results in less radiation exposure to the patient and technical personnel and allows the use of relatively low-output x-ray machines to make radiographs of large body parts, such as the equine stifle or the equine thorax.

Intensifying screens originally incorporated calcium tungstate ($CaWO_4$) as the phosphor, but new phosphors have replaced $CaWO_4$. These new phosphors are termed rare-earth phosphors, not because the components are uncommon but because some of the components come from the rare-earth series of elements, which includes elements of atomic numbers 57 through 71. The x-ray/light conversion of these rare-earth intensifying screens is significantly greater than that of $CaWO_4$. For example, one x-ray absorbed in $CaWO_4$ produces approximately 1000 light rays versus approximately 4000 produced by a rare-earth phosphor. Thus, by using rare-earth intensifying screens, radiographs at milliamperage settings lower than ever before can be produced.

In some instances in which outstanding detail is desired, radiographs are produced without the use of intensifying screens. This "nonscreen" technique requires much higher

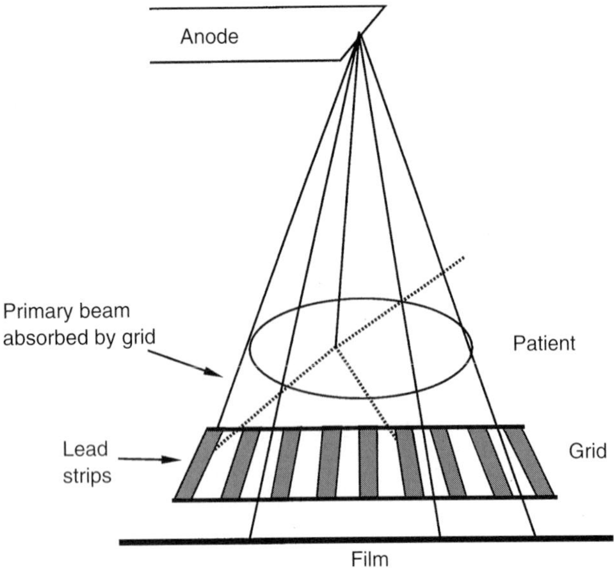

Fig. 1-28 How a grid works. The grid is placed between the patient and the film. Its purpose is to absorb scattered radiation. The lead strips in the grid are shown as stippled regions. Between the lead strips are strips made from some low atomic number, low physical density material such as aluminum. This allows a portion of the primary x-ray beam to reach the film, which is necessary for patient information to be recorded. The scattered photons, shown as *dashed lines,* that hit the grid are likely to be absorbed by the grid because their angle is such that they do not pass between the lead strips.

milliamperage values than screen techniques. However, radiographic detail is superior in nonscreen techniques because the distance that light diffuses from a crystal in an intensifying screen is larger than the size of the silver halide crystals in the film. With nonscreen techniques, sliver halide crystals are exposed directly by x-rays without conversion to visible light. Therefore information from the patient is spread out over a smaller area of x-ray film than with screen techniques.

Grids

Scattered photons originating from coherent or Compton scattering produce a generalized fog (grayness) on the film that reduces both detail and contrast (Fig. 1-28). Photon scattering is directly related to the physical density of the patient, the total volume of tissue irradiated, and the energy of the x-ray beam (kilovoltage peak). Scattered radiation, being undesirable, can be removed by a grid before it strikes the patient. A grid is a flat, rectangular plate with alternating lead and aluminum foil strip (see Fig. 1-28). Some x-rays passing through the patient will be aligned with the aluminum strips and reach the film. Some x-rays hitting the patient will be scattered and absorbed in the grid, preventing them from reaching the film (see Fig. 1-28). These scattered x-rays represent useless information and would only contribute to film fogging if the grid were not present. Some primary x-rays not scattered by the patient also are absorbed in the grid. Therefore the number of x-rays generated must be increased when grids are used. In general, milliamperage values two to three times as large are needed when grids are used. Because small patients do not scatter many x-rays, grids are used only for patients with a thickness greater than approximately 10 cm.

The size of each lead strip in Figure 1-28 has been exaggerated. Typically each linear inch of grid width contains approximately 80 to 160 lead lines; thus the lead strips are very thin. Note that in Figure 1-28 the more peripheral lead strips are progressively angled such that planes drawn through each lead strip will intersect at a point. The distance from the surface of the grid to the point of intersection of these planes is called the focal distance of the grid. The purpose of this focusing is to maximize the number of the diverging primary x-rays passing through the grid. In the previous example, if the lead strips were parallel to each other, a large portion of the periphery of the diverging x-ray beam would be "cut off" by the grid.

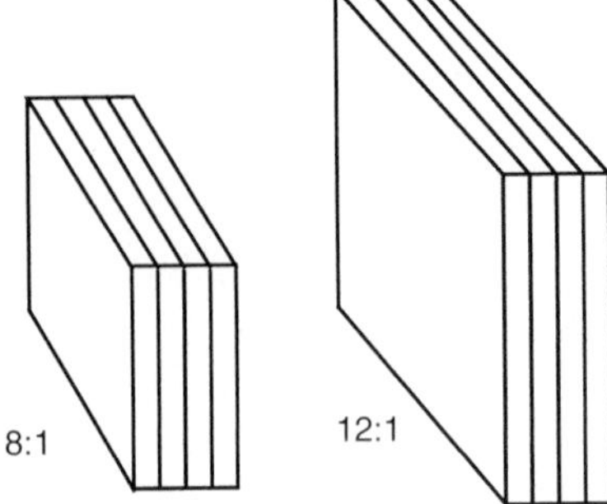

Fig. 1-29 A grid ratio. The lead strips are represented as the *thin black lines.* The grid ratio is the ratio of the height of the lead strips to the distance between them.

The grid ratio is another parameter used to describe a grid. Grid ratio is the relation of the height of the lead strips to the distance between them; that is, if lead strips are five times as high as the space between them, the grid ratio is 5:1 (Fig. 1-29). The larger the grid ratio, the more effective the grid is in absorbing scatter but the more difficult it will be for primary x-rays to pass through it. This should be apparent by comparing the 8:1 and 12:1 grids in the previous figure. Thus the higher the grid ratio, the more milliamperage needed to produce a diagnostic radiograph.

Whenever a grid is used, each lead strip casts a linear opaque shadow. If the grid is stationary during the exposure, the shadows may be visible, particularly if few lead lines are present per inch of grid. If, however, the grid can oscillates during the exposure in a direction perpendicular to the lead strips, the shadows cast by the lead strips are blurred and cannot be identified. One disadvantage of an oscillating grid is that it may make noise or vibrate during a radiographic exposure, causing the patient to move unexpectedly.

When the primary x-ray beam is not properly aligned with the grid, particularly a focused grid, artifacts result (Figs. 1-30 to 1-33).

DISTORTION

Distortion is caused by unequal magnification of the part being radiographed. This results from one part of the object being closer to the x-ray tube than is the rest of the object (Fig. 1-34). Interpretation of radiographs can be compromised if the patient is not kept in proper relation with the primary x-ray beam.

FACTORS AFFECTING CONTRAST

Radiographic contrast refers to the difference in film blackness between areas in the image. If no contrast were present, all parts of the patient would be of the same opacity and no individual structures would be visible. Radiographic contrast depends on three factors: subject contrast, film contrast, and fog and scatter.

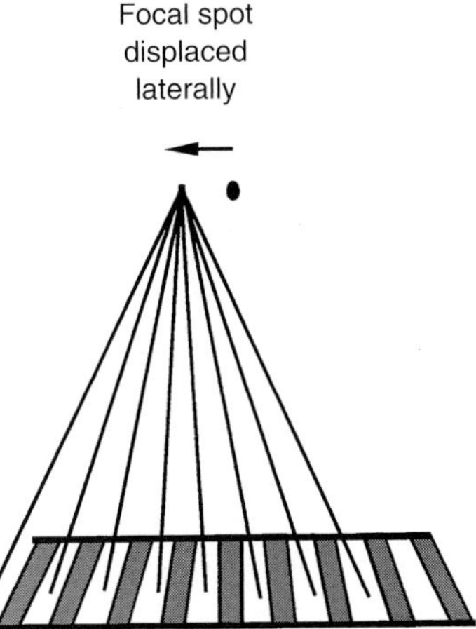

Fig. 1-30 Lateral decentering. When the central ray is centered over the grid, the shadow of the lead strips will be very narrow. When the central ray is laterally decentered, the divergence of the beam no longer matches the divergence of the lead strips in the grid, and the lead strips will absorb more of the primary beam, reducing film blackness. Grid lines may also be visualized depending on the grid ratio and number of grid lines per inch. Lateral decentering is the most common type of grid-induced artifact.

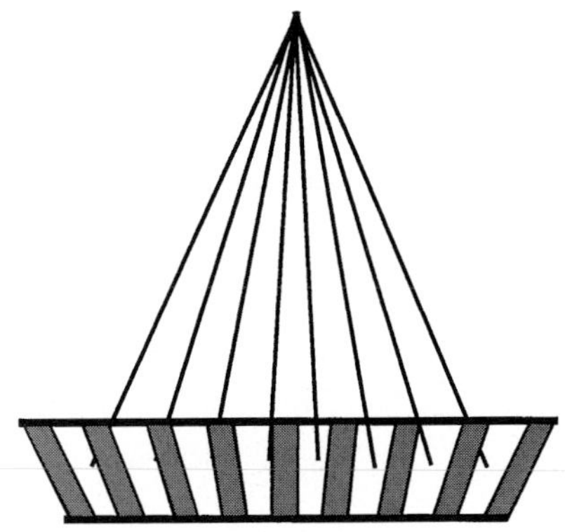

Fig. 1-31 Upside-down grid. If a focused grid is used upside down, the primary x-ray beam will be nearly completely absorbed, except in the exact center of the grid.

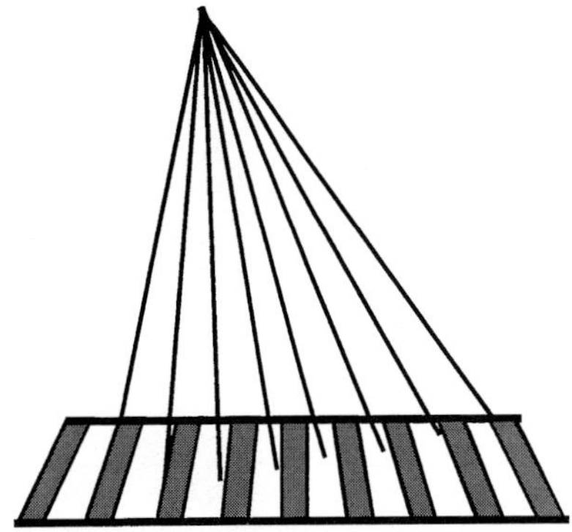

Fig. 1-32 The primary x-ray beam is not perpendicular to the grid. This could occur if using a grid that is not affixed to the x-ray table or if the x-ray tube housing is tilted. This results in cut-off of the primary beam and visualization of grid lines.

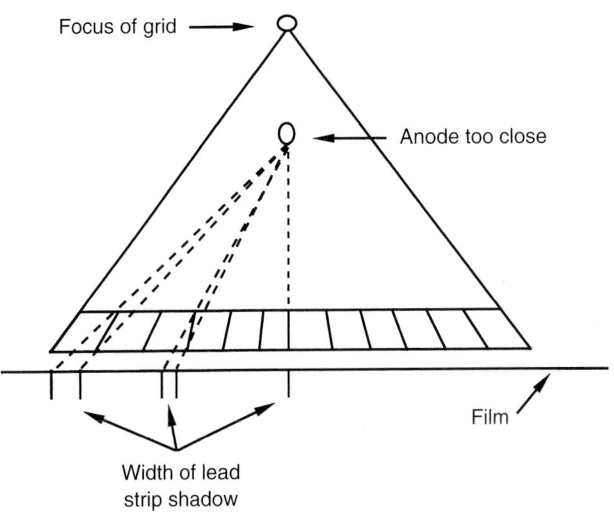

Fig. 1-33 Because of the fixed relation of the lead strips in a focused grid, it will only function properly over a fixed range of FFDs. The grid focus, the point from which the diverging x-rays exactly match the divergence pattern of the lead strips in the grid, is shown. The anode should obviously be located near the grid focal point. If the focal spot is too close, the divergence of the x-ray beam will no longer match the divergence of the lead strips, and cut-off will occur. Note that even though the focal spot is too close, the shadows of the lead strips remain acceptable in the center of the grid. Progressing toward the periphery of the grid, however, the shadows of the lead strips become progressively larger, and cut-off becomes severe.

Subject Contrast

Subject contrast is the difference in x-ray absorption through one part of the subject compared with another. Subject contrast is affected by thickness differences, physical density differences, atomic number differences, and x-ray beam energy (kilovoltage peak). Thickness, physical density, and atomic number effects on radiographic opacity and intensity have been discussed previously. The effect of x-ray beam energy (kilovoltage peak) control on contrast has not been discussed but is important.

The ability of an x-ray to penetrate tissue depends on its energy (see Fig. 1-18). X-rays generated at higher kilovoltage peak values have higher energy. Selecting the proper kilovoltage peak is one of the most important factors to consider in choosing the exposure factors. If the kilovoltage peak is too low, too few x-rays penetrate the patient (the radiograph is underexposed). If the kilovoltage peak is too high, too many x-rays penetrate the patient (the radiograph is overexposed). The kilovoltage peak also has an effect on subject contrast. To understand how kilovoltage peak affects contrast, it is important to realize that numerous combinations of milliamperage and kilovoltage peak will result in an acceptable radiograph (acceptable film blackness). The major factor in producing an acceptable radiograph is the right intensity of x-rays (x-rays/unit area) at the film. This can be achieved by many combinations of milliamperage and kilovoltage peak; if high milliamperage values are used (many x-rays generated), then low kilovoltage peak values must also be used to prevent too many of the x-rays from penetrating the patient and reaching the film. If low milliamperage values are used, then high kilovoltage peak values must be used so that more of the x-rays penetrate the patient and reach the film (Fig. 1-35).

Even though multiple combinations of milliamperage and kilovoltage peak will result in a satisfactory radiograph, the

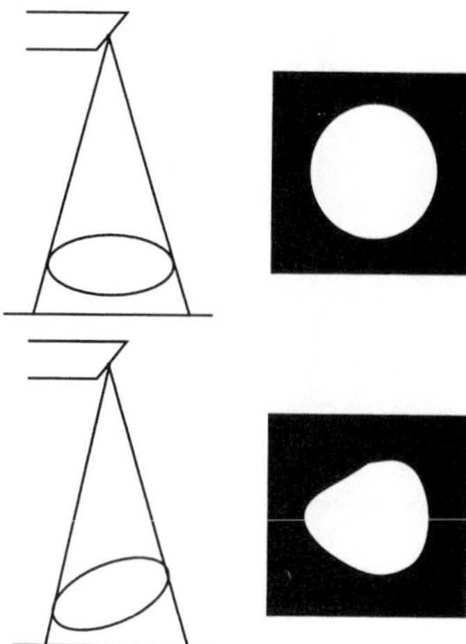

Fig. 1-34 At the top of this figure, a circular object is radiographed, and all parts of the circle are the same distance from the anode. The resulting radiograph represents the true shape of the object. At the bottom of this figure, some of the circle is closer to the anode than is the rest of the circle. The resulting radiographic image of the object does not represent the true shape of the circle; it has been distorted and is now teardrop shaped.

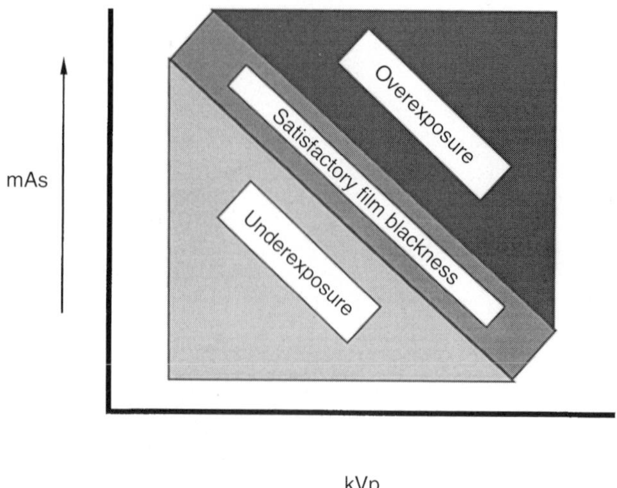

Fig. 1-35 A range of milliampere seconds/kilovoltage peak (mAs/kVp) combinations will produce a satisfactory radiograph. When low numbers of x-rays are generated, their energy must be high (high kilovoltage peak) so that sufficient numbers reach the film. When many x-rays are generated (high milliamperage), their energy must not be too great or too many will reach the film.

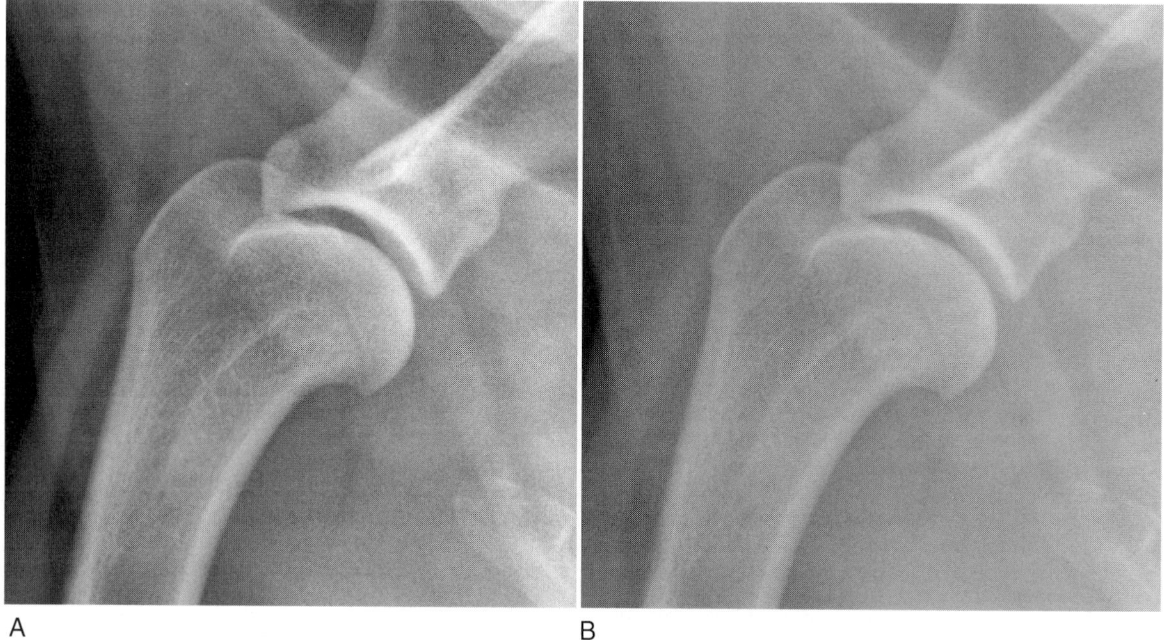

Fig. 1-36 A high-contrast (A) and low-contrast (B) radiograph of a the same canine shoulder. The high-contrast radiograph would be made using a low kilovoltage peak and high milliamperage technique, whereas the low-contrast radiograph would be made with a high kilovoltage peak and low milliamperage technique. Both radiographs are of acceptable overall film blackness, but the high-contrast image is more useful for assessment of osseous structures. In areas of the body with high subject contrast, such as the thorax, radiographic contrast can be controlled by using a high kilovoltage peak and low mAs technique.

contrast of the image will depend on whether the kilovoltage peak is high or low relative to the milliamperage. As previously noted, contrast refers to the magnitude of the gradation of film blackness in the radiograph. In a high-contrast radiograph, mostly black and white opacities and very few shades of gray are present. High-contrast radiographs are also referred to as having a "short scale" of contrast because everything is either black or white. Low-contrast radiographs have few blacks and whites but many shades of gray; low-contrast radiographs are referred to as having a "long scale" of contrast because a long scale of shades of gray is present between the lightest and darkest portions of the image (Fig 1-36).

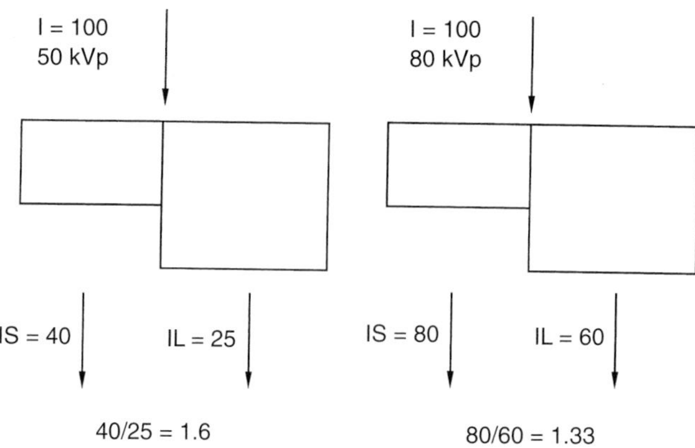

Fig. 1-37 Assume that an x-ray beam with an intensity of 100 x-rays/unit area strikes an object composed of two distinct regions with different thickness. *IS* (thin) and *IL* (thick) are the intensities of the beam after being transmitted through small (IS) and large (IL) regions of the object, respectively. Contrast is defined as the ratio of the intensity of the x-ray beam after passing through the thin/thick regions of the object (i.e., IS/IL). On the left, most of the low-energy x-rays are attenuated by the thick part, but quite a few can penetrate the thin part. Therefore subject contrast for 50 kVp is 40/25 = 1.6. This means that the thin part transmits 60% more x-rays than does the thick part at 50 kVp. If the kilovoltage peak is increased to 80, more x-rays will get through both the thick and the thin parts. Both IS and IL will increase, but IL will increase proportionally more than IS because the higher energy of the x-rays allows them to penetrate the thick part with greater ease. The ratio IS/IL becomes smaller, and subject contrast decreases; that is, 80/60 = 1.33, or only 33% difference exists in the transmitted radiation intensity. Structures of high atomic number (bone) are also more easily penetrated by higher energy x-rays. Therefore the thick part in this illustration could also be something of high atomic number and the same principle would apply. (Modified from Curry TS III, Dowdey JE, Murry RC Jr: The radiographic image. In Curry TS III, editor: Christensen's physics of diagnostic radiology, ed 4, Philadelphia, 1990, Lea & Febiger.)

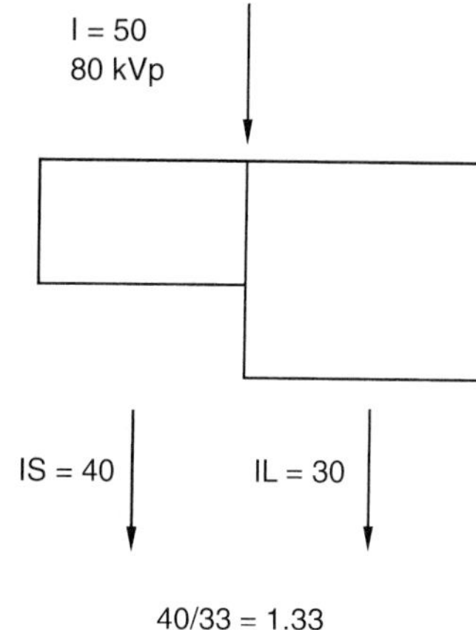

Fig. 1-38 In Figure 1-37, the quality of the radiograph was acceptable when 50 kVp was used. When the setting was increased to 80 kVp, contrast decreased but the entire radiograph was overexposed. Thus, to obtain a satisfactory exposure, an intensity of 40 x-rays/unit area beneath the thin part of the object is needed, but 80 kVp is continued because of the need for lower contrast in this instance. To reduce the intensity under the thin part from 80 to 40 kVp, the original intensity (milliamperage) can be reduced by half. The intensity under the thin and thick parts of the object is thereby reduced to 40 and 30 kVp, respectively, and the contrast remains at 1.33 (i.e., 40/30). (Reprinted with permission from Curry TS III, Dowdey JE, Murry RC Jr: The radiographic image. In Curry TS III, editor: *Christensen's physics of diagnostic radiology*, ed 4, Philadelphia, 1990, Lea & Febiger.)

In general terms, the reason why low kilovoltage peak produces greater subject contrast than high kilovoltage peak can be explained by a simple example (Fig. 1-37). The radiograph on the right in Figure 1-36 has increased film blackness, and it is overexposed if the radiograph on the left is satisfactory. This results from the intensity of x-rays (x-rays/unit area) being too high beneath the object on the right. This can be corrected by using a lower milliamperage with a higher kilovoltage peak setting (Fig. 1-38).

Film Contrast

Radiographic contrast is also a function of the type of x-ray film in use. X-ray film exaggerates subtle changes in subject contrast. This is an inherent property of the film and cannot be varied. For general use, extremely high- or low-contrast film should not be used; a midrange contrast film is satisfactory.

Fog and Scatter

The effect of fog is to reduce radiographic contrast. Fog produced by scattered radiation can be prevented by a grid. Therefore radiographs made with a grid have higher contrast than those that are not. Film can also become fogged by exposure to pressure or high temperature, or by accidental exposure to light, such as results from a defective darkroom safelight or a faulty light seal around the darkroom door. X-ray film also becomes fogged over time; therefore an expiration date is provided by the x-ray film manufacturer. X-ray film should not be stored in the x-ray room. Film should be kept in a lead-lined container.

FILM PROCESSING

Many errors made in radiography of animals are related to the processing of radiographic film. If using manual processing, the darkroom should be clean, dry, lightproof, and uncluttered. It is difficult to encourage a technician to perform a radiographic examination carefully if the quality of the study is lowered by poor darkroom facilities. Despite the increased use of automatic processors, many radiographs in veterinary medicine are still processed manually. Regardless, the principles of each of the following steps apply to both manual and automatic film processing.

Developing

The developer reduces exposed silver halide crystals to metallic silver by supplying electrons to the positively charged silver ions in exposed silver halide crystals. Film developing is a chemical process and therefore depends on both time and temperature, and the efficiency of the developer chemicals, which become exhausted with use and must be replenished. In the darkroom, replenishment must be manual while this is done automatically in an automatic processor. Because development in an automatic processor is shorter than when done manually, the temperature of the developer must be higher in an automatic processor.

Table • 1-4

Appearance, Cause, and Correction for Common Technical Errors

APPEARANCE	CAUSE	CORRECTION
Too dark	Incorrect machine setting	Lower kilovoltage peak, milliamperage, or time
	FFD too short	Increase FFD
	Wrong screen/film	Check screen/film
	Overdeveloped	Check developer temperature/time
Too light	Incorrect machine setting	Increase kilovoltage peak, milliamperage, or time
	FFD too long	Decrease distance
	Wrong screen/film	Check screen/film
	Underdeveloped	Check developer temperature/time
Gray/loss of contrast	Film stored improperly	Check storage conditions
	Film exposed to light	Check storage conditions
	Old film	Discard film
	Incorrect machine setting	Decrease kilovoltage peak, increase milliamperage
	Film processed improperly	Check age, temperature of chemicals
Crescent-shaped black marks	Film bent during handling	Handle film more gently
Sharp, linear black marks	Film scratched before processing	Handle film more gently
Edge of film black	Film fogged	Check for light leak in cassette or film bin
Black water spots or fingerprints	Developer on film before development	Do not contaminate darkroom work surface or hands
White fingerprints	Fixer on hands before development	Do not contaminate darkroom work surface or hands
White "hair" marks	Hair in cassette	Clean cassette
Sharp white specks	Dirt in cassette	Clean cassette
Sharp white lines or marks	Emulsion scratched off	Handle film with care when wet
Blurred image	Patient motion	Use chemical restraint
	Tube motion	Secure tube
	Cassette motion	Secure cassette
Yellow-brown film	Insufficient washing	Wash completely
Treelike black marks	Static electricity	Move film slowly

Fixing

The fixer converts undeveloped silver halide crystals on the film into a soluble compound. Fixer clears undeveloped, unexposed silver crystals from the film. This leaves the silver as a permanent image on the film. Areas where no or minimal silver halide exposure occurred are clear (appear white). Insufficient fixation leads to incomplete removal of undeveloped emulsion and consequently, a cloudy or milky-appearing radiograph.

Final Wash

The film should be washed after fixing to remove excess chemicals and any residual silver halide still on the film. Failure to wash adequately results in retained fixer chemicals reacting with silver in the film, forming silver sulfide, which causes the film to turn brown as it ages. When films are processed by hand, they should wash for 30 to 40 minutes. The wash cycle in an automatic processor is much shorter. Excessive washing or washing in water that is too warm will result in the emulsion becoming soft and the entire image "slipping" off the film.

TECHNICAL ERRORS

Technical errors are common in radiography. These errors are irritating when reviewing a radiograph, and at worst can result in the radiograph being useless. A complete discussion of technical errors is beyond the scope of this text. In Table 1-4, the appearance and causes of, as well as methods to correct, some of the more common technical errors are presented.

REFERENCES

1. Roentgen WC: On a new kind of rays, *Vet Radiol Ultrasound* 36:371, 1995.
2. Widmer WR, Shaw SM, Thrall DE: Effects of low-level exposure to ionizing radiation: current concepts and concerns for veterinary workers, *Vet Radiol Ultrasound* 37:227, 1996.
3. National Council on Radiation Protection and Measurements: *NCRP report no. 82—SI units in radiation protection and measurements,* Bethesda, MD, 1985, National Council on Radiation Protection and Measurements.
4. Title 10, Chapter 1, Code of federal regulations—energy. Part 20, standards for protection against radiation. In *United States Nuclear Regulatory Commission rules and regulations,* Washington, DC, 1995, U.S. Government Printing Office, pp 20-27.
5. Hall EJ: Radiation protection. In Hall EJ, editor: *Radiobiology for the radiologist,* ed 5, Philadelphia, 2000, Lippincott, Williams & Wilkins, pp 234-248.
6. National Council on Radiation Protection and Measurements: NCRP report no. 107—implementation of the

principle of as low as reasonably achievable (ALARA) for medical and dental personnel, Bethesda, MD, 1990, National Council on Radiation Protection and Measurements.
7. Committee on the Biological Effects of Ionizing Radiations: *Health effects of exposure to low levels of ionizing radiation*, Washington, DC, 1990, National Academy Press.
8. National Council on Radiation Protection and Measurements: NCRP report no. 91—recommendations on limits for exposure to ionizing radiation, Bethesda, MD, 1987, National Council on Radiation Protection and Measurements.
9. National Council on Radiation Protection and Measurements: NCRP report no. 93—ionizing radiation exposure of the population of the United States, Bethesda, MD, 1987, National Council on Radiation Protection and Measurements.
10. Curry TS III, Dowdey JE, Murry RC Jr: The production of x rays. In Curry TS III, Dowdey JE, Murry RC Jr, editors: *Christensen's physics of diagnostic radiology*, ed 4, Philadelphia, 1990, Lea & Febiger, 1990, pp 10-35.
11. Curry TS III, Dowdey JE, Murry RC Jr: X-ray generators. In Curry TS III, Dowdey JE, Murry RC Jr, editors: *Christensen's physics of diagnostic radiology*, ed 4, Philadelphia, 1990, Lea & Febiger, pp 36-53.
12. Siebert JA: The AAPM/RSNA physics tutorial for residents: x-ray generators, *Radiographics* 17:1533, 1997.

ELECTRONIC RESOURCES evolve

Additional information related to the content in Chapter 1 can be found on the companion Web site at evolve http://evolve.elsevier.com/Thrall/vetrad/

- Key Points
- Chapter Quiz

CHAPTER • 2
Digital Images and Digital Radiographic Image Capture

Laura J. Armbrust

Since the discovery of x-rays, radiographic images have been produced by exposing silver-containing film to ionizing radiation or light from an intensifying screen. Within the past decade, transition from film-based radiographic image capture to the direct production of digital radiographic images has been rapid. Today, virtually all types of medical images can be produced in digital format, including images generated by computed radiography, direct digital radiography, nuclear medicine, computed tomography (CT), ultrasound, and magnetic resonance (MR) imaging. Although the physics underlying the formation of digital images from these modalities varies markedly, an understanding of digital image formation, viewing, manipulation, storage, and transfer of data is essential.

Conventional film-screen radiography remains widely used in veterinary medicine; however, the transformation to digital radiography is currently underway, and film-screen radiographic systems will likely become obsolete.[1-3] The term *digital radiography* is used in reference to the two main systems in use today, computed radiography (CR) and direct digital radiography (DDR).

CR systems were introduced to the medical market in the early 1980s by Fuji Medical Corporation.[1-4] DDR was introduced after CR and is currently marketed for human and veterinary imaging.

The following is an overview of the basics of digital image formation, types of digital radiography products available, and the physics of image capture. Additionally, the advantages and disadvantages, artifacts, viewing, and archival and retrieval of digital radiographic images is described.

BASICS OF DIGITAL IMAGING

Analog to Digital Conversion

Most diagnostic imaging modalities such as nuclear medicine, CT, MR imaging, ultrasound, and digital radiography acquire information in analog, or signal, format. Analog information is transferred by a voltage or voltage pulse. The disadvantages of the analog format include electronic noise that can distort the signal and the necessity of converting the electrical information into numbers (digital) that a computer can understand. The analog signals that are acquired by medical imaging equipment are converted to digital data, that is, numbers, by an analog to digital converter (ADC). ADCs take samples of the continuous flow of the analog signal and convert these signals to a digital (numeric) form by the binary system (Fig. 2-1).[5]

Computers operate by using the base-2 number system, also known as the binary system. Computers use the base-2 system because it is easier to implement with current electronic technology. In the binary system, the only integers used are 0 and 1.

Disadvantages of digital data are the potential for information loss from sampling and quantization. ADCs have different sampling rates. For medical imaging the sampling rates are very high; therefore, sampling error is negligible. Quantization occurs because an analog signal is continuous, whereas digital data have a finite limit of possibilities. The digital data therefore represent the "rounded-off" form of the analog signal. The ADCs for medical imaging have sufficient output to minimize quantization error. When digital data are converted back to analog signals for display on a video monitor by a digital to analog converter (DAC), the original analog signal cannot be restored because of the sampling and quantization loss that has occurred (see Fig. 2-1).[5]

Computer Processing in Digital Imaging

Computers are required to handle the large amount of digital data that form a digital image. Each digital number is represented in a gray-scale image on a computer/video screen in the form of tiny squares called pixels, or picture elements (Fig. 2-2). The computer assigns a shade of gray to each pixel depending on the numeric value of the number represented by that pixel. To determine the shade of gray that is assigned to a pixel, a basic understanding of computer memory, or storage, is required. Computer memory consists of bits (binary digits) that are grouped into bytes (1 byte = eight bits). Bit depth represents the number of values available to define each pixel.[5,6] For example, a computer whose pixels were defined with one-bit depth could only have binary values of 0 or 1 (on or off), representing black (0) or white (1); this would not produce a useful image (see Fig 2-2).

For representing imaging data, in which multiple shades of gray are required, a higher bit number, called bit depth, is able to accommodate more information and thus more shades of gray. For example, N bits have 2^N possibilities for representing data (Table 2-1). For the purposes of digital medical imaging, this means that eight bits can represent a gray-scale range with 256 (2^8) shades of gray, ranging from 0 (black) to 255 (white) (Fig. 2-3). Because the human eye only discerns a limited number of shades of gray, excessive bit depth results in large file sizes without providing added information.[6] Many texts are available for further information on the components of a basic computer and computers in medical imaging.[5,6]

Digital Image Display

All digital images, whether from a digital camera or a medical imaging device, are composed of a grid of rows and columns of tiny picture elements called pixels (see Fig. 2-2). Pixel size plays an important role in spatial resolution, the ability to define or separate two objects close together, of digital images. Better (higher) spatial resolution is obtained by increasing the number of pixels without changing the field of view, thereby decreasing pixel size and increasing matrix size (Fig. 2-4). For CT and MR imaging, 512 × 512 or 1024 × 1024 matrix sizes

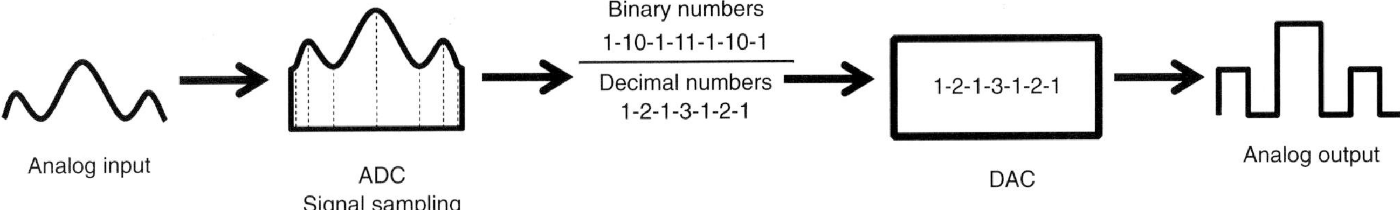

Fig. 2-1 An analog voltage waveform is converted to digital information (shown as corresponding binary and decimal numbers) by the ADC. If this digital information is converted back to an analog signal, it is evident that the information is representative but not identical to the original analog waveform.

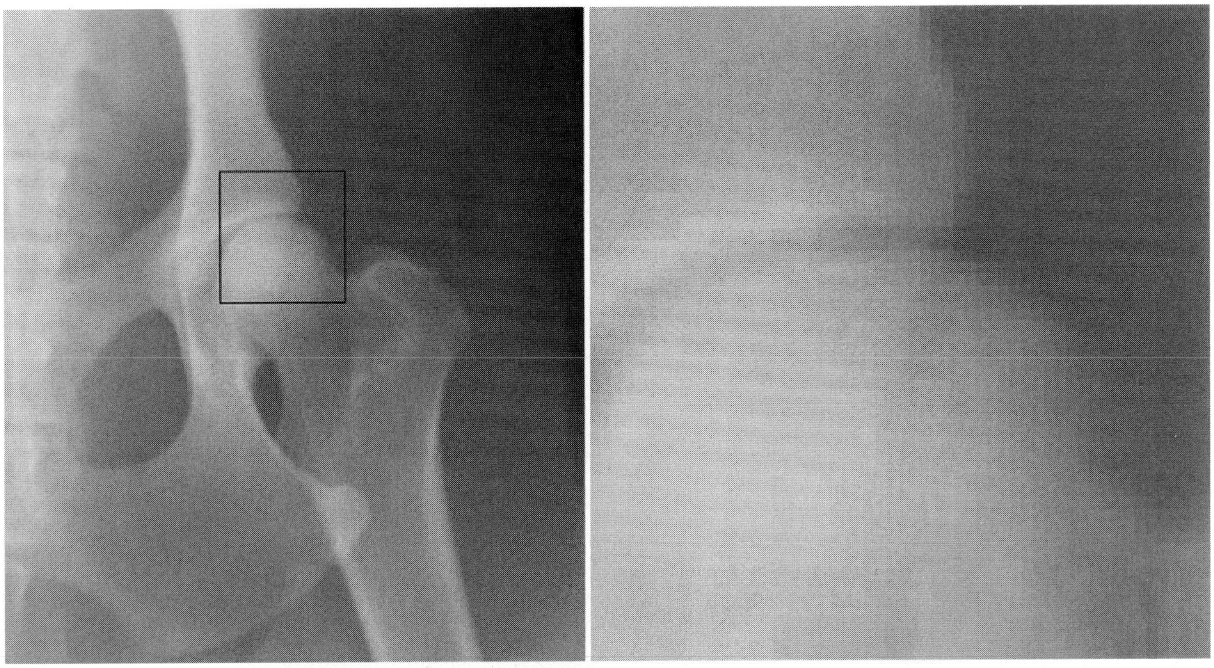

A

B

C

Fig. 2-2 A, The digital image viewed on a computer monitor is a composite of tiny squares arranged in rows and columns. These tiny squares are termed pixels. The close-up (B) is so highly magnified that individual pixels become visible. Note the various shades of gray of individual pixels. The number of gray shades available is determined by the bit depth of the image. (C) This is the same image as (A) but at a bit depth of one. Thus the only allowable gray shades are black and white. This image has no diagnostic value and more gray shades are needed, that is, a higher bit depth.

are used. This means a 512 × 512 image has 512 columns with 512 pixels in each column (262,144 total pixels). For digital radiography a 2048 × 2048 (2-K) matrix or higher is preferred because of the need for higher spatial resolution.[2]

Pixel size is also related to the field of view. The field of view is the actual physical area that is being included, or captured, by the image modality. Pixel size is determined by dividing the size of the field of view by the matrix size (number of pixels across the image).[5] For example, if the field of view for a CT acquisition is 30 cm and a 512 × 512 matrix is used, then the pixel size is equal to 300 mm/512 = 0.58 mm (Fig. 2-5).

The pixel matrix represents an array of numbers with a minimal and maximal value corresponding to the darkest and brightest light intensities of the computer or video monitor. The number of shades of gray depends on the bit depth of the image (number of bytes), as discussed above. The appearance of a digital image, in terms of blackness and contrast, can be changed after it is obtained; this is one of the main advantages of a digital radiographic image compared with a film image.[1,2,5]

Table • 2-1

Influence of Bit Depth on Number of Gray Shades Possible per Pixel

BIT DEPTH	SHADES OF GRAY
1	2
2	4
3	8
8	256
16	65,536

Changing the appearance of a digital image is achieved by a process called *windowing*. A windowing function should be available on all digital imaging software. Windowing is achieved through variation in the window width and window level (or window center). The window width determines the range of exposures that can be assigned to a shade of gray. Pixels above the range will all be white, whereas pixels with a value below the range will be black. The window level represents the center point of the window width (Fig. 2-6).

Computer Storage

Computer storage is quantified in terms of bytes. Because the byte is a very small unit, storage capability and file size are typically expressed in terms of kilobytes, megabytes, or gigabytes. For storage purposes the total number of bytes required to store an image is determined by the number of pixels in the image multiplied by the number of bytes per pixel. For example if the image matrix is 256 × 256 and there is one byte (eight-bit depth) per pixel, then 65,536 bytes of storage would be required. If this number is divided by 1024 bytes per kilobyte (kB), then 64 kB of storage space is needed for the image. Thus if pixel size decreases (image resolution improves) increases in both storage and processing requirements occur. Likewise, if bit depth (number of bytes per pixel) increases, file size and storage requirements will also increase.[5]

DIGITAL RADIOGRAPHY IMAGING EQUIPMENT AND PHYSICS OF IMAGE CAPTURE

General Equipment

An x-ray generator similar to that used for conventional film-screen radiography is used for both CR and DDR digital imaging systems. With CR systems, modification of the original radiographic system is not required because the only change is use of a different type of cassette. CR cassettes are

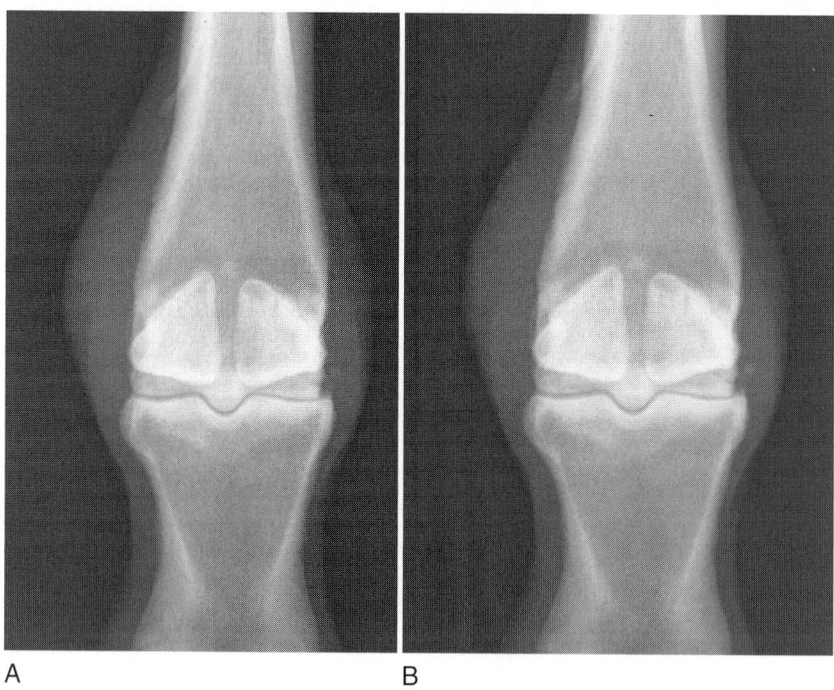

Fig. 2-3 Dorsopalmar digital radiographs of an equine metacarpal phalangeal joint using different bit depth. **A** is 16-bit depth with a file size of 805 kB, whereas **B** is an 8-bit depth with a file size of 398 kB. Sixteen-bit depth provides 65,536 shades of gray compared with 256 shades of gray with 8-bit images. However, the human eye cannot discern this difference, as noted by the similar appearance of the images. As bit depth decreases, however, the fewer number of gray shades becomes apparent.

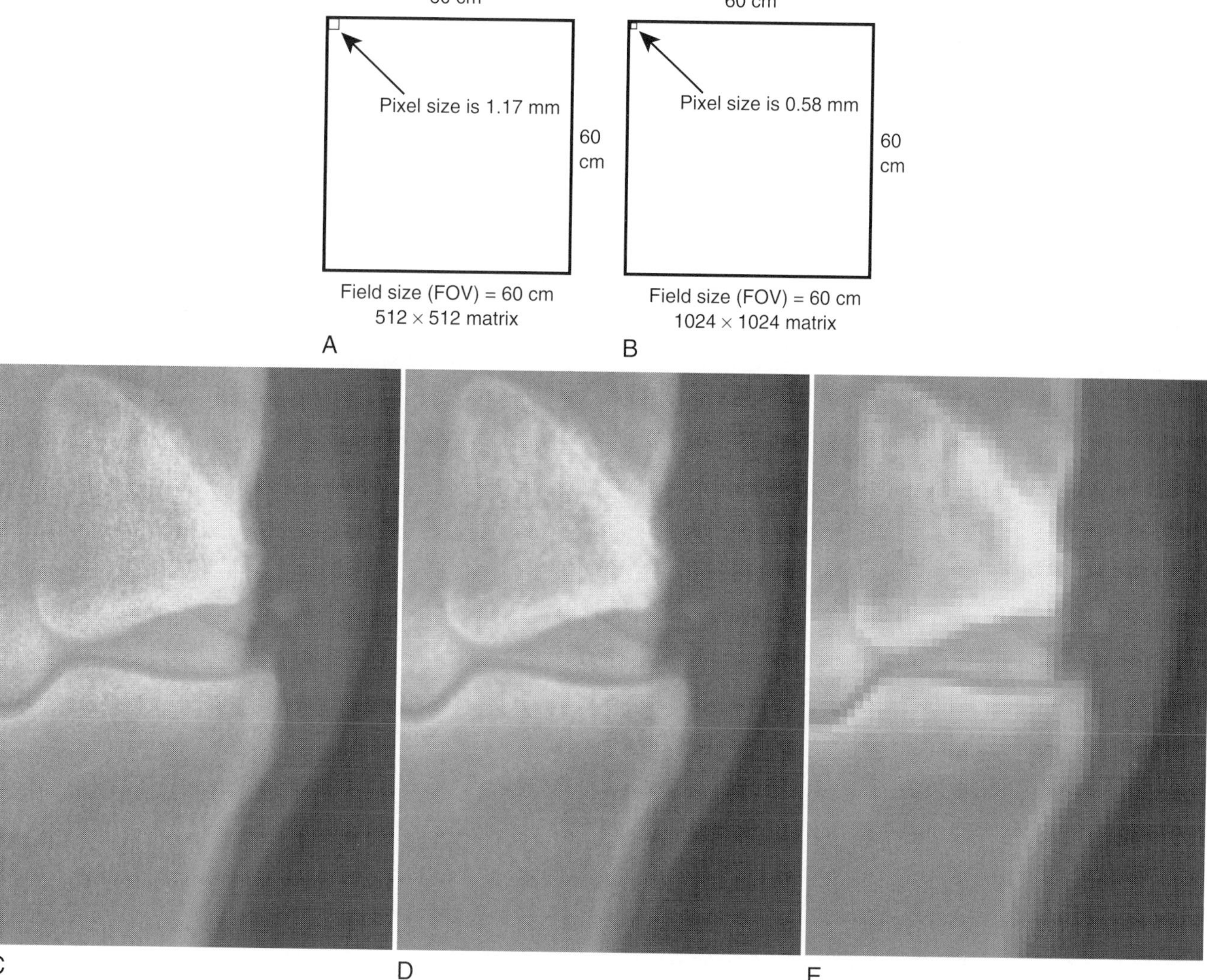

Fig. 2-4 A change in matrix size of the display monitor results in a change in pixel size. If the field size or field of view (FOV) stays the same (60 cm in this example), then the pixel size will decrease with an increase in matrix size. In **A** the matrix size is 512 × 512, resulting in a pixel size of 1.17 mm. In **B** a 1024 × 1024 matrix has a pixel size of 0.58 mm on the same monitor. The remaining images, **C** through **E,** are a close-up region from Figure 2-3, *B* shown at varied resolution. The image resolution in **C** is 72 pixels/in, in **D** 36 pixels/in, and in **E** 18 pixels/in. Note the decreased resolution as the size of the pixels increases.

physically similar to film cassettes but contain an imaging plate rather than intensifying screens and film. For DDR the imaging plate is independent of any cassette. CR imaging plates must be "read" in a plate reader before the x-ray exposure information is sent to the computer. On the other hand, DDR imaging plates send the signal measured from the x-ray beam directly to a computer without a "read" step and therefore result in faster image generation. Some vendors use entirely new radiographic systems for the transition to DDR, whereas other vendors can retrofit existing x-ray tables to allow for insertion of the DDR imaging plate.[1,4,5]

The aluminum filters and collimator used to prevent scatter radiation are similar in digital radiography to traditional film-screen radiography. Grids are also used in CR and DDR; however, they may have to be modified depending on the digital equipment (higher grid ratio or more line pairs per inch may be needed). With either CR or DDR, a user interface, or computer workstation, is needed to enter and link the patient information with the digital image and review the digital images before final acceptance.

The main difference between film-screen systems and digital systems (CR and DDR) is the method by which the radiation is detected after the x-rays pass through the patient. Principles of image formation using a film-screen system are discussed in Chapter 1.

A popular misconception is that digital radiographic systems require less radiation for image production; this is not true. Although exposures vary between CR and DDR systems, they are roughly comparable to exposures used with 200-speed film-screen systems.[3,4] A major advantage of CR and DDR systems, however, is the wide range of exposure factors that can be used without compromising the diagnostic value of the image.[1,2,4] Thus overexposure and underexposure problems that are so common when using a film-based system are much less problematic in the digital environment. Also, processing errors that can render an excellent quality radiograph nondiagnostic are not issues in digital radiography because the images are processed electronically by a computer rather than physically in the darkroom.

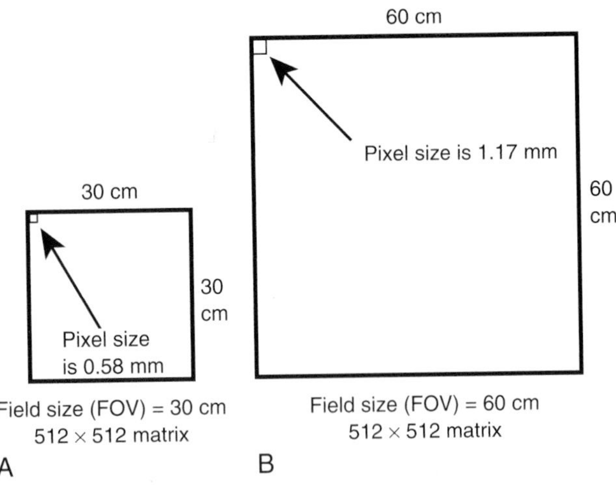

Fig. 2-5 A change in the field size results in a change in spatial resolution. For example, in **A** if a 512 × 512 matrix is used with a 30-cm field of view (FOV), the area displayed per pixel would be 0.58 mm. If the matrix size stays the same (512 × 512) but field size doubles to 60 cm, the area displayed per pixel doubles to 1.17 mm, thus decreasing spatial resolution.

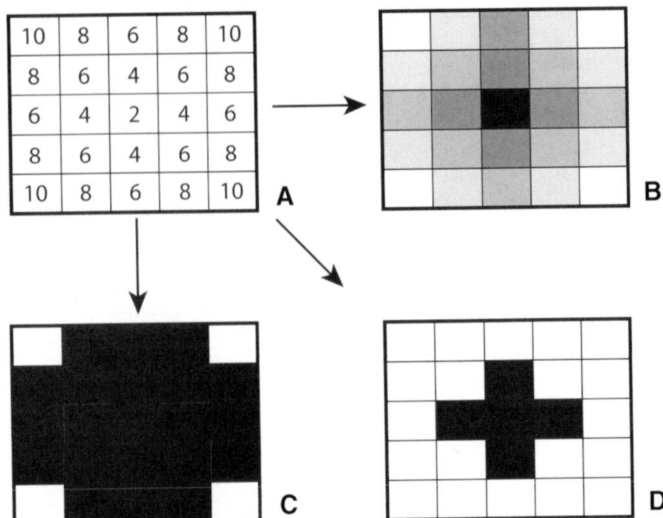

Fig. 2-6 The shade of gray displayed for each pixel is based on the digital information (number) acquired for that specific location. Once the information is acquired, changes can be made after the fact; this is called postprocessing. **B** shows the original representation of the image (wide window width with the window level in the mid-range of the numbers). For **C** a narrow window width, level 9, was used. This results in all pixels that are equal or less than 9 being black. For **D** a narrow window width was also used (level 5). This results in numbers equal to or less than 5 being black, whereas all other pixels are white. Postprocessing changes are important to allow for variation in contrast that will be important in assessing bone (high-contrast window needed) versus soft tissue (low contrast window needed), for example.

CR and DDR systems require computer hardware and software to view the images for interpretation.[1-4] This equipment is separate from that needed to capture the image and make it viewable for quality control (Fig. 2-7). Captured images that are acceptable are generally transferred to a storage device and then interpreted by using a separate workstation, occasionally outfitted with high-quality monitors capable of displaying images in high resolution. An interface that allows the imaging system to connect with the hospital network is also necessary. Many vendors sell complete packages that include both x-ray equipment and the computer hardware and software.

Computed Radiography

In CR, an imaging plate rather than conventional x-ray film is used to record the latent image. The imaging plate, which is stored in a cassette that has an outward appearance similar to a conventional cassette, is coated with photostimulable phosphors (layer of crystals). As x-rays strike the imaging plate, electrons in the crystals are energized to a higher level and stored in electron traps, thereby forming the latent image.[1-4]

CR requires a specialized plate reader. The exposed cassette is placed in the plate reader (Fig. 2-8). The plate reader extracts the imaging plate from the cassette and scans the plate with a red laser. During the scanning process the electrons that were trapped in a higher energy state during x-ray exposure are released into a lower energy state. As the electrons undergo this transition, they stimulate phosphorescence (emission of visible light). The light that is produced is detected by photomultiplier tubes in the reader. The light energy is amplified and converted to an electric signal that is proportional to the light intensity released from the plate. This analog signal is converted into digital data (numbers) by an ADC, as previously described. These digital data are transferred to a computer, and the image can then be displayed on a computer monitor or printed on film. The image represents the collected data for each specific pixel that has a shade of gray corresponding to the degree of attenuation of the imaged part.[2,3]

Direct Digital Radiography

DDR uses an imaging plate designed with an array of detector elements. Two main types of detectors exist: direct and indirect. Indirect detectors convert the x-ray energy into light, which is then converted to an electrical signal. Direct detectors convert the x-ray energy directly to an electrical pulse.[4] The imaging plate for DDR is built directly into the x-ray table or is portable, thus eliminating all use of cassettes (Fig. 2-9). The DDR plate must be connected directly to a computer. The intensity of the light or electrical pulse is immediately digitized, and the digital image is available for almost immediate viewing (4 to 10 seconds) on a monitor for quality control. If acceptable, the image is transferred to the storage computer, where it is available for viewing and interpretation on a workstation, as with CR.

In both CR and DDR, whether to print the digital image on film for viewing and storage or whether to view the digital image directly with storage on a suitable digital medium (hard disc, magnetic tape, optical disc) is optional. Film printing requires acquisition of a suitable printer and, unless the original digital data file is archived, problems with film loss and damage, as with conventional radiographs, will still be an issue. Viewing, interpreting, and storing the digital data directly increases flexibility and eliminates the need to acquire and maintain a film printer.

Portable Computed Radiography and Direct Digital Radiography Equipment

In addition to in-house systems, portable CR and DDR systems have been developed. The portable units are particularly valuable for equine ambulatory practices, allowing images to be viewed in the field and eliminating the requirement to return to the hospital for film developing.[2]

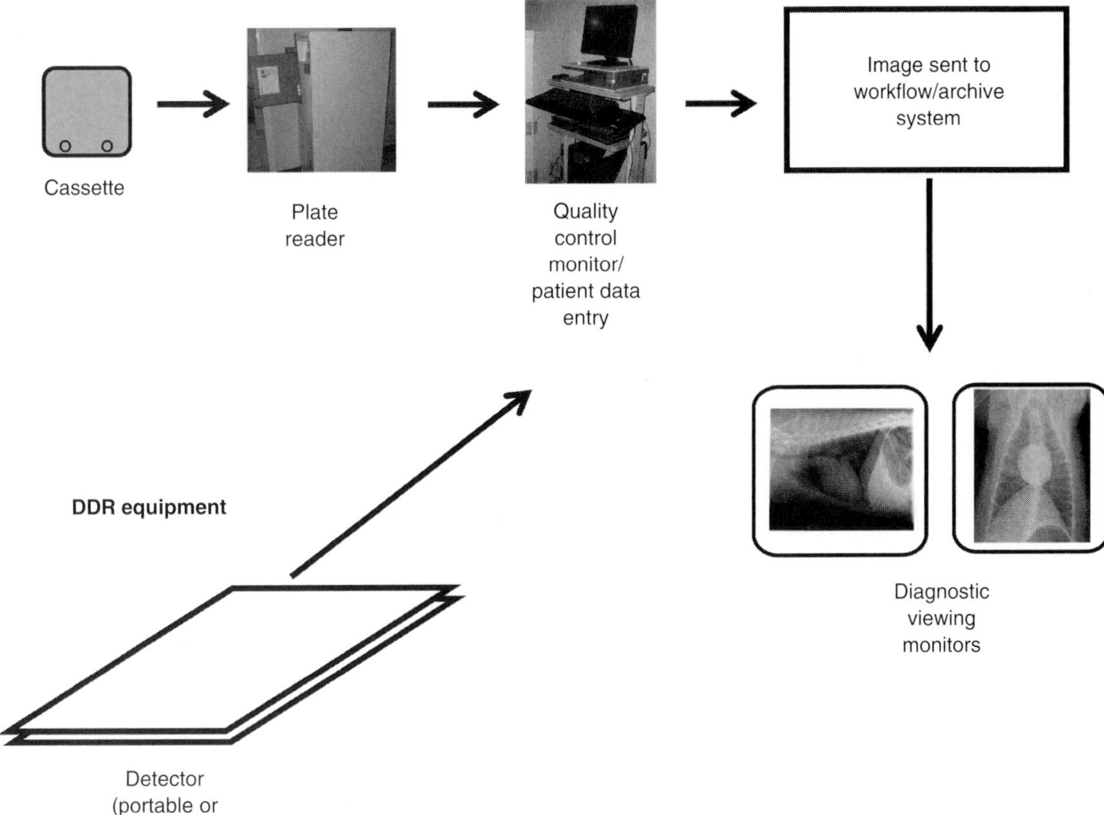

Fig. 2-7 CR equipment uses a conventional x-ray tube and table with a specialized plate in a cassette (the cassette outwardly appears similar to a traditional film cassette). A plate reader is required to read the image off the plate. A DDR system consists of either all new equipment or the same x-ray tube and table retrofitted with an imaging plate. With both systems, after the image is acquired it is displayed on a quality control workstation to determine that adequate exposure and positioning were used.

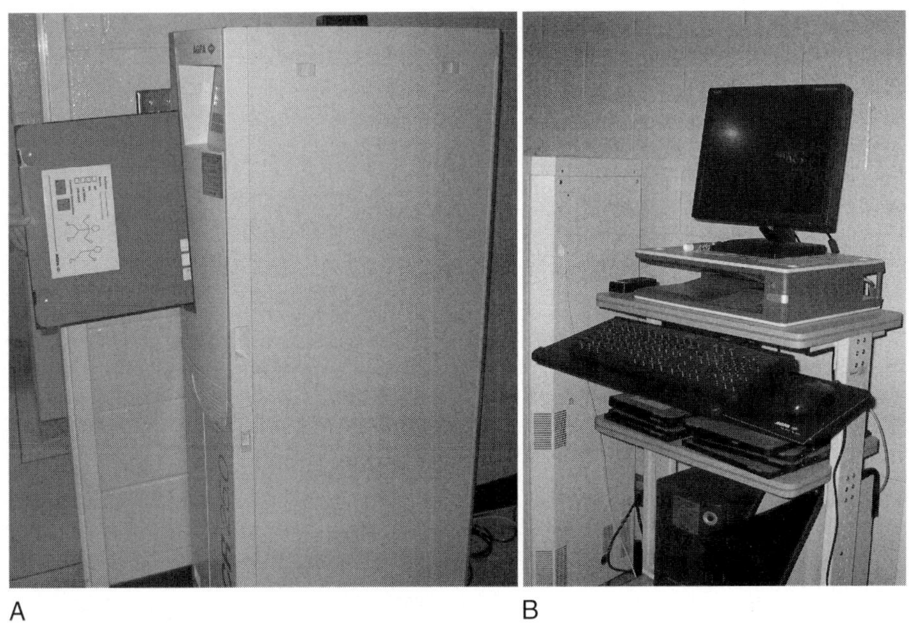

Fig. 2-8 A CR cassette is placed in the plate reader **(A)**. Once inside, the imaging plate is extracted from the cassette and scanned with a red laser that leads to the emission of trapped energy in the plate as visible light. The light that is produced is detected by photomultiplier tubes in the plate reader and is converted to an electric signal, and then into digital data. These digital data can then be displayed on the quality control monitor **(B)**.

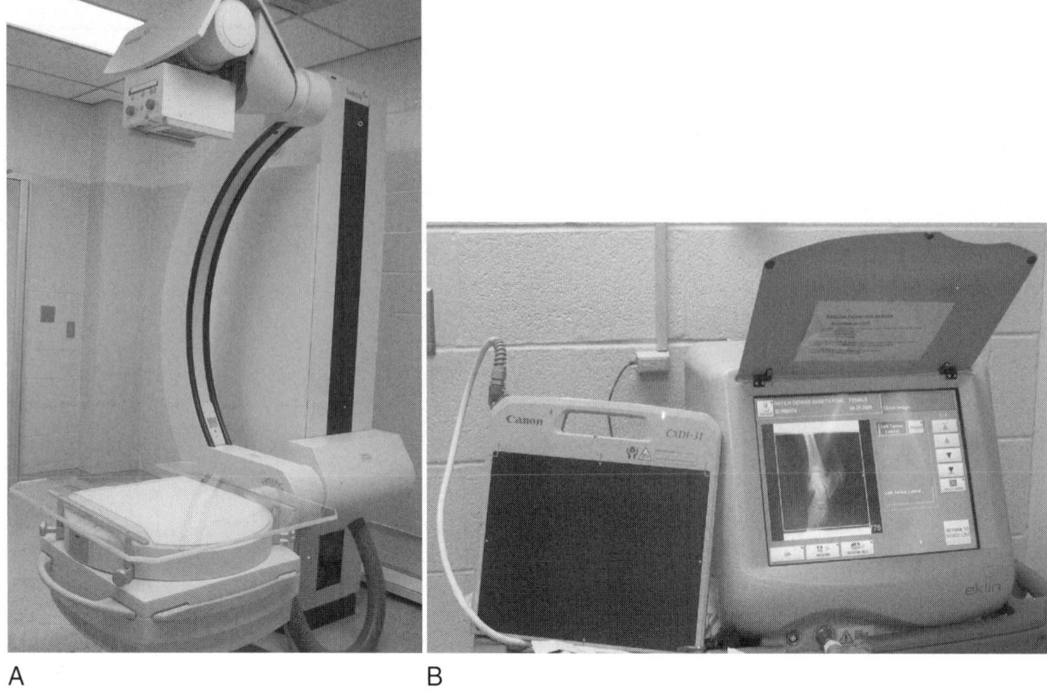

Fig. 2-9 Different DR systems. **A** is a SwissRay DR system used for small animal radiography (Swissray International, Inc., Elizabeth, NJ). **B** is a portable Eklin DR system used for equine radiography (Eklin Medical Systems, Inc., Santa Clara, Calif.).

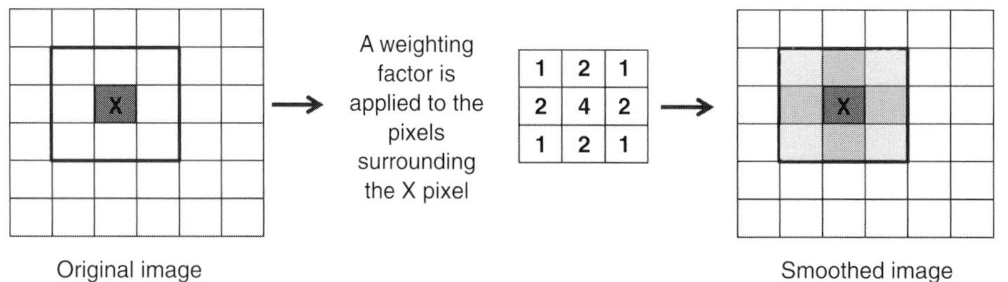

Fig. 2-10 Smoothing is a postprocessing change that blends the adjacent pixels to create a more uniform image without a large change in information between adjacent pixels. In this example the pixel marked with the *X* is used as the center of the smoothing process. A weighting factor is applied to the adjacent pixels, resulting in the adjacent pixels becoming more uniform with respect to the pixel marked X. Although only shown for a single pixel in this example, the same process would occur for the entire image, resulting in a smoothed image.

IMAGE PROCESSING AND IMAGE QUALITY IN DIGITAL RADIOGRAPHY

Image Processing

Digital data from the CR or DDR plate are sent to a processing computer, where they are evaluated and manipulated by vendor-specific software before the image is displayed on the monitor. Specific computer algorithms are defined by the vendor and user on the basis of body region examined. These algorithms define contrast resolution, optical density, contrast type (linear or nonlinear), spatial and frequency resolution, and the degree of edge enhancement.[1,2] The computer forms an image histogram that identifies a value for each pixel. This is compared to the ideal histogram that has been specified for a particular processing algorithm. This processing attempts to adjust the image blackness to compensate for overexposure and underexposure, making CR and DDR systems more forgiving in terms of radiographic exposure factors, as previously mentioned.[1-4] Digital radiographic systems store the raw data so that new algorithms can be applied if the wrong one was initially selected.

Different filters can also be applied in digital imaging.[5] A spatial filtering operation called smoothing can decrease the mottled appearance of a digital image. Smoothing an image is essentially blurring an image. This is performed by using a weighted average of a number of pixels (filter kernel) surrounding a particular pixel (Fig. 2-10). If too much smoothing occurs, the image can be blurred to the extent that spatial resolution is decreased and clinically significant detail is lost (Fig. 2-11). The weighting factors in the filter kernel can also be modified to enhance the edges of structures in the image. This is called edge enhancement and actually increases the statistical noise in the image (Fig. 2-12).

The digital images can then be adjusted for contrast enhancement. The two most common methods of contrast enhancement on medical imaging devices are windowing and translation table selection. The translation table is a look-up table that the video interface uses to modify each pixel value

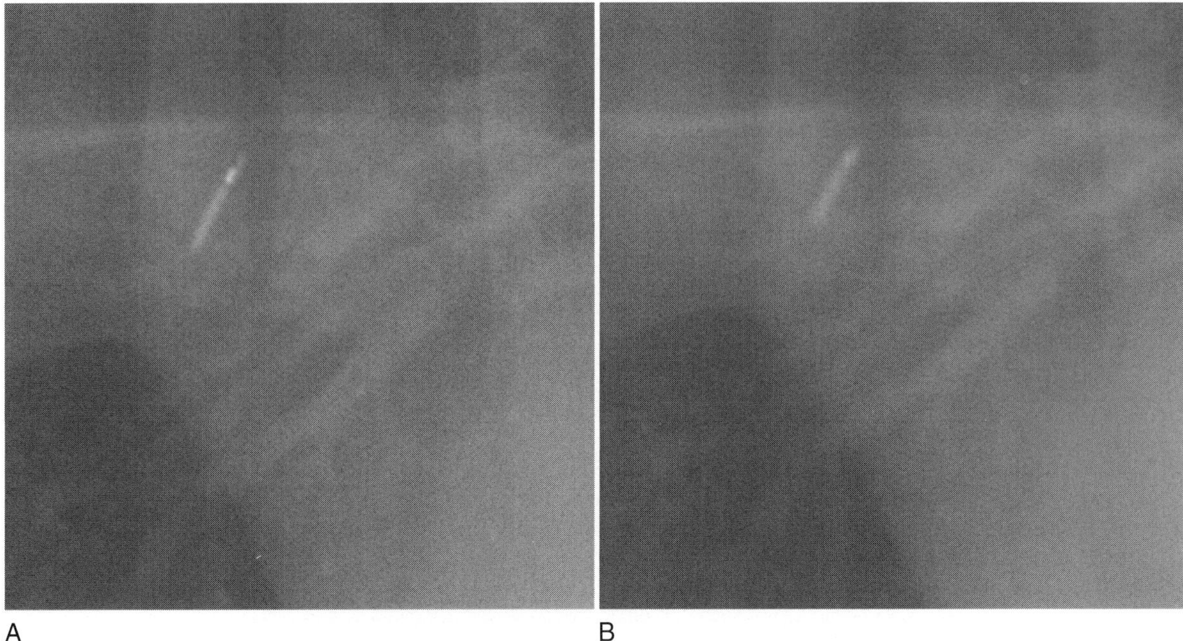

Fig. 2-11 Smoothing can create blurring if an image is processed improperly. Compare the close-up view from a thoracic radiograph. **A** used a proper smoothing algorithm but in **B** the image has been overly smoothed, resulting in blurring.

before it is sent to the DAC and becomes an analog signal.[5]

Image Quality

The image quality of a digital radiograph depends on proper patient positioning and beam angle.[1,2] Image quality related to spatial resolution depends on matrix or pixel size, as previously discussed. It is recommended that a minimum of a 2-K matrix with a 12-bit depth be used for digital radiography.[2,6,7] Recall that this large matrix size will result in large file sizes that are a consideration for file transfer and storage.[1,3,6] The American College of Radiology specifies that the spatial resolution of CR images should be at least 2.5 line pairs/mm and 10 bits/pixel or greater.[7] This spatial resolution is less than that achieved with film screen radiography; however, the improved contrast resolution and latitude described below overcome this limitation.

Image contrast and latitude are major advantages of digital radiography compared with traditional film-screen systems. Latitude, termed dynamic range in the digital world, is the range of exposures that results in a useable, or diagnostic, image. The latitude of digital radiography is much greater than that of film-screen systems.[1-4,6] Film-screen systems typically have either good latitude or good contrast, but not both. Once a film is exposed and processed, the image contrast or blackness cannot be adjusted. In a digital image, both the contrast and blackness can be adjusted by using the concept of windowing. Digital radiography systems can capture a much wider range of x-ray energies compared with film-screen systems (Fig. 2-13).[1-4,6] With film-screen systems a narrow range of x-ray intensities appear as different shades of gray. Most of the x-ray intensities are black or white, making them useless for tissue resolution.

Digital images can be adjusted to display high-contrast (few shades of gray) or wide latitude (many shades of gray). The wide latitude, or dynamic range, of digital radiographs enables the viewing of both soft tissues and bone on the same image without repeat exposures at different techniques, as would be needed for a film-screen system (Fig. 2-14).

Image noise is caused by quantum mottle as a result of too few x-ray photons striking the imaging plate (CR) or detector (DDR). In digital systems, the milliamperes per second (mAs) setting is not related to blackness as with film-screen systems because digital systems compensate for overexposure and underexposure to provide optimal viewing quality. Although digital imaging is much more forgiving to underexposure than are film-screen systems, severe underexposure will result in a mottled or coarsely stippled image (Fig. 2-15).[2]

Digital images are viewed on computer monitors for diagnosis; therefore careful consideration must be given to the quality of the monitor. High-quality monitors have been designed for viewing digital radiographs; these monitors are expensive but provide an environment to maximize identification of lesions.[7] Monitor resolution, brightness (luminance), and contrast should all be considered. Recommendations for display workstations where interpretation of images is performed include the use of gray-scale monitors with at least 50-foot lamberts for maximum luminance.[7] Some standard monitors will not be adequate for diagnosis of digital images, having less than the recommended 2000 × 2000 pixels.[6] Standard computer monitors do provide sufficient quality to use for reviewing digital radiographs.

When an image is magnified, as often occurs during interpretation of digital images, pixel/matrix size becomes an important factor. For example, if an image is enlarged to twice its original size, the information that was originally in one pixel is displayed in four pixels. This results in pixilation, in which the pixels appear larger with magnification with a resultant degradation of image quality (Fig. 2-16).[6]

Collimation is used for digital radiography, as in film-screen radiography, to lessen the effects of scatter radiation on image quality and for safety reasons. For CR systems used for imaging equine extremities, the primary x-ray beam should extend to the edge of the imaging plate where bone crosses the plate. This is recommended for improved and consistent image quality.[2] Collimation can be used parallel to the long axis of the bone.

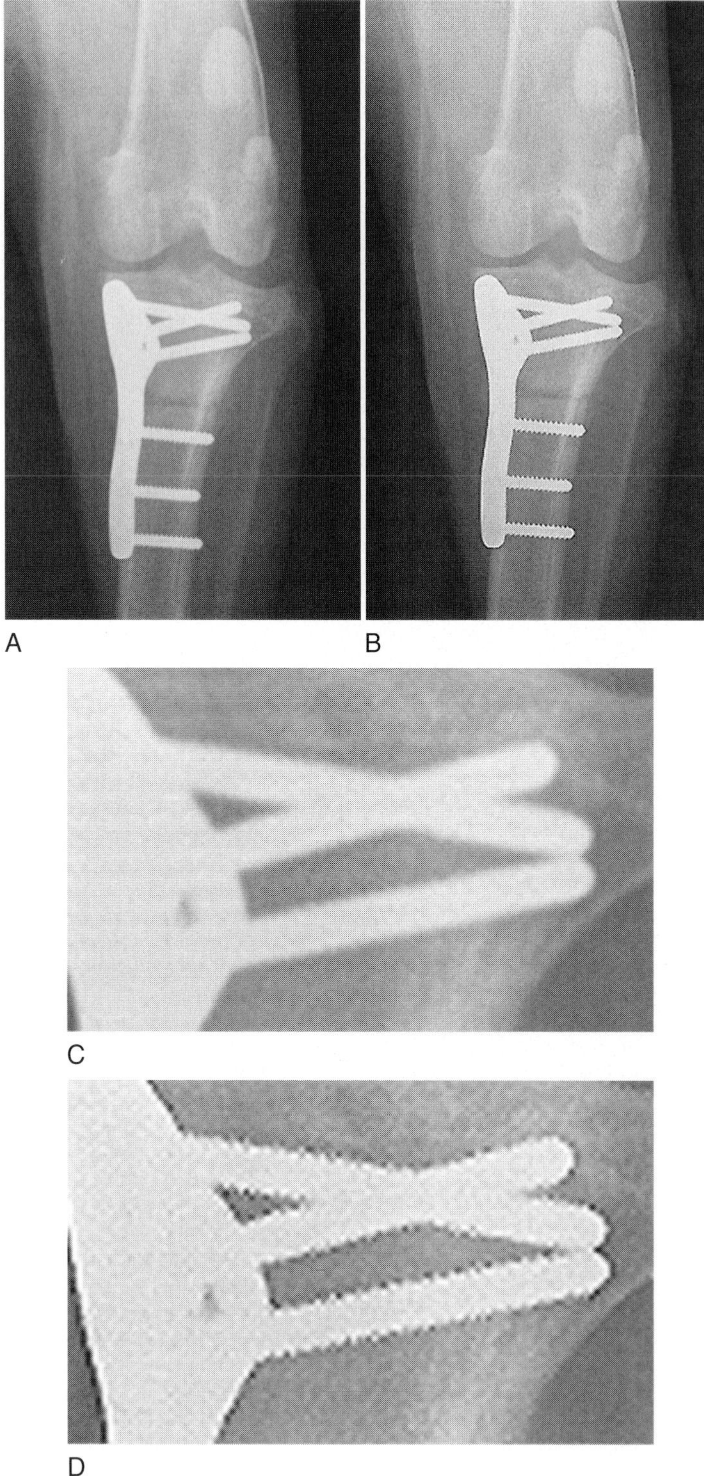

Fig. 2-12 Edge enhancement is a postprocessing function that can enhance the edges of structures on the radiograph. Compare the two images of a craniocaudal tibia. **A** was made with the original presets, whereas postprocessing edge enhancement has been used for **B.** The edge enhancement results in visualization of a black halo surrounding the metal implant seen in the close-ups of the proximal tibia (**C** and **D**); this is an artifact and should not be confused with bone lysis from movement or infection.

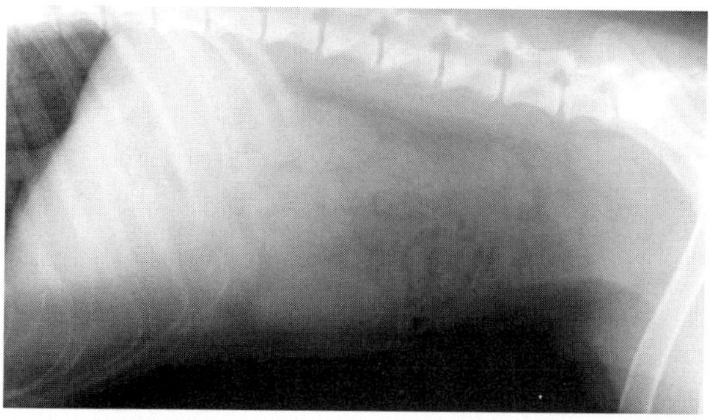

A

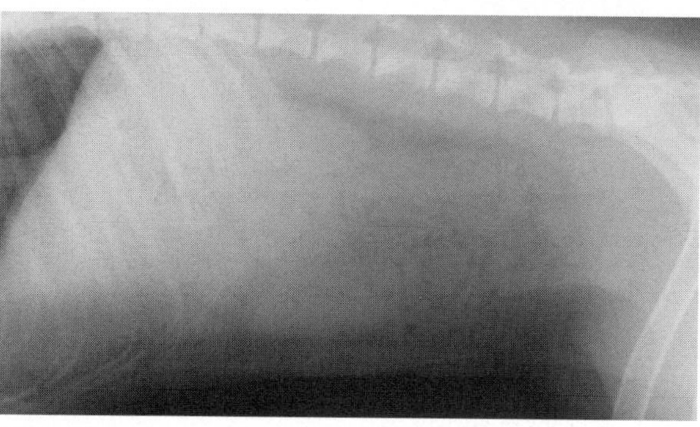

B

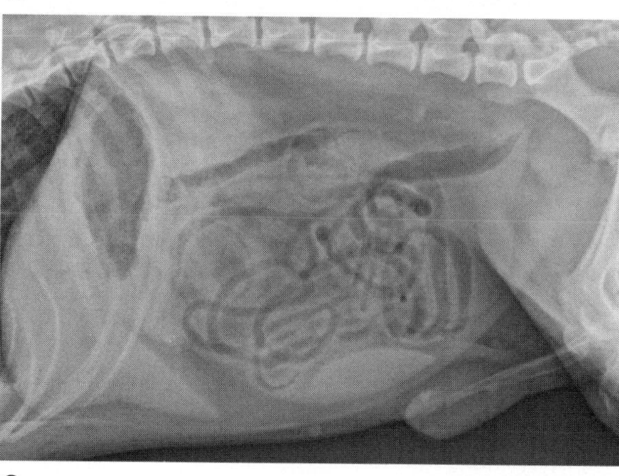

C

Fig. 2-13 A is a conventional radiograph with good contrast (black and white). B is a conventional radiograph with good latitude (many shades of gray). C is a digital radiograph with both good contrast and latitude (able to define both bone and soft tissue).

ADVANTAGES AND DISADVANTAGES OF DIGITAL RADIOGRAPHY

Advantages of Digital Radiography Systems

Digital radiography has numerous advantages compared with traditional film-screen radiography. One of the major advantages is the linear response to x-ray intensity over a wide latitude (dynamic range), as previously discussed (Fig. 2-17). Additional advantages include a decreased number of retakes attributable to technical errors (underexposure or overexposure), computed image enhancement (edge and contrast), image manipulation tools, digital storage, and transmission to the outside.[1-4,6]

Digital radiography compensates for improper exposure techniques. For example, a film that was underexposed by 15% to 20% would be nondiagnostic, but in digital radiography this error could still result in a diagnostic image. With digital imaging systems underexposure results in image noise and loss of detail (see Fig. 2-15).[3,8] The recognition of underexposure is extremely important in digital imaging. Even though consistent global optical density is achieved over a wide range of exposures, detection of low-contrast objects is decreased on underexposed digital images, reducing the overall diagnostic quality.[9]

Most manufactures have an optimal exposure index expressed as a range of numbers that determines whether the exposure is adequate.[3] Overexposure can result in the loss of ability to see thinner soft tissue areas. This is most problematic in large-breed dogs, in which the lung lobes or body wall may be overexposed when trying to penetrate the thicker portions of the patient (Fig. 2-18). Retakes are reduced with digital imaging systems; however, retakes are not eliminated because many are a result of poor positioning, lack of inclusion of the entire area of interest, and motion.[1,3] Technologist time spent on radiology has decreased by using digital imaging, resulting in increased productivity.[10]

Computed image enhancement provides both edge and contrast enhancement. As previously discussed, various algorithms can be used and changed for different body areas to enhance the images.

Image windowing is one of the biggest advantages of a digital imaging system. With windowing, the blackness and contrast of an image can be manipulated after the image has been acquired. This postprocessing is impossible when using a radiographic film-screen system; if a radiographic image is not optimal, it must be repeated. Windowing allows accurate assessment of both bone and soft tissue in the same image (see Chapter 4). Many other image manipulation tools are available depending on the software system used for image viewing. These include, but are not limited to, magnification, measurement tools, ratios, and angle measurements.[1,3]

Digital storage becomes advantageous for practices with limited capacity for film storage and is beneficial in viewing images at various locations throughout the clinic. The problem of lost or damaged film is also no longer relevant. Transmission to the outside (consultation, owner, colleague) is becoming more important as many teleradiology and specialty services are becoming readily available. This makes obtaining a second opinion easier and faster.[1-3,6]

Although the initial investment in equipment is considerable, high-volume practices may recognize savings from eliminating the cost of film, processor maintenance, and chemicals.[1-3]

Disadvantages of Digital Radiography Systems

Digital imaging systems still do not have the degree of spatial resolution possible with film-screen radiography; however, this is of little clinical relevance and is overcome by its advantages.[2] CR systems have a spatial resolution of approximately 2.5 line pairs/mm, whereas film-screen systems range from 6 to 10 line pairs/mm. Studies have shown that digital radiography systems (both CR and DDR) are the same or better than film-screen systems in diagnostic image quality for the thorax.[11,12] In fact, the perceived quality of the image depends more on contrast and other postprocessing functions than on spatial resolution.

The initial investment in digital radiography can be considerable. Annual maintenance of the system should be determined because it can add considerably to the cost. In general most CR systems or DDR systems that use the same x-ray

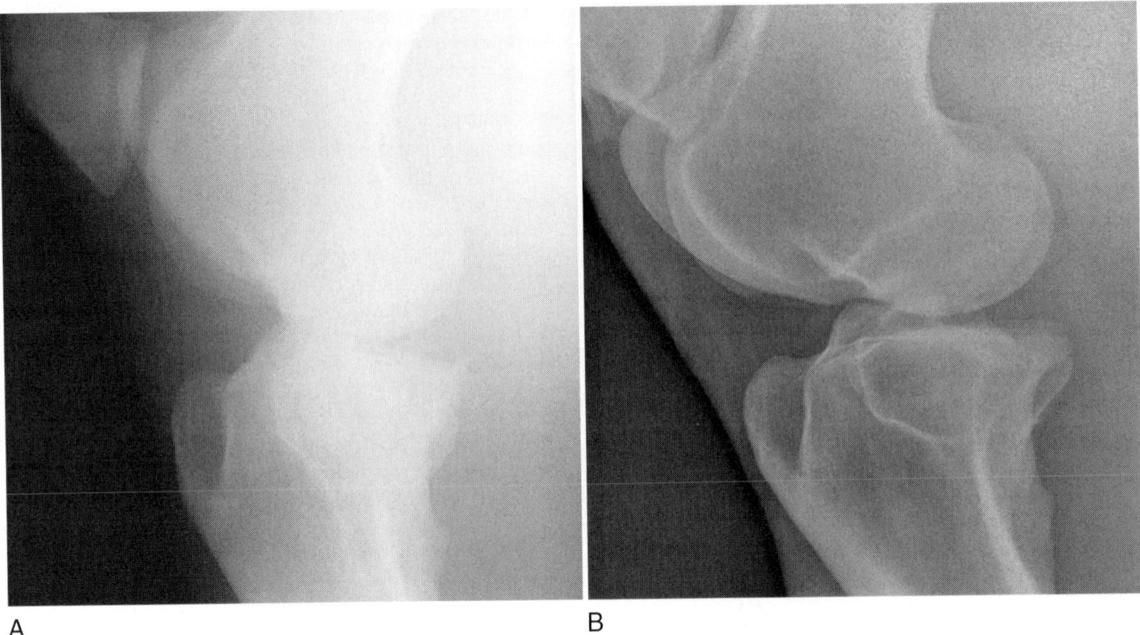

Fig. 2-14 Compare the conventional radiograph (A) of the equine stifle to the digital radiograph (B). In A the soft tissues are overexposed cranial to the stifle joint and underexposed caudal to the stifle joint. On the digital radiograph the soft tissues can be clearly visualized.

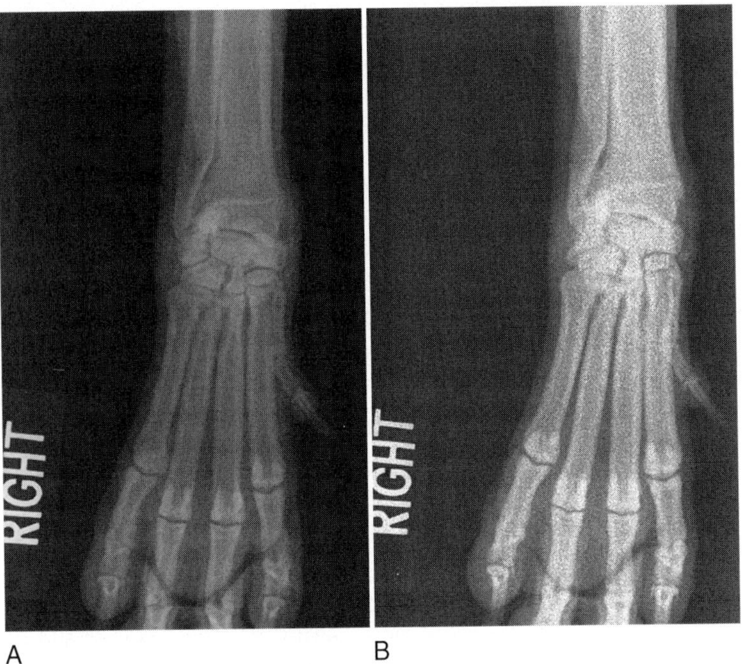

Fig. 2-15 An underexposed digital radiograph will still have adequate brightness and contrast because of postprocessing algorithms. However, compare the properly exposed digital radiograph of the carpus (A) to the underexposed image of the same carpus (B) that was made by decreasing the kilovoltage peak by 30% compared with the original image. The underexposed radiograph maintains adequate brightness and contrast but is extremely mottled.

generator are a lower initial investment than DDR systems in which all equipment needs to be replaced.

Many different CR and DDR products are available but must be compatible with the rest of the hospital system. This may increase the cost in other areas, for example, requiring a computer in the examination room where a view box would have previously sufficed.

ARCHIVING AND RETRIEVAL OF IMAGES

Digital Image Storage

Storage of digital data is an important consideration because it is part of the medical record. A wide range of storage devices differ in storage capacity, data access, transfer rates, and cost. Off-site storage is also available. For local on-site storage, hard

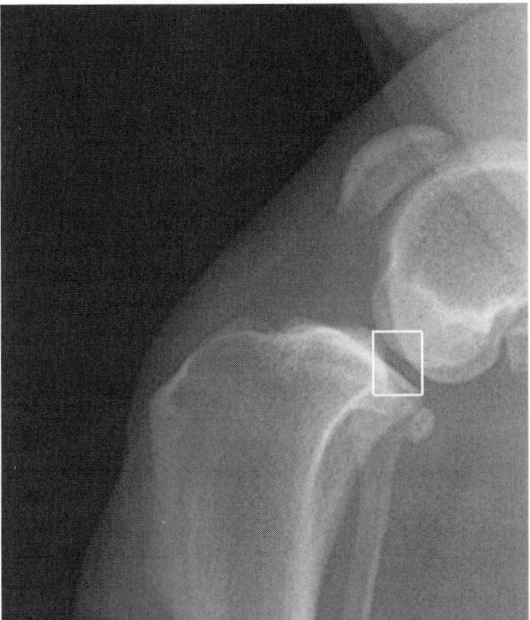

A

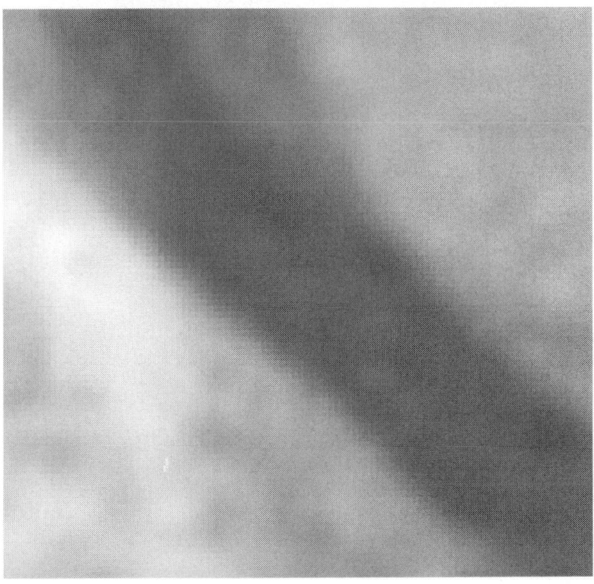

B

Fig. 2-16 Magnifying an image on the monitor will result in the ability to see individual pixels. The *white box* on the image at *left* shows the area of the stifle joint that is magnified on the right side. Note the tiny pixels (squares) that are particularly noticeable at the bone surface.

disk drives, removable disks, magnetic tape drives, and optical (laser) disks are options. Transfer of images can also be done by e-mail, CD, or DVD.[3]

Picture Archiving and Communication System

A complete system of hardware and software designed for digital radiographic systems is known as a picture archiving and communication system (PACS) (Fig. 2-19).[13] PACS provides image capture, display, annotation, storage, and communication functions. Useful features include zooming, contrast and brightness adjustments, annotations and marking, and measuring functions. PACS are used by larger hospitals for archival, retrieval, and transport to multiple viewing stations around the hospital.[3] Mini-PACS are also provided for smaller clinics that allow viewing in examination rooms and surgery. The software is often a major part of the cost for PACS.

Digital Imaging Communications in Medicine

Digital imaging communications in medicine (DICOM) is a specific image file format analogous to JPEG and TIF formats commonly used in manipulation and storage of digital camera images. DICOM was conceived to provide connectivity between medical imaging devices (CT, MR imaging, ultrasound, nuclear medicine, and digital radiography) and PACS systems.[14] This connectivity requires that a standard file format be used for all medical images. Consider if each vendor made its digital images proprietary. This would mean that a CT image from vendor A and ultrasound images from vendor B could not be viewed with software from vendor C; this would create a system of great inconvenience and inflexibility.

In addition to standardizing connectivity, DICOM format provides important security features to help ensure the images are authentic. DICOM conformance is currently not required in veterinary medicine, but all systems should provide a DICOM conformance statement. PACS should transport the images in DICOM format and meet the Food and Drug Administration standards for security.

Hospital and Radiology Information System

A Radiology Information System (RIS) is a software program that coordinates manipulation, distribution, and storage of patient radiologic data and images. The system generally incorporates patient scheduling, generation of reports, and image tracking. A hospital information system (HIS), on the other hand, is a software program that coordinates all aspects, including administrative, financial, and clinical functions, of a hospital. Each of these systems assumes great importance in a paperless, or filmless, environment. Integration between the RIS and HIS is important for maximizing efficiency and for linking image information to other patient data. Attention must be paid to these aspects of electronic business when considering a switch to a digital (filmless) environment.

ARTIFACTS IN DIGITAL RADIOGRAPHY

Digital radiography can compensate for a wide range of exposures. If underexposure occurs the resultant digital image appears grainy (pixilated). In an overexposed image thin, soft tissue structures are not visible.

Processing artifacts can be seen with both DR and CR.[3,8,15] For example, improper use of edge enhancement may result in the lung fields appearing to have an interstitial pattern (Fig. 2-20). If correct processing parameters are established at the commissioning of the new system, they will rarely need to be manipulated in the future.

Artifacts unique to CR include image plate and plate reader artifacts.[3,8,15] As plates become worn over time they can crack on the edges, resulting in white linear artifacts on the image. If a CR plate is incompletely erased before the next exposure, then portions of the previous image or scatter radiation may be present (Fig. 2-21). If the light guide on the plate reader needs to be cleaned, a white line artifact will appear on the image (Fig. 2-22). Lack of primary beam collimation and failure to center the area of interest on the cassette may result in artifacts.

Similar to traditional film-screen radiography, any debris on an imaging plate will result in a sharp white artifact. Backscatter, images of objects behind the cassette, can also be seen with CR plates.[3,15] High line ratio grids should be used for digital imaging and are specified or provided by the manufacturer of the digital imaging equipment. Low line grids will result in a moiré pattern if the grid lines are parallel to the reader's scan lines.[3,15]

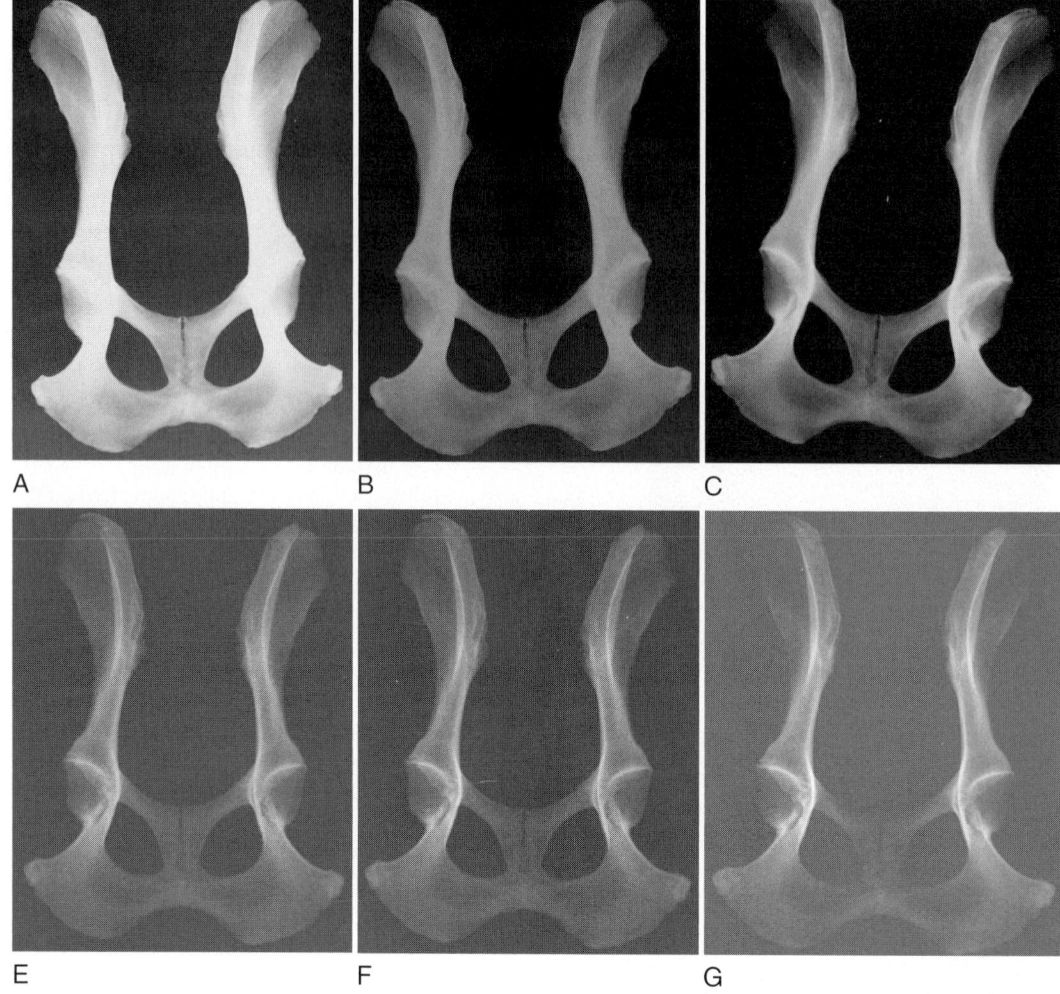

Fig. 2-17 A through C were made with conventional x-ray equipment. The exposure for B was the correct exposure. A had the exposure technique decreased by 20% (underexposed), whereas C had the technique increased by 20% (overexposed). D through F are digital images showing the proper technique (E) and a decrease in technique by 20% (D) and an increase in technique by 20% (F). The digital images provide a much wider range of exposures to achieve an acceptable image compared with conventional radiography.

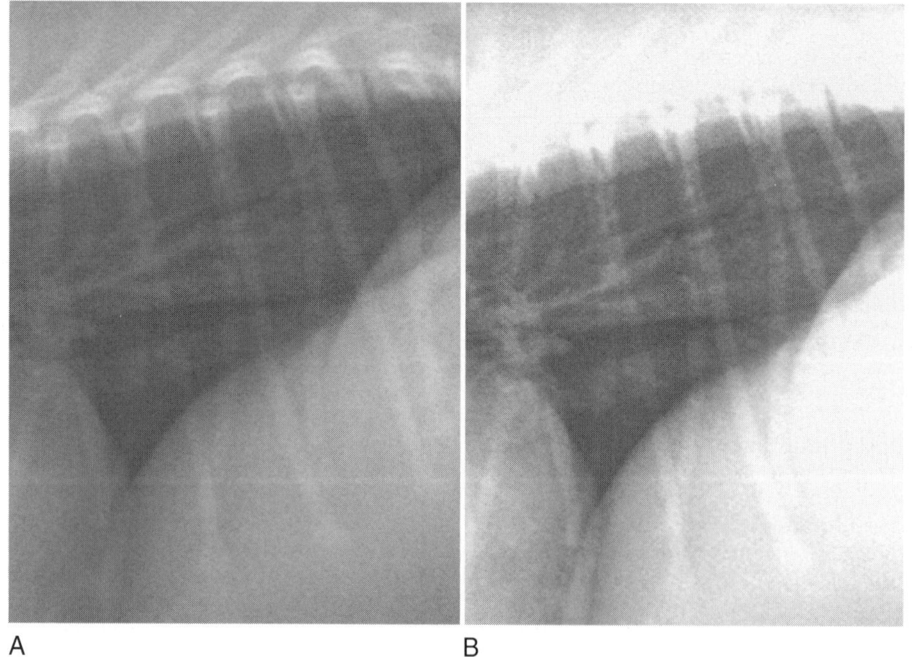

Fig. 2-18 Overexposure of the thorax resulted in a black area surrounding the caudal vena cava (A). Even with adjustments in brightness (B) the overexposed area remains black.

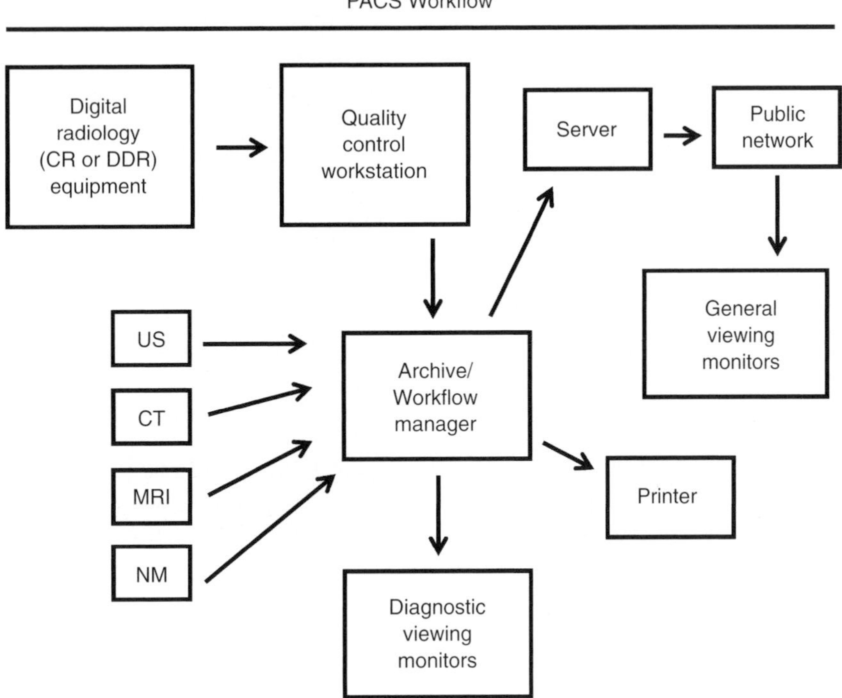

Fig. 2-19 Diagram of general workflow for PACS. All imaging modalities should be connected to a central workflow computer that can then disseminate the information for backup storage and retrieval, viewing on diagnostic workstations and computers around the hospital, and sending to off-site locations or printout.

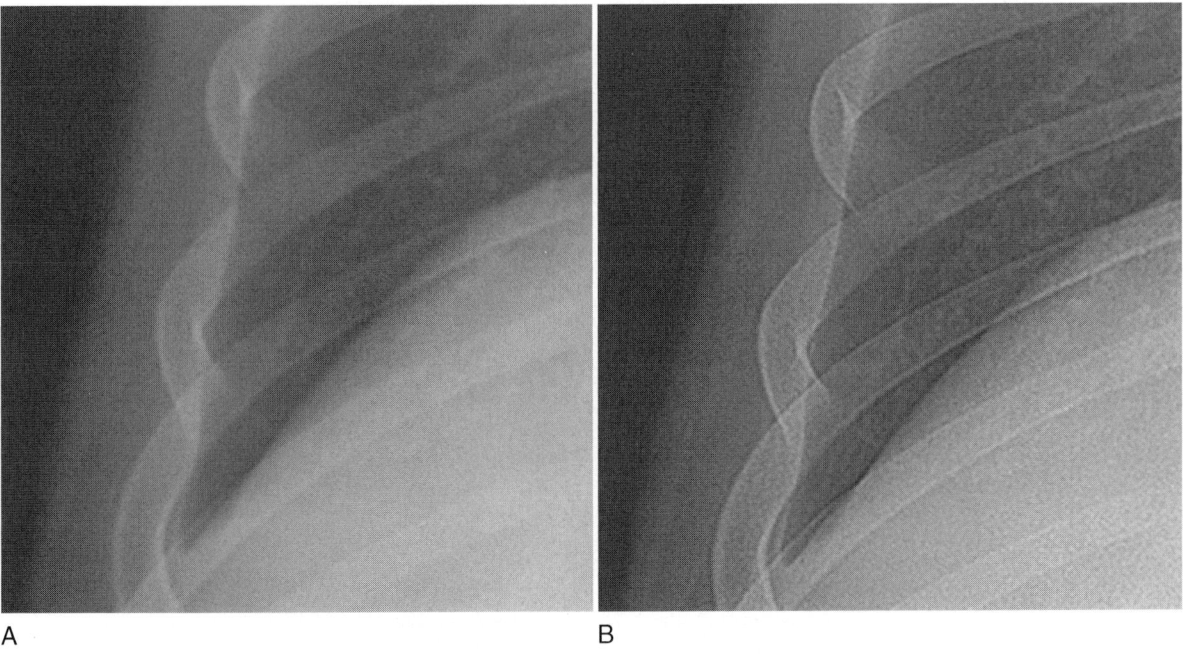

Fig. 2-20 Close-up of the right caudal lung lobe from a ventrodorsal thoracic radiograph with standard processing (A) and an overly edge enhanced algorithm (B).

DIGITIZING CONVENTIONAL FILM-SCREEN RADIOGRAPHS

Handheld digital cameras and flat-bed CCD scanners have been used to convert film-based images to a digital format for the purposes of teleradiology and teaching.[6,16] This may be a feasible option for those who cannot afford primary digital radiography systems. The concern with digitizing radiographs with cameras or scanners is that file type, image compression, and dynamic range are highly variable and may result in poor-quality digital images.[6] With rapidly changing technology, by the time a digital camera is tested a new and improved model is available. Although some previous digital cameras were shown to be adequate by the American College of Radiology

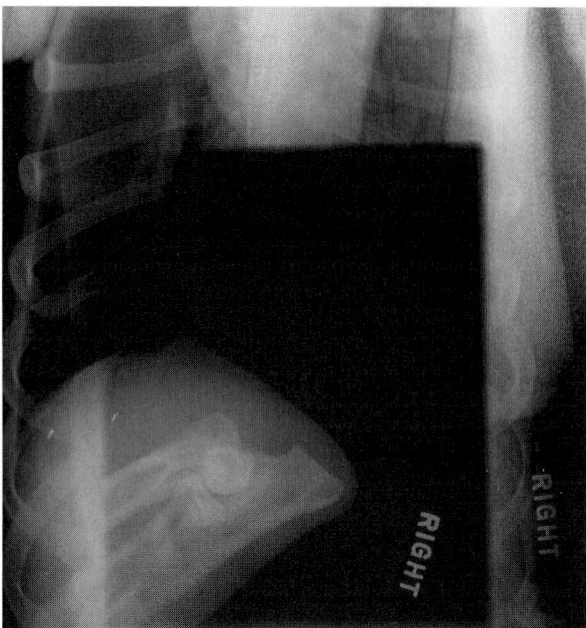

Fig. 2-21 A double-exposure artifact on a CR plate. The image of the lateral elbow was made first. The plate was not erased and a second image of a thorax was made. The thorax is visible only on the area of the plate that was not already exposed for the elbow.

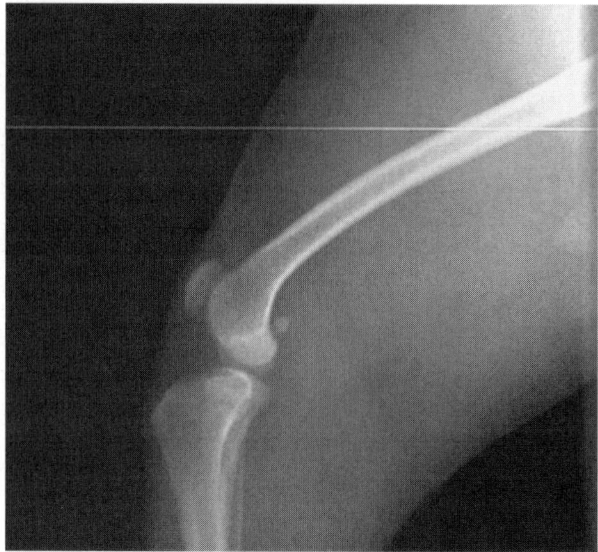

Fig. 2-22 A plate reader artifact caused by dirt on the plate reader's light guide. This resulted in the *white line* that extends across this image of a lateral stifle.

standards for line pair and contrast resolution,[17] these same cameras did not perform as well as conventional film-screen radiographs for detection of lung nodules.[18] The poor performance of digital cameras is not a result of their pixel/matrix size, but their lack of adequate dynamic range (ability to demonstrate many shades of gray).[6,18] Proper use of the digital camera is imperative, and several sources describe how to maximize the image quality.[6,19] Hybrid digital radiography systems containing CCD imaging devices for image capture are also not recommended because of their lack of dynamic range and overall image quality.

DETERMINING WHICH DIGITAL SYSTEM TO USE

CR, DDR, and film-screen radiography have been compared in many studies.[20-22] In an experimental study comparing bone lesions, no difference in image quality and lesion detection was noted among the three modalities.[20] In another study, film-screen radiography was compared with CR (both hard copy and soft copy viewed on computer monitors) for the detection of foreign bodies in hands, and soft copy CR was found to be superior.[21] This occurred because the dynamic range provided the ability to enhance differences in contrast in the soft copy images. Some concern still may arise in veterinary medicine in terms of spatial resolution; however, in a study looking at a comparison of human hands, CR was found to be at least as good as or better in terms of image quality compared with film-screen radiography.[22] Ultimately the needs of the practice and the equipment available must be considered in a rapidly changing market.

ACKNOWLEDGMENT

The author acknowledges the valuable assistance of Mal Hoover in the production of Figures 2-1, 2-4, 2-5, 2-7, 2-10, and 2-19.

REFERENCES

1. Mattoon JS, Smith C: Breakthroughs in radiography: computed radiography, *Compendium* 17:1, 2004.
2. Roberts GD, Graham JP: Computed radiography. In Kraft SL, Roberts GD, editors: *Modern diagnostic imaging, veterinary clinics of North America: equine practice,* Philadelphia, 2001, Saunders.
3. Stearns ED: Computed radiography in perspective, *NAVTA Journal* Summer:53, 2004.
4. Digital x-ray systems, part 1: an introduction to DX technologies and an evaluation of cassette DX systems, *Health Devices* 30:273, 2001.
5. Bushberg JT, Seibert JA, Leidholdt EM et al: Computers in medical imaging. In Passano WM, editor: *The essential physics of medical imaging,* Baltimore, 1994, Williams & Wilkins.
6. Papageorges M: Image capture devices. In Papageorges M, editor: *Understanding and using telemedicine: how to harness the telecommunication revolution,* Clackamas, OR, 1999, Veterinary Diagnostic Imaging and Cytopathology Publishing, Inc.
7. American College of Radiology: *2005 ACR technical standard for teleradiology,* Reston, VA, 2005, American College of Radiology.
8. Solomon SL, Jost RG, Glazer HS et al: Artifacts in computed radiography, *AJR* 157:181, 1991.
9. Kimme-Smith C, Aberle D, Sayre JW et al: Effects of reduced exposure on computed radiography: comparison of nodule detection accuracy with conventional and asymmetric screen-film radiographs of a chest phantom, *AJR* 165:269, 1995.
10. Reiner BI, Siegel EL: Technologists' productivity when using PACS: comparison of film-based versus filmless radiography, *AJR* 179:33, 2002.
11. Ganten M, Radeleff B, Kampschulte A et al: Comparing image quality of flat-panel chest radiography with storage phosphor radiography and film-screen radiography, *AJR* 181:171, 2003.

12. Fink C, Hallscheidt PJ, Noeldge G et al: Clinical comparative study with a large-area amorphous silicon flat-panel detector: image quality and visibility of anatomic structures on chest radiography, *AJR* 178:481, 2002.
13. Oosterwijk H: *PACS fundamentals*, Aubrey, TX, 2004, Otech.
14. Oosterwijk H, Gihring PT: *DICOM basics*, ed 3, Aubrey, TX, 2005, Otech.
15. Cesar LJ, Schueler BA, Zink FE et al: Artefacts found in computed radiography, *Br J Radiol* 74:195, 2001.
16. Sistrom CL, Gray SB: Digital cameras for reproducing radiologic images: evaluation of three cameras, *AJR* 170:279, 1998.
17. Brault B, Hoskinson J, Armbrust L et al: Comparison of seven digital cameras for digitizing radiographs, *Vet Radiol Ultrasound* 45:298, 2004.
18. Armbrust LJ, Hoskinson JJ, Biller DS et al: Comparison of digitized and direct viewed (analog) radiographic images for detection of pulmonary nodules, *Vet Radiol Ultrasound* 46:361, 2005.
19. Whitehouse RW: Use of digital cameras for radiographs: how to get the best pictures, *J R Soc Med* 92:178, 1999.
20. Ludwig K, Link TM, Fiebich M et al: Selenium-based digital radiography in the detection of bone lesions: preliminary experience with experimentally created defects, *Radiology* 216:220, 2000.
21. Reiner B, Siegel E, McLaurin T et al: Evaluation of soft-tissue foreign bodies: comparing conventional plain film radiography, computed radiography printed on film, and computed radiography displayed on a computer workstation, *AJR* 167:141, 1996.
22. Swee RG, Gray JE, Beabout JW et al: Screen-film versus computed radiography imaging of the hand: a direct comparison, *AJR* 168:539, 1997.

ELECTRONIC RESOURCES evolve

Additional information related to the content in Chapter 2 can be found on the companion Web site at evolve http://evolve.elsevier.com/Thrall/vetrad/

- Key Points
- Chapter Quiz

CHAPTER • 3
Basic Ultrasound Physics

Wm. Tod Drost

A basic understanding of the physics of ultrasound is important because it helps explain some of the limitations and artifacts encountered. Medical sonography uses sound wave echoes to create images and is the only diagnostic imaging modality that does not use electromagnetic radiation. In this chapter, the basic physical principles of gray-scale ultrasonography are discussed.

PHYSICAL PRINCIPLES OF ULTRASOUND WAVES

Sound travels in waves and carries information from one location to another. It transmits energy by alternating regions of low pressure (rarefaction) and high pressure (compression).[1-4] Unlike light and radio waves, sound waves require a medium through which to travel; they cannot be propagated in a vacuum.[5] Frequency, wavelength, and velocity are parameters used to describe sound waves; these terms are also used in reference to electromagnetic radiation (see Chapter 1).

Frequency is the number of times a wave is repeated per second. One wave or cycle occurs when pressure starts at a normal value, increases to a high-pressure value, decreases (passing the normal value) to a low-pressure value, and then returns to normal (Fig. 3-1). A cycle may also be defined as the combination of compression and successive rarefaction.[4] Frequency is expressed in hertz (Hz), where 1 Hz equals 1 cycle/sec. Diagnostic ultrasound typically uses frequencies between 2 megahertz (MHz) and 13 MHz (1 MHz = 1,000,000 Hz). The audible range of sound for human beings is 20 Hz to 20,000 Hz; sound less than 20 Hz is infrasound, and sound greater than 20,000 Hz (0.02 MHz) is ultrasound.[5,6]

Wavelength is the distance traveled by a sound wave in one cycle. In ultrasonography, wavelength is expressed in millimeters (mm). Wavelength is important for image resolution and is discussed later.

Velocity is the rate at which sound travels through an acoustic medium; it is determined by the physical density (mass per unit volume) and stiffness (hardness) of the transmitting medium.[1,2,5] The velocity of sound in some commonly encountered tissues is listed in Box 3-1. If physical density remains constant, velocity increases as stiffness increases. If the stiffness remains constant, velocity decreases as physical density increases. As a general rule, velocity is highest in solids, lower in liquids, and the lowest in gases.[7] In solids, molecules are closer together, so sound waves are transmitted faster; in gases, the molecules are far apart and sound waves travel more slowly.[5] Medically, sound waves travel the fastest in bone and the slowest in gas-filled lungs. This causes a problem for diagnostic ultrasound machines because they use the average velocity of sound in soft tissue (1.54 mm/μs) for computations performed in the computer of the ultrasound machine. However, because sound waves do not penetrate lung or bone well (almost all sound is reflected because of high differences in acoustic impedance), the velocity of sound within these tissues is not a factor in diagnostic ultrasound. Velocity is related to frequency and wavelength of a sound wave in the following equation:

$$\text{Velocity (mm/}\mu\text{s)} = \text{Frequency (MHz)} \times \text{Wavelength (mm)} \qquad \text{(Eq 1)}$$

For a constant velocity, frequency and wavelength have an inverse relationship so that as frequency increases, wavelength decreases, and vice versa. Within soft tissue, the average velocity of sound is 1.54 mm/μs (1540 m/s).[2,5] The velocity of sound in soft tissue is important because, as noted above, ultrasound machines use this constant velocity for all calculations.

ULTRASOUND WAVE INTERACTION WITH MATTER

The principle of echo formation is important because echoes contain the information about the structures being imaged. The interface that causes the echo reflection and the angle at which the sound wave strikes the reflector, or the angle of incidence, should both be considered.

Acoustic impedance of a tissue is the product of the tissue's physical density and sound velocity within the tissue.[5,8]

$$\text{Acoustic impedance (Z)} = \text{Velocity } (\upsilon) \times \text{Tissue density (p)} \qquad \text{(Eq 2)}$$

Changes in acoustic impedance from one tissue to another determine how much of the sound wave is reflected and how much is transmitted into the second tissue. The amplitude of the returning echo is proportional to the difference in acoustic impedance. If two tissues have no difference in acoustic impedance, then no echo is created. If a large difference in acoustic impedance exists between two tissues, then almost all the sound is reflected.[5] To calculate the percentage of the sound wave that is reflected and transmitted, the following formulas are used[1]:

$$\% \text{ reflected} = (Z_2 - Z_1)/(Z_2 + Z_1) \times 100 \qquad \text{(Eq 3)}$$

$$\% \text{ transmitted} = 100 - \% \text{ reflected} \qquad \text{(Eq 4)}$$

In Eq2, Z_2 is the acoustic impedance of the second tissue, and Z_1 is the acoustic impedance of the first tissue. The approximate acoustic impedance of commonly encountered tissues is listed in Box 3-2. By the values in Box 3-2, the largest difference in acoustic impedance is shown to occur at interfaces with bone and gas. These interfaces, soft tissue/gas and soft tissue/bone, reflect almost all the sound wave; thus little or no sound wave passes these boundaries. Hence the speed of sound in bone and gas-filled lung is not clinically important. This nearly total reflection creates an acoustic void or shadow deep to the tissue interface. Without placement of

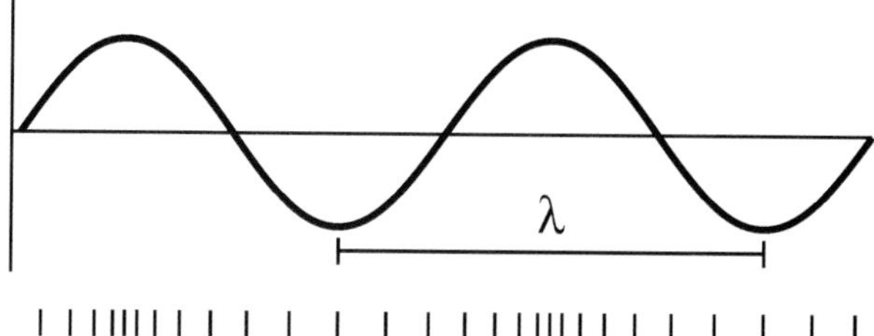

Fig. 3-1 An ultrasound wave depicted as a sine wave *(top)* and as a series of compressions and rarefactions *(bottom)*. One wavelength (λ) is the distance between two successive peaks or valleys of the sine wave or between two successive compression or rarefaction events.

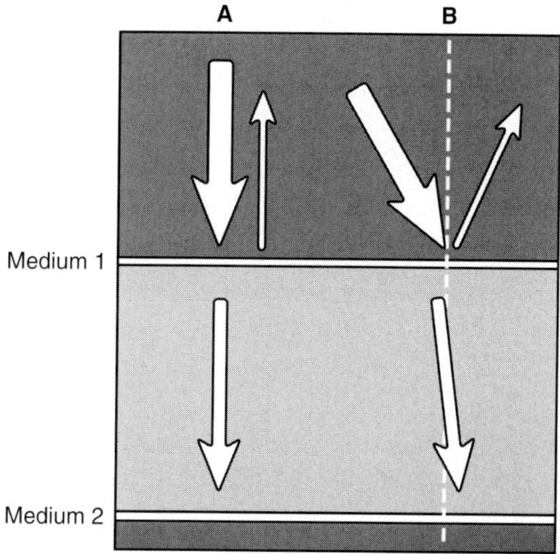

Fig. 3-2 The angle of incidence is the angle at which a sound wave encounters a medium. If the angle of the sound wave is perpendicular (90 degrees) to the reflector **(A)**, the reflected portion of the sound wave travels opposite (180 degrees) to the direction of the initial sound wave, and the transmitted portion of the sound wave continues in the same direction as the initial sound wave. If the angle of incidence is not perpendicular **(B)**, then the angle of reflectance equals the angle of incidence; the angle of transmittance depends on the difference in acoustic impedance of *medium 1* versus *medium 2*.

Box 3-1

Velocity of Sound in Commonly Encountered Tissues[5]

Tissue	*Velocity (mm/μs)*
Air	0.331
Fat	1.450
Water (50° C)	1.540
Soft tissue	1.540
Brain	1.541
Liver	1.549
Kidney	1.561
Blood	1.570
Muscle	1.585
Lens of eye	1.620
Bone (skull)	4.080

Box 3-2

Approximate Acoustic Impedance in Commonly Encountered Tissues[1,5]

Tissue	*Acoustic Impedance (in Rayls)*
Air	0.0004
Fat	1.38
Water (50° C)	1.54
Brain	1.58
Blood	1.61
Kidney	1.62
Liver	1.65
Muscle	1.70
Lens of eye	1.84
Bone (skull)	7.80

acoustic coupling gel between the patient and the transducer, the soft tissue/gas interface (created principally by gas trapped between the skin and transducer) would prevent imaging because of reflection of all the oncoming sound waves.

Angle of incidence is the angle at which a sound wave encounters a medium. If the angle of the sound wave is perpendicular (90 degrees) to the reflector, the reflected portion of the sound wave travels opposite (180 degrees) to the direction of the initial sound wave, and the transmitted portion of the sound wave continues in the same direction as the initial sound wave (Fig. 3-2, *A*). If the angle of incidence is not perpendicular, then the angle of reflectance equals the angle of incidence (Fig. 3-2, *B*). If a sound wave strikes a reflector farther than 3 degrees from perpendicular, then the reflected sound will likely not reach the transducer.[5] The angle of transmission on a nonperpendicular sound wave depends on the relative acoustic impedance of the two media. Any sound wave that is not reflected toward the transducer will not be recorded. Remember that the amount of reflected and transmitted sound depends on the differences in acoustic impedance of the two media.

As an ultrasound beam travels through a medium, it is attenuated. In other words, it loses strength as it travels through tissue. The amount of attenuation is determined by the distance traveled and the frequency of the sound wave. The amount of attenuation approximates 0.5 decibels (dB)/cm per MHz over a round-trip distance.[8] If a reflector is 3 cm from the transducer, the round trip distance is 6 cm and the attenuation of the sound beam is 3 dB/MHz. Sound beams of higher frequency are attenuated more than are lower frequency sound waves. Attenuation of the sound wave involves three components: absorption, reflection, and scattering.[3,5]

The conversion of a sound wave's mechanical energy to heat is called absorption.[2] It is the dominant component of attenuation in soft tissue.[6] The conversion of sound waves to heat occurs primarily by frictional forces.[8] With diagnostic ultrasound machines, the relative amount of sound absorbed is quite low and the temperature change is insignificant and imperceptible.

Reflection of the sound beam contributes to attenuation. As the sound wave encounters tissue interfaces of different acoustic impedance, a reflection is generated. Only reflections that return to the transducer are used for image formation. The scanning of structures from different angles may enhance image quality if more echoes are returned to the transducer from different angles.

Scattering occurs when sound waves encounter small, irregular surfaces. This occurs mainly within the parenchyma of organs and is responsible for the texture of the internal organs.[2] As the frequency of a sound beam increases, the incidence of scattering increases.

TRANSDUCERS

A transducer is a device that converts one form of energy to another.[1,5,9] In ultrasound imaging, this means converting electric activity into sound waves, and vice versa. This conversion is accomplished in a piezoelectric crystal. As an electric charge is applied to a piezoelectric crystal, the material deforms and creates a sound wave.[9] Conversely, when sound waves are applied to piezoelectric crystals, they produce an electric signal. Therefore the same crystal is used to send and receive sound waves but it cannot send and receive signals at the same time.[5] A typical ultrasound transducer emits sound waves less than 1% of the time and receives sound waves more than 99% of the time.[3,8]

Ultrasound transducers come in many shapes and sizes. The selection of the proper transducer depends on the physical properties of the transducer and the characteristics of the anatomic region to be imaged.

Mechanical transducers are either single- or multiple-crystal devices in which movement of the crystal(s) actually affects the coverage (and imaging) of a volume of tissue. The crystal elements oscillate back and forth or are continuously rotated within the head of the transducer. The elements are immersed in acoustic coupling medium within the transducer assembly so that only the internal parts of the transducer move while the outer surface remains stationary against the patient. Mechanical transducers produce sector (pie)-shaped images. Because of their moving parts, mechanical transducers are subject to wear.[8]

Electronic transducers, also called array transducers, are composed of several small elements in various arrangements. The elements may be arranged in a line or rectangle (linear array), in a curved line (convex array), or in concentric ring fashion (annular array).[9] The elements that compose these transducers are electronically fired in various sequences to create different-shaped images or to focus the sound beam at specific depths. Electronic transducers do not have moving parts and do not need an internal acoustic coupling medium. The most commonly used type of transducer in current ultrasound machines is the electronic transducer.

Two basic shapes of ultrasound images are commonly encountered. Images made in sector fashion are pie shaped (see Fig. 3-7), and images made in linear fashion are rectangular (see Fig. 3-4). Sector images are often produced from transducers with small footprints (the amount of transducer that makes contact with the patient); linear transducers usually have larger footprints. For thoracic imaging, sector-shaped transducers are preferable because images must be acquired from within the intercostal spaces. For abdominal imaging, the use of sector or linear transducers is often dictated by the personal preference of the sonographer.

Transducers are classified by the location of the crystals on the scan head. In end-fire transducers, the elements are located on the end of the probe, but side-fire transducer elements are found on the side of the probe, 90 degrees from the end. End-fire transducers are used in cardiac and abdominal imaging; side-fire transducers are used for intracavitary imaging such as large animal (per rectum) reproductive examinations.

Diagnostic ultrasound machines operate in pulsed mode for imaging.[7] This means that the ultrasound machine sends only a few cycles of a sound wave into a tissue and then spends the rest of the time listening for returning echoes. The pulse repetition frequency (PRF) is the number of times this pattern of sending and listening is repeated within 1 second.[6] The length of space in one pulse of ultrasound is called the spatial pulsed length. If a sound wave has a wavelength of 0.5 mm and three pulses are sent each time, the spatial pulsed length is 1.5 mm. Spatial pulsed length is important for axial resolution.

Resolution is the ability of an ultrasound machine to distinguish echoes on the basis of space, time, and strength.[9] The better the resolution, the more likely the sonographer will identify abnormalities. As the frequency of an ultrasound transducer increases, the resolution increases. Sonographers want to use transducers of the highest possible frequency for imaging to get the best possible resolution.

Axial resolution is the resolution of two separate reflectors along the direction in which the sound wave is traveling.[3,4,9] It is equal to half the spatial pulse length. As previously mentioned, spatial pulsed length is the length of space over which the pulse of a sound wave travels. When two reflectors are separated by a distance that is greater than half the spatial pulsed length, the echoes from these two reflectors do not overlap as they return to the transducer and are interpreted as separate echoes (Fig. 3-3). If the distance between the reflectors is less than half the spatial pulsed length, the returning echoes overlap and are interpreted as a single echo. Because transducers with higher frequency have shorter spatial pulsed length, axial resolution is improved.

Lateral resolution is the resolution of two separate reflectors perpendicular to the direction in which the sound wave is traveling.[4,9] This is determined by the ultrasound beam

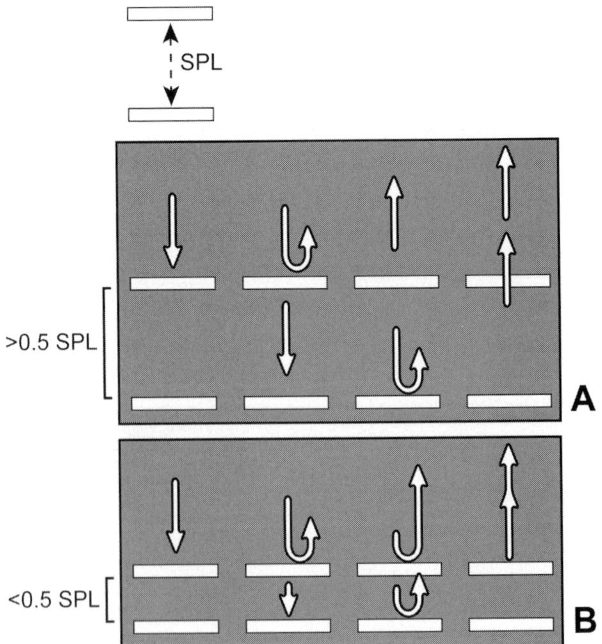

Fig. 3-3 Axial resolution depends on the spatial pulse length *(SPL)* of the sound wave and the amount of separation of the reflectors. If the reflectors are greater than 0.5 times the SPL **(A)**, the structures return two discrete echoes, as shown by the two *separate arrows.* If the reflectors are less than 0.5 times the SPL **(B)**, the structures return only one echo, as illustrated by the *overlapping arrows.*

width.[4] To recognize the objects discretely, the beam must be narrower than the distance between the objects. The width of an ultrasound beam decreases with increasing frequency. In a focused ultrasound beam, where the width of the beam is restricted, the lateral resolution is best at the focal point of the ultrasound beam because this is the narrowest part of the beam.

Depth of sound wave penetration varies inversely with frequency.[4] Higher-frequency transducers are best for structures that are close to the surface; lower-frequency transducers are best for deeper structures. The choice of ultrasound transducer varies with the experience of the sonographer. As a guide, begin with a higher-frequency transducer (because it has better resolution) and switch to a lower-frequency transducer if deeper structures are not well imaged.

DISPLAY

Image formation for ultrasonography is based on the pulse echo principle.[7] A small burst of sound waves is sent into a structure by a transducer, and the transducer becomes an echo receiver. In between, the transducer is dampened to stop the piezoelectric crystal from vibrating. The electric signals generated from the returning echoes are amplified to form the final image. When the initial burst of sound is sent into the tissue, a timer is started to determine the amount of time it takes to receive echoes. The elapsed time from sending to receiving is directly related to the distance traveled by the sound wave.

$$\text{Rate (mm/}\mu\text{s)} \times \text{Time (}\mu\text{s)} = \text{Distance (mm)} \qquad \text{(Eq 5)}$$

The ultrasound machine assumes a constant rate for the velocity of sound (1.54 mm/μs), and because time is recorded, distance can easily be calculated.[7] Remember that the trip from the transducer to the reflector and back is twice the actual distance from the reflector to the transducer. This assumes that the sound wave travels in a straight line with no side trips along the way.

Two modes of echo display are commonly used in ultrasonography: brightness mode (B-mode, B scan, or gray scale) and motion mode (M-mode). B-mode is the most commonly used format and is used in both abdominal and cardiac imaging. M-mode is used only for echocardiography.

B-mode images are composed of a collection of dots that correspond to the amplitude or strength of the returning echo.[3,10] These dots are displayed on a black background, and the brightness or gray scale of the dot is highest (whitest) for the strongest returning echoes. The depth of the structure returning the echoes determines the position of the dots relative to the position of the transducer. Multiple thin scan lines make up a complete image so that B-mode images look like a slice of tissue.[5]

M-mode records a thin section of an ultrasound image over time. By using the B-mode image, the region for M-mode imaging is chosen; this is usually represented on the screen as a line. Once the M-mode cursor is in the desired location, M-mode is activated. On an M-mode image, the depth of the image is displayed on the vertical axis, and time is displayed on the horizontal axis. The brightness of the dots is proportional to the strength of the returning echoes, as it is in B-mode. When holding the transducer stationary, the examiner can evaluate how structures move over a particular amount of time.[10,11] M-mode sonography is most commonly used in echocardiography to quantitatively evaluate the function of both the ventricles and the cardiac valves.

Image orientation varies with the structure that is being imaged. For cardiac imaging, the right side of the screen is cranial (toward the patient's head) with long axis images. For all other structures, the left side of the screen is cranial and the top of the screen is dorsal (toward the patient's spine) for longitudinal images. For transverse images, the left side of the screen is dorsal. The portion of the image closest to the transducer, usually the top of the screen, is called the near field and the opposite side is called the far field.

BASIC SCANNER CONTROLS

The power control modifies the intensity of sound output by the transducer.[8] This is accomplished by adjusting the voltage applied to the piezoelectric crystal. Increasing the power leads to a uniform increase in the amplitude of returning echoes and thereby increases overall image echogenicity (brightness). Keeping the power level low helps improve image resolution and helps prevent artifacts.[8]

Gain affects the amplification of the returning echoes within the receiver. Increasing or decreasing the gain increases or decreases the brightness of the image displayed on the screen. If the gain is too low, the subtle parenchymal detail of tissue is lost. If the gain is too high, the image is too bright and contrast resolution is lost. A common analogy is to compare the gain knob on the ultrasound machine with the volume knob on a stereo. At low settings, subtle music cannot be heard, and at high settings, the music is too offensive to be enjoyed.

Because sound waves lose intensity (attenuation) as they travel in tissue, echoes returning from deeper tissues are weaker than echoes returning from tissues closer to the ultrasound transducer. To make an image uniform in brightness, amplification of the echoes from deeper tissues to a greater degree than echoes from shallow tissues is helpful.[10] The time gain compensation controls allow the user to adjust the gain in selected regions of the image.[3]

The reject function of an ultrasound machine is a method of reducing unwanted, low-amplitude noise. This noise, electronic or acoustic, is not useful and can subtly degrade the image. Many machines allow the user to select how much of the low-level noise is filtered from the image. If the reject is set too high, some of the subtle parenchymal echotexture is removed from the image.

PRINCIPLES OF INTERPRETATION

Echogenicity relates to the relative brightness of a structure. Anechoic structures have no echoes within them and appear black. When the echogenicity of two structures is compared, the darker structure is hypoechoic and the brighter structure is hyperechoic. If the structures have the same degree of brightness, they are isoechoic to one another. Because tissue derangements result in changes in echogenicity, it is important to know the relative echogenicity of each abdominal organ. Box 3-3 lists abdominal organs in order of their relative echogenicity.[12,13] Detecting diffuse changes in echogenicity of a whole organ is difficult, and accurate detection is related to the experience of the sonographer. Multiple abdominal organs should be compared to determine which are truly abnormal. Additional complexity results from the fact that machine settings may alter the echogenicity of an organ. Focal changes in echogenicity are easier to detect because the adjacent, normal parenchyma can be compared.

ARTIFACTS

Misrepresentation of structures caused by some characteristic of the imaging technique is an artifact. In diagnostic radiology, artifacts hinder evaluation of the image and are undesirable. Ultrasound artifacts are not always undesirable and may actually enhance evaluation of structures by providing insight regarding the composition of the structures. For instance, sonographic imaging of a fluid-filled structure (versus a hypoechoic tissue mass) reveals enhancement of soft tissues distal to the fluid-filled structure. Some basic ultrasound artifacts are discussed in this section of the text.

Box • 3-3

Relative Echogenicity of Commonly Encountered Structures in Order of Decreasing Echogenicity[8,13]

- Bone, gas, organ boundaries
- Structural fat, vessel walls
- Renal sinus
- Prostate
- Spleen
- Storage fat
- Liver
- Renal cortex
- Muscle
- Renal medulla
- Bile, urine

Reverberation artifacts are multiple hyperechoic foci that occur at regular intervals on the image. Reverberation occurs when the sound wave encounters an area of high reflectivity and the sound wave is reflected back toward the transducer.[13] When the reflected sound wave encounters the transducer, most of it is reflected back into the tissues where it again encounters the area of high reflectivity. This cycle of bouncing between the transducer and the patient continues many times, resulting in the regularly spaced hyperechoic foci on the screen (Fig. 3-4) (Video 3-1; see http://evolve.elsevier.com/Thrall/vetrad). The distance between the transducer and the highly reflective surface determines the spacing of the hyperechoic foci. A common cause of reverberation artifacts in abdominal sonography is intestinal gas.

Mirror-image duplicate structures normally present on one side of a strong reflector sometimes also appear on the other side of the reflector (Fig. 3-5). This is most commonly encountered when the liver is imaged with the diaphragm/lung interface acting as a highly reflective structure.[14] "Duplication" of the gallbladder is an example that can be used to explain the artifact. Normally the sound wave is sent toward the gallbladder, is reflected back toward the transducer, and is recorded on the screen according to how long it took the echoes to return to the transducer. For the artifactual gallbladder, the sound wave is sent from the transducer, bounces off the diaphragm/lung interface toward the gallbladder, and echoes off the gallbladder back toward the diaphragm/lung interface, where it is reflected toward the transducer. Because some of the sound must bounce off the diaphragm/lung interface, the sound takes longer to return to the transducer; thus the position of the artifactual gallbladder is misrepresented on the screen.

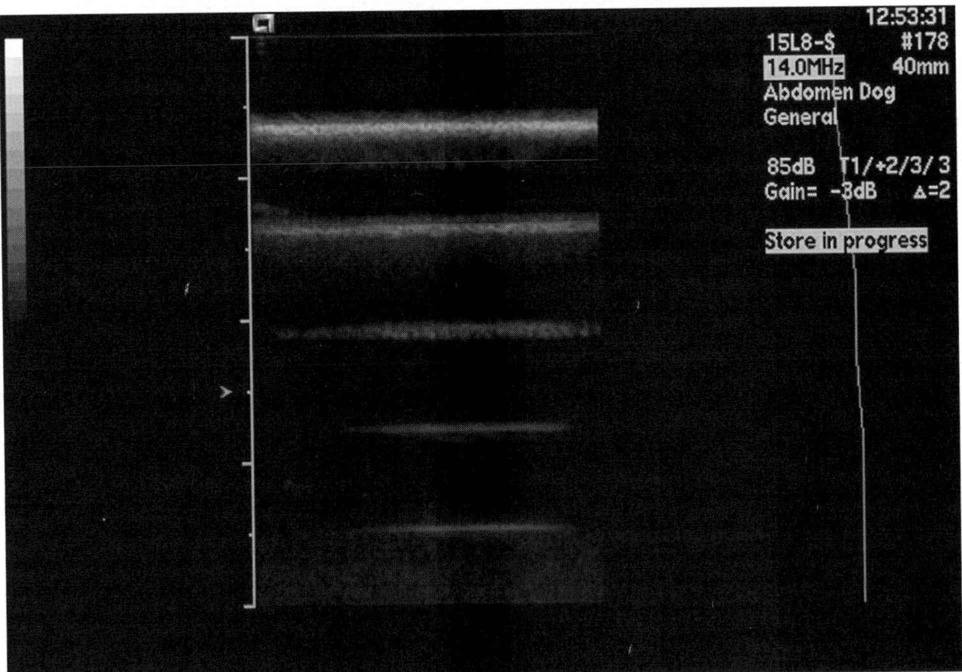

Fig. 3-4 A reverberation artifact was created by submerging a tongue depressor in a water bath. The actual tongue depressor is the uppermost hyperechoic line, closest to the transducer, and the four other hyperechoic lines are artifactual tongue depressors. Some of the sound waves reflected by the tongue depressor are reflected by the transducers (instead of being recorded by the transducer) and then again reflected by the tongue depressor. The ultrasound machine interprets the twice-reflected signals at a depth of twice the actual distance of the transducer and tongue depressor because the echoes took twice as long to return. The deeper three artifactual tongue depressors took 3, 4, and 5 times as long, respectively, to be recorded by the ultrasound machine and are recorded further from the transducer.

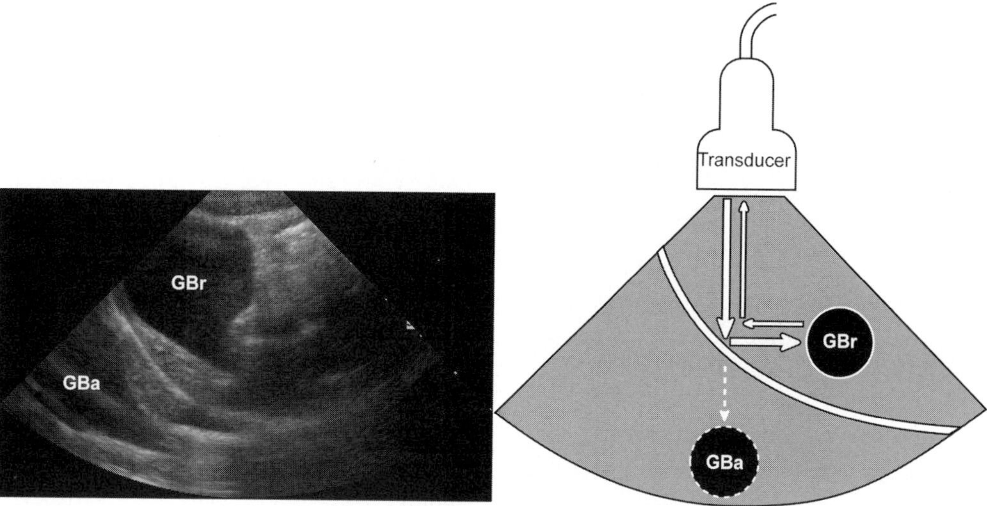

Fig. 3-5 A mirror image artifact of a dog's gallbladder was created at the lung/diaphragm interface. The real gallbladder (GBr) is in the near field and the artifactual gallbladder is in the far field (GBa). The lung/diaphragm interface is the *curved, thin white line* separating the two gallbladders. The schematic shows the route that the sound wave travels *(white arrows)* to create the image of the artifactual gallbladder. Because the ultrasound machine cannot detect that the sound wave changed direction during its travel, the ultrasound machine assumes another gallbladder (GBa) is present below the lung/diaphragm interface.

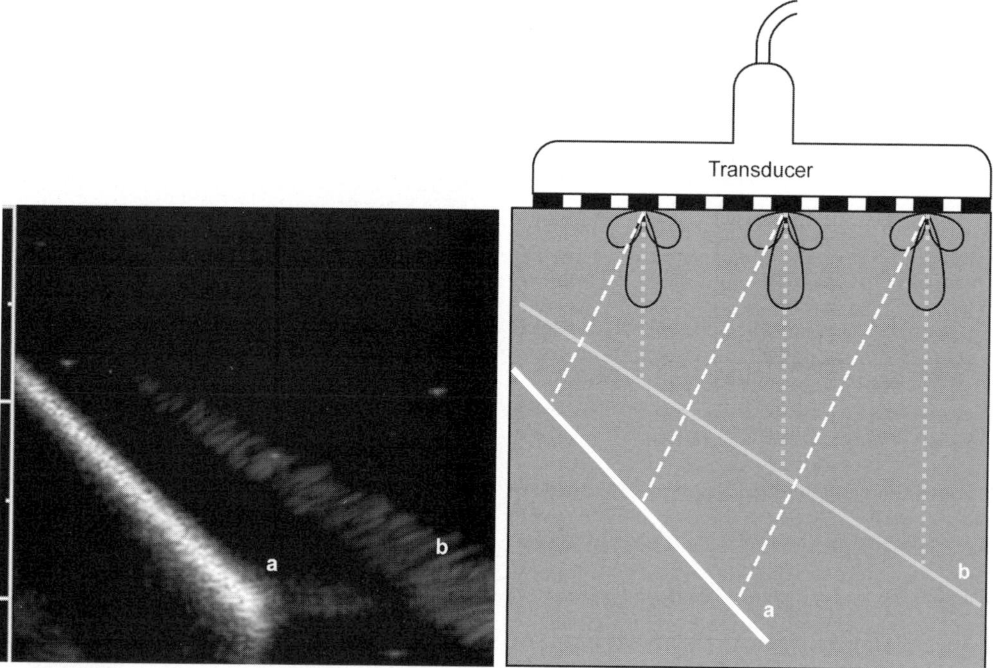

Fig. 3-6 The ultrasonographic image on the left was created in a water bath by using a linear array transducer and a tongue depressor. The tongue depressor is the *bright linear structure* closer to the *bottom left* of the image *(a)*. The grating lobe artifacts *(b)* are between the transducer *(top right)* and the tongue depressor. The schematic on the right shows the grating lobes emitted from selected elements of a linear transducer and how they interact with the tongue depressor *(a)* and create the artifact *(b)*. The *angled dotted lines* show the actual path of the grating lobes, and the *vertical dotted lines* illustrate where the ultrasound machine places the image. (Modified from Barthez PY, Leveille R, Scrivani PV: Side lobes and grating lobes artifacts in ultrasound imaging, *Vet Radiol Ultrasound* 38:387, 1997.)

Side lobes and grating lobes are secondary sound beams that emanate in a different direction than the primary sound beam.[15,16] Side lobes are associated with all transducers and originate from additional mode vibrations of the piezoelectric crystal; grating lobes emanate from array transducers. In each instance these lobes result in an error in positioning of the returning echo (Fig. 3-6). The side or grating lobes are weaker than the primary sound beam; these lobes must encounter a highly reflective surface and be of sufficient intensity to be noticed.[17,18]

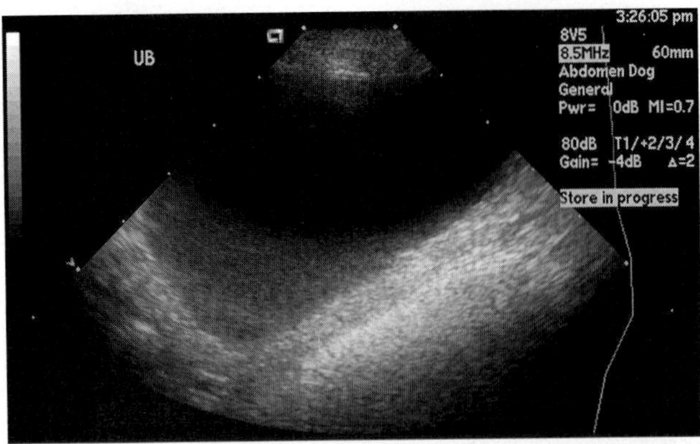

A

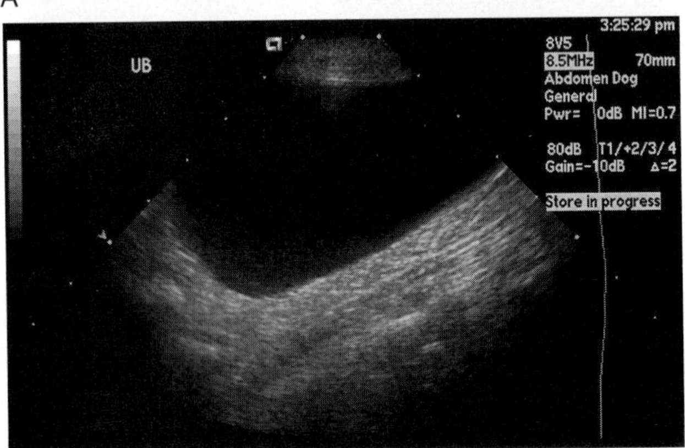

B

Fig. 3-7 **A,** An ultrasound image of a dog's urinary bladder illustrating slice thickness artifacts. The hypoechoic region in the urinary bladder (left ventral aspect) is created when part of the ultrasound beam images the anechoic urine and part images the isoechoic urinary bladder wall. The two parts of the beam are averaged together to create the hypoechoic region that could be confused with sediment. **B,** An ultrasound image of the same dog's urinary bladder after slightly altering the angle of insonation from **A.** The artifact was eliminated.

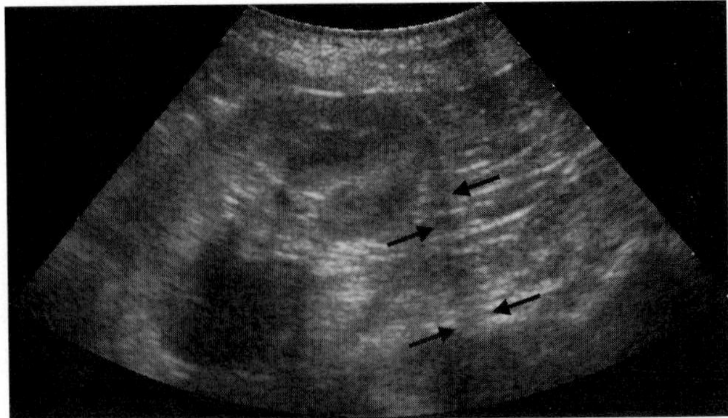

Fig. 3-8 Ultrasound image of a dog's kidney illustrating an edge-shadowing artifact caused by sound wave refraction. As sound waves tangentially encounter curved surfaces, they are bent so that no sound wave is transmitted into the tissues distal to the curved surface. The triangular black areas *(arrows)* distal to the caudal aspect of the kidney are edge-shadowing artifacts.

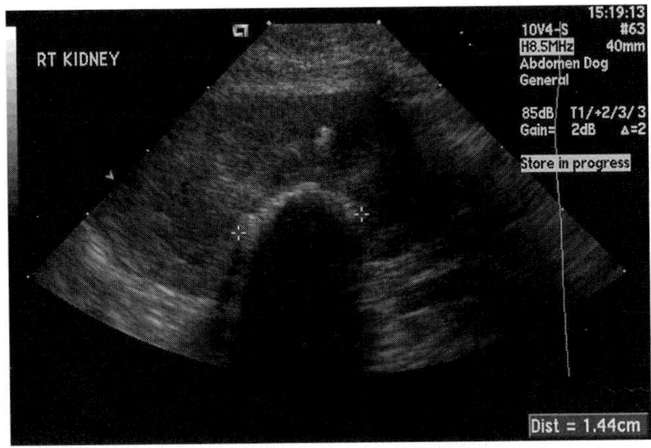

Fig. 3-9 An ultrasound image of a dog's right kidney illustrating acoustic shadowing caused by a renal calculus. The calculus is the curvilinear hyperechoic structure in the central aspect of the kidney. The *black area* below the calculus represents the acoustic shadowing.

Slice thickness artifacts are most commonly noticed in association with the urinary bladder and the gallbladder. In these structures slice thickness artifacts mimic the presence of sludge or sediment (Fig. 3-7). A primary sound beam, which is three dimensional, has thickness. When the periphery of the urinary bladder is imaged, for example, part of the thickness of the primary sound beam is involved in imaging the urinary bladder wall while the other part is imaging the anechoic urine. The computer averages these two parts to create the pseudo-sludge artifact. The surface of the pseudo-sludge is usually curved, but the surface of real sludge is flat.[18] Imaging the structure from a slightly different angle usually eliminates the artifact (Fig. 3-7, *B*).

Refraction occurs as the sound wave traverses tissues of different acoustic impedance. As the sound wave moves to the new medium, it is bent. The bending of the sound wave may result in the display of organs in incorrect locations. Although organ duplication caused by refraction artifacts has been described in human beings,[19] it does not commonly occur in animals. Refraction artifacts may lead to measurement errors.

Edge-shadowing artifacts are refraction artifacts that are created when sound waves are bent as they tangentially encounter a curved surface (Fig. 3-8).[13,20] Anechoic regions are present distal to the curved surfaces to which the bent sound waves should have traveled. This artifact commonly occurs when the kidneys, urinary bladder, or gallbladder is imaged.

Acoustic shadows are regions of decreased echogenicity distal to structures of high reflectivity (Fig. 3-9).[13,17,18] In these situations, the primary sound beam is almost completely reflected or absorbed. An insufficient quantity of echoes returned from the location distal to the strong reflector make these regions appear anechoic (black).[3] Naturally occurring acoustic shadows are found at soft tissue/gas (bowel, lung) and soft tissue/bone interfaces; pathologic acoustic shadows are most common with renal, cystic, or cholecystic calculi.

Acoustic enhancement is a region of increased echogenicity behind structures of low attenuation (Fig. 3-10).[17,18] This results in areas of increased echogenicity distal to these areas of low attenuation. The two most common sites for acoustic enhancement are distal to the gallbladder and the urinary bladder. To better understand this artifact, the acoustic shadowing caused by the gallbladder must be considered. Sound wave 1 travels through the liver and the bile within the gallbladder, then back into the liver. Sound wave 2 travels only through liver tissue. As sound wave 1 passes through the bile,

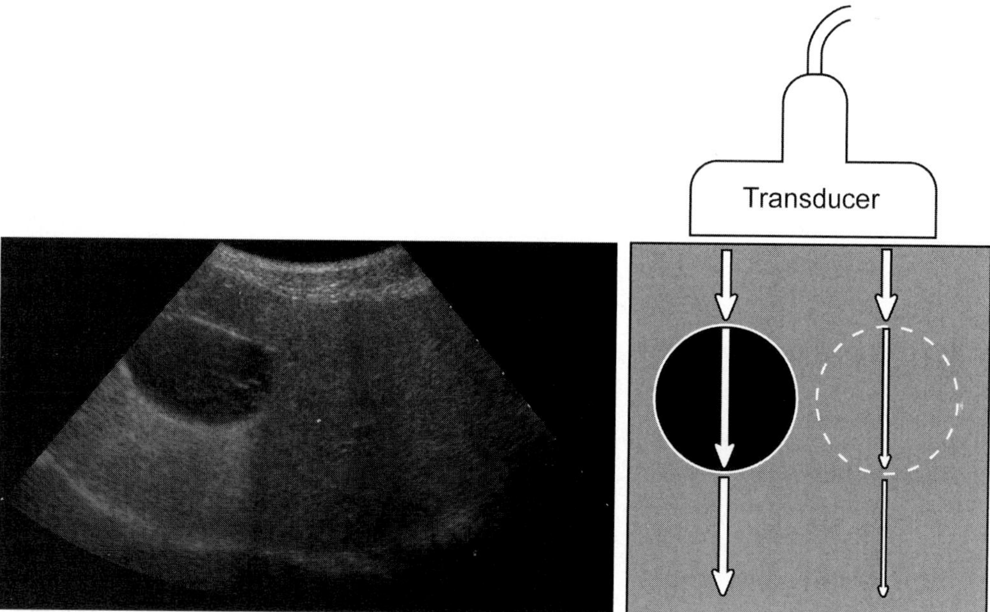

Fig. 3-10 Acoustic enhancement is a region of increased echogenicity behind structures of low attenuation. In the sonographic image on the left, bile in the gallbladder *(black circular structure)* does not attenuate the sound wave as much as the equivalent amount of liver tissue, creating acoustic enhancement (*bright area* distal to the gallbladder). The *black linear area* on the right aspect of the region of acoustic enhancement is an edge-shadowing artifact (see Fig. 3-8). In the schematic on the right, the left sound wave travels through the liver bile within the gallbladder *(white circle)*, and then back into the liver. The right sound wave travels only through liver tissue. As the left sound wave passes through the bile, it is attenuated less than the right sound wave as it travels through the liver. Thus when the left sound wave reenters the liver it has a higher intensity; it returns stronger echoes to the transducer, creating the distal acoustic enhancement.

it is less attenuated than sound wave 2 (as it passes through liver). Thus when sound wave 1 reenters the liver, it has a higher intensity and returns stronger echoes to the transducer.

DOPPLER TECHNIQUES

The pitch of a train's whistle or a siren changes as it approaches or moves away from the listener. The apparent change in pitch, or sound wave frequency, is called the Doppler shift. This principle has been applied to medical sonography, allowing imaging of the direction and velocity of blood flow.

The Doppler effect is named for Johann Christian Andreas Doppler, an Austrian mathematician and physicist, who first proposed the effect in 1842.

A moving object that is emitting sound is enveloped by "ring" of sound. In the direction of object movement toward a reference point, such as the listener, the sound waves are compressed, causing an increased frequency of the sound wave and a higher pitch.[2] As the object moves away from the listener, the sound waves are expanded, the frequency of the sound wave decreases, and the pitch becomes lower.[2] For example, when waiting at a train crossing, the pitch of the whistle gets higher as the train approaches the crossing. As the train moves away from the crossing, the pitch of the whistle gets lower.

In ultrasonography, the change in the frequency of the ultrasound wave is caused by a moving reflector, most commonly red blood cells.[2] The Doppler shift is the frequency difference between the incident sound waves and the reflected sound waves and is described by the following formula[21]:

$$f_D \approx (2 \times f_O \times \upsilon_{RBC})/c \qquad \text{(Eq 6)}$$

where f_D is the frequency of Doppler shift, f_O is the original frequency; υ_{RBC} is the velocity of red blood cells; and c is the speed of sound in soft tissue. The frequency of Doppler shift, recorded in hertz (versus megahertz used for sonographic imaging), is in the audible range. Hence ultrasound machines emit sound related to the Doppler shift (Audio 3-1; see http://evolve.elsevier.com/Thrall/vetrad).

Equation 6 assumes that the sound waves are parallel to the direction of blood flow. Realistically, when sound waves strike blood vessels, the sound waves are rarely parallel to the direction of blood flow. The Doppler angle is the angle between the blood flow direction and the sound wave direction.[2] Without accounting for the Doppler angle, the Doppler shift is underestimated.[2] This is very important for quantification of blood flow. Accounting for the Doppler angle, the velocity of blood flow is calculated by the following formula[2]:

$$\upsilon_{RBC} = (f_D \times c)/(2 \times f_O \times \cos\theta) \qquad \text{(Eq 7)}$$

where υ_{RBC} is the velocity of red blood cells, f_D is the frequency of Doppler shift, c is the speed of sound in soft tissue, f_O is the original frequency, cos is cosine, and θ is the Doppler angle.

Doppler shift cannot be measured if the Doppler angle is 90 degrees because cos 90 degrees = 0, thus making Equation 6 invalid (cannot divide by 0). The optimal Doppler angle is 30 to 60 degrees.[8]

DOPPLER MODES

Four Doppler modes are discussed below: (1) continuous-wave Doppler, (2) pulsed-wave Doppler, (3) color Doppler, and (4) power Doppler.

Continuous-wave Doppler is performed by using two separate crystals housed in one transducer.[2,21] One crystal continuously emits a sound wave, and the second crystal continuously receives echoes. Continuous-wave Doppler is highly accurate for measuring the Doppler shift. With continuous-wave Doppler, much higher velocities can be recorded (compared with pulsed-wave Doppler) because of the continuous signal sampling. The crystal sending the sound waves does not have to wait to receive echoes because the second crystal handles the echo-receiving task. However, continuous-wave Doppler measures all Doppler shifts along the path of the sound wave, making differentiation of blood flow velocity from two blood vessels in the path of the sound wave impossible.

Pulsed-wave Doppler is performed by using the same crystal for sending and receiving sound waves.[2,21] Pulsed-wave Doppler is used in combination with B-mode imaging; this is termed duplex Doppler (Fig 3-11).[2,8] With B-mode imaging, a blood vessel is selected for Doppler interrogation, and an electronic region of frequency sampling, called the gate, is positioned over the blood vessel. In Figure 3-11, the gate, two parallel lines, is positioned on the anechoic, tubular blood vessel (aorta in this example). The electronic gate effectively tells the ultrasound machine to accept only echoes from within this region on the basis of how long it takes for sound to reach the structure within the gate and for echoes to return to the transducer. Being able to select a blood vessel for interrogation visually is a benefit of pulsed-wave Doppler.

Continuous- and pulsed-wave Doppler both produce a spectral tracing. The tracing records the velocity and direction of blood flow as a function of time (see Fig. 3-11). Tracing above baseline (if baseline = 0 m/s) represents blood flow toward the transducer. Tracing below baseline (if baseline = 0 m/s) represents blood flow away from the transducer. Spectral broadening refers to the "thickness" of the spectral tracing. If a large range of blood flow velocity is present within the sample area, the spectral tracing will be broad. If the blood flow velocity within the sample area is homogenous, the spectral tracing will be thin (see Fig. 3-11).

Color Doppler is a variation of pulsed-wave Doppler.[2,8,21] Blood flow velocity is recorded in multiple regions within an image, and the velocities are color-coded. The user determines the size and location of the color Doppler region of interest. Color-coded information is superimposed on the gray-scale B-mode image, and a color-coded reference scale is displayed on the ultrasound machine monitor when operating the machine in color Doppler mode (Figs. 3-12 and 3-13). Red and blue hues are commonly used for color Doppler, but other variations exist depending on the manufacturer of the ultrasound machine. One color indicates net blood flow toward the transducer and the other color in the reference scale indicates net blood flow away from the transducer. Velocity of blood flow is indicated by the intensity or hue of the color. Limitations of color Doppler include that only mean velocity is displayed and that the maximum velocity that can be displayed is limited.[8] Color Doppler is angle dependent so that no Doppler shift is recorded when blood flow is 90 degrees to the transducer. In this instance, no color is recorded at this location; this should not be interpreted as lack of blood flow.

Power Doppler is a signal-processing method that analyzes the total strength of the Doppler signal while ignoring direction.[2] This method creates a color map of the Doppler shift where the hue and brightness of the color represent

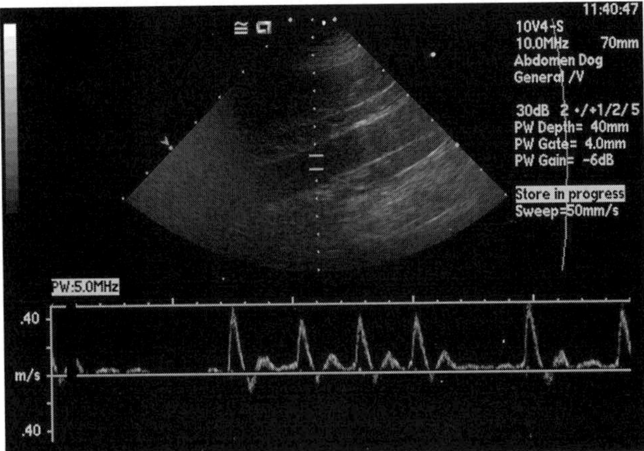

Fig. 3-11 Duplex Doppler image illustrating pulsed-wave Doppler interrogation of a dog's distal aorta. The B-mode image, in the near field, shows placement of the Doppler gate within the central aspect of the aorta. The *parallel white lines* displayed within the aorta are the pulsed-wave Doppler gate. This is the region of the aorta in which blood flow velocity is measured. The pulsed-wave Doppler spectral tracing is in the far field. The *white line* in the center of the spectral tracing represents the baseline; blood flow = 0 m/s. Signal above baseline represents blood flow toward the transducer, whereas signal below the baseline represents blood flow away from the transducer. The velocity scale on the left aspect of the spectral tracing ranges from 0 to 0.50 m/s toward the transducer and from 0 to 0.50 m/s away from the transducer. The pulsatile velocity tracing in this figure is typical of an artery.

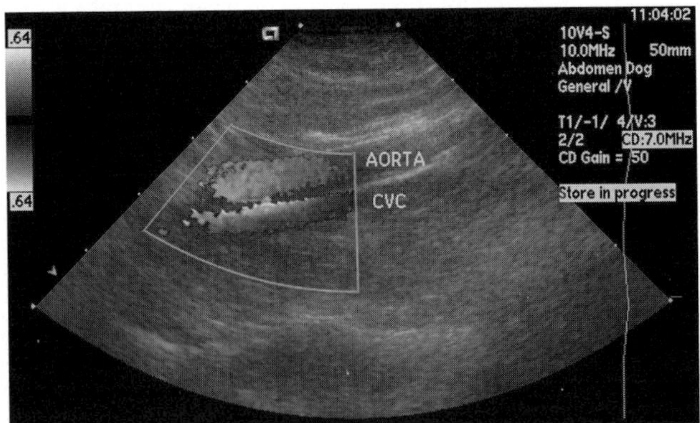

Fig. 3-12 Doppler image of the distal aorta and caudal vena in a dog. The aorta is in the near field and is red. The caudal vena cava is in the far field and is blue. According to the color scale, red represents blood flowing toward the transducer and blue represents blood flowing away from the transducer. The colors are assigned by the ultrasound machine and are related to the direction of blood flow. In other words, arteries will not always be red and veins will not always be blue. Blood flow velocity ranges from 0.64 m/s toward the transducer (red/yellow) to 0.64 m/s away from the transducer (blues). The *black bar* in the middle of the scale represents 0 m/s. Yellow and light blue represent faster velocities in their respective directions. (See Color Plate 1.)

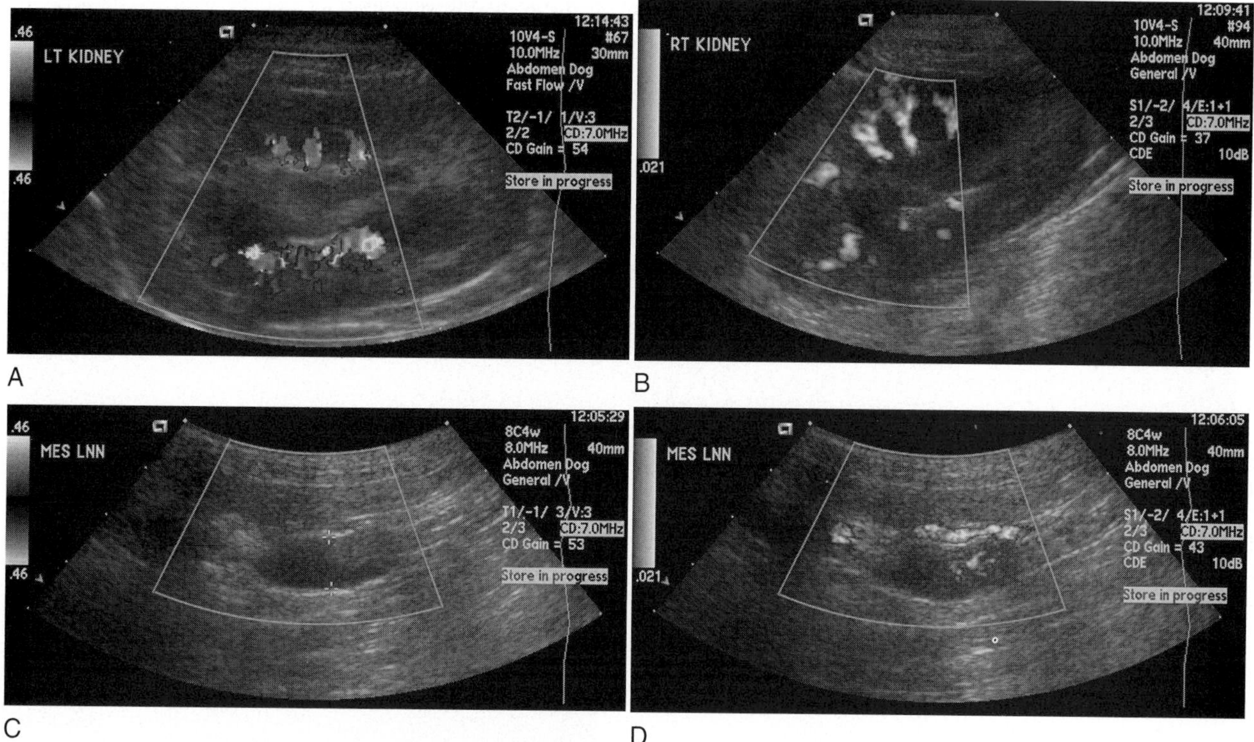

Fig. 3-13 Images of the left kidney in a dog. **A,** Color Doppler image showing blood flow within the kidney. Red hues indicate blood flow toward the transducer and blue hues, away from the transducer. Note the color scale at *left*. **B,** Power Doppler image showing blood flow in the same kidney. Because power Doppler is not direction dependent, only one hue is used (orange in this case). Lower-velocity blood flow can be detected with power Doppler compared with color Doppler. Compared to **A,** blood flow is noted further into the renal cortex by using power Doppler. **C,** Image of a mesenteric lymph node in a dog with color Doppler (note color scale). No blood flow is noted by color Doppler in or around the mesenteric lymph node. **D,** Image of a mesenteric lymph node in a dog with power Doppler active. A blood vessel is noted in the immediate near field to the lymph node and blood flow is noted within the lymph node. (See Color Plate 1.)

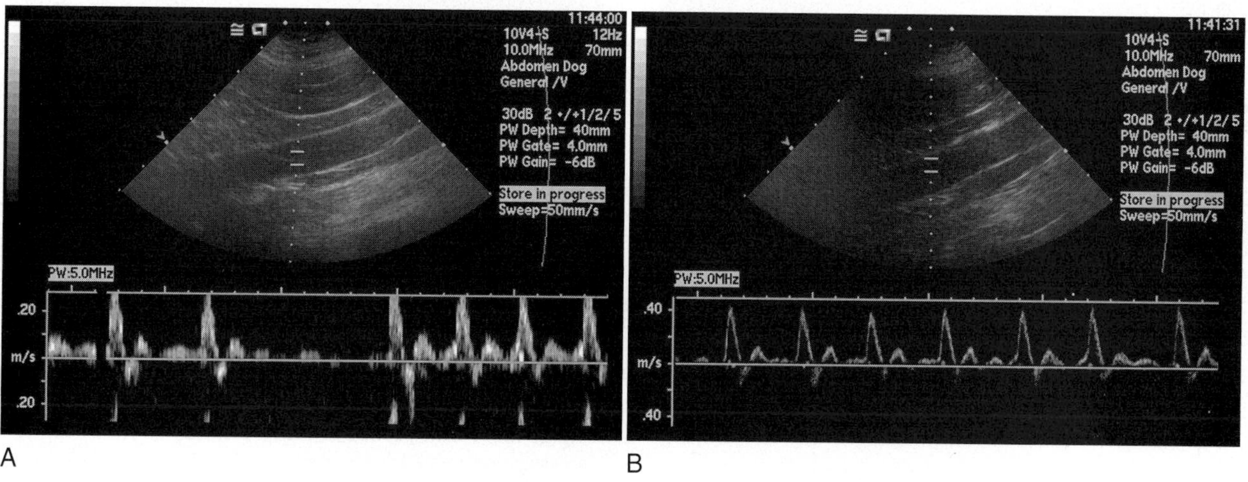

Fig. 3-14 Duplex Doppler image from a pulsed-wave Doppler interrogation of a dog's distal aorta. **A,** Aliasing of the spectral tracing is noted by the peaks of the tall "spikes" being displayed on the bottom of the spectral tracing. The scale (*left* of the spectral tracing) indicates that the highest velocity is 0.30 m/s. Because the peak velocity of blood flow within the aorta is greater than 0.30 m/s, the computer displays the tracing on the other end of the scale. **B,** Aliasing is corrected by increasing the scale, which increases the PRF. The maximum velocity is now 0.50 m/s. Note that the width of the spectral tracing in **A** is wider than in **B.** This is caused by more homogenous velocity of blood flow within the pulsed-wave Doppler gate.

the power of the Doppler signal. Power Doppler information is superimposed on the gray-scale B-mode image, and a color-coded reference scale is displayed on the ultrasound machine monitor when the machine is in power Doppler mode. Orange hues are commonly used for power Doppler, but other variations exist depending on the manufacturer of the ultrasound machine. Compared with color Doppler, power Doppler detects very-low-velocity blood flow; it is essentially angle independent and not prone to aliasing artifact.[22]

DOPPLER ARTIFACTS

Aliasing occurs when the pulse repetition frequency (PRF) is too low when using pulsed-wave Doppler. On the spectral tracing of the Doppler signal (Fig. 3-14), a portion of the tracing "wraps around" to the opposite direction and is therefore displayed on the wrong side of baseline.[2,8] On a color Doppler image (Fig 3-15), aliasing is seen as the addition of color from the opposite end of the color scale. The sampling rate of the ultrasound machine needs to be twice the highest frequency as the returning blood flow.[8] To correct aliasing, the PRF is increased.

Typically the velocity scale may be widened because many ultrasound machines have the PRF of the Doppler unit linked to the scale setting.[2] When using pulsed-wave Doppler, if most of the spectral tracing is on one side of baseline, the baseline can be adjusted to eliminate the aliasing (Fig. 3-16). However, increasing PRF may lead to another artifact called range ambiguity.

Range ambiguity occurs when the PRF is high enough that not all the returning echoes are received before the next sound wave pulse is sent.[8] As a result, the lagging echoes are misinterpreted as being closer to the transducer than they actually are. This creates "ghost" images between the structure of interest and the skin surface. These ghost images may not interfere with image interpretation, especially if the user is aware they exist.

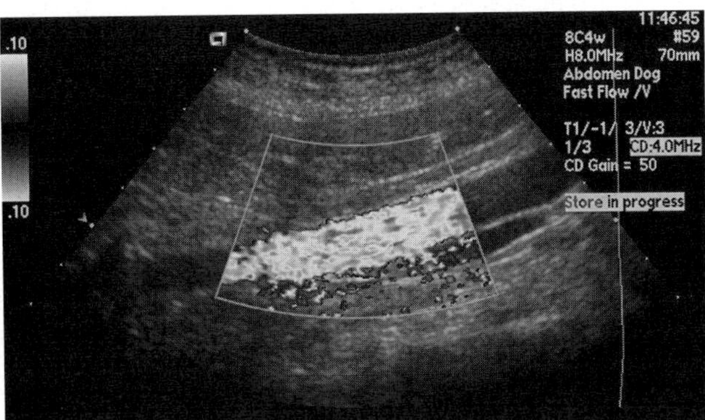

A

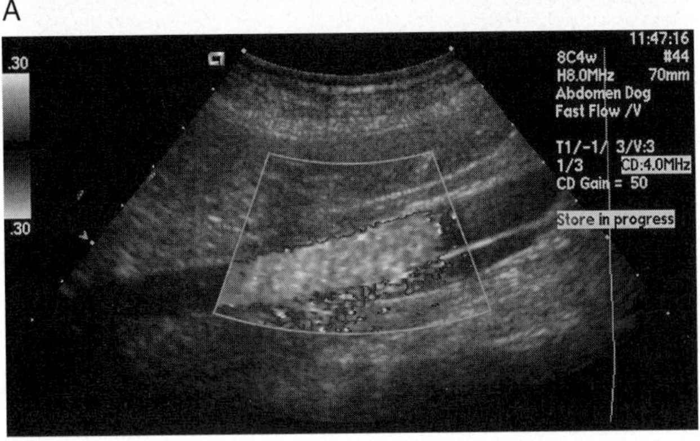

B

Fig. 3-15 Color Doppler image of the distal aorta in a dog. **A,** Color Doppler aliasing is seen as a mixture of red and blue hues. As the blood flow velocity exceeds 0.10 m/s toward the transducer, the computer changes the color coding from yellow to light blue. **B,** The aliasing was corrected by increasing the velocity scale to 0.30 m/s. Increasing the velocity scale increased PRF. The mixture of red and yellow hues within the aorta represents different velocity of blood flow. (See Color Plate 2.)

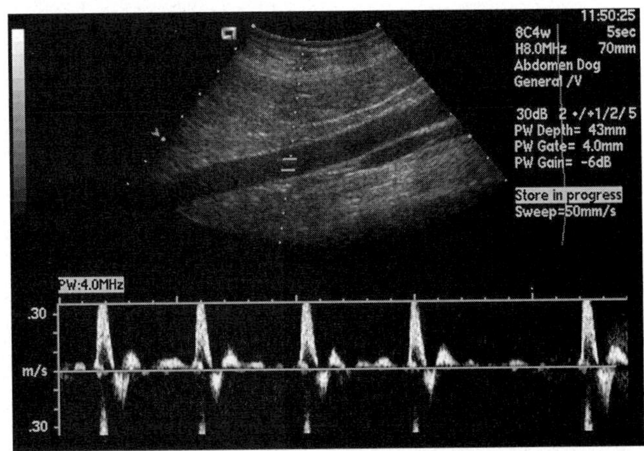

A

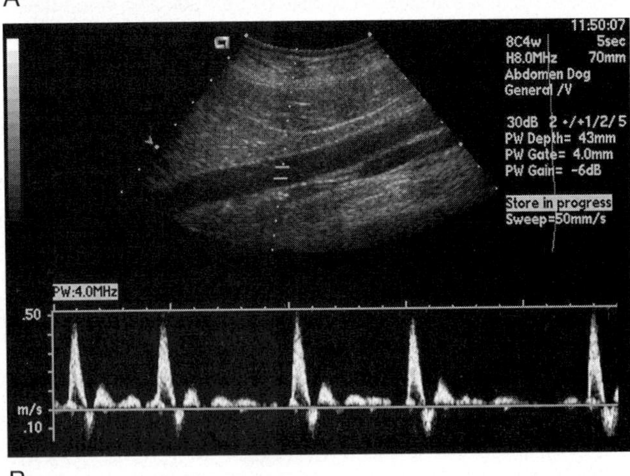

B

Fig. 3-16 Duplex Doppler image from a pulsed-wave Doppler interrogation of the distal aorta in a dog. **A,** Aliasing of the spectral tracing is noted by the peaks of the tall "spikes" displayed on the bottom of the spectral tracing. The scale (*left* of the spectral tracing) indicates that the highest velocity is 0.40 m/s. Because the peak velocity of blood flow within the aorta is greater than 0.40 m/s, the computer displays the tracing on the other end of the scale. **B,** Aliasing is corrected by changing the range of velocities displayed (also called adjusting the baseline). The velocity range displayed is from 0.20 m/s away from the transducer to 0.60 m/s toward the transducer.

REFERENCES

1. Buddemeyer EU: The physics of diagnostic ultrasound, *Radiol Clin North Am* 13:391, 1975.
2. Bushberg JT, Seibert JA, Leidholdt EM Jr et al: Ultrasound. In Bushberg JT, Seibert JA, Leidholdt EM Jr, et al, editors: *The essential physics of medical imaging,* ed 2, Philadelphia, 2002, Lippincott Williams & Wilkins, p 469-554.
3. Herring DS, Bjornton G: Physics, facts, and artifacts of diagnostic ultrasound, *Vet Clin North Am Small Anim Pract* 15:1107, 1985.
4. Powis RL: Ultrasound science for the veterinarian, *Vet Clin North Am Equine Pract* 2:3, 1986.
5. Curry TS III, Dowdy JE, Murry RC Jr: Ultrasound. In Curry TS III, Dowdy JE, Murry RC Jr, editors: *Christensen's physics of diagnostic radiology,* ed 4, Philadelphia, 1990, Lea & Febiger, p 323-371.
6. Kremkau FW: Ultrasound. In *Diagnostic ultrasound—principles and instrumentation,* ed 5, Philadelphia, 1998, WB Saunders, p 19-78.
7. Carlsen EN: Ultrasound physics for the physician. A brief review, *J Clin Ultrasound* 3:69, 1975.
8. Nyland TG, Mattoon JS, Herrgesell EJ et al: Physical principles, instrumentation, and safety of diagnostic ultrasound. In Nyland TG, Mattoon JS, editors: *Small animal diagnostic ultrasound,* ed 2, Philadelphia, 2002, WB Saunders, p 1-18.
9. Kremkau FW: Transducers. In *Diagnostic ultrasound—principles and instrumentation,* ed 5, Philadelphia, 1998, WB Saunders, p 79-140.
10. Rantanen NW, Ewing RL: Principles of ultrasound application in animals, *Vet Radiol* 22:196, 1981.
11. Leo FP, Rao GU: The technology of diagnostic ultrasound, *Radiol Clin North Am* 13:403, 1975.
12. Nyland TG, Park RD, Lattimer JC et al: Gray-scale ultrasonography of the canine abdomen, *Vet Radiol* 22:220, 1981.
13. Park RD, Nyland TG, Lattimer JC et al: B-mode gray-scale ultrasound: imaging artifacts and interpretation principles, *Vet Radiol* 22:204, 1981.
14. Gardner FJ, Clark RN, Kozlowski R: A model of hepatic mirror-imaging artifact, *Med Ultrasound* 4:19, 1980.
15. Laing FC, Kurtz AB: The importance of ultrasonic side-lobe artifacts, *Radiology* 145:763, 1982.
16. Barthez PY, Leveille R, Scrivani PV: Side lobes and grating lobes artifacts in ultrasound imaging, *Vet Radiol Ultrasound* 38:387, 1997.
17. Kremkau FW: Artifacts. In *Diagnostic ultrasound—principles and instrumentation,* ed 5, Philadelphia, 1998, WB Saunders, p 377-436.
18. Penninck DG: Artifacts. In Nyland TG, Mattoon JS, editors: *Small animal diagnostic ultrasound,* ed 2, Philadelphia, 2002, WB Saunders, p 19-29.
19. Middleton WD, Melson GL: Renal duplication artifact in US imaging, *Radiology* 173:427, 1989.
20. Sommer FG, Filly RA, Minton MJ: Acoustic shadowing due to refractive and reflective effects, *Am J Roentgenol* 132:973, 1979.
21. Boote EJ: AAPM/RSNA physics tutorial for residents: topics in US: Doppler US techniques: concepts of blood flow detection and flow dynamics, *Radiographics* 23:1315, 2003.
22. Rubin JM, Bude RO, Carson PL et al: Power Doppler US: a potentially useful alternative to mean frequency-based color Doppler US, *Radiology* 190:853, 1994.

ELECTRONIC RESOURCES evolve

Additional information related to the content in Chapter 3 can be found on the companion Web site at evolve http://evolve.elsevier.com/Thrall/vetrad/

- Key Points
- Chapter Quiz
- Video 3-1: Depiction of a reverberation artifact
- Audio 3-1: Sound of Doppler signal from an artery
- Audio 3-2: Sound of Doppler signal from a vein

CHAPTER • 4
Principles of Computed Tomography and Magnetic Resonance Imaging

Amy S. Tidwell

The physical principles of computed tomography (CT) and magnetic resonance (MR) imaging are complex. However, these modalities are now mainstream components of veterinary imaging. Thus image interpreters, at all skill levels, must have a basic understanding of their fundamental concepts.

Although CT and MR imaging have the ability to aid in the diagnosis of an almost endless list of diseases, the possible manifestations of these diseases in the images is, fortunately, limited. This is caused in part by the limited number of basic pathologic reactions of tissue to disease as well as the finite, and sometimes characteristic, responses at the underlying atomic and subatomic level. For example, on a CT image, increased water content associated with necrosis, edema, inflammation, and many types of tumors typically reduces a tissue's electron density and its ability to attenuate x-rays, making the tissue appear predictably darker than normal. These same pathologic processes, by virtue of increased water content and altered molecular binding, also affect the nucleus of the hydrogen atom, usually resulting in a relative increase in hydrogen proton mobility and thereby imparting a relatively bright appearance on some MR images and a dark appearance on others. Therefore when formulating a diagnosis based on these imaging responses, assumptions can be based on expected atomic behavior. This concept is more easily applied to CT, in which a single physical parameter, x-ray attenuation, determines a tissue's appearance. With MR imaging, on the other hand, a host of factors contributes to the appearance of the image, including the intrinsic properties of hydrogen mobility and binding as well as factors that are not proton related, such as instrument-dependent pulse sequences, timing parameters, and the local magnetic environment. The complex, multifaceted nature of MR imaging makes interpretation less amenable to simple generalizations and predictions. For this reason, MR imaging, perhaps more than any other imaging technique, demands a thorough understanding of the physical interactions of tissue at the atomic level and how the instrumentation creates and manipulates these interactions and ultimately records the results.

ADVANTAGES OF COMPUTED TOMOGRAPHY AND MAGNETIC RESONANCE IMAGING

The objective of most medical imaging procedures is to distinguish normal from pathologic tissue and, if possible, to differentiate among various diseases. How well this objective is accomplished depends on the imaging technique's localizing and resolving capabilities. One of the main advantages of CT and MR imaging over conventional radiography is that the images are tomographic in nature. That is, CT and MR imaging allow sectional or slice-oriented imaging of the patient, thereby eliminating the problem of depth perception loss associated with radiography. Anatomic localization of an abnormality is therefore more accurate in a tomographic image than in a conventional radiograph. Another main advantage of both CT and MR imaging is increased contrast resolution. Contrast resolution refers to the ability to discriminate tissues of different composition and faithfully display these differences with various shades of gray or brightness levels in the image. In CT, contrast resolution is enhanced over that achieved in radiographs because differences in x-ray attenuation between tissues are optimized by computerization. In MR imaging, contrast resolution is enhanced because image contrast arises from multiple parameters relating to a tissue's biochemical environment. Furthermore, image contrast in MR can be manipulated to accentuate tissue differences through the use of instrument-controlled techniques.

Importantly, beginning interpreters of CT and MR images may think that their benefits are related to improved spatial resolution; that is, the ability to see small detail. In actuality, both CT and MR imaging have poorer spatial resolution than either film-screen or digital radiography. The limiting spatial resolution is the size of the smallest object that an imaging system can resolve.[1] An imaging system has better spatial resolution if it can demonstrate the presence of smaller objects in the image. As noted in Table 4-1, the limiting spatial resolutions for CT and MRI are actually larger than those for both film-screen and digital radiography.[1] This implies that, when compared with radiography, fine details will be poorly resolved on a CT or MR image. This disadvantage, however, is nearly always outweighed by the exceptional contrast resolution in images free of superimposed anatomy.

IMAGE FORMATION

CT and MR imaging are electronic imaging technologies. This means that information about the imaged subject is carried by flowing electrons, or current. When an electronic image is viewed on a monitor, light emits from the screen with varying intensities of brightness. The degree of illumination determines the perceived black, white, and gray shades composing the image and is regulated by the strength of the supplied current. This measured current, or signal, conveys information about the composition and location of the tissue in question and therefore lies at the heart of image formation and interpretation.

So, how are electrical signals delivered to the imaging system from the patient? With MR imaging, the hydrogen protons within the patient, by virtue of possessing magnetic fields, directly induce voltage in a coiled conductor by a process known as electromagnetic induction. With CT, the process is indirect; x-ray photons that have passed through the patient are converted to electrical signals by a panel of detectors. Because the initial x-ray intensity is a known value, the degree of x-ray attenuation by the patient can be inferred by

Table • 4-1

Limiting Spatial Resolutions of Selected Medical Imaging Modalities

MODALITY	LIMITING SPATIAL RESOLUTION (MM)
Film-screen radiography	0.08
Digital radiography	0.17
CT	0.40
MR	1.00

Modified from Bushberg JT, Seibert JA, Leideholt EM et al: Introduction to medical imaging. In Bushberg JT, Seibert JA, Leidholt EM, et al, editors: *The essential physics of medical imaging,* ed 2, Philadelphia, 2002, Lippincott Williams & Wilkins.

the transmitted intensity at the detectors and thus by the strength of the resultant signal. Because the signals created during the scanning process are numerous and complex, they must first be sampled and digitized by an analog-to-digital converter (ADC) and then processed by a computer that, in turn, constructs and sends the image to the display device in a digital format.

The concepts of CT and MR image formation are summarized in Figure 4-1 and are discussed throughout this chapter. For optimal understanding of this material, readers are encouraged to develop a basic understanding of the physical concepts of digital images as presented in Chapter 2.

Computed Tomography

Contrast in CT images arises from tissues differing in their ability to attenuate x-rays. Attenuation is simply the removal

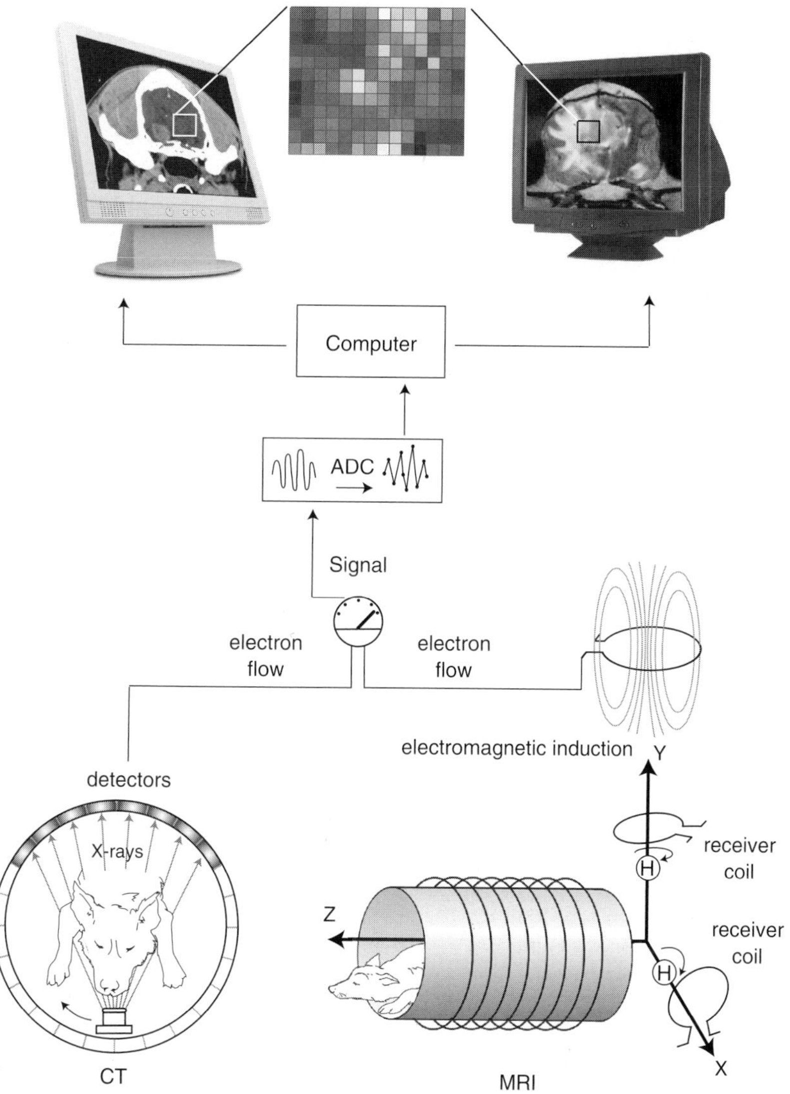

Fig. 4-1 Overview of CT and MR image formation. The signals used to reconstruct a CT image come from detectors that convert transmitted x-ray photons into electrical current. Because the original x-ray intensity is known, attenuation by the patient can be calculated from the transmitted x-ray intensity or the strength of the resultant current. With MR imaging, current is induced in a coiled conductor by the magnetic fields of hydrogen protons in the patient in a process called electromagnetic induction. The signals for both CT and MR imaging must be digitized by an analog-to-digital converter and sent to a computer for processing. The digital electronic images appear as varying intensities of light within pixels on a monitor.

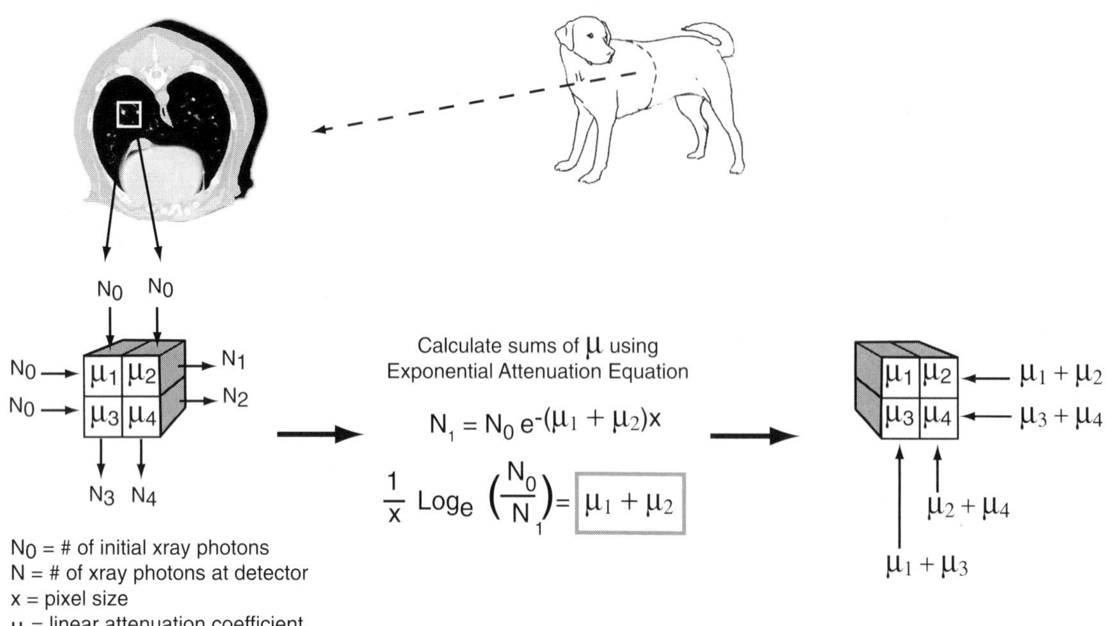

Fig. 4-2 Example of how attenuation is calculated along the path of the x-ray beam. A CT slice of the thorax is acquired. For this example, only a small portion of the image, consisting of a 2 × 2 matrix, is examined. During the acquisition of the image, x-rays are projected through the patient from multiple angles. All structures residing in the path of the x-ray beam contribute to attenuation. The sums of μ (or $\mu_1 + \mu_2$, $\mu_3 + \mu_4$, etc.) can be calculated by the exponential attenuation equation, as all other values are known. To determine attenuation from each individual voxel, the μ sums are backprojected onto the image. This is denoted on the *far right* in the figure, where *arrows* point from the μ sums back to the 2 × 2 matrix. In actuality, the situation is much more complex because hundreds of voxels may be in the path of the x-ray beam. (See the text for a detailed explanation of the principles behind backprojection.)

of x-ray photons from the beam as it passes through the patient, either by scatter or absorption. Attenuation depends on photon interactions with the electrons of the patient's atoms; these interactions depend on photon energy and the physical characteristics of the tissue. A tissue's physical density, atomic number, and electrons per gram govern photon interactions (see Chapter 1), with physical density being one of the most important factors contributing to attenuation.[2] Because physical density determines the number of electrons present in a given thickness, electron density (physical density multiplied by the electrons per gram) becomes the key contributor to attenuation.

The x-ray attenuation properties of a material can be described by the linear attenuation coefficient, denoted by the Greek symbol μ. The linear attenuation coefficient describes the fraction of x-rays removed per unit thickness of tissue. As x-ray photons are attenuated, they are removed from the beam according to the law of exponential decay or attenuation according to the following equation:

$$N = N_o e^{-\mu x} \qquad \text{(Eq 1)}$$

where N_o is the number of initial photons (measured at the tube), N is the number of photons transmitted (measured at the detecting device), e is the base of the natural logarithm (2.718), x is the thickness of the absorber, and μ is the linear attenuation coefficient. Because all factors in the equation, except for μ, are known or can be measured, μ can be calculated for any tissue or substance having a thickness of x.

As with film-screen radiography, all structures residing in the path of the x-ray beam contribute to attenuation during the acquisition of a CT image. With both CT and radiography, attenuation from these structures is therefore summed. In other words, instead of attenuation being dependent on the μ of a single homogenous tissue, it is attributable to the sum of μ for all tissues along the x-ray beam's path, or $\mu_1 + \mu_2 + \ldots \mu_n$ (Fig. 4-2).

With conventional radiography, the composite of these attenuation sums forms the actual image, which is a two-dimensional summation image (see Chapter 1). With CT, the sum of the linear attenuation coefficients along the path of an x-ray beam through multiple voxels is instead used to calculate the individual contributions from each voxel. This process is based on a mathematic principle theorized by J. H. Radon in 1917 long before the invention of tomographic imaging.[3,4] According to this principle, an object can be perfectly reconstructed from an infinite set of projections taken at an infinite number of angles. Relating this to CT, if the attenuation sums of rays projected through the object at different angles are known, then the individual components of the sums, the attenuation values from each voxel, and their spatial distribution can be determined. Because the x-ray tube rotates around the object and projection data are collected for numerous angles, this principle of projection reconstruction can be applied to assemble a spatial plot of individual attenuation values for the object in the CT image. Although an infinite number of measurements and a perfect reconstruction are not attainable, the CT image nevertheless represents an excellent approximation of the scanned subject. Unencumbered by summation effects, the CT image can faithfully represent tissue composition without the visual perception problems occurring with radiography (Fig. 4-3).

The process of acquiring the attenuation sums from multiple projection angles and reconstructing the image from

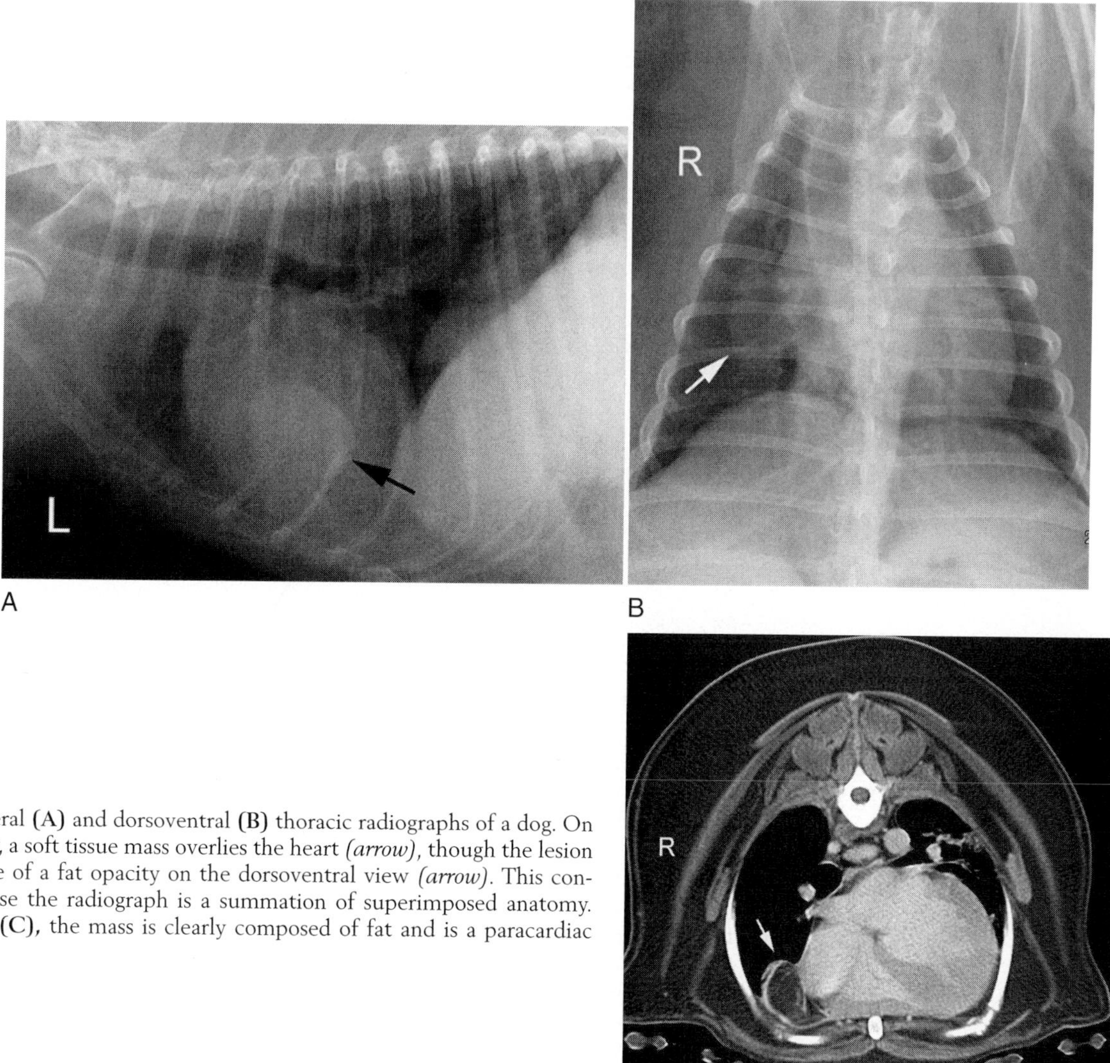

Fig. 4-3 Left lateral (A) and dorsoventral (B) thoracic radiographs of a dog. On the left lateral view, a soft tissue mass overlies the heart *(arrow)*, though the lesion appears to be more of a fat opacity on the dorsoventral view *(arrow)*. This confusion arises because the radiograph is a summation of superimposed anatomy. On the CT image (C), the mass is clearly composed of fat and is a paracardiac lipoma *(arrow)*.

these sums is summarized in the following six steps and illustrated in Figures 4-4 and 4-5.

(1) Contemporary single-slice scanners that acquire slices one at a time are described as being either third- or fourth-generation scanners. Although more sophisticated scanners that acquire multiple slices simultaneously are making their way into veterinary imaging, the basic principles of CT physics are adequately explained based on these third- or fourth-generation scanners. In these scanners, the x-ray tube produces a fan-shaped, thinly collimated x-ray beam that rotates around the patient during the acquisition of one slice. Collimation determines the thickness of the slice, and thus the voxel. In a third-generation scanner, the x-rays are directed to an array of detectors that rotate in concert with the x-ray tube. During the rotation, measurement of the transmitted x-ray beam by the detectors occurs incrementally as the tube-detector assembly position changes by small angles. In a fourth-generation scanner, instead of a row of detectors that moves with the tube, the detectors are stationary and line the entire 360 degrees of the gantry.

(2) The beam is attenuated by the patient and the transmitted photons fall on the detectors. The intensity of the beam before it strikes the patient is also measured. With scintillation crystal-photomultiplier tube–type detectors, x-ray photons fall on scintillation crystals, which in turn emit light. The amount of light produced by a detector depends on the number of photons striking it and the energy of each photon.[5] Light then strikes the photocathode of the photomultiplier tube, which in turn releases electrons. These electrons, after passing through a series of dynodes, create a weak electrical current.

(3) The electrical current is then measured, amplified, and converted to digital numbers by the ADC in the data acquisition system. Relative transmission or attenuation for each ray striking a detector (or the μ sums, $\mu_1 + \mu_2 + \ldots \mu_n$, for each ray) can be calculated because N and N_o are known (see Fig. 4-4). A profile of attenuation for each sampling period is created from a set of rays known as a "ray projection" or "view."[6] The total number of data samples composing the raw data for each slice is therefore equal to the number of views multiplied by the number of rays per view (see Fig. 4-4).[7]

In a third-generation scanner, each ray of the fan beam strikes a single detector in the array. A view is the set of rays striking the detectors with the tube in one position.[8] More views can be obtained by moving the tube-detector assembly over a smaller distance (angle) before taking more samples.[6]

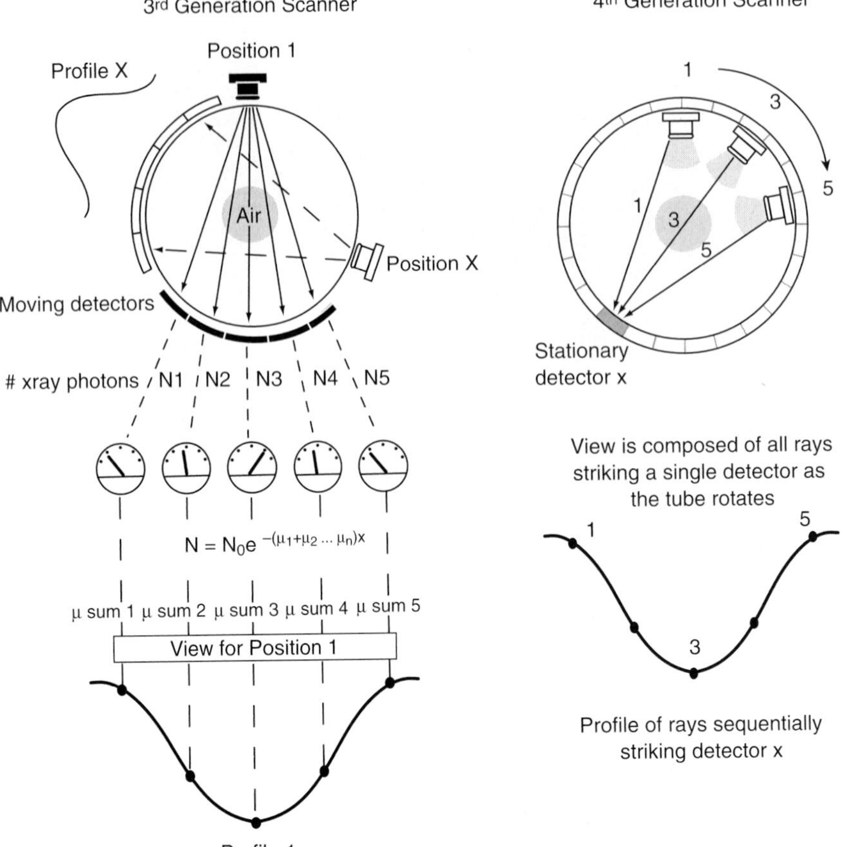

Fig. 4-4 How views and attenuation profiles are determined for a block of tissue with an air-filled hole in the center. A third-generation scanner is depicted on the *left*. With the x-ray tube in position 1, each ray of the fan beam strikes a single detector. In this simplified example, five rays fall onto five detectors. *N1-N5* represent the transmitted x-ray intensities for each ray. With scintillation crystal-photomultiplier tube type detectors, transmitted x-ray photons are converted to light that, in turn, is converted to electrical current. As depicted by the meters, current will be greatest in the center because the x-ray path traverses a greater thickness of air. The attenuation sums for each ray are calculated from the transmission measurements by the exponential attenuation equation. A profile of attenuation is then obtained from the set of rays, or the view, for position 1. In this phantom the attenuation profile for position X will be identical to that for position 1 because the object is homogeneous except for the air cavity. In a patient, all profiles will be different. All attenuation profiles will then be backprojected to reconstruct the CT image. The *right panel* compares measurement of the transmitted x-rays in a fourth-generation scanner. In this situation, the view is the set of rays striking a single detector as the tube rotates. A profile of attenuation is obtained from this set of x-rays.

Thus the number of samples of information for each slice depends on the number of detectors multiplied by the number of views, the latter being determined by the angle between each tube position. In a fourth-generation scanner, a view is composed of all the rays striking a single detector as the tube rotates around the patient.[8] The total number of samples of information therefore depends on the number of detectors (views) multiplied by the number of rays a detector sees (see Fig. 4-4).

(4) The raw data are then processed by the computer to reconstruct the image from the attenuation profiles, usually by a process called filtered backprojection. This is not a trivial exercise; a CT image may contain more than 200,000 individual pixels (512 × 512 matrix = 262,144 pixels in a square image field), and the object has multiple images. Backprojection has its mathematic foundation in the principle of projection reconstruction previously discussed. During backprojection, all the sampled projection measurements are added "back" to the pixels in the image along the lines of the original projection paths. As illustrated in Figure 4-5, simple backprojection results in a blurring effect because all the data are projected back across the entire image and therefore affect values at other pixel locations. Where these data overlap, streaks appear. With few backprojections, the overlap appears as the arms of a star. As more backprojections are added, the arms become blurred around the edges of the object, eventually affecting its appearance in the final image. A process called convolution, or filtering, remedies this problem. Although many types of filters are available, an edge-enhancing filter applied to the attenuation profile before backprojection prevents blurring. During convolution, the predesigned filter is passed over the profile at multiple points; the filter and the profile are combined to form a new filtered profile. When the new profiles are backprojected, overlap and the blurring effect are eliminated (see Fig. 4-5).

(5) Once attenuation has been numerically mapped within pixels, the values are standardized with a scale by which they can be expressed relative to the attenuation of

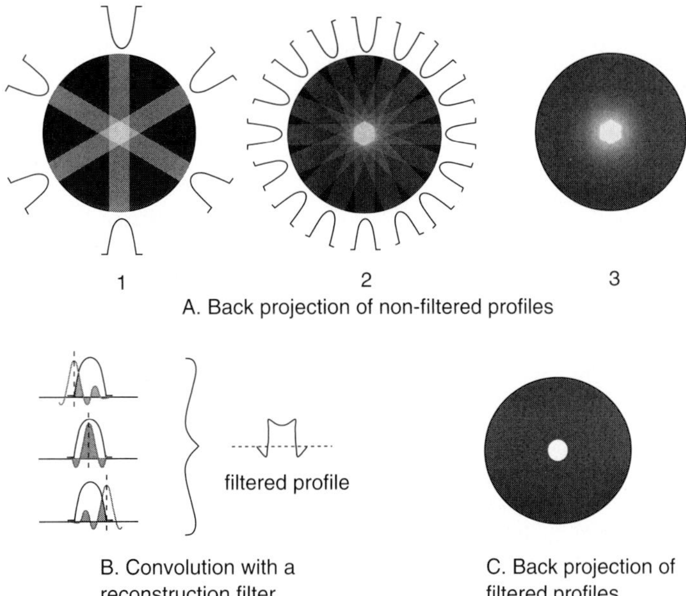

Fig. 4-5 **A,** Backprojection of the attenuation profiles of a round, dense object without filtering results in a blurring effect because all the data are projected back across the entire image, affecting values at other pixel locations. Where these data overlap, streaks appear. With few backprojections *(1)*, the overlap appears as the arms of a star. When more profiles are backprojected *(2)*, the arms of the star become increasingly overlapped and blurred, resulting in an object with a blurred shadow in the final image *(3)*. **B,** A predesigned, edge-enhancing filter (waveform with *dotted line*) is passed over the profile at multiple points; the filter and the profile are combined to form a new filtered profile. Note that the new filtered profile has negative lobes. When these profiles are backprojected, the negative lobes remove the overlapping data, or arms of the star, resulting in an image without blurred edges, as seen in **C.**

water. Tissues are assigned Hounsfield units (HU) or CT numbers. Hounsfield units are named after Sir Godfrey Newbold Hounsfield, who in 1972 built the prototype for the first CT scanner, which originally was designed to produce detailed images of cross-sections of the human head. Hounsfield's research resulted in the development of a clinically useful CT scanner for imaging the brain.[3] For this innovation he shared the 1979 Nobel Prize in Physiology or Medicine with Allan Macleod Cormack, who had independently derived and published the mathematic basis of CT scanning in 1963-1964. Hounsfield units are based on the following relation:

$$\text{HU of a tissue} = [(\mu_{\text{tissue}} - \mu_{\text{water}})/\mu_{\text{water}}] \times 1000\ \text{HU} \quad \text{(Eq 2)}$$

According to Equation 2, water has a Hounsfield unit value of zero. At the low end of the scale, air has a Hounsfield unit value of negative 1000 (−1000). With modern scanners having 12-bit pixel depth, or 4096 different gray levels, the upper end of the scale is therefore greater than 3000. The Hounsfield units of various tissues are listed in Table 4-2.

(6) Pixels are assigned relative gray shades and monitor brightness levels on the basis of the Hounsfield units of the tissues within their voxels. Application of a gray scale to Hounsfield unit values is illustrated in Figure 4-6. Images are then displayed on a monitor.

Windowing allows the operator to apply the gray scale to a specified range of pixel values. For example, if the tissues to be imaged are diverse and have a large range of pixel values, but only a small range of tissues are of interest, then applying the entire gray scale to the entire range of pixels values would, in effect, waste many of the gray levels. In other words, the tissues of interest would be assigned their proportion of the gray scale, but the remaining gray levels would be assigned to tissues not needing such discrimination. This problem is compounded by the fact that the human eye perceives far fewer gray shades than those provided by the imaging systems,[7] so the effective gray scale is even smaller. Narrowing the window to only include the area of interest would allow better gray level discrimination of small differences in tissue composition. When a large range of tissues needs to be discriminated, a wide window should be applied. Figure 4-6 and Video 4-1 illustrate the concept of windowing for CT. Video 4-1 can be found on

Table • 4-2

Hounsfield Unit Measurements for Various Substances

SUBSTANCE	HOUNSFIELD UNITS
Air	−1000
Lung	−845 (mean) For dog with 15 cm water, positive pressure ventilation[11]
Fat	−100 (approximately)[10]
Water	0
Brain	30-40
Kidney	30
Liver, spleen, muscle	50-70
Acute to subacute clotted blood	60-100[9]
Mineral	Variable; e.g., 100 to 1000
Bone	Variable; e.g., 100 to 1000
Metal (e.g., iodine)	Variable, depends on dilution; e.g., 100 to 3000

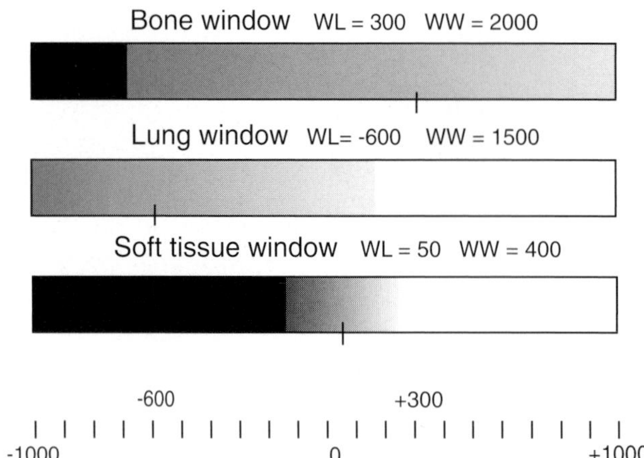

Fig. 4-6 Three common CT window settings. The numbers along the bottom of the image represent HU. The window levels *(WL, tick marks)* are centered near the tissues of interest and the window width *(WW)* determines the range of tissues encompassed by the gray scale. Below this range tissues appear black, and above this range tissues appear white. With a soft tissue window, a narrow WW is used to improve density discrimination. With bone and lung windows, a wide WW is needed to encompass the potential range of HUs found within bone and lung, respectively.

the accompanying Evolve site at http://evolve.elsevier.com/Thrall/vetrad.

Substances that can be discriminated on a CT image (from black to white on the monitor) include gas, lung, fat, water or other fluids, normal and abnormal soft tissues, mineral, dense bone, and metal. Soft tissues that appear less opaque than normal (hypoattenuating) may be cystic, necrotic, edematous (Fig. 4-7, *A*), or have fatty infiltration (Figs. 4-3, C, and 4-8). Soft tissues that appear more opaque than normal (hyperattenuating) may contain hemorrhage (because of the globin in hemoglobin, fibrin and clot retraction; Fig. 4-9),[9] mineral, or metal (e.g., iodinated contrast medium; Figs. 4-7, *B*, and 4-8) or are densely cellular (Fig. 4-7, *A*), particularly those tissues with cells having a high nuclear/cytoplasmic ratio or are densely fibrotic.[10]

Hounsfield units may be obtained from CT images by using region of interest measurements, a feature available in the computer software of most CT scanners.[11] This quantification of the Hounsfield unit value of a tissue may provide a guide regarding the identification of the tissue (see Table 4-2) and also an aid to determining if a tissue is normal (Fig. 4-10). However, Hounsfield units are not specific for any tissue type or substance; they are simply a quantification of the x-ray attenuation characteristics of a thickness of tissue. Just because a substance has a Hounsfield unit value consistent with hemorrhage, for example, does not mean that the substance is actually hemorrhage. All that can really be concluded is that the x-ray attenuation of the substance is similar to that expected from hemorrhage. Many combinations of various tissue types and substances, at least theoretically, will yield the same Hounsfield unit value.

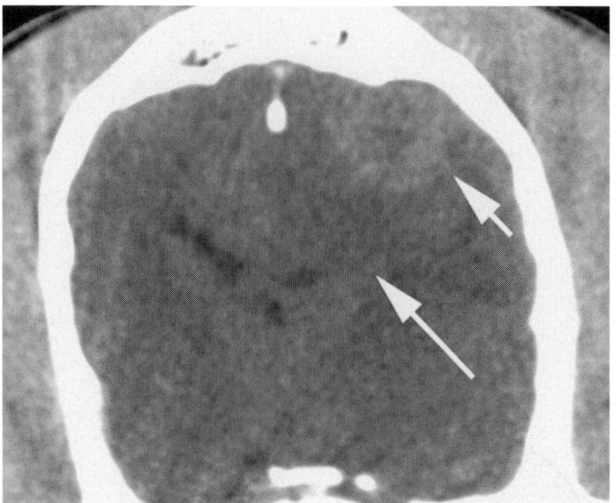

A

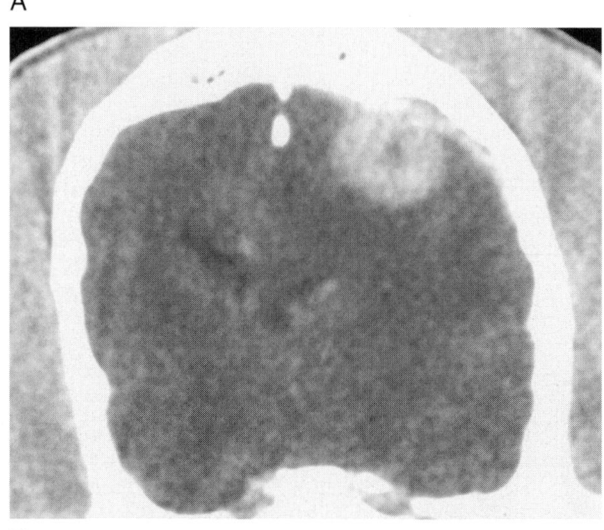

B

Fig. 4-7 Noncontrast (**A**) and postcontrast (**B**) CT images of the brain in a dog with a malignant meningioma in the left parietal lobe. **A** shows a hyperattenuating mass (*short arrow,* 59 HU) causing a mass effect and surrounding hypoattenuating vasogenic edema (*long arrow,* 26 HU). After administration of iodinated contrast medium **(B),** the mass enhanced (103 HU) and adjacent dural enhancement occurred. Histopathologically, the tumor cells were densely packed and some fibrous tissue response was present. The hyperattenuation seen in the noncontrast image may have resulted from this dense cell packing because no mineralization was present within the meningioma.

Magnetic Resonance Imaging

Signals generated during MR imaging come from the hydrogen nucleus, or proton. Although various atomic nuclei can be imaged, hydrogen protons are the basis of medical MR imaging because they are much more numerous than other atoms and have favorable magnetic properties.

With CT, electron density, and therefore x-ray attenuation, determines signal intensity and differences of such contribute to tissue contrast. With MR imaging, however, proton density, or the number of protons per unit volume of tissue, is only one of four major factors contributing to signal, with the others being T1, T2, and T2*.[12] These factors will be defined and discussed in more detail but for now can be loosely thought of as properties reflecting the interactions of hydrogen protons with other hydrogen protons and with their environment when the environment is disturbed during the MR process.

Hydrogen atoms exist within the body in molecules such as water and lipids that, in turn, comprise liquids or solid tissues.[13] The differences in intramolecular and intermolecular relations, along with proton density, make the hydrogen-based substances within the body biochemically different. During the MR process, the environment of the hydrogen proton can be perturbed in some fashion and the responses

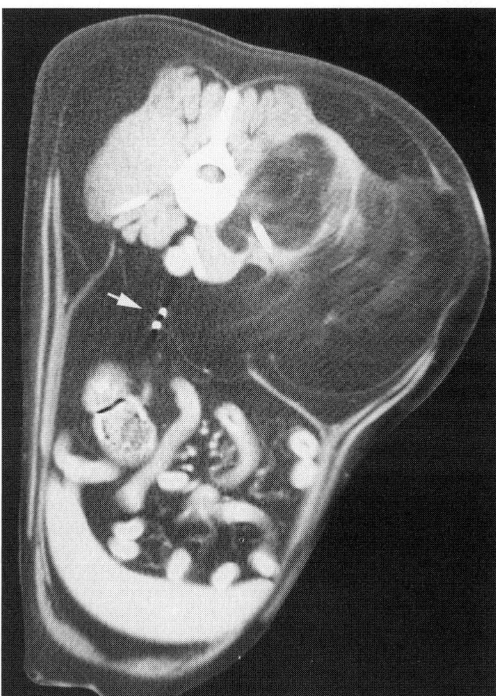

Fig. 4-8 CT intravenous urogram of a dog with an infiltrating lipoma of the body wall that invades muscle and the retroperitoneal space. The ureters are filled with iodinated contrast medium, allowing for their identification *(arrow)*. HU of the lipoma was −105.

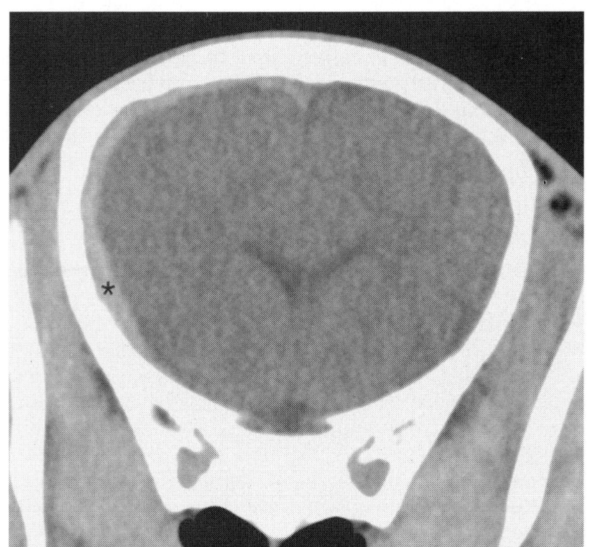

Fig. 4-9 Noncontrast CT image of a subdural hematoma in a foal. The hematoma *(asterisk)* is hyperattenuating and has a HU value of 76.

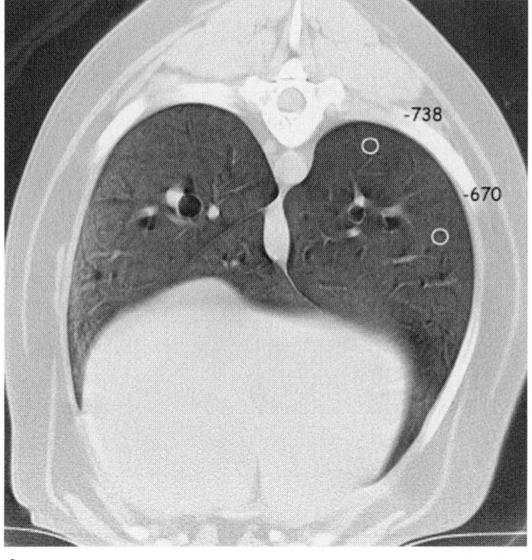

A

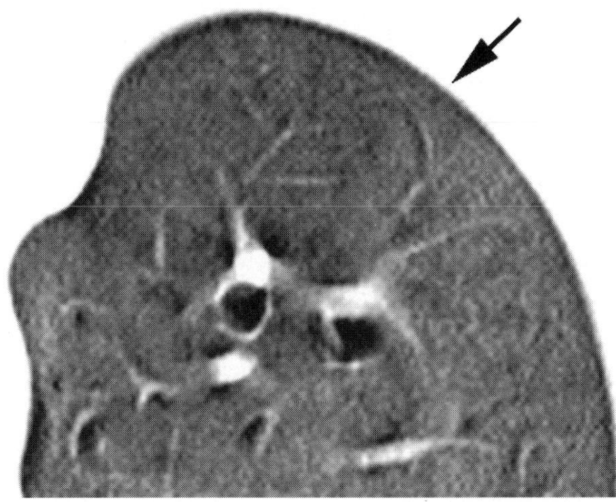

B

Fig. 4-10 Thoracic CT image **(A)** in a dog with a postmortem diagnosis of diffuse alveolar damage. A bilateral, diffuse mild increase in lung opacity is present with preservation of bronchial and vascular margins. The distribution in the left lung is slightly uneven, as illustrated in the magnified view (*arrow* in **B**), and is compatible with acute respiratory distress syndrome. Because the opacity is mild and diffuse, the lungs could be erroneously interpreted as normal. Region of interest evaluation *(circular cursors)*, however, confirms the increased lung attenuation (despite positive pressure ventilation), with −738 HU and −670 HU readings for the dorsal and ventral cursors, respectively. The mean HU value for normal lung inflated to 15 cm of water should be approximately −845.

by different tissues measured, compared, and recorded. More specifically, hydrogen protons are energized by exposure to a strong magnetic field and radiofrequency waves. The response of different tissues or substances to this disturbance can be manipulated to accentuate the signal they emit by using instrument controls. Contrast in an MR image is therefore a reflection of proton density, the response of protons to magnetic and radiofrequency fields, and technical manipulation. It is the multiparametric nature of the MR signal that imparts such good contrast resolution to the MR image but also makes MR physics the most difficult imaging concept to grasp.

A hydrogen proton is a positively charged particle, spinning about its own axis, randomly oriented within the body. Because moving electrical charges create magnetic fields, each proton possesses its own magnetic field and can be thought of as a tiny bar magnet with lines of magnetic force or flux emanating from its poles.

The lines of the magnetic field of one proton in a molecule can cross neighboring protons in the same molecule, as well as those in surrounding ones (Fig. 4-11). Protons spin

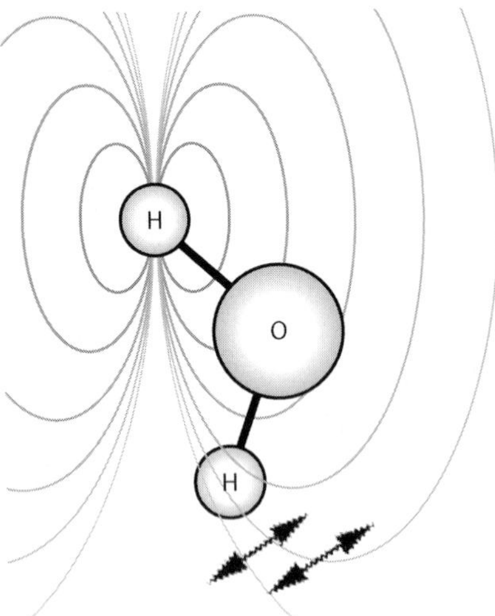

Fig. 4-11 Intramolecular proton-proton interaction. Magnetic lines of flux from one hydrogen proton in a water molecule cross the other proton. This relation changes as the molecule rotates and vibrates *(arrows)* and translates, resulting in a magnetic field that fluctuates in the "eyes" of the bottom proton.

about their own axes and also move in accordance with the motion of their host molecules, which are in a constant state of tumbling (rotating, vibrating, and translating) and colliding with other molecules. Because these protons are in constant motion, their magnetic fields fluctuate, causing random effects in their neighbors. Therefore the magnetic field experienced by a proton will fluctuate with a frequency that depends on the tumbling rate of the host and surrounding molecules.[14-18] The frequency of these random fluctuations in magnetic field—governed by a substance's molecular motions—influence how the protons in a substance will behave during the scanning process. Also affecting this behavior are nonrandom or static magnetic fields within the proton's local environment. These behaviors, known as T1, T2, and T2* relaxation, will be described in more detail later in the chapter.

Excitation

As previously mentioned, hydrogen protons within the patient induce signal in a coiled conductor in a process known as electromagnetic induction (see Fig. 4-1). The concept of Faraday's law of induction is critical to the generation of a useful signal by hydrogen protons. This law states that any change in the magnetic environment of a coil of wire will cause a voltage to be induced in the coil. In other words, if the net amount of magnetic force or flux passing through a coiled wire changes, current will be induced in the coil.[19] The change could be produced, for example, by moving a magnet toward or away from a coil, moving a coil into or out of a magnetic field, or by rotating the coil of wire relative to a magnet. In MR imaging, the magnetic fields of hydrogen protons are made to pass into and out of coils of wire, the receiver coils, thus generating a current. This current is measured as the MR signal (see Fig. 4-1).[19-22]

At the heart of an MR scanner is a magnet producing a powerful magnetic field. Various types of magnets are used for MR imaging but are not described here. The magnetic field associated with the main magnet, termed B_0, can be quite large. Many clinical imaging magnets producing fields have a strength of 1.5 Tesla (1 Tesla = 10,000 gauss). A refrigerator magnet has a magnetic strength of less than 100 gauss, emphasizing how strong the magnetic field is in an imaging magnet. Although a clinical imaging magnet has no ionizing radiation

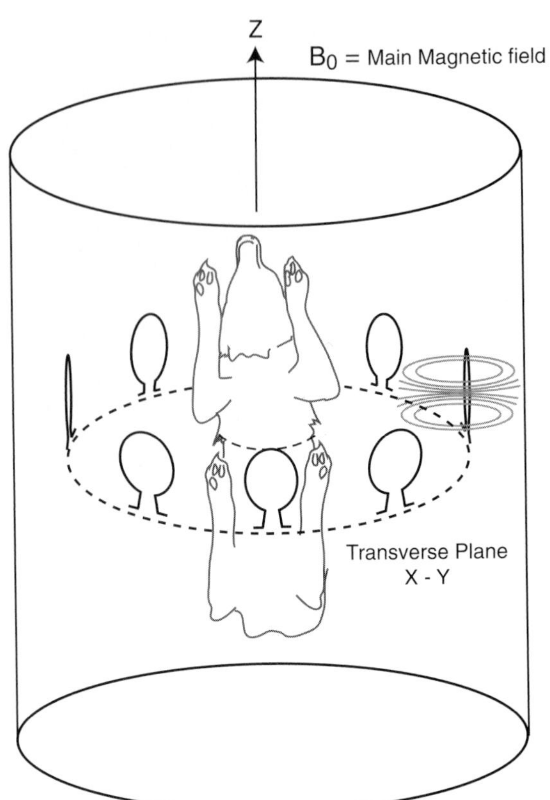

Fig. 4-12 Orientation of the main magnetic field and receiver coils. The patient is in the center of the magnet, with the long axis parallel to the direction of the main magnetic field, B_0, termed the Z direction. The magnetic field of the protons is aligned parallel to Z. For a signal to be measured, the magnetic field of the protons must oscillate into and out of the receiving coils. Receiver coils are oriented so that the signal from protons can only be measured if they are oriented perpendicular to the Z axis in the X-Y plane.

danger (ionizing radiation is not used in the MR imaging process), these strong magnetic fields still necessitate rigorous safety procedures because ferromagnetic objects (wrenches, oxygen tanks, floor polishers, etc.) can become lethal projectiles in the vicinity of the strong magnetic field. Also, once lodged against a strong magnet, an object such as a wrench cannot be removed by hand and the magnet may have to be turned off for its removal; this procedure is complex and can be quite expensive.

For imaging, the patient lies within the center of the magnet and experiences the force of the magnetic field, which is usually aligned along the long axis of the magnet (Fig. 4-12). The magnetic fields of the hydrogen protons within the body then align with B_0. To produce current in the receiver coils, the magnetic flux of the protons must pass though a receiving coil according to Faraday's law, as previously described. Because electrical systems that function with alternating current require an oscillating signal, a receiver coil placed at the end of the magnet would not "see" a continuous *change* in magnetic flux of the protons, so no signal would be sustained.[21] Although many receiver coils give the outward impression that B_0 runs through them, they are in reality composed of loops of wire oriented alongside B_0 and the patient (see Fig. 4-12). Therefore, to induce signal, the protons must somehow be forced perpendicular to the main magnetic field and must oscillate when getting there. In MR imaging, the direction of the main magnetic field is termed the longitudinal plane, Z plane, or Z direction, and the plane perpendicular to the Z plane is the transverse plane, X-Y plane, or X-Y direction. This rotation of the proton magnetic field from the Z plane into the X-Y plane is accomplished by excitation.

In addition to spinning about their own axes and randomly tumbling along with their host molecules, hydrogen protons exhibit a third type of motion known as precession when exposed to B_0. Proton precession is often likened to the wobbling of a spinning top or a gyroscope as it experiences the pull of gravity. Inside the magnet, protons precess, or wobble, around B_0. Precession occurs because the protons have a property called angular momentum. Angular momentum is the tendency of a moving object to continue moving in the same direction. If disturbed by a force, the object will respond to that force but will stay in motion. When the protons experience B_0, angular momentum prevents them from simply lining up with B_0; instead they precess about it a few degrees off the Z axis. The rate at which the protons precess is called the angular precessional frequency and is determined by the strength of the magnetic field being applied to them. The Larmor equation describes the relation between the strength of the main magnetic field and the precessional frequency as is shown below (Fig. 4-13):

$$\omega = \gamma \times B \qquad \text{(Eq 3)}$$

where ω is the angular precessional frequency expressed in MHz, γ is the gyromagnetic ratio expressed in MHz/Tesla, and B is the magnetic field strength expressed in Tesla. γ is unique to each element. The main contributor to the magnetic field strength is the main magnet, but the overall magnetic field is also influenced by slight imperfections in the equipment, the presence of encoding gradients, magnetic substances in the nearby tissues, and of course by the random fluctuating fields created by the protons themselves (see Fig. 4-13).

Hydrogen protons also exhibit another property called spin quantum number, also called nuclear spin or simply spin.[15,18,23] This is a quantum mechanical description that determines the number of measurable discrete energy levels for a nucleus when experiencing an external magnetic field. Because of this property, protons or spins within the main magnetic field tend to align either parallel (spin-up, low-energy state) or antiparallel (spin-down, high-energy state) with respect to the main magnetic field. This does not imply that the spins exist exclusively in one state or the other but that the measuring process allows observation of only one of the principle states on a given occasion.[15] As illustrated in Figure 4-14, the lower-energy state will always demonstrate a slight excess of spins; the difference between the number of protons in the spin-up state versus the spin-down state results in the spin excess. The relative difference in spin-up versus spin-down protons may only be three protons out of 1 million protons at a magnetic field strength of 1.0 T. However, with 10^{21} total protons in an MR image voxel, approximately 3×10^{15} more protons may be present in the low-energy state (spin-up) in each voxel![12] The spin excess results in a net longitudinal, or Z axis, magnetization termed M_0. However, although each spin is precessing at the Larmor frequency, each one is out of phase with the others, effectively canceling out precession of the net magnetization. In other words, M_0 does not initially precess and points mainly in the Z direction.[21]

As previously mentioned, if magnetization from the spins is to create current in the receiver coils, it must be oscillating and have a component in the X-Y or transverse plane because of the orientation of the coils, as mandated by Faraday's law. The objective therefore becomes to synchronize the spin excess into phase and energize or excite the spins enough to create a precessing net vector of magnetization that points in the X-Y or transverse plane. This oscillating net transverse magnetization, termed $M_{x\text{-}y}$, creates alternating current in the receiver coils (Figs. 4-14 and 4-15) and the signal for image formation.

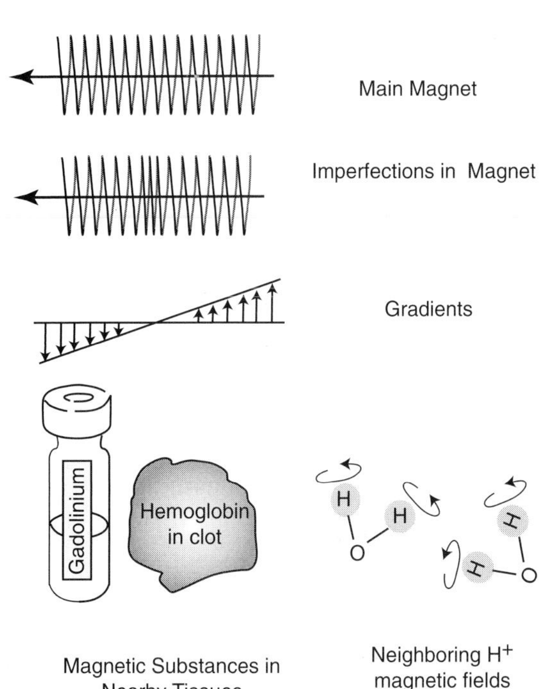

Fig. 4-13 The Larmor equation and contributors to it. The precessional frequency of a proton is related to the magnetic field strength and the gyromagnetic ratio, which is atom specific. For hydrogen, the value of the gyromagnetic ratio is 42.58 MHz/T. Thus the precessional frequency of hydrogen protons in a 1.0 T magnetic field is 42.58 MHz and is 64 MHz in a 1.5 T magnet. By using the Larmor equation, the precessional frequency of hydrogen at other magnetic field strengths can be calculated. The main determinant of the precessional frequency is the strength of the main magnetic field. However, this is altered by imperfections in the magnet itself, applied gradients, magnetic substances in nearby tissues such as hemoglobin or paramagnetic contrast media, and the magnetic field of neighboring protons.

To synchronize precession of the protons aligned with B_0 and create a magnetic vector in the X-Y plane, energy in the form of radiofrequency (RF) current at the Larmor frequency is applied perpendicular to Z (see Fig. 4-14). An RF pulse is a form of electromagnetic radiation. As the name implies, it is made up of an electrical field and a magnetic field. The mag-

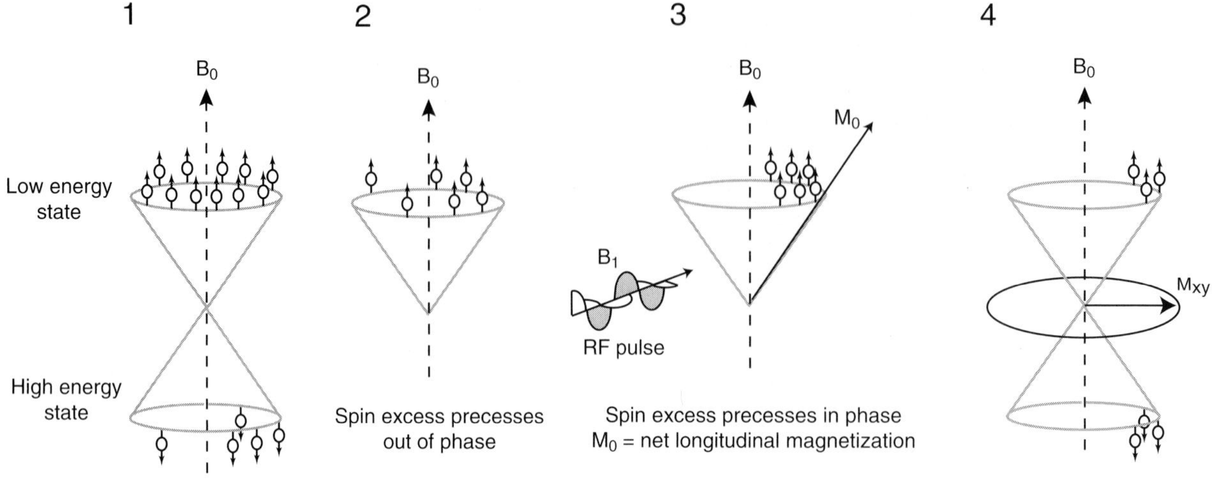

Fig. 4-14 Energy states and excitation with RF pulse. *1*, In a strong magnetic field, protons either align in the direction of the main magnetic field or directly opposite to the main magnetic field. Because aligning opposite to the magnetic field requires more energy, a majority of protons align with the direction of B_0. *2*, This panel illustrates just the excess number of protons aligning with B_0 as the effects of the others cancel out. Note that the position of the protons is random. Although the protons are precessing, they are out of phase with each other, so no net precessing longitudinal magnetization occurs. *3*, If an external RF pulse at the Larmor frequency is applied, M_0 will begin to precess in resonance with the RF pulse. The RF pulse provides the precise amount of energy to cause a transition of protons from the low-energy state to the high-energy state. *4*, With continued application of the RF pulse, more and more protons will assume the antiparallel, or higher-energy, orientation. This causes M_0 to begin to rotate downward toward the X-Y plane. When the vector reaches the X-Y plane, the external RF pulse can be turned off; a pulse of RF that allows for rotation of the magnetic vector into the X-Y plane is called a 90-degree pulse. By adjusting the time that the external RF pulse is applied, the magnetic vector can be moved any number of degrees away from Z that is desired.

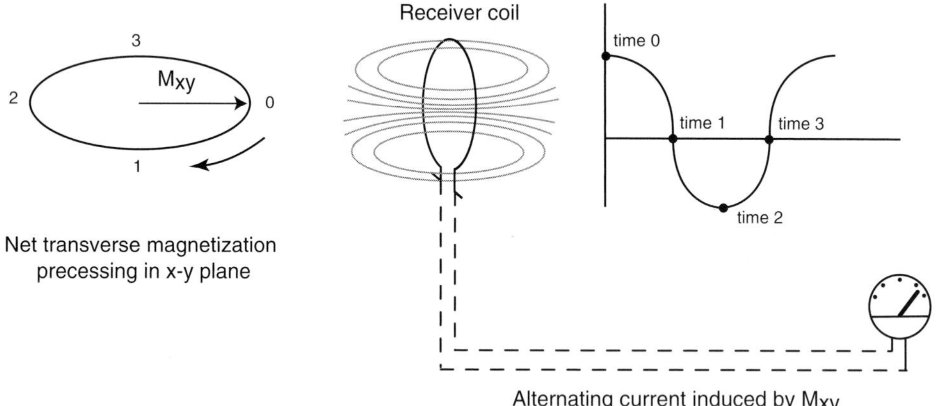

Fig. 4-15 Precessing transverse magnetization induces current in receiver coil. As the magnetic vector in the X-Y plane precesses into and out of the region of the receiver coil, an alternating current is produced according to Faraday's law.

netic field of the RF is denoted B_1 and is relatively weak when compared with B_0. Application of the RF pulse causes M_0 to precess in the Y-Z plane around the magnetic field (B_1) of the RF wave in the X axis while still precessing at the Larmor frequency around B_0 in the Z axis. Because B_1 is much smaller than B_0, precession in the Y-Z plane around B_1 will be quite slow, whereas precession around B_0 will be fast. The combination of these simultaneous precessions causes a downward spiraling of M_0 toward the X-Y plane; this process is sometimes referred to as nutation. Although this sounds complicated, an animation nicely illustrates what is occurring; see Video 4-2 on the Evolve site at http://evolve.elsevier.com/Thrall/vetrad/.

The principle of nutation can also be demonstrated in an easy exercise modified from a description by Pipe.[19] In a standing position, raise the left arm above the head. The left arm represents M_0 and the body represents B_0 and the Z axis. Point horizontally straight out in front with the right arm. The right arm represents B_1 in the X axis. Now begin spinning around. Simultaneously rotate the left arm downward toward the left side, a direction identical to the Y-Z plane in the magnet, to mimic precession around B_1. However, because B_1 is quite small, move the left arm downward more slowly compared with the spinning motion. The path the left arm takes during these simultaneous motions mimics the nutation of M_0. Spinning until the left arm is level with the right arm mimics a 90-degree RF pulse. Stopping any time before this point mimics an RF pulse duration that creates a deviation of the magnetic vector of less than 90 degrees. The number of degrees that the main magnetic vector is displaced from the Z axis by the pulsed RF current is termed the flip angle and is often denoted by the symbol α or θ.

Depending on the duration (or strength) of the RF pulse, spiraling can occur until M_0 is any number of degrees away from Z. For example, an RF pulse can cause nutation of M_0 90 degrees or 180 degrees or can cause a "flip" of the magnetization vector of any degree. As will be discussed later in this chapter, spin-echo pulse sequences use 90- and 180-degree pulses, whereas gradient-echo pulse sequences often use flip angles of less than 90 degrees. With a flip angle smaller than 90 degrees, the entirety of the main magnetic field vector, M_0, will not "point" directly toward the receiver coil, but some component of magnetization in the transverse plane always will. In fact, the magnitude of $M_{x\text{-}y}$ after a partial flip can be determined by using simple trigonometry. According to the relation $M_{x\text{-}y} = M_0 \sin\theta$, transverse magnetization ($M_{x\text{-}y}$) will always be smaller than the original longitudinal magnetization (M_0) after a partial flip because the sine of any angle less than 90 degrees is less than 1.0.[21]

For nutation to occur, however, the frequency of the applied RF pulse must match the Larmor frequency of the hydrogen protons. In other words, for M_0 to precess around B_1 in the X axis, M_0 and B_1 must be in sync as they precess around B_0 in the Z axis (see Video 4-2 at http://evolve.elsevier.com/Thrall/vetrad.). If the rate of rotation did not match, M_0 would be alternately in and out of phase with B_1 and could not effectively rotate around it.[15] B_1 therefore could not effectively "torque" the spins into the transverse X-Y plane. The requirement that the RF and M_0 must precess in harmony is based on the phenomenon of resonance. Resonance is the tendency of a system to absorb more energy when the energizer's frequency matches the system's natural or resonant frequency. Outside of MR imaging, resonance explains why a tuning fork will vibrate in the presence of another vibrating fork tuned to the same pitch or frequency and explains the enhanced efficiency of pushing a child on a swing when the frequency of pushing matches the natural mechanical frequency of the swinging child. If the frequency of the actions match, then energy is added and the child swings higher.[21] In MR imaging, the required applied RF energy is the precise amount that will cause a transition of spins in the spin excess from the low-energy state to the high-energy state, thus creating transverse magnetization. A critical point is that the only signal measured when acquiring an MR image comes from the X-Y plane; magnetic vectors in any other plane do not induce a signal in the receiving coil. Because this transverse X-Y magnetization is needed to create the signal for MR images, MR imaging would not be possible without resonance.

T1, T2, and T2 Relaxation Processes*

Once magnetization is rotated into the X-Y plane it immediately begins to decay according to T1, T2, and T2* relaxation processes. As the magnetization in the X-Y plane decays, the signal recorded in the receiving coil also decays. Therefore, to induce enough signal in the receiving coil to create an image, the magnetization in the Z direction must be reoriented into the X-Y plane multiple times by using multiple applied external RF pulses. The time between each successive RF excitation pulse is termed the repetition time, or TR. However, if no longitudinal magnetization (M_0) were present at the time of subsequent externally applied RF pulses, nothing would be available for reorientation into the X-Y plane. Therefore subsequent TRs must be timed to be delivered after some magnetization has been restored in the Z plane.

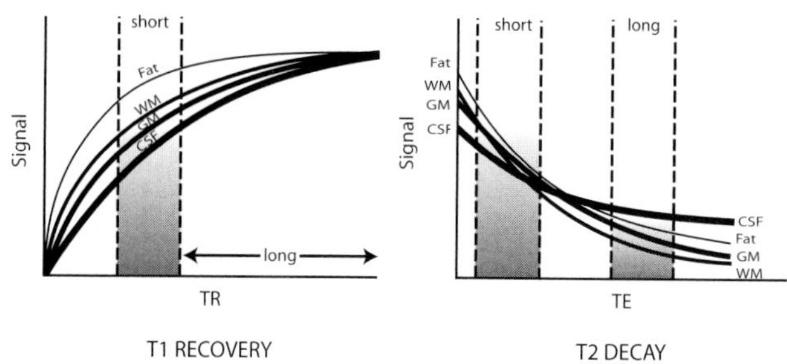

Fig. 4-16 T1 recovery and T2 decay curves. *Left,* The magnitude of T1 relaxation for cerebrospinal fluid *(CSF),* gray matter *(GM),* white matter *(WM),* and fat as a function of time after turning off the external RF pulse. As can be seen, fat is quicker at returning its magnetic vector to the Z direction than are the other tissues. If T1 differences need to be optimized, a short TR (time between two RF pulses) is selected because this is when the greatest tissue-dependent difference in magnetization occurs in the Z direction. The gray-scale gradient indicates that in a T1-weighted image, tissues with short T1 relaxation (fat) will be bright, whereas tissues with long T1 relaxation (CSF) will be dark. *Right,* Loss of the magnetization vector in the X-Y plane can also occur from T2 decay. As with T1 relaxation, the rate of T2 relaxation varies between tissues. The T2 relaxation of WM is shorter than the T2 relaxation rate of other tissues. By selecting a long TE, the T2 relaxation characteristics of tissues can be best discriminated. The long TE gray-scale gradient indicates that, in T2-weighted images, tissues with a long T2 relaxation time (CSF) will have a high signal, whereas tissues with rapid T2 relaxation (WM) will be dark. Fat will have an intermediate signal intensity. The short TE gray-scale gradient reflects contrast in one type of PD-weighted image. In this instance, CSF has low signal intensity.

Magnetization is restored in the Z direction by a process called T1 relaxation. Once a transverse magnetization vector is produced in the X-Y plane, the external RF pulse is turned off and the spins begin to relax and release the absorbed RF energy. T1 relaxation is the return of magnetization from the transverse plane to the Z-axis and is measured by the time it takes for regrowth of magnetization in the Z direction. The timing of magnetization's return to the Z direction, termed T1 recovery, follows logarithmic kinetics (Fig. 4-16). The T1 recovery rate determines how much longitudinal magnetization will be available to be moved into the transverse plane by the next RF pulse. Most importantly, because the rate of T1 relaxation is an intrinsic property that differs in different substances, measuring and comparing the extent of T1 relaxation is one way of providing tissue contrast to the image. Looking at Figure 4-16, tissues such as fat have short T1 relaxation or recovery times, brain tissue is intermediate, and cerebrospinal fluid (CSF) has a long T1 relaxation time. T1 relaxation is related to the physical characteristics of the tissues. (The effect of these tissue characteristics on relaxation rates will be discussed later.) By using a procedure called weighting, the MR technician can control contrast in the image by selecting a TR that optimizes signal and maximizes differences in T1 recovery rates. As the T1 recovery curves indicate in Figure 4-16, the best way to differentiate these tissues is by using a short TR. For example, with a short TR, most of the magnetization in the Z direction will have come from relaxation of protons in fat molecules. Thus upon reorientation of this magnetic vector into the X-Y plane after subsequent RF pulses, most of the signal measured in the receiving coil will come from fat. This is an example of controlling image contrast by varying the machine parameters. Further, as the gray-scale gradient in Figure 4-16 implies,

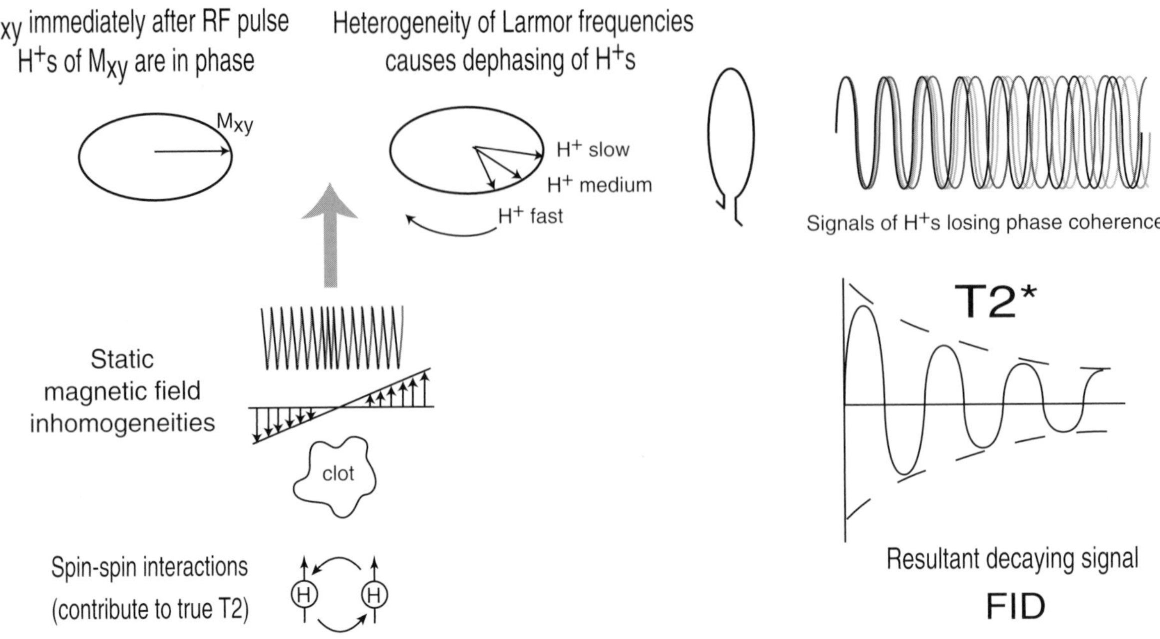

Fig. 4-17 Dephasing and T2* relaxation. Immediately after excitation, the protons precess in the X-Y plane in unison and create a relatively large magnetic vector. The Larmor frequencies of the protons are influenced by (1) static magnetic field inhomogeneities created by defects in the magnet, applied gradients, and magnetic substances such as those found in blood clot; and (2) the magnetic fields of other protons (which contribute to true T2 relaxation). This results in heterogeneity in the rates of proton precession, which causes dephasing and decay of the signal in the receiving coil. The decaying signal is known as the FID.

substances with short T1 relaxation times (such as fat) will have high signal on a T1-weighted image and will be relatively hyperintense or brighter in the image; substances with long T1 relaxation times (such as CSF) will be relatively hypointense on a T1-weighted image and appear relatively darker in the image.

T1 relaxation is not the only type of relaxation that occurs. Another relaxation process occurs within the X-Y plane and is called T2 relaxation. T2 relaxation occurs simultaneous to T1 relaxation but is completely independent from it. T2 relaxation occurs much faster than T1 relaxation and is caused by a loss of coherence or uniformity of precession rates of the spins in the X-Y plane. Because the protons start to spin at different rates, they no longer spin in phase; this loss of coherence is called dephasing.

As illustrated in Figure 4-17, protons in $M_{x\text{-}y}$ dephase because their Larmor frequencies are heterogeneous. This heterogeneity of precession rates is caused by variations within the local magnetic environment. As demonstrated in Figure 4-13, Larmor frequency depends on magnetic fields in the proton's environment. Static fields arise from the magnet, slight imperfections in the equipment, the applied gradient fields, and magnetic substances in the nearby tissues; these fields indiscriminately affect the Larmor frequencies of the protons in all types of substances or tissues. The magnetic fields that a proton "sees" from its neighboring protons, on the other hand, depend on the binding and motion characteristics of the molecules within a particular substance. The contribution of proton-proton or "spin-spin" interactions to dephasing is therefore characteristic for a substance and, in actuality, represents the true T2 relaxation properties of that substance. The initial decay of X-Y or transverse magnetization immediately after the RF pulse is removed is therefore, in actuality, a combination of true T2 relaxation and relaxation influenced by static field inhomogeneities; for this reason the initial decay is more accurately termed T2* (pronounced "T2 star") relaxation.[13,15,18,25]

Beginning students of MR physics often express confusion over the differences between T2 relaxation and T2* relaxation. As stated above, T2* relaxation occurs immediately after removal of the RF pulse and is simply the combined effect of spin-spin interactions and static inhomogeneities on dephasing (Fig. 4-17).[13,15,18,25] During T2* relaxation, the current induced in the receiver coil by $M_{x\text{-}y}$ decays; this decaying signal is called the free induction decay (FID). Because the FID is fast and short lived, some means of rebuilding the signal in the coil is necessary to produce images. Likewise, because true T2 relaxation is characteristic of a tissue or substance and dephasing caused by static inhomogeneities is nonspecific, some means of minimizing or canceling out the contribution to T2* by the static inhomogeneities is required to produce images that truly reflect differences in T2. As illustrated in Figure 4-18, *A*, an MR technique producing a "spin echo" accomplishes both these objectives in the following manner:

After the 90-degree RF pulse is removed, the dephasing spins of $M_{x\text{-}y}$ are reoriented 180 degrees through the application of another RF pulse, this time a pulse that flips the spins 180 degrees across the transverse plane. In Figure 4-18, *A*, this is denoted by the large arrow along the dotted line. After the 180-degree flip, faster spins, whose Larmor frequencies are greater because they experienced stronger local magnetic fields, become reoriented behind slower spins; as the faster spins catch up with slower ones, the spins rephase. The rephased spins reform transverse magnetization and recreate signal in the receiver coil. This refocused signal is an "echo" of the FID. The time from the initial 90-degree RF pulse and the echo is called the echo time (TE). The 180-degree RF pulse is applied at precisely TE/2.

However, as previously discussed, the effect of one proton's magnetic field on another, or spin-spin interactions, is random and fluctuating; its contribution to dephasing therefore cannot be reversed with this process. Thus only the effect of static magnetic field inhomogeneities on dephasing is reversed during this process. As seen in Figure 4-18, *A*, the spins are therefore only partially rephased, and the resultant echo is weaker than the original FID. Because the only factor not reversed by this process is the spin-spin interaction, the difference in the height of the FID and the echo is a reflection of a substance's true T2 relaxation. If a curve is used to connect the FID to sequential echoes (that is, after repetitive 90-degree, then 180-degree, pulses), it would reveal that T2 decay occurs exponentially. The curves can be used to compare tissues or substances having different (true) T2 relaxation rates. Looking at Figure 4-16, the exponential decay curves show the relative T2 relaxation times for 4 substances. T2-weighting capitalizes on differences in T2 relaxation rates for different substances by using a long TE in a pulse sequence employing spin echoes. As the long TE gray-scale gradient in the figure implies, substances with long relaxation rates (such as CSF) are hyperintense on a T2-weighted image and appear relatively bright, and substances with short relaxation rates (such as brain white matter) are hypointense on a T2-weighted image and appear relatively dark.

Pulse Sequences

Spin Echo Pulse Sequence In the process described above, creation of a spin echo occurs when 90- and 180-degree RF pulses are used to move the magnetic vector from the Z direction into the X-Y plane and refocus it, respectively. This sequence of events, that is, the application of a 90-degree, then 180-degree, RF pulse followed by an echo is called a spin-echo pulse sequence. Pulse sequences are often annotated as lines showing chronologic events. In the top line of the top panel in Figure 4-19, the spin-echo sequence is displayed. To provide sufficient signal (echoes) to construct an image, the pulse sequence must be repeated multiple times for one image slice. A medical MR imaging study consists of many image slices; not surprisingly, faster variations called fast spin-echo pulse sequences have been developed. Nevertheless, the conventional spin-echo pulse sequence is still used routinely.

Although the earlier discussion of spin echoes was made in reference to T2 relaxation, spin-echo pulse sequences can be weighted to produce contrast, reflecting either T1 relaxation or T2 relaxation by selecting the appropriate TR and TE. Producing an image that reflects mainly the spatial concentration of protons, or a proton density image, is also possible. These images are usually referred to, respectively, as a T1-weighted image, a T2-weighted image, and a proton density (PD)–weighted image. Looking at the T2 decay graph in Figure 4-16, the short TE gray-scale gradient represents image contrast in one type of PD-weighted spin-echo image, and the long TE gray scale gradient represents contrast in a T2-weighted spin-echo image.

The effect of timing parameters on image weighting in spin echo pulse sequences is summarized in the left panel of Figure 4-20.

Gradient Echo Pulse Sequence In gradient echo pulse sequences, an RF pulse is used to move the magnetic vector out of the Z direction, but this is usually not a 90-degree pulse. In fact, the amount that the vector rotates toward the X-Y plane can be accurately controlled, and this distance, the flip angle, can either be small or large, approaching 90 degrees. The advantage of small flip angles is that less longitudinal magnetization in the Z direction is lost during excitation, so less longitudinal recovery time is needed before the next RF pulse. Shorter TRs can therefore be used. As previously defined, TR is the time between two successive RF excitation pulses and is therefore the time necessary to run through the pulse sequence one time. Because TR contributes the most to scanning time, gradient-echo sequences are faster than spin-echo sequences. The gradient-echo pulse sequence is annotated in the top line of the bottom panel in Figure 4-19. Note the absence of a 180-degree refocusing RF pulse. Instead, echo formation is through the application of externally applied gradients whose polarity is reversed at TE/2. As seen in Figure 4-18, *B*, protons dephase in a gradient-echo pulse sequence because some are close to the strong end of the gradient, making those protons spin faster, whereas others are near the opposite end. By reversing the gradient polarity, this relation is reversed, allowing for rephasing. However, as with spin-echo pulses, true T2 relaxation cannot be reversed. Furthermore, the gradient reversal used to form the echo only serves to eliminate the gradient's contribution to dephasing, and unlike the spin-echo sequence, does nothing to cancel the effects of other local static inhomogeneities. T2 contrast in gradient-echo images, in reality, therefore reflects tissues or substances differing in T2* relaxation rates. Note, however, that this does not mean that the image is formed only from the FID; echoes make up the signal just as they did in spin-echo pulse sequences. Nevertheless, because true T2 contributes to T2*, the basic contrast between tissues differing in T2 relaxation is still maintained in gradient-echo images (e.g., intensity of CSF is greater than gray matter, which is greater than white matter).[13]

As seen in Figure 4-18, C, gradient-echo images are especially prone to signal losses in the presence of increased magnetic inhomogeneity. This can create signal void artifacts at diverse tissue interfaces or when magnetically susceptible substances (that is, substances that locally alter [increase, in this instance] the magnetic field strength such as paramagnetic deoxyhemoglobin and methemoglobin in blood clot) are nearby. Nevertheless, as seen in Figure 4-18, *D*, this phenomenon can be purposefully exploited to increase the detection of such substances by lengthening TE. When the time before the gradient polarity reversal is prolonged, more time is allowed for initial dephasing, and therefore more unrecoverable signal loss occurs in the presence of susceptible substances. By using this technique, acute hemorrhage will appear as a signal void and can be detected earlier than on spin-echo sequences.[18,26] The purposeful use of a gradient-echo pulse sequence with a long TE is called susceptibility weighting or T2* weighting.

By using various combinations of flip angle and TE, gradient-echo images can be created that are T1 weighted, T2* weighted, or PD weighted. The effect of timing parameters and flip angles on image weighting in gradient-echo pulse sequences is summarized in the right panel of Figure 4-20.

Inversion Recovery Pulse Sequence Inversion recovery pulse sequences are performed by using a 180-degree pulse before the first 90-degree pulse of a spin-echo sequence. The time between this 180-degree pulse and the 90-degree pulse is defined as inversion time (TI). By selecting the appropriate TI, image contrast can be altered and selective tissues suppressed as desired. As illustrated in Figure 4-21, inversion recovery pulse sequences manipulate T1 relaxation. When the 180-degree pulse is applied, the magnetization vector in the Z direction will be relocated to the negative Z direction. As soon as the 180-degree pulse is turned off, magnetization will begin regrowing toward the positive Z direction. The rate at which this magnetization regrows is tissue dependent; tissues with short T1 relaxation times will have their magnetization vector regrow the fastest. Thus applying the 90-degree pulse when the tissue needing to be nulled or suppressed has its magnetization vector near zero (as it regrows from negative Z toward positive Z) will result in that tissue having no available longitudinal magnetization to create transverse magnetization and signal in the receiver coil in response to the 90-degree pulse. For example, fat can be suppressed when using a short TI because of its rapid T1 relaxation time.

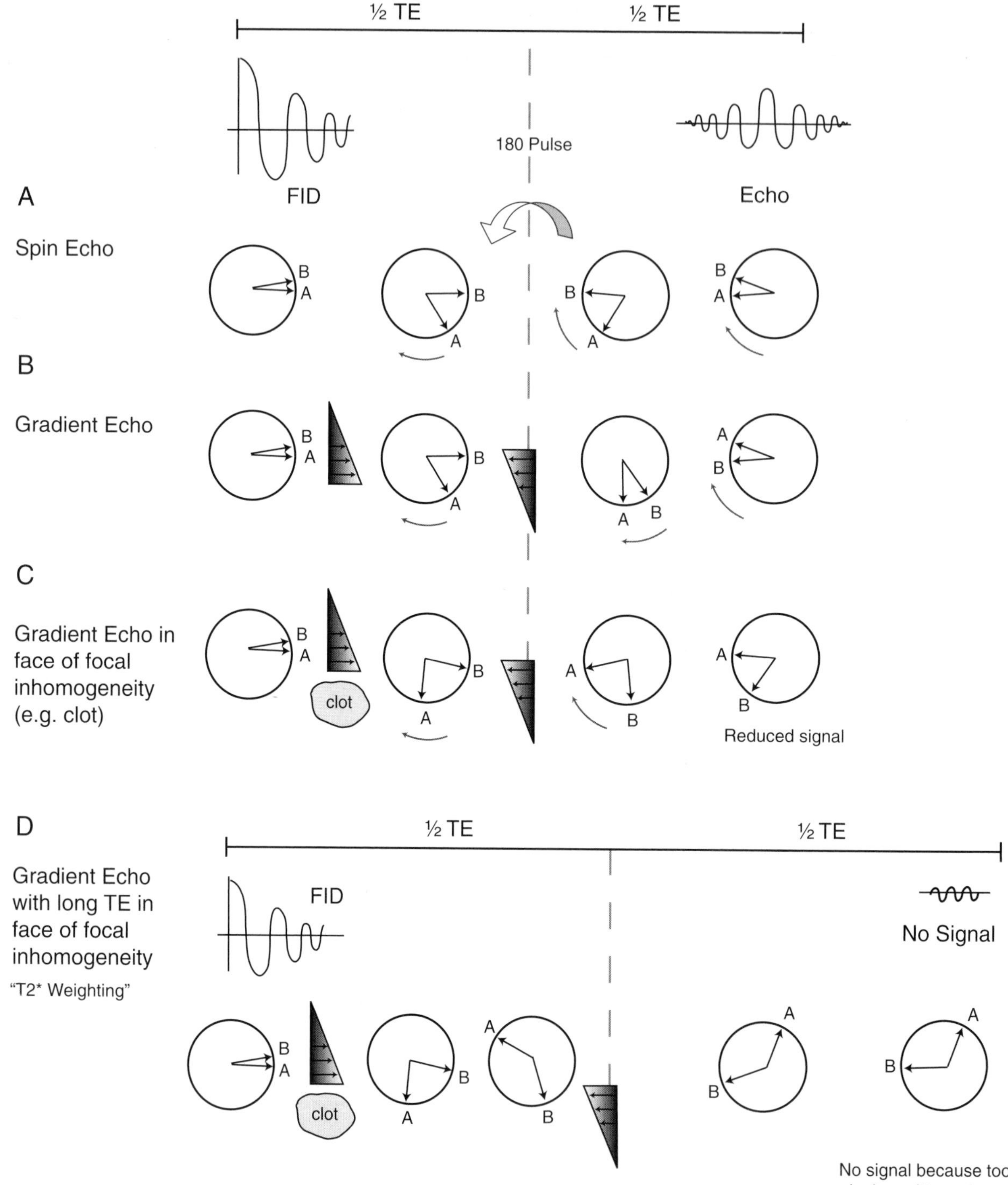
Echo Formation
½ TE
½ TE
180 Pulse
FID
Echo
A
Spin Echo
B
Gradient Echo
C
Gradient Echo in face of focal inhomogeneity (e.g. clot)
clot
Reduced signal
D
Gradient Echo with long TE in face of focal inhomogeneity
"T2* Weighting"
FID
No Signal
No signal because too dephased to rephase

Fig. 4-18 Two methods of echo formation. **A,** Spin echo. **B** to **D,** gradient echo. Because the FID is short lived, an echo must be created to provide signal for image construction. In **A,** immediately after the RF pulse is turned off, the protons begin to dephase because some protons (A) spin faster than others (B) because they experienced stronger local magnetic fields. This is depicted by the separation of A and B as they spin clockwise in the transverse plane. The *arrow* on the *dotted line* represents application of another RF pulse, a 180-degree refocusing pulse, which serves to flip the protons 180 degrees across the transverse plane. The flip can be likened to flipping a pancake over one time, so that the positions of A and B (different blueberries in the pancake) after the flip are a mirror image of A and B before the flip. After the 180-degree flip, faster spins (A) are now behind slower spins (B); as the faster spins catch up with the slower ones, the spins rephase. The rephased spins reform transverse magnetization and recreate signal in the receiver coil. The time from the initial 90-degree RF pulse and the echo is known as the TE. The 180-degree RF pulse is applied at precisely TE/2. In the last circle of **A,** note that A and B are still slightly separated. This occurs because the refocusing pulse cannot reverse the effect of spin-spin interactions on dephasing, so only partial rephasing occurs. This is why the echo height is less than the original FID. In **B,** in a gradient-echo pulse sequence, echo formation is through the application of externally applied gradients whose polarity is reversed at TE/2. Protons dephase in this sequence because some are close to the strong end of the gradient (A), making those protons spin faster, and others are near the opposite end (B). By reversing the gradient polarity, this relation is reversed, allowing for rephasing. However, the gradient reversal used to form the echo only serves to eliminate the gradient's contribution to dephasing, and unlike the spin-echo sequence, does nothing to cancel the effects of other local static inhomogeneities. As seen in **C,** the images are especially prone to signal losses in the presence of magnetically susceptible substances such as hemoglobin in a blood clot. Magnetic substances within the blood clot locally alter (in this instance, increase) the magnetic field strength, thus affecting the Larmor frequency of the nearby protons. In **C,** the faster protons (A) are faster because they are near the strong end of the gradient *and* because they are near the clot. The added effect of the clot imparts exceptional speed to A relative to B, so by the time the gradient polarity is reversed, B can only partially catch up with A. This results in reduced signal near the clot, as indicated in the last circle of **C.** In **D,** this phenomenon is purposefully exploited to increase the detection of such substances by lengthening TE. When the time before the gradient polarity reversal is prolonged, more time is allowed for initial dephasing, and therefore more unrecoverable signal loss occurs in the presence of susceptible substances found in the clot. In other words, B can never catch up with A despite the gradient reversal because it is too late. This results in a signal void near the clot, allowing for its identification.

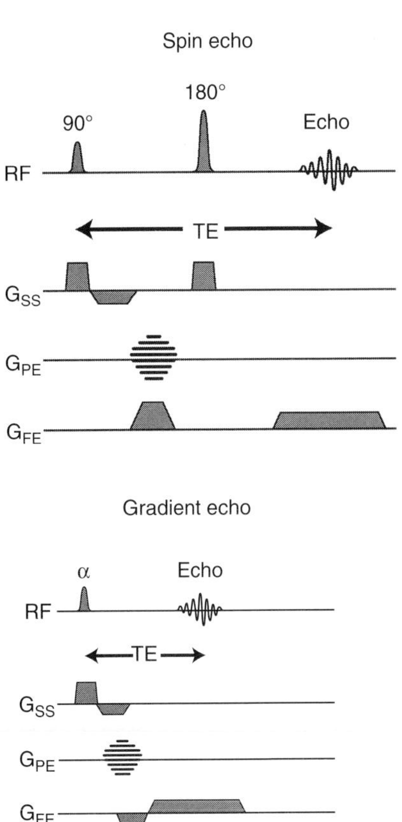

Fig. 4-19 Pulse sequence annotations for spin-echo and gradient-echo sequences. The narrow spikes represent RF pulses. α is the flip angle. TE is the time to echo. G_{ss} is the slice selection gradient, G_{PE} is the phase-encoding gradient, and G_{FE} is the frequency encoding gradient. The *gray boxes* represent the chronologic application of the gradients during the pulse sequence. The *symbol* along the G_{PE} direction indicates the multiple steps of phase encoding. G_{ss} is turned on simultaneously with the RF pulses. The G_{PE} is turned on soon after excitation. During the readout of the echo, the G_{FE} stays turned on, as indicated by the *long gray box* along the G_{FE} line.

Sequences to suppress fat that use inversion recovery techniques are called STIR sequences (***s**hort **t**au [for TI] **i**nversion **r**ecovery*). By using a longer TI, the signal can be nulled from free fluids. The T1 relaxation time of fluids is relatively long, necessitating a long TI before their magnetization vector approaches the zero value. Sequences to null the signal from free fluid are called FLAIR sequences (***fl**uid **a**ttenuated **i**nversion **r**ecovery*) (see Fig. 4-21).

Chemical Fat Saturation Pulse The resonant frequencies of the protons in water and fat differ by 3.5 ppm. This difference is known as chemical shift. By limiting the transmitting

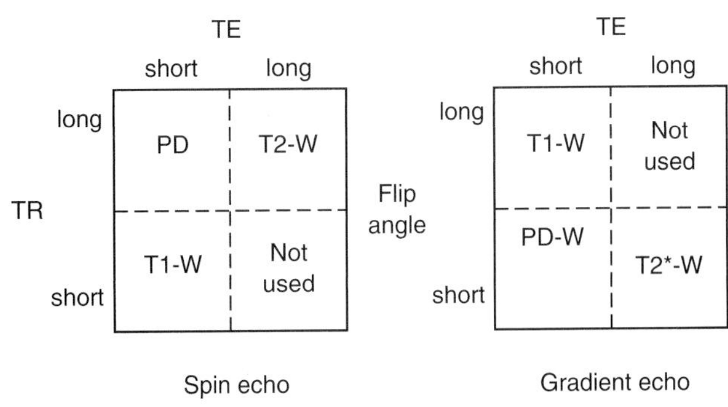

Fig. 4-20 Timing and flip angle parameters for spin-echo and gradient-echo pulse sequences.

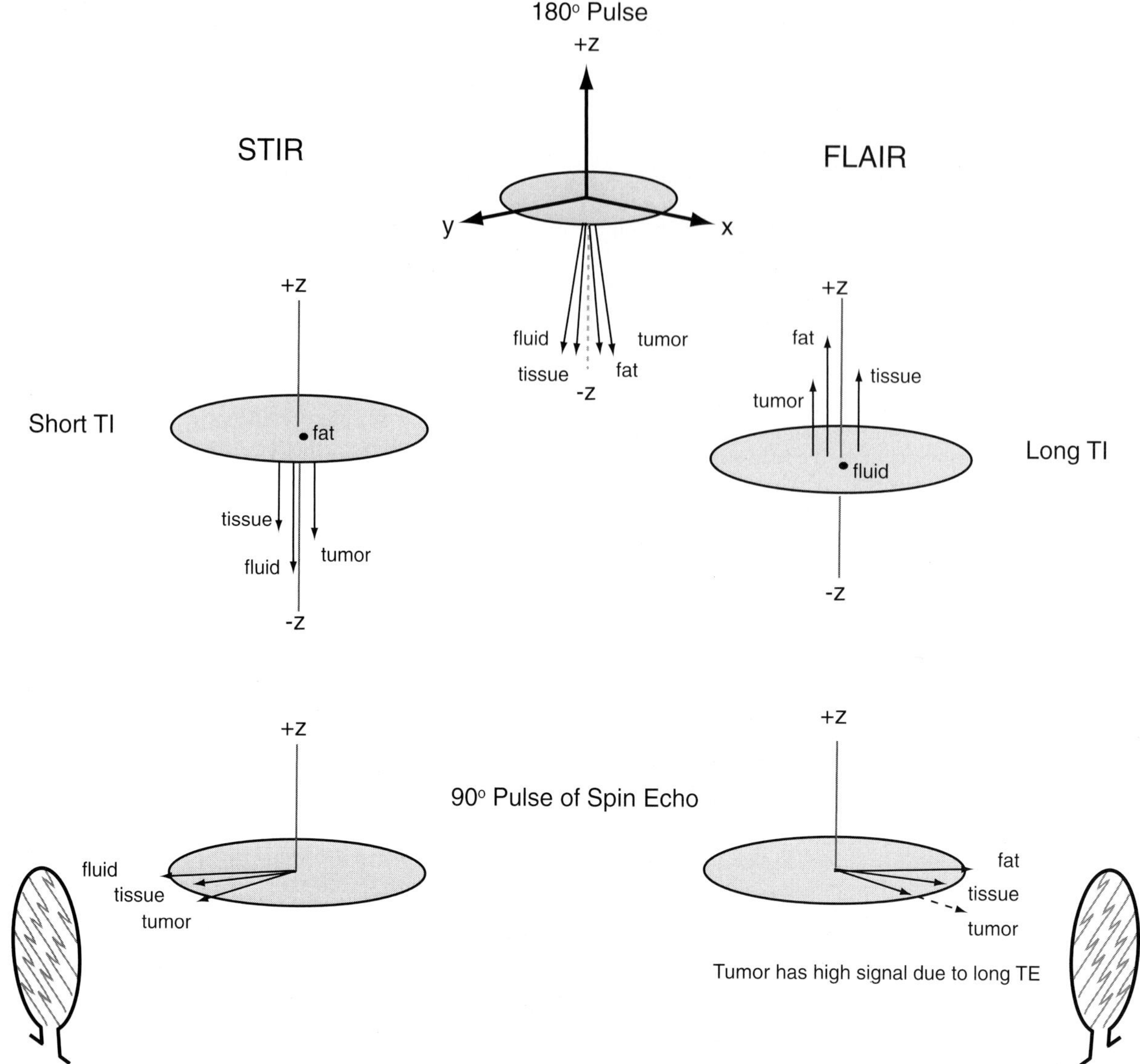

Fig. 4-21 Inversion recovery vector diagrams. Inversion recovery sequences apply a 180-degree pulse before a spin-echo pulse sequence to manipulate T1 relaxation. The time between the 180-degree pulse and the 90-degree pulse of the spin-echo pulse sequence is the TI. The 180-degree pulse relocates the Z magnetization vector to the negative Z direction. As soon as the 180-degree pulse is turned off, magnetization begins regrowing toward the positive Z direction. Sequences used to suppress fat are called STIR sequences and are depicted on the *left side* of the figure. Sequences to null the signal from free fluid are called FLAIR sequences and are depicted on the *right side.* In a STIR sequence, the 90-degree pulse is applied after a short time (short TI) precisely when fat has no longitudinal magnetization to create subsequent transverse magnetization and signal in the receiver coil. In a FLAIR sequence, a longer time passes before the 90-degree pulse is applied so that fluid has no longitudinal magnetization to create subsequent transverse magnetization. In both STIR and FLAIR, solid but "juicy" tissues such as tumor are hyperintense. In the STIR sequence, this is because tumor still has a fair amount of (negative) Z magnetization to create subsequent transverse magnetization and signal at the 90-degree pulse. In the FLAIR sequence this is also true, but tumor appears brighter than normal tissues because the sequences use very long TEs and are therefore heavily T2 weighted.

bandwidth of the RF pulse of a spin-echo pulse sequence, the signal from fat can be selectively excited and then spoiled, that is, forced to decay. This technique leaves the protons in water untouched, so the subsequent signals creating the image come only from water, and the signals from fat are suppressed.

Tissue Contrast Mechanisms

As previously mentioned, the frequency of the random fluctuations in magnetic field—governed by a substance's molecular motions—influence how the protons in a substance will behave during the scanning process, or more specifically, how they will relax after excitation. T1 relaxation occurs most efficiently when the frequency of this fluctuating field is near the Larmor frequency of the proton.[14-18,24] Just as resonance was needed for excitation, T1 relaxation is enhanced when the fluctuating field resonates with the precessing proton and provides the stimulus for movement of spins back to the spin-up state, thus promoting regrowth of longitudinal magnetization.[14] As shown in Figure 4-22, different tissues, based on their molecular motions, binding, and size, will relax at different rates depending on how close their natural motional frequencies or tumbling rates are to the Larmor frequency. The fat stores of adipose and marrow tissues, which are mostly triglycerides, have short T1 relaxation times because the motional frequencies of the carbons around the terminal C-C bond are quite close to the Larmor frequency. They therefore appear bright on a T1-weighted image (Figs. 4-23, *A*, and 4-24, *C* and *D*). Bulk-free water molecules are small and tumble rapidly, much faster than the Larmor frequency, and therefore have long relaxation times and appear dark on a T1-weighted image (Figure 4-24, *D*). On the opposite end of the scale, large macromolecules such as protein and membrane phospholipids (such as those found in myelin) are rigidly bound, making their motions much slower than the Larmor frequency; their T1 relaxation times are therefore also relatively long.[14,15]

Most cellular soft tissues have abundant surface area on organelles for intracellular binding of water.[27] Binding slows the molecular motions of water molecules, bringing the motions closer to the Larmor frequency relative to free water. Cellular tissues therefore have shorter T1 relaxation than water and appear gray (see Fig. 4-24, *C* and *D*) compared with pure fluids, which are dark gray to black on T1-weighted images.[27] Likewise, when fluids become bound to protein, as in mucin, water molecules become more structured and T1 relaxation is shortened (see Fig. 4-23, *A*).[15,24,27,28] Note that protein itself does not contribute to the MR signal,[27] but its presence in solutions shortens T1 relaxation[15,24,27,28] because the molecular motions of the water molecules are lowered to a rate closer to the Larmor frequency.[15,24,28]

T2 relaxation also depends on the frequencies of the fluctuating magnetic fields experienced by the protons of a substance (see Fig. 4-22) because these interactions contribute to dephasing. When motional frequencies are rapid, the magnetic fields "seen" by a proton fluctuate quite rapidly and effectively average, making the local environment homogeneous. This homogeneity of the field results in little dephasing.[14,15] This process is termed motional averaging and accounts for the long T2 relaxation times of bulk-free water.[14] Bulk-free water is therefore hyperintense on a T2-weighted image (see Fig. 4-24, *B*). On the other hand, rigidly bound substances tumbling much slower than the Larmor frequency are almost static and influence dephasing to a much greater degree; they are therefore associated with extremely short T2 relaxation times.[14,15] Macromolecules such as proteins and membrane phospholipids are examples of rigidly bound tissues. The phospholipids' protons behave differently from the protons in triglycerides of adipose tissue. If macromolecules and membrane phospholipids are isolated, their T2 relaxation times are so short that no signal is produced, so they are MR "invisible."[14,15] Myelin contains membrane phospholipids. The myelinated white matter of the brain has shorter T2 relaxation times and appears relatively dark compared with gray matter on a T2-weighted image (see Figs. 4-16 and 4-24, *A*). (White matter also has shorter T1 relaxation time than gray matter.[17,24,29]) Because the hydrogen protons in isolated phospholipids do not contribute to the MR signal or are MR invisible, the differences in signal intensity of white and gray matter have been attributed to the lower water content of white matter[17] and other mechanisms involving the immobilization of nearby water molecules by the lipid protons.[29]

Finally, note in Figure 4-22 that the molecules in the triglycerides of fat stores have intermediate T2 relaxation[15,24,28] and therefore have intermediate intensity on a T2-weighted image (see Figs 4-24, *A* and *B*, and 4-23, C).[24,28] The degree or intensity of fat's signal on T2-weighted images depends on the type of spin echo sequence used. The signal from fat is more intense on fast spin echo T2-weighted images compared with conventional spin-echo images.

Slice and Pixel Localization

Although the MR image has the same technical features (matrix, slice, voxels, and pixels) as other digital images such as CT, image construction is unique. MR imaging uses three encoding gradients that purposefully alter magnetic field strength (and therefore the Larmor frequencies) of protons in one of the three imaging axes and selective radiofrequency transmitting bandwidths to determine slice and pixel location. The process is summarized below, but this discussion begins with how gradients and selective RF bandwidths work.

A slice selection gradient is applied along the Z axis, for example, to produce transverse images, or slices, of the patient. This means that, in this example, the strength of the magnetic field is intentionally varied linearly along the Z direction. Typically, the center of the gradient is null, so no change in net magnetic field strength (and Larmor frequency) occurs in the center of the magnet when the gradient is turned on. Away from the center, the gradient's amplitude increases but with opposite polarity in opposite directions, so that the gradient field adds to or subtracts from the main magnetic field.[30] If a 1.5 T magnet is used, the field strength could be 1.5 T at the center but slightly more than 1.5 T at the head of the magnet and slightly less than 1.5 T at the foot of the magnet. Here is where the Larmor phenomenon becomes important. If an RF pulse at the Larmor frequency of hydrogen at 1.5 T (approximately 64 MHz) is transmitted, only those protons in a 1.5 T magnetic field (at the center of the magnet in this example) precessing at 64 MHz will undergo excitation as a result of the resonance phenomenon. Therefore only these protons (residing along the center slice) will contribute to the signal and image formation. Protons at other locations will not contribute to the image. This is just one example of how spatial information can be encoded into the MR image.

Because of the complexity of the echoes or signals, MR imaging uses a temporary data storage map called K space (Fig. 4-25)[31-33] and the mathematical tool known as Fourier transformation[31,34,35] (Fig. 4-26) to assign signal amplitudes to individual pixels within a slice. (Each image slice has its own K space.) Although K space sounds like a cosmic phenomenon, it is a manmade method of storing the numerous complex signals as a set of complex numbers eventually contributing to the image.[31] Each line of data is filled with the received echo for an entire image slice in an organized fashion; once the data are sampled, digitized, and mathematically converted to the spatial frequency domain, K space is formed.[33] Fourier transformation is then applied to K space to form the final image. Although the number of steps along an axis in K space is the same as the number of pixels along that axis in the image, no direct physical relation exists between individual points in K space and in the image. In fact, the center of K space provides information about signal and contrast throughout the image, and the periphery of K space provides information about spatial resolution.

The process for one image slice is summarized in the following steps and demonstrated in Video 4-3 on the Evolve site (http://evolve.elsevier.com/Thrall/vetrad/) and in Figures 4-19 and 4-25.

(1) A slice selection gradient (G_{ss}) is turned on to alter Larmor frequencies of protons along the Z axis in a graded linear fashion. An RF pulse whose frequency matches the

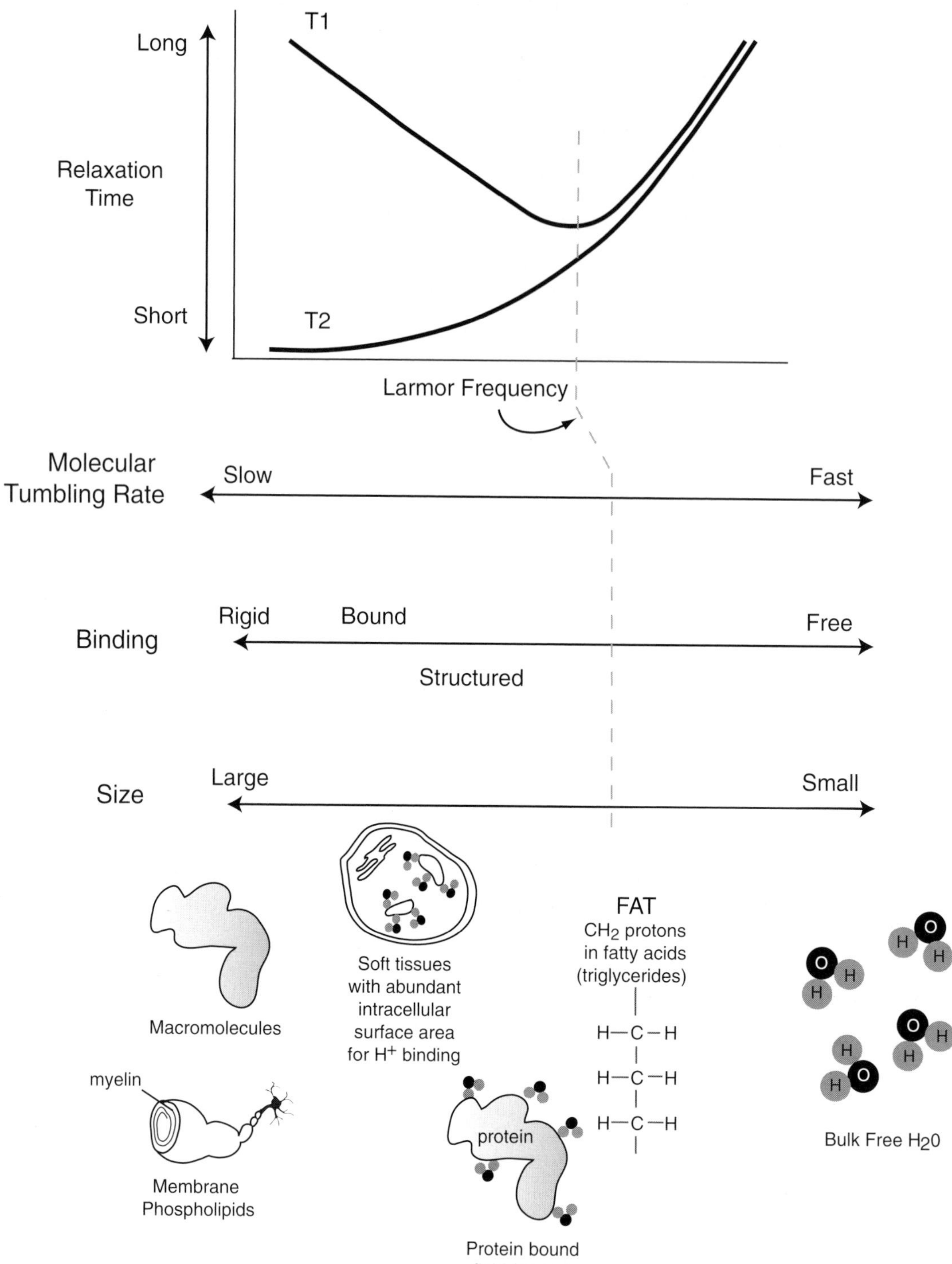

Fig. 4-22 Relation of T1 and T2 with various tissues differing in molecular motions, binding, and size. At the *bottom* are four different groups of tissues: bulk-free water, fat, structured or bound water in the form of cells and proteinaceous fluid, and rigidly bound large macromolecules and membrane phospholipids. At the right extreme are bulk water molecules that are small and free to tumble rapidly. At the left extreme are large macromolecules, such as proteins, and membrane phospholipids, which comprise myelin. These large molecules are rigidly bound, making their motions very slow. Between the extremes are the triglycerides of fat tissue, cells, and protein-bound substances. Fat molecules are intermediate in size and, because of the rotation of the terminal C-C bond, their molecular motions are close to the Larmor frequency *(dotted line)*. Following the *dotted line* up to the T1 and T2 curves shows that T1 relaxation is enhanced (shortened) if molecular motions are close to the Larmor frequency. This is why fat has such short T1 relaxation. Note also the relation of fat to the T2 curve. This illustrates that fat has intermediate T2 relaxation. When free water molecules become structured or bound, either to cell membranes and organelles or to macromolecules such as protein, their molecular motions are slowed. For this reason the water molecules in cells and proteinaceous or mucinous fluids have shorter T1 and T2 relaxation rates compared with bulk-free water molecules. This is evident by comparing their positions relative to the T1 and T2 curves.

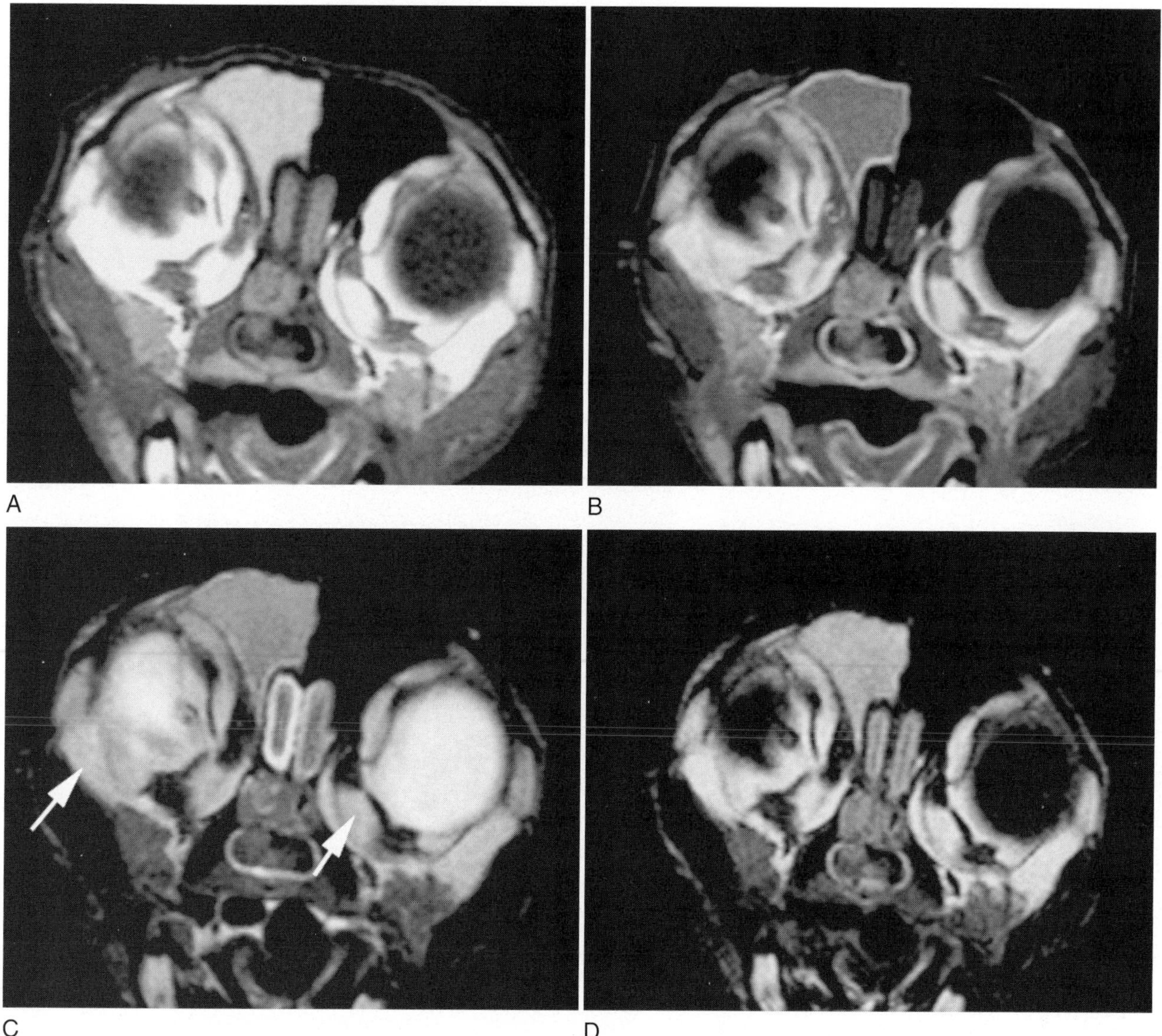

Fig. 4-23 Precontrast **(A)** and postcontrast **(B)** T1-weighted spin-echo, T2-weighted fast spin-echo **(C)**, and FLAIR **(D)** images of a cat with a nasal adenocarcinoma. Right is to the left side in each image. A portion of the tumor can be seen ventral to the olfactory lobes of the brain on all views. In the T2-weighted image **(C)**, the normal orbital fat *(arrows)* has intermediate intensity. The normal left frontal sinus appears as a signal void because no hydrogen protons are in the air. In the T1-weighted image **(A)** a mass appears to be in the right frontal sinus. After contrast medium administration **(B)**, no central enhancement is visible, but the lining of the sinus enhances; this indicates that the material in the sinus is not a mass but more likely fluid. Note, however, that the fluid is hyperintense to the vitreous of the eye in the T1-weighted images and hypointense to the vitreous in the T2-weighted image. These characteristics indicate that the fluid is protein bound because it has shorter T1 and T2 relaxation times than would be expected for pure simple fluid. In the FLAIR image **(D)** the presumed fluid does not attenuate, again indicating it is more likely to be proteinaceous. These are fairly characteristic intensities of protein-laden or mucinous fluids in the nasal and paranasal sinuses and tympanic bullae.

Larmor frequencies of the protons in the desired slice location is simultaneously applied to limit excitation to that slice. The thickness of the slice is determined by the range of frequencies in the transmitting radiofrequency bandwidth. All the protons within that slice will precess with the same frequency.

(2) The phase encoding gradient (G_{PE}) is turned on soon after the RF pulse to alter the frequencies for each row within the slice. As soon as the gradient is turned off, protons will resume precessing as before, but now each row of protons will have a different phase. This creates a phase shift between rows; the magnitude of this phase shift depends on the strength of the gradient.

(3) During the echo, the frequency encoding gradient (G_{FE}) is turned on to alter Larmor frequencies for each column within the slice. Protons in each pixel in the slice now

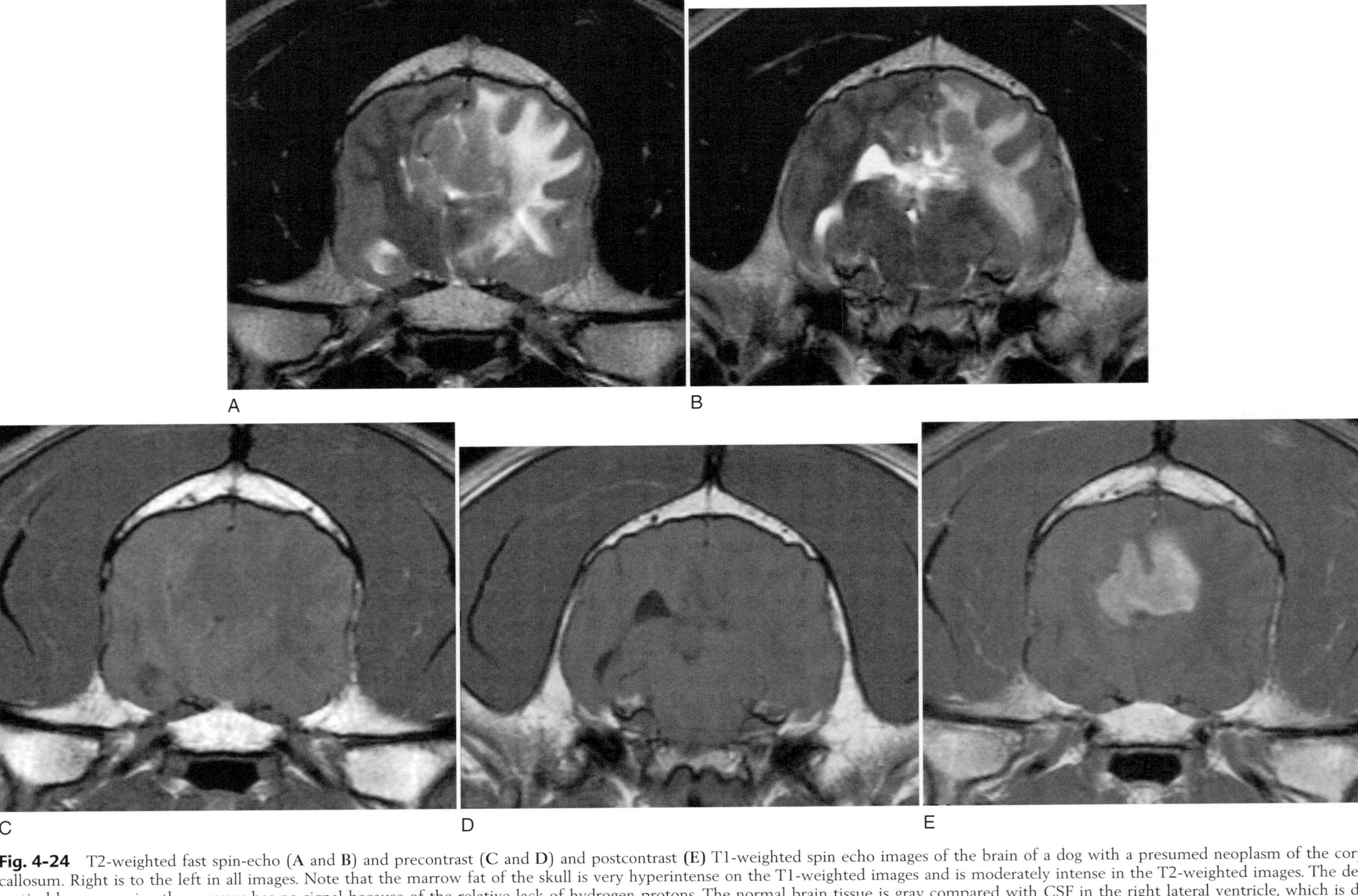

Fig. 4-24 T2-weighted fast spin-echo (**A** and **B**) and precontrast (**C** and **D**) and postcontrast **(E)** T1-weighted spin echo images of the brain of a dog with a presumed neoplasm of the corpus callosum. Right is to the left in all images. Note that the marrow fat of the skull is very hyperintense on the T1-weighted images and is moderately intense in the T2-weighted images. The dense cortical bone covering the marrow has no signal because of the relative lack of hydrogen protons. The normal brain tissue is gray compared with CSF in the right lateral ventricle, which is dark gray or black in the T1-weighted image **(D)**. CSF, a form of free fluid, is very hyperintense in the lateral ventricle in the T2-weighted image **(B)**. In the T2-weighted images, the normal myelinated white matter of the right cerebrum is hypointense to the gray matter. Vasogenic edema is also present in the left cerebral white matter. This has prolonged T1 and T2 relaxation times, making the white matter hypointense on T1-weighted images and hyperintense on T2-weighted images. In **A** and **C,** noncontrast images, the borders of the mass are difficult to distinguish from the white matter vasogenic edema in the left cerebrum. However, with the use of gadolinium **(E),** marked enhancement of the mass appears, consistent with vascularization and lack of a functional blood-brain barrier. The gadolinium shortens the T1 relaxation time of protons in the mass, leading to a drastic increase in signal.

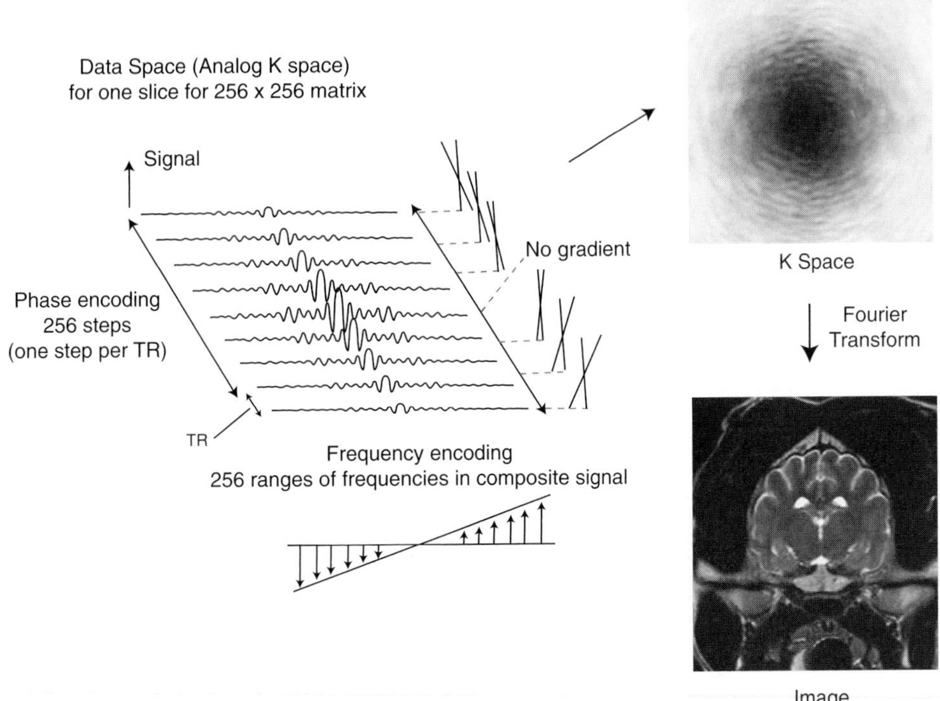

Fig. 4-25 Data space, K space for one image having a 256 × 256 matrix. K space is a temporary data storage map for the numerous complex echoes collected from the patient for one image slice. True K space is filled with signals that have been digitized and mathematically converted to the spatial frequency domain. However, illustration of the process of image reconstruction is easier with an analog version called data space. Each line of data space is filled with the received signal in an organized fashion. Although the number of steps along an axis in the K space image (in this example, 256) is the same as the number of pixels along that axis in the final image, no direct physical relation exists between individual points in the two images. For the initial steps of spatial encoding, refer to Video 4-3 (http://evolve.elsevier.com/Thrall/vetrad). During the application of the frequency encoding gradient, the MR receiver samples or takes discrete measurements of the echo signal induced in the receiver coil. In this example, 256 ranges of frequencies are in the frequency-encoding direction and 256 samples are obtained. Unlike the process in the phase direction, only one gradient strength is used for encoding in the frequency direction. This is indicated by the single gradient along the frequency-encoding direction at the bottom of the data space map. Typically, the first readout of the echo is performed with no phase-encoding gradient. This signal fills the center line of data space. Then the entire process is repeated for every TR and echo, but each time with a different gradient strength in the phase direction. Changes in gradient strength in the phase direction are depicted by the tall *Xs* on the right of the data space map. The phase shifts between rows created for every TR (review Video 4-3 if necessary [http://evolve.elsevier.com/Thrall/vetrad]) will alter the signal that is received during readout of corresponding echoes. Note that a single conglomerate echo signal is recorded from the entire slice for each phase-encoding step. These echoes are represented in the data space map as the squiggly waveforms. The echoes for each TR are continually stored along the 256 lines of K space in the phase axis until K space is filled. Because the composite signals are complex and contain numerous frequencies, Fourier transformation is needed to decipher the signal amplitudes or intensities for each range of frequencies to assign the proper signal amplitudes to the proper pixels. When K space is transformed by Fourier transformation, the final image is constructed.

precess at a frequency determined by the G_{FE} and with phases determined by the G_{PE}.

(4) While the G_{FE} is being applied, the MR receiver samples or measures the echo signal induced in the receiver coil. This sampled composite signal is therefore composed of numerous frequencies.

(5) Once the sampled signal is digitized and mathematically converted to a map in the spatial frequency domain, one line of K space is filled.

(6) The entire process is repeated for every TR and echo, but each time with a different gradient strength in the phase direction. The phase shifts between rows created by the different phase gradients alter the signal that is received during readout of corresponding echoes. (Note that a single conglomerate echo signal is recorded from the entire slice for each phase encoding step.[31]) The signals for each TR are continually stored along the lines of K space in the phase axis until K space is filled. The location that the signal is placed along

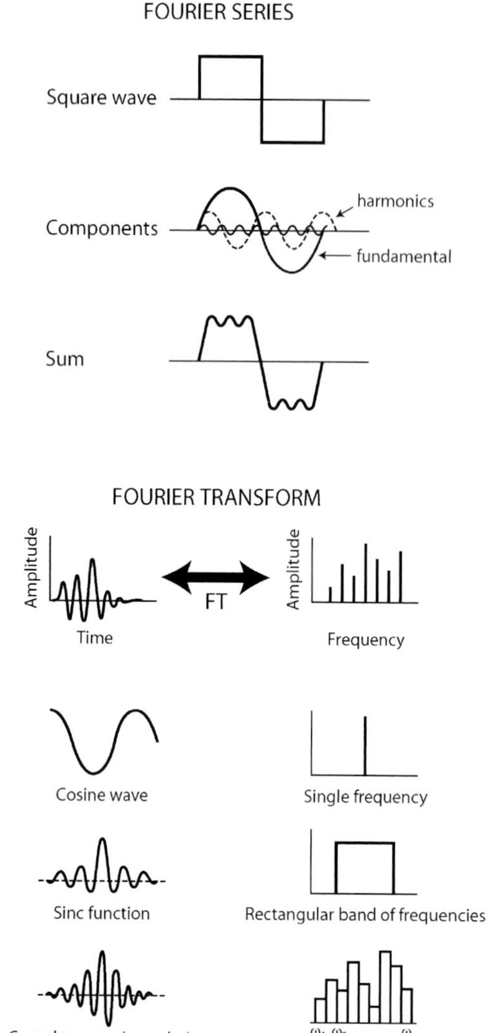

Fig. 4-26 The Fourier series *(top)* and the Fourier transform *(bottom)*. The Fourier series is the breakdown of a periodic wave into a series of harmonically related sine or cosine waves. Harmonics are integer multiples (two times, three times, etc.) of the lowest or fundamental frequency. In this example, a square wave is broken into its harmonic components, which can be summed to re-form an approximation of the square wave. Fourier transformation allows a signal in the time domain (i.e., relating amplitude over time) to be transformed to the frequency domain (i.e., relating amplitude over frequency). The Fourier transformation of a cosine or sine wave is a single frequency, whereas most signals are transformed into a spectrum or range of frequencies. The Fourier transformation of a sinc function is a rectangular band of frequencies; because the rectangle has the ideal geometry for MR image slices, many RF pulses are sinc functions. The most important application of Fourier transformation in the MR process is to decipher the amplitudes of the various frequencies in the composite echo signals stored in K space *(bottom transform)*. This allows the appropriate signal intensities or amplitudes to be localized to appropriate pixels in the final image.

the phase-encoding direction of K space will depend on the strength of the G_{PE} for a given RF pulse and echo. When no gradient is used, the signal is typically placed in the center line of K space.

(7) Recall that TR is the time between two successive RF excitation pulses and is therefore the time necessary to run through the pulse sequence one time. The number of times the encoding process, and therefore the pulse sequence, must be repeated depends on the number of rows of data (in the phase axis) needed to reconstruct the image. For example, if 256 rows are desired, the pulse sequence must be repeated 256 times.[36]

(8) Because the composite signals are complex and contain numerous frequencies, Fourier transformation is needed to decipher the signal amplitudes or intensities for each range of frequencies. The concept behind Fourier transformation is that a complex wave can be broken into its individual component frequencies. For example, in music, although a note will be heard as a certain pitch, the sound is actually composed of multiple frequencies, the fundamental frequency and its harmonics. In Figure 4-26, the Fourier series is the breakdown of a periodic wave (in this example, a square wave) into a series of harmonically related sine or cosine waves.[35] Fourier transform allows a signal in the time domain (i.e., relating amplitude over time) to be transformed to the frequency domain (i.e., relating amplitude over frequency).[31,35] The Fourier transformation of a cosine or sine wave is a single frequency, whereas most signals are transformed into a spectrum or range of frequencies.[31,35] Recall, in step 4 above, that G_{FE} application and echo sampling occur simultaneously. This permits a direct correlation between the frequencies in the received signal and the protons' position along the frequency encoding direction. However, because the echo was stored in K space as a single conglomerate or composite signal, Fourier transformation is required to determine the amplitudes for each range of frequencies in that composite signal. Fourier transformation therefore allows the appropriate signal intensities or amplitudes to be localized to appropriate pixels in the final image. Thus, the Fourier transformation of K space is the final image (see Fig. 4-25).

(9) Finally, the signal intensities determine brightness or gray levels for each pixel in the image, as viewed on the monitor (see Fig. 4-1).

Interpretation: Bringing It Back to Reality

Because tissue contrast in MR imaging is multifactorial, a single or universal gray scale cannot be applied to the images.[17] Interpretation of signal intensities is therefore not amenable to simple generalizations. Nevertheless, some basic rules of thumb should serve both novice and seasoned interpreters of MR images fairly well.

(1) Substances having minimal or no hydrogen protons have no signal. These include gas, dense cortical bone, calcification, fibrous tissue, implanted materials and, in some instances, rapidly flowing blood.[28] Arterial blood vessels will appear as a signal void on spin-echo images because the blood does not stay in the slice long enough to create an echo. The lack of signal in the dense cortical bone of the skull and the air of the frontal sinus is illustrated in Figures 4-24 and 4-23, respectively.

(2) Fluid and solid, but "juicy" water-based tissues (edema, necrosis, inflammation, and many tumors) have opposite intensities on T1-weighted compared with T2-weighted images (see Fig. 4-24, *A-D*).

(3) Fat stores often do not have opposite intensities on T1-weighted compared with T2-weighted images. In other words, although fat appears very bright on T1-weighted images, it may not appear very dark on T2-weighted images, instead

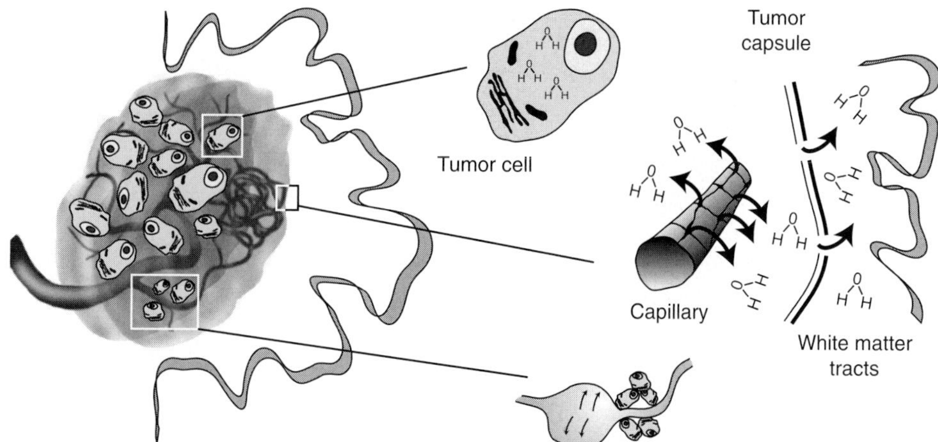

Fig. 4-27 Causes of prolonged relaxation times associated with a brain tumor. This figure corresponds to the suspected tumor in the dog of Figure 4-24. The tumor and surrounding white matter have prolonged relaxation, most likely because of an increase in intracellular and extracellular free (unbound) water. The tumor has large, disorganized cells, with disrupted organelle membranes that have released their intracellular water molecules. Hypervascularization of the mass is present from the tumor angiogenesis. Tumor vessels are known to have a nonfunctional or poorly functional blood-brain barrier, so water leaks from the capillaries into the tumor and across the capsule into the adjacent white matter tracts, causing vasogenic edema. Cell growth inside a confined space occludes or compresses vessels, leading to further leakage of fluid from capillaries. As seen in Figure 4-24, prolonged relaxation times cause the abnormalities to appear hyperintense on a T2-weighted image and hypointense on a T1-weighted image.

appearing intermediate gray (see Figs. 4-24, *A* and *B*, and 4-23, C). This is especially evident in fast spin-echo T2-weighted images. The simple explanation for this observation is that fat in adipose stores has short T1 but intermediate T2 relaxation rates.[15,24,28]

(4) Most solid, but "juicy" water-based tissues have long relaxation times.[15] Because these lesions are hyperintense against a background of darker normal tissues on a T2-weighted image and are usually fairly conspicuous, T2-weighted images are often called "pathology" scans[13] whereas T1-weighted images are considered better "anatomy" scans.

(5) Many soft tissue tumors are "juicy" because they have more intracellular and extracellular unbound water. Tumor cells are often larger and disorganized, with cell and organelle membranes releasing their bound intracellular water molecules (Fig. 4-27).[27,28] Often poor lymphatic drainage creates more extracellular or interstitial fluid.[37] Tumor angiogenesis leads to increased vascularization[38]; these vessels may be compressed or occluded by cells growing in a confined space, causing transudation from increased pressure (see Fig. 4-27).[37] Likewise, cellular hypoxia may lead to poor osmotic regulation. In neural tissue, tumor capillaries are often more permeable because of the lack of a functional blood-brain barrier.[38] This causes vasogenic edema, which often migrates down adjacent white matter tracts (Figs. 4-24, *A-D*, and 4-27). The loss of the blood-brain barrier is responsible for contrast enhancement of the vascularized portions of the lesion (Fig. 4-24, *E*).

(6) A contrast medium enhanced lesion appears bright on both CT and T1-weighted MR images. Be aware, however, that the mechanism of contrast enhancement in the two modalities is different. A lesion enhances when its altered vascularity allows the contrast medium to accumulate after intravenous injection. On a CT image, a lesion appears bright because of increased attenuation of x-rays by the accumulated iodinated contrast medium. With MR imaging, paramagnetic gadolinium-based agents have no signal of their own, but instead increase the relaxation efficiency of the protons in solution and cause shortening of T1 and T2 relaxation. At the low concentrations found in tissues with gadolinium accumulation, T1 shortening predominates, so enhancing lesions appear bright on T1-weighted images. Occasionally lesions do not have a signal intensity that differs significantly from adjacent normal tissue on noncontrast images or their boundaries are obscured by surrounding edema (see Fig. 4-24, *A* and C). After administration of contrast medium, however, the lesion becomes conspicuous (see Fig. 4-24, *E*).

(7) If a substance is hyperintense on a T1-weighted image, it usually contains either fat, gadolinium contrast medium, blood clot or hematoma containing methemoglobin, or melanin, or it is protein bound.

(8) Protein bound or mucinous fluids do not behave as simple fluids; that is, they have shorter T1 relaxation. They appear hyperintense on T1-weighted images when compared with simple fluids and do not fully attenuate on FLAIR images. Mucinous fluids are frequently found in the nasal and paranasal sinuses (see Fig. 4-23) or tympanic bullae.

(9) Brain hemorrhage can be identified earlier on T2*- or susceptibility-weighted gradient-echo images than on spin-echo images. Within a few hours of the onset of bleeding, deoxyhemoglobin causes susceptibility losses so the hematoma will appear black on T2*-weighted images.[26] Although deoxyhemoglobin is paramagnetic, it will not cause a hematoma to appear bright on a T1-weighted spin-echo image; conversion to methemoglobin in the subacute stage (a few days after the onset of bleeding) is required for T1 shortening to occur (Figs. 4-28 and 4-29).

(10) Inversion recovery pulse sequences suppress pure fluid (with FLAIR) or fat (with STIR), but they have the added benefit of depicting solid, "juicy" lesions as hyperintense.[39] The heavy T2-weighting of FLAIR images allows improved conspicuity of such hyperintensities (Fig. 4-30),[40] especially around sulci and in the periventricular white matter. The other use of a FLAIR sequence is to distinguish cystic (low signal) from solid "juicy" tissues (high signal). On

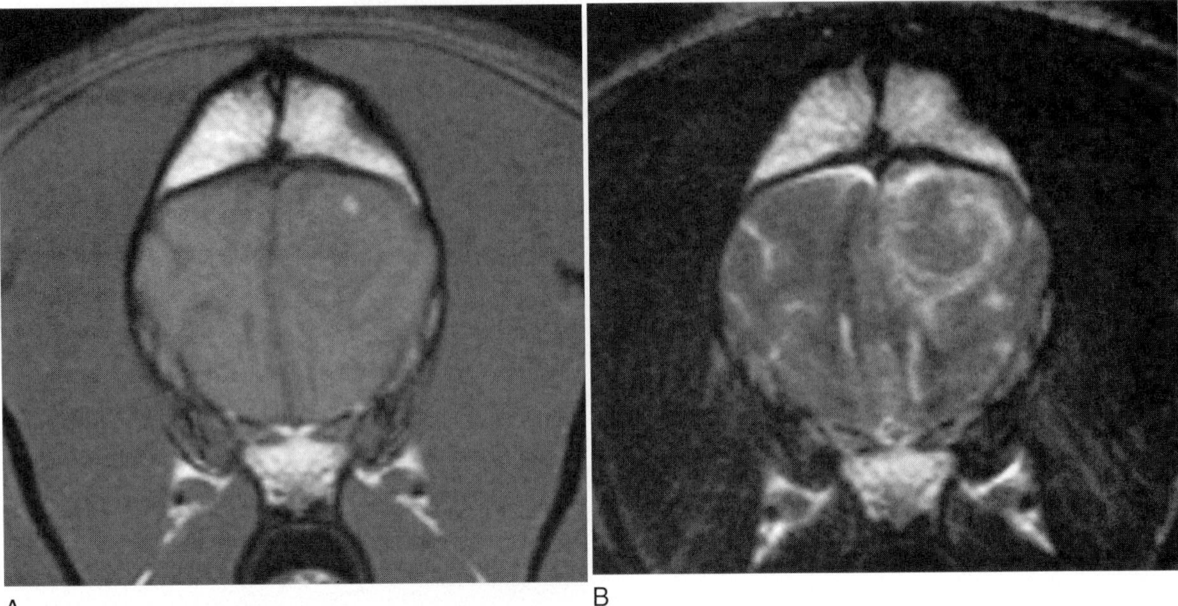

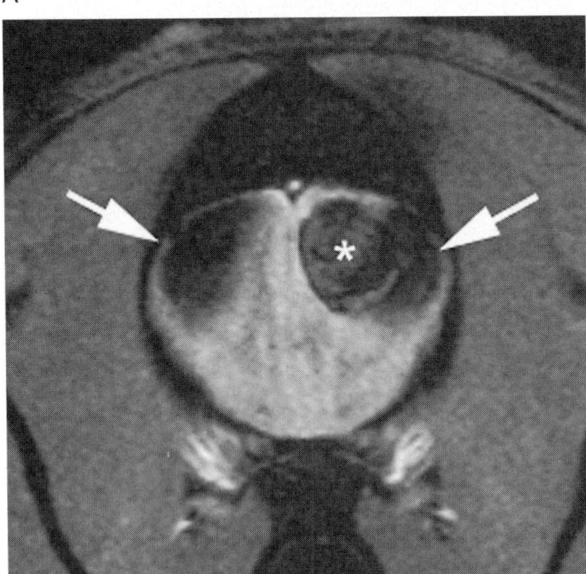

Fig. 4-28 T1-weighted spin-echo (**A**), T2-weighted fast spin-echo (**B**), and T2*-weighted gradient-echo (**C**, flip angle 20, TE = 26) images in a dog with acute seizures occurring within 2 days of the MR images. A mass is present in the left frontal lobe that is inhomogeneously hypointense to normal brain, with surrounding hyperintense edema on the T2-weighted spin-echo image. The mass is slightly hypointense to isointense to normal brain on the T1-weighted image, although a faint hyperintensity is also noted. In the gradient-echo image the mass appears as a signal void *(asterisk)* because of susceptibility loss, most likely attributable to the presence of hemorrhage with its attendant magnetic properties. (Also note the bilateral signal void artifacts *[arrows]* caused by the magnetically inhomogeneous tissue-frontal sinus interface.) Based on the T2*-weighted images, a hematoma was suspected. The time course and the spin-echo images suggested it to be in the deoxyhemoglobin stage, with some conversion to methemoglobin suspected because of the hyperintensity on the T1-weighted image. On follow-up MR images 2 months later, the lesion was smaller. The dog died for unrelated reasons and a postmortem confirmed the presence of a resolving hemorrhagic stroke (hematoma) and the absence of neoplasia.

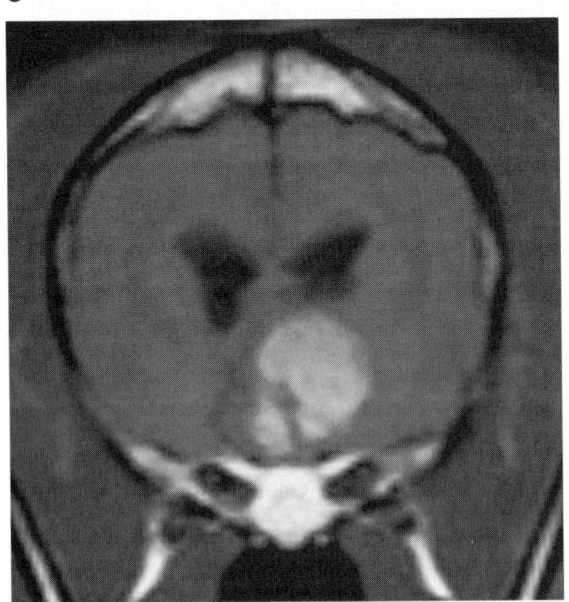

Fig. 4-29 Noncontrast T1-weighted spin-echo image in a dog with a postmortem diagnosis of pituitary adenocarcinoma with hemorrhage. The mass is hyperintense, indicating shortened T1 relaxation time, most likely caused by methemoglobin within blood clot in the tumor.

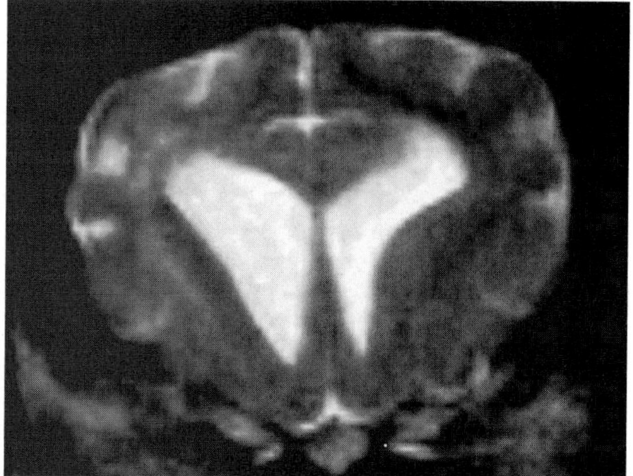

A

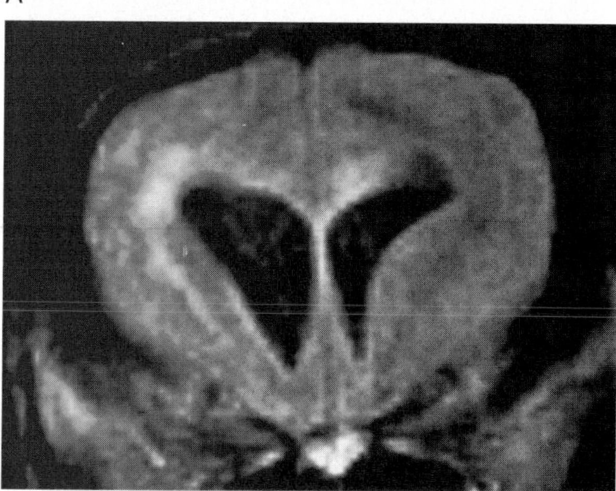

B

Fig. 4-30 T2-weighted fast spin-echo (A) and FLAIR (B) images in a Yorkshire Terrier with necrotizing leukoencephalitis. Note the attenuated CSF in the ventricles on the FLAIR image and how the periventricular white matter hyperintensities are more conspicuous. FLAIR images are usually more heavily T2 weighted than spin-echo images because longer TEs are used, thereby increasing lesion signal intensity. Note how partial volume averaging produces a "smeared" appearance of the sulci on the spin-echo image. Because fluid is attenuated on the FLAIR image, the artifact is eliminated, helping raise the conspicuity of the lesions.

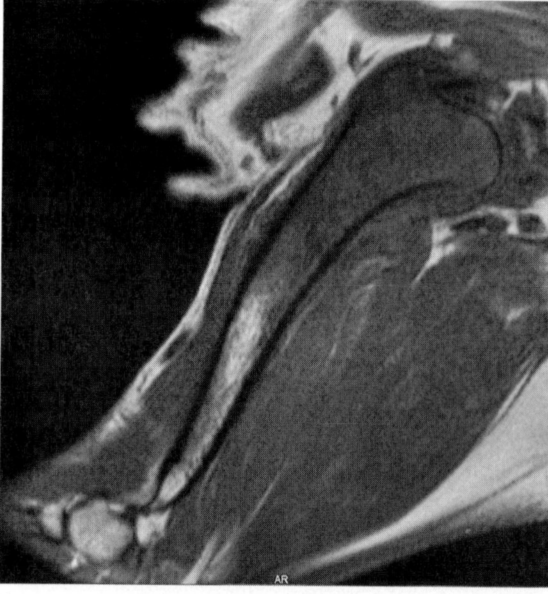

A

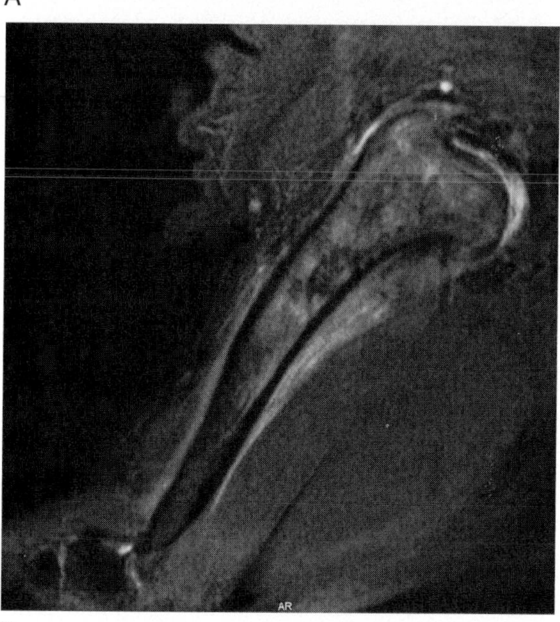

B

Fig. 4-31 Noncontrast T1-weighted spin-echo (A) and STIR (B) image of the humerus of a dog with osteosarcoma. On the T1-weighted image, the normally hyperintense marrow fat in the proximal half of the humerus has been replaced by tumor, leading to reduced signal in this area. In the STIR image, the signal from the normal marrow fat of the distal humerus and subcutaneous tissues has been suppressed, with the tumor appearing inhomogeneous but predominantly hyperintense. Also note the hyperintense periosteal response along the entire shaft that was not seen in the T1-weighted noncontrast image. Clearly the STIR image was more valuable for assessing the extent of the tumor than the T1-weighted spin-echo image.

STIR images, hyperintense fluid or "juicy" lesions are conspicuous because the signals from background fat are suppressed. STIR pulse sequences are especially useful to screen for tumors and evaluate lesions in the bone marrow (Fig. 4-31), optic cone, and fascial regions.

(11) Use chemical fat saturation pulses to make gadolinium contrast-enhanced (hyperintense) lesions more conspicuous. If the background fat (which is also hyperintense) in a postcontrast T1-weighted image is not suppressed, an enhancing lesion may become lost in the surrounding fat. By suppressing the signal from fat, any tissue maintaining an intense signal in the image will contain gadolinium (e.g., contrast-enhancing tumors, vessels [Fig. 4-32]). Fat saturation pulses are occasionally used to suppress fat in noncontrast T1-, PD-, and T2-weighted images and may be used to confirm the fatty composition of a substance. In other words, if a substance is suppressed by this method, it is fat, assuming the technique worked properly.

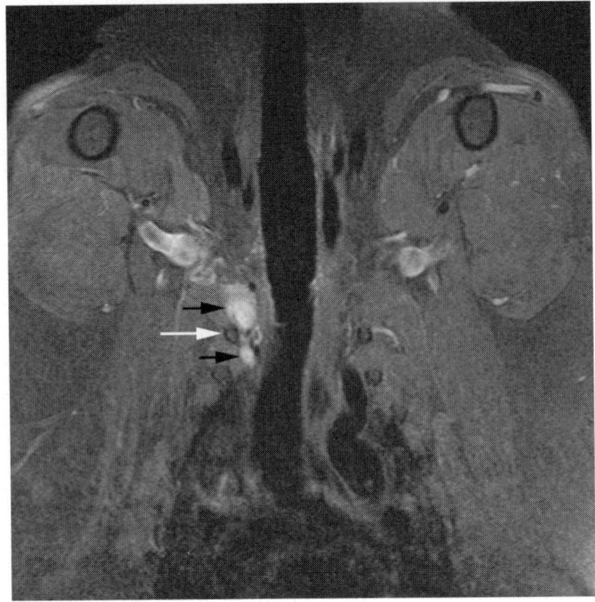

Fig. 4-32 Dorsal plane postcontrast T1-weighted image, with chemical fat saturation, of the brachial plexus region of a dog with a nerve sheath tumor involving the right C8 (cranial *black arrow*) and T1 (caudal *black arrow*) nerves on each side of the first rib *(white arrow)*. Note how the fat saturation technique has suppressed background fat, leaving only the gadolinium-enhancing tumor and vessels to appear hyperintense.

REFERENCES

1. Bushberg JT, Seibert JA, Leideholt EM et al: Introduction to medical imaging. In Bushberg JT, Seibert JA, Leidholt EM et al, editors: *The essential physics of medical imaging,* ed 2, Philadelphia, 2002, Lippincott Williams & Wilkins, p 1-15.
2. Curry TS, Dowdey JE, Murry RC: Attenuation. In Curry TS, Dowdey JE, Murry RC, editors: *Christensen's physics of diagnostic radiology,* ed 4, Philadelphia, 1990, Lea and Febiger, p 70-86.
3. Seeram E: Computed tomography. In Seeram E, editor: *Computed tomography physical principles, clinical applications, and quality control,* ed 2, Philadelphia, 2001, WB Saunders, p 1-19.
4. Kalender WA: Principles of computed tomography. In Kalender WA, editor: *Computed tomography fundamentals, system technology, image quality, applications,* Erlangen, 2005, Publicis Corporate Publishing, p 1-35.
5. Curry TS, Dowdey JE, Murry RC: Computed tomography. In Curry TS, Dowdey JE, Murry RC, editors: *Christensen's physics of diagnostic radiology,* ed 4, Philadelphia, 1990, Lea and Febiger, p 289-322.
6. Berland LL: Selectable scan factors: routine scanning. In Berland LL, editor: *Practical CT technology and techniques,* New York, 1987, Raven Press, p 45-69.
7. Seeram E: Physical principles of computed tomography. In Seeram E, editor: *Computed tomography physical principles, clinical applications, and quality control,* ed 2, Philadelphia, 2001, WB Saunders, p 59-74.
8. Berland LL: Image creation and refinement. In Berland LL, editor: Practical CT technology and techniques, New York, 1987, Raven Press, p 77-87.
9. Parizel PM, Makkat S, Van Miert E et al: Intracranial hemorrhage: principles of CT and MRI interpretation, *Eur Radiol* 11:1770, 2001.
10. Woodruff WW: Anatomy and general approach. In Woodruff WW, editor: *Fundamentals of neuroimaging,* Philadelphia, 1993, WB Saunders, p 33-70.
11. Morandi F, Mattoon JS, Lakritz J et al: Correlation of helical and incremental high- resolution thin-section computed tomographic imaging with histomorphometric quantitative evaluation of lungs in dogs, *Am J Vet Res* 64:935, 2003.
12. Bushberg JT, Seibert JA, Leideholt EM et al: Nuclear magnetic resonance. In Bushberg JT, Seibert JA, Leidholt EM et al, editors: *The essential physics of medical imaging,* ed 2, Philadelphia, 2002, Lippincott Williams & Wilkins, p 373-413.
13. McRobbie DW, Moore EA, Graves MJ et al: Seeing is believing: introduction to image contrast. In McRobbie DW, Moore EA, Graves MJ et al, editors: *MRI from picture to proton,* Cambridge, 2003, Cambridge University Press, p 27-45.
14. McRobbie DW, Moore EA, Graves MJ et al: Getting in tune: resonance and relaxation. In McRobbie DW, Moore EA, Graves MJ et al, editors: *MRI from picture to proton,* Cambridge, 2003, Cambridge University Press, p 135-163.
15. Elster AD, Burdette JH: Introduction to nuclear magnetic resonance. In Elster AD, Burdette JH, editors: *Questions and answers in magnetic resonance imaging,* ed 2, St Louis, 2001, Mosby, p 19-53.
16. Gore JC, Kennan RP: Contrast agents and relaxation effects. In Atlas SW, editor: *Magnetic resonance imaging of the brain and spine,* ed 2, Philadelphia, 1996, Lippincott and Raven, p 89-107.
17. Wehrli FW, McGowan JC: The basis of MR contrast. In Atlas SW, editor: *Magnetic resonance imaging of the brain and spine,* ed 2, Philadelphia, 1996, Lippincott and Raven, p 29-48
18. Weisskoff RM, Edelman RR: Basic principles of MRI. In Edelman RR, Hesselink JR, Zlatkin MB, editors: *Clinical magnetic resonance imaging,* ed 2, Philadelphia, 1996, WB Saunders, p 3-51.
19. Pipe JG: Basic spin physics, *MRI Clin North Am* 7:607, 1999.
20. Lufkin RB: Magnetic resonance physics. In Lufkin RB, editor: *The MRI manual,* ed 2, St Louis, 1998, Mosby, p 3-19.
21. Hashemi RH, Bradley WG: Radiofrequency pulse. In Hashemi RH, Bradley WG, editors: *MRI the basics,* Baltimore, 1997, Williams & Wilkins, p 32-40.
22. Mitchell DG, Cohen MS: From protons to images. In Mitchell DG, Cohen MS, editors: *MRI principles,* ed 2, Philadelphia, 2004, Saunders, p 9-20.
23. Hashemi RH, Bradley WG: Basic principles of MRI. In Hashemi RH, Bradley WG, editors: *MRI the basics,* Baltimore, 1997, Williams & Wilkins, p 17-31.
24. Hashemi RH, Bradley WG: Tissue contrast: some clinical applications. In Hashemi RH, Bradley WG, editors: *MRI the basics,* Baltimore, 1997, Williams & Wilkins, p 32-40.
25. Hashemi RH, Bradley WG: T1, T2, and T2*. In Hashemi RH, Bradley WG, editors: *MRI the basics,* Baltimore, 1997, Williams & Wilkins, p 41-48.
26. Patel MR, Edelman RR, Warach S: Detection of hyperacute primary intraparenchymal hemorrhage by magnetic resonance imaging, *Stroke* 27:2321, 1996.
27. Mitchell DG, Cohen MS: Proton environments and T1 relaxation. In Mitchell DG, Cohen MS, editors: *MRI principles,* ed 2, Philadelphia, 2004, Saunders, p 21-33.
28. Lufkin RB: Magnetic resonance contrast mechanisms. In Lufkin RB, editor: *The MRI manual,* ed 2, St Louis, 1998, Mosby, p 21-40.

29. Edwards-Brown MK, Bonnin JM: White matter diseases. In Atlas SW, editor: *Magnetic resonance imaging of the brain and spine,* ed 2, Philadelphia, 1996, Lippincott and Raven, p 649-706.
30. Bushberg JT, Seibert JA, Leideholt EM et al: Magnetic resonance imaging, In Bushberg JT, Seibert JA, Leidholt EM et al, editors: *The essential physics of medical imaging,* ed 2, Philadelphia, 2002, Lippincott Williams & Wilkins, p 415-467.
31. Elster AD, Burdette JH: Making a picture. In Elster AD, Burdette JH, editors: *Questions and answers in magnetic resonance imaging,* ed 2, St. Louis, 2001, Mosby, p 72-101.
32. McRobbie DW, Moore EA, Graves MJ et al: The devil's in the detail: pixels, matrices and slices. In McRobbie DW, Moore EA, Graves MJ, et al, editors: *MRI from picture to proton,* Cambridge, 2003, Cambridge University Press, p 46-62.
33. Hashemi RH, Bradley WG: Data space. In Hashemi RH, Bradley WG, editors: *MRI the basics,* Baltimore, 1997, Williams & Wilkins, p 137-154.
34. McRobbie DW, Moore EA, Graves MJ et al: Spaced out: spatial encoding. In McRobbie DW, Moore EA, Graves MJ, et al, editors: *MRI from picture to proton,* Cambridge, 2003, Cambridge University Press, p 106-134.
35. Hashemi RH, Bradley WG: Fourier transform. In Hashemi RH, Bradley WG, editors: *MRI the basics,* Baltimore, 1997, Williams & Wilkins, p 82-87.
36. Pooley RA: AAPM/RSNA physics tutorial for residents: fundamental physics for MR imaging, *Radiographics* 25:1087, 2005.
37. Steen RG: Edema and tumor perfusion: characterization by quantitative ^{1}H MR imaging, *AJR* 158:259, 1992.
38. DelMaestro RF: Angiogenesis. In Berger MS, Wilson CB, editors: *The gliomas,* Philadelphia, 1999, WB Saunders, p 87-106.
39. Elster AD, Burdette JH: Miscellaneous advanced MR imaging techniques. In Elster AD, Burdette JH, editors: *Questions and answers in magnetic resonance imaging,* ed 2, St Louis, 2001, Mosby, p 235-247.
40. DeCoene B, Hajnal JV, Gatehouse P et al: MR of the brain using fluid-attenuated inversion recovery (FLAIR) pulse sequences, *Am J Neuroradiol* 13:1555, 1992.

ELECTRONIC RESOURCES evolve

Additional information related to the content in Chapter 4 can be found on the companion Web site at evolve http://evolve.elsevier.com/Thrall/vetrad/

- Key Points
- Chapter Quiz
- Video 4-1: Example of soft-tissue windowing in the abdomen and lung windowing in the thorax
- Video 4-2: Rotation of main magnetic vector into X-Y plane
- Video 4-3: Example of spatial signal encoding within one image slice

CHAPTER • 5
Introduction to Radiographic Interpretation

Clifford R. Berry
Donald E. Thrall

X-RAYS AND RADIOGRAPHS

A radiograph is possible because of the ability of x-rays to penetrate matter. When a patient is struck by an x-ray beam, some x-rays are absorbed, some are scattered, and others pass through unchanged (see Chapter 1). Therefore a radiograph is an image of the number and distribution of x-rays that pass through the patient and strike the cassette. Production of a digital radiographic image follows these same principles, but in this chapter the emphasis is on film-screen systems. Principles of digital imaging are covered in Chapter 2. Jargon terms such as *x-ray, film, plate,* and *picture* are sometimes used as names for a radiograph, but this is incorrect and should be avoided.

The blackness of a radiograph depends on the amount of light emitted by the intensifying screen; light production is related to the number of x-rays striking the cassette and intensifying screen. Areas of the film exposed to a large number of light photons are black (radiolucent) after film processing. Conversely, areas struck by fewer light photons are translucent or appear white (radiopaque). Between these two extremes is a range of gray film tones, the blackness of which is directly related to the number of x-rays that penetrate the patient and reach the intensifying screen (Figs. 5-1 and 5-2).

The degree of blackening of the film is measured in terms of optical density. Optical density, also called film blackness, is directly related to the x-ray exposure of the cassette (Fig. 5-3). The term *density* is sometimes used to describe the degree to which a patient or object absorbs incident x-rays. For example, in Figure 5-2, some would say that the bones and fishhook foreign objects are more dense than adjacent soft tissue. Use of density in this context is confusing because the *optical* density of the bones and fishhooks is low, whereas the *radiographic* density is high. Further confusion arises when the added variable of physical density (in grams per cubic centimeter) of the patient or object is considered. As the physical density of the patient or object increases, the optical film density decreases and the radiographic density increases. This confusing terminology can be eliminated by avoiding use of the term *density* to describe radiographic changes (Fig. 5-4). The degree of blackness or whiteness of the patient should be referred to in terms of radiolucency or radiopacity. For example, in Figure 5-2, soft tissues of the coelom are less radiopaque than the bones; both are more radiolucent than the fishhooks. It may also be said that the fishhooks are more radiopaque than the remainder of the turtle. Describing radiographic appearance in terms of one of five radiographic opacities—air, fat, water, bone, and metal—would eliminate the confusion associated with use of the word density.

IMAGE FORMATION AND DIFFERENTIAL ABSORPTION

X-rays can produce an image of a patient on film because some x-rays are absorbed by the patient and some pass through unchanged, thus producing film blackening (see Fig. 5-1). Of particular importance is the fact that x-rays are not absorbed homogeneously by the body, but differentially depending on the makeup of the tissue. If absorption of x-rays were uniform, the resulting radiographic image would be homogeneously gray or white. If no absorption occurred, the resulting radiograph would be homogeneously black. The effect of differential absorption is illustrated in Figure 5-2, in which areas peripheral to the turtle are black because no x-rays were absorbed before reaching the intensifying screen. Soft tissues of the turtle are visible because they have absorbed some x-rays from the primary beam. Bones of the turtle are more radiopaque than soft tissues; the bones have absorbed more x-rays, and thus that part of the intensifying screen under the bones was struck by fewer x-rays than the areas of the turtle adjacent to the bones. The fishhooks are nearly totally radiopaque because essentially no x-rays were able to pass through them. The degree of differential absorption of x-rays by a patient or an object depends on the energy of the x-rays and the composition of the patient or object, as discussed in detail in Chapter 1.

IMPORTANCE OF TISSUE COMPOSITION

X-ray absorption by a body part is determined by the effective atomic number of its elements and the physical density of the object being radiographed (Table 5-1). The effect of tissue composition on x-ray absorption allows radiographic images of patients to be produced. Based on the relationship between the absorption of x-rays, physical density, and effective atomic number, the substances in Table 5-1 may be ranked in order of increasing radiopacity. Even though the effective atomic number of air is higher than that of fat, air is the most radiolucent because of its low physical density (i.e., fewer molecules per unit area absorb x-rays). If air were compressed until its physical density equaled that of fat, it would be more radiopaque because of its higher atomic number.

The next most radiopaque substance is fat. Although the effective atomic number of fat is less than that of air, its physical density is greater, making fat more radiopaque. Next, consider the physical density and effective atomic number of water and muscle. Theoretically, muscle should be more radiopaque than water because of its higher physical density

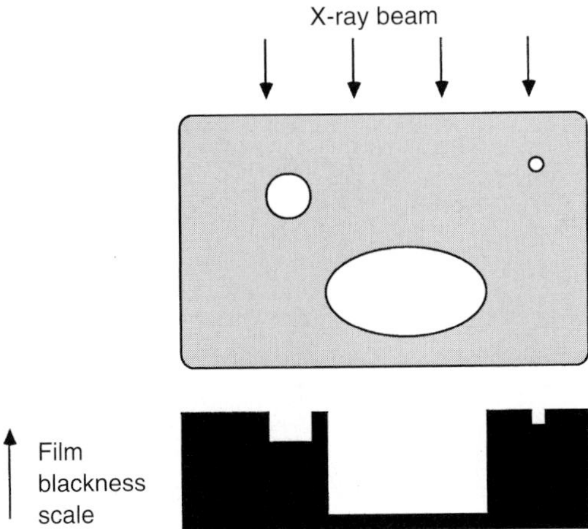

Fig. 5-1 The effect of tissue composition on absorption of x-rays. X-rays strike an object containing three regions of higher physical density, illustrated by the *two circles* and the *ellipse*. Beneath the object is a scale of film blackness. Film blackness will be the greatest when the x-ray beam does not hit one of the regions of higher physical density. If the x-ray beam hits one of the regions of higher physical density, film blackness will be less because of absorption of some of the x-rays by these objects. The degree to which film blackness decreases is a function of the thickness of the objects because they are all homogeneous and of the same physical density. The *small circle* on the right affects film blackness only minimally, whereas beneath the *ellipse* film blackness is decreased considerably because it is thicker.

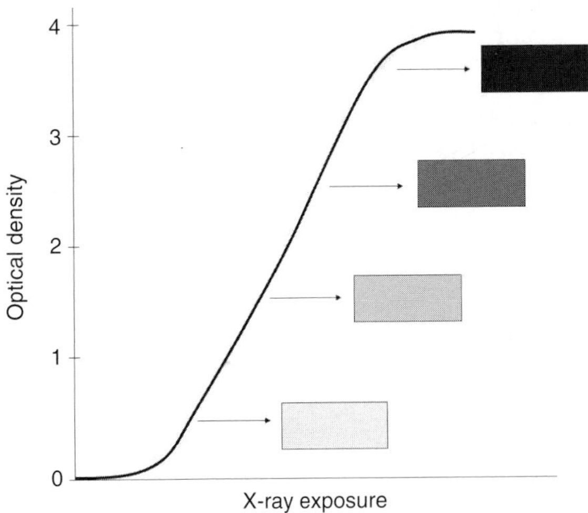

Fig. 5-3 Optical density (y axis) plotted as a function of x-ray exposure. As radiation exposure increases, so does optical film density (film blackness). The optical density scale is logarithmic. Going from an optical density reading of 1 to 2 increases film blackness by a factor of 10. This type of curve is called a characteristic curve, or H & D curve, and is unique for every film type.

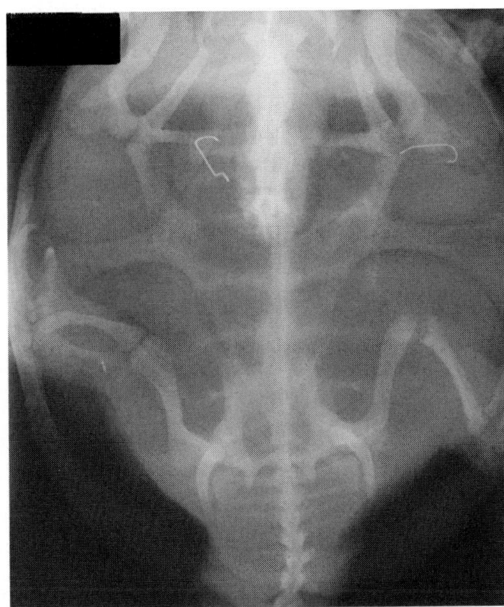

Fig. 5-2 Radiograph of a sea turtle that ingested two fishhooks. *Black regions* represent film areas where no x-rays were absorbed from the x-ray beam before reaching the intensifying screens. *Intensely white areas,* such as the fishhooks, are areas where essentially all x-rays were absorbed from the incident x-ray beam before their interaction with the intensifying screen. Between these two extremes are many shades of gray resulting from various degrees of x-ray absorption from the primary beam by the turtle. The bones absorbed more x-rays (and are thus more radiopaque) than did the other parts of the turtle.

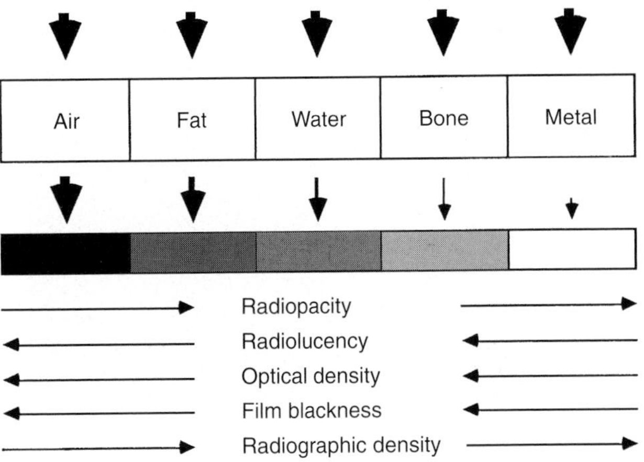

Fig. 5-4 Identical thicknesses of five substances are struck by an equal number of x-rays. Not all substances absorb x-rays with the same efficiency. In this example, as the physical density and effective atomic number increase (from *left* to *right*), the number of x-rays penetrating the substance decreases. This dependency of differential absorption on the basis of a material's physical density and atomic number is what allows x-rays to be useful for producing radiographs. As the number of x-rays passing through the object changes, the blackness of the radiograph also changes. Note the changes in radiopacity that occur with each object. Use of the term "radiographic density" is not recommended but is included in this figure for comparison.

and effective atomic number. However, film-screen radiographic imaging systems are not sensitive enough to allow discrimination between the radiopacity of substances with such small differences in physical density and effective atomic number. Thus the radiopacity of most fluids (e.g., blood, urine, transudates, exudates, bile, and cerebrospinal fluid) and tissues (e.g., cartilage, muscle, fascia, tendons, ligaments, and parenchymal organs) is the same. The radiopacity of these fluids and tissues is collectively referred to as soft-tissue radiopacity. The next most radiopaque substance is bone; its

Table • 5-1

Physical Density and Effective Atomic Number of Various Substances

SUBSTANCE	PHYSICAL DENSITY (G/CM³)	EFFECTIVE ATOMIC NUMBER
Air	0.001	7.8
Fat	0.92	6.5
Water	1.00	7.5
Muscle	1.04	7.6
Bone	1.65	12.3
Lead	8.70	82.0

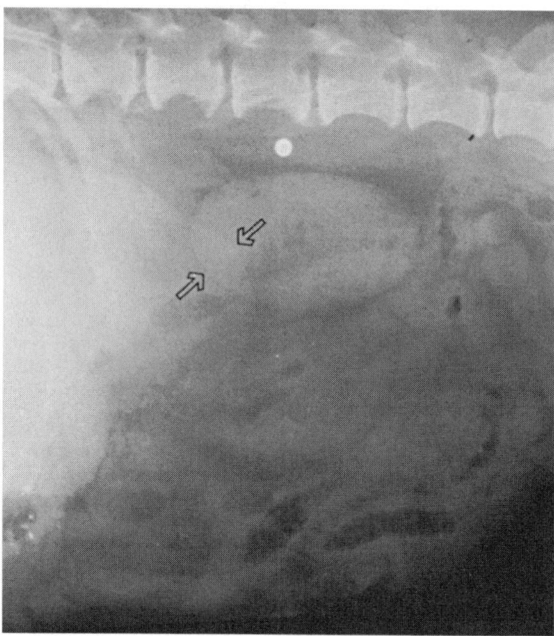

Fig. 5-5 Lateral view of abdomen in which the five different radiopacities are represented. Air: gas in the bowel. Fat: adipose tissue in the retroperitoneal space. Fat is more radiopaque than gas but less radiopaque than the kidneys. Soft tissue: the kidneys. Note the summation shadow created by the overlapping of the caudal pole of the right kidney and the cranial pole of the left kidney *(arrows)*. Bone: the vertebrae. Metal: the shotgun pellet. The exact location of the pellet cannot be determined from this lateral view alone. It could be in the skin, the intraperitoneal space, or the retroperitoneal space, or it could be lying on top of the x-ray table. Two views, at 90 degrees to each other, are necessary to identify the precise location of any object.

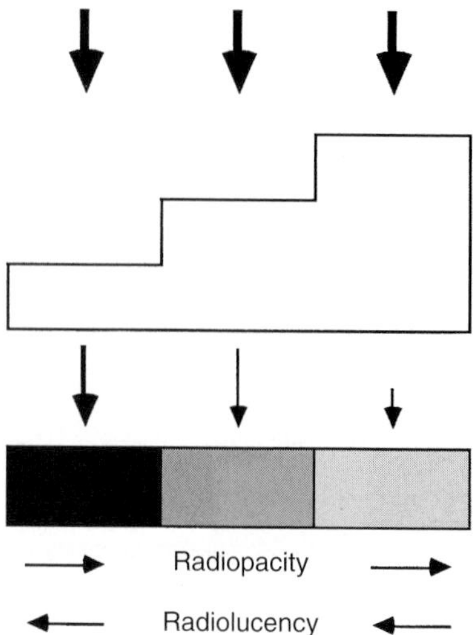

Fig. 5-6 The effect of thickness on radiographic opacity. Increasing the thickness of the object in the path of the x-ray beam will reduce the number of x-rays that reach the film and therefore film blackness.

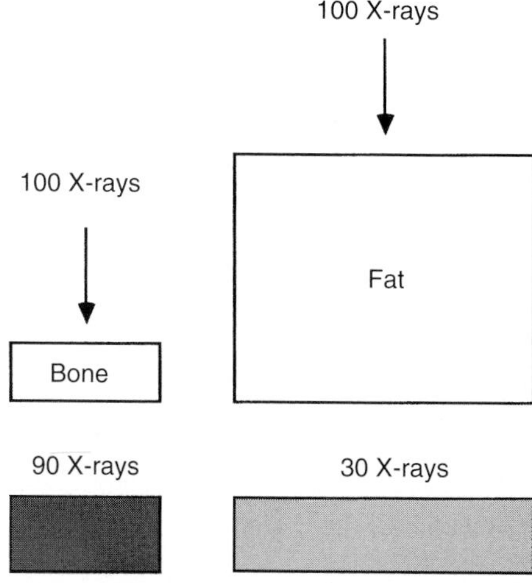

Fig. 5-7 Bone has greater inherent radiopacity than fat (see Figs. 5-4 and 5-5). However, inherent radiopacities are relative, and thickness can cause substances with higher inherent radiopacity to appear less opaque. In this example, 100 x-rays hit a thin piece of bone and a thick piece of fat. More x-rays are absorbed in the fat because of its greater thickness, and in the resulting radiograph the fat will appear more opaque than bone even though its inherent radiopacity is less.

physical density and effective atomic number are higher than those of air, fat, water, and muscle. The most radiopaque substance in Table 5-1 is lead (other metals could also have been used as an example). Lead and other metals have high physical density and effective atomic number, making them extremely radiopaque. Thus five perceivable degrees of inherent radiopacity exist: air, fat, soft tissue, bone, and metal (Figs. 5-4 and 5-5).

In any discussion of relative inherent radiopacities, thickness must also be considered. Thickness and radiopacity are interrelated; as thickness increases, radiopacity increases (Fig. 5-6). Thus the five basic inherent radiopacities (air, fat, soft tissue, bone, and metal) are relative, assuming that the object's thickness is approximately the same. For example, although fat is inherently more radiolucent than bone, if a large thickness of fat is next to a small thickness of bone, the fat will be more radiopaque (i.e., its total radiopacity would be greater) (Fig. 5-7). Thus total radiopacity is determined by object thickness *and* inherent radiopacity.

RADIOGRAPHIC GEOMETRY AND THINKING IN THREE DIMENSIONS

Because a radiograph is a two-dimensional image of a three-dimensional object, the appearance of a radiographic image

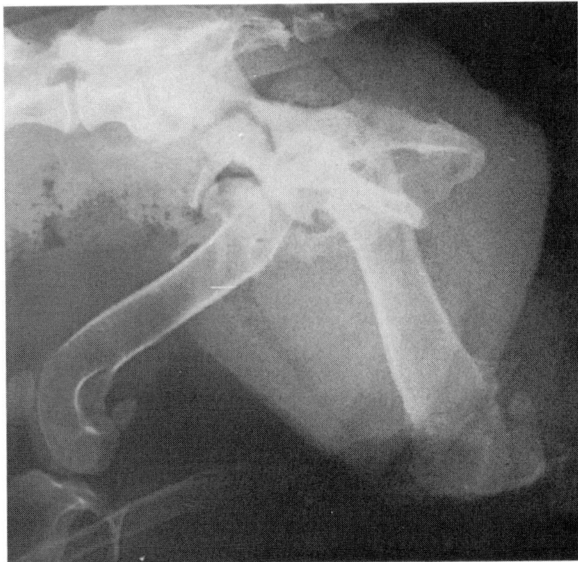

Fig. 5-8 Lateral view of the pelvis of a dog in right lateral recumbency. The right pelvic limb was pulled cranially, the left pelvic limb, caudally. Notice the increased diameter of the left femur compared with the right because of *magnification*—the left femur is farther from the cassette. Margins of the magnified left femur are also less sharp than those of the right.

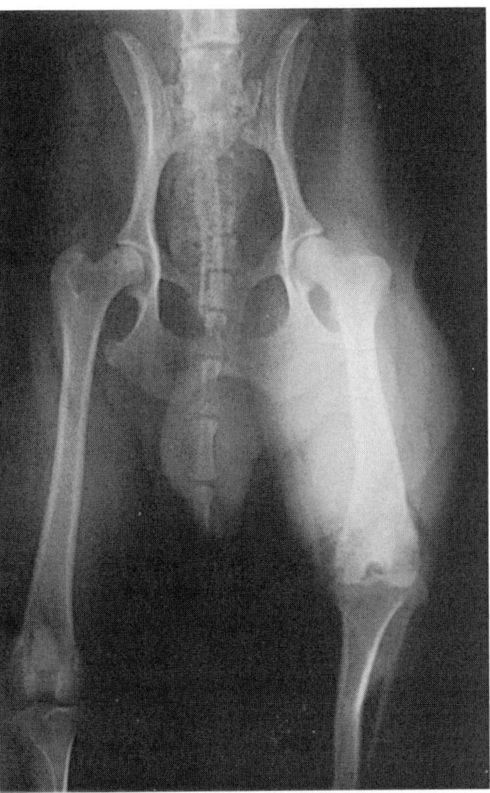

Fig. 5-9 Ventrodorsal view of the pelvis. The right femur was held parallel to table top; the left femur was positioned with the stifle slightly flexed. This results in the left femur being angled in relation to the primary x-ray beam. Thus the left femur appears shorter than the right and is asymmetrically magnified because of *distortion;* that is, it was not struck perpendicularly by the x-ray beam. The left thigh also appears more radiopaque than the right because the tissue traversed by the x-ray beam was thicker on the left because of the leg angulation.

varies with the patient's orientation in relation to the primary x-ray beam. Consequences of radiographs being two dimensional are (1) magnification and distortion, (2) image of a familiar part appearing unfamiliar, (3) loss of depth perception, and (4) presence of summation shadows.

Magnification and Distortion

Magnification refers to the enlargement of the image relative to its actual size. Magnification varies with the object-film distance and the focal spot–film distance. In clinical practice, object-film distance affects magnification more than focal spot–film distance does because focal spot–film distance is typically constant. When object-film distance increases, magnification increases. In the magnified image, each bit of visual information is spread over a larger area of the film, which reduces image detail. Some parts of the patient are always farther from the film than other parts (Fig. 5-8). Thus, whenever possible, the area of primary interest should be placed closest to the cassette to avoid magnification. The only exception to this rule is in radiography of the small animal thorax in which lesions in the dependent lung are commonly not visualized because the border of the lesion is effaced by the atelectatic dependent lung.

Distortion occurs when the image misrepresents the true shape or position of the object. Distortion results from unequal magnification of different parts of the same object; it can be minimized by keeping the object and film planes parallel. Some distortion occurs in every radiograph because parts of the patient are always not parallel to the film plane. Severe distortion, however, may limit the diagnostic quality of the radiograph (Fig. 5-9).

Unfamiliar Image

An *unfamiliar image* of a familiar object sometimes results in the object not being identifiable (Fig. 5-10). Therefore patient positioning for radiography must be standardized. Clinicians become familiar with the radiographic appearance of patients as a result of positioning them in standard fashions.

Loss of Depth Perception

Depth perception is lost in radiographs. To evaluate depth radiographically, two radiographs of the object are necessary, with one at a 90-degree angle to the other. Depth can then be mentally reconstructed (see Fig. 5-5). In addition, some lesions are apparent in only one radiographic projection (Fig. 5-11). Thus for each patient a minimum of two views should be obtained 90 degrees to each other. Views made 90 degrees to each other are called *orthogonal projections.*

Summation Sign

The *summation sign* results when parts of a patient or object in different planes (i.e., not in contact with each other) are superimposed (see Fig. 5-5). The result is a summation image representing the degree of x-ray absorption by all superimposed objects. For example, consider a block of Swiss cheese. Holes on the exterior of the block are caused by the cheese being sliced through gas cavities that formed as the cheese fermented. Inside the block of cheese are more gas cavities, some of which overlap when viewed from the perspective of the x-ray tube. If the block of Swiss cheese were to be radiographed, fewer x-rays would be absorbed by the cheese in areas where cavities overlap. The more overlapping cavities present, the greater the number of x-rays that penetrate the cheese and reach the film (Figs. 5-12 and 5-13). In the example of Swiss cheese, the resulting summation is radiolucent because it represents summation of multiple, adjacent, or superimposed air

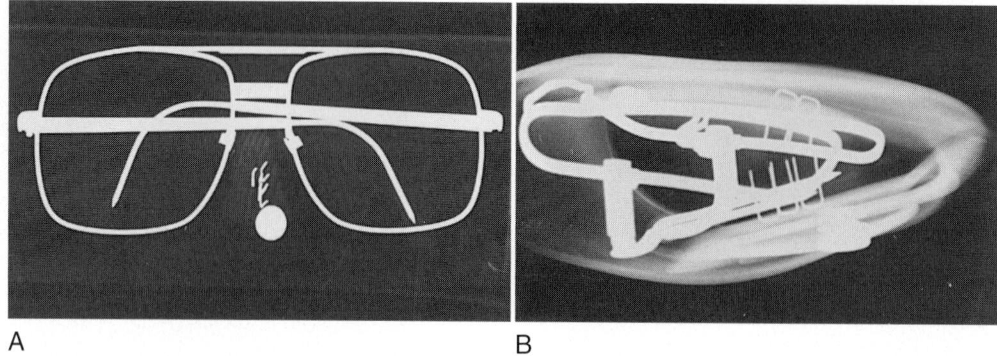

Fig. 5-10 How recognizable an object or a body part is from its radiograph depends on its relation to the primary x-ray beam. The object in **A** is easily recognizable. The object in **B** is difficult to recognize as the same pair of eyeglasses unless the identity of the object is known before radiography and that the glasses and their case were radiographed on end (parallel to the primary beam).

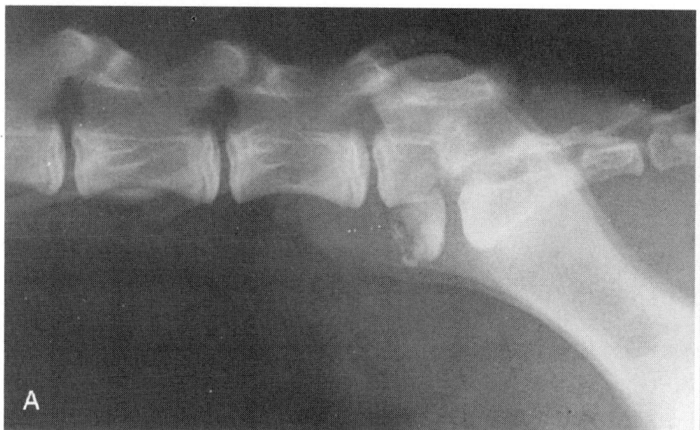

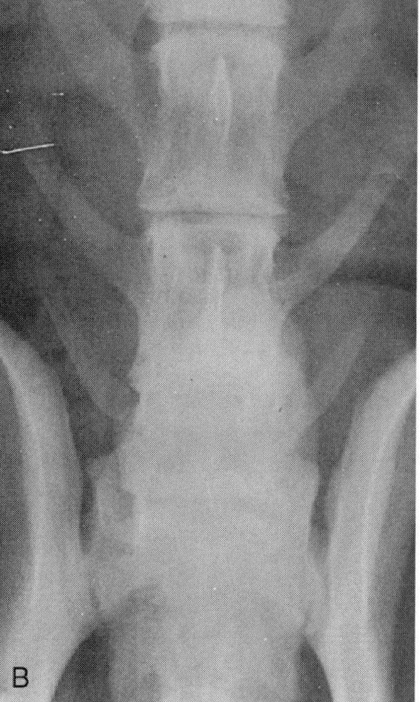

Fig. 5-11 Lateral **(A)** and ventrodorsal **(B)** radiographs of a canine lumbar spine. **A,** A displaced fracture of L7 is visible. **B,** The fracture itself cannot be seen; however, L7 appears short. Some lesions are more apparent on one radiographic projection than on others. At least two orthogonal projections of a body part should routinely be made.

spaces. Summation shadows can also be radiopaque (see Fig. 5-5). When a suspicious radiopacity or radiolucency is identified, the possibility must be considered that it represents a summation shadow produced by overlapping structures. A typical example occurs when a pulmonary vessel is viewed end on, or when a pulmonary vessel overlaps a rib, creating a summation shadow that is more radiopaque than the adjacent pulmonary vessel. This summation "nodule" should not be mistaken for a true pulmonary nodule.

Border Effacement (Silhouette Sign)

Border effacement occurs when two structures of the same radiopacity are in contact, leading to the inability to distinguish their margin. Another term for this phenomenon is "silhouette sign." Conversely, if two structures of the same radiopacity are separated by a substance of a differing radiopacity, their borders can be distinguished radiographically.

For example, consider Figure 5-14. The drawing represents a thoracic cavity containing the heart, a lung, a coronary artery, and pulmonary arteries. When radiographed, the coronary artery is not visible because it has the same radiographic opacity as the heart, and no intervening tissue of a different radiographic opacity is present. The pulmonary arteries are visible even though they are of the same radiographic opacity as the heart because they do not touch the heart and an intervening tissue (lung) of a different opacity (gas) is present.

Border effacement often results in diseases masking normal radiographic structures. For example, in a patient with pleural effusion, the pooling of fluid around the heart when the patient is radiographed in sternal recumbency (dorsoventral radiograph) renders the heart margin invisible (see Chapter

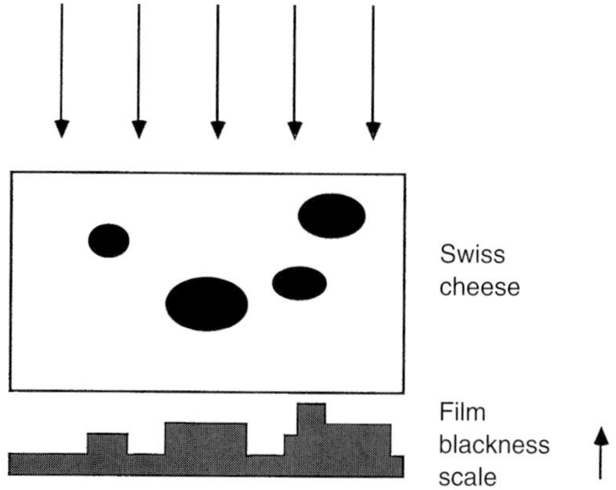

Fig. 5-12 The summation shadow effect. A block of Swiss cheese is struck by an x-ray beam. Gas cavities in the cheese may not be superimposed from the vantage point of the x rays. The two on the left are not, and the resultant increase in film blackness beneath the bubbles is caused by the individual absorption characteristics of each bubble. The two bubbles on the right, however, are partially overlapped from the perspective of the x-ray beam. In this region of overlap, film blackness is increased as a result of decreased x-ray absorption in the region of bubble overlap.

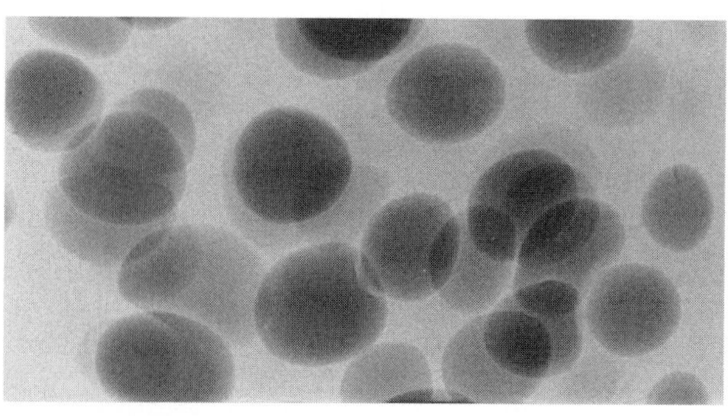

Fig. 5-13 Radiograph of a block of Swiss cheese. Gas-filled cavities in the cheese are apparent. Areas in which cavities overlap are more radiolucent than are areas in which no overlapping has occurred. Increased radiolucency is caused by decreased x-ray absorption in areas where cavities overlap. Areas where none, two, three, and four cavities have overlapped are visible. These summation shadows are negative because they result in increased radiolucency. See Figure 5-5 for an example of a positive summation shadow.

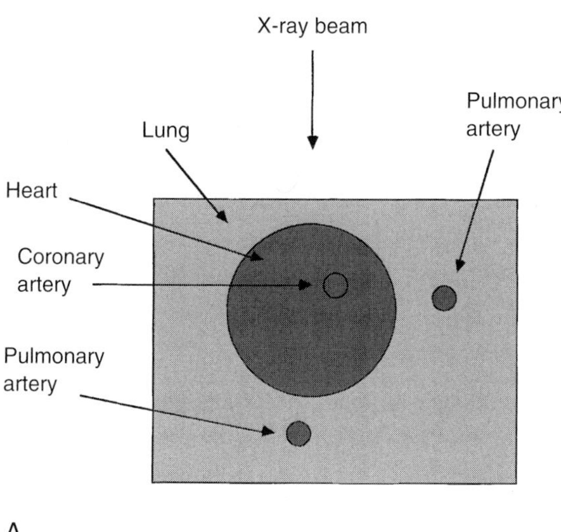

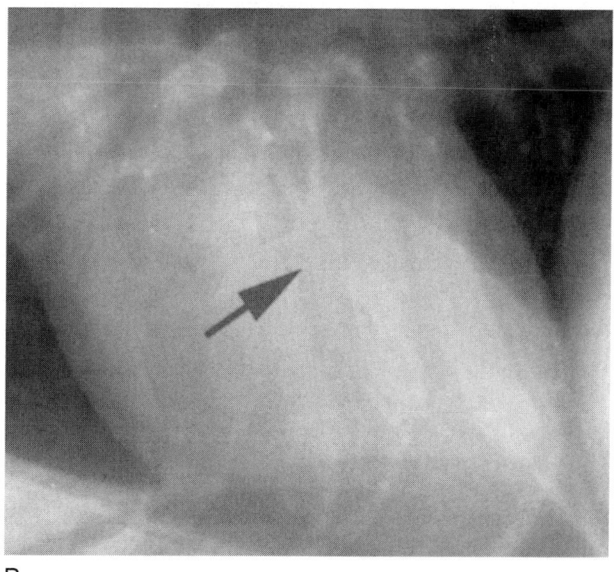

Fig. 5-14 Border effacement or the silhouette sign. **A,** Illustration of a lung with two pulmonary arteries and the heart with one coronary artery. In a radiograph of this specimen, the coronary artery will not be visible, but the two pulmonary arteries will be clearly seen. **B,** Lateral thoracic radiograph. The vessel superimposed on the heart *(arrow)* is occasionally mistaken for a coronary artery, but this is not possible; it must be a pulmonary vessel. See text for details.

29). Another example is noted in patients with peritoneal fluid because of diminished organ and bowel serosal margins (see Chapter 35).

IMPORTANCE OF A CONTRASTING SUBSTANCE

Just as the lack of a contrasting material prevents distinction between two structures of the same opacity, the presence of a contrasting material allows some structures to become exquisitely visible in radiographs. This is particularly true when the contrasting material is air and the object in question is on the surface of the body. For example, in many patients nipples and the prepuce are clearly visible in ventrodorsal radiographs of the body. These structures are not particularly large, but they cast a disproportionately opaque shadow because they are surrounded by air and their margins are parallel to the central x-ray beam, thus providing optimal geometry for visualization (Fig. 5-15).

ROLE OF PERCEPTION IN INTERPRETATION

When interpreting radiographs, clinicians rely on their eyes to detect abnormalities. Unfortunately, the eyes and brain do not always perceive appearances accurately. For example, examine

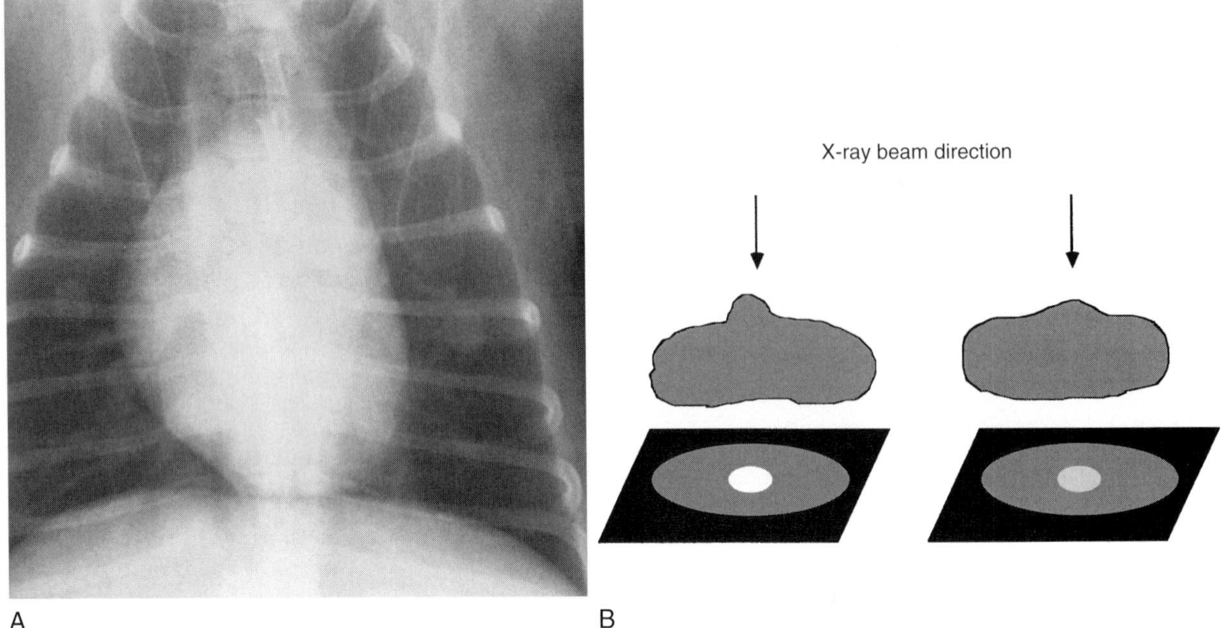

Fig. 5-15 Ventrodorsal (A) thoracic radiograph of a dog in which two soft tissue opacities are apparent lateral to the heart. These are nipples but could be confused with lung nodules. Why are nipples so opaque? **B,** Diagram illustrating why small superficial masses cast such apparent radiographic shadows. On the *left*, the mass has perpendicular sides and is surrounded on all sides by air. This creates a situation in which the x-ray beam strikes the mass/air interface in a parallel fashion, optimizing contrast. On the *right*, a comparably sized mass has sloping sides that are not in a parallel relation to the primary beam, and this mass, if seen at all, will not appear nearly as opaque because its sides will not be projected as distinctly.

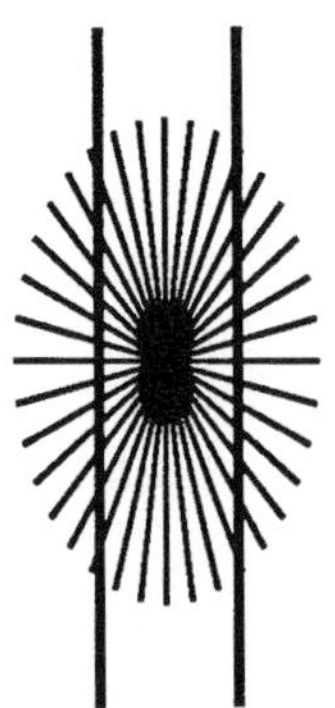

Fig. 5-16 *Perception* artifact. The two *vertical lines* appear curved. A ruler placed next to them will reveal they are straight. This optical illusion is created by the radiating lines on which the *curved lines* are superimposed. Perception can be a source of error in assessing radiographic abnormalities.

Figure 5-16. The two vertical lines appear curved, but when a straight edge is placed next to them, both horizontal lines are obviously straight. The curving nature of these lines is an optical illusion created by the radiating lines on which they are superimposed. Therefore what appears as concrete visual evidence is not always such. Perception is an important part of radiographic interpretation. What appears as an obvious finding to beginning radiologists may be an incorrect assessment because of perception. Only by viewing many radiographs, with the continual feedback of experienced interpreters, can perceptual inaccuracies be minimized. An excellent discussion of how perception influences radiographic interpretation prepared by Dr. Marc Papageorges is available on the Evolve Web site (http://evolve.elsevier.com/Thrall/vetrad).

Naming of Radiographic Projections

Radiographic projections are named according to the direction in which the central ray of the primary x-ray beam penetrates the body part of interest, from *point-of-entrance* to *point-of-exit*. Directional terms listed in the *Nomina Anatomica Veterinaria* should be used to describe radiographic views. An abdominal radiograph made with the dog in dorsal recumbency and with the use of an overhead, vertically directed x-ray beam is a ventrodorsal view; with the dog in ventral recumbency, it is a dorsoventral view. The same method is used for other body parts, with the appropriate directional term applied (Fig. 5-17).

Oblique projections should be named by using the same method as standard views (i.e., by anatomically designating the points of entrance and exit) (Fig. 5-18). Angles of obliquity can also be designated by inserting the number of degrees of obliquity between the directional terms involved. If the dorsolateral palmaromedial oblique (DLPaMO) projection in Figure 5-18 were made by positioning the x-ray tube 60 degrees laterally with respect to dorsal, the designation would be D60LPaMO. This term implies that, beginning dorsally, proceed 60 degrees to the lateral side to locate the point of entrance of the x-ray beam.

Names of lateral radiographs of the abdomen and thorax are abbreviated relative to the recumbency of the patient lying on the x-ray table or, in a standing patient, relative to the side of the patient closest to the cassette. For example, the radiograph of a canine abdomen made with the dog lying on the left side is referred to as a left lateral rather than the more correct right-left lateral.

Viewing Radiographs

To assist in developing a mental picture of normal radiographic anatomy, and also in detecting abnormalities, radiographs should always be placed on the illuminator (or screen

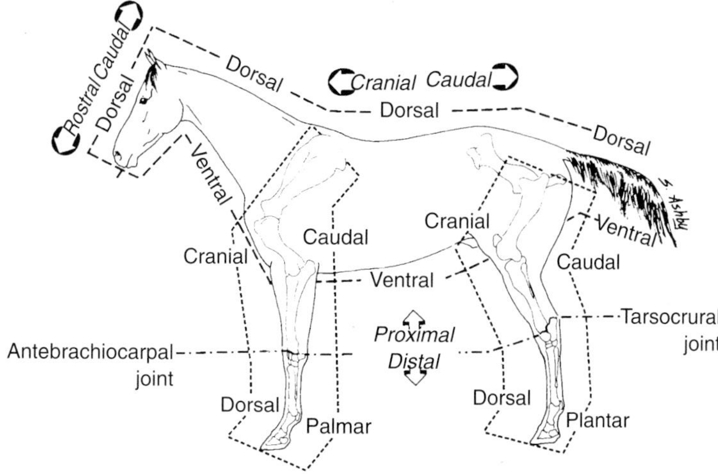

Fig. 5-17 Proper anatomic directional terms as they apply to various parts of the body. (Courtesy of Dr. J. E. Smallwood.)

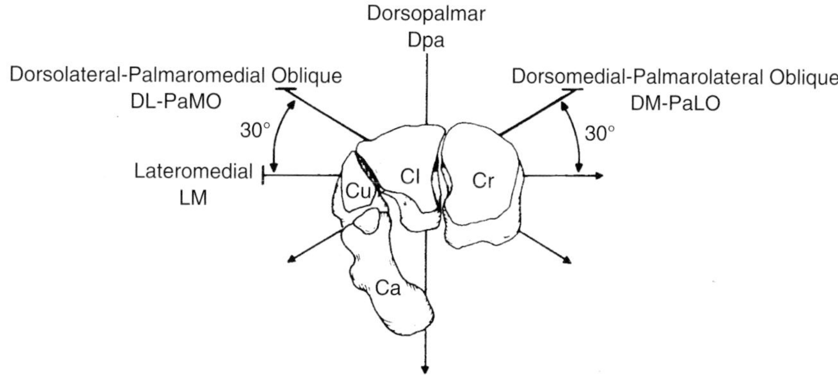

Fig. 5-18 Description of radiographic projections by the direction of the primary x-ray beam from the point of reference to the point of exit (proximal view of the equine carpal bones). (Courtesy of Dr. J. E. Smallwood.)

if using computed or digital radiography) in a standard manner.

- Lateral views of any part should be viewed with the cranial (rostral) aspect of the animal to the viewer's left.
- Ventrodorsal or dorsoventral radiographs of the head, neck, or trunk should be placed with the cranial (rostral) part of the animal pointing up and with the left side of the animal to the viewer's right.
- When viewing lateromedial or mediolateral radiographs of the extremities, including oblique projections, the radiograph should be placed on the illuminator with the proximal aspect of the limb pointing up and the cranial or dorsal aspect of the limb to the viewer's left.
- Caudocranial (plantarodorsal, palmarodorsal) or craniocaudal (dorsopalmar, dorsoplantar) radiographs of the extremities should be placed on the illuminator with the proximal end of the extremity at the top. No convention exists regarding whether the medial or lateral side of the extremity is placed to the viewer's right or left. However, consistency is important, so a suggested format is that the lateral aspect of the limb (craniocaudal or dorsopalmar/plantar radiograph) be placed on the viewer's left.

Radiographic Interpretation

Routine evaluation of radiographs begins with assessing the technical aspects of the images to the final conclusions or impressions based on the noted changes. Evaluation of poor-quality radiographs is at best inconclusive and at worst misleading.

This section defines a framework that can be used to formulate a systematic approach for radiographic evaluation. Systematic interpretation is paramount in the process. Lack of a systemic approach will result in the introduction of errors that may result in false-positive or false-negative findings.

The clinician must decide, on the basis of physical findings, the signalment, and the history, which imaging examination is the correct one to perform. Radiographic examinations must not be limited to a single lateral radiograph of a given area. Typically two orthogonal views are acquired, but for complex structures with bones that are superimposed and overlap, such as the skull, carpus, or tarsus, supplementary oblique radiographs are necessary for complete evaluation.

Radiographic interpretation need not be mysterious or difficult as long as the appropriate amount of time and the right environment are provided.[1-3] Over time, beginning interpreters will learn specific radiographic patterns of clinical disorders. Initially, however, the task of interpretation is overwhelming because each radiograph contains a lot of information. Within the context of normal and abnormal radiographic patterns, knowledge is required of normal radiographic anatomy and the possible anatomic and age-related variants that might occur. An additional requirement is to know information regarding specific radiographic

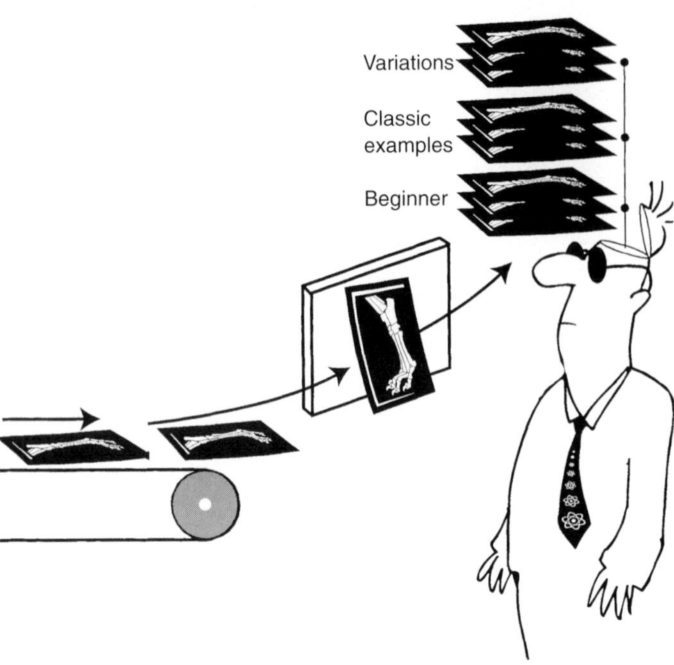

Fig. 5-19 Initially, a reader will learn what a particular disease process looks like in the classic or textbook example. As readers evaluate more radiographic examples of the disease, their experience and ability to understand the variations are increased, which expands their interpretative skills.

abnormalities associated with a particular disease process or syndrome. For example, the identification of pleural fissure lines and retraction of the lung from the thoracic wall would lead to the conclusion that a pleural disorder exists. If the opacity between the lung and thoracic wall is soft tissue, then pleural effusion and/or a pleural mass would be considered. Reading about a particular disorder and its associated radiographic changes can help develop two fundamental understandings of the disease process. The first is *pattern recognition*.[1-3] The recognition of a radiographic change is an important first step in determining the presence of an abnormality. Second, specific locations are emphasized about the distribution of specific abnormalities on the radiograph. For example, pleural fissure lines are expected to be in the region between the normal divisions of the lung lobes. Knowledge of lung lobe anatomy (even though lung lobes are usually not apparent as distinct structures on normal radiographs) is necessary for deciding whether pleural effusion is present or absent.

This approach, however, assumes the knowledge of how to assess the entire radiograph, not just a particular section such as the pleural space. Although the division of material within this text into chapters based on regional anatomy may not facilitate the collective approach needed to become a proficient radiologist, it does provide a framework of abnormalities on which to build. However, illustration of all radiographic variations of an abnormality is impossible. In reality, a spectrum of radiographic appearances for a given disease category will serve as a foundation for future performance. For example, bone infections have a spectrum of appearances. Different experiences of what bone infections can look like will help the reader over the long term (Fig. 5-19). Continually looking at radiographs will facilitate long-term memory of these patterns; gaps in radiographic interpretation will necessitate some "relearning" of information. A systematic review of radiographs after specific feedback based on pathologic findings (histology or necropsy) should be done so as not to continue to view specific roentgen abnormalities in the wrong fashion.

When beginning to evaluate radiographs, an expectation of being able to identify the primary abnormalities exists. This also assumes that the viewer is able to discriminate abnormalities from normal structures and that the change seen on the radiograph fits into the preconceived context of what the lesion is expected to look like. As the reader sees more and more radiographs, this basic knowledge expands, thereby providing a degree of confidence that facilitates further learning.[1]

A Systematic Approach to Interpretation

This edition of *Textbook of Veterinary Diagnostic Radiology* provides introductory chapters to each major anatomic region. These chapters include a basic approach or interpretation paradigm for evaluating each region. A *paradigm* is an example or a model. In radiology, interpretation paradigms are a reflection of the reader's approach to reviewing a radiograph systematically on the basis of experience. The interpretive paradigms presented are not the only model of interpretation for evaluating radiographs. These models, however, provide a basic framework on which a systematic approach to radiographic evaluation can be built. Because the radiograph is a two-dimensional presentation of regional anatomy, one must have an understanding of the inherent limitations of visual acuity in identifying specific anatomic structures and derangements. As noted earlier, an excellent overview of the role of visual perception in diagnostic imaging is available on the Evolve Web site (http://evolve.elsevier.com/Thrall/vetrad). The reader is encouraged to digest this information to assist in understanding the limitations of evaluating two-dimensional survey radiographs. Limitations specific to a given location are stressed within individual chapters.

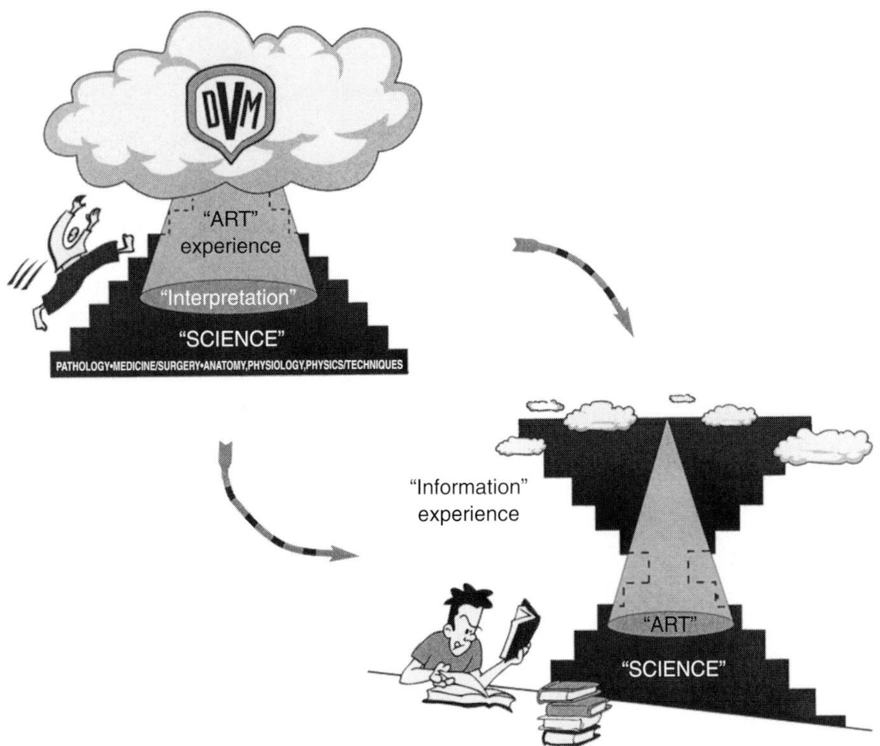

Fig. 5-20 Initial radiographic evaluation depends on the reader's knowledge base of anatomy and pathophysiology, radiographic physics, and basic principles of medicine and surgery. Progression up the mountain for evaluation of the radiographs provides more information gained through experience; this is the art of radiology.

A basic approach to each radiograph is to ask a series of questions about the structures present on the radiograph. To ensure inclusion of all the structures, basic checklists can be placed next to the view box as a reminder for the clinician while reviewing the radiographs. The question approach may seem cumbersome at first, but the goal is to create a systematic review of each radiograph. A final question in any imaging study is, "What have I missed?"

Interpreting images is a balance between science and art. The science involves knowledge of radiographic production and the identification of abnormalities on the basis of the details of radiographic anatomy, pathophysiology, medicine, and surgery. The art is a function of the viewer's experience (Fig. 5-20). As new information is brought to the forefront, these new findings must be incorporated into the clinician's scientific database, and this information must be correlated with personal experience. As the clinician gains experience with radiographic studies, he or she sees the great variety that can take place within the context of the "art" of radiographic interpretation and thereby acquires a better understanding of the clinical significance of certain radiographic abnormalities. As mentioned earlier, initial pattern recognition is important, but all the possible radiographic patterns that a disease entity may have cannot be experienced. Thus the expectation is that even experienced radiologists will regularly review radiographs that contain new information. This new information cannot always be interpreted correctly.

The basic tools for radiographic interpretation include knowledge of normal anatomy, a systematic approach to radiographic interpretation, and use of the basic radiographic signs, then tying all these together to formulate a differential diagnosis list. Once a differential list is established and prioritized on the basis of signalment, physical examination findings, and other clinical data, the next step should be to establish a definitive diagnosis (Fig. 5-21).

EVALUATING RADIOGRAPHIC ABNORMALITIES

After systematically evaluating a radiograph, compile a basic description of the abnormalities. This step is often skipped by inexperienced interpreters. The ability to describe the appearance, severity, and location of the lesions, and the roentgen sign changes, will lead to a conclusion regarding the differential diagnoses, possibly even a primary differential diagnosis for the radiographic abnormalities.

A radiographic abnormality can be viewed as a window, a mirror, or a picture (Fig. 5-22). As a window, the abnormality is considered to have happened in the past. These historical changes may or may not be important or related to the reason why the patient is being radiographed. For example, spondylosis deformans is often assessed as an abnormality of the past and is usually not related to the immediate problem. This information, however, should not be ignored; it should simply be placed lower on the priority list of the described radiographic abnormalities. As a mirror, it is assumed that the abnormality is important and is a reflection of the current problem. A femoral fracture would be an example of an abnormality being a mirror. As a picture, the radiographic abnormality is assumed to be significant currently and also as a predictor of future events. For example, canine lymphoma patients with radiographically detectable cranial mediastinal lymph node enlargement have been shown to have a poorer prognosis than dogs without cranial mediastinal lymphadenopathy.[4]

Bayes' theorem is a method of evaluating whether a diagnostic test should be used on the basis of clinical history and signs. In other words, if the patient has the disease and the test is run, the test is likely to be positive.[2] Certain clinical tests such as survey radiographs are highly sensitive and specific for different diseases in human beings, but the same statistical scrutiny has not been applied to veterinary medicine. In part,

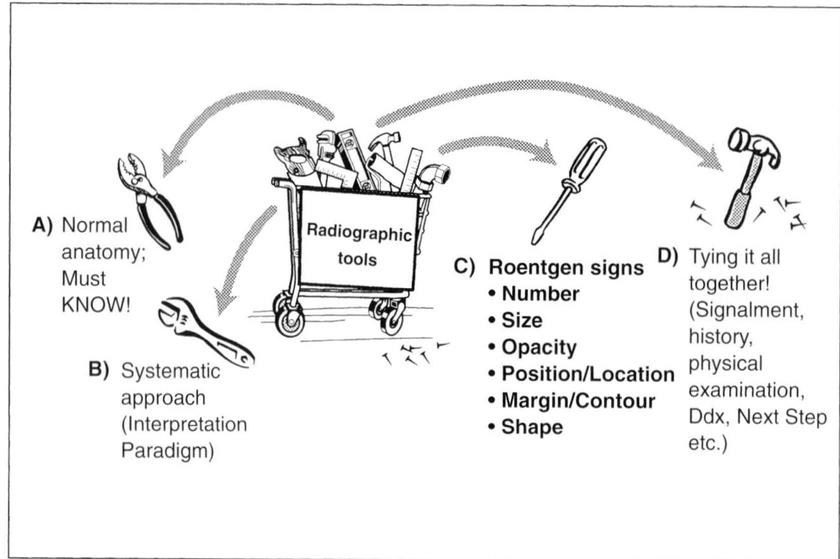

Fig. 5-21 The basic radiographic tools for interpretation. The end point of interpretation is tying together all radiographic abnormalities and formulating a differential diagnosis that takes these abnormalities into account within the clinical context of the patient. A final decision tree is established regarding whether additional testing is required to confirm the top differential consideration.

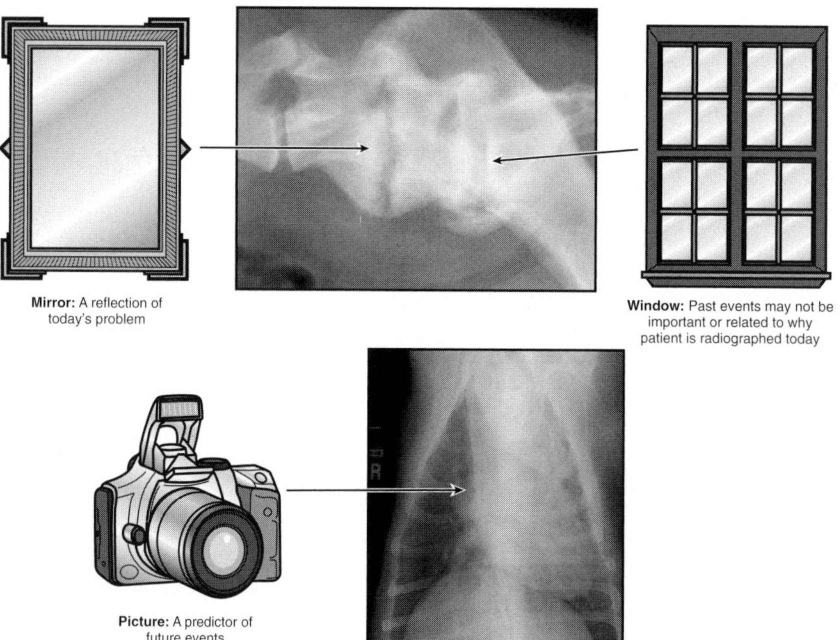

Fig. 5-22 Each radiographic abnormality can be viewed as a *window* (past change that may or may not be important today), *mirror* (a reflection of the current problem), or a *picture* (a predictor or prognosticator). The spondylosis deformans at L7-S1 represents a window of past instability at the lumbosacral junction. However, the end-plate lysis at L6-L7, which signifies discospondylitis, reflects the reason for the dog's current problem (a mirror). The cranial mediastinal lymph node enlargement in a dog with lymphoma represents a future outcome, a picture, because this finding has been defined as an independent negative predictor for response to chemotherapy.[4]

this is because studying the large numbers of animals needed to make statistically valid conclusions is impossible. Regardless, experience has provided information about situations in which radiography is useful in veterinary medicine. Each chapter of this text provides discussions regarding certain radiographic signs or abnormalities related to the presence or absence of a particular disease.

If the sensitivity of a given radiographic abnormality is considered by itself, a list of differential diagnostic considerations can be formulated on the basis of signalment and history. The radiographic abnormality (such as an interstitial lung pattern) may be neither sensitive nor specific for a particular disorder. No radiographic abnormality is going to be 100% sensitive, or its absence 100% specific, regarding whether a particular

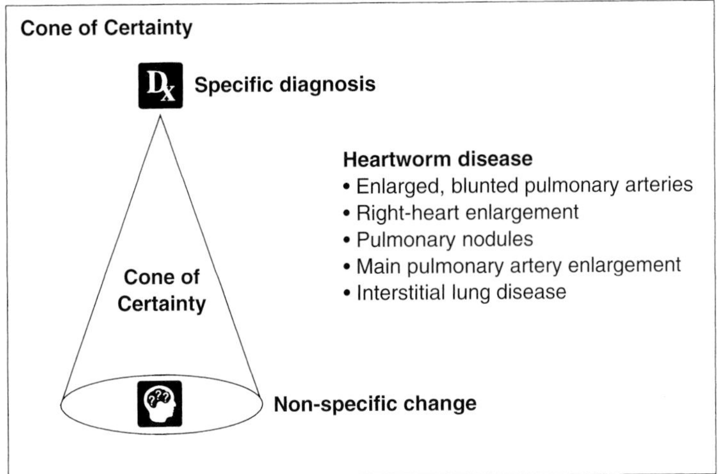

Fig. 5-23 The cone of certainty represents the degree of confidence a reader can place on a given radiographic diagnosis on the basis of identified radiographic abnormalities. For example, a generalized interstitial lung pattern can have many causes ranging from technical to age-related to disease specific, and one would be in the widest portion of the cone of certainty. Other radiographic abnormalities such as enlargement and tortuosity of the pulmonary arteries, blunting of the pulmonary arteries, right ventricular enlargement, and enlargement of the main pulmonary artery segment would increase confidence that the interstitial lung pattern is related to heartworm infection and secondary eosinophilic pneumonitis. Specific conclusions have been made relating the radiographic abnormalities that are high in the cone of certainty to the radiographic diagnosis of heartworm infection.

disease is present. In thinking about this, we use all the radiographic data collectively to build support for a given radiographic diagnosis. This concept can be thought of as an inverted ice cream cone, called the *cone of certainty* (Fig. 5-23).* At the bottom of the cone are a number of diagnostic considerations for a given radiographic abnormality. As more radiographic evidence is found for a given disease, the confidence regarding a specific radiographic diagnosis increases. If specific and sensitive radiographic abnormalities are identified, the top of the cone is reached and a high degree of confidence exists that a specific disease is present.

The clinical context and signalment become important in establishing a list of differential diagnoses. If formulating a reasonable list of differential diagnoses is difficult, aids such as the mnemonic acronym CITIMITV (*c*ongenital, *i*nflammatory, *t*umor, *i*nfectious, *m*etabolic, *i*atrogenic, *t*raumatic, and *v*ascular) can be used. This approach should provide at least one specific etiology for a given radiographic abnormality. For example, a solitary lung mass in a 10-year-old Doberman pinscher is most likely a primary lung tumor. Other diagnoses could be considered, but common sense leads to this conclusion. For example, other considerations in this dog are granuloma (parasitic, eosinophilic, or tuberculous) or abscess. However, conditions included in the differential diagnosis list must be prioritized. Without prioritization (based on experience, continuing education, and feedback), *a laundry list of possible diagnoses becomes a roadblock to efficient attainment of the definitive diagnosis.* When differential diagnosis lists are formulated, some ordering of possibilities, based on the radiographic abnormalities present and the probability of occurrence, is critical.

When interpreting radiographs, remember that the radiographic appearance represents only a snapshot of the disease (Fig. 5-24). Clinical signs often precede radiographic changes. Therefore, even though radiographs are normal, rapid changes could develop and would be apparent if repeat radiographs were made within a short period. Additionally, assessment of how a patient is responding to therapy can be done by using sequential radiographs. Is the therapeutic intervention having any effect on the radiographic appearance of the disease? If the radiographic changes detected on a recheck examination have not resolved, then the differential diagnosis or the therapy being used should be reconsidered. Finally, if a radiographic abnormality is present and a long differential list exists, a "next step" is usually necessary because most radiographic changes are nonspecific. For example, hepatomegaly may warrant evaluation of serum chemistry and/or an ultrasound examination. Being able to know what to do next and how to continue to assess the patient for a particular disease is just as important as being able to interpret radiographic abnormalities correctly. In essence, radiology can be thought of as a screening test for abnormalities, similar to evaluation of a blood count. How the information is handled in establishing the cause of the abnormality becomes part of the art of radiographic interpretation.

Errors in Interpretation

Radiographic information can easily be misinterpreted.[2] Subtle changes can be overvalued or undervalued in the interpretive process. Sometimes subtle clues are most important in formulating the correct differential diagnosis. Several types of errors need to be considered: errors of searching or scanning, errors of recognition, decision-making errors, and egocentric errors.[1,2]

Searching or Scanning Errors

Errors of searching or scanning result when the reader fails to search the image in a systematic fashion and completely misses the lesion. Sometimes these errors are called "corner" errors because of the tendency to overlook lesions located at the periphery of the radiograph. There is also a "satisfaction of search" error that occurs when the reader has preconceived ideas regarding what should be found. Once the reader has assessed the radiograph for the preconceived conclusion, the

*The concept of the cone of certainty has been adopted from Dr. Richard Pratt's (Old Testament scholar) lecture notes. See *Introduction to Pastoral and Theological Studies*, Reformed Theological Seminary, Orlando, FL.

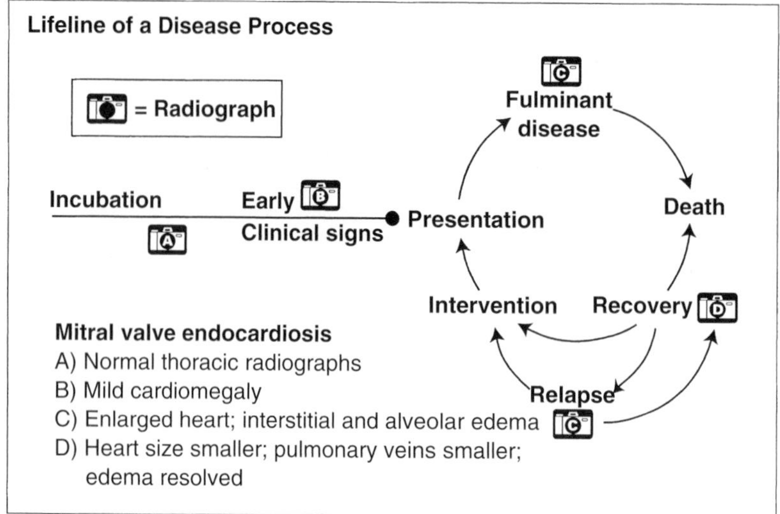

Fig. 5-24 Lifeline of a disease. The camera represents a radiograph made at a particular stage of mitral valvular endocardiosis. At point *A*, the thoracic radiographs are often normal in spite of murmur being auscultated. If the radiographs are made at point *B*, there may be mild to moderate cardiomegaly with left atrial dilation causing compression of the mainstem bronchi and resulting in a cough. In *C*, the dog may have dyspnea, and radiographic features of left heart failure with pulmonary edema are seen. In *D*, after treating the dog with appropriate medications, the pulmonary edema resolves and the cycle continues with the next exacerbation of heart failure (*C*, relapse).

reader becomes content that the remainder of the radiograph is normal, and the search is stopped.

Recognition Errors

In a recognition error the abnormality is identified but is either not taken into account in the final analysis or is given too much weight and a misinterpretation results. For example, small discrete nodules in the thorax caused by osseous metaplasia or "end on" pulmonary vessels are misinterpreted as pulmonary metastatic disease. This error is based on the reader's previous experience and the art of radiographic interpretation. Again, understanding normal radiographic anatomy, normal anatomic variations, pathophysiology, and the myriad of ways a particular disorder may appear radiographically is critical.

Decision-Making Errors

Decision-making errors involve how radiographic information is interpreted and which radiographic abnormalities are assumed to be important. Some findings fall into a gray zone in which clinical significance may or may not be known, even with knowledge of the clinical information about a given patient. In these instances, waiting and repeating radiographs may be in order or, on the basis of the clinical context, a definitive biopsy may be the next step.

Egocentric Errors

By overestimating personal grasp of the truth and misapplying the information that is known, the clinician can make an egocentric error. Additionally, certain radiographic abnormalities may be ignored that contradict basic assumptions and assessments. Egocentric errors can be avoided by not reviewing radiographs in a sterile, single-person environment and seeking second opinions. In most settings, radiology rounds can be established in which multiple individuals can review the radiographic images; this allows for quality control.

The following process can be used to evaluate a radiographic study. It can be modified and tailored to individual preferences so that it works for many different situations.

PROCESS FOR RADIOGRAPHIC EVALUATION

Preliminary Work: Diagnostic Quality

Review all radiographs in an appropriate environment. An appropriate environment means a quiet, dark area that is free from distractions and that has adequate viewing facilities so that the entire study can be viewed simultaneously. At all cost, avoid holding the images up to a room light and attempting to interpret them. A "hot" light should be accessible. The hot light serves two functions. The first is to provide additional illumination for evaluation of overexposed or high-contrast areas (e.g., lung fields, soft tissue/bone interfaces); the second function is that it forces the reader to focus on small sections of the radiograph. The reader is not overwhelmed by looking at the entire radiograph and can systematically review all parts of the radiograph in a bite-size, section-by-section manner. In evaluating radiographs, all overhead lighting and other view boxes not being used should be turned off. These external light sources distract the visual cortex from the purpose at hand: evaluating just the radiograph(s) in question.

Hang the radiographs the same way (including the order) each time a particular radiographic examination is reviewed. Pattern recognition within the viewer's visual cortex becomes a key player in the recognition of abnormalities. If the radiographs are consistently viewed in a specific manner, the viewer will start to identify abnormalities before the systematic review begins because the brain recognizes that something is not normal for that particular study. This system of pattern recognition does not replace a systematic approach to reviewing the radiographs; however, it does provide the groundwork for organization and the foundation for a systematic evaluation of all radiographic images.

Ensure that all the views for a given radiographic examination have been made. For example, a thoracic radiographic study consists of a right lateral, a left lateral, and a ventrodorsal or dorsoventral view. If views are missing, the interpretive accuracy is compromised. The missing views should be acquired before formulating a radiographic impression unless the patient is at risk for respiratory or cardiovascular compromise. Repeat radiographs can be made after the patient has been stabilized.

Evaluate patient positioning. This should include the anatomic boundaries of the area of interest (e.g., is the entire thorax included in the study?) and any obliquity that may hinder accurate interpretation of a given radiograph.

Evaluate the radiographic technique. Are the images too light or too dark? If yes, is the problem caused by a disease? If so, do not attempt to adjust the technical factors, but treat the patient and repeat the radiographic study. For example, in a dog with pneumothorax, thoracic radiographs will possibly appear too dark. Or, in a dog with pleural effusion, the radiographs will appear too light. Repeat radiographs should not be attempted in these dogs until they have undergone thoracocentesis.

If technical problems have resulted in the image being too dark, a starting point is to decrease the peak kilovolt by 15% or decrease the milliamperage by 50%. If the radiograph is too light, increase the peak kilovolt by 15% or increase the milliamperage by a factor of two. The adjustments used will depend on the type of study (anatomic region), consideration of contrast, and technical factors that could limit these adjustments based on the type of x-ray generator. Manipulation of both the peak kilovolt and milliamperage at the same time should be avoided.

Evaluate for other technical errors and artifacts that may hinder the interpretation of the radiographs. Processing artifacts and technical errors can hinder radiographic interpretation. Technical errors in the darkroom can destroy a high-quality radiograph. Be sure to maintain consistent darkroom technique so that high-quality radiographs can be obtained on a consistent basis. An overview of darkroom technique is provided in Chapter 1. More detailed information is available elsewhere.[5-7]

Continuously review normal radiographic anatomy present on the radiographs. Review the entire radiograph and review each radiograph using the same process. Refer to anatomic aids and textbooks when reviewing radiographs. Familiarization with normal anatomy is required to identify radiographic abnormalities.

Disease Detection and Description

Identify the radiographic abnormalities. Determine that a structure is abnormal by noting variation from the expected radiographic appearance of a given structure (see Fig. 5-21). Roentgen signs include changes from the expected size, shape, number, location, margination, and/or opacity.

At this point, the viewer must determine if the abnormality identified is relevant. Do not discount any abnormality until all radiographs are evaluated and a list of abnormalities has been established. Remember that the descriptions used to characterize radiographic abnormalities may be subjective (e.g., mild interstitial lung pattern). Also remember that the existence of a radiographic abnormality does not mean that it is clinically relevant. The abnormality may be an anatomic variant or reflect a past event (window).

Differential Diagnosis/Radiographic Diagnosis

Establish a list of differential diagnoses for the radiographic findings. The determination of whether any of the radiographic abnormalities that have been identified are consistent with one disease or a group of diseases is important. For example, many considerations exist for right ventricular enlargement; however, in conjunction with enlarged, blunted, and tortuous pulmonary arteries, heartworm infection becomes a likely possibility. The history and signalment can be used to establish and prioritize the differential diagnosis. The pathophysiologic basis of the radiographic changes must be understood so that different radiographic abnormalities can be tied together as a single disease entity. The goal of clinical medicine, in addition to establishing a radiographic diagnosis, is to bring all available information together and settle on one or two conditions that are consistent with all the abnormalities. All differentials listed for an interstitial lung pattern are not relevant to every patient in which such is diagnosed. The clinical context of the patient's signalment and history must be considered before the differential diagnosis list is prioritized. If the radiographic abnormalities are specific and are high in the cone of certainty, than a diagnosis becomes more likely. Recognize that this will not be common and that a well-thought-out differential diagnostic list is often a necessity. Again, however, this differential list should not be a laundry list but should include real possibilities for a given patient.

Make a radiographic diagnosis. Incorporate the clinical history, physical examination findings, and signalment when making a radiographic diagnosis. This radiographic diagnosis must incorporate all the radiographic abnormalities identified and try to tie them into one clinical disease entity. For example, the radiographic abnormalities of tracheobronchial and sternal lymphadenopathy, an interstitial lung pattern, hepatosplenomegaly, and medial iliac lymph node enlargement most likely represent lymphoma. The reader may discover something on the radiographs that is clinically important but that may not have anything to do with the current clinical history or presentation. Do not ignore these radiographic abnormalities; instead, pursue these changes as part of the patient's diagnostic workup by adding them to the working problem list of the patient.

Next Step Recommendation

Make a recommendation or give thought to the next step in patient management. This could include or involve (1) additional imaging studies that would confirm the presence or absence of a disease (e.g., a suspected pyloric-region mass may be confirmed in a left lateral radiograph, leading to accumulation of air in the pyloric outflow tract that would outline the mass); (2) special oblique radiographs that may allow better visualization of a suspected abnormality (e.g., oblique views of the carpus to detect a carpal bone fracture); or (3) special procedures, such as ultrasound, nuclear medicine, computed tomography, or magnetic resonance imaging, that may confirm the presence or absence of a disease. Additionally, other clinical tests may be needed to establish the definitive diagnosis, such as needle aspiration or biopsy, or repeat radiographs over time to see how a lesion is responding or is not responding to therapy.

In summary, radiographic interpretation is a systematic process of reviewing a radiograph in a preestablished manner. Once an abnormal pattern is recognized and described, a rational thought process leads to reasonable differential diagnostic considerations from the standpoint of known pathophysiologic processes that occur within the species in question. Figure 5-25 shows several points. The life of a given patient or the entire diachronic trace can be viewed over time. Within this lifeline is the course of a disease that undergoes a preclinical incubation period before illness develops in the patient. At this time a synchronic slice is obtained (e.g., blood work and radiographs are performed to give a snapshot of the disease at that time), the process of interpretation is followed, and the radiographs are reviewed. A basic understanding of radiographic anatomy and normal physiology, as well as the pathophysiologic basis of the radiographic changes that are seen in a given disease process, is required.

The approach to radiographic interpretation depends on the use of specific tools. These include a basic systematic approach or interpretation paradigm and a method for evaluating each structure according to the six basic roentgen signs. Once radiographic abnormalities have been established, a list of differential diagnoses is formulated and a possible radiographic

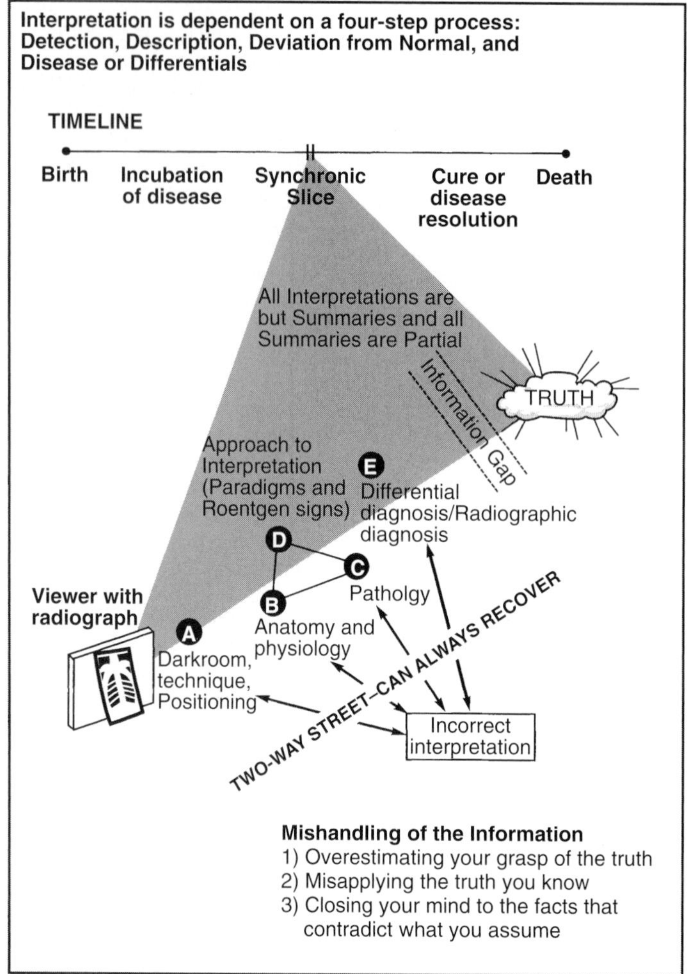

Fig. 5-25 Summary of radiographic interpretation. Interpretation depends on *A*, technical considerations, darkroom, and positioning; *B*, normal radiographic anatomy and physiology; *C*, pathophysiology and expected radiographic changes associated with disease; *D*, interpretation paradigms and approach to review of the radiographs; and *E*, differential diagnostic considerations. Errors at any one of these points result in incorrect interpretation and an incorrect diagnosis.

diagnosis is established on the basis of the abnormalities present. More importantly, the next step in working up a patient is determined. This step should move through the information gap to the truth regarding what the disease actually is.

At this point, step back and look at the process (see Fig. 5-25, *A* through *E*). Each step has the potential for error, whether poor radiographic technique or overlooking important radiographic abnormalities. These can result in an incorrect interpretation and thereby move the viewer farther from the truth. Human beings are not perfect, and everyone will make mistakes. The goal is to minimize these mistakes and remember that at each of these decision points, recovery is possible and the path to the truth can be found. Only the interpretation of the radiograph can lead the viewer astray because all the information is correct and true on the radiograph (within the limitations of what a radiograph represents). Determining the truth on the basis of correct interpretation of the radiograph is the goal.

REFERENCES

1. Novelline RA: *Squire's fundamentals of radiology,* ed 5, Cambridge, MA, 1999, Harvard University.
2. Gunderman RB: *Essential radiology: clinical presentation, pathophysiology and imaging,* New York, 1998, Thieme.
3. Suter PF: *Thoracic radiography: a text atlas of thoracic diseases of the dog and cat,* Wettswil, Switzerland, 1984, Peter F. Suter.
4. Starrak GS, Berry CR, Page RL et al: Correlation between thoracic radiographic changes and remission/survival duration in 270 dogs with lymphosarcoma, *Vet Radiol Ultrasound* 38:411, 1997.
5. Eastman Kodak Company: *The fundamentals of radiography,* ed 12, Rochester, NY, 1980, Eastman Kodak.
6. Morgan JP, Silverman S: *Techniques in veterinary radiography,* ed 5, Ames, IA, 1997, Iowa State University.
7. Ticer JW: *Radiographic technique in small animal practice,* Philadelphia, 1980, W.B. Saunders.

ELECTRONIC RESOURCES evolve

Additional information related to the content in Chapter 5 can be found on the companion Web site at evolve http://evolve.elsevier.com/Thrall/vetrad/

- Key Points
- Chapter Quiz

SECTION II

The Axial Skeleton

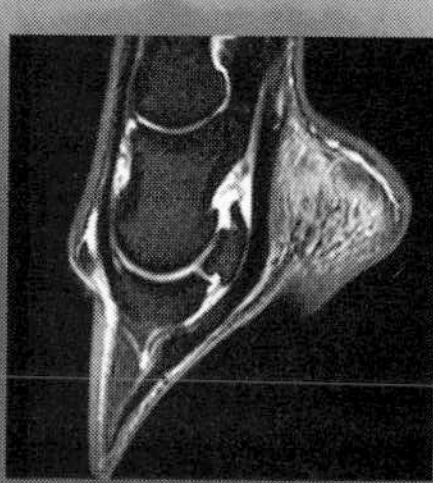

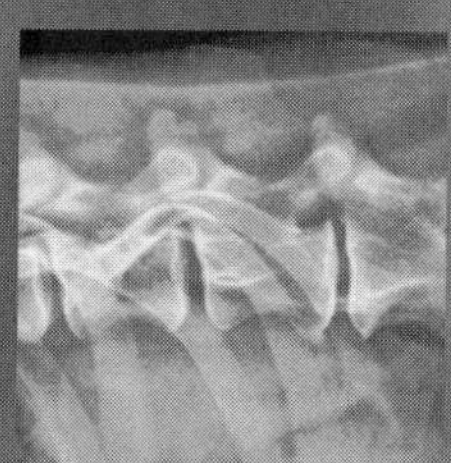

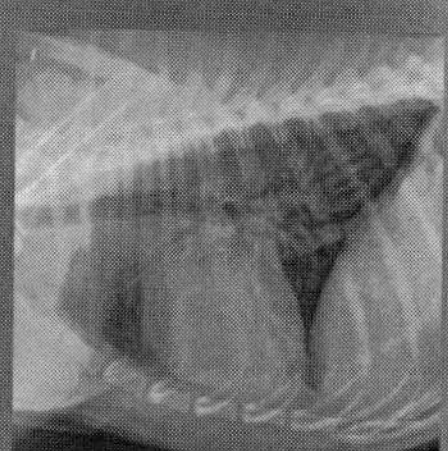

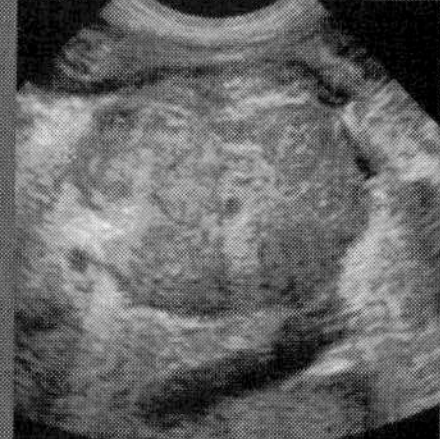

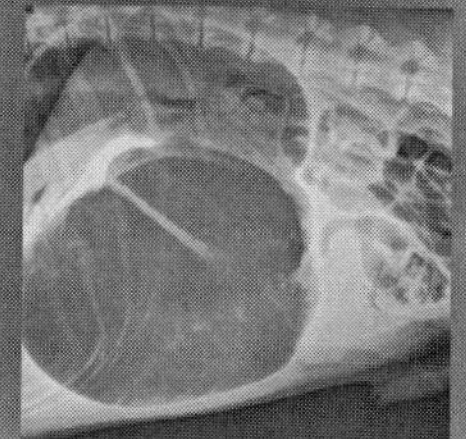

CHAPTER • 6
Technical Issues and Interpretation Principles Relating to the Axial Skeleton

Eric A. Ferrell
Clifford R. Berry
Donald E. Thrall

This chapter is intended to provide a framework for beginning interpreters of radiographs of the axial skeleton. Basic information on how to produce a diagnostic radiograph, recommend views, and a structure for interpretation are presented. This chapter is not intended to be a standalone resource for axial skeletal image interpretation. Rather, it is an overview of some important principles that will assist the reader in the evaluation of the more detailed chapters that focus on individual regions and diseases.

The axial skeleton consists of the skull and vertebral column, areas characterized by complex three-dimensional structures. For complete evaluation, multiple oblique and/or special radiographic projections or alternate imaging techniques (magnetic resonance imaging and computed tomography) are required so that different areas can be viewed.[1-3] An understanding of the anatomy of the axial skeleton is necessary; see Chapter 7 for further anatomic review and details. The radiographic anatomy of the skull and vertebral column is unique for the dog compared with the cat and horse.[4] As such, being able to recognize the similarities and differences among species is important.

ANATOMY OF THE SKULL

The skull of the dog, cat, and horse is made up of the nasal cavity, paranasal sinuses, cranial cavity, maxilla, mandible, pharynx, hyoid apparatus, and the larynx. The larynx and pharynx are reviewed with the upper respiratory system in Chapters 10 and 27. A thorough knowledge of the basic radiographic anatomy of the small animal and equine skull is critical for interpretation. Because the skull has many superimposed structures, the ability to recognize summation shadows and mentally reconstruct a three-dimensional structure is essential. For this, review of normal cross-sectional anatomy is helpful.[5,6] Also, anatomic references should be readily available when reviewing skull radiographs.

Before making radiographs of the skull, an index of suspicion must be present of what structures may be involved to decide what radiographic views to obtain initially. Additional radiographs can be made as needed on the basis of radiographic abnormalities identified during the study. After the appropriate radiographs are obtained, a systematic review of the structures of the skull begins. If dealing with radiographic film, hanging the films in a specific order is critical. In the system described, the dorsoventral (DV) view is hung in the upper left hand corner and any open-mouth ventrodorsal (VD) radiographs are hung next to it. The lateral, oblique, and any special oblique tangential radiographs are placed below these radiographs for further evaluation. The availability of a hot light is useful so that each radiograph can be individually reviewed. A magnifying glass can be useful, particularly for evaluating skull radiographs of small dogs and cats.

SKULL

Technical Considerations

Skull radiographs for small animals should be made with the patient under general anesthesia. This way open-mouth and oblique radiographs can be easily made. Also, properly positioned radiographs can be obtained without unnecessary personnel exposure. If nonscreen film is used, anesthesia is critical because exposure factors between 150 and 200 mAs are needed, necessitating long exposure times. Skull radiographs in the horse are made with the horse standing. Correctly marking the film (right versus left) is critical for oblique and DV or VD radiographs. If properly positioned radiographs cannot be obtained, the interpreter will struggle with image distortion and unfamiliar summation shadows. Standard radiographic views for various areas of interest of the skull are summarized in Table 6-1.

When imaging the skull, a consistent film-marking system that is understood by all personnel must be used, particularly for oblique views. One system needs to be adopted as the norm for the practice and embraced by all personnel. This will ensure that the right and left sides of the skull are correctly identified when evaluating oblique radiographs. Also, if the images will be referred to a specialist, some explanation of the marking system is needed to avoid confusion on the part of the specialist.

Multiple positioning and image-marking systems are used; one system for maxillary and mandibular radiography in small animals is explained.

When obtaining oblique radiographs of either the maxilla or mandible, a set of various-sized radiolucent triangular sponges should be used to elevate the maxilla or mandible off the table in a consistent manner with an angle of approximately 25 to 30 degrees. The mouth should be restrained in an open position so that the mandible and maxilla, or the associated dental arcades, do not overlap when being projected onto the final radiographic image. A dental mouth gag placed on a canine tooth can be used if this will not overlap the area of interest. Begin by placing the dog or cat in right lateral recumbency with the mouth open, as described.

First ask the question, "Am I trying to image the mandible or the maxilla?" To image the right maxilla (remember, the dog is in right recumbency), place the sponge under the

Table • 6-1

Radiographic Projections Involved in Various Types of Routine Evaluations of the Skull for Small and Large Animals

TYPE OF EXAMINATION (AREA OF INTEREST)	BASIC RADIOGRAPHIC VIEWS	SPECIAL RADIOGRAPHIC VIEWS*	COMMENTS
Small Animal			
Routine examination	Right lateral and VD or DV		
Nasal cavity (including frontal sinuses)	Right lateral, VD/DV, open-mouth VD	Rostrocaudal radiograph of the frontal sinuses; open-mouth VD with nonscreen film is an additional optional radiograph that provides the best detail of the nasal passages	The patient's nose will be pointing to the x-ray tube with the dog or cat in dorsal recumbency. Frontal sinuses will be small to nonexistent in brachiocephalic dogs and cats. Evaluate the lateral radiograph first to see if they are present. If not, do not attempt the rostrocaudal radiograph.
Tympanic bullae	Right lateral and VD/DV	Open-mouth rostrocaudal radiograph of the bullae; left rostral-right caudal oblique and right rostral/left caudal oblique for evaluation of each bulla	On the oblique radiographs, the skull is maintained in a straight lateral position and the nose is elevated 30 degrees away from the table. The beam is centered between the caudal mandibular ramus and the base of the ear. This will displace the nondependent bulla caudally and the dependent bulla rostrally. The dog or cat is then repositioned into opposite recumbency for evaluation of the opposite bulla. In brachiocephalic dogs and cats, opening the mouth may not be necessary, but tip the nose dorsally slightly and center the x-ray beam just dorsal to the hyoid apparatus and the larynx. The patient's nose is pointing toward the x-ray tube.
Temporomandibular joint	Right lateral and DV	Open-mouth and closed-mouth left dorsal/right ventral and right dorsal/left ventral obliques	For the oblique radiographs, follow the directions for the tympanic bullae.
Maxillary series for fracture or dental arcade evaluation	Right lateral and VD/DV	Intraoral DV for evaluation of the rostral maxillary teeth or intraoral VD radiograph for evaluation of the rostral mandible; left dorsal/right ventral oblique and right dorsal/left ventral obliques	See text for details of labeling and positioning the oblique radiographs.
Mandibular series for fracture or dental arcade evaluation	Right lateral and VD/DV	Intraoral VD for evaluation of the rostral teeth; left dorsal/right ventral oblique and right dorsal/left ventral obliques	See text for details of labeling and positioning the oblique radiographs.
Equine			
Nasal series and frontal sinuses	Right lateral and DV	Left dorsal/right ventral oblique and right dorsal/left ventral obliques	If a specific area has a focal soft tissue swelling or drainage, a radiographic view tangential to the area of interest can help highlight the area. Also, a small external radiopaque marker can be used to help rapidly assess the area of interest.
Maxillary sinuses and teeth	Right lateral and DV	Left dorsal/right ventral oblique and right dorsal/left ventral obliques	If a specific area has a focal soft tissue swelling or drainage, a radiographic view tangential to the area of interest can help highlight the area. Also, a small external radiomarker can be used to help rapidly assess the area of interest. See text for details of labeling and positioning the oblique radiographs.
Temporomandibular joint evaluation	Right lateral and DV	Lateral oblique radiographs; left rostral/right caudal and right rostra/left caudal obliques	See text for details of labeling and positioning the oblique radiographs.
Guttural pouch evaluation	Right lateral and DV	Lateral oblique radiographs; left rostral/right caudal and right rostral/left caudal obliques	See text for details of labeling and positioning the oblique radiographs.

*Special radiograph views are additional radiographs to the basic examination that are still required as part of a routine study for that particular area.

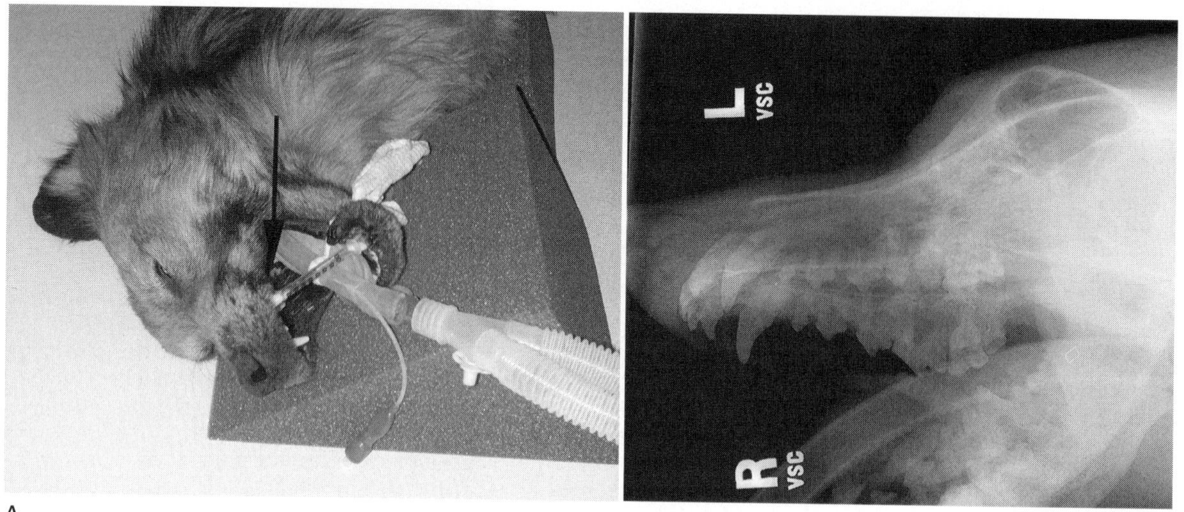

A B

Fig. 6-1 A dog positioned for the lateral oblique view of the right maxilla **(A)** and the corresponding radiograph **(B)**. Note that the dog is under general anesthesia, the mouth is held open with a plastic syringe, and the endotracheal tube is tied to the mandible so that it is not superimposed over the maxilla. The arrow indicates the direction of the x-ray beam.

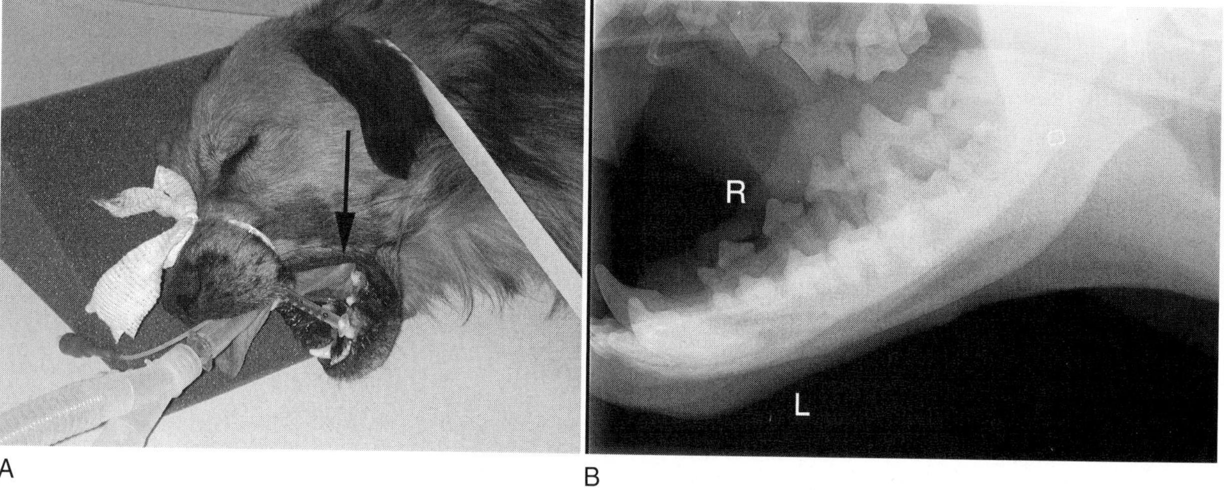

A B

Fig. 6-2 A dog positioned for the lateral oblique view of the right mandible **(A)** and the corresponding radiograph **(B)**. From a technical standpoint, the mandible could have been obliqued more to separate fully the right from the left mandibular arcade. The *arrow* indicates the direction of the primary x-ray beam.

mandible so that the left (nondependent) side of the dog or cat rotates dorsally (Fig. 6-1). Tie the endotracheal tube and tongue to the mandible so no overlap with the maxilla occurs. Place the *L* marker above the nose and the *R* marker beneath the maxilla. This means that the left maxilla is dorsal relative to the right maxilla. The L and R have nothing to do with the fact that the dog is in right lateral recumbency, only the relative position of the left to the right maxillary dental arcades!

To image the left side of the maxilla, place the patient in left recumbency with the sponge under the mandible so that the right (nondependent) side of the dog or cat rotates dorsally. Place the *R* marker above the nose and the *L* marker beneath the maxilla. This means that the right maxilla is dorsal relative to the left maxilla. Again, the L and R have nothing to do with the fact that the dog or cat is now in left recumbency.

For imaging the right mandible, place the dog or cat in right recumbency with the mouth held open (Fig. 6-2). Place the sponge under the maxilla so that the left (nondependent) side of the dog or cat rotates ventrally. Place the *L* marker below the dog or cat's mandible and the *R* marker dorsal to the mandible. This means that the left mandible is ventral relative to the right mandible that has been displaced dorsally by the positioning sponge. Again, the L and R have nothing to do with the fact that the dog or cat is in right recumbency. To image the left mandible, place the patient in left recumbency with the sponge under the maxilla so the right (nondependent) side of the dog or cat rotates ventrally. Place the *R* marker below the dog or cat's mandible and the *L* marker dorsal to the mandible. This means that the right mandible is ventral relative to the left mandible that has been displaced dorsally by the positioning sponge.

Individual tympanic bulla can be imaged with a similar technique as described for the maxilla, except the R or L marker now specifies the side that is recumbent (Fig. 6-3). In either right or left recumbency, the down (dependent) tympanic bulla is ventrally displaced, whereas the up (nondependent) bulla will be displaced dorsally and superimposed over the ventral aspect of the cranial cavity and cannot be evaluated.

Similar oblique projections of the temporomandibular joints can be obtained by using the positioning just described for the tympanic bulla; however, even though the joint space is obliqued, the radiograph provides a unique view of the entire mandibular condyle from a different perspective than on either a lateral or DV/VD radiographs. Another way to view a temporomandibular joint (or a tympanic bulla) is achieved by positioning the dog or cat in right lateral recumbency with the sponge under the rostral aspect of the nose so that the nose is elevated off the table by 25 to 30 degrees from horizontal.[1] This will position the down (dependent) temporomandibular joint rostrally and the up (nondependent) temporomandibular joint caudally (Fig. 6-4). The rostral joint will be more clearly visualized; typically the joint space and the retroarticular process of the temporal bone can be visualized. The disadvantage of this positioning is that the entire length of the mandibular condyle cannot be evaluated.

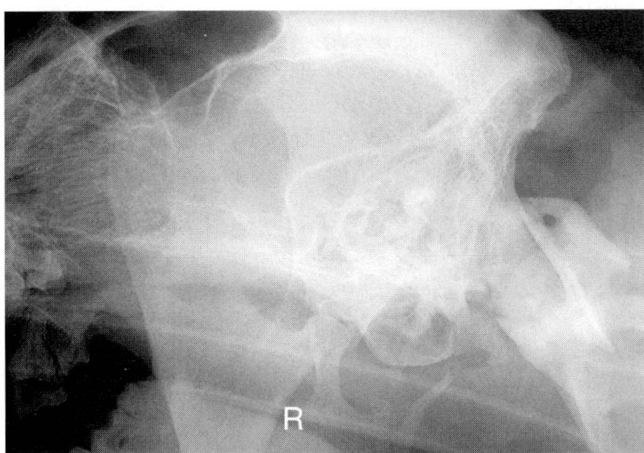

Fig. 6-3 Lateral radiograph of the right tympanic bulla and temporomandibular joint, with the dog being positioned in the same manner as the patient in Fig. 6-1, *A*.

Additional views that can be used are the rostrocaudal tangential views. If the dog is a mesaticephalic or a dolichocephalic breed, place the dog in a positioning trough in dorsal recumbency. The dog's nose is then pointed toward the x-ray tube, perpendicular to the long axis of the body. The x-ray beam is centered between the eyes for evaluation of the frontal sinuses (Fig. 6-5). For evaluation of the tympanic bullae in this position, the mouth is opened and the endotracheal tube and tongue are moved with the mandible, being careful to avoid kinking the endotracheal tube. The x-ray beam is centered just dorsal to the tongue and endotracheal tube at the level of the soft palate.

In brachiocephalic dogs and cats, the mouth can be kept closed and the head angled dorsally from the perpendicular position. Center the x-ray beam just dorsal to the hyoid apparatus for the rostro-10 degrees ventral to caudodorsal oblique radiograph (Fig. 6-6).[7]

For evaluation of the equine skull, standard radiographic views depend on the area of interest (see Table 6-1).[1,2] A vertically oriented radiolucent suture is normally present between the basioccipital and basisphenoid bones in horses

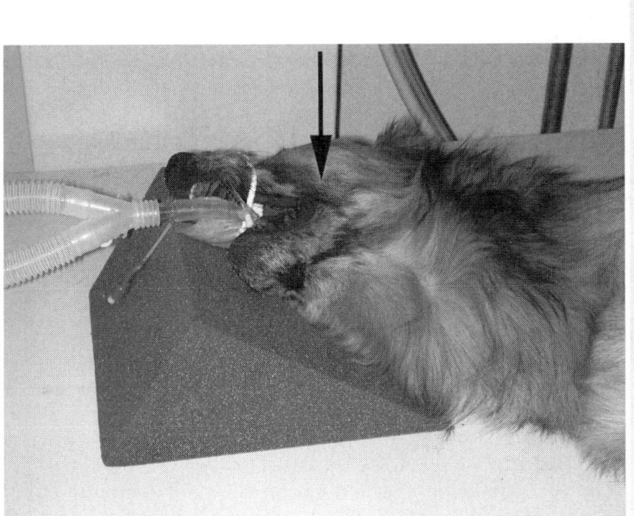

A

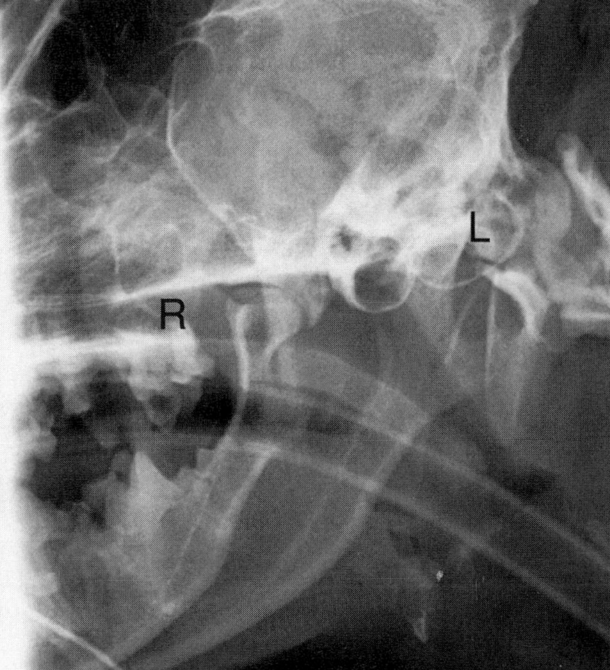

B

Fig. 6-4 A dog positioned for evaluation of the right temporomandibular joint **(A)** with the corresponding radiograph **(B)**. The dog is positioned in right lateral recumbency with the nose dorsally displaced by the positioning sponge. This will rotate the dependent (right) temporomandibular joint rostrally *(R)* and superimpose the left *(L)* temporomandibular joint over the caudoventral aspect of the skull. The *arrow* indicates the direction of the primary x-ray beam. The position of the "R" and "L" markers designates the relative position of each joint and bulla.

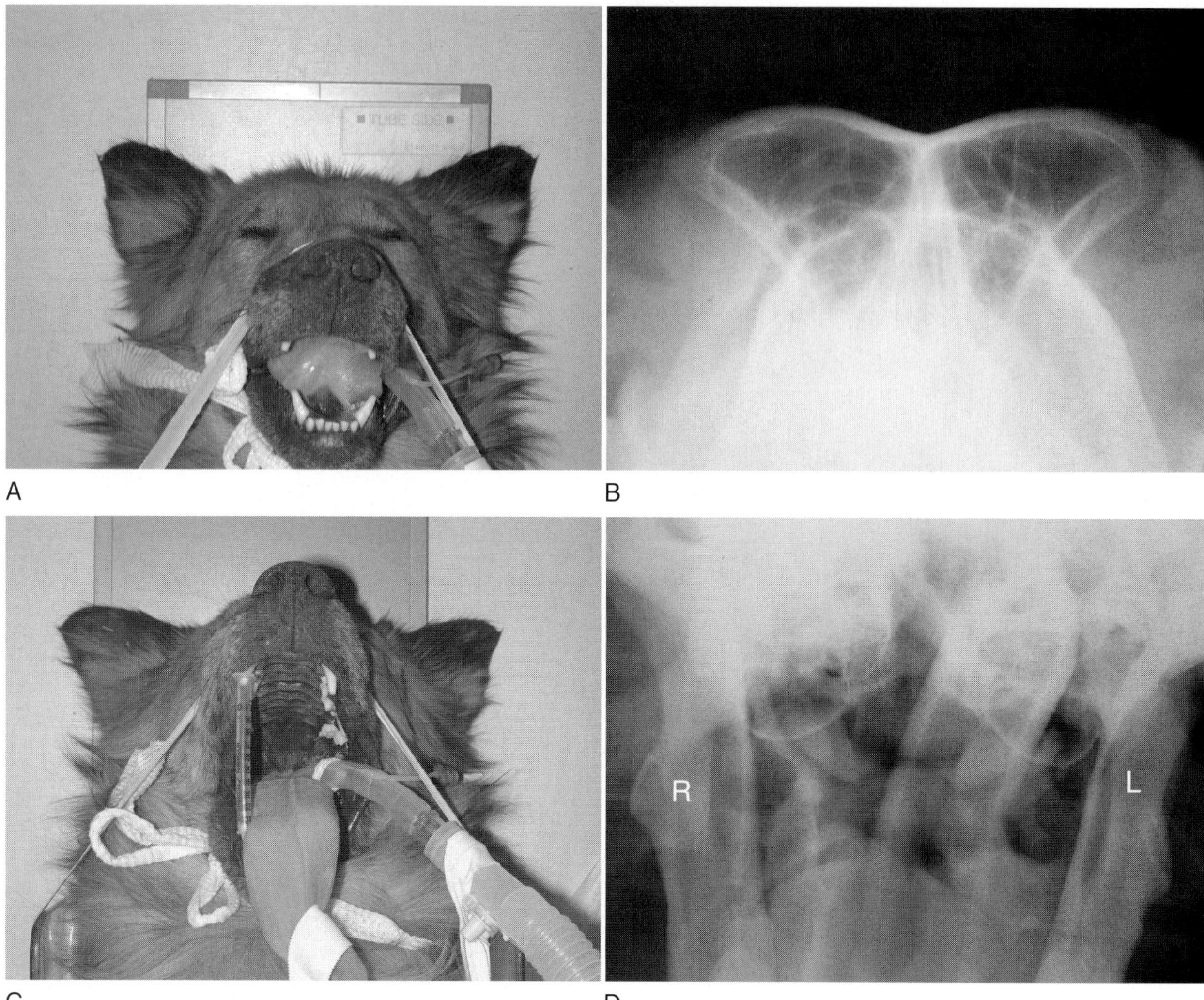

Fig. 6-5 A dog positioned for a rostrocaudal tangential radiograph of the frontal sinuses **(A)** with the corresponding radiograph of the frontal sinuses **(B).** On the radiograph, the frontal sinuses are shown in their entirety. The x-ray beam is centered dorsally to the level of the eyes between the frontal sinuses. A dog positioned for the rostrocaudal tangential radiograph of the tympanic bullae **(C)** with the corresponding radiograph of the tympanic bullae **(D).** Note that the endotracheal tube is inappropriately positioned toward the left and is superimposed over the left tympanic bulla. The tube should be secured to the mandible along midline with the patient's tongue.

up to 4 years of age (Fig. 6-7).[2] When evaluating the maxillary and frontal sinuses the x-ray tube is positioned dorsolaterally and angled ventromedially at a 45-degree angle. The cassette is perpendicular to the x-ray beam on the opposite side of the head. If the x-ray tube is on the left side of the horse and the beam centered on the dorsal aspect of the maxilla, the right sides of the maxillary and frontal sinuses and nasal cavity are projected dorsal to other skull structures. If the x-ray beam is centered in the middle of the mandible, the left hemimandible is projected ventral to the right side of the mandible.

For evaluation of a tympanic bulla, guttural pouch, or temporomandibular joint, the horse is positioned next to a cassette holder that fixes the cassette in a vertical plane and the nose is angled toward the x-ray tube; the caudal aspect of the mandible remains next to the cassette. The most caudal guttural pouch or temporomandibular joint region can be assessed with this technique. To assess the contralateral side, the horse is then turned around and the same position repeated. Often because the rostral nasal passages are predominantly air and the cranial cavity is predominantly soft tissue and bone, two radiographs may have to be made so that each area is properly exposed.

Variants

Mesaticephalic and dolichocephalic dogs typically have well-developed frontal sinuses. Brachycephalic breeds will not have a frontal sinus that is recognizable on a lateral radiograph; useful rostrocaudal radiographs of the frontal sinuses are therefore not possible in these dogs.

The largest variation in overall radiographic opacity and appearance is in the immature skull of dogs, cats, and horses. This is because immature teeth have a large radiolucent pulp cavity and are less opaque than mature teeth.[8] As the adult teeth are developing within the maxilla or mandible, multiple radiopaque curvilinear tooth buds will be seen. Radiopaque structures of the teeth include the dentin, enamel, and lamina dura that surround each tooth root (Fig. 6-8). The soft tissue components of the teeth include the pulp cavity and periodontal membrane. As the cat or dog grows older, the periodontal membrane will decrease in width.

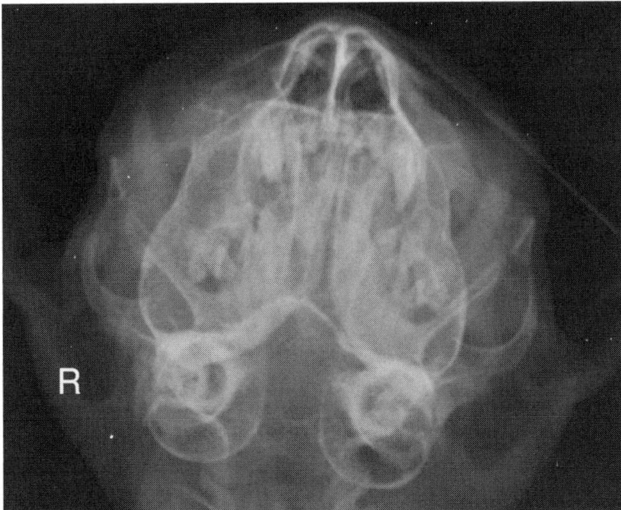

Fig. 6-6 Another radiograph that can be used for evaluation of the tympanic bulla is a rostro-10-degree ventral to caudodorsal oblique radiograph of the tympanic bulla from a cat. The mouth is not opened but both the mandible and maxilla are displaced dorsally 10 degrees. *R*, right side.

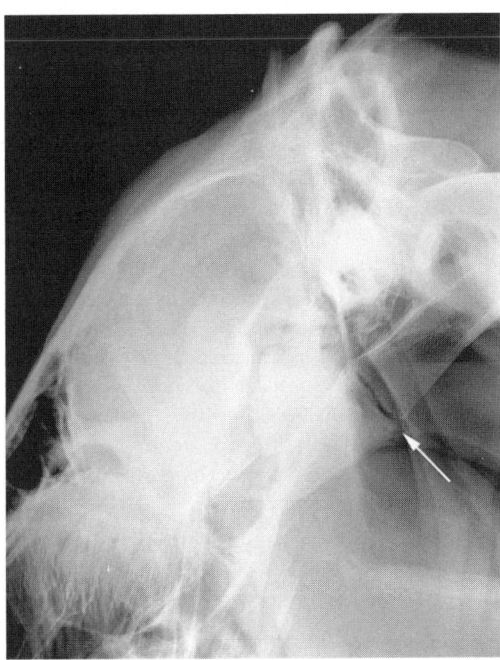

Fig. 6-7 The open basioccipital-basisphenoid suture *(arrow)* of a horse.

In horses, if fluid is present within the paranasal sinuses, an air-fluid level will be seen because of the gravity-dependent distribution of the fluid and the fact that the radiographs were made with the horse standing and a horizontally directed x-ray beam was used (Fig. 6-9). Typically a grid is used for equine skull radiographs, which means artifacts must be avoided because correctly positioning a horizontally oriented x-ray beam with reference to the grid is more difficult than positioning a vertically directed beam from a column-mounted x-ray tube.

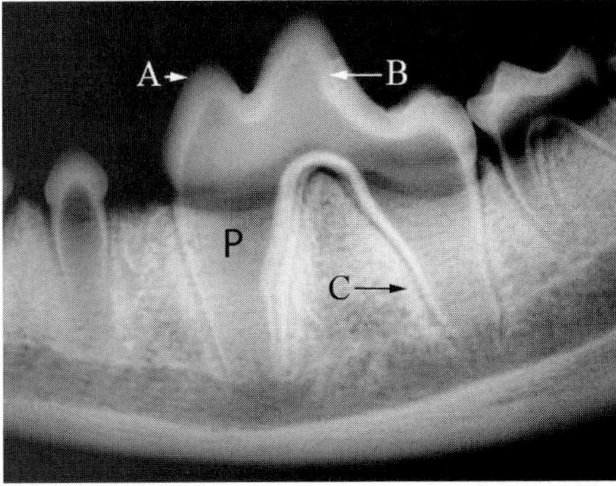

Fig. 6-8 A specimen radiograph of a first mandibular molar in which the enamel *(A)*, dentin *(B)*, and lamina dura *(C)* are labeled. Note the large radiolucent pulp cavity *(P)* consistent with a young dog.

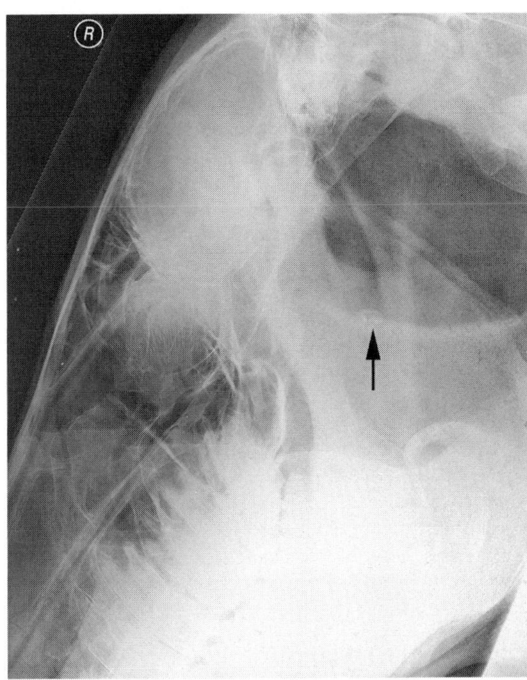

Fig. 6-9 A standing right lateral radiograph of a horse. Multiple horizontal air-fluid lines are visible in the frontal and maxillary sinuses. A partially mineralized chondroid within one of the guttural pouches is present *(arrow)*. The "R" indicates that the right side of the head is against the cassette.

Interpretation Paradigm

The skull is anatomically complex, and thereby visually complex, when evaluated on a two-dimensional radiographic image. This limitation may be overcome if the interpreter is familiar with the anatomy, the patient was positioned correctly, and proper radiographic technique was used. Do not become overwhelmed by skull images. If this happens, identify one structure and think of the relation of this structure to other structures. If the VD/DV radiograph is straight, the right and left sides can be compared for structural and opacity symmetry because most disease processes are asymmetric. Applying past experience to the current patient can lead to errors in interpretation because of the complex skull anatomy and the variation in skull size and shape across breeds.

Radiographic interpretation of the skull can be approached in many ways. The model presented is an approach that starts rostrally and works caudally through the level of C1-C2. Once the interpreter is convinced the study is complete and the radiographic views are of diagnostic quality, then images are reviewed individually and then collectively. A hot light is critical for viewing to ensure that all bone and soft tissues are assessed. If an abnormality is seen in a specific location, a mental note should be made so that the area can be evaluated on all radiographs collectively to gain a three-dimensional perspective of the lesion. Initially this approach may seem cumbersome, but over time the review process will become second nature. An easy mnemonic to remember is "***n**o **e**ager **m**an **m**isses **o**ther **c**aveats of the **s**kull*," where *n* stands for nasal/paranasal passages, *e* stands for ethmoid region, *m* stands for maxillary bones and dental arcade, *m* stands for mandibular bones and dental arcade, *o* stands for orbital structures, *c* stands for cranial cavity extending into the cervical vertebrae, and *s* stands for soft tissues (Table 6-2). In the horse, the soft tissues also include the guttural pouches.

Fortunately, the skull is a bilaterally symmetric structure so that if the VD or DV views are straight, or the oblique views are obtained at the same angle, an immediate contralateral (presumed normal) comparison is possible. When evaluating symmetry on an open-mouth VD radiograph of the nasal passages, the overall nasal opacity and turbinate detail are expected to be the same on both sides (Fig. 6-10).

The hyoid bones should not be overlooked, especially in horses. The mnemonic *the **s**ick **e**lephant **c**an **b**e **t**reated* can be used to remember the order of the hyoid bones (Fig. 6-11). The tympanohyoid articulates with the tympanic bulla of the petrous portion of the temporal bones, but it is cartilaginous and not seen on radiographs. The stylohyoid, epihyoid, ceratohyoid, basihyoid (unpaired), and thyrohyoid bones are the remaining parts of the hyoid apparatus. The basihyoid bone is the only bone that is unpaired and courses in a transverse plane from one side of the pharynx to the other. In the horse, the basihyoid bone has a cranial extension toward the tongue called the lingual process. The thyrohyoid bones articulate with the thyroid cartilage of the larynx. The stylohyoid bones are the largest bones of the hyoid apparatus in the horse and course through the cranial aspect of the guttural pouches, resulting in a division of each pouch into a larger medial and a smaller lateral compartment.

VERTEBRAL COLUMN

Vertebrae are divided into five regions: cervical (C), thoracic (T), lumbar (L), sacral (S), and caudal (Cd). The vertebral formula for the dog and cat is C7, T13, L7, S3, and Cd20-Cd24. The vertebral formula for the horse is C7, T18, L6, S5, and Cd15-Cd20.[4] In general each vertebral body is made up of a body, vertebral arch, articular processes, and various bony processes.[4] Each region of the vertebral column has distinguishing characteristics that aid in the identification of the specific region of the spine being evaluated (Table 6-3). A thorough understanding of these characteristics is necessary.

Radiographic Technique and Positioning

Radiographically, the vertebral column is complex. Vertebral radiographs must be correctly exposed and positioned.[1] Intervertebral disc space narrowing and abnormalities of normal vertebral structures can easily be misinterpreted on marginal or poor-quality images. For these reasons, sedation or general anesthesia is generally required when making radiographs of the spine. Routinely, two orthogonal (right or left lateral and VD) radiographs are made of the cervical, cervicothoracic, thoracic, thoracolumbar, lumbar and/or sacral vertebrae (10 total images). The beam should be tightly collimated and centered in the middle of the region of interest, including centering over C3-C4 for the cervical spine, T6-T7 for the thoracic spine, and L3-L4 for the lumbar spine. The spine should be parallel to the table. To accomplish this for a lateral radiograph of the cervical spine, a sponge or radiolucent positioning device is placed under the neck so that the neck does not sag and cause the intervertebral disc spaces to appear narrow. Also, to align the cervical spine to the long axis of the cassette, the pelvic region of the dog or cat should be pushed dorsally. The thoracic limbs should be pulled ventrally and caudally so that overlap of the caudal cervical vertebrae with the scapula is minimized. If using film, the highest detail

Table • 6-2

Mnemonic for Interpretation and Evaluation of the Skull: "No Eager Man Misses Other Caveats of the Skull"

AREA EVALUATED	STRUCTURES EVALUATED
Nasal passages and paranasal sinuses	Maxillary, nasal, incisive, and palatine bones. Nasal turbinates and passages, vomer bone, frontal sinuses, and sphenoid sinuses. In the horse, other sinuses such as the maxillary sinuses and dorsal and ventral conchal sinus.
Ethmoid and ethmoid turbinate region	Ethmoid bone and ethmoid turbinates.
Maxilla	Maxillary dental arcade, including the incisors, canine, premolars, and molars of the right and left maxillae.
Mandible	Mandibular dental arcade, including the incisors, canine, premolars, and molars of the right and left maxilla. Horizontal and vertical aspects of the right and left hemimandibles. Coronoid process of the hemimandibles and the temporomandibular joints.
Orbital region	Orbital area including the zygomatic arch; frontal process of the zygomatic bone; zygomatic process of the frontal bone and frontal sinus.
Cranial cavity	All bones of the cranial cavity, starting rostrally with the ethmoid region, moving dorsally and laterally with the frontal and parietal bones, and extending caudally to the occipital bones, occipital condyles, and articulation with C1 (atlas) and the foramen magnum. Ventral and lateral extent of the temporal bones and sphenoid bones.
Skull soft tissues	Soft tissues surrounding the skull, including the planum nasale, soft palate, nasopharynx, oropharynx, tongue, submandibular soft tissues, hyoid apparatus, and the larynx.

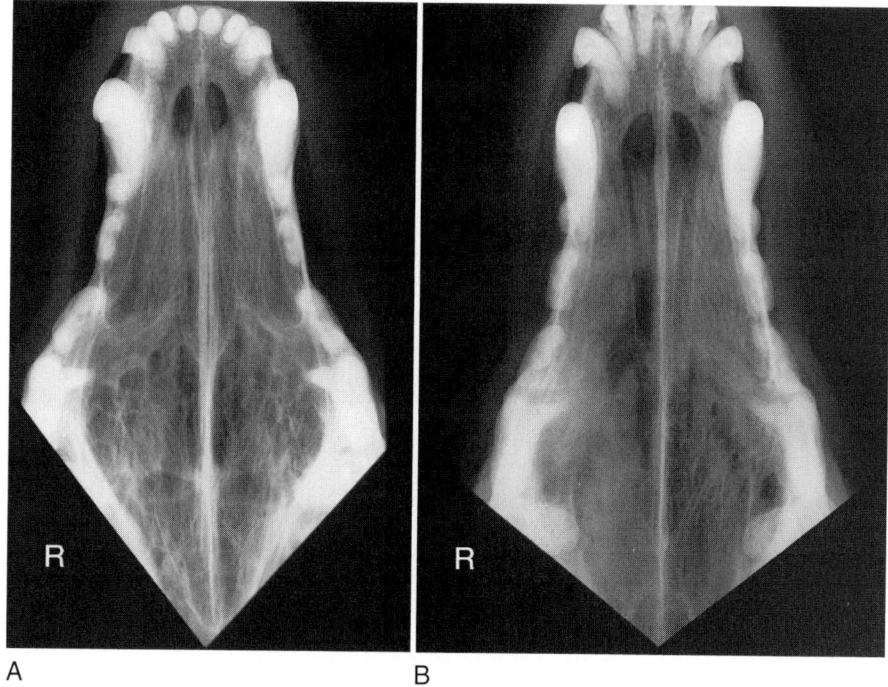

Fig. 6-10 Open-mouth VD radiographs of the nasal cavities from a normal dog (A) and a dog with a right-sided destructive fungal rhinitis (B).

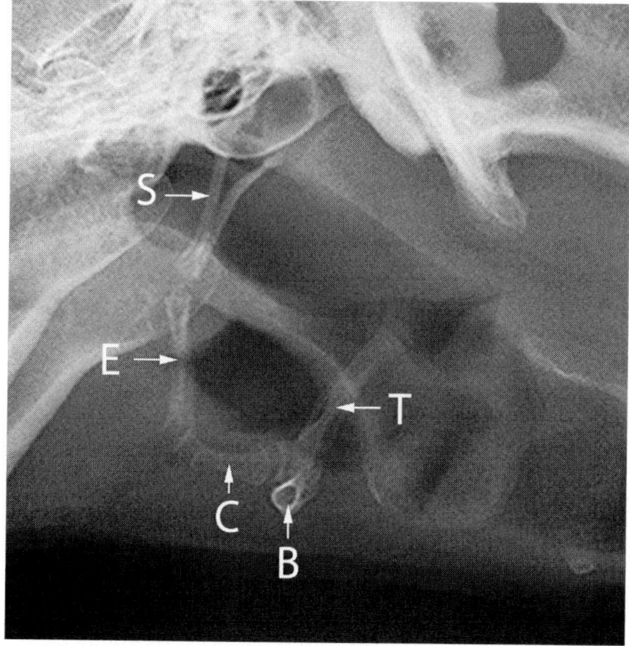

Fig. 6-11 A lateral radiograph of the larynx from a dog in which the stylohyoid *(S)*, epihyoid *(E)*, ceratohyoid *(C)*, basihyoid *(B)*, and thyrohyoid *(T)* bones are labeled. The laryngeal cartilages are also mineralized. The small tympanohyoid is not visible.

x-ray cassette/film combination, and a grid, should be used (100 to 200 speed system). A low kVp and high mAs technique is used for better radiographic contrast. When evaluating the cervical spine on the lateral radiograph, the transverse processes should be superimposed. A separate image of the cervicothoracic junction is obtained to evaluate this region better.

When positioning the patient for a lateral radiograph of the thoracic vertebrae, the pelvis is repositioned ventrally so that all the thoracic vertebrae are aligned with the long axis of the cassette because dogs and cats have a natural area of kyphosis in the mid to caudal thoracic region. Also, the rib heads should be superimposed and the thoracic limbs pulled cranially. To get the rib heads superimposed in some barrel-chested and deep-chested dogs, a triangular sponge may be placed under the sternum. The x-ray beam is centered at T6-T7 or just caudal to the dorsal border of the scapula. Another radiograph is made, centered at the thoracolumbar junction. For the lateral radiograph of the lumbar vertebral column, the x-ray beam should be centered between the last rib and the coxal joint (usually at L3-L4). The pelvis is typically lined up in a neutral position as the dog or cat is lying on the table. When evaluating the lumbar radiographs for positioning, the transverse processes should be superimposed. These look like the Swoosh logo for Nike footwear and athletic equipment, and the transverse processes should be superimposed when correctly positioned (Fig. 6-12). Also, the intervertebral foramina should be superimposed and be of consistent size from the thoracolumbar junction to the sacrum. On VD radiographs, alignment of the spinous processes and symmetry noted to the ribs (thoracic vertebrae) and transverse processes is normally present (lumbar vertebrae). Also, in the thoracic region the sternum should be superimposed over the thoracic vertebrae.

On the basis of evaluation of the initial survey radiographs, other views may be needed that are specific to suspected or visualized radiographic abnormalities. With the patient in dorsal recumbency as positioned for a VD, the sternum can be rotated, first to one side and then the other, to make oblique radiographs. For a suspected vertebral body fracture, a horizontal beam VD radiograph should be made with the patient in lateral recumbency. Additionally, dynamic flexed or extended views of an area of interest (not in traumatized patients) can be obtained (Fig. 6-13). Dynamic flexed or extended views are sometimes used to evaluate the lumbosacral junction and the caudal aspect of the cervical spine.

Table • 6-3

Unique Characteristics of Individual Vertebral Segments for Dogs, Cats, and Horses

ANATOMIC SEGMENT	DOG	CAT	HORSE
Cervical: Dogs, cats, and horses have seven cervical vertebrae.			
Atlas (C1)	No spinous process; articulates by a right and left condyle with the occipital condyles cranially, which are synovial joints; articulates caudally with C2 by a synovial joint; has two large wings (lateral processes).	Similar anatomy to the dog.	Similar anatomy to the dog.
Axis (C2)	Has a large elongated spinous process that should overlap and come just dorsal to the caudal vertebral arch of C1; has a large bone extension along the cranial aspect of the vertebral body called the dens (odontoid process); articulates caudally with C3 by an intervertebral disc (fibrocartilaginous joint) and synovial joints at the articular processes dorsally.	As in the dog.	As in the dog; Arabian horses have genetic breed predisposition to atlantooccipital malformations that can include the occipital bone of the skull, C1, and C2.
C6	Has large transverse processes (ventral lamina).	As in the dog.	As in the dog.
Thoracic vertebrae	The dog has 13 thoracic vertebrae, 13 pairs of ribs, large spinous processes; T11 is also called the anticlinal vertebra; T10-T11 is the anticlinal intervertebral disc space and the narrowest intervertebral disc space; intercapital ligaments are present extending from one rib head dorsal to the intervertebral disc space to the other rib head from T2 through T11.	The cat has 13 thoracic vertebrae; rib heads are cranial to their corresponding thoracic vertebral body.	The horse has 18 thoracic vertebrae, 18 pairs of ribs; because of the large size of adult horses, generally only the spinous processes can be imaged on a lateral radiograph; irregular margination of the dorsal aspect of the spinous process is normal and a result of incomplete mineralization of a secondary center of ossification.
Lumbar vertebrae	The dog has seven lumbar vertebrae; short spinous processes; and large, cranially angulated lateral processes; the ventral margins of L3 and L4 may be irregular or more ill defined because of the attachment of the diaphragmatic crura; has a straight or a kyphotic curvature.	The cat has seven lumbar vertebrae; the cat's lumbar vertebral bodies are longer when compared with the dog (ratio of the vertebral body length to height is greater in the cat than in the dog; also has a lordotic curve to the lumbar spine).	The horse has six lumbar vertebrae.
Sacrum	The dog has three sacral vertebrae that are fused.	The cat has three sacral vertebrae that are fused.	The horse has five sacral vertebrae that are fused.
Caudal vertebrae	20 to 25 caudal vertebrae; may have hemal arches ventral to the cranial caudal vertebral bodies.	20 to 25 caudal vertebrae; may have hemal arches ventral to the first several caudal vertebral bodies and are more commonly seen in cats than dogs.	15 to 20 caudal vertebrae; usually has hemal arches ventral to the first few caudal vertebrae.

In the cervical region, flexed or extended radiographs may be made after a myelogram to evaluate for signs of ligamentous hypertrophy, as in cervical vertebral malformations (see Chapter 11). In dogs with cervical vertebral malformation, a neutrally positioned traction radiograph may also be obtained in which the radiograph is made while longitudinal traction is placed on the cervical vertebrae. This will allow assessment of whether compression can be alleviated by surgical procedures to increase the distance between adjacent vertebrae.

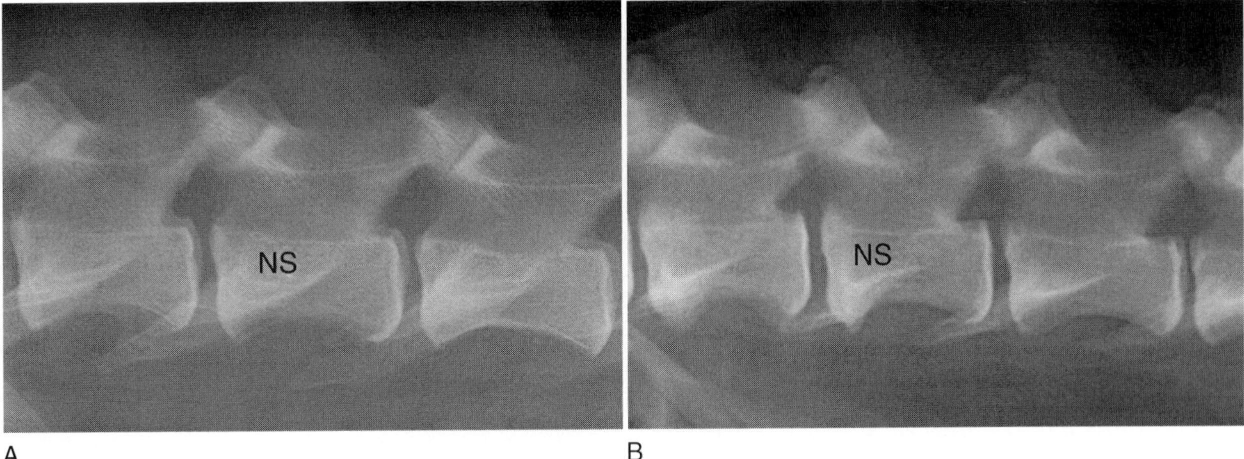

Fig. 6-12 A lateral radiograph from a dog centered over the second, third, and fourth lumbar vertebrae **(A)**. The Nike Swoosh *(NS)* is seen superimposed over the dorsal aspect of the vertebrae. *NS* represents the origin of the transverse process at the vertebral body. In this radiograph, the vertebrae are rotated slightly so that two "Swooshes" are present. The ventral cortex of L3 is thin relative to that of L2 and L4. **B,** The lateral radiograph is straight and only one "Swoosh" is visible superimposed over the second through fifth vertebral bodies.

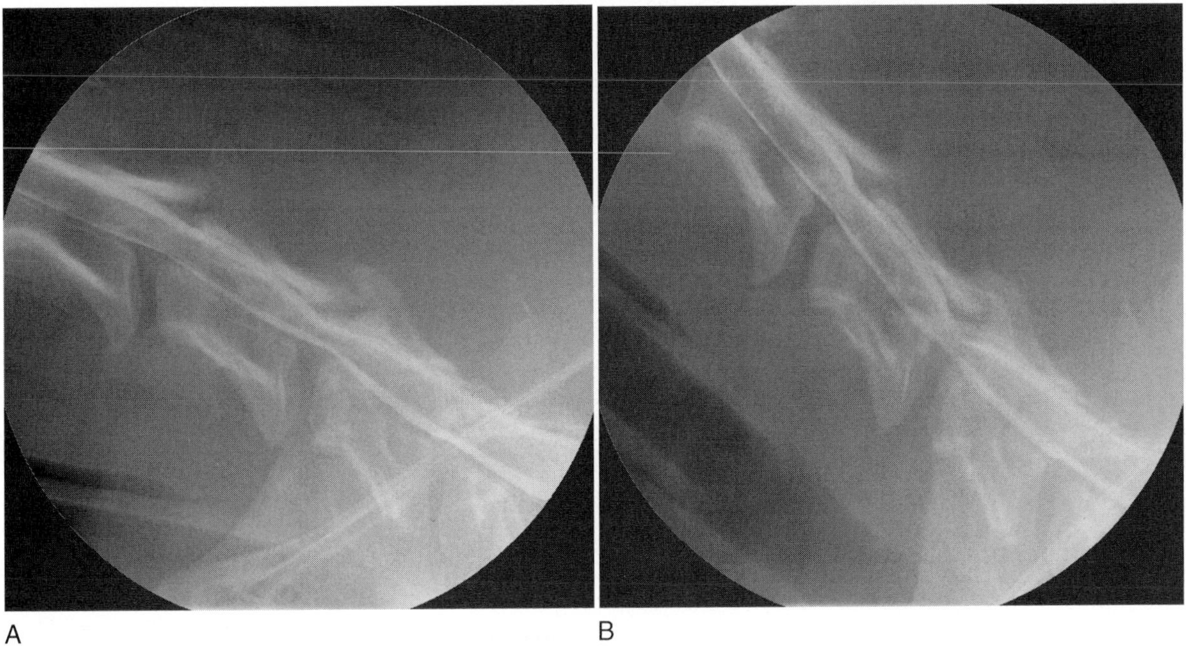

Fig. 6-13 Neutral lateral **(A)** and dorsal flexed lateral **(B)** radiographs of a caudal cervical myelogram from a dog with a cervical spondylomyelopathy. Notice the dynamic spinal cord compression demonstrated on the dorsal flexed image **(B)**. This is evidenced by more severe attenuation of the dorsal aspect of the contrast medium column.

In horses, the cervical spine is the spinal region radiographed most commonly. Cervical radiography can be performed in the standing (tranquilized) horse or with the horse in lateral recumbency under general anesthesia.[1] At least three 14-inch × 17-inch images are required to radiograph the entire adult equine cervical spine. External markers can be taped at several points on the neck so that repeat evaluation of specific areas can be done with relative ease knowing the position of the specific marker relative to where the radiograph is to be obtained. The third, fourth, and fifth cervical vertebrae in the horse have a similar appearance. The sixth cervical vertebra is unique given its enlarged ventral processes (Fig. 6-14). If the horse is anesthetized, then VD radiographs can be made of the middle and cranial aspects of the cervical spine if warranted.

Anatomic Variants

The anatomic variants of the vertebral bodies can be complex and predominantly involve abnormal vertebral body numbers (one additional or one less vertebral body in a specific vertebral segment) and abnormal shape (maldevelopment such as hemivertebrae, or butterfly vertebrae; see Chapter 11). Additionally, the ventral cortex of the L3 and L4 vertebral bodies may be thin or have a decreased opacity (see Fig. 6-12).

This is caused by normal muscular attachments of the left and right diaphragmatic crura. Transitional vertebral body segments are also apparent where the last or first vertebral body of a specific vertebral segment has the characteristics of both the cranial and caudal vertebral joints (see Chapter 11).

Interpretation Paradigm

Many ways are possible to approach radiographic interpretation of the vertebrae. The steps provided are one approach that may provide a foundation to develop an individual approach or help the reader become more organized in the evaluation of vertebral radiographs. The largest obstacles to overcome when evaluating vertebral radiographs are the shear number of radiographs and the number of individual vertebral bodies to evaluate. The acronym "A SPINE" can be used to help in the evaluation process. A SPINE stands for ***a***lignment, ***s***oft tissues, ***p***rocesses, ***i***nternal, ***n***erves, and ***e***xternal (Table 6-4). First, ensure that the appropriate number of images have been acquired to include all vertebrae and that they are of diagnostic quality. Assess overall alignment by tracing three lines on the lateral radiograph. The first line starts at the most cranial aspect of the dorsal part of the vertebral canal. This line is then traced caudally to the end of the image. The second line is along the ventral aspect of the vertebral canal. The third line is the ventral aspect of each vertebral body (Fig. 6-15). On the VD radiograph, again assess the alignment of the vertebral column by tracing three lines. The first is along the left pedicles of the vertebrae; the second is along the spinous processes centrally on each vertebrae; and the third is along the right pedicles of each vertebrae.

After this initial assessment, evaluate the ***s***oft tissues and paraspinal structures surrounding the vertebrae. The ***p***rocesses from each vertebral body should then be evaluated for normal size, shape, margin, and opacity. As the spinous processes are being evaluated, count the vertebrae. Vertebral anomalies at

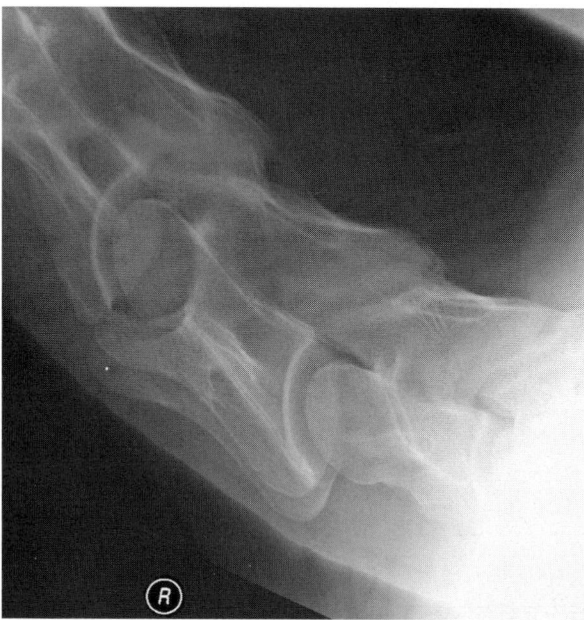

Fig. 6-14 A lateral caudal cervical radiograph of a horse. Note the normal large transverse processes of the sixth cervical vertebra.

Table • 6-4

Mnemonic for the Interpretation Paradigm for Evaluation of the Vertebral Column: "A SPINE"

DEFINITION	AREA EVALUATED
Alignment	Evaluation of the dorsal and ventral aspects of the vertebral canal and the ventral margins of the vertebral bodies on the lateral radiograph(s) and the right and left pedicles and central vertebral canal on the VD radiographs.
Soft tissues	Evaluation of the soft tissues immediately adjacent to the vertebral bodies (and other regions seen on the radiographs).
Processes	Evaluation of the spinous and transverse processes for each vertebral body. Evaluation of all articular processes, starting in sequence from the most cranial vertebral body to the most caudal vertebral body on the radiographic examination.
Internal	Evaluation of the internal size, margin, and opacity of the vertebral arches.
Nerves / spinal cord	Evaluation of the vertebral canal with all aspects of the intervertebral foramina being reviewed. Evaluation for enlargement or collapse of the intervertebral foramina.
External	Evaluation of the vertebral bodies for shape, margin, and opacity, including areas of spondylosis deformans. Evaluation of the intervertebral disc spaces for width and opacity.

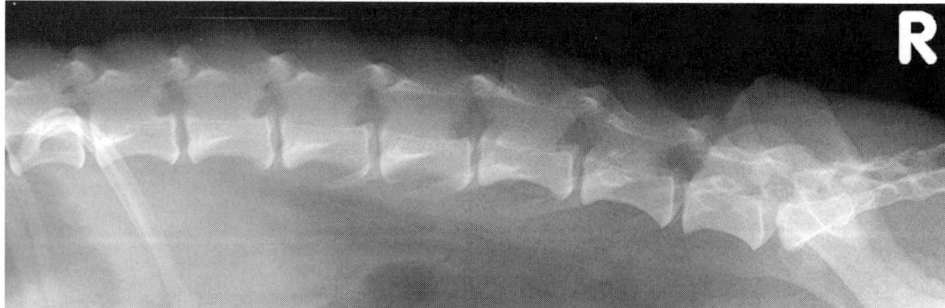

Fig. 6-15 A lateral radiograph of a dog lumbar spine. Mild L4-L5 subluxation is present where L5 is dorsally displaced in relation to L4. Note how the Nike "Swooshes" are superimposed for the first four lumbar vertebrae, whereas the transverse processes are rotated and not superimposed from L5-L7. This would imply some degree of rotational malalignment as well as VD malalignment. Focal mineralized opacities are visible at L2-L3 and superimposed over the vertebral canal at L6.

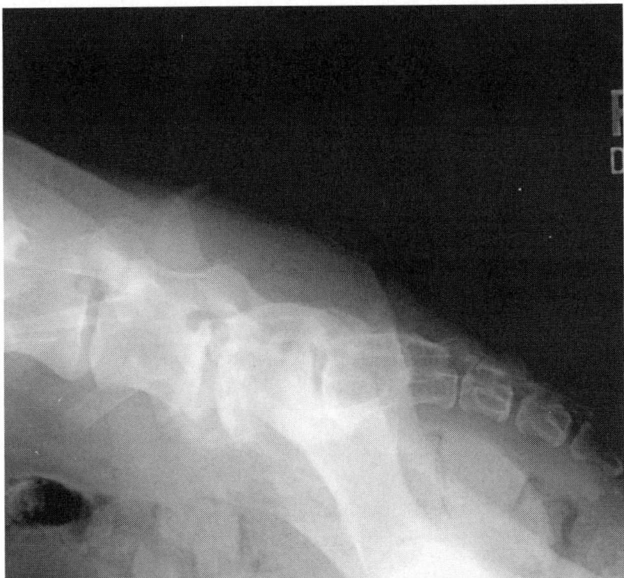

A

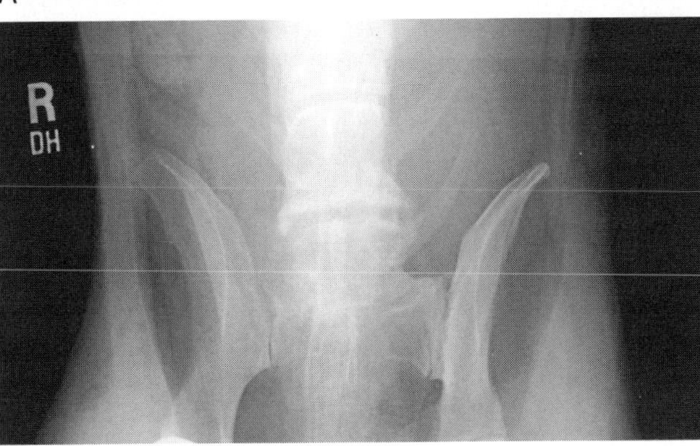

B

Fig. 6-16 Right lateral (A) and VD (B) radiographs of a dog's pelvis. A transitional lumbosacral segment is present with a normal transverse process of a lumbar vertebrae *(left)* and a normal wing of the sacrum *(right)*. The cranial sacral vertebral segment has not fused with the rest of the sacral segments, and an intervertebral disc space is present between the presumed first and second sacral segments.

the cervicothoracic, thoracolumbar, and lumbosacral junctions, called transitional segments, are not uncommon and will have external processes that are characteristic of both the cranial and caudal vertebral segments (Fig. 6-16).

Evaluation of the ***i***nterior involves a critical look at the vertebral canal, its diameter, and overall opacity, which provides a second opportunity to evaluate the alignment of the vertebrae relative to each other. The vertebral canal will widen at the brachial (C5-T2) and lumbosacral (L3-S3) intumescences. The sagittal vertebral canal diameter is larger in the lumbar spine of the cat when compared with the dog. Evaluate the ***n***erves by looking at the intervertebral foramina. The foramina should be relatively similar in size in adjacent vertebrae, with the exception of C2-C3 and L7-S1, which are typically larger than the rest. Look for any widening or collapse of the foramina. Again, counting from cranial to caudal helps in the evaluation. Finally, evaluate the ***e***xterior. The exterior refers to the vertebral bodies and the intervertebral disc spaces. Typically, adjacent intervertebral disc spaces are of approximately equal width and adjacent vertebral bodies are of similar size, shape, and radiopacity. Peripheral to the central axis of the x-ray beam, the intervertebral disc spaces will appear narrowed as a result of beam divergence. If areas of interest are away from the central axis, then the radiograph should be recentered and repeated to ensure no artifacts related to beam divergence are present.

A similar approach is used for the evaluation of the equine cervical spine, recognizing that usually only lateral radiographs are evaluated. Use of the mnemonic A SPINE will be similar to that described above.

REFERENCES

1. Morgan JP: *Techniques of veterinary radiography,* ed 5, Ames, Iowa, 1993, Iowa State University Press.
2. Butler JA, Colles CM, Dyson SJ et al: *Clinical radiology of the horse,* ed 2, Oxford, 2000, Blackwell Scientific.
3. Kus SP, Morgan JP: Radiography of the canine head: optimal positioning with respect to skull type, *Vet Radiol* 26:196, 1985.
4. Dyce KM, Sack WO, Wensing JG: Textbook of veterinary anatomy, ed 3, Philadelphia, 2002, WB Saunders.
5. George FT, Smallwood JE: Anatomic atlas for computed tomography in the mesaticephalic dog: head and neck, *Vet Radiol Ultrasound* 33:217, 1992.
6. Morrow KL, Park RD, Spurgeon TL et al: Computed tomographic imaging of the equine head, *Vet Radiol Ultrasound* 41:491, 2000.
7. Hofer P, Meisen N, Bartholdi S et al: Radiology corner: a new radiographic view of the feline tympanic bullae, *Vet Radiol Ultrasound* 36:14, 1995.
8. Zontine WJ: Canine dental radiology: radiographic technic, development, and anatomy of the teeth, *Vet Radiol* 16:75, 1975.

ELECTRONIC RESOURCES evolve

Additional information related to the content in Chapter 6 can be found on the companion Web site at evolve http://evolve.elsevier.com/Thrall/vetrad/

- Key Points
- Chapter Quiz

CHAPTER • 7
Radiographic Anatomy of the Axial Skeleton

James E. Smallwood
Kathy A. Spaulding

To use the roentgen sign method of recognizing abnormal radiographic findings effectively, an understanding of normal radiographic anatomy for the specific area of interest is necessary. Within the space constraint of a comprehensive veterinary radiology text, this chapter provides a limited reference for the radiographic anatomy of the axial skeleton. For more detailed information, readers are referred to comprehensive texts on radiographic anatomy.[1,2] The radiographic nomenclature used in this chapter was approved by the American College of Veterinary Radiology in 1983.[3]

REFERENCES

1. Schebitz HCH: *Atlas of radiographic anatomy of the dog*, Parey Verlag, 2005, Stuttgart, Germany.
2. Schebitz H, Wilkens H: *Atlas of radiographic anatomy of the horse*, ed 4, Philadelphia, 2005, WB Saunders.
3. Smallwood JE, Shively MJ, Rendano VT et al: A standardized nomenclature for radiographic projections used in veterinary medicine, *Vet Radiol* 26:2, 1985.

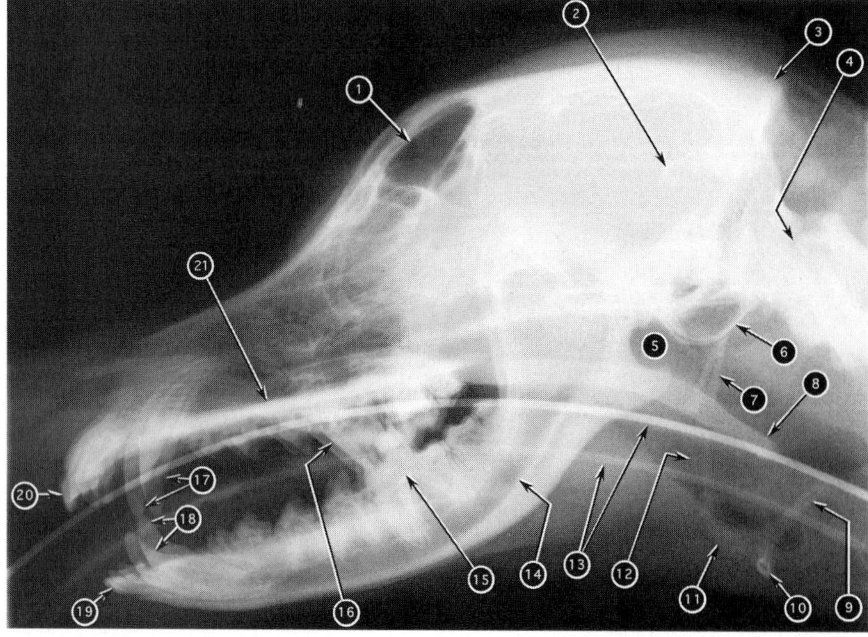

Fig. 7-1 Left-Right Lateral Radiograph of Canine Head.
1. Frontal sinuses
2. Tentorium osseum cerebelli
3. External occipital protuberance
4. Atlantooccipital joints
5. Air in nasopharynx
6. Tympanic bullae
7. Stylohyoid bones
8. Soft palate
9. Thyrohyoid bones
10. Basihyoid bone
11. Ceratohyoid bones
12. Epihyoid bones
13. Endotracheal tube
14. Inferior alveolar canals of mandibles
15. Inferior first molar teeth
16. Superior fourth premolar teeth
17. Superior canine teeth
18. Inferior canine teeth
19. Inferior incisor teeth
20. Superior incisor teeth
21. Hard palate

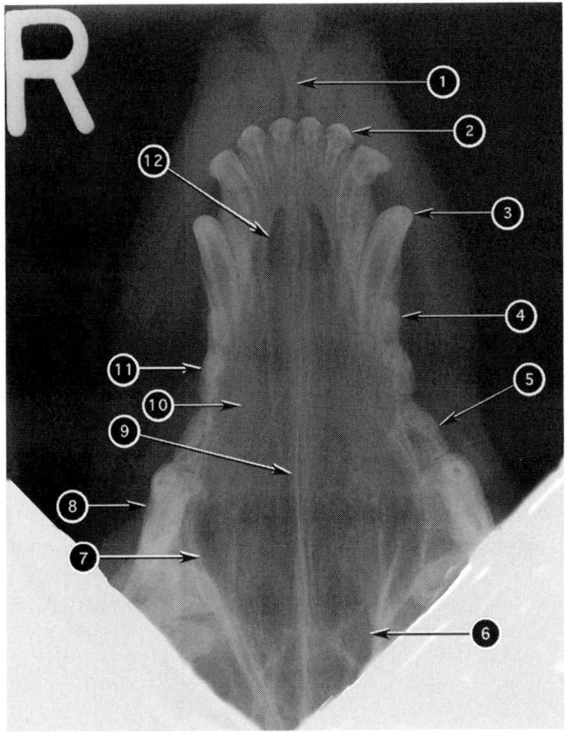

Fig. 7-2 Intraoral Dorsoventral Radiograph of Canine Nasal Cavity.

1. Cartilaginous nasal septum
2. Superior incisor 2
3. Superior canine tooth
4. Superior premolar 1
5. Superior premolar 3
6. Ethmoidal conchae
7. Maxillary recess
8. Superior premolar 4
9. Nasal septum
10. Dorsal and ventral nasal conchae
11. Superior premolar 2
12. Palatine fissure

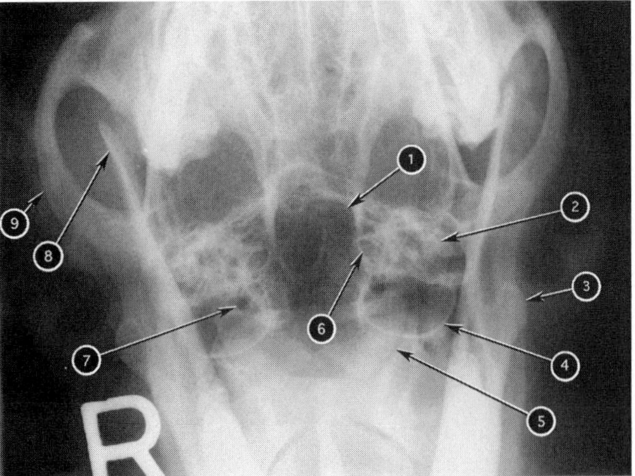

Fig. 7-4 Rostroventral-Caudodorsal Oblique (Open-Mouth) Radiograph of Canine Tympanic Bullae.

1. Nasopharynx
2. Petrous temporal bone
3. Angular process of mandible
4. Tympanic bulla
5. Atlantooccipital joint
6. Foramen lacerum
7. Jugular foramen
8. Coronoid process of mandible
9. Zygomatic arch

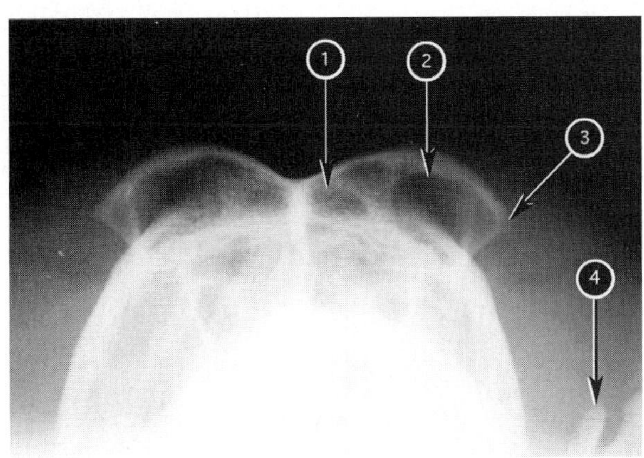

Fig. 7-3 Rostrodorsal-Caudodorsal Oblique Radiograph of Canine Frontal Sinuses.

1. Medial frontal sinus
2. Lateral frontal sinus
3. Zygomatic process of frontal bone
4. Coronoid process of mandible

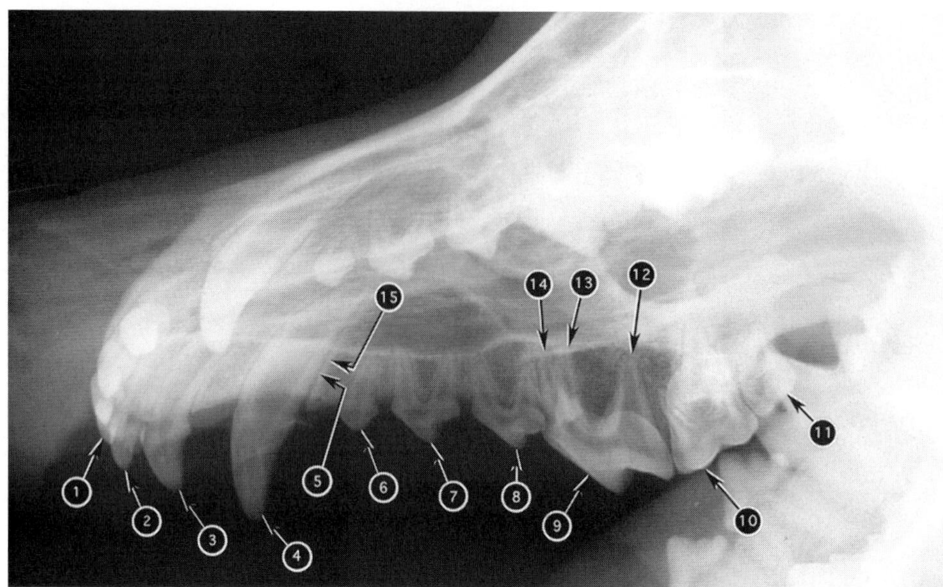

Fig. 7-5 Left Ventral/Right Dorsal Oblique Radiograph of Canine Superior Teeth.
1. Superior incisor 1
2. Superior incisor 2
3. Superior incisor 3
4. Superior canine tooth
5. Periodontal ligament
6. Superior premolar 1
7. Superior premolar 2
8. Superior premolar 3
9. Superior premolar 4
10. Superior molar 1
11. Superior molar 2
12. Caudal root of PM 4
13. Rostromedial root of PM 4
14. Rostrolateral root of PM 4
15. Cortical bone forming wall of alveolus

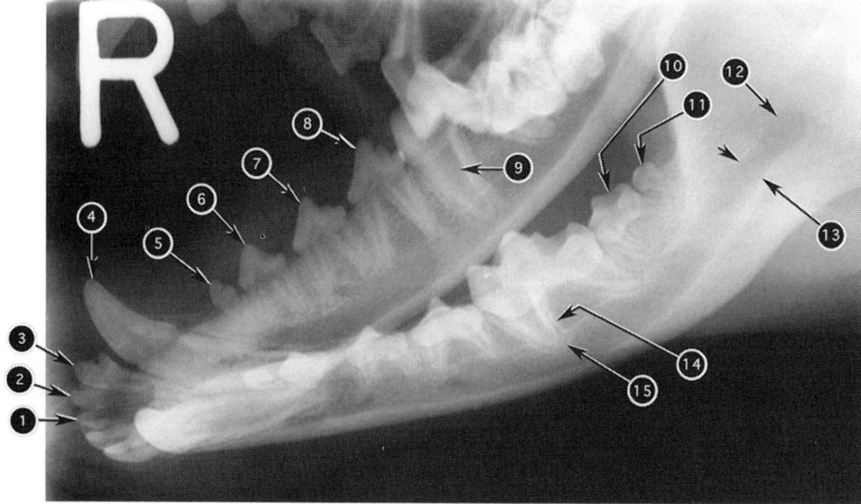

Fig. 7-6 Left Ventral/Right Dorsal Oblique Radiograph of Canine Superior Teeth.
1. Inferior incisor 1
2. Inferior incisor 2
3. Inferior incisor 3
4. Inferior canine tooth
5. Inferior premolar 1
6. Inferior premolar 2
7. Inferior premolar 3
8. Inferior premolar 4
9. Dental cavity of inferior molar 1
10. Inferior molar 2
11. Inferior molar 3
12. Mandibular foramen
13. Mandibular canal
14. Cortical bone forming wall of alveolus
15. Periodontal ligament

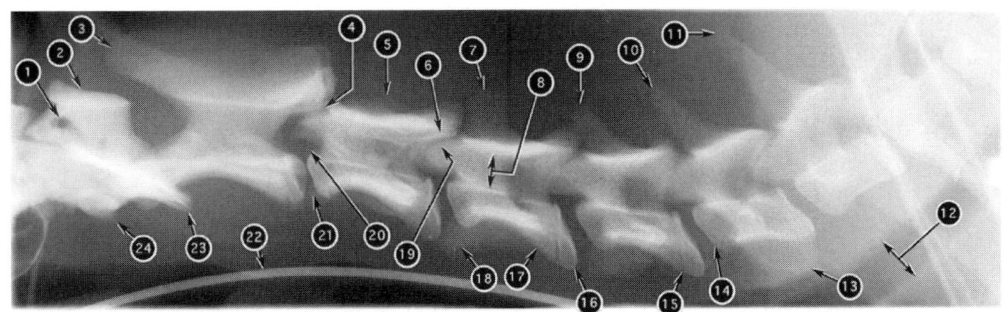

Fig. 7-7 **Left-Right Lateral Radiograph of Canine Cervical Vertebrae.**

1. Lateral vertebral foramina (left and right) of atlas; emergence of cervical nerve 1
2. Dorsal arch of atlas (C1)
3. Spinous process of axis (C2)
4. Synovial joints between articular processes of C2 and C3
5. Spinous process of C3
6. Caudal articular processes of C3
7. Spinous process of C4
8. Vertebral canal of C4
9. Spinous process of C5
10. Spinous process of C6
11. Spinous process of C7
12. Trachea
13. Expanded ventral laminae of transverse processes of C6
14. Cranial extremity (head) of C6
15. Caudal physis of C5
16. Caudal extremity (fossa) of C4
17. Body of C4
18. Transverse processes of C4
19. Cranial articular processes of C4
20. Intervertebral foramina between C2 and C3
21. Intervertebral space (disk) between C2 and C3
22. Endotracheal tube
23. Wings (transverse processes) of atlas
24. Ventral tubercle of atlas

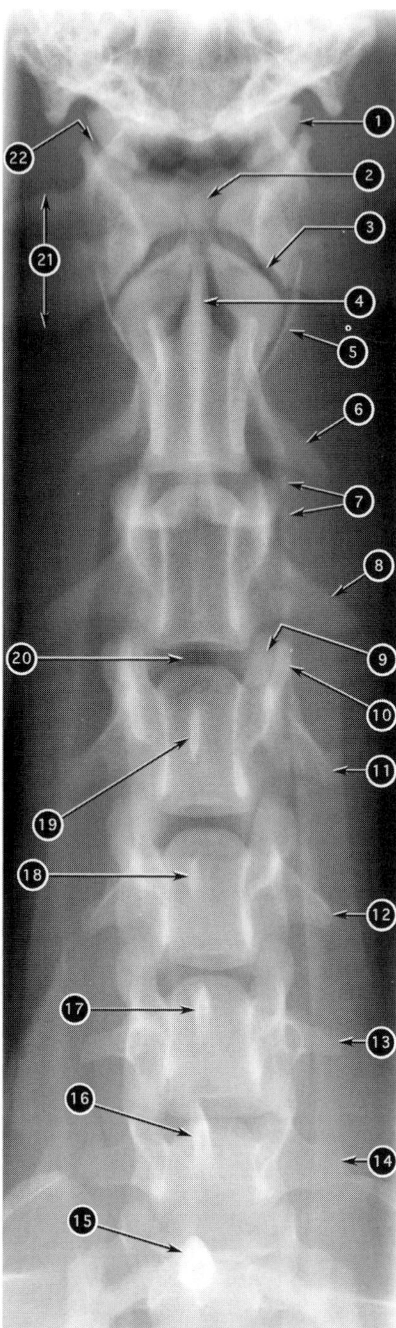

Fig. 7-8 Ventrodorsal Radiograph of Canine Cervical Vertebrae.

1. Left occipital condyle
2. Dens of axis
3. Atlantoaxial joint
4. Spinous process of axis
5. Left thyrohyoid bone
6. Left transverse process of axis
7. Tracheal cartilages
8. Left transverse process of C3
9. Left caudal articular process of C3
10. Left cranial articular process of C4
11. Left transverse process of C4
12. Left transverse process of C5
13. Left transverse process of C6
14. Left transverse process of C7
15. Spinous process of T1
16. Spinous process of C7
17. Spinous process of C6
18. Spinous process of C5
19. Spinous process of C4
20. Intervertebral space (disk) between C3 and C4
21. Right wing of atlas
22. Right atlantooccipital joint

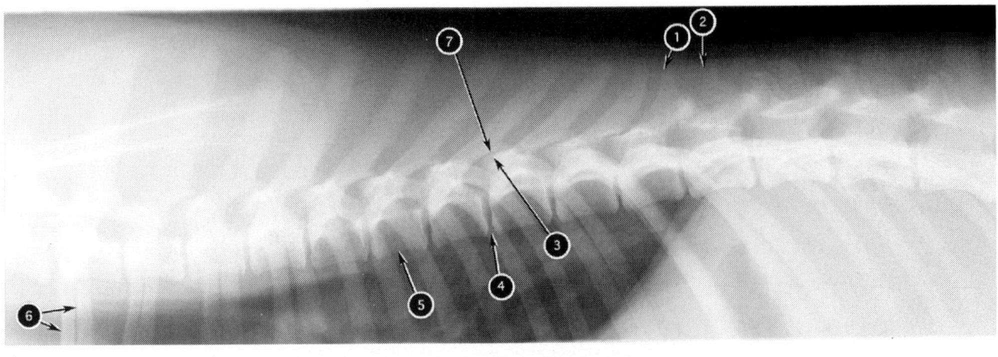

A

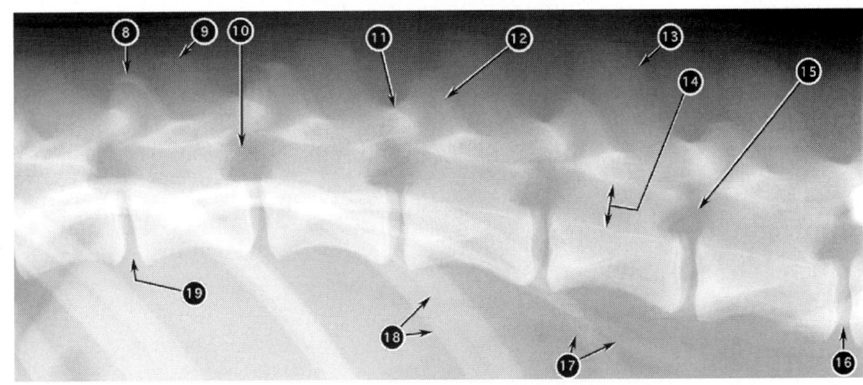

B

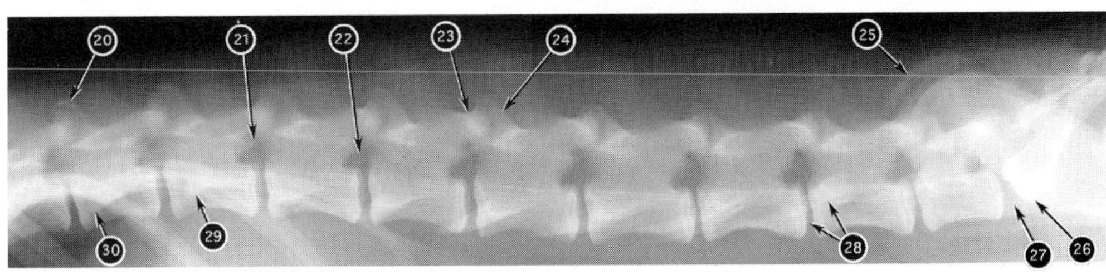

C

Fig. 7-9 Left-Right Lateral Radiographs of Canine Thoracic and Lumbar Vertebrae.

A, Left-right *(Le-Rt)* lateral radiograph of thoracic spine.

1. Spinous process of T10
2. Spinous process of T11 (anticlinal vertebra)
3. Cranial articular processes of T8
4. Intervertebral space (disk) between T7 and T8
5. Body of T6
6. First pair of ribs
7. Caudal articular processes of T7

B, Left-right *(Le-Rt)* lateral radiograph of thoracolumbar spine.

8. Mamillary processes atop cranial articular processes of T12
9. Spinous process of T12
10. Accessory processes of T12
11. Caudal articular processes of T13
12. Cranial articular processes of L1
13. Spinous process of L2
14. Vertebral canal of L2
15. Intervertebral foramina between L2 and L3
16. Transverse processes of L4
17. Thirteenth pair of ribs
18. Twelfth pair of ribs
19. Intervertebral space (disk) between T11 and T12

C, Left-right *(Le-Rt)* lateral radiograph of lumbar spine.

20. Mamillary processes atop cranial articular processes of T12
21. Accessory processes of T13
22. Intervertebral foramina between L1 and L2
23. Caudal articular processes of L2
24. Cranial articular processes of L3
25. Secondary ossification center for crest of ilium
26. Promontory of sacrum
27. Intervertebral space (disk) between L7 and S1
28. Transverse processes of L6
29. Heads of thirteenth ribs superimposed on body of T13
30. Heads of twelfth ribs superimposed on body of T12

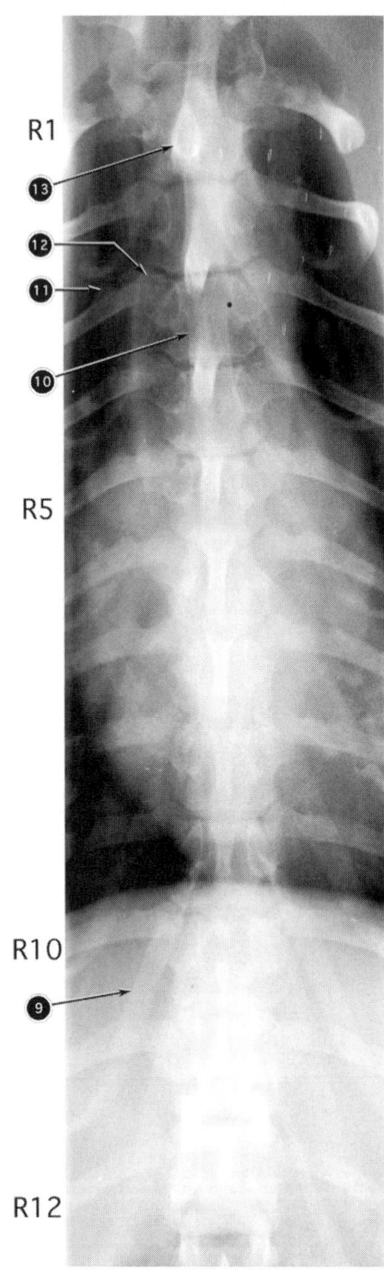

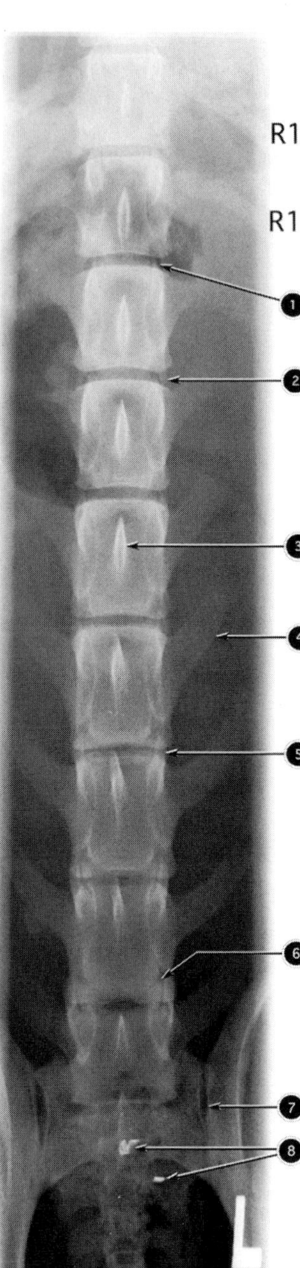

Fig. 7-10 Ventrodorsal Radiographs of Canine Thoracic and Lumbar Vertebrae (*R* = Rib).

1. Intervertebral space (disk) between T13 and L1
2. Left accessory process of L2
3. Spinous process of L3
4. Left transverse process of L4
5. Left cranial articular process of L5
6. Left caudal articular process of L6
7. Left sacroiliac joint
8. Metallic foreign bodies in descending colon
9. Costal cartilage of right rib 11
10. Sternum superimposed over vertebrae
11. Tubercle of right rib 3
12. Head of right rib 3, articulating with bodies of vertebrae T2 and T3
13. Spinous process of T1

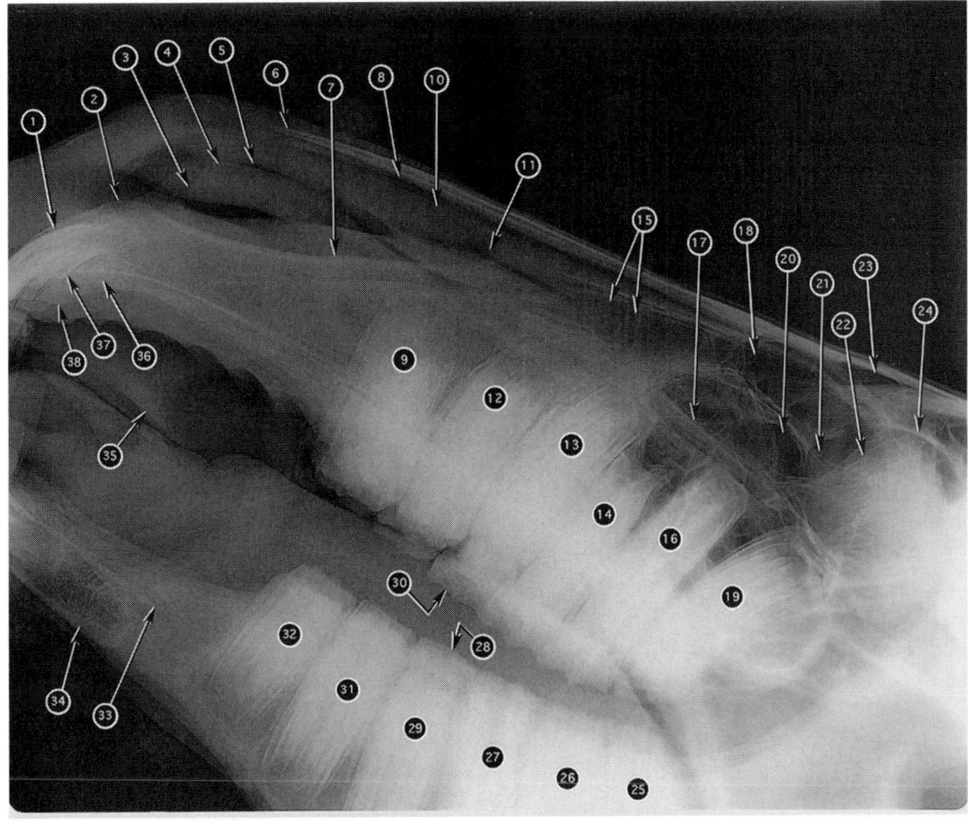

Fig. 7-11 Left-Right Lateral Radiograph of Rostral Part of Equine Head (3 Years Old).

1. Superior incisor 1
2. Body of incisive bone
3. Lateral border of nostril
4. Alar fold of ventral nasal concha
5. Middle nasal meatus
6. Nasal bone
7. Nasal process of incisive bone
8. Dorsal nasal meatus
9. Superior premolar 2
10. Dorsal nasal concha
11. Nasoincisive notch
12. Superior premolar 3
13. Superior premolar 4
14. Superior molar 1
15. Dorsal conchal bulla
16. Superior molar 2
17. Infraorbital canal
18. Dorsal conchal sinus
19. Superior molar 3
20. Frontomaxillary opening
21. Lacrimal canal
22. Ethmoidal conchae
23. Frontal sinus
24. Dorsal border of orbit
25. Inferior molar 3
26. Inferior molar 2
27. Inferior molar 1
28. Deciduous inferior premolar 4
29. Inferior premolar 4
30. Deciduous superior premolar 4
31. Inferior premolar 3
32. Inferior premolar 2
33. Mental foramen
34. Intermandibular joint (fused)
35. Mouth gag used to separate teeth
36. Developing superior incisor 3
37. Nonerupted superior incisor 2
38. Deciduous superior incisor 3

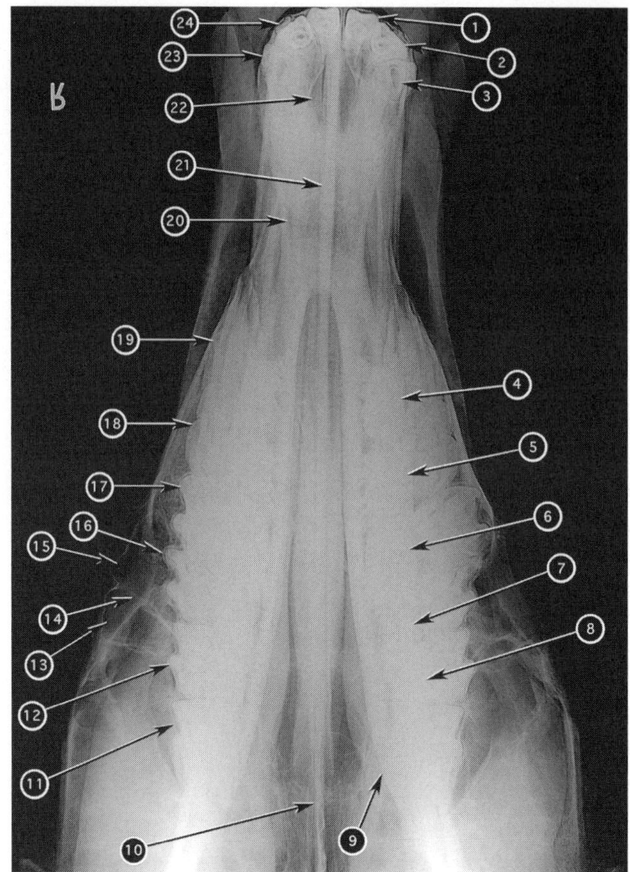

Fig. 7-12 Dorsoventral Radiograph of Rostral Part of Equine Head (3 Years Old).

1. Left superior incisor 1
2. Left superior incisor 2
3. Left superior incisor 3
4. Left inferior premolar 2
5. Left inferior premolar 3
6. Left inferior premolar 4
7. Left inferior molar 1
8. Left inferior molar 2
9. Body of left mandible
10. Vomer
11. Right superior molar 3
12. Right superior molar 2
13. Right caudal maxillary sinus
14. Oblique septum between 13 and 15
15. Right rostral maxillary sinus
16. Right superior molar 1
17. Right superior premolar 4
18. Right superior premolar 3
19. Right superior premolar 2
20. Right mental foramen
21. Nasal septum
22. Right palatine fissure
23. Right deciduous superior incisor 3
24. Right deciduous superior incisor 2

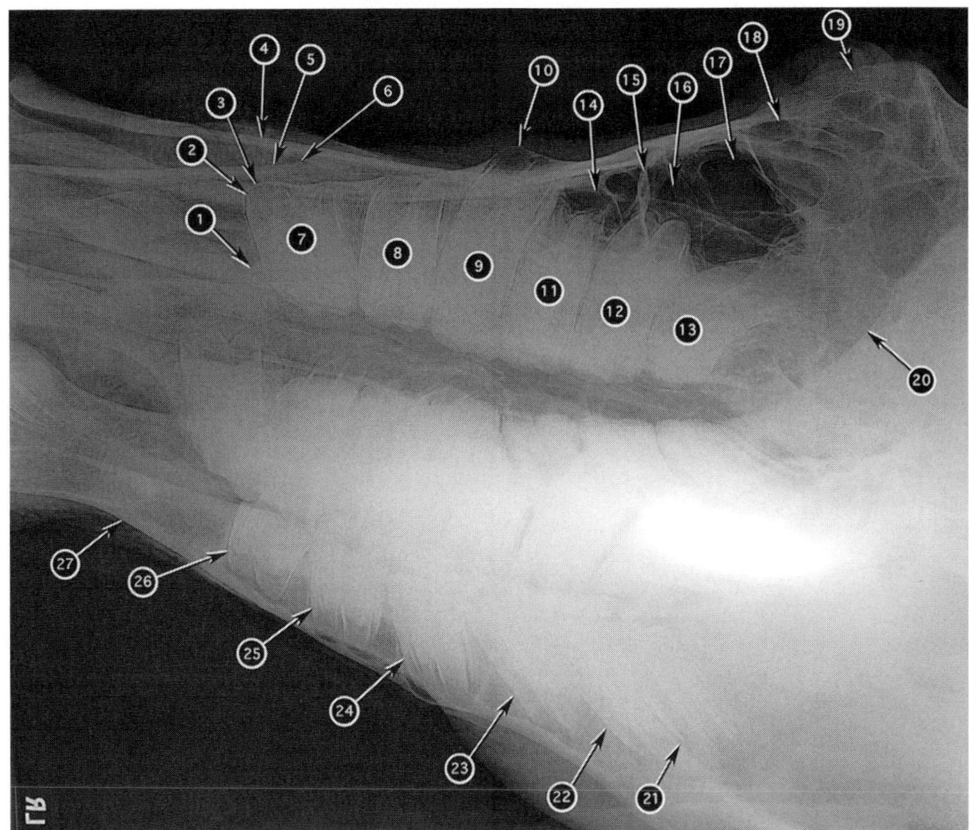

Fig. 7-13 Left Ventral-Right Dorsal Oblique Radiograph of Rostral Part of Equine Head (3 Years Old).

1. Left superior premolar 1
2. Periodontal ligament
3. Cortical bone forming wall of alveolus
4. Left nasal bone
5. Nasal process of left incisive bone
6. Nasoincisive notch
7. Left superior premolar 2
8. Left superior premolar 3
9. Left superior premolar 4
10. Left maxillary bone
11. Left superior molar 1
12. Left superior molar 2
13. Left superior molar 3
14. Left rostral maxillary sinus
15. Oblique septum between 14 and 16
16. Left caudal maxillary sinus
17. Left frontomaxillary opening
18. Left conchofrontal sinus
19. Left frontal bone forming dorsal wall of orbit
20. Ramus of left mandible
21. Right inferior molar 3
22. Right inferior molar 2
23. Right inferior molar 1
24. Right inferior premolar 4
25. Right inferior premolar 3
26. Right inferior premolar 2
27. Body of right mandible

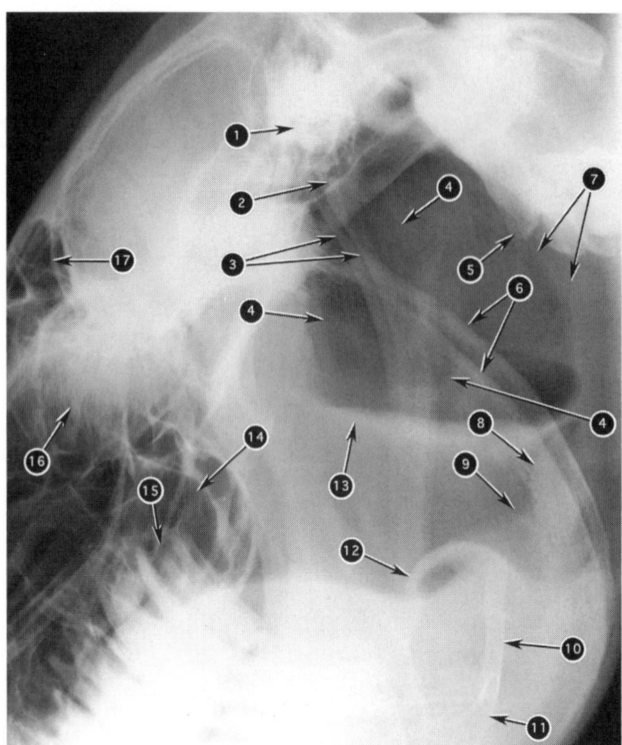

Fig. 7-14 Left-Right Lateral Radiograph of Guttural Pouch Region of Equine Head.

1. Petrous temporal bones
2. Tympanohyoid cartilage
3. Stylohyoid bones
4. Lateral compartments of guttural pouches
5. Ventral tubercle of atlas
6. Caudal borders of mandibles
7. Medial compartments of guttural pouches
8. Corniculate process of arytenoid cartilage
9. Aryepiglottic fold
10. Thyrohyoid bone
11. Basihyoid bone
12. Epiglottis
13. Dorsal wall of nasopharynx
14. Caudal maxillary sinus
15. Superior molar 3
16. Ethmoidal conchae
17. Conchofrontal sinus

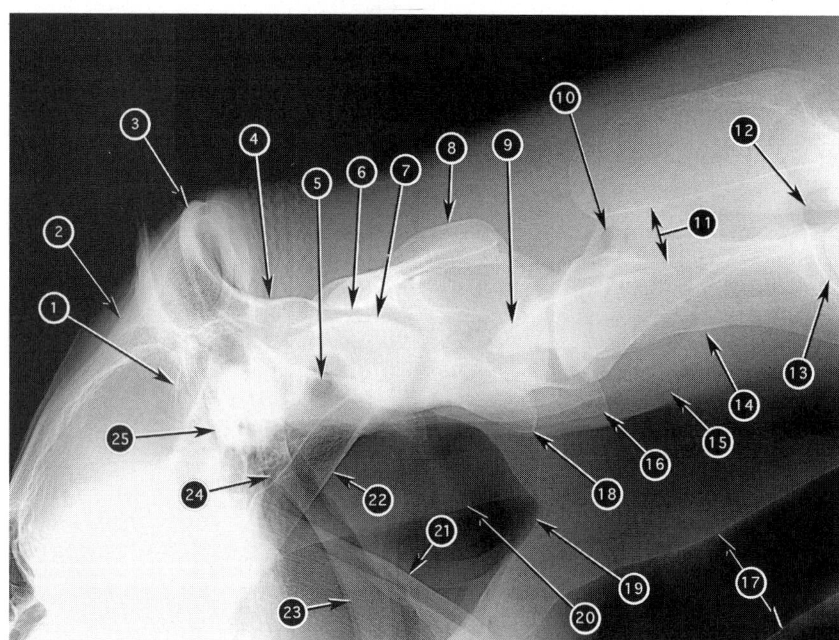

Fig. 7-15 Left-Right Lateral Radiograph of Occipital Region of Equine Head.

1. Osseous tentorium cerebelli
2. Parietal bones
3. Nuchal crest
4. Squamous part of occipital bone
5. Hypoglossal canals
6. Atlantooccipital joint
7. Occipital condyles
8. Dorsal arch of atlas
9. Dens of axis
10. Lateral vertebral foramen of axis
11. Vertebral canal
12. Intervertebral foramina between C2 and C3
13. Intervertebral space (disk) between C2 and C3
14. Body of axis
15. Longus colli muscles
16. Wings of atlas
17. Trachea
18. Ventral tubercle of atlas
19. Medial compartments of guttural pouches
20. Longus capitis muscles
21. Caudal borders of mandibles
22. Basal part of occipital bone
23. Stylohyoid bones
24. Tympanohyoid cartilage
25. Petrous parts of temporal bones

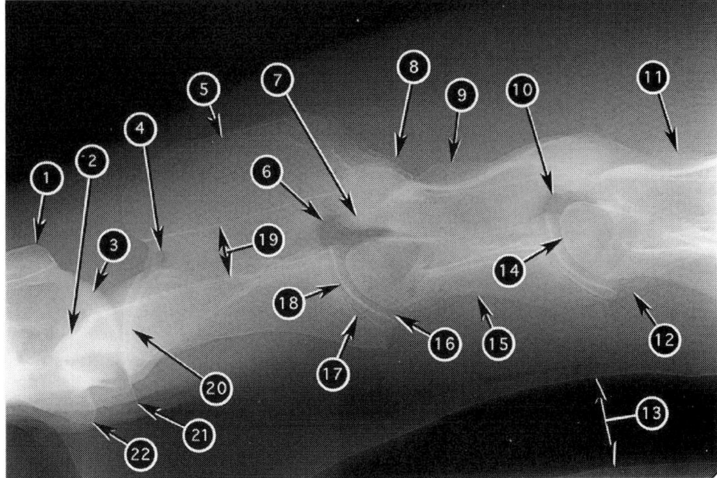

Fig. 7-16 Left-Right Lateral Radiograph of Equine Cranial Cervical Vertebrae.

1. Dorsal arch of atlas
2. Dens of axis
3. Caudal articular fovea of atlas
4. Lateral vertebral foramina of axis
5. Spinous process of axis
6. Intervertebral foramina between C2 and C3
7. Cranial articular processes of C3
8. Caudal articular processes of C2
9. Spinous process of C3
10. Intervertebral foramina between C3 and C4
11. Spinous process of C4
12. Transverse processes of C4
13. Trachea
14. Cranial extremity (head) of C4
15. Body of C3
16. Intervertebral space (disk) between C2 and C3
17. Caudal physis of C2
18. Caudal extremity (fossa) of C2
19. Vertebral canal of C2
20. Cranial articular processes of axis
21. Wings of atlas
22. Ventral tubercle of atlas

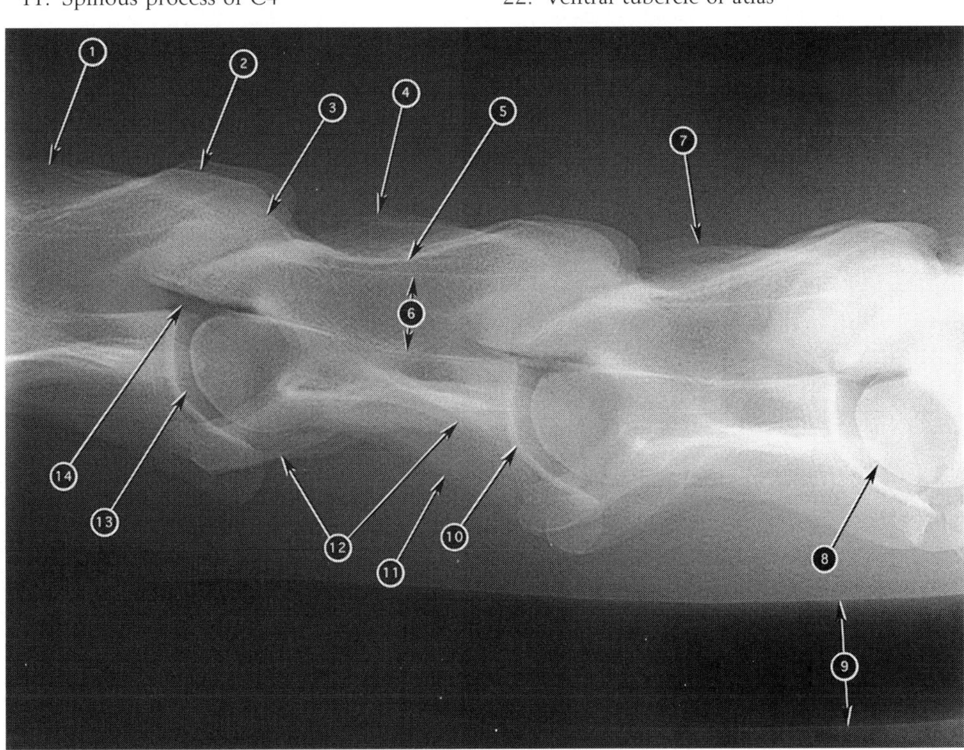

Fig. 7-17 Left-Right Lateral Radiograph of Equine Middle Cervical Vertebrae.

1. Spinous process of C3
2. Caudal articular processes of C3
3. Cranial articular processes of C4
4. Spinous process of C4
5. Vertebral arch laminae of C4
6. Vertebral canal of C4
7. Spinous process of C5
8. Cranial extremity (head) of C6
9. Trachea
10. Caudal extremity (fossa) of C4
11. Body of C4
12. Transverse processes of C4
13. Intervertebral space (disk) between C3 and C4
14. Intervertebral foramina between C3 and C4

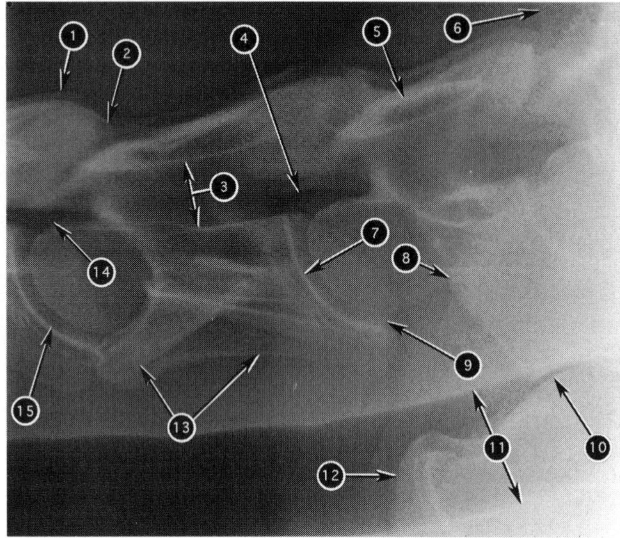

Fig. 7-18 Left-Right Lateral Radiograph of Equine Caudal Cervical Vertebrae.

1. Caudal articular processes of C5
2. Cranial articular processes of C6
3. Vertebral canal of C6
4. Intervertebral foramina between C6 and C7
5. Vertebral arch laminae of C7
6. Spinous process of T1
7. Caudal extremity (fossa) of C6
8. Supraglenoid tubercle of scapula
9. Intervertebral space (disk) between C6 and C7
10. Shoulder joint
11. Trachea
12. Intermediate tubercle of humerus
13. Transverse processes of C6
14. Intervertebral foramina between C5 and C6
15. Intervertebral space (disk) between C5 and C6

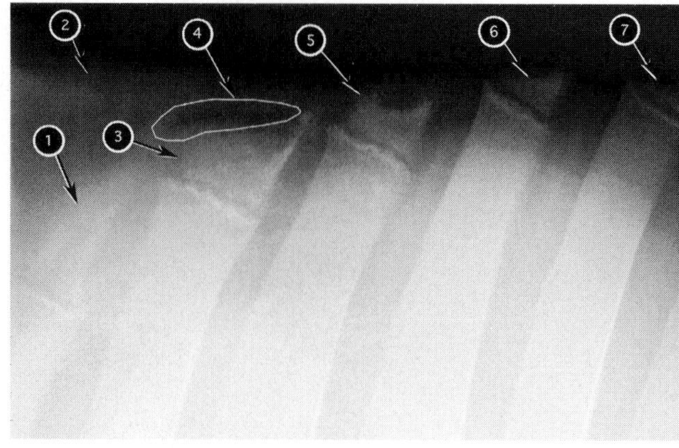

Fig. 7-19 Left-Right Lateral Radiograph of Equine Withers Region.

1. Spinous tuberosity of T2
2. Funiculus nuchae
3. Spinous tuberosity of T3
4. Approximate location of supraspinous bursa
5. Spinous tuberosity of T4
6. Spinous tuberosity of T5
7. Spinous tuberosity of T6

ELECTRONIC RESOURCES evolve

Chapter 7 can also be found on the companion Web site at evolve http://evolve.elsevier.com/Thrall/vetrad/

CHAPTER • 8

Cranial and Nasal Cavities: Canine and Feline

Lisa J. Forrest

NORMAL ANATOMY

The skull encompasses the brain and houses the sense organs for hearing, equilibrium, sight, smell, and taste. The skull provides attachment sites for the teeth, tongue, larynx, and muscles.[1] Variation in the shape of the skull is pronounced in the canine species. Three terms are used to designate the different shapes. *Dolichocephalic* breeds, such as the collie and Russian wolfhound, have long, narrow heads with an extensive nasal cavity from rostral to caudal. *Mesaticephalic* breeds, such as the German shepherd and Beagle, have heads of medium proportion (Fig. 8-1). *Brachycephalic* breeds, such as the Boston terrier and Pekingese, have short, wide heads. Cats are more uniform in their skull conformation. However, Siamese tend to have longer heads compared with Himalayan and Persian breeds.

Calvaria and Associated Structures

The calvarium comprises the bones of the brain case, with the occipital bone forming the base of the skull. The occipital crest is the most dorsocaudal aspect of the skull (see Fig. 8-1), and the occipital condyles are caudoventral as seen on lateral radiographs. The foramen magnum, centered between the occipital condyles, forms an orifice for passage of the spinal cord.

Nasal Passages and Paranasal Sinuses

The nasal passage extends caudally from the external nares to the cribriform plate and nasopharynx. The cribriform plate is a sievelike partition between the olfactory bulbs and the nasal passage. The nasal passage is divided in half by the nasal septum and is filled with thinly scrolled conchae. Caudally, the nasal septum is bony and fuses with the cribriform plate; it becomes cartilaginous as it extends rostrally.[1] The vomer bone is unpaired and forms the caudoventral bony part of the nasal septum; it can be seen radiographically.[2] The cartilaginous nasal septum cannot be seen in radiographs, though it can be distinguished in computed tomographic and magnetic resonance images. Both dogs and cats have frontal sinuses (see Fig. 8-1), lateral maxillary recesses, and small sphenoidal sinuses. These are named for the bones in which they are located.

Tympanic Bullae and Temporomandibular Joint

The tympanic bullae (see Fig. 8-1) form the ventral part of the temporal bone. These air-filled cavities of the middle ear communicate with the nasopharynx by the auditory tube. The temporal bone consists of the petrosal, tympanic, and squamous sections, which are fused in the adult. The petrosal portion is medial and dorsal to the tympanic bulla and is composed of dense bone in the mature animal. The squamous portion of the temporal bone extends rostrally and laterally to form the zygomatic arch.

The temporomandibular joint is a condylar joint. The temporal portion consists of the zygomatic process of the squamous temporal bone, which forms the mandibular fossa and the retroarticular process. The retroarticular process is the ventral extension of the squamous temporal bone. The mandibular aspect of the joint includes the condyloid process, which articulates with the mandibular fossa.

Teeth

The teeth are anchored in alveoli within the mandible and maxilla. The dental formulas for the dog and cat are provided in Box 8-1. Components of the tooth include the root (embedded in bone) and the crown (within the oral cavity); the bone between teeth is referred to as the alveolar crest. The dentin, enamel, and lamina dura of the tooth are radiopaque. The pulp cavity and periodontal membrane are of soft tissue opacity (Fig. 8-2). The size of the pulp cavity changes with maturity, becoming smaller with age.[3] Specifics on radiographic technique and positioning for tooth evaluation can be found elsewhere.[4-7]

Cross-Sectional Imaging

Cross-sectional imaging techniques, computed tomography (CT) and magnetic resonance (MR) imaging, are increasingly available for imaging of the head. CT and MR technology provides images without superimposition of structures and better soft tissue delineation compared with radiography (Fig. 8-3).[8-14] Several references describe the normal CT and MR image anatomy of the dog and cat head.[9,15-22]

CONGENITAL ANOMALIES

Hydrocephalus

Hydrocephalus is excessive accumulation of cerebrospinal fluid within the ventricular system of the brain. Congenital hydrocephalus may occur as a result of structural defects that either obstruct cerebrospinal fluid outflow or impede its absorption. Canine breeds affected with congenital hydrocephalus include the Maltese, Yorkshire terrier, English bulldog, Chihuahua, Lhasa Apso, Chinese pug, Toy Poodle, Pomeranian, Pekingese, Cairn terrier, and Boston terrier.[23] Hydrocephalus is much less common in cats.[24-26]

Radiographic signs associated with hydrocephalus include doming of the calvaria and cortical thinning, persistent fontanelles, and a homogeneous appearance to the brain resulting from the loss of normal convolutional skull markings (Fig. 8-4). Radiographs are insensitive for detection of hydrocephalus. Previously, diagnosis of hydrocephalus was made by ventriculography,[27] but this invasive procedure has been replaced primarily by CT and MR imaging. With persistent fontanelles, ultrasound can also be used to assess ventricular

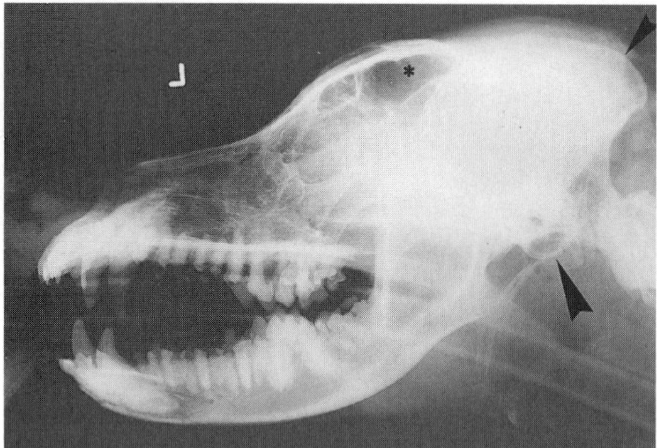

Fig. 8-1 Lateral skull radiograph of a German shepherd dog, which is a mesaticephalic breed. Note the occipital crest *(small arrowhead)*, superimposed frontal sinuses *(asterisk)*, and tympanic bullae *(large arrowhead)*.

Box 8-1

Dental Formulas for the Dog and Cat

Dental Formula: Cat
Deciduous teeth
2 × (I 3/3, C 1/1, P 3/2) = 26
Permanent teeth
2 × (I 3/3, C 1/1, P 3/2, M 1/1) = 30

Dental Formula: Dog
Deciduous teeth
2 × (I 3/3, C 1/1, P 3/3) = 28
Permanent teeth
2 × (I 3/3, C 1/1, P 4/4, M 2/3) = 42

I, Incisor teeth; *C,* canine teeth; *M,* molar teeth; *P,* premolar teeth.

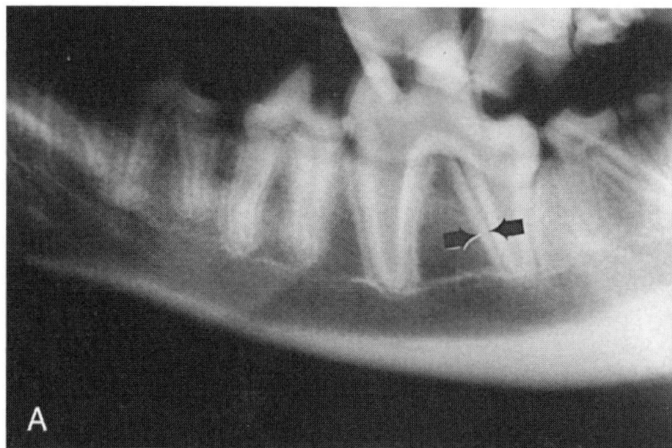

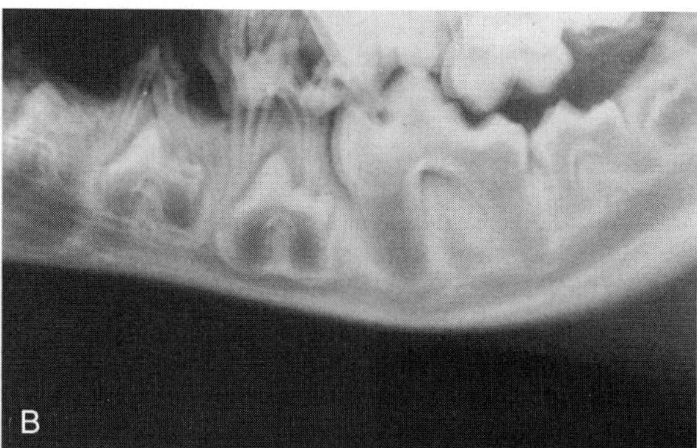

Fig. 8-2 **A,** Lateral radiograph of the mandible of a mature dog. Note the well-defined lamina dura *(arrows)*, which mark the dental alveolus. **B,** Lateral radiograph of the mandible of a 4-month-old dog. Note the open apical foramina of the teeth, the large pulp cavity, and the location of permanent premolars ventral to the deciduous precursors. (Courtesy of Dr. Wendy Myer, Ohio State University, Columbus, Ohio.)

size,[28-35] and normal appearance and size has been quantified in the dog.[28,29,36,37] The advantage of CT and MR imaging for evaluating ventricular size is the ability to assess the entire brain for causes of hydrocephalus (Fig. 8-5). Asymmetry in ventricular size is often normal in dogs, and correlation between ventricular size and clinical signs is poor.[28,29,31,34,35]

Occipital Dysplasia

Occipital dysplasia is the dorsal extension of the foramen magnum as a result of a developmental defect in the occipital bone[38]; it has been related to clinical signs of neurologic disease and is usually identified in miniature and toy breeds.[39-41] Foramen magnum size and shape can be evaluated in the rostrodorsal-caudoventral skull radiograph. The anesthetized patient is placed in dorsal recumbency with the neck flexed so that the nose is angled toward the sternum. The central x-ray beam is directed between the eyes and exits through the foramen magnum. The beam is angled 25 to 40 degrees from the vertical axis, depending on calvarial shape.[42] Figure 8-6 represents both the normal and the abnormal appearance of the foramen magnum as seen on the rostrodorsal-caudoventral skull radiograph. The characteristics of the foramen magnum can be assessed more accurately by CT than by radiographs (Fig. 8-7). That occipital dysplasia may not cause neurologic signs and is a normal morphologic variation in brachycephalic dogs has been suggested.[43-45]

Occipital Bone Malformation and Syringomyelia (Chiari I–Like Malformation)

Occipital bone malformation may result in overcrowding of the caudal fossa, leading to obstruction of cerebral spinal fluid (CSF) flow, hydrocephalus, and secondary syringomyelia. This hereditary defect, termed Chiari I–like malformation, is identified in the Cavalier King Charles spaniel but is seen in other brachycephalic breeds as well.[46-49] CSF flow is obstructed by the malformation, and the cerebellum may be herniated through the foramen magnum with dorsal deviation of the brainstem.[48] Clinical signs vary in severity and usually are seen in dogs between the age of 6 months and 2 years; however, neurologic signs may not manifest until late in life.[48] Neurologic signs are consistent with a central spinal cord lesion, and clinically dogs often present with persistent scratching of the shoulder region, with no dermatologic cause, that is thought to be a paraesthesia as a result of syringomyelia.[46]

Radiographs are not useful for diagnosis of Chiari I–like malformation. Definitive diagnosis is made by MR imaging, whereby crowding of the cerebellum in the caudal fossa can be detected.[48] Cervical syringohydromyelia is also commonly encountered. Herniation of a portion of the vermis of the cerebellum may be present (see Fig. 10-28).

Temporomandibular Joint Dysplasia

Open-mouth jaw locking is the clinical sign associated with temporomandibular joint (TMJ) dysplasia. This congenital condition is uncommon; it is most frequently reported in the Basset hound but has also been seen in Irish setters.[50] The open-mouth jaw locking occurs after hyperextension of the jaw, excessive lateral movement of the condyloid process, and subsequent entrapment lateral to the zygomatic arch. Physical entrapment usually occurs on the contralateral side from the joint with the most severe dysplastic changes (Fig. 8-8). Yawning often precipitates jaw locking when it results in extreme opening of the mouth.[50] In spaniels, Pekingese, and Dachshunds, TMJ dysplasia is an asymptomatic anatomic anomaly.[22,51,52]

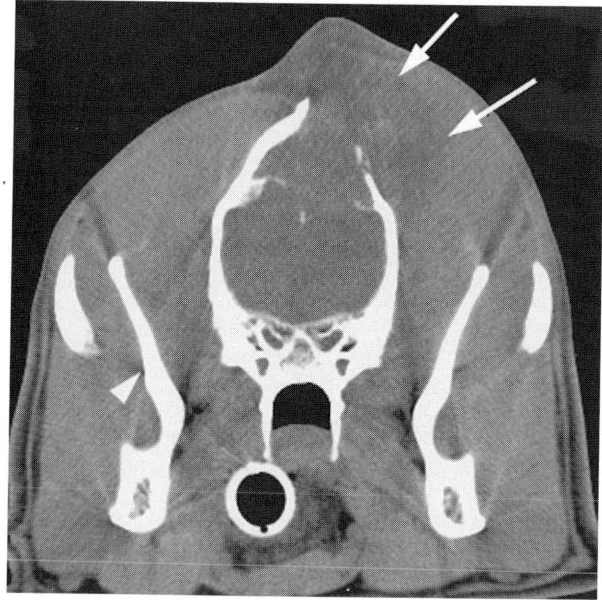

Fig. 8-3 Transverse CT image at the level of the brain and caudal frontal sinus of a 5-year-old male Rottweiler dog with an osteosarcoma of the frontal bone. The *white arrows* delineate the soft tissue component of the tumor, which is destroying the right frontal bone and compressing the brain. The *white arrowhead* marks the normal left ramus of the mandible.

Mucopolysaccharidosis

Mucopolysaccharidoses are a group of hereditary disorders of lysosomal storage that occur in human beings, dogs, cattle, and cats.[53] Mucopolysaccharidosis VI (MPS VI) is an autosomal recessive lysosomal storage disease recognized in Siamese cats.[54-56] Radiographic skeletal changes in cats with MPS VI include epiphyseal dysplasia, generalized osteoporosis, pectus

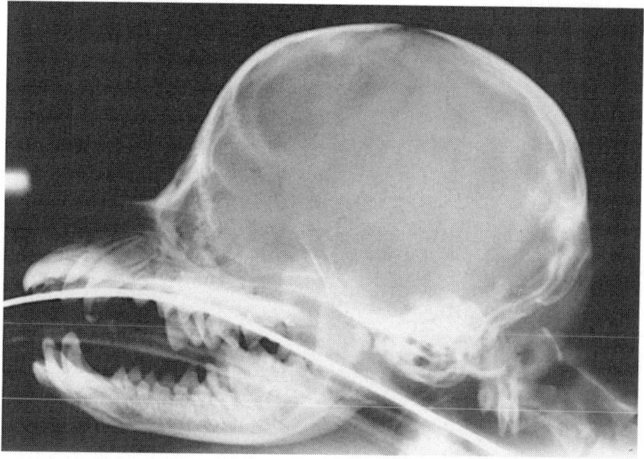

Fig. 8-4 Lateral radiograph of a 1-year-old male Chihuahua with severe hydrocephalus. Note the homogeneous appearance of the calvaria caused by a loss of the normal convolutional skull markings. (Courtesy of Dr. Wendy Myer, Ohio State University, Columbus, Ohio.)

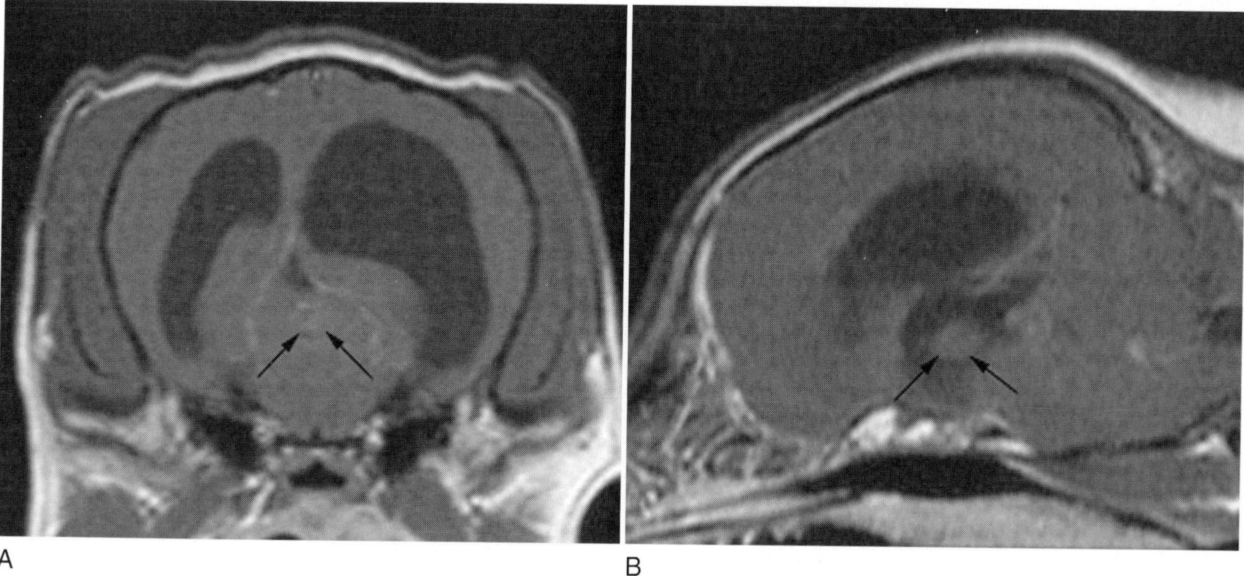

Fig. 8-5 Transverse (A) and sagittal (B) spin-echo T1-weighted postcontrast MR images of the brain of a dog with a small mass in the third ventricle *(arrows)*. This mass has resulted in obstruction to CSF flow and secondary obstructive hydrocephalus. The lateral ventricles (black in this MR sequence) are dilated, with the left being larger than the right.

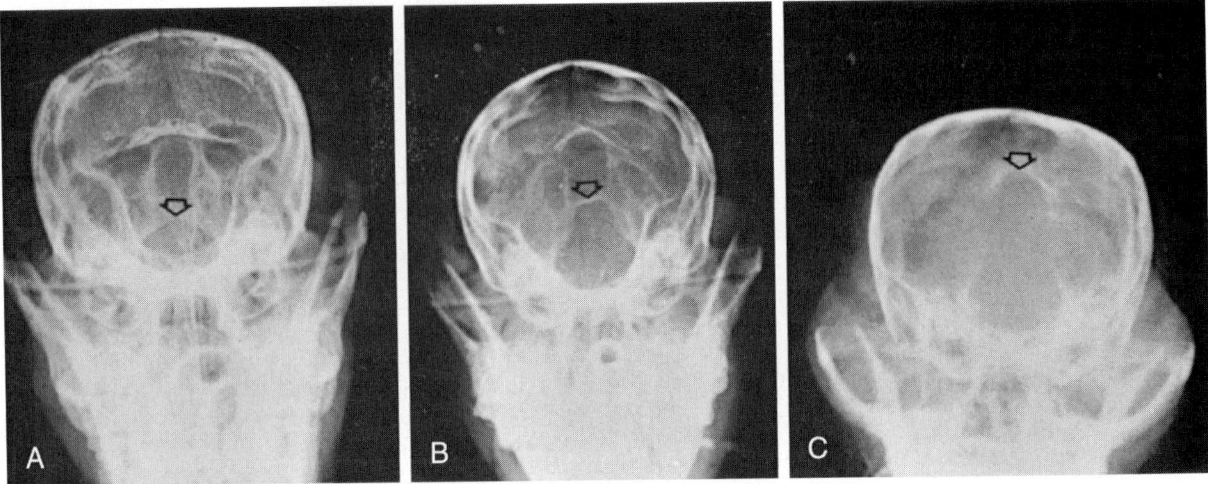

Fig. 8-6 Rostrodorsal-caudoventral oblique radiograph of the skull in three small-breed dogs. Note the appearance of the foramen magnum; *arrows* indicate the dorsal extent. **A,** Normal foramen magnum. **B,** Moderate occipital dysplasia. **C,** Severe occipital dysplasia. (Courtesy of Dr. Wendy Myer, Ohio State University, Columbus, Ohio.)

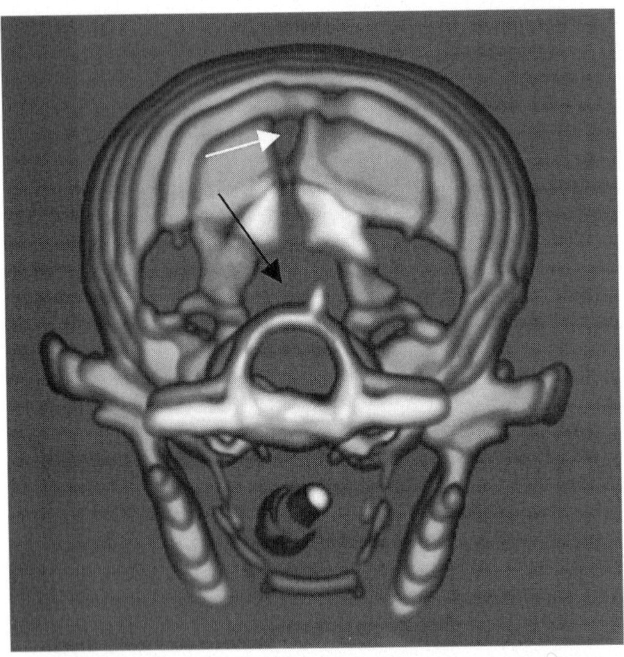

Fig. 8-7 Caudal view of a three-dimensional volume rendering obtained from transverse CT images of the skull. The foramen magnum should be the approximate size of the vertebral canal of C1. Note the extension of the foramen magnum dorsal to C1 *(black arrow)* and a vertical cleft extending even further dorsally *(white arrow)*. Two large dysplastic areas are also visible in the occipital bone to either side of the foramen magnum.

excavatum, and vertebral and skull changes.[57] Specific skull changes seen on radiographs include shortened nasal conchae, aplasia and hypoplasia of the frontal and sphenoid sinuses, and shortened dimensions to the incisive and maxillary bones.[57] Another form of mucopolysaccharidosis, MPS I, has been documented in the domestic shorthaired cat,[58] with radiographic skeletal changes similar to those in MPS VI; however, the facial dysmorphia may not be as pronounced as it is in the Siamese.[56,59] MPS in animals has clinical and pathologic manifestations similar to human beings and therefore represents an excellent model for studying approaches to therapy and care.[55,60]

METABOLIC ANOMALIES

Primary or secondary hyperparathyroidism can result in an overall decreased opacity of the entire skeleton, often easily noted in the skull. A solitary parathyroid adenoma or carcinoma, or adenomatous hyperplasia of one or both parathyroid glands, causes primary hyperparathyroidism. This results in excessive synthesis and secretion of parathyroid hormone, which leads to hypercalcemia and subsequent bone resorption.[61,62] Secondary hyperparathyroidism, which includes renal and nutritional secondary hyperparathyroidism, is subsequent to nonendocrine alterations in calcium and phosphorus homeostasis that lead to increased levels of parathyroid hormone and ultimate bone resorption.[61]

An early radiographic sign of hyperparathyroidism (primary and secondary) is loss of the lamina dura. This will be followed by overall demineralization of the skull bones as the disease progresses (Fig. 8-9). In fact, loss of the lamina dura is not commonly noted without some concurrent generalized demineralization of the skeleton. The level of cortical thinning and degree of overall osteolysis and osteomalacia depend on duration and severity of the hyperparathyroidism. Also, because young animals are growing and have rapid skeletal turnover, they are more severely affected than older animals. In extreme hyperparathyroidism, demineralization is followed by fibrous tissue hyperplasia, termed fibrous osteodystrophy. This uncommon development leads to a floating appearance to the teeth and thickening of the affected part of the skull (Fig. 8-10).

Ultrasound evaluation of the cervical region can be used to evaluate dogs with hypercalcemia to search for a parathyroid mass. In 210 dogs with primary hyperparathyroidism, masses were identified in 129 of 130 dogs that were imaged sonographically with a size range of 3 to 23 mm in diameter.[62] Thirty-one percent of the dogs in this study had cystic calculi either identified on abdominal radiographs or abdominal ultrasound; all calculi were either calcium phosphate or calcium oxalate (radiopaque).[62]

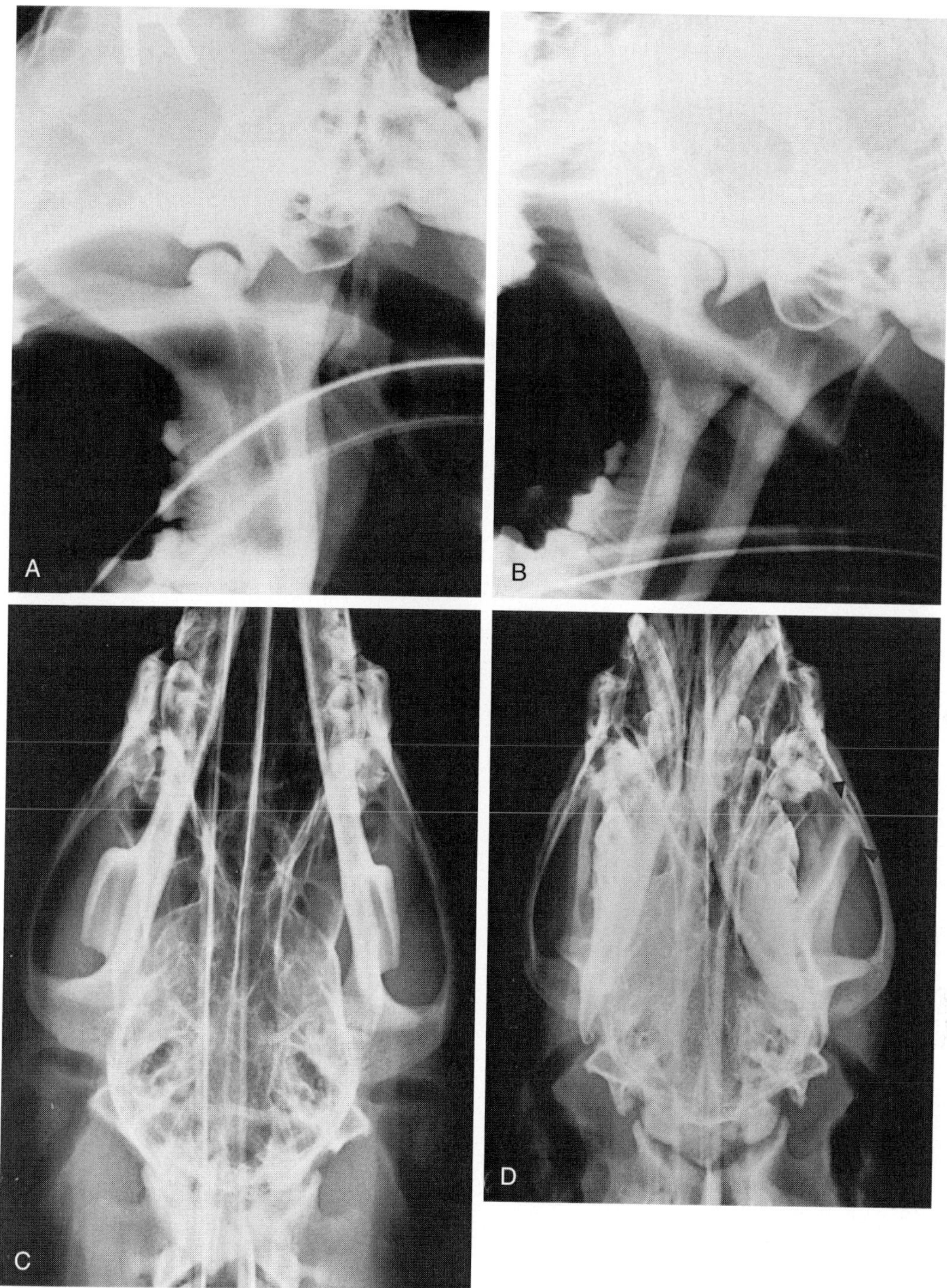

Fig. 8-8 Open-mouth, left dorsal/right ventral (A); open-mouth, right dorsal/left ventral (B); closed-mouth, ventrodorsal (C); and open-mouth, ventrodorsal (D) radiographs of the TMJs of a 2-year-old female Gordon setter with a history of chronic intermittent jaw locking. Subluxation of the right TMJ is present (A) compared with the more normal appearance of the left TMJ (B). Radiographs were made after the jaw was locked. Note the difference in the relation of the coronoid process of the mandible and the zygomatic arch on the closed-mouth, ventrodorsal radiograph (C) compared with the open-mouth, ventrodorsal view (D) after the jaw has been locked in the open position. When the jaw is locked, the coronoid process shifts laterally and is in contact with the zygomatic arch (D, *arrowheads*). (Courtesy of Dr. Wendy Myer, Ohio State University, Columbus, Ohio.)

NEOPLASTIC ABNORMALITIES

Nasal Tumors

Tumors of the nasal cavity in dogs and cats account for approximately 1% to 2% of all neoplasms.[63-65] These tumors occur in older dogs and cats; approximately two thirds of nasal tumors are carcinomas (adenocarcinoma, squamous cell carcinoma, undifferentiated carcinoma), and the other one third are sarcomas (fibrosarcoma, chondrosarcoma, osteosarcoma, undifferentiated sarcoma).[66-68] Intranasal lymphoma can also occur, with a higher prevalence in cats.[67-71] Tumors of the nasal cavity are locally invasive but have a relatively low metastatic

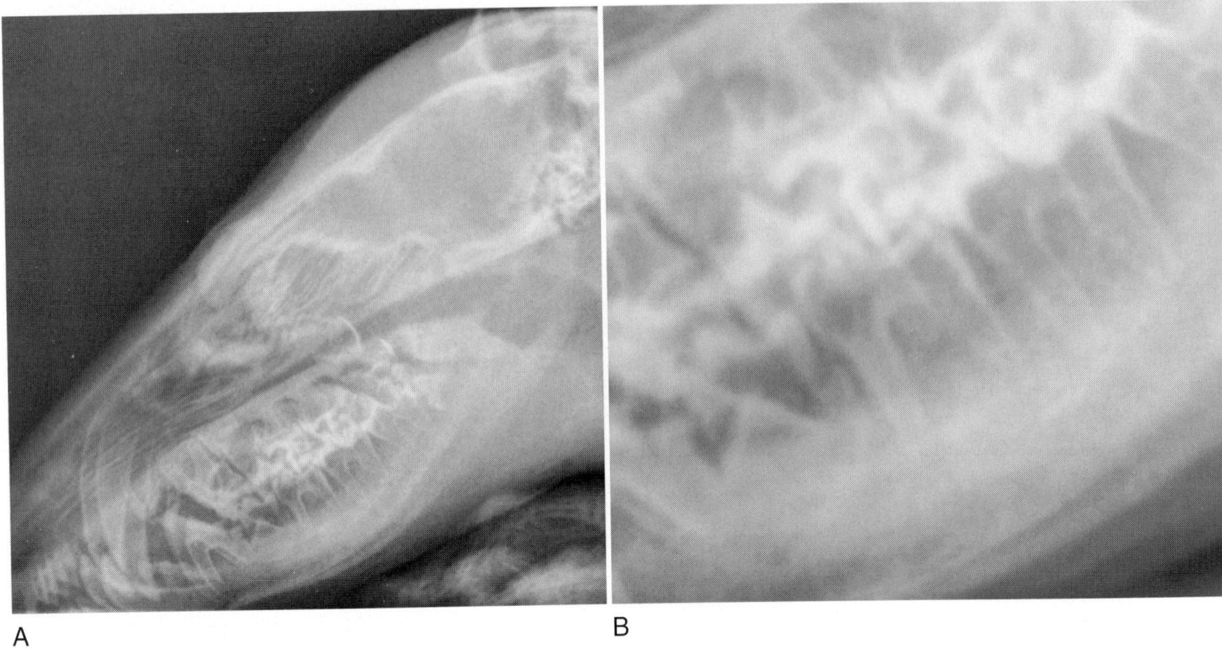

Fig. 8-9 **A,** Lateral skull radiograph of an opossum with nutritional secondary hyperthyroidism. Note the decreased opacity and poor delineation of the skull. This is especially noticeable in the caudal mandibular region, where it is difficult to differentiate the mandible from adjacent soft tissue. **B,** Close-up of mandibular teeth. Note the lack of visualization of the lamina dura.

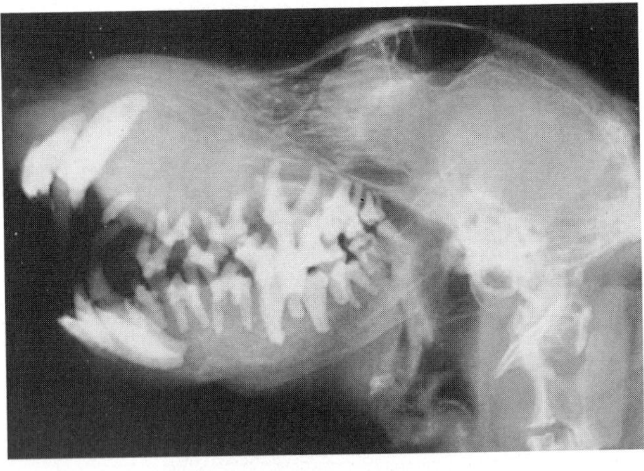

Fig. 8-10 Lateral skull radiograph of a 12-year-old female Scottish terrier with primary hyperparathyroidism and severe fibrous osteodystrophy causing thickening of the maxilla and displacement of teeth. Note the absence of the lamina dura around the tooth roots. (Courtesy of Dr. Wendy Myer, Ohio State University, Columbus, Ohio.)

potential. External-beam radiotherapy is the current treatment of choice.[70,72-75] Unfortunately, diagnosis of these tumors often occurs late in the course of disease, resulting in a poor prognosis in many patients.

Nasal cavity tumors have an aggressive radiographic appearance, with bony invasion and loss of conchal detail being common radiographic features.[14,71,76-78] Tumors may be unilateral or bilateral and cause an increased soft-tissue opacity in the nasal cavity with underlying conchal destruction. Destruction of bones adjacent to the nasal cavity is also common in advanced tumors. Nasal tumors may result in increased opacity within the frontal sinus[71,77-79]; determining whether this frontal sinus opacification is caused by tumor extension or occlusion of the nasofrontal communication with subsequent mucus accumulation in the sinus is impossible from radiographs. Making this distinction can be important for treatment planning options. MR imaging, which is based on the chemical composition of the tissue rather than the electron density of the tissue, is helpful in distinguishing tumor from mucus in the frontal sinus (Fig. 8-11).

The most useful radiographic views for evaluating nasal disease include the intraoral dorsoventral and the open-mouth ventrodorsal view for detailed evaluation of the nasal cavity without superimposition of the mandible (Fig. 8-12). The open-mouth ventrodorsal view is better for cribriform plate assessment because radiographic film cannot physically be positioned to include the cribriform plate in the intraoral view. The cribriform plate is represented by a **V**-shaped to **C**-shaped bony opacity on radiographs, varying according to skull shape (dolichocephalic versus mesaticephalic and brachycephalic).[80] Evaluation of the cribriform plate is important because nasal tumors often originate from the ethmoid conchae and cribriform plate,[66] and bony lysis detected on radiographs indicates potential tumor extension into the brain (see Fig. 8-12). The rostrocaudal frontal sinus projection is necessary for evaluation of individual frontal sinuses (Fig. 8-13) and is a useful radiographic view especially if cross-sectional imaging techniques are not available.[81] However, as previously noted, MR imaging is much more sensitive for assessing the frontal sinus for tumor versus fluid collection.

General anesthesia is an absolute requirement for achieving accurate radiographic positioning, and it facilitates evaluation and comparison of the complex nasal passages. Techniques for obtaining radiographic views of the nasal cavity and paranasal sinuses can be found elsewhere.[82]

The radiographic appearance of nasal tumors varies with histologic type and duration. Aggressive tumors and those with a prolonged duration are more destructive and less confined radiographically, often exhibiting an external soft-tissue mass that represents tumor extension through overlying bone.

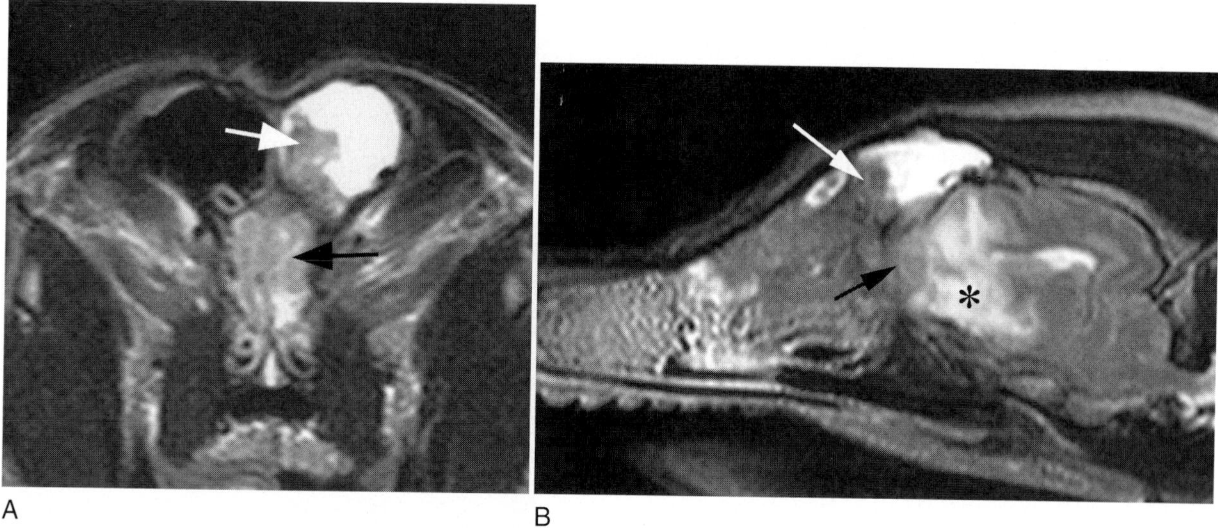

Fig. 8-11 Transverse (A) and parasagittal (B) fast spin-echo T2-weighted MR images of a dog with a malignant nasal tumor. In B the amorphous tumor mass can be seen in the caudal aspect of the nasal cavity. The tumor has invaded the frontal sinus *(white arrows)*, causing obstruction of the nasofrontal communication and resulting in mucus collection in the sinus dorsal to the tumor. In these T2-weighted images this mucus has high signal intensity (appears white) and the tumor has less signal intensity. In radiographs the frontal sinus, the tumor, and the mucus would have the same opacity, making distinction impossible. This tumor has also invaded the cranial cavity *(black arrows)*, leading to extensive white matter edema (streaky white signal, *asterisk*) caudal to the tumor in the sagittal view.

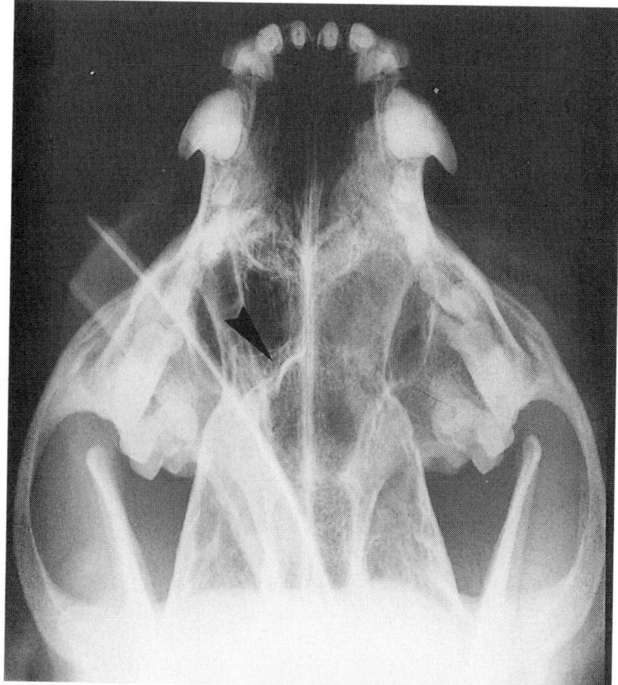

Fig. 8-12 Open-mouth, ventrodorsal radiograph of the nasal cavity of a 7-year-old female Chow Chow with a 1-week history of left-sided facial swelling and nasal discharge. Note the increased opacity, loss of conchal detail, and bony destruction of the cribriform plate of the left nasal passage. The right side of the cribriform plate is intact *(arrowhead)*. Unilateral involvement and bony destruction are suggestive of a nasal cavity tumor. The diagnosis of adenocarcinoma was made histologically.

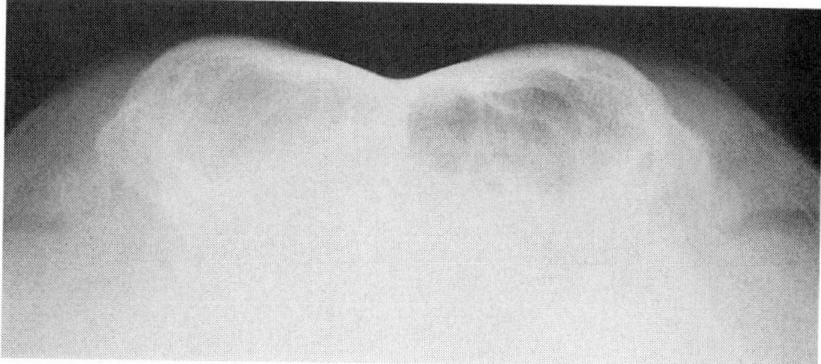

Fig. 8-13 Rostrocaudal frontal sinus radiograph of a 7-year-old German shepherd with a history of epistaxis. Note the increased opacity to the right frontal sinus compared with the left. The increased opacity is consistent with obstructive, neoplastic, fungal, or infectious sinusitis.

Conchae destruction and deviation and destruction of the bony nasal septum are apparent on radiographs. Radiographic evidence of bony destruction is an important prognostic sign; aggressive bony lysis is associated with a poor outcome.[67,78,79,83] Less-aggressive tumors and ones that are detected early are difficult to differentiate from rhinitis on radiographs.[78] Radiographic detection of bony lysis of the cribriform plate and nasoorbital wall is difficult radiographically and better suited to cross-sectional imaging techniques.[84]

CT of the nasal passage is superior to routine radiography for accurate tumor staging (Figs. 8-14 and 8-15) and is useful for attempting to differentiate infectious rhinitis from neoplasia.[8,10,12-14,85,86] Adequately determining the stage of a nasal mass from radiographs is impossible; CT imaging, if available, is the preferred screening modality for nasal disease. The presence of a mass effect (increased soft tissue in the nasal cavity) along with bone destruction is a hallmark sign of nasal neoplasia (see Fig. 8-15). A destructive pattern without a marked mass effect is more typical of aspergillus infection, whereas a mass effect without turbinate destruction is also more typical of infection, though usually not aspergillus. CT images of patients with nasal cancer are also used in computerized radiation therapy planning systems. Use of this sophisticated anatomic information allows optimization of dose distribution across the tumor volume and probable improved survival.[73]

Mandibular and Maxillary Tumors

Tumors of the oral cavity account for approximately 6% of all canine cancers and 3% of feline cancers.[87,88] Squamous cell carcinoma tumors commonly affect the mandible or maxilla in both the dog and cat. Fibrosarcoma, malignant melanoma, and tumors of the periodontal ligament (epulis) are common in the dog but rarely occur in cats.[89,90]

In the dog, the rostral mandible is a common site for oral squamous cell carcinoma. This tumor has variable bony lysis, and regional or distant metastasis is rare.[91] Oral fibrosarcoma tumors in dogs can affect the maxilla or mandible, with a predilection for the palate.[91] In a report of maxillary and incisive tumors in dogs, 82% of squamous cell carcinomas and 78% of fibrosarcomas were characterized radiographically by

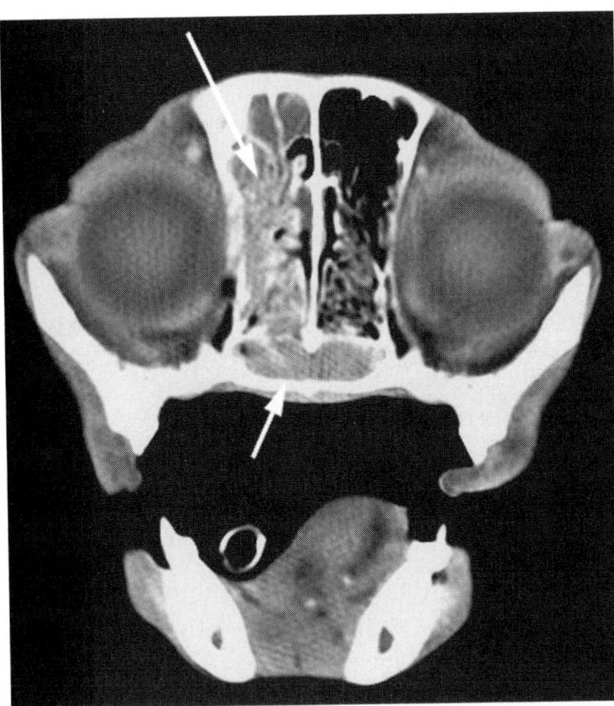

Fig. 8-14 Transverse CT image of the nasal cavity of a cat with nasal lymphoma at the level of the eyes. Tumor is visible within the nasopharynx *(short white arrow)* and the left nasal cavity *(long white arrow)*.

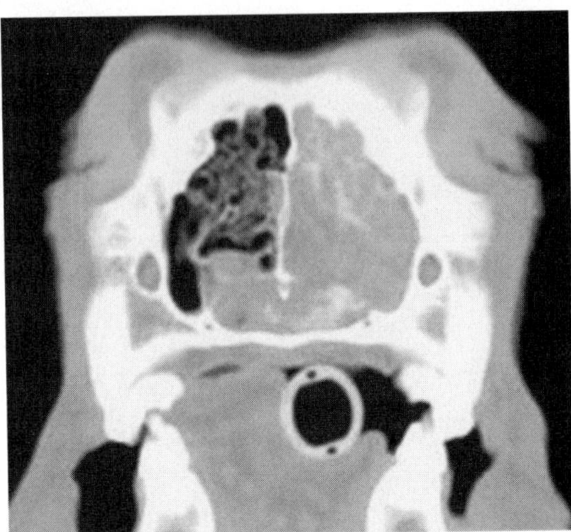

A

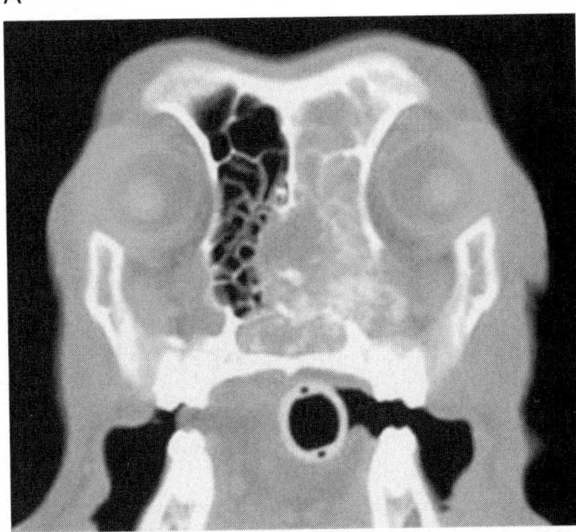

B

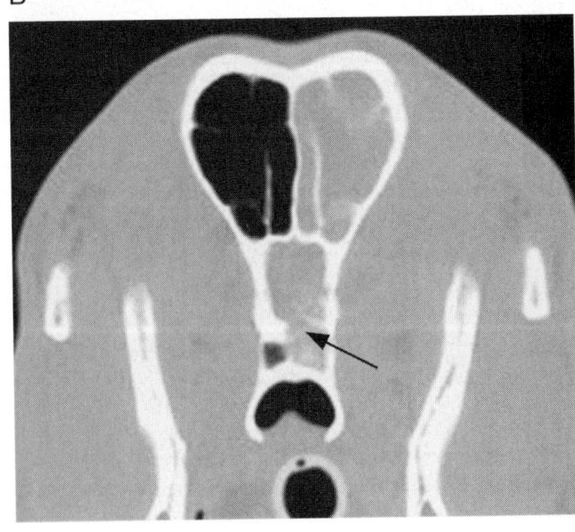

C

Fig. 8-15 Three transverse CT images from a dog with a malignant nasal tumor. **A,** Erosion of the vomer with extension of the tumor to the right nasal cavity. **B,** Extension into the left pterygopalatine fossa, across the midline to the right nasal cavity and tumor in the nasopharynx. **C,** Erosion of the cranial vault with intracranial extension *(arrow)*. Hyperattenuating material is also present in the left frontal sinus; CT images cannot distinguish tumor extension from fluid/mucus collection caused by obstruction of the nasofrontal communication. This combination of CT abnormalities is characteristic of a malignant nasal tumor. The tumor extensions visible in these CT images would not have been detected in radiographs.

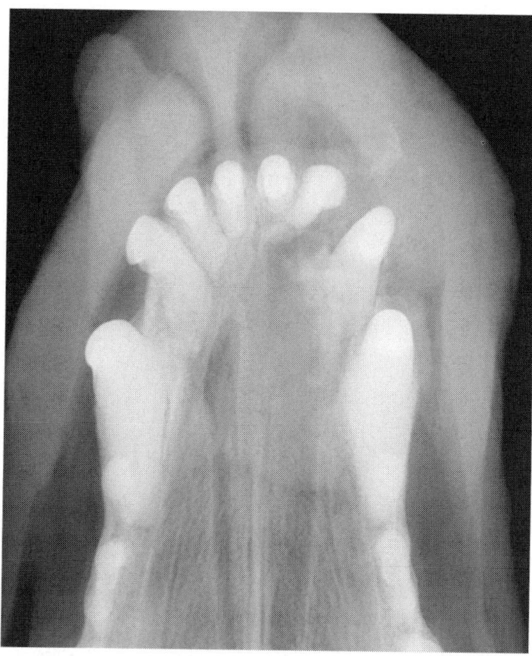

Fig. 8-16 Intraoral dorsoventral radiograph of the maxilla of a dog with a left maxillary gingival mass. In radiographs the mass is visible and contains foci of mineralization. Distortion of the left incisors and marked bone lysis are also present in this area. Lysis extends caudally and blends into normal-appearing conchae. Accurately determining the caudal extent of this tumor with radiographs is impossible; if treatment is undertaken, a CT study of the maxilla should be acquired to stage the extent of this tumor's involvement more accurately. Determination of the tumor type from radiographs is also impossible and a biopsy is needed; however, the appearance of this lesion is most consistent with a malignant gingival tumor. The histologic diagnosis was fibrosarcoma.

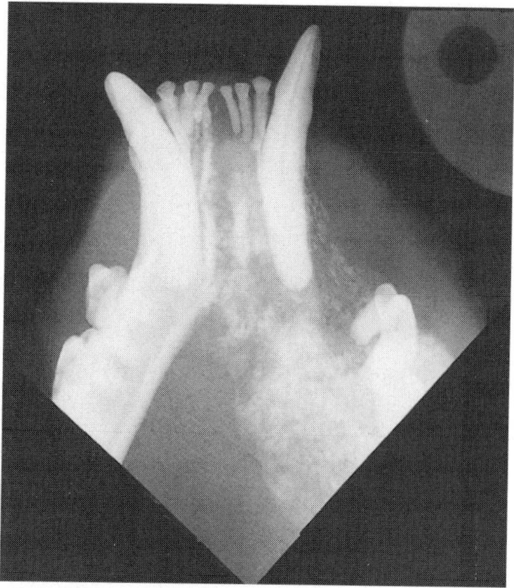

Fig. 8-17 Intraoral ventrodorsal radiograph of a 12-year-old domestic medium-hair cat with a swelling of the left mandible. Note the aggressive mottled appearance of the left rostral mandible. The diagnosis of squamous cell carcinoma was made histologically.

bone involvement.[83] Often, oral fibrosarcoma appears benign histologically, but biologic activity is aggressive. These tumors, often found in the maxilla and mandible of large-breed dogs and commonly in Golden retrievers, are histologically low-grade yet are biologically high-grade aggressive tumors. Bone lysis is a common feature.[92] Dogs with oral fibrosarcoma have a lower median survival rate compared with those with soft-tissue sarcomas at other sites (Fig. 8-16).[93] In contrast, malignant melanoma tends to occur in smaller breed dogs, commonly metastasizes to regional lymph nodes and lungs, and has variable bony lysis radiographically.[91] Squamous cell carcinoma in cats affects the mandible or maxilla, causing sclerotic and/or lytic changes to bone (Fig. 8-17). Flea control products and diet may play a role in the development of squamous cell carcinoma in cats.[94] Unlike squamous cell carcinoma in the dog, these tumors have a poor prognosis in the feline species.[91]

The epulides of periodontal origin have been divided into three categories: fibromatous epulis, ossifying epulis, and acanthomatous epulis.[95] Fibromatous and ossifying epulides are similar benign growths cured by surgical excision; the distinctive feature of ossifying epulis is the histologically large segments of osteoid matrix.[89] The predominant feature of acanthomatous epulis is the sheets of acanthomatous epithelial tissue noted histologically[89] and the local invasion, which often causes bony destruction on radiographs. Although rare, multiple epulides in cats have been reported and tend to recur after surgical excision yet do not exhibit metastatic behavior.[90]

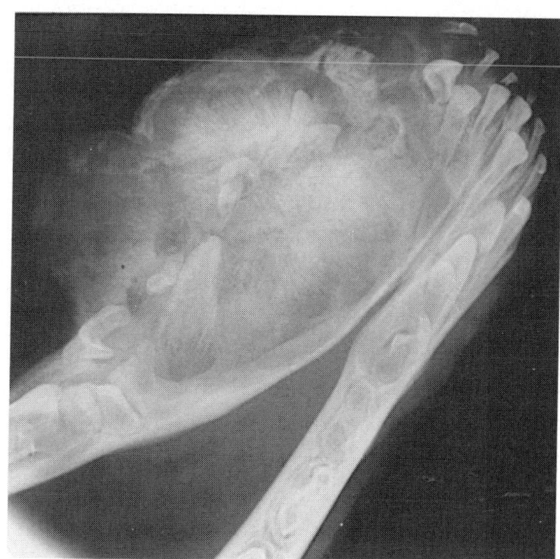

Fig. 8-18 Intraoral ventrodorsal radiograph of a 3-month-old male collie with a complex odontoma. The irregularly marginated, heterogeneously mineralized mass has caused destruction of the rostral mandible and displaced teeth. The soft tissue component of the mass extends across the midline. (Courtesy of Dr. Wendy Myer, Ohio State University, Columbus, Ohio).

Canine epulides are radiosensitive, with few complications.[96-98] Tumors originating from dental laminar epithelium in dogs and cats include ameloblastoma, odontoma (Fig. 8-18), and inductive fibroameloblastoma. Although rare, ameloblastoma is the most common tumor of dental origin in the dog and presents as a slowly growing, expansile mass.[89] Inductive fibroameloblastoma is a rare tumor of the rostral maxilla found in young cats.[89,99]

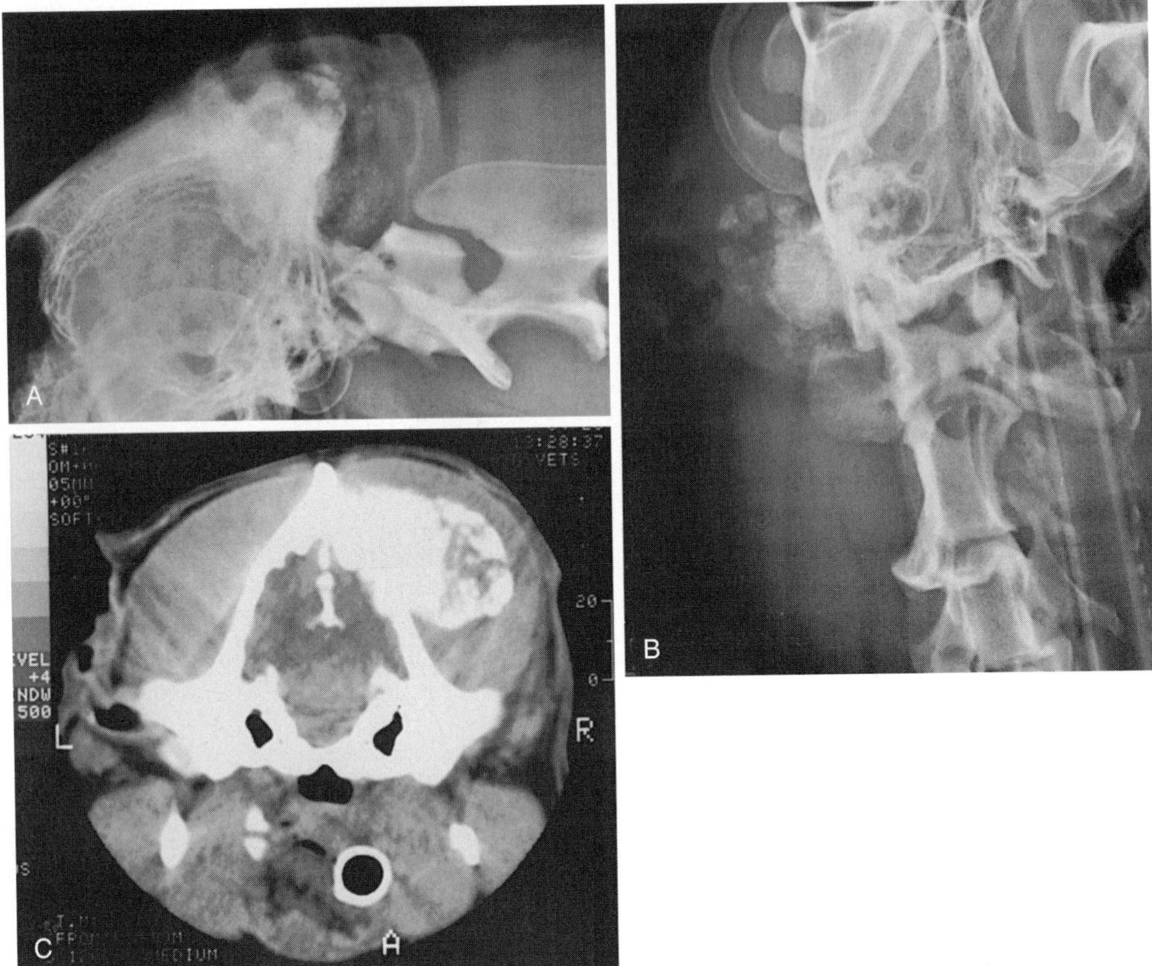

Fig. 8-19 Lateral (A) and right ventral/left dorsal (B) radiographs and CT image (C) of the skull of a 9-year-old boxer with multilobular osteochondrosarcoma of the right occipital bone. Note the granular mineral mass opacity on radiographs (B) and the superior tumor size estimation and degree of brain compression (minimal) evident in the CT image (C). (Courtesy of Dr. Wendy Myer, Ohio State University, Columbus, Ohio.)

Determining the histologic type of tumor from radiographs is impossible. Radiographic changes do not depend on tumor type; some tumors will be lytic, some osteoproductive, and some characterized by a combination of these changes. A sense of biologic aggressiveness can be obtained on the basis of radiographic changes, but a biopsy is necessary for definitive diagnosis. Determining the extent of normal tissue involvement of a tumor from radiographs is also impossible. If therapy is being considered, either CT or MR imaging should be used to determine the extent of tumor involvement more accurately.

Treatment options for oral tumors consist of surgical excision alone, radiotherapy alone, or a combination of surgery and radiotherapy.[92,96,97,100-102] In a study of 100 dogs with oral tumors treated by mandibulectomy or maxillectomy, excellent survival rates were achieved for carcinomas, acanthomatous epulides, and squamous cell carcinomas, with poorer outcomes noted for sarcomas (fibrosarcoma, osteosarcoma, and malignant melanoma).[100] Adjuvant chemotherapy in addition to surgery and/or radiotherapy should be considered for oral tumors with the propensity to metastasize.[103]

Multilobular Osteochondrosarcoma

Multilobular osteochondrosarcoma (MLO) is a rare tumor that arises from the skull of dogs. Other names for this tumor include chondroma rodens and multilobular osteoma. These tumors often arise from the temporooccipital area of the skull, although involvement of the orbit, maxilla, mandible, tympanic bulla, and zygomatic arch has been reported.[104-110] These tumors have characteristic radiographic features. The margins of MLO are well defined, and lysis of adjacent bone is limited.[111] The central core of the tumor is composed of a coarse, granular mineral opacity throughout (Fig. 8-19). Dogs with MLO are typically older, large-breed dogs.[105,111] Approximately 50% of dogs have local recurrence after treatment (surgical excision alone or surgery and radiotherapy), and approximately half have metastatic disease develop.[105,108,111] CT is superior for the detection of cranial vault invasion, which was a common feature in five of seven patients recently described.[112] MRI features of MLO have been described in three dogs, all of which had a similar appearance of heterogeneous signal intensity with large regions of contrast enhancement; tumor invasion of soft tissues and brain was well delineated.[113]

Other Tumors of the Cranium

Other primary tumors of the cranium include osteosarcoma, osteoma, and osteochondroma. Osteosarcoma is the most common primary bone tumor, with 10% to 15% arising from

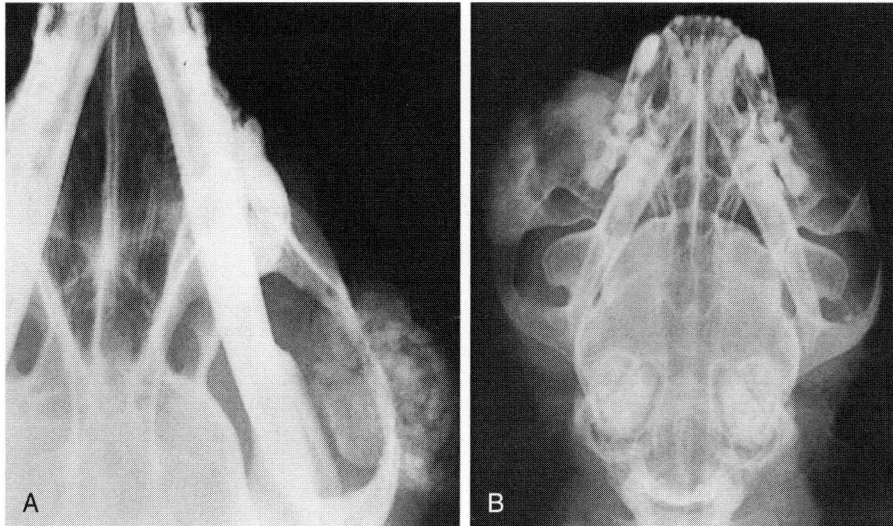

Fig. 8-20 A, Ventrodorsal radiograph of a 9-year-old female mixed-breed dog with an osteoma of the left zygomatic arch. B, Ventrodorsal radiograph of an aged cat (with an osteoma of the rostral portion of the right zygomatic arch). Note the smooth, well-defined margins of these tumors and the lack of bony destruction, which suggest a relatively nonaggressive process. (Courtesy of Dr. Wendy Myer, Ohio State University, Columbus, Ohio.)

the skull (see Fig. 8-3). Distribution of canine skull osteosarcoma in one report included cranial vault in 37%, facial bone in 36%, and mandible in 27% of patients.[114] Osteosarcomas arising from the cranial vault do not resemble those from the appendicular skeleton or other skull sites because they tend to be osteoblastic, have well-defined borders, and contain granular areas of calcification.[20] Osteoma is a slow-growing, benign tumor that has a smooth, well-defined border on radiographs (Fig. 8-20). These tumors can arise from the mandible, cranial vault, or sinuses.[20]

Most brain tumors do not have associated survey radiographic findings and are best identified with MR imaging.[115-117] Occasionally sclerosis of the adjacent calvarium may be noted on routine skull radiographs in cats with meningioma (Fig. 8-21). These tumors may calcify and cause sclerosis and/or lysis of the adjacent bony calvaria.[118]

INFECTIOUS DISORDERS

Nasal Aspergillosis

Nasal aspergillosis is a destructive rhinitis involving the nasal cavity and paranasal sinuses of the dog; it affects younger (less than 4 years of age), nonbrachycephalic breeds more frequently than other breeds.[119,120] *Aspergillus* species (primarily *Aspergillus fumigatus*) are common saprophytic fungal organisms found in the environment.[119] Destructive rhinitis caused by other fungal agents, such as *Penicillium* species, is less common.[119,121] Nasal blastomycosis can occur in endemic areas. The most common radiographic appearance of nasal aspergillosis includes lysis of conchae with punctate lucencies of bone (Fig. 8-22).[77,120,122] Increased localized soft-tissue opacity of the nasal cavity is also seen, but frontal sinus involvement is variable and consists of sinus opacity with or without mottled bony thickening.[77,120,122] Bony nasal septum erosion or deviation is uncommon except in advanced disease. *Cryptococcus neoformans,* a fungal infection more commonly seen in cats, can infect the nasal passages but generally causes a nondestructive hyperplastic rhinitis (Fig. 8-23).[123,124]

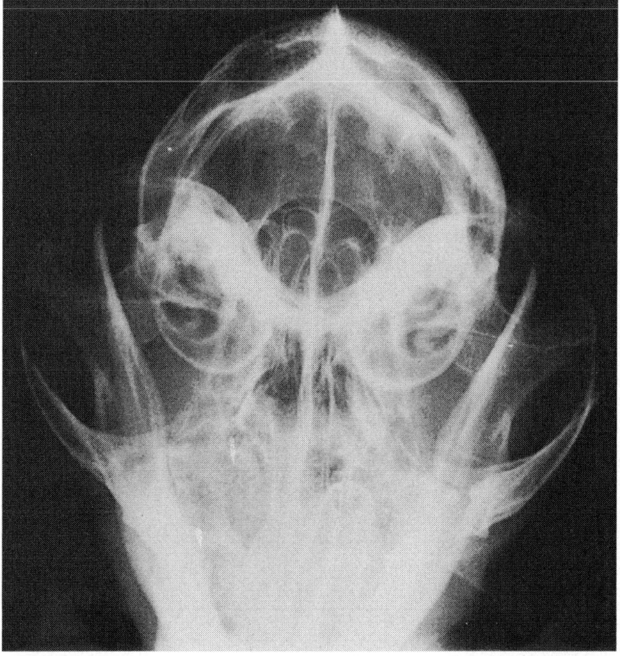

Fig. 8-21 Rostrodorsal–caudoventral oblique radiograph of the skull of a 12-year-old domestic shorthair cat with a left cerebral meningioma. Note the bony thickening (hyperostosis) of the left side of the calvarium.

Destructive rhinitis as a result of fungal disease can be difficult to differentiate radiographically from neoplasia. Both diseases cause loss of conchal detail, but a nasal cavity mass effect and invasion of bones surrounding the nasal cavity are more common features of nasal cavity neoplasia.[77,122] CT and MR imaging have been used to evaluate nasal aspergillosis, with the cross-sectional imaging modalities superior to radiography because of the greater contrast resolution and

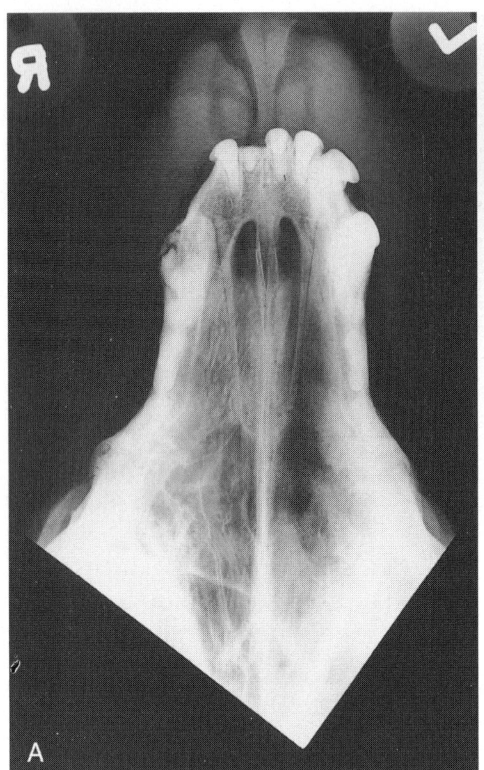

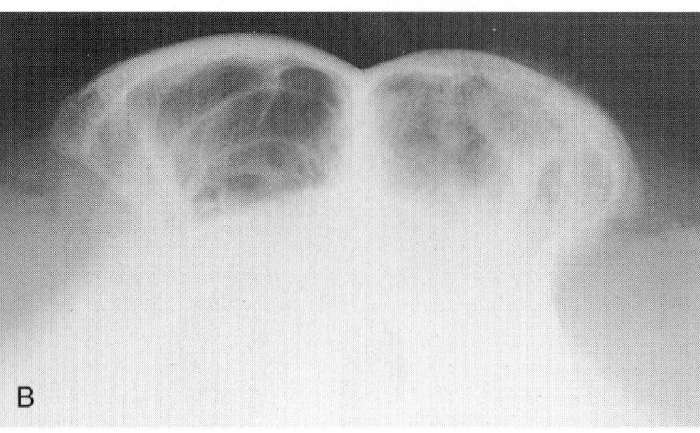

Fig. 8-22 Open-mouth, ventrodorsal **(A)** and rostrocaudal–frontal sinus **(B)** radiographs of a 9-year-old female Labrador retriever with a 3-month history of nasal discharge. Note the destruction of the nasal conchae in the midportion of the left nasal cavity **(A)** and the increased opacity to the left frontal sinus **(B)**. Evidence of frontal-bone irregularity is also present, indicating destructive sinusitis **(B)**. Destructive rhinitis secondary to *Aspergillus fumigatus* was diagnosed by culture.

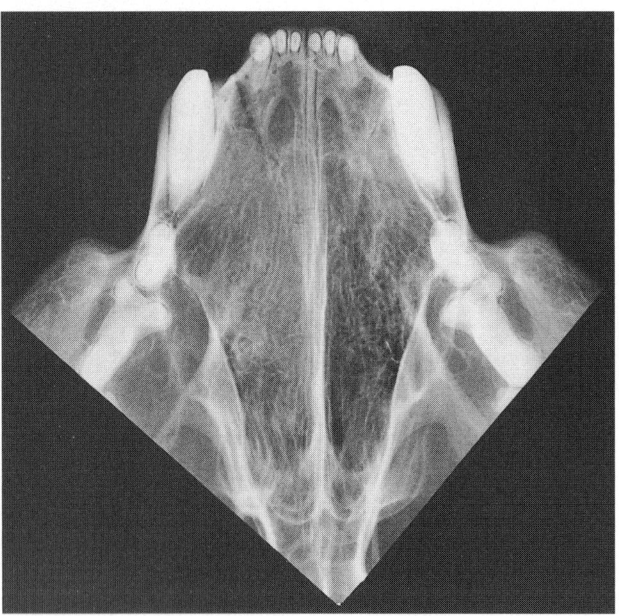

Fig. 8-23 Intraoral, dorsoventral radiograph of a 4-year-old domestic shorthair cat with a history of nasal discharge. Note the increased opacity to the right nasal cavity without loss of conchal detail. *Cryptococcus neoformans* was diagnosed by culture.

cross-sectional nature (Fig. 8-24).[11-13,86] Regardless of the imaging presentation of aggressive nasal disease, a biopsy sample for histopathologic evaluation is necessary for diagnosis.

Nasal Rhinitis and Foreign Bodies

Rhinitis as a result of bacterial infection, or corticosteroid-responsive rhinitis with lymphoplasmacytic infiltrates, can have a variable radiographic appearance in dogs and cats. Depending on the chronicity and severity of rhinitis, evidence of destruction of conchae and of bony erosion may be present.[13,71] Chronic rhinitis and sinusitis in cats are common sequelae to viral upper respiratory tract disease (Fig. 8-25). Radiographic changes can range from none in mild infections to an increased opacity of the nasal cavity and frontal sinuses, with conchae and vomer bone destruction in severe infections (Fig. 8-26).[71,125]

In five dogs with lymphoplasmacytic rhinitis, the radiographic appearance varied from increased opacity without bony destruction to nasal conchae and vomer bone lysis.[126] Destruction of conchae is more frequently observed in destructive rhinitis caused by aspergillosis or neoplasia but can also occur in other forms of rhinitis.[71,126,127]

Intranasal foreign bodies can occur in dogs, and inhalation of foreign plant matter is common in certain areas, such as inhalation of grass awns in California. Affected dogs have an acute onset of sneezing and pawing at the nose, and they often have a unilateral nasal discharge.[127,128] Radiopaque foreign bodies are obvious in radiographs (Fig. 8-27). Localization of nonopaque foreign bodies may be suspected in radiographs on

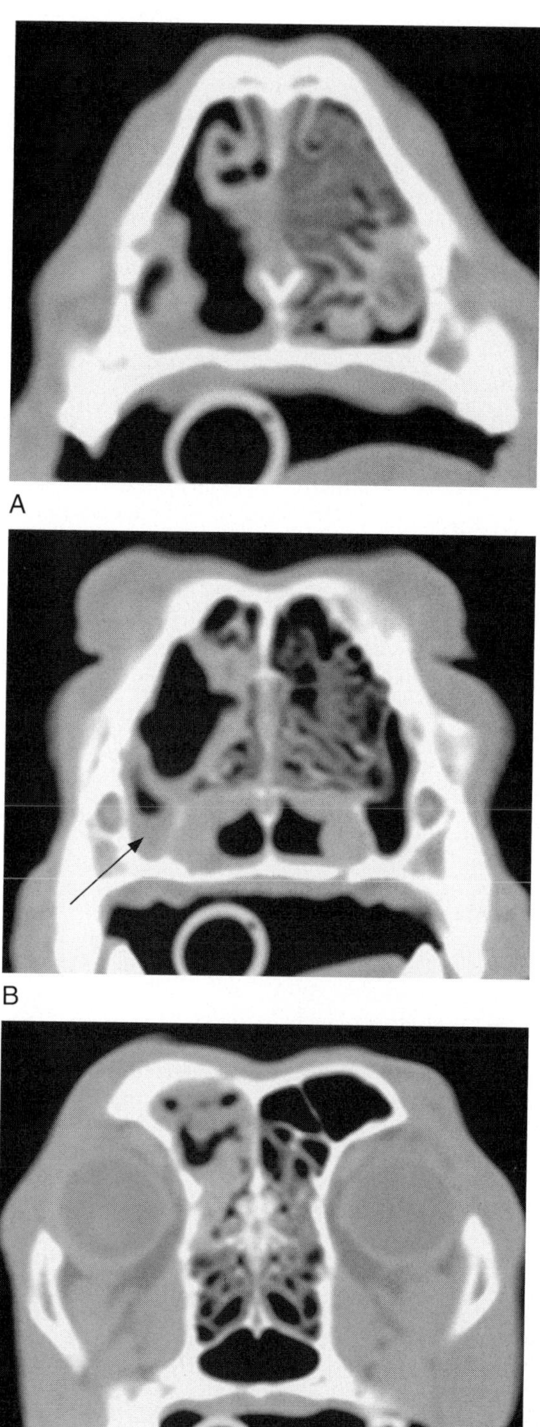

Fig. 8-24 Computed tomographic images of the nasal cavity from a dog with nasal aspergillosis. **A** and **B,** Destruction of conchae on the right side. Note the normal-appearing left conchae. Residual conchae on the right appear thickened and irregular. **B,** A small amount of fluid (note the meniscus effect, *arrow*) in the ventral aspect of the nasal cavity. **C,** Irregular masses in the right frontal sinus without fluid accumulation, hyperostosis of the lateral aspect of the right frontal sinus, and erosion of the dorsomedial aspect of the right frontal sinus. The finding of conchal destruction and irregular frontal sinus mass effect is much more consistent with nasal aspergillosis than a tumor.

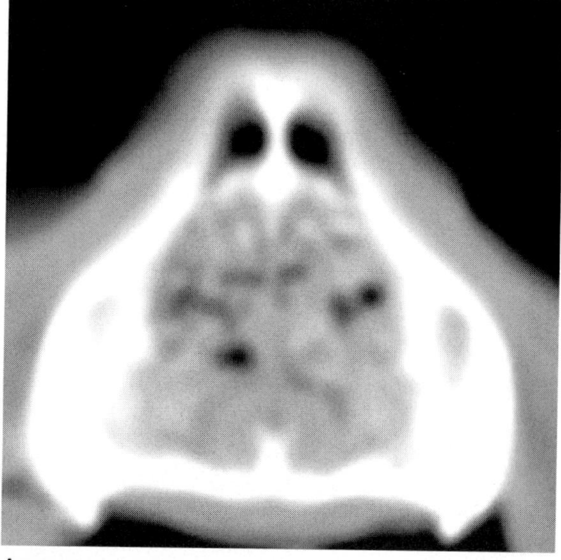

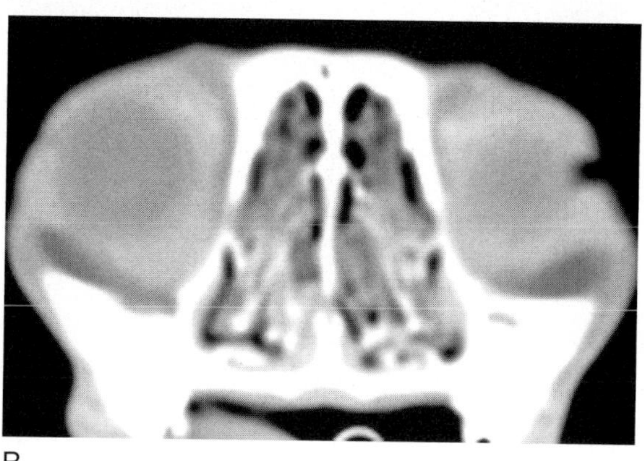

Fig. 8-25 CT images of the nasal cavity from a cat with chronic nasal discharge and presumed lower respiratory infection. Amorphous increased opacity in the nasal cavity is visible with indistinct conchal detail (**A** and **B**) likely caused by edema. This change, without a defined mass effect, and lack of turbinate destruction (**B**) is much more typical of an inflammatory process than a tumor. In radiographs, this change may not have been detected because of its minor nature.

the basis of the presence of inflammation and mucopurulent material, which appear as increased soft-tissue opacity. CT is more sensitive for identification of foreign bodies than is radiography, but unfortunately not all foreign objects are hyperattenuating in CT images.

Otitis

Radiographs are an integral part of the diagnostic workup of a dog or cat with ear disease for evaluation of otitis media. Diagnosis of otitis interna is made on the basis of clinical signs because it does not reliably produce radiographic changes.[129] However, external ear canal stenosis and mineralization can often be identified in ventrodorsal radiographs.

Otitis media is often caused by chronic otitis externa. Evaluation of tympanic bullae for the presence of increased opacity or thickening of the osseous bulla, indicating otitis media, is best seen on lateral oblique and open-mouth radiographic projections (Fig. 8-28). Otitis media can be unilateral; when this occurs, the diagnosis is simplified by a comparison between the two tympanic bullae (see Fig. 8-28). In advanced disease, exuberant bony proliferation may involve the petrous temporal bone or the temporomandibular joint. Positioning is crucial when radiography of the bullae is performed; general anesthesia facilitates proper positioning and allows personnel to vacate the room during radiographic exposure. A review of imaging techniques for middle ear disease can be found elsewhere.[130-133]

When radiographic and surgical findings of otitis media were compared, all cases with abnormal radiographic findings were surgically confirmed. However, 25% of patients with normal radiographs of the middle ear were abnormal at surgery.[134] CT is a more sensitive test for evaluation of otitis media,[135] but proper imaging technique is necessary to avoid artifactual wall thickening of the bulla on CT images (Fig. 8-29).[136] Middle ear changes in MR images of dogs with neurologic disease were assessed, and no correlation between the signal intensity of material within the middle ear and final diagnosis was noted.[137] Additionally evidence of material within the middle ear in MR images of dogs without clinical signs of otitis media was thought to represent subclinical otitis media or fluid accumulation without inflammation.[137]

Feline nasopharyngeal polyps are nonneoplastic growths originating from the mucous membrane of the auditory tube or middle ear.[138] Nasopharyngeal polyps generally occur in younger cats and can extend into the external ear canal, the osseous bulla, or the nasopharynx. Cats may have signs of middle ear disease, rhinitis, or upper airway disease caused by the space-occupying polyp. Signs of otitis media (increased soft-tissue opacity of the affected bulla) or nasopharyngeal obstruction (Fig. 8-30) may be noted on radiographs. In a study of 31 cats with nasopharyngeal polyps, a radiographic diagnosis of otitis media was made in 26, and nasopharyngeal masses were detected in 30.[139] CT and MR imaging can also be used to identify inflammatory polyps in cats (Fig. 8-31).[140,141]

Ear canal tumors occur in dogs and cats. Most often, these soft-tissue neoplasms are squamous cell carcinoma or mucinous gland adenocarcinoma.[142] These masses obliterate the external ear canal and can cause aggressive bony lysis of the adjacent calvaria and osseous bulla (Fig. 8-32).

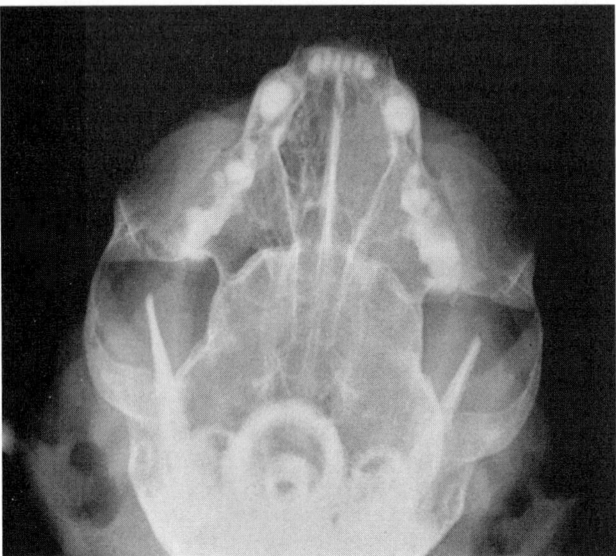

Fig. 8-26 Open-mouth, ventrodorsal radiograph of a 13-year-old castrated male domestic shorthair cat with a 4-week history of primarily left-sided nasal discharge and anorexia. Note the diffuse increase in opacity of the left nasal cavity with loss of conchal detail. Severe subacute pyogranulomatous rhinitis secondary to *Pasteurella multocida* was diagnosed after nasal curettage and culture. A tumor would also have to be considered on the basis of this radiographic appearance. (Courtesy of Dr. Wendy Myer, Ohio State University, Columbus, Ohio.)

Periapical (Tooth Root) Abscess

Periapical infection has a typical radiographic appearance of a radiolucent halo around the affected tooth root with destruction of alveolar bone (Fig. 8-33). Other radiographic signs seen with periapical abscess include widening of the periodontal space surrounding the apex, bone lysis or sclerosis adjacent to the apex, loss of the lamina dura, and resorption of the tooth root. Periapical infections are common in older animals and may be a result of periodontal disease or fracture of the affected tooth. In dogs, infections of the fourth maxillary premolar (carnassial tooth) often result in a draining fistula below the eye on the affected side.

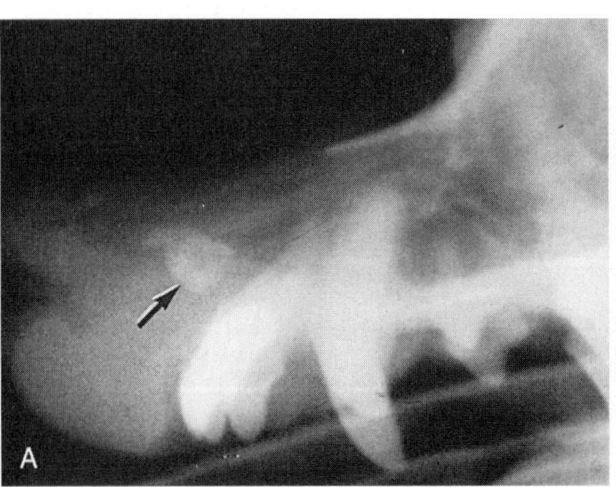

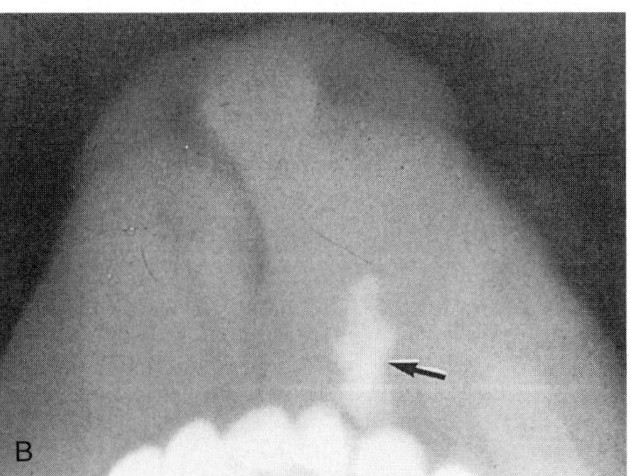

Fig. 8-27 Lateral (A) and close-up ventrodorsal, open-mouth (B) radiographs of a 9-year-old female Poodle with a 3-week history of unilateral nasal discharge and sneezing. A radiopaque foreign body *(arrows)* is present in the left nostril. Note the loss of aeration of the left nostril. (Courtesy of Dr. Wendy Myer, Ohio State University, Columbus, Ohio.)

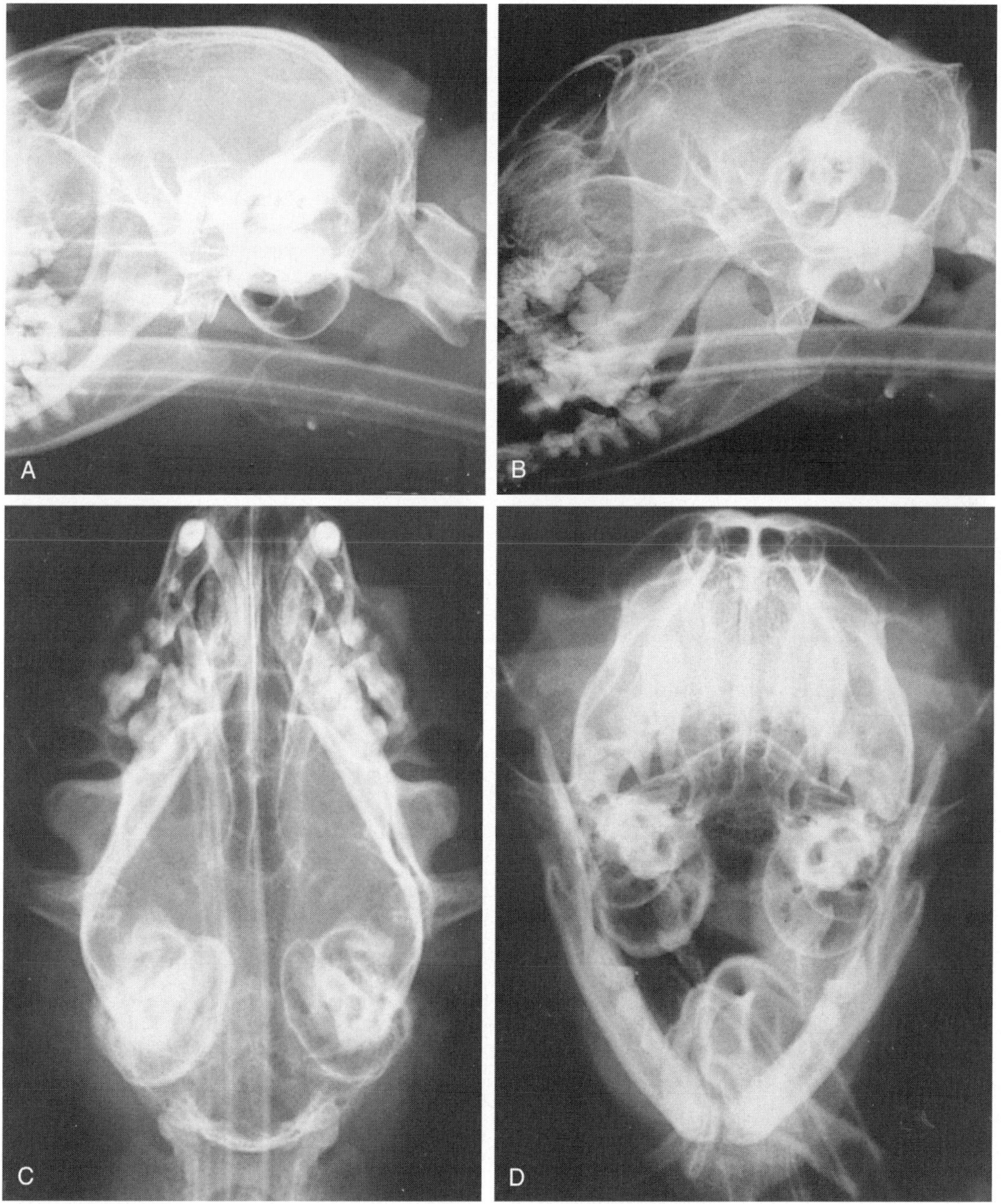

Fig. 8-28 Tympanic bulla radiographs of a 6-year-old female domestic shorthair cat with chronic otitis externa and media. Compare the normal left bulla (air-filled, thin, bony rim) seen in the right dorsal/left ventral oblique radiograph **(A)** with the thickened right bulla seen in the left dorsal/right ventral oblique **(B)**, ventrodorsal **(C)**, and open-mouth rostrocaudal **(D)** radiographs. (Courtesy of Dr. Wendy Myer, Ohio State University, Columbus, Ohio.)

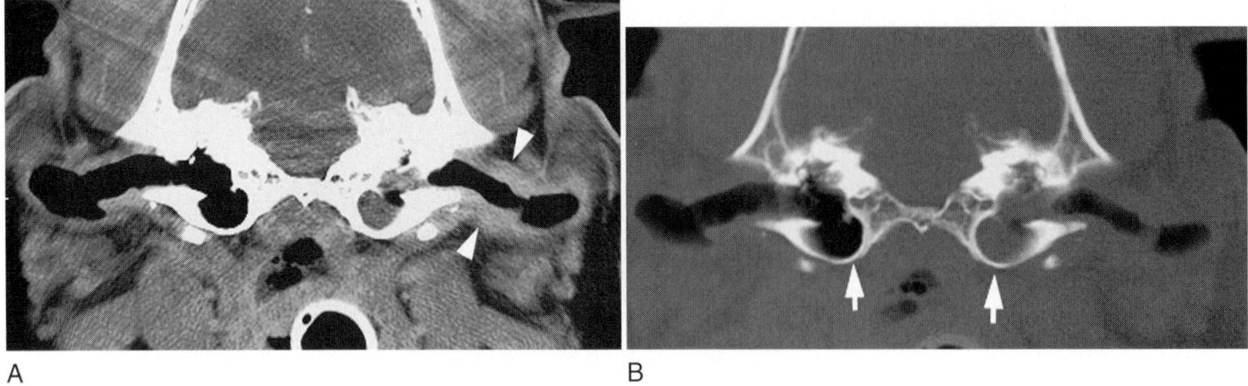

Fig. 8-29 Transverse CT image **(A)** at the level of the ears using a soft tissue window (W 350, L 90) of a 6-year-old dog with a slight head tilt to the right. Note the thickened external ear canal *(white arrowheads)* and the soft tissue attenuating material in the right tympanic bulla. With a bone window (W 2500, L 480) for the same image **(B)**, the bone thickness is more accurate. Note the tympanic bullae are the same thickness *(white arrows)*.

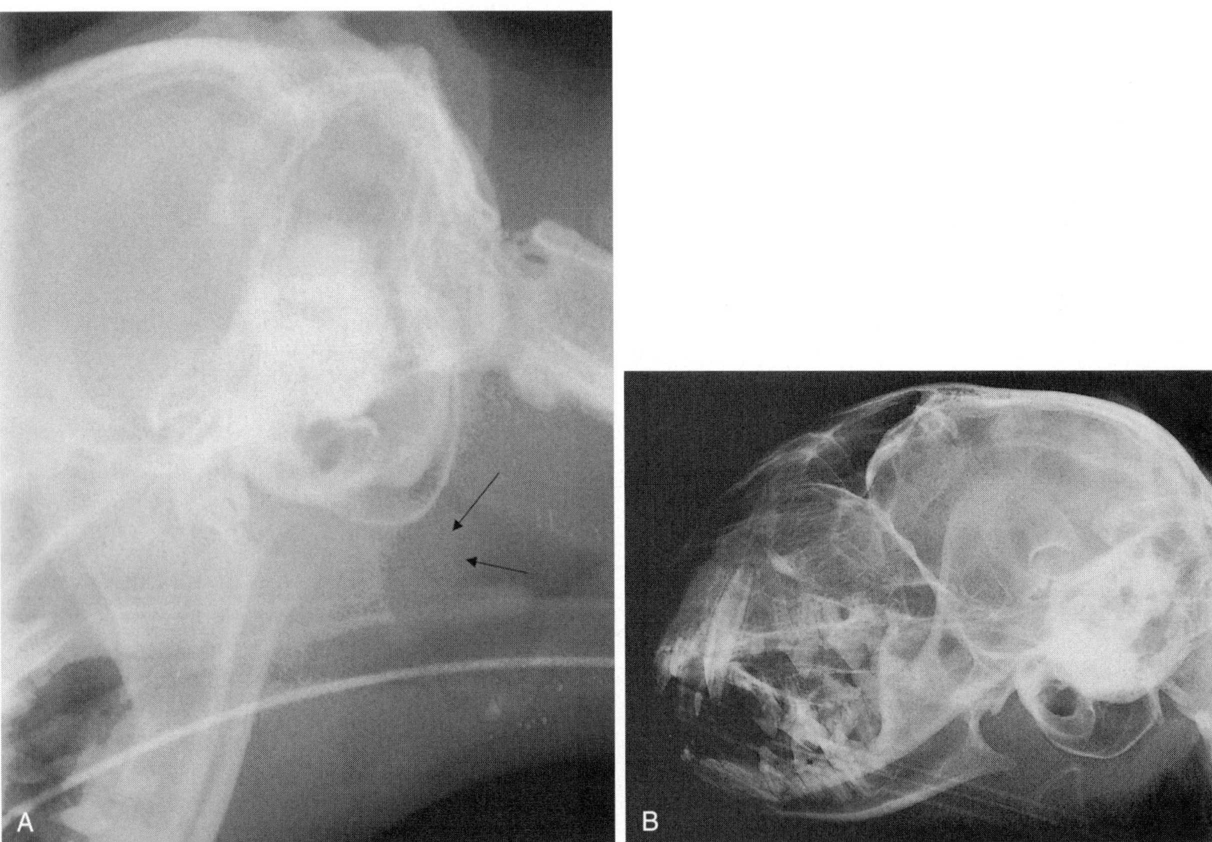

Fig. 8-30 Lateral **(A)**, right dorsal/left ventral oblique **(B)**, left dorsal/right ventral oblique **(C)**, and 10-degree ventrodorsal **(D)** radiographs of a 1-year-old domestic shorthair cat with a history of inspiratory dyspnea. Note the increased soft tissue opacity filling the pharyngeal region on the lateral projection (**A,** *arrows*). Compare the left and right bullae on the lateral obliques **(B, C)**, and 10-degree ventrodorsal radiographs **(D)** and note the increased opacity and bony thickening of the right bulla. Nasopharyngeal polyps involving the right bulla and nasopharynx were removed surgically.

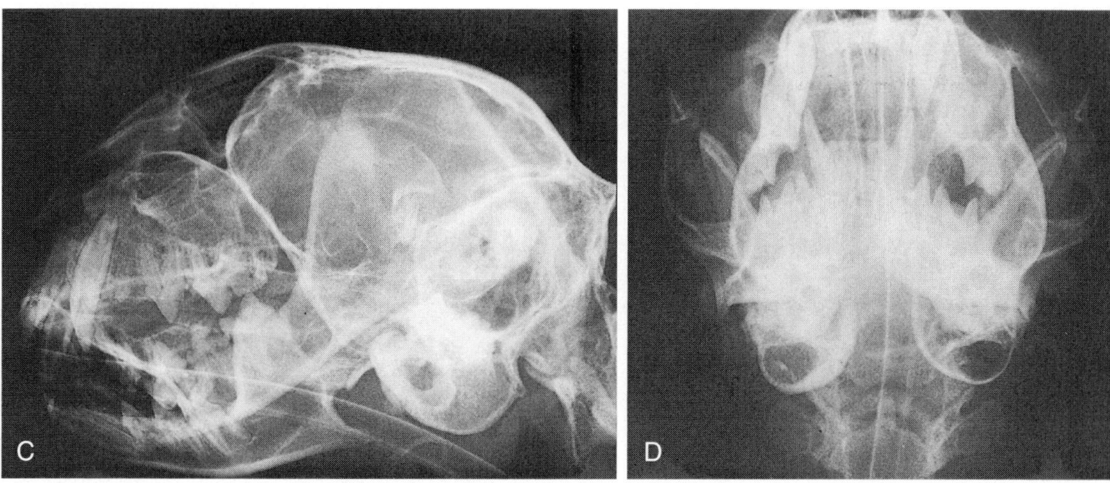

Fig. 8-30, cont'd For legend see opposite page.

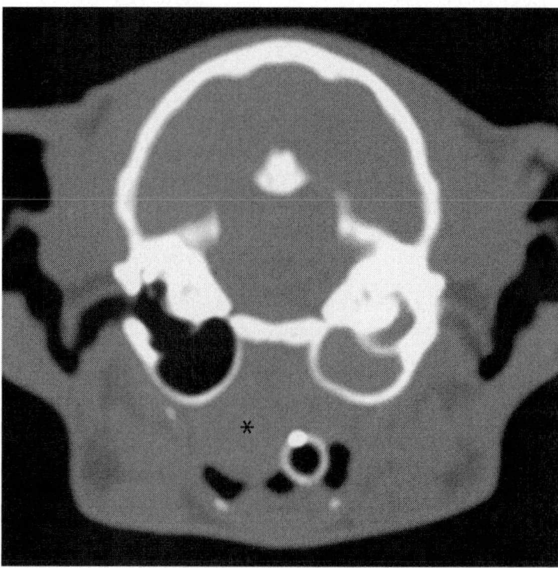

Fig. 8-31 CT image of the pharyngeal region of a cat with a nasopharyngeal polyp (*asterisk*). Fluid is present in the left tympanic bulla, as is a large mass effect in the nasopharynx. This CT appearance is typical of nasopharyngeal polyps in cats.

Dental radiographs can be obtained by conventional x-ray equipment and film-screen combinations, which consist of open-mouth oblique views of the dental arcades. A dental x-ray machine provides enhanced flexibility in adjustment of focal film distance, angulation, and collimation, and it enables the use, with improved accuracy, of small, intraoral dental film.[4] Since the recognition of the American Veterinary Dental College by the American Veterinary Medical Association in 1988, the number of specialists in veterinary dentistry has increased. These dentists commonly perform endodontal and periodontal procedures to treat dental disease in dogs and cats.[4]

TRAUMATIC INJURIES

TMJ luxation can occur in both dogs and cats after external trauma. In the cat, TMJ luxation often occurs after the cat has jumped from a height; in both dogs and cats, dislocation can result from being hit by a car.[143] The TMJ is capable of luxation without fracture because it has considerable lateral sliding movement, and the synchondrosis of the mandibular symphysis allows independent movement of the mandibular rami.[52] Dislocation of the TMJ tends to be in the rostrodorsal direction (Fig. 8-34) because ventrocaudal luxation is prevented by the retroarticular process of the temporal bone.[52] Dogs and cats with TMJ dislocation are unable to completely close the mouth, have dental malocclusion with the mandible displaced to one side, and display excessive salivation.[52,143] Luxation is most often unilateral; it may occur alone or with concomitant fractures of the retroarticular process, mandibular fossa, and zygomatic process of the squamous temporal bone, or with the condyloid process of the mandible.[143]

Radiographic views necessary for evaluating the TMJ include ventrodorsal and 20-degree lateral oblique views in the cat.[22,143] These views are useful in the dog, but the angle of rotation will vary depending on head conformation.[22,144] A sagittal oblique radiograph, in which the nose is elevated with a foam wedge so that the head is at a 20-degree angle to the cassette from a lateral position, is suggested in dogs as an alternative to lateral oblique views.[22,82,144] CT imaging provides superior images of the TMJ.

MISCELLANEOUS DISEASES

Craniomandibular Osteopathy

Craniomandibular osteopathy (CMO) is a proliferative bone disease that occurs mainly in young West Highland White, Scottish, Cairn, Boston, and other terriers; it is occasionally seen in nonterrier breeds such as the Labrador retriever, Doberman pinscher, and bullmastiff.[145] A known autosomal recessive inheritance occurs in West Highland White terriers.[146] CMO is usually seen in young dogs aged 3 to 8 months; affected dogs have mandibular swelling, prehension difficulties, pain on opening the mouth or with mastication, pyrexia, or combinations of these clinical signs.[59,147]

On radiographic evaluation of the skull, an increased bony opacity is present in affected areas, primarily the mandible, the tympanic bulla, and the petrous temporal bone (Fig. 8-35). Bony proliferation is somewhat irregular and often bilateral and may be asymmetrical, although unilateral presentation can occur. Bony proliferation can involve the TMJ and can affect jaw movement. Diagnosis is based on signalment and on radiographic findings. Bone biopsy is helpful in

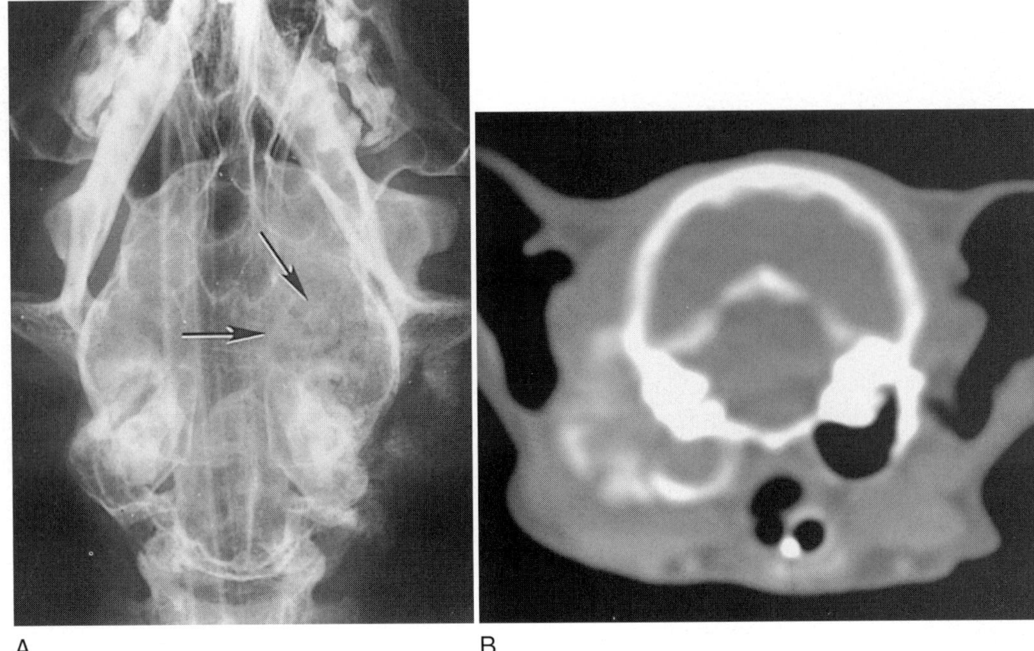

Fig. 8-32 A, Ventrodorsal skull radiograph of a 12-year-old domestic shorthair cat with squamous cell carcinoma of the left ear canal. Note the lysis of the skull *(arrows)* and lateral aspect of the left tympanic bulla. **B,** CT image of the tympanic bulla region of a cat with a malignant tumor of the left middle ear. Increased tissue or fluid is present in the left tympanic bulla and erosion and expansion of the lateral aspect of the left tympanic bulla. This aggressive appearance is typical of a malignant process and should not occur as a result of infection. (**A** Courtesy of Dr. Wendy Myer, Ohio State University, Columbus, Ohio.)

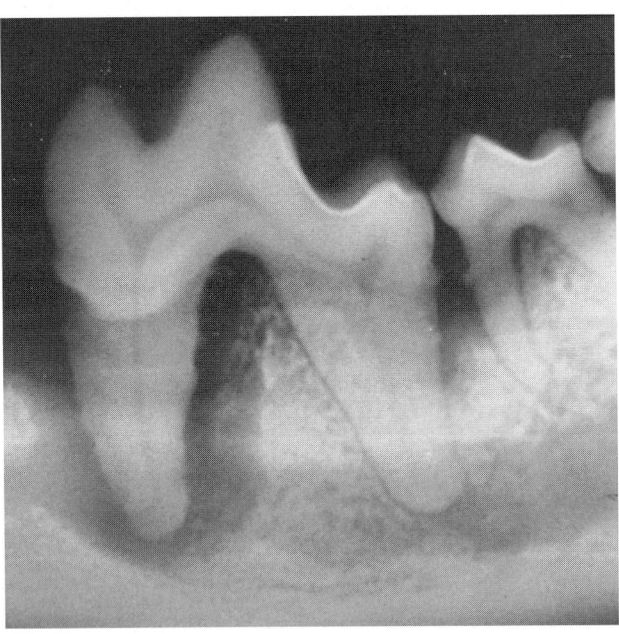

Fig. 8-33 Close-up lateral dental radiograph of a periapical abscess of the rostral root of the first mandibular molar. Note the lysis of alveolar bone, loss of lamina dura, and erosion of the tooth root. (Courtesy of Dr. Wendy Myer, Ohio State University, Columbus, Ohio.)

nonterrier breeds with unilateral involvement. Concurrent metaphyseal long-bone changes similar to hypertrophic osteodystrophy have been seen in dogs with CMO, but this is uncommon.[59] CMO is a self-limiting disease with unknown etiology. Bony proliferation generally ceases with skeletal maturation.

Periodontal Disease

The structures that support the teeth include the cementum, the periodontal ligament, the alveolar bone, and the gingiva. Periodontal disease involves both hard tissue (cementum, alveolar bone) and soft tissue (periodontal ligament, gingiva) that surrounds the teeth; it commonly affects dogs and cats.[4,148,149] Gingival recession or hyperplasia and bony resorption in periodontal disease lead to ultimate loss of tooth support. Although radiography provides little information about gingival tissues, it is an important part of the evaluation of bony structures in periodontal disease.

Early radiographic signs of periodontal disease include an irregular surface and bone loss in the alveolar crest. The lamina dura may be ill defined or may lack continuity.[4] As the disease progresses, horizontal bone loss of a group of teeth occurs so that alveolar bone resorption develops away from the tooth crown, thus exposing tooth roots. Widening of the periodontal space is also seen. Alveolar bone recession exposes root surfaces, which can lead to root caries and root resorption, seen radiographically as radiolucent defects (Fig. 8-36).[150]

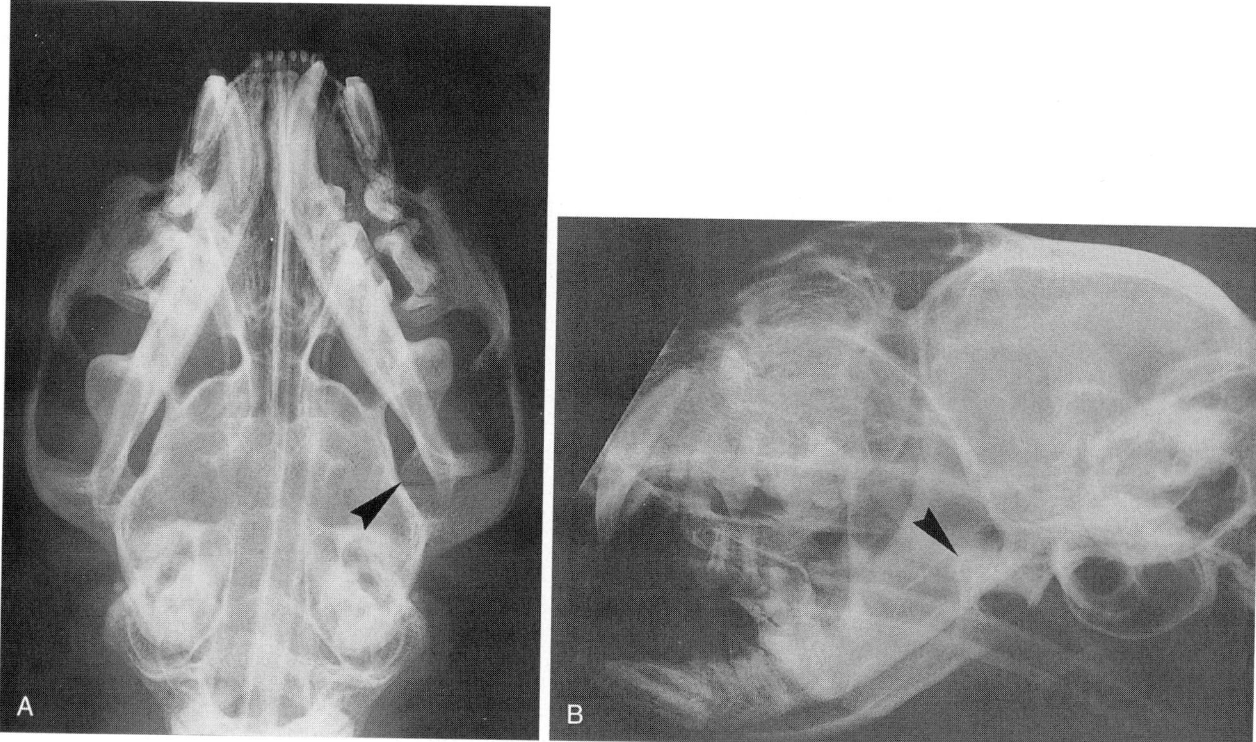

Fig. 8-34 Ventrodorsal (A) and right dorsal/left ventral oblique (B) radiographs of a 1-year-old domestic shorthair cat with a left temporomandibular joint luxation. Note the rostral location of the left mandibular condylar process *(arrowhead)* in the ventrodorsal radiograph (A). In the lateral oblique radiograph (B), note the rostral and dorsal luxation of the mandibular condylar process *(arrowhead)*.

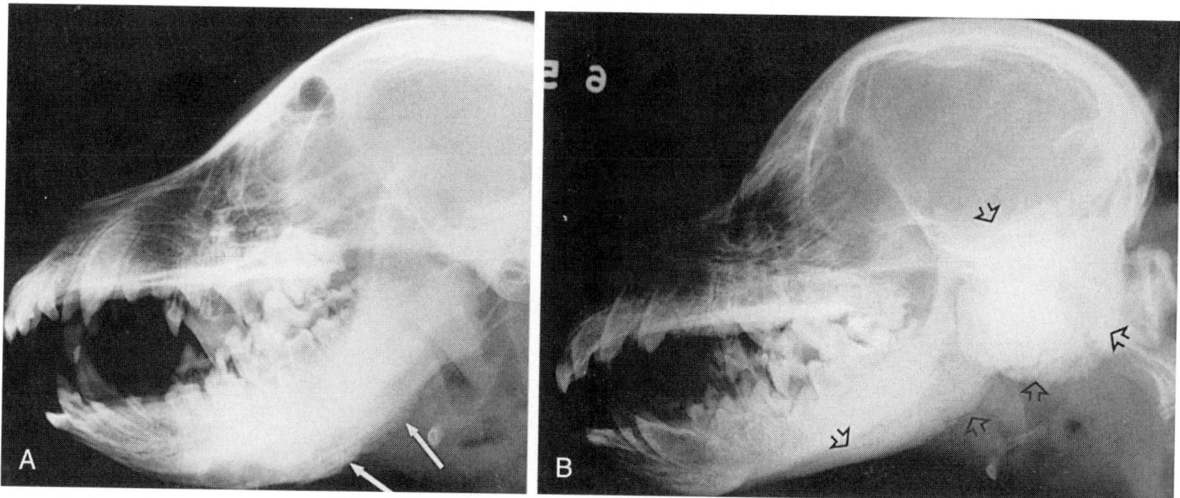

Fig. 8-35 Lateral skull radiographs of two West Highland white terrier dogs with craniomandibular osteopathy. A, The proliferation is primarily on the mandibular ramus *(white arrows)*. B, Bony proliferation involving the tympanic bullae and TMJs as well as the mandibular ramus *(open arrows)*. (Courtesy of Dr. Wendy Myer, Ohio State University, Columbus, Ohio.)

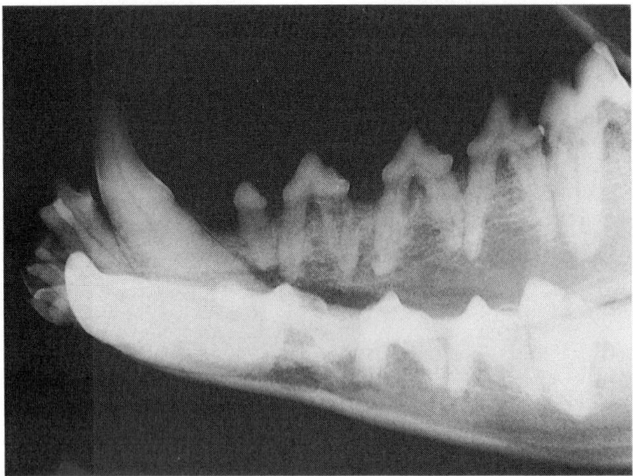

Fig. 8-36 Oblique radiograph of the rostral mandible of a 14-year-old mixed-breed dog with severe dental disease. Note the irregularity of the alveolar crest between the second and third premolar teeth. Also note the lysis of the caudal root of the first premolar and the rostral root of the third premolar, changes consistent with dental root caries.

REFERENCES

1. Miller ME, Evans HE: *Miller's anatomy of the dog*, ed 3, Philadelphia, 1993, WB Saunders, pp. 128-166.
2. Harvey CE: The nasal septum of the dog: is it visible radiographically? *Vet Radiol* 20:88-90, 1979.
3. Morgan JP, Miyabayashi T: Dental radiology: aging changes in permanent teeth of beagle dogs, *J Small Anim Pract* 32:11-18, 1991.
4. Mulligan TW, Aller MS, Williams CA: *Atlas of canine and feline dental radiography*, Trenton, 1988, Veterinary Learning Systems, p. 246.
5. San Roman F, Llorens MP, Peña MT et al: Dental radiography in the dog with a conventional x-ray device, *Vet Radiol* 31:235-238, 1990.
6. Zontine WJ: Dental radiographic technique and interpretation, *Vet Clin North Am* 4:741-762, 1974.
7. Zontine WJ: Canine dental radiology: radiographic technique, development, and anatomy of the teeth, *J Am Vet Rad Soc* 16:75-82, 1975.
8. Codner EC, Lurus AG, Miller JB et al: Comparison of computed tomography with radiography as a noninvasive diagnostic technique for chronic nasal disease in dogs, *J Am Vet Med Assoc* 202:1106-1110, 1993.
9. De Rycke LM, Saunders JH, Gielen IM et al: Magnetic resonance imaging, computed tomography, and cross-sectional views of the anatomy of normal nasal cavities and paranasal sinuses in mesaticephalic dogs, *Am J Vet Res* 64:1093-1098, 2003.
10. Park RD, Beck ER, LeCouteur RA: Comparison of computed tomography and radiography for detecting changes induced by malignant nasal neoplasia in dogs, *J Am Vet Med Assoc* 201:1720-1724, 1992.
11. Saunders JH, Clercs C, Snaps FR et al: Radiographic, magnetic resonance imaging, computed tomographic, and rhinoscopic features of nasal aspergillosis in dogs, *J Am Vet Med Assoc* 225:1703-1712, 2004.
12. Saunders JH, van Bree H: Comparison of radiography and computed tomography for the diagnosis of canine nasal aspergillosis, *Vet Radiol Ultrasound* 44:414-419, 2003.
13. Saunders JH, van Bree H, Gielen I et al: Diagnostic value of computed tomography in dogs with chronic nasal disease, *Vet Radiol Ultrasound* 44:409-413, 2003.
14. Thrall DE, Robertson ID, McLeod DA et al: A comparison of radiographic and computed tomographic findings in 31 dogs with malignant nasal cavity tumors, *Vet Radiol* 30:59-66, 1989.
15. Burk RL: Computed tomographic anatomy of the canine nasal passages, *Vet Radiol Ultrasound* 33:170-180, 1992.
16. Assheuer J, Sager M: Head. In Assheuer J, Sager M, editors: *MRI and CT atlas of the dog*, Berlin, 1997, Blackwell Science, p. 50-57.
17. Feeney D, Fletcher T, Hardy R: *Atlas of correlative imaging anatomy of the normal dog, ultrasound and computed tomography*, Philadelphia, 1991, WB Saunders.
18. George TF, Smallwood JE: Anatomic atlas for computed tomography in the mesaticephalic dog: head and neck, *Vet Radiol Ultrasound* 33:217-240, 1992.
19. Lasonsky JH, Abbott LC, Kuriashkin IV: Computed tomography of the normal feline nasal cavity and paranasal sinuses, *Vet Radiol Ultrasound* 38:251-258, 1997.
20. Myer W: Cranial vault and associated structures. In Thrall DE, editor: *Textbook of veterinary diagnostic radiology*, Philadelphia, 1998, WB Saunders, p. 45-59.
21. Kneissl S, Probst S, Konar M: Low-field magnetic resonance imaging of the canine middle and inner ear, *Vet Radiol Ultrasound* 45:520-522, 2004.
22. Schwarz T, Weller R, Dickie AM et al: Imaging of the canine and feline temporomandibular joint: a review, *Vet Radiol Ultrasound* 43:85-97, 2002.
23. O'Brien DP, Axlund TW: Brain disease. In Ettinger SJ, Feldman EC, editors: *Textbook of veterinary internal medicine*, St Louis, 2005, Elsevier Saunders, p. 803-835.
24. Burt JK, Bhargava AK, Prynn RB: Unilateral hydrocephalus with cranial distortion in a cat, *Vet Med Clin North Am (Small Anim Pract)* 65:979-982, 1970.
25. Krum S, Johnson K, Wilson J: Hydrocephalus associated with the noneffusive form of feline infectious peritonitis, *J Am Vet Med Assoc* 167:746-748, 1975.
26. Shell LG: Congenital hydrocephalus, *Feline Pract* 24:10-11, 1996.
27. Hoerlein BF: *Canine neurology*, Philadelphia, 1978, WB Saunders, pp. 560-569.
28. Spaulding KA, Sharp NJH: Ultrasonographic imaging of the lateral cerebral ventricles in the dog, *Vet Radiol* 31:59-64, 1990.
29. Hudson JA, Simpson ST, Buxton DF et al: Ultrasonographic diagnosis of canine hydrocephalus, *Vet Radiol* 31:50-58, 1990.
30. Vite CH, Insko EK, Schotland HM et al: Quantification of cerebral ventricular volume in English bulldogs, *Vet Radiol Ultrasound* 38:437-443, 1997.
31. Vullo T, Korenmann E, Manzo RP et al: Diagnosis of cerebral ventriculomegaly in normal adult beagles using quantitative MRI, *Vet Radiol Ultrasound* 38:277-281, 1997.
32. Kuwamura M, Hattori R, Yamate J et al: Neuronal ceroid-lipofuscinosis and hydrocephalus in a Chihuahua, *J Small Anim Pract* 44:227-230, 2003.
33. Thomas WB: Nonneoplastic disorders of the brain, *Clin Techniques Small Anim Pract* 14:125-147, 1999.
34. Kii S, Uzuka Y, Taura Y et al: Developmental change of lateral ventricular volume and ratio in beagle-type dogs up to 7 months of age, *Vet Radiol Ultrasound* 39:185-189, 1998.
35. De Hann CE, Kraft SL, Gavin PR et al: Normal variation in size of the lateral ventricles of the Labrador

retriever dog as assessed by magnetic resonance imaging, *Vet Radiol Ultrasound* 35:83-86, 1994.
36. Hudson JA, Cartee RE, Simpson ST et al: Ultrasonographic anatomy of the canine brain, *Vet Radiol* 30:13-21, 1989.
37. Hudson JA, Simpson S, Cox NR et al: Ultrasonographic examination of the normal canine neonatal brain, *Vet Radiol* 32:50-59, 1991.
38. Watson AG, de Lahunta A, Evans HE: Dorsal notch of foramen magnum due to incomplete ossification of supraoccipital bone in dogs, *J Small Anim Pract* 30:666-673, 1986.
39. Bardens JW: Congenital malformation of the foramen magnum in dogs, *SW Vet* 18:295, 1965.
40. Kelly JH: Occipital dysplasia and hydrocephalus in a toy poodle, *Vet Med Small Anim Clin* 70:940-941, 1975.
41. Parker AJ, Park RD: Occipital dysplasia in the dog, *J Am Anim Hosp Assoc* 10:520, 1974.
42. Ticer JW: *Radiographic technique in veterinary practice,* Philadelphia, 1984, WB Saunders, p. 256.
43. Watson AG: *The phylogeny and development of the occipito-atlas-axis complex in the dog,* Ithaca, NY, 1981, Cornell University.
44. Wright JA: A study of the radiographic anatomy of the foramen magnum in dogs, *J Small Anim Pract* 20:501-508, 1979.
45. Simoens P, Poels P, Lauwers H: Morphometric analysis of the foramen magnum in Pekingese dogs, *Am J Vet Res* 55:34-39, 1994.
46. Rusbridge C, MacSweeny JE, Davies JV et al: Syringohydromyelia in Cavalier King Charles spaniels, *J Am Anim Hosp Assoc* 36:34-41, 2000.
47. Rusbridge C, Knowler SP: Hereditary aspects of occipital bone hypoplasia and syringomyelia (Chiari type I malformation) in Cavalier King Charles spaniels, *Vet Record* 153:107-112, 2003.
48. Rusbridge C: Neurological diseases of the Cavalier King Charles spaniel, *J Small Anim Pract* 46:265-272, 2005.
49. Rusbridge C, Knowler SP: Inheritance of occipital bone hypoplasia (Chiari type I malformation) in Cavalier King Charles spaniels, *J Vet Intern Med* 18:673-678, 2004.
50. Robbins G, Grandage J: Temporomandibular joint dysplasia and open-mouth jaw locking in the dog, *J Am Vet Med Assoc* 171:1072-1076, 1977.
51. Dickie AM, Schwarz T, Sullivan M: Temporomandibular joint morphology in Cavalier King Charles spaniels, *Vet Radiol Ultrasound* 43:260-266, 2002.
52. Lane JG: Disorders of the canine temporomandibular joint, *Vet Ann* 21:175-186, 1982.
53. Cowell KR, Jezyk PF, Haskins ME et al: Mucopolysaccharidosis in a cat, *J Am Vet Med Assoc* 169:334-339, 1976.
54. Haskins ME, Gustavo DA, Jezyk PF et al: The pathology of the feline model of mucopolysaccharidosis VI, *Am J Pathol* 101:657-674, 1980.
55. Haskins ME, Casal M, Ellinwood NM et al: Animal models for mucopolysaccharidoses and their clinical relevance, *Acta Paediatr Suppl* 91:88-97, 2002.
56. Crawley AC, Muntz FH, Haskins ME et al: Prevalence of mucopolysaccharidosis type VI mutations in Siamese cats, *J Vet Intern Med* 17:495-498, 2003.
57. Konde LJ, Thrall MA, Gasper P et al: Radiographically visualized skeletal changes associated with mucopolysaccharidosis VI in cats, *Vet Radiol* 28:223-228, 1987.
58. Haskins ME, Aguirre GD, Jezk PF et al: The pathology of the feline model of mucopolysaccharidosis I, *Am J Pathol* 112:27-36, 1983.
59. Johnson KA, Watson ADJ: Skeletal diseases. In Ettinger SJ, Feldman EC, editors: *Textbook of veterinary internal medicine,* St Louis, 2005, Elsevier Saunders, pp. 1965-1992.
60. Crawley A, Ramsay SL, Byers S et al: Monitoring dose response of enzyme replacement therapy in feline mucopolysaccharidosis type VI by tandem mass spectrometry, *Ped Research* 55:585-591, 2004.
61. Feldman EC: Disorders of the parathyroid glands. In Ettinger SJ, Feldman EC, editors: *Textbook of veterinary internal medicine,* St Louis, 2005, Elsevier Saunders, pp. 1508-1535.
62. Feldman EC, Hoar B, Pollard R et al: Pretreatment clinical and laboratory findings in dogs with primary hyperparathyroidism: 210 cases (1987-2004), *J Am Vet Med Assoc* 227:756-761, 2005.
63. Brodey RS: Canine and feline neoplasia, *Adv Vet Sci Comp Med* 14:309-354, 1970.
64. Engle GC, Brodey RS: A retrospective study of 395 feline neoplasms, *J Am Anim Hosp Assoc* 5:21-31, 1969.
65. Madewell BR, Priester WA, Gillette EL et al: Neoplasms of the nasal passages and paranasal sinuses in domesticated animals as reported by 13 veterinary colleges, *Am J Vet Res* 37:851-856, 1976.
66. Bright RM, Bojrab MJ: Intranasal neoplasia in the dog and cat, *J Am Anim Hosp Assoc* 12:806, 1976.
67. Cox NR, Brawner WR, Powers RD et al: Tumors of the nose and paranasal sinuses in cats: 32 cases with comparison to a national database (1977-1987), *J Am Anim Hosp Assoc* 27:339-347, 1991.
68. Legendre AM, Krahwinkel DJ, Spaulding KA: Feline nasal and paranasal sinus tumors, *J Am Anim Hosp Assoc* 17:1038-1039, 1981.
69. Allen HS, Broussard J, Noone K: Nasopharyngeal diseases in cats: a retrospective study of 53 cases (1991-1998), *J Am Anim Hosp Assoc* 35:457-461, 1999.
70. Evans SM, Hendrick MJ: Radiotherapy of feline nasal tumors: a retrospective study of nine cases, *Vet Radiol* 30:128-132, 1989.
71. O'Brien RT, Evans SM, Wortman JA et al: Radiographic findings in cats with intranasal neoplasia or chronic rhinitis: 29 cases (1982-1988), *J Am Vet Med Assoc* 208:385-389, 1996.
72. LaDue TA, Dodge R, Page RL et al: Factors influencing survival after radiotherapy of nasal tumors in 130 dogs, *Vet Radiol Ultrasound* 40:312-317, 1999.
73. McEntee MC, Page RL, Heidner GL et al: A retrospective study of 27 dogs with intranasal neoplasms treated with cobalt radiation, *Vet Radiol* 32:135-138, 1991.
74. Adams WM, Withrow SJ, Walshaw R et al: Radiotherapy of malignant nasal tumors in 67 dogs, *J Am Vet Med Assoc* 191:311-315, 1987.
75. Adams WM, Miller PE, Vail DM et al: An accelerated technique for irradiation of malignant canine nasal and paranasal sinus tumors, *Vet Radiol Ultrasound* 39:475-481, 1998.
76. Harvey CE, Biery DN, Morello J et al: Chronic nasal disease in the dog: its radiographic diagnosis, *Vet Radiol* 20:91-98, 1979.
77. Russo M, Lamb MA, Jakovljevic S: Distinguishing rhinitis and nasal neoplasia by radiography, *Vet Radiol and Ultrasound* 41:2118-2124, 2000.
78. Morgan JP, Suter PF, O'Brien TR et al: Tumors in the nasal cavity of the dog: a radiographic study, *J Am Vet Radiol Soc* 13:18-26, 1972.
79. Morris JS, Dunn KJ, Dobson JM et al: Radiological assessment of severity of canine nasal tumours and relationship with survival, *J Small Anim Pract* 37:1-6, 1996.

80. Schwarz T, Sullivan M, Hartung K: Radiographic anatomy of the cribriform plate (lamina cribrosa), *Vet Radiol Ultrasound* 41:220-225, 2000.
81. Kirberger RM, Fourie SL: An investigation into the usefulness of a rostrocaudal nasal radiographic view in the dog, *J S Afr Vet Assoc* 73:171-176, 2002.
82. Morgan JP, Silverman S: *Techniques of veterinary radiography,* ed 4, Davis, CA, 1984, Veterinary Radiology Associates, pp. 169-174.
83. Frew DG, Dobson JM: Radiological assessment of 50 cases of incisive or maxillary neoplasia in the dog, *J Small Anim Pract* 33:11-18, 1992.
84. Schwarz T, Sullivan M, Hartung K: Radiographic detection of defects of the nasal boundaries, *Vet Radiol Ultrasound* 41:226-230, 2000.
85. Burk RL: Computed tomographic imaging of nasal disease in 100 dogs, *Vet Radiol Ultrasound* 33:177-180, 1992.
86. Saunders JH, Zonderland J-L, Clercx C et al: Computed tomographic findings in 35 dogs with nasal aspergillosis, *Vet Radiol Ultrasound* 43:5-9, 2002.
87. Hoyt RF, Withrow SJ: Oral malignancy in the dog, *J Am Anim Hosp Assoc* 20:83-92, 1984.
88. Stebbins KE, Morse CC, Goldschmidt MH: Feline oral neoplasia: a ten-year survey, *Vet Pathol* 26:121-128, 1989.
89. Dubielzig RR: Proliferative dental and gingival diseases of dogs and cats, *J Am Anim Hosp Assoc* 18:577-584, 1982.
90. Colgin LM, Schulman FY, Dubielzig RR: Multiple epulides in 13 cats, *Vet Pathol* 38:227-229, 2001.
91. Withrow SJ: Cancer of the gastrointestinal system: cancer of the oral cavity. In MacEwen EG, Withrow SJ, editors: *Small animal clinical oncology,* Philadelphia, 2001, WB Saunders, pp. 305-318.
92. Ciekot PA, Powers BE, Withrow SJ et al: Histologically low-grade, yet biologically high-grade, fibrosarcomas of the mandible and maxilla in dogs: 25 cases (1982-1991), *J Am Vet Med Assoc* 204:610-615, 1994.
93. Forrest LJ, Chun R, Adams WM et al: Postoperative radiotherapy for canine soft tissue sarcoma, *J Vet Intern Med* 14:578-582, 2000.
94. Bertone ER, Snyder LA, Moore AS: Environmental and lifestyle risk factors for oral squamous cell carcinoma in domestic cats, *J Vet Intern Med* 17:557-562, 2003.
95. Dubielzig RR, Goldschmidt MH, Brodey RS: The nomenclature of periodontal epulides in dogs, *Vet Pathol* 16:209-214, 1979.
96. Langham RF, Mostosky UV, Schirmer RG: X-ray therapy of selected odontogenic neoplasms in the dog, *J Am Vet Med Assoc* 170:820-822, 1977.
97. Thrall DE: Orthovoltage radiotherapy of acanthomatous epulides in 39 dogs, *J Am Vet Med Assoc* 184:826-829, 1984.
98. McEntee MC, Page RL, Theon A et al: Malignant tumor formation in dogs previously irradiated for acanthomatous epulis, *Vet Radiol Ultrasound* 45:357-361, 2004.
99. Dubielzig RR, Adams WM, Brodey RS: Inductive fibroameloblastoma, an unusual dental tumor of young cats, *J Am Vet Med Assoc* 174:720-722, 1979.
100. White RAS: Mandibulectomy and maxillectomy in the dog: long term survival in 100 cases, *J Small Anim Pract* 32:69-74, 1991.
101. Bateman KE, Catton PA, Pennock PW et al: 0-7-21 Radiation therapy for the treatment of canine oral melanoma, *J Vet Intern Med* 8:267-272, 1994.
102. Blackwood L, Dobson JM: Radiotherapy of oral malignant melanomas in dogs, *J Am Vet Med Assoc* 209:98-102, 1996.
103. Klein MK: Multimodality therapy for head and neck cancer, *Vet Clin North Am Small Anim Pract* 33:615-628, 2003.
104. Pletcher JM, Koch SA, Stedhem MA: Orbital chondroma rodens in a dog, *J Am Vet Med Assoc* 175:187-190, 1979.
105. Dernell WS, Straw RC, Cooper MF et al: Multilobular osteochondrosarcoma in 39 dogs: 1979-1993, *J Am Anim Hosp Assoc* 34:11-18, 1998.
106. Zaki FA, Liu S-K, Kay WJ: Calcifying aponeurotic fibroma in a dog, *J Am Vet Med Assoc* 166:384-387, 1975.
107. Selcer BA, McCracken MD: Chondroma rodens in dogs: a report of two case histories and a review of the veterinary literature, *J Vet Orthop* 2:7-11, 1981.
108. McLain DL, Hill JR, Pulley LT: Multilobular osteoma and chondroma (chondroma rodens) with pulmonary metastasis in a dog, *J Am Anim Hosp Assoc* 19:359-362, 1983.
109. Groff JM, Murphy CJ, Pool RR et al: Orbital multilobular tumour of bone in a dog, *J Small Anim Pract* 33:597-600, 1992.
110. McCalla TL, Moore CP, Turk J et al: Multilobular osteosarcoma of mandible and orbit in a dog, *Vet Pathol* 26:92-94, 1989.
111. Straw RC, LeCouter RA, Powers BE et al: Multilobular osteochondrosarcoma of the canine skull: 16 cases (1978-1988), *J Am Vet Med Assoc* 195:1764-1769, 1989.
112. Hathcock JT, Newton JC: Multilobular tumor of bone involving the cranium in 7 dogs and zygomatic arch in 2 dogs, *Vet Radiol Ultrasound* 41:214-217, 2000.
113. Lipsitz D, Levitski RE, Berry WL: Magnetic resonance imaging features of multilobular osteochondrosarcoma in 3 dogs, *Vet Radiol Ultrasound* 42:14-19, 2001.
114. Hardy WD, Brodey RS, Riser WH: Osteosarcoma of the canine skull, *J Am Vet Radiol Soc* 8:5-16, 1967.
115. LeCouteur RA: Current concepts in the diagnosis and treatment of brain tumours in dogs and cats, *J Small Anim Pract* 40:411-416, 1999.
116. Polizopoulou ZS, Koutinas AF, Souftas VD et al: Diagnostic correlation of CT-MRI and histopathology in 10 dogs with brain neoplasms, *J Vet Med* 51:226-231, 2004.
117. Kraft SL, Gavin PR: Intracranial neoplasia, *Clin Techniques Small Anim Pract* 14:112-123, 1999.
118. Lawson C, Burk RL, Prata RG: Cerebral meningioma in the cat: diagnosis and surgical treatment of 10 cases, *J Am Anim Hosp Assoc* 20:333-342, 1984.
119. Sharp NJH, Harvey CE, Sullivan M: Canine nasal aspergillosis and penicilliosis, *Comp Contin Ed Pract Vet* 13:41-48, 1991.
120. Sullivan M, Lee R, Jakovlijevic S et al: The radiological features of aspergillosis of the nasal cavity and frontal sinuses in the dog, *J Small Anim Pract* 27:167-180, 1986.
121. Harvey CE, O'Brien JA, Felsburg PJ et al: Nasal penicilliosis in six dogs, *J Am Vet Med Assoc* 178:1084-1087, 1981.
122. Gibbs C, Lane JG, Denny HR: Radiological features of intra-nasal lesions in the dog: a review of 100 cases, *J Small Anim Pract* 20:515-535, 1979.
123. Malik R, Martin P, Wigne DI et al: Nasopharyngeal cryptococcosis, *Aust Vet* 75:483-488, 1997.
124. Wilkinson GT: Feline cryptococcosis: a review and seven case reports, *J Small Anim Pract* 20:749-768, 1979.
125. Hawkins EC: Chronic viral upper respiratory disease in cats: differential diagnosis and management, *Comp Contin Ed Pract Vet* 10:1003-1012, 1988.
126. Burgener DC, Slocombe RF, Zerbe CA: Lymphoplasmacytic rhinitis in five dogs, *J Am Anim Hosp Assoc* 23:565-568, 1986.

127. Tasker S, Knottenbelt CM, Munro EAC et al: Aetiology and diagnosis of persistent nasal disease in the dog: a retrospective study of 42 cases, *J Small Anim Pract* 40:473-478, 1999.
128. Gartrell CL, O'Handley PA, Perry RL: Canine nasal disease: part II, *Comp Contin Ed Pract Vet* 17:539-546, 1995.
129. Gibbs C: The head—part III: ear disease, *J Small Anim Pract* 19:539-545, 1978.
130. Hoskinson JJ: Imaging techniques in the diagnosis of middle ear disease, *Sem Vet Med Surg* 8:10-16, 1993.
131. Hofer P, Meisen N, Bartoldi S et al: Radiology corner: a new radiographic view of the feline tympanic bullae, *Vet Radiol Ultrasound* 36:14-15, 1995.
132. Bischoff MG, Kneller SK: Diagnostic imaging of the canine and feline ear, *Vet Clin Small Anim Pract* 34:437-458, 2004.
133. Garosi LS, Dennis R, Schwarz T: Review of diagnostic imaging of ear diseases in the dog and cat, *Vet Radiol Ultrasound* 44:137-146, 2003.
134. Remedios AM, Fowler JD, Pharr JW: A comparison of radiographic versus surgical diagnosis of otitis media, *J Am Anim Hosp Assoc* 27:183, 1991.
135. Love NE, Kramer RW, Spodnick GJ et al: Radiographic and computed tomographic evaluation of otitis media in the dog, *Vet Radiol Ultrasound* 36:375-379, 1995.
136. Barthez PY, Koblik PD, Hornof WJ et al: Apparent wall thickening in fluid filled versus air filled tympanic bulla in computed tomography, *Vet Radiol Ultrasound* 37:95-98, 1996.
137. Owen MC, Lamb CR, Lu D et al: Material in the middle ear of dogs having magnetic resonance imaging for investigation of neurologic signs, *Vet Radiol Ultrasound* 45:149-155, 2004.
138. Stanton MLE: Feline nasopharyngeal and middle ear polyps. In Bojrab MJ, editor: *Disease mechanisms in small animal surgery,* Philadelphia, 1993, Lea and Febiger, pp. 128-129.
139. Kapatkin AS, Matthiesen DT, Noone KE et al: Results of surgery and long-term follow-up in 31 cats with nasopharyngeal polyps, *J Am Anim Hosp Assoc* 26:387-392, 1990.
140. Seitz SE, Lasonsky JM, Marretta SM: Computed tomographic appearance of inflammatory polyps in three cats, *Vet Radiol Ultrasound* 37:99-104, 1996.
141. Kudnig ST: Nasopharyngeal polyps in cats, *Clin Techniques Small Anim Pract* 14:174-177, 2002.
142. London CA, Dubilzeig RR, Vail DM et al: Evaluation of dogs and cats with tumors of the ear canal: 145 cases (1978-1992), *J Am Vet Med Assoc* 208:1413-1418, 1996.
143. Ticer JW, Spencer CP: Injury of the feline temporomandibular joint: radiographic signs, *J Am Vet Radiol Soc* 19:146-156, 1978.
144. Dickie AM, Sullivan M: The effect of obliquity on the radiographic appearance of the temporomandibular joint in dogs, *Vet Radiol Ultrasound* 42:205-217, 2001.
145. Huchkowsky SL: Craniomandibular osteopathy in a bullmastiff, *Can Vet J* 43:883-885, 2002.
146. Padgett GA, Mostosky UV: The mode of inheritance of craniomandibular osteopathy in West Highland White terrier dogs, *Am J Med Genet* 25:9-13, 1986.
147. Riser WH, Parkes LJ, Shirer JF: Canine craniomandibular osteopathy, *J Am Vet Radiol Soc* 8:23-31, 1967.
148. Roudebush P, Logan E, Hale FA: Evidence-based veterinary dentistry: a systematic review of homecare for prevention of periodontal disease in dogs and cats, *J Vet Dent* 22:6-15, 2005.
149. Harvey CE: Management of periodontal disease: understanding the options, *Vet Clin North Am Small Anim Pract* 35:819-836, 2005.
150. Grove TK: Periodontal disease. In Harvey CE, editor: *Veterinary dentistry,* Philadelphia, 1985, WB Saunders, pp. 59-77.

ELECTRONIC RESOURCES evolve

Additional information related to the content in Chapter 8 can be found on the companion Web site at evolve http://evolve.elsevier.com/Thrall/vetrad/

- Key Points
- Chapter Quiz
- Case Study 8-1

CHAPTER 9
Magnetic Resonance Imaging Features of Brain Disease in Small Animals

Ian D. Robertson

Magnetic Resonance (MR) imaging is the imaging modality of choice for evaluation of brain morphology. The superior soft tissue contrast resolution afforded by MR imaging and the lack of bone-hardening artifacts commonly seen with computed tomography (CT), particularly in the caudal fossa, make it a superior modality when imaging almost all aspects of intracranial disease. This chapter presents a basic overview of the most common intracranial disorders amenable to MR imaging.

High-field magnets of 1.5 T (so-called superconducting magnets) are usually able to generate thin-slice tomographic images of the brain at higher resolution and in a shorter time than low-field (0.3 T) permanent magnets. However, high-field magnets are expensive and have significant ongoing maintenance costs compared with low-field permanent magnets. Both magnet types are becoming more available to the pet-owning community, particularly in larger cities. As magnet and computer technology continues to improve, veterinary systems will become more affordable and accessible.

BASIC MAGNETIC RESONANCE EXAMINATION OF THE BRAIN

A standard MR examination of a canine or feline brain usually involves multiple sequences designed to optimize signal from a particular tissue type or obtain images in various anatomic planes. Images are usually acquired in the transverse plane (typically at right angles to the hard palate), sagittal plane, and dorsal plane (parallel to the base of the brain) (Fig. 9-1).

Tissues emitting a high signal in a pulse sequence appear white in an MR image. This is often referred to as being "bright." Bright lesions or tissues can also be described as being hyperintense or as having T2-weighted (or T1-weighted, or whatever sequence is being viewed) hyperintensity. Tissues not emitting a high signal in a pulse sequence appear dark; these dark tissues may be described as dark, hypointense, or as having T2-weighted (or T1-weighted, or whatever sequence is being viewed) hypointensity.

Conventional fast (turbo) spin-echo T2-weighted sequences are useful for detecting regions of increased fluid within tissues. In T2-weighted sequences, free fluid (e.g., cerebrospinal spinal fluid) is extremely bright. Most common pathologic processes, whether neoplastic or inflammatory, result in increased fluid within tissues. This is manifest as an increase in brightness of the abnormal tissue relative to the surrounding tissue; the term "increased T2-weighted signal intensity" is commonly used to describe this effect.

Sometimes it is difficult to identify lesions resulting in an increase in T2 signal intensity when the lesion is adjacent to normal regions of high signal, such as adjacent to cerebrospinal fluid (CSF) within the ventricles. An inversion pulse can be added the basic sequence, which causes free fluid to be "nulled out," causing it to be dark on a T2-weighted sequence. This sequence, known as a fluid attenuation inversion recovery (FLAIR) sequence, makes CSF and other true fluids dark.[1] This may make the detection of subtle lesions adjacent to regions of fluid accumulation, such as the ventricles and brain periphery, easier. A FLAIR sequence may also provide additional information about T2 hyperintense lesions that must be distinguished from CSF, such as cystic meningioma, dermoid and epidermoid cysts, and arachnoid cysts (Fig. 9-2).[2]

T1-weighted sequences accentuate the T1 recovery characteristics of tissue and are quicker to acquire than T2-weighted sequences. In a T1 sequence protocol, fluid and overhydrated lesions have reduced signal intensity, appearing dark. A T1-weighted sequence is excellent for evaluation of anatomy, but on its own it is poor in allowing detection of lesions. However, regions of disruption to the blood-brain barrier and regions of altered perfusion can often be differentiated on T1-weighted images made after the administration of an MR imaging contrast medium. The most common MR contrast medium is a chelated form of gadolinium, a transitional compound with paramagnetic properties that shortens the T1 relaxation time of tissue in which the material accumulates.[3] In regions of higher gadolinium concentration, signal will therefore be increased in T1-weighted images.

Many pathologic processes in the brain result in some disruption to the blood-brain barrier, often resulting in an accumulation of contrast medium and thereby increased signal intensity (brightness on T1 images after contrast medium sequences). After gadolinium administration, T1-weighted images are usually acquired in the transverse, dorsal, and sagittal planes. Contrast medium is usually administered after all other imaging sequences have been acquired because the presence of contrast medium can sometimes affect the appearance of images from other sequences. In addition to the sequences mentioned above, a T2-weighted sagittal sequence should be performed. This sequence allows better evaluation of the anatomy of the cerebellum and brainstem and is important in the assessment of increased intracranial pressure (Fig. 9-3).[4]

Putting It All Together

By using a selection of pulse sequences, the different imaging characteristics of a disease process can be characterized. By evaluating the imaging characteristics of the lesion(s) on the various sequences, a more accurate assessment of the underlying cause can be established than in CT images, for example, in which the image appearance is based solely on the x-ray attenuation characteristics of the tissue. In MR imaging, chemical characteristics of the tissue determine the signal intensity.

The T2-weighted image in Figure 9-4, *A*, contains a region of abnormally high signal in the right temporal lobe, extending into the white matter lateral to the right lateral ventricle. In Figure 9-4, *B*, a T1-weighted image made after the administration of contrast medium, the same level is characterized

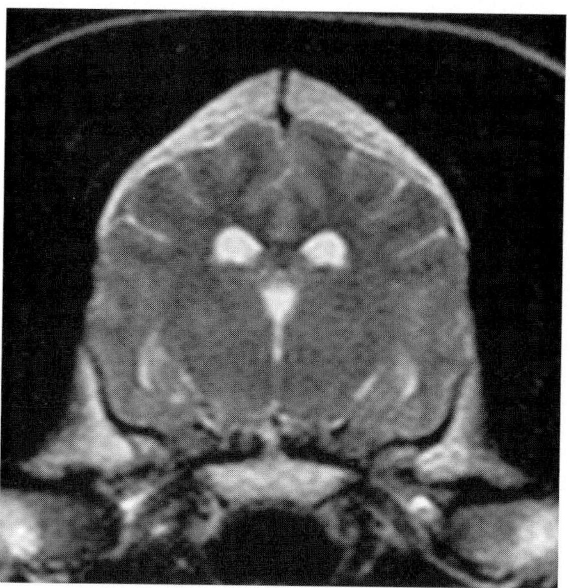

Fig. 9-1 A transverse T2-weighted image of a normal canine brain at the level of the ventricles. True fluid (CSF within the ventricles) is bright in this sequence.

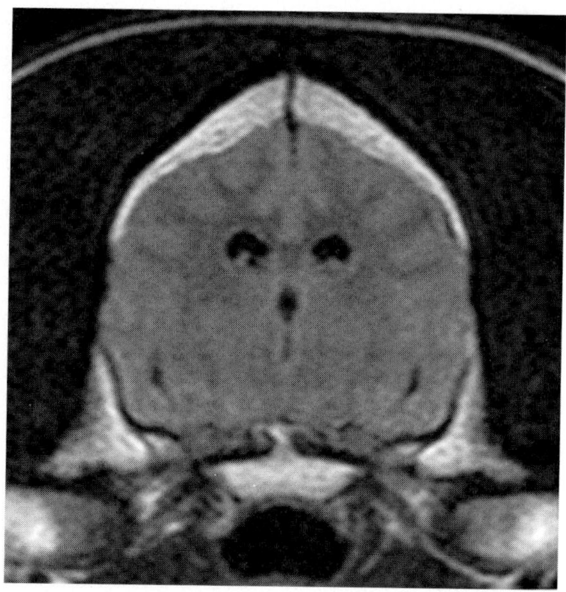

Fig. 9-2 A transverse FLAIR image at the same level, and in the same normal brain, as in Figure 9-1. In this sequence, CSF and other true fluids appear dark, but the image maintains a T2 weighting. This often allows easier visualization of lesions adjacent to regions of fluid accumulation, such as the ventricles and brain periphery.

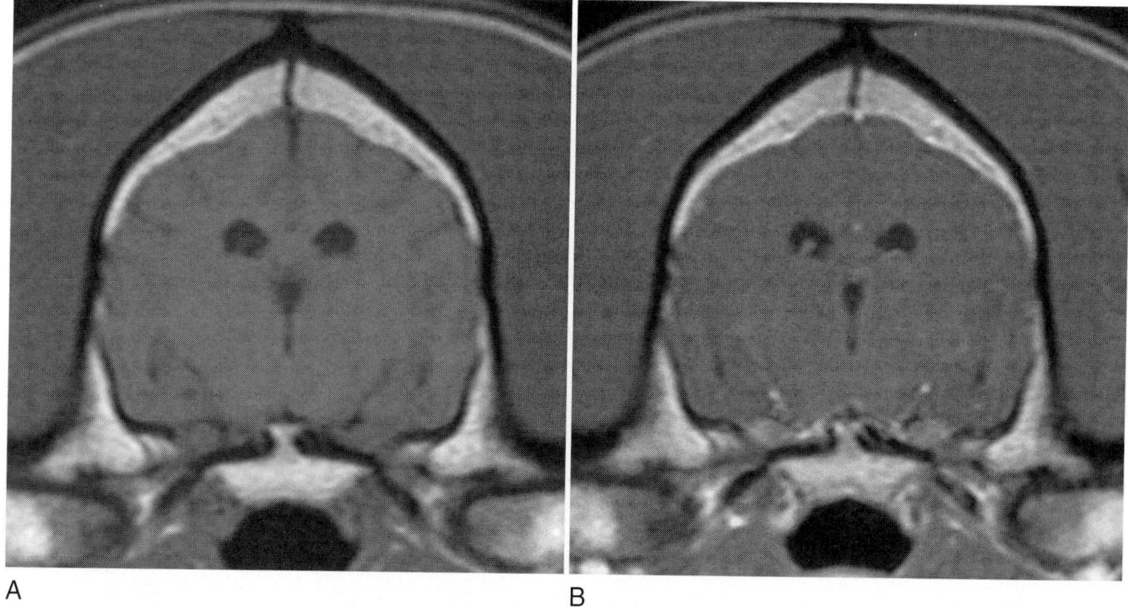

Fig. 9-3 **A,** T1-weighted image in the same normal brain, and at the same level, as Figures 9-1 and 9-2. In this sequence, true fluid and overhydrated tissue are dark. **B,** The same imaging parameters were used as in **A,** but the sequence was acquired after intravenous administration of gadolinium, an MR contrast medium. MR contrast media are paramagnetic and result in an increase in signal intensity (brightness) on T1-weighted images. The bright regions in the lateral ventricles represent normal enhancement of the choroid plexus, and the linear opacities in the brain represent normal enhancing vascular structures.

by a peripherally enhancing mass with a T1 hypointense center within the ventrolateral aspect of the right temporal lobe. The bright ring was not apparent on T1-weighted images made before the administration of contrast medium. The center of the mass does not enhance, indicating a lack of blood supply to deliver the contrast medium. Additionally, the tissue adjacent to the mass does not enhance. The most likely explanation for the imaging characteristics is that the center of the mass is devoid of blood supply and the high T2 signal in the adjacent white matter is edema caused by the presence of the mass. This patient could be expected to have a marked, albeit transient, improvement in neurologic status if the peripheral edema can be resolved with medial management.

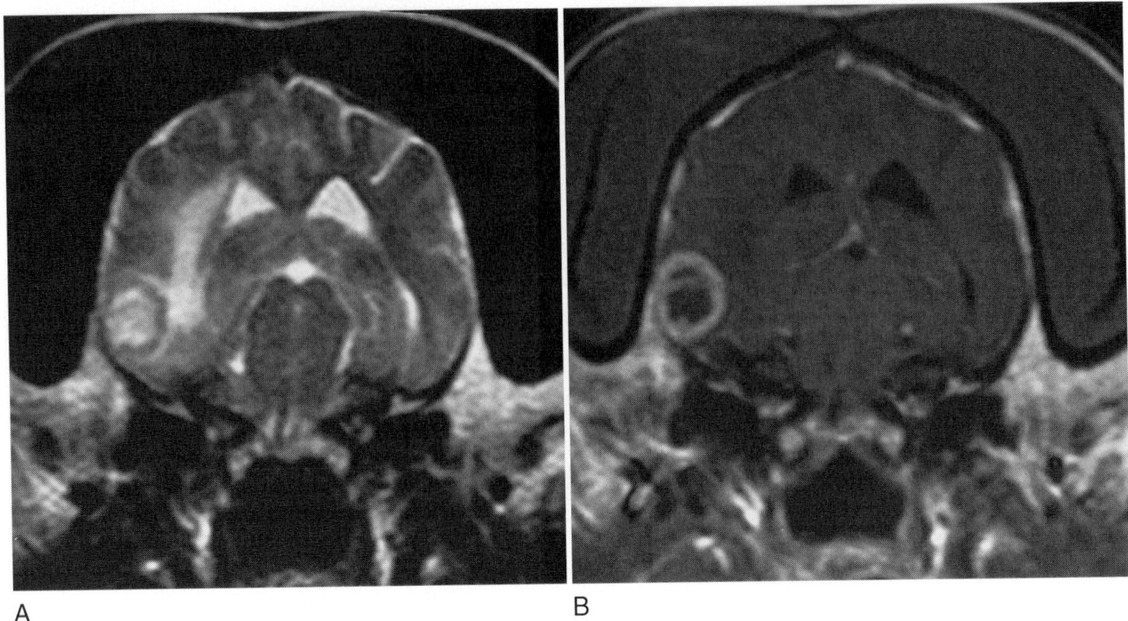

Fig. 9-4 A, T2-weighted image. A focal T2 hyperintense mass is present with a hypointense border surrounded by adjacent wispy regions of high signal consistent with white matter edema. B, T1-weighted image acquired after contrast medium administration. A mass with marked ring enhancement is present in the right temporal lobe. A shift of midline structures to the left is visible (contralateral or paradoxical shift) as a result of the mass and associated peripheral edema. The center of the mass does not enhance. Final diagnosis was a hemangiosarcoma brain metastasis.

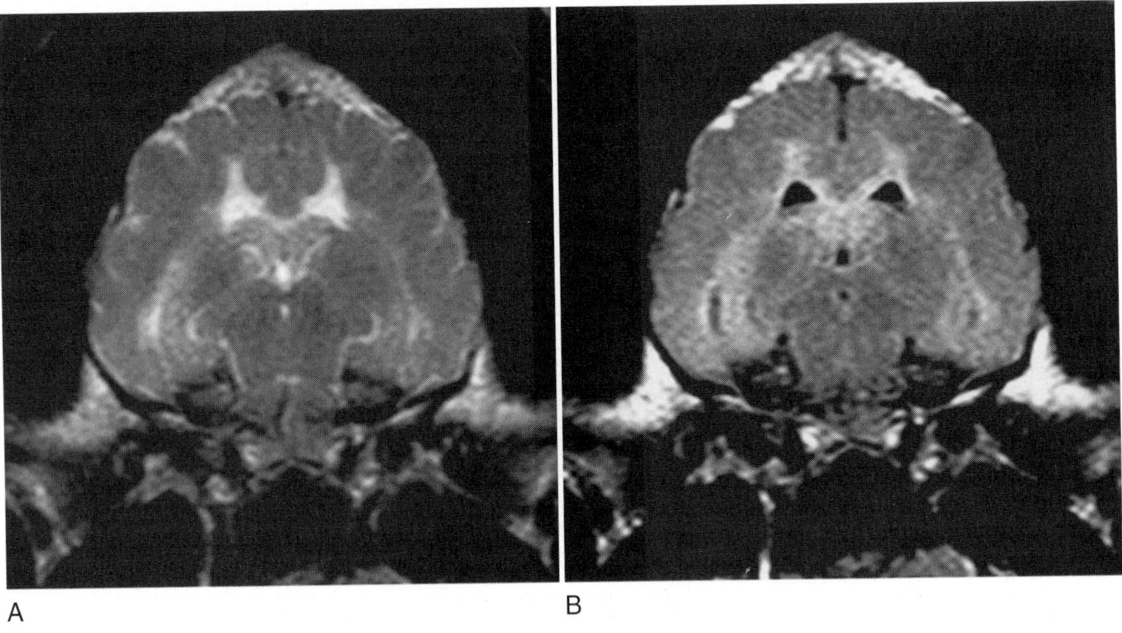

Fig. 9-5 Comparison of T2 (A) and FLAIR (B) images for periventricular lesions in a dog with leukoencephalitis. The increased T2 signal intensity within the white matter adjacent to the ventricles has increased conspicuity on the FLAIR sequence compared with the T2-weighted sequence as a result of removal (nulling) of the high signal from the CSF.

In another example, whether the signal coming from the brain is caused by normal fluid, such as CSF, or concurrent brain edema sometimes cannot be determined. In Figure 9-5, *A*, a large amount of high signal seems to be present, but perhaps this is simply caused by the characteristics of the ventricular system. In the FLAIR sequence in Figure 9-5, *B*, however, the signal from CSF has been removed and considerable high signal remains in the region adjacent to the ventricular system. It can be concluded with high accuracy that an abnormal amount of fluid is present in the neuropil.

Secondary Effects of Focal Intracranial Disease

In addition to altering local signal intensity, brain masses can also cause major changes to brain morphologic characteristics depending on their location and size. Many masses and associated peripheral edema result in brain compression, with a contralateral shift of midline structures, obstruction of the ventricular system, and ultimately brain herniation. These secondary signs should not be overlooked, particularly brain herniation (Fig. 9-6).

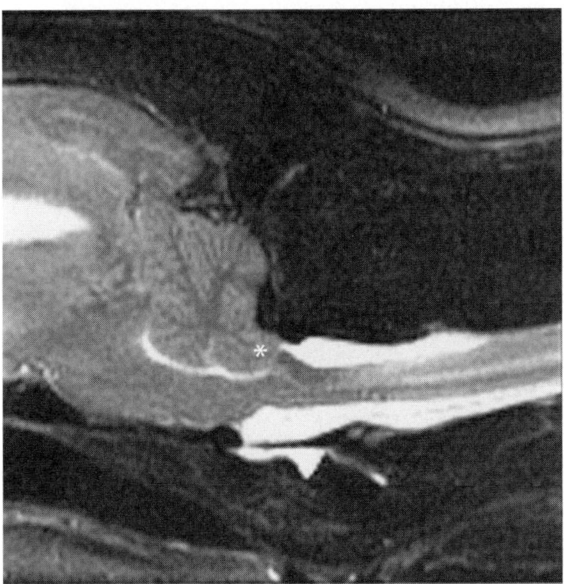

Fig. 9-6 Sagittal T2-weighted image of the caudal fossa and cranial portion of the cervical spinal cord of a dog with a large forebrain mass. Marked compression of the cerebellum and herniation of the cerebellar vermis *(asterisk)* into the cervical vertebral canal are visible as a result of pressure from the intracranial mass. The wispy T2 hyperintensity in the spinal cord is syringohydromyelia, likely a result of altered CSF flow dynamics as a result of brainstem compression. The cranial aspect of the spinal cord is bounded dorsally and ventrally by the highly conspicuous subarachnoid space.

COMMON INTRACRANIAL CONDITIONS IN SMALL ANIMALS AND THEIR MAGNETIC RESONANCE IMAGING CHARACTERISTICS

Developmental Conditions of the Brain

Hydrocephalus

A complete review of all the developmental disorders of the brain that can be documented by MR imaging is beyond the scope of this chapter; only hydrocephalus, the most common developmental anomaly, is discussed. Hydrocephalus is the excessive accumulation of CSF within the ventricular system that occurs when normal flow is obstructed, preventing fluid from being absorbed, or a disparity between fluid production and absorption exists. The most common form of hydrocephalus is congenital hydrocephalus. In congenital hydrocephalus, the excess fluid accumulates before or soon after birth. An inherited malformation of the fluid pathway may be present, or infection or injury around the time of birth leads to scarring that affects CSF reabsorption. Less commonly, hydrocephalus occurs in adult patients, usually the result of tumor or infection, which obstructs CSF flow as a result of compression or inflammation (Fig. 9-7).

Hydrocephalus is readily apparent as an increase in size of the ventricular system. The lateral ventricles are usually relatively symmetrical, but considerable variation exists in what is considered "normal" ventricular size, particularly in small-breed dogs.[5]

Inflammatory Conditions of the Brain

Inflammatory conditions of the brain can often be detected by MR imaging. Most commonly an analysis of CSF, including cytology and immunologic testing, is required to help establish a definitive diagnosis. In some patients with meningitis, increased enhancement of the meninges occurs after contrast medium administration (Fig. 9-8).[6] This is best detected when comparing T1-weighted images acquired before and after contrast medium administration. Some clinicians, in the interest of time, may bypass the precontrast study, which complicates the objective assessment of meningeal enhancement.

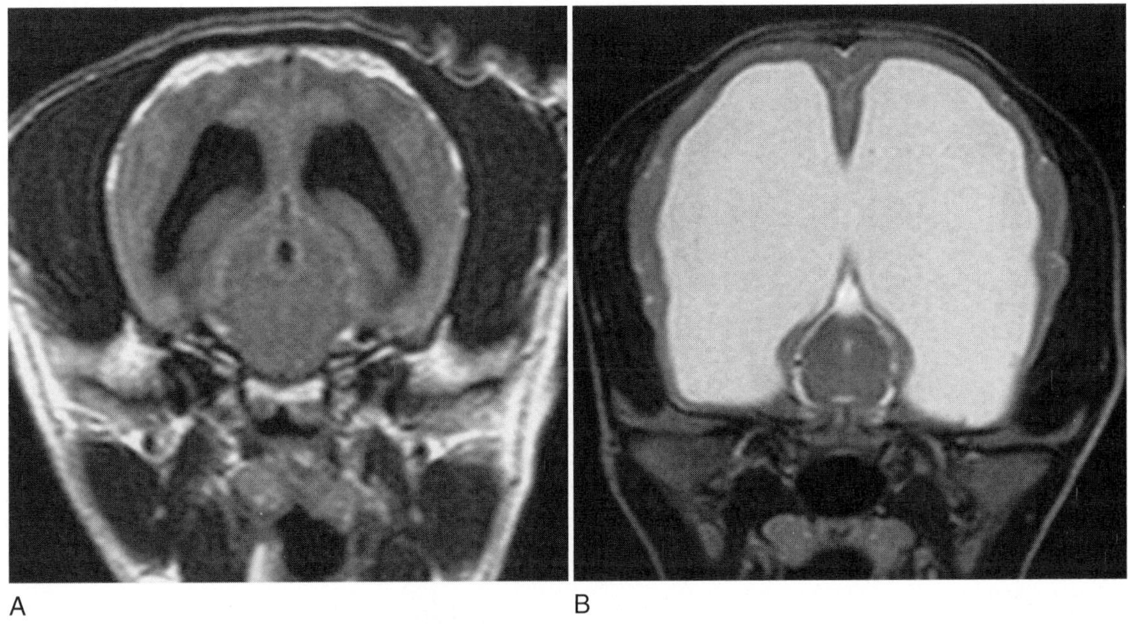

Fig. 9-7 Transverse FLAIR (A) and T2-weighted (B) images from two dogs with congenital hydrocephalus. Note the varying degree of ventricular enlargement.

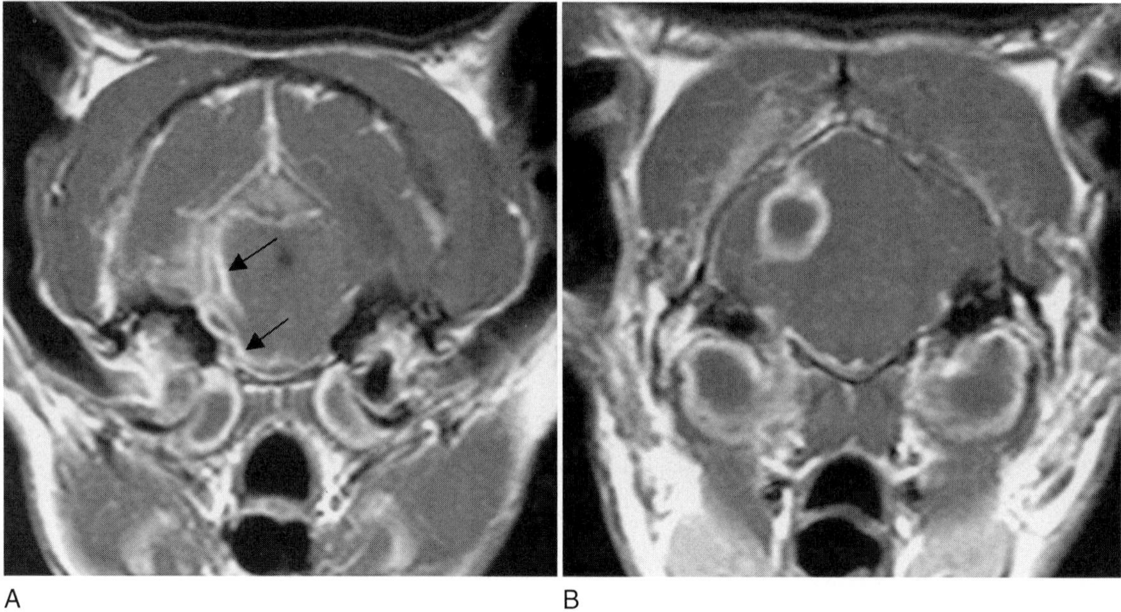

Fig. 9-8 Adjacent transverse plane T1-weighted postcontrast images in a 5-year-old cat with a head tilt and otitis externa. Increased signal intensity in both tympanic bullae is visible. The lining of the bullae is enhanced, but material within either bulla does not enhance. This is consistent with inflammation (exudate in bullae). The meninges and brain parenchyma adjacent to the right tympanic bulla are markedly enhanced (*arrows* in **A**), and a ring-enhancing mass is present in the right aspect of the cerebellum. The imaging findings are attributable to aggressive otitis media/interna that has progressed to meningoencephalitis and cerebellar abscess.

Encephalitis is sometimes characterized by a patchy increase in parenchymal T2 signal intensity, often more apparent on a FLAIR sequence. These regions are usually isointense or hypointense on T1-weighted images and have variably increased signal intensity on T1-weighted images made after contrast medium administration. Granulomatous meningoencephalitis (GME) can appear as ill-defined focal regions of T2 hyperintensity with minimal or variable patchy enhancement after contrast medium administration (Fig. 9-9). Some GME lesions have minimal parenchymal enhancement after contrast medium administration and as a result can appear similar to infarcts.

Intracranial feline infectious peritonitis usually causes an ependymitis, resulting in an increase in T2 signal intensity (often best appreciated on the FLAIR sequence) and an increase in T1 signal intensity in the lining of the ventricular system after contrast medium administration (Fig. 9-10).

Many inflammatory conditions of the brain have abnormal findings on a standard MR examination. Parasitic migration tracts and parenchymal and subdural abscess have all been reported (see Fig. 9-8). The necrotizing encephalitides (Yorkshire Terrier and Pug) are characterized by minimal contrast enhancement, and regions of brain necrosis may be present, sometimes manifesting as compensatory hydrocephalus depending on the maturity of the lesion (Fig. 9-11). These lesions often have no or minimal mass effect. Normal MR images do not rule out the possibility of inflammatory disease, and a CSF tap is required to assist in establishing the diagnosis. In one study of 25 patients with CSF alterations consistent with inflammatory brain disease, 24% of the MR studies were considered normal.[6]

BRAIN NEOPLASIA

Extraaxial Tumors

Meningiomas are extraaxial tumors (meaning outside the brain parenchyma) that arise from dural elements within the calvarium. They are the most commonly reported brain tumors in cats and one of the most common intracranial tumors in dogs. Meningiomas in dogs and cats are usually benign and tend to grow slowly under the dura mater. They are variable in size and shape and may be irregular, nodular, ovoid, lobulated, or plaquelike, ranging from a few millimeters to several centimeters in diameter. Meningiomas are often firm and encapsulated, usually discrete, and may contain mineralization. A significant number of basal and plaquelike meningiomas occur in the floor of the cranial cavity, especially in the optic chiasm and suprasellar region. They also commonly occur over the cerebral hemispheres, less commonly in the cerebello-pontomedullary region, and rarely in the retrobulbar space, arising from the optic nerve. The presence of multiple meningiomas is not uncommon in cats. Thickening of bone adjacent to meningiomas, termed hyperostosis, may occur, especially in cats (Fig. 9-12). Meningiomas can usually be distinguished from tumors within the brain parenchyma (intraaxial) because they are usually broad based, peripherally located, or falx-associated masses that homogeneously enhance after contrast medium administration (Fig. 9-13). Meningiomas are often associated with a "dural tail," a linear enhancement of thickened dura mater adjacent to an extraaxial mass seen on contrast medium–enhanced, T1-weighted images. In one study the predictive value of the dural tail sign for meningioma was 94%.[4] Whether the dural tail represents neoplastic infiltration beyond the margins of the meningioma or a manifestation of associated inflammation is uncertain. The amount of adjacent parenchymal enhancement and disruption to normal parenchymal symmetry caused by meningiomas is variable. Some tumors have minimal peripheral edema, whereas others may have extensive peripheral edema and an associated "mass" effect.

Choroid Plexus Papillomas and Ependymomas

Choroid plexus papillomas are common in dogs, occurring in almost all components of the intracranial ventricular system but most commonly in the third ventricle and the lateral

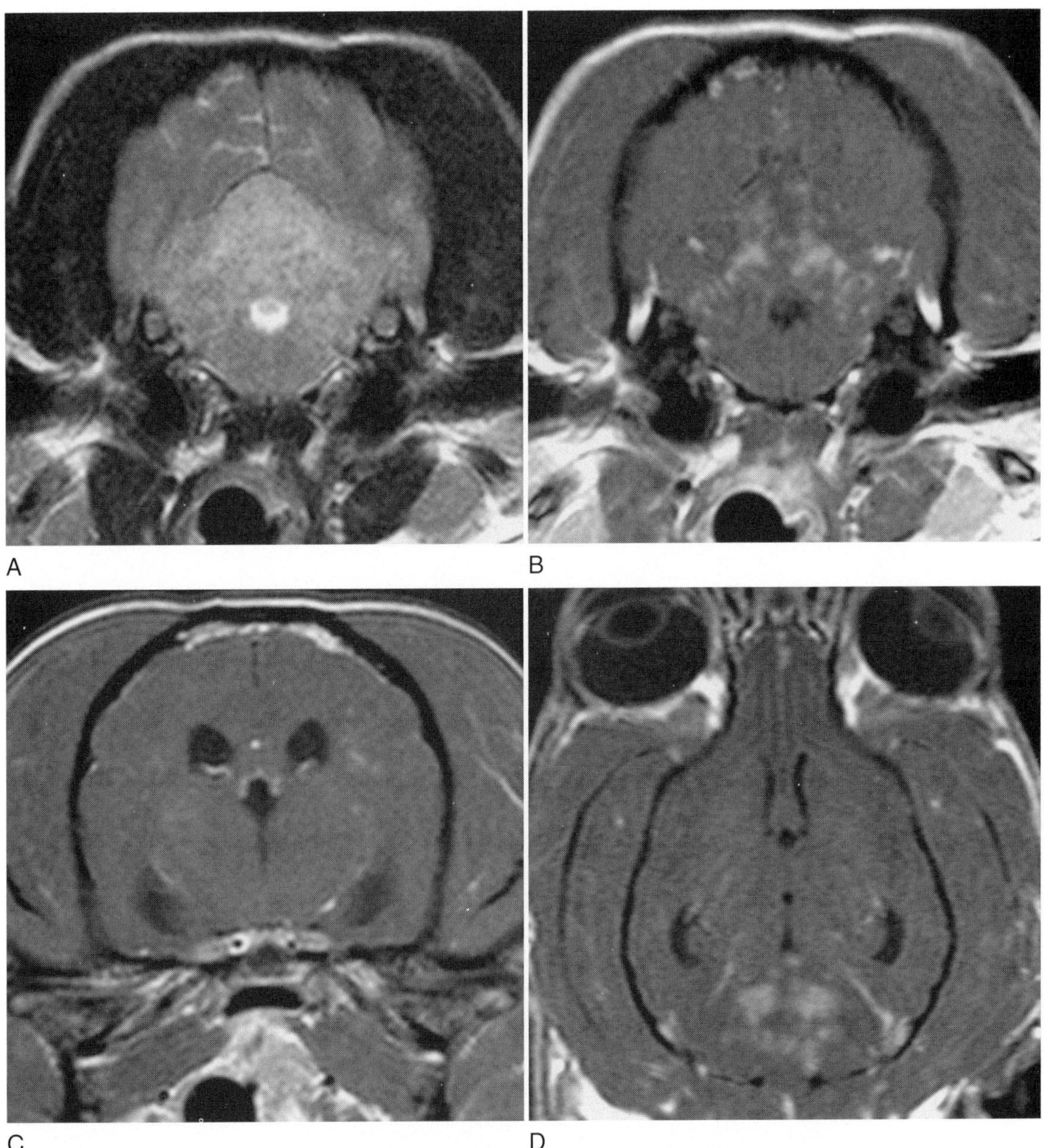

Fig. 9-9 A T2-weighted transverse image (**A**) at the level of the cerebellum and T1-weighted postcontrast transverse image (**B**) made at the same level as **A**. **C** and **D** are transverse and dorsal plane T1-weighted postcontrast images, respectively. This is a 9-year-old Miniature Poodle with confirmed GME presenting with progressive tetraparesis and truncal ataxia. An ill-defined region of T2 hyperintensity is visible within the central aspect of the cerebellum. After contrast medium administration, multiple patchy regions of contrast enhancement are visible within the cerebellum, as are additional multifocal regions of contrast enhancement, primarily within the corona radiata. The MR findings with GME are variable, and some lesions have minimal enhancement after contrast medium administration.

recess of the fourth ventricle. The choroid plexus epithelium originates from differentiation of the primitive medullary epithelium and is embryologically related to ependymal cells. Choroid plexus papillomas have a tendency to bleed, and exfoliation of choroid plexus papilloma cells (benign and malignant variants) may occur with subsequent tumor seeding to other areas of the brain or spinal cord by way of the CSF. Obstructive hydrocephalus may be life threatening if the primary or any disseminated tumor causes CSF obstruction. An important distinguishing feature of choroid plexus tumors in MR images is that they are located within a ventricle (Fig. 9-14). Like meningiomas, these tumors usually have marked contrast enhancement after gadolinium administration and sometimes have evidence of hemorrhage and dystrophic mineralization.[7] The MR characteristics of central ependymomas are probably similar to choroid plexus papillomas, but ependymomas are much less common.

Pituitary Tumors

Pituitary tumors are common in dogs but uncommon in cats. They may be nonfunctional or functional. Functional pituitary tumors associated with the adenohypophysis are typically

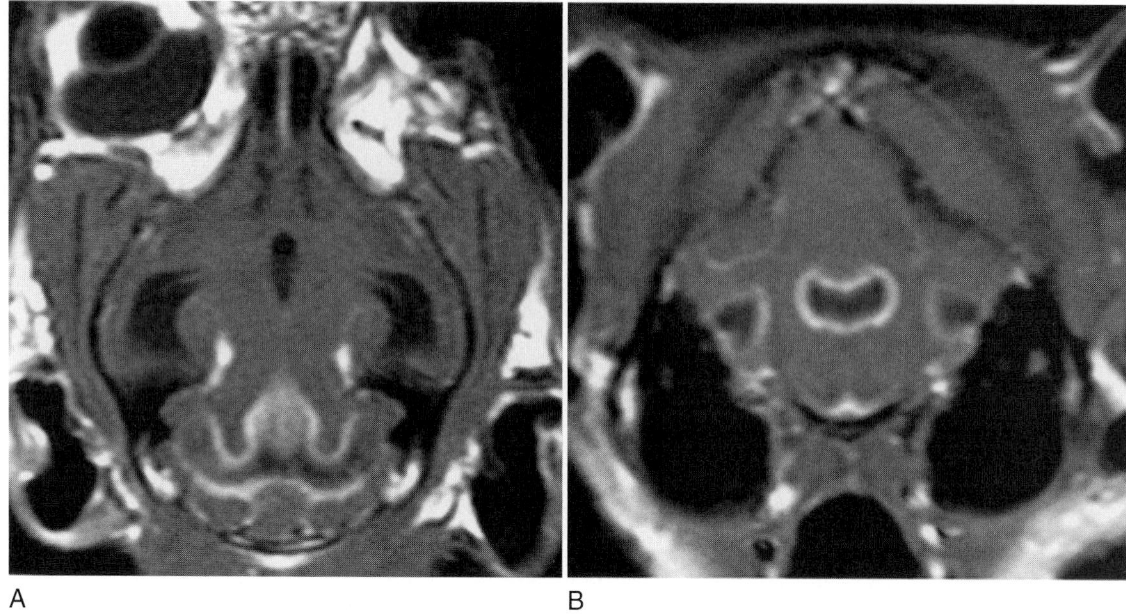

Fig. 9-10 Dorsal (A) and transverse plane (B) T1-weighted postcontrast images of a cat with feline infectious peritonitis. Intense contrast enhancement of the lining of the ventricular system is visible. This is consistent with ependymitis, a common finding in feline infectious peritonitis. The left eye is absent, removed as a result of trauma.

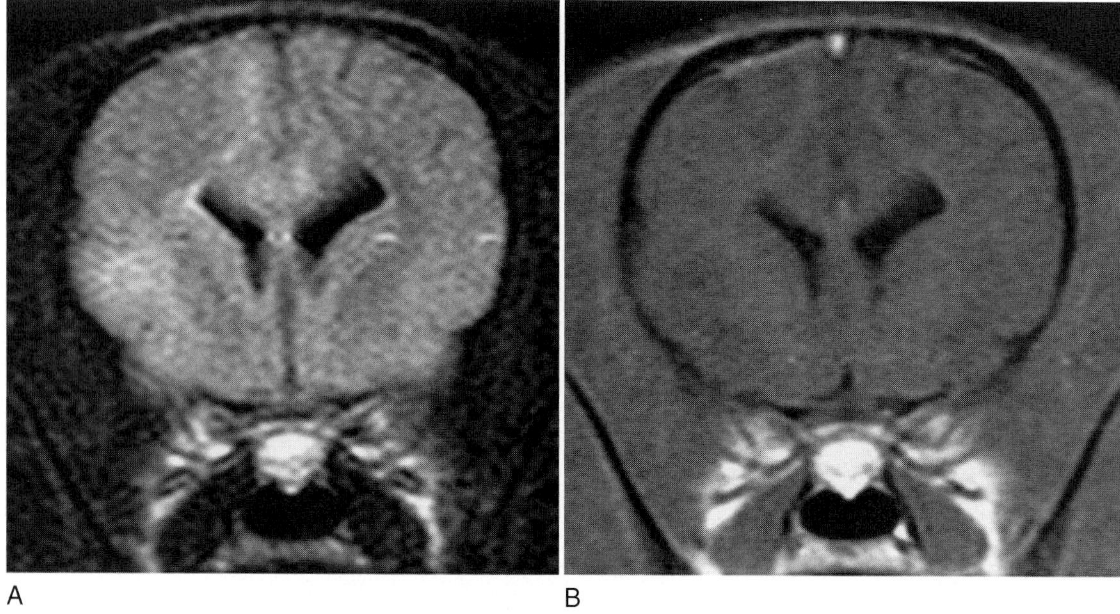

Fig. 9-11 A FLAIR (A) and T1-weighted image made after administration of contrast medium (B) of a 4-year-old Pug with a history of seizures of progressing severity over a 4-day period. Patchy, ill-defined regions of increased T2 signal intensity are visible within the right cerebral cortex, most severe in the temporal and parietal lobes. Minimal mass effect is present. These regions are mildly hypointense on a T1-weighted sequence and do not enhance after gadolinium administration. The most common differential diagnoses for these findings include encephalitis, necrotizing encephalitis, and cerebral infarct. On the basis of breed, progressive clinical signs, multifocal distribution of lesions, CSF analysis, and MR findings, a necrotizing encephalitis is the most likely diagnosis.

characterized by pituitary-dependent hyperadrenocorticism (PDH). Based on MR imaging studies, up to 60% of dogs with PDH but without neurologic signs have a pituitary tumor 4 to 12 mm in diameter (at greatest vertical height).[7] Most pituitary tumors tend to grow dorsocaudally, leading to compression and obliteration of the infundibulum, ventral aspect of the third ventricle, hypothalamus, and thalamus and eventually impinge on internal capsules and optic tracts. MR imaging is useful for visualizing the presence of pituitary tumors in dogs with PDH, with or without neurologic signs,

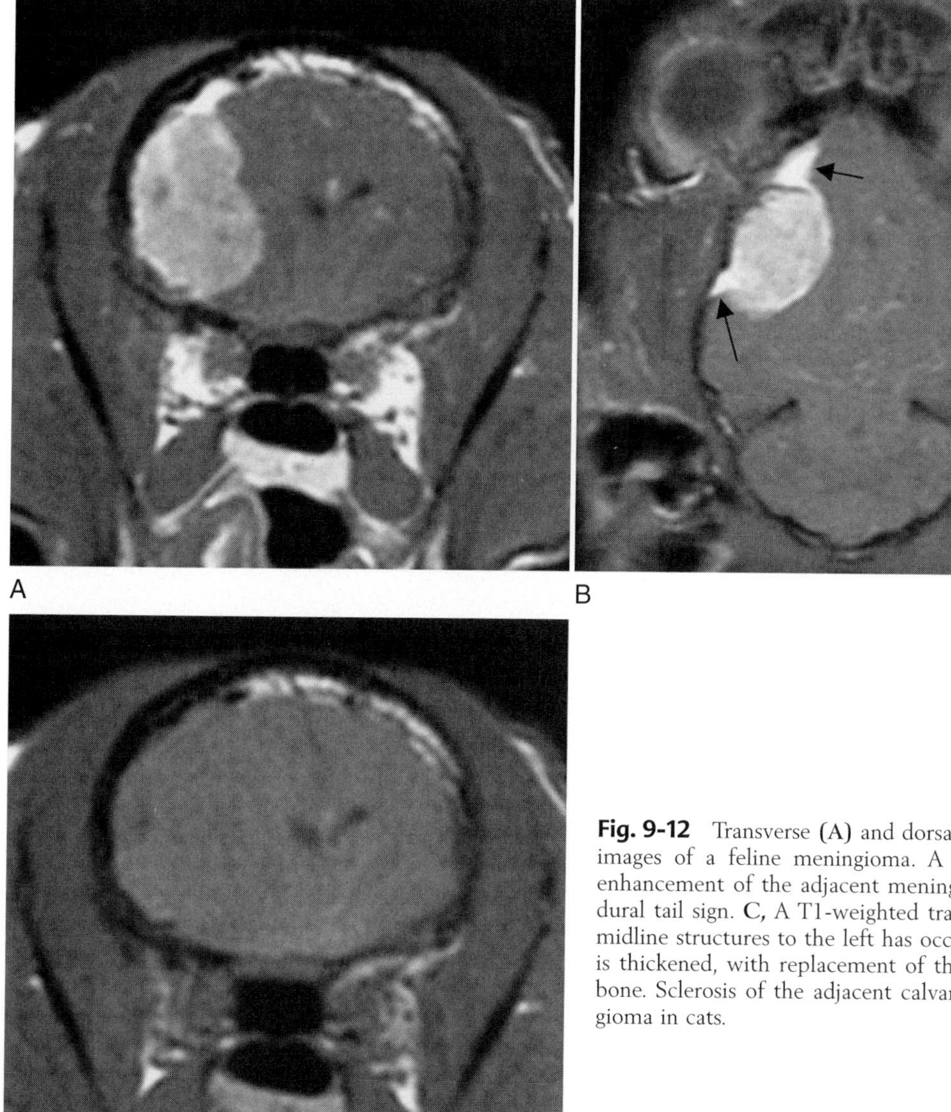

Fig. 9-12 Transverse (A) and dorsal (B) plane T1-weighted postcontrast images of a feline meningioma. A broad peripheral base and contrast enhancement of the adjacent meninges are visible *(arrows):* the so-called dural tail sign. C, A T1-weighted transverse precontrast image. A shift of midline structures to the left has occurred and the calvarium on the right is thickened, with replacement of the bright marrow fat with low signal bone. Sclerosis of the adjacent calvarium is commonly seen with meningioma in cats.

especially when endocrine test results are equivocal. Tumors are always better visualized after contrast medium administration. These tumors usually have minimal peritumoral edema, uniform contrast enhancement, and well-defined margins (Fig. 9-15).

Sometimes cystic regions, or evidence of hemorrhage, may be present. Pituitary tumors less than 3 mm in diameter may not be visible by MR imaging.[7]

Intraaxial Tumors

Glioma

The term glioma is used to describe tumors that arise from the neuropil. These tumors arise from the supporting cells of the brain and include astrocytomas, oligodendrogliomas, glioblastoma multiforme, and ependymomas. They are common in certain breeds of dog, in particular the brachycephalic breeds such as Boxer, Boston Terrier, and the French and English bulldogs. Gliomas can range in malignancy from low grade and slow growing to high grade, poorly differentiated, highly malignant tumors.

Glial cell tumors vary widely in their MR features. These tumors are often difficult to detect on contrast-enhanced CT examinations of the brain because, unlike meningiomas, many have minimal enhancement after contrast medium administration. These tumors are more easily detected with MR imaging, which is one of the many reasons why MR imaging is so clinically superior to CT imaging when evaluating the brain. Gliomas are often ill defined, have variable degrees of peripheral edema, and show variable contrast medium enhancement (Fig. 9-16). Occasionally gliomas have no contrast enhancement. Gliomas can be difficult to differentiate from brain abscess and other focal inflammatory conditions of the brain parenchyma,[4] or even from infarcts, which are massive vasoocclusive events. The patient's history with a massive infarct is usually different than in a patient with a glioma.

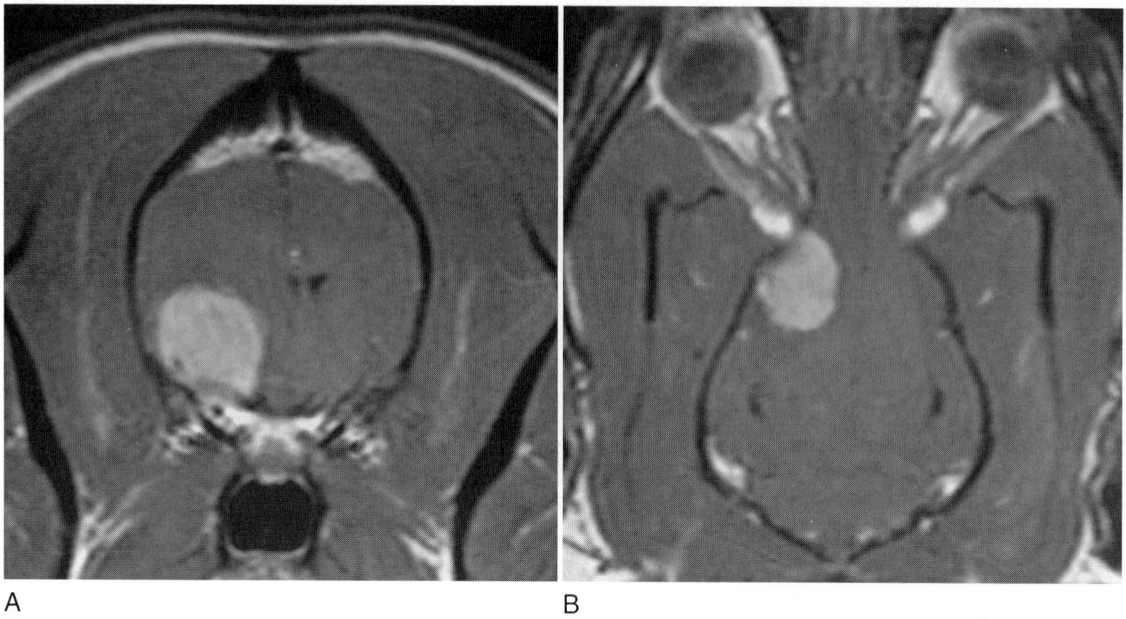

Fig. 9-13 Transverse (A) and dorsal (B) plane T1-weighted postcontrast images of a canine meningioma. A broad peripheral base and relatively intense homogeneous contrast medium enhancement are visible. These findings are commonly associated with a meningioma.

INVASIVE EXTRACRANIAL TUMORS

Nasal Tumors

Aggressive nasal tumors can extend through the cribriform plate, caudal nasal region, or frontal sinuses into the cranial vault. When imaging the brain, including the caudal aspect of the nasal cavity is important, particularly when clinical signs are consistent with a lesion in the olfactory region or abnormal image findings in the olfactory region are present. Extension of primary nasal cavity tumors into the cranial vault may lead to seizures, behavior changes, paresis, circling, and visual deficits. Respiratory signs such as sneezing, nasal discharge, epistaxis, stertor, dyspnea, and mouth breathing are often present but may not be clinically apparent in a patient with caudal nasal or frontal sinus neoplasia (Fig. 9-17). Brain tumors do not commonly extend through the cribriform plate and calvarium into the nasal cavity; the usual course of progression is intracranial invasion of nasal tumors.

Cranial Nerve Tumors

Tumors of cranial and spinal nerves and nerve roots are common in dogs. The terminology given to these tumors is confusing because of differing opinions regarding their cell of origin. Although schwannoma, neurilemmoma, and neurofibroma are used interchangeably, the designation *malignant peripheral nerve sheath tumors* is recommended because many of these tumors are malignant, and determining the cell of origin (Schwann cell, perineurial cell, fibroblast, etc.) is often not possible. Of the cranial nerves, malignant peripheral nerve sheath tumors commonly involve the trigeminal nerve (cranial nerve V), leading to signs of unilateral trigeminal nerve dysfunction (e.g., unilateral temporalis and masseter muscle atrophy). Cranial nerve sheath tumors are either isointense or hyperintense on T2-weighted sequences and enhance intensely after gadolinium administration.[8] The trigeminal nerve arises at the level of the pons and caudal part of the mesencephalon. The nerve courses cranially and branches to the various divisions (mandibular, maxillary, ophthalmic), which continue to course cranially to exit their respective foramen. Depending on the location of the tumor, foraminal enlargement as a result of pressure remodeling from the expanding tumor can sometimes be seen; this is an important secondary sign associated with cranial nerve sheath tumors (Fig. 9-18).

VASCULAR DISRUPTIONS

Occlusive Infarcts

Occlusive cerebral infarcts, long thought not to be a clinical entity in dogs, are being diagnosed with increasingly frequency by MR imaging. Infarcts occur most commonly in the cerebellum but also in the brainstem and forebrain.

Patients with brain infarction are usually older and typically have acute, nonprogressive focal neurologic signs. When the brainstem or cerebellum is involved, an important clinical differential is idiopathic peripheral vestibular disease, in which no abnormal MR findings are present. The typical MR characteristics of a cerebellar infarct include a triangular or segmental region of T2 hyperintensity that is often most apparent on the FLAIR sequence. The shape of the signal change usually closely reflects the regional distribution of the compromised artery.

With a cerebral infarct, the MR findings may overlap with those of a glioma. A cerebral infarct usually has ill-defined T2 hyperintensity, T1 hypointensity, and little to no initial contrast enhancement (Fig. 9-19). As the infarct matures, typically after 3 days, regional vascularity increases, particularly at the periphery of the lesion. One differentiating feature between infarct and glioma is the initial lack of a mass effect with an infarct. Later, however, a mass effect may develop 3 to 5 days after infarction because of vasogenic edema.[10] One of the characteristic findings of infarction is that the mass effect usually resolves before the development of contrast enhancement. A definitive distinction between cerebral infarct and glioma may not be possible in some patients, and a biopsy may be necessary.

Text continued on p. 156

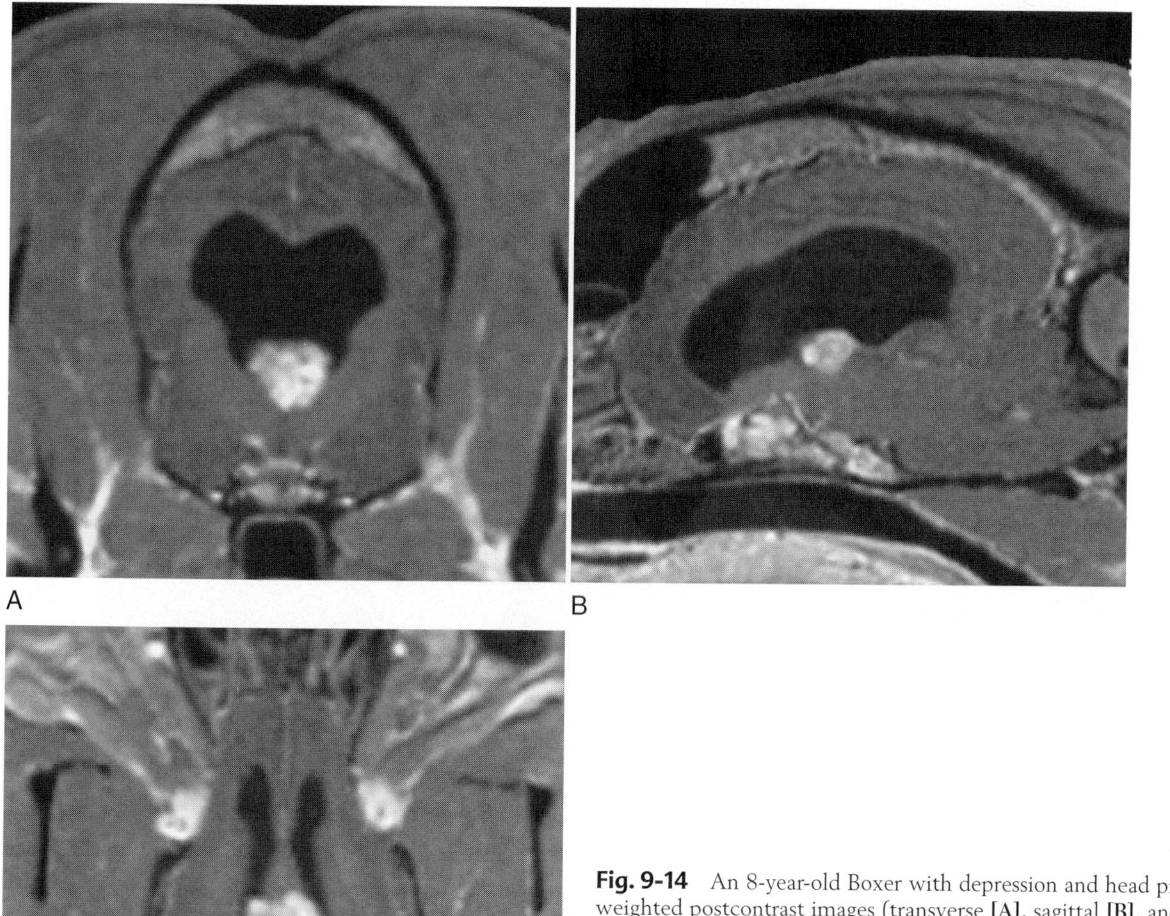

Fig. 9-14 An 8-year-old Boxer with depression and head pressing. In T1-weighted postcontrast images (transverse [A], sagittal [B], and dorsal plane [C]), a contrast-enhancing mass in the third ventricle is visible that is resulting in obstructive hydrocephalus. The lateral ventricles are enlarged, causing an increase in intracranial pressure and the associated clinical signs.

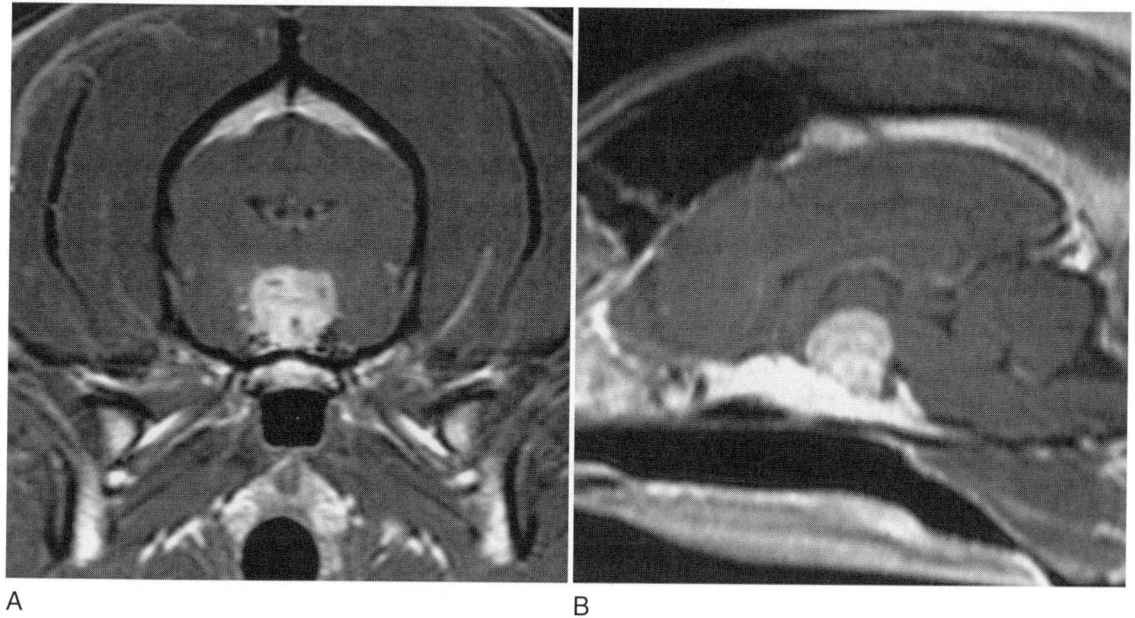

Fig. 9-15 Transverse (A) and sagittal (B) plane T1-weighted postcontrast images. A large, relatively homogeneous, contrast-enhancing mass is visible on the floor of the calvarium at the level of the sella turcica. This is typical of a pituitary tumor.

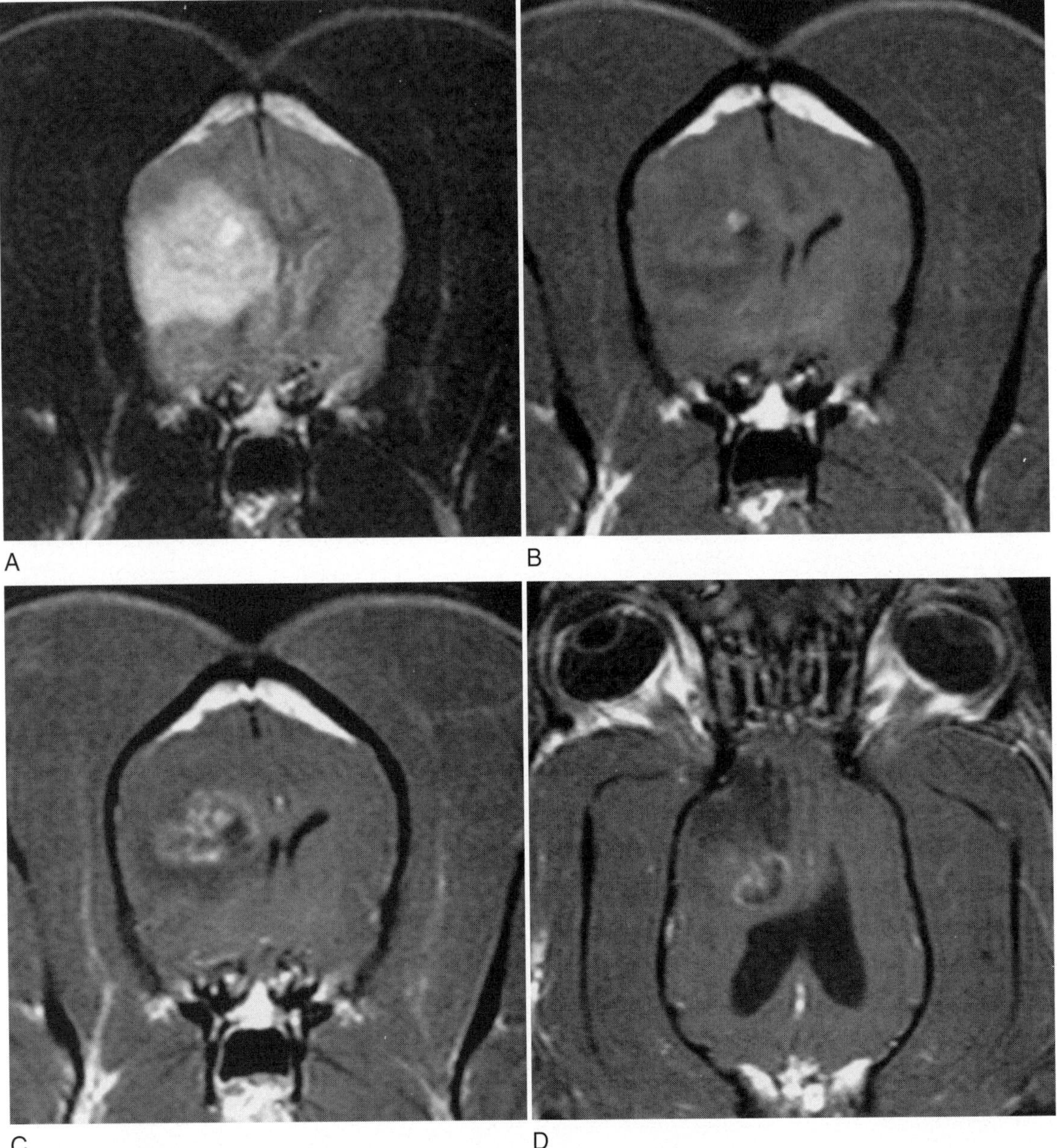

Fig. 9-16 T2-weighted transverse (A) and T1-weighted images made before (B) and after (C and D) contrast medium administration in a 7-year-old Boxer with seizures and behavioral changes. These images are at the level of the center of a large mass effect, which is causing a leftward midline shift and compression of the ventricular system. The hyperintensity in the T2-weighted image is caused by the increased brain water content associated with this tumor. The hyperintense focus on the T1 precontrast image (B) is likely a focus of recent hemorrhage (methemoglobin, occurring approximately 3 days after a hemorrhagic event, is highly paramagnetic and acts like gadolinium in shortening T1 relaxation time). The wispy contrast medium enhancement, ill-defined margin, and peripheral edema (most apparent on the T2 sequence [A]) are consistent with a glioma.

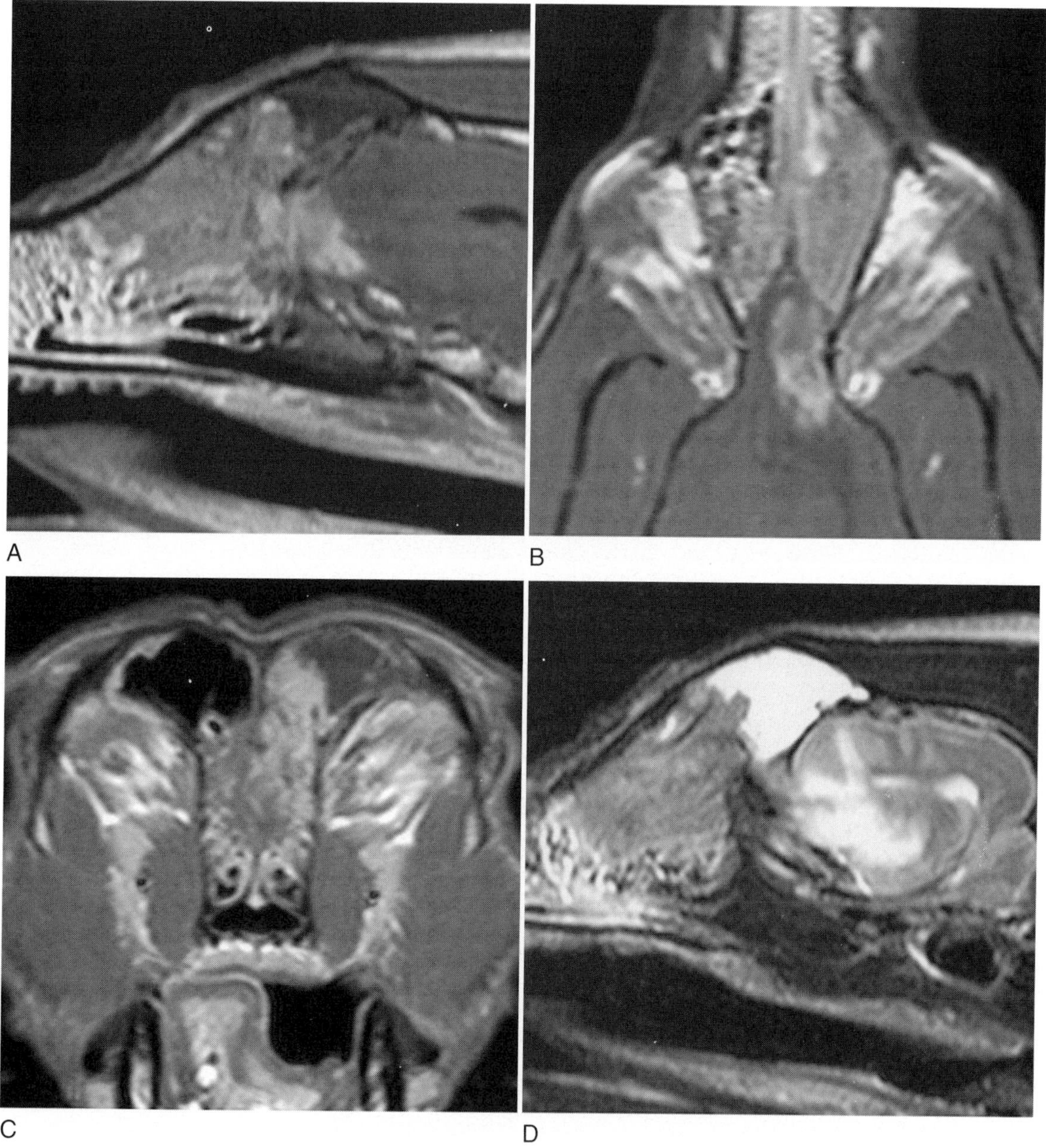

Fig. 9-17 T1-weighted sagittal (A), dorsal (B), and transverse (C) plane post contrast images and a T2-weighted sagittal plane image (D) of an elderly dog with intermittent epistaxis. A mass is evident in the caudal aspect of the left nasal cavity, which is extending into the right nasal cavity and also into the cranial fossa. The increased signal in the left frontal sinus is bright on the T2-weighted sequence (D) and dark on the T1-weighted sequence and does not enhance after contrast medium administration. On the basis of signal characteristics, the frontal sinus lesion is largely trapped fluid rather than all tumor mass. Distinguishing mass from trapped fluid often cannot be made as easily with contrast-enhanced CT. In the T2-weighted image, extensive white matter edema is visible as a result of the intracranial extension. Histologic diagnosis was carcinoma.

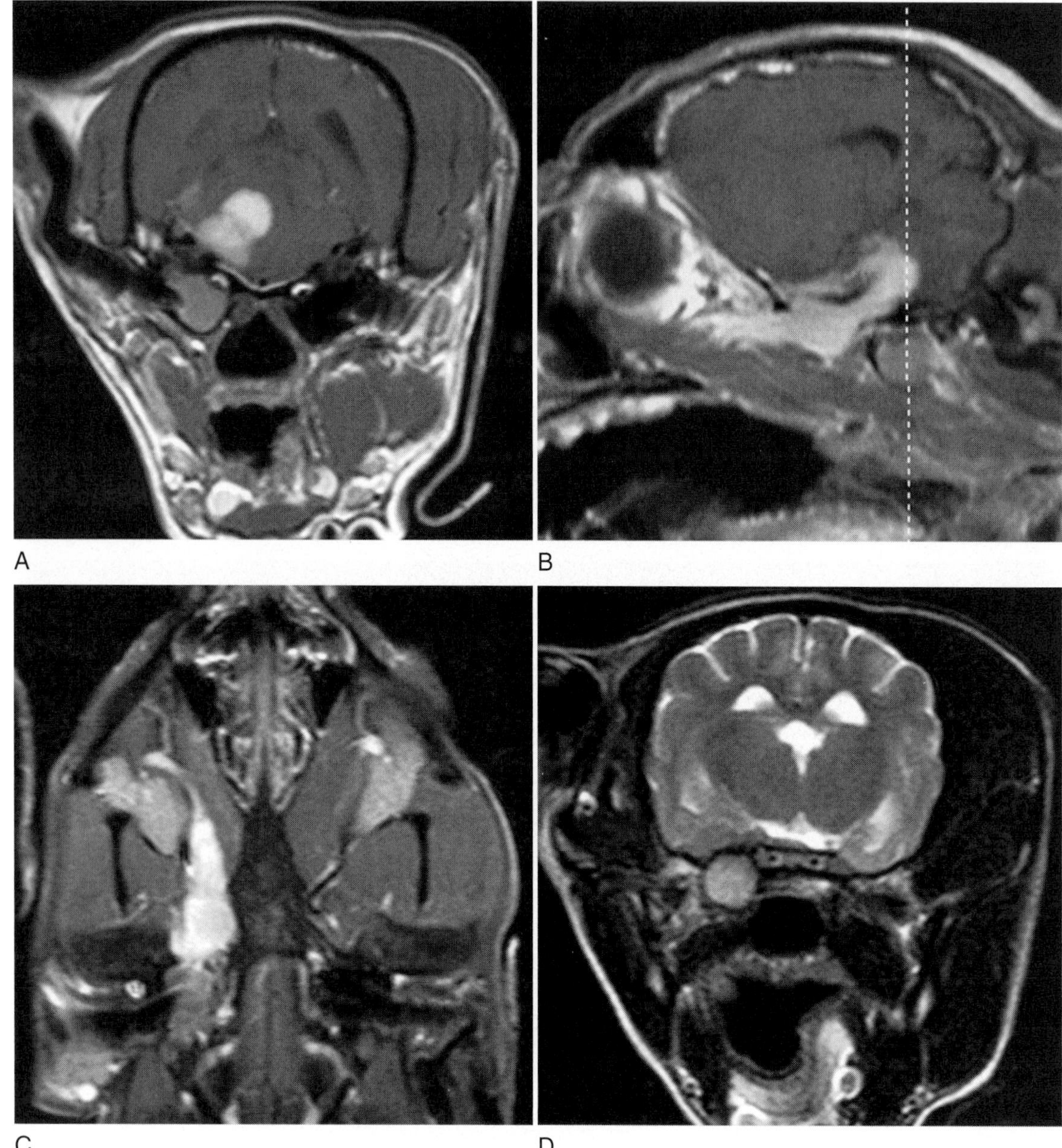

Fig. 9-18 Transverse (A), sagittal (B), and dorsal plane (C) T1-weighted post contrast images, and a transverse T2-weighted image (D). Marked atrophy of the temporal musculature on the right side is present and an intensely contrast enhancing tubular structure is emanating from the right ventral pons and coursing cranially through an enlarged cranial foramen to the retrobulbar region. The vertical *dashed line* in **B** designates the location of the transverse image seen in **A**. Final diagnosis was trigeminal nerve sheath tumor. Incidentally, fluid is visible in the right tympanic cavity.

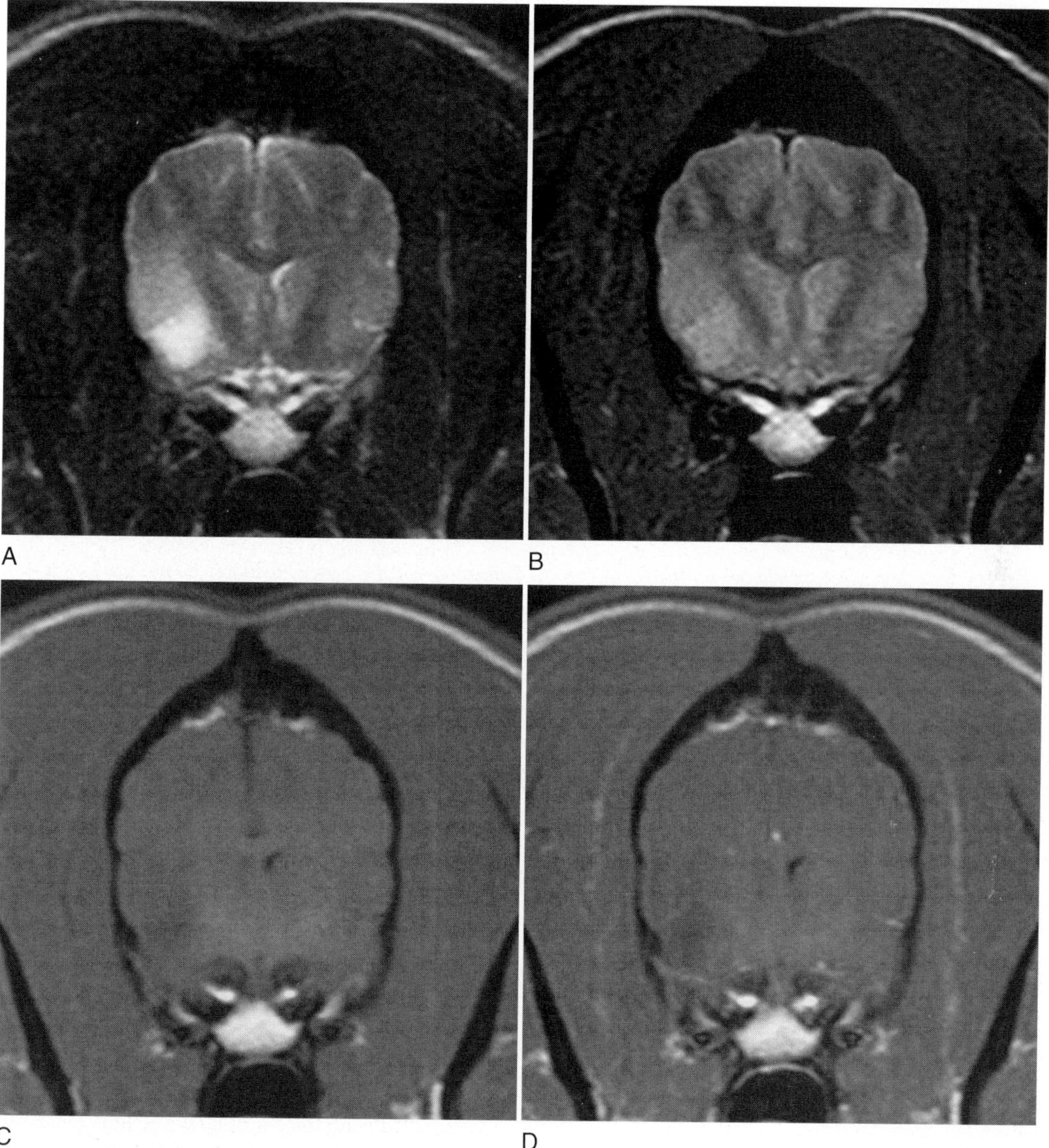

Fig. 9-19 Transverse T2-weighted (A), proton density weighted (B) and T1-weighted images made before (C) and after (D) contrast medium administration in a 10-year-old Labrador retriever with an acute onset of seizures that began 5 days previously. An ill-defined region of T2 hyperintensity is visible in the right piriform lobe. The region is hypointense on T1-weighted images, no associated mass effect is present, and only scant peripheral enhancement occurred after gadolinium administration. These findings are most commonly associated with an infarct. The sudden onset of nonprogressive signs is important collaborating history in these patients and helps decide the likelihood of infarction versus glioma. Other considerations for the findings as seen in this patient include necrotizing encephalitis and GME (sometimes minimal enhancement). Diffusion-weighted imaging can be used to help differentiate these conditions more accurately in the acute stage of an infarct; that is, the first 1 to 3 days.

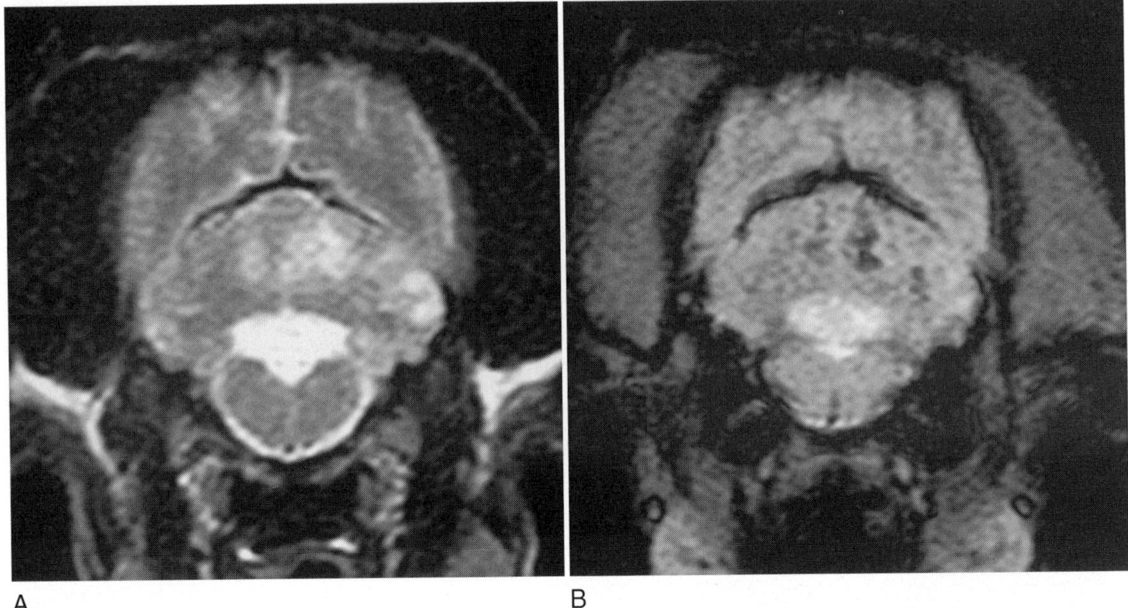

Fig. 9-20 A T2-weighted transverse image (A) at the level of the cerebellum. A region of increased signal intensity is visible in the central and left aspect of the cerebellum. B, T2-weighted gradient echo T2* sequence at the same level. Hemorrhage is best detected on a gradient echo sequence because of the magnetic susceptibility effect of hemoglobin breakdown products. The focal regions of signal void are the result of local disruption to the magnetic field and do not truly reflect the size of the hematoma.

One way to be more confident that a cerebral lesion is an infarct is through the use of diffusion-weighted imaging. Diffusion imaging uses the variability of Brownian motion of water molecules in brain tissue. Brownian motion refers to the random movement of molecules. Water molecules are in constant motion, and the rate of movement or diffusion depends on the kinetic energy of the molecules and temperature. The diffusion imaging protocol, usually only available on high-field magnets, uses the fact that infarcted brain cells become overhydrated from failure of the adenosine triphosphate pump, resulting in "restricted" movement of water. In tumors, water movement is less restricted and tumors will therefore have a different appearance in the diffusion image. However, restricted movement of water in an infarct typically lasts only 1 to 3 days after infarction, so after this time the value of using diffusion-weighted imaging to distinguish infarction from glioma is decreased.

Patients in whom an occlusive infarct is suspected should be evaluated for conditions resulting in a hypercoagulable state (e.g., Cushing's disease) and loss of antithrombin III.

Hemorrhagic Infarcts

Hemorrhagic infarcts are most commonly associated with hypertension, thrombocytopenia, or other coagulopathies. The MR imaging characteristics may be similar to those for an occlusive infarct (Fig. 9-20). However, hemorrhage in the brain has a particular appearance in MR images that changes as the hematoma matures (Table 9-1). The use of standard spin-echo sequences sometimes allows a rough estimate of the age of a hemorrhagic lesion on the basis of the signal characteristics of the lesion. The change in appearance of a hematoma on different sequences over time is related to the magnetic properties of iron within hemoglobin as it transitions through intracellular deoxyhemoglobin to methemoglobin and finally extracellular hemosiderin.

Compared with fast (turbo) spin-echo sequences, gradient recalled echo sequences are more susceptible to magnetic field inhomogeneity created by hemoglobin. Hemorrhage acts like ferromagnetic material, causing minute distortions in the local magnetic field resulting in a signal void (Figs. 9-20 to 9-22). Gradient recalled echo sequences can be acquired in addition to standard spin-echo sequences when hemorrhage is suspected. Low signal on T2-weighted spin echo and gradient recalled echo images is, however, not specific for hemorrhage but may also be seen with mineralization, gas, fibrous tissue, or iron deposits.[8] Such findings must be interpreted in light of information gained from all other sequences in the study and the available clinical information.

ACKNOWLEDGMENT

Many of the images in this chapter are courtesy of the IAMS Pet Imaging Center Database.

Table • 9-1

Classic MR Appearance of a Maturing Hematoma in Human Central Nervous System Tissue

PHASE	TIME	HEMOGLOBIN	T1	T2
Hyperacute	<24 hours	Oxyhemoglobin (intracellular)	Isointense or hypointense	Hyperintense
Acute	1-3 days	Deoxyhemoglobin (intracellular)	Isointense or hypointense	Hypointense
Early subacute	>3 days	Methemoglobin (intracellular)	Hyperintense	Hypointense
Late subacute	>7 days	Methemoglobin (extracellular)	Hyperintense	Hyperintense
Chronic	>14 days	Hemosiderin (extracellular)	Isointense or hypointense	Hypointense

Modified from Bradley WG Jr: MR appearance of hemorrhage in the brain, *Radiology* 189:15-26, 1993.
There is considerable variation in the appearance of hematomas, and these observations have not been fully clinically validated in dogs. This table should act as guide only.

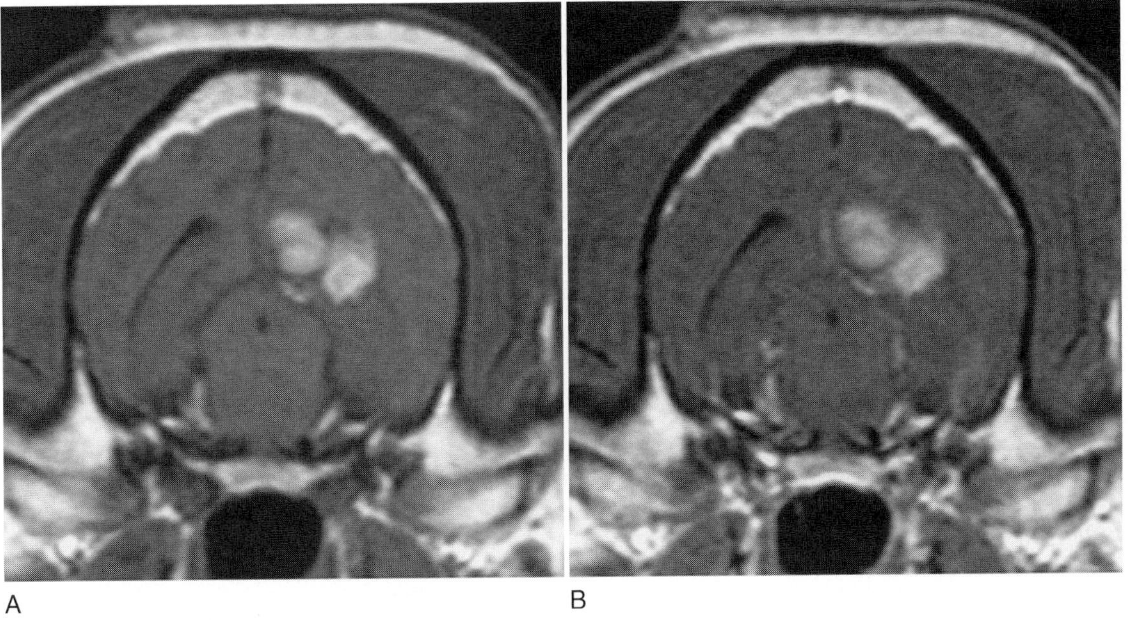

Fig. 9-21 T1-weighted images of a 10-year-old spaniel with acute-onset seizures. **A** is without contrast medium. The T1 hyperintense region is hemorrhage of at least 3 days' duration (both intracellular and extracellular methemoglobin are hyperintense on T1-weighted sequences, as is fat, melanin, and proteinaceous fluids). **B** was acquired after contrast medium administration. No enhancement of the lesion is visible, but normal vascular enhancement is apparent adjacent to the lesion.

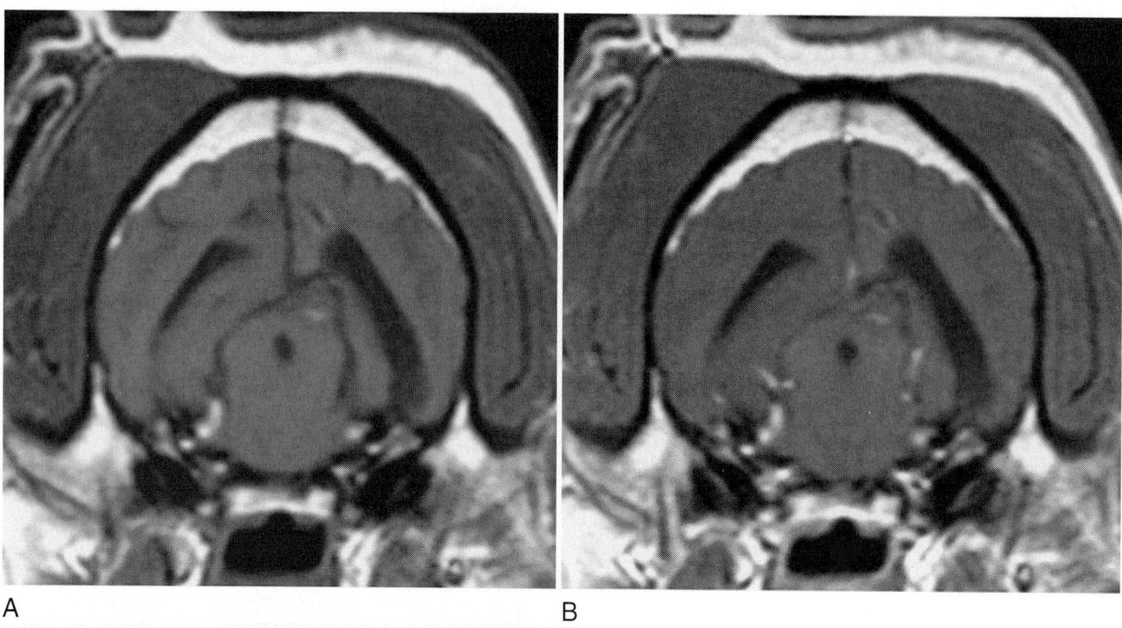

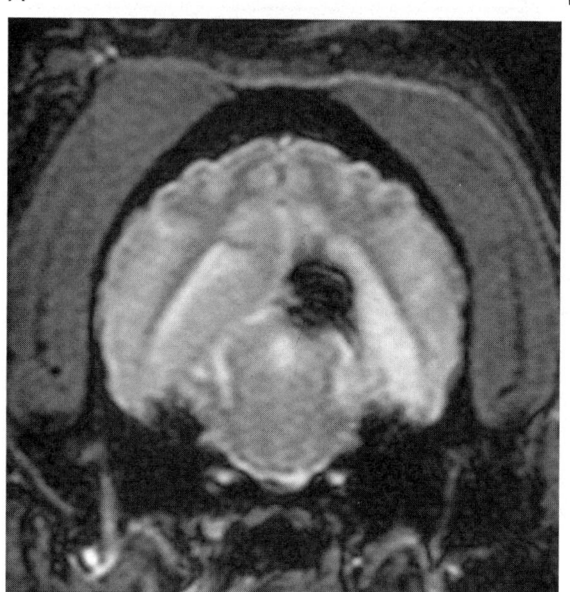

Fig. 9-22 The same dog in Figure 9-21 imaged 9 months later. The dog has seizures controlled by medication and is otherwise normal. T1-weighted images made before **(A)** and after **(B)** contrast medium administration. The high T1 signal previously seen is almost completely resolved, indicating a significant reduction in methemoglobin. Focal parenchymal distortion is visible in the region of presumed hemorrhage and adjacent mild left hydrocephalus. The left ventricle may be larger than the right as a result of adjacent parenchymal necrosis/atrophy—so-called compensatory hydrocephalus. No abnormal contrast medium enhancement **(B)** is present. **C** is a T2-weighted gradient echo sequence in which a large susceptibility artifact is visible as a result of residual hemosiderin. The presumptive diagnosis is intracranial hemorrhage of undetermined etiology. The final diagnosis was hemorrhage associated with a cavernous angioma.

REFERENCES

1. Westbrook C, Kaut Roth C: Pulse sequences. In *MRI in practice, vol 3*, Malden, MA, 2005, Blackwell, p. 165.
2. Benigni L, Lamb CR: Comparison of fluid-attenuated inversion recovery and T2-weighted magnetic resonance images in dogs and cats with suspected brain disease, *Vet Radiol Ultrasound* 46:287, 2005.
3. Westbrook C, Kaut Roth C: Contrast media. In *MRI in practice, vol 3*, Malden, MA, 2005, Blackwell, p. 352.
4. Cherubini GB, Mantis P, Martinez TA et al: Utility of magnetic resonance imaging for distinguishing neoplastic from non-neoplastic brain lesions in dogs and cats, *Vet Radiol Ultrasound* 46:384, 2005.
5. Esteve-Ratsch B, Kneissl S, Gabler C: Comparative evaluation of the ventricles in the Yorkshire Terrier and the German Shepherd dog using low-field MRI, *Vet Radiol Ultrasound* 42:410, 2001.
6. Lamb CR, Croson PJ, Cappello R et al: Magnetic resonance imaging findings in 25 dogs with inflammatory cerebrospinal fluid, *Vet Radiol Ultrasound* 46:17, 2005.
7. Braund KG, editor: *Clinical neurology in small animals: localization, diagnosis and treatment*, Ithaca, NY, 2003, International Veterinary Information Service. Available at www.ivis.org.
8. Bagley RS, Wheeler SJ, Klopp L et al: Clinical features of trigeminal nerve-sheath tumor in 10 dogs, *Am Anim Hosp Assoc* 34:19, 1998.

9. Marks MP: Cerebral ischemia and infarction. In Atlas SW, editor: *Magnetic resonance imaging of the brain and spine,* Philadelphia, 2002, Lippincott Williams & Wilkins, pp. 919-980.
10. Mulkern RV: Fast imaging techniques. In Atlas SW, editor: *Magnetic resonance imaging of the brain and spine.* Philadelphia, 2002, Lippincott Williams & Wilkins, p. 178.

ELECTRONIC RESOURCES evolve

Additional information related to the content in Chapter 9 can be found on the companion Web site at evolve http://evolve.elsevier.com/Thrall/vetrad/
- Key Points
- Chapter Quiz

CHAPTER • 10
The Equine Head

Anthony P. Pease

RADIOGRAPHY VERSUS OTHER IMAGING MODALITIES

Until recently, the primary imaging modalities available to assess abnormalities of the equine head were radiographs and nuclear medicine. The equine head is a complex structure to evaluate with radiographs because of the numerous overlying structures, thick bone, and relatively complex anatomy; detection of small areas of lysis or soft tissue lesions is sometimes impossible in the equine head. Nuclear medicine provides valuable information on various functional parameters but has poor spatial resolution. In the last several years, cross-sectional imaging techniques such as computed tomography (CT), magnetic resonance (MR) imaging, and ultrasound have become more readily available. Such techniques have greatly simplified identification of abnormalities of the equine head. In addition, postprocessing programs allowing multiplanar and three-dimensional reconstruction of CT and MR images have greatly simplified surgical planning.[1,2] Despite the enhanced capabilities provided by these other imaging modalities, conventional radiography is still the main modality used to evaluate the equine head.[3-6]

The large gas-filled structures of the equine head, such as the guttural pouches, larynx, pharynx, nasal cavity, and paranasal sinuses, enable portable radiographic units to provide diagnostic-quality radiographs. The main limitation of radiography is the superimposition of structures. In addition, despite the difficulties associated with the interpretation of conventional radiographs, they are generally considered helpful in providing diagnostic information in a majority of diseases that occur in the head, though the true extent of the disease may be underestimated.[7] Nevertheless, other techniques often provide more detailed or specific information.

Nuclear medicine has been primarily applied to localize sites of bone remodeling. When using bone-seeking radiopharmaceuticals, such as technetium-99m methylene diphosphonate, the image is generated by the radiopharmaceutical binding to the hydroxyapatite crystals in regions of osteoblastic activity. In the head, the main use for nuclear medicine is evaluating dental disease and differentiating sinusitis of dental origin from other causes.[8] This can be particularly difficult radiographically because lesions of the teeth may not be detected as a result of the superimposition of numerous bone and soft tissue structures, minimal bone lysis, or superimposition of overlying disease within the paranasal sinuses. In addition, scintigraphy is also useful for identifying regions of bone remodeling caused by degenerative joint disease within the temporomandibular and temporohyoid joints, which may not be evident on radiography (Fig. 10-1).

Radioactive labeling of white blood cells has also been used in the evaluation of tooth abnormalities. However, the overall low level of radioactivity in sites of abnormal white cell accumulation causes poor resolution and does not provide adequate landmarks, making this technique inaccurate.[9]

The primary limitation of scintigraphy is that spatial resolution is poor, and the bloom of activity detected signifies only a general area of abnormality rather than a specific site. Thus nuclear medicine has a high sensitivity for detection of bone destruction and remodeling though scintigraphy is not as specific in detecting the cause of remodeling compared with radiology.[9] The sensitivity of conventional radiography for equine dental disease is only approximately 50%,[9-11] but when used in combination with scintigraphy this figure increases to 97.7% and the specificity to 100%.[9]

The use of cross-sectional imaging eliminates the problem of overlying structures. Computed tomography and MR imaging allow the evaluation of slices of the head that are generally 1 mm to 1 cm thick in the transverse plane. These images provide great anatomic localization (Fig. 10-2). In addition, acquiring CT images lends itself well to three-dimension reconstructions that can aid in surgical planning and visualizing lesions not easily identified on transverse images (Fig. 10-3). CT and MR imaging require specialized equipment, including custom tables and hoists (Fig. 10-4) and a purpose-built room to accommodate the size of the horse. Many sources provide CT and MR imaging of normal anatomy.[12-14]

Ultrasonography has been used to evaluate skull fractures as well as temporomandibular joints, retrobulbar masses, and jugular vein thrombosis.[15] Ultrasonography is also useful for evaluation of the superficial soft tissue structures of the head, with the major limitations being the contour of the head, which prevents adequate transducer-skin contact, and the inability of sound to penetrate bone. The most useful application of ultrasound is evaluating soft tissue structures where the bone is not obstructing the region of interest, such as in the guttural pouches to look for fluid, and allowing the evaluation of draining tracts associated with atlantoaxial septic bursitis ("poll evil") (Fig. 10-5). Ultrasound can also help evaluate the size and appearance of lymph nodes in horses afflicted with *Streptococcus equi*. In addition, the use of ultrasound has been suggested as an aid in the evaluation of the larynx.[16]

With all these modalities being available, the main consideration when selecting one is the level of invasiveness, the speed of acquisition, and the type of lesion being evaluated. If general anesthesia is possible, CT should be used to evaluate lesions of the skull that involve bone, such as tooth root abscesses, fractures from trauma, or temporohyoid osteoarthropathy. MR imaging is extremely useful for evaluating the equine brain, sinuses, or the surrounding soft tissue structures of the head. Ultrasound can be used to evaluate superficial soft tissue structures in the standing horse, whereas radiography remains the mainstay for rapid evaluation of the

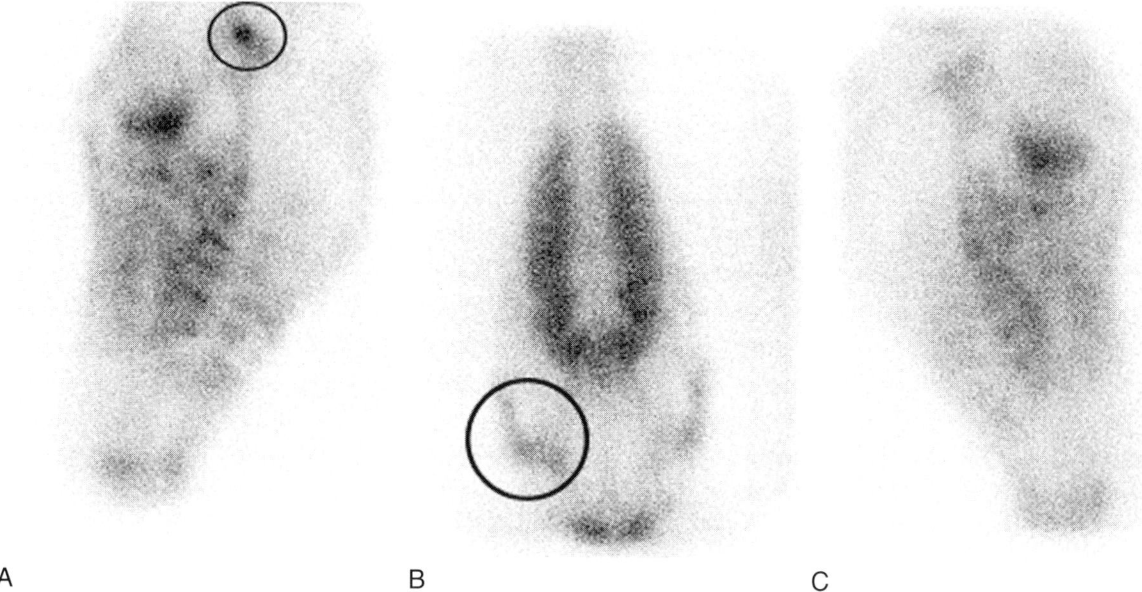

Fig. 10-1 Bone phase scintigrams of an equine head with technetium-99m methylene diphosphonate. The left lateral (A) and dorsal projections (B) show a focal increased activity in the region of the temporomandibular joint *(circles)*. The same area of activity is not visible in the right lateral projection (C).

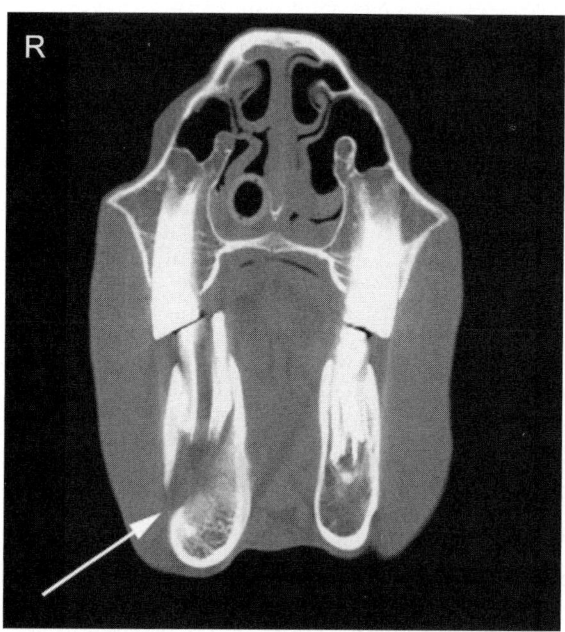

Fig. 10-2 A transverse CT image at the level of the maxillary first molar. Note the tract extending out of the lateral aspect of the mandible from an apical tooth root abscess *(arrow)*.

equine head, with only minimal sedation needed. Nuclear medicine has generally been replaced by the other modalities described above; however, when appropriate, scintigraphic evaluation can aid in the diagnosis of disease involving the paranasal sinuses as well as the teeth, especially when used in combination with radiography.

ABNORMALITIES OF THE EQUINE HEAD

One approach for beginning a radiographic assessment of the equine head is to divide the head into general locations and then address the diseases that occur at these sites. Although overlap will undoubtedly occur, this method seems appropriate and image acquisition and special views should be focused on when appropriate.

Rostral Head (Incisive Region and Rostral Mandible)

The rostral aspect of the head is the area rostral to the premolars. The standard radiographic projections to evaluate this region include a lateral and a dorsoventral projection. Intraoral radiographs are useful to eliminate superimposition of structures and are accomplished by placing a plastic bag over a radiographic cassette and then inserting the cassette into the horse's mouth (Fig. 10-6). A dorsoventral projection is used to evaluate the incisive bone, and a ventrodorsal projection allows assessment of the rostral aspect of the mandible.

Diseases that involve the rostral equine head include fractures, neoplasia, and cyst formation.[3,4,6] Fractures generally occur in young, inquisitive animals that become startled while chewing or playing with a fixed object.[6] This causes a displaced fracture involving the incisive teeth with extension into the diastema (the portion of the body of the mandible without teeth). These fractures are usually moderately displaced and easily identified; however, radiographs tend to underestimate the extent of incomplete fracture lines that may extend into the mandible or involve premolar tooth roots. Involvement of tooth roots by the fracture increases the complications of surgical repair because of the increased likelihood of tooth root infection and abscess formation.

Tumors that occur on the rostral head are rare and generally benign. Osteoma is a benign tumor that can affect the mandible, maxilla, paranasal sinuses, and nasal cavity. The main feature of an osteoma is that it has an intense, well-demarcated mineral opacity and is usually midline in the rostral mandible.[4] Adamantinomas (also known as epidermoid

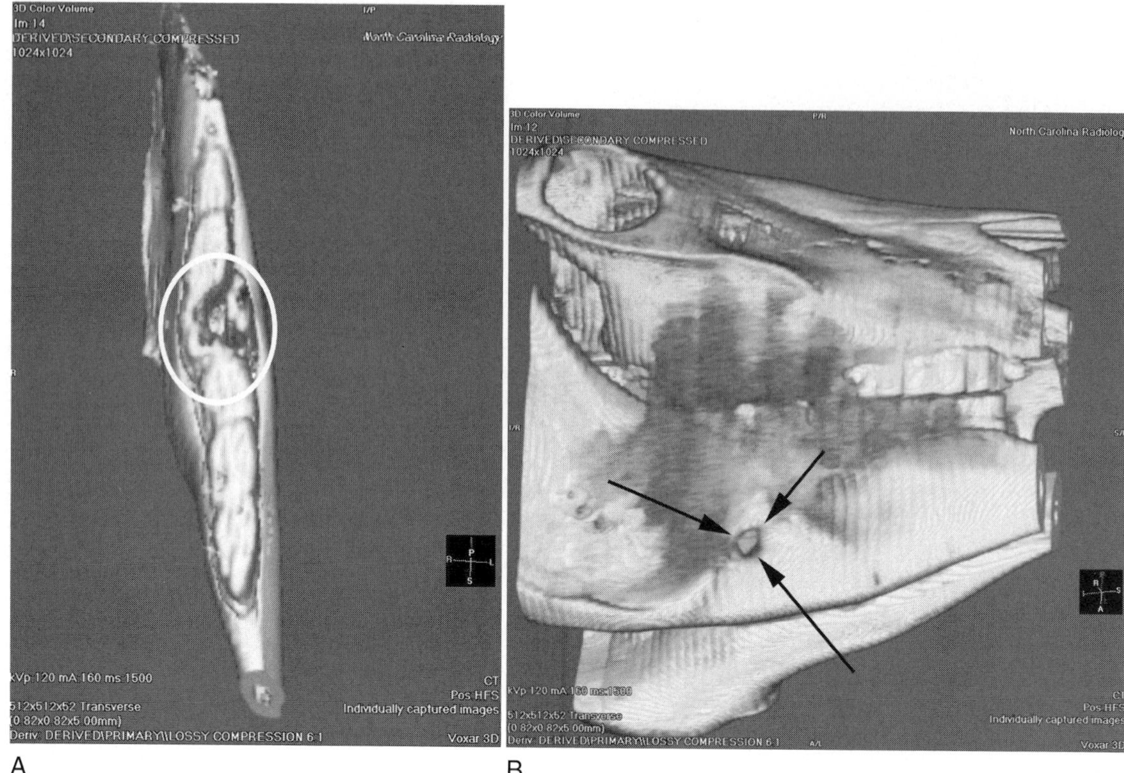

Fig. 10-3 Three dimensional reconstructions of the apical tooth root abscess in Figure 10-2. Note the fracture of the first molar along the sagittal plane (A, *circle*) as well as the defect in the mandible (B, *arrows*). (See Color Plate 3.)

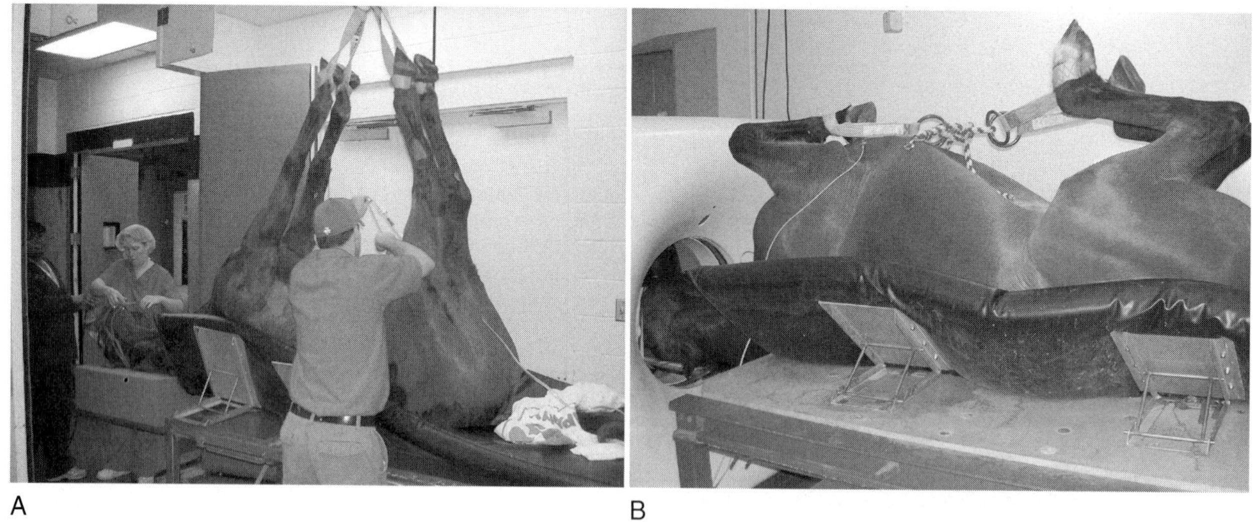

Fig. 10-4 A, The hoist required to place a horse on the specialized table for CT or MR examination. B, A horse positioned for a CT examination of the head.

cysts) result in a unilateral enlargement of the rostral mandible or ventral aspect of the body of the mandible in young animals.[3,4,6] This lesion causes an expansile mass that can look clinically similar to osteosarcoma.[3] Another cause of cystlike enlargement and septation in the mandible of a young horse is nutritional hyperparathyroidism.[3] Large aneurismal bone cysts are also possible in the rostral mandible of a young horse (Fig. 10-7). Soft tissue tumors have also been described as expansile lesions that cause bone lysis and displace the incisor teeth but generally consist of a large soft tissue mass with secondary bone involvement.[17]

Mandible

The mandible is a difficult structure to examine in its entirety because of the superimposition of the contralateral mandible and parts of the skull. Evaluation of the temporomandibular joints and the rami of the mandible requires oblique radiographs, CT imaging, or MR imaging. Standard radiographic

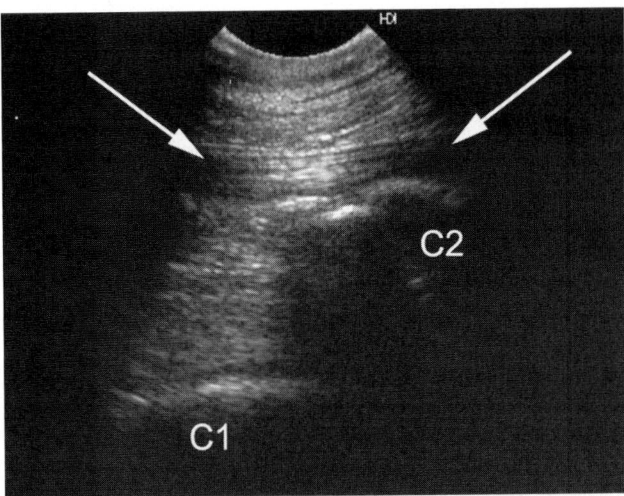

A

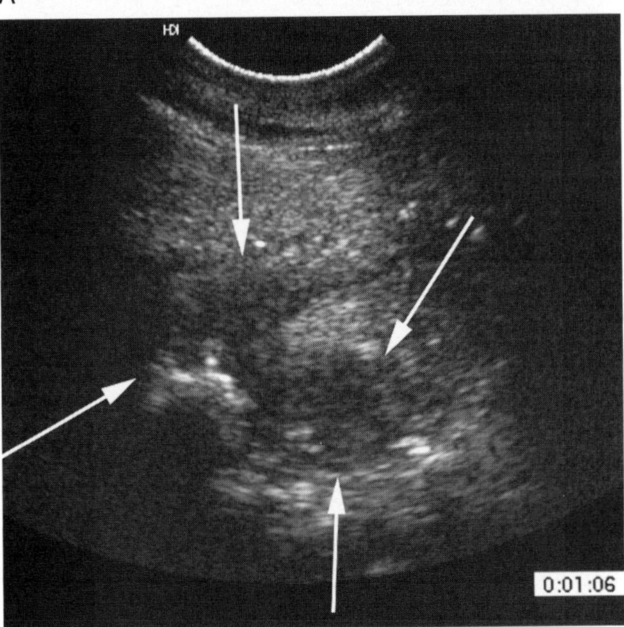

B

Fig. 10-5 A, Longitudinal sonogram of the region of the poll at the level of C1. No abnormalities are seen, and the *arrows* indicate the normal fiber pattern of the nuchal ligament. **B,** Longitudinal sonogram of the left craniodorsal aspect of the neck at the level of C1 in the same horse. Note the large hypoechoic cavity *(arrows)* near the bone from an abscess in the nuchal bursa, also called "poll evil." (Courtesy Cornell University, Ithaca, NY.)

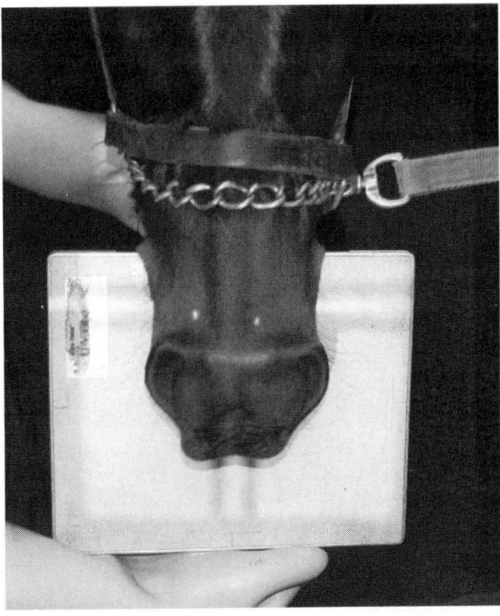

Fig. 10-6 The position for an intraoral, dorsoventral radiograph to evaluate the rostral aspect of the incisive bone.

views for the mandible include lateral, dorsoventral, and two oblique projections. The goal of an oblique radiograph is to offset the two sides of the mandible to allow each ramus or body to be individually evaluated.[4,6] Thus a right 45-degree dorsal-left ventral oblique (RDLVO) radiograph and a left 45-degree dorsal to right ventral oblique (LDRVO) radiograph should be obtained. When obtaining oblique radiographs, care should be taken to place the appropriate radiographic marker to identify the image; this is discussed in detail in Chapter 6. For example, with a LDRVO radiograph, the image will cause the left ventral aspect of the ramus of the mandible to be projected in an unobstructed manner. Therefore a left marker should be placed on the ventral aspect of the image to indicate that the left ramus of the mandible is being viewed. Additionally, a right marker can be placed on the dorsal aspect of the image to indicate that the right dorsal aspect of the skull is being accentuated.

Radiographs of the mandible are usually performed to evaluate the mandibular tooth roots or the body of the mandible for fractures. Mandibular tooth root infections are suspected when swelling is present in the mandibular region that frequently manifests itself as a sinus tract draining from the ventral aspect of the ramus.[6] Evaluation of the extent of this tract can be performed by a metallic probe or injection of contrast medium. This contrast procedure is performed while obtaining an oblique radiograph to further isolate the involved area of the mandible while eliminating superimposition. The goal of adding the contrast medium or metallic probe is to trace the sinus tract to the source of the infection, which often centers on the apical aspect of the infected tooth root. The radiographic findings of apical tooth root abscesses include indistinct margins of the lamina dura, loss of the normal outline of the tooth root, blunting of the tooth root, widening of the periodontal membrane and, frequently, an associated lytic tract extending out of the ventral cortex of the mandible (Figs. 10-8 and 10-9).[4,6] In chronic infections, the mandible may have a periosteal reaction associated with the defect and extension of the infection into the soft tissues. Bone formation can extend on the medial and lateral borders of the mandible and obscure the mandible and cause a loss of detail on the radiographs because of superimposition.[6]

Fractures of the caudal aspect of the mandible may be unilateral or bilateral. Because of the superimposition of the teeth, mandibular fractures are difficult to evaluate without the use of oblique radiographic projections.[4,6] Caudal mandibular fractures are usually incomplete and have a worse prognosis if the fracture line involves a tooth root because that extension may lead to a tooth root infection.[4]

Subluxation and osteoarthropathy of the temporomandibular joint is also difficult to assess on conventional radiographs because of the superimposition of the petrous temporal bone. One technique is to acquire a right 30-degree caudal to left cranial oblique radiograph to examine the left temporomandibular joint and a left 30-degree caudal to right cranial oblique radiograph to examine the right

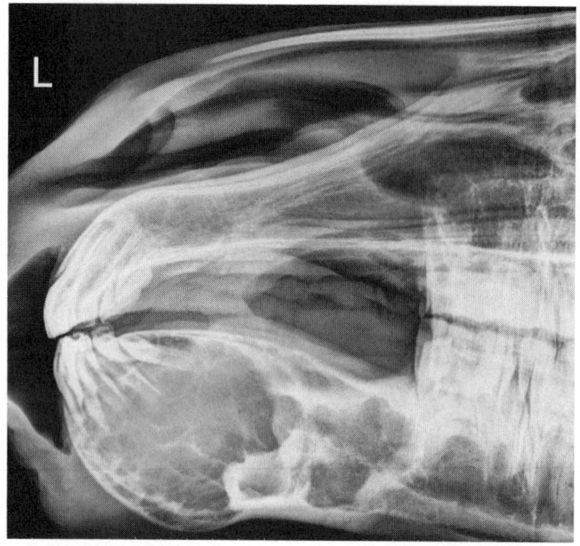

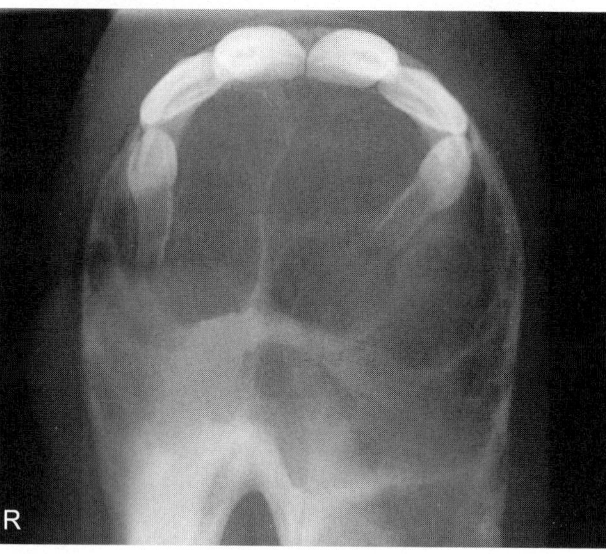

Fig. 10-7 Lateral (A) and ventrodorsal intraoral (B) radiographs of the rostral aspect of the mandible in a 7-month-old thoroughbred with a rapidly enlarging mass. Biopsies were obtained, and this expansile mass of the rostral mandible was diagnosed as an aneurismal bone cyst.

temporomandibular joint; see Chapter 6 for more details. Moving the tube cranial or caudal to the temporomandibular joint will separate the joints without projecting them on the petrous temporal bone. Because the petrous temporal bone is superimposed on the temporomandibular joint, sometimes the projection is also obliqued ventrodorsally. However, when multiple planes are obliqued, interpretation of the image is difficult because distortion of the normal anatomy will occur.

Dorsoventral radiographs can be acquired in the standing horse, but care needs to be used because the x-ray tube is difficult to move out of the way rapidly if the horse becomes startled; this could cause injury to personnel, equipment, and the patient.[18] Recently, more emphasis on the ultrasonographic appearance of the temporomandibular joint has been reported, including the normal anatomy.[19] After comparing radiography, scintigraphy, and ultrasound to diagnose temporomandibular arthropathy in a horse, ultrasound was considered the least expensive and technically easiest and yielded the most information.[20] However, this technique is useful only if applied by trained sonographers.

CT and MR imaging are quite useful to assess the mandible and temporomandibular joint. In terms of assessing tooth root abscesses, the same changes described with radiography can be identified with CT; however, CT is also able to assess whether fragmentation or lucencies within the tooth are present (see Fig. 10-2).[1] In addition, CT can better evaluate mandibular fractures and allow detection of subtle fracture lines obscured by superimposition on conventional radiographs. For the temporomandibular joint, both CT and MR imaging allow evaluation of the surrounding soft tissues for evidence of infection or swelling, determine if the joint is misaligned, and identify bone lysis associated with the mandibular condyle or mandibular fossa.

Nasal Cavity, Paranasal Sinuses

Because horses are obligate nasal breathers, the nasal cavity and paranasal sinuses are very large to provide adequate airflow during exercise. The extensive sinus system occupies the majority of the head and has an intricate communication system within the sinuses as well as in the nasal cavity (Fig. 10-10). On each side of the horse are a frontal, caudal maxillary, rostral maxillary, and sphenopalatine sinuses. The unique characteristics of this sinus system is that among domestic species the horse is the only species in which the frontal sinus communicates indirectly with the nasal cavity through the caudal maxillary sinus; in other species the communication is direct.[21]

The frontal sinus, more correctly the conchofrontal sinus, is in the caudodorsal aspect of the head and overlies the rostral portion of the calvaria, medial to the orbits and extending rostrally as the closed portion of the dorsal concha. On the rostrolateral aspect of the conchofrontal sinus is the frontomaxillary opening that allows communication between the conchofrontal and caudal maxillary sinuses. The caudal maxillary sinus and the rostral maxillary sinus are in the lateral aspect of the caudal head and overlie the maxillary cheek teeth. These two sinuses are divided from each other by an oblique septum that varies in position. Both sinuses communicate with the nasal cavity by a small, shared communication called the nasomaxillary opening that extends to the middle nasal meatus.[21] This opening bifurcates to allow the communication with the rostral and caudal maxillary sinuses while preventing direct communication between the two maxillary sinuses.[22] The sphenopalatine sinus communicates rostrally with the caudal maxillary sinus and infrequently has direct communication with the ventral nasal meatus.[22] This sinus is located ventrally to the cranial vault within the sphenoid bone, and the lateral wall is associated with the pterygoid fossa. The septum between the right and left sides of the sphenoid varies in position, and the two sides are never equal size.[22] This sinus is closely associated with the ethmoid labyrinth and optic canal; therefore disease such as infection or ethmoid hematomas can result in vision loss.

Because of the large network of sinuses and meatuses within the nasal cavity, assessing the location of lesions can be difficult with conventional radiography. Because all the structures are superimposed, determining whether a soft tissue structure is present within a sinus, the nasal cavity, or both is sometimes impossible. In addition, the primary limitation of both CT and conventional radiography is that soft tissue and fluid have the same relative attenuation/opacity. Some have suggested the use of intravenous contrast medium–enhanced CT to help differentiate soft tissue from fluid because the soft tissue of a mass or nasal mucosa should enhance with contrast medium administration, whereas fluid would not. This

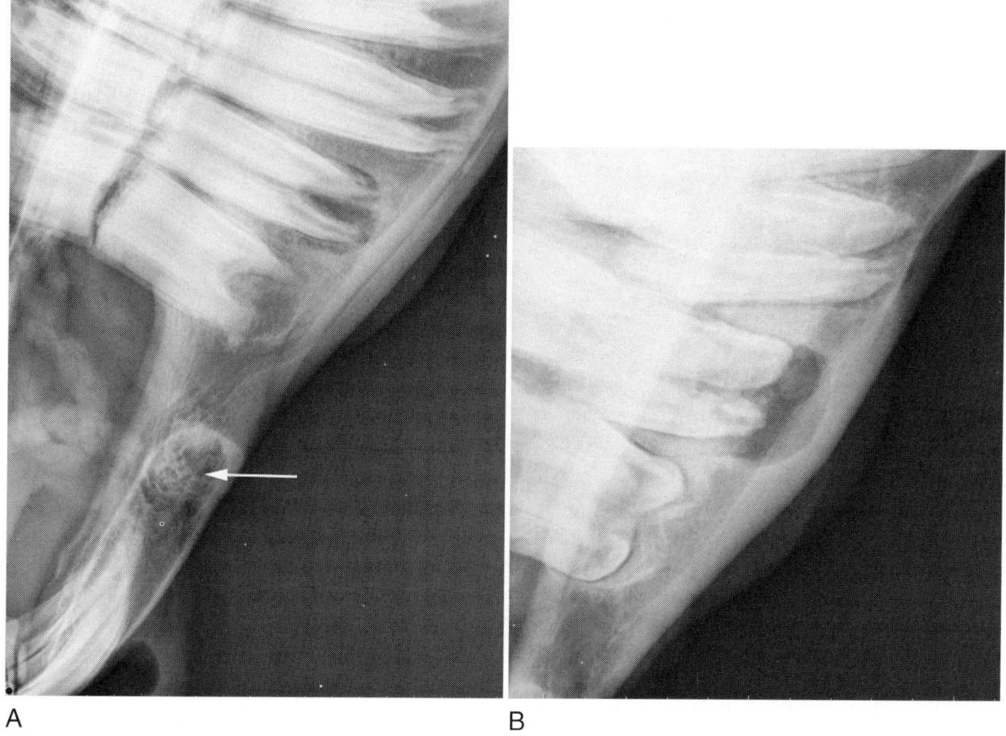

Fig. 10-8 Lateral (A) and RDLVO (B) radiographs of the rostral aspect of the head of a horse with a tooth root abscess. **A,** A region of lucency can be seen around the roots of one of the third mandibular premolars. Determining whether the affected tooth is on the left or the right is impossible. Also note the heterogeneous appearance of the mandibular symphysis *(arrow)*; this is often misinterpreted as an aggressive lesion. The rope halter can be seen superimposed over the symphyseal region; care must be taken to avoid misinterpretation of a halter as a lesion. **B,** The lysis is clearly localized to the right arcade. Note the irregularity of the rostral root of the right third mandibular premolar.

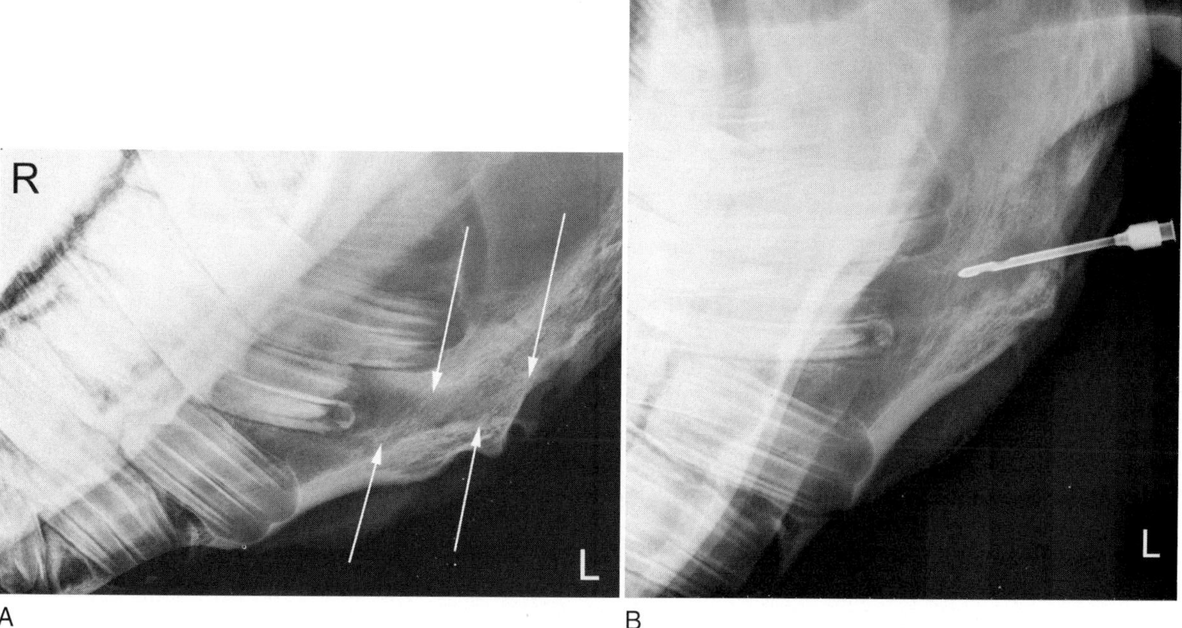

Fig. 10-9 RDLVO projection without (A) and with (B) a cannula present in a draining tract from the ventral aspect of the mandible. The caudal tooth root of the left mandibular first molar is radiolucent, and a well-margined radiolucent tract is visible within the body of the mandible *(arrows)*. This is an example of a mandibular apical tooth root abscess with an associated draining tract.

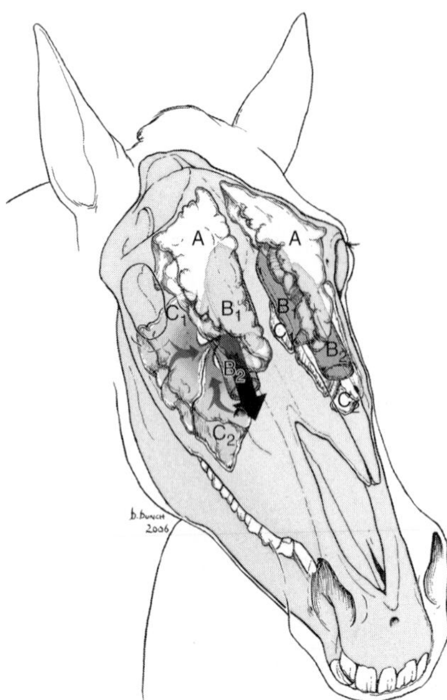

Fig. 10-10 A schematic representation of the equine nasal sinuses and their communications. *A*, Conchofrontal sinus; B_1, dorsal nasal meatus; B_2, middle nasal meatus; C_1, caudal maxillary sinus; C_2, rostral maxillary sinus.

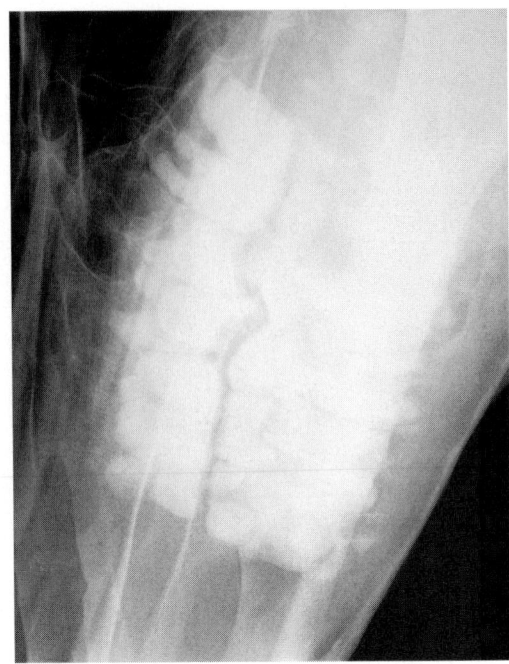

Fig. 10-11 LDRVO radiograph of the head of a 41-year-old pony. Note the irregular occlusive surface of the teeth, termed "wave mouth." This is usually seen in older animals as a result of improper dental care.

problem of differentiation is negated with MR imaging. With MR imaging, focus is possible on the T2 characteristics of fluid, both with T2 and fluid attenuating inversion recovery (FLAIR) sequences, to see the difference between fluid and soft tissue. This fundamental principle of MR imaging makes it the modality of choice when evaluating soft tissue structures of the head.

For radiography of the nasal cavity and paranasal sinuses, the acquisition of left to right and right to left lateral radiographs is important, as well as dorsoventral, LVRDO, and LDRVO radiographs, to maximize the chance of detecting abnormalities such as fluid lines and determine if bilateral disease is present.[23] When performing oblique radiographic projections, the angle should be approximately 60 degrees in the dorsal or ventral direction to try to minimize the superimposition of the contralateral sinus.[4] The oblique radiographs can also be acquired with a speculum placed within the horse's mouth so that the occlusive surface of the teeth can be better evaluated.[24]

To understand the development and association of disease processes in the sinuses and teeth, an understanding of the normal anatomy of the equine head is important. The main point to note is that the maxillary cheek teeth are embedded within a thin rim of alveolar bone that separates the teeth from the overlying paranasal sinuses. This close association changes throughout the life of the horse. In young foals, the last premolar and first molar project into the rostral and caudal maxillary sinuses, respectively. As the horse grows, the teeth migrate forward so that the rostral maxillary sinus makes contact with the last premolar and first molar, and the caudal maxillary sinus makes contact with the second and third molar. As the horse continues to age the tooth roots regress, and by 20 years of age a limited amount of the tooth root is embedded in the maxillary sinus cavity.[21] This constant growth can cause abnormal wear to occur to some teeth compared with others. Without proper dental care, an undulating pattern to the teeth can occur, usually in older horses. These will cause a malocclusion, or "wave mouth" (Fig. 10-11) that results in dropping feed during mastication, called quidding.

Another variation in normal dental anatomy is seen in horses aged approximately 2 to 4 years. At this time, the alveolus surrounding the tooth roots in the mandible expand and distort the ventral margin of the mandible. These "eruption bumps" are a transient finding but generally occur because of remnants of the deciduous tooth that prevent the normal eruption of the permanent teeth (Fig. 10-12). These remnants, often referred to as caps, are usually shed and the mandible remodels to the point that the swellings are no longer detected.[21] Occasionally the tooth root continues to grow ventrally, and this distortion can lead to a tooth root infection.

A final note is that the first premolar teeth are usually absent. However, in the rare instance in which they are present, these "wolf teeth" can generally only be detected with radiography or palpation because they rarely erupt through the mucosa (Fig. 10-13).[25] The first premolar teeth can be a cause for horses resisting a bit or tossing their heads under the saddle and may require extraction.

The most common diseases of the nasal cavity and paranasal sinuses include fractures, primary sinusitis, sinusitis from dental disease, dentigerous cysts, maxillary sinus cysts, ethmoid hematomas, and neoplasia.[4,25] These diseases are usually detected with conventional radiography; however, they are difficult to differentiate because of the superimposition of structures as well as the similar opacity between soft tissue and fluid.

Fractures of the nasal cavity and sinuses are frequently the result of direct trauma that causes displacement of bone into the air-filled spaces.[4] These depression fractures can be difficult to assess with radiographs because the radiographic projection needs to be tangential to the fracture to see the defect (Fig. 10-14).[4,5] Care must be taken to evaluate fracture fragments for sequestrum formation from a loss of blood supply and infection of the bone fragment.[4,25]

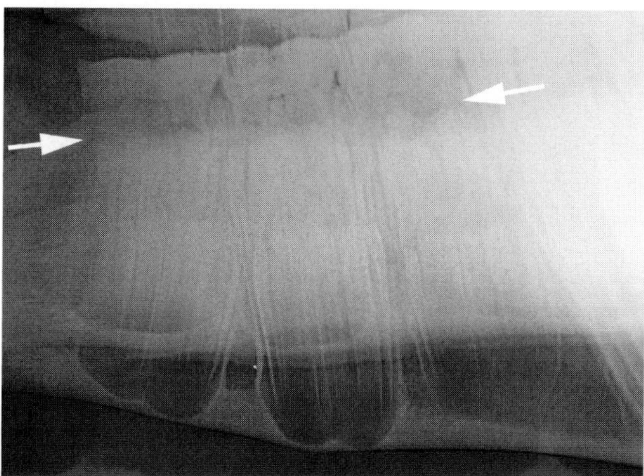

Fig. 10-12 Left 10° dorsal–right ventral radiograph of the rostral premolar area of a 2-year-old Oldenberg. The deciduous premolars have not yet been shed. The arrow indicates the plane between the deciduous and permanent premolars, and the deciduous premolars are visible dorsal to the plane indicated by the *arrows*. These deciduous premolars are termed "caps." Note the bulbous, radiolucent region around the roots of the permanent premolars. This is a normal appearance. These regions are termed "eruption bumps" and may be palpable along the ventral aspect of the mandible. They will remodel as the deciduous teeth are shed and the permanent premolars erupt. They are often misinterpreted as abscesses but are a normal finding.

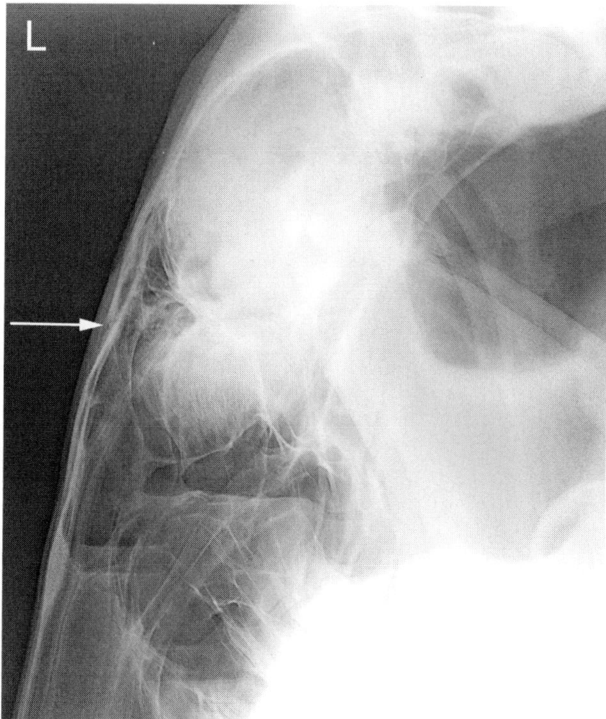

Fig. 10-14 Right-left lateral radiograph of a depression fracture of the frontal bone (*arrow*). Also note the multiple fluid lines in the conchofrontal, caudal maxillary, and rostral maxillary sinuses.

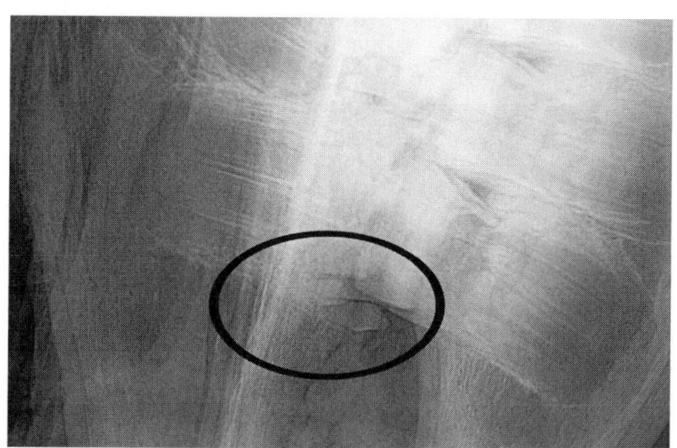

Fig. 10-13 Right-left lateral radiograph of the head showing the first maxillary premolars, also known as "wolf teeth" *(circle)*.

Sinusitis in horses is characterized by the accumulation of fluid in one of the many nasal sinuses. Although sinusitis can occur from a respiratory tract disease, it is also almost equally associated with other conditions such as tooth root abscesses.[4,10,23,25-27] Tooth root abscesses can cause sinusitis because certain caudal maxillary cheek teeth are surrounded by the rostral and caudal maxillary sinuses, with only a narrow portion of bone separating the two structures. In the standing horse, fluid within the sinuses will be in the dependent portion of the involved sinus cavity and will form an air-fluid interface (Fig. 10-15). If the horse is recumbent, note that this gas-fluid interface will not be seen because the x-ray beam will not strike the gas-fluid interface in a parallel orientation. Because fluid is generally uniform in opacity and, if heterogeneous, inspissation of the purulent material or mineralization should be considered.[25] Care should also be used to determine if multiple fluid lines are present. The location of fluid lines within specific sinuses can help with the differential diagnosis. In addition, removing fluid from the sinuses and then repeating radiographs may aid in identifying tooth root abscesses, cysts, or tumors that were previously masked by the fluid.[4,25]

A dentigerous cyst, also called temporal teratoma or "ear tooth," can vary in shape but generally has the appearance of a tooth near the region of the external acoustic meatus; an associated draining tract usually is present.[4,25,28] The cyst is believed to be caused by a failure of the first branchial cleft to close during development.[29] Radiographs tangential to the lesion are helpful to confirm the diagnosis (Fig. 10-16).[4]

Maxillary sinus cysts and progressive ethmoid hematomas appear similar on radiographs and may have a common origin.[27,30] They are both well-margined, round, soft tissue opacities that appear within the equine sinuses. Maxillary sinus cysts generally occur rostral to the ethmoid turbinates and are superimposed on the rostral or caudal maxillary sinus. These cysts are usually found in young horses less than 1 year of age or horses older than 9 years (Fig. 10-17).[27]

Ethmoid hematomas usually involve horses older than 7 years, and Arabians and Thoroughbreds appear to be overrepresented.[30,31] A progressive ethmoid hematoma is generally in contact with the ethmoid region; however, they have been reported in the frontal, maxillary, and sphenopalatine sinuses.[30,32,33] Progressive ethmoid hematomas are usually unilateral,[25,30,34] though they may grow large enough to cross the ethmoidal septum (Fig. 10-18).[30] These lesions may result in secondary fluid accumulation within the sinuses because of physical obstruction of normal drainage of the

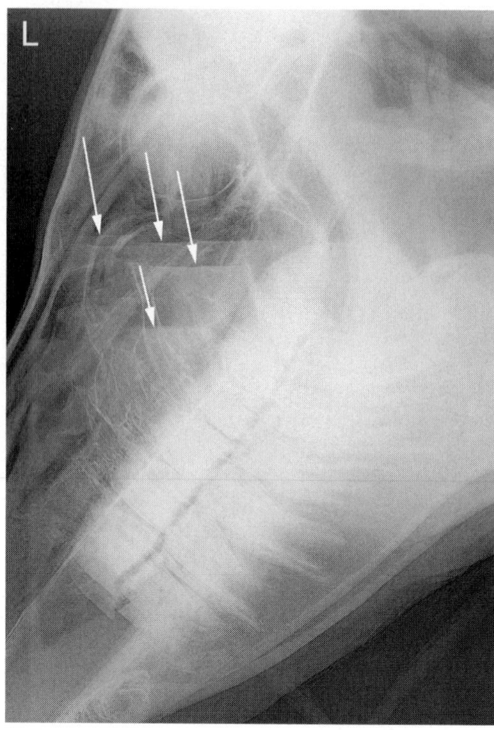

Fig. 10-15 Right-left standing lateral radiograph of the head of a 20-year-old Arabian with sinusitis. Multiple fluid lines within the conchofrontal, caudal maxillary, and rostral maxillary sinuses are present *(arrows)*.

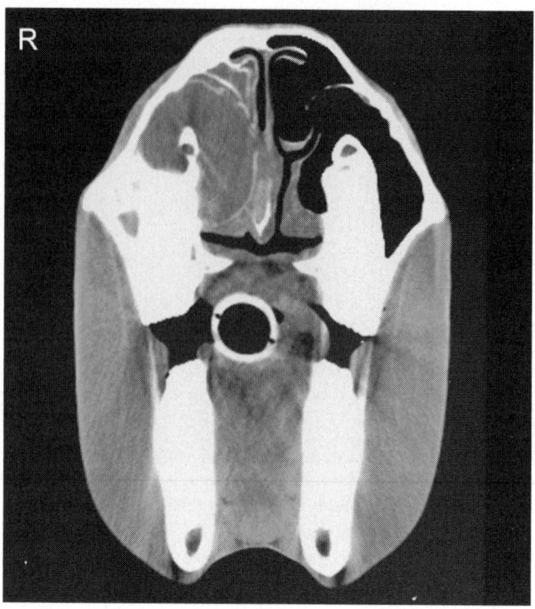

Fig. 10-17 Transverse CT image of the caudal aspect of the nasal cavity displayed in a soft tissue window. A region of soft tissue/fluid surrounds the infraorbital canal and creates a mass effect. After contrast medium administration, no enhancement supported the abnormality as being a fluid-filled cyst within the caudal maxillary sinus.

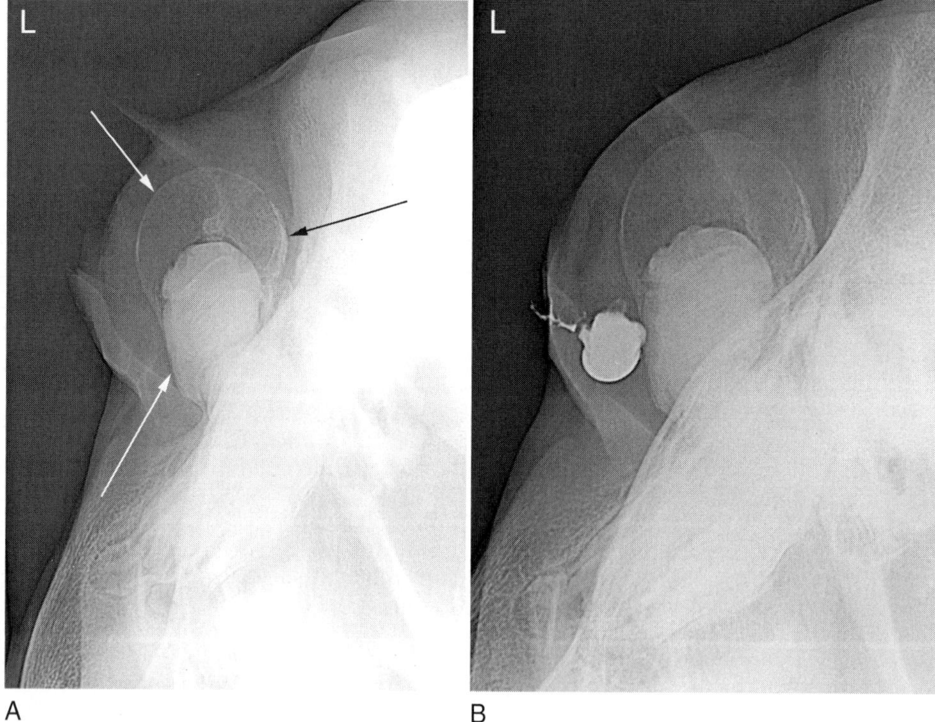

Fig. 10-16 Oblique radiographs of the left temporal region in a 3-year-old quarter horse with swelling and a draining tract in this region. Note that the mineral opacity in the region of the temporal bone on the survey radiographs **(A)** has the appearance of a tooth *(arrows)*. Contrast medium was placed into the draining tract and makes contact with this mineral opacity **(B)**.

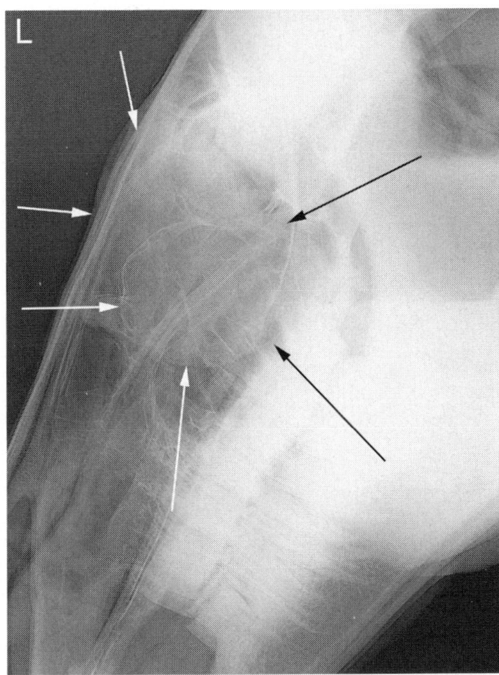

A

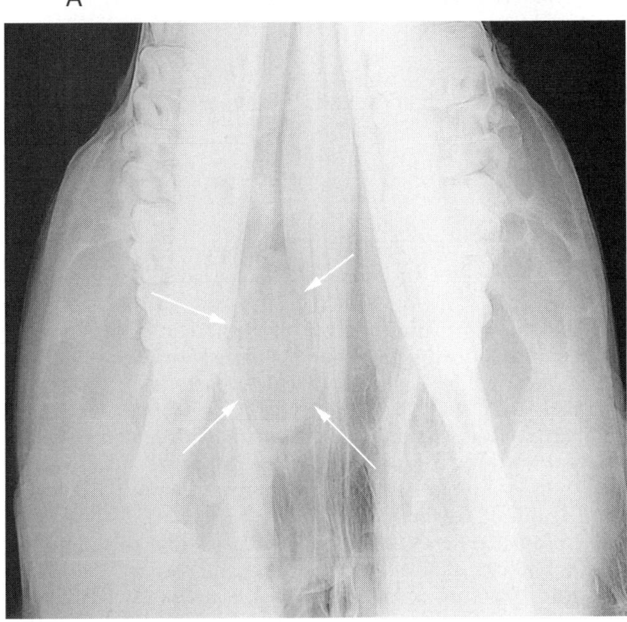

B

Fig. 10-18 A, Right-left lateral radiograph of the head. A soft tissue opacity is visible in the region of the ethmoid labyrinth from an ethmoid hematoma. **B,** Dorsoventral skull radiograph, where the typical location of an ethmoid hematoma can be seen *(arrows)*.

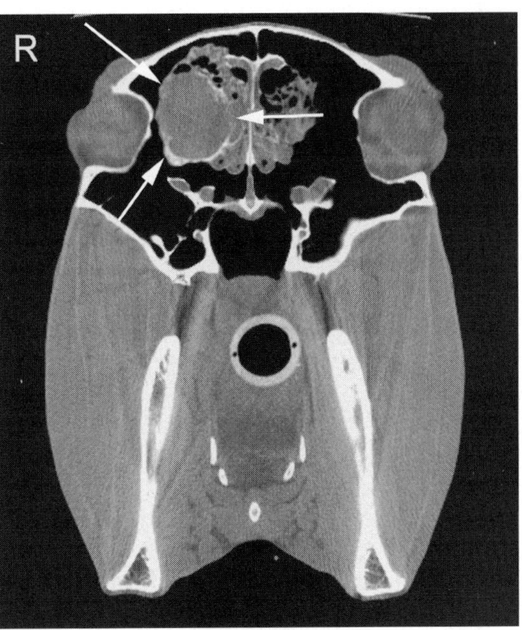

Fig. 10-19 Transverse CT image of the region of the ethmoid labyrinth displayed in a soft tissue window. Note the mass extending into the right frontal sinus that has an attenuation consistent with either soft tissue or fluid. This is an ethmoid hematoma.

sinus cavities. In addition, sinus cysts and neoplasia are the sinonasal disorders that most frequently cause deformation of the skull.[26]

Although neoplasia does occur in the equine nasal passage, it is rare, being reported in 7.6% of 277 horses in one study.[26] Tumors are generally advanced at the time of diagnosis; however, metastasis of nasal tumors is considered uncommon.[30] The most common nasal tumor in horses is squamous cell carcinoma, and whether it originates from the nasal or oral cavity is unclear.[30,34,35] Other tumors have been reported, including adenocarcinoma,[36,37] fibrosarcoma, osteoma, lymphosarcoma, hemangiosarcoma, myxoma, osteosarcoma, ameloblastic odontoma, and dentigerous cysts, but generally these are single-patient reports.[30,34,38] The two tumors most distinct on radiographs are the osteoma[25,39] and dentigerous cyst.[25] Osteomas are mineral opacities that are smoothly margined and protrude from the bone surface.[30,39] Osteomas are believed to be hamartomas, which are malformations characterized by increased production of normal tissue that stops growing when the animal reaches adulthood.[30] Osteomas are generally monostotic and cause adjacent bones to undergo pressure necrosis.[30]

Although determining the difference between a neoplasm and a cyst may not be possible with CT, the location of the mass can be accurately identified, which may guide the most advantageous approach to remove the lesion (Fig. 10-19). MR imaging, or administration of contrast medium during CT evaluation, should help differentiate between a fluid-filled cyst and a neoplastic mass and generally provides more information than does conventional radiography alone (Fig. 10-20).[40,41]

Skull and Hyoid Apparatus

When examining the skull, a dorsoventral view and right and left lateral radiographs are required. Further evaluation depends on what portion of the skull is being examined. If an orbital fracture is suspected, then oblique projections are highly recommended. Unlike the oblique radiographs for sinus evaluation, the oblique radiographs for the orbit require a steeper angle. If a right orbital fracture is suspected, then a right 70-degree ventral to left dorsal oblique radiograph allows the rim of the frontal bone to be visible with minimal superimposition of other structures (Fig. 10-21).

Other fractures involving the skull include nasofrontal suture separation, occipitosphenoid suture separation, and

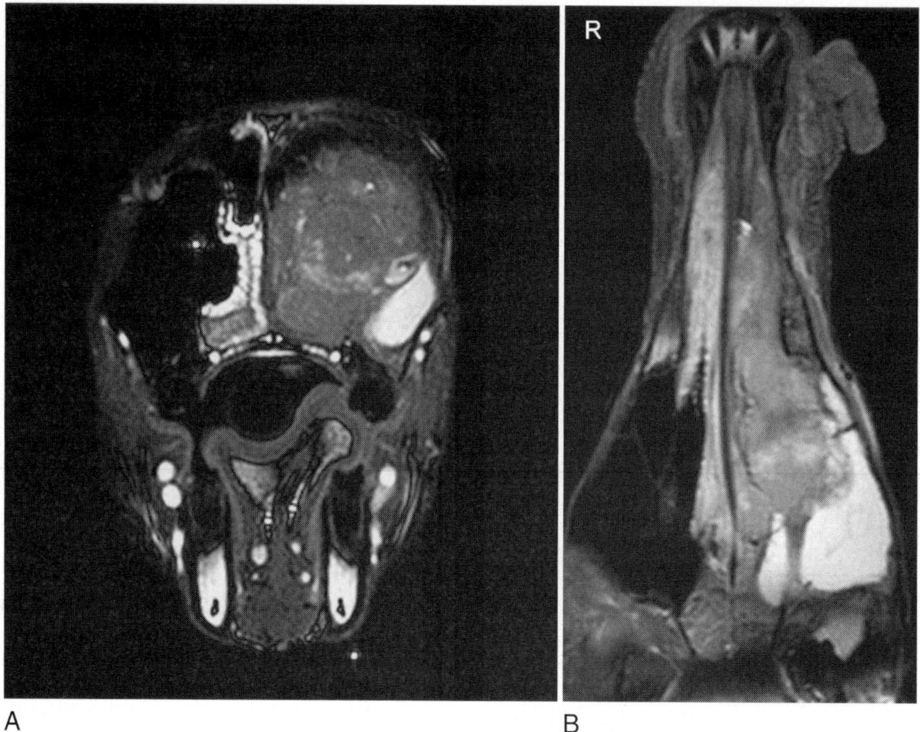

Fig. 10-20 T2-weighted MR images in the transverse (A) and dorsal (B) planes. Note the high signal area on the periphery of the gray, soft tissue, intense mass. This is fluid within the sinus outlining a nasal lymphoma.

fractures of the stylohyoid and petrous temporal bone caused by temporomandibular osteoarthropathy.[7,25] Nasofrontal suture separation is considered a periostitis and is usually not associated with trauma. Nasofrontal suture separation has been called "horns" because it generally causes firm bumps to appear where the frontal bone contacts the nasal bone. On lateral or oblique radiographs, nasofrontal suture separation appears as a periostitis with smoothly margined new bone formation causing a raised area. A suture line can usually be seen that should not be mistaken for a fracture line. Nasofrontal suture separation is usually not clinically important, though it often leaves permanent disfigurement (Fig. 10-22).[25]

Occipitosphenoid suture separation generally occurs when a horse falls backwards. When the nuchal crest hits the ground it acts as a pivot point, causing the head to hyperextend.[7] This extension stretches the rectus capitus ventralis minor and the longus capitus muscles and can cause a fracture of the basisphenoid bone or avulsion of the muscular attachment site.[7,42] Because the dorsal aspect of the guttural pouch is adjacent to these muscles, damage to the muscles can lead to hemorrhage within the guttural pouch or the retropharyngeal space (Fig. 10-23).[7,42] Because the suture of the basisphenoid bone fuses between 2 and 5 years of age, older horses are believed to be less prone to separation of the occipitosphenoid bones.[7,42,43]

Temporohyoid osteoarthropathy is a disease characterized by fusion of the stylohyoid bone to the temporal bone at the level of the tympanic bulla. The hyoid apparatus in the horse consists of paired stylohyoid bones, paired ceratohyoid bones, a single basihyoid bone, a lingual process, and paired thyrohyoid bones. This apparatus serves to support the tongue, pharynx, and larynx.[44-46] Temporohyoid osteoarthropathy causes ankylosis of the temporohyoid joint, which puts abnormal force on the petrous temporal bone as well as the stylohyoid bone when the horse swallows or moves its tongue.[44-47] Temporohyoid osteoarthropathy has been reported to cause clinical signs of vestibular disease and/or facial paresis as well as behavioral changes; however, it has also been diagnosed in clinically normal horses at postmortem examination.[44,45,47,48] Varying causes have been suggested, ranging from extension of otitis media/externa or guttural pouch infection to a nonseptic osteoarthritis.[44,46-48] To diagnose temporohyoid osteoarthropathy, endoscopy,[46] radiography,[44,48] and CT examination[45] have been used. Although all these modalities are useful, only CT was able to determine the presence of fluid within the tympanic cavity.[45] In severe afflictions, fracture of the stylohyoid bone will occur, which can be detected with conventional radiography or CT examination (Fig. 10-24).

Brain

Cholesterol granulomas, pituitary tumors, hydrocephalus, brain tumors, and brain abscess have all been reported in horses. The diagnosis, extent of disease, and surgical treatment plan for various disease processes can all be determined by CT and MR imaging.

Brain tumors are considered uncommon, with the most recognized disorder centered on the accumulation of cholesterol crystals, breakdown products, red blood cells in the ventricular system.[49] These lesions appear as high attenuating, roughly circular lesions within the lateral ventricles that create a mass effect (Fig. 10-25). Other tumors, such as nasal adenocarcinoma, may arise from the nasal cavity and extend into the brain, but this is considered rare. These soft tissue tumors generally arise from or involve the cribriform plate and then extend into the cranial vault.[36]

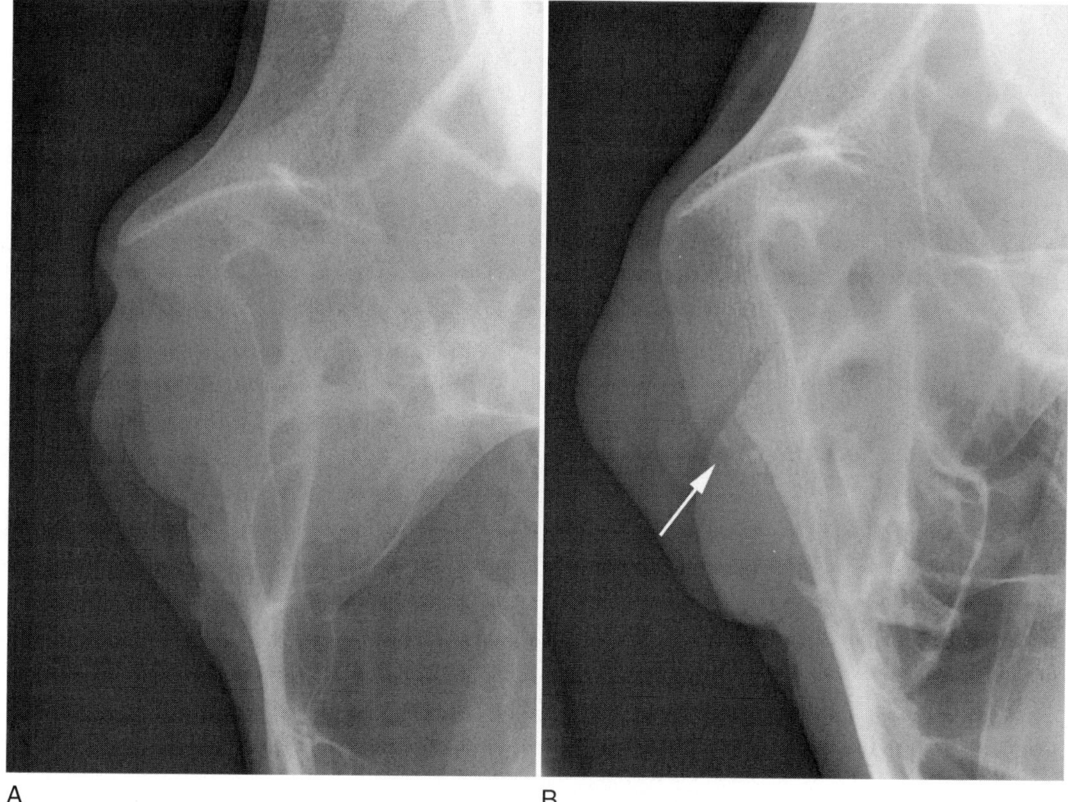

Fig. 10-21 Oblique radiographs of a normal left supraorbital process (A) and a right (B) supraorbital process that has sustained fractures *(arrow)* from a horse kick. These images are from the same horse.

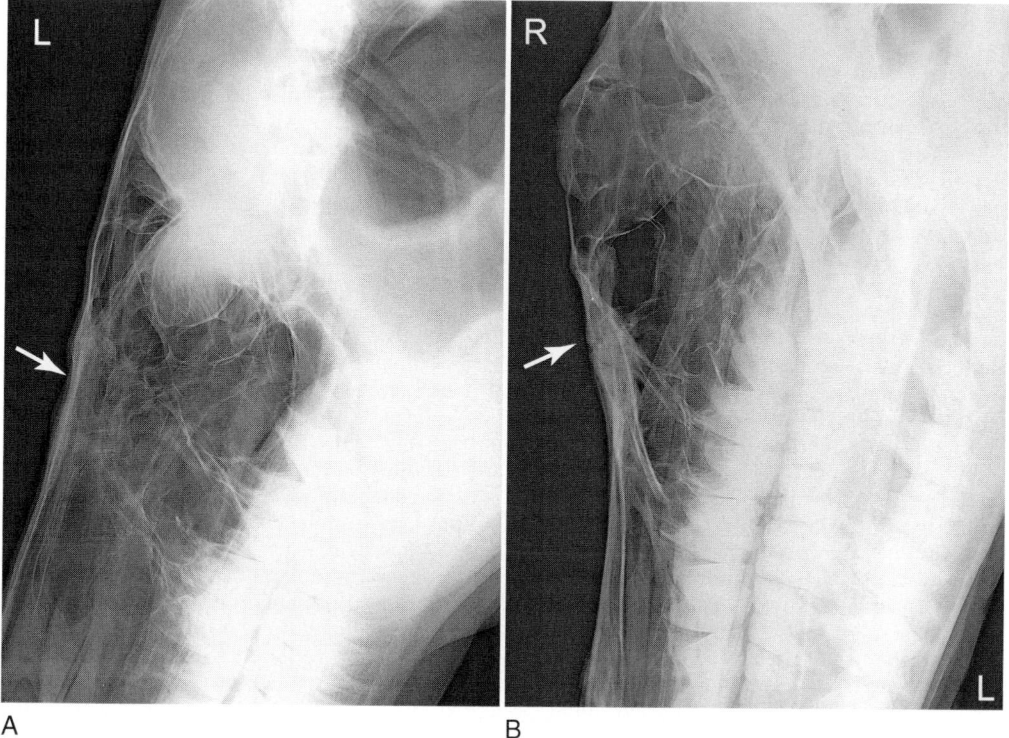

Fig. 10-22 Theses are right-left lateral (A) and left rostrodorsal/right caudoventral oblique radiographs of the head. Note the area of increased bone opacity at the rostral aspect of the frontal bone. This is an example of nasofrontal suture separation, also known as "horns."

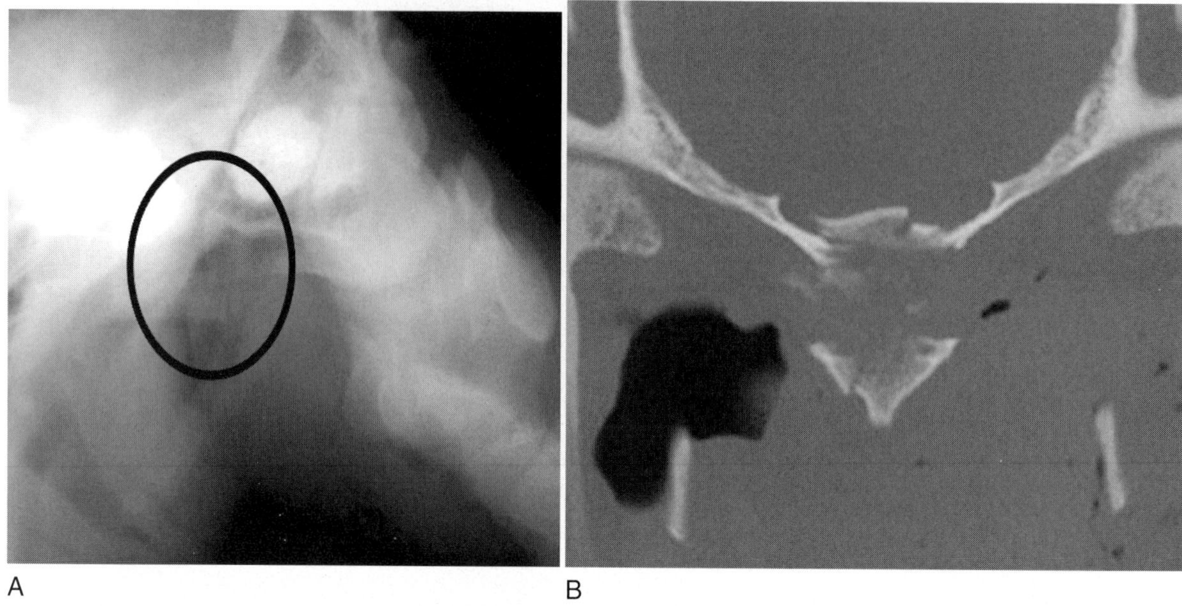

Fig. 10-23 Left-right lateral radiograph of the head **(A)** in a thoroughbred colt that fell backwards. The basisphenoid bone is displaced ventrally in relation to the basioccipital bone *(circle)*. The guttural pouch is filled with a soft tissue/fluid opacity that displaces and compresses the nasopharynx ventrally. This is caused by hemorrhage and hematoma formation likely a result of avulsion of the longus capitus and/or rectus capitus ventralis muscles and fracture of the basisphenoid and basioccipital bones. A CT examination thorough the basisphenoid region **(B)** shows the severely displaced and comminuted fracture of the basisphenoid bone.

Brain abscesses are also rare but can be seen after severe head trauma and open fractures of the calvaria. Abscess lends itself well to evaluation with CT or MR imaging, but these modalities require general anesthesia, which is complicated in head trauma patients. On CT images, brain abscesses appear as low attenuating regions that create a mass effect and have ring enhancement after contrast medium administration (Fig. 10-26). With MR imaging, the lesion will have low signal intensity on T1-weighted images but high signal on T2-weighted images, including FLAIR. The contrast medium enhancement pattern seen is similar to CT, with a low signal region surrounded by a ring of contrast medium enhancement.

Guttural Pouch and Larynx

The large air-filled spaces of the larynx and guttural pouch make examination of these regions amenable to radiography. In fact, radiography should be considered a complement to endoscopic evaluation of the equine head.[50] Evaluation of the guttural pouches and larynx generally consists of a lateral radiograph. Dorsoventral projections can be accomplished with the patient standing, but obtaining an image sufficiently far caudally is difficult without having motion artifacts occur. For this reason, a ventrodorsal radiograph under general anesthesia is required to produce an image of the caudal aspect of the skull and the cranial cervical region of a horse.[50,51] Acquiring right-to-left and left-to-right lateral radiographs has been suggested to avoid the ventrodorsal view.[18] Another method involves acquiring a right 30-degree caudal to left rostral oblique radiograph and a left 30-degree caudal to right rostral oblique radiograph to separate the guttural pouches.[18] Although this would not result in an orthogonal projection of the larynx or guttural pouches, it would help separate the guttural pouches enough to establish whether unilateral or bilateral disease was present (Fig. 10-27).

The goal of radiography of the guttural pouch is generally to identify the presence of soft tissue opacity in the usually gas-filled structure (Fig. 10-28). The appearance of this opacity varies depending on the disease, such as multiple smoothly margined, irregularly shaped masses caused by chronic guttural pouch mycosis and chondroids. (Fig. 10-29). In addition, fluid lines that indicate an air-fluid interface do not provide any information regarding the nature of the fluid in the guttural pouch (hemorrhage, empyema, or diverticulitis) but may be used to determine if unilateral or bilateral disease is present.[50,51] Areas that surround the guttural pouch, such as the wall of the pharynx (ventral border of the guttural pouch), may appear thick or irregular when pharyngeal lymphoid hyperplasia is present. In addition, in foals the guttural pouch can be diffusely gas filled, tympanic, and extend beyond the level of the first cervical vertebrae (the atlas) (Fig. 10-30).[25,51]

Tumors or cervical masses in, or encroaching on, the guttural pouch are rare; however, structures displacing the guttural pouch include masses of the parotid salivary gland or retropharyngeal lymph nodes, or a primary tumor of the guttural pouch, usually squamous cell carcinoma.[51] Differentiating masses from fluid, and whether the mass is within or adjacent to the guttural pouch, is difficult and usually requires endoscopy or ultrasonography.[18] Because the parotid salivary gland can sometimes cause guttural pouch lesions, contrast medium can be placed into the salivary gland to produce a sialogram. However, sialography is rarely performed because of the risk of damaging the salivary gland with the hyperosmolar contrast medium.[50] Scintigraphy can also be used to assess salivary gland function. By administering technetium-

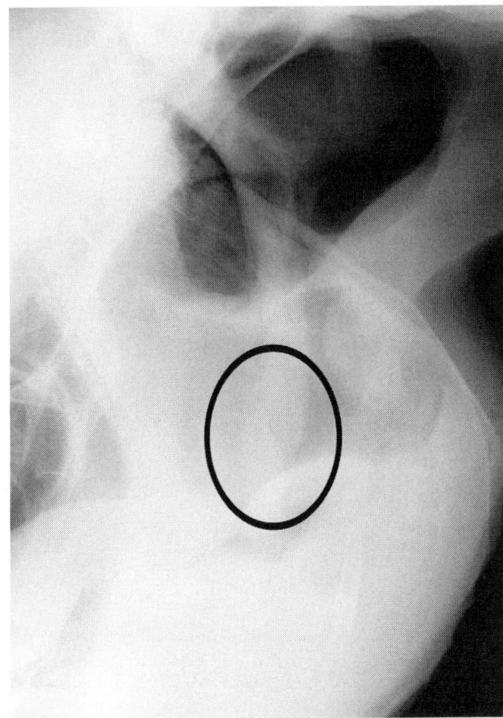

A

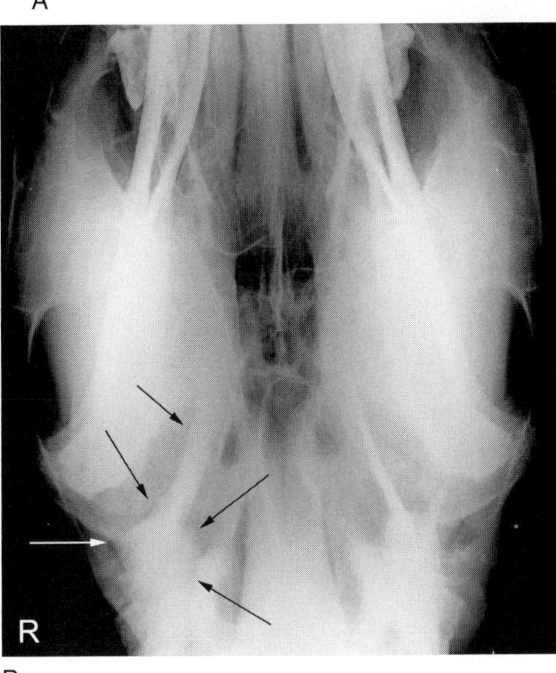

B

Fig. 10-24 Lateral (A) and dorsoventral (B) radiographs of the head. The right stylohyoid bone is fractured *(circle)* and *(arrow)* thick compared with the left. The area of the petrous temporal bone on the right is also more opaque and larger than the left. This fracture and increased size is a result of temporohyoid osteoarthropathy.

99m pertechnetate, which accumulates in salivary glands, documentation of the approximate size of the parotid salivary gland and the function and patency of the parotid salivary duct is possible. After adequate activity is detected in the salivary gland, the duct can be imaged after offering a piece of food (such as a mint or a carrot) and obtaining a static acquisition of the head in both lateral and ventral planes (Fig. 10-31).

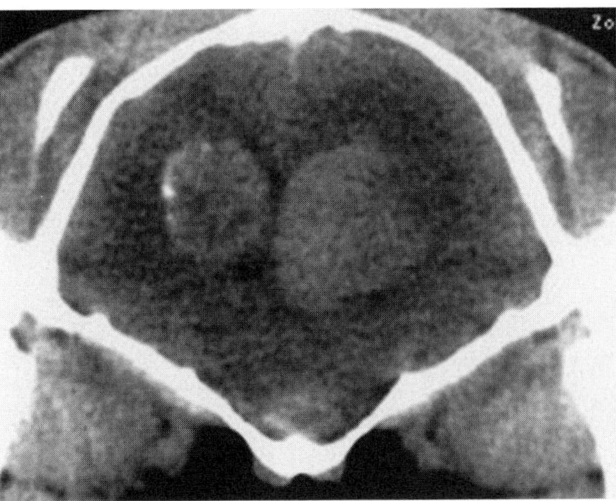

Fig. 10-25 Transverse CT image of the brain and surrounding structures displayed in a soft tissue window. Note the two large, circular, mineral-attenuating structures in the region of the lateral ventricles. This is an example of cholesterol granulomas. (Courtesy Cornell University, Ithaca, NY.)

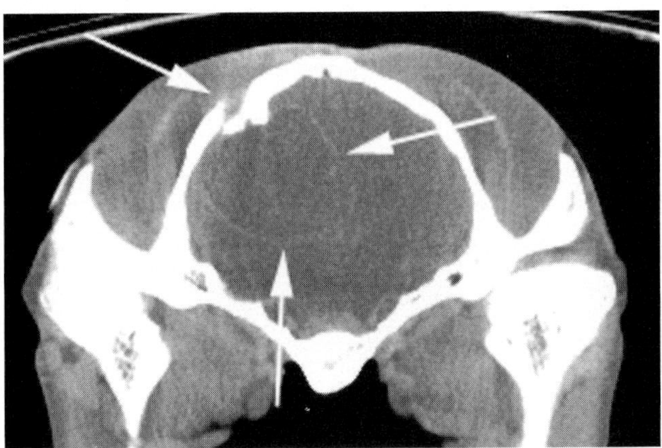

Fig. 10-26 Transverse CT image of the brain and surrounding structures after contrast medium administration and displayed in a soft tissue window. A depression fracture of the right parietal bone and a ring-enhancing lesion within the brain are visible. This ring-enhancing lesion is the vascular capsule of a brain abscess caused by penetrating trauma to the calvaria. (Courtesy Dr. Nathan Dykes, Cornell University, Ithaca, NY.)

CT has not been reported as an aid to diagnosing guttural pouch disease in the horse, but it has been used to determine the anatomy of the guttural pouch.[14,52] CT may help identify bone lesions, such as avulsion fractures, or petrous temporal bone fractures that may cause hemorrhage into the guttural pouches.[7] Blood has been reported to accumulate in the guttural pouch as a result of avulsion of the longus capitis muscle[42] and with fracture of the stylohyoid bone. However, because of the vasodilatory effects of anesthetics and manipulation of the patient for CT examination, the risk of complications outweighs the benefits of the procedure. Therefore surgical exploration is still the diagnostic modality of choice.[18]

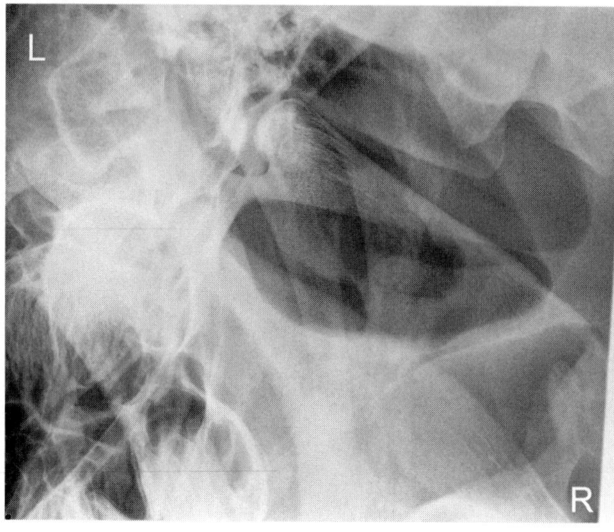

Fig. 10-27 Left caudoventral/right rostrodorsal oblique radiograph of the temporomandibular and guttural pouch regions in a normal horse. Note that right and left guttural pouches can be seen individually and the right temporomandibular joint is clearly identified. The left temporomandibular joint is superimposed on the petrous temporal bone. An artifact from superimposition of a rope halter is superimposed on the guttural pouches.

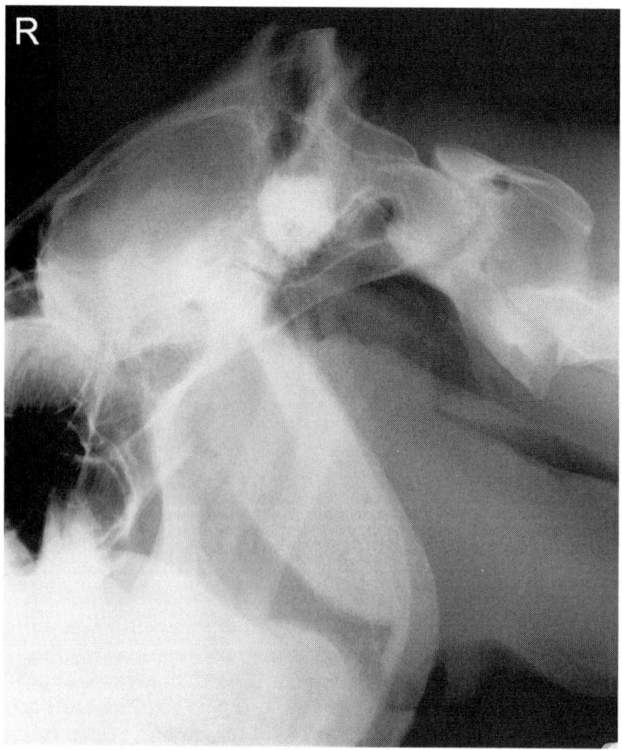

Fig. 10-28 Right-left lateral radiograph of the laryngeal region of an 11-year-old Arabian with bilateral purulent nasal discharge. In the region of the guttural pouch and extending caudally into the retropharyngeal region is a large, heterogeneous soft tissue opacity with multiple small gas opacities. This lesion creates a mass effect that displaces the larynx and trachea ventrally. This patient was diagnosed with guttural pouch empyema and retropharyngeal lymph node enlargement.

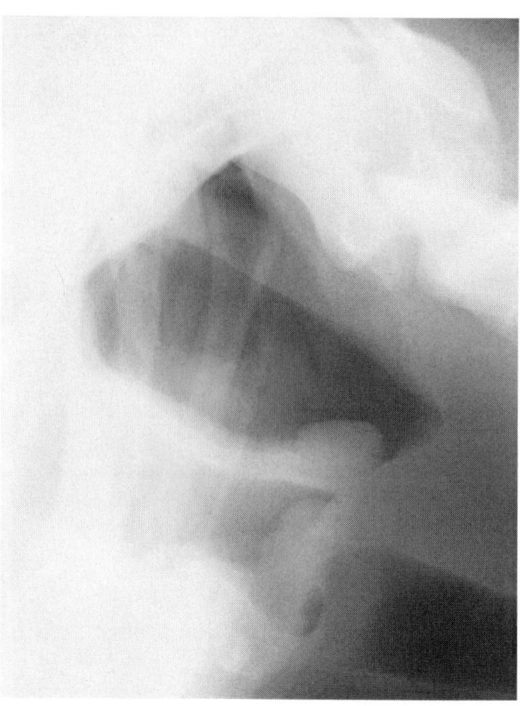

Fig. 10-29 Left-right lateral radiograph of the head. A solitary, smooth-margined soft tissue opacity is in the guttural pouch. This is a focus of inflammatory debris called a chondroid.

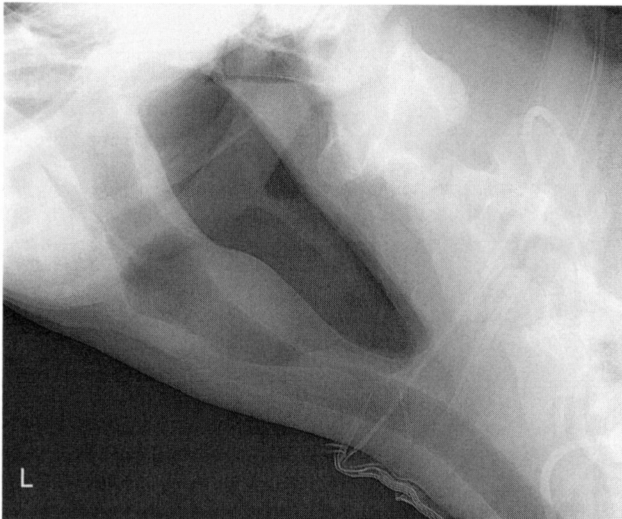

Fig. 10-30 Right-left lateral radiograph of the cranial cervical region in a 2-month-old quarter horse with guttural pouch tympany. Note the elongated appearance of the guttural pouch. Also observe how the guttural pouch extends beyond the caudal margin of the first cervical vertebra, beyond its normal anatomic limit.

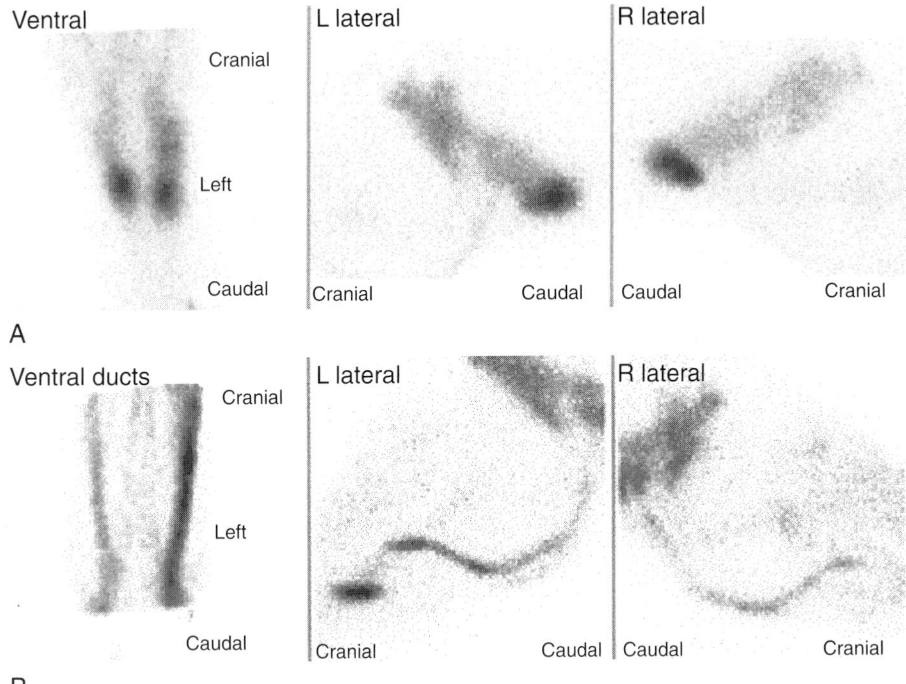

Fig. 10-31 A, Scintigraphic images acquired 20 minutes after 50 mCi of technetium-99m pertechnetate was administered intravenously. The parotid salivary glands are shown, with the right having slightly less activity then the left. **B,** The same horse after being fed a peppermint. Activity is detected within the left parotid salivary duct to a greater degree than the right parotid salivary duct. (Images courtesy of Dr. Nathan Dykes, Cornell University, Ithaca, NY.) (See Color Plate 4.)

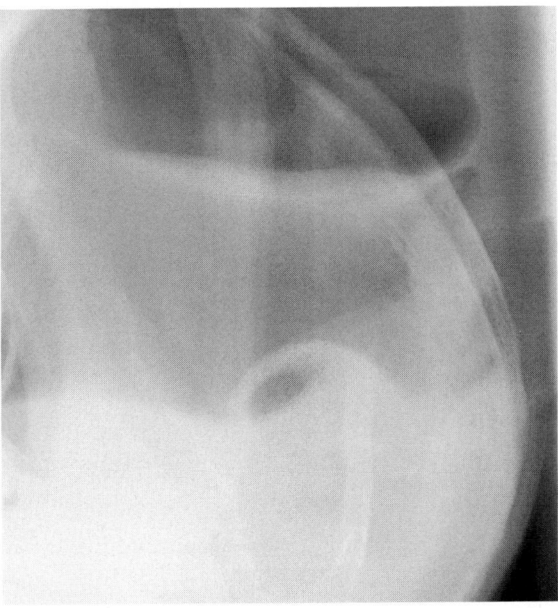

Fig. 10-32 Right-left lateral radiograph of the laryngeal region in a normal horse. Note the sharp, thin appearance of the epiglottis and its position dorsal to the soft palate.

The primary diseases of the larynx identified by conventional radiography include dorsal displacement of the soft palate, aryepiglottic fold entrapment, subepiglottic cyst, and arytenoiditis. All these diseases can be readily identified on a lateral radiograph if the reader has a general understanding of the normal anatomy of the equine epiglottis (Fig. 10-32). Because horses are obligate nasal breathers, no gas should be identified in the oral cavity of a horse except if it is heavily sedated. The epiglottis should be identified dorsal to the soft palate. If the epiglottis is ventral to the soft palate, then the soft palate is considered dorsally displaced and abnormal (Fig. 10-33). The epiglottis contains a thin piece of cartilage

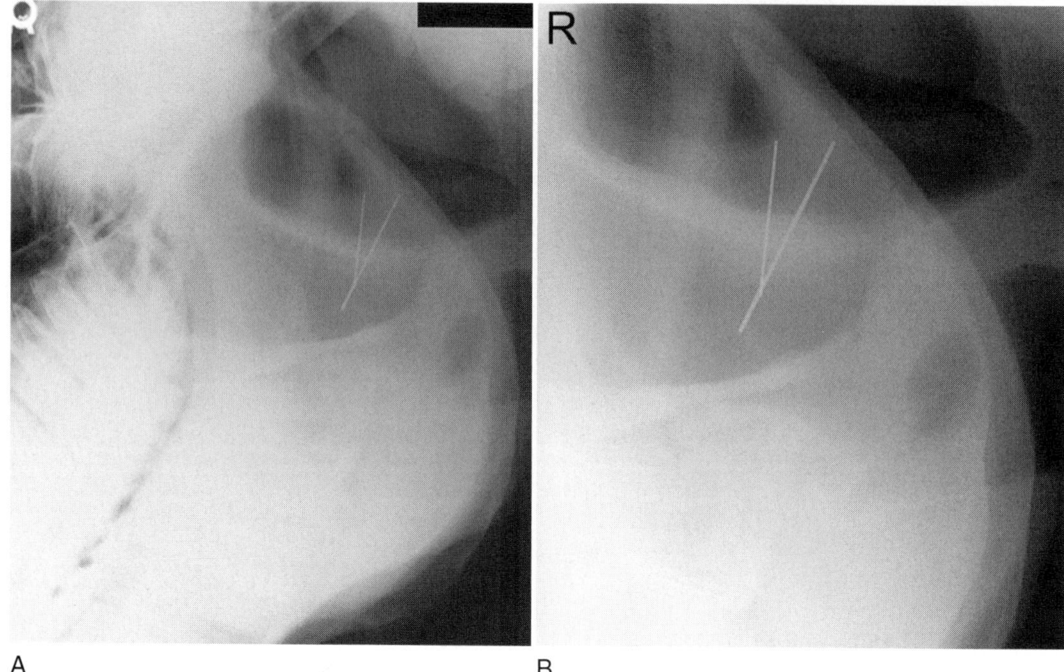

Fig. 10-33 Left-right lateral radiograph of the laryngeal region (A) and a close-up image of the epiglottis from the same radiograph (B). The epiglottis is ventral to the soft palate, indicating a dorsally displaced soft palate. Two metal opaque wires of known length are present to determine the magnification factor at the level of the epiglottis. A Mitchell marker is present in the *upper left corner* of the radiograph to verify that the exam was performed on a standing horse. (Image courtesy of Dr. Nathan Dykes, Cornell University, Ithaca, NY.)

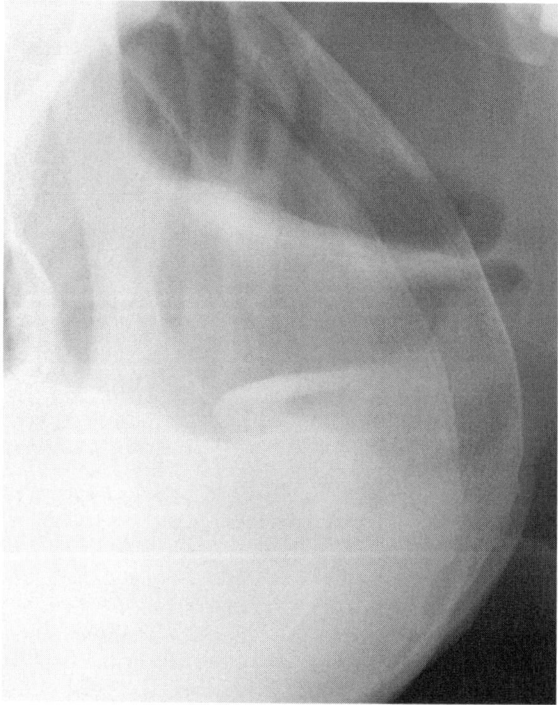

Fig. 10-34 The laryngeal region of a horse. Note the blunt appearance of the epiglottis and the prominent aryepiglottic fold. This is an example of aryepiglottic entrapment.

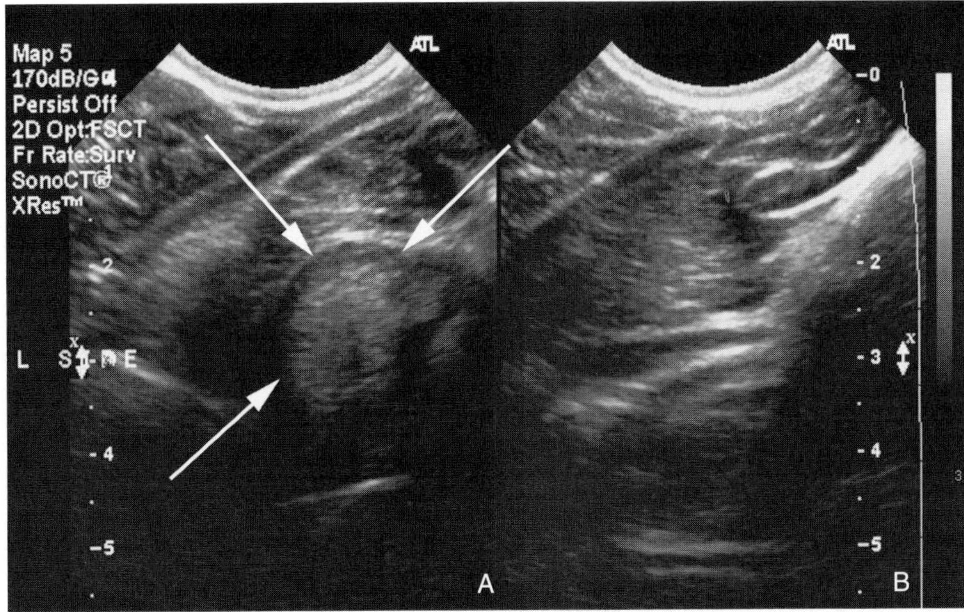

Fig. 10-35 Ultrasound images acquired from the left (A) and right (B) lateral windows of the laryngeal region of a 4-year-old female thoroughbred. An endoscopic diagnosis of left arytenoid chondritis was made characterized by incomplete abduction of the left arytenoid cartilage and enlargement of the arytenoid body and corniculate process. The ultrasound image depicts that the left arytenoid cartilage is thick and has a smoothly margined 1.7-cm bulge on the lateral surface. The right arytenoid cartilage is normal and shown for comparison. (Images courtesy of Dr. Heather Chalmers, Cornell University, Ithaca, NY.)

covered by a mucosal surface. This surface is thin, smooth, and comes to a definitive point rostrally. If the rostral aspect of the epiglottis appears blunted, then the primary differential diagnosis is an aryepiglottic fold entrapment (Fig. 10-34). A subepiglottic cyst is suspected when the epiglottis is dorsally displaced by a well-margined soft tissue/fluid opacity centered just rostroventral from the larynx. All these lesions can be confirmed by endoscopy; however, care should be taken when evaluating for dorsal displacement of the soft palate because this is a transient condition that can spontaneously correct itself.

Arytenoiditis is more difficult to identify by radiography because it generally causes a subtle irregularity in the margin of the arytenoid cartilage. The use of ultrasound to identify arytenoid cartilages in the horse has recently been presented as a technically easy method to identify arytenoiditis (Fig. 10-35); however, laryngoscopy remains the gold standard.[16]

REFERENCES

1. Henninger W, Frame EM, Willmann M et al: CT features of alveolitis and sinusitis in horses, *Vet Radiol Ultrasound* 44:269, 2003.
2. Tietje S, Becker M, Bockenhoff G: Computed tomographic evaluation of head diseases in the horse: 15 cases, *Equine Vet J* 28:98, 1996.
3. Cook W: Skeletal radiology of the equine head, *J Am Vet Radiol Soc* 11:35, 1970.
4. Park RD: Radiographic examination of the equine head, *Vet Clin North Am Equine Pract* 9:49, 1993.
5. Wyn-Jones G: Interpreting radiographs 6: the head, *Equine Vet J* 17:274, 1985.
6. Wyn-Jones G: Interpreting radiographs 6: radiology of the equine head (part 2), *Equine Vet J* 17:417, 1985.
7. MacKay RJ: Brain injury after head trauma: pathophysiology, diagnosis, and treatment, *Vet Clin North Am Equine Pract* 20:199, 2004.
8. Barakzai S, Tremaine H, Dixon P: Use of scintigraphy for diagnosis of equine paranasal sinus disorders, *Vet Surg* 35:94, 2006.
9. Weller R, Livesey L, Maierl J et al: Comparison of radiography and scintigraphy in the diagnosis of dental disorders in the horse, *Equine Vet J* 33:49, 2001.
10. Gibbs C, Lane JG: Radiographic examination of the facial, nasal and paranasal sinus regions of the horse. II. Radiological findings, *Equine Vet J* 19:474, 1987.
11. Tremaine WH, Dixon PM: A long-term study of 277 cases of equine sinonasal disease. Part 1: details of horses, historical, clinical and ancillary diagnostic findings, *Equine Vet J* 33:274, 2001.
12. Arencibia A, Vazquez JM, Jaber R et al: Magnetic resonance imaging and cross sectional anatomy of the normal equine sinuses and nasal passages, *Vet Radiol Ultrasound* 41:313, 2000.
13. Barbee DD, Allen JR, Gavin PR: Computed tomography in horses. Technique, *Veterinary Radiology & Ultrasound* 28:144, 1987.
14. Morrow KL, Park RD, Spurgeon TL et al: Computed tomographic imaging of the equine head, *Vet Radiol Ultrasound* 41:491, 2000.
15. MacDonald MH: Clinical examination of the equine head, *Vet Clin North Am Equine Pract* 9:25, 1993.
16. Chalmers H, Cheetham J, Yeager A et al: *Ultrasonography of the equine laryngeal region: technique, normal appearance, and clinical applications,* American College of Veterinary

Radiology Annual Scientific Conference Proceedings, Chicago, IL, 2005, p 36.
17. Barber SM, Clark EG, Fretz PB: Fibroblastic tumor of the premaxilla in two horses, *J Am Vet Med Assoc* 182:700, 1983.
18. Perkins G, Pease A, Fubini S: Part I: diagnosis and medical management of guttural pouch disease, *Compendium for Continuing Education* 25:966, 2003.
19. Weller R, Taylor S, Maierl J et al: Ultrasonographic anatomy of the equine temporomandibular joint, *Equine Vet J* 31:529, 1999.
20. Weller R, Cauvin ER, Bowen IM et al: Comparison of radiography, scintigraphy and ultrasonography in the diagnosis of a case of temporomandibular joint arthropathy in a horse, *Vet Rec* 144:377, 1999.
21. Dyce K, Sack W, Wensing C: The head and ventral neck of the horse. In Dyce K, Sack W, Wensing C, editors: *Veterinary anatomy,* Philadelphia, 2002, WB Saunders, p 488.
22. Schummer A, Nickel R, Sack W: Respiratory organs of the horse. In Schummer A, Nickel R, Sack W, editors: *The viscera of the domestic mammals,* ed 2, Berlin, 1979, Verlag Paul Parey, p 274.
23. Lane JG, Gibbs C, Meynink SE et al: Radiographic examination of the facial, nasal and paranasal sinus regions of the horse: I. Indications and procedures in 235 cases, *Equine Vet J* 19:466, 1987.
24. Barakzai S, Dixon P: A study of open-mouthed oblique radiographic projections for evaluating lesions of the erupted (clinical) crown, *Equine Vet Educ* AE:183, 2003.
25. Butler JA, Colles CM, Dyson SJ et al: The head. In Butler JA, Colles CM, Dyson SJ et al, editors: *Clinical radiology of the horse,* ed 2, London, 2000, Blackwell Science, pp 327-401.
26. Allen JR, Barbee DD, Boulton CR et al: Brain abscess in a horse: diagnosis by computed tomography and successful surgical treatment, *Equine Vet J* 19:552, 1987.
27. Lane JG, Longstaffe JA, Gibbs C: Equine paranasal sinus cysts: a report of 15 cases, *Equine Vet J* 19:537, 1987.
28. Provost P: Skin conditions amenable to surgery. In Auer J, Stick J, editors: *Equine surgery,* Philadelphia, 1999, WB Saunders, pp 174-175.
29. DeBowes RM, Gaughan EM: Congenital dental disease of horses, *Vet Clin North Am Equine Pract* 14:273, 1998.
30. Head KW, Dixon PM: Equine nasal and paranasal sinus tumours. Part 1: review of the literature and tumour classification, *Vet J* 157:261, 1999.
31. Specht TE, Colahan PT, Nixon AJ et al: Ethmoidal hematoma in nine horses, *J Am Vet Med Assoc* 197:613, 1990.
32. Freeman DE, Orsini PG, Ross MW et al: A large frontonasal bone flap for sinus surgery in the horse, *Vet Surg* 19:122, 1990.
33. Sullivan M, Burrell MH, McCandlish IA: Progressive haematoma of the maxillary sinus in a horse, *Vet Rec* 114:191, 1984.
34. Nickels F: Nasal passages In Auer J, Stick J, editors:. *Equine surgery,* ed 2, Philadelphia, 1999, WB Saunders, pp 334-335.
35. Walker MA, Schumacher J, Schmitz DG et al: Cobalt 60 radiotherapy for treatment of squamous cell carcinoma of the nasal cavity and paranasal sinuses in three horses, *J Am Vet Med Assoc* 212:848, 1998.
36. Davis JL, Gilger BC, Spaulding K et al: Nasal adenocarcinoma with diffuse metastases involving the orbit, cerebrum, and multiple cranial nerves in a horse, *J Am Vet Med Assoc* 221:1460, 2002.
37. Hepburn RJ, Furr MO: Sinonasal adenocarcinoma causing central nervous system disease in a horse, *J Vet Intern Med* 18:125, 2004.
38. Dixon PM, Head KW: Equine nasal and paranasal sinus tumours. Part 2: a contribution of 28 case reports, *Vet J* 157:279, 1999.
39. Schumacher J, Smith BL, Morgan SJ: Osteoma of paranasal sinuses of a horse, *J Am Vet Med Assoc* 192:1449, 1988.
40. Saunders JH, Van Bree H: Comparison of radiography and computed tomography for the diagnosis of canine aspergillosis, *Vet Radiol Ultrasound* 44:414, 2003.
41. Tucker R, Farrell E: Computed tomography and magnetic resonance imaging of the equine head, *Vet Clin North Am Equine Pract* 17:131, 2001.
42. Sweeney CR, Freeman DE, Sweeney RW et al: Hemorrhage into the guttural pouch (auditory tube diverticulum) associated with rupture of the longus capitis muscle in three horses, *J Am Vet Med Assoc* 202:1129, 1993.
43. Ramirez O 3rd, Jorgensen JS, Thrall DE: Imaging basilar skull fractures in the horse: a review, *Vet Radiol Ultrasound* 39:391, 1998.
44. Blythe LL, Watrous BJ: Temporohyoid osteoarthropathy. In Robinson NE, editor: *Current therapy in equine medicine IV,* Philadelphia, 1997, WB Saunders, pp 323-325.
45. Pease AP, van Biervliet J, Dykes NL et al: Complication of partial stylohyoidectomy for treatment of temporohyoid osteoarthropathy and an alternative surgical technique in three cases, *Equine Vet J* 36:546-550, 2004.
46. Walker AM, Sellon DC, Cornelisse CJ et al: Temporohyoid osteoarthropathy in 33 horses (1993-2000), *J Vet Intern Med* 16:697, 2002.
47. Blythe LL, Watrous BJ, Shires GMH, et al: Prophylactic partial stylohyoidostectomy for horses with osteoarthropathy of the temporohyoid joint, *J Equine Vet Sci* 14:32, 1994.
48. Power HT, Watrous BJ, deLahunta A: Facial and vestibulocochlear nerve disease in six horses, *J Am Vet Med Assoc* 183:1076, 1983.
49. Jackson CA, deLahunta A, Dykes NL et al: Neurological manifestation of cholesterinic granulomas in three horses, *Vet Rec* 135:228, 1994.
50. Cook WR: The auditory tube diverticulum (guttural pouch) in the horse: its radiographic examination, *J Am Radiol Soc* 14:41, 1973.
51. Butler JA, Colles CM, Dyson SJ et al: Pharynx, larynx and eustachian tube diverticulum. In Butler JA, Colles CM, Dyson SJ et al, editors: *Clinical radiology of the horse,* ed 2, London, 2000, Blackwell Science, pp 384-393.
52. Sasaki M, Hayashi Y, Koie H et al: CT examination of the guttural pouch (auditory tube diverticulum) in Przewalski's horse (Equus przewalskii), *J Vet Med Sci* 61:1019, 1999.

ELECTRONIC RESOURCES evolve

Additional information related to the content in Chapter 10 can be found on the companion Web site at evolve http://evolve.elsevier.com/Thrall/vetrad/
- Key Points
- Chapter Quiz
- Case Study 10-1

CHAPTER • 11
The Vertebrae

Anne Bahr

Radiographic evaluation of the vertebrae is focused primarily on changes in bone opacity, shape, and angulation of the vertebrae or vertebral column. These changes may or may not be the cause of clinical signs. Illustrations of the radiographic anatomy of the vertebral column can be found in Chapter 7. Vertebral changes can be attributed to a variety of diseases or abnormalities that can be assigned to the following categories: congenital, developmental, degenerative, and other anomalies. These categories are used in this chapter to discuss the common radiographic changes seen in the vertebrae.

CONGENITAL VERTEBRAL ANOMALIES

Congenital vertebral anomalies are common in dogs and cats; however, many do not cause clinical signs unless they result in deformity of the vertebral canal with resultant spinal cord or nerve root impingement. Congenital anomalies result from disturbances in embryonic development.[1] Vertebrae develop from the mesoderm. The mesodermal layer separates into dermatomes, myotomes, and sclerotomes. The vertebrae are formed from sclerotomes, which separate into cranial and caudal halves. Each vertebra is formed by the caudal portion of one sclerotome and the cranial portion of the adjacent caudal sclerotome. Incorrect combination of sclerotome segments results in vertebral abnormalities, including transitional vertebra, hemivertebra, butterfly vertebra, and block vertebrae. More complex anomalies can occur, including spina bifida. Many congenital anomalies are heritable and are often found in brachycephalic breeds (pugs, bulldogs, etc.); however, they can occur spontaneously in any animal.[2]

Changes in the Number of Vertebrae

Deviation from the normal vertebral number is most commonly seen as the presence of transitional vertebrae. This can result in a deviation from the normal number of cervical, thoracic, lumbar, or sacral vertebrae. Vertebrae that have the characteristics of two sections of the vertebral column, such as thoracic and lumbar, are called transitional vertebrae.[3] They occur most frequently in the thoracolumbar and lumbosacral regions. Examples include the last thoracic vertebra having a transverse process instead of a rib (Fig. 11-1, *A*) or the last lumbar vertebra having a transverse process fused to the ilium (Fig. 11-1, *B* and *C*).

Asymmetric morphologic characteristics of the last thoracic vertebra are clinically important because the last pair of ribs is often used as a physical landmark to plan surgical compression of the spinal cord. Thus knowing whether the T13 ribs are asymmetric ensures that the correct decompression site is located on the patient. Asymmetric morphologic characteristics of the lumbosacral junction are also clinically important because they have been associated with predisposition to cauda equina syndrome with hyperostosis and disc degeneration from the altered biomechanics, leading to nerve root compression.

Block vertebrae are most commonly recognized when development of the intervertebral disc is incomplete, with complete or partial fusion of two adjacent vertebrae. Some evidence of partial development of the disc may be present, or it may be completely obliterated. Of note, the intervertebral disc spaces immediately adjacent to a block vertebrae may be predisposed to degeneration and subsequent herniation from the altered forces placed on them (fulcrum effect) (Figs. 11-2 and 11-3).[1]

Changes in Vertebral Shape

Hemivertebrae occur with inappropriate recombination of somites and/or failure of formation of one portion of the vertebrae during development. Depending on which portion is affected, the end result can be a unilateral, dorsal, or ventral hemivertebrae.[4] Hemivertebrae are typically wedge shaped and often result in angulation of the vertebral column (scoliosis, kyphosis, or lordosis). Radiographically, hemivertebrae have a smooth, normal-appearing cortex but the body is malformed. The disc spaces are also well formed but may be wider than normal. The main differential diagnosis for hemivertebrae is a vertebral body fracture. However, because hemivertebrae are commonly seen in screw-tailed breeds (Bulldogs, Pugs, and Boston Terriers), the signalment can be useful in distinguishing between hemivertebra and fracture. Failure of formation of the central portion of the vertebra occurs may result in two hemivertebrae (a right and left side), termed a "butterfly" vertebrae (Figs. 11-4 and 11-5).

Spina bifida, another defect in formation of the vertebral body, is failure of fusion of the vertebral arches with or without protrusion or dysplasia of the spinal cord and/or meninges. Spina bifida is part of a more general defect called spinal dysraphism (lack of fusion of parts that normally unite). Spina bifida occulta is a subcategory of spina bifida where the spinal cord and meninges are normal but there is failure of fusion of the vertebral arches. Radiographically, spina bifida is seen as absence of the vertebral arch or failure of fusion of the spinous processes in one or more vertebrae (Fig. 11-6). Spina bifida is often seen in Bulldogs and Manx cats, which suggests a heritable basis.[5] Cross-sectional imaging, such as computed tomography (CT) or magnetic resonance imaging (MRI), can provide more detailed evaluation of the defects associated with spina bifida because it allows visualization of soft tissues such as the spinal cord and meninges (Fig. 11-7).

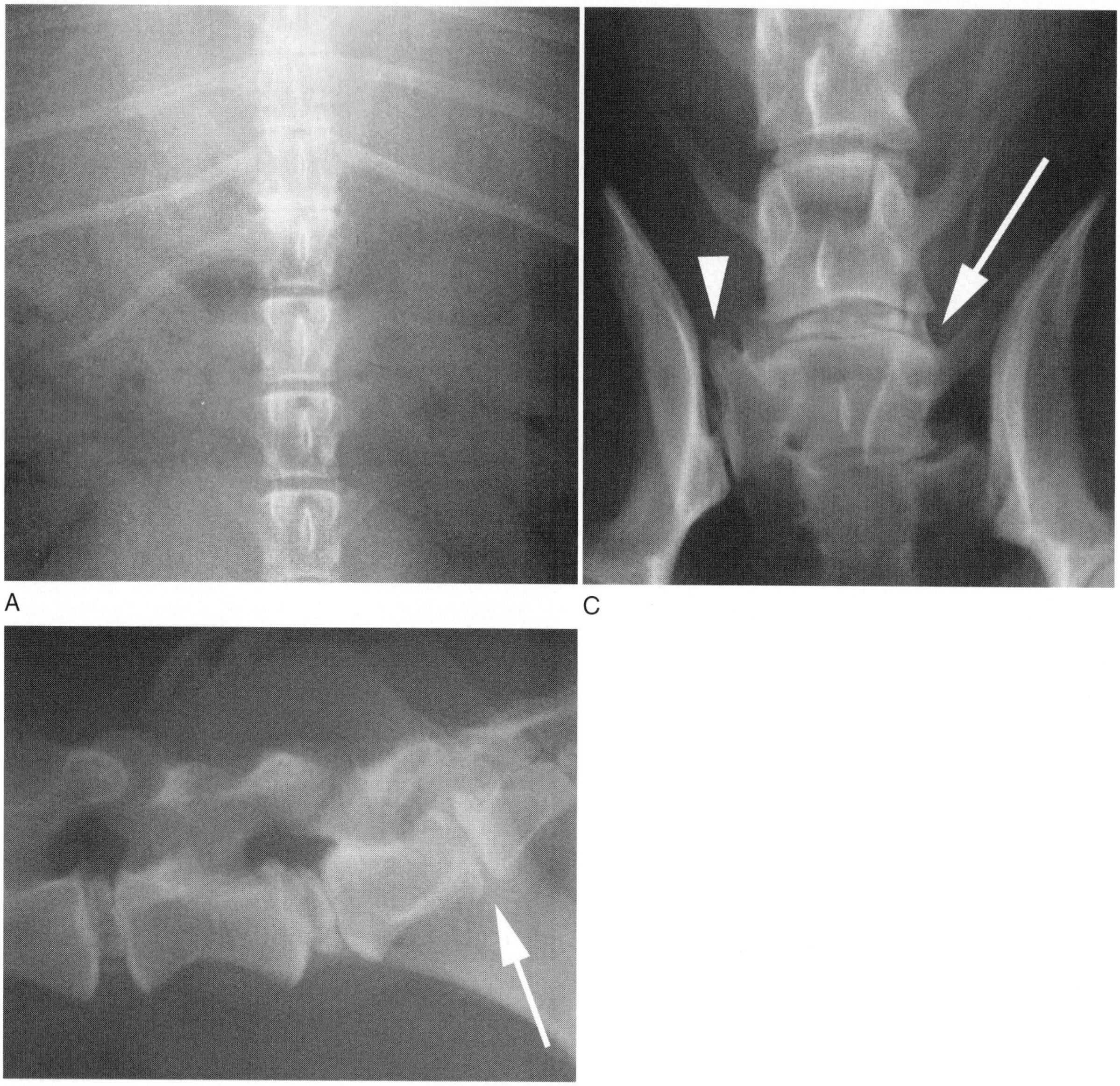

A

C

B

Fig. 11-1 A, Ventrodorsal view of the thoracolumbar region. T13 has no left rib, and on the right is a transverse process rather than a rib. If this asymmetry is not recognized, it could lead to incorrect localization of a planned surgical site depending on which side is used as the reference point. **B,** Lateral view of the lumbosacral junction in a dog with lumbarization of the sacrum. A small disc space is noted *(arrow)*. **C,** Ventrodorsal view of the lumbosacral junction. A transverse process is on the left *(arrow)* and fusion of the right side of the transitional vertebra to the wing of the ileum *(arrowhead)* is visible. This anomaly may predispose to development of cauda equine syndrome.

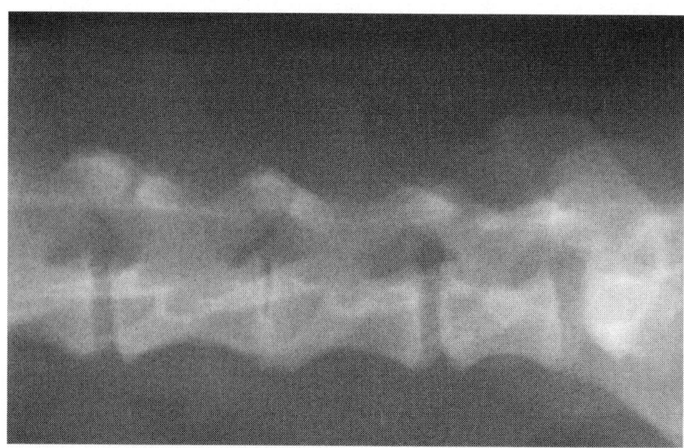

Fig. 11-2 Lateral view of the caudal lumbar spine. Note the fusion of the fifth and sixth lumbar vertebrae and the greatly decreased disc space, creating a block vertebra.

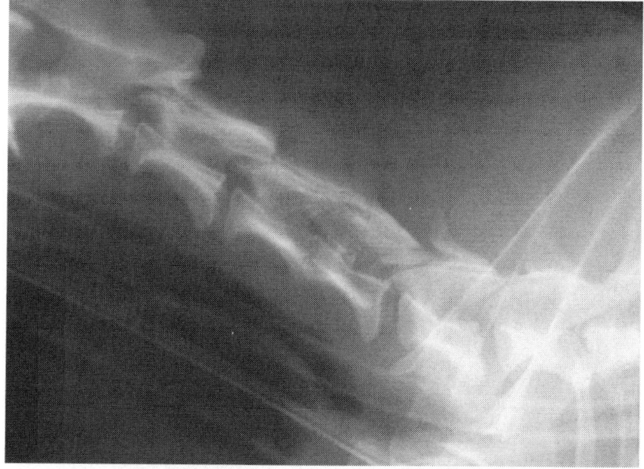

A

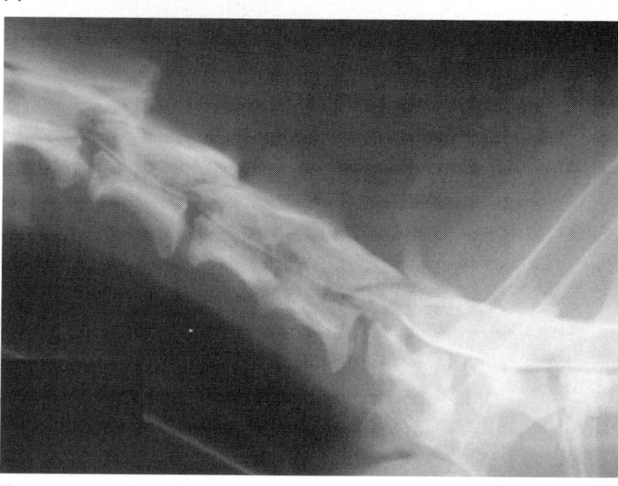

B

Fig. 11-3 A, Lateral view of the cervical spine. A block vertebra has formed between segments C4-C5. **B,** Lateral view of cervical myelogram in the same dog. Extradural compression is caused by disc herniation at C5-C6. Disc herniation adjacent to a block vertebra is commonly seen from the altered biomechanics resulting from the fusion.

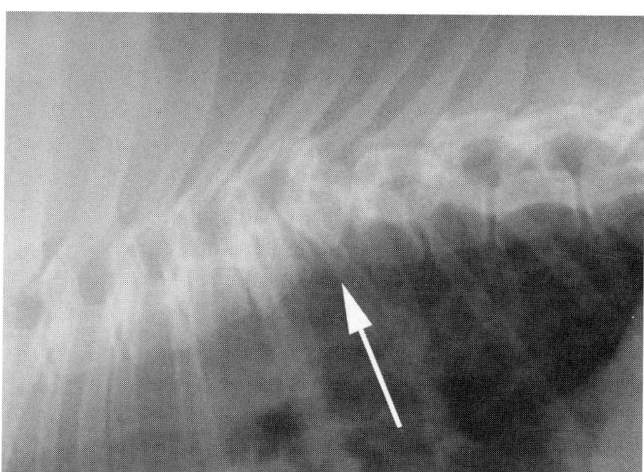

Fig. 11-4 Lateral view of the caudal thoracic spine. Notice the hemivertebra that is causing kyphosis of the spine *(arrow)*. Also note the wedging of the adjacent vertebrae but the sparing of the disc spaces.

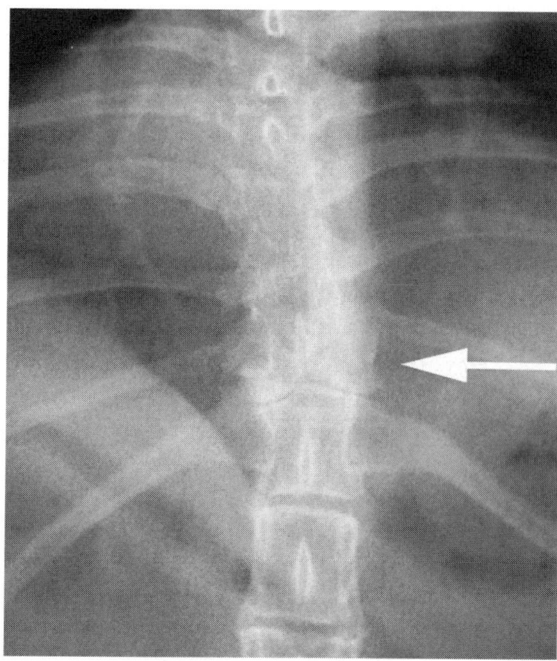

Fig. 11-5 Ventrodorsal view of the caudal thoracic spine. A butterfly vertebra is causing scoliosis of the spine *(arrow)*.

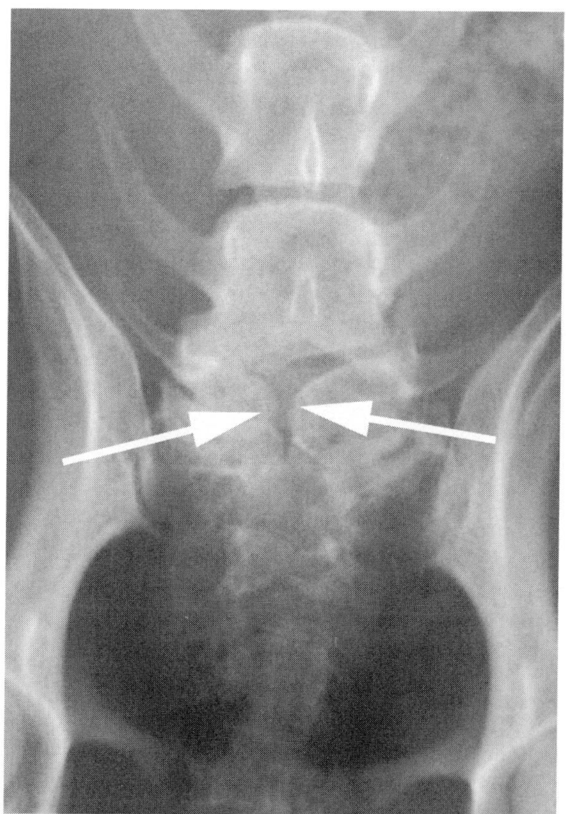

Fig. 11-6 Ventrodorsal view of the lumbosacral spine. A cleft in the vertebral arch consistent with spina bifida is present *(arrows)*.

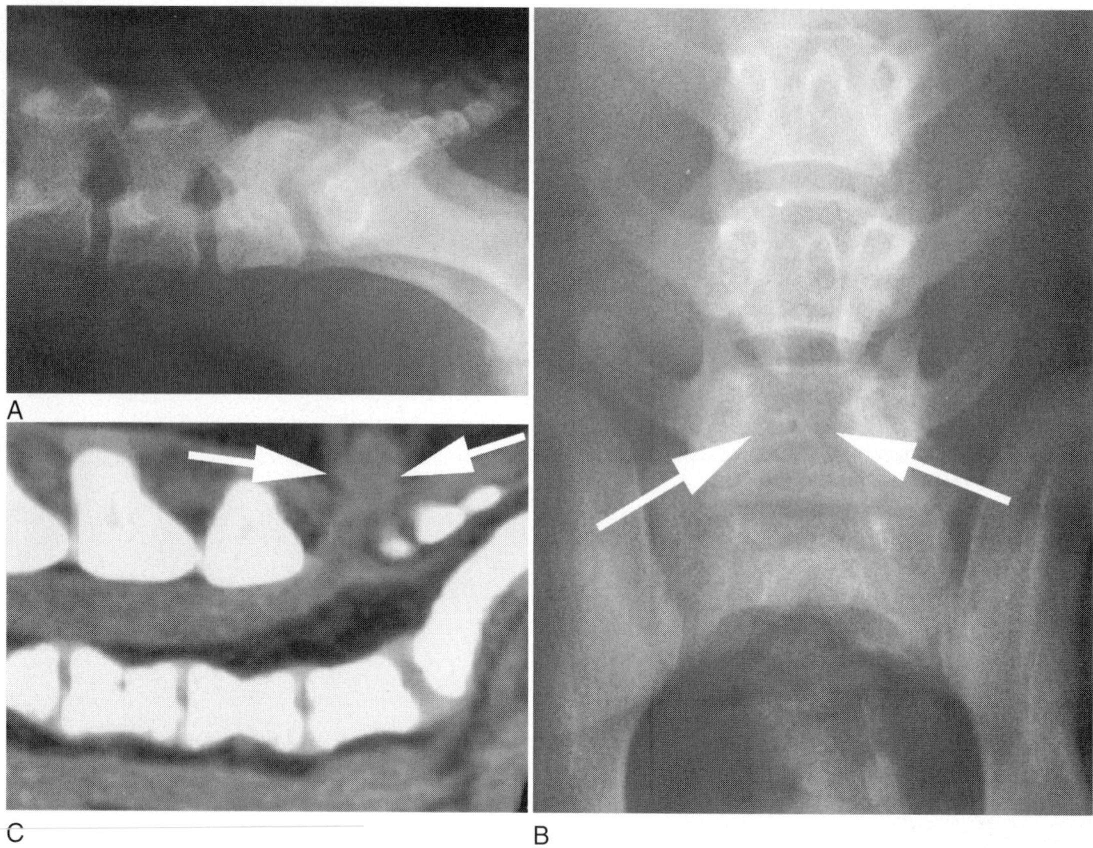

Fig. 11-7 A, Lateral radiograph of the lumbosacral spine. No spinous process exists on L7. B, Ventrodorsal radiograph of the same dog as in A. A large cleft in the dorsal arch of L7 *(arrow)* is present. C, Sagittally reconstructed CT image of the same dog. Extension of the cauda equina through the defect in the vertebral arch (spina bifida aperta) is visible *(arrows)*.

DEVELOPMENTAL VERTEBRAL ANOMALIES

Atlantoaxial subluxation or atlantoaxial instability, which can be congenital or acquired, occurs with the following conditions: excessive motion of the atlantoaxial joint from agenesis or hypoplasia of the dens, absence of the transverse ligament (see Fig. 6-11), nonunion of the dens, or trauma. Atlantoaxial instability allows compression of the cranial cervical spinal cord; it is most commonly seen in young, small-breed dogs.[6,7] Often such dogs appear normal until a traumatic event causes clinical signs. Radiographically, atlantoaxial subluxation is diagnosed by identification of increased space between the dorsal arch of C1 and the spinous process of C2 (Fig. 11-8). Atlantoaxial subluxation also results in angulation between the dorsal aspects of the vertebral canal over C1 compared with C2; these portions of the vertebral canal are usually nearly parallel. In addition, if the problem is caused by an abnormality of the dens, agenesis or separation of the dens may be noted. The most useful radiographic view for evaluation of atlantoaxial subluxation is the lateral or lateral oblique projection of the cervical spine. In the past, an open-mouth view was recommended for optimal visualization of the dens; however, this requires flexion of the head with respect to the spine, which could potentially cause catastrophic damage to the spinal cord if atlantoaxial instability exists.

Cervical spondylomyelopathy, often called Wobbler syndrome, is a condition typically seen in large to giant-breed dogs, particularly Doberman Pinschers and Great Danes.[8] Typically, affected animals have ataxia and/or tetraparesis. The changes found in dogs with cervical spondylomyelopathy include malformation/malarticulation of the cervical vertebrae, cervical instability, and cervical vertebral canal stenosis (static or dynamic). In survey radiographs this is manifest as (1) premature disc calcification, (2) articular process degenerative joint disease, (3) spondylosis deformans, (4) flattening (remodeling) of the cranioventral aspect of one or more vertebral bodies, (5) vertebral malalignment, and (6) narrowing of the vertebral canal. The C5-C6 and C6-C7 disc spaces are most commonly affected (Fig. 11-9). Survey radiographs are not sufficient for assessing of the degree of spinal cord compression associated with the bone changes; spinal cord compression can only be assessed by myelography, CT, or MRI. CT and MRI are also valuable for more accurately assessing malformed or hyperostotic articular processes, and MRI has the added advantage of being able to assess the spinal cord parenchyma (Fig. 11-10). Dynamic radiographs (flexion, extension, traction) may show subluxation not present on neutral views (Fig. 11-11).[9] Traction views, where firm traction is placed on the neck during the exposure of a lateral radiograph, or even during CT or MR imaging, can help delineate between a protruding annulus fibrosus or ligamentous hypertrophy versus a more static extradural compression such as seen with disc extrusion (Fig. 11-12). Cross-sectional imaging also allows visualization of the shape of the vertebral canal (Fig. 11-13).[10] Functional vertebral canal stenosis may occur as a result of soft tissue changes such as hypertrophy of the ligamentum flavum or secondary intervertebral disc herniation, both of which result from instability.

Spinal curvature can develop as a result of congenital or developmental anomalies of the vertebrae. Although the

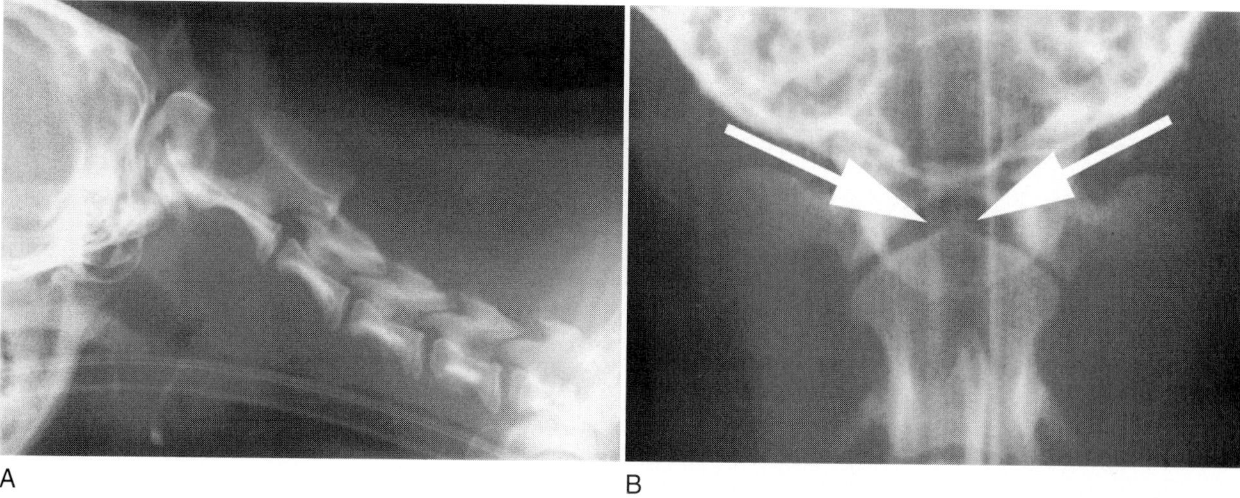

Fig. 11-8 A, Lateral radiograph of the cervical spine. Increased space is visible between the dorsal aspect of C1 with respect to the dorsal spinous process of C2. Also, the dorsal aspect of the vertebral canal over C1 is not parallel to the dorsal aspect of the vertebral canal over C2. **B,** The dens is visible *(arrows)* on the ventrodorsal view of the same patient as seen in **A.** Thus ligamentous damage/laxity is the likely cause of the instability.

vertebrae normally move to allow bending of the vertebral column, the ventral aspect of the vertebral canal from one vertebra to the next should form a smooth, sweeping line. Scoliosis, kyphosis, or lordosis can occur when the vertebrae do not line up; this is often attributable to congenital or developmental anomalies. Scoliosis refers to a lateral deviation of the spinal column; kyphosis indicates a dorsal deviation, and lordosis indicates a ventral deviation of the vertebral column (Fig. 11-14).

DEGENERATIVE VERTEBRAL ANOMALIES

Spondylosis deformans is a common condition characterized by formation of osteophytes on the vertebral endplates from degeneration of the intervertebral discs.[11] Radiographically, spondylosis deformans appears as smooth, bony proliferation centered at the disc space that bridges (or almost bridges) the ventral aspect of the vertebral bodies (Fig. 11-15). It can also occur on the lateral aspect of the disc space. It can occur across normal width as well as narrowed disc spaces. The caudal thoracic, lumbar, and lumbosacral regions are most commonly affected, which may be from the increased motion that often occurs in these regions. Typically, no clinical significance is applied to the presence of this bony proliferation. However, if spondylosis deformans is excessive and extends along the dorsolateral margin of the vertebral bodies, nerve root impingement may occur (Fig. 11-16). In addition, the presence of spondylosis deformans may indicate instability; however, its presence cannot be used to confirm this diagnosis.

Diffuse idiopathic skeletal hyperostosis (DISH) is a diffuse ossifying condition of young dogs and cats. Radiographically, it may appear similar to extensive spondylosis deformans. However, it has several other findings that distinguish it from spondylosis. Four of the following five conditions must be present to confirm a diagnosis of DISH: (1) flowing calcification and ossification along ventral and lateral aspects of three contiguous vertebral bodies; (2) relative preservation of intervertebral disc width; (3) periarticular osteophytes surrounding the articular process joints; (4) formation of pseudoarthrosis between the bases of spinous processes; (5) periarticular osteophytes and calcification and ossification of soft tissue attachments (enthesophytes) in the axial and peripheral skeleton. The etiology of DISH is not known.[12,13]

Spondylitis is a generic term that implies inflammation of the vertebrae. It may or may not be associated with infection. Radiographically, spondylitis usually appears as an active periosteal/bony proliferation often involving the body of the vertebrae. *Spirocerca lupi* infection can cause spondylitis of the ventral aspect of the T8-T11 vertebrae. Infection is the most common cause of spondylitis. Migrating grass awns ("foxtails") can cause an infectious spondylitis of the ventral aspect of the L3-L4 vertebral bodies. This occurs because the foreign body follows the path of least resistance along the diaphragmatic crura and lodges at their attachment site (Fig. 11-17).

Discospondylitis is caused by bacterial or fungal infection of the intervertebral discs and adjacent vertebral bodies/endplates. It may occur as a result of migrating plant awns, a penetrating wound, previous surgery in the area or, most commonly, hematogenous spread of infection. Some common sources of hematogenous spread include urinary tract infection, dental disease, and endocarditis. The most common organism isolated from animals with discospondylitis is *Staphylococcus* spp. However, evaluation for *Brucella canis* should always be performed in these cases because of the zoonotic potential.[14]

Typical radiographic findings of discospondylitis include destruction of vertebral endplates, intervertebral disc collapse, and varying degrees of sclerosis and/or new bone formation around the disc space (Fig 11-18). Lysis of the endplates tends to be seen earlier in the disease process, whereas bone formation is seen later. In addition, more than one site within the vertebral column may be affected. The radiographic findings may continue to deteriorate despite appropriate therapy before radiographic signs of recovery are noted.[15] Cross-sectional imaging, such as CT, allows visualization of these changes without superimposition of other structures (transverse processes, articular processes, and spondylosis deformans) and may be preferable to survey radiography for evaluation of discospondylitis (Fig. 11-19). MR imaging shares this advantage and also is useful for assessing the extent of

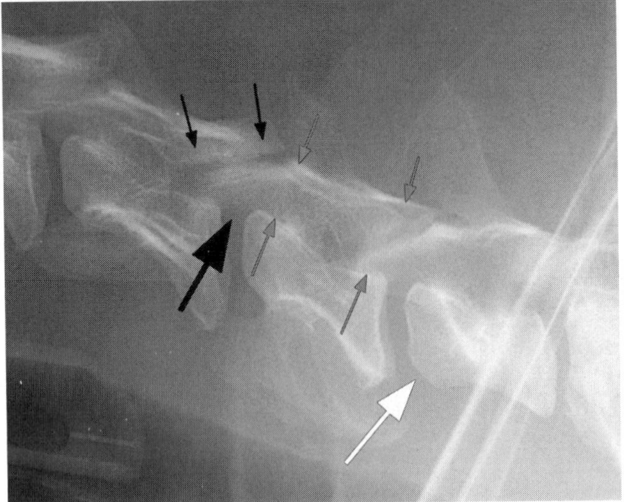

A

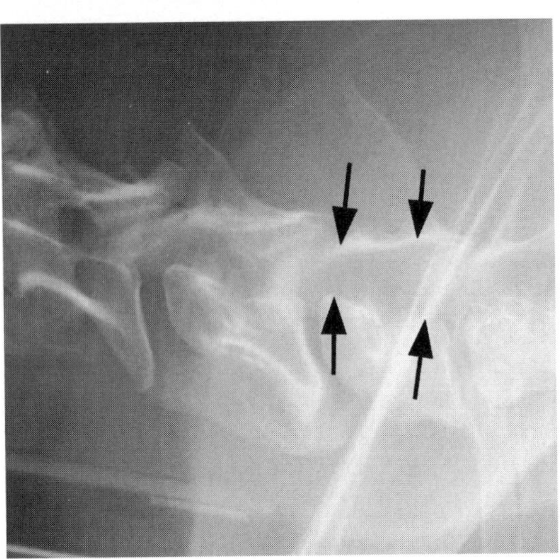

B

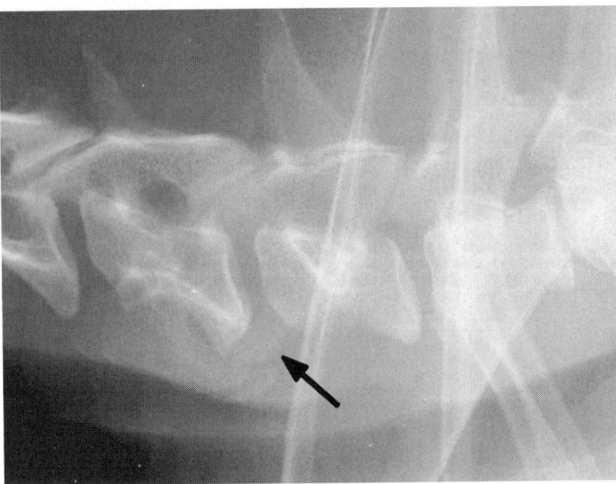

C

Fig. 11-9 Cervical spine radiographs of dogs with cervical spondylopathy. **A,** This dog has remodeling of the cranioventral aspect of C7 *(large white arrow)*, articular process degenerative joint disease at C5-C6 *(small black arrows)*, stenosis of the vertebral canal over C6 *(open arrows)*, and malalignment at C5-C6 *(large black arrow)*. **B,** This dog has similar changes to the dog in **A** except the vertebral canal stenosis over C7 is more pronounced *(black arrows)*, and disc space narrowing at C6-C7 is marked. **C,** This dog has less severe bone changes but has evidence of malalignment at C5-C6, flattening of the cranioventral aspect of C6 and, to a lesser extent, C7. This dog also has spondylosis at C6-C7 *(arrow)*.

adjacent soft tissue involvement or multiplicity of involvement (see Fig 11-18, *B*). Bone scintigraphy may also be used as a screening tool in the evaluation of multiple lesions.

Vertebral neoplasia can be primary or metastatic from another site. Typical primary tumors include osteosarcoma, lymphoma, and chondrosarcoma. Typical secondary tumors include adenocarcinoma and hemangiosarcoma. A benign neoplasm sometimes seen is osteoma. Radiographic findings of vertebral neoplasia are dependent somewhat on the type of tumor but cannot be used for tumor type diagnosis; a cytologic evaluation is necessary. Common radiographic changes of vertebral tumors include a sclerotic reaction within the bone, bone lysis with resultant pathologic fracture, collapse of the body, and destruction of the endplates (Fig. 11-20). Collapse of the disc space, bone sclerosis, and bone proliferation also can be seen. Typically, primary bone tumors involve only one vertebra and secondary tumors involve more than one vertebra. However, this is not a defining characteristic that can be used to determine tumor type. In some instances, other differentials such as spondylitis and discospondylitis could be considered.[16,17]

Because of overlapping rib and soft tissue opacities in radiographs, the detection of subtle changes of vertebral neoplasia may be difficult. Cross-sectional imaging eliminates this superimposition and provides a more detailed view of the changes that occur in vertebral neoplasia as well in paraspinal soft tissue (Fig. 11-21).

Degenerative lumbosacral stenosis causing cauda equina syndrome as a result of nerve root compression can have numerous etiologies. These include, but are not limited to, lumbosacral instability, lumbosacral spondylosis, lumbosacral canal stenosis (congenital or acquired), herniated intervertebral disc disease, osteochondrosis-like lesions of the cranial aspect of the sacrum, or proliferation surrounding the intervertebral foramen.[18,19,20] All these etiologies ultimately cause compression or impingement of the nerve roots that form the cauda equina, thus the name of the syndrome. Survey radiographs may be used to assess some of these problems, especially spondylosis (see Fig. 11-15), but radiography cannot be used to assess nerve root compression. Myelography is often inadequate in evaluating the lumbosacral vertebral canal because the dural sac frequently does not extend that far caudally. Epidurography, a procedure in which contrast medium is injected into the epidural space in the caudal spine, can be helpful in identifying some compressive lesions at the lumbosacral junction, but epidurography is not very sensitive for assessing nerve root compression. CT and MR imaging are becoming standard for assessing the lumbosacral junction. The superior contrast resolution of MR imaging is helpful in assessing the lumbosacral vertebral canal (Fig. 11-22). However, until more experience is gained with lumbosacral MR

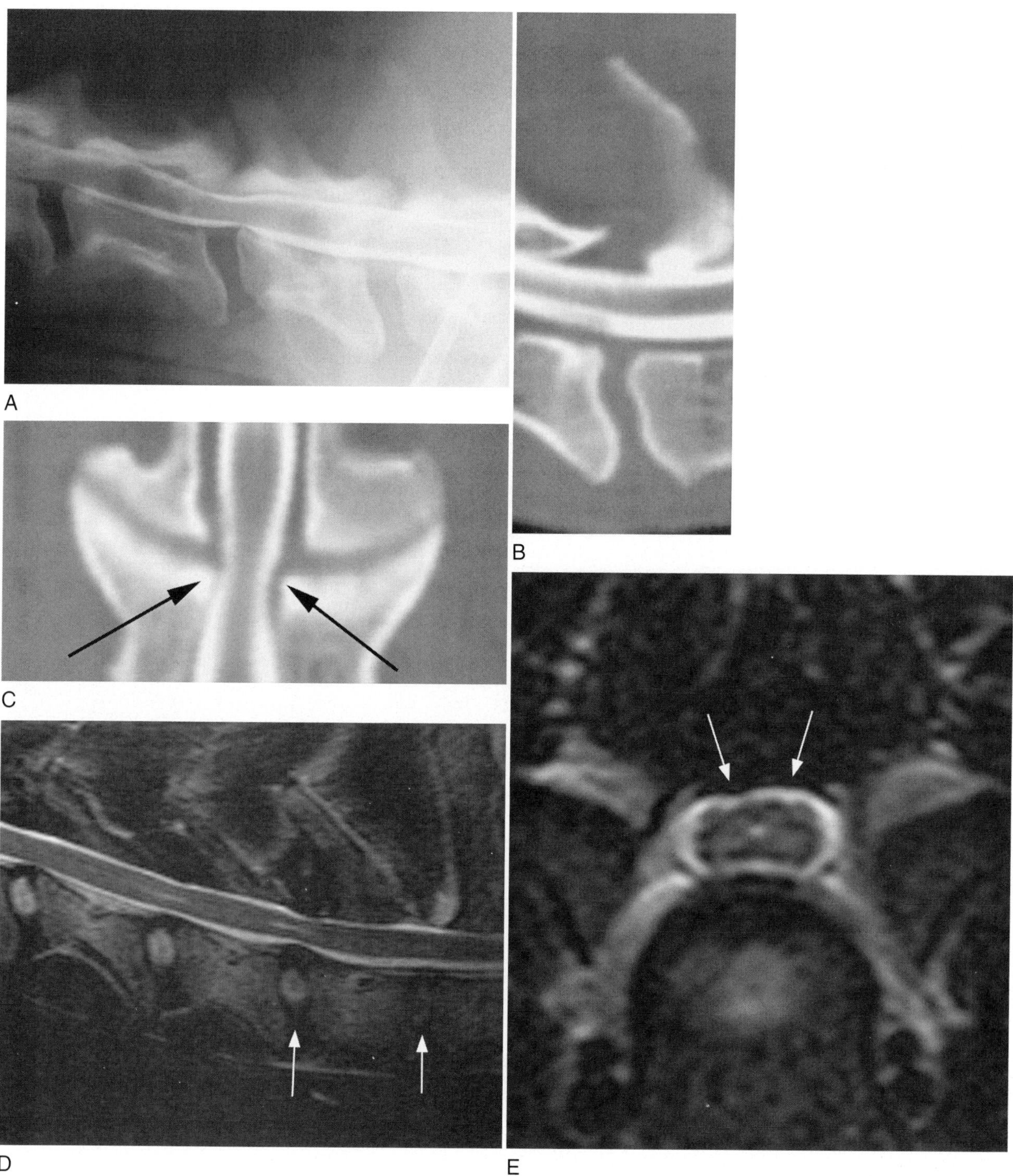

Fig. 11-10 A, Lateral radiograph of a cervical myelogram of a young Great Dane. Notice the dorsal subluxation of the cranial aspect of C6 with respect to C5. This dog has a mild ventral extradural compression from this subluxation. Also note the dorsal extradural compression from the articular processes at C5-C6. **B,** Sagittal CT reconstruction at C6-C7 with contrast medium in the subarachnoid space. No obvious extradural compression is noted in this plane. **C,** Dorsal plane CT reconstruction of the same site as in **B.** Note the lateral impingement of the spinal cord by the malformed articular processes *(arrows)*. **D,** Sagittal T2-weighted fast spin-echo MR image of a dog with cervical spondylomyelopathy. The discs at C6-C7 and C7-T1 are partially (C6-C7) or extensively (C7-T1) dehydrated *(arrows)*. Dorsal and ventral compression of the spinal cord is visible at C6-C7. Important information that cannot be obtained by other imaging modalities relates to the spinal cord itself; here, foci of increased signal within the spinal cord at C5-C6 and C6-C7 indicate spinal cord edema, likely caused by repeated dynamic compression at these sites. **E,** Transverse T2-weighted fast spin-echo image of the spine at C6-C7; this is the same dog as in **D.** Note the asymmetric dorsal compression of the spinal cord from articular process hyperostosis *(arrow)*; this is a common finding in dogs with cervical spondylomyelopathy.

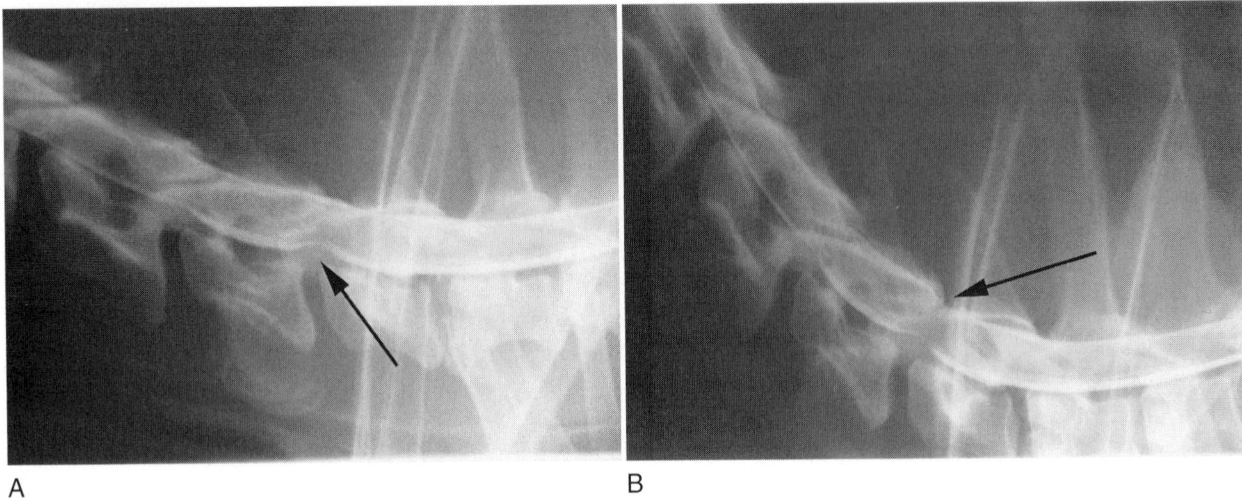

Fig. 11-11 A, Lateral view of a myelogram in a neutral position in which ventral extradural compression from disc herniation is apparent. **B,** Lateral view in an extended position in which dorsal extradural compression is apparent *(arrow)*. This is an example of dynamic impingement of the spinal cord.

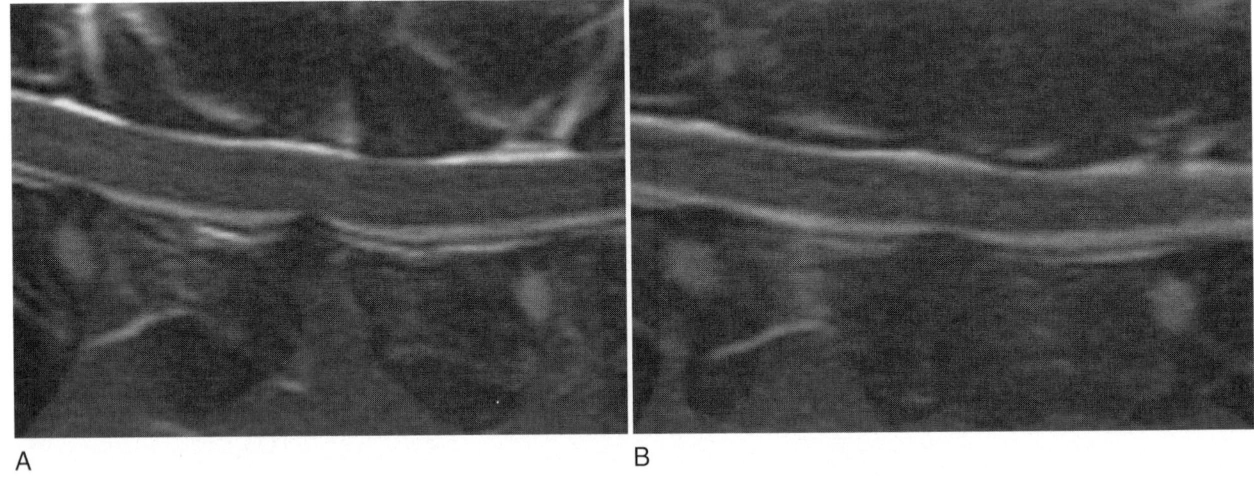

Fig. 11-12 A, Sagittal T2-weighted fast spin-echo MR image of the cervical spine of a dog with cervical spondylomyelopathy. Dehydration of the disc at C6-C7 is present with compression of the ventral aspect of the spinal cord. Traction was placed on the neck and the image acquisition repeated **B.** The amount of spinal cord compression is reduced. Although distinguishing between compressions from disc protrusion and ligamentous hypertrophy is not possible in these images, the reduced compression with traction suggests that surgery to distract the affected vertebrae may result in clinical improvement. If no reduction in compression had been seen in the traction view, the indication for such a surgical procedure would have been more questionable.

imaging, determination of the clinical significance of abnormalities detected may be difficult; the sensitivity of MR imaging is so great that many more abnormalities are being detected, and these may not always correlate with the clinical signs.[21]

Of the causes of acquired lumbosacral vertebral canal stenosis, instability is one of the most difficult to diagnose. It occurs when the sacrum subluxates with respect to the last lumbar vertebra (retrolisthesis). Images (including survey radiographs, myelograms, and cross-sectional images) obtained in a neutral or flexed position may not reveal any abnormality. Imaging in an extended position is often necessary to detect the presence of retrolisthesis. This can result in compression of the nerve roots because it effectively creates a stenotic vertebral canal. Intervertebral disc protrusion is also a common component of any cause of lumbosacral canal stenosis (Figs. 11-23 and 11-24).

The dorsal joints between vertebrae, the articular process joints, are small diarthrodial joints. As with other diarthrodial joints, the dorsal articular process joints can degenerate and become characterized by typical changes of subchondral sclerosis and osteophytosis. This has already been mentioned with reference to cervical spondylomyelopathy. Articular process degenerative joint disease may affect other portions of the spine as well (Fig. 11-25). These degenerative changes may be painful because of the joint abnormality or if the hyperostosis extends ventromedially to compress the spinal cord; neural signs or pain may also result from that complication (see Fig 11-25, C).

Text continued on p. 191

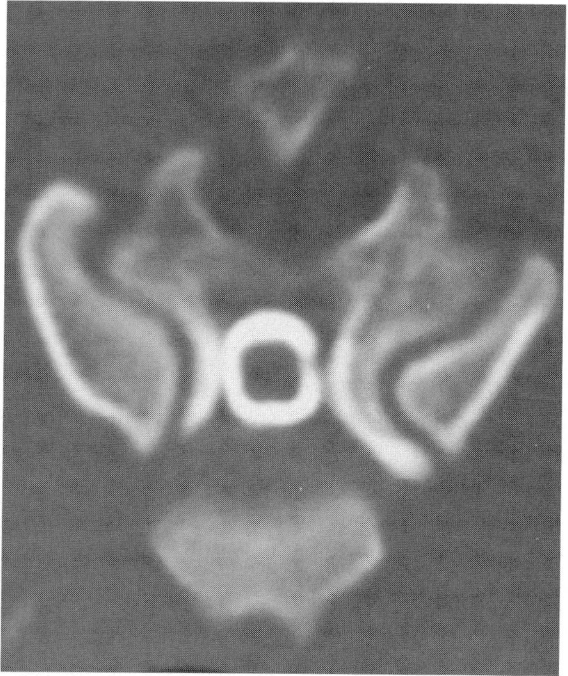

Fig. 11-13 Transverse CT image showing lateral impingement of the spinal cord from narrowing of the vertebral canal.

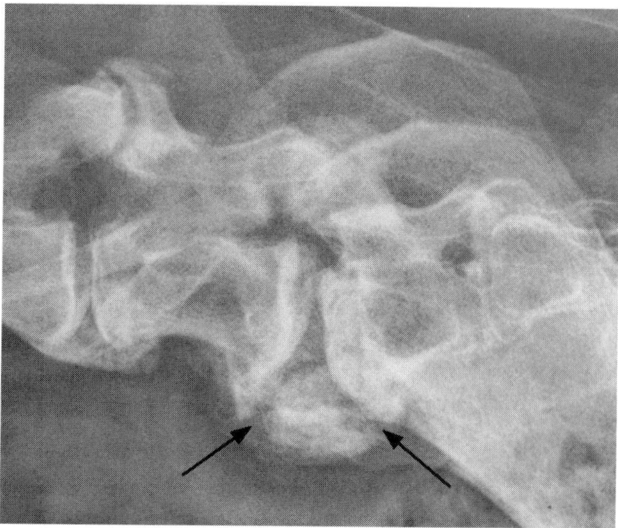

Fig. 11-15 Lateral radiograph of the lumbosacral junction. Ventral spondylosis deformans is noted *(arrow)*. Notice the small lucent gap at the edges of the spondylosis deformans *(arrows)*, which is a typical finding and is due to incomplete mineralization, not a fracture. A transitional sacral segment is also evidenced by the vertical radiolucent line in the cranial aspect of the sacrum, and there is articular process degenerative joint disease at L6-L7.

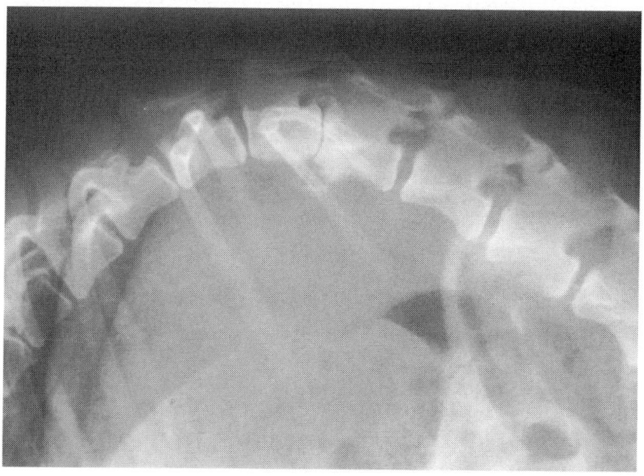

Fig. 11-14 Lateral radiograph of a dog with severe kyphosis.

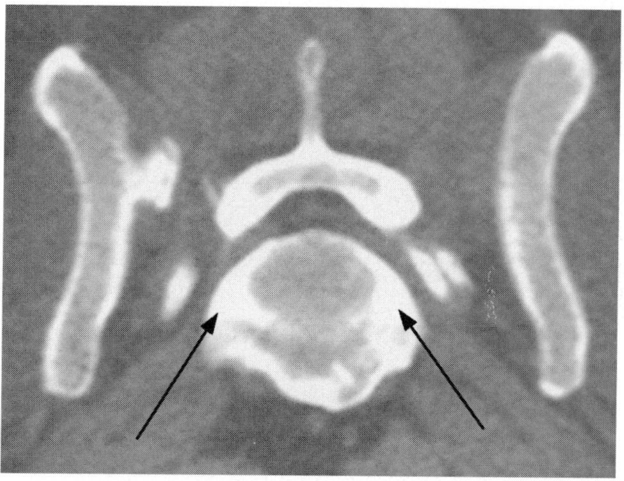

A

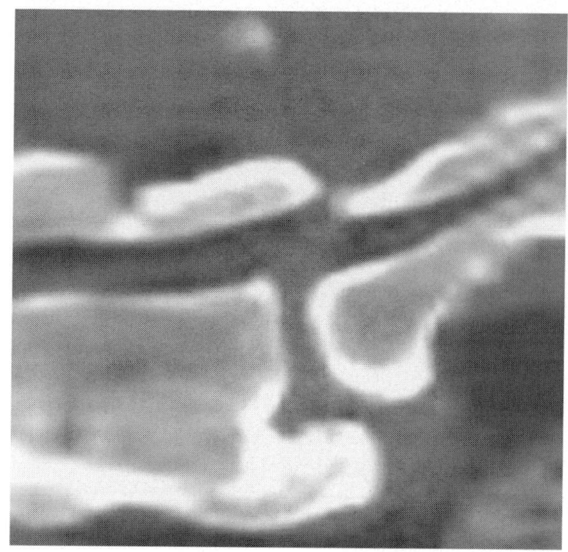

B

Fig. 11-16 **A,** Transverse CT image of the lumbosacral junction of a dog with marked lumbosacral spondylosis. The new bone formation has extended laterally and dorsally along the endplate of L7 *(arrows)*, causing bilateral encroachment on the intervertebral foramina. **B,** Sagittal reconstruction of the caudal aspect of the lumbar spine from the same dog as in **A.** The spondylosis at L7-S1 is apparent. The degree of lateral extension of spondylosis is hard to assess from radiographs and cannot be assessed in this midsagittal CT reconstruction. The L7-S1 disc also protrudes into the vertebral canal.

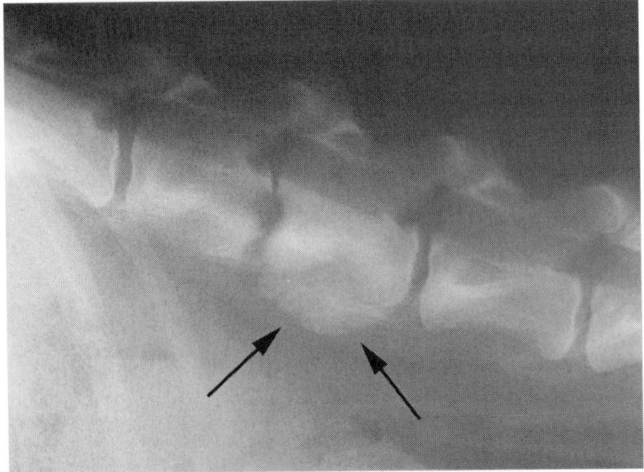

Fig. 11-17 Lateral radiograph of the lumbar spine. Active periosteal proliferation is present along the ventral aspect of L3. This reaction is caused by spondylitis from a migrating foreign body. Note the endplate lysis at L2-L3 from discospondylitis.

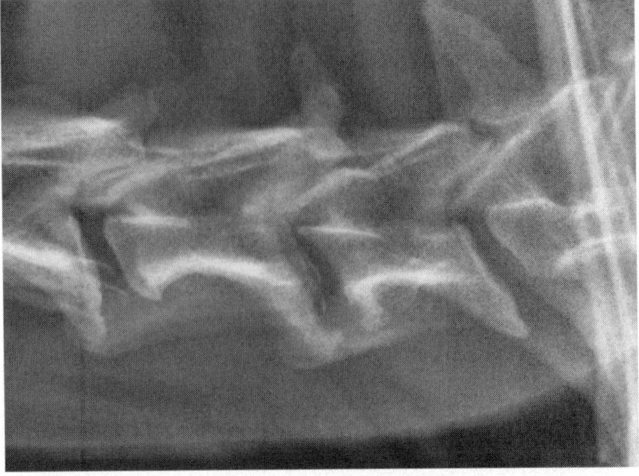

A

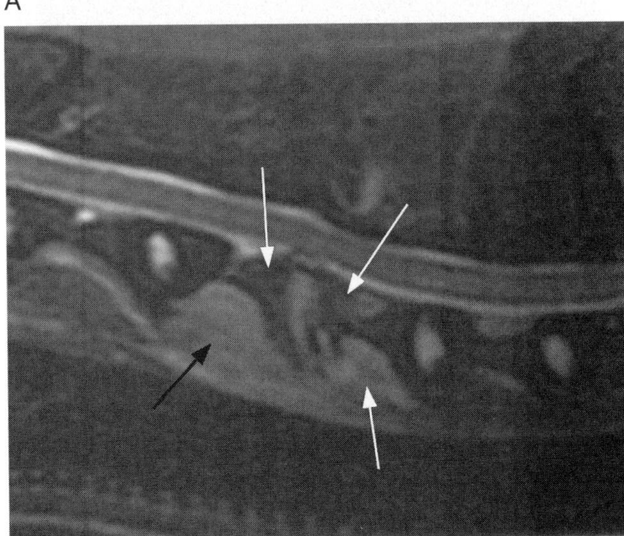

B

Fig. 11-18 A, Lateral cervical radiograph of a dog with discospondylitis at C4-C5. Concave lysis of the cranial endplate of C5 and vertically oriented lysis of the caudal endplate of C4 are present. These changes are typical of infection of the disc and adjacent vertebrae. **B,** Short tau inversion recovery (STIR) sagittal MR image of the cervical spine of the same dog as in **A.** STIR images are designed to have no signal from fat, allowing sites of abnormal tissue water, such as accompanies inflammation, to be conspicuous hyperintensities. Note the increased signal in the affected vertebrae *(white arrows)*, the abnormally shaped disc at C4-C5, and the relatively extensive ventral paraspinal hyperintensity, signifying paraspinal cellulitis from the discospondylitis. This paraspinal involvement cannot be detected radiographically or by CT imaging, which illustrates the value of MR imaging for more accurate disease staging.

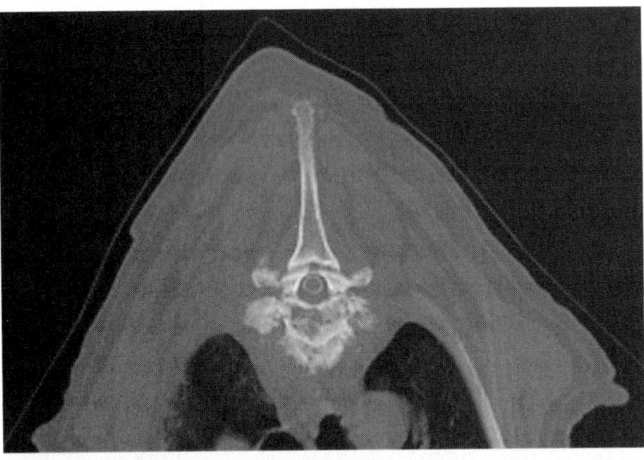

A

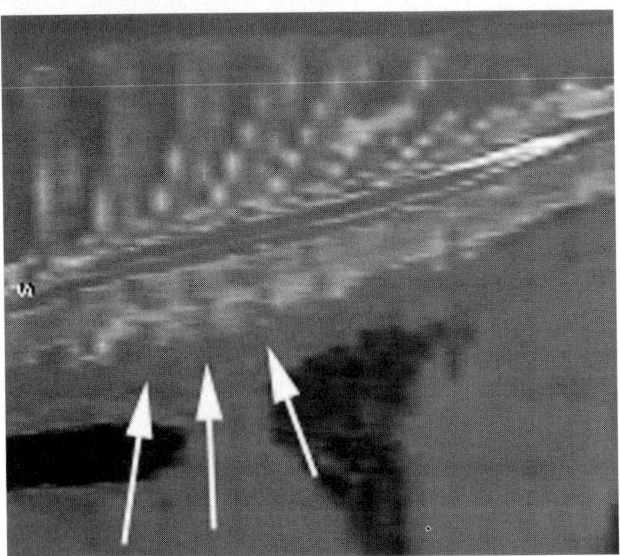

B

Fig. 11-19 A, Transverse CT image of the thoracic spine. There is endplate lysis and active periosteal proliferation surrounding the body of the vertebra. **B,** Sagittal reformatted CT image of the same dog as in **A.** Multiple sites of endplate lysis are present *(arrows)* from discospondylitis. (Courtesy Dr. Robert Bergman.)

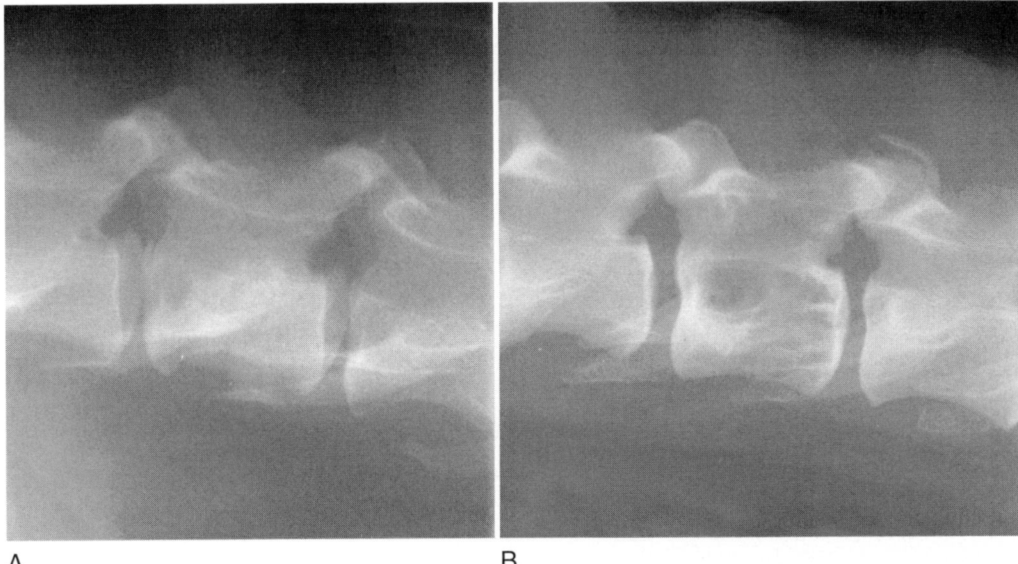

Fig. 11-20 A, Lateral lumber spine radiograph of a dog with an osteosarcoma of L3. Mixed lysis and sclerosis are present in the body and pedicle. These changes are typical of an aggressive bone lesion. Diagnosis of primary versus metastatic tumor cannot be determined from this image, but these changes are typical of primary mesenchymal vertebral tumors. **B,** Lateral lumbar spine radiograph of a dog with a plasma cell tumor of L4. A primarily lytic, somewhat expansile, lesion is present in the body involving the pedicle and lamina. Mostly lytic vertebral lesions such as this are consistent with vertebral reticuloendothelial tumors such as plasma cell tumors and lymphoma, but a metastatic tumor or a lytic primary tumor cannot be ruled out.

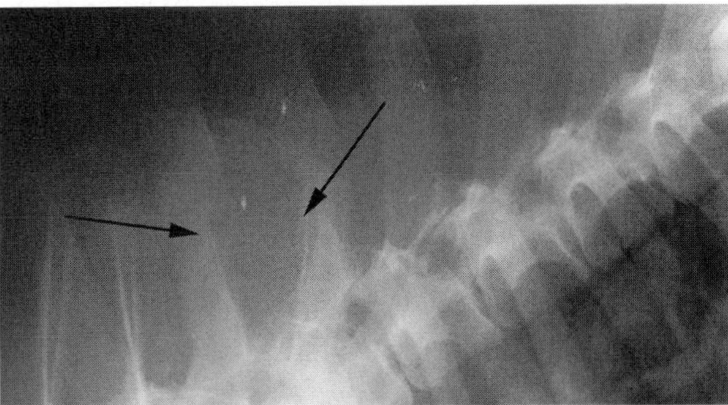

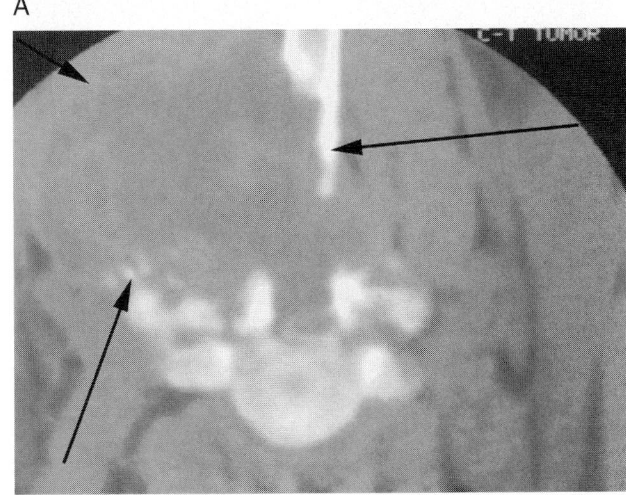

Fig. 11-21 A, Lateral radiograph of the thoracic spine. Lysis of the spinous processes of T1 and T2 is present *(arrows)*. **B,** Contrast-enhanced CT image of the same area as in **A.** A large soft tissue mass and extensive lysis of spinous process and laminae of the vertebra are visible. The mass has also invaded the vertebral canal to cause extradural compression of the spinal cord.

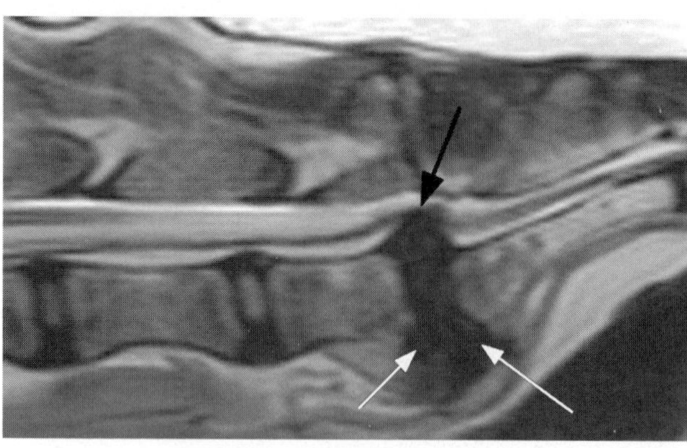

A

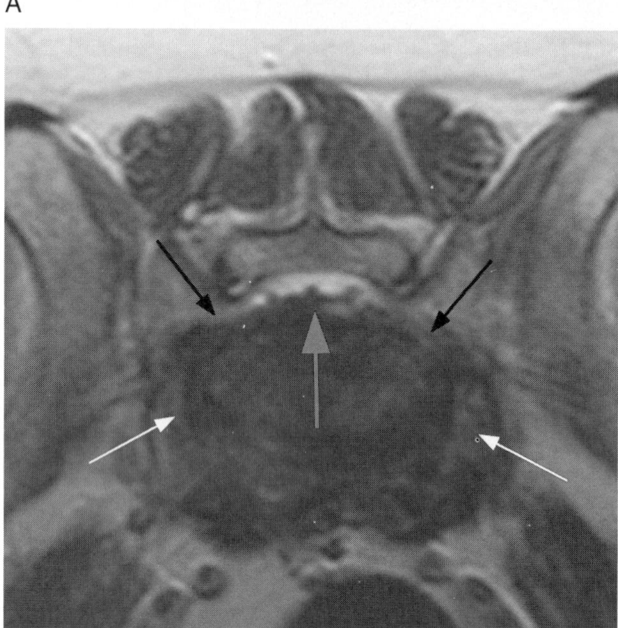

B

Fig. 11-22 T2-weighted fast spin-echo images of a dog with caudal equina syndrome. **A,** Sagittal view. Marked dehydration (*black;* no signal) of the disc at L7-S1 is present with dorsal protrusion and nerve root compression *(black arrow)*. Note the normally hydrated *(white)* discs at L4-L5 and L5-L6. Ventral spondylosis is also present at L7-S1 *(white arrows)*. **B,** Transverse view. Marked lateral spondylosis *(white arrows)* is impinging on both intervertebral foramina *(black arrows)*. Disc protrusion is causing marked crowding of nerve roots in the vertebral canal *(large grey arrow)*.

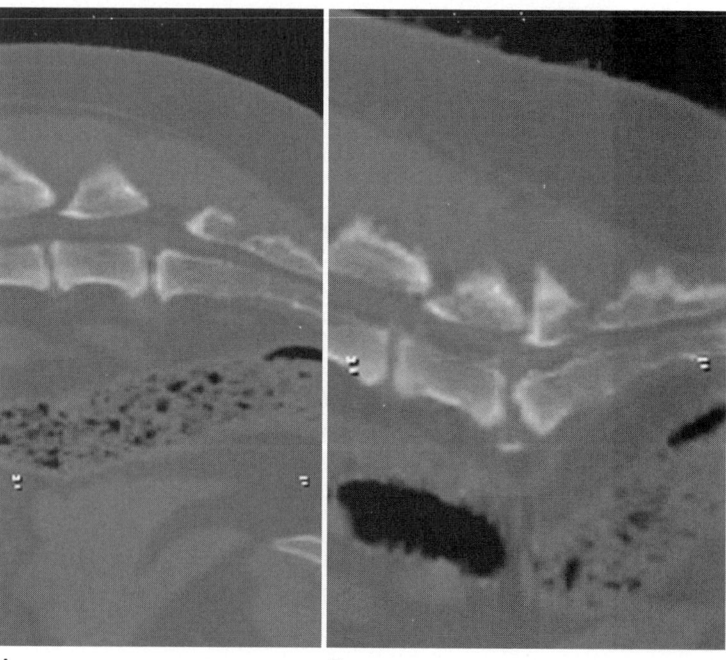

A B

Fig. 11-23 **A,** Sagittal reformatted CT image of the lumbosacral junction with the pelvis and limbs in a flexed position. No malalignment or compression of the cauda equina is noted. **B,** Sagittal reformatted CT image of the lumbosacral junction of the same animal as in **A** obtained with the pelvis and limbs in an extended position. Note the subluxation of the sacrum with respect to L7 and the concurrent stenosis and compression that occurs in the vertebral canal at the level. (Courtesy Dr. Robert Bergman.)

OTHER

Diseases that cause changes in overall bone mass (osteopenia) can be seen but are less common than the diseases previously discussed. Osteopenia (overall decrease in bone mass or radiographic opacity) can result from a variety of causes. Hyperparathyroidism (either nutritional or renal origin) is commonly seen in young animals, particularly cats. Other diseases that can cause osteopenia include hyperadrenocorticism, hypothyroidism, pseudohyperparathyroidism, osteogenesis imperfecta, and disuse atrophy.[22,23] If osteopenia is severe, weakening of the vertebrae may be noted, with evidence of pathologic fractures or changes in the shape of the vertebrae (Fig. 11-26).

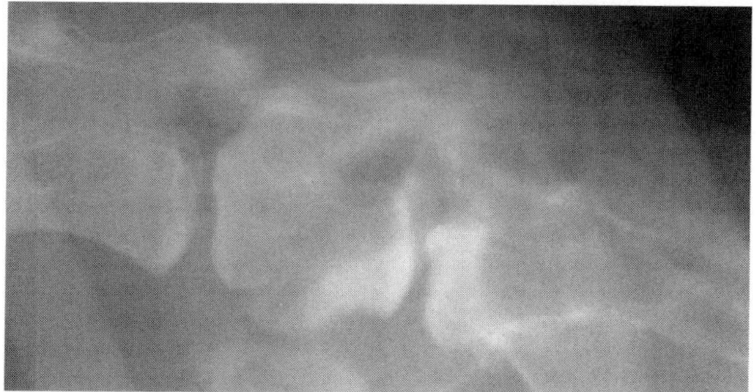

Fig. 11-24 Lateral radiograph of a dog. Subluxation of the sacrum with respect to L7 (retrolisthesis) is present, effectively creating a stenotic vertebral canal.

Another disease that can cause a change in the appearance of the spine is mucopolysaccharidosis. This is a group of genetic diseases that result from defects in the metabolism of glycosaminoglycans. The pertinent change that occurs is fusion of the vertebrae with proliferation that may ultimately cause spinal cord compression. Variations of this disease have been documented in Siamese and domestic shorthair cats as well as a dog, and not all types cause the described vertebral changes.[24]

Trauma to the vertebrae can result in fractures of any portion. This is commonly seen in vehicular trauma, gunshot injury, falls from high places, or falling objects such as garage doors. Most spinal fractures occur at the junction of a mobile and immobile segment (e.g., lumbosacral, thoracolumbar, cervicothoracic).[25] Radiographic changes include malalignment of the vertebral column, narrowing of the intervertebral disc

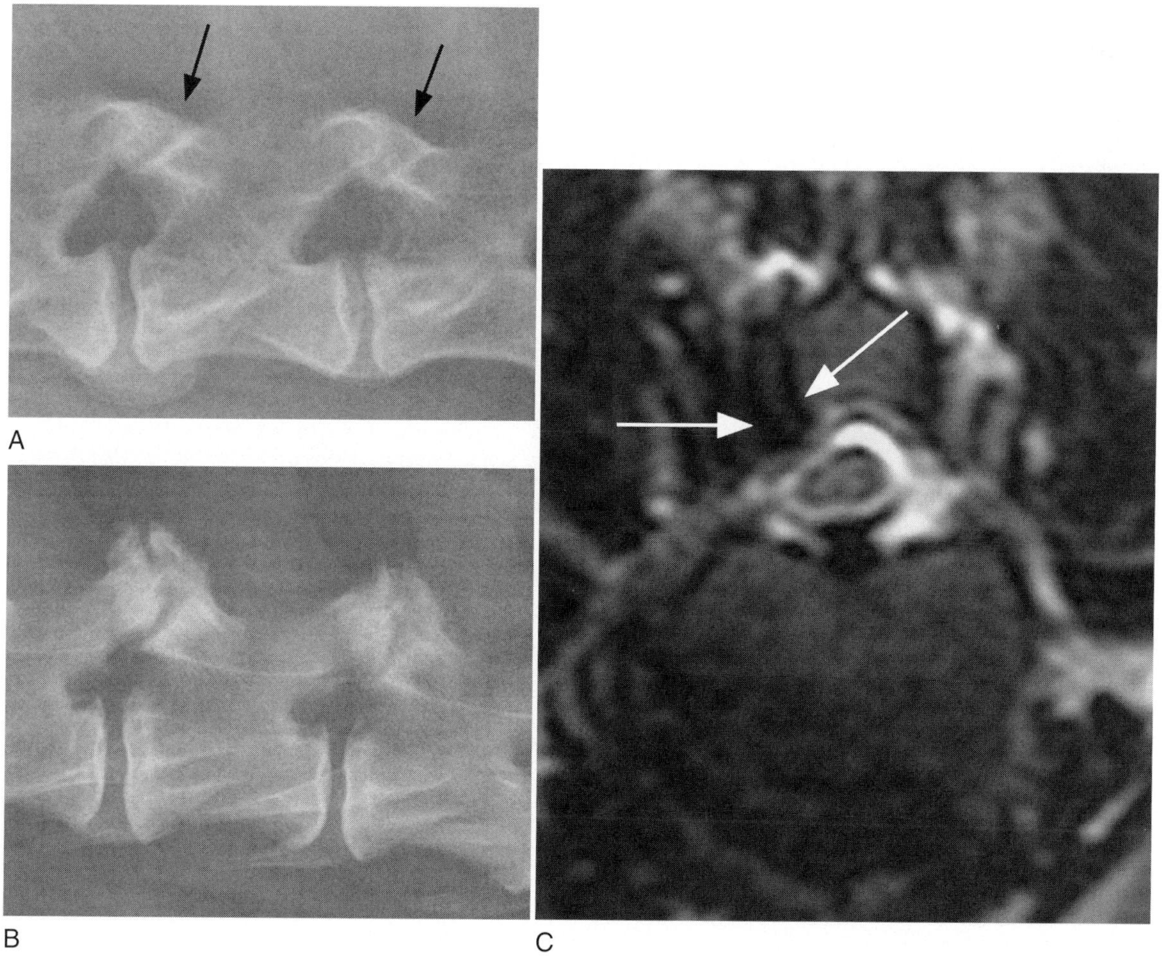

Fig. 11-25 Lateral radiographs of the lumbar spine of two dogs. **A,** Relatively normal-appearing dorsal articular process joints *(arrows)*. **B,** Marked dorsal articular process degenerative joint disease characterized by subchondral sclerosis and marked periarticular osteophytosis. **C,** Transverse T2-weighted fast spin-echo MR image of the T13-L1 interspace in a dog with articular process degenerative joint disease. A large hyperostotic *(black)* articular process is causing dorsolateral compression of the spinal cord.

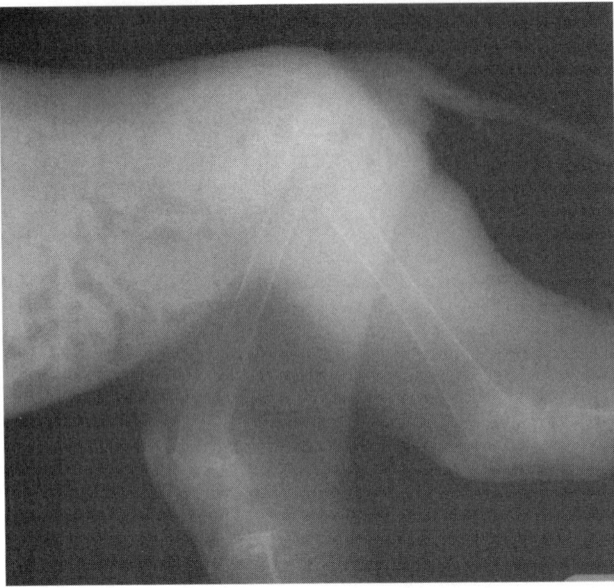

Fig. 11-26 Lateral pelvic radiograph of a felidae. Extreme osteopenia is present from nutritional secondary hyperparathyroidism.

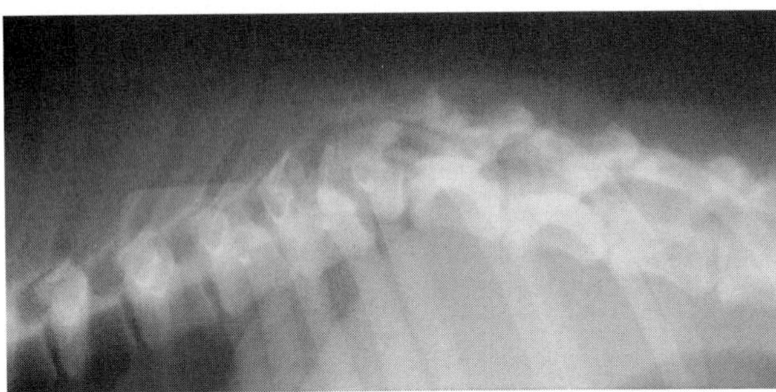

Fig. 11-27 Lateral radiograph of the thoracolumbar spine. A fracture/subluxation is present at T10-T11. Notice the disruption of the integrity of the vertebral canal.

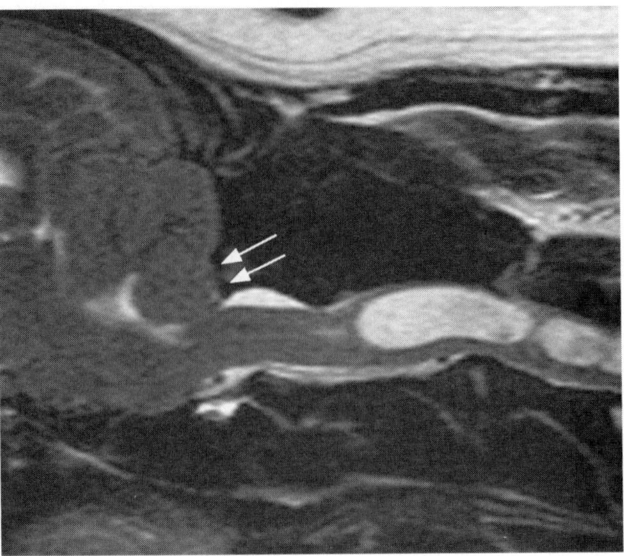

Fig. 11-28 Sagittal T2-weighted fast spin-echo image of a dog with a Chiari I–like malformation. Marked crowding of the cerebellum in the caudal fossa is visible *(arrows)*. This crowding leads to altered cerebrospinal fluid dynamics commonly associated with development of syringohydromyelia in the cervical spinal cord, as seen here.

space, and disruption of the cortical margin of the affected area. Care should be taken when performing radiography in these patients because instability may be exaggerated during radiography, leading to worsening of neural compression (Fig. 11-27).

A syndrome of occipitocervical malformation, sometimes called Chiari I–like malformation, is seen in Cavalier King Charles Spaniels and many other Terrier breeds. Occipital bone malformation causes crowding of the cerebellum in the caudal fossa, sometimes with partial herniation of the cerebellum. Occassionally there are also sites of subarachnoid impingement in the cranial aspect of the cervical spine. This malformation results in an alteration of flow of cerebrospinal fluid and often leads to syringohydromyelia in the cervical spinal cord and hydrocephalus. This syndrome is best imaged by cross-sectional techniques, particularly MR imaging. No correlation of the severity of the imaging signs with the clinical signs exhibited by the patient seems to exist (Fig. 11-28).[26,27]

REFERENCES

1. Bailey CS, Morgan JP: Congenital spinal malformations, *Vet Clin North Am* 22:985, 1992.
2. Morgan JP: Congenital anomalies of the vertebral column of the dog: a study of the incidence and significance based on a radiographic and morphologic study, *J Am Vet Radiol Soc* 9:21, 1968.
3. Morgan JP, Bahr A, Franti CE: Lumbosacral transitional vertebrae as a predisposing cause of cauda equina syndrome in German Shepherd Dogs: 161 cases (1987-1990), *J Am Vet Med Assoc* 202:1877, 1993.
4. Bailey CS: An embryological approach to the clinical significance of congenital vertebral and spinal cord anomalies, *J Am Anim Hosp Assoc* 11:426, 1975.
5. Wilson JW: Spina bifida in the dog and cat, *Comp Cont Educ Pract Vet* 8:626, 1982.
6. Havig Me, Cornell KK, Hawthorne JC et al: Evaluation of nonsurgical treatment of atlantoaxial subluxation in dogs: 19 cases (1992-2001), *J Am Vet Med Assoc* 227:257, 2005.
7. Beaver DP, Ellison GW, Lewis DD et al: Risk factors affecting the outcome of surgery for atlantoaxial subluxation in dogs: 46 cases (1978-1998), *J Am Vet Assoc* 216:1104, 2000.
8. Trotter EJ, deLahunta A, Geary JC et al: Caudal cervical malformation: malarticulation in Great Danes and Doberman Pinschers, *J Am Vet Med Assoc* 168:10, 1976.
9. Penderis J, Dennis R: Use of traction during magnetic resonance imaging of caudal cervical spondylomyelopathy ("Wobbler syndrome") in the dog, *Vet Radiol Ultrasound* 45: 216, 2004.
10. Sharp NJH, Cofone M, Robertson ID et al: Computed tomography in the evaluation of caudal cervical spondylomyelopathy of the Doberman pinscher, *Vet Radiol Ultrasound* 36:100, 1995.
11. Carnier P, Gallo L, Sturaro E et al: Prevalence of spondylosis deformans and estimates of genetic parameters for the degree of osteophytes development in Italian Boxer dogs, *J Anim Sci* 82:85, 2004.
12. Woodard JC, Poulos PW Jr, Parker RB et al: Canine diffuse skeletal hyperostosis, *Vet Pathol* 22:317, 1985.
13. Morgan JP, Stavenborn M: Disseminated idiopathic skeletal hyperostosis (DISH) in a dog, *Vet Radiol* 32:65, 1991.

14. Burkert BA, Kerwin SC, Hosgood GL et al: Signalment and clinical features of discospondylitis in dogs: 513 cases (1980-2001), *J Am Vet Med Assoc* 15:268, 2005.
15. Shamir MH, Tavor N, Aizenberg T: Radiographic findings during recovery from discospondylitis, *Vet Radiol Ultrasound* 42:496, 2001.
16. Levy MS, Katapkin AS, Patnaik A et al: Spinal tumors in 37 dogs: clinical outcome and long-term survival (1987-1994), *J Am Anim Hosp Assoc* 33:307, 1997.
17. Drost WT, Love NE, Berry CR: Comparison of radiography, myelography and computed tomography for the evaluation of canine vertebral and spinal cord tumors in sixteen dogs, *Vet Radiol Ultrasound* 37:28, 1996.
18. Ferguson HR: Conditions of the lumbosacral spinal cord and cauda equina, *Semin Vet Med Surg* 11:185, 1996.
19. Palmer RH, Chambers JN: Canine lumbosacral diseases. Parts I & II, *Comp Contin Educ* 13:16, 1991.
20. Hanna FY: Lumbosacral osteochondrosis: radiological features and surgical management in 34 dogs, *J Small Anim Pract* 42:272, 2001.
21. Mayhew PD, Kapatkin AS, Wortman JA et al: Association of cauda equina compression on magnetic resonance images and clinical signs in dogs with degenerative lumbosacral stenosis, *J Am Anim Hosp Assoc* 38:555, 2002.
22. Schwarz T, Stork CK, Mellor D et al: Osteopenia and other radiographic signs in canine hyperadrenocorticism, *J Small Anim Pract* 41:491, 2000.
23. Saunders Hm, Jezyk PF: The radiographic appearance of canine congenital hypothyroidism: skeletal changes with delayed treatment, *Vet Radiol* 32:171, 1991.
24. Wilkerson MJ, Lewis DC, Marks SL et al: Clinical and morphologic features of mucopolysaccharidosis type II in a dog: naturally occurring model of Hunter syndrome, *Vet Pathol* 35:230, 1998.
25. Shores A: Spinal trauma: pathophysiology and management of traumatic spinal injuries, *Vet Clin North Am* 22:859, 1992.
26. Rusbridge C, Knowler SP: Inheritance of occipital bone hypoplasia (Chiari type I malformation) in Cavalier King Charles Spaniels, *J Vet Intern Med* 18:673, 2004.
27. Lu D, Lamb CR, Pfeiffer DU et al: Neurological signs and results of magnetic resonance imaging in 40 Cavalier King Charles Spaniels with Chiari type1-like malformations, *Vet Rec* 30:260, 2003.

ELECTRONIC RESOURCES evolve

Additional information related to the content in Chapter 11 can be found on the companion Web site at evolve http://evolve.elsevier.com/Thrall/vetrad/

- Key Points
- Chapter Quiz
- Case Study 11-1
- Case Study 11-2

CHAPTER • 12
Canine and Feline Intervertebral Disc Disease, Myelography, and Spinal Cord Disease

William R. Widmer
Donald E. Thrall

Intervertebral disc disease is a degenerative condition of unknown cause that results in protrusion of the disc or disc material into the vertebral canal, compressing the spinal cord or spinal nerve roots.[1-3] Intervertebral disc disease affects all breeds of dogs; the chondrodystrophic breeds are overrepresented, with the highest prevalence in the Dachshund (45% to 65% of affected dogs).[1-4] Beagles, Cocker Spaniels, Toy Poodles, and Pekingese also have a high prevalence. Doberman Pinschers afflicted with cervical vertebral instability/malformation,[5] German shepherds,[6] and mixed-breed dogs also develop intervertebral disc disease.

Neural signs of intervertebral disc disease generally manifest after 3 years of age; however, in chondrodystrophic breeds, disc degeneration begins before 1 year of age. No gender predilection has been identified.[1] Common sites of disc protrusion are T12-T13 and T13-L1 in the thoracolumbar region, and C2-C3 and C3-C4 in the cervical region.[1,3] Although clinical signs of intervertebral disc disease are uncommon in cats, cervical disc degeneration frequently occurs in cats older than 6 years.[1,2]

Suspected intervertebral disc disease is one of the most important indications for imaging the vertebral column of small animals. Accurate imaging can establish the presence and severity of disc disease, allowing clinicians to determine prognosis and proceed with treatment. Because many imaging signs of disc disease are subtle and other spinal conditions may be the cause of clinical signs, accurate image interpretation requires a thorough knowledge of anatomy, physiology, and neurology.

ANATOMIC AND PHYSIOLOGIC CONSIDERATIONS

The intervertebral disc is composed of a tough outer annulus fibrosus, which contains the gelatinous, inner nucleus pulposus (Fig. 12-1).[7,8] The annulus has several concentric fibrocartilaginous layers, which are firmly attached to adjacent vertebral end plates.[1,8] The nucleus pulposus is eccentrically located in the disc; thus the annulus is thinner dorsally and thicker ventrally. This partially explains the tendency for dorsal herniation of diseased discs. A mixture of proteoglycans, collagen fibers, mesenchymal cells, and water makes up the normal jellylike nucleus. Only the outermost layers of the annulus have a neurovascular supply.[1]

The disc forms a cartilaginous joint between vertebral segments (except at C1-C2 and the sacrum, where intervertebral discs are not present) and thus functions as a hydraulic shock absorber. Shock absorption depends on a hydrated, deformable nucleus and an intact, elastic annulus.[7]

The longitudinal ligaments of the vertebral column provide dorsal and ventral support for the intervertebral discs.[8] The dorsal longitudinal ligament lies on the floor of the vertebral canal (see Fig. 12-1). In the cervical region, the dorsal ligament is wide and thick; consequently, lateral extrusion of disc material and radiculopathy (root signature) are more common than dorsal extrusion of the disc and severe cord compression.[9] In comparison, the dorsal longitudinal ligament is thin in the thoracolumbar region, predisposing to dorsal protrusion and spinal cord compression. The intercapital ligaments are short, transverse fibrous bands that lie ventral to the dorsal longitudinal ligament, joining the rib heads between T2 and T11. These ligaments buttress the dorsal part of the annulus cranial to T11 and help resist dorsal disc protrusion.[8,10,11] The ventral longitudinal ligament spans the ventral surface of the vertebral column, offering ventral support.

The vertebral canal of the dog is crowded, and the epidural space is small. Therefore the canine spinal cord is subject to compression by epidural masses, including disc protrusion. The Dachshund, compared with the German Shepherd, has a very high spinal cord/canal ratio; that is, a small epidural space.[12] This may explain the severe neurologic signs seen in the Dachshund after disc protrusion. Owing to a larger epidural space, small protrusions causing minimal cord compressions are less significant in large-breed dogs. The ratio of spinal cord to vertebral canal is lowest in the cervical area; therefore neurologic signs tend to be less severe with cervical versus thoracolumbar disc protrusion.[3,9,11]

The spinal cord and the spinal nerve roots lay within the bony vertebral canal, which consists of the individual vertebral foramina (see Fig. 12-1). Paired intervertebral foramina serve as windows, allowing exit of the spinal nerves and blood vessels. The meninges surround the spinal cord and consist of the inner pia-arachnoid membrane and the tough, outer dura (Fig. 12-2). The cervical and lumbar intumescences are normal enlargements of the spinal cord and should not be confused with cord swelling in image modalities in which spinal cord diameter can be assessed (myelography, computed tomography [CT], magnetic resonance [MR] imaging).

The spinal cord begins at the foramen magnum and, depending on the breed of dog, terminates at the conus medullaris, near the level of L6. In small-breed dogs, the spinal cord ends caudal to L6 and in large breeds it ends cranial to L6, an important consideration when lumbar subarachnoid puncture is performed. In the cat, the spinal cord extends slightly beyond L6.[13]

The spinal cord segments and vertebrae have the same numeric designation (with the exception of cord segment C8), but the location of each cord segment is rarely found within the corresponding vertebra.[10] The reasons are twofold.

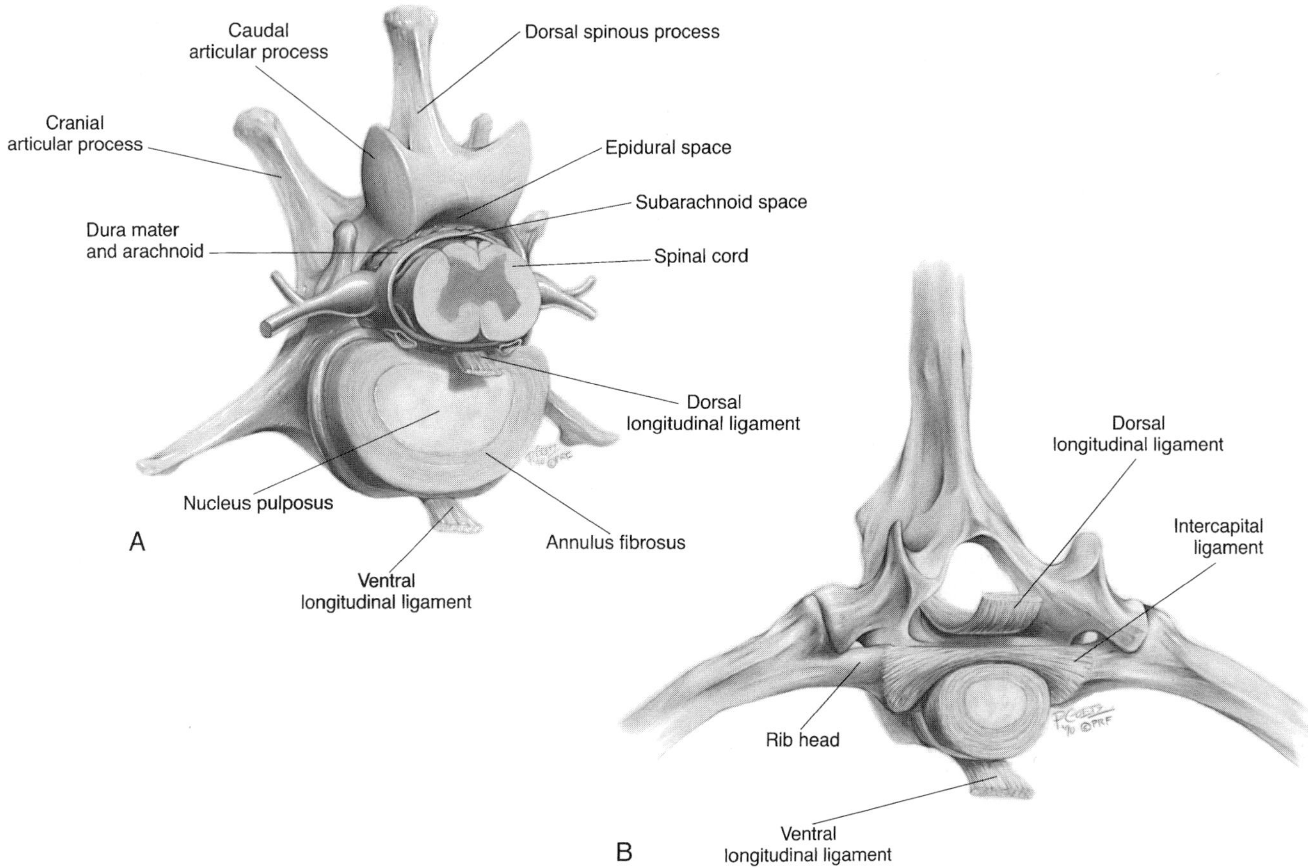

Fig. 12-1 Anatomic components of a typical lumbar vertebra (A) and an intervertebral disc (B). (Modified from Evans HE, Christensen JC: *Miller's anatomy of the dog*, ed 2, Philadelphia, 1979, WB Saunders.)

First, the spinal cord is shorter than the vertebral column because of differential fetal growth rates. Second, many of the spinal cord segments are shorter than the vertebral segments. Therefore spinal cord segments are located cranial to their respective vertebrae, and the spinal nerves must course caudally and obliquely within the vertebral canal over a short distance before exiting their respective intervertebral foramina. The collection of spinal nerve roots in the lumbosacral region is known as the cauda equina. These nerves, like the spinal cord, are subject to compressive injury caused by disc protrusion.

The subarachnoid space lies between the arachnoid membrane and the pia mater, which surrounds the spinal cord and spinal nerve roots. Cerebrospinal fluid (CSF) fills the subarachnoid space. The spinal subarachnoid space begins at the foramen magnum, where it communicates with the subarachnoid space of the cranial cavity, and ends caudally at the filum terminale, near the lumbosacral junction.[8] The central canal of the spinal cord is filled with CSF and communicates rostrally with the ventricular system. In most dogs, the central canal terminates blindly at the conus medullaris; however, in some dogs the canal is continuous with the lumbar subarachnoid space.

PATHOPHYSIOLOGIC CONSIDERATIONS

The nomenclature used to describe intervertebral disc lesions is confusing and inconsistent.[1] *Protrusion* is a nonspecific term that defines any discal mass that is impinging on the spinal cord or spinal nerve roots. Herniation implies that the nucleus pulposus is causing a bulge by stretching an intact annulus. An extruded, prolapsed, or blown-out disc is one in which the nucleus has broken through the annulus into the epidural space. Unfortunately, these terms are often used interchangeably. The distinction between protrusion, herniation, and extrusion is not always evident with conventional radiography, or even with CT and MR imaging. In human beings a consensus has been reached regarding the imaging description of lumbar disc disease.[14]

Classically, two forms of disc degeneration result in different types of protrusion.[1,7] Chondroid degeneration occurs in chondrodystrophic breeds and is typified by dehydration and mineralization of the nucleus pulposus. The annulus fibrosus also degenerates and loses its capacity to contain the diseased nucleus. Consequently, the weakened disc cannot withstand dynamic forces applied by the vertebral column, and protrusion ensues. Type I protrusion follows chondroid degeneration and is a result of extrusion of dehydrated nuclear material into the vertebral canal. Fibroid degeneration is frequently recognized in old, nonchondrodystrophic breeds and is characterized by fibrous metaplasia of the nucleus pulposus. The annulus fibrosus may stretch, partially rupture, or hypertrophy and protrude into the vertebral canal, thereby compressing the spinal cord. Type I lesions tend to be acute and forceful, causing compressive myelopathy and severe neurologic signs.[9] Type II lesions are associated with a chronic, progressive course and mild neurologic signs, even though significant spinal cord compression may be present.[9] This is because the spinal cord can better sustain the slow deforma-

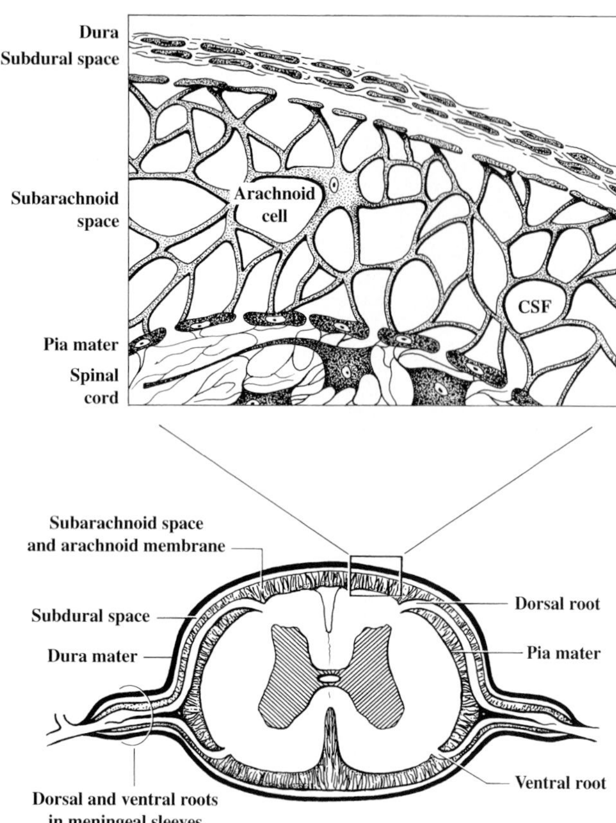

Fig. 12-2 Anatomic relation (transverse plane) of spinal cord, meningeal layers, and subarachnoid space. *Inset* shows microscopic structure of a segment of the meninges and cord. (Modified from Hoerlein BF: *Canine neurology: diagnosis and treatment*, ed 3, Philadelphia, 1978, WB Saunders.)

tion of a type II lesion than it can the explosive concussion and compression of a type I lesion.[7]

A variant of a type I lesion may occur in healthy, nondegenerate discs when the disc is subjected to extreme supraphysiologic pressure. The result is extrusion of normal nuclear material between intact annular fibers into the vertebral canal leading to severe myelitis. This type of herniation has been referred to by a variety of terms, including type III herniation and "missile" disc. Some controversy exists regarding which term to use to describe this uncommon type of disc herniation.

Spinal cord compression by protruded discs causes a closed type of injury that alters spinal cord function and structure.[7,9,11,15-17] Factors contributing to the pathologic changes of closed spinal cord injury are (1) mechanical disruption caused by compression and concussion and (2) chemical and vascular changes within the spinal cord. Severity depends on the dynamic force, duration and amount of compression, and degree of concussion associated with the initial injury. Spinal cord compression restricts the local arteriovenous supply, and severe arterial compromise may cause infarction. Ischemia of the spinal cord induces the release of potent vasoactive amines, including norepinephrine, serotonin, and dopamine, which leads to hematomyelia and myelomalacia.[15]

SURVEY RADIOGRAPHY

Radiographic signs consistent with intervertebral disc protrusion include (1) narrowing of the disc space, (2) narrowing of the dorsal intervertebral articular process joint space, (3) a small intervertebral foramen, (4) increased opacity in the intervertebral foramen, and (5) extruded, mineralized disc material within the vertebral canal (Fig. 12-3).

Importantly, survey radiographs are not sufficiently sensitive or specific to determine the site for spinal decompression to treat disc protrusion. Although some radiographic signs are associated with disc protrusion, radiographs often fail to allow identification of the site of protrusion responsible for the clinical signs. Spinal decompression should never proceed without definitive evidence of spinal cord compression obtained by myelography, CT, or MR imaging.

Disc space narrowing must be assessed in view of the animal's age and the presence or lack of secondary bony changes.[18] Narrowing may be caused by acute (type I) disc protrusion in young to middle-aged dogs when no secondary bony changes are present. In older dogs, narrowing may represent chronic (type II) disc disease, and only a bulging annulus fibrosus is present. Spondylosis deformans often accompanies chronic protrusion and reflects poor shock absorption by the diseased disc (see Fig. 12-3, *A*).

Discal mineralization indicates intervertebral disc degeneration but not always disc protrusion (see Fig. 12-3, C and *D*).[18] Dystrophic mineralization of a degenerating disc usually begins in the center of the nucleus pulposus and extends peripherally. The annulus may undergo mineralization separately. Not all mineralized discs will prolapse, and not all prolapsed disc material is mineralized. Extruded mineralized disc material can sometimes be seen on survey radiographs (see Fig. 12-3, *B* and *E*). With acute prolapse, mineralized disc material is dispersed by local inflammation. Therefore the opacity of disc material in the vertebral canal is nearer that of soft tissue than of mineral. As inflammation subsides, the extruded mass of disc material contracts and becomes more opaque. In addition, chronically extruded disc material may undergo mineralization or ossification.

Lateral and intraforaminal protrusions of the cervical discs may escape detection when standard ventrodorsal and lateral projections are used. Because of the relatively large extradural space in the cervical region, protrusions may not cause an extradural myelographic lesion. Oblique radiographic projections (V45°L-DR or V45°R-DL) allow assessment of the left and right foramina, respectively, enabling identification of an opaque foramen. This procedure aids the surgeon because the animal may otherwise fall into the nonsurgical treatment category.[19]

After hemilaminectomy, the disc space often remains narrow. The hemilaminectomy site can be identified by unilateral absence of the articular processes (Fig. 12-4). The thoracolumbar region should always be scrutinized for this finding because historic information regarding previous surgical decompression may be lacking. If complete laminectomy has been performed, the absence of the lamina and spinous processes is easily recognized. Fenestrations generally result in disc space narrowing and occasionally discospondylitis.[17]

MYELOGRAPHY

Myelography, which is radiography after injection of contrast medium into the spinal subarachnoid space, is useful for evaluating the spinal cord and cauda equina. Indications for myelography include (1) confirming a spinal lesion seen or suspected on survey radiographs, (2) defining the extent of a survey lesion, (3) finding a lesion not observed on survey radiographs, and (4) identifying patients that are likely to benefit from surgery. A disadvantage of myelography is that it may cause intensification of preexisting neurologic signs.[20]

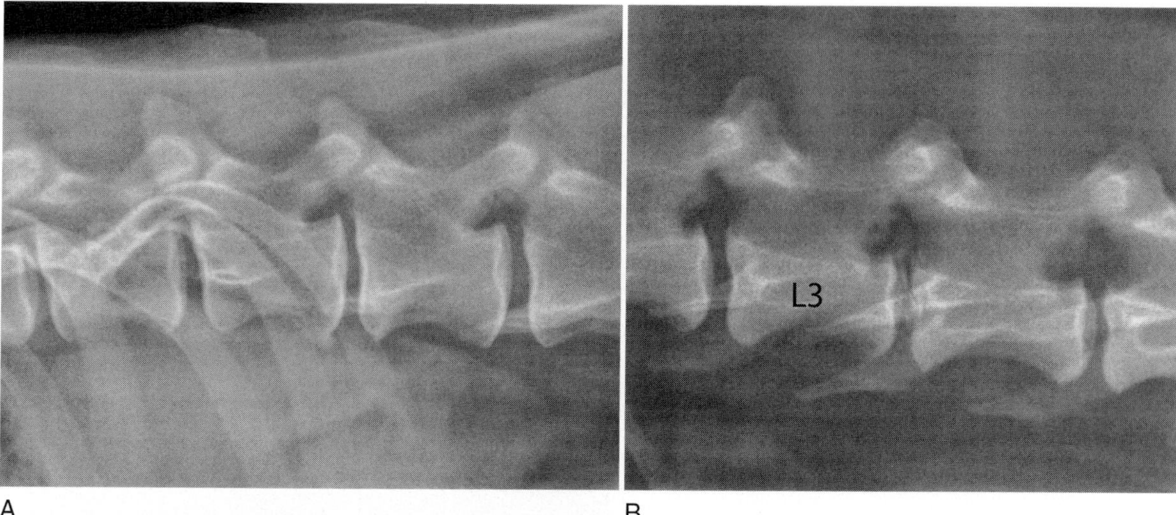

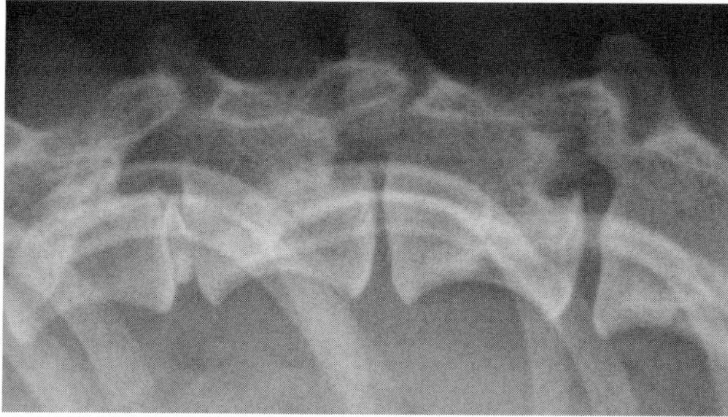

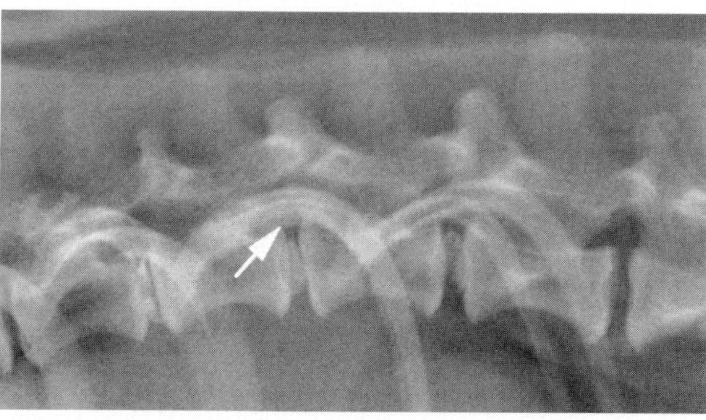

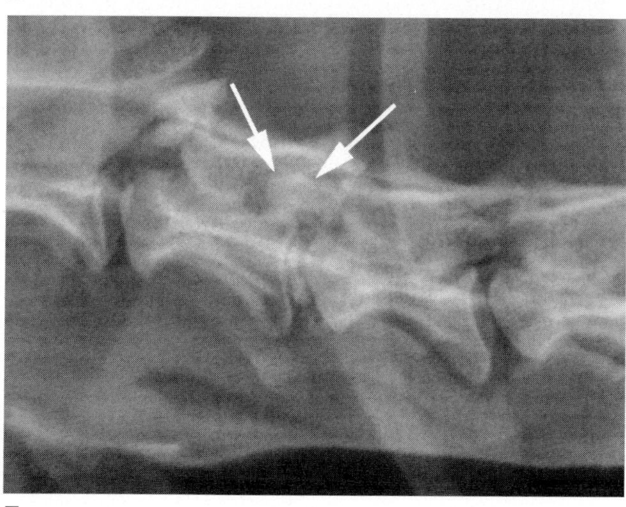

Fig. 12-3 Survey radiographic signs of intervertebral disc disease. **A,** The intervertebral disc space, intervertebral foramen, and dorsal articular process joint space at L1-L2 are all decreased in size compared with adjacent vertebrae. These signs are typically found with a protruding disc as vertebrae adjacent to the affected disc move closer together. Mild spondylosis deformans at L1-L2 is consistent with chronic disc protrusion with loss of normal shock absorption at this site. **B,** Mineralization of the disc at L3-L4 as well as mineralized material superimposed over the intervertebral foramen; this is consistent with the presence of mineralized disc material in the vertebral canal. This emphasizes that a disc may not herniate completely; in this dog residual disc material is between the vertebral end plates. It cannot be determined with certainty from this lateral view alone that the mineralization presumed to be within the vertebral canal is not lateral to the vertebral canal. The intervertebral foramen at L3-L4 is also slightly smaller than the foramen at L4-L5. **C,** The intervertebral disc space, intervertebral foramen, and dorsal articular process joint space at T12-T13 are all decreased in size compared with adjacent vertebrae. As in **A,** these signs are typically found with a protruding disc caused by the vertebrae adjacent to the affected disc moving closer together. In situ mineralization of the disc is present at T11-T12. This mineralization is not clinically important and only signifies degeneration of the disc. **D,** Mineralized discs are seen in situ at T11-T12, T12-T13, and T13-L1. As noted for in **C,** in situ mineralization is not clinically significant. However, even though ribs are superimposed on the foramen at T12-T13, it is smaller than adjacent foramina and the dorsal articular process joint space at T12-T13 appears narrow. A suggestion of a focal mineralization superimposed on the intervertebral foramen *(arrow)* is also present. This close inspection raises suspicion for partial extrusion of the disc at T12-T13, which was confirmed in subsequent CT images. **E,** Mineralization of the disc at C3-C4, with a narrow disc space. In the cervical vertebral column, the articular processes are larger than in the thoracolumbar region and are typically superimposed on the intervertebral foramina, making assessment of the foramina more difficult in the cervical vertebral column. However, in this dog a large mineralized opacity is visible in a position consistent with it being in the vertebral canal *(arrows)*. Confirmation that this opacity is within the vertebral canal requires additional images or modalities.

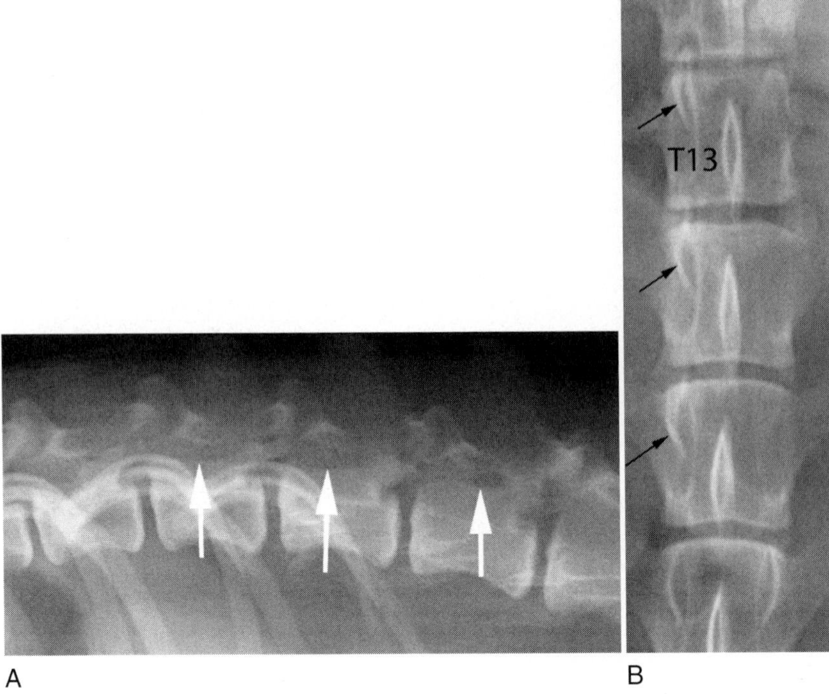

Fig. 12-4 A, Laminectomy sites are recognized because some lamina have been removed *(arrows)*. B, Unilateral absence of articular processes after left hemilaminectomy; compare with the intact processes on the right *(arrows)*.

Myelography, or another modality capable of assessing spinal cord compression, is absolutely necessary before surgical decompression of the spinal cord. In studies of dogs with surgically confirmed disc disease, survey radiographs were only 68% to 72% accurate in identifying the site of disc protrusion; the accuracy of myelography was 86% to 97%.[4,21] In a more recent study accuracy of multiple observers for determining sites of disc protrusion on survey radiographs was only 51% to 61%.[22] The authors concluded that recognition of multiple signs of disc protrusion increased accuracy at a particular site, but accuracy was still unacceptable for surgical treatment. Myelography also provides evidence for whether a hemilaminectomy should be performed on the left or the right side of the affected disc space.

Technique

For decades, myelography was the technique of choice for determining sites of spinal cord compression and other spinal cord lesions. However, CT and MR imaging are replacing the use of myelography in many practice settings because they are quicker and noninvasive and, in the case of MR imaging, capable of assessing the integrity of the spinal cord itself. However, myelography remains a valuable tool for assessing the spinal cord.

Myelographic technique is well described[19-29]; therefore only a brief summary is presented. Myelography is always performed under aseptic conditions and with the animal under general anesthesia. An accurate survey radiographic study serves as a baseline and must precede myelography. Iohexol (Omnipaque, 240 mgI/mL) and iopamidol (Isovue, 200 mgI/mL) are safe and efficacious and are the nonionic contrast media of choice for small animal myelography. The full-spine dosage is approximately 0.45 mL/kg and the regional dosage is approximately 0.30 mL/kg. These dosages are guidelines; administering sufficient contrast medium to fill the subarachnoid space in the region of interest is important. A 22-gauge spinal needle with stylet is preferred for myelography because it has a short bevel, which increases the likelihood that the needle will be positioned in the thin subarachnoid space. The stylet is kept in place during subarachnoid puncture to minimize damage if the spinal cord is accidentally pierced and to prevent tissue from clogging the needle lumen.

Cervical myelography can be performed by injecting contrast medium into the cerebellomedullary cistern through the atlantooccipital space (Fig. 12-5). Puncture can be accomplished with the animal in either sternal or lateral recumbency. The head is flexed ventrally, and the needle is carefully inserted on the midline near the center of a triangle formed by the external occipital protuberance and the wings of the atlas.[23] As the needle is advanced, a distinct "pop," followed immediately by loss of resistance, is often felt as the needle traverses the dorsal atlantooccipital membrane and dura. This classic sensation is less obvious or absent in small dogs and should not be relied on as evidence of cisternal entry. During puncture, the myelographer should frequently stop, withdraw the stylet, and check for evidence of CSF flow out the needle. A radiograph can also be made with the needle in place for orientation purposes.

Lumbar myelography is performed by puncture of the subarachnoid space, preferably at L5-L6, but L4-L5 can be used if injection at L5-L6 or L6-L7 cannot be made successfully. Injection at L4-L5 should be avoided unless absolutely necessary because of the greater chance for injury to the spinal cord by the needle (Fig. 12-6). The animal is placed in lateral recumbency and either of two methods can be used to punc-

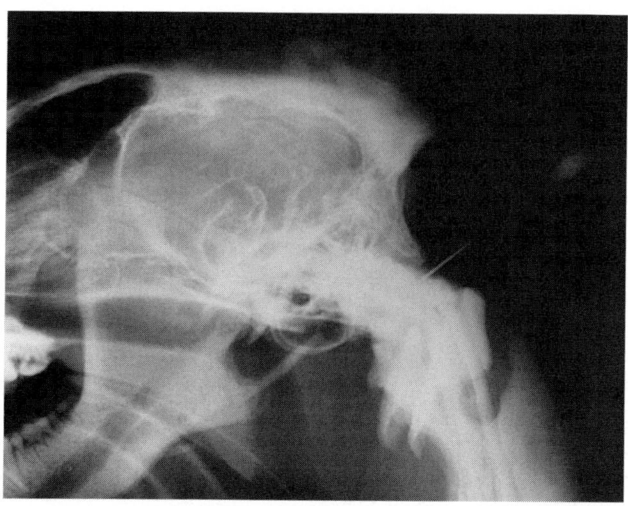

Fig. 12-5 Technique of cervical myelography. After the occipital bone is located, the needle can be "walked" caudally and inserted into the cerebellomedullary space. Contrast medium has been injected into the subarachnoid space, and some contrast medium is present in the cranial cavity.

ture the subarachnoid space.[20] With the paramedian approach, the needle is inserted slightly caudolateral to the spinous process of L6 or L7 and is directed cranioventrally at a 45-degree angle through the interarcuate space. The median approach requires insertion of the needle just cranial to the spinous process of L5 or L6 at a 90-degree angle to the vertebral column.

Because the lumbar subarachnoid space ends blindly in most dogs, contrast medium can be forced cranially past an area of intramedullary swelling, allowing evaluation of the cranial and caudal aspects of a compressive lesion. However, with cervical injection, contrast medium tends to flow rostrally into the ventricular system when resistance to caudal flow is encountered; thus only the cranial margin of a compressive lesion may be identified.[30] Cervical myelography is rarely of value when severe thoracolumbar cord swelling is present. In many instances, myelography from a lumbar injection is the best way to evaluate a cervical spinal cord lesion.

Because locating the dorsal subarachnoid space is difficult, most myelographers choose to position the needle bevel in the ventral aspect of the subarachnoid space (Fig. 12-7). Less risk of intramedullary injection of contrast medium exists when the needle is on the floor of the vertebral canal. However, although positioning the needle bevel in the dorsal aspect of the subarachnoid space is technically more difficult, such placement causes less mechanical damage to the spinal cord (see Fig. 12-6, C).

Transneural passage of the needle is necessary for needle placement on the ventral aspect of the subarachnoid space and invariably damages the spinal cord or nerve roots. This can be minimized by keeping the stylet in place and avoiding horizontal movement of the needle during puncture. However, the dorsal aspect of the spinal cord is compressed 2 to 3 mm ventrally as the needle tip is resisted by the tough dura (see Fig. 12-7).[31] Therefore the spinal cord can be injured by compression as well as by the needle. Obviously, with placement of the needle in the dorsal aspect of the subarachnoid space, the spinal cord is only compressed, not penetrated. Whether aiming for the dorsal or the ventral aspect of the subarachnoid space, correct needle placement should be confirmed by fluoroscopy or radiography after a test injection of a small volume (0.5 to 1.0 mL) of contrast medium; otherwise, intramedullary injection may occur. Positioning the needle in the dorsal aspect of the subarachnoid space is technically superior because only one puncture of the subarachnoid space is made, thus decreasing the likelihood of extradural leakage of contrast medium. Regardless of the approach used, multiple needle punctures should be avoided because the risk of epidural leakage is increased with each attempt.[23]

Interpretive Principles

Knowledge of the relation of the spinal cord to the meninges, epidural space, and vertebral canal is essential for accurate myelographic interpretation (see Fig. 12-2). This relation is important for proper localization of vertebral canal mass lesions with respect to the dura, whether interpreting a myelogram or CT/MR images.

The normal myelogram is typified by a sharply marginated, thin column of contrast medium in the subarachnoid space (Fig. 12-8).[23-25] Small-breed dogs and cats (see Fig. 12-8, *C* and *D*) tend to have relatively large spinal cords and, as a result, a thin subarachnoid space.[24] The ventral aspect of the epidural (extradural) space is normally wide in the caudal cervical region, giving the false impression of cord displacement. The dorsal aspect of the subarachnoid space is widest at the C1-C2 level and tends to be wider than the corresponding ventral aspect of the subarachnoid space in the thoracolumbar region. Small filling defects often seen dorsal to the cervical discs are caused by hypertrophy of the ligamentum flavum or the annulus fibrosus. Clinically significant subarachnoid space filling defects should be accompanied by thinning of the opposite aspect of the contrast medium column or evidence of spinal cord compression. The thoracic spinal cord lacks an intumescence and is smaller than the cervical and lumbosacral regions of the spinal cord. Although the canine spinal cord terminates at L5-L6, the contrast medium–filled dural sac may extend beyond the lumbosacral junction (see Fig. 12-6, *B*).[23]

The abnormal myelogram is characterized by changes in the size and location of the contrast medium–filled subarachnoid space and in the width and opacity of the spinal cord. Myelographic lesions can be grouped into the following patterns: extradural lesions, intradural-extramedullary lesions, intramedullary swelling, and intramedullary opacification (Fig. 12-9 and Box 12-1).[23,32-34] As previously noted, these same principles apply to interpretation of CT and MR images.

Several technical factors affect myelographic quality and interpretation (Fig. 12-10).[28] Air bubbles cause circular or oval filling defects that are potentially confusing; however, their location is usually variable on subsequent radiographs.[23] Subdural leakage may occur if the needle bridges the subdural and the subarachnoid spaces, causing irregular margination and poor filling of the contrast medium columns. Epidural leakage of contrast medium should be avoided because it adds unwanted opacity, obscuring the subarachnoid contrast medium column.[23] Gravity affects the distribution of contrast medium, reducing subarachnoid opacification in nondependent regions. On the ventrodorsal projection, dependency causes contrast medium to pool cranially, thereby reducing the opacity of the caudal cervical subarachnoid space. The opposite situation occurs with the dorsoventral projection; therefore both projections should be obtained routinely. On the lateral projection, contrast medium pools cranial to and caudal to the thoracic region. The effect of pooling can be overcome by elevating the rear and forequarters of the animal, filling the thoracic subarachnoid space. Pooling becomes more of a problem with hyperosmolar, high–iodine content contrast media.[28]

Visualization of contrast medium in the central canal occurs when the needle shaft is placed in the central canal or

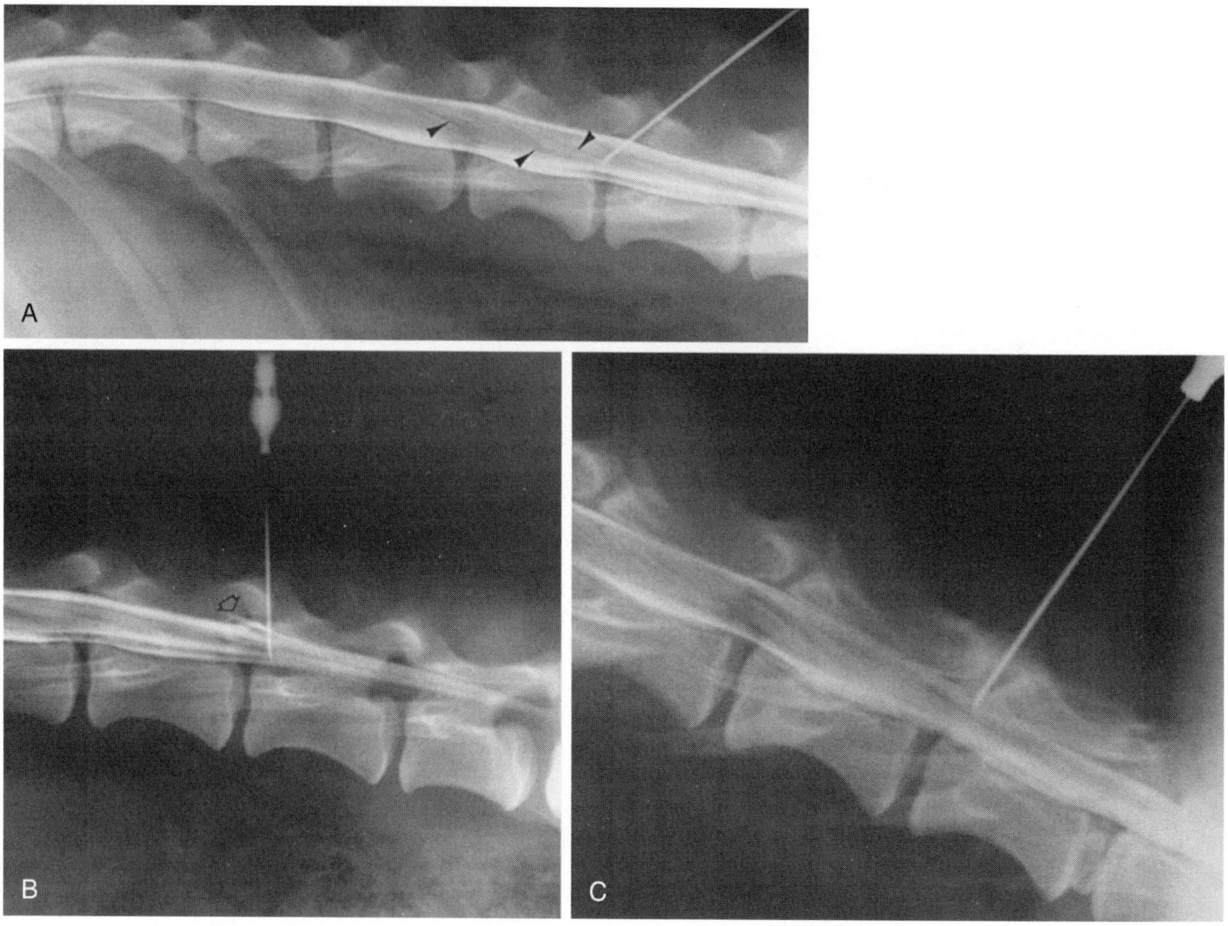

Fig. 12-6 Technique of lumbar myelography. **A,** Lumbar myelogram obtained by the paramedian approach. The needle tip is in the ventral aspect of the subarachnoid space at L4-L5, and the needle shaft is at an approximately 45-degree angle to the spinal cord and parallel to the plane of the dorsal intervertebral articular process joints. Filling defects *(arrowheads)* are caused by the spinal nerve roots of the lumbar cord segments. Note the sharply marginated contrast medium column, which indicates subarachnoid injection. **B,** Lumbar myelogram obtained by the median approach at L5-L6. The needle tip is in the ventral aspect of the subarachnoid space, and the needle shaft is perpendicular to the spinal cord. Slight epidural leakage has occurred around the needle tract *(arrow)*. The dural sac is opacified, ending at L7-S1. **C,** Lumbar myelogram with the needle tip in the dorsal aspect of the subarachnoid space at L5-L6. Note the disc mineralization at L6-L7.

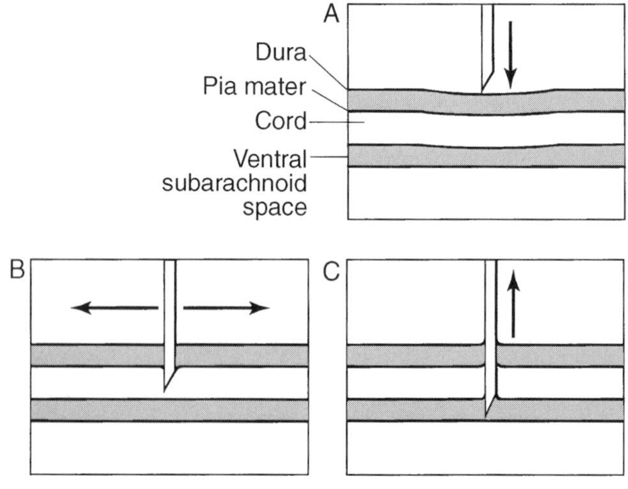

Fig. 12-7 Lumbar puncture may cause mechanical damage to the neural tissue. **A,** Compression of the spinal cord by resistance of the tough dura. **B,** The compression is released as the needle tip passes through the dura, entering the spinal cord. Horizontal movement should be minimized to avoid spinal cord damage. **C,** The needle is retracted slightly (1 to 2 mm) after it has reached the ventral aspect of the vertebral canal, reducing the chance of epidural injection. (Reprinted from Widmer WR, Blevins WE: Veterinary myelography: a review of contrast media, adverse effects, and technique, *J Am Anim Hosp Assoc* 19:755, 1991.)

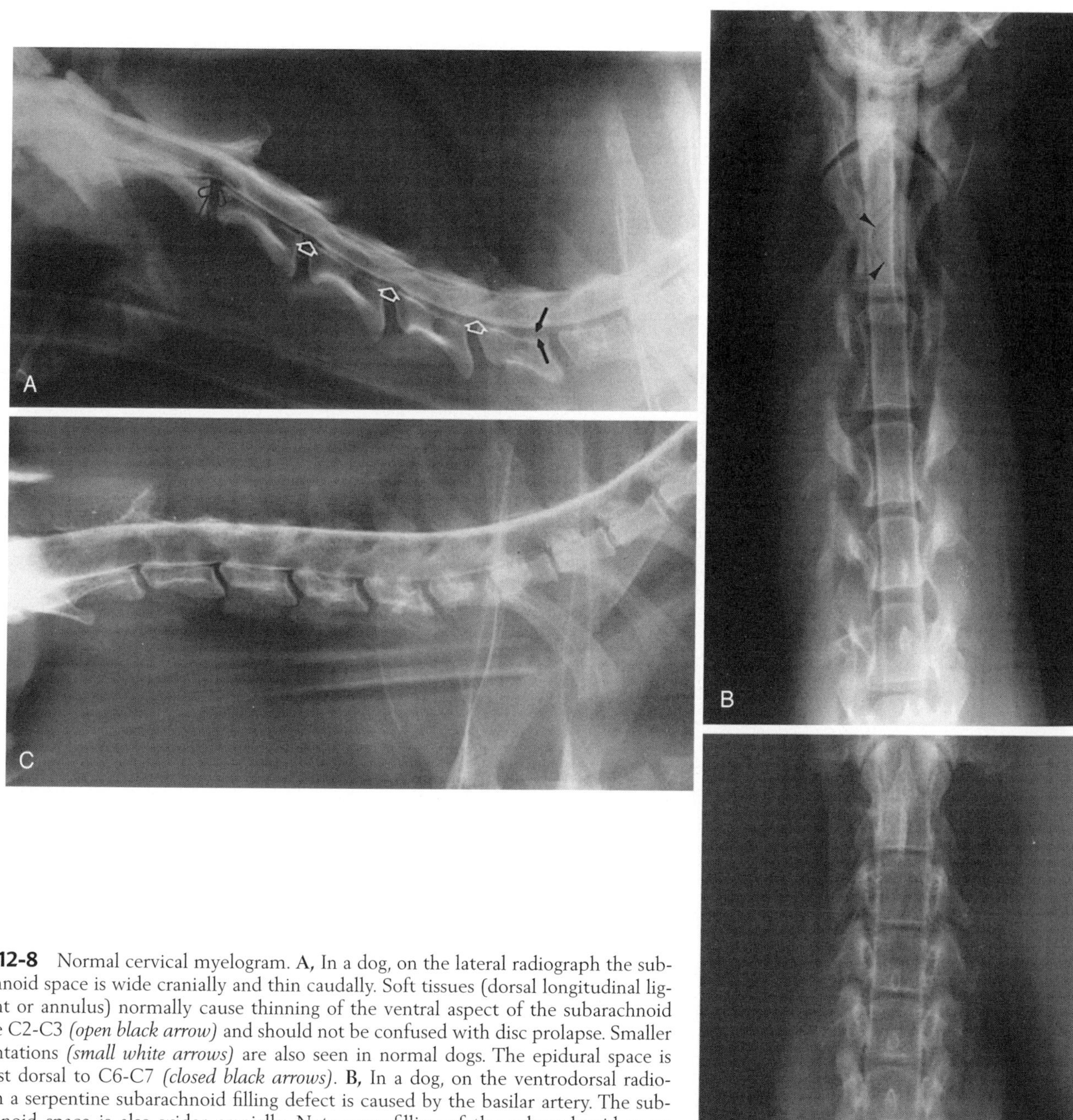

Fig. 12-8 Normal cervical myelogram. **A,** In a dog, on the lateral radiograph the subarachnoid space is wide cranially and thin caudally. Soft tissues (dorsal longitudinal ligament or annulus) normally cause thinning of the ventral aspect of the subarachnoid space C2-C3 *(open black arrow)* and should not be confused with disc prolapse. Smaller indentations *(small white arrows)* are also seen in normal dogs. The epidural space is widest dorsal to C6-C7 *(closed black arrows)*. **B,** In a dog, on the ventrodorsal radiograph a serpentine subarachnoid filling defect is caused by the basilar artery. The subarachnoid space is also wider cranially. Note poor filling of the subarachnoid space in the caudal cervical region, which is caused by the effect of dependency. **C** and **D,** In the cat, the spinal cord is relatively wide and occupies a large percentage of the vertebral canal. As a result, the subarachnoid space is thin and conforms closely to the margins of the vertebral canal; this can give a false impression of cord swelling.

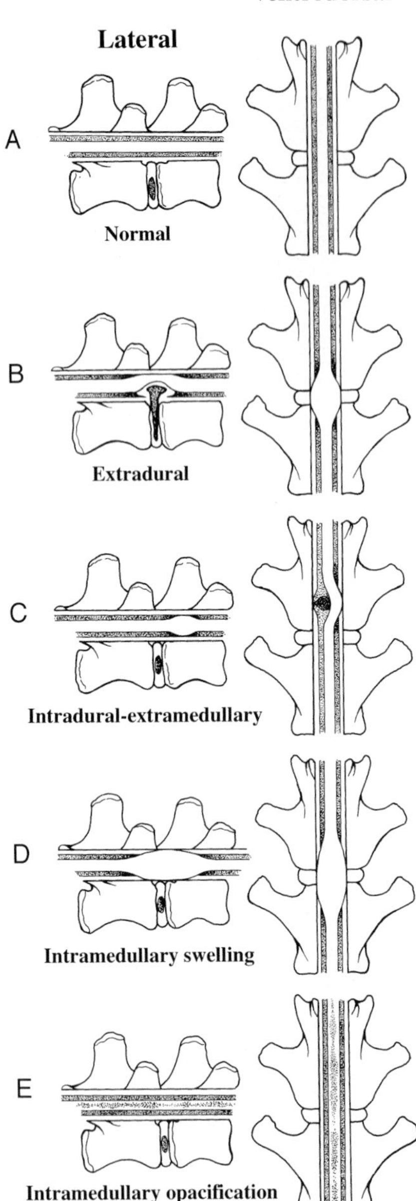

Fig. 12-9 Classification of myelographic lesions. A, Normal. B, Extradural. An aspect of the contrast medium column is displaced toward the center of the vertebral canal and often thinned or obliterated on one radiographic projection. On the orthogonal projection the spinal cord may appear widened with peripheral displacement of the subarachnoid space because of an increase in spinal cord diameter caused by the compression. C, Intradural-extramedullary mass lesion within the subarachnoid space causes a filling defect in at least one projection. On the orthogonal projection, spinal cord swelling may be present depending on the size of the mass. As the contrast medium abuts the mass in the subarachnoid space, it flares around the mass and has been described as having the appearance of a golf tee. D, Intramedullary swelling. The spinal cord is swollen, causing thinning and obliteration of the subarachnoid space on both myelographic projections. E, Intramedullary opacification. Opacification of the spinal cord parenchyma is caused by the presence of contrast medium. This may be secondary to myelomalacia, which allows intramedullary diffusion of contrast medium. Opacification of the central canal differs and should not be confused with myelomalacia (see Fig. 12-11).

Box • 12-1

Diagnostic Possibilities Associated with Myelographic Patterns

Pattern	*Diagnosis*
Extradural	Intervertebral disc protrusion Ligamentous hypertrophy Hematoma/hemorrhage Neoplasia (vertebral or epidural soft tissue) Vertebral fracture/dislocation
Intradural-extramedullary	Neoplasia (neurofibroma, neurofibrosarcoma, and meningioma) Lateralized extradural masses, such as discs, may give the appearance of an intradural-extramedullary lesion
Intramedullary swelling	Spinal cord edema Neoplasia (neural, metastatic discrete cell, e.g., granulomatous meningoencephalitis) Ischemic myelopathy
Intramedullary opacification	Myelomalacia Hematomyelia
Normal	Degenerative myelopathy* Ischemic myelopathy Myelitis Meningitis

*It is the authors' opinion that spinal cord size may be decreased in dogs with degenerative myelopathy; however, this has not yet been proved by scientific investigation.

when the central canal communicates with the subarachnoid space at the level of the conus medullaris (Fig. 12-11, *A*).[35] In the former instance, contrast medium is presumed to leak back along the needle, especially during rapid injection.[35] Canalograms are most likely to occur when puncture is made at L4-L5, where the spinal cord/vertebral canal ratio is large. The presence of contrast medium in a normal-appearing central canal should not be confused with spinal cord opacification caused by myelomalacia (Fig. 12-12, *B*). Enlargement of the central canal is associated with hydromyelia. The central canal may also become opacified when severe trauma or neoplasia disrupts the spinal cord parenchyma.

Intervertebral Disc Protrusion

Either an extradural or an intramedullary pattern may result from disc protrusion (Box 12-2).[23,24,36-38] Disc protrusion typically causes an extradural lesion characterized by thinning and dorsal deviation of the ventral aspect of the subarachnoid space in the lateral radiograph and compensatory widening of the spinal cord in the ventrodorsal radiograph (see Fig. 12-12).[28] On the lateral radiograph, the spinal cord is compressed and is deviated away from the site of disc protrusion. The aspect of the contrast medium column adjacent to the

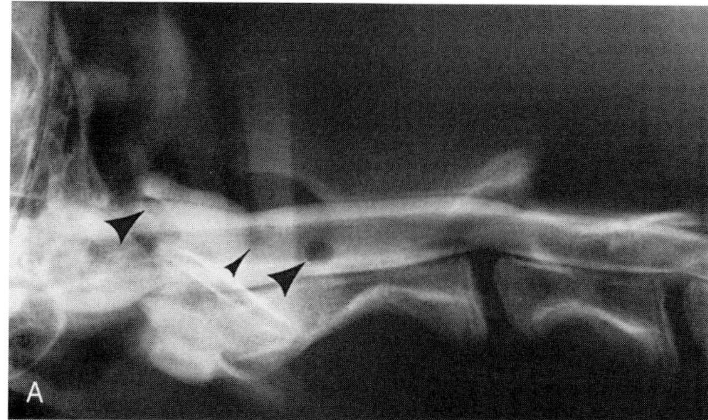

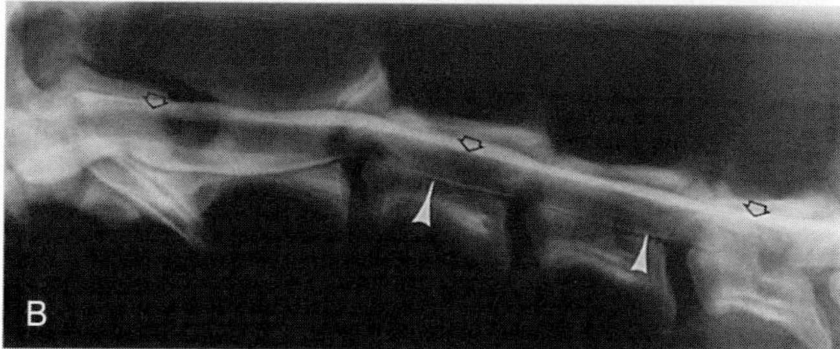

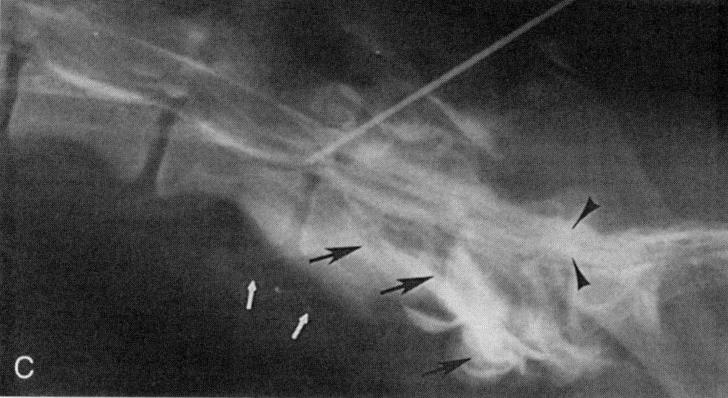

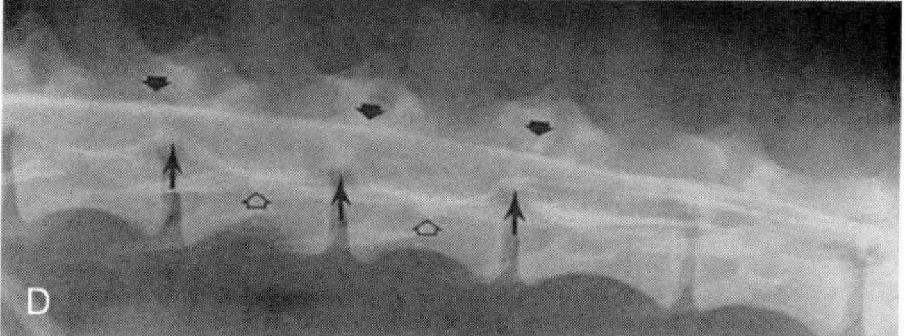

Fig. 12-10 Myelograms with artifacts caused by technical errors. **A,** Air bubbles *(arrowheads)* create circular or oval filling defects; their location varies from radiograph to radiograph, unlike a filling defect caused by a lesion. Air bubbles can be eliminated by filling the plastic extension tube with contrast medium before injection of contrast medium. **B,** Injection of contrast medium into the subdural space may occur if the needle bevel bridges the subdural and subarachnoid spaces. Note wavy and irregularly marginated appearance of the dorsal aspect of the contrast medium *(open arrows)* and incomplete filling of the ventral aspect of the subarachnoid space *(arrowheads)*. **C,** Severe epidural leakage caused by improper needle placement. Contrast medium has spilled into the epidural space of the intervertebral canal and that which surrounds the sacral nerve roots *(black arrows)*. **D,** Moderate epidural leakage after lumbar myelography at L5-L6. Epidural contrast medium can be recognized ventrally by the appearance of opacified vertebral venous sinuses *(large closed arrows)* and dorsally by opacification dorsal to the subarachnoid space *(small closed arrows)*. Opacified depressions in the vertebral bodies contain the basivertebral veins *(open black arrows)*.

Box • 12-2

Myelographic Signs of Intervertebral Disc Disease

Extradural Pattern

Deviation and thinning of subarachnoid contrast medium column at intervertebral disc space (ventral, dorsal, or lateral)
Forked subarachnoid contrast medium column (false intradural-extramedually sign) if disc is lateralized
Spinal cord displacement
Spinal cord compression (compensatory displacement flattens cord owing to extradural mass, mimics cord swelling)
"Hourglass" subarachnoid space filling defect

Intramedullary Pattern

Uniform spinal cord swelling caused by edema; subarachnoid contrast medium column displaced, thin, or absent
Opacification of spinal cord parenchyma

protrusion tends to be dome shaped, and the opposite side of the contrast medium column is narrowed by the displaced spinal cord. When disc protrusion is slightly lateral to the midline a split, or forked, appearance to the contrast medium column may be seen on the lateral projection (see Fig. 12-12, C). This finding should not be confused with an intradural-extramedullary lesion (see Fig. 12-9).[4,28]

In a type I protrusion an intramedullary pattern frequently predominates as a consequence of severe spinal cord swelling (Fig. 12-13). This swelling masks the classic extradural appearance of an extruded disc. Spinal cord swelling is caused by edema of one to three vertebral segments cranial or caudal to the site of protrusion as a result of acute injury, but it is not a feature of chronic disc protrusion. With intramedullary swelling, the subarachnoid space is thin and displaced peripherally in the vertebral canal (see Fig. 12-13). In some instances, severe spinal cord swelling may completely obliterate the subarachnoid space (see Fig. 12-13, C).

Evidence of intramedullary swelling is typically visible on both the lateral and ventrodorsal radiographic projections. Compensatory extradural compression of the spinal cord causes focal spinal cord widening on a single radiographic projection, usually the ventrodorsal, that extends over a shorter length than *bona fide* intramedullary swelling. Also, extradural signs of disc protrusion are seen on the orthogonal projection. In some instances acutely extruded disc material may disperse around the cord and prevent the subarachnoid space from filling mimicking cord swelling.[39]

If intramedullary swelling is present but no signs of extradural compression are obvious, careful scrutiny of the myelogram may identify the site of disc protrusion. Slight central deviation of the subarachnoid space somewhere within the region of spinal cord swelling suggests the site of an extradural discal mass (see Fig. 12-13, *B*). This important clue is often found on only one radiographic projection but can help determine the site for surgical exploration and decompression. On the other hand, if CT is available, postmyelographic imaging can accurately depict the exact site of extradural compression when severe intramedullary swelling is present.

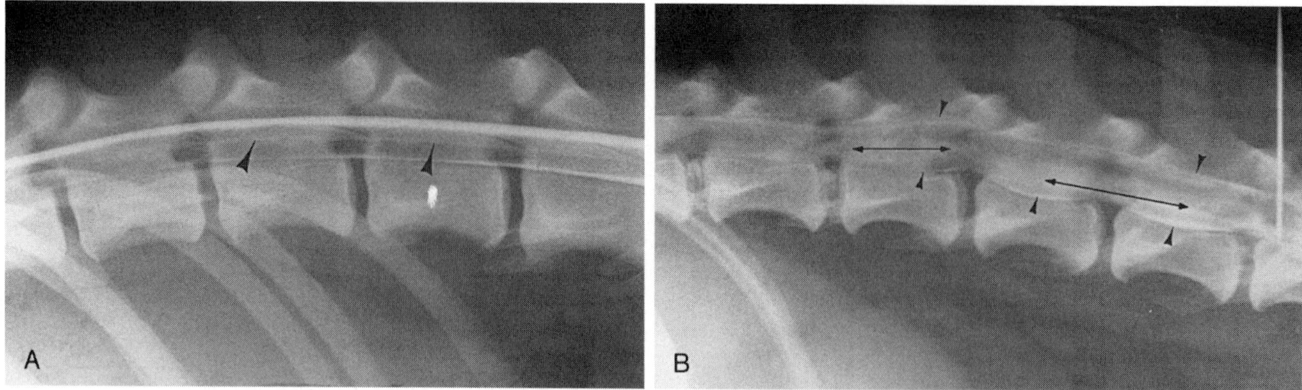

Fig. 12-11 A, Opacification of the central canal *(arrows)* occurs when communication exists between the central canal and the subarachnoid space. **B,** Myelomalacia is typified by diffusion of contrast medium into the spinal cord parenchyma *(double-headed arrows)*. Intramedullary swelling is also present and the subarachnoid space is thin *(arrowheads)*.

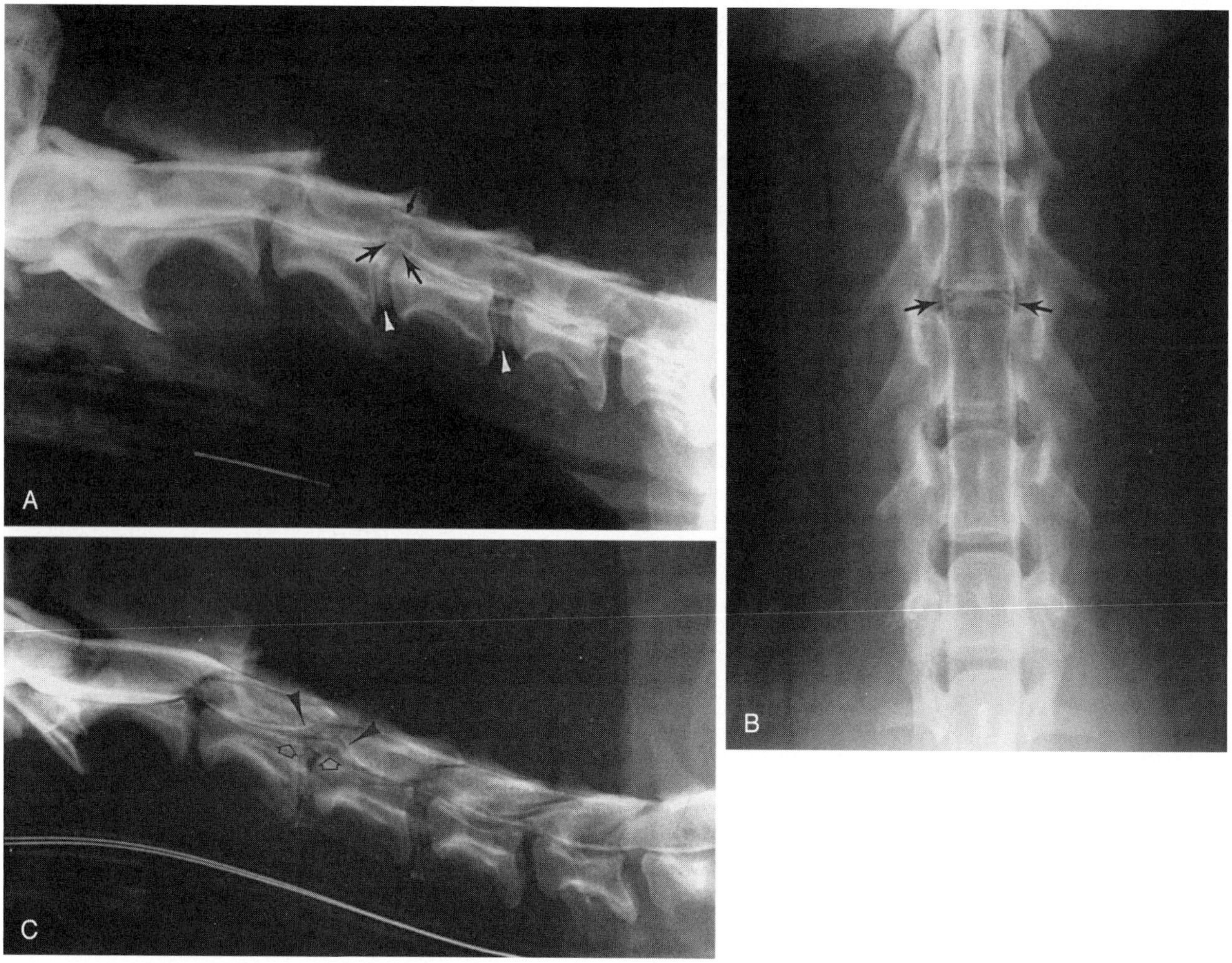

Fig. 12-12 Cervical myelogram. Typical extradural lesions caused by intervertebral disc prolapse at C3-C4 are visible. **A,** Lateral radiograph. Dorsal deviation of the ventral aspect of the subarachnoid space is visible *(large arrows)*. The dorsal aspect of the subarachnoid space is thin owing to displacement of the spinal cord *(small arrow)*. Note mineralized disc material remaining in situ *(white arrowheads)*. **B,** On the ventrodorsal radiograph, spinal cord widening is typified by thinning and peripheral deviation of the subarachnoid space at C3-C4 *(arrows)*. **C,** Forked appearance of the ventral aspect of the subarachnoid space is caused by the x-ray beam striking two tangents of the subarachnoid space. The extruded disc material is located lateral to the midline, causing the ventral aspect of the contrast medium column to appear as a *double line* on the lateral radiograph *(open arrows)*. The double line is not seen in **A** because of a slight difference in patient positioning.

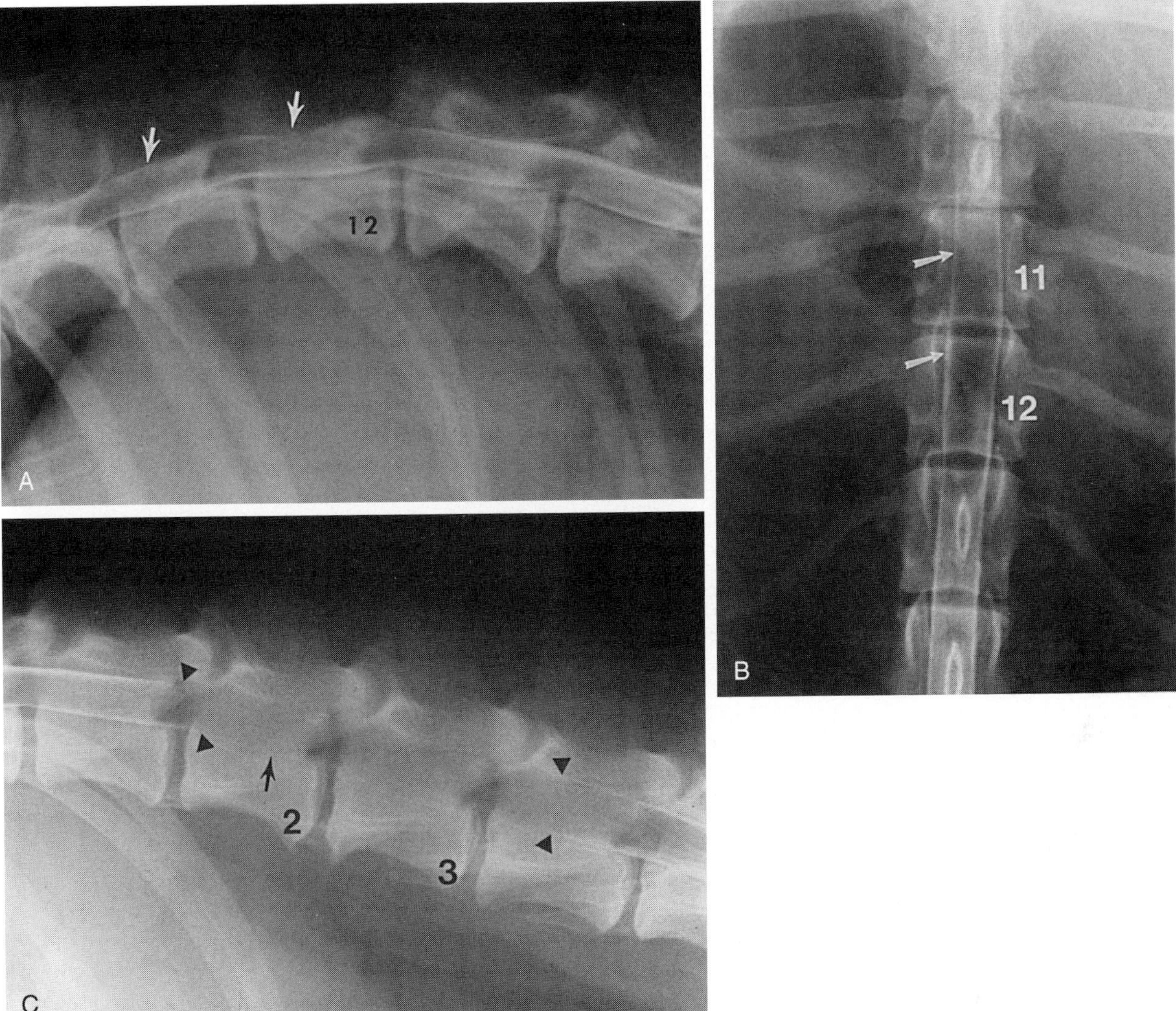

Fig. 12-13 Type I disc prolapse with intramedullary pattern. **A,** Lateral myelogram. Intramedullary swelling and a thin subarachnoid space *(arrows)* at T11-T12 are visible. **B,** Ventrodorsal myelogram of the dog in **A.** The spinal cord is wide at T11-T12; note central shift of the right aspect of the contrast medium column *(arrows)*, which indicates lateralization of the prolapse. In this instance, the surgeon may elect to perform a right hemilaminectomy. Intervertebral disc prolapse at T11-T12 was confirmed at surgery. **C,** With severe intramedullary swelling, the contrast medium column may be totally obliterated *(arrowheads)*, masking the extradural component of the lesion. Intervertebral disc prolapse at L2-L3 was confirmed at surgery.

Technical considerations play an important role in the myelographic diagnosis of intervertebral disc disease. The extradural component of disc protrusion and the extent of spinal cord swelling may both be more conspicuous in radiographs made immediately after injection of contrast medium.[4,36] The use of oblique radiographic projections should be considered during every myelographic study because they frequently provide useful information. If disc material is located lateral to midline, the lateral and ventrodorsal radiographs will be characterized by only a widened appearance to the spinal cord, whereas in oblique radiographic projections (VL-DR and VR-DL) an extradural pattern will be seen (Fig. 12-14). In some instances, both left and right lateral radiographic projections are needed for accurate identification of an extradural lesion.[40]

The gradual onset of type II disc protrusion tends to minimize spinal cord swelling, resulting in an extradural myelographic pattern (Fig. 12-15). Long-term changes, including hypertrophy of the annulus fibrosus, ligamentum flavum, and joint capsule of the dorsal intervertebral articular process joint, cause circumferential compression of the spinal cord ("hourglass appearance"). Type II protrusion is part of the cervical spondylomyelopathy (wobbler) and lumbosacral instability (caudal equina) syndromes of large-breed dogs.[5,6]

Diagnosis of lumbosacral disc protrusion presents a special problem.[41] Although disc space narrowing, end-plate sclerosis, and spondylosis deformans are associated with L7-S1 disc protrusion, these changes can also occur in asymptomatic dogs.[6] In addition, some dogs with L7-S1 protrusion have no

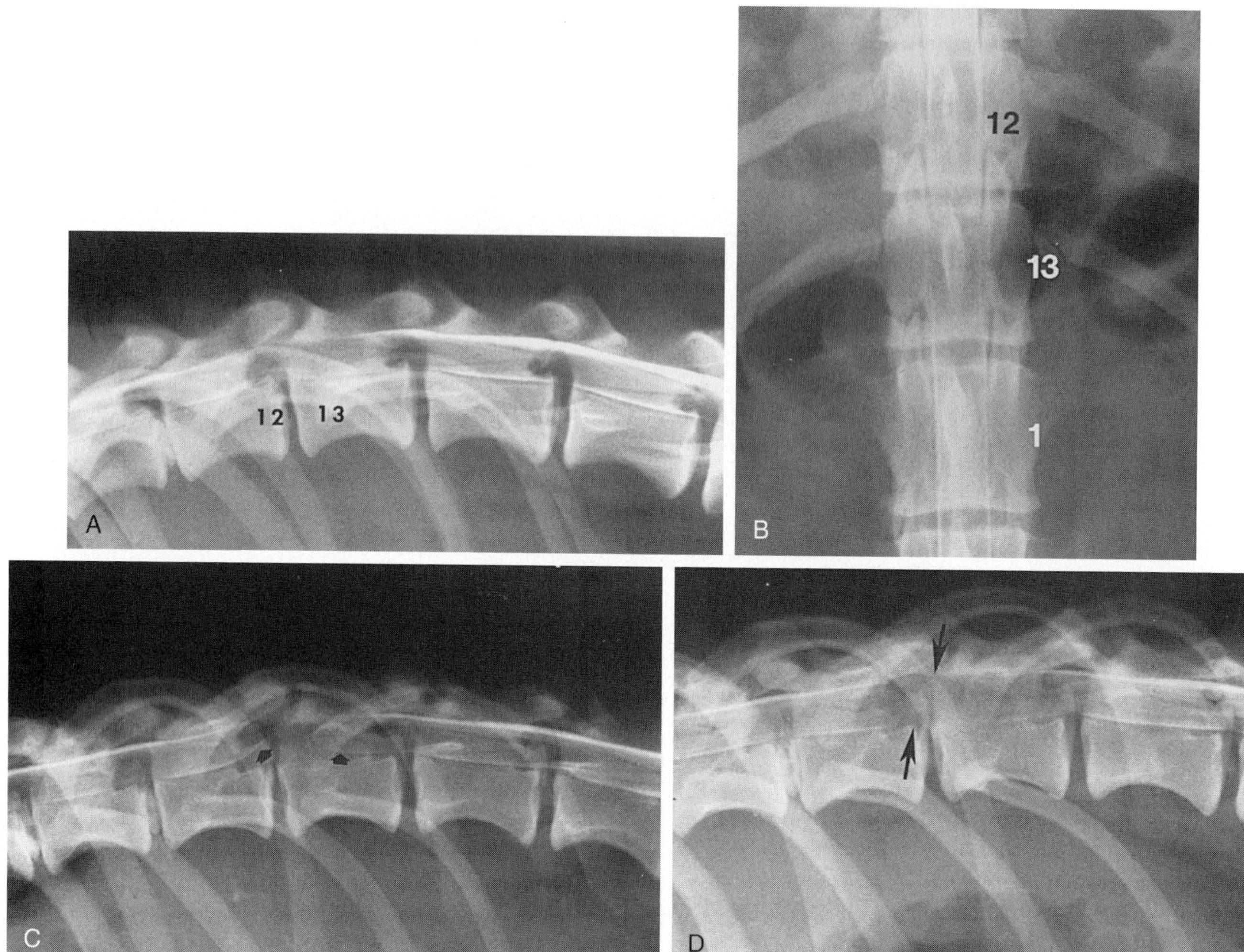

Fig. 12-14 Ventrolateral disc protrusion. A and B, Lateral and ventrodorsal myelograms showing signs of mild spinal cord widening, but the site of disc protrusion is not evident. C, In a ventral 65-degree right dorsal to left oblique projection an extradural mass effect is visible, typified by subarachnoid space thinning and deviation from disc prolapse. D, In a ventral 65-degree left dorsal to right oblique projection (orthogonal to C), marked spinal cord widening is visible. The extradural and intramedullary lesions are best recognized on the oblique projections because the x-ray beam is striking each lesion tangentially.

radiographic changes.[23] Lateral radiographic projections of the lumbosacrum in both flexion and extension help in the evaluation of the dynamics of lumbosacral instability, but results are often misleading.[6] Radiographic contrast procedures routinely used to evaluate the lumbosacral region include flexion-extension myelography[42] and epidurography.[43] Myelography may reveal evidence of disc protrusion, providing the dural sac extends beyond the lumbosacral joint and the myelogram is technically adequate.

Epidurography is performed by placing a spinal needle into the vertebral canal between S3 and C3 and injecting contrast medium into the epidural space.[43] Dorsal displacement of the ventral aspect of the epidural space and complete obstruction to cranial flow of contrast medium are the most consistent epidurographic findings of lumbosacral stenosis (compression).[43] However, the normal contour of the epidural space, unlike the subarachnoid space, is undulating and subject to misinterpretation. Myelography should always precede epidurography because the latter obscures the subarachnoid space. Epidurography has essentially been replaced by CT and MR imaging.

COMPUTED TOMOGRAPHY

The main advantages of CT over conventional radiography are its tomographic nature and improved contrast resolution. In the past decade, availability of third- and fourth-generation single-slice and helical (spiral) CT scanners has greatly facilitated the evaluation of dogs and cats with conditions affecting the vertebral column, spinal cord, and intervertebral discs. These scanners provide thin image slices that give good spatial resolution and allow reformatting of images in sagittal and dorsal planes. CT examination is performed with and without intravenous contrast medium administration or after a conventional myelogram. Indications for CT are essentially the same as for conventional myelography. When the neurologic examination provides compelling anatomic localization,

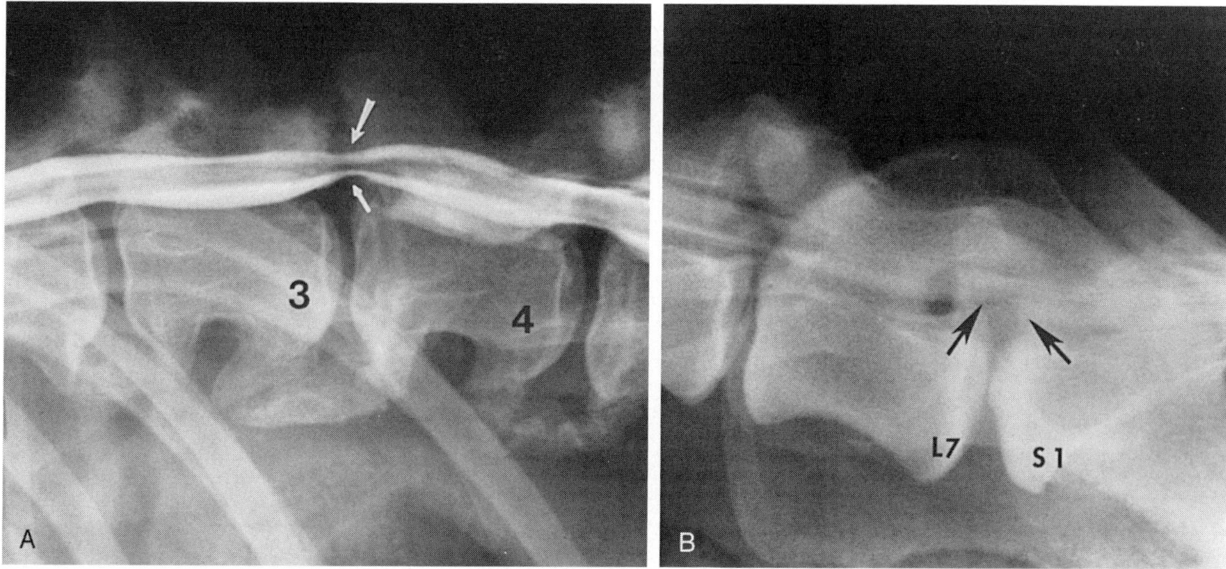

Fig. 12-15 Type II disc protrusion. **A,** Extradural mass effect caused by disc protrusion at L3-L4 *(arrows)*. The hourglass appearance, a long-term change, is a result of disc protrusion and hypertrophy of the ventral longitudinal ligament, the annulus fibrosus, and the ligamentum flavum. Long-term degenerative changes of the vertebra are also present (spondylosis and articular process degenerative joint disease). **B,** Disc protrusion at L7-S1. Note the narrowed intervertebral disc space and deviation of the dural sac *(arrows)*.

survey radiographs of the vertebral column may be unnecessary. However, survey radiography is generally recommended.

Postmyelographic CT is useful when conventional myelography does not clearly demonstrate a suspected extradural lesion caused by disc protrusion (Fig. 12-16).[44-46] Spinal cord swelling and intervertebral foraminal changes are accurately diagnosed with CT myelography, especially when the subarachnoid space is minimally distended. Because the contrast resolution of CT is superior to that of conventional radiography, extradural compressive lesions caused by lesions other than disc protrusion (ligamentous hypertrophy, hematoma, tumor, etc.) can also be identified. For example, in Doberman Pinschers with cervical spondylomyelopathy, CT findings provide prognostic information regarding paraspinal soft tissue structures that cannot be obtained with conventional radiography.[47]

CT has greatly facilitated the assessment of the lumbosacral junction of dogs.[48] Pelvic limb pain and weakness commonly result from compression of nerve roots in the vertebral canal or in the intervertebral foramina at the lumbosacral junction. This compression is often caused by a combination of disc protrusion and osseous changes associated with spondylosis deformans. As with intervertebral disc protrusion in the thoracolumbar spine, disc disease at the lumbosacral junction cannot be accurately assessed from survey radiographs. Also, as previously mentioned, neither myelography nor epidurography is adequate for assessing the lumbosacral junction. This meant that for many years accurate evaluation of dogs with suspected lumbosacral disc disease was difficult. However, the advent of CT and MR imaging has led to much greater accuracy for detecting neural compressive lesions at the lumbosacral junction. This increased accuracy has resulted from the tomographic nature of these modalities, along with their increased contrast resolution. Particularly with reference to CT imaging, the multiplanar reconstruction capabilities have allowed greatly increased accuracy for assessing the lumbosacral disc (Fig. 12-17), and MR has provided more accurate assessment of the disc as well as nerve root compression in the foramina (see Fig. 11-22).

Conventional CT imaging without contrast medium in the subarachnoid space may also be used in lieu of myelography for the assessment of suspected acute disc extrusion.[49] CT can usually be completed in a shorter time than myelography and negates injection of contrast medium into the subarachnoid space. For example, in a chondrodystrophic dog with acute neurologic impairment consistent with a T3-L3 myelopathy caused by disc protrusion, the relevant region of the vertebral column can be imaged by CT within a few minutes. Given the high-contrast resolution of CT images, the site of disc herniation may be quickly identified in many such patients (Fig. 12-18). Additionally, CT images often allow differentiation between herniated disc material and vertebral canal hemorrhage based on the Hounsfield units of the material in the vertebral canal (Fig. 12-19). (See Chapter 4 for an explanation of Hounsfield units.) Distinguishing between disc material and hemorrhage is important because decompression must encompass the site of herniated disc material but it may not always be necessary to decompress regions of hemorrhage. In a myelogram, distinguishing disc material from hemorrhage as a cause of an extradural mass may not be possible.

If disc herniation is not identified in such a screening CT study, a myelogram can be performed to assess other regions of the spine. Because of the high-contrast resolution of CT images, rarely will a CT screening examination fail to reveal the site(s) of disc herniation if that is the problem causing the clinical signs.

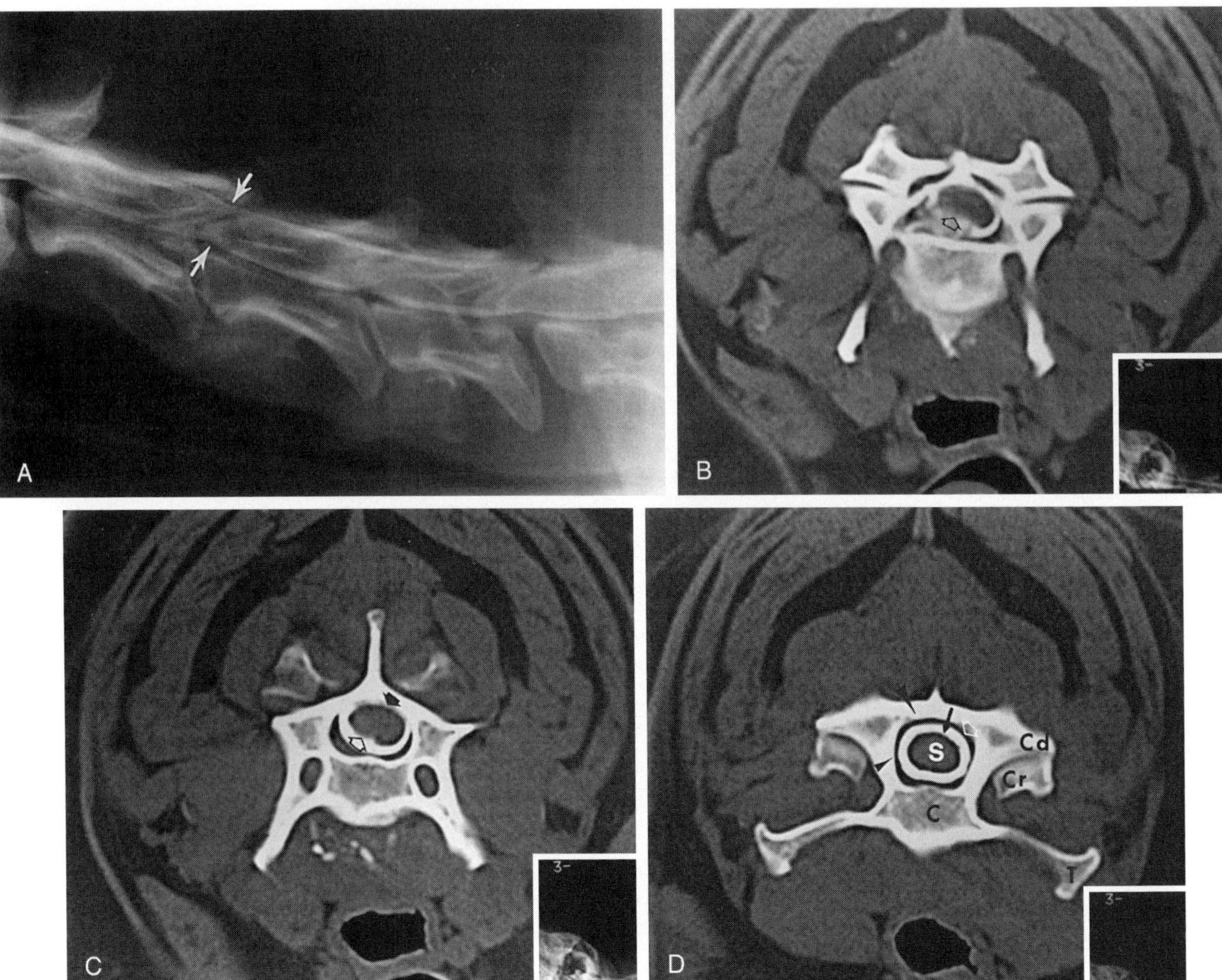

Fig. 12-16 Myelography and CT image of a cervical disc prolapse. **A,** The lateral cervical myelogram shows a slight annular extradural compression of the subarachnoid space at C3-C4 *(arrows)*. **B,** The transverse CT image shows ventrolateral spinal cord compression at C3-C4 *(open arrow)* caused by extruded disc material. Dorsolaterally, the subarachnoid space is thin. Only a small margin of the intervertebral disc can be seen because the image plane is oblique with respect to the disc space. **C,** A contiguous 3-mm slice caudal to **B;** spinal cord compression *(open arrow)* and thinning of the dorsolateral aspect of the subarachnoid space *(closed arrow)* are visible. **D,** A slice made at the caudal aspect of C4 is within normal limits. *Arrow,* Subarachnoid space with contrast medium; *black arrowheads,* vertebral arch; *C,* centrum of vertebra; *Cd,* caudal articular process; *Cr,* cranial articular process; *open arrow,* epidural space; *T,* transverse process; *S,* spinal cord.

MAGNETIC RESONANCE IMAGING

MR imaging is becoming increasingly important for spinal imaging in dogs and cats. In veterinary practices where MR is available, routine myelography is no longer performed in animals with neural signs relating to the spinal cord. MR imaging affords superior soft tissue contrast compared with both radiography and CT imaging and provides insight regarding changes in the soft tissue components of the vertebral column, including the spinal cord, ligaments, and intervertebral discs, that is unmatched by other imaging modalities.[50] The ability to acquire primary images in any plane also increases the value of MR imaging for intervertebral disc assessment. Discs can be assessed for changes in signal intensity relating to stage of degeneration, and annular tears, hernias, and extrusions can be documented (Fig. 12-20).[51,52] An additional advantage of MR over radiography and CT is that inherent contrast of the CSF makes myelography unnecessary.

MR changes of cartilage end plates and adjacent marrow have been extensively studied in human beings with low back pain.[53,54] Three types of change have been described: (1) Modic 1, hypointense signal in T1-weighted sequences and hyperintense signal in T2-weighted sequences corresponding

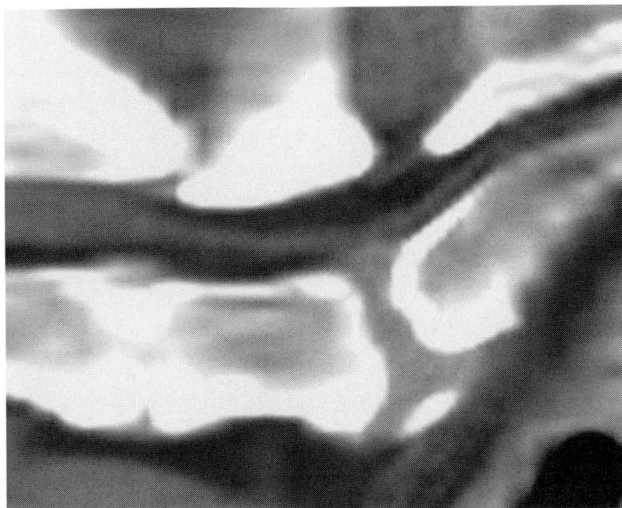

A

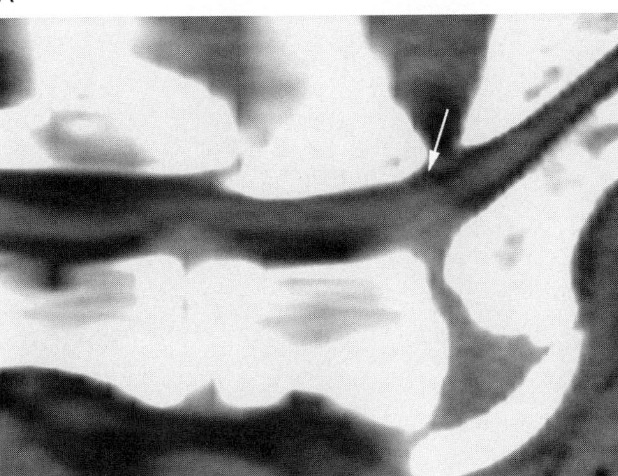

B

Fig. 12-17 Reconstructed sagittal CT images of the lumbosacral region in two dogs with lumbosacral disc disease (soft tissue window). **A** shows a mild protrusion of the intervertebral disc at L7-S1 and mild to moderate spondylosis. The disc protrusion is not causing displacement of nerve roots in the vertebral canal. In **B** the disc disease is more severe, as is the spondylosis. Protrusion is more marked at L7-S1 and disc protrusion at L6-L7 is also present. Nerve roots are displaced at both sites. Some fat (fat is less attenuating than muscle or nerve and appears black in this image) remains in the vertebral canal dorsal to the nerve roots at L7-S1 *(arrow)*, indicating that outright nerve root compression against the dorsal aspect of the vertebral canal has not occurred. Nevertheless, the irritation of the nerve roots from the displacement may be problematic.

to edema, end plate fissures, and hypervascularity; (2) Modic 2, hyperintense signal in T1-weighted sequences and hyperintense signal in T2-weighted sequences corresponding to fatty marrow degeneration and end plate disruption (Fig. 12-21); and Modic 3, hypointense signal in T1-weighted sequences and hypointense signal in T2-weighted sequences corresponding to sclerosis of the end plates. This classification is believed to represent a longitudinal spectrum of pathologic alteration of the vertebral end plates and adjacent marrow. The Modic classification is useful in predicting outcome from surgical arthrodesis in persons with chronic back pain; those with type I lesions have a greater success rate. These changes also occur in dogs with intervertebral disc disease; however, the exact relation between MR signal and clinical signs is unclear.[52]

Pathologic changes in the spinal cord after disc protrusion such as hemorrhage, edema, myelomalacia, and cavitary lesions are easily seen with MR imaging (Fig. 12-22).[55,56] Data have attributed prognostic value to the characteristics of spinal cord signal intensity in dogs with herniated intervertebral discs; in one study, dogs without deep pain but no spinal cord signal alteration had a better prognosis than dogs without deep pain but T2-weighted hyperintensity in the spinal cord.[56]

SPINAL CORD DISEASES

Selected conditions of the spinal cord that are amenable to evaluation by myelography, CT, or MR imaging are considered in this section. Because of their limited contrast resolution, survey radiography and myelography provide only indirect evidence of pathologic changes of the spinal cord. However, CT and MR can directly image pathologic changes because of their extensive image contrast.

Spinal Cord Neoplasia

Tumors affecting the spinal cord may have intramedullary or extramedullary origin. Intramedullary tumors are located within the cord and cause spinal cord swelling and disruption of neural pathways. They are primary, developing from neural elements, or metastatic. Extramedullary tumors arise from within the meninges (intradural) or from any tissue found within the vertebral column (extradural), including the vertebrae. Extradural and intradural-extramedullary tumors involve the spinal cord secondarily, causing compression.

Intramedullary tumors are relatively uncommon in the dog and cat. Glial cell tumors, including astrocytomas and oligodendrogliomas, are the most common primary neoplasms of the spinal cord in dogs.[57] Ependymomas and medulloepitheliomas have also been reported and arise from the neuroepithelium.[58,59] Lymphosarcoma is the most frequent intramedullary tumor of cats. Intramedullary spinal cord metastasis is seldom diagnosed in dogs and cats; lymphosarcoma and hemangiosarcoma are the predominant cell types.[60] Primary lymphosarcoma of the cord (i.e., no evidence of extraneural involvement) has been reported in dogs.[61]

Extradural tumors are the most common tumor affecting the spinal cord. These tumors lie within the vertebral canal and include vertebral-origin osteosarcomas, myelomas, lymphosarcomas, meningiomas, and metastatic tumors (Fig. 12-23).

Intradural-extramedullary tumors are located within the dural sheath; neurofibrosarcomas, meningiomas, and lymphosarcomas are the predominant cell type. In a myelogram, these tumors cause a filling defect because they are actually located in the subarachnoid space (Fig. 12-24). The advantage of CT or MR imaging for assessing these tumors is that the paravertebral extent of tumor involvement can be assessed; this is not possible with a myelogram (Fig. 12-25).

Unfortunately, the clinical presentation of animals with spinal cord tumors often mimics that of disc protrusion and other nonmalignant causes. Pain and neural dysfunction are usually present. Although gradual onset is expected with intramedullary tumors, some animals may manifest acute signs.[58,59]

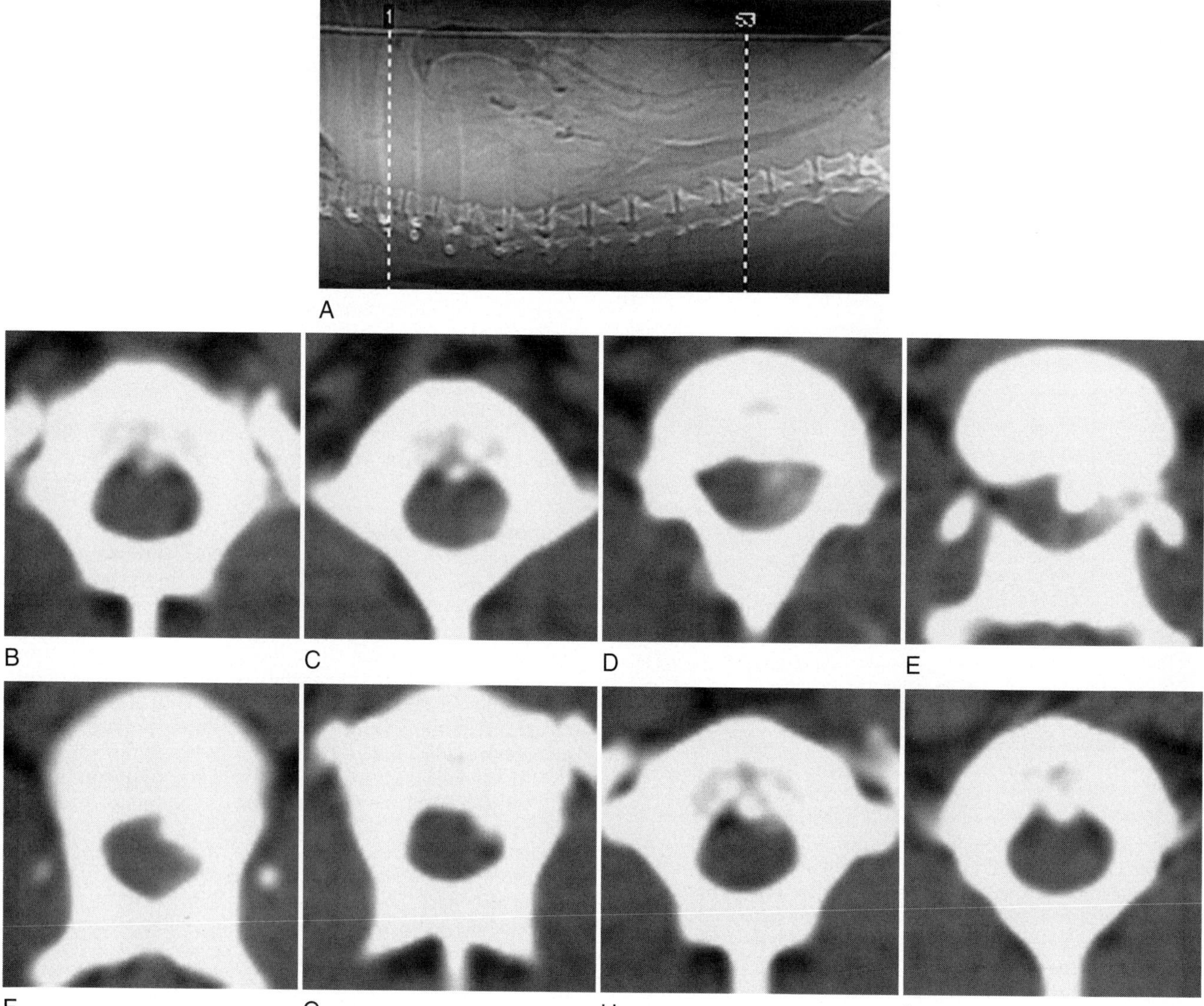

Fig. 12-18 A, Lateral locator image of the spine of a 7-year-old Dachshund with acute pelvic limb paralysis and no deep pain sensation. This is the same dog as in Fig. 12-3, *D*. The vertical lines represent the region over which 53 contiguous CT slices were acquired from mid T9 caudally to mid L5; each slice was 3 mm thick (soft tissue window). In contiguous images **B** to **I**, which represent the region from the cranial aspect of the T12 vertebral body **(B)** caudally to the caudal aspect of the T13 vertebral body **(I)**, a hyperattenuating mass can be seen in the vertebral canal on the left side (on the right in the image), causing compression of the spinal cord. At surgery this mass was determined to be extruded disc material. Because the material spans the T12-T13 interspace, that is the likely site of origination. Images were not acquired cranial to T9 in this dog because of the rare occurrence of disc herniation in that region of the spine. Localization of the herniated disc material on the left side was useful to the surgeon so that the spinal decompression could be lateralized appropriately.

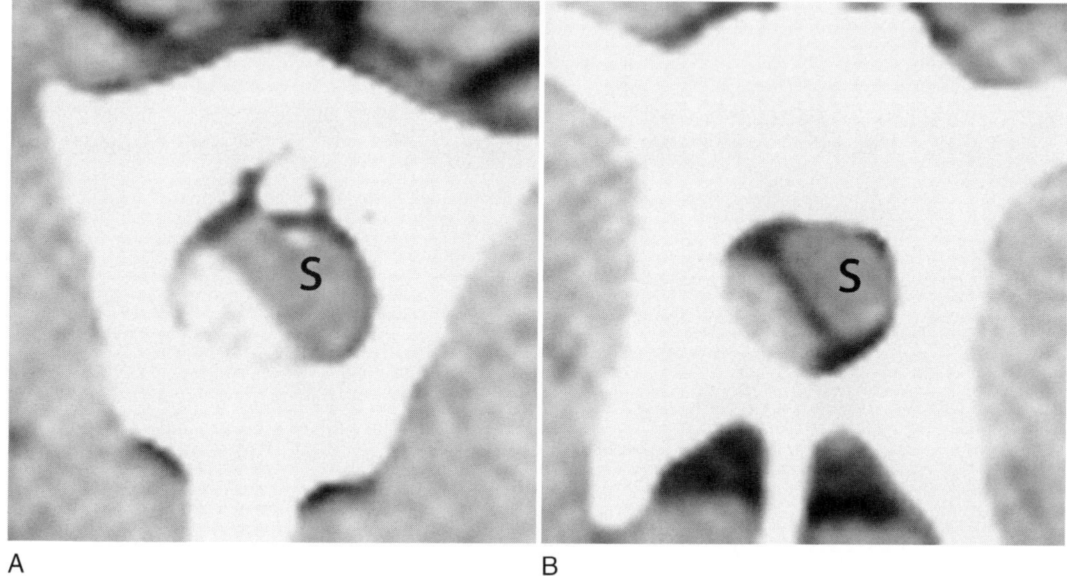

Fig. 12-19 **A,** Transverse CT image (soft tissue window) at the level of the cranial aspect of L4. A mineralized mass in the right (on the left in the image) dorsolateral aspect of the vertebral canal is compressing the spinal cord *(s)*. This mass represents mineralized disc material that has migrated from its more typical ventral location. The Hounsfield unit value of this mass is 111. **B,** Transverse CT image at the level of the cranial aspect of L3 shows a mass in a similar location to that seen in **A** that is also compressing the spinal cord *(s)*, but the Hounsfield unit value of this mass is 63; in other words, it is less attenuating. This signifies that this mass is consistent with hemorrhage. Use of Hounsfield unit values of vertebral canal masses can be helpful in deciding whether the mass is disc material or another type of lesion.

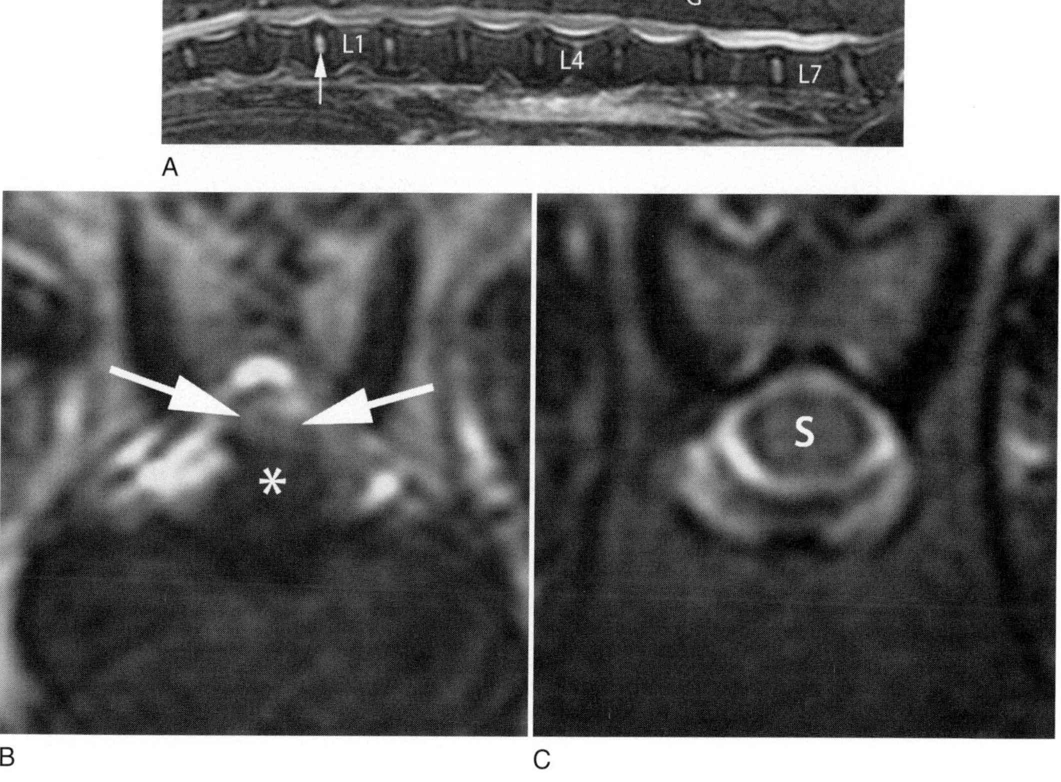

Fig. 12-20 MR images from a 14-year-old Dalmatian with multifocal disc disease illustrating the spectrum of changes that can be seen. **A,** Sagittal short tau inversion recovery (STIR) image of the thoracolumbar and lumbar regions. The disc at T13-L1 *(arrow)* has a high signal characteristic of a normally hydrated disc. All other discs have lower signal, indicating they are dehydrated to some degree. Most, but not all, discs are dehydrated before they prolapse.

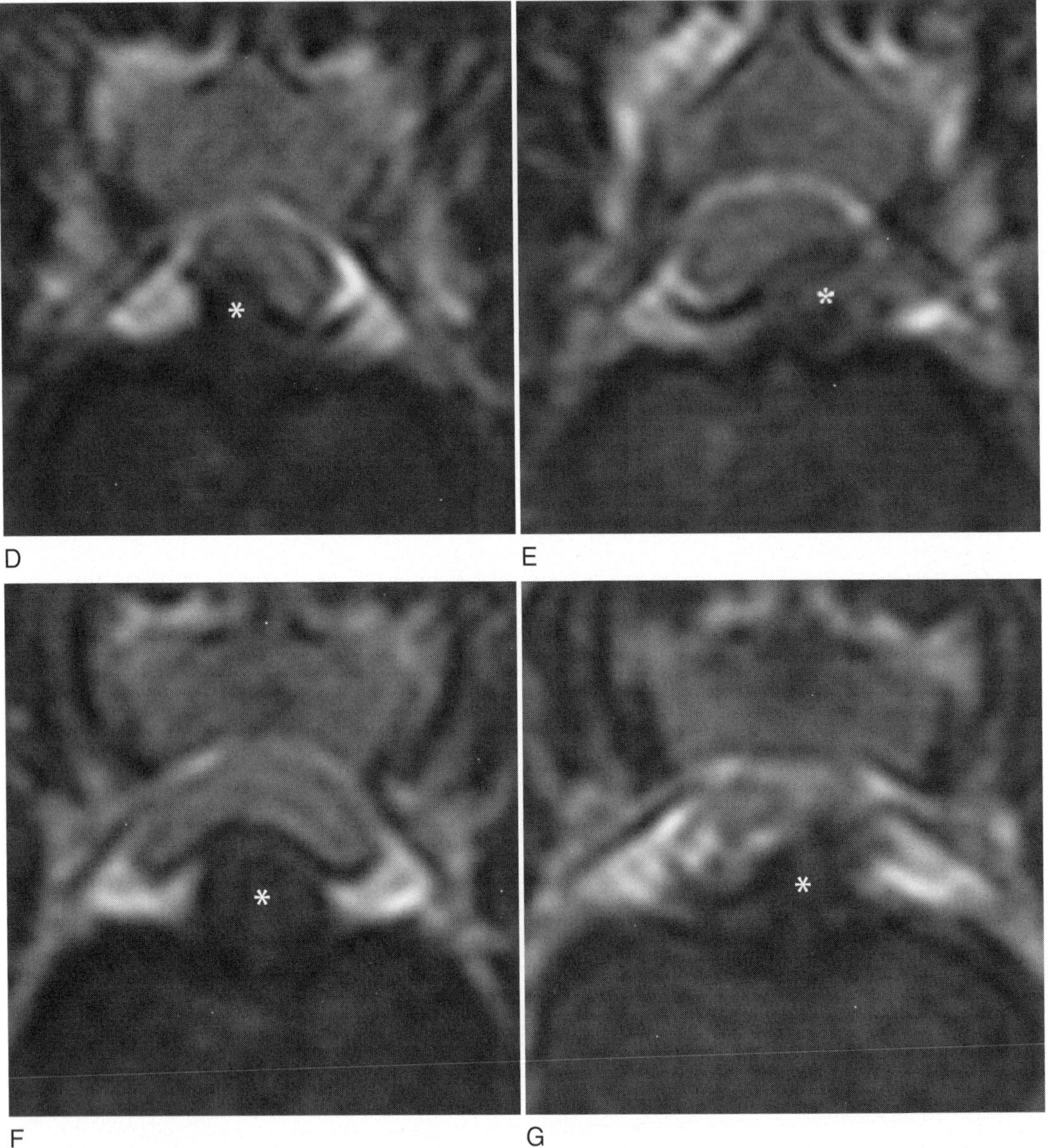

Fig. 12-20, cont'd B through G indicate where the subsequent transverse fast spin-echo T2-weighted images were acquired. In all transverse images, the patient's right side is on the left of the image. B was acquired at T12-T13. Extrusion of mineralized disc material *(asterisk)* is compressing the spinal cord *(arrows)*. Mineralized disc material is hypointense in MR images because calcium does not produce an MR signal (see Chapter 4). C was acquired at the cranial aspect of L2 and is a normal-appearing transverse image of the canine spine. The spinal cord *(s)* is surrounded by epidural fat and CSF creating a hyperintense (white) ring. Interpreting the white ring as CSF is tempting, but in a fast spin-echo T2-weighted image fat also has high signal and cannot be differentiated from fluid. D was acquired at L2-L3. Right-sided disc herniation *(asterisk)* is causing compression of the spinal cord. E was acquired at L3-L4. A left-sided disc herniation *(asterisk)* is causing compression of the spinal cord. F was acquired at L4-L5. Central disc herniation *(asterisk)* is causing compression of the spinal cord. G was acquired at L5-L6. A left-sided disc herniation *(asterisk)* is causing compression of the spinal cord.

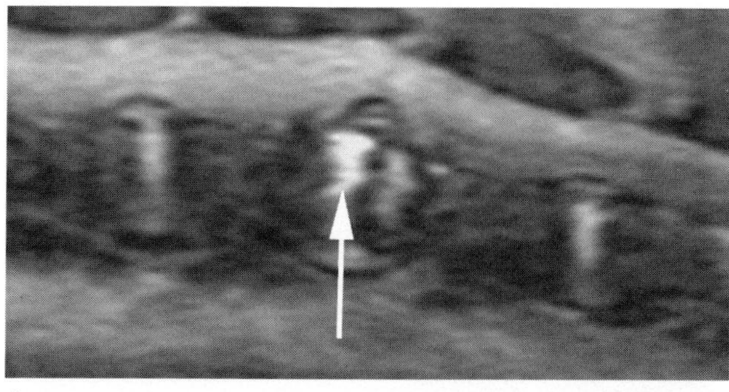

A

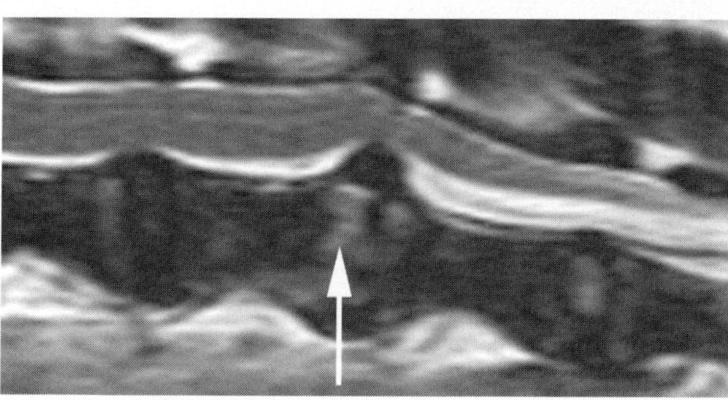

B

Fig. 12-21 Sagittal noncontrast, fat-suppressed, T1-weighted image (A) and sagittal T2-weighted fast spin-echo image (B) of the caudal lumbar region of a dog with chronic disc herniation at L4-L5. A T1-weighted hyperintense and T2-weighted hyperintense region in the caudal aspect of L4 corresponds to a Modic type 2 lesion *(arrows)*. The significance of these vertebral body changes in dogs with chronic disc herniation is not understood, but they may certainly contribute to the clinical discomfort.

Intramedullary Cavitary Disease

Conditions typified by cavitation of the cord parenchyma are often included under the general classification of spinal dysraphism.[62] This all-inclusive term relates to failure of the neural tube to close. Cavitary diseases of the cord reported in dogs and cats include hydromyelia, syringomyelia, and myelomeningocele. Hydromyelia pertains to dilation of the central canal and may be congenital or acquired. Congenital hydromyelia is thought to be associated with malformations of the ventricular system that cause altered CSF flow and increased CSF pressure. In fact, hydrocephalus is often present when hydromyelia is identified.[63] With acquired hydromyelia, dilation may occur subsequent to increased CSF pressure associated with infection, trauma, or neoplasia affecting the ventricular system.[63] Myelographically, hydromyelia is typified as a wide, contrast medium–filled central canal (see Fig. 12-11, *A*). Filling usually results from leakage around the needle, but in some instances the dilation of the canal is so large that it is accidentally punctured during a cerebellomedullary tap. Saccular or smoothly marginated widening of the canal may occur. Clinical signs associated with hydromyelia may result from dilation and loss of cord parenchyma or from the condition causing the hydromyelia (e.g., feline infectious peritonitis). Frequently, hydromyelia is an incidental finding and is not accompanied by clinical signs.

Syringomyelia refers to cavitation of the cord parenchyma, which may or may not communicate with the central canal.[62] When communication is present, contrast medium fills the cavitations and can be seen on myelography. However, distinguishing cavitation of the spinal cord parenchyma from hydromyelia is difficult because the cavitations tend to merge with the dilated central canal.[63] Because the cord parenchyma is directly affected, animals with syringomyelia frequently have clinical signs. Syringomyelia is overrepresented in Weimaraners and is a common sequel to the occipitocervical malformation syndrome (Fig. 12-26).

Myelomeningoceles are associated with spina bifida and consist of protrusion of the cord and meninges through a defect in the vertebral arch.[62] Close examination of survey radiographs often reveals duplication or attenuation of the spinous processes of the affected vertebra (see Chapter 11). Myelographically, dorsal displacement of the meningeal sac and the conus medullaris of the spinal cord is present. The meningeal sac is dilated and various abnormalities, including hydromyelia and syringomyelia, may occur cranial to the myelomeningocele. Spina bifida frequently affects the lumbar and sacral vertebrae and is common in the English Bulldog and the Manx cat.

Fibrocartilaginous Embolism

Fibrocartilaginous embolism is a syndrome of acute infarction of the spinal cord caused by the release of small fibrocartilaginous emboli from intervertebral discs, which lodge in the cord parenchyma. Infarction and ischemia occur, and cord swelling may be present. Thus intramedullary swelling may be seen on myelography. In one report narrowing of the intervertebral disc space associated with fibrocartilaginous embolism was described.[64] However, with fibrocartilaginous embolism, frequently no changes are seen with radiography or myelography. With increased use of MR imaging for assessment of spinal cord disease in animals, localized T2-weighted hyperintensity has been recognized as an MR imaging finding consistent with fibrocartilaginous embolism.[65] However, accurate anamnesis and neurologic examination remain important because imaging alone cannot rule out acute disc protrusion (Fig. 12-27).

Nerve Root Neoplasia

Neurofibromas, neurofibrosarcomas, meningiomas, and schwannomas are the primary neoplasms that involve the nerve roots. Neurofibromas and neurofibrosarcomas arise from the nerve parenchyma, whereas schwannomas are encapsulated and distinct from the nerve.[66] Meningiomas originate from the adjacent meningeal covering and may compress nerve roots. Nerve root tumors are most commonly associated with the cervical and thoracic cord segments. After myelography, an intradural-extramedullary sign is seen when a tumor lies within the subarachnoid space. However, if invasion of the dura or cord occurs, or if the tumor lies outside of the dura, a classic intradural-extramedullary lesion is absent. In the latter instance, the tumor mass may cause compression of the cord (see Figs. 12-24 and 12-25). For paravertebral nerve root tumors, such as brachial plexus tumors, CT or MR imaging is necessary for identification.

Arachnoid Cysts

Benign, cystlike areas in the subarachnoid space may cause extramedullary compression and neural signs. Histologically, these are not true cysts because they are not lined with epithelial cells.[67,68] The cause of arachnoid cysts is unknown, but

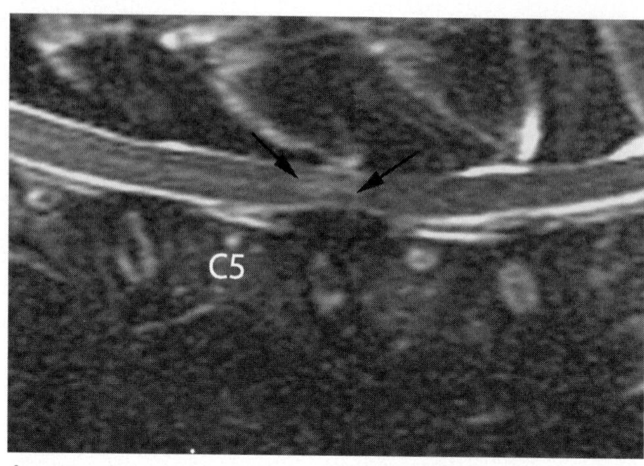

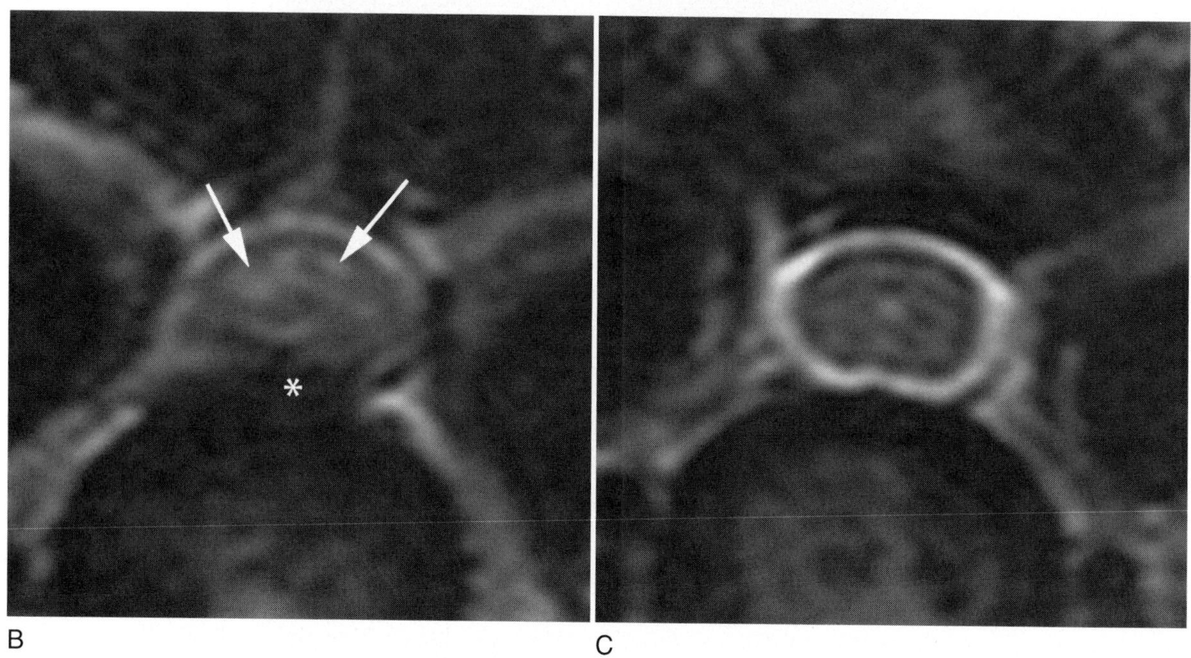

Fig. 12-22 Cervical T2-weighted fast spin-echo images from a 9-year-old German Shepherd with forelimb paraplegia and pelvic limb paresis. The sagittal view **(A)** shows compression of the ventral aspect of the subarachnoid space at C5-C6. Additionally a focal region of T2-hyperintensity within the spinal cord *(arrow)* is consistent with edema and/or focal inflammation. The central region of discs is hypointense, suggesting central dehydration and/or mineralization. In the transverse image at C5-C6 **(B)**, the herniated mineralized material can be seen *(asterisk)* and the T2-weighted hyperintensity within the spinal cord is also apparent *(arrows)*. A transverse image through C4-C5 **(C)** where no abnormality exists is provided for comparison. Spinal cord hyperintensity such as this, being associated with disc herniation, may signify a less-than-optimal prognosis; more work is needed to characterize the significance of this relation.

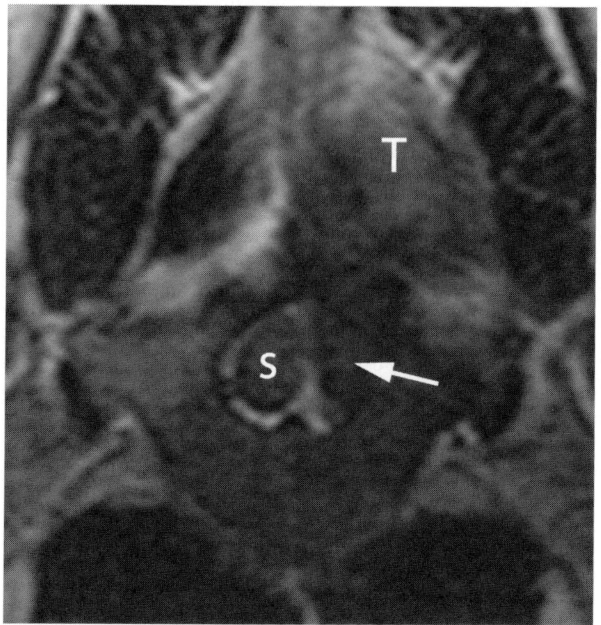

Fig. 12-23 Transverse T2-weighted fast spin-echo image of T2 in a dog with a vertebral osteosarcoma. The tumor *(T)* extends into the vertebral canal *(arrow)* and causes extradural compression of the spinal cord *(S)*.

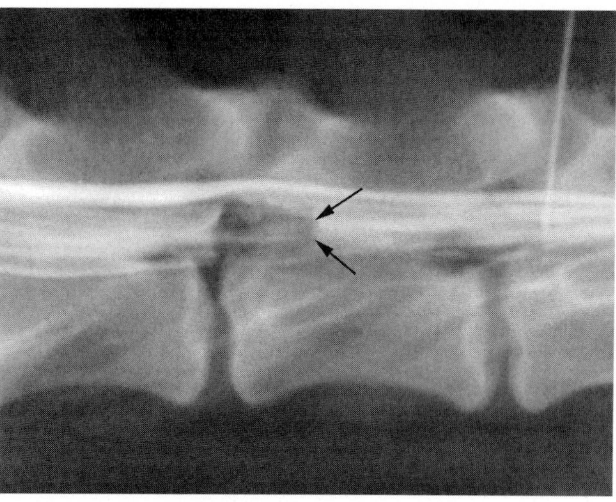

Fig. 12-24 Lumber myelogram of a dog with a nerve root tumor at L4-L5. Contrast medium has been injected at L5-L6 and the needle remains in place. At L4-L5 a filling defect is present caused by the mass in the subarachnoid space displacing contrast medium from around it. As the contrast medium abuts the cranial and caudal aspect of the mass *(arrows)*, a concave region of contrast medium forms; this has been called the "golf tee sign" because of its visual similarity to a golf tee.

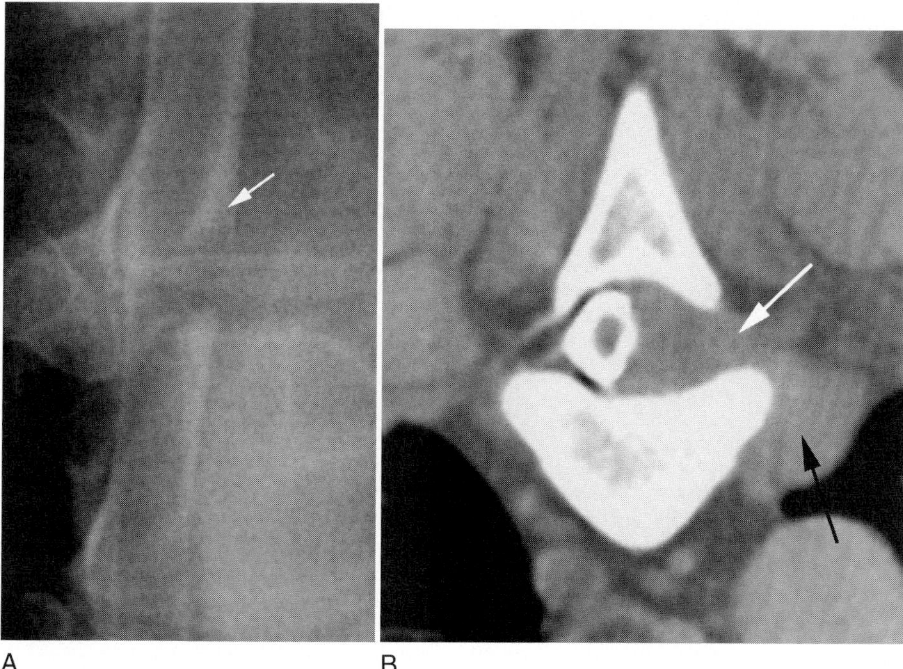

Fig. 12-25 A, Ventrodorsal image from a myelogram with the dog's sternum rotated slightly to the left. A filling defect with a "golf tee sign" *(arrow)* is visible in the vertebral canal at T7-T8. This is consistent with a nerve root tumor. In a CT image at the same site **(B)**, the vertebral canal mass causing spinal cord displacement is seen, but enlargement of the left intervertebral foramen and extension of the mass through the foramen *(white arrow)* form a paraspinal mass that indents the parietal pleura *(black arrow)*. The information gained from CT is valuable from staging purposes and was not obtainable from the myelogram.

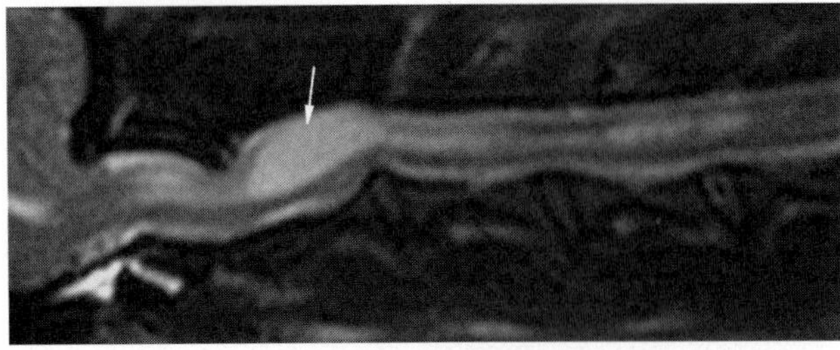

Fig. 12-26 Sagittal T2-weighted fast spin-echo image of the cranial aspect of the cervical vertebral column of a Cavalier King Charles Spaniel with occipitocervical malformation, also referred to as Chiari I–like malformation. Multiple osseous impingements on the subarachnoid space typify this condition. These impingements, along with cerebellar crowding and/or herniation, are thought to cause modification of CSF flow with secondary dilation of the central canal and the formation of cavitations in the spinal cord. Lumped together these spinal cord changes are termed syringohydromyelia and can be seen here as regions of T2-hyperintensity within the cervical spinal cord. The syringohydromyelia is most extensive over the body of C2 *(arrow)*.

because they are usually seen in young dogs, a congenital etiology is likely. Resistance to CSF flow, possibly induced by trauma, resulting in back pressure and dilation of the subarachnoid space, has also been implicated as a cause. With arachnoid cysts, survey radiographic examination is usually normal. After myelography, contrast medium fills the "cystic" area, defining abrupt dilation of the subarachnoid contrast medium column and compression of the adjacent spinal cord (Fig. 12-28). Recognition of the intradural-extramedullary location of arachnoid cysts is important so that they can be differentiated from nonsurgical intramedullary lesions such as hydromyelia or syringomyelia. The intramedullary-extramedullary sign in this instance differs from that of a mass lesion (e.g., neurofibroma) in which a filling defect is present as well as subarachnoid dilation. Arachnoid cysts that arise from causes other than previous trauma or surgery are commonly located in the dorsal aspect of the cervical subarachnoid space.[67,68]

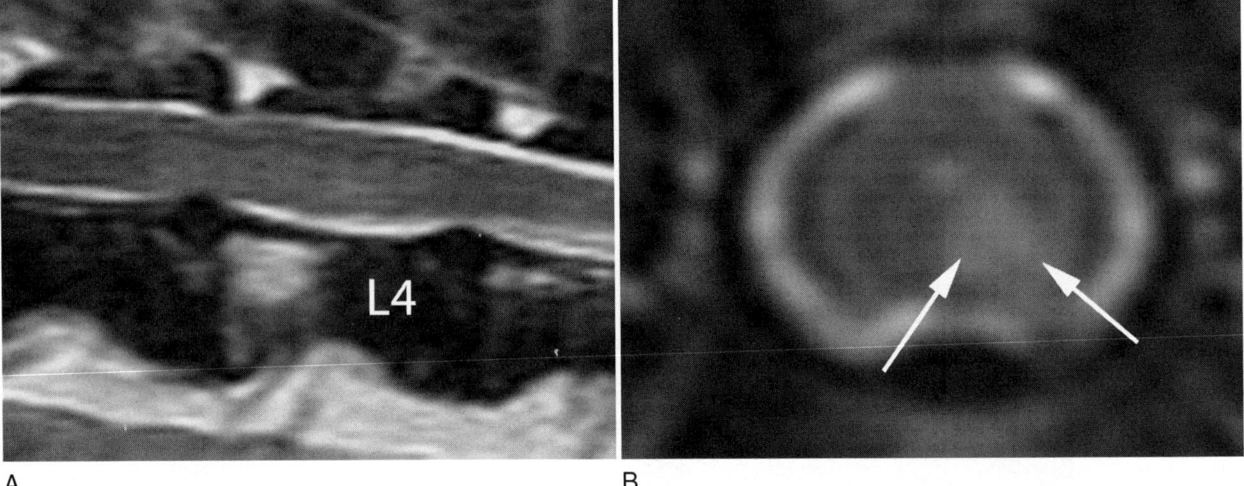

Fig. 12-27 Sagittal (A) and transverse (B) T2-weighted fast spin-echo images of the lumbar spine of a 12-year-old Chihuahua with acute pelvic limb paraparesis. An ill-defined region of T2-hyperintensity is visible within the spinal cord over the L4 vertebral body. In the transverse image (B), acquired near the cranial aspect of L4, a region of T2 hyperintensity can be seen in the ventral left aspect of the spinal cord. Although discs in the caudal lumbar spine are desiccated, no evidence of an extradural mass was present, as might occur with disc herniation. Therefore the primary consideration was fibrocartilaginous embolism. The T2 hyperintense region in the cranial aspect of the L4 vertebral body is normal and is attributable to an accumulation of fat in this region.

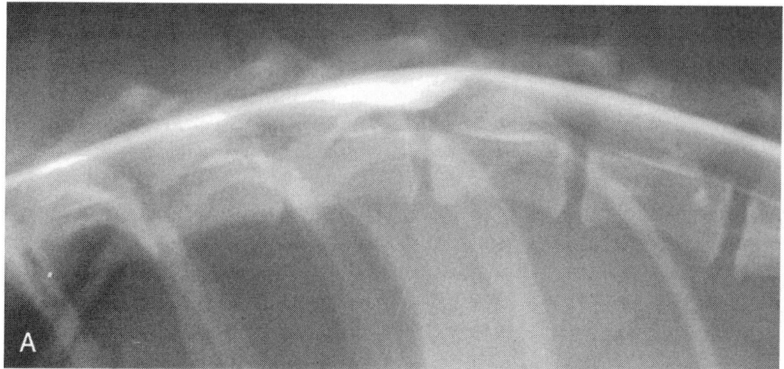

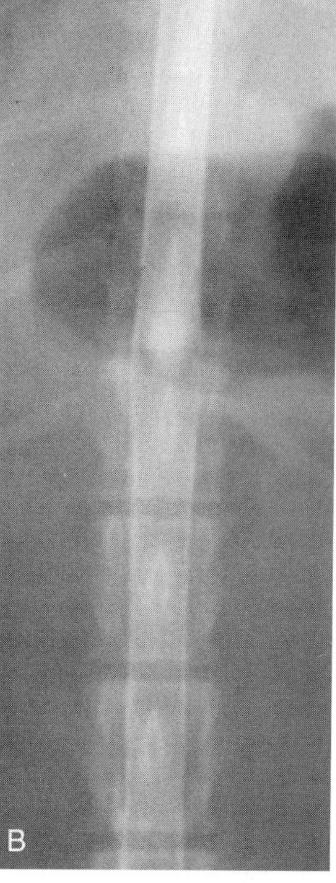

Fig. 12-28 Lateral (A) and ventrodorsal (B) projections of the spine of a 1-year-old Chihuahua after subarachnoid contrast medium instillation. Focal dilation of the subarachnoid space over T12 and the cranial part of T13 is visible. This appearance is typical of arachnoid cysts. Note the widening of the cord in the ventrodorsal view from cord compression by the cyst. Myelographically, determining whether arachnoid cysts are congenital or the result of prior surgery or trauma is usually not possible.

REFERENCES

1. Hoerlein BF: *Canine neurology: diagnosis and treatment,* ed 3, Philadelphia, 1978, W.B. Saunders, pp 470-560.
2. DeLahunta A: *Veterinary neuroanatomy and clinical neurology,* ed 2, Philadelphia, 1983, W.B. Saunders, pp 186-188.
3. Trotter EJ: Canine intervertebral disc disease. In Kirk RW, editor: *Current veterinary therapy VI,* Philadelphia, 1977, WB Saunders, pp 841-848.
4. Kirberger RM, Roos CJ, Lubbe AM: The radiological diagnosis of thoracolumbar disc disease in the dachshund, *Vet Radiol Ultrasound* 33:255, 1992.
5. Seim HB, Withrow SJ: Pathophysiology and diagnosis of caudal cervical spondylo-myelopathy with emphasis on the Doberman pinscher, *J Am Anim Hosp Assoc* 18:241, 1982.
6. Wheeler SJ: Lumbosacral disease, *Vet Clin North Am Small Anim Pract* 22:859, 1992.
7. Thatcher CT: Neuroanatomic and pathophysiologic aspects of intervertebral disc disease in the dog, *Probl Vet Med Intervert Disc Dis* 1:337, 1989.
8. Evans HE, Christensen JC: *Miller's anatomy of the dog,* ed 2, Philadelphia, 1979, WB Saunders.
9. Toombs JT: Cervical intervertebral disc disease in dogs, *Compend Contin Edu Pract Vet* 14:1477, 1992.
10. Shores A: Intervertebral disc syndrome in the dog. Part I. Pathophysiology and management, *Compend Contin Edu Pract Vet* 7:639, 1981.
11. Simson S: Intervertebral disc disease, *Vet Clin North Am Small Anim Pract* 22:889, 1992.
12. Morgan JP, Atilola M, Bailey CS: Vertebral canal and spinal cord mensuration. A comparative study and its effect on lumbosacral myelography in the Dachshund and German shepherd dog, *J Am Vet Med Assoc* 191:951, 1987.
13. Pardo AD, Morgan JP: Myelography in the cat: a comparison of cisternal versus lumbar puncture, using metrizamide, *Vet Radiol* 29:89, 1988.
14. Fardon DF, Milette PC: Nomenclature and classification of lumbar disc pathology. Recommendations of the combined task forces of the North American Spine Society, American Society of Spine Radiology, and American Society of Neuroradiology, *Spine* 26: E93, 2001.
15. Shores A: Spinal trauma: pathophysiology and management of traumatic spinal injuries, *Vet Clin North Am Small Anim Pract* 22:859, 1992.
16. Prata R: Neurosurgical treatment of thoracolumbar discs: the rationale and value of laminectomy and concomitant disc removal, *J Am Anim Hosp Assoc* 17:17, 1981.
17. Griffiths IR: The extensive myelopathy of intervertebral disc protrusion in dogs ("the ascending syndrome"), *J Small Anim Pract* 13:425, 1972.
18. Morgan JP, Miyabayashi T: Degenerative changes in the vertebral column of the dog: a review of radiographic findings, *Vet Radiol* 29:72, 1988.
19. Felts JF, Prata RG: Cervical disc disease in the dog: intraforaminal and lateral extrusions, *J Am Anim Hosp Assoc* 19:755, 1983.

20. Widmer WR, Blevins WE: Veterinary myelography: a review of contrast media, adverse effects and technique, *J Am Anim Hosp Assoc* 27:163, 1991.
21. Olby NJ, Dyce J, Houlton JEF: Correlation of plain radiographic and lumbar myelographic findings in thoracolumbar disc disease, *J Small Anim Pract* 35:345, 1994.
22. Lamb CN, Nichols A, Targett P et al: Accuracy of survey radiographic diagnosis of intervertebral disc protrusion in dogs, *Vet Radiol Ultrasound* 43:222, 2002.
23. Roberts RE, Selcer BA: Myelography and epidurography, *Vet Clin North Am Small Anim Pract* 23:307, 1993.
24. Burk RL: Problems in the radiographic interpretation of intervertebral disc disease in the dog, *Probl Vet Med Intervert Disc Dis* 1:381, 1989.
25. Sande R: Radiography, myelography, computed tomography and magnetic resonance imaging of the spine, *Vet Clin North Am Small Anim Pract* 22:811, 1992.
26. Wood AKW: Iohexol and iopamidol: new non-ionic contrast media for myelography in dogs, *Comp Contin Edu Pract Vet* 10:32, 1988.
27. Widmer WR, Blevins WE, Cantwell HD et al: Iohexol and iopamidol myelography in the dog: a clinical trial comparing adverse effects and myelographic quality, *Vet Radiol* 33:327, 1992.
28. Lamb CR: Common difficulties with myelographic diagnosis of acute intervertebral disc disease in the dog, *J Small Anim Pract* 35:549, 1994.
29. Weber WJ, Berry CR: Radiology corner: determining the location of contrast medium on the canine lumbar myelogram, *Vet Radiol Ultrasound* 35:430, 1994.
30. McKee WM, Penderis J, Dennis R: Radiology corner. Contrast medium flow during cervical myelography, *Vet Radiol Ultrasound* 41:342, 2000.
31. Tilmant L, Ackerman N, Spencer CP: Mechanical aspects of subarachnoid space puncture in the dog, *Vet Radiol* 25:227, 1984.
32. Wright JA, Jones DGC: Metrizamide myelography in sixty-eight dogs, *J Small Anim Pract* 22:415, 1981.
33. Adams WM: Myelography, *Vet Clin North Am* 12:295, 1971.
34. Suter PF, Morgan JP, Holliday TA et al: Myelography of the dog: diagnosis of tumors of the spinal cord and vertebrae, *Vet Radiol* 12:29, 1971.
35. Kirberger RM, Wrigley R: Myelography in the dog: a review of patients with contrast medium in the central canal, *Vet Radiol* 3:253, 1993.
36. Funquist B: Thoraco-lumbar myelography with water-soluble contrast medium in dogs. I. Technique of myelography; side effects and complications, *J Small Anim Pract* 3:53, 1962.
37. Funquist B: Thoraco-lumbar myelography with water-soluble contrast medium in dogs. II. Appearance of the myelogram in disc protrusion and its relation to functional disturbances and pathoanatomic changes in the epidural space, *J Small Anim Pract* 3:67, 1962.
38. Ticer J, Brown SJ: Water-soluble myelography in canine intervertebral disc protrusion, *Vet Radiol* 15:3, 1974.
39. Morgan JP, Suter PF, Holliday TA: Myelography with water-soluble contrast medium: radiographic interpretation of disc herniation in dogs, *Acta Radiol* 319(suppl): 217, 1972.
40. Matteucci ML, Ramirez O 3rd, Thrall DE: Radiographic diagnosis: effect of right vs. left lateral recumbency on myelographic appearance of a lateralized extradural mass, *Vet Radiol Ultrasound* 40:351, 1999.
41. Mattoon JS, Koblik PD: Quantitative survey radiographic evaluation of the lumbosacral spine of normal dogs and dogs with degenerative lumbosacral stenosis, *Vet Radiol Ultrasound* 34:194, 1993.
42. Lang J: Flexion-extension myelography canine caudal equina, *Vet Radiol* 29:242, 1988.
43. Selcer BA, Chambers JN, Schwensen K et al: Epidurography as a diagnostic aid in canine lumbosacral compressive disease: 47 cases (1981-1986), *Vet Comp Orthop Trauma* 29:97, 1988.
44. Stickle RL, Hathcock JT: Interpretation of computed tomographic images, *Vet Clin North Am* 23:417, 1993.
45. Feeney DA, Fletcher TF, Hardy RM: *Atlas of correlative imaging anatomy of the normal dog*, Philadelphia, 1991, W.B. Saunders.
46. Bagley RS, Tucker RL, Moore MP et al: Radiographic diagnosis. Intervertebral disk extrusion in a cat, *Vet Radiol Ultrasound* 36:380, 1995.
47. Sharp NJ, Cofone M, Robertson ID et al: Computed tomography in the evaluation of caudal cervical spondylomyelopathy of the Doberman pinscher, *Vet Radiol* 36:100, 1995.
48. Jones JC, Wilson ME, Bartels JE: A review of high resolution computed tomography and a proposed technique for regional examination of the lumbosacral spine, *Vet Radiol* 35:339, 1994.
49. Olby NJ, Munana KR, Sharp NJ et al: The computed tomographic appearance of acute thoracolumbar intervertebral disc herniations in dogs, *Vet Radiol Ultrasound* 41:396, 2000.
50. Levetisk RE, Lipstiz D, Chauvet AE: Magnetic resonance imaging of the cervical spine in 27 dogs, *Vet Radiol Ultrasound* 40:332, 1999.
51. Sether JA, Nguyen C, Yu S et al: Canine intervertebral disks: correlation of anatomy and MR imaging, *Radiology* 175:207, 1990.
52. Besalti O, Pekcan Z, Sirin Y et al: Magnetic resonance imaging findings in dogs with intervertebral disk disease: 69 cases (1997-2005), *J Am Vet Med Assoc* 228:902, 2006.
53. Modic MT, Steinberg PM, Ross JS et al: Degenerative disk disease: assessment of changes in vertebral marrow with MR imaging, *Radiology* 166:193, 1988.
54. Vital JM, Pointillart GV, Pedram M et al: Course of Modic 1 six months after lumbar posterior osteosynthesis, *Spine* 28:715, 2003.
55. Platt SR, McConnell JF, Bestbier M: Magnetic resonance imaging characteristics of ascending hemorrhagic myelomalacia in a dog, *Vet Radiol Ultrasound* 47:78, 2006.
56. Ito D, Matsunaga S, Jefery ND et al: Prognostic value of magnetic resonance imaging in dogs with paraplegia caused by thoracolumbar intervertebral disk extrusion: 77 cases (2000-2003), *J Am Vet Med Assoc* 227:1454, 2005.
57. Morrison WB: Cancer affecting the nervous system. In Morrison WB, editor: *Cancer in dogs and cats—medical and surgical management*, Philadelphia, 1998, Williams & Wilkins, pp 655-666.
58. Luttgen PJ, Braund KG, Brawner WR et al: A retrospective study of twenty-nine spinal tumours in the dog and cat, *J Small Anim Pract* 21:213, 1980.
59. Luttgen PJ: Neoplasms of the spinal cord, *Vet Clin North Am Small Anim Pract* 22:973, 1992.
60. Waters DJ, Hayden DW: Intramedullary spinal cord metastasis in the dog, *J Vet Intern Med* 4:207, 1990.
61. Dallman MJ, Saunders GK: Primary spinal cord lymphosarcoma in a dog, *J Am Vet Med Assoc* 189:1348, 1986.
62. Oliver JE, Lorenz MD, Kornegay JN, editors: *Handbook of veterinary neurology*, ed 3, Philadelphia, 1997, WB Saunders, pp 162-163.
63. Kirberger RM, Jacobson LS, Davies JV et al: Hydromyelia in the dog, *Vet Radiol Ultrasound* 38:30, 1997.
64. Cook JR Jr: Fibrocartilaginous embolism, *Vet Clin North Am Small Anim Pract* 18:581, 1988.

65. Grünenfelder FI, Weishaupt D, Green R et al: Magnetic resonance imaging findings in spinal cord infarction in three small breed dogs, *Vet Radiol Ultrasound* 46:91, 2002.
66. Oliver JE, Lorenz MD, Kornegay JN, editors: *Handbook of veterinary neurology,* ed 3, Philadelphia, 1997, W.B. Saunders, p 122.
67. Cambridge AJ, Bagley RS, Britt LG et al: Radiographic diagnosis: arachnoid cyst in a dog, *Vet Radiol Ultrasound* 38:434, 1997.
68. Bentley JF, Simpson ST, Hathcock JT: Spinal arachnoid cyst in a dog, *J Am Anim Hosp Assoc* 27:549, 1991.

ELECTRONIC RESOURCES evolve

Additional information related to the content in Chapter 12 can be found on the companion Web site at evolve http://evolve.elsevier.com/Thrall/vetrad/

- Key Points
- Chapter Quiz
- Case Study 12-1
- Case Study 12-2

SECTION III

The Appendicular Skeleton

CHAPTER • 13
Interpretation Paradigms for the Appendicular Skeleton

Eric A. Ferrell
Clifford R. Berry
Donald E. Thrall

This chapter provides a framework for beginning interpreters of radiographs of the appendicular skeleton. Basic information on how to produce a diagnostic radiograph, recommended standard radiographic views and a simple approach for interpretation are presented. This chapter is not intended to be a stand-alone resource for musculoskeletal radiographic interpretation. Rather, it is an overview of some important principles that will assist the reader in the evaluation of the more detailed chapters that focus on individual regions and diseases.

Radiographic evaluation of the appendicular skeleton of small and large animals is based on the basic four-step process (detection, description, differential for abnormal or deviation from normal, and diagnosis) outlined in Chapter 5. The reader should be able to apply the basic interpretation paradigm or models presented in this chapter to any radiographic study of the appendicular skeleton. A fundamental concept is the fact that bone is continuously remodeling throughout the animal's life and, under normal circumstances (appropriate stresses and biomechanics), bone remodeling is a balance between production and resorption.

Radiographic examination is a standard of practice for evaluation of many small animal and equine orthopedic conditions. Increased emphasis has been placed on obtaining correct diagnoses as well as using follow-up radiographic studies for evaluating response to therapy. Determining the extent of a lesion and the involvement of adjacent soft tissue and bone is an important aspect of the radiographic examination. Additionally, in equine practice, performing multiple joint examinations in a prepurchase examination is common.

TECHNICAL CONSIDERATIONS

Accurate radiographic evaluation of small animal and equine skeletal disorders requires precise technique, positioning, and image processing along with a sound, systematic approach to the review and interpretation of the images. This is especially true for equine radiography, in which expertise in positioning the standing horse relative to the primary x-ray beam for various radiographic projections is essential. Because of the complexity of equine joints, oblique (dorsolateral to palmaromedial [or plantaromedial] and dorsomedial to palmarolateral [or plantarolateral]) projections are often required in addition to lateromedial and dorsopalmar (or dorsoplantar) views. This is done in the thoracic and pelvic limbs from the carpus and tarsus distally. Additional oblique projections for evaluation of areas on specific bones are detailed in individual chapters with regard to the specific joint being evaluated. These projections, such as tangential views designed to project the dorsal surface of the carpus, however, are considered essential for the specific bones evaluated and would be part of a routine examination.

For the best radiographic detail when using film-screen systems, the radiographer should use the slowest film-screen combination consistent with the capabilities of the x-ray machine. Low-output, portable x-ray machines are satisfactory for distal limb radiographs of the horse but are problematic for evaluation of the upper limb, neck, or trunk. Additional safety considerations are also important. Most radiation laws mandate routine use of lead gloves, aprons, thyroid shields, and lead-impregnated glasses for individuals involved in the production of radiographs. In addition, cassette holders allow added distance between the holder and x-ray beam, resulting in reduced exposure. Other important technical factors include the removal of any external skin debris, removal of horseshoes, proper foot cleaning, and sulcus packing of the sole of the hoof with soft tissue–equivalent material (e.g., modeling compound) before radiography.

Additional oblique projections may be required for further assessment of either small-animal or equine orthopedic problems, particularly occult fracture evaluation or the evaluation of complex fractures. For small-animal musculoskeletal radiography, aside from oblique projections, the most common additional radiographic views include the following:

- Cranioproximal to craniodistal tangential projection of the greater tubercle and glenohumeral joint
- Flexed mediolateral radiograph of the elbow joint
- "Frog-leg" or flexed ventrodorsal radiograph of the coxofemoral joints and pelvis
- Cranioproximal to craniodistal tangential projection of the patella and trochlear groove of the stifle joint
- Flexed dorsoplantar projection of the trochlear ridges of the talus
- Distraction radiographic projections of the coxofemoral joints and pelvis for PennHIP (University of Pennsylvania Hip Improvement Program) evaluation

Labeling of radiographs must be done in a systematic and meticulous fashion. Right/left markers should always be used. In the horse, the right/left marker should be placed on the lateral side of the limb for the dorsopalmar (or dorsoplantar) and oblique radiographs, and on the dorsal aspect of the limb for lateromedial radiographs. From the mid-metacarpus and mid-metatarsus distally, the lateral and medial aspects of the limb are axially symmetric; therefore lateral and medial cannot be differentiated on images that do not contain a marking system. Permanent image labeling with animal and owner identification as well as the date of the study must also be present.

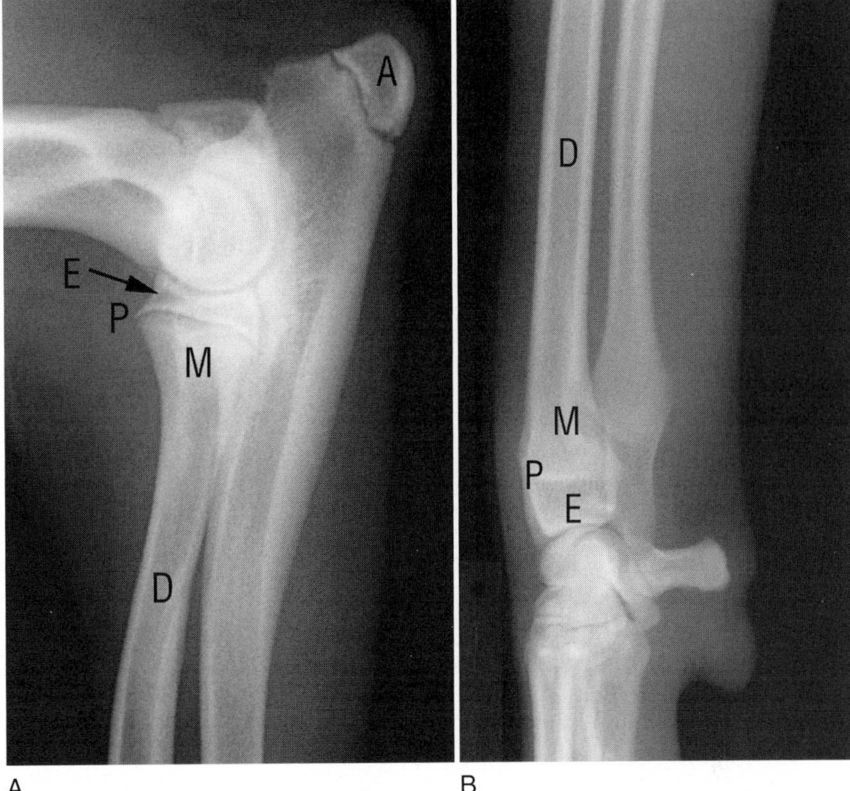

Fig. 13-1 **A,** Mediolateral radiograph of the elbow joint of a 10-month-old dog. The mid-shaft of the radial and ulnar long bones is called the diaphysis *(D)*. The section where growth of the long bone is taking place is the metaphysis *(M)*. The radiolucent zone is the endochondral ossification center, the physis *(P)*. The part of the bone between the physis and the joint is the epiphysis *(E)*. The end of the epiphysis is covered by hyaline cartilage and articulates with the next bone at the synovial joint. In the case of the radius this would be the antebrachiocarpal joint distally and the humeroradial joint proximally. The olecranon apophysis *(A)* or separate center of ossification is present in the proximal ulna. **B,** Mediolateral radiograph from a normal 14-month-old dog in which the physis is closed. The distal ulnar and radial physeal scars *(P)* are radiopaque lines across the long bone at the junction between the epiphysis and the metaphysis.

Before reviewing the study for abnormalities, the radiographs should be assessed for quality and positioning. If exposure, positioning, or other factors are not suitable the study should be repeated. A complete set of radiographs is imperative for basic review of the joint or area in question. Follow-up radiographic evaluation of certain joints may require additional radiographs at a slightly different angle to ensure that abnormalities (e.g., fracture line) have been adequately projected. Follow-up radiographs may include evaluation of the contralateral limb because developmental abnormalities can be bilaterally symmetric but acquired diseases are usually asymmetric.

The availability of portable fluoroscopic units in the equine market should not supplant the radiographic study of a given joint. A negative fluoroscopic study does not equate a normal radiographic evaluation of the particular area in question. The contrast and spatial resolution of routine radiographs are superior to images obtained during fluoroscopic examination.

The brain can only process a certain amount of information simultaneously, so it is better to review one joint completely rather than get overwhelmed with radiographs of multiple joints simultaneously. Once an interpretation is rendered on a given joint, remove the radiographs from the viewer and then assess the next joint. Making notes or voice dictation of each joint will aid in summarizing all abnormalities identified.

BONE ANATOMY AND FORMATION

Bone is formed through a process of mesenchymal models.[1-5] One model is endochondral ossification, in which mesenchymal progenitor cells first differentiate into a cartilaginous model that forms the framework from which bone is formed. During endochondral ossification cartilage cells (chondrocytes) mature, hypertrophy, undergo mineralization within the matrix secreted by the chondrocytes, and ultimately die. This area of cell death forms the scaffolding for ingrowth of blood vessels (angiogenesis) and osteoprogenitor cells that differentiate into osteoblasts. In a long bone, the model of endochondral ossification is located in the physis and metaphysis, where active bone formation takes place. The metaphysis is also called the primary center of ossification.

In a typical long bone, the shaft is termed the diaphysis. Progressing away from the diaphysis is the metaphysis, the physis, and then the epiphysis (Fig. 13-1). The physis is the cartilaginous model that leads to the development of metaphyseal bone. Within each epiphysis, a secondary center of ossification develops from a cartilaginous model. As this secondary center of ossification develops, the physis is essentially trapped between the epiphysis and metaphysis. The physis and metaphysis contribute to increased length and width of the bone toward the diaphysis, whereas the epiphysis contributes to increased length and width of the end of the bone distant to the physis. Osteoprogenitor cells in the epiphysis form the subchondral bone, articular cartilage, and surface for articulation with the adjacent bone. These areas of active bone remodeling and new bone formation, particularly the metaphysis, are the predominant sites of origin for primary bone tumors.

The physis is important from a radiographic standpoint in that it is radiolucent relative to the mineralized osteoid of the epiphysis and metaphysis.[6-9] The physis is also susceptible to injury and is a weak link when long bones are traumatized.

If a physeal fracture is suspected but not identified on initial radiographs, the patient should undergo repeat radiography every 4 to 7 days for the next several weeks to ensure that the physis has not been damaged and that bone is elongating normally. Failure to detect a physeal growth anomaly early will lead to a deformity that will be difficult to repair.

As the physis closes, the radiolucent gap between the metaphysis and epiphysis narrows and becomes nonexistent. Initially, a radiopaque line called the physeal scar develops. As

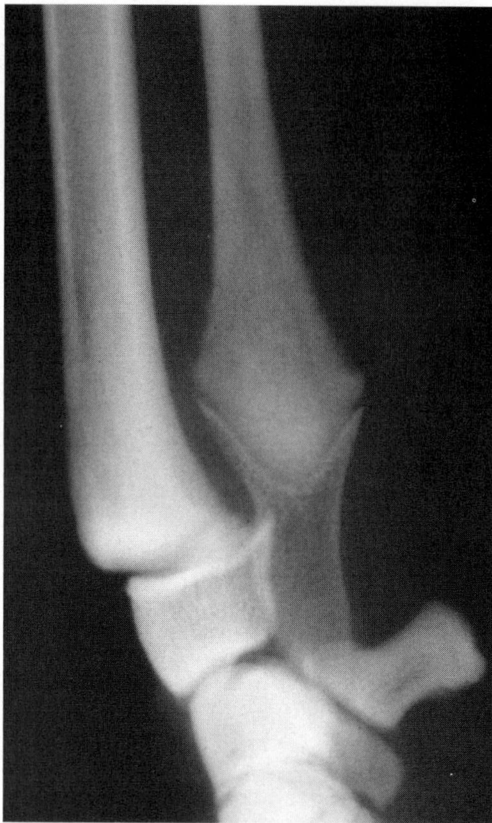

Fig. 13-2 Close-up mediolateral radiograph of the distal antebrachium. Note the unique conical appearance of the ulnar physis. This physis is susceptible to premature closure as a result of compaction injuries. The irregular cortical margination of the distal ulnar metaphysis represents a normal "cut-back" zone. Step malalignment of the distal radial physis is present. This is a result of a type II Salter-Harris fracture of the distal radial physis.

the animal ages, the physeal scar undergoes remodeling and disappears, making the cancellous, intramedullary area of the epiphysis continuous with the metaphysis. On average, the physis of long bones closes between 8 and 14 months of age in dogs and between 24 and 48 months in horses. Large-breed dogs tend to have later physeal closure times than small dogs. Some physes, such as the physis associated with the wing of the ilium, may remain open for the life of the dog.

The distal ulnar physis is unique and warrants separate discussion. The distal ulnar physis has a conical shape, with the point extending distally into the epiphysis. A transverse radiolucent line is also present across the ulnar metaphysis corresponding to the flared rim of the physis that is parallel to the primary x-ray beam (Fig. 13-2). Because of the unique anatomic arrangement of the distal ulnar physis, it is particularly susceptible to compaction injuries and premature closure.

An apophysis is a secondary center of ossification in areas of ligamentous or tendinous attachments to bone. Examples are the greater tubercle of the humerus, greater trochanter of the femur, and the anconeal process of the ulna. Occasionally the apophysis and the parent bone may not fuse. For example, the anconeal process is expected to fuse with the ulna by 6 months of age at the latest in the dog. Thus the diagnosis of an ununited anconeal process would be made if a radiolucent line is present between the anconeal process and the ulnar olecranon after 6 months of age.

A working knowledge of the time and pattern of physeal closure is necessary when evaluating radiographs of the appendicular skeleton. If a question exists about a long bone abnormality, radiographs should be made of the contralateral limb because physes are bilaterally symmetric. Physeal closure times are also affected by hormones such as somatotropin (growth hormone), thyroxine, and tri-iodothyronine. Failure of normal hormonal interactions with the chondrocytes of the physis will result in abnormal development and delayed closure.[3]

Osteoprogenitor cells are also present in the inner cambium layers of the periosteum and endosteum. These cells, which allow for growth and remodeling of the cortex of the bone, remain active beyond the growth period of the animal and are a primary source for osteogenesis during fracture repair.[2,4]

Another model for bone formation is intramembranous ossification, in which mesenchymal progenitors differentiate into a layer of fibrous tissue that then undergoes further differentiation into osteoblasts.[2,4] The bones of the skull undergo intramembranous ossification. Of note, ossification is a process by which the organic matrix is produced with subsequent mineralization of the inorganic matrix.

As the primary spongiosa (metaphysis) is replaced by new bone through the remodeling process, a more organized pattern of collagen and inorganic matrix deposition occurs; this layered appearance can be seen histologically. This type of bone is called lamellar bone. Lamellar bone is divided into four types: circumferential (found just beneath the periosteum and endosteum), concentric lamellae (around which haversian canals and systems are formed), interstitial lamellae (found between concentric lamellar or haversian systems), and trabecular lamellae. Radiographically, the bone cortex is composed of circumferential (outer and inner layers), concentric, and interstitial lamellae. Within the cortex, or the intramedullary space, are trabecular lamellae that can be seen radiographically. In the young animal trabecular lamellae are present in the epiphysis and metaphysis and extend toward the central diaphysis. As the animal ages and growth stops, this trabecular pattern recedes from the diaphysis and metaphysis. The trabecular pattern will often thicken toward the end of the epiphysis, just beneath the articular cartilage. This thicker area of bone beneath the articular cartilage is called subchondral bone. These patterns of cancellous bone development are specific to the bone, species, age of the animal, and the individual depending on the abnormal stresses applied to the bone. These cancellous patterns will continue to change as the animal matures, with a lack of cancellous bone in the diaphysis in an adult long bone.

Detailed concepts of calcium and phosphorus metabolism are beyond the scope of this chapter. Of note, multiple hormonal regulatory mechanisms are responsible for homeostasis of calcium and phosphorus metabolism.[3] Bone represents the storehouse for 99% of the body's calcium and 85% of the body's phosphorus. The primary organs and glands involved in regulation of calcium are the kidneys, liver, intestinal tract, and parathyroid glands.

Two pairs of parathyroid glands exist; an internal gland is embedded in caudal pole of the thyroid gland, and an external gland is located along the cranial aspect of the thyroid gland.[3] The major hormone produced by the parathyroid glands is parathormone. Parathormone increases the plasma calcium levels by the following actions:

- Activating osteoclasts and thereby mobilizing calcium from bone
- Increasing renal tubular reabsorption of calcium and renal tubular secretion of phosphorus
- Increasing conversion of vitamin D_3 to the active dihydroxy form
- Increasing calcium absorption from the gastrointestinal tract[3,4]

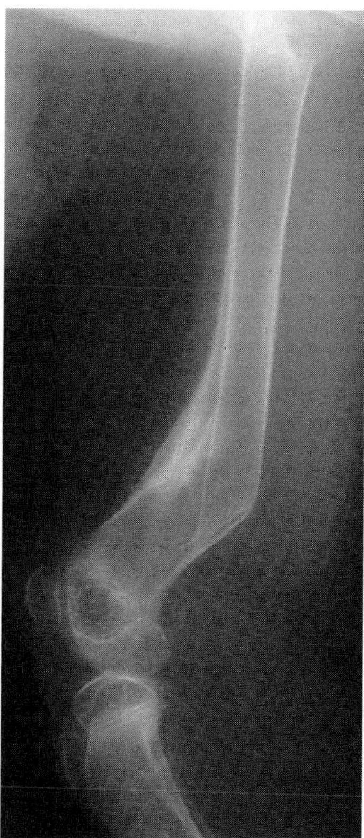

Fig. 13-3 Folding pathologic fractures of the femur caused by nutritional hyperparathyroidism. This cat was raised on a raw meat diet, and thus the calcium/phosphorus ratio was abnormal. The relative osteopenic appearance and the folding cortical fractures are caused by a lack of normal inorganic osteoid within the bones.

Enhanced secretion of parathyroid hormone (primary hyperparathyroidism, nutritional/renal secondary hyperparathyroidism) or parathyroid-like hormone (lymphosarcoma, anal sac carcinoma) leads to skeletal demineralization, with radiographic visualization of generalized skeletal radiolucency and subsequent pathologic folding or compression fractures (Fig. 13-3).[10]

Calcitonin, in essence an antagonist to the effect of parathyroid hormone, is secreted by the C-cells of the thyroid gland. Calcitonin inhibits further calcium reabsorption from bone and in the short term promotes bone formation. Calcitonin also stimulates phosphorus excretion. 1,25-dihydroxyvitamin D_3 is responsible for calcium absorption from the gastrointestinal tract.[3]

Response of Bone

Bone can respond to injury in a limited number of ways. After maturity the skeletal system continues to remodel, but the rates of resorption and production are equal so no net gain or loss of bone occurs. According to Wolff's law, bone will respond according to the principal stresses and strains placed on the bone. This includes periosteal, cortical, subchondral, endosteal, and cancellous remodeling according to new stresses and strains placed on, or removed from, the bone.[5] In a diseased bone, the response is typically a combination of bone lysis (leading to radiolucency on the radiograph), and bone formation (leading to sclerosis on the radiograph). Lysis or sclerosis results from a local imbalance in the ratio of bone production to bone removal. Because bone response to many diseases is similar, a specific diagnosis is usually not possible strictly on the basis of the radiographic abnormalities present.

Normal or Abnormal Findings

When reviewing bone radiographs, the first question to answer is whether a particular finding is normal, a projection artifact based on positioning of the bone relative to the primary x-ray beam, a normal variant, or a true abnormality.[6,11] The opposite limb can be radiographed for anatomic comparison. If suspicious of a long bone lesion in a small animal that may be polyostotic, survey mediolateral radiographs of all four limbs should be acquired.

Normal Variations

Radiolucent lines are expected as a normal part of the bone, particularly in young animals.[7-9] These radiolucencies include the physis and the nutrient canal and foramina. The physis can be complex and result in superimposed radiolucent lines that are often confusing. Several examples include the distal femoral and distal ulnar physes. These normal anatomic radiolucencies should not be mistaken for a fracture. The nutrient canals and foramina are typically found in the diaphysis and are present along the caudal cortex. Some variation may be seen, but these structures are usually bilaterally symmetric.

Sesamoid bones, multipartite sesamoid bones, and accessory centers of ossification are seen in and around a number of joints and should not be mistaken for avulsion fractures or fracture fragments (see Chapter 18 for a review of normal sesamoid location and appearance). In young, rapidly growing dogs, particularly larger breeds, periosteal remodeling occurs along the metaphysis of the long bones as it grows in length into the diaphysis. This zone is called the cut-back zone and is the area of active osteoclastic activity where the width of the metaphysis remodels and reduces to the width of the diaphysis. This area can appear irregular, scalloped, and with a degree of periosteal reaction (see Fig. 13-2). This is most pronounced along the distal ulnar metaphysis.

Anticipated radiolucencies within equine bones include the physis and the nutrient canal. However, certain areas, especially in the distal phalanx and the proximal and distal sesamoid bones, will have conspicuous vascular and synovial channels with expected normal patterns and numbers within the specific bone. The pattern of vascular channel development in the distal phalanx varies by the breed of horse and even over the life of an individual horse. These vascular channels can also change in size and number in diseases such as laminitis or pedal osteitis. Small radiolucent synovial invaginations in the distal border of the navicular bone are normal. Radiolucent channels along the abaxial margin of the proximal sesamoid bones are caused by blood vessels in the area where the suspensory ligament attaches. Improper packing of the sole for radiographs of the hoof is a common source of a radiolucency that is commonly misdiagnosed as a fracture. Reimaging the foot after proper packing or noting whether the radiolucent line extends beyond the edge of the distal phalanx are ways to know that the radiolucent line is not a fracture.

When a horse does not bear weight on a limb, a dramatic decrease in overall bone opacity occurs within several weeks as a result of disuse osteopenia (atrophy). The osteopenia may be so severe that radiographic exposure factors need to be reduced to get the proper exposure of the image.

The chestnut and ergot result in radiopacities superimposed over the metacarpus (or metatarsus), and the metacarpophalangeal (or metatarsophalangeal) joints, respectively. Miscellaneous debris on the skin can also create artifacts superimposed over underlying bone that need to be correctly identified as artifactual.

Aggressive versus Benign Bone Lesions

When a bone is determined to be abnormal, the next step should be assessing the aggressiveness of the lesion. Lesions that are not aggressive may represent a window or a past event that is unrelated to the current condition. Invasive procedures aimed at identifying the specific cause of a benign lesion may not be necessary. Whether a lesion is aggressive or not is based on the specific appearance of the osteolytic and osteoproductive responses. In a nonaggressive or benign lesion the radiographic changes are chronic, degenerative, or benign. In an aggressive lesion, specific bone responses indicate an active, ongoing process.

The distinction between nonaggressive and aggressive lesions is important because of the potentially life-threatening consequences of aggressive lesions, such as neoplasia and infection. When an aggressive bone lesion is identified, the next steps are obtaining thoracic radiographs and open biopsy with histopathologic and microbiologic evaluations of the sample.

The following parameters are evaluated in distinguishing a benign lesion from an aggressive lesion:

- Presence of bone disruption, particularly involving a cortex
- Pattern of bone lysis
- Type of periosteal reaction
- Characteristics of the zone of transition[12,13]

Patterns of bone destruction should be categorized according to the following criteria:

- Localized or generalized
- Presence and degree of cortical destruction
- Presence of intramedullary lysis
- Pattern of lysis (any or all of these can be associated with a single aggressive bone lesion in a given patient)
  - Geographic
  - "Moth eaten"
  - Permeative

Characterization of the lesion location within the bone as epiphyseal, physeal, metaphyseal, or diaphyseal is also important.

Regarding patterns of lysis, focal geographic areas of lysis tend to have well-defined margins and are the least aggressive form of lysis. Geographic lysis is caused by a lesion such as a bone cyst (Fig. 13-4) or abscess. With geographic lysis the cortex may be expanded but it usually has not been destroyed (is not lytic). "Moth-eaten" lysis shows multiple discrete areas of lysis of variable size; the cortex may or may not be lytic. Moth-eaten lysis is typically seen in small animals with bone tumors and infection (Fig. 13-5). The most aggressive pattern of bone lysis is permeative lysis, in which focal areas of ill-defined osteolysis are present throughout a region of a bone (Fig. 13-6). Moth-eaten and permeative lysis are indicative of an aggressive process, and the lesion should be biopsied and assessed for microorganisms for complete evaluation.[14-16]

Bone osteolysis represents a continuum of change, and several patterns may be present in the bone or bones depending on whether the disease is monostotic or polyostotic. The most aggressive pattern identified should be used to characterize the lesion. A "wait and see" approach can be taken with follow-up radiographs. However, if an aggressive component is present, radiographic reevaluation should be within 4 to 10 days because aggressive lesions typically change quickly (Fig. 13-7).

Production of new bone can be encountered as a response to bone disease and can be either adjacent to or away from the joint. Bone production adjacent to a joint is discussed later in this chapter. Bone production away from the joint is either

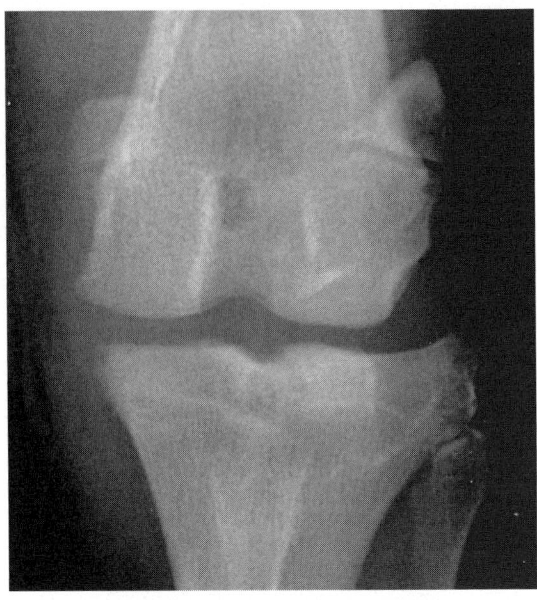

Fig. 13-4 Geographical osteolysis within the intercondylar fossa in a dog with synovial hyperplasia and chronic ligamentous instability. Note the sclerotic margins surrounding the synovial induced "cystic" lesion.

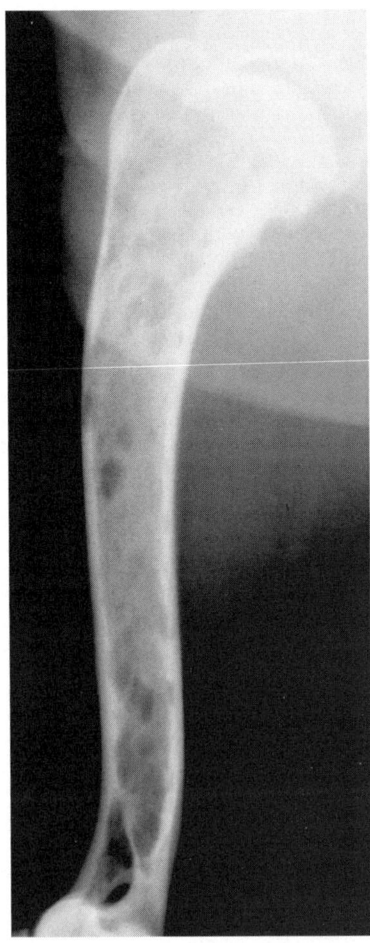

Fig. 13-5 Moth-eaten osteolysis in a dog with metastatic neoplasia of the humerus.

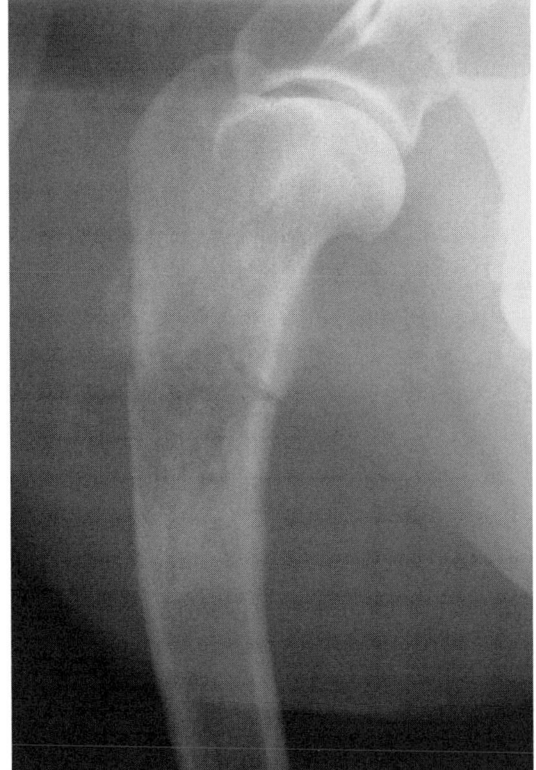

Fig. 13-6 Permeative osteolysis in a dog with a primary bone tumor of the proximal humerus with a transverse pathologic fracture. Amorphous new bone formation is noted surrounding the cranial and caudal aspects of this bone tumor. The histologic diagnosis was osteosarcoma.

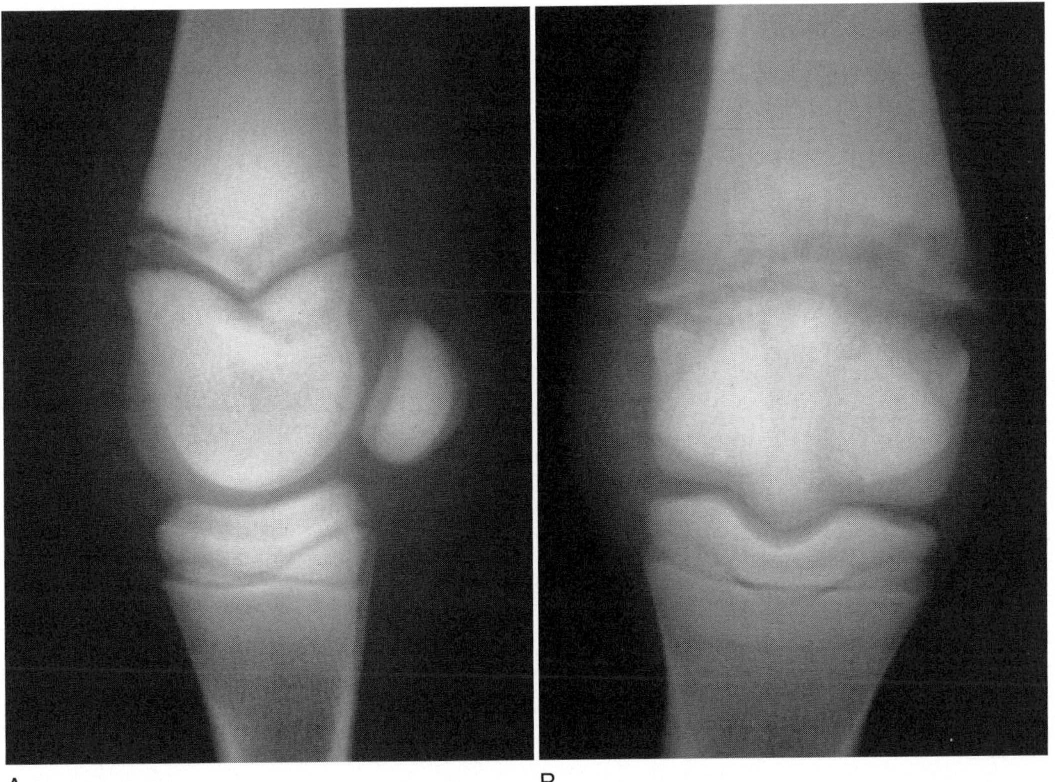

Fig. 13-7 A, Mediolateral radiograph of the distal metaphysis of the metacarpus in a foal with hematogenous osteomyelitis. Irregular focal areas of osteolysis reflect bone destruction without surrounding bone production. This indicates an aggressive osteomyelitis within the bone. **B,** Dorsopalmar radiographs of the same foal 48 hours after initial evaluation. Dramatic areas of progressive osteolysis are visible. These changes were caused by hematogenous osteomyelitis. *Pseudomonas* spp. and *Klebsiella* were isolated from these lesions at surgery.

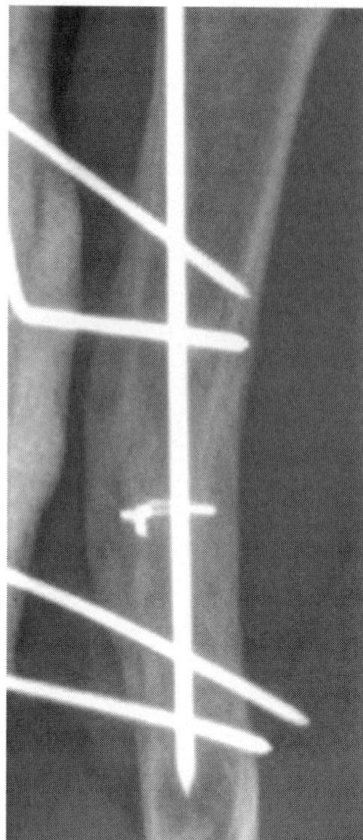

Fig. 13-8 Smooth periosteal new bone formation along the cranial and caudal aspects of the humerus of a cat as a result of a previous fracture. Over time this periosteal reaction became smooth and contiguous with the cortex of the humerus. An external fixation device is present.

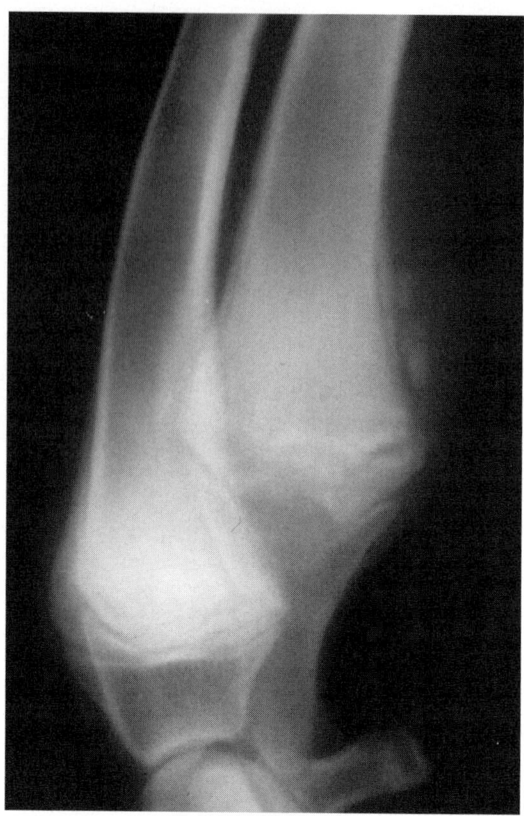

Fig. 13-9 Periosteal cuffing in the region of the metaphysis in a young dog with hypertrophic osteodystrophy. A retained cartilage core associated with the distal ulnar physis is identified, represented by the radiolucency extending proximally into the metaphysis.

periosteal or endosteal proliferation and is usually located along the metaphyseal and diaphyseal regions of the bone. As with osteolysis, periosteal reaction comes in different types. These reactions depend on local factors that stimulate new bone formation and the degree to which the periosteal or endosteal layers of osteoprogenitor cells respond to the stimulus. The characteristics of periosteal and endosteal new bone formation are a continuum, as noted for osteolytic lesions. The following are different types of periosteal reactions, listed in order of increasing aggressiveness:

- Smooth, solid bone formation
- Multilayered or lamellar bone formation
- Spiculated, columnar bone formation
- "Sunburst" bone formation
- Amorphous new bone

Smooth new bone formation is typical of focal trauma in which a subperiosteal hematoma or part of the periosteum has been elevated away from the cortex. Smooth new bone production is not a sign of an aggressive bone lesion (Fig. 13-8).

Multiple layers of new bone formation along a cortex can have the appearance of a multilayered onion skin and can be seen in a variety of conditions ranging from focal trauma to infection to neoplasia. A thick lamellar periosteal reaction that appears separated from the cortex can be seen in the metaphysis of the distal radius and ulna in immature dogs with hypertrophic osteodystrophy (Fig. 13-9).[17] As with smooth periosteal reactions, lamellar periosteal reactions are usually associated with less-aggressive diseases, although bone tumors occasionally result in a lamellar periosteal reaction.

A spiculated periosteal reaction is new bone formation radiating perpendicularly from the long bone cortex as is typically seen along the diaphysis of long bones with hypertrophic osteopathy (Fig. 13-10) and occasionally in bacterial osteomyelitis. A "sunburst" pattern is new bone formation in which long rays of new bone radiate from a central, aggressive osteolytic or osteoproductive lesion, such as a primary bone tumor.

Amorphous new bone formation occurs when new bone is being deposited within soft tissues surrounding the bone, but the new bone is haphazard and does not have a functional or organized shape (Fig. 13-11).[12,13]

Another term used to describe periosteal bone formation is Codman's triangle. The periosteum adjacent to the lesion is elevated away from the cortex (Fig. 13-12) and a triangle of smooth bone is formed. Codman's triangle is a nonspecific periosteal reaction and can occur with both benign and aggressive processes.[17]

Intramedullary and endosteal bone production should be assessed; however, it may be difficult to identify because of superimposed cortical bone or a periosteal reaction. Focal areas of bone sclerosis within the medullary cavity are a typical manifestation of canine panosteitis but can also be seen with systemic fungal disease or bone metastasis.

When evaluating the spectrum of periosteal reactions and osteolysis, the most aggressive part of the lesion should define whether the lesion has an aggressive or benign character. An example of a benign bone lesion is one in which the periosteal reaction is smooth and solid in appearance. The lesion may be somewhat expansile, but no cortex destruction or radiographic evidence of permeative or moth-eaten lysis is present. An aggressive lesion has aggressive osteolytic and osteoproliferative radiographic features. Whether a bone lesion is primarily

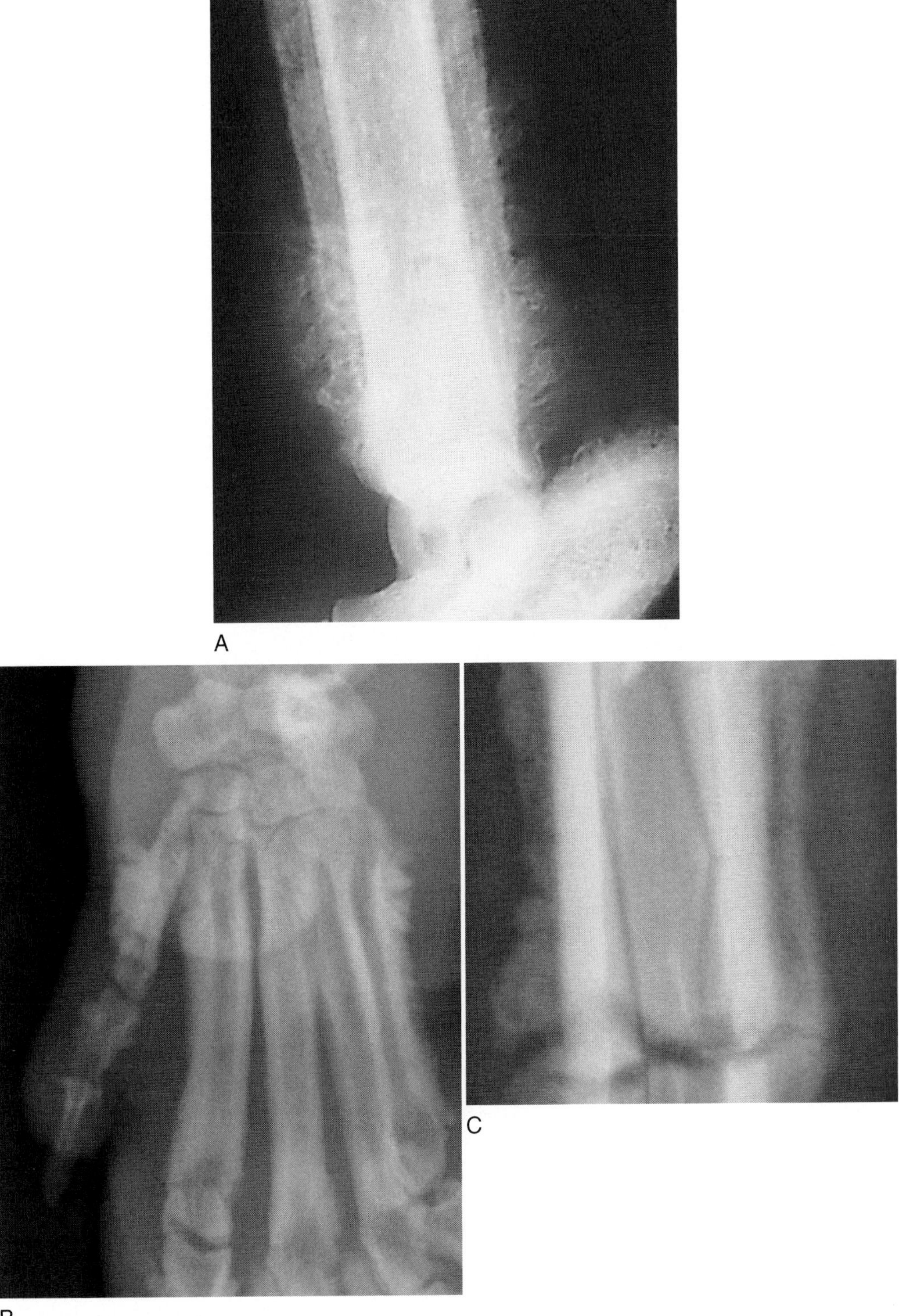

Fig. 13-10 Spiculated, or columnar, periosteal reaction. **A,** This dog had a primary lung tumor and the periosteal reaction is consistent with hypertrophic osteopathy. **B,** The manus of another dog, also with hypertrophic osteopathy. **C,** The metatarsus of a goat with bacterial osteomyelitis.

lytic or primarily productive has nothing to do with its aggressiveness.

A final characteristic that may help assess the aggressiveness of a lesion is the appearance of the region of transition between the lesion and adjacent normal bone. Benign lesions or lesions that are not particularly aggressive will have a relatively abrupt demarcation of the edge of the lesion. The edge of the disease process in the bone can be delineated from adjacent unaffected bone fairly precisely. This is called a distinct transition zone. With aggressive lesions, the growth or

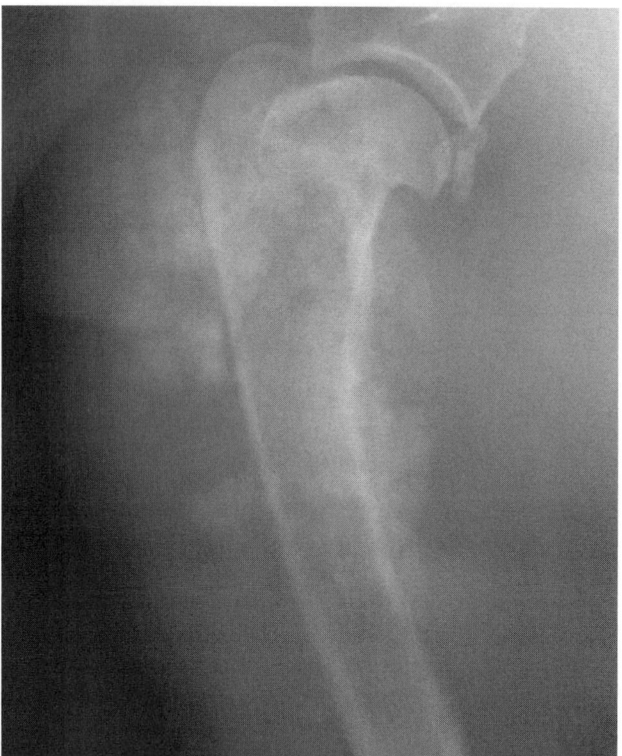

Fig. 13-11 Amorphous new bone formation within the soft tissues adjacent to a an osteolytic lesion of the proximal humerus caused by a primary bone tumor.

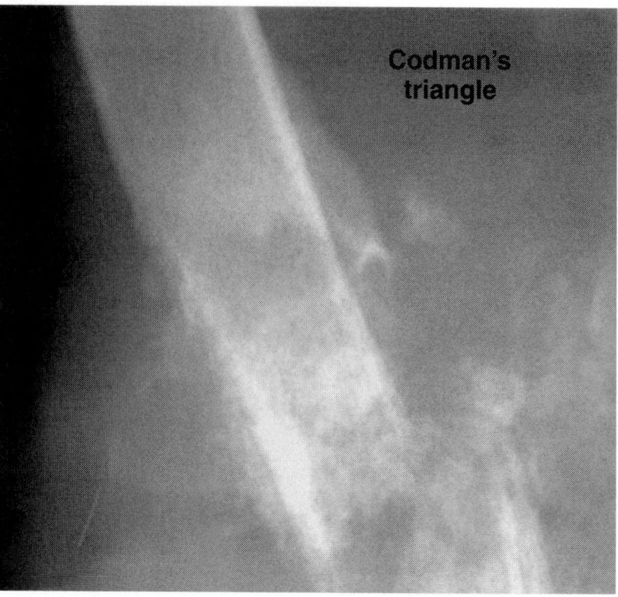

Fig. 13-12 Periosteal elevation from any cause can result in smooth new bone formation. This triangle of new bone formation is called Codman's triangle as seen in this distal humeral lesion. In this dog, the periosteal elevation was caused by an osteosarcoma.

extension of the lesion in the bone makes identification of the edge of the lesion imprecise, determining the limits of the lesion in the bone is impossible. This is called an indistinct transition zone. Figure 13-4 shows a well-defined transition zone at the edge of the lesion. Figure 13-11 has no sharp demarcation that defines the extent of involvement of the bone.

All these patterns fall along a continuum and need to be considered when deciding whether a lesion is aggressive. If the answer is still unclear, thoracic radiographs can be obtained and the lesion can be radiographed again in 10 to 14 days. If the lesion has changed, the aggressive character of the lesion may be more obvious.

Aside from whether a lesion is aggressive, its location and number of bones involved are important factors in establishing the differential diagnoses. Whether a bone disease is monostotic (one bone) or polyostotic (multiple bones) drastically influences the considerations. For example, a monostotic metaphyseal aggressive long bone lesion should be considered a primary bone tumor until proven otherwise. But a primary bone tumor would not be considered for multiple metaphyseal aggressive lesions; infection or metastatic neoplasia are more likely. Specific disease entities occur within specific locations (Table 13-1).

The Synovial Joint

Radiographic evaluation of a joint in small animals consists of two orthogonal radiographs, usually a mediolateral and a craniocaudal (or caudocranial) or dorsopalmar (plantar). Because joint radiographs in small animals are usually obtained in a non-weight-bearing patient, joint space width cannot be assessed unless overtly subluxated, luxated, or collapsed with radiographic features of subchondral sclerosis and eburnation.

The synovial joint is composed of hyaline cartilage covering the epiphyseal subchondral bone, the joint capsule, and the synovial fluid that bathes the cartilage with nutrients and oxygen. Normal hyaline cartilage is a well-organized layer of chondrocytes with surrounding type II collagen fibers forming a meshwork for proteoglycans, mucopolysaccharides, and water.[4-6]

The response of the joint and surrounding structures to damage is complex, and this process is simplified in the following discussion. New molecular factors that affect joint response are being identified almost daily.

Degenerative joint disease, osteoarthritis, and osteoarthrosis are generic terms used to summarize radiographic changes involving a joint. In primary degenerative joint disease no inciting factor can be established. This is seen as an age-related change in the shoulder joint of dogs. Secondary degenerative joint disease is a condition in which an inciting etiology is present, such as an osteochondrosis lesion or previous articular fracture.

The radiographic changes accompanying degenerative joint disease can be characterized by the soft tissue and bone responses to the degenerative process. First, because of either a biochemical or biomechanical abnormality, the hyaline cartilage is damaged and joint instability develops. Inflammation and synovitis result in periarticular soft tissue swelling or intraarticular effusion that may be seen radiographically. The joint attempts to stabilize itself by thickening the supporting ligaments and synovial hyperplasia. Radiographically, bone changes are the most commonly identified changes noted in association with degenerative joint disease. These changes include osteophyte formation, enthesopathy, and subchondral bone thickening.

Over time, the remodeling becomes advanced. If articular cartilage becomes fragmented in the joint and embedded in synovium, it can undergo endochondral ossification and appear radiographically as a mineralized intraarticular or juxtaarticular fragment. As articular cartilage thins and fissures develop, synovial fluid may be forced between the fissures and cause pressure atrophy of subchondral bone, resulting in synovial cyst–like lucencies.

Table • 13-1

Common Causes of Joint Disease of Small Animals

JOINT	DISEASE	SPECIES	SITE
Shoulder	Osteochondrosis	C	Caudal humeral head (best evaluated on lateral radiograph)
	Bicipital tenosynovitis	C, F	Bicipital tendon sheath and the intertubercular groove (arthrogram may be helpful for evaluation)
	Trauma	C, F	Any site
	Congenital luxation	C, F	Abnormal development of humeral head and glenoid cavity
	Primary DJD	C	Idiopathic; osteophyte formation at periarticular locations such as glenoid cavity and humeral head
	Synovial cell sarcoma	C, F	Osteolysis along joint capsule insertion sites
Elbow	Feline progressive polyarthritis	F	Osteoproliferative DJD of both elbows
	Ununited anconeal process	C	Anconeal fails to fuse with olecranon by 6 months of age
	Osteochondrosis of medial aspect of distal humeral condyle	C	On cranial caudal radiograph, radiolucent defect in medial aspect of distal humeral condyle
	Fragmented medial coronoid process	C	Blunting, fragment, or absence of medial coronoid process
	Premature closure of distal radial or ulnar physis	C, F	DJD and subluxation of the elbow joint
	Synovial cell sarcoma	C, F	Osteolysis along joint capsule insertion sites
	Septic arthritis	C (young)	Osteolysis and remodeling of bones of elbow joint
Carpus	Repetitive trauma	C, F	Osteoproliferative DJD; enthesopathy of the accessory carpal bone
	Rheumatoid arthritis, SLE	C, F (less common in F)	Resorption of bone at areas of pannus and synovial proliferation
	Synovial cell sarcoma	C, F	Osteolysis along joint capsule insertion sites
	Premature closure of distal radial or ulnar physis	C, F	DJD of the carpal joint(s)
Coxofemoral joint	Hip dysplasia	C, F (much less common in F)	Subluxation, luxation, and DJD of coxofemoral joints
	Bilateral slipped capital physeal fractures (atraumatic history)	F	Widened capital physis or step malalignment with "apple core" appearance of the femoral neck over time
	Trauma	C, F	Physeal or femoral neck fractures
	Aseptic necrosis of the femoral head	C (small breeds)	Remodeling of head and neck, fragmentation of femoral head, thickening of femoral neck
	Synovial cell sarcoma	C	Osteolysis along joint capsule insertion sites
	Osteochondrosis	C	Radiolucent defect of femoral head
Stifle joint	Ligamentous instability	C, F (less common in F)	Joint effusion and DJD of femoropatellar and femorotibial joints
	Patellar luxations	C, F	Joint effusion and DJD of femoropatellar and femorotibial joints
	Osteochondrosis	C	Lateral femoral condyle
	Trauma	C, F	Any location
	Synovial cell sarcoma	C, F	Osteolysis along joint capsule insertion sites
Tarsus	Osteochondrosis	C	Medial trochlear and lateral trochlear ridges
	Trauma	C, F	Any location
	Synovial cell sarcoma	C, F	Osteolysis along joint capsule insertion sites
	Rheumatoid arthritis, SLE	C, F (less common in F)	Resorption of bone at areas of pannus and synovial proliferation

C, Dog; *F,* cat; *DJD,* degenerative joint disease; *SLE,* systemic lupus erythematosus.

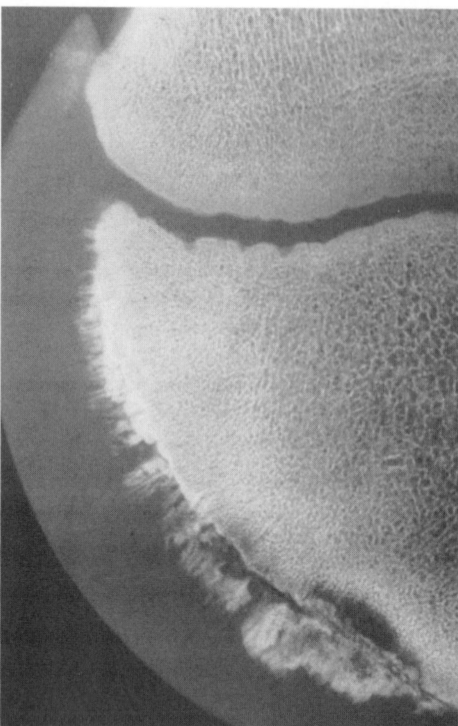

Fig. 13-13 Microradiograph of the medial trochlear ridge of the distal femur from a newborn foal that was euthanized for unrelated reasons. The microradiograph shows the irregular pattern of incomplete ossification within the normal femoral trochlear ridge. (Courtesy Dr. Roy Pool, Texas A&M University, College Station, Texas.)

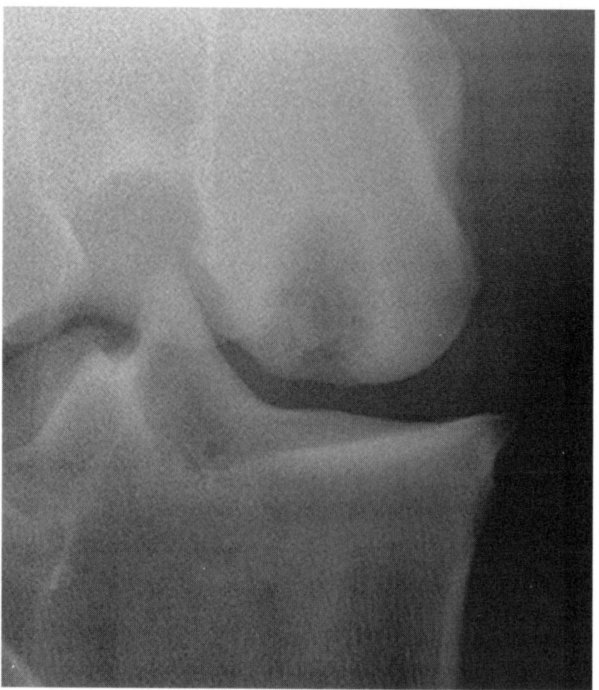

Fig. 13-14 A caudocranial radiograph of the left stifle joint of a horse. A focal circular area of lucency is visible within the medial femoral condyle with surrounding subchondral sclerosis, consistent with a subchondral cystlike lesion.

Differences Between Large and Small Animals

Physeal blood vessels cross the physis from the metaphysis to the epiphysis in young horses. These transphyseal vascular loops form complex capillary networks with a high density on the metaphyseal side of the physis and within the epiphysis beneath the articular cartilage. This anatomic difference, not present in small animals, is important in hematogenous osteomyelitis where bacteria lodge in the physis, metaphysis, and epiphysis.

In the neonate certain epiphyses can be immature, with incomplete endochondral ossification resulting in a highly irregular bone margin (Fig. 13-13). This is particularly true for the trochlear ridges of the distal femur and the talus. This incomplete ossification cannot be differentiated radiographically from bacterial osteomyelitis.

The nutrient foramina and canals form diaphyseal lines that can be mistaken for incomplete fractures. The position of the nutrient canal in the proximal phalanx is variable and can be located dorsally in a mid-diaphyseal position. The proximal fibula in the horse is also characterized by transverse radiolucent lines representing regions of fibrous/cartilaginous union that should not be mistaken for a fracture. Important anatomic consideration should be given to the radiographic variations within the equine third metacarpal and metatarsal bones. These bones have variable cortical thickness within the diaphysis at different locations, with the thickest portion of the cortex being within the middle of the diaphysis.

The location of the lesion in the bone is as important in horses as it is in small animals. Traumatic injury to bone, periosteum, or soft tissues can occur at any location in the bone, so complete evaluation of each radiograph is necessary. Epiphyseal disorders usually include disorders specific to the growing horse or degenerative joint disease. Physeal and metaphyseal disorders include angular limb deformities, growth-related abnormalities (aseptic physitis), septic bacterial emboli with physeal and metaphyseal osteomyelitis, and trauma (fracture). Diaphyseal disorders tend to be confined to traumatic injuries (stress fractures, fractures, etc.).

In horses, particularly neonates, osteolysis will supersede osteoproliferation in inflammatory diseases, particularly hematogenous osteomyelitis or septic arthritis. A moth-eaten or permeative appearance to the bone may be present without adjacent areas of osteosclerosis. This helps differentiate benign lesions such as a subchondral cyst with surrounding sclerosis from an osteolytic lesion of the subchondral bone as a result of septic arthritis (Fig. 13-14). Dramatic osteolytic lesions can develop within 24 to 48 hours within the bone in foals with hematogenous osteomyelitis. The bone response in the neonate has a more lamellar appearance, whereas in the adult new bone proliferation (periosteal) appears more spiculated or smooth. Subperiosteal hematomas can mineralize and also appear as focal smooth bone exostoses along a diaphyseal cortex. The response of the bone depends on many factors, and a continuum exists between the appearance of an aggressive lesion and a benign lesion. Also of note, bone reactions take time to develop, even after a penetrating wound. An acute bursal infection of the distal sesamoid bone or an acute septic arthritis may not initially have any radiographic evidence of bone change.

PRINCIPLES OF OBLIQUE RADIOGRAPHS

As noted above, oblique projections of a bone or joint are often necessary for complete assessment. This is especially true in complex joints such as the equine carpus. In addition to lateromedial and dorsopalmar radiographs, dorsolateral-

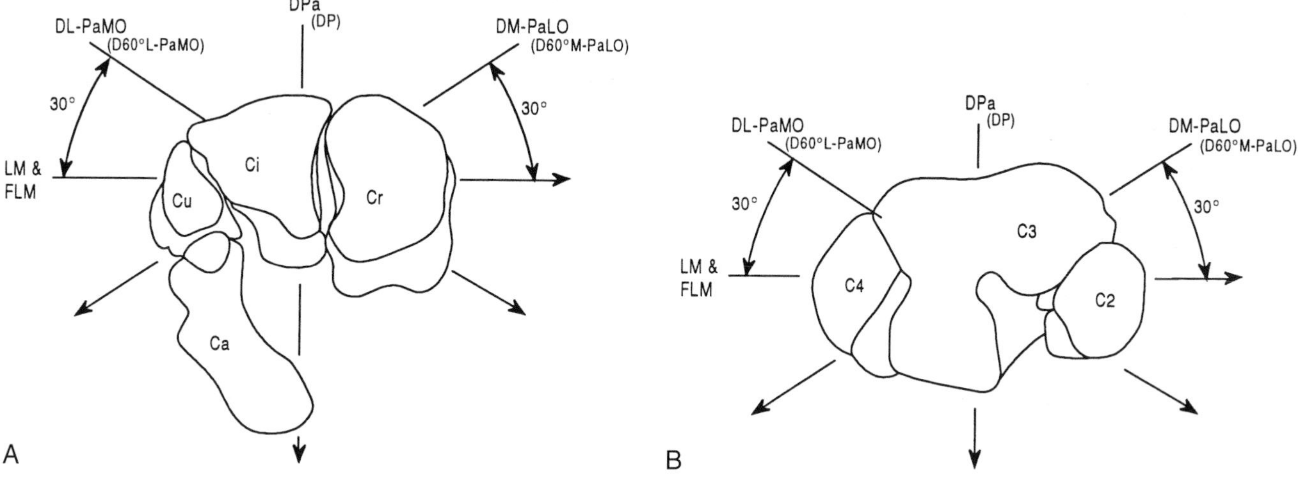

Fig. 13-15 X-ray beam direction for various views of the equine carpus. Diagrams of the proximal (A) and distal (B) row of carpal bones. Directional terms describing the point of entrance to the point of exit of the primary x-ray beam are designated. The terminology shown in parentheses describes the angulation of the x-ray beam. *Ca,* Accessory carpal; *Ci,* intermediate carpal; *Cr,* radial carpal; *Cu,* ulnar carpal. (Courtesy Dr. Lisa Neuwirth, Lexington, Kentucky, and Dr. Gregg Boring, Mississippi State University.)

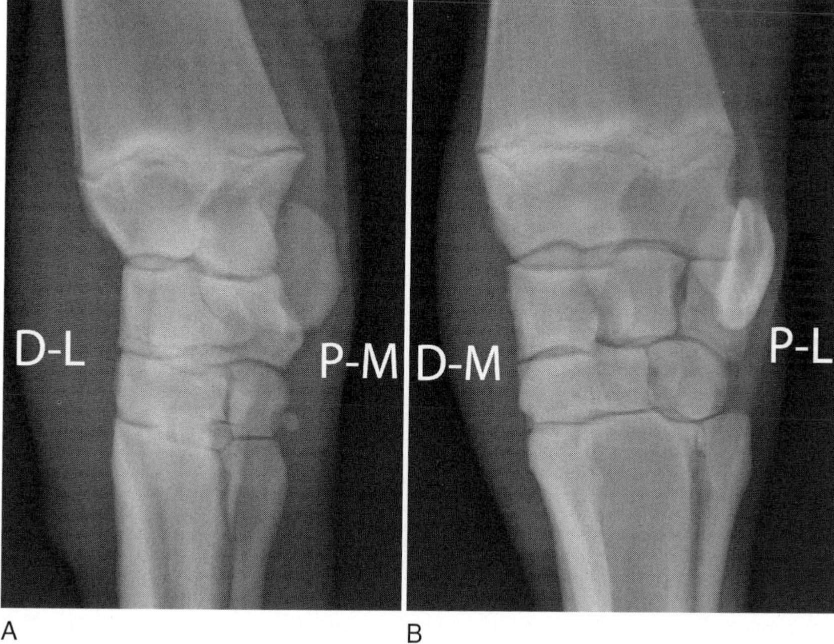

Fig. 13-16 Dorsomedial-palmarolateral (A) and dorsolateral-palmaromedial (B) radiographs of an equine carpus. In A, the dorsolateral *(D-L)* and palmaromedial *(P-M)* surfaces are projected, whereas in B, the dorsomedial *(D-M)* and palmarolateral *(P-L)* surfaces are projected.

palmaromedial and dorsomedial-palmarolateral oblique projections are often acquired. Understanding which bone surfaces are being projected in such oblique views is important. The equine carpus is used as an example.

In a dorsolateral-palmaromedial view of the equine carpus, the x-ray beam strikes the dorsolateral surface and exits the palmaromedial surface (Fig. 13-15). In the resulting radiograph (Fig. 13-16, *B*), the dorsomedial and palmarolateral surfaces of the carpus are projected. In a dorsomedial-palmarolateral view of the equine carpus, the x-ray beam strikes the dorsomedial surface and exits the palmarolateral surface. In the resulting radiograph (Fig. 13-16, *A*), the dorsolateral and palmaromedial surfaces of the carpus are projected. The specific anatomy of bone location in each of these views can be found in Chapter 14. The principles of surface projection as dependent on x-ray beam direction described here for the carpus are the same as for similar oblique projections of other joints or parts.

Interpretation Paradigm

The interpretation paradigm for reviewing musculoskeletal radiographs should be based on the mnemonic "ABCs," standing for ***a***lignment, ***b***one, ***c***artilage, and ***s***oft tissue. Alignment implies the appearance of the way the bones line up at the joint and along the bone itself. The alignment of the joint or bone in question should be evaluated from all available radiographs. Alignment can be misinterpreted if oblique radiographs have been made and not centered correctly or a limb

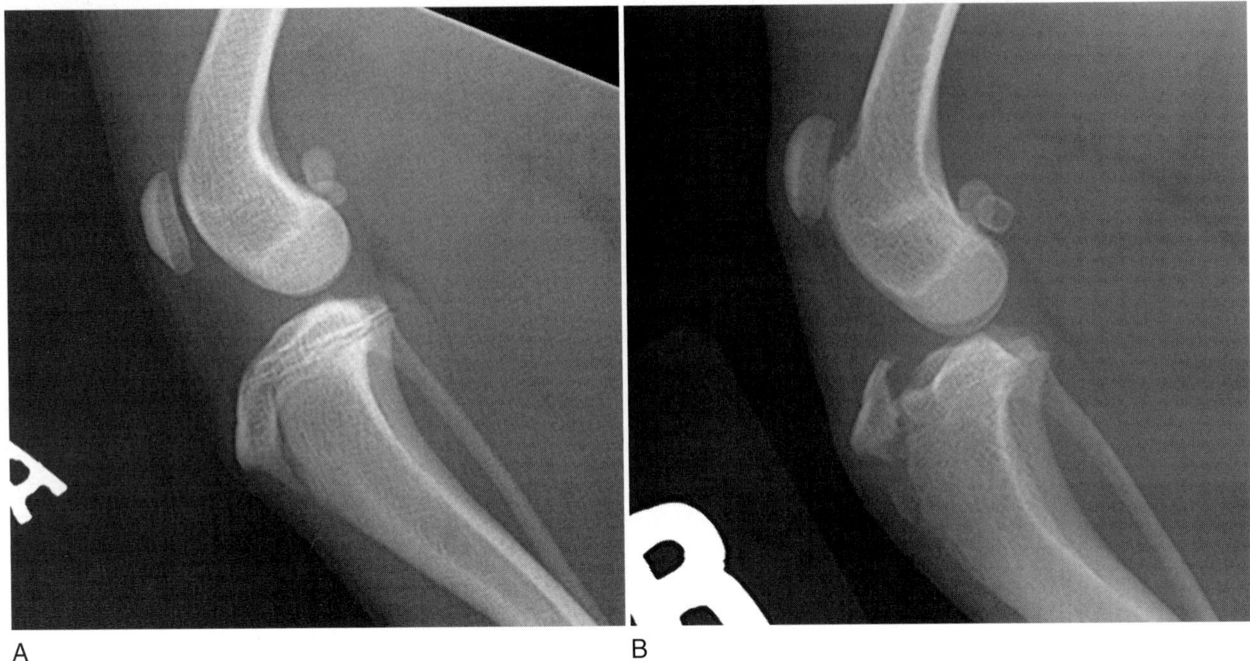

Fig. 13-17 A, Normal open tibial tuberosity apophysis in a dog that should not be mistaken for an avulsion fracture. **B,** An avulsion fracture of the tibial tuberosity as a result of trauma in a dog. Note the proximal displacement of the fracture fragment along with the similar displacement of the patella. The proximal tibial epiphysis is closed.

is malpositioned in a non-weight-bearing radiograph. The experienced radiographer will develop an expected appearance of joint space width and bone-to-bone congruity. Radiographic anatomy textbooks are helpful for comparison, as are the normal labeled radiographs in this text. Malalignment within a bone can be caused by fractures or developmental abnormalities (premature physeal closure or inherited metabolic bone diseases).

Radiographic evaluation of bones can be time consuming. This implies evaluation from cortex to cortex from the proximal to the distal end of each bone on the radiograph. An expected size, shape, position (location), opacity, margin, and number are associated with each bone. Each roentgen sign must be assessed with each bone. Also, the bone must be assessed from cortex to cortex, which includes the periosteum, cortex, endosteum, medullary cavity (with or without cancellous bone depending on location), endosteum, cortex, and finally periosteum. The endosteum and periosteum have a soft tissue opacity that is contiguous with the overlying musculature, tendons, or ligaments and cannot be seen as a distinct structure. These margins should be evaluated for the possibility of new bone formation or osteolysis (change in margin and opacity).

The cartilage is of soft tissue opacity unless it has become mineralized. A typical degree of widening should be mentally noted for each joint and each physis. To a certain extent, joint space width is slightly variable for some joints (such as the glenohumeral joint) in small animals because the radiographs are not weight bearing. Stress views and radiographs of the opposite limbs may be beneficial to confirm or deny joint space widening. The pattern of physeal development is important to keep in mind, particularly when assessing a physeal injury. One of the most common areas of concern is the proximal tibial physis and the appearance of the tibial tuberosity. On a lateral radiograph, the apophysis of the tibial tuberosity fuses with the epiphysis of the tibial plateau; the physis then closes in a caudal-to-cranial direction, with the cartilage associated with the tibial tuberosity being the last to close. This radiolucent region is commonly misdiagnosed as an avulsion fracture (Fig. 13-17). Beneath articular cartilage is the subchondral bone plate. This thickened area of bone can provide clues that abnormalities are present within the joint or a particular location of the joint. The subchondral bone plate should be of uniform thickness; however, it will change if degenerative changes are present within the joint.

Finally, evaluation of the extracapsular and intracapsular soft tissues is performed. With film, this usually requires a hot light. Any soft tissue swelling is a potential site of underlying bone injury. The area of the bone beneath the soft tissue swelling should be critically evaluated for subtle periosteal reactions, areas of osteolysis, or articular subchondral bone changes. Whether additional radiographs are required to evaluate the areas in question better should be evaluated.

Radiographs of the opposite limb serve as a valuable point of reference when a specific question arises about a possible abnormality being a normal anatomic variant. When an abnormality is detected, a description of the abnormal roentgen signs should be written. In private practice this step is often skipped, but it forces the reader to evaluate the radiograph more critically. The next question to be answered is whether the abnormalities identified are normal anatomic variants or true abnormalities. From here a diagnosis or differential diagnosis can be established. Pitfalls in interpretation of musculoskeletal radiographs include the following:

- Poor technique
- Lack of systematic review
- Not obtaining an orthogonal radiograph
- Failure to obtain radiographs of the contralateral limb
- Failure to use a hot light
- Failure to consult normal radiographic anatomy sources

Within the process of radiographic evaluation, as the interpretation paradigm of the ABCs is applied, roentgen signs must be used as the tools to describe the abnormality. This assumes a working knowledge of normal radiographic

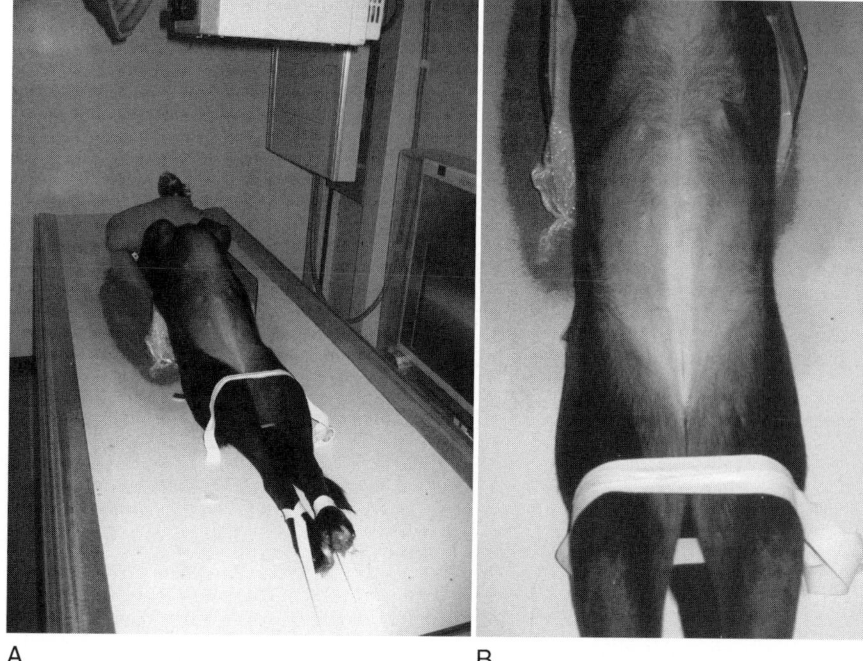

Fig. 13-18 Correct positioning of a dog for obtaining a ventrodorsal extended-leg pelvic radiograph (A) and a close-up (B).

anatomy and possible normal anatomic variations. Additionally, the astute equine practitioner will memorize the specific areas on the radiograph to assess specific disease processes. These areas are not meant to limit the extent of the radiographic examination. For example, a false sense of security can arise that nothing must be wrong with the tarsus because typical areas have been found free of osteochondrosis. This type of satisfaction of search error (stopping too soon), is a common mistake and should be avoided. The use of the hot light for evaluating each radiograph forces the interpreter to look at each radiograph individually and focus on specific areas.

Once roentgen abnormalities have been detected and described, a reasonable differential diagnostic list or a specific diagnosis can be compiled on the basis of the abnormalities present, signalment, clinical history, and presentation. When tying all facts together, several caveats exist to musculoskeletal imaging. The first is that a normal radiographic study does not equate with the absence of bone abnormalities. Thirty percent to 50% of the total bone mass must change before a lesion can be detected radiographically. Second, radiographic abnormalities may or may not correlate with clinical lameness or the absence of a lameness. Finally, further diagnostic testing should include nerve blocks and/or other imaging modalities (if available) if multiple radiographic lesions are identified.

THE PELVIS

The pelvis makes up the proximal extent of the pelvic limb appendicular skeleton and is composed of the paired ilium, acetabulum, pubis, and ischium. In small animals, evaluation of the pelvis is frequently performed to assess dysplastic and degenerative changes of the coxofemoral joints or document pelvic fractures or suspected joint-associated neoplasia or septic arthritis.

Canine hip dysplasia is the abnormal development of the coxofemoral joint that results from a lack of conformity between the acetabulum and the femoral head. The most common radiographic procedure for evaluation of canine hip dysplasia is the ventrodorsal extended-limb projection, developed by the American Veterinary Medical Association, Council of Veterinary Science, Panel on Canine Hip Dysplasia in 1961.[18-24] This radiographic procedure was subsequently adopted for use by the Orthopedic Foundation for Animals and continues to be one of the most commonly used procedures today for canine coxofemoral joint certification. The positioning of the pelvic limbs in this conventional procedure has been shown to have a tightening effect on the joint capsule and surrounding soft tissues.[18,22,24] This tightening may subsequently mask evidence of joint laxity in mild to moderate hip dysplasia. As a result, during the past 15 years dynamic pelvic radiographic studies have received increased attention as a result of their ability to document the degree of laxity of a specific patient's coxofemoral joints.

Evaluation of the equine pelvis is pursued most often for assessing stress fractures or abnormalities of the sacroiliac joint. Given the potential complications associated with general anesthesia in horses, skeletal scintigraphy and ultrasound are more commonly used to evaluate potential pelvic trauma in horses.

Radiographic Technique and Positioning

The radiographic techniques for evaluation of the small animal pelvis use high milliampere seconds and moderate kilovoltage peaks, similar to that for the skull and spine. The examination should be performed on an appropriately sized radiographic cassette, routinely a 14 × 17 inch cassette for a ventrodorsal extended-leg projection of an average-sized to large-breed dog. In small animals, the radiographic examination of the pelvis commonly requires use of sedation or anesthesia to ensure that a quality radiographic study can be obtained.

The ventrodorsal extended-leg projection remains the most frequent means of evaluating the pelvis in dogs and cats.[19,20] In this study, the patient may be positioned manually and have the hindlimbs extended by the examiner, or the patient may be appropriately positioned with a radiographic trough and tape (Fig. 13-18). With this projection, symmetric positioning of the pelvis is assessed by a comparative evaluation of the size and shape of the right and left obturator foramen and pelvic bones, parallelism of the femoral diaphy-

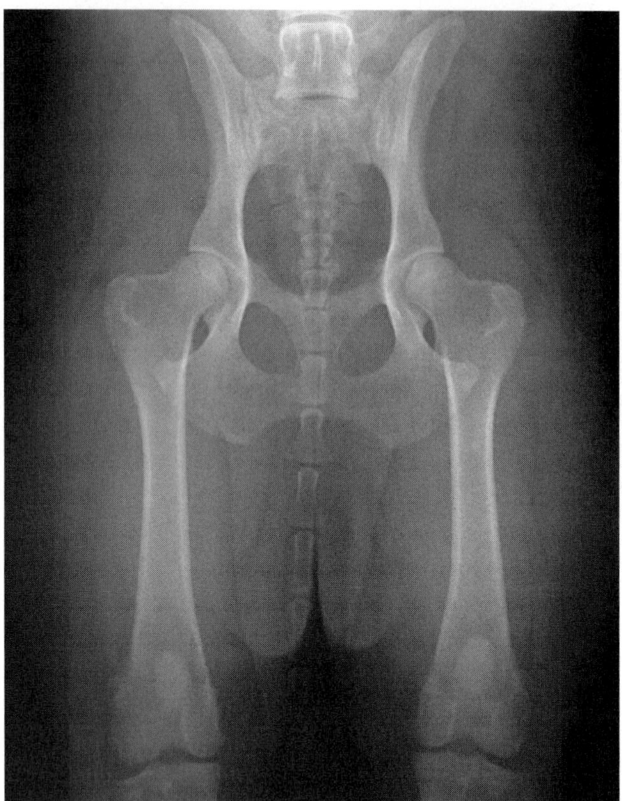

Fig. 13-19 A correctly positioned, normal ventrodorsal extended-leg pelvic radiograph. Notice the symmetry of the sacroiliac joints, pelvic inlet, obturator foramina, coxal joints, femurs, and stifle joints.

ses, and superimposition of the patellae over the center of the femoral condyles (Fig. 13-19). The obturator foramen, being of unequal size, indicates that one side of the pelvis is elevated in relation to the other. The side of the pelvis with the larger foramen is the more ventrally positioned (Fig. 13-20). Such knowledge allows for greater ease of positioning corrections.

A lateral radiograph of the pelvis should be performed routinely to accompany the ventrodorsal projection. Correct positioning should be evaluated by anatomic symmetry and by ensuring that the femoral head, ileal wing, and caudal lumbar vertebrae transverse processes are as superimposed as possible. Lateral and ventrodorsal extended-leg radiographs comprise the standard views used to evaluate the pelvis of small animals, particularly in suspected trauma.

Additional projections may be required to evaluate the pelvis for unique fractures or when the patient is in pain and will not tolerate a ventrodorsal extended-leg radiograph. A ventrodorsal flexed-leg (frog-leg) radiograph can routinely be made on a patient that is in too much pain for positioning with the pelvic limbs in extension.[20] This frog-leg projection is also useful for assessing the coxofemoral joints in suspected capital physeal or femoral neck fractures. On routine ventrodorsal extended-leg radiographs, the presence of a capital physeal fracture is often masked by the tightening of the joint capsule and surrounding tissues. The ventrodorsal flexed-leg radiograph allows relaxation of the periarticular soft tissues and rotation of the distal femoral fracture fragment away from the epiphyseal fragment (Fig. 13-21).

The PennHIP radiographic method is a type of dynamic radiographic examination of the pelvis used specifically to assess for canine hip dysplasia.[18] This study was developed to provide an objective means of assessing coxofemoral joint laxity. This procedure requires special certification of the examiner. A PennHIP study requires the same dorsal recumbent positioning of the patient and quality control assessment of the pelvis as for conventional canine pelvic radiographs. However, the femurs are positioned at approximately 80 degrees perpendicular to the surface of the radiographic table. This limb position is described as the point of maximal passive laxity. Once the femurs are in this position, the examiner manually applies an axial compressive force to the femurs against a distraction device placed between the femurs along the ventral aspect of the pelvis. This maneuver functions as a fulcrum and forces the femoral heads in an abaxial direction, allowing assessment of coxofemoral joint laxity. The radiographic exposure is obtained during application of the compressive force, termed a distraction view (Fig. 13-22). A distraction index, or a measure of passive laxity, can be calculated by the PennHIP Analysis Center from the distraction view. In addition to the distraction view, PennHIP requires that a ventrodorsal extended-leg and ventrodorsal compression view of the pelvis be submitted with the study.

Another radiographic stress technique for evaluation of coxofemoral joint laxity has been described.[22] This procedure uses patient and pelvic limb positioning that is different from the PennHIP procedure. This dynamic pelvic study does not require certification or a special distraction device. This stress technique requires that the femurs be positioned at 60 degrees to the radiographic table with the stifles adducted and manually pushed in a craniodorsal direction. The application of the craniodorsal force promotes subluxation of the femoral heads in a joint with some degree of laxity.

Another radiographic procedure has been developed to quantify the degree of passive femoral head laxity when the coxofemoral joints are placed in simulated weight-bearing position.[23] The radiographic procedure is called the dorsolateral subluxation method. With this method the anesthetized patient is positioned into a customized foam pad in sternal recumbency with their stifles in contact with the radiographic table. Once positioned appropriately, a dorsoventral pelvic radiograph is obtained.

The radiographic examination of the equine pelvis requires general anesthesia and the use of an x-ray machine with high-output milliampere second capabilities. Ventrodorsal flexed-leg radiographs are the routine views used for assessment of the pelvis. Lateral pelvic radiographs can be obtained in foals and small horses. Horses are commonly placed on a custom-built radiographic table with a cassette tunnel that aids in the alignment of the grid, x-ray cassette, and x-ray tube head. Given the discrepancy in size between radiographic cassettes and the equine pelvis, a sufficient number of overlapping radiographs of the pelvis is required. In an adult horse, five to seven projections, using 14 × 17 inch cassettes, may be necessary.[20] As with small animals, evaluation of symmetric positioning is critical when evaluating the equine pelvis.

Interpretation Paradigm

Regardless of the radiographic technique, ideal patient position is crucial to obtaining pelvic radiographs of diagnostic quality. Without such attention to detail additional unnecessary difficulties will be encountered in determining the presence or absence of early radiographic evidence of canine hip dysplasia, pelvic trauma, or other pelvic pathologic changes. The pelvis of small animals or the horse should be examined as any other radiographic examination, by assessment of symmetry and evaluation of roentgen signs. A routine pattern of examination should be adapted to limit the potential of overlooking important pathologic changes. For example, the examiner could review each hemipelvis in a cranial-to-caudal (sacroiliac joint, ilium, acetabulum, pubis, and ischium) fashion on all radiographs of the study.

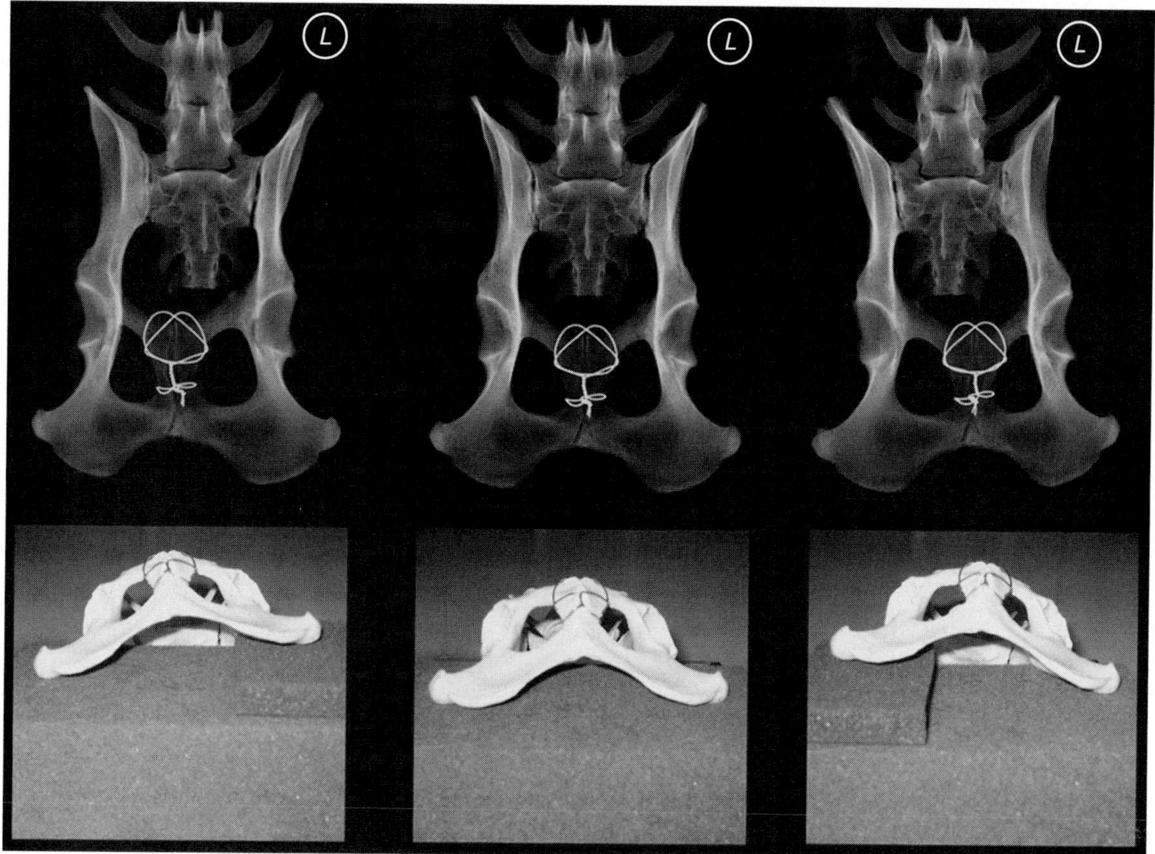

Fig. 13-20 Radiographic positioning of a pelvic anatomy specimen. *Top row,* ventrodorsal pelvic radiographs. *Bottom row,* photographs from a caudal perspective (ischiatic arch and tuberosities are located in the near field of view) of the pelvic anatomy specimen positioned for a ventrodorsal radiograph. The images in the left column demonstrate ventral elevation of the left hemipelvis that results in the obliquity of the radiograph, evidenced by the larger, circular, left obturator foramen. The right column of images demonstrate the appearance of a rotated pelvis in which the right hemipelvis is ventrally elevated. The central images show a correctly positioned pelvic anatomy specimen and the resultant symmetry and oval shape of each obturator foramina.

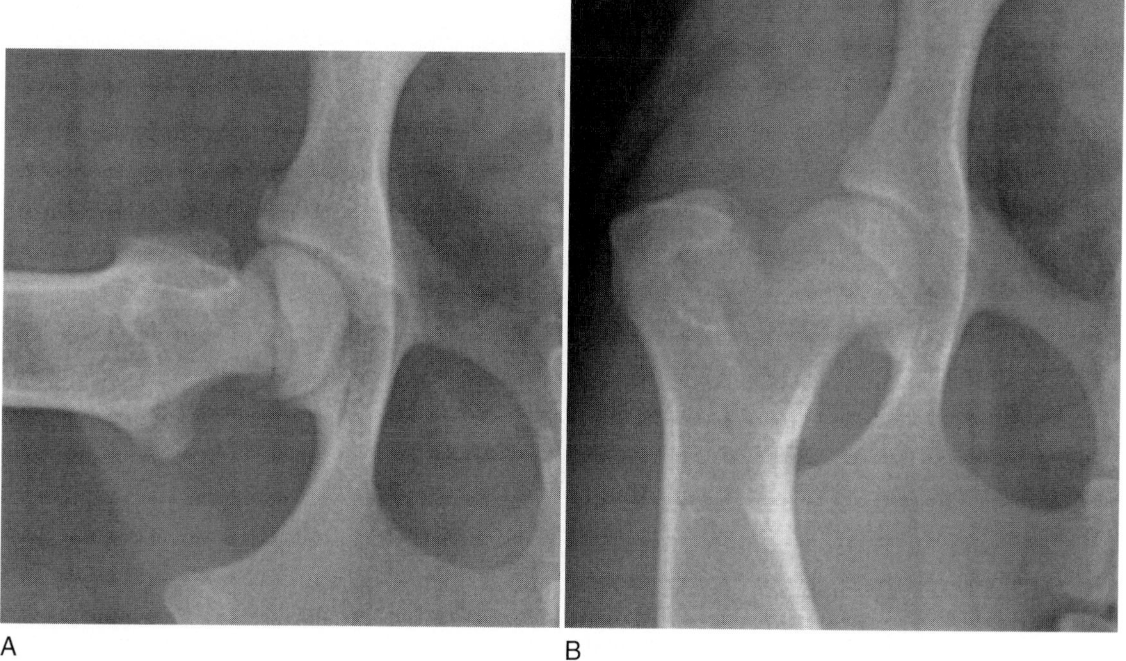

Fig. 13-21 This dog's right capital physeal fracture is more readily identified on the frog-leg ventrodorsal pelvic radiograph (A) than on the extended-leg ventrodorsal pelvic radiograph (B).

In canine hip dysplasia, the subtleties of mildly affected patients can make the early diagnosis of this disease challenging. Only after obtaining diagnostic-quality pelvic radiographs can these early changes of canine hip dysplasia be assessed. Because of the joint capsule tightening encountered on the extended ventrodorsal projection, careful scrutiny must be paid to the congruence between the acetabulum and femoral head (Fig. 13-23). A lack of parallelism between these two structures is the first indication of coxofemoral joint laxity. Ultimately this laxity can progress to femoral head subluxation and the appearance of inadequate acetabular coverage. Given the inherent difficulties of assessing the coxofemoral joints for early incongruency, a distraction view may be applied so that subluxation may be quantified, as with the PennHIP technique (see Fig. 13-23).

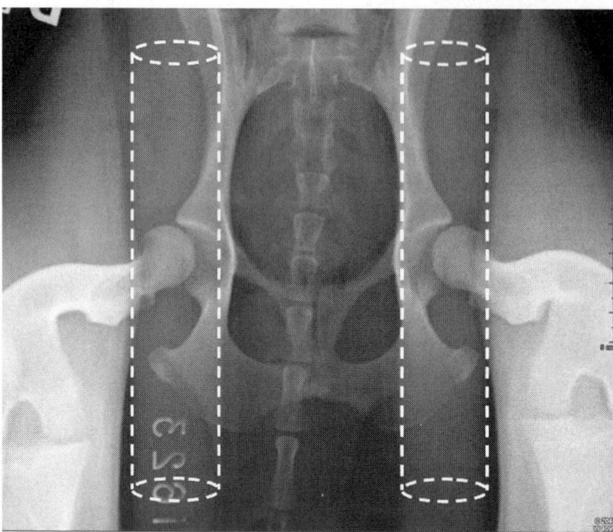

Fig. 13-22 PennHIP radiographic procedure, distraction view. Note the vertically oriented radiopaque rods of the distraction device superimposed over the coxofemoral joints and femoral heads *(dashed lines)*.

The PennHIP distraction radiograph allows for repeated objective assessment of coxofemoral joint laxity. From this distraction radiograph, a distraction index *(DI)* is calculated by the equation DI = d/r, where *d* is the distance between the centers of geometric circles of the acetabulum and femoral head and *r* is the measurement of the radius of the femoral head.[18,24] These measurements are obtained and reported only by the PennHIP Analysis Center, which provides a comparative analysis of a submitted individual patient to that of an establish breed-specific distraction index score. In general, a lower distraction index correlates with less coxofemoral joint laxity and lesser probability of developing degenerative joint disease from hip dysplasia. The PennHIP analysis also allows for assessment of patients from 4 months of age. The stressed pelvic radiographic technique allows the examiner to perform a maneuver similar to the first part of an Ortolani test. The induced joint luxation, if present, is measured to obtain a subluxation index. The subluxation index is calculated in the same manner that the PennHIP distraction index is derived. The normal subluxation index values for the canine have been published as 0.3, where a subluxation index value of greater than 0.5 has been shown to correlate with canine hip dysplasia 95% of the time.[22]

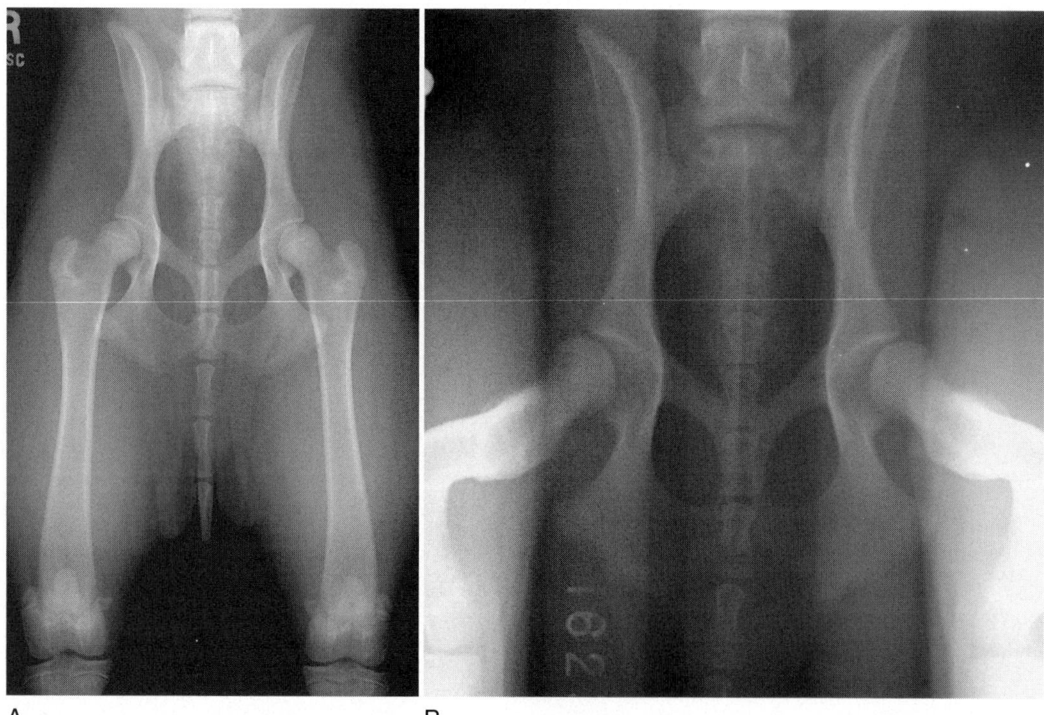

Fig. 13-23 Mild bilateral coxofemoral joint incongruity is noted on the extended-leg ventrodorsal pelvic radiograph of this 8-month-old Golden Retriever **(A)**. This subtle change is important to detect because it is the early radiographic finding of hip dysplasia. A PennHIP radiographic series was performed on this dog, and from the distraction view **(B)**, distraction index measurements of 0.58 and 0.50 were determined for the right and left coxofemoral joints, respectively. These measurements, when compared with other Golden Retrievers, placed this dog in the 40th percentile, with 60% of Golden Retrievers having "tighter" hips.

SUMMARY

Small animal musculoskeletal radiography presents a challenge to the reviewer in that overlap exists in the radiographic appearance of a variety of diseases. An adequate physical examination with sufficient lameness localization allows more accurate radiographic assessment of specific joints and/or areas rather than general limb surveys that are of nondiagnostic quality. Technical considerations include the use of orthogonal views (with or without oblique radiographs), a detail film-screen combination, and a low kilovoltage peak and relatively high milliampere second technique. Comparison of possible radiographic abnormalities with radiographs of the opposite limb and/or anatomy references, such as those included in this text, can be important for accurate assessment of roentgen abnormalities. Characterization of lesion location, number of bones involved, involvement of a joint, and the spectrum of lytic and productive bone features of aggressive or benign bone disease can lead to formulation of a specific primary differential diagnostic consideration or a list of differentials. By using the mnemonic of the ABCs, the reviewer should evaluate all aspects of the bones and soft tissues on the radiographs.

REFERENCES

1. deKleer VS: Development of bone. In Sumner-Smith G, editor: *Bone in clinical orthopedics: a study in comparative osteology,* Philadelphia, 1982, WB Saunders, p 1-80.
2. Olsson SE: Morphology and physiology of the growth cartilage under normal and pathologic conditions. In Sumner-Smith G, editor: *Bone in clinical orthopedics: a study in comparative osteology,* Philadelphia, 1982, WB Saunders, pp 159-196.
3. Capen CC, Weisbrode SE: Hormonal control of mineral metabolism and bone cell activity. In Sumner-Smith G, editor: *Bone in clinical orthopedics: a study in comparative osteology,* Philadelphia, 1982, WB Saunders, pp 197-252.
4. Rosenberg A: Bones, joints and soft tissue tumors. In Cotran RS, Kumar V, Collins T, editors: *Robbins pathologic basis of disease,* ed 6, Philadelphia, 1999, WB Saunders, pp 1215-1268.
5. Lanyon LE: Mechanical function and bone remodeling. In: Sumner-Smith G. *Bone in clinical orthopedics: a study in comparative osteology,* Philadelphia, 1982, WB Saunders, pp 305-334.
6. Pennock PW: Radiologic interpretation of bone. In: Sumner-Smith G, editor: *Bone in clinical orthopedics: a study in comparative osteology,* Philadelphia, 1982, WB Saunders, pp 253-260.
7. Grandage J: Interpretation of bone radiographs: some hazards for the unwary, *Aust Vet J* 52:305, 1976.
8. Campbell JR: Radiology of the epiphysis, *J Am Vet Radiol Soc* 9:11, 1968.
9. Riser WH: Radiographic differential diagnosis of skeletal diseases of young dogs, *J Am Vet Radiol Soc* 5:15, 1964.
10. Buckley JC: Pathophysiologic considerations of osteopenia, *Compend Contin Educ Small Anim Pract* 6:552, 1984.
11. Losonsky JM, Kneller SK: Misdiagnosis in normal radiographic anatomy: eight structural configurations simulating disease entities in dogs and cats, *J Am Vet Med Assoc* 191:109, 1987.
12. Konde L: Interpretation of aggressive musculoskeletal lesions. In Thrall DE, editor: *Textbook of veterinary radiology,* ed 3, Philadelphia, 1997, WB Saunders.
13. Thrall DE: Infection versus neoplasia of bones. In Thrall DE, editor: *Textbook of veterinary radiology,* ed 3, Philadelphia, 1997, WB Saunders.
14. Goedegebuure SA: Secondary bone tumors in the dog, *Vet Pathol* 16:520, 1979.
15. Rogers KS, Janovitz EB, Fooshee SK et al: Lymphosarcoma with disseminated skeletal involvement in a pup, *J Am Vet Med Assoc* 95:1242, 1989.
16. Hahn KA, Matlock CL: Nasal adenocarcinoma metastatic to bone in two dogs, *J Am Vet Med Assoc* 197:491, 1990.
17. Susaneck SJ, Macy DW: Hypertrophic osteodystrophy, *Compend Contin Educ Small Anim Pract* 4:689, 1982.
18. Smith GK, Beiry DN, Gregor TP: New concepts of coxofemoral joint stability and the development of a clinical stress-radiographic method for quantitating hip joint laxity in the dog, *J Am Vet Med Assoc* 196:59, 1990.
19. Rendano VT, Ryan G: Canine hip dysplasia evaluation: a positioning and labeling guide for radiographs to be submitted to the orthopedic foundation for animals, *Vet Radiol* 26:170, 1985.
20. Morgan JP: *Techniques of veterinary radiography,* ed 5, Ames, IA, 1993, Iowa State University.
21. Crawford JT, Manley PA, Adams WM: Comparison of computed tomography, tangential view radiography, and conventional radiography in evaluation of canine pelvic trauma. *Vet Radiol Ultrasound* 44:619, 2003.
22. Flückiger MA, Friedrich GA, Binder H: A radiographic stress technique for evaluation of coxofemoral joint laxity in dogs, *Vet Surg* 28:1, 1999.
23. Farese JP, Todhunter RJ, Lust G et al: Dorsolateral subluxation of hip joints in dogs measured in a weight-bearing position with radiography and computed tomography, *Vet Surg* 27:393, 1998.
24. Smith GK, Gregor TP, Rhodes H et al: Coxofemoral joint laxity from distraction radiography and its contemporaneous and prospective correlation with laxity, subjective score and evidence of degenerative joint disease from conventional hip-extended radiography in dogs, *Am J Vet Res* 54:1021, 1993.

ELECTRONIC RESOURCES evolve

Additional information related to the content in Chapter 13 can be found on the companion Web site at evolve http://evolve.elsevier.com/Thrall/vetrad/

- Key Points
- Chapter Quiz

CHAPTER • 14
Radiographic Anatomy of the Appendicular Skeleton

James E. Smallwood
Kathy A. Spaulding

To use the roentgen sign method of recognizing abnormal radiographic findings effectively, an understanding of normal radiographic anatomy for the specific area of interest is necessary. The purpose of this chapter is to provide a limited reference for the radiographic anatomy of the appendicular skeleton. Refer to comprehensive textbooks on radiographic anatomy for more detailed information.[1,2]

The radiographic nomenclature used in this chapter was approved by the American College of Veterinary Radiology in 1983.[3] Some equine images in this chapter (Figs. 14-30 through 14-49 and 14-54 through 14-57) have been taken from previous publications and are reproduced here with permission of the journals and author.[4-6]

REFERENCES

1. Waibl H, Mayrhofer, E, Matis U et al: *Atlas of radiographic anatomy of the dog,* Stuttgart, 2005, Parey Verlag.
2. Schebitz H, Wilkens H: *Atlas of radiographic anatomy of the horse,* ed 3, Philadelphia, 1978, W.B. Saunders.
3. Smallwood JE, Shively MJ, Rendano VT et al: A standardized nomenclature for radiographic projections used in veterinary medicine, *Vet Radiol* 26:2, 1985.
4. Smallwood JE, Shively MJ: Radiographic and xeroradiographic anatomy of the equine carpus, *Equine Pract* 1:22, 1979.
5. Smallwood JE, Holladay SD: Xeroradiographic anatomy of the equine digit and metacarpophalangeal region, *Vet Radiol* 28:166, 1987.
6. Shively MJ, Smallwood JE: Radiographic and xeroradiographic anatomy of the equine tarsus, *Equine Pract* 2:19, 1980.

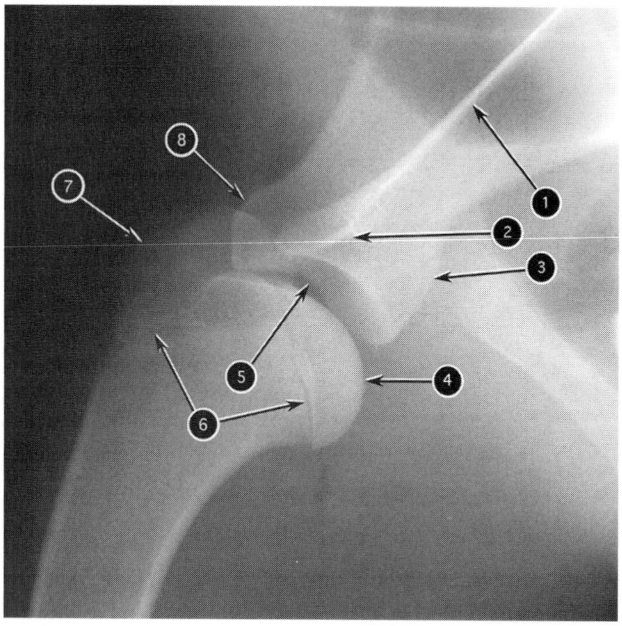

Fig. 14-1 Mediolateral Radiograph of Canine Shoulder Joint.
1. Spine of scapula
2. Acromion of scapula
3. Infraglenoid tubercle of scapula
4. Head of humerus
5. Glenoid cavity of scapula
6. Proximal physis of humerus
7. Greater tubercle of humerus
8. Supraglenoid tubercle of scapula

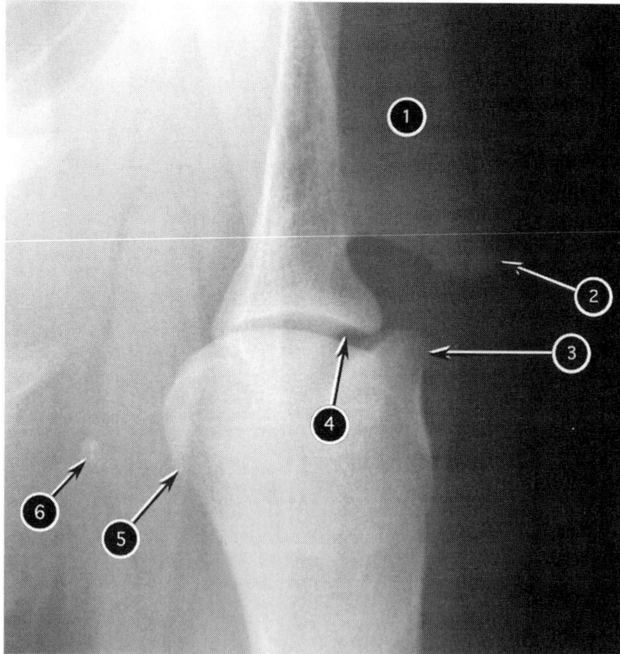

Fig. 14-2 Caudocranial Radiograph of Canine Shoulder Joint.
1. Spine of scapula
2. Acromion of scapula
3. Greater tubercle of humerus
4. Humeral (scapulohumeral) joint
5. Lesser tubercle of humerus
6. Clavicle

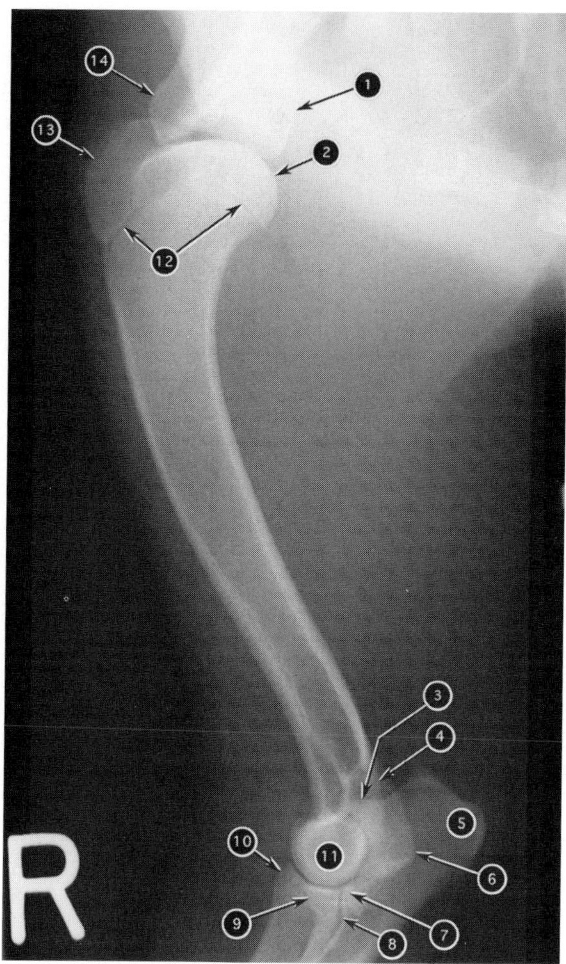

Fig. 14-3 Mediolateral Radiograph of Canine Humerus.

1. Infraglenoid tubercle of scapula
2. Head of humerus
3. Anconeal process of ulna
4. Lateral epicondyle of humerus
5. Tuber olecrani
6. Medial epicondyle of humerus
7. Lateral coronoid process of ulna
8. Proximal radioulnar joint
9. Medial coronoid process of ulna
10. Head of radius
11. Condyle of humerus
12. Proximal physis of humerus
13. Greater tubercle of humerus
14. Supraglenoid tubercle of scapula

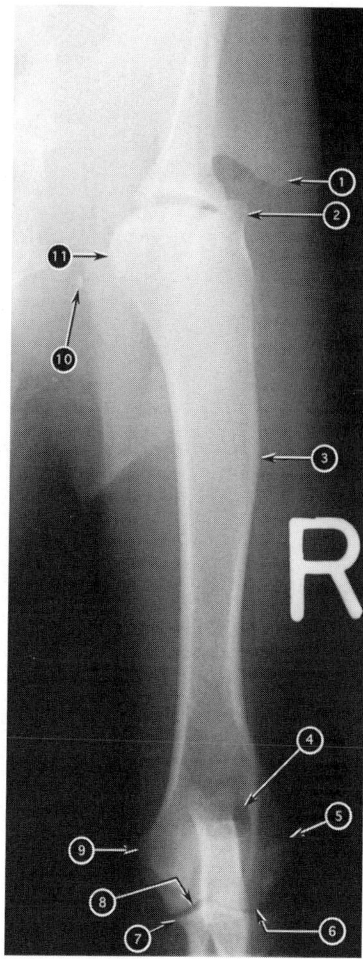

Fig. 14-4 Caudocranial Radiograph of Canine Humerus.

1. Acromion of scapula
2. Greater tubercle of humerus
3. Deltoid tuberosity
4. Supratrochlear foramen of humerus
5. Lateral epicondyle of humerus
6. Capitulum of humeral condyle
7. Medial coronoid process of ulna
8. Trochlea of humeral condyle
9. Medial epicondyle of humerus
10. Clavicle
11. Lesser tubercle of humerus

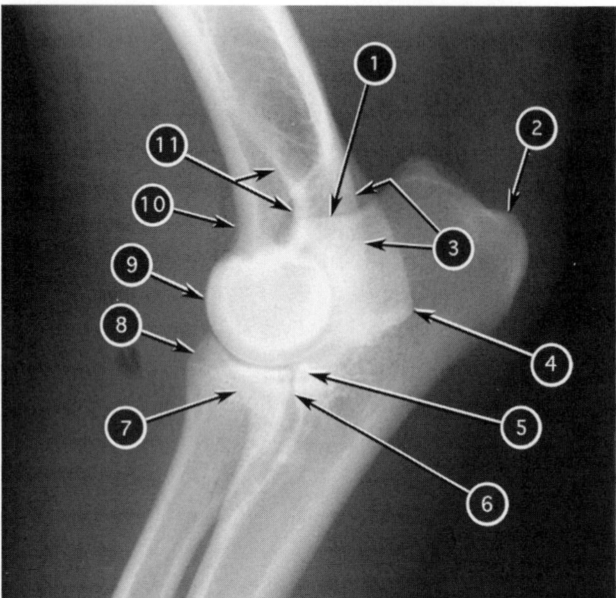

Fig. 14-5 Mediolateral Radiograph of Canine Elbow Joint.
1. Anconeal process of ulna
2. Tuber olecrani of ulna
3. Caudal border of lateral epicondyle of humerus
4. Caudal border of medial epicondyle of humerus
5. Lateral coronoid process of ulna
6. Proximal radioulnar joint
7. Medial coronoid process of ulna
8. Head of radius
9. Condyle of humerus
10. Cranial border of medial epicondyle of humerus
11. Cranial border of lateral epicondyle of humerus

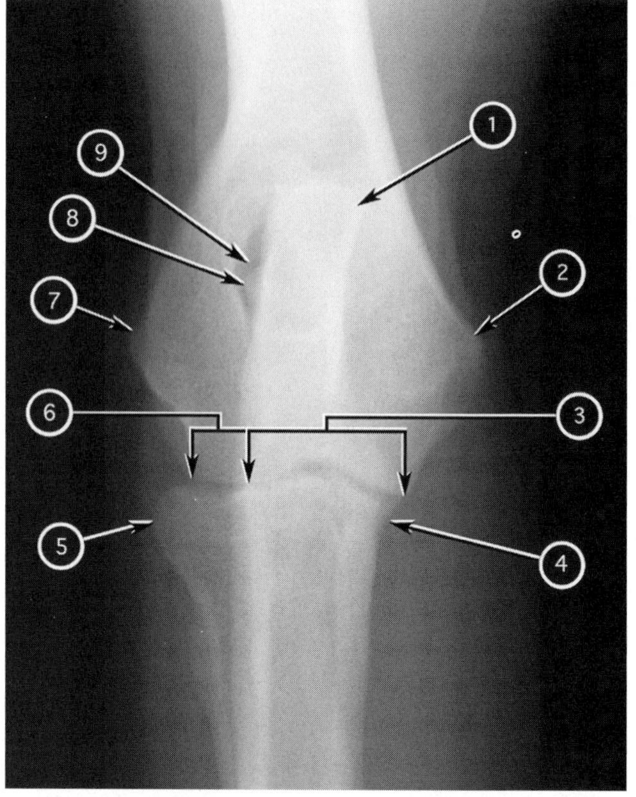

Fig. 14-7 Craniocaudal Radiograph of Canine Elbow Joint.
1. Tuber olecrani of ulna
2. Medial epicondyle of humerus
3. Trochlea of humeral condyle
4. Medial coronoid process of ulna
5. Head of radius
6. Capitulum of humeral condyle
7. Lateral epicondyle of humerus
8. Anconeal process of ulna
9. Supratrochlear foramen of humerus

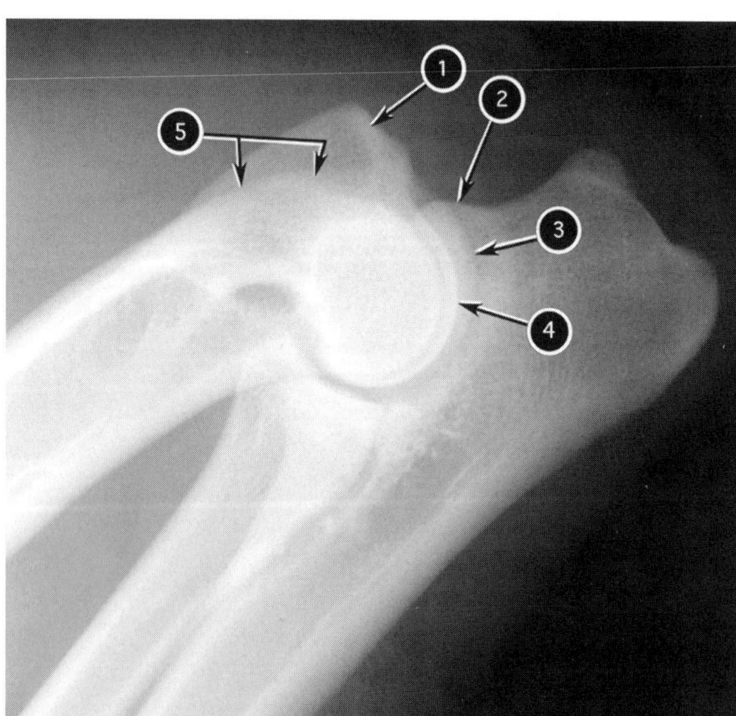

Fig. 14-6 Mediolateral Radiograph of Flexed Canine Elbow Joint.
1. Medial epicondyle of humerus
2. Anconeal process of ulna
3. Medial part of humeral condyle
4. Lateral part of humeral condyle
5. Caudal border of lateral epicondyle of humerus

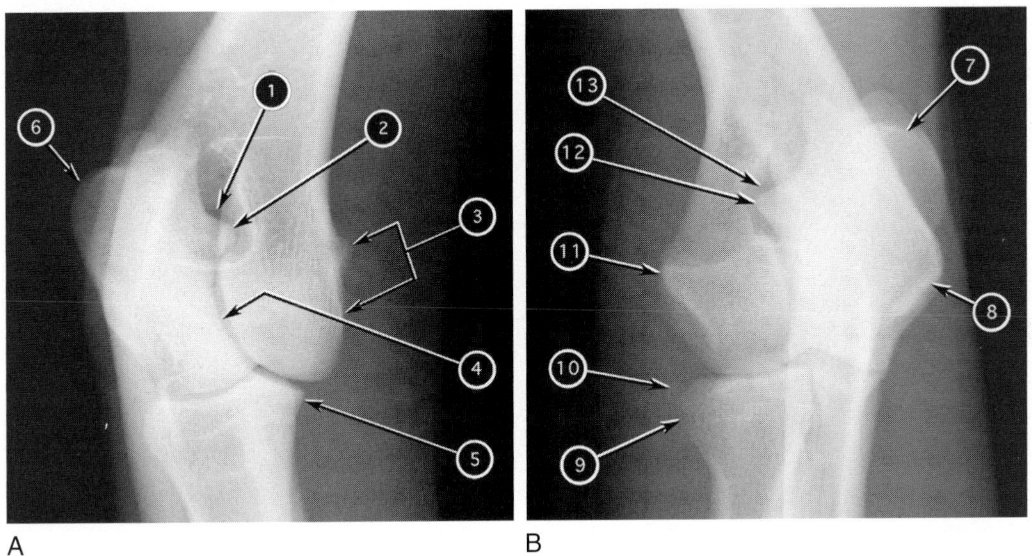

Fig. 14-8 Craniolateral-Caudomedial Oblique (A) and Craniomedial-Caudolateral Oblique (B) Radiographs of Canine Elbow Joint.

1. Supratrochlear foramen of humerus
2. Anconeal process of ulna
3. Medial epicondyle of humerus
4. Trochlear notch of ulna
5. Medial coronoid process of ulna
6. Tuber olecrani of ulna
7. Tuber olecrani of ulna
8. Medial epicondyle of humerus
9. Head of radius
10. Sesamoid bone of supinator muscle (inconstant)
11. Lateral epicondyle of humerus
12. Anconeal process of ulna
13. Supratrochlear foramen of humerus

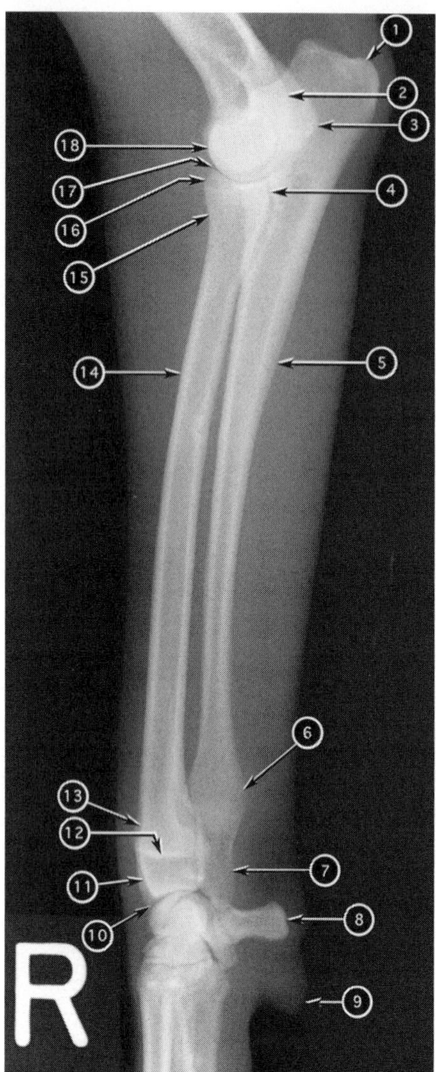

Fig. 14-9 Mediolateral Radiograph of Canine Antebrachium.

1. Tuber olecrani of ulna
2. Lateral epicondyle of humerus
3. Medial epicondyle of humerus
4. Proximal radioulnar joint
5. Body of ulna
6. Distal metaphysis of ulna
7. Distal epiphysis of ulna
8. Accessory carpal bone
9. Carpal pad
10. Antebrachiocarpal joint
11. Distal epiphysis of radius
12. Distal physis of radius
13. Distal metaphysis of radius
14. Body of radius
15. Neck of radius
16. Head of radius
17. Elbow (cubital) joint
18. Condyle of humerus

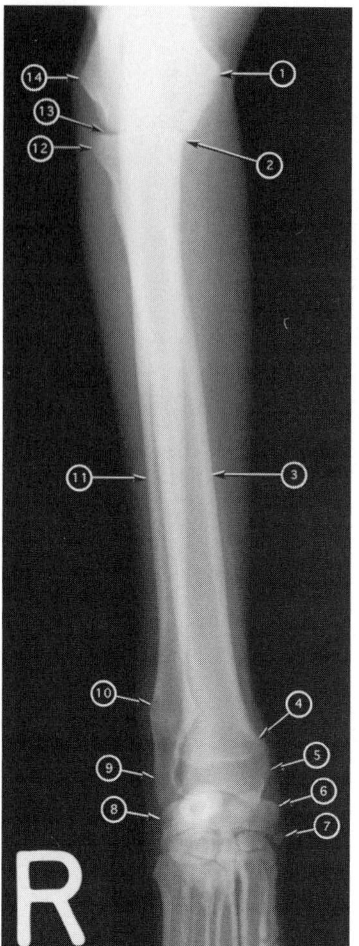

Fig. 14-10 Craniocaudal Radiograph of Canine Antebrachium.

1. Medial epicondyle of humerus
2. Medial coronoid process of ulna
3. Body of radius
4. Distal metaphysis of radius
5. Distal epiphysis of radius
6. Intermedioradial carpal bone
7. Sesamoid bone of abductor pollicis longus
8. Ulnar carpal bone
9. Distal epiphysis (styloid process) of ulna
10. Distal metaphysis of ulna
11. Body of ulna
12. Head of radius
13. Elbow (cubital) joint
14. Lateral epicondyle of humerus

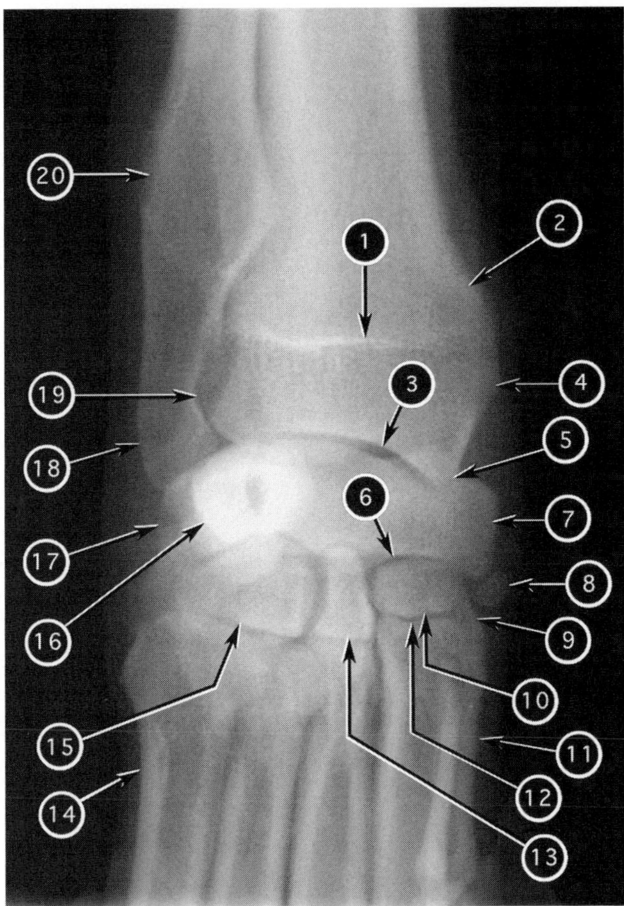

Fig. 14-11 Dorsopalmar Radiograph of Canine Carpus.

1. Distal physis of radius
2. Distal metaphysis of radius
3. Antebrachiocarpal joint
4. Distal epiphysis of radius
5. Styloid process (medial) of radius
6. Middle carpal joint
7. Intermedioradial carpal bone
8. Sesamoid bone of abductor pollicis longus
9. First carpal bone (C1)
10. Second carpal bone (C2)
11. First metacarpal bone (Mc1)
12. Carpometacarpal joint
13. Third carpal bone (C3)
14. Fifth metacarpal bone (Mc5)
15. Fourth carpal bone (C4)
16. Accessory carpal bone
17. Ulnar carpal bone
18. Distal epiphysis (styloid process) of ulna
19. Distal radioulnar joint
20. Distal metaphysis of ulna

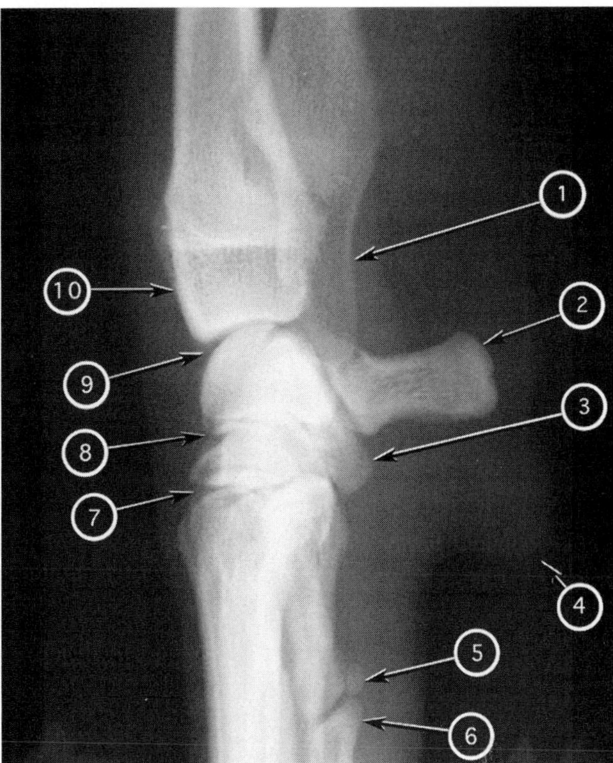

Fig. 14-12 Mediolateral Radiograph of Canine Carpus.

1. Distal epiphysis (styloid process) of ulna
2. Accessory carpal bone
3. Ulnar carpal bone
4. Carpal pad
5. Proximal sesamoid bone of first digit
6. Proximal phalanx (Pp) of first digit
7. Carpometacarpal joint
8. Middle carpal joint
9. Antebrachiocarpal joint
10. Distal epiphysis of radius

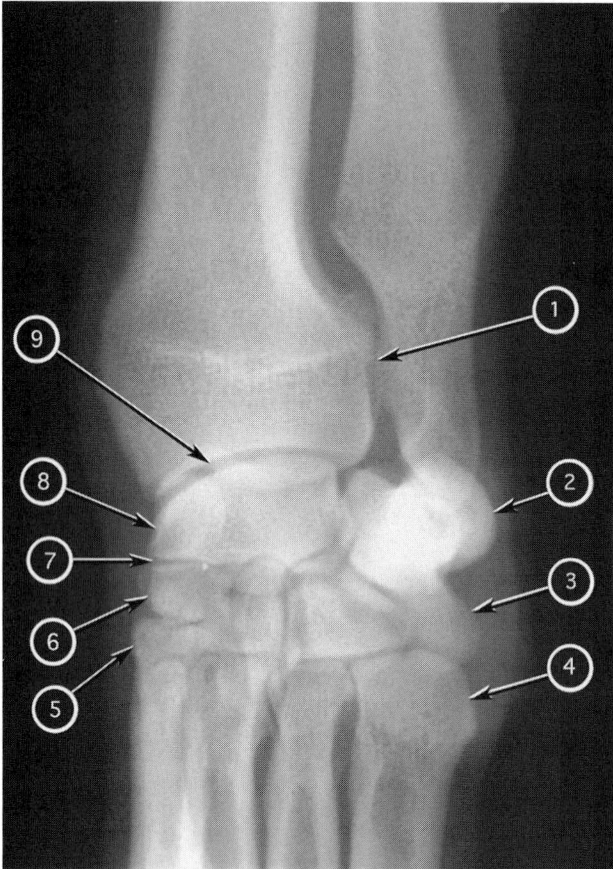

Fig. 14-13 Dorsolateral-Palmaromedial Oblique Radiograph of Canine Manus.

1. Distal radioulnar joint
2. Accessory carpal bone
3. Ulnar carpal bone
4. Base of Mc5
5. C1
6. C2
7. Middle carpal joint
8. Intermedioradial carpal bone
9. Antebrachiocarpal joint

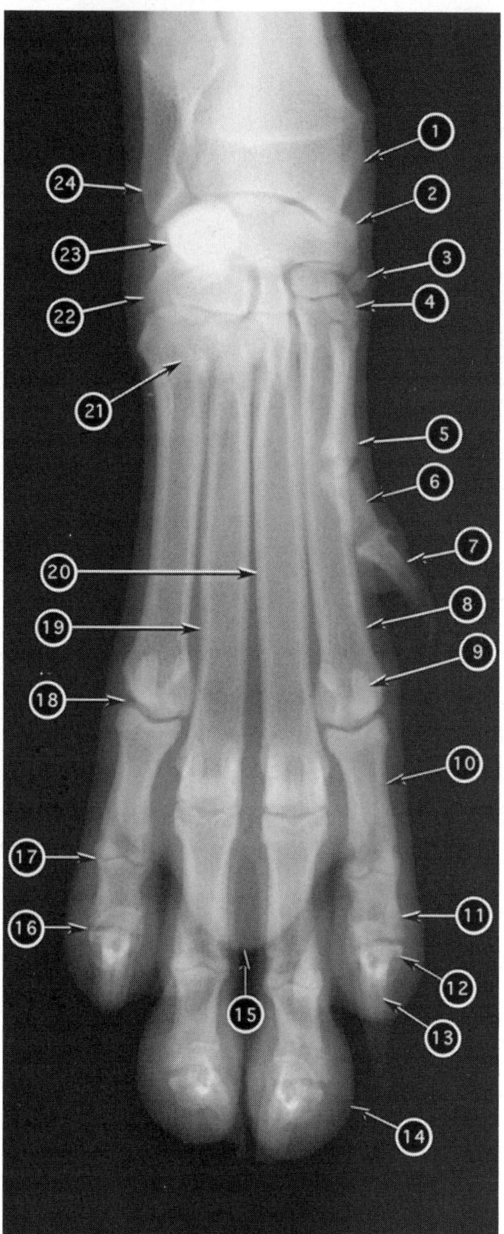

Fig. 14-14 Dorsopalmar Radiograph of Canine Manus.

1. Distal epiphysis of radius
2. Intermedioradial carpal bone
3. Sesamoid bone of abductor pollicis longus
4. C1
5. Mc1
6. Pp of digit 1
7. Distal phalanx (Pd) of digit 1
8. Mc2
9. Abaxial proximal sesamoid bone of digit 2
10. Pp of digit 2
11. Middle phalanx (Pm) of digit 2
12. Unguicular crest of Pd of digit 2
13. Unguicular process of Pd of digit 2
14. Digital pad of digit 3
15. Metacarpal pad
16. Distal interphalangeal joint (DIJ) of digit 5
17. Proximal interphalangeal joint (PIJ) of digit 5
18. Metacarpophalangeal joint of digit 5
19. Mc4
20. Mc3
21. Carpal pad
22. Ulnar carpal bone
23. Accessory carpal bone
24. Distal epiphysis (styloid process) of ulna

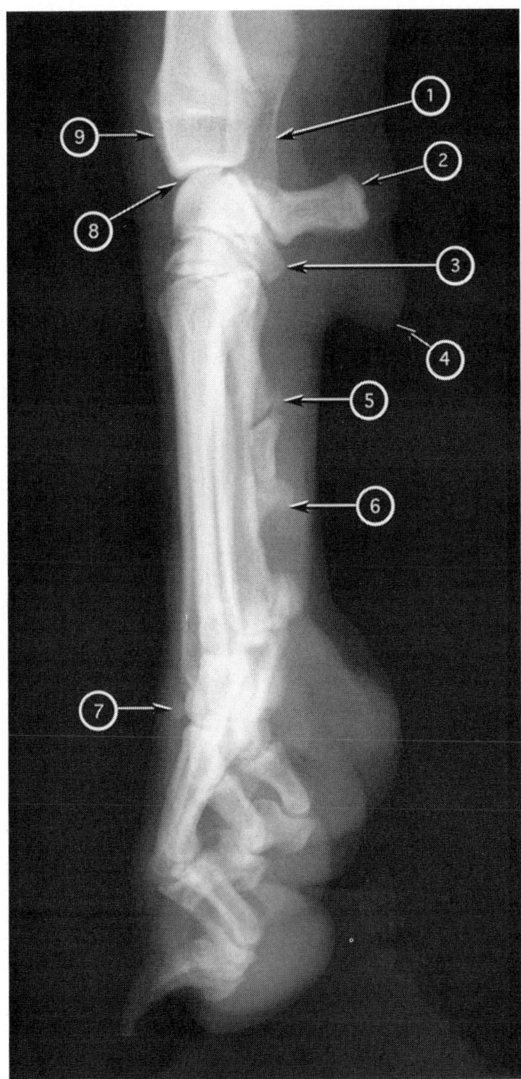

Fig. 14-15 Mediolateral Radiograph of Canine Manus.
1. Distal epiphysis (styloid process) of ulna
2. Accessory carpal bone
3. Ulnar carpal bone
4. Carpal pad
5. Proximal sesamoid bone of digit 1
6. Pd of digit 1
7. Dorsal sesamoid bone
8. Antebrachiocarpal joint
9. Distal epiphysis of radius

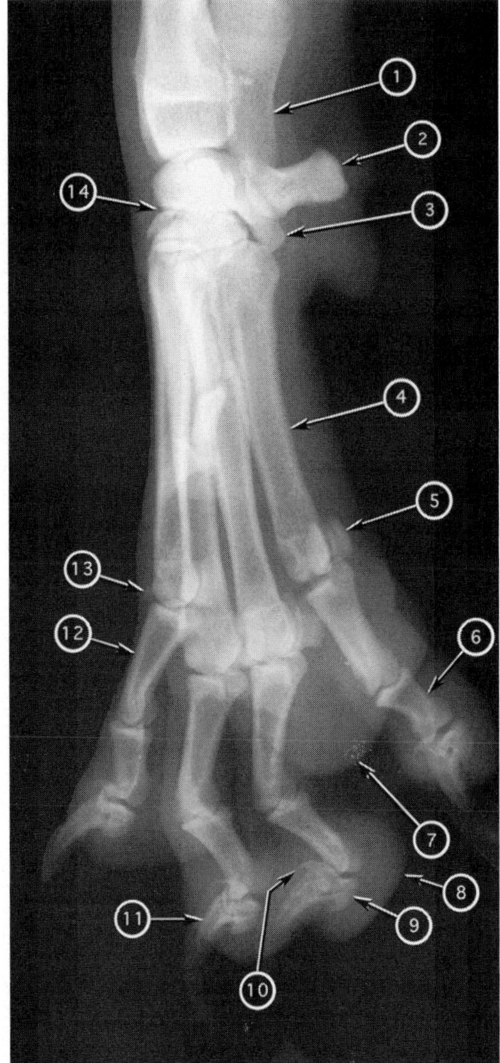

Fig. 14-16 Palmaromedial-Dorsolateral Oblique Radiograph of Canine Manus.
1. Distal epiphysis (styloid process) of ulna
2. Accessory carpal bone
3. Ulnar carpal bone
4. Body of Mc5
5. Abaxial proximal sesamoid bone of digit 5
6. Pm of digit 5
7. Metacarpal pad
8. Digital pad of digit 4
9. Flexor tubercle of Pd of digit 4
10. Unguicular crest of Pd of digit 4
11. Unguicular process of Pd of digit 3
12. Pp of digit 2
13. Dorsal sesamoid bone of digit 2
14. Middle carpal joint

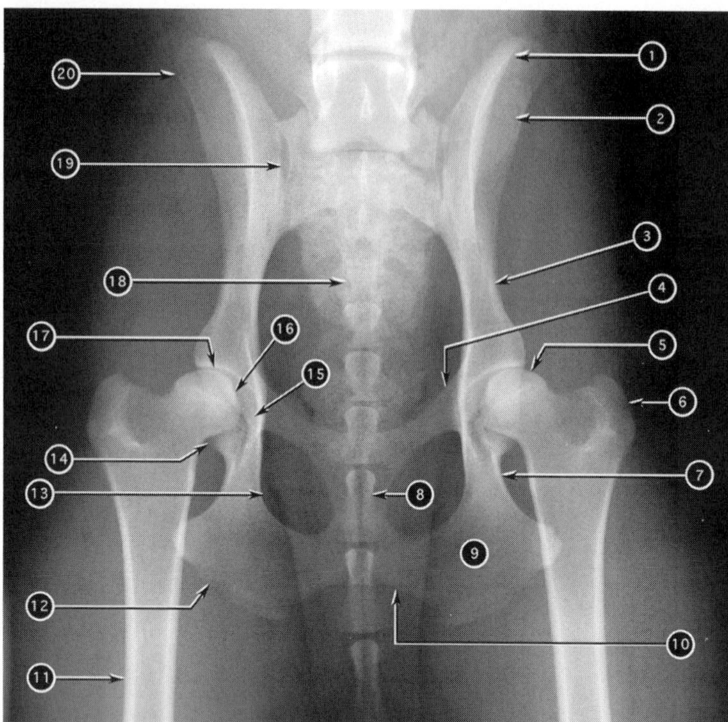

Fig. 14-17 Ventrodorsal Radiograph of Canine Pelvis.
1. Crest of left ilium
2. Wing of left ilium
3. Body of left ilium
4. Body of left pubis
5. Head of left femur
6. Greater trochanter of left femur
7. Body of left ischium
8. Caudal vertebra 4
9. Table of left ischium
10. Ischial arch
11. Body of right femur
12. Right tuber ischiadicum (ischiatic tuberosity)
13. Right obturator foramen
14. Caudodorsal aspect of lunate surface of acetabulum
15. Acetabular fossa
16. Fovea capitis of right femur
17. Cranioventral aspect of lunate surface of acetabulum
18. Sacral vertebra 3
19. Right sacroiliac joint
20. Right tuber coxae (cranioventral iliac spine)

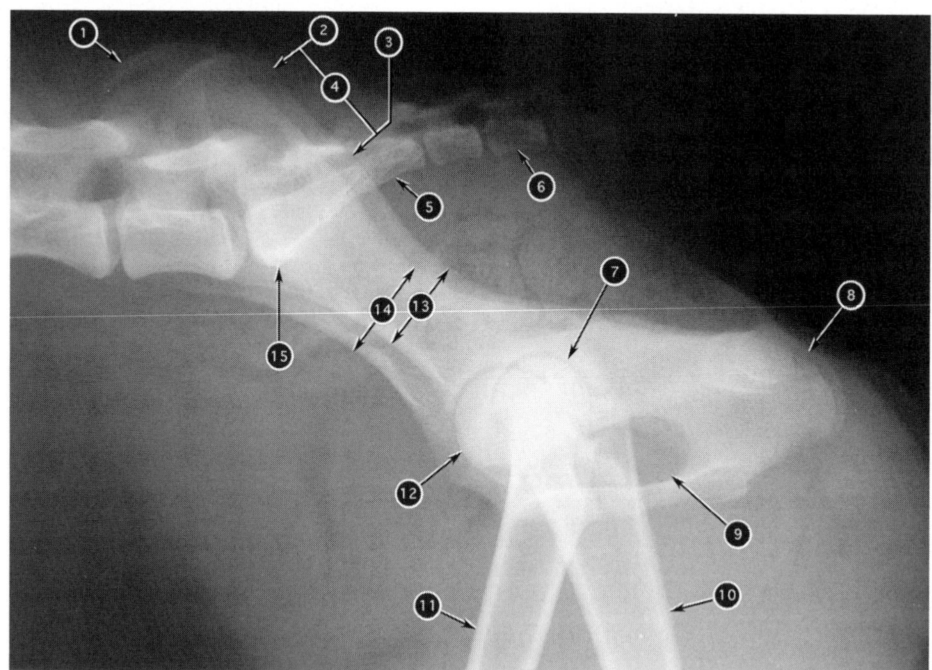

Fig. 14-18 Right-Left Lateral Radiograph of Canine Pelvis.
1. Crest of right ilium (more magnified)
2. Craniodorsal iliac spine
3. Caudodorsal iliac spine
4. Left tuber sacrale (less magnified)
5. Sacral vertebra 3
6. Caudal vertebra 2
7. Left coxal joint (less magnified)
8. Superimposed right and left tubera ischiadica
9. Superimposed right and left obturator foramina
10. Body of right femur (more magnified)
11. Body of left femur (less magnified)
12. Head of right femur (more magnified)
13. Body of left ilium (less magnified)
14. Body of right ilium (more magnified)
15. Promontory of sacrum

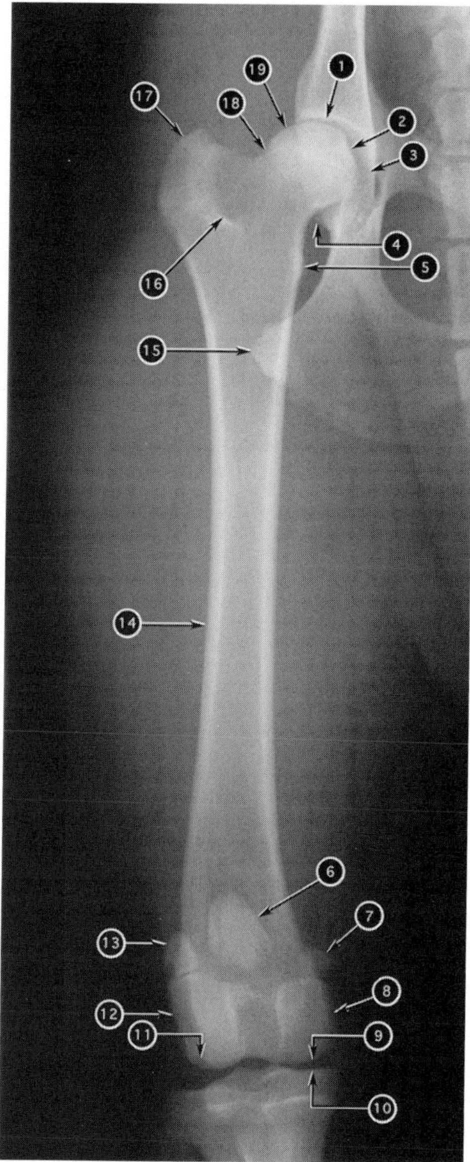

Fig. 14-19 Craniocaudal Radiograph of Canine Femur.
1. Cranioventral aspect of lunate surface of acetabulum
2. Fovea capitis of femur
3. Acetabular fossa
4. Caudodorsal aspect of lunate surface of acetabulum
5. Lesser trochanter of femur
6. Patella
7. Medial sesamoid of gastrocnemius muscle
8. Medial epicondyle of femur
9. Medial condyle of femur
10. Medial condyle of tibia
11. Extensor fossa of femur
12. Lateral epicondyle of femur
13. Lateral sesamoid of gastrocnemius muscle
14. Body of femur
15. Tuber ischiadicum
16. Trochanteric fossa of femur
17. Greater trochanter of femur
18. Neck of femur
19. Head of femur

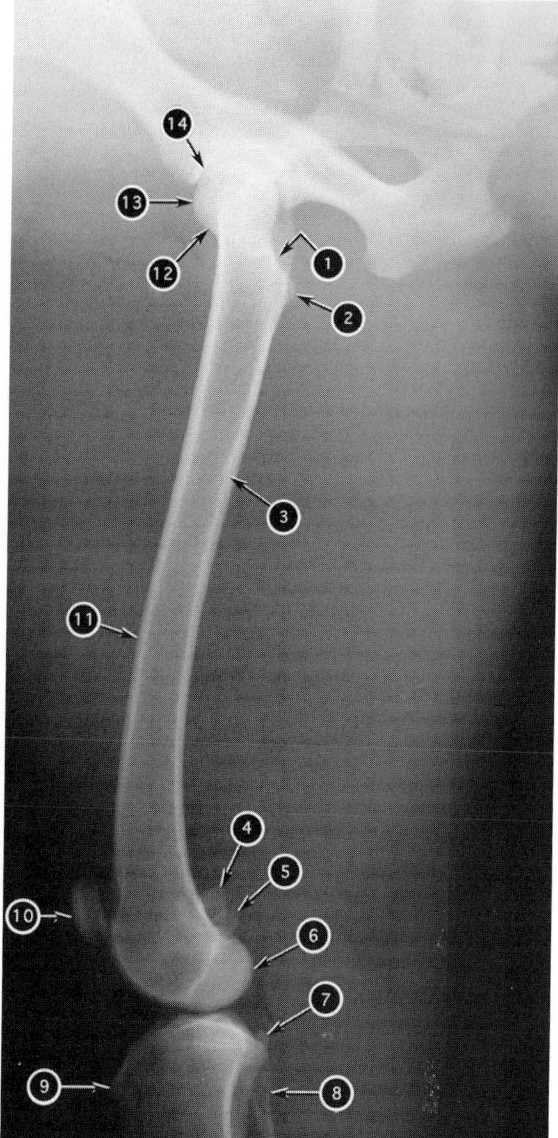

Fig. 14-20 Mediolateral Radiograph of Canine Femur.
1. Trochanteric fossa of femur
2. Lesser trochanter of femur
3. Nutrient canal of femur
4. Lateral sesamoid of gastrocnemius muscle
5. Medial sesamoid of gastrocnemius muscle
6. Medial and lateral condyles of femur
7. Sesamoid bone of popliteus muscle
8. Fibula
9. Tibial tuberosity
10. Patella
11. Body of femur
12. Neck of femur
13. Head of femur
14. Craniodorsal aspect of lunate surface of acetabulum

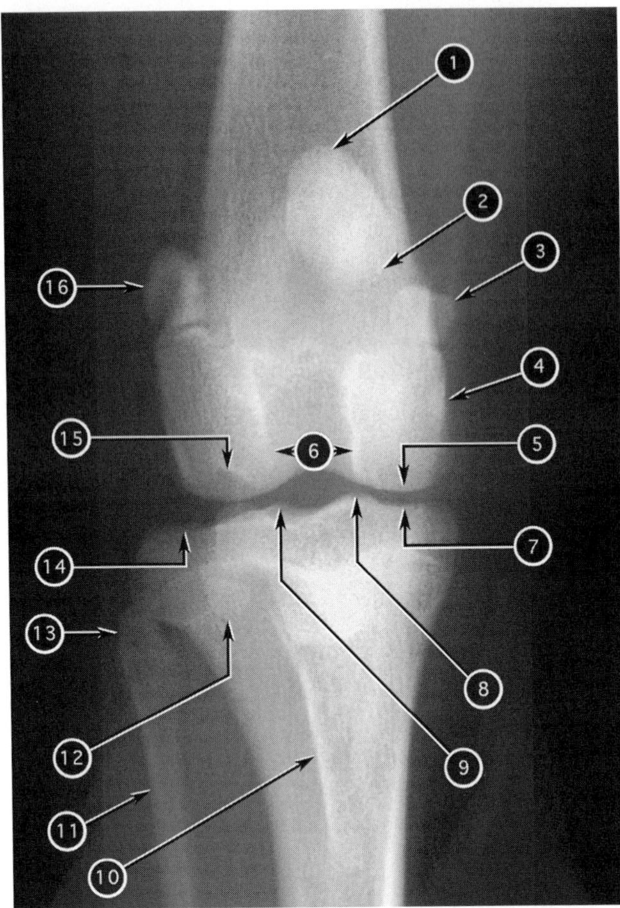

Fig. 14-21 Craniocaudal Radiograph of Canine Stifle Joint.
1. Base of patella
2. Apex of patella
3. Medial sesamoid of gastrocnemius muscle
4. Medial epicondyle of femur
5. Medial condyle of femur
6. Intercondylar fossa of femur
7. Medial condyle of tibia
8. Medial tubercle of intercondylar eminence
9. Lateral tubercle of intercondylar eminence
10. Cranial border of tibia
11. Body of fibula
12. Sesamoid bone of popliteus muscle
13. Head of fibula
14. Lateral condyle of tibia
15. Extensor fossa of femur
16. Lateral sesamoid of gastrocnemius

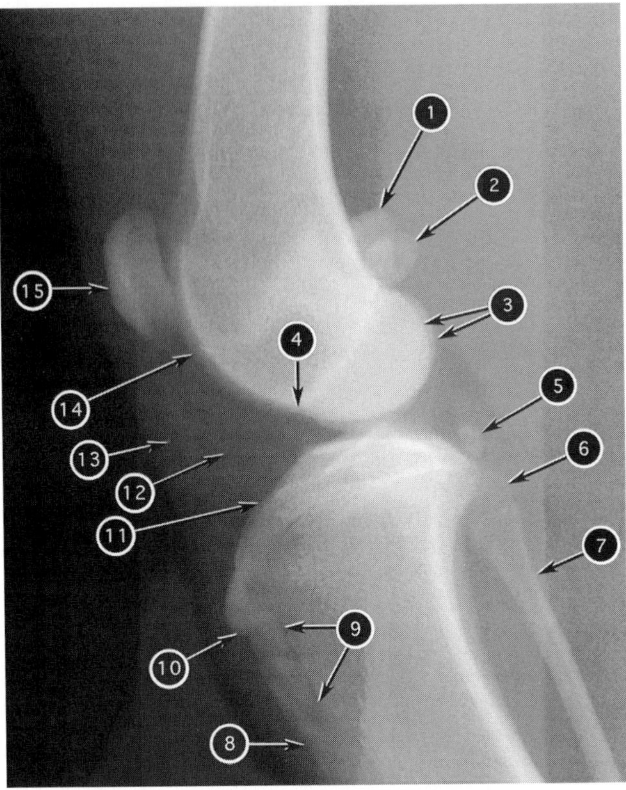

Fig. 14-22 Mediolateral Radiograph of Canine Stifle Joint.
1. Lateral sesamoid of gastrocnemius muscle
2. Medial sesamoid of gastrocnemius muscle
3. Medial and lateral condyles of femur
4. Extensor fossa of femur
5. Sesamoid bone of popliteus muscle
6. Head of fibula
7. Body of fibula
8. Cranial border of tibia
9. Cartilage between tibial tuberosity and body of tibia
10. Tibial tuberosity
11. Cranial intercondylar area of tibia
12. Infrapatellar fat body
13. Patellar ligament
14. Superimposed ridges of femoral trochlea
15. Patella

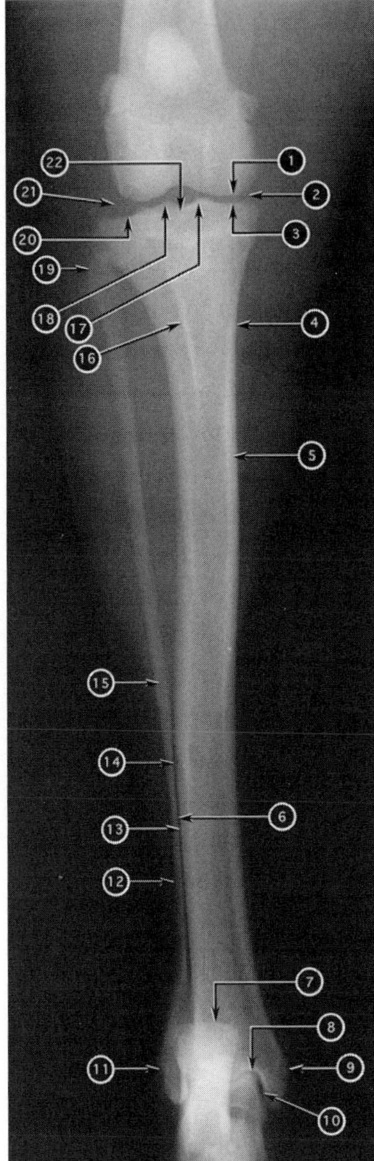

Fig. 14-23 Craniocaudal Radiograph of Canine Crus.
1. Medial condyle of femur
2. Medial meniscus
3. Medial condyle of tibia
4. Medial border of tibia
5. Body of tibia
6. Medial surface of fibula (faces tibia)
7. Tuber calcanei
8. Medial groove of tibial cochlea
9. Medial malleolus of tibia
10. Medial aspect of tarsocrural joint
11. Lateral malleolus of fibula
12. Lateral surface of fibula
13. Lateral border of tibia (faces fibula)
14. Interosseous membrane
15. Body of fibula
16. Cranial border of tibia
17. Medial tubercle of intercondylar eminence
18. Lateral tubercle of intercondylar eminence
19. Head of fibula
20. Lateral condyle of tibia
21. Lateral meniscus
22. Central intercondylar area of tibia

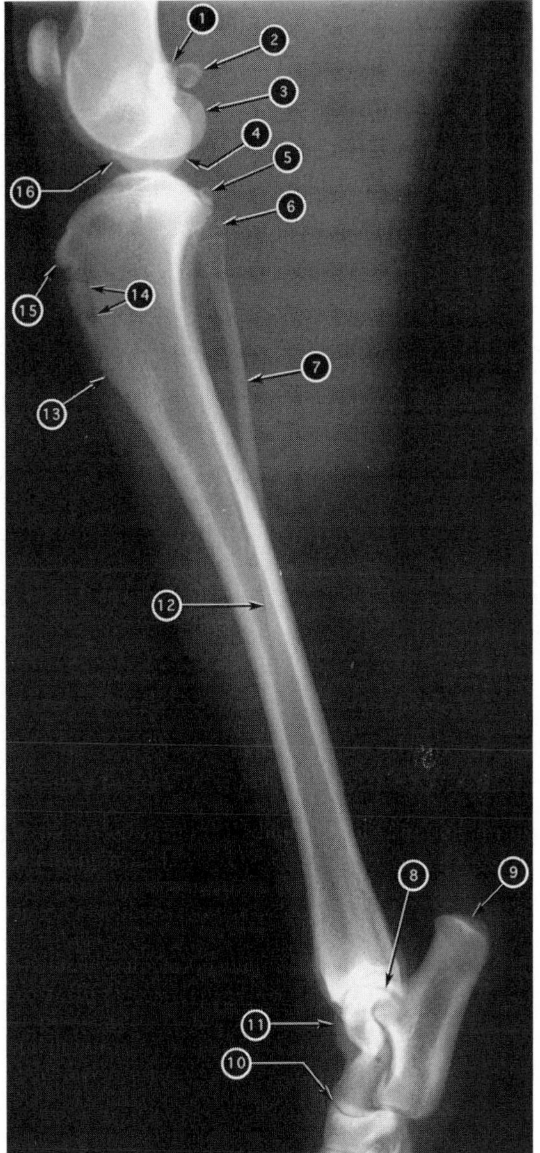

Fig. 14-24 Mediolateral Radiograph of Canine Crus.
1. Lateral sesamoid of gastrocnemius muscle
2. Medial sesamoid of gastrocnemius muscle
3. Medial condyle of femur
4. Lateral condyle of femur
5. Sesamoid bone of popliteus muscle
6. Head of fibula
7. Body of fibula
8. Tarsocrural joint
9. Tuber calcanei
10. Proximal intertarsal joint
11. Trochlea of talus
12. Body of fibula superimposed on tibia
13. Cranial border of tibia
14. Cartilage between tibial tuberosity and body of tibia
15. Tibial tuberosity
16. Extensor fossa of femur

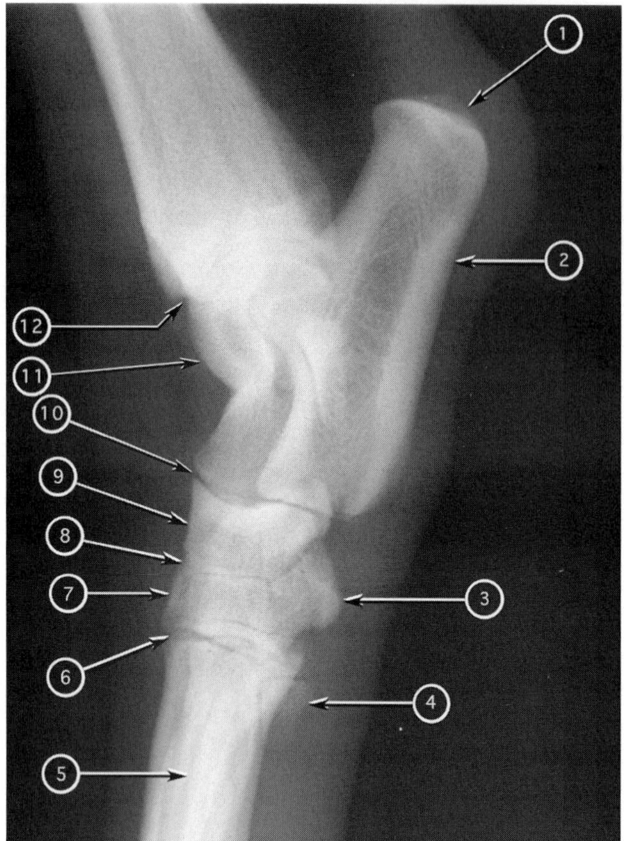

Fig. 14-25 Mediolateral Radiograph of Canine Tarsus.

1. Tuber calcanei
2. Body of calcaneus
3. Fourth tarsal bone (T4)
4. Metatarsal bone 1 (Mt1)
5. Superimposed Mt2 through Mt5
6. Tarsometatarsal joints
7. Third tarsal bone (T3)
8. Distal intertarsal joint
9. Central tarsal bone (Tc)
10. Proximal intertarsal joint
11. Trochlea tali
12. Tarsocrural joint

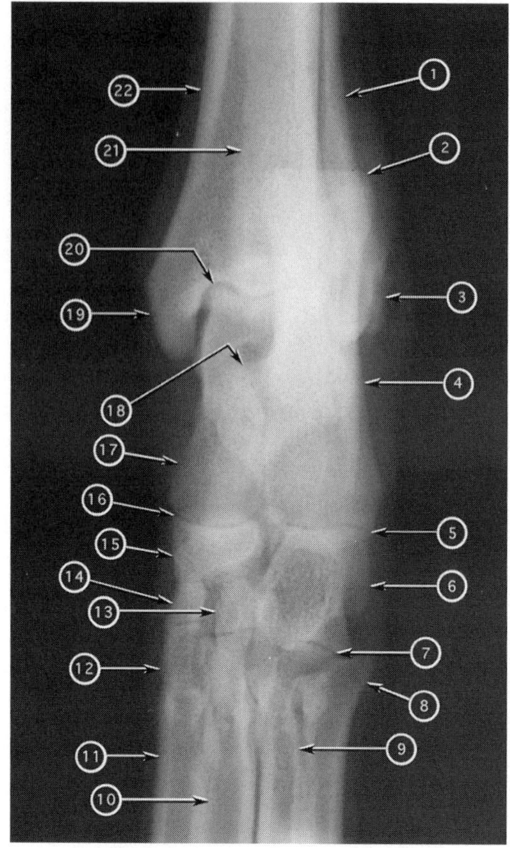

Fig. 14-26 Dorsoplantar Radiograph of Canine Tarsus.

1. Body of fibula
2. Tuber calcanei
3. Lateral malleolus of fibula
4. Body of calcaneus
5. Proximal intertarsal (calcaneoquartal) joint
6. T4
7. Tarsometatarsal joints
8. Base of Mt5
9. Mt4
10. Mt3
11. Mt2
12. Mt1
13. T3
14. Superimposed T1 and T2
15. Tc
16. Proximal intertarsal (talocalcaneocentral) joint
17. Talus
18. Sustentaculum tali of calcaneus
19. Medial malleolus of tibia
20. Tarsocrural joint
21. Common calcanean tendon superimposed on tibia
22. Body of tibia

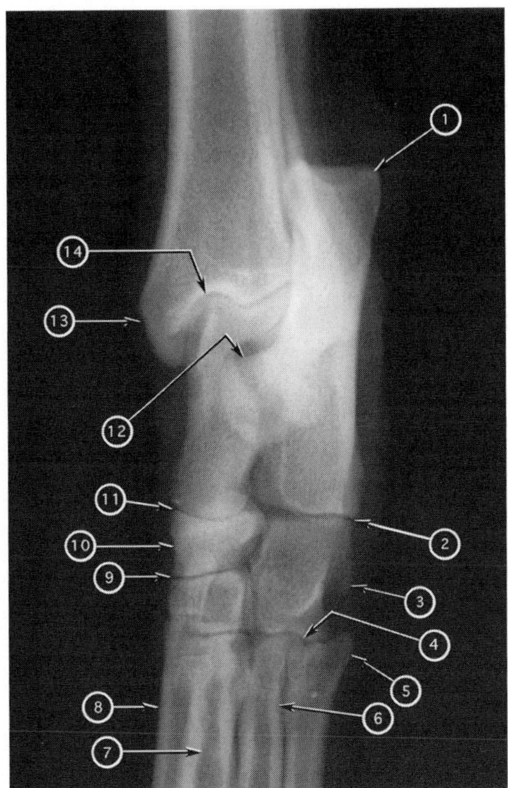

Fig. 14-27 Dorsolateral-Plantaromedial Oblique Radiograph of Canine Tarsus.

1. Tuber calcanei
2. Proximal intertarsal (calcaneoquartal) joint
3. T4
4. Tarsometatarsal joints
5. Base of Mt5
6. Mt4
7. Mt3
8. Mt2
9. Distal intertarsal joint
10. Tc
11. Proximal intertarsal (talocalcaneocentral) joint
12. Sustentaculum tali of calcaneus
13. Medial malleolus of tibia
14. Tarsocrural joint

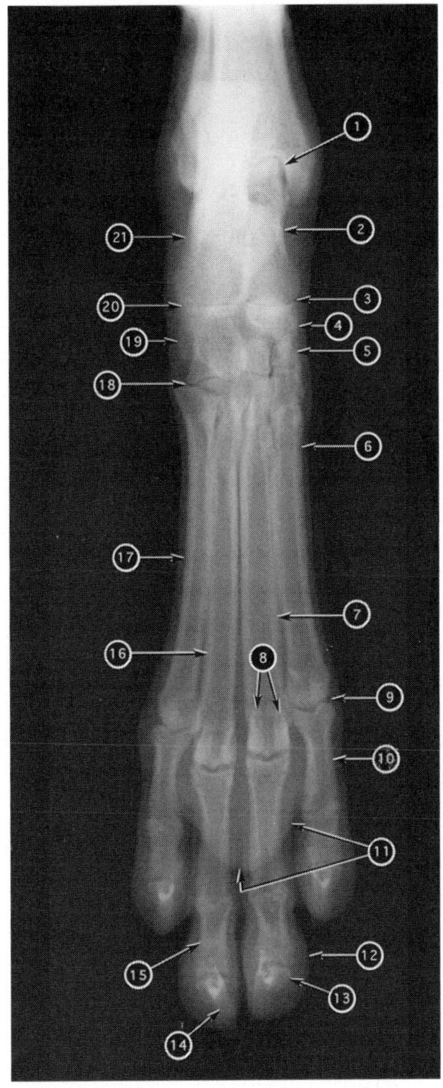

Fig. 14-28 Dorsoplantar Radiograph of Canine Pes.

1. Tarsocrural joint
2. Talus
3. Proximal intertarsal (talocalcaneocentral) joint
4. Tc
5. Superimposed T1 and T2
6. Mt2
7. Mt3
8. Proximal sesamoid bones of digit 3
9. Metatarsophalangeal joint of digit 2
10. Pp of digit 2
11. Metatarsal pad
12. Digital pad of digit 3
13. Pd of digit 3
14. Unguicular process of Pd of digit 4
15. Pm of digit 4
16. Mt4
17. Mt5
18. Tarsometatarsal joints
19. T4
20. Proximal intertarsal (calcaneoquartal) joint
21. Calcaneus

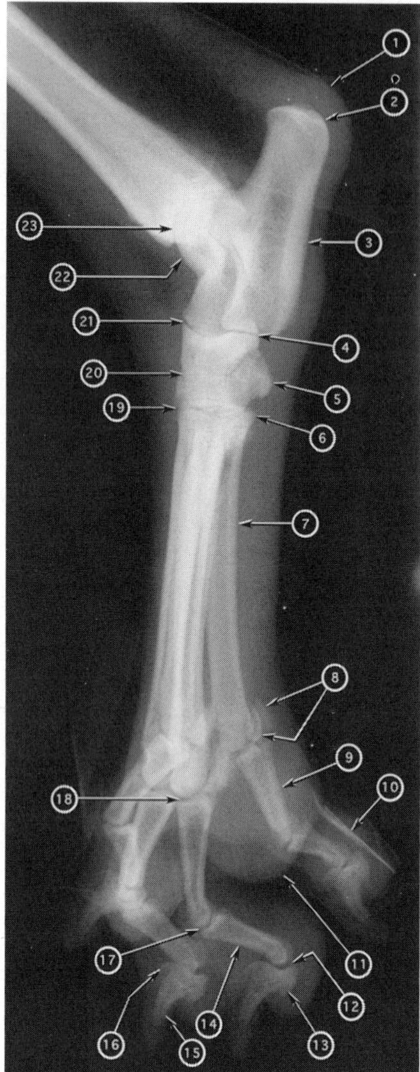

Fig. 14-29 Mediolateral Radiograph of Canine Pes with Digits Spread.

1. Superficial digital flexor (SDF) tendon
2. Tuber calcanei
3. Calcaneus
4. Proximal intertarsal (calcaneoquartal) joint
5. T4
6. Base of Mt5
7. Body of Mt5
8. Proximal sesamoid bones of digit 5
9. Pp of digit 5
10. Tape used in positioning
11. Metatarsal pad
12. DIJ of digit 4
13. Flexor tubercle of Pd of digit 4
14. Pm of digit 4
15. Unguicular process of Pd of digit 3
16. Unguicular crest of Pd of digit 3
17. PIJ of digit 4
18. Metatarsophalangeal joint of digit 4
19. Tarsometatarsal joints
20. Distal intertarsal joint
21. Proximal intertarsal (talocalcaneocentral) joint
22. Trochlea of talus
23. Tarsocrural joint

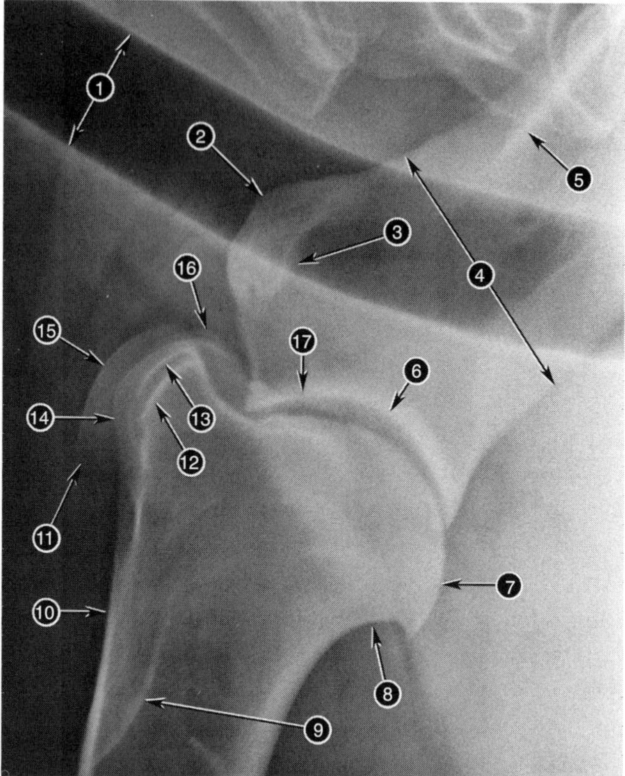

Fig. 14-30 Mediolateral Radiograph of Equine Shoulder Joint.

1. Air in trachea
2. Supraglenoid tubercle of scapula
3. Coracoid process of scapula
4. Neck of scapula
5. Spine of scapula
6. Medial edge of glenoid fossa
7. Head of humerus
8. Neck of humerus
9. Deltoid tuberosity of humerus
10. Cranial surface of humerus
11. Pointed distal end of intermediate tubercle
12. Floor of lateral part of intertubercular groove
13. Floor of medial part of intertubercular groove
14. Cranial part of lesser tubercle
15. Intermediate tubercle of humerus
16. Cranial part of greater tubercle
17. Glenoid notch in medial edge of glenoid fossa

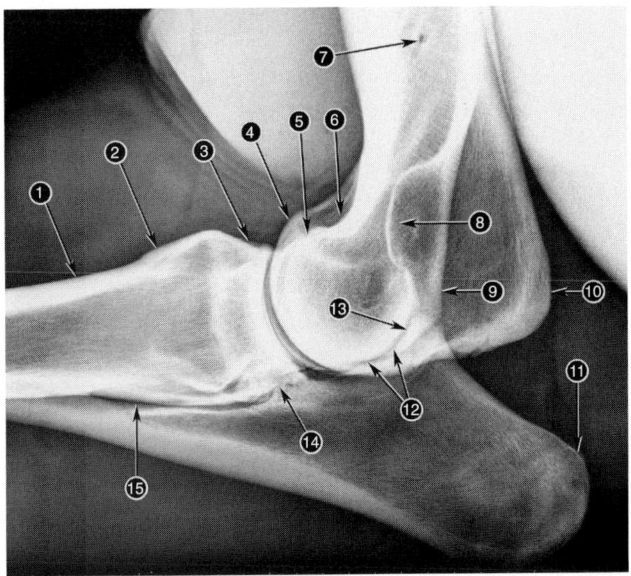

Fig. 14-31 Mediolateral Radiograph of Equine Elbow Joint.
1. Body of radius
2. Radial tuberosity
3. Head of radius
4. Trochlea of humeral condyle (medial)
5. Capitulum of humeral condyle (lateral)
6. Radial fossa of humerus
7. Nutrient canal of humerus (medial)
8. Olecranon fossa of humerus
9. Lateral epicondyle of humerus
10. Medial epicondyle of humerus
11. Tuber olecrani
12. Trochlear notch of ulna
13. Anconeal process of ulna
14. Proximal radioulnar joint
15. Proximal interosseous space

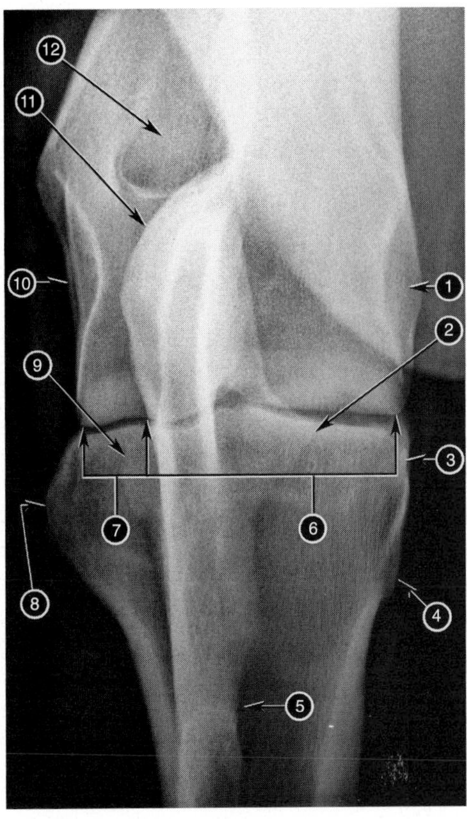

Fig. 14-32 Craniocaudal Radiograph of Equine Elbow Joint.
1. Medial epicondyle of humerus
2. Medial coronoid process of ulna
3. Head of radius
4. Radial tuberosity
5. Proximal interosseous space
6. Trochlea of humeral condyle
7. Capitulum of humeral condyle
8. Eminence for lateral collateral ligament
9. Lateral coronoid process of ulna
10. Lateral epicondyle of humerus
11. Tuber olecrani
12. Olecranon fossa of humerus

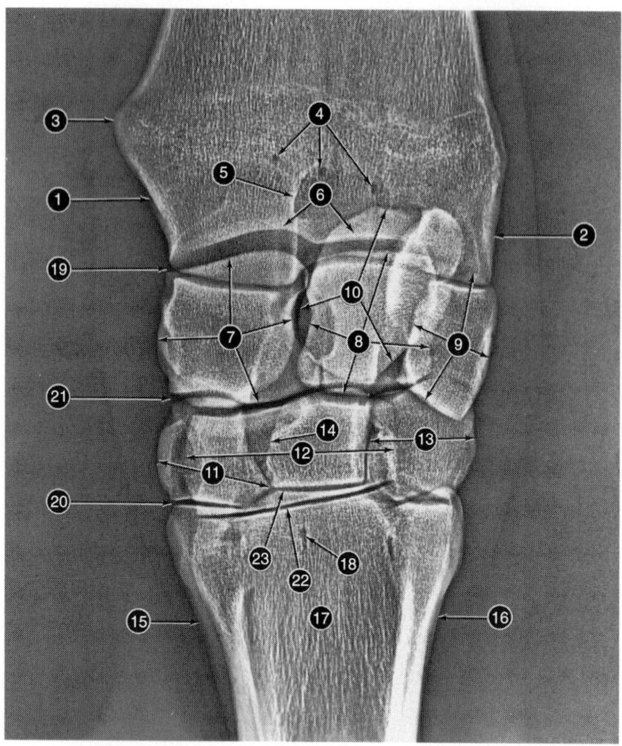

Fig. 14-33 Dorsopalmar Radiograph of Left Equine Carpus.
1. Medial styloid process of radius
2. Lateral styloid process of ulna
3. Projection at proximomedial aspect of medial styloid process of radius
4. Vascular channels
5. Caudolateral border of medial styloid process of radius
6. Junction of carpal articular surface with cranial surface of radius
7. Radial carpal bone
8. Intermediate carpal bone
9. Ulnar carpal bone
10. Accessory carpal bone
11. C2
12. C3
13. C4
14. Medial border of palmar process of C3
15. Mc2
16. Mc4
17. Mc3
18. Vascular channel
19. Antebrachiocarpal joint
20. Carpometacarpal joints
21. Middle carpal joint
22. Shadow cast by dorsal aspects of carpometacarpal joints
23. Shadow cast by palmar aspects of carpometacarpal joints

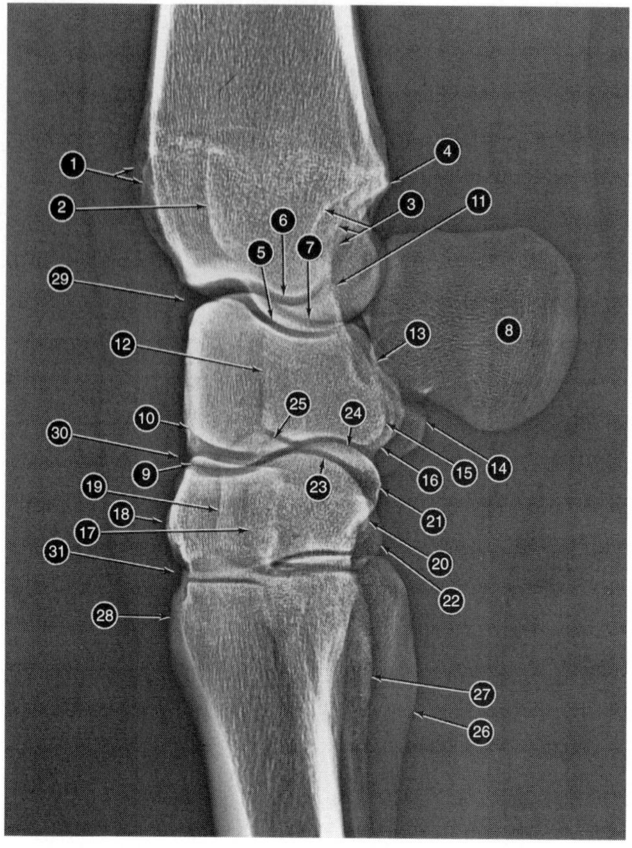

Fig. 14-34 Lateromedial Radiograph of Left Equine Carpus.
1. Ridges on cranial surface of radius
2. Ridge adjacent to lateral border of common digital extensor tendon
3. Caudal border of radial trochlea
4. Transverse crest of radius
5. Medial part of carpal articular surface
6. Intermediate part of carpal articular surface
7. Lateral part of carpal articular surface
8. Accessory carpal bone
9. Dorsodistal border of radial carpal bone
10. Dorsodistal border of intermediate carpal bone
11. Proximal process of Ci
12. Dorsal surface of ulnar carpal bone
13. Articulation of Ca with Cu
14. Palmar border of Cu
15. Palmar border of Ci
16. Palmar border of Cr
17. Dorsal border of C2
18. Dorsal border of C3
19. Dorsal border of C4
20. Palmar border of C2
21. Palmar border of C3
22. Palmar border of C4
23. Proximal border of C2
24. Proximal border of C3
25. Proximal border of C4
26. Mc4
27. Mc2
28. Metacarpal tuberosity
29. Antebrachiocarpal joint
30. Middle carpal joint
31. Carpometacarpal joints

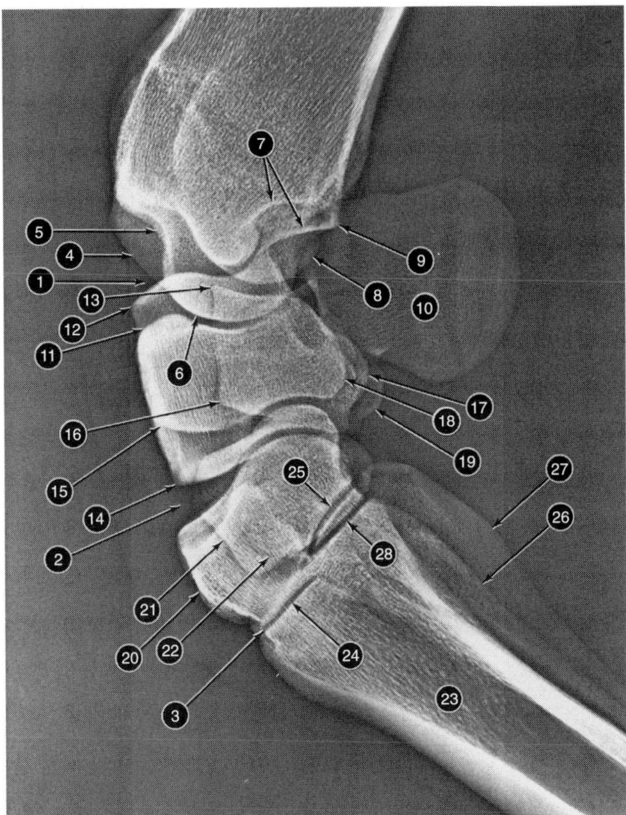

Fig. 14-35 Lateromedial Radiograph of Flexed Left Equine Carpus.

1. Antebrachiocarpal joint
2. Middle carpal joint
3. Carpometacarpal joints
4. Medial border of medial part of carpal articular surface
5. Lateral border of medial part of carpal articular surface
6. Medial styloid process
7. Shadows from caudal aspect of intermediate part of radial trochlea
8. Lateral styloid process
9. Transverse crest of radius
10. Accessory carpal bone
11. Dorsoproximal border of Cr
12. Dorsoproximal border of Ci
13. Dorsoproximal border of Cu
14. Dorsodistal border of Cr (isolated)
15. Dorsodistal border of Ci
16. Dorsodistal border of Cu
17. Palmar border of Cr
18. Palmar border of Ci
19. Palmar border of Cu
20. Dorsal border of C3
21. Dorsal border of C4
22. Dorsal border of C2
23. Mc3
24. Third carpometacarpal joint
25. Second carpometacarpal joint
26. Mc2
27. Mc4
28. Fourth carpometacarpal joint

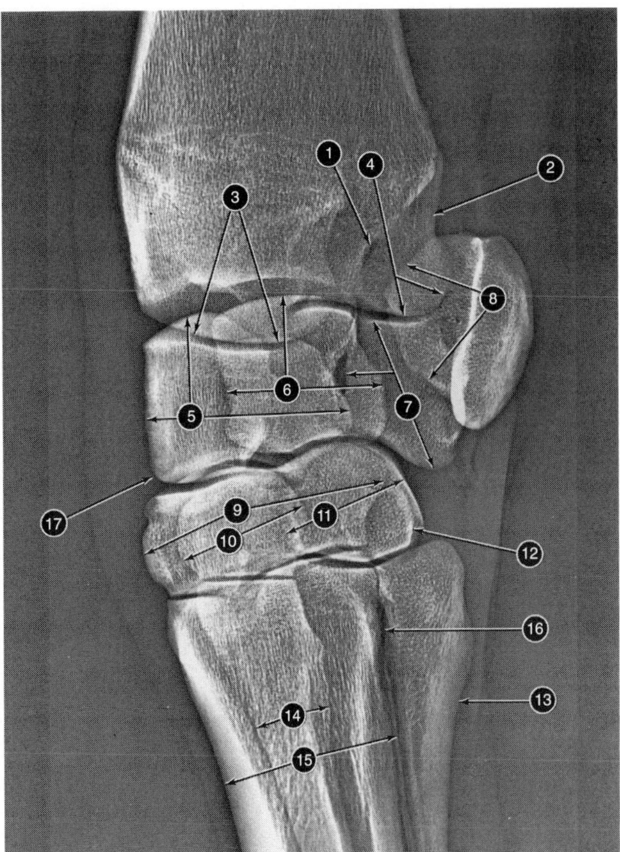

Fig. 14-36 Dorsolateral-Palmaromedial Oblique Radiograph of Left Equine Carpus.

1. Radiolucent area at line of fusion between lateral styloid process and radius
2. Lateral styloid process
3. Medial part of radial trochlea
4. Lateral styloid process
5. Radial carpal bone
6. Intermediate carpal bone
7. Ulnar carpal bone
8. Articulations of accessory carpal bone with lateral styloid process and ulnar carpal bone
9. C3
10. C2
11. C4
12. Palmar projection of C4
13. Mc4
14. Mc2
15. Mc3
16. Location of metacarpal interosseous ligaments
17. Distal aspect of dorsomedial border of Cr (isolated)

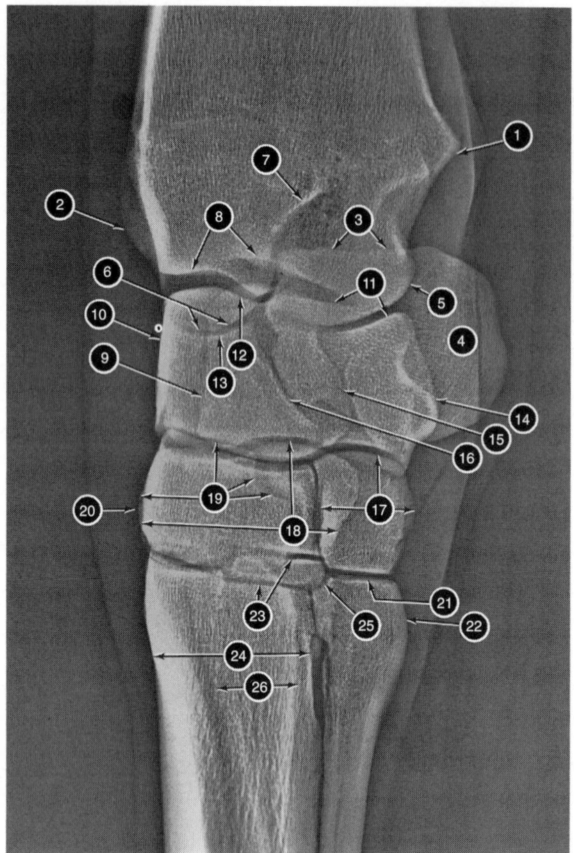

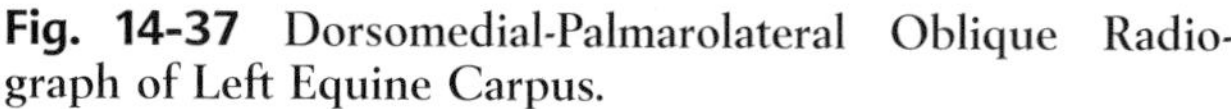

Fig. 14-37 Dorsomedial-Palmarolateral Oblique Radiograph of Left Equine Carpus.

1. Projection of radius for attachment of medial collateral ligament
2. Ridge that forms lateral border of groove for common digital extensor tendon
3. Proximal border of accessory carpal bone
4. Accessory carpal bone
5. Medial styloid process of radius
6. Lateral styloid process
7. Ridge on caudal aspect of radius
8. Ridge at junction of cranial surface of radius with carpal articular surface
9. Dorsolateral border of Cr
10. Dorsolateral borders of Cu and Ci
11. Proximal surface of Cr
12. Proximal surface of Ci
13. Proximal surface of Cu
14. Palmaromedial border of Cr
15. Palmaromedial border of Ci
16. Palmaromedial border of Cu
17. C2
18. C3
19. C4
20. Dorsolateral borders of C3 and C4
21. Articulation between C2 and Mc2
22. Mc2
23. Articulation between C3 and Mc3
24. Mc3
25. Inconstant articulation between C3 and Mc2
26. Mc4

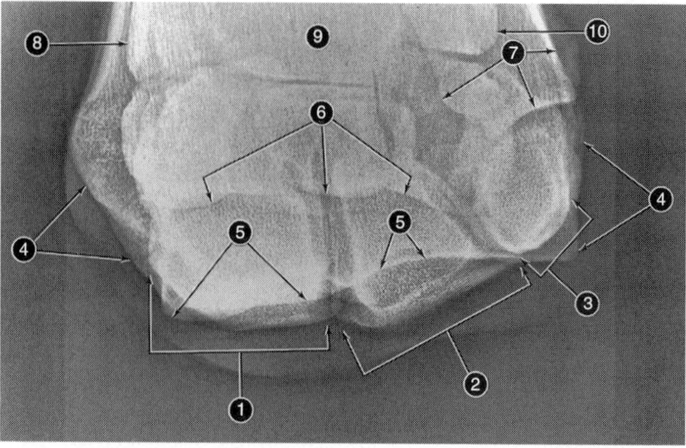

Fig. 14-38 Dorsoproximal-Dorsodistal Oblique Radiograph of Proximal Row of Equine Carpal Bones.

1. Dorsal surface of radial carpal bone
2. Dorsal surface of intermediate carpal bone
3. Dorsal surface of ulnar carpal bone
4. Radius
5. Carpal articular surface of radial trochlea
6. Dorsal surfaces of distal carpal bones
7. Accessory carpal bone
8. Mc2
9. Mc3
10. Mc4

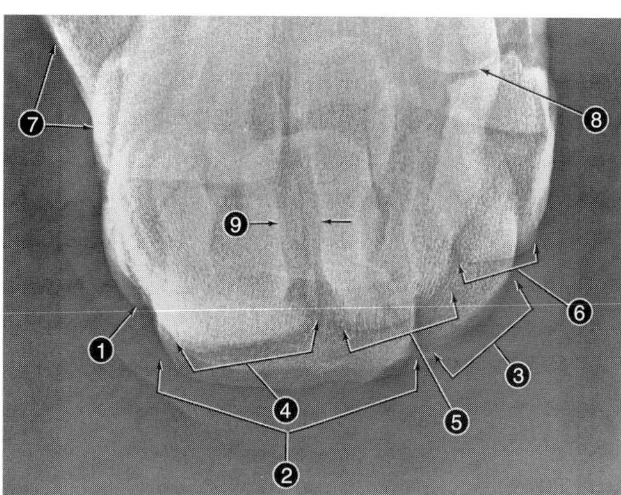

Fig. 14-39 Dorsoproximal-Dorsodistal Oblique Radiograph of Distal Row of Equine Carpal Bones.

1. Dorsal surface of C2
2. Dorsal surface of C3
3. Dorsal surface of C4
4. Dorsal surface of radial carpal bone
5. Dorsal surface of intermediate carpal bone
6. Dorsal surface of ulnar carpal bone
7. Radius
8. Accessory carpal bone
9. Interosseous space between Cr and Ci

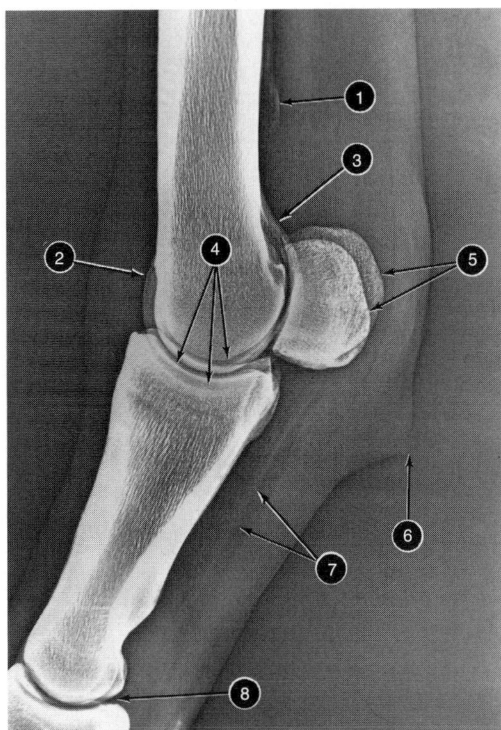

Fig. 14-40 **Lateromedial Radiograph of Left Equine Metacarpophalangeal Joint.**

1. Distal end (head) of small metacarpal bone
2. Dorsal part of sagittal ridge of Mc3
3. Palmar part of sagittal ridge of Mc3
4. Metacarpophalangeal joint
5. Proximal sesamoid bones
6. Ergot
7. Straight sesamoid ligament
8. Proximal interphalangeal joint

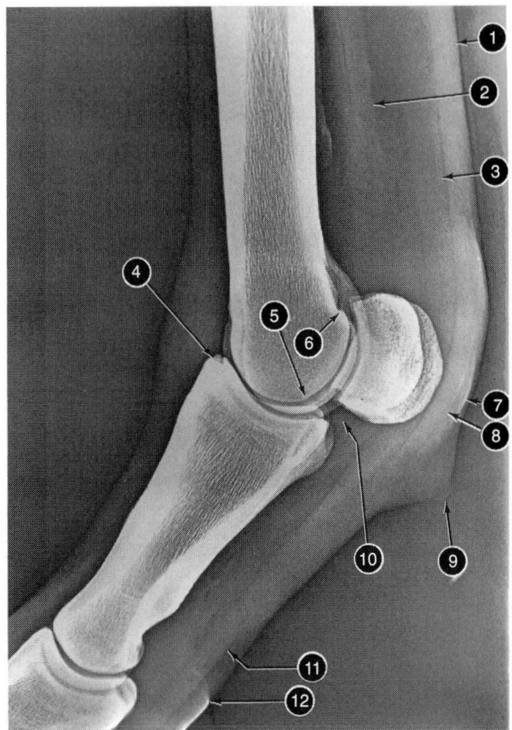

Fig. 14-41 **Lateromedial Radiograph of Left Equine Metacarpophalangeal Joint with Right Limb Lifted to Increase Weight on Left Limb.**

1. SDF tendon
2. Interosseus
3. Deep digital flexor (DDF) tendon
4. Dorsoproximal aspect of Pp
5. Subtle transverse ridge on head of Mc3
6. Distinct transverse ridge at palmar edge of articular surface
7. Palmar annular ligament of metacarpophalangeal joint
8. SDF tendon
9. Ergot
10. Increased distance between proximal sesamoid bones and Pp (see Fig. 14-40)
11. DDF tendon
12. Distal digital annular ligament

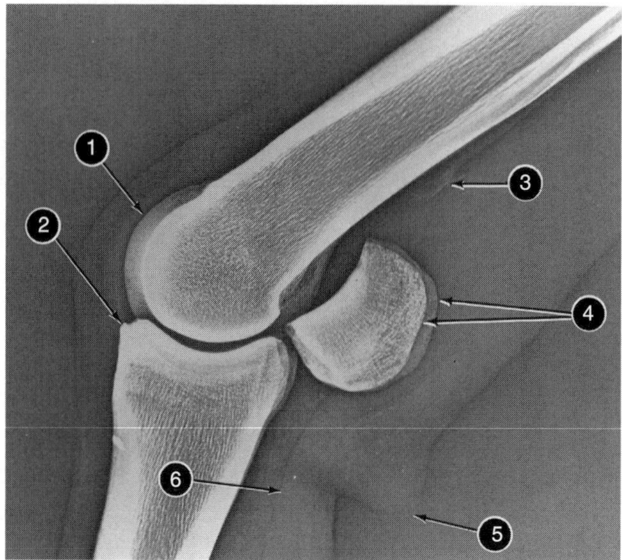

Fig. 14-42 **Lateromedial Radiograph of Flexed Left Equine Metacarpophalangeal Joint.**
1. Sagittal ridge on head of Mc3
2. Dorsoproximal aspect of Pp
3. Distal end of small metacarpal bone
4. Proximal sesamoid bones
5. Ergot
6. DDF tendon

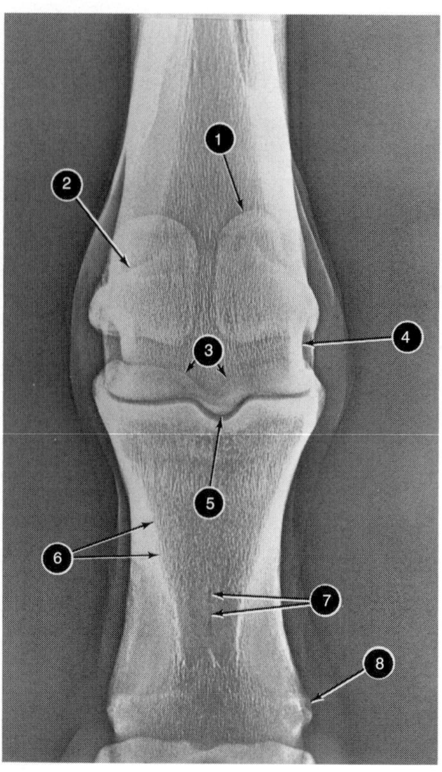

Fig. 14-43 **Dorsoproximal-Palmarodistal Oblique Radiograph of Left Equine Metacarpophalangeal Joint.**
1. Lateral proximal sesamoid bone
2. Depression in interosseus (abaxial) surface of medial proximal sesamoid bone for attachment of interosseus tendon
3. Palmaroproximal edge of Pp
4. Depression in Mc3 for attachment of lateral collateral ligament of metacarpophalangeal joint
5. Sagittal ridge on head of Mc3
6. Area of oblique ridge on palmar surface of Pp for attachment oblique sesamoid ligament
7. Nutrient canal through dorsal cortex of Pp
8. Lateral distal collateral tubercle of Pp

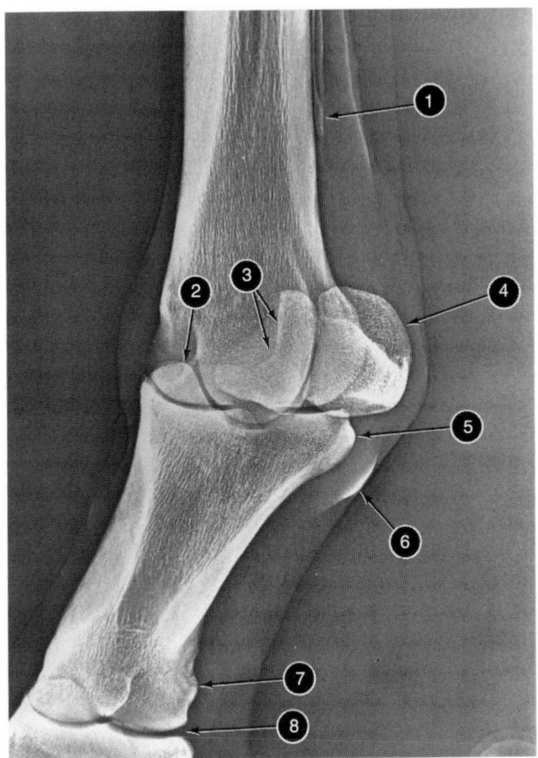

Fig. 14-44 **Dorsolateral-Palmaromedial Oblique Radiograph of Left Equine Metacarpophalangeal Joint.**

1. Distal end of Mc4
2. Dorsoproximal aspect of Pp
3. Depression in interosseus surface of medial proximal sesamoid bone for attachment of interosseus tendon
4. Palmaroabaxial border of lateral proximal sesamoid bone
5. Lateral proximal collateral tubercle of Pp
6. Ergot
7. Lateral distal collateral tubercle of Pp
8. Proximal interphalangeal joint

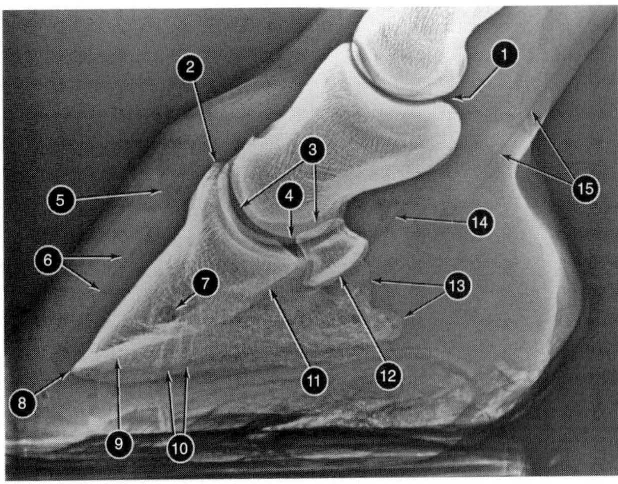

Fig. 14-45 **Lateromedial Radiograph of Left Equine Foredigit.**

1. PIJ
2. Extensor process of Pd
3. DIJ
4. Part of DIJ that extends between Pd and the distal sesamoid (navicular) bone
5. Proximal extent of tubular horn forming stratum medium of hoof wall
6. Junction of stratum medium and laminar horn of stratum internum
7. Transverse part of sole canal of Pd; accommodates terminal arch of digital vessels
8. Sole border of Pd
9. Planum cuneatum (sole surface) of Pd
10. Vascular channels extending from sole canal to sole border of Pd
11. Flexor surface of Pd
12. Flexor surface of navicular bone
13. Superimposed medial and lateral palmar processes of Pd
14. Radiolucent areas created by fat within synovial folds
15. Borders of DDF tendon; defined by fat within synovial folds of digital sheath

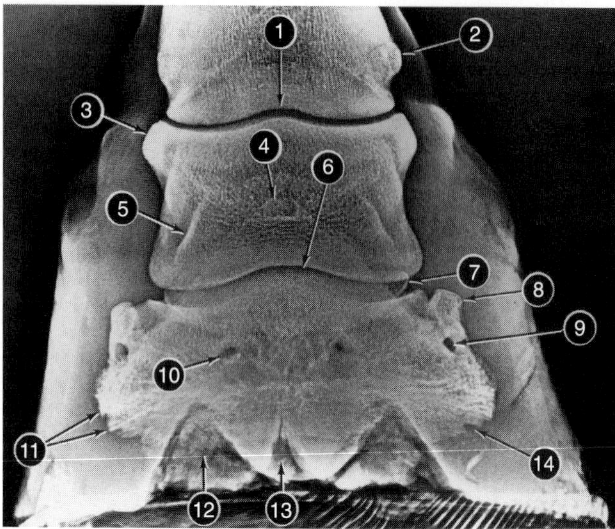

Fig. 14-46 Dorsopalmar Radiograph of Left Equine Foredigit.

1. PIJ
2. Lateral distal collateral tubercle of Pp
3. Medial proximal collateral tubercle of Pm
4. Extensor process of Pd
5. Wall of depression in Pm for attachment of medial collateral ligament of DIJ
6. DIJ
7. Lateral extremity of navicular bone
8. Lateral palmar process of Pd
9. Foramen in lateral palmar process of Pd that accommodates dorsal branches of digital vessels
10. Medial sole foramen of Pd; receives digital vessels as they enter sole canal
11. Sole border of Pd; typically irregular because of notches for vascular channels
12. Medial collateral groove of frog
13. Central groove of frog
14. Notch in sole border associated with vascular channel from sole canal of Pd

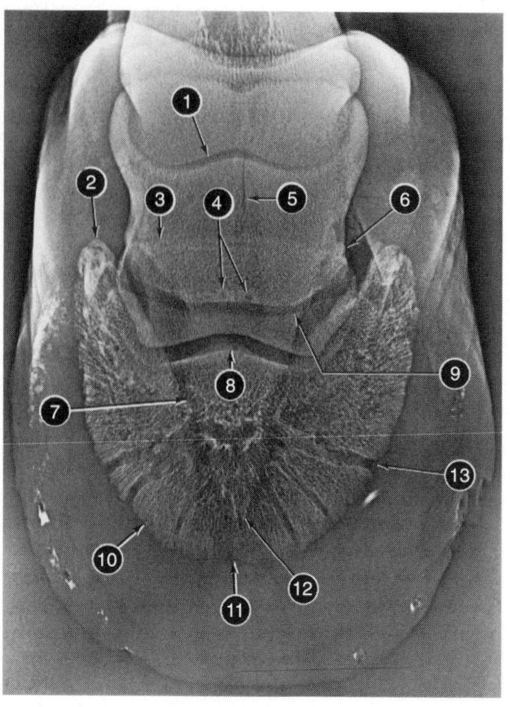

Fig. 14-47 Dorsal 65-Degree Proximal-Palmarodistal Oblique Radiograph of Left Equine Foredigit.

1. PIJ
2. Medial palmar process of Pd
3. Proximal border of navicular bone
4. Vascular foramina and synovial fossae along distal border of navicular bone
5. Air within central groove of frog
6. Lateral extremity of navicular bone
7. Sole canal of Pd
8. DIJ
9. Articulation of Pd with navicular bone; part of DIJ
10. Sole border of Pd
11. Crena marginis solaris
12. Apex of frog
13. Vascular channel from sole canal to sole border of Pd

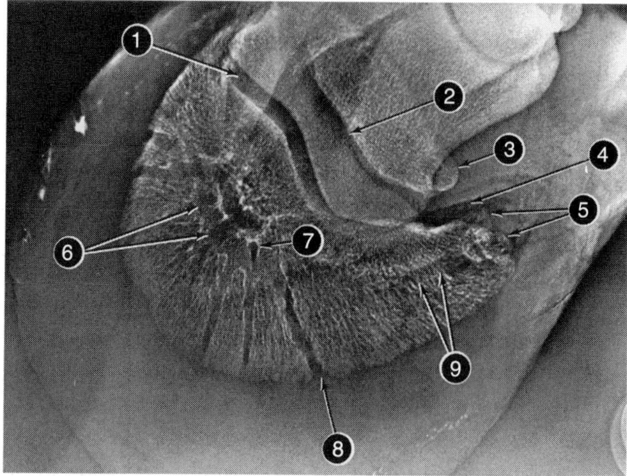

Fig. 14-48 Dorsoproximolateral-Palmarodistomedial Oblique Radiograph of Left Equine Foredigit.

1. DIJ
2. Articulation of Pd with navicular bone; part of DIJ
3. Lateral extremity of navicular bone
4. Air within lateral collateral groove of frog
5. Lateral palmar process of Pd
6. Sole canal of Pd
7. End-on perspective of vascular channel from sole canal to parietal surface of Pd
8. Vascular channel from sole canal to sole border of Pd
9. Lateral parietal groove of Pd; accommodates dorsal branches of digital vessel

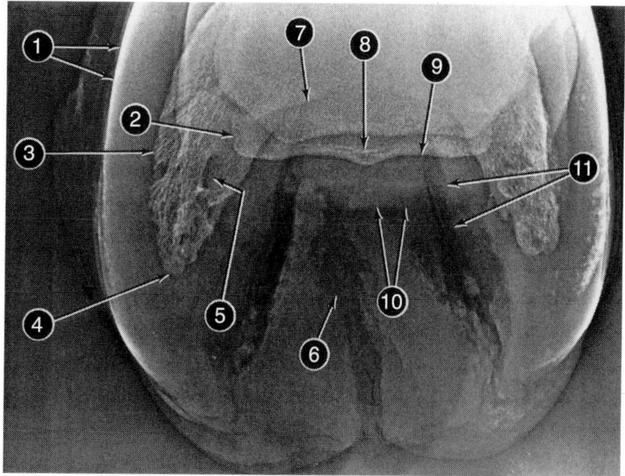

Fig. 14-49 Palmaroproximal-Palmarodistal Oblique Radiograph of Left Equine Foredigit.

1. Proximal border of hoof wall
2. Lateral extremity of navicular bone
3. Sole border of Pd
4. Lateral palmar process of Pd
5. Foramen of lateral palmar process
6. Air within central groove of frog
7. Articulation of Pm with navicular bone; part of DIJ
8. Sagittal ridge of navicular bone
9. Flexor surface of navicular bone
10. DDF tendon
11. Air within medial collateral groove of frog

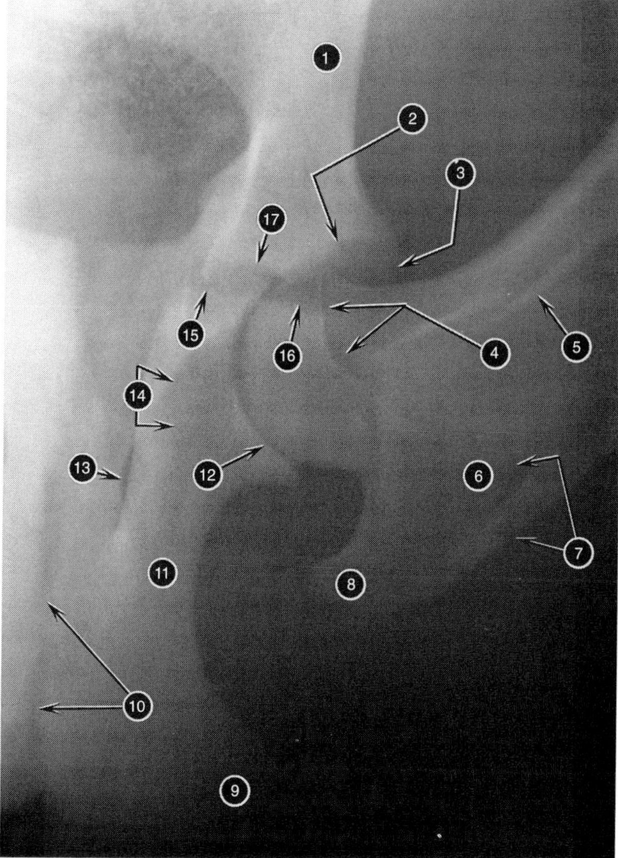

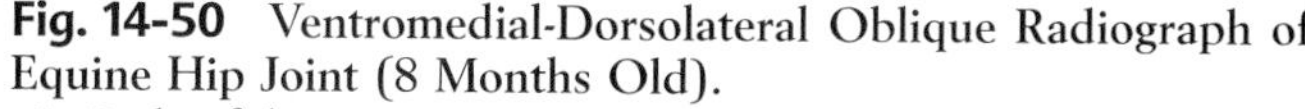

Fig. 14-50 Ventromedial-Dorsolateral Oblique Radiograph of Equine Hip Joint (8 Months Old).

1. Body of ilium
2. Cranioventral border of acetabulum
3. Craniodorsal border of acetabulum
4. Proximal physis (epiphyseal cartilage) of femur
5. Shadow created by caudal edge of lesser trochanter
6. Radiolucent area created by trochanteric fossa of femur
7. Cartilaginous junction between greater trochanter and femoral body
8. Greater trochanter of femur, caudal part
9. Tuber ischiadicum
10. Cartilaginous pelvic symphysis
11. Body of ischium
12. Caudoventral border of acetabulum
13. Obturator foramen
14. Radiolucent area created by acetabular fossa
15. Radiolucent area created by groove on ventral surface of pubis for accessory ligament of femoral head
16. Radiolucent area created by fovea capitis of femoral head
17. Cranial edge of acetabular notch

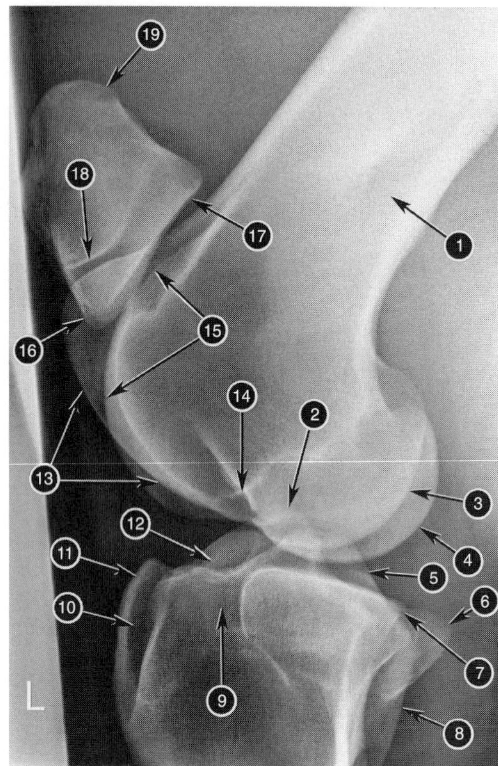

Fig. 14-51 Lateromedial Radiograph of Equine Stifle Joint.
1. Supracondylar fossa of femur for SDF
2. Medial tubercle of intercondylar eminence
3. Lateral condyle of femur
4. Medial condyle of femur
5. Lateral tubercle of intercondylar eminence
6. Lateral condyle of tibia
7. Medial condyle of tibia
8. Fibula
9. Extensor groove of tibia
10. Groove for intermediate patellar ligament
11. Lateral part of tibial tuberosity
12. Cranial intercondylar area of tibia
13. Medial ridge of femoral trochlea
14. Extensor fossa of femur
15. Lateral ridge of femoral trochlea
16. Apex of patella
17. Articular surface of patella, gliding part
18. Articular surface of patella, resting part
19. Base of patella

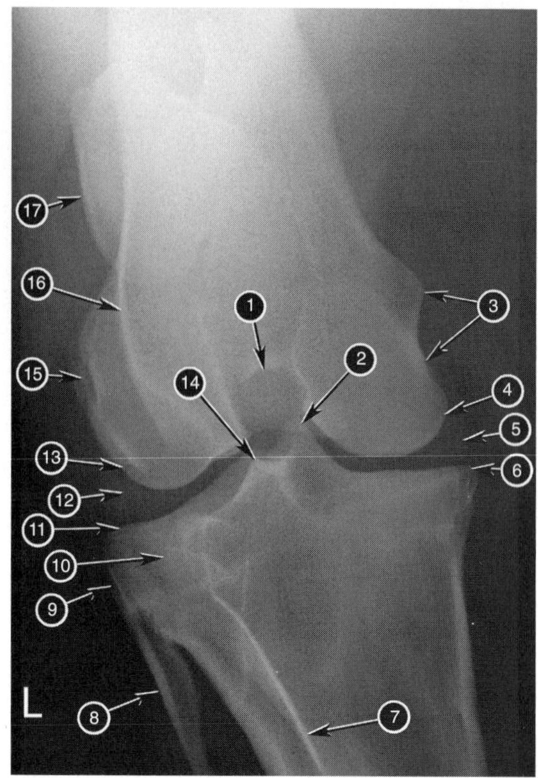

Fig. 14-52 Caudocranial Radiograph of Equine Stifle Joint.
1. Intercondylar fossa of femur
2. Medial tubercle of intercondylar eminence
3. Medial epicondyle of femur
4. Medial condyle of femur
5. Medial meniscus and femorotibial joint
6. Medial condyle of tibia
7. Cranial margin of tibia
8. Body of fibula
9. Head of fibula
10. Lateral part of tibial tuberosity
11. Lateral condyle of tibia
12. Lateral meniscus and femorotibial joint
13. Depression for origin of popliteus muscle
14. Lateral tubercle of intercondylar eminence
15. Lateral epicondyle of femur
16. Lateral ridge of femoral trochlea
17. Patella

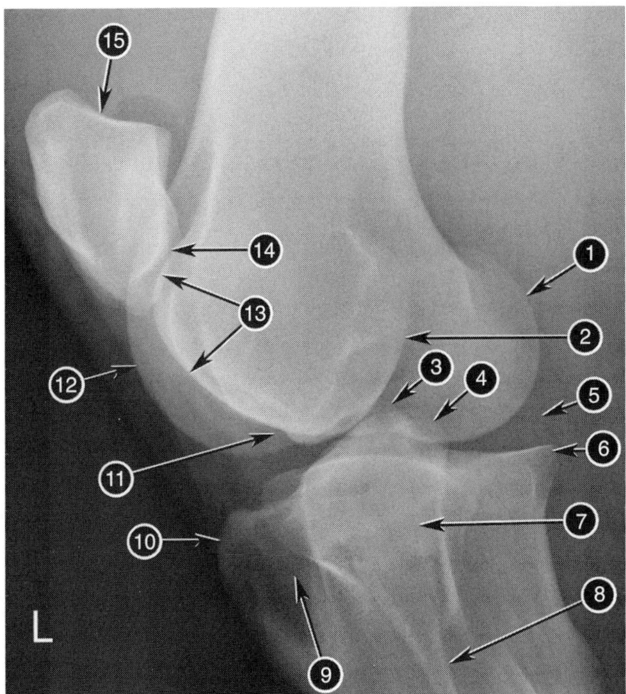

Fig. 14-53 Caudolateral-Craniomedial Oblique Radiograph of Equine Stifle Joint.

1. Medial condyle of femur
2. Lateral condyle of femur
3. Medial tubercle of intercondylar eminence
4. Lateral tubercle of intercondylar eminence
5. Medial meniscus and femorotibial joint
6. Medial condyle of tibia
7. Head of fibula
8. Body of fibula
9. Extensor groove of tibia
10. Tibial tuberosity
11. Extensor fossa of femur
12. Lateral ridge of femoral trochlea
13. Groove of femoral trochlea
14. Femoropatellar joint
15. Patella

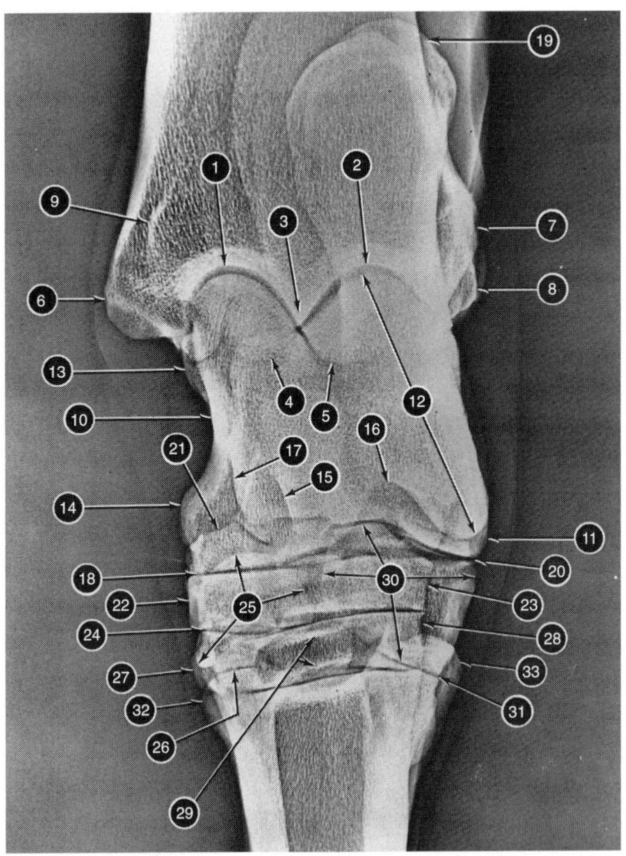

Fig. 14-54 Dorsoplantar Radiograph of Left Equine Tarsus.

1. Medial groove of tibial cochlea
2. Lateral groove of tibial cochlea
3. Oblique ridge separating medial and lateral grooves of tibial cochlea
4. Pointed caudal end of oblique ridge
5. Rounded cranial end of oblique ridge
6. Medial malleolus
7. Caudal part of lateral malleolus
8. Cranial part of lateral malleolus
9. Radiopaque shadow
10. Talus
11. Calcaneus
12. Lateral ridge of trochlea tali
13. Proximal tubercle of talus
14. Distal tubercle of talus
15. Medial ridge of trochlea tali
16. Groove between lateral and medial ridges of trochlea tali
17. Medial edge of sustentaculum tali
18. Proximal intertarsal (talocalcaneocentral) joint
19. Tuber calcanei
20. Proximal intertarsal (calcaneoquartal) joint
21. Proximoplantar aspect of Tc
22. Medial aspect of Tc
23. Lateral aspect of Tc
24. Distal intertarsal (centrodistal) joint
25. Fused first and second tarsal bones (T1+2)
26. Articulation between T1+2 and Mt2
27. Medial aspect of T3
28. Lateral aspect of T3
29. Radiopaque lines produced by walls of nonarticular depressions on T3
30. T4
31. Tarsometatarsal joints (also articulation between T1+2 and Mt2)
32. Base of Mt2
33. Base of Mt4

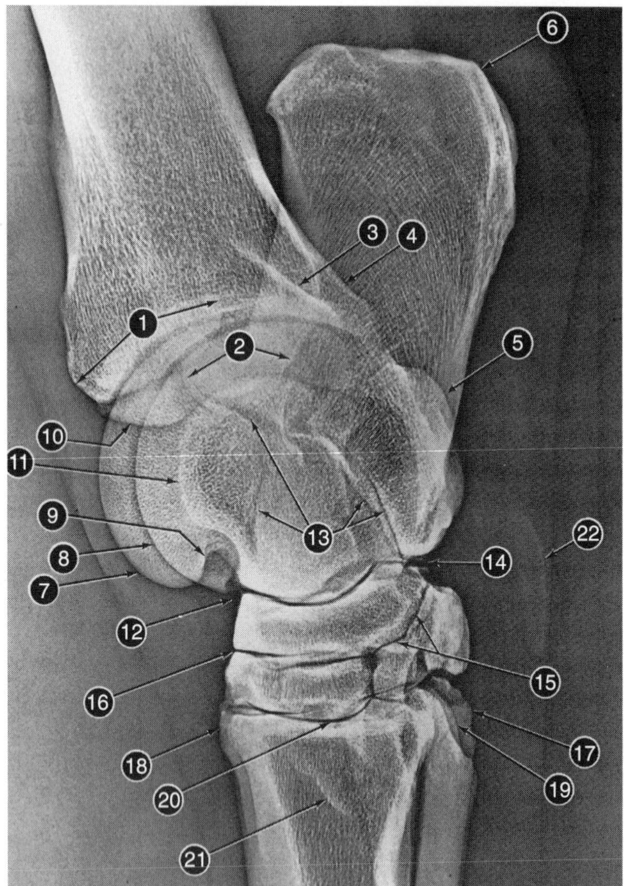

Fig. 14-55 Lateromedial Radiograph of Left Equine Tarsus.

1. Lateral malleolus
2. Medial malleolus
3. Radiopaque line produced by ridge on caudal surface of tibia
4. Medial part of caudal surface of tibia
5. Sustentaculum tali
6. Tuber calcanei
7. Lateral ridge of trochlea tali
8. Medial ridge of trochlea tali
9. Larger notch associated with lateral ridge of trochlea tali
10. Intermediate part of tibial cochlea
11. Groove of trochlea tali
12. PIJ
13. Articular facets between talus and calcaneus
14. Plantar aspect of PIJ
15. Articulation between Tc and T1+2
16. Distal intertarsal joint
17. Base of Mt2
18. Base of Mt3
19. Base of Mt4
20. Tarsometatarsal joint
21. Groove on Mt3 for dorsal metatarsal artery 3
22. Chestnut (torus tarseus)

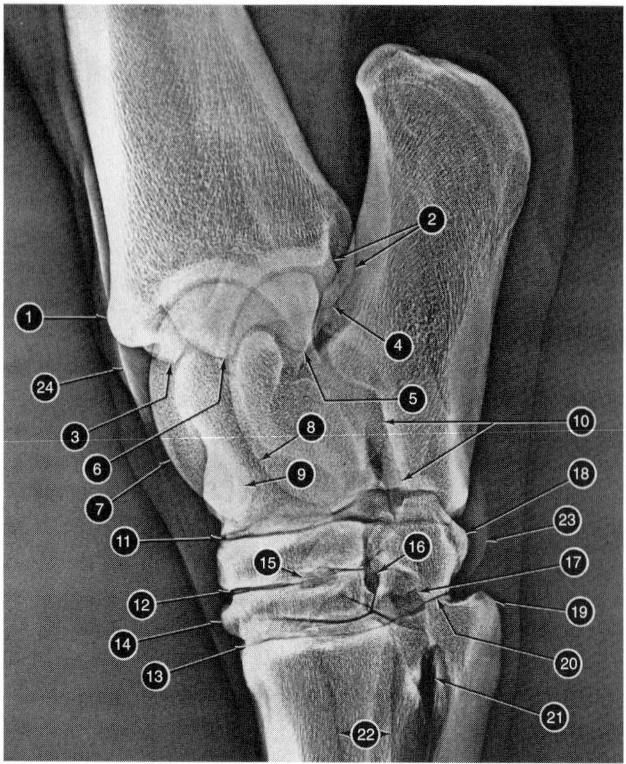

Fig. 14-56 Dorsolateral-Plantaromedial Oblique Radiograph of Left Equine Tarsus.

1. Cranial aspect of medial malleolus
2. Shadows produced by borders of groove in lateral malleolus
3. Distal projection of medial malleolus
4. Distal projection of lateral malleolus
5. Caudal aspect of intermediate ridge of tibial cochlea
6. Cranial aspect of intermediate ridge of tibial cochlea
7. Medial ridge of trochlea tali
8. Lateral ridge of trochlea tali
9. Radiopaque area produced by distal tubercle of talus
10. Sinus tarsi
11. Dorsomedial aspect of PIJ
12. Dorsomedial aspect of DIJ
13. Dorsomedial aspect of third tarsometatarsal joint
14. Ridge on dorsomedial aspect of T3
15. Nonarticular area between Tc and T3
16. Dorsal opening of tarsal canal
17. Plantar opening of tarsal canal
18. Plantar tuberosity on T4
19. Base of Mt4
20. Articulation between T4 and Mt4
21. Interosseous space between Mt3 and Mt4
22. Mt2
23. Chestnut
24. Tendons crossing flexor surface of tarsus

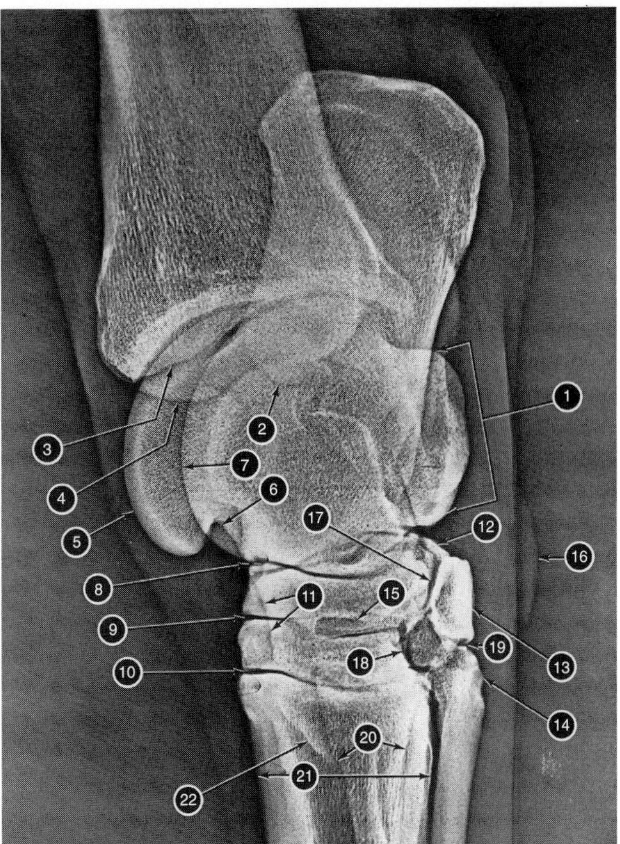

Fig. 14-57 Dorsomedial-Plantarolateral Oblique Radiograph of Left Equine Tarsus.

1. Sustentaculum tali
2. Distal extremity of medial malleolus
3. Distal extremity of lateral malleolus
4. Intermediate ridge of tibial cochlea
5. Lateral ridge of trochlea tali
6. Notch distal to lateral ridge of trochlea tali
7. Medial ridge of trochlea tali
8. Dorsolateral aspect of proximal intertarsal joint
9. Dorsolateral aspect of distal intertarsal joint
10. Dorsolateral aspect of third tarsometatarsal joint
11. Dorsal aspect of T4
12. Plantaromedial aspect of Tc
13. Plantaromedial aspect of T1+2
14. Plantaromedial aspect of Mt 2
15. Nonarticular depression between Tc and T3
16. Chestnut
17. Articulation between T1+2 and Tc
18. Articulation between T1+2 and T3
19. Articulation between T1+2 and Mt 2
20. Mt4
21. Mt3
22. Radiopaque line produced by border of groove for dorsal metatarsal artery 3

ELECTRONIC RESOURCES evolve

Chapter 14 can also be found on the companion Web site at evolve http://evolve.elsevier.com/Thrall/vetrad/

CHAPTER • 15

Orthopedic Diseases of Young and Growing Dogs and Cats

Erik R. Wisner
Rachel E. Pollard

The radiographic aspects of developmental skeletal disease are as varied as the causes of the disorders themselves. Box 15-1 lists some common and uncommon disorders of the immature skeleton. It is intended to provide some structure to this chapter and should not be considered a definitive classification scheme.

Developmental lesions may be solitary and localized but are often multifocal or generalized. Localized lesions, such as those seen with osteochondrosis, are often bilateral. Lesion location can be predicted on the basis of the characteristic anatomic distribution of many of these diseases. Although radiographic features of the various developmental skeletal diseases vary widely, they generally appear nonaggressive.

Secondary degenerative joint disease is a common sequela to developmental disorders of the immature skeleton, particularly when the primary lesion involves joints or produces limb deformity. Often the most pronounced radiographic findings are those of the secondary degenerative changes, which can mask the original developmental lesion. To reach an accurate radiographic diagnosis, differentiation of the cause (developmental lesion) from the effect (degenerative lesion) is important whenever possible.

DISORDERS PRIMARILY AFFECTING JOINTS

Osteochondrosis and Osteochondritis Dissecans

Osteochondrosis is a common cause of lameness in young, rapidly growing, large-breed dogs. Clinical signs usually develop between 6 and 9 months of age. Osteochondrosis occurs from epiphyseal cartilage necrosis, resulting in a failure of normal endochondral ossification.[1] If the vascular bed of the adjacent subchondral bone can envelop and bypass the region of cartilage necrosis, endochondral ossification may resume without development of a clinical lesion. Otherwise, progressive chondromalacia leads to development of clefts or fissures extending from the surface of the cartilage to the subchondral bone. When a chondral or osteochondral fragment separates from adjacent subchondral bone, the disorder technically should be referred to as *osteochondritis dissecans.*[1] However, in most patients, determination of whether a cartilage fragment exists is impossible from survey radiographs; thus osteochondrosis is an acceptable term.

In dogs, osteochondrosis occurs in specific anatomic locations and often involves weight-bearing articular surfaces. It occurs most frequently in the caudal aspect of the proximal humeral head (Fig. 15-1) but also occurs in the distomedial aspect of the humeral trochlea (Fig. 15-2), the lateral and medial femoral condyles (Fig. 15-3), the femoral trochlea, and the medial and lateral trochlear ridges of the talus (Fig. 15-4).[2-9] Osteochondrosis is frequently bilateral, but affected animals may have clinical signs in only one limb. Large subchondral defects are frequently associated with the presence of separate osteochondral fragments, which tends to increase the severity of clinical signs.[10]

Radiographic Signs

Typical radiographic findings of osteochondrosis include flattening or concavity of the affected subchondral bone surface with surrounding subchondral bone sclerosis. This may result in nonuniformity and apparent widening of the joint space. When mineralized, a cartilage flap is sometimes seen within the subchondral defect, and separate osteochondral fragments (joint mice) may migrate within the joint space. Fragments that have migrated often adhere to the synovial lining and may become vascularized and continue to mineralize and enlarge over time. Joint effusion, or joint capsule thickening, may appear as a localized region of soft-tissue swelling centered on the affected joint. A subchondral bone defect is occasionally seen involving the articular surface opposite the primary lesion. These defects are called "kissing lesions." Secondary degenerative joint disease is a common sequela to osteochondrosis.

Gas is occasionally present within the joint space of dogs with shoulder osteochondrosis. This finding is referred to as *the vacuum phenomenon* and is caused by the intraarticular accumulation of nitrogen gas from negative pressure induced by traction on the joint during positioning (see Fig. 15-1).

With osteochondrosis of the lateral trochlea of the talus, the superimposed calcaneus may obscure the lesion in the dorsoplantar view. In this instance, a dorsolateral-plantaromedial oblique, or a flexed dorsoplantar, view can be acquired to provide an unobstructed view of the lesion. Similarly, supinated projections of the shoulder may help with visualization of lesions on the caudal aspect of the humeral head. In the stifle, the fossa for the origin of the long digital extensor muscle is sometimes mistaken for a lateral femoral condyle osteochondrosis lesion because it is superimposed on the dorsolateral aspect of the condyle on both the lateromedial and the caudocranial views.

Cartilage flaps are not visible on survey radiographs unless calcification or ossification of the fragment has occurred. When a nonmineralized cartilage fragment is present, an arthrogram can be used to outline the flap if contrast medium dissects between the fragment and the underlying subchondral bone. Arthrography may also define migrating intraarticular cartilage fragments (see Fig. 15-1, C).[11,12] Newer nonionic and low–osmolar-contrast media provide significantly better arthrographic quality than hyperosmolar, ionic contrast media do because the contrast medium is not diluted as quickly from fluid flux into the joint space.[13] However, because arthroscopy has gained acceptance for the diagnosis and definitive treat-

Box • 15-1

Disorders of the Immature Appendicular Skeleton

Disorders Primarily Affecting Joints

- Osteochondrosis, osteochondritis dissecans
- Elbow dysplasia
  - Ununited coronoid process
  - Fragmented medial coronoid process
  - Osteochondrosis of the medial humeral condyle
- Hip dysplasia
- Aseptic necrosis of the femoral head (Legg-Calvé-Perthes disease)

Disorders Primarily Affecting Bone

- Malformation or agenesis of single or multiple bones
  - Amelia, hemimelia
  - Ectrodactyly, polydactyly
  - Syndactyly
- Skeletal disorders of unknown cause
  - Panosteitis
  - Hypertrophic osteodystrophy
- Metabolic and other generalized disorders
  - Nutritional secondary hyperparathyroidism
  - Congenital hypothyroidism
  - Pituitary dwarfism
  - Mucopolysaccharidosis
  - Osteogenesis imperfecta
  - Osteopetrosis
- Metaphyseal and epiphyseal dysplasias
  - Osteochondrodysplasias
  - Chondrodysplasia: Alaskan Malamute, Norwegian Elkhound, Cocker Spaniel, English Pointer, Great Pyrenees
  - Oculoskeletal dysplasia: Labrador Retriever, Samoyed
  - Osteochondral dysplasia: Scottish Fold cats, Scottish Deerhounds, Bull Terriers
  - Hypochondroplasia: Irish Setters
  - Multiple epiphyseal dysplasia: Beagles
  - Multiple cartilaginous exostoses
  - Retained cartilage cores
  - Incomplete ossification of the humeral condyle: Spaniels, other breeds

ment of osteochondrosis, arthrography is now used less commonly.[14,15]

Elbow Dysplasia

Elbow dysplasia is a nonspecific term referring to a triad of developmental lesions that include ununited anconeal process, fragmented medial coronoid process of the ulna, and osteochondrosis of the distomedial aspect of the humeral trochlea. Although osteochondrosis has previously been implicated as the cause of all three disorders, asynchronous growth of the radius and ulna and proximal ulnar dysplasia resulting in an elliptically shaped ulnar notch have more recently been suggested as implicating factors.[3,16-20] Elbow joint incongruity may result in nonuniform contact of articulating surfaces, leading to nonunion of the anconeal process or separation or fragmentation of the medial coronoid process.[19,21] Although severe incongruity can be seen radiographically, computed tomography of the elbow seems to be more sensitive.[22,23] One, two, or all three of the primary lesions may be present in the same animal, and both elbow joints are commonly affected.

Ununited Anconeal Process

Large-breed dogs that normally have a separate anconeal ossification center early in development are at greater risk for ununited anconeal process (Fig. 15-5). German shepherd dogs are overrepresented, although the lesion occurs in other breeds as well. The anconeal process should normally be fused to the olecranon of the ulna by 150 days of age. The anconeal center of ossification fails to fuse by this time in dogs with ununited anconeal process. A flexed lateral radiograph in addition to routine lateral and craniocaudal views of the elbow should be included in the radiographic examination. The flexed lateral view displaces the medial epicondylar physis away from the anconeus, thereby decreasing the possibility that an overlying epicondylar physeal line may be confused with an ununited anconeal process margin.

Radiographic Signs

The primary radiographic finding is best seen on the lateral view and consists of a radiolucent line separating the anconeal process from the olecranon in dogs older than 150 days. This lucent line can be sharply defined, or it may appear irregular and of variable width. Degenerative joint disease of the elbow is a common sequela, and periarticular new bone production from osteoarthrosis may partially obscure the lucency between the ulna and the anconeal process.[24-26]

Fragmented Medial Coronoid Process

Fragmented medial coronoid process is the most common developmental disorder involving the elbow joint. It primarily affects medium- and large-breed dogs and has a significantly higher incidence in males. Clinical signs may be apparent as early as 4 to 6 months of age. Radiographic visualization of the coronoid fragment is usually not possible because of superimposition of the medial coronoid process on the radius, superimposition of proliferative new bone from degenerative joint disease on the coronoid fragment, or failure of the x-ray beam to strike the fragment plane in a parallel fashion (Fig. 15-6). In addition, coronoid fragments that consist mostly of cartilage or that are still partially attached cannot be seen. In most instances, the radiographic diagnosis of fragmented medial coronoid process is indirectly made through the recognition of secondary degenerative changes that accompany the primary lesion.

Both a neutral lateral and a craniocaudal radiograph of both elbow joints should be made. In addition, a flexed lateral radiograph facilitates visualization of new bone formation on the proximal margin of the anconeal process. Flexing the elbow, however, induces a mild degree of rotation that can partially obscure the medial coronoid margin. A cranial 25-degree lateral-caudomedial oblique view can also be obtained to highlight the medial coronoid region and fragmented coronoid process.[27] Although joint incongruity can be seen in association with fragmented coronoid process, caution should be used to prevent overreading of this finding. On the lateral view, the normal overlapping lucent lines representing the complex elbow joint margins can be confused with joint incongruity when even mild positioning obliquity is present. Computed tomography is now being regularly used to diagnose fragmented medial coronoid process and is more sensitive than survey radiography for detecting the coronoid fragment.[28-30]

Radiographic Signs

Primary radiographic signs include an abnormal contour, or poor definition, of the cranial margin of the medial coronoid process on the lateral view. Often the margin, which is

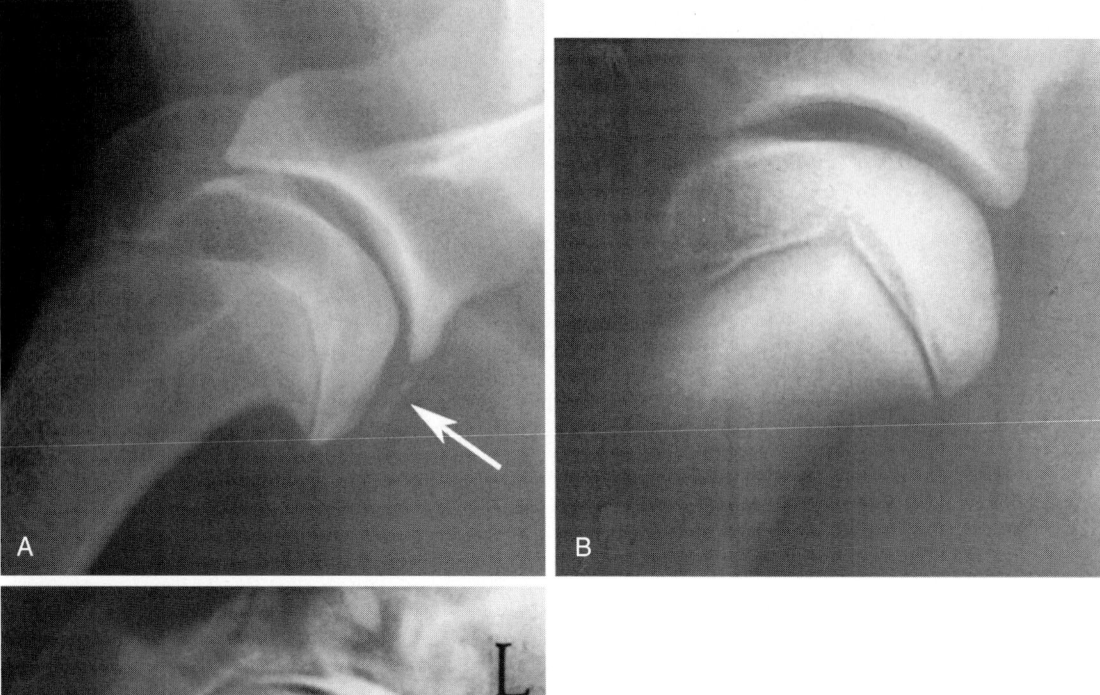

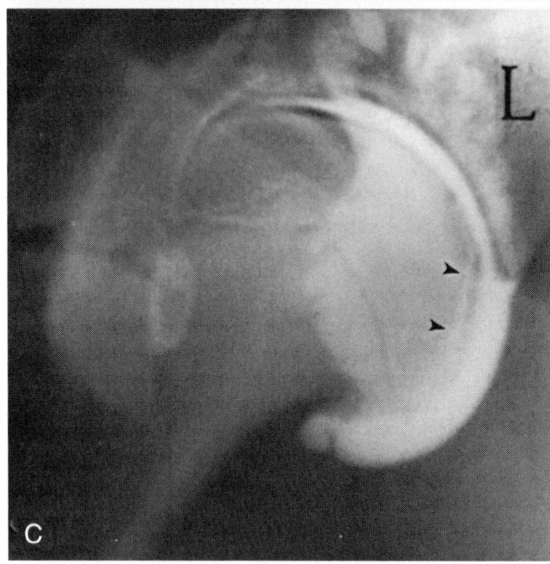

Fig. 15-1 Osteochondrosis of the shoulder. **A,** An ill-defined, mineralized cartilage flap adjacent to the caudal humeral head *(arrow)*. The subchondral bone is nonuniformly sclerotic and has an irregular flattened margin. **B,** A slightly flattened caudal humeral head but no obvious flap. In an arthrogram **(C)** on the same shoulder as that in **B,** contrast medium dissects beneath a cartilage flap *(arrows)*.

radiographically distinct in normal dogs, cannot be followed proximally to the articular surface in affected animals. On the craniocaudal view, the medial margin of the medial coronoid process may appear blunted or rounded. A separate osseous body, representing the fractured coronoid process, is rarely seen. Joint incongruity or subluxation may also be present and appears as a "stair step" lesion between the ulna and the radial head on the lateral view. Secondary radiographic signs include osteophyte formation on the proximal margin of the anconeal process as one of the earliest signs of degenerative joint disease. Similar new bone is often present on the caudal surface of the lateral epicondyle. Subchondral bone sclerosis also develops adjacent to the trochlear notch and the proximal radioulnar articulation near the lateral coronoid process. These secondary findings are best appreciated on the lateral view. A large osteophyte may arise from the medial coronoid margin on the craniocaudal view in addition to the more generalized degenerative periarticular osteophyte production.[21,26,29,31,32]

Aseptic Necrosis of the Femoral Head (Legg-Calvé-Perthes Disease)

Aseptic necrosis of the femoral head occurs in adolescent toy and small-breed dogs (Fig. 15-7). Compromised blood supply to the femoral capital epiphysis causes necrosis of subchondral bone while overlying articular cartilage continues to grow. Revascularization occurs in an attempt to repair the defect and removal of necrotic bone cause decreased opacity in the affected femoral head. Incomplete removal of necrotic bone and invasion of granulation tissue interfere with healing, resulting in a misshapen femoral head of nonuniform opacity.[33,34]

Radiographic Signs

As with many of the other developmental skeletal disorders, the radiographic findings of aseptic necrosis of the femoral head vary with the duration of the lesion. Radiographs of the hip joints may appear normal early in the course of the disease. Early in the progression of the disease, linear lucencies can be detected within the subchondral bone deep within the femoral head. Areas of decreased opacity may also appear in both the femoral epiphysis and the metaphysis. Flattening and irregularity of the femoral head and neck become apparent as the affected bone remodels and collapses on itself. Remodeling of the femoral head may cause coxofemoral joint space widening and subluxation. Fragmentation of the femoral head may eventually occur from pathologic fracture. Muscle atrophy and radiographic findings associated with degenerative joint disease

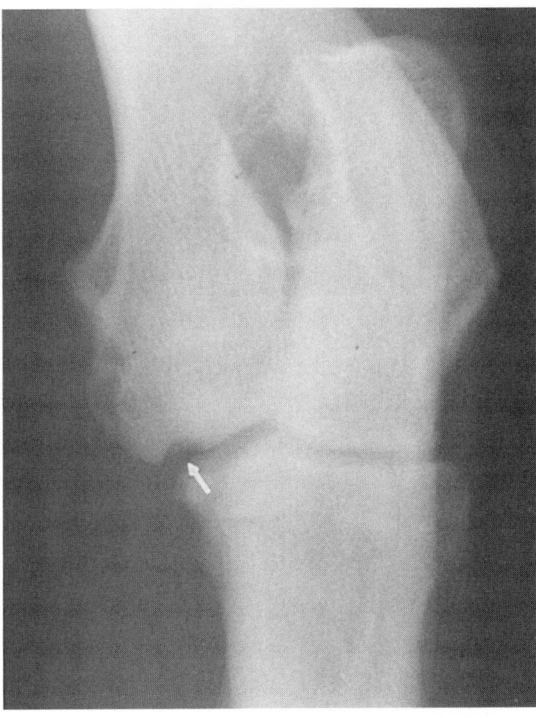

Fig. 15-2 Osteochondrosis of the medial humeral condyle. A well-defined lucent concavity in the subchondral bone of the medial humeral condyle *(arrow)* can be visualized.

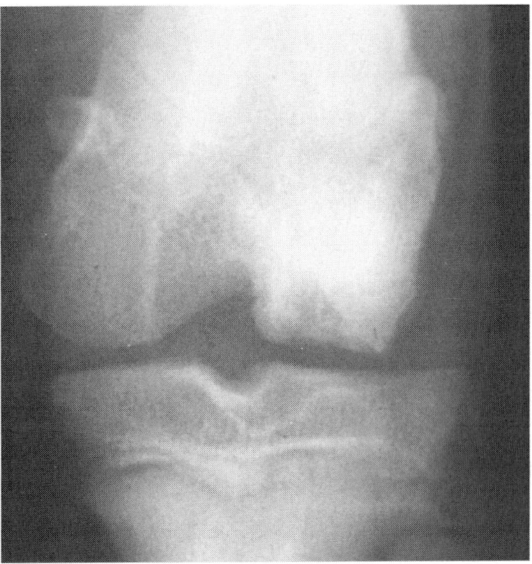

Fig. 15-3 Osteochondrosis of the lateral femoral condyle. The subchondral bone of the lateral femoral condyle is flattened. Irregular lucent areas in the condyle are surrounded by sclerosis.

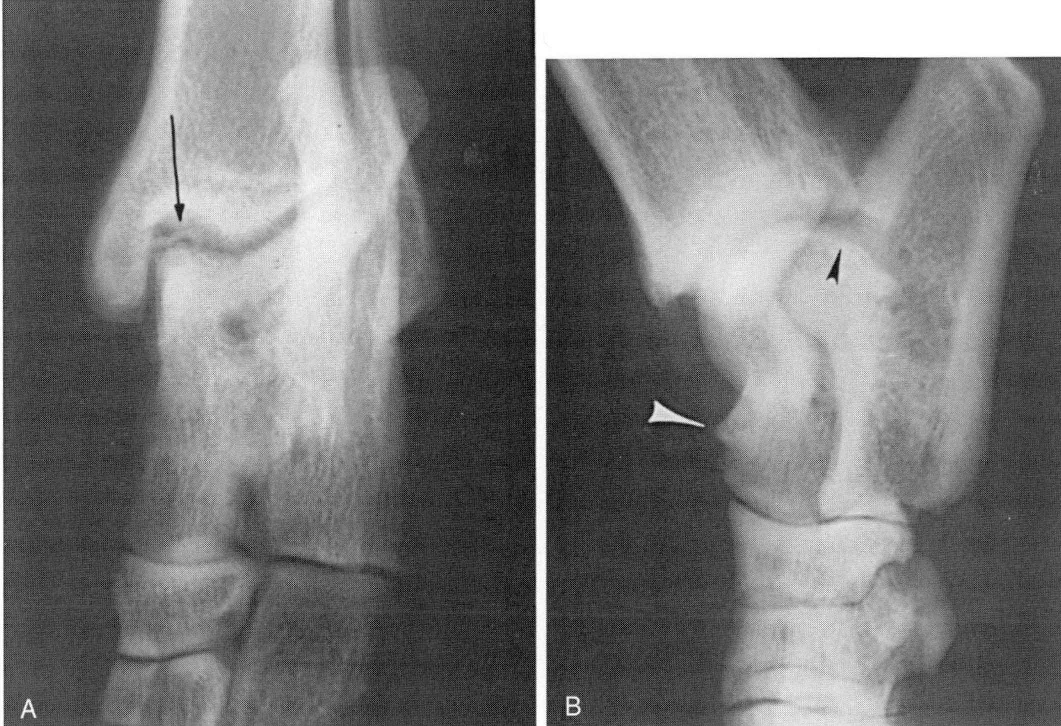

Fig. 15-4 Osteochondrosis the medial trochlea of the talus. On the dorsoplantar view **(A)**, a small bone flap is present proximal to the medial trochlear ridge of the talus *(arrow)*. Adjacent to the flap the bone is irregular in contour, with lucency surrounded by sclerosis. Flattening of the trochlear ridge and concurrent widening of the tarsocrural joint *(black arrow)* are seen on the lateral view **(B)**. Osteophyte formation is present on the cranial and caudal margins of the distal tibia and on the dorsal surface of the talus *(white arrow)*.

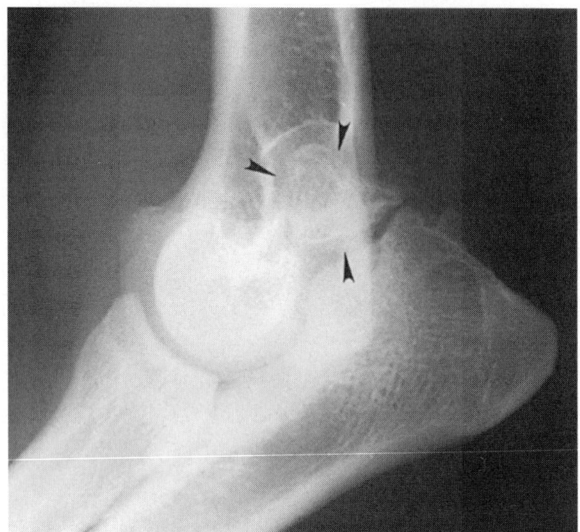

Fig. 15-5 Ununited anconeal process. *Arrows* outline the anconeal process, which is separate from the proximal ulna. The bone margins at the site of separation are smooth and sclerotic, suggesting chronicity.

usually develop. Radiographic evaluation of both hips is indicated because this disease may be bilateral.

DISORDERS PRIMARILY AFFECTING BONE

Agenesis or Malformation of Single or Multiple Bones

Agenesis and Hypoplasia

Complete agenesis, partial agenesis, or hypoplasia of a long bone may occur (Fig. 15-8). The radius, tibia, and ulna are most often involved, although the metacarpal and metatarsal bones can also be affected. These anomalies, which can usually be detected at or shortly after birth, may be inherited but are more often a result of in utero environmental factors.

Radiographic Signs The affected bone or bones are conspicuously absent and the limb is usually malformed and shorter than normal. Limb curvature and joint malformation may also be present.

Polymelia

This general term denotes supernumerary limbs or parts of a limb. Polydactyly, the presence of an excess number of digits, is the most common form of polymelia and is most often seen in cats. A few breeds of dogs, such as the Great Pyrenees, have also been bred to retain this trait. The anomaly is generally clinically insignificant.

Radiographic Signs Radiographic signs of polymelia vary according to the bone or bones involved. Findings of polydactyly include a greater-than-normal number of digits, usually arising on the medial side of the limb. Supernumerary digits may include complete or partial metacarpal/metatarsal bones and variable numbers of phalanges.

DISORDERS OF UNKNOWN ETIOLOGY

Panosteitis

Panosteitis is a self-limiting disease that affects the long bones of primarily young, large-breed dogs (Fig. 15-9). Males are affected four times more often than are females, and the lesion is most common in German Shepherd dogs. Dogs between the ages of 5 and 12 months are most often affected; however, afflicted dogs as young as 2 months and as old as 7 years have been reported. Panosteitis lesions may be solitary, affect multiple sites in a single bone, or be multifocal in multiple bones. Although the lesions can affect any part of the diaphysis of a long bone, they often originate and are most pronounced near the nutrient foramen. Bone involvement is often sequential, and the disease may be protracted over several months, with lesions resolving in some areas while developing in others. Severity and location of radiographic lesions do not necessarily correlate with the severity of clinical signs, and the most clinically affected limb may not have the most pronounced radiographic lesions.[35,36] The term *panosteitis* is a misnomer in that histologically no evidence of an inflammatory response is present. Microscopically, medullary, endosteal, and periosteal osteoblastic and fibroblastic activity is increased.

Radiographic Signs

Early in the course of the disease, blurring and accentuation of trabecular bone of the affected long bone are noted. Circumscribed nodular opacities similar in opacity to cortical bone form within the diaphyseal medullary cavity of long bones, often near nutrient foramina. As the lesion progresses, medullary opacities become more diffuse and homogeneous. Smooth, continuous periosteal new bone formation develops in the diaphysis of affected bones in one third to one half of dogs. Late in the disease opacities resolve, leaving coarse, thickened trabecular bone that eventually assumes a normal appearance. Cortical thickening may persist as periosteal new bone remodels. These findings should not be confused with the metaphyseal irregularities recently reported as a common incidental lesion in young Newfoundlands. Radiolucent zones surrounded by radiopaque osseous trabeculae have been described in the distal radius and ulna of 46% of asymptomatic Newfoundlands.[37]

Hypertrophic Osteodystrophy

Hypertrophic osteodystrophy is a systemic illness that usually affects large- and giant-breed dogs between the ages of 2 and 7 months. The cause is unknown, but oversupplementation of minerals and vitamins, hypovitaminosis C, and suppurative inflammation without isolation of infectious agents have all been proposed.[38-44] More recently, canine distemper virus has been isolated from metaphyseal bone cells in affected animals and has been suggested as a causative factor.[45-47] Clinical signs, including marked pyrexia, diarrhea, footpad hyperkeratosis, leukocytosis, anemia, and pneumonia, are occasionally seen with hypertrophic osteopathy, lending credibility to the possibility of a systemic infection as a cause for this disease.[44]

Resulting bone lesions are generally bilaterally symmetric and involve the metaphyses of long bones, particularly the distal radius, ulna, and tibia (Fig. 15-10). The costochondral junctions, the metacarpal/metatarsal bones, and the craniomandibular region may also be involved. Craniomandibular osteopathy may, in fact, be a different clinical manifestation of hypertrophic osteodystrophy.

Although hypertrophic osteodystrophy is usually self-limiting and resolves after a few weeks, more severe involvement can ultimately result in abnormal/premature physeal closure and subsequent skeletal deformity. Histologically, lesions in the metaphyses consist of a neutrophilic inflammatory response associated with necrosis, hemorrhage, and increased osteoclast numbers. Collapse of necrotic metaphyseal trabecular bone and subperiosteal hemorrhage are also seen.[44]

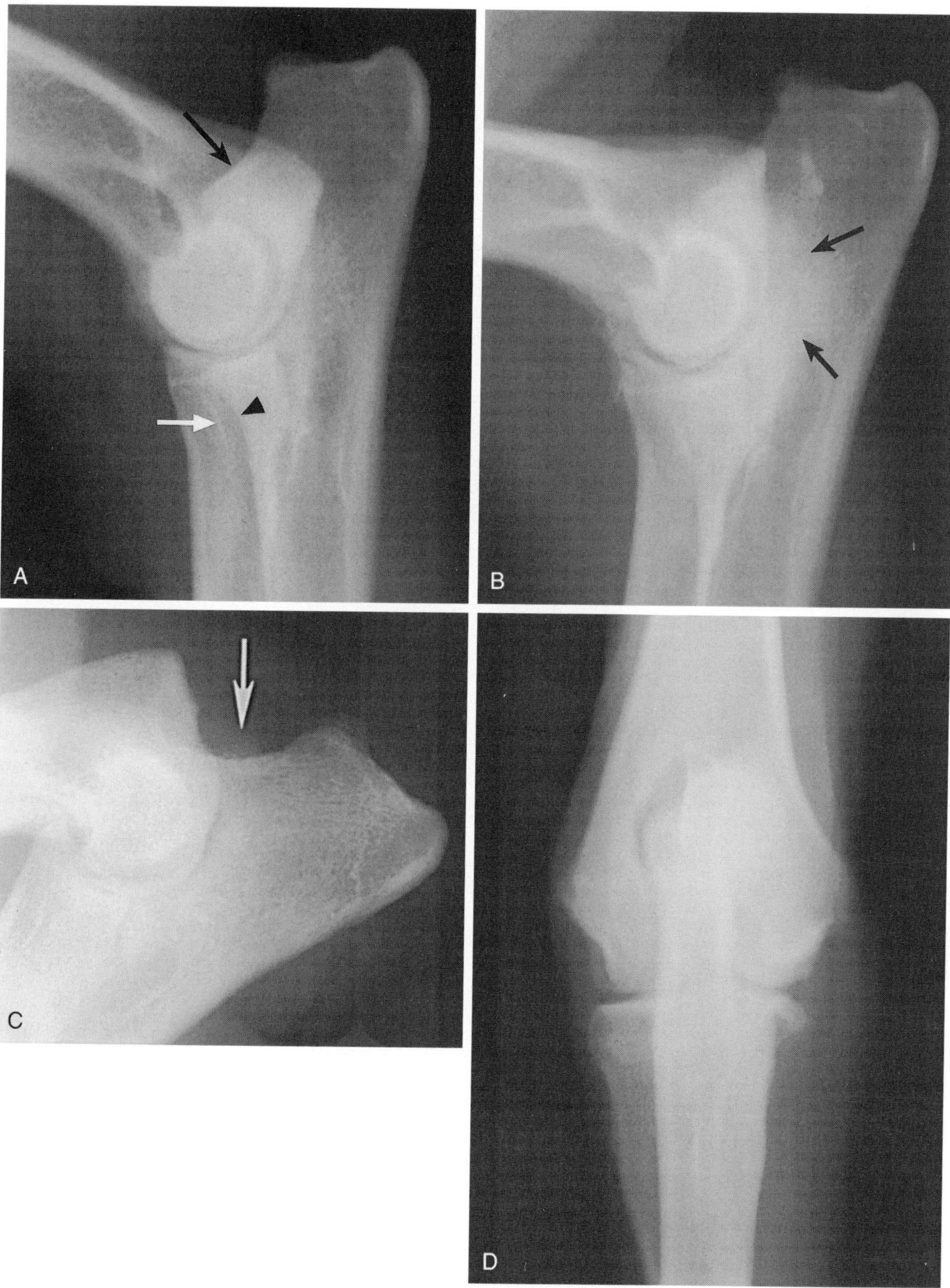

Fig. 15-6 Fragmented medial coronoid process. **A,** Lateral view of a normal elbow. The cranial edge of the medial coronoid process *(black arrowhead)* has a distinct margin that is superimposed on the head of the radius. The adjacent thin opaque line represents the radial tuberosity *(white arrow)*. The proximal margin of the anconeal process *(black arrow)* is also distinct despite being superimposed on the medial and lateral epicondyles of the humerus. **B,** Fragmented medial coronoid process with secondary degenerative changes. The margins of the medial coronoid and anconeal processes are indistinct compared with those in Figure 15-6, *A*. Subchondral bone sclerosis is also present adjacent to the ulnar notch *(arrows)*. Periarticular osteophyte formation is evident on the cranial margin of the radial head. **C,** Visualization of periosteal new bone on the proximal margin of the anconeal process *(arrow)* is facilitated by flexing the elbow joint. **D,** A large osteophyte arises from the medial margin of the ulna on a craniocaudal view. This osteophyte should not be misinterpreted as the coronoid fragment.

Continued

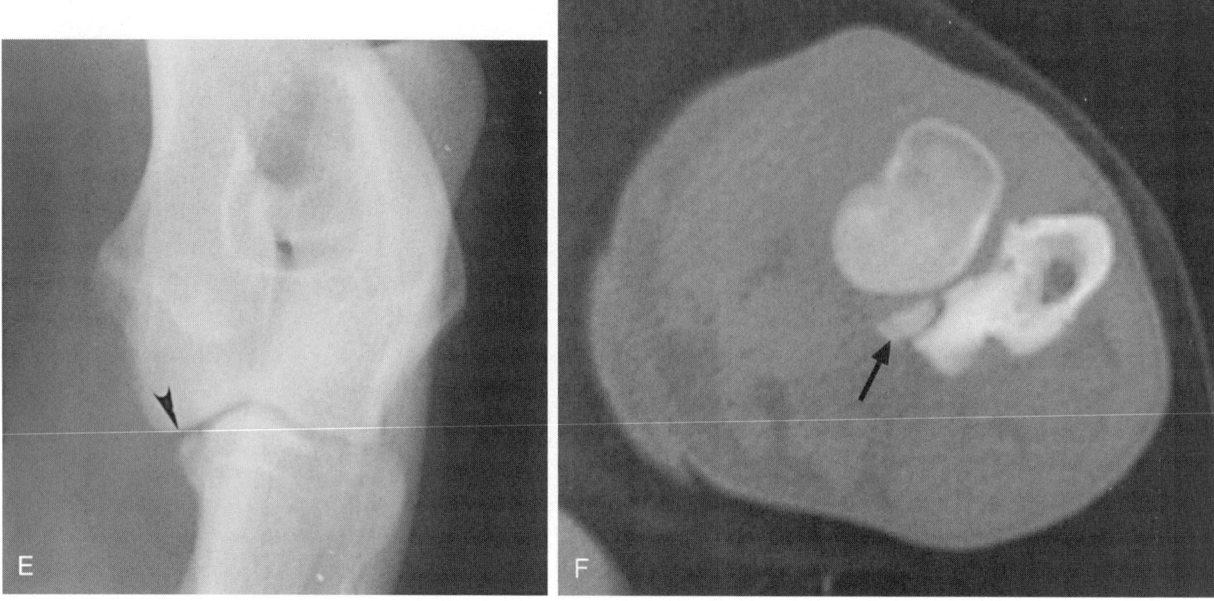

Fig. 15-6, cont'd E, Fragmentation of the coronoid process can occasionally be seen on a craniolateral, caudomedial, oblique view *(arrow)*. F, A computed tomography image of the elbow from a dog with a fragmented medial coronoid process and degenerative joint disease. The fragmented coronoid process *(arrow)* is easily seen. In addition, the basilar part of the coronoid process is sclerotic and remodeled.

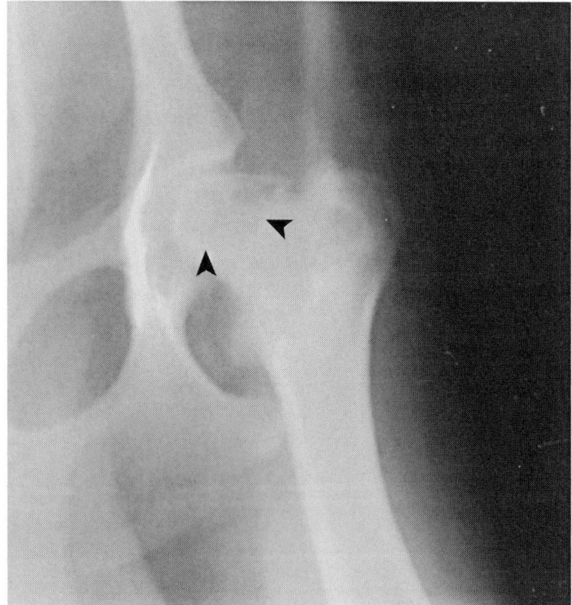

Fig. 15-7 Aseptic necrosis of the left femoral head. The femoral head contains a large radiolucent area with surrounding sclerosis *(arrows)*. Flattening of the weight-bearing surface of the femoral head is visible, and the joint space is widened. Osteophytes are present on the femoral neck.

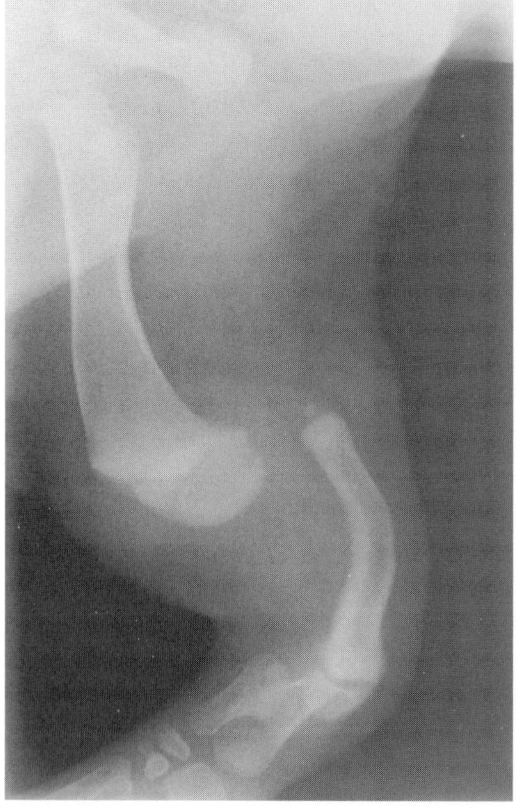

Fig. 15-8 Tibial agenesis in a young dog. The tibia is not formed and the fibula is misshapen. The proximal fibular epiphysis is hypoplastic and poorly mineralized. Tibial agenesis has led to stifle and tarsocrural joint malformation as well as limb shortening and angular deformity.

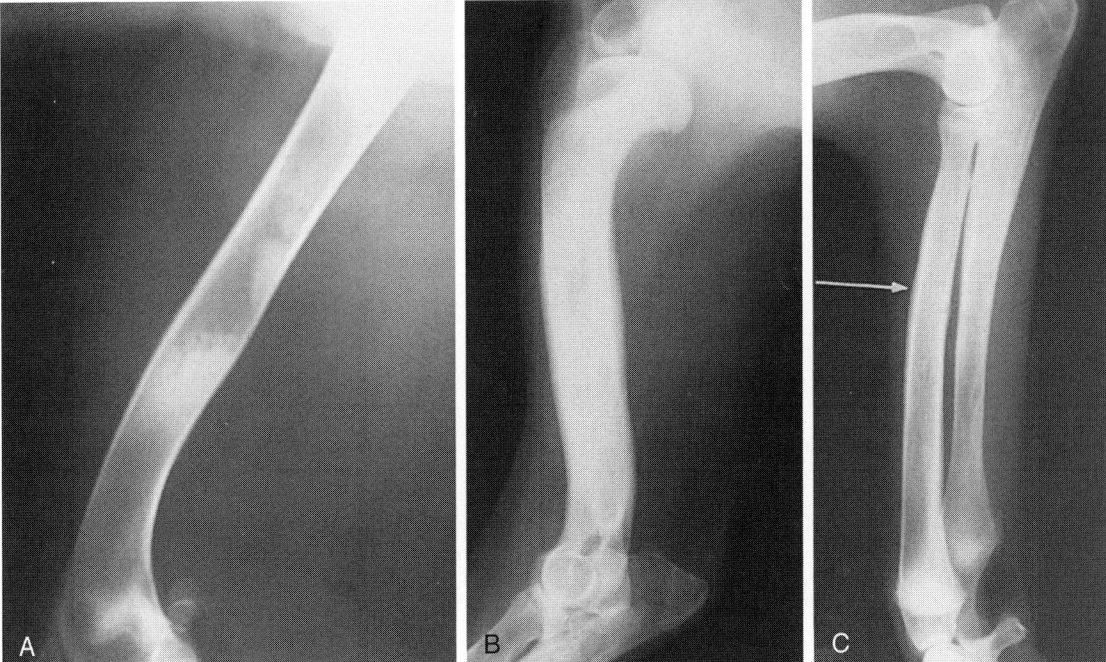

Fig. 15-9 Stages of panosteitis. **A,** Early stage in a femur. Circumscribed increased opacity is visible in the mid-diaphysis and the proximal diaphysis. **B,** Middle stage in a humerus. Diffuse increased opacity of the entire diaphysis and a continuous periosteal new bone formation on the diaphysis are present. **C,** Later stage in radius and ulna. Less-intense but still apparent increased opacity is visible, primarily in the proximal radius and ulna. Mild periosteal new bone formation is present on the cranial radius *(arrow)*.

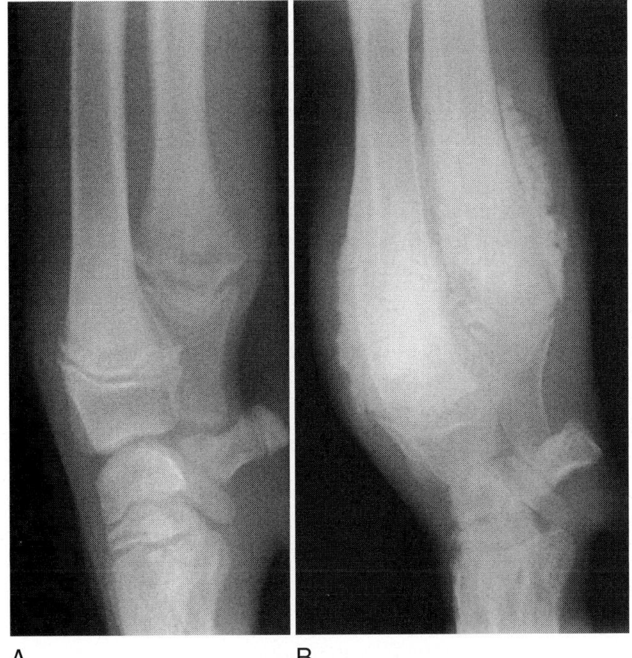

Fig. 15-10 Hypertrophic osteodystrophy. **A,** Acute phase. Irregular radiolucent regions are evident in the distal radial and ulnar metaphyses, proximal to the physis. **B,** Chronic phase. An irregular, pallisading periosteal productive response surrounds the radial and ulnar metaphyses. The physes are relatively unaffected.

Radiographic Signs

Early radiographic signs include transversely oriented lucent zones within the metaphysis that are parallel and adjacent to the physes (see Fig. 15-10, *A*). These are usually best seen in the distal radius and ulna, and this appearance is sometimes referred to as the "double physis" sign. A thin margin of subchondral bone sclerosis may parallel the lucent zone and is caused by collapse of necrotic trabecular bone. Irregular periosteal new bone forms around the metaphysis and is usually distinct and separate from the underlying cortex in the earlier stages of the disease. The extent of new metaphyseal bone formation depends on the severity and duration of the disorder, and such formation may extend to the diaphysis in severely affected dogs (see Fig. 15-10, *B*). Diffuse soft-tissue swelling can be seen centered on the metaphyseal regions. Widening, concavity, and increased opacity of the distal rib ends may be present in some dogs.

METABOLIC AND GENERALIZED BONE DISORDERS

Nutritional Secondary Hyperparathyroidism

Nutritional secondary hyperparathyroidism is caused by a diet that is either calcium deficient or calcium/phosphorus imbalanced. Inadequate dietary calcium intake causes an increase in parathyroid hormone. This, in turn, results in bone calcium resorption and generalized osteomalacia (Fig. 15-11). The skeletal changes are diffuse and generalized.[38,48,49]

Radiographic Signs

Bone opacity is generally decreased, and cortices may appear abnormally thin. In severely affected animals, bone opacity

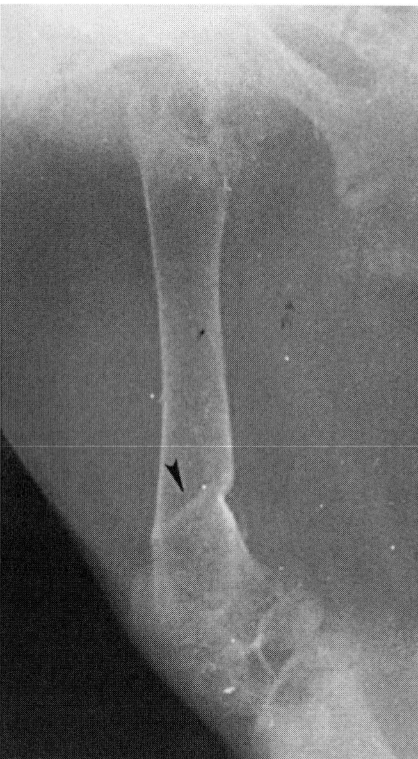

Fig. 15-11 Nutritional secondary hyperparathyroidism. Overall bone opacity of the femur is decreased and cortices are thin. An opaque line in the distal femur *(arrow)* with angulation at this site indicates a pathologic folding fracture.

may be similar to that of soft tissue. A loss of definition of the normally dense dental lamina may also occur. Spinal deformity and pathologic folding fractures of the appendicular and the axial skeleton are common.

Congenital Hypothyroidism

Congenital hypothyroidism is an uncommon developmental disorder that has been reported in Boxers, Scottish Deerhounds, Giant Schnauzers, Affenpinschers, and Great Danes and is caused by thyroid aplasia or hypoplasia (Fig. 15-12).[50-53] Clinically the dogs are disproportionate, short-limbed dwarves with bowed limbs and long necks and trunks.

Radiographic Signs

Radiographic findings consist of epiphyseal dysplasia that appears as reduced or delayed ossification of the epiphyseal cartilage model. This is most easily seen in the proximal tibia and the humeral and femoral condyles. Cuboid bone ossification in the carpus and tarsus is also delayed. Vertebral bodies appear shorter than normal as a result of endplate dysplasia. The skull may appear shorter and broader than normal. Secondary degenerative joint disease may be seen.

Mucopolysaccharidosis

Mucopolysaccharidosis represents a loosely related group of uncommon autosomal recessive inherited disorders that result in a reduction or absence of glycosaminoglycan catabolism (Fig. 15-13). Lysosomal degradation of these mucopolysaccharides is necessary for normal growth in developing animals, and the abnormal metabolism leads to chronic, progressive, multisystemic disease. More than 10 forms are recognized in human beings, each produced by a different enzyme defect. Many of these have also been identified in dogs and cats.[54-61]

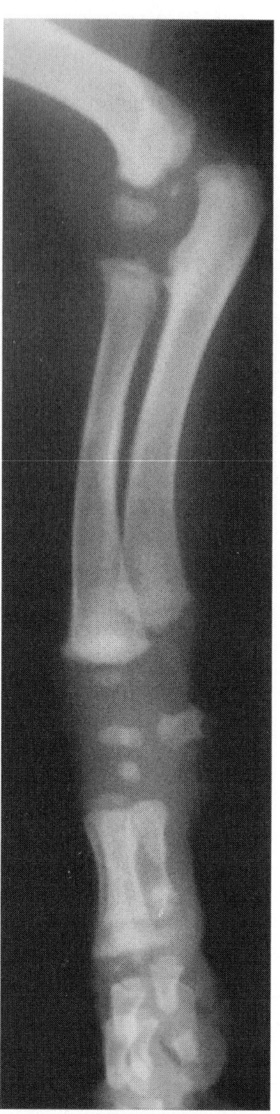

Fig. 15-12 Congenital hypothyroidism in a skeletally immature dog. Mineralization of the long bone epiphyses and cuboid bones of the carpus is markedly reduced. (From Saunders H: The radiographic appearance of canine congenital hypothyroidism: skeletal changes with delayed treatment, *Vet Radiol* 32:171, 1991.)

The most pronounced clinical manifestations involve the musculoskeletal, ocular, neurologic, hepatic, and cardiovascular systems. Affected animals are often stunted and lame and have visual deficits. Clinical manifestations include disproportionate dwarfism and facial dysmorphia, which includes a broad maxilla, widespread eyes, a flat nose, and short ears. Hyperextension of the distal extremity joints occurs as a result of joint laxity.

Radiographic Signs

Radiographic changes of mucopolysaccharidosis involve both the axial and the appendicular skeleton. Generalized epiphyseal dysplasia is present, involving long bones and vertebral endplates. Findings include delayed and incomplete mineralization of the epiphyseal cartilage model. Ossified regions of the epiphyses are smaller than normal and have a nonuniform opacity with a granular appearance. Vertebral bodies appear cuboid and shorter than normal. The maxilla is short and flattened; the frontal sinuses may be small or absent. Progressive degenerative joint disease occurs as a result of the epiphyseal

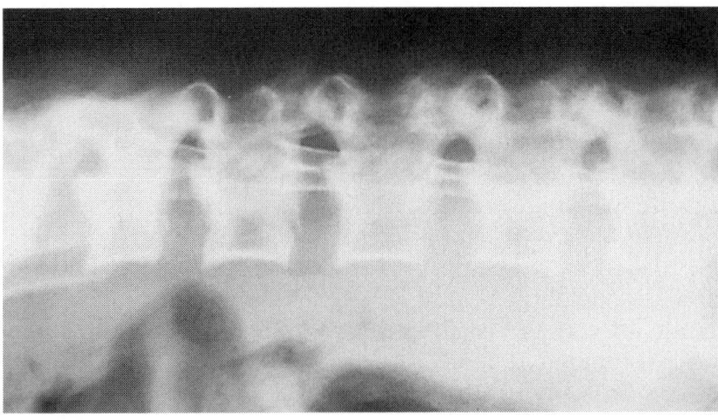

Fig. 15-13 Lateral lumbar spine of a cat with mucopolysaccharidosis. The vertebral bodies are short and intervertebral disk spaces are wider than normal as a result of delayed endplate mineralization from epiphyseal dysplasia. Similar findings were present in the epiphyses of long bones.

malformations. Hip subluxation or luxation may result from femoral head epiphysis remodeling. Ventral, bridging spondylosis is seen in older animals.[58]

Osteogenesis Imperfecta

Osteogenesis imperfecta is a rare, generalized multisystemic heritable disease caused by a structural defect in type 1 collagen, which constitutes the majority of the nonmineral bone matrix.[62-64] Affected animals have stunted growth, generalized muscle atrophy, and weakness and are at risk for pathologic fractures. Teeth may also appear pink. Affected animals may have a recurring history of fractures.

Radiographic Signs

A generalized decrease in bone opacity is present, and long bone cortices are thin. Pathologic fractures are common and may be associated with excessively opaque callus formation and medullary sclerosis. Findings are similar to and can be confused with generalized bone mineral loss from secondary hyperparathyroidism.

Osteopetrosis

Osteopetrosis is a rare, inherited metabolic bone disease that is presumed to be caused by abnormal osteoclast function (Fig. 15-14).[65] Affected animals have a generalized increase in bone opacity specifically affecting medullary cavities. A resulting decrease in the number of normal hematopoietic cells subsequently occurs, leading to myelophthisic anemia.

In cats, varying degrees of osteosclerosis with nonregenerative anemia induced by feline leukemia virus have also been reported, and the radiographic appearance is identical to that described for osteopetrosis.[66,67] Other reports describe generalized osteosclerosis as possibly being a paraneoplastic phenomenon.[68]

Until more information is obtained, the finding of generalized osteosclerosis in cats should be considered nonspecific, but the fact that the bone changes may be attributable to a more serious condition should be considered.

Radiographic Signs

Bone opacity is generally increased, particularly in medullary cavities. The normal trabecular pattern is diminished as a result of the uniform increase in bone opacity, and the internal cortical margins become indistinct. In some animals, the medullary cavity retains normal opacity in the central diaphyseal region.

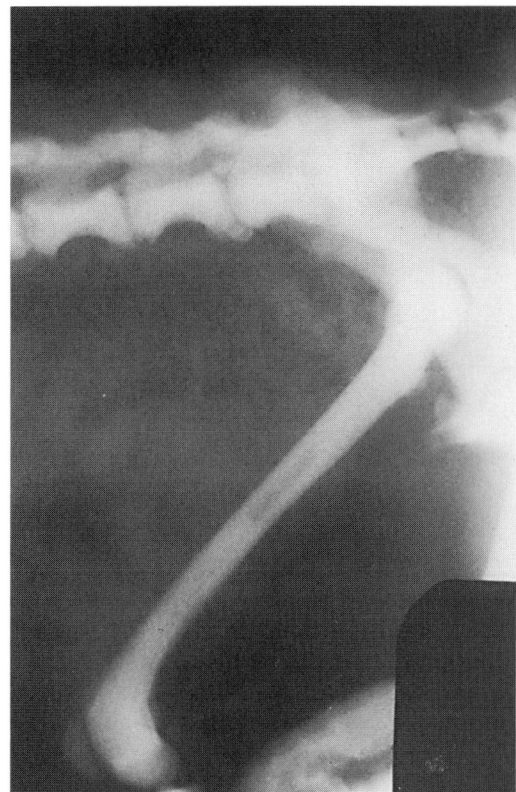

Fig. 15-14 Osteopetrosis in a cat. A generalized increase in bone opacity is visible involving the appendicular and the axial skeleton. A loss of corticomedullary junction definition is attributable to increased medullary opacity. In this example, a small central diaphyseal region of the femoral medullary cavity is not yet affected and appears less opaque than surrounding bone.

METAPHYSEAL AND EPIPHYSEAL DYSPLASIAS

Osteochondral Dysplasias

Osteochondral dysplasias include chondrodysplasia, osteochondrodysplasia, enchondrodystrophy, multiple enchondromatosis, oculoskeletal dysplasia, hypochondroplasia, multiple epiphyseal dysplasia, and pseudoachondroplasia. Chondrodysplasia and osteochondrodysplasia result in disproportionate dwarfism and have been reported in a number of breeds, including Alaskan Malamutes, Norwegian Elkhounds, Great Pyrenees, Scottish Deerhounds, Bull Terriers, and Scottish Fold cats.[69-76] Similar disorders have been described in Irish Setters (hypochondroplasia), English Pointers (enchondrodystrophy), and Miniature Poodles (multiple enchondromatosis). Chondrodysplasia associated with ocular defects has been described in Labrador retrievers, Samoyeds, and German Shepherd dogs. Although these disorders may sometimes appear clinically and radiographically similar, they represent a histologically and biochemically heterogeneous group of diseases. Characterization is further complicated by the variety of classification systems that were used to describe these lesions when they were originally reported.

In almost all instances in which microscopic findings have been described, marked alterations in chondrocyte morphologic characteristics and cartilage architecture are present. Although many of these disorders are inherited and known to be single autosomal recessive defects, others have not been

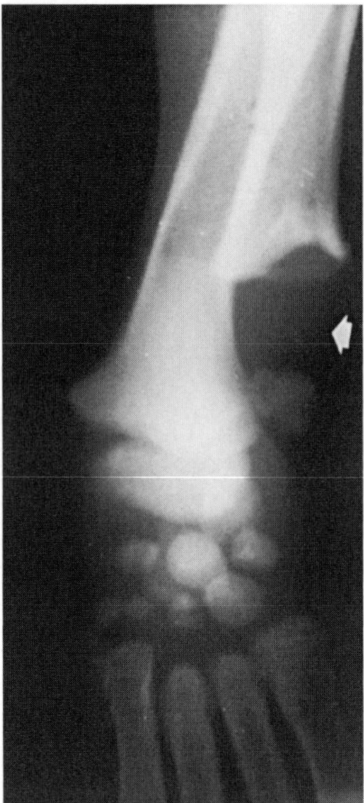

Fig. 15-15 Chondrodysplasia in an Alaskan Malamute. The distal ulnar metaphysis is flattened and the physis is much wider than normal *(arrow)*. The carpal bones are smaller in size than those in normal littermates.

adequately characterized. In some instances, the genetic defect can also be variably expressed, resulting in a wide variation in severity of clinical signs. Distinguishing between chondrodystrophoid dogs, those that have been bred for many generations to establish a defect as a breed characteristic, and chondrodysplastic dwarves that sporadically arise from normal parents is important. Following are representative descriptions of some of these latter disorders.

Chondrodysplasia of Alaskan Malamutes

This disorder is transmitted by an autosomal recessive gene, and skeletal abnormalities are accompanied by a macrocytic hemolytic anemia (Fig. 15-15). Limb shortening with cranial and lateral deviation of the forelimbs and enlarged carpi are common clinical signs. Abnormalities appear to be limited to the long bones and the cuboid bones. The skull and spine are radiographically unaffected.

Radiographic Signs

All appendicular growth plates can be affected, but lesions are best seen in the distal ulnar physis and the metaphysis. The distal metaphysis of the radius is flared, and the border is irregular. Trabecular bone is coarse and disorganized, and cortices appear thin. Asynchronous growth of the radius and ulna produces angular limb deformities. Radiographic changes may be detected in dogs as early as 7 to 10 days of age but can be more definitively diagnosed between 5 and 12 weeks of age.[70,72,74,77]

Chondrodysplasia of Norwegian Elkhounds

This is an autosomal recessive disorder of variable expressivity that appears to be fairly widespread.[71,72,74] As with other forms of chondrodysplasia, this disorder produces disproportionate dwarfism but the front limbs may be more affected than the hindlimbs. Unlike the disorder affecting Alaskan Malamutes, this disease also affects the axial skeleton.

Radiographic Signs

Long-bone abnormalities may appear similar to those of Alaskan Malamute chondrodysplasia. Forelimb curvature may be evident by 5 weeks of age. Spinal changes include lipping and pleating of the ventral vertebral body margins and delayed union of vertebral endplates. Costochondral junctions may be prominently flared and cupped. The skull appears radiographically unaffected.

Osteochondrodysplasia of Scottish Fold Cats

This disorder is probably caused by a simple autosomal dominant trait that is expressed to some degree in cats displaying the characteristic folding of the pinna. Affected animals are shorter than normal and have difficulty supporting their weight, gait abnormalities, and a thick, inflexible tail base. Lesions are radiographically evident by 7 weeks of age.

Radiographic Signs

Metaphyses of the metatarsals and metacarpals are distorted and physes are widened. Similar but less pronounced abnormalities are seen involving the phalanges. Shortening of the metacarpi, metatarsi, and phalanges results in decreased limb length. Punctate lucencies within the carpal and tarsal bones may also be seen. Caudal vertebrae are reduced in length and have widened endplates. Secondary degenerative joint disease invariably develops and leads to carpal or tarsal ankylosis in severely affected cats (Fig. 15-16).[78,79]

Ocular Chondrodysplasia of Labrador Retrievers

Ocular chondrodysplasia also appears to be an uncommon autosomal recessive inherited chondrodysplasia.[69,72,75] In addition to typical skeletal changes, ocular manifestations include cataracts, retinal dysplasia, and retinal detachment.

Radiographic Signs

Long-bone shortening is seen, specifically involving the radius and ulna, and is associated with delayed growth of the anconeal and coronoid processes of the ulna and the medial epicondyle of the humerus. Cortical opacity and thickness are reduced, and a retained cartilage core is sometimes present in the distal ulna. Flaring of the ulnar metaphysis and widening of the adjacent growth plate occur. The opacity of the primary spongiosa is increased in all metaphyses. Retarded and asynchronous radial and ulnar elongation leads to the development of radius curvus. The cuboid bones and the epiphyses are misshapen and larger than normal. Ribs are wider than normal, with prominent flaring at the costochondral junction. Hip dysplasia is a common sequel of this disorder. The skull and spine appear to be spared.

Multiple Epiphyseal Dysplasia of Beagles

Multiple epiphyseal dysplasia is a rare hereditary disorder of variable expression that is characterized by a failure of normal epiphyseal ossification (Fig. 15-17). *Pseudoachondroplasia*, reported in young Miniature Poodles, is also considered by some to be a form of multiple epiphyseal dysplasia.[80] Affected individuals have delayed growth and never reach normal size.

Radiographic Signs

Stippling of the epiphyses and irregular epiphyseal margins are evident by 3 weeks of age, with the most pronounced changes in the humeral condyles at 1 to 3 months of age. Epiphyseal alterations are identified in the humerus, femur,

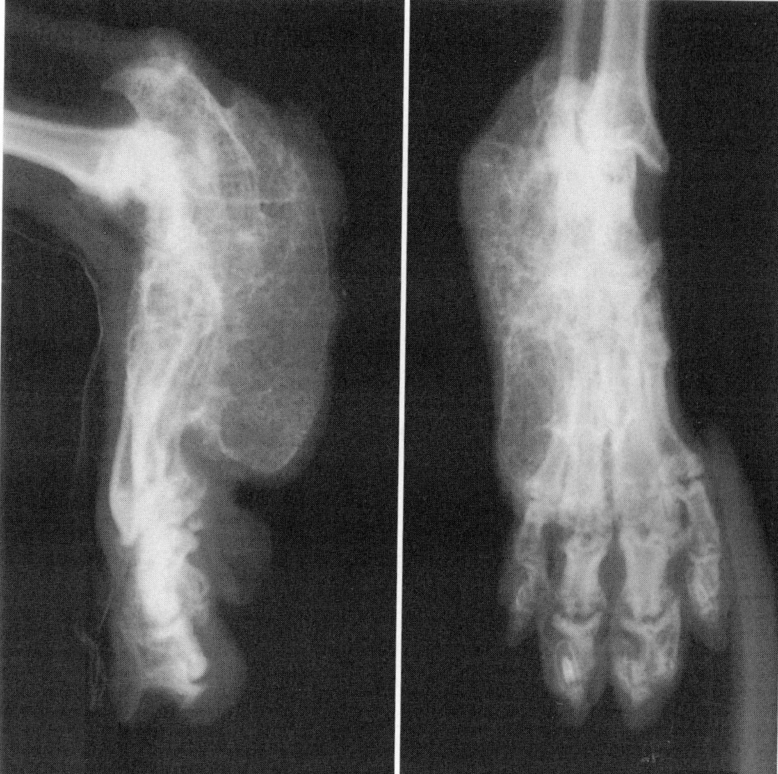

Fig. 15-16 Scottish Fold osteochondral dysplasia. Metatarsal bones are short and misshapen. Phalanges also appear to be affected. Marked secondary degenerative changes are present at all levels from the tarsocrural joint distally. The large mass of new bone in the plantarolateral aspect of the limb contributes to cuboidal bone fusion and tarsal ankylosis.

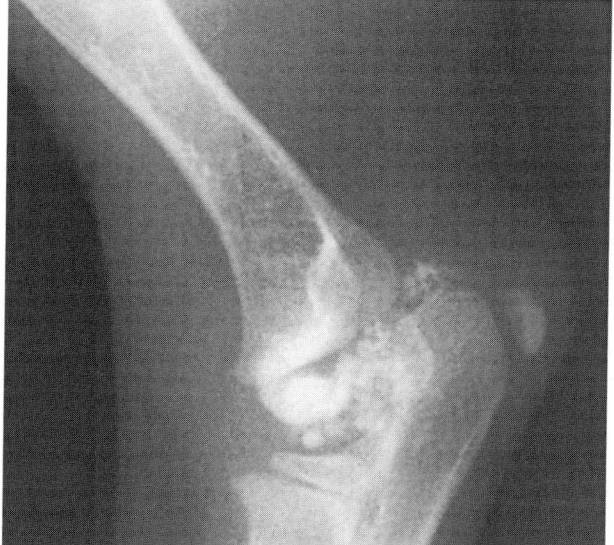

Fig. 15-17 Epiphyseal dysplasia in a 2-month-old Beagle. The distal humeral epiphysis consists of rounded, sclerotic centers of bone formation. The proximal radial and olecranon physes have a normal appearance.

metacarpal and metatarsal bones, and occasionally the vertebrae. Similar stippling may also be seen in the carpal and tarsal bones in some dogs. Affected epiphyses eventually mineralize but are moderately deformed. Aberrant separate centers of ossification that eventually fuse with the normal ossification centers have also been described. Hip dysplasia appears to develop in most affected dogs, and degenerative joint disease of other joints is a typical sequel to the primary disease.[81-83]

Multiple Cartilaginous Exostosis

Multiple cartilaginous exostosis is a benign proliferative disease of bone and cartilage (Fig. 15-18). Hereditary transmission of the disease is suspected in dogs.[84] Any bone that develops by endochondral ossification may be affected, and simultaneous involvement in multiple bones is common. Chondrocytes are pushed into the metaphyses and do not differentiate into osteoblasts. Instead, these cartilage islands continue to proliferate as cartilaginous masses that eventually ossify. Growth usually ceases once the animal has reached maturity, resulting in nonpainful bony protuberances throughout the skeleton. The bone lesions are of no clinical significance unless they arise in an area in which function could be compromised, such as the spinal canal and the trachea. Most exostoses remain inert once the dog has matured, but malignant transformation has been reported.[85,86] Several atypical examples of multiple cartilaginous exostoses have been reported.[87] One was a 2-year-old Great Dane who developed multiple cartilaginous exostoses after reaching skeletal maturity. The exostoses continued to grow, with some bridging of physeal regions and irregular margins. Another was a 4-month-old Border Collie that had tumors with a stippled appearance that were not contiguous with adjacent bone. The microscopic appearance in both dogs was consistent with multiple cartilaginous exostoses. More recently, three mixed-breed dogs from the same litter developed symmetrical, semiannular, and annular osteochondromas that accompanied limb shortening and angular deformity.[88] A similar disorder is seen in mature cats, and a viral etiology has been proposed.[79,89] In cats, however, the disorder tends to be progressive, resulting in clinical signs related to pain and loss of function.

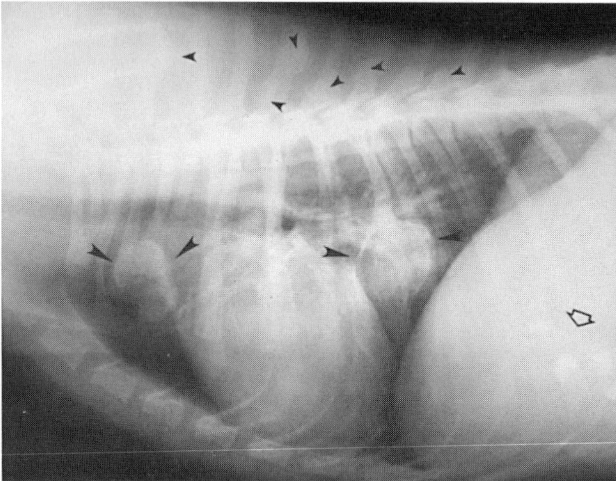

Fig. 15-18 Multiple cartilaginous exostosis. Two large, expansile lesions are present involving the third and seventh ribs *(large arrowheads)*. The opacity is mixed bone and soft tissue. Multiple nodular bone masses deform the shape of the thoracic spinous processes *(small arrowheads)*. An incidental finding is the presence of rocks in the stomach *(open arrow)*.

Radiographic Signs

Rib masses are an amorphous mixture of radiolucency and bone opacity with irregular contours. Long-bone and vertebral masses tend to be more organized in appearance, with radiolucent cartilage and trabecular bone. Cortical bone in the area of the lesion may be present or absent; the bone may be deformed or the exostosis may project externally. The size and shape of exostoses vary.

Retained Cartilage Core

Retained cartilage cores are primarily seen in the distal ulnar metaphysis of large-breed dogs, although they are occasionally seen in the lateral femoral condyle.[90,91] The lesion is caused by a disruption of the normal progression of endochondral ossification with retention of hypertrophied cartilage cells in the central metaphysis. Cartilage retention may cause angular limb deformity from retardation of distal ulnar growth and a resulting mismatch in radial and ulnar elongation, but the lesion is sometimes an incidental finding in otherwise normal dogs.

Radiographic Signs

Primary radiographic findings include the presence of a cone-shaped radiolucent area in the distal ulnar metaphysis or lateral femoral condyle (Fig. 15-19). A narrow zone of sclerosis may surround the radiolucent area. Additional radiographic findings may include angular limb deformity and degenerative joint disease of the elbow and carpal joints.

Incomplete Ossification of the Humeral Condyle

Incomplete ossification of the humeral condyle is a heritable condition of pure-bred and cross-bred Spaniels, resulting in a higher-than-normal incidence of humeral condylar fractures associated with normal physical activity (Fig. 15-20).[92] The incidence of the disorder appears to be higher in males. Sporadic reports have been made of other medium- and large-breed dogs affected by this disorder.[93] Two separate centers of ossification in the humeral condyle typically appear by approximately 22 days after birth. The medial and lateral centers of the condyle should fuse by approximately 84 days after birth. Incomplete ossification leads to the presence of a

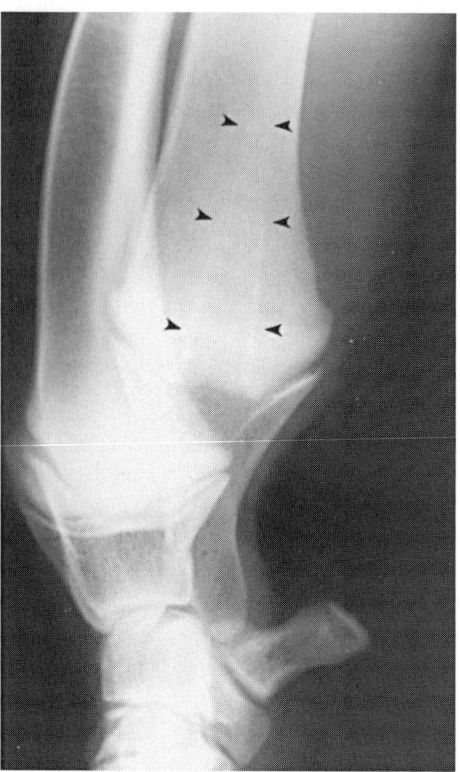

Fig. 15-19 Retained cartilage core in the distal ulna. A triangular radiolucent region is present in the distal ulnar metaphysis *(arrows)*. A thin rim of bone sclerosis is present next to the radiolucency. Slight cranial bowing of the radius and a thick caudal radial cortex are caused by mild angular limb deformity resulting from delayed ulnar growth.

thin fissure separating the medial and lateral halves of the humeral condyle in skeletally mature dogs. When pathologic fractures occur, approximately half are Y- or T-type fractures affecting the entire epicondylar region; the remainder are limited to fractures of the lateral (35%) or medial (15%) condyle.[92] The incidence of incomplete humeral condylar ossification is high enough that bilateral elbow radiographs should be obtained in any Spaniel with a unilateral condylar fracture. An increased incidence of fragmented coronoid processes also appears to be associated with this disorder.

Radiographic Signs

The primary radiographic finding in dogs with incomplete humeral condylar ossification is a vertically oriented radiolucent line in the central region of the condyle that may extend from the subchondral bone margin of the trochlea to the distal margin of the supratrochlear foramen. This lucency is evident only on the craniocaudal view and may be better seen when the view is obliqued approximately 15 degrees craniomedial to caudolateral, which positions the fissure parallel to the x-ray beam angle. Secondary radiographic signs include smooth periosteal new bone formation along the lateral and caudal aspect of the humeral epicondylar region. This finding may be a response to chronic instability or incomplete, nondisplaced fracture through the nonossified region. Overt, displaced, pathologic condylar fractures may be present in one or both limbs.

Radiographic evidence of concurrent fragmented medial coronoid process may be present.

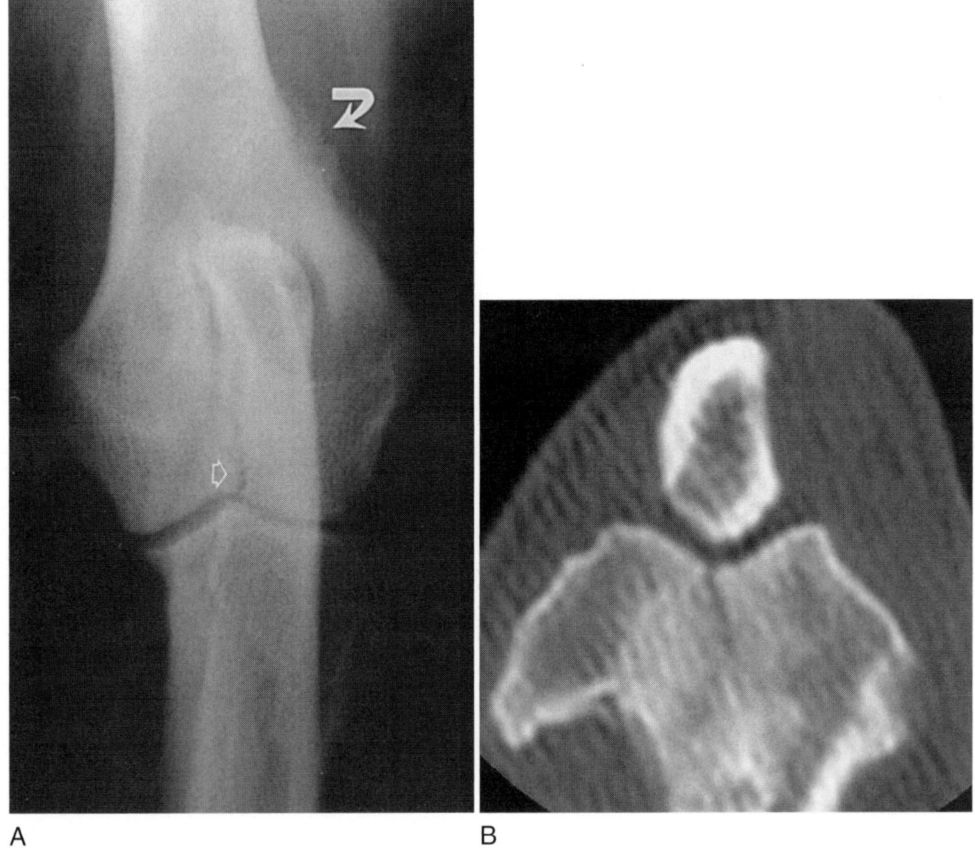

Fig. 15-20 A, Incomplete ossification of the humeral condyle. A vertical radiolucent line is present in the distal humeral condyle *(open arrow)*. Periosteal new bone formation is present on the distal lateral humerus *(curved arrow)*, probably as a result of motion from an incomplete fracture extending laterally from the supracondylar foramen. **B,** Computed tomography image of the distal humerus of a Cocker Spaniel with incomplete humeral condylar ossification. An ill-defined sagittally oriented lucent line is evident surrounded by sclerosis of adjacent bone.

REFERENCES

1. Ekman S, Carlson CS: The pathophysiology of osteochondrosis, *Vet Clin North Am Small Anim Pract* 28:17, 1998.
2. Smitach L, Stowater T: Osteochondritis dissecans of the shoulder joint: a review of 35 cases, *J Am Anim Hosp Assoc* 11:658, 1975.
3. Olsson S-E: The early diagnosis of fragmented coronoid process and osteochondritis dissecans of the canine elbow joint, *J Am Anim Hosp Assoc* 19:616, 1983.
4. Alexander J, Richardson D, Selcer B: Osteochondritis dissecans of the elbow, stifle and hock—a review, *J Am Anim Hosp Assoc* 17:51, 1981.
5. Denny H, Gibbs C: Osteochondritis dissecans of the canine stifle joint, *J Small Anim Pract* 21:317, 1980.
6. Fitch RB, Beale BS: Osteochondrosis of the canine tibiotarsal joint, *Vet Clin North Am Small Anim Pract* 28:95, 1998.
7. Harari J: Osteochondrosis of the femur, *Vet Clin North Am Small Anim Pract* 28:87, 1998.
8. Poulos PW Jr: Canine osteochondrosis, *Vet Clin North Am Small Anim Pract* 12:313, 1982.
9. Wisner ER, Berry CR, Morgan JP et al: Osteochondrosis of the lateral trochlear ridge of the talus in seven Rottweiler dogs, *Vet Surg* 19:435, 1990.
10. van Bree H: Evaluation of subchondral lesion size in osteochondrosis of the scapulohumeral joint in dogs, *J Am Vet Med Assoc* 204:1472, 1994.
11. van Bree H: Evaluation of the prognostic value of positive-contrast shoulder arthrography for bilateral osteochondrosis lesions in dogs, *Am J Vet Res* 51:1121, 1990.
12. van Bree H: Comparison of the diagnostic accuracy of positive-contrast arthrography and arthrotomy in evaluation of osteochondrosis lesions in the scapulohumeral joint in dogs, *J Am Vet Med Assoc* 203:84, 1993.
13. van Bree H, Van Rijssen B, Tshamala M et al: Comparison of the nonionic contrast agents, iopromide and iotrolan, for positive-contrast arthrography of the scapulohumeral joint in dogs, *Am J Vet Res* 53:1622, 1992.
14. Bertrand SG, Lewis DD, Madison JB et al: Arthroscopic examination and treatment of osteochondritis dissecans of the femoral condyle of six dogs, *J Am Anim Hosp Assoc* 33:451, 1997.
15. van Bree HJ, Van Ryssen B: Diagnostic and surgical arthroscopy in osteochondrosis lesions, *Vet Clin North Am Small Anim Pract* 28:161, 1998.
16. Boudrieau R, Hohn R, Bardet J: Osteochondritis dissecans of the elbow in the dog, *J Am Anim Hosp Assoc* 19:627, 1983.
17. Goring R, Bloomberg M: Selected developmental abnormalities of the canine elbow: radiographic evaluation and

surgical management, *Compend Cont Ed Pract Vet* 5:178, 1983.
18. Mason T, Lavelle S, Skipper S et al: Osteochondrosis of the elbow joint in young dogs, *J Small Anim Pract* 21:641, 1980.
19. Wind A: Elbow incongruity and developmental elbow diseases in the dog: I, *J Am Anim Hosp Assoc* 22:711, 1986.
20. Wind A: Elbow incongruity and developmental elbow diseases in the dog: II, *J Am Anim Hosp Assoc* 22:725, 1986.
21. Boulay J: Fragmented medial coronoid process of the ulna in the dog, *Vet Clin North Am Small Anim Pract* 28:51, 1998.
22. Blond L, Dupuis J, Beauregard G et al: Sensitivity and specificity of radiographic detection of canine elbow incongruence in an in vitro model, *Vet Radiol Ultrasound* 46:210, 2005.
23. Holsworth IG, Wisner ER, Scherrer WE et al: Accuracy of computerized tomographic evaluation of canine radio-ulnar incongruence in vitro, *Vet Surg* 34:108, 2005.
24. Battershell D: Ununited anconeal process, *J Am Vet Med Assoc* 155:35, 1969.
25. Sjostrom L: Ununited anconeal process in the dog, *Vet Clin North Am Small Anim Pract* 28:75, 1998.
26. Tirgari M: Clinical, radiographical and pathological aspects of ununited medial coronoid process of the elbow joint in dogs, *J Small Anim Pract* 21:595, 1980.
27. Berzon J, Quick C: Fragmented coronoid process: anatomical, clinical, and radiographic considerations with case analyses, *J Am Anim Hosp Assoc* 16:241, 1980.
28. Braden T, Stickle R, Dejardin L et al: The use of computed tomography in fragmented coronoid disease: a case report, *Vet Comp Orthop Trauma* 7:40, 1994.
29. Hornof WJ, Wind AP, Wallack ST et al: Canine elbow dysplasia. The early radiographic detection of fragmentation of the coronoid process, *Vet Clin North Am Small Anim Pract* 30:257, 2000.
30. Reichle JK, Park RD, Bahr AM: Computed tomographic findings of dogs with cubital joint lameness, *Vet Radiol Ultrasound* 41:125, 2000.
31. Berry C: Evaluation of the canine elbow for fragmented medial coronoid process, *Vet Radiol Ultrasound* 33:273, 1992.
32. Read R, Wind A, Morgan J et al: Fragmentation of the medial coronoid process of the ulna in dogs: a study of 109 cases, *J Small Anim Pract* 31:330, 1990.
33. Lee R: A study of the radiographic and histological changes occurring in Legg-Calvé-Perthes disease (LCP) in the dog, *J Small Anim Pract* 11:621, 1970.
34. Lee R: Legg-Perthes disease in the dog: The histological and associated radiological changes, *J Am Vet Radiol Assoc* 15:24, 1974.
35. Burt JK, Wilson GP: A study of eosinophilic panosteitis (enostosis) in German shepherd dogs, *Acta Radiol Suppl* 319:7, 1972.
36. Bohning RH Jr, Suter PF, Hohn RB et al: Clinical and radiologic survey of canine panosteitis, *J Am Vet Med Assoc* 156:870, 1970.
37. Trangerud C, Sande RD, Rorvik AM et al: A new type of radiographic bone remodeling in the distal radial and ulnar metaphysis in 54 Newfoundland dogs, *Vet Radiol Ultrasound* 46:108, 2005.
38. Grundalen J: Metaphyseal osteopathy (hypertrophic osteodystrophy) in growing dogs. A clinical study, *J Small Anim Pract* 17:721, 1976.
39. Bennett D: Nutrition and bone disease in the dog and cat, *Vet Rec* 98:313, 1976.
40. Alexander JW: Selected skeletal dysplasias: craniomandibular osteopathy, multiple cartilaginous exostoses, and hypertrophic osteodystrophy, *Vet Clin North Am Small Anim Pract* 13:55, 1983.
41. Woodard JC: Canine hypertrophic osteodystrophy: a study of the spontaneous disease in littermates, *Vet Pathol* 19:337, 1982.
42. Watson AD, Blair RC, Farrow BR et al: Hypertrophic osteodystrophy in the dog, *Aust Vet J* 49:433, 1973.
43. Olsson S-E: Radiology in veterinary pathology. A review with special reference to hypertrophic osteodystrophy and secondary hyperparathyroidism in the dog, *Acta Radiol Suppl* 319:255, 1972.
44. Muir P, Dubielzig R, Johnson K et al: Hypertrophic osteodystrophy and calvarial hyperostosis, *Compendium* 18:143, 1996.
45. Baumgartner W, Boyce RW, Weisbrode SE et al: Histologic and immunocytochemical characterization of canine distemper-associated metaphyseal bone lesions in young dogs following experimental infection, *Vet Pathol* 32:702, 1995.
46. Abeles V, Harrus S, Angles JM et al: Hypertrophic osteodystrophy in six Weimaraner puppies associated with systemic signs, *Vet Rec* 145:130, 1999.
47. Mee AP, Gordon MT, May C et al: Canine distemper virus transcripts detected in the bone cells of dogs with metaphyseal osteopathy, *Bone* 14:59, 1993.
48. Riser W: Radiographic differential diagnosis of skeletal diseases of young dogs, *J Am Vet Radiol Soc* 145:5, 1964.
49. Voorhout G: Radiographic features of nutritional secondary hyperparathyroidism in the growing dog and cat [in German], *Tijdschr Diergeneeskd* 106:317, 1981.
50. Greco DS, Feldman EC, Peterson ME et al: Congenital hypothyroid dwarfism in a family of giant schnauzers, *J Vet Intern Med* 5:57, 1991.
51. Lieb AS, Grooters AM, Tyler JW et al: Tetraparesis due to vertebral physeal fracture in an adult dog with congenital hypothyroidism, *J Small Anim Pract* 38:364, 1997.
52. Robinson WF, Shaw SE, Stanley B et al: Congenital hypothyroidism in Scottish deerhound puppies, *Aust Vet J* 65:386, 1988.
53. Saunders H: The radiographic appearance of canine congenital hypothyroidism: skeletal changes with delayed treatment, *Vet Radiol* 32:171, 1991.
54. Haskins M, Jezyk P, Desnick R et al: Alpha-L-iduronidase deficiency in a cat: a model of mucopolysaccharidosis: I, *Pediatr Res* 13:1294, 1979.
55. Haskins ME, Aguirre GD, Jezyk PF et al: Mucopolysaccharidosis type VII (sly syndrome). Beta-glucuronidase-deficient mucopolysaccharidosis in the dog, *Am J Pathol* 138:1553, 1991.
56. Haskins ME, Jezyk PF, Desnick RJ et al: Animal models of mucopolysaccharidosis, *Prog Clin Biol Res* 94:177, 1982.
57. Haskins ME, Otis EJ, Hayden JE et al: Hepatic storage of glycosaminoglycans in feline and canine models of mucopolysaccharidoses I, VI, and VII, *Vet Pathol* 29:112, 1992.
58. Konde L, Thrall M, Gasper P et al: Radiographic changes associated with muco-polysaccharidosis in the cat, *Vet Radiol* 28:223, 1987.
59. Shull RM, Helman RG, Spellacy E et al: Morphologic and biochemical studies of canine mucopolysaccharidosis: I, *Am J Pathol* 114:487, 1984.
60. Shull RM, Munger RJ, Spellacy E et al: Canine alpha-L-iduronidase deficiency. A model of mucopolysaccharidosis: I, *Am J Pathol* 109:244, 1982.
61. Wilkerson MJ, Lewis DC, Marks SL et al: Clinical and morphologic features of mucopolysaccharidosis type II in a dog: naturally occurring model of hunter syndrome, *Vet Pathol* 35:230, 1998.

62. Campbell BG, Wootton JA, Krook L et al: Clinical signs and diagnosis of osteogenesis imperfecta in three dogs, *J Am Vet Med Assoc* 211:183, 1997.
63. Potena A: On osteogenesis imperfecta. Studies of some cases observed in dogs [in Italian], *Acta Med Vet (Napoli)* 14:79, 1968.
64. Schmidt V: Osteogenesis imperfecta in 2 collie litter siblings [in German], *Wien Tierarztl Monatsschr* 54:92, 1967.
65. Lees GE, Sautter JH: Anemia and osteopetrosis in a dog, *J Am Vet Med Assoc* 175:820, 1979.
66. Hoover EA, Kociba GJ: Bone lesions in cats with anemia induced by feline leukemia virus, *J Natl Cancer Inst* 53:1277, 1974.
67. Onions D, Jarrett O, Testa N et al: Selective effect of feline leukaemia virus on early erythroid precursors, *Nature* 296:156, 1982.
68. Hanel RM, Graham JP, Levy JK et al: Generalized osteosclerosis in a cat, *Vet Radiol Ultrasound* 45:318, 2004.
69. Carrig CB, MacMillan A, Brundage S et al: Retinal dysplasia associated with skeletal abnormalities in Labrador retrievers, *J Am Vet Med Assoc* 170:49, 1977.
70. Terpin T, Roach MR: Chondrodysplasia in the Alaskan malamute: involvement of arteries, as well as bone and blood, *Am J Vet Res* 42:1865, 1981.
71. Bingel SA, Sande RD: Chondrodysplasia in the Norwegian elkhound, *Am J Pathol* 107:219, 1982.
72. Sande RD, Bingel SA: Animal models of dwarfism, *Vet Clin North Am Small Anim Pract* 13:71, 1983.
73. Bingel SA, Sande RD, Wight TN: Chondrodysplasia in the Alaskan malamute. Characterization of proteoglycans dissociatively extracted from dwarf growth plates, *Lab Invest* 53:479, 1985.
74. Minor RR, Farnum CE: Animal models with chondrodysplasia/osteochondrodysplasia, *Pathol Immunopathol Res* 7:62, 1988.
75. Carrig CB, Sponenberg DP, Schmidt GM et al: Inheritance of associated ocular and skeletal dysplasia in Labrador retrievers, *J Am Vet Med Assoc* 193:1269, 1988.
76. Breur GJ, Zerbe CA, Slocombe RF et al: Clinical, radiographic, pathologic, and genetic features of osteochondrodysplasia in Scottish deerhounds, *J Am Vet Med Assoc* 195:606, 1989.
77. Sande RD, Alexander JE, Padgett GA: Dwarfism in the Alaskan malamute: its radiographic pathogenesis, *J Am Vet Radiol Soc* 15:10, 1974.
78. Malik R, Allan GS, Howlett CR et al: Osteochondrodysplasia in Scottish Fold cats, *Aust Vet J* 77:85, 1999.
79. Allan GS: Radiographic features of feline joint diseases, *Vet Clin North Am Small Anim Pract* 30:281, 2000.
80. Riser WH, Haskins ME, Jezyk PF et al: Pseudoachondroplastic dysplasia in miniature Poodles: clinical, radiologic, and pathologic features, *J Am Vet Med Assoc* 176:335, 1980.
81. Rasmussen PG: Multiple epiphyseal dysplasia in a litter of Beagle puppies, *J Small Anim Pract* 12:91, 1971.
82. Rasmussen PG: Multiple epiphyseal dysplasia in Beagle puppies, *Acta Radiol Suppl* 319:251, 1972.
83. Rasmussen PG, Reimann I: Multiple epiphyseal dysplasia, with special reference to histological findings, *Acta Pathol Microbiol Scand (A)* 81:381, 1973.
84. Gambardella PC, Osborne CA, Stevens JB: Multiple cartilaginous exostoses in the dog, *J Am Vet Med Assoc* 166:761, 1975.
85. Doige C, Pharr J, Withrow S: Chondrosarcoma arising in multiple cartilaginous exostoses in a dog, *J Am Anim Hosp Assoc* 14:605, 1978.
86. Owen L: Multiple cartilaginous exostoses with development of a metastasizing osteosarcoma in a Shetland sheepdog, *J Small Anim Pract* 12:507, 1971.
87. Jacobson LS, Kirberger RM: Canine multiple cartilaginous exostoses: unusual manifestations and a review of the literature, *J Am Anim Hosp Assoc* 32:45, 1996.
88. Mozos E, Novales M, Ginel PJ et al: A newly recognized pattern of canine osteochondromatosis, *Vet Radiol Ultrasound* 43:132, 2002.
89. Pool R, Harris J: Feline osteochondromatosis, *Feline Pract* 5:24, 1975.
90. Johnson KA: Retardation of endochondral ossification at the distal ulnar growth plate in dogs, *Aust Vet J* 57:474, 1981.
91. Riser W, Lincoln J, Rhodes W et al: Genu valgum: a stifle deformity of giant dogs, *J Am Vet Radiol Assoc* 10:28, 1969.
92. Marcellin-Little DJ, DeYoung DJ, Ferris KK et al: Incomplete ossification of the humeral condyle in spaniels, *Vet Surg* 23:475, 1994.
93. Rovesti GL, Fluckiger M, Margini A et al: Fragmented coronoid process and incomplete ossification of the humeral condyle in a Rottweiler, *Vet Surg* 27:354, 1998.

ELECTRONIC RESOURCES evolve

Additional information related to the content in Chapter 15 can be found on the companion Web site at evolve http://evolve.elsevier.com/Thrall/vetrad/

- Key Points
- Chapter Quiz
- Case Study 15-1
- Case Study 15-2

CHAPTER • 16
Fracture Healing and Complications

George A. Henry

BONE TISSUE

Bone is a specialized form of connective tissue that functions as an integral part of the locomotor system. Bones act as lever arms during motion, provide resistance to the effects of gravitational force on the body, and provide protection and support to adjacent structures. Bone also serves as a reservoir of mineral for systemic mineral homeostasis.[1,2]

Bones differ in shape and function and include long, flat, intramembranous, woven, and compact bones. Specialized connective tissue called periosteum surrounds the outside surface of the bones and provides protection and nutrition. Long bones are divided into epiphyseal, physeal, metaphyseal, and diaphyseal regions. Woven, cancellous, and lamellar bone is found adjacent to the physis in the epiphyseal and metaphyseal regions; compact or cortical bone surrounds the marrow cavity in the diaphyseal region.[1,2]

Bones contain three principal cell types: osteoblasts, osteocytes, and osteoclasts. Osteoblasts synthesize the osteoid bone matrix. Following mineralization of the osteoid, the osteoblasts become osteocytes. Osteoclasts are larger cells that reside on the surface of the mineralized matrix and remove both mineral and matrix by secretion of acids and enzymes. In normal bone the activities of osteoblasts and osteoclasts are coordinated and occur in response to stress on the bone. The bone pattern and shape of the bone adapt to withstand the stresses placed on it.

The regulation of mineral ions in the serum is controlled mainly by parathyroid hormone, calcitonin, and vitamin D. Parathyroid hormone increases resorption of bone by stimulating osteoblastic activity to increase serum calcium. Calcitonin inhibits the activity of osteoblasts. Vitamin D acts on the intestine to increase absorption of calcium and phosphorous and directly on bone by both mobilization of calcium and phosphorous from previously formed bone and promotion of maturation and mineralization of bone matrix. Bone is an active living tissue that is able to adapt and react, although somewhat slowly, to forces applied to the musculoskeletal system. Although bone can react to external stimuli or forces, it has limited methods of reaction: bone production, bone resorption, or a combination of production and resorption.[1,2]

Bone is formed and grows by intramembranous ossification, endochondral ossification, or both. *Intramembranous* bone formation begins with proliferation of mesenchymal cells that transform into osteoblasts that form matrix, which is then calcified. A fibrovascular layer develops on the internal and external surfaces of the bone to provide nutrition and osteogenic cells to allow the continued production and resorption of the bone. Intramembranous bone formation occurs primarily in the bones of the calvarium and mandible. The bones of the extremities, spine, and pelvis form by both intramembranous and endochondral ossification, with endochondral ossification predominant in the long bones. *Endochondral* (intracartilaginous) ossification progresses by the formation of a cartilage model derived from the mesenchyma that is then replaced with bone. Long (tubular) bones begin by a primary center of ossification in the center of the cartilaginous model and grow by intramembranous ossification, with secondary centers appearing later at the ends within the epiphyses and apophyses that continue the growth by endochondral ossification. The physis is organized into five clearly demarcated histologic zones: (1) resting zone containing immature cells on the epiphyseal side of the physis, (2) cell growth or proliferation, (3) cell hypertrophy, (4) provisional calcification, and (5) ossification. The weakest zone is in the area of the hypertrophied cartilage cells; this is the most common area of physeal fracture after trauma.[1,2] Bone healing is similar to the endochondral growth process.[2]

BONE HEALING

Bone healing is a normal ongoing process throughout all bones as a result of aging of the bone that requires replacement of bone over time and healing of microfractures, which if not repaired could result in structural failure of the bone and clinical fracture. Disease processes that interfere with normal bone metabolism or physical trauma that stresses the bone beyond its structural capacity can result in fractures. Fracture healing may occur by two basic methods: *direct* and *indirect* bone healing. *Distraction osteogenesis* is a third type of bone healing that is associated with bone lengthening techniques, which are being used more frequently.[2-5]

Indirect (secondary) bone healing is the most common type of healing observed in animals and occurs in fractures in which some movement is possible between fracture fragments because of a lack of rigid fixation. Motion between fragments produces strain on the tissues attempting to heal the fracture and causes tissue disruption if the strain is excessive. Initially the fracture gap is bridged by tissues that are more stress tolerant, with replacement of each tissue type by a more rigid type of tissue until a rigid bridge is formed between the fragments. Granulation tissue can withstand 100% stretching before failure, whereas fibrous tissue can withstand only 10% and bone only 2% deformation before failure.[2] The initial hematoma at a fracture site is replaced by granulation tissue followed by fibrous connective tissue that is replaced by fibrocartilage and then endochondral ossification to produce a bony union. The initial bony bridging callus is woven bone that is remodeled over time to produce compact cortical bone (see Fig. 16-11).[2,5]

Direct (primary) bone healing is defined as healing that occurs directly between fracture fragments without a cartilaginous stage and no observable callus. Excellent anatomic reduction and alignment of the fracture fragments with rigid fixation are required. The fracture gap must be quite small—

no more than 150 to 300 μm. The gap is initially filled with fibrous bone followed by remodeling and reconstruction of the haversian systems across the fracture to provide a stronger union.[3-5]

Distraction osteogenesis results from gradual distraction of the bone segments, often after osteotomy. The gradual widening of the gap, ideally 1 mm/day, allows deposition of parallel columns of osteoid leading to formation of lamellar bone within these columns if sufficient stability is present at the osteotomy gap (Fig. 16-1). If stability is insufficient, formation of fibrous or cartilaginous tissue that becomes ossified occurs.

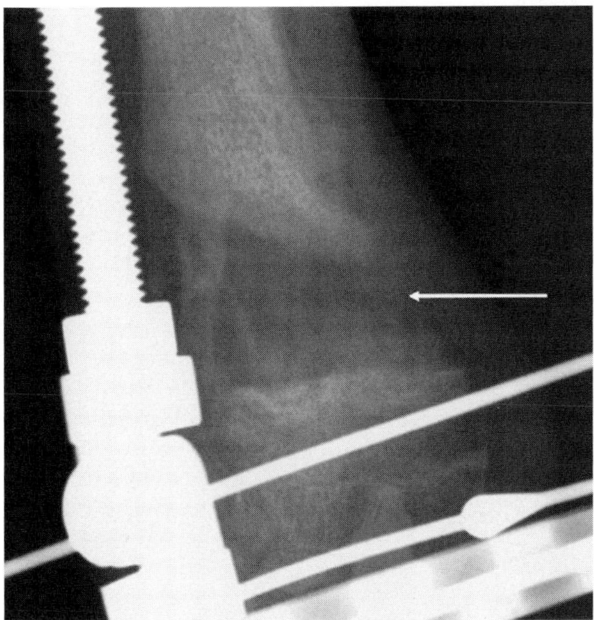

Fig. 16-1 Osteotomy performed to correct angular limb deformity and lengthen the limb. Note the columns of lamellar bone formation typically seen with distraction osteogenesis *(white arrow)*.

The goal of this technique is to lengthen a bone that is too short as a result of premature growth cessation, loss of a segment of the bone, or overriding malunion caused by previous trauma.[3,6]

FACTORS AFFECTING BONE HEALING

Many factors individually or in combination can have a marked effect on the success or failure of fracture healing. The time required to achieve clinical union adequate to change or remove orthopedic fixation devices varies significantly depending on these factors. Many variables are known to influence fracture healing adversely. These include age of the patient, weight of the patient, quality of anatomic reduction, stability of fracture (poor fixation or excessive patient activity), extent of local blood supply, type of fracture, bone involved, presence of infection, iatrogenic interference, systemic diseases such as metabolic and endocrine diseases, pathologic fracture, corticosteroids, use of nonsteroidal anti-inflammatory drugs, and other less well-documented variables.[2-4,7-9]

Anatomic reduction with a narrow fracture gap will improve the chance of direct or rapid indirect bone healing. Large fracture gaps or missing bone fragments require more and larger callus formation and a longer period for bridging of the fracture. In addition, anatomic reduction allows the apposition of the bone fragments to enhance the stability of the fracture. Positioning of fracture ends should have at least 50% contact to expect healing of the fracture. However, fracture healing is more likely with anatomic reduction. Anatomic reduction is critical with articular fractures to prevent long-term cartilage damage and degenerative changes from abnormal pressure distribution.[2]

Stability is a key factor in successful healing of a fracture; motion at the fracture site is the most common cause of poor fracture healing in animals. Motion caused by poor fixation or excessive patient activity is a significant contributing factor. Strain produced by movement in the fracture gap can disrupt the tissues, including the new blood vessels required for proper healing. Lack of stability delays healing until more stable tissues can form in the fracture gap and produce sufficient stability for osteogenesis (Fig. 16-2).[10]

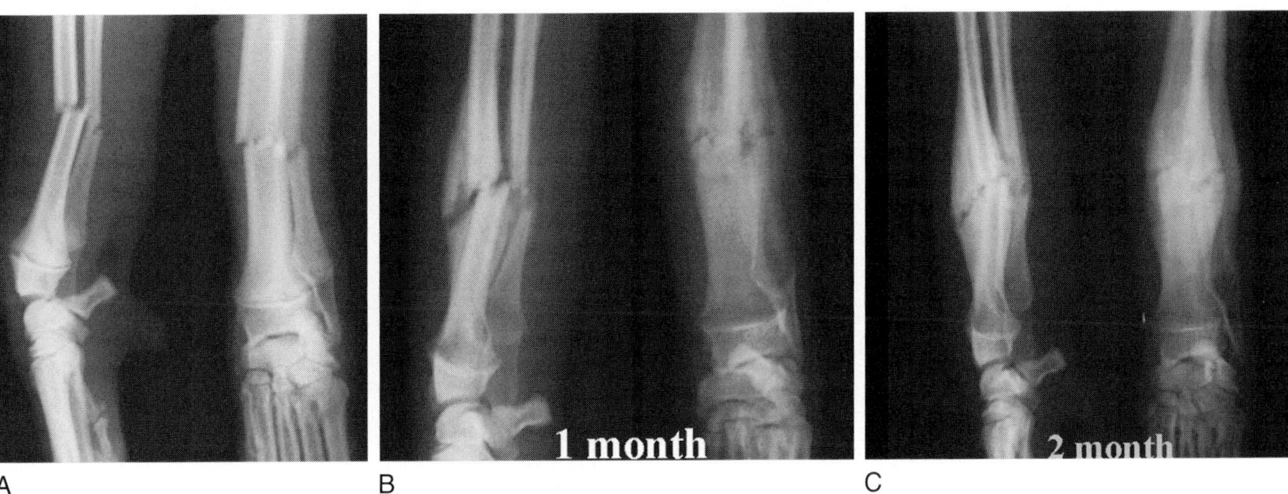

Fig. 16-2 Transverse diaphyseal fractures of the radius and ulna of an immature dog with 1-month and 2-month follow-up radiographs. The lack of good fracture stabilization resulted in delayed secondary healing with exuberant callus. A radiolucent fracture line is still visible at 2 months, indicating the fracture is not completely healed.

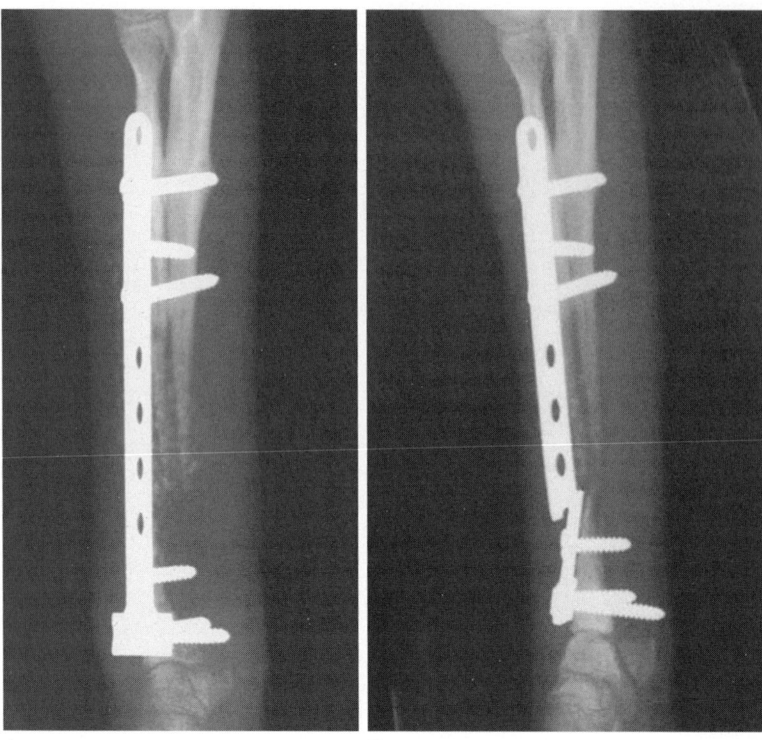

Fig. 16-3 A, This Toy Poodle has atrophic nonunion radial and ulnar fractures at 3 months after the original injury. Note the lack of callus and atrophy of the adjacent ends of the fracture fragments. The small mineral foci overlying the fragments are small islands of cancellous bone graphs placed during fixation. Poor soft tissue environment, including poor blood supply, at the fracture site prevented the formation of callus. **B,** At 4.5 months after the initial injury, bone plate failure from metal fatigue is evident.

Viability of the surrounding soft tissues has a significant effect on the ability of the bone to heal.[9,11] Viable adjacent soft tissue provides protection for the bone fragments and a source of extraosseous blood supply that is vital in the healing process. Disruption of the normal blood supply to the fracture zone inhibits the repair process. Blood vessels from surrounding tissues are recruited to provide adequate oxygen and nutrients for fracture repair. When the fracture is healed these extraosseous vessels become dormant as the normal blood supply to the bone is revitalized. Severe damage or loss of surrounding soft tissues decreases the rate of fracture repair and may prevent healing in some patients. Fracture fragments that are denuded of soft tissue and bone grafts require adequate stabilization to allow early revascularization of the bone and healing of the fracture. Without revascularization of these bone fragments, healing will not occur.

The *specific bone involved* in the fracture can affect the outcome of fracture healing. Some bones have less adjacent soft tissue to supply temporary vasculature for healing. Some small canine breeds have delayed healing of antebrachial factures with higher complication rates than those observed in larger breeds (Fig. 16-3).[12,13] Stabilization of the calcaneus is more difficult because of the normally higher stress on this bone.

Infection of the bone or surrounding tissues can have a profound effect on the healing process. The recognition and aggressive treatment of infection is important for successful bone healing. Infection can disrupt the healing process in the fracture gap directly and indirectly by causing loosening of the fixation devices attached to the bone fragments, allowing the facture to become unstable (Fig.16-4).

Proper selection and application of fixation devices has a significant effect on the rate and success of fracture repair. The fixation device must provide stabilization of the fracture and not interfere with the tissue environment conducive to the healing process. Common problems include inadequate size

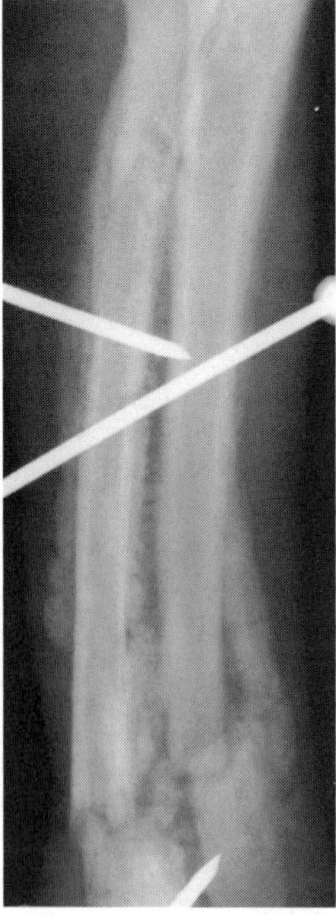

Fig. 16-4 Advanced bacterial osteomyelitis after fixation of a distal antebrachial fracture with an external fixator. Note the active periosteal reaction that extends the entire length of the diaphysis and metaphysis. Soft tissue swelling is also present and is important in differentiating septic versus nonseptic periosteal new bone. Also, the irregular margins of the periosteal reaction are atypical for callus and suggest an aggressive process.

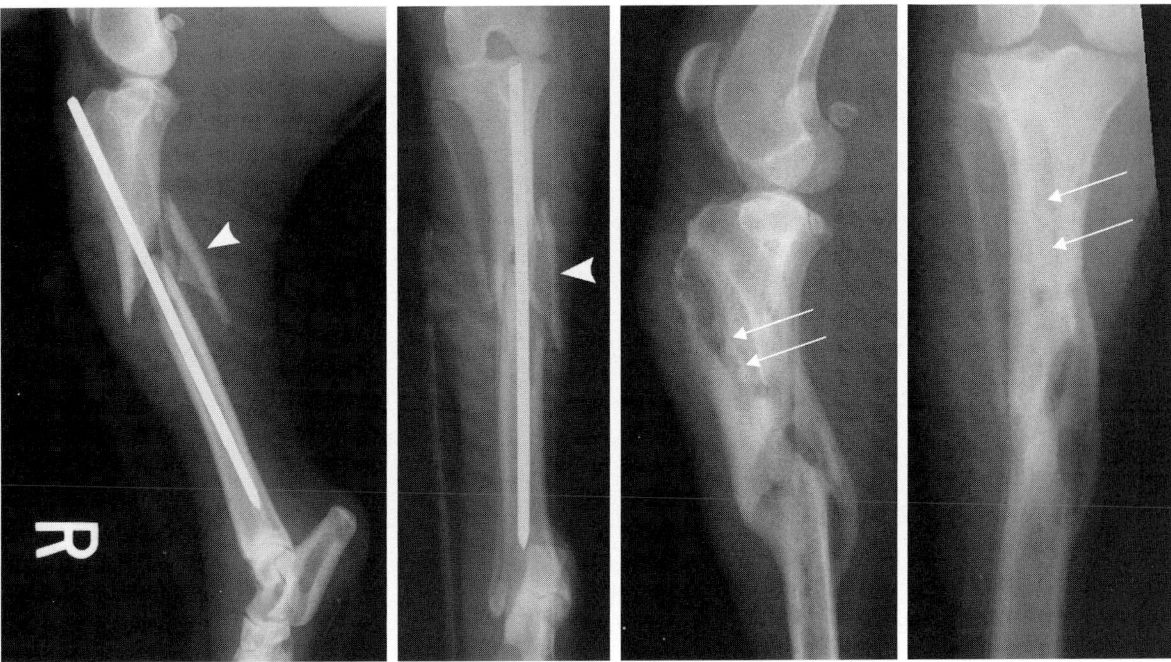

Fig. 16-5 Poor postoperative alignment and fixation resulted from use of a single intramedullary pin. A large butterfly fragment is not incorporated into the fixation *(arrowhead)*. The result is a malunion and large callus. A segment of the proximal fracture fragment lost blood supply and became devitalized, resulting in a sequestrum *(arrows)*. A draining fistula (not observable on radiographs) was associated with the sequestrum. The sequestrum required surgical removal. (Courtesy Dr. Gregory Daniel, University of Tennessee, Knoxville, Tennessee.)

and placement of intramedullary pins or insufficient number of plate-associated screws on each side of a fracture that allow fracture instability as well as excessive soft tissue disruption that delays or prevents revascularization (Fig. 16-5). Adequate knowledge, experience, and skills are necessary for the appropriate treatment of the many varieties of bone fractures.

Metabolic factors, including species, breed, age of the patient, nutritional status, and presence or absence of systemic metabolic disease, can affect the duration and success of fracture healing. Some species such as horses require longer healing times for clinical fracture repair because of their greater weight and slower metabolism compared with the average dog and heal more slowly with less callus. Fractures in younger animals heal faster than those in older animals of the same species.[14] Hypothyroidism, hyperparathyroidism, diabetes mellitus, and some paraneoplastic syndromes can delay bone healing.[15]

PROMOTING FRACTURE HEALING

Bone grafting is commonly used to promote healing of fractures with missing fragments or in the treatment of nonunion fractures. Other techniques that may promote healing of fractures include the use of electrical fields, low-intensity pulsed ultrasound, demineralized bone matrix, growth factors, autologous bone marrow, extracorporeal shock wave treatment, and gene therapy. A discussion of these new techniques is beyond the scope of this chapter, and the reader is referred to other publications.[2,4,16-21]

FRACTURE IDENTIFICATION

Physical examination is an essential first step in evaluating fractures and possible complicating factors in addition to identifying bone injury. Dealing with immediate life-threatening injuries takes precedence over imaging to look for fractures. Careful systematic palpation of the entire skeleton is warranted in patients suspected of having a fracture. Obvious abnormalities must not distract from a through examination for less-obvious but significant fractures. Identification of open fractures, spinal fractures, and skull fractures requires careful evaluation with temporary stabilization. Appropriate treatment of open wounds associated with fractures prevents further injury and bacterial contamination that can negatively affect the outcome. Although the overall condition of the patient must be considered, unnecessary delay of treatment is undesirable because delaying fracture stabilization for more than 48 hours after injury is associated with a poorer functional outcome.[2,22]

Diagnostic imaging provides valuable information concerning the location, type, complexity, and potential complications associated with fractures. Imaging also provides a basis for planning appropriate fracture reduction and stabilization. Appropriate pain management, tranquilization, physical restraint, and anesthesia commensurate with the patient's status are necessary for obtaining high-quality images for evaluation and planning. Motion is the most common cause of inferior images in animals. Motion leads to degraded images in which important smaller fractures or fissures vital for planning reduction and stabilization of the fracture may be overlooked.

Knowledge of normal anatomy and normal variations or aberrant anatomic change is critical for accurate interpretation of images. Normal and accessory ossification centers and normal or aberrant nutrient foramina can mimic fractures.[23,24] Anatomic references and skeletal models are invaluable and should be readily available.

Radiography remains the most commonly used imaging tool for fracture evaluation in veterinary medicine. Two orthogonal views of the area in question are essential for

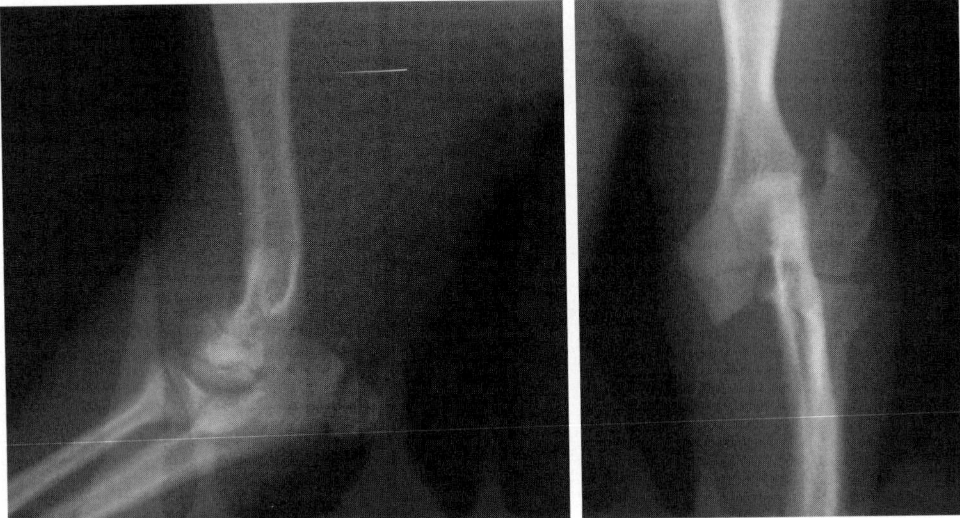

Fig. 16-6 Salter-Harris type IV intercondylar fracture of the distal humerus with the fracture line passing through the lateral metaphysis, physis, and epiphysis. The fracture is difficult to identify on the lateral view. At least two views of a suspected fracture area should be made. With some intercondylar fractures an oblique view is necessary for identification of the fracture.

adequate evaluation of a potential fracture. A single view does not allow complete assessment of the fracture fragments and can be misleading, possibly causing disastrous results. In some patients oblique views are necessary to define or identify a subtle or complex fracture. With minimal displacement, the fracture line must be parallel to the x-ray beam for the radiolucent fracture line to be seen (Fig. 16-6).

If the severity of signs found on physical examination indicates a high probability of fracture and no fractures are identified on initial views, oblique radiographs should be made in addition to the routine two orthogonal views. Some small stress fractures or incomplete fractures may not have sufficient displacement immediately after the injury to allow their detection. Follow-up radiographs in 7 to 10 days are recommended to check for these fractures. The normal healing process begins with some resorption of the ends of the fracture fragments. This normal osteolysis enlarges the fracture line to a sufficient degree to allow observation on a radiograph. Sometimes early callus formation is the only finding that allows identification of a stress fracture. In some patients, other anatomic structures may obscure a fracture on some views, and multiple views may be required to detect the fracture.[25]

For extremity fractures in small animals, the joint(s) proximal and distal to the fracture should be included on the radiograph for assessment of possible joint involvement or preconditions that may alter the treatment or outcome. The radiographic technique should be excellent for bone and ideally allow evaluation of the adjacent soft tissues as well. One of the distinct advantages of new digital radiography systems is the increased dynamic range that allows optimizing the same image for viewing bone and soft tissues.

Computed tomography (CT) is becoming more available in veterinary practice. CT is especially useful in detection and description of fractures in regions with complex anatomy such as the nose, skull, and pelvis (Fig. 16-7). Detail of both cortical and trabecular bone is excellent, and fractures and fissures that are not observed on radiographs are readily apparent in CT images.[26,27] In addition, some adjacent soft tissue injuries can be observed as well as improved identification of underlying conditions contributing to a pathologic fracture such as neoplastic invasion of bone.[28] Postoperative assessment of articular fractures with CT improves the detection of step deformities compared with survey radiography.[29]

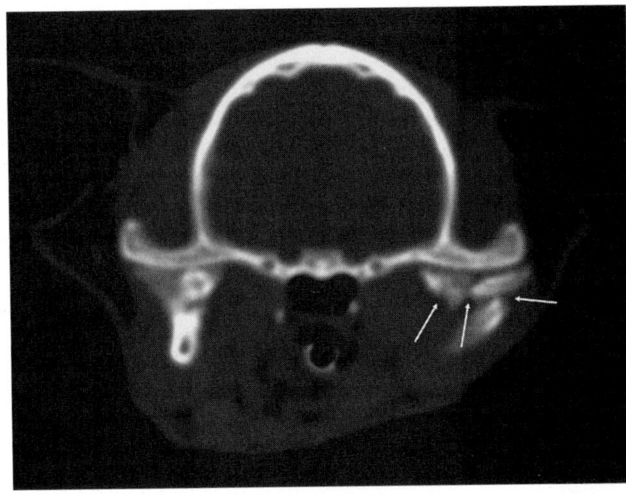

Fig. 16-7 Transverse CT image through the level of the temporomandibular joints. A comminuted articular fracture of the articular condyle of the mandible is visible *(arrows)*. The severity of the fracture was not observable on radiographs.

Scintigraphy is a sensitive method to detect stress fractures and other occult fractures not identified on radiography. Increased uptake of a bone-seeking radiopharmaceutical is related to osteoblastic activity. Bone scintigraphy is very sensitive, being able to detect a stress fracture in an equine metacarpal bone within 24 to 72 hours of injury.[30,31] However, its specificity is low because of other factors and diseases that can cause increased radiopharmaceutical uptake. The history, degree of uptake, degree of lameness, and information from other imaging modalities must be considered in determining a probable diagnosis of fracture.[30,32,33] Scintigraphy does require patient isolation for radiopharmaceutical clearance after the procedure. Scintigraphy in orthopedic patients is primarily used to identify possible sites of occult fracture or bone pathology not detected by other imaging means.

Magnetic resonance imaging (MRI) is the modality of choice for the diagnosis of many musculoskeletal disorders in human beings.[1] MRI provides significantly more information than radiography in evaluation of the extent of injury to an open physis and the extent of physeal closure after injury.[1] MRI is used to a lesser extent in veterinary orthopedics, mainly because of limited availability. However, the number of veterinary imaging centers that provide MRI is increasing. MRI is most notable for its detailed imaging of soft tissues with significantly better contrast resolution than CT. MRI is especially useful for detecting abnormal changes in muscles, tendons, ligaments, and cartilage. MRI is sensitive to changes in the bone marrow that can aid in the identification of bone lesions that would not be otherwise detected. Radiography is ineffective in the differentiation and identification of soft tissue injuries, and although CT has improved soft tissue contrast resolution, neither modality provides the exquisite images of soft tissues possible with MRI. As availability increases and cost decreases, MRI will be used to a greater extent for evaluating musculoskeletal injuries, especially those involving joints.[28,34]

Ultrasound examination of musculoskeletal injuries is becoming more common, primarily for evaluating the soft tissue component. Evaluation of tendons and ligaments with ultrasound is common.[35,36] The integrity of bone surfaces can be evaluated with ultrasound with some success in observing occult fractures and sequestra.[37] However, sonographic skill and familiarity with the bone anatomy are required. Although ultrasound has been reported to be useful in the evaluation of fracture healing, this is not a common practice, possibly because of the high-quality equipment and advanced sonographer expertise required.[38]

Although other imaging modalities are being used to provide additional information on musculoskeletal injury, radiography remains the mainstay for initial evaluation of most of these injuries.

FRACTURE CLASSIFICATION

Fracture classifications serve to standardize language to improve communication. Some are developed to organize fractures into clinically useful groups that help guide treatment options and prognosis.[4,28] Fractures are commonly classified according to location, direction, complete or incomplete status, number of fracture lines, displacement, and open or closed status. Additional descriptive terms are used in combination with the basic classification to further describe a fracture or describe a specific type of fracture.[3,25]

Location is the first descriptor used in describing a fracture and includes the bone involved and location in the bone.

Diaphyseal fractures of long bones may be described with the diaphysis divided into thirds: *proximal, distal,* or *mid-diaphyseal.*

Metaphyseal fractures of long bones are described as involving the proximal or distal metaphysis.

Epiphyseal fractures commonly involve the adjacent joint and physis. If the physis is open, the Salter-Harris classification system is used to describe the fracture (see below).

Articular fractures consist of any fracture that enters a joint. Important aspects to describe with an articular fracture are extent and location of the articular surface involved and if free fragments are present within the joint.

Physeal fractures involving an open physis are described with the *Salter-Harris* classification system.[39] Five classes were originally described on the basis of involvement of the epiphysis, physis, and metaphysis (Fig. 16-8).

Salter-Harris Type I fractures are fractures through the physis (Fig. 16-9).

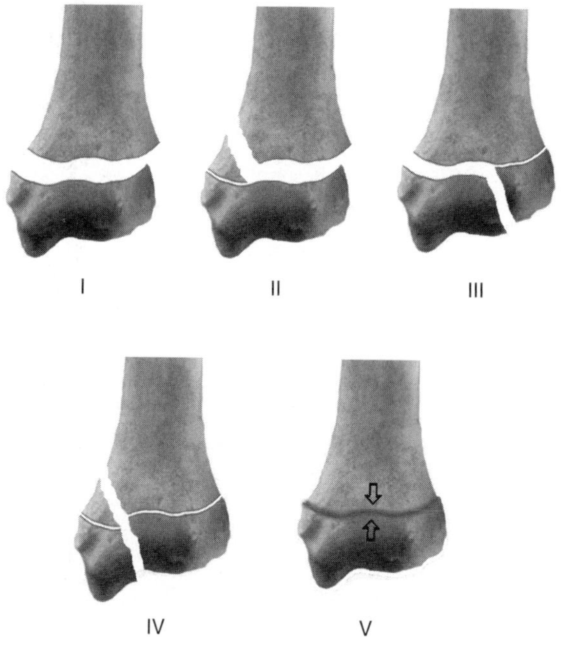

I II III

IV V

Fig. 16-8 Salter-Harris physeal fracture classification.

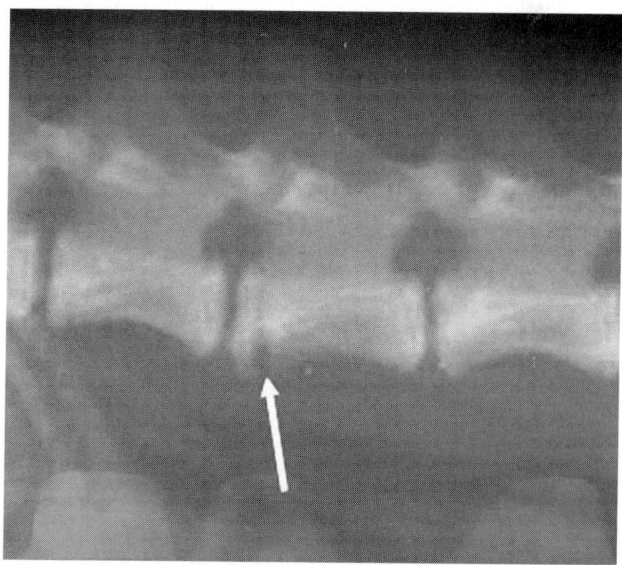

Fig. 16-9 Minimally displaced Salter-Harris type I fracture of the cranial physis of L3.

Salter-Harris Type II fractures are fractures through the physis and a portion of the metaphysis (Fig. 16-10).

Salter-Harris Type III fractures are fractures through the physis and through the epiphysis and are usually articular fractures.

Salter-Harris Type IV fractures are fractures through the epiphysis, across the physis, and through the metaphysis. These are usually articular fractures (see Fig. 16-6).

Salter-Harris Type V fractures are crushing- or compression-type fractures that involve the physis. Increased opacity of the physis is the only radiographic sign observed in the acute injury; however, the change is often not recognizable on initial radiographs. Comparison with the normal opposite limb may aid in identifying subtle changes. Salter-Harris type V fractures frequently cause premature closure of all or a portion of the physis, leading to growth deformities.

A Salter-Harris type VI group was added later by others and is described as a partial physeal closure resulting from damage to only a portion of the physis, leading to asymmetric closure. However, this description suggests this is a sequel of physeal injury rather than the initial injury and is not universally used.[1]

Direction of the fracture is a description of the direction of the fracture line relative to the long axis of the bone and is typically described as *transverse, oblique,* or *spiral.*

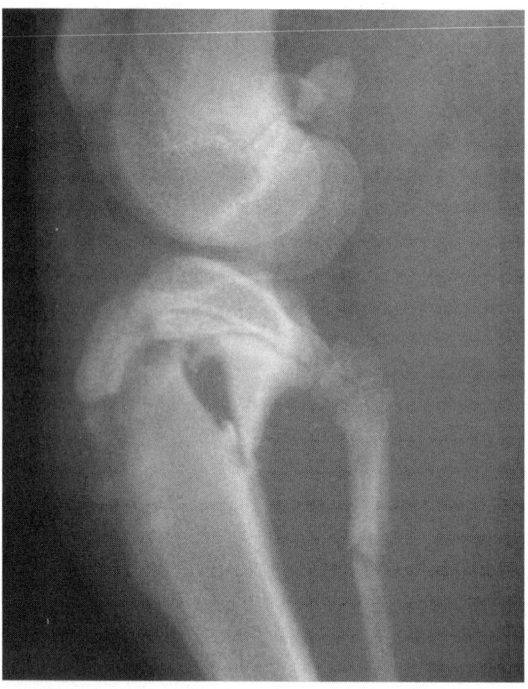

Fig. 16-10 Salter-Harris type II fracture of the proximal tibia.

Transverse fractures run perpendicular to the long axis of the bone (see Fig. 16-2).

Oblique fractures run at less than 90 degrees to the long axis with fractures equal to or less than 45 degrees (described as *long oblique*) and factures that are greater than 45 degrees (described as *short oblique*) (see Fig. 16-13).[3]

Spiral fractures are usually associated with significant torsional trauma and are an oblique fracture that wraps around the long axis of the long bone (Figs. 16-11 and 16-12).

Complete fractures extend through the entire bone and are more common than incomplete fractures. The term "complete" is not commonly used in fracture description because a fracture is assumed to be complete unless the description states that it is an incomplete fracture.

Incomplete fractures have lines that involve only a single bone cortex or small portion of a bone and do not cause separation of the bone into two or more fragments. A *greenstick* fracture usually occurs in young animals and is an incomplete fracture of one side of the bone with bending of the opposite cortex (plastic deformation) (Fig. 16-13). *Fatigue* or *stress* fractures are another type of incomplete fracture. They are typically microfractures caused by repeated trauma over time that slightly exceeds the load capacity of the bone. Stress fractures may not be seen radiographically or may appear as faint, linear, incomplete fractures involving one portion of a bone. Scintigraphy can be used to identify the presence of stress fractures when radiographs are normal or inconclusive. Radiographic changes observed in addition to linear or curvilinear radiolucencies in a focal aspect of the cortex are increased bone opacity and early periosteal new bone production.

Number of fracture lines is generally defined as simple or comminuted.

Simple fractures are those that have only one fracture line and divide the bone into only two main fragments. Generally, if the fracture is not stated to be comminuted, a simple fracture is assumed and the term "simple" is not included in the description.

Comminuted fractures have more than one fracture line that communicates to a single point or plane and divides the bone into three or more fragments. Comminuted fractures with three large fragments often have a triangular-shaped fragment called a *butterfly fragment* (see Fig. 16-5). Fractures that

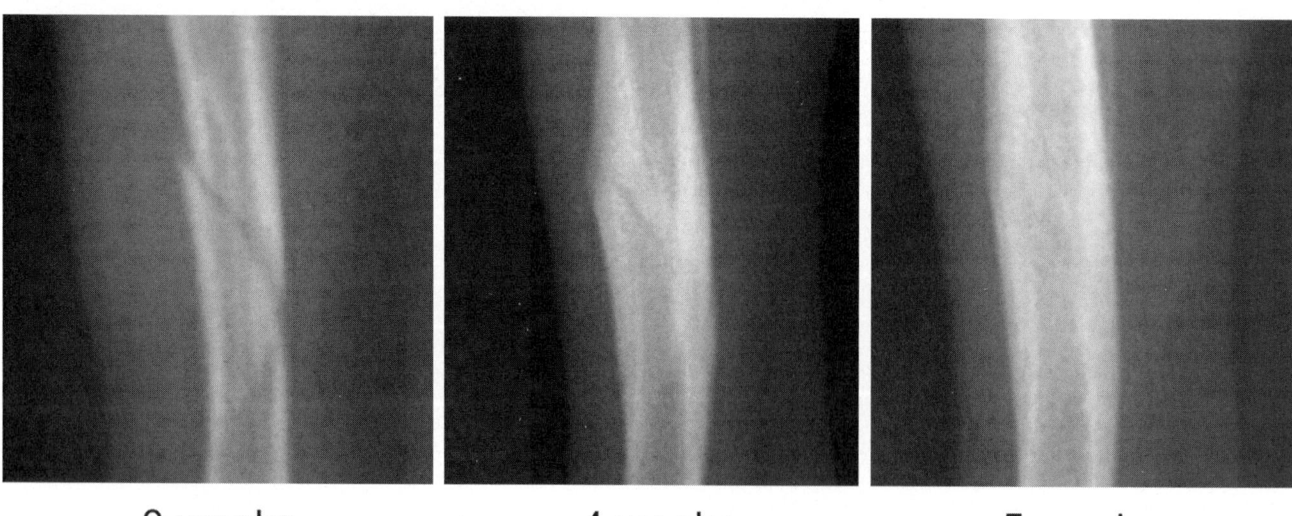

Fig. 16-11 Mildly displaced spiral fracture with good stability leading to indirect (secondary) healing by 5 weeks.

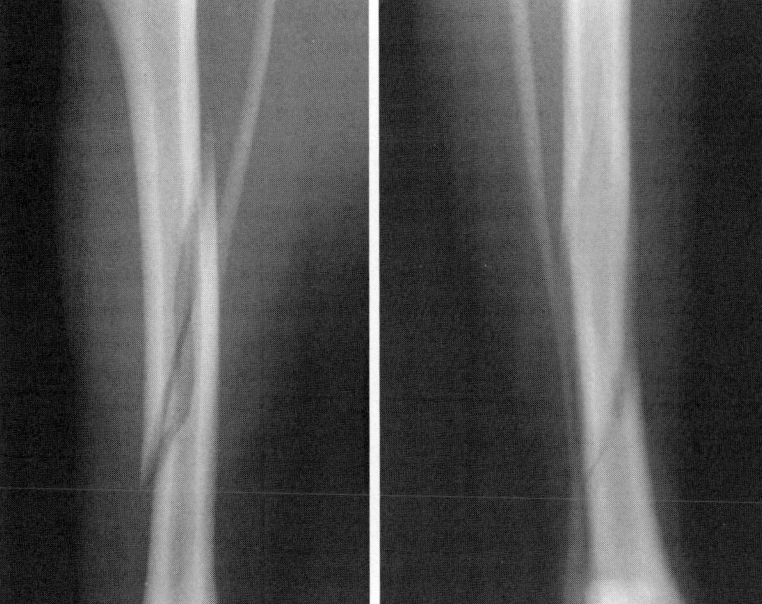

Fig. 16-12 Mid-diaphyseal spiral fracture of the tibia.

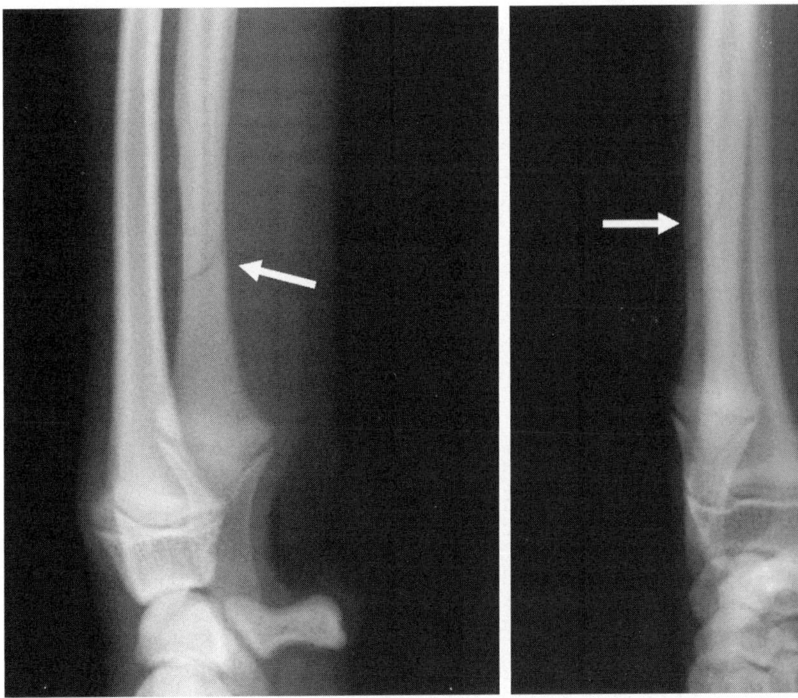

Fig. 16-13 Incomplete short oblique fracture of the distal diaphysis of the ulna *(arrows)*.

divide the bone into five or more fragments are *severely* or *highly* comminuted (Fig. 16-14).

Open or *closed* are descriptive terms that indicate whether the fracture is exposed to the outside environment. Open fractures can be classified according to the mechanism of puncture and severity of soft tissue injury (Fig. 16-15).[2-4] Typically the term "closed" is not used in a description because a fracture is assumed to be closed unless the description states the fracture is open. The terms *type, grade,* and *degree* have been used somewhat interchangeably for this classification system.

Type I: Open fracture with small puncture wound in the skin close to the fracture caused by one of the bone fragments penetrating the skin. The wound is less than 1 cm long.

Type II: Variable-sized skin wound associated with the fracture as a result of external trauma. Type II has more soft tissue damage than does type I.

Type III: Severe bone fragmentation associated with extensive soft tissue injury with or without skin loss. Type III can be subdivided into the following categories:

Type IIIa: Requires no major soft tissue reconstruction procedures such as skin flaps or graphs to cover the wound.

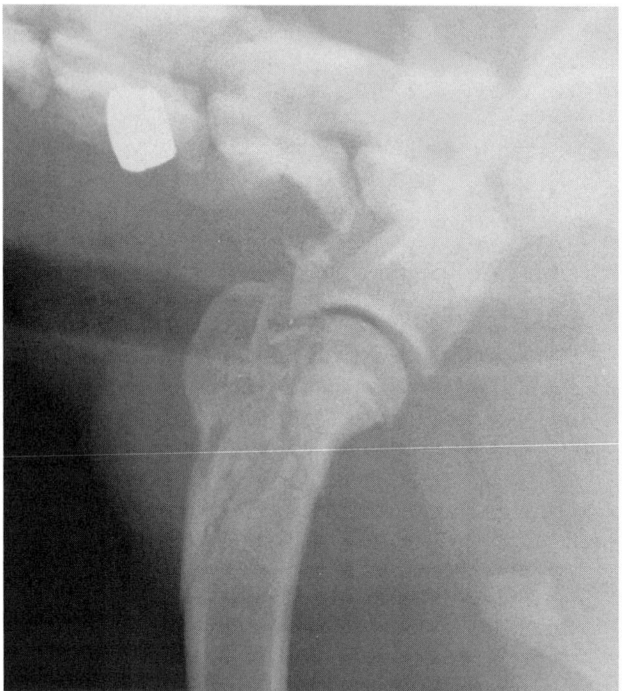

Fig. 16-14 Severely comminuted articular fracture of the proximal humerus; this fracture was caused by a ballistic injury. High-velocity projectiles cause severe soft tissue injury in addition to fractures if they interact with bone. Projectiles made of softer materials will fragment on contact with bone, and numerous small metal fragments will be seen in association with the fracture site. This patient has only a few small metal fragments, indicating the bullet was made of harder metal. The main metal fragment is adjacent to C4.

Type IIIb: Requires reconstructive soft tissue procedures because of insufficient viable soft tissue to cover the wound.

Type IIIc: Open fractures that have major arterial injuries that must be repaired for viability of the tissues.

Type IV: Open fractures that involve amputation or near amputation of the limb. These fractures have severe soft tissue and neurovascular injuries.[2]

Displacement of a fracture is described in terms of the distal or caudal fracture fragment. In some fractures the fragments are freely moveable and easily change positions. The importance of displacement is related to interference with or extent of injury to other structures. For example, medial displacement of pelvic fractures suggests acute injury to the lower urinary tract or possible interference with defecation or parturition after healing if not corrected.[25] Displacement is usually defined in terms of shortening or lengthening, angular displacement, and torsional displacement. Shortening of the length of the bone is most commonly a result of traction by surrounding musculature and may be caused by *collapse* of multiple fragments or *overriding* of the main fracture fragments. Lengthening of the bone caused by *distraction* of the fragments, resulting in widening of the fracture gap, is uncommon except with *avulsion* fractures (Fig. 16-16). *Angular displacement* is described as the direction taken by the distal or caudal fragment relative to the proximal or cranial fragment. *Torsional displacement* describes inward or outward rotation of the distal or caudal fragment.

Other descriptive terminology and classifications can be used to describe specific fractures further.

Pathologic fractures occur without abnormal or overt trauma as a result of secondary weakening of the bone by a disease process. Pathologic fractures are commonly seen with neoplastic weakening of the bone (Fig. 16-17). However, other diseases such as hyperparathyroidism are also associated with these fractures (Fig. 16-18). Pathologic fractures are important

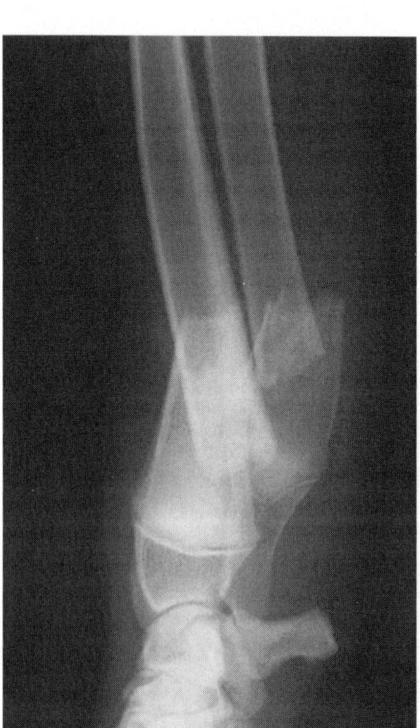

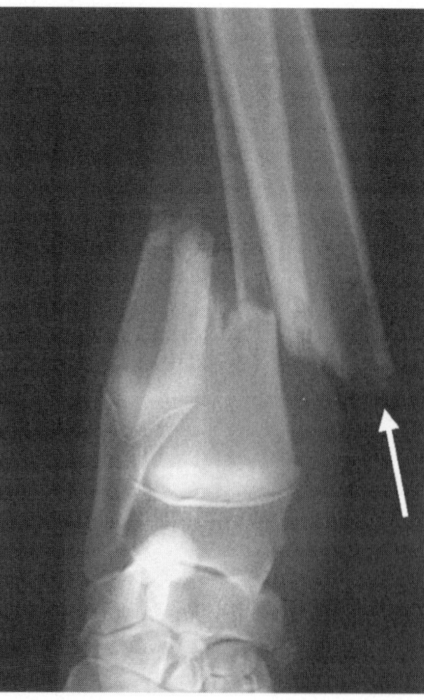

Fig. 16-15 Open transverse distal diaphyseal fractures of the radius and ulna with lateral displacement and mild overriding. The distal end of the proximal radial fracture fragment is seen outside the soft tissues on the cranial-caudal view, indicating that it is an open fracture *(arrow)*.

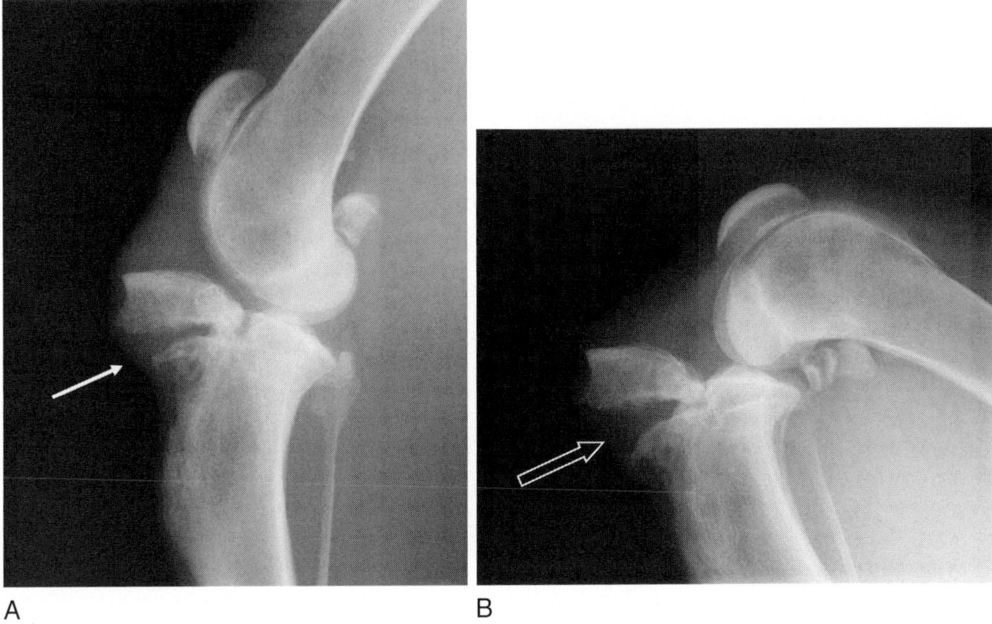

Fig. 16-16 A, Four-day-old avulsion fracture of tibial tuberosity *(solid arrow)*. B, In a flexed view, widening of the fracture gap indicates dynamic instability *(open arrow)*.

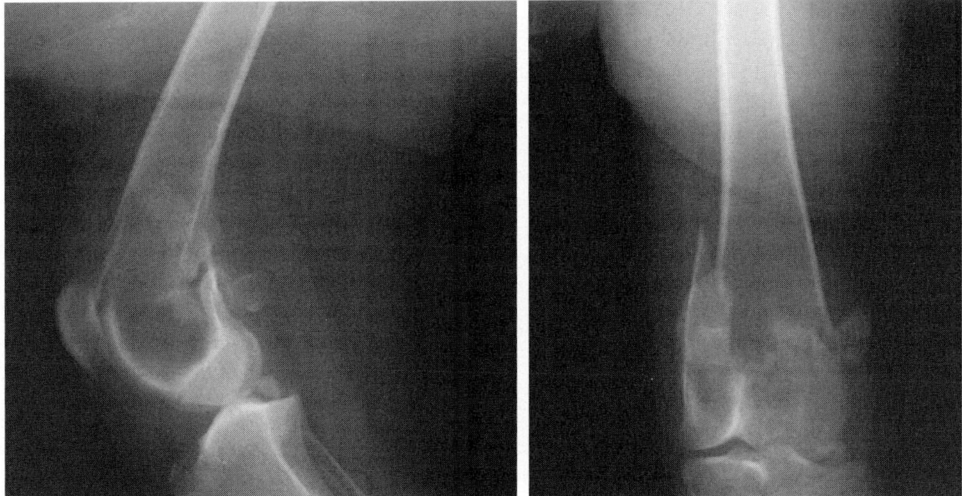

Fig. 16-17 Pathologic fracture of distal metaphysis of the femur. Note the thinning and loss of dense cortical bone at the fracture site and the lack of normal opaque cancellous bone in the metaphysis proximal to the physeal scar. The fracture occurred without a history of trauma. A primarily osteolytic osteosarcoma was diagnosed following biopsy.

to recognize to make an informed assessment of treatment options and prognosis.

Chip fractures are typically small fragments of bone that are broken off of a bone as a result of direct trauma. The presence of a fracture bed helps differentiate chip fractures from accessory ossification centers and dystrophic soft tissue mineralization.

Slab fractures are typically seen in cuboidal bones of the joints and are fractures that run from one joint surface of the bone to the opposite joint surface. A fracture of a cuboidal bone that involves just one joint surface would be a *chip* fracture.

Avulsion fractures occur at attachment sites of tendons, ligaments, or joint capsules and are caused by excessive forces placed on these structures that result in a piece of bone being pulled off of the parent bone. These fractures should have observable fracture beds (see Fig. 16-16).

Multiple or *segmental* fractures have more than one fracture line, but they do not communicate as in comminuted fractures.

Compression or *impacted* fractures occur from trauma that crushes the bone, thus decreasing one or more dimensions of the bone. This is most commonly seen in vertebral bodies and cuboidal bones.

Depression fractures occur in the skull, sinuses, and nose, with fracture fragments displaced below the normal surface.

Condylar, bicondylar, and *supracondylar, T,* and *Y* fractures are terms used to describe fractures involving the metaphysis

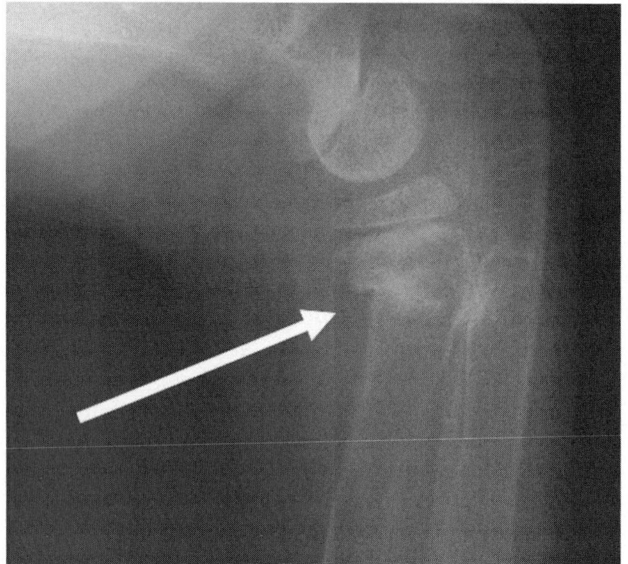

Fig. 16-18 Incomplete folding pathologic fracture of proximal radial metaphysis *(arrow)* due to inadequate bone mineralization caused by nutritional secondary hyperparathyroidism.

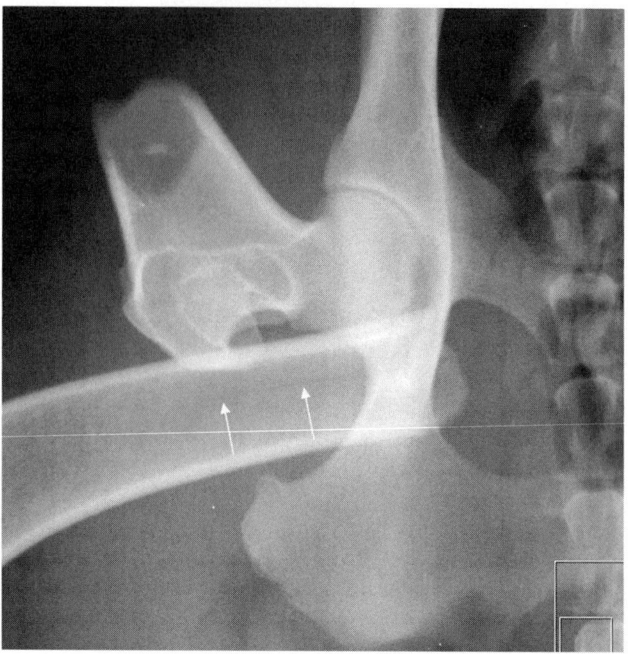

Fig. 16-19 Short oblique proximal diaphyseal fracture of the femur with a single fissure fracture in the proximal aspect of the distal fracture fragment *(arrows)*. This fissure fracture was not recognized on presurgical radiographs. In postoperative radiographs made the day after surgery, the fissure fracture had developed into a complete fracture that required a second surgery for fixation.

and condyles. Fractures between the condyles as well as through the epicondyles or metaphysis can be described as a T or Y fracture. Fracture of a condyle only from the parent bone is termed a *condylar* fracture.

Osteochondral fractures are defined as a disruption of articular cartilage along with a portion of subchondral bone. If the fracture fragment is loose within the joint, it is termed a *loose body* or *joint mouse*.[28]

Fissure fractures are incomplete fractures that appear as thin radiolucent lines often arising from a complete fracture (Fig. 16-19). Fissure fractures must be identified because they often develop into complete fractures during reduction and fixation and compromise the repair. Identification during initial imaging provides the information necessary for adequate planning.

Abrasion or *shearing fractures* are caused by loss of soft tissue and bone as a result of friction or glancing trauma. The most common cause is abrasion of extremities being pulled along asphalt or concrete surfaces when the animal is hit by a moving vehicle. A portion of soft tissue and bone is lost from the abrasive effect of the rough surfaces. These type fractures are always open fractures and commonly involve joints (Fig. 16-20).

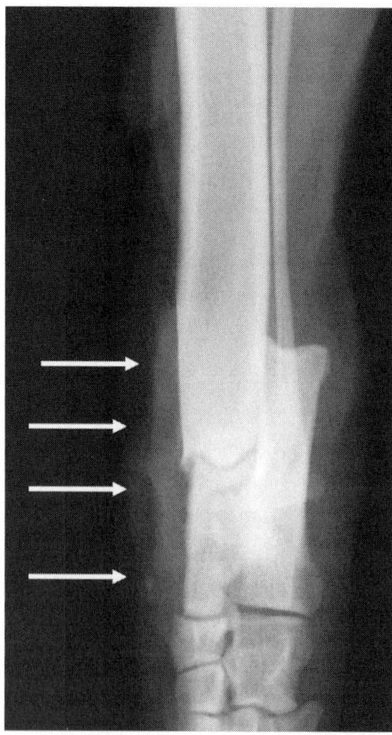

Fig. 16-20 Abrasion-type open articular fractures of the distal tibia and talus *(arrows)*. The medial malleolus and a portion of the medial aspect of the talus are missing because of the abrasive action of the road pavement as the dog was dragged for a short distance after being hit by a car. The soft tissues on the medial aspect are irregular, indicating loss of the soft tissue as well. The tarsocrural joint is open to the environment. These fractures are typically open fractures. Blood supply and supportive ligaments in these areas can be severely compromised.

RADIOGRAPHIC EVALUATION OF BONE HEALING

Postoperative imaging is essential for proper evaluation of the reduction and alignment of the fracture as well as placement of orthopedic devices (Fig. 16-21). The importance of good-quality postoperative radiographs to serve as a baseline for future imaging evaluation cannot be overemphasized. At least two orthogonal views are required to interpret the location of bony structures and orthopedic devices accurately. Radiographs should be repeated every 4 to 6 weeks unless clinical signs indicate a possible acute change in condition.[3]

An organized paradigm is required for evaluating radiographs of orthopedic procedures. One commonly used system

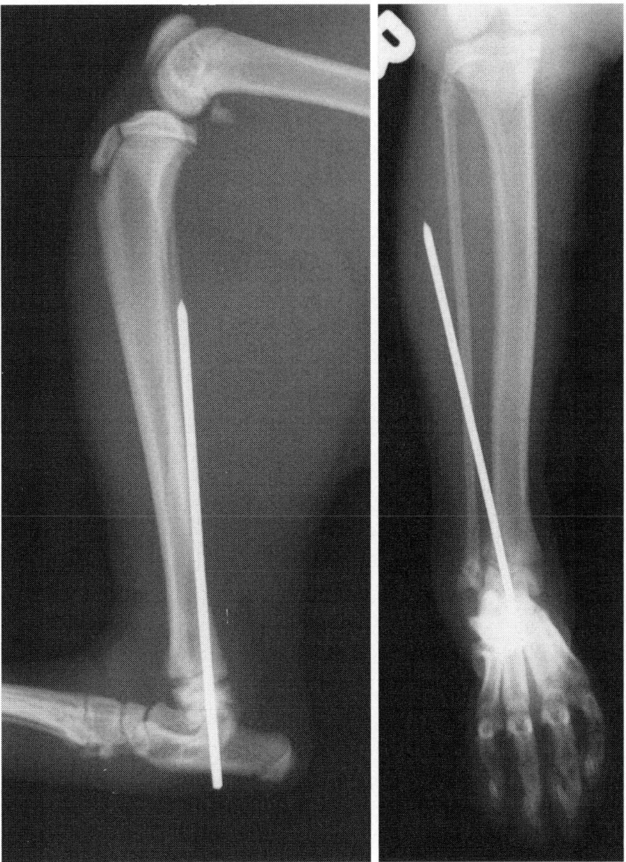

Fig. 16-21 Inadequate closed pinning of a Salter-Harris type II fracture of the distal tibia. In the lateral radiograph the pin appears to be passing through the epiphysis and metaphysis exiting the caudal diaphyseal cortex. In the cranial-caudal radiograph the intramedullary pin engages only a small portion of the metaphysis and extends laterally into the soft tissues of the limb. Two orthogonal views are required for accurate evaluation of the placement of the fixation devices.

Box • 16-1

Radiographic Signs of Secondary Bone Healing

5-10 Days after Reduction
Fracture fragments lose sharp margins
Demineralization of fracture fragment ends results in slight fracture line widening

10-20 Days after Reduction
Formation of endosteal and periosteal callus
Decreasing size of fracture gap
Variable loss in opacity of free fracture fragments

≥30 Days after Reduction
Fracture lines gradually disappear
External callus increases in opacity and remodels

≥3 Months after Reduction
Continued remodeling of external calluses
Trabecular pattern may develop within the callus
Cortical shadow becomes visible through the callus
Medullary cavity continuity gradually reestablished
Cortical remodeling along the lines of stress

goes by the mnemonic ABCDS, standing for ***a***lignment, ***b***one, ***c***artilage, ***d***evice, and ***s***oft tissues.

Alignment is evaluated for any change in fracture fragment alignment since the previous radiographs, with changes indicating possible instability of the fixation. Two orthogonal views are necessary for a thorough evaluation. The positioning of the recheck radiographs should be as close as possible to the previous radiographs to compare the images accurately. The previous radiographs should be reviewed and compared with the current images before the patient is dismissed so that views can be retaken if necessary for accurate evaluation. Minor changes in angle of view can make dramatic changes in the appearance of the bone fragment and orthopedic devices position.

The *bone* is evaluated for evidence of progression of the healing process on the basis of radiographic changes (Box 16-1). Early healing is observed as slight widening of the fracture line and callus formation. Later phase healing is observed as opaque, mature callus and increasing mineral opacity within the fracture line. Bone fragments that retain sharp margins and do not participate in the callus may indicate devitalization. If a fragment fails to revascularize, it may develop into a *sequestrum* (see Fig. 16-5). Excessive callus and periosteal new bone may be seen with fracture instability, infection, and periosteal injury at the time of the fracture or during surgery (Fig. 16-22). History and clinical signs may help differentiate these possibilities.

The amount of callus is related to the type of fracture, degree of reduction, and fixation.[3,25] Comminuted fractures require a larger callus to achieve adequate stabilization for healing. Fractures that have large gaps either because of less-than-anatomic reduction or missing fragments will heal with a larger callus. Fractures with anatomic reduction and rigid fixation may heal with little or no visible callus. The lack of callus in some of these fractures can be differentiated from an atrophic nonunion by clinical signs, history, and serial radiographs.

Cartilage refers to evaluation of the joints directly involved in a fracture (articular) or joints proximal or distal to the fracture. The apposition of articular fracture fragments as indicated by alignment of the subchondral bone is an important radiographic sign. Placement or migration of orthopedic devices into a joint can also indicate a complication in fracture healing (Fig. 16-23). The presence of joint effusion with subchondral bone lysis and periosteal new bone may indicate a septic joint.

Next is evaluation of placement and alignment of the *orthopedic devices*. This step is essential because these changes may signal loosening of the stabilizing devices that could delay or compromise healing of the fracture. Migration (movement) of an orthopedic device indicates loosening and must be correlated with the clinical signs and history to determine if corrective intervention is necessary. Bending of a fixation device can also indicate instability of the orthopedic repair. Breakage of pins, screws, wires, and plates indicates significant past, current, or chronic stress on the orthopedic devices (Fig. 16-24). Evaluation for signs of healing, including bridging or nonbridging callus, and clinical signs are used to decide if corrective action is necessary or if healing is occurring in a reasonable manner. Patients with loose orthopedic devices and unstable factures usually have signs of pain and disuse of the affected structures (Fig. 16-25).

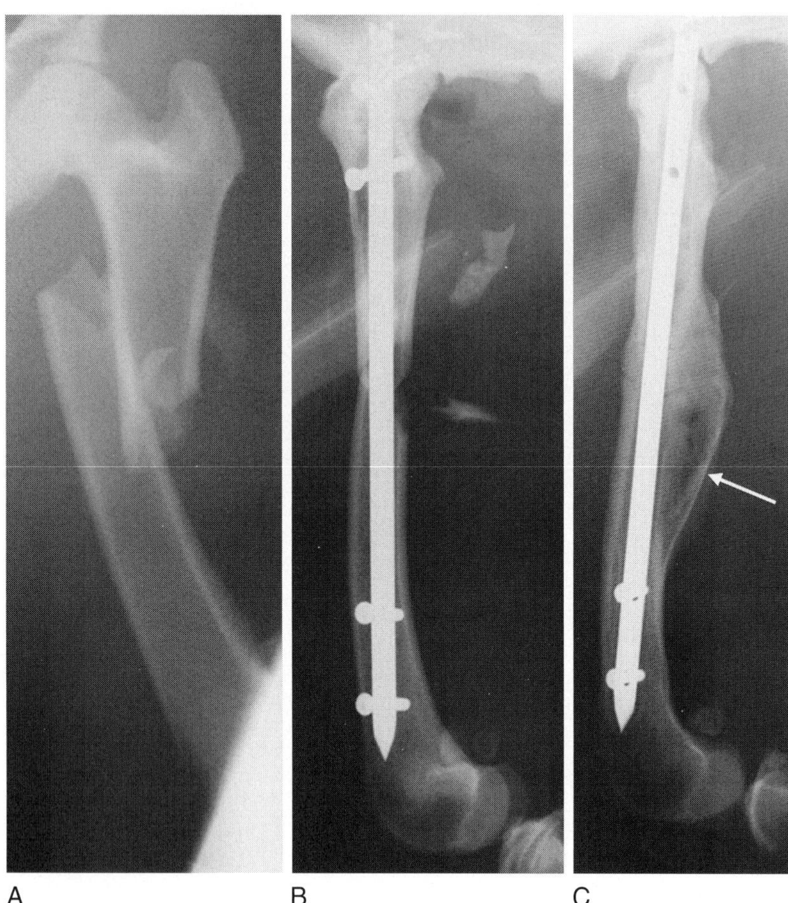

Fig. 16-22 A, Comminuted diaphyseal fracture of the femur. B, Reduction and fixation with an interlocking nail. C, Subsequent indirect (secondary) healing. The convex callus and new bone on the caudal aspect of the femur *(arrow)* is caused by periosteal stripping at the time of the fracture and is commonly seen with diaphyseal femoral fractures. (Courtesy Dr. Gregory Daniel, University of Tennessee, Knoxville, Tennessee.)

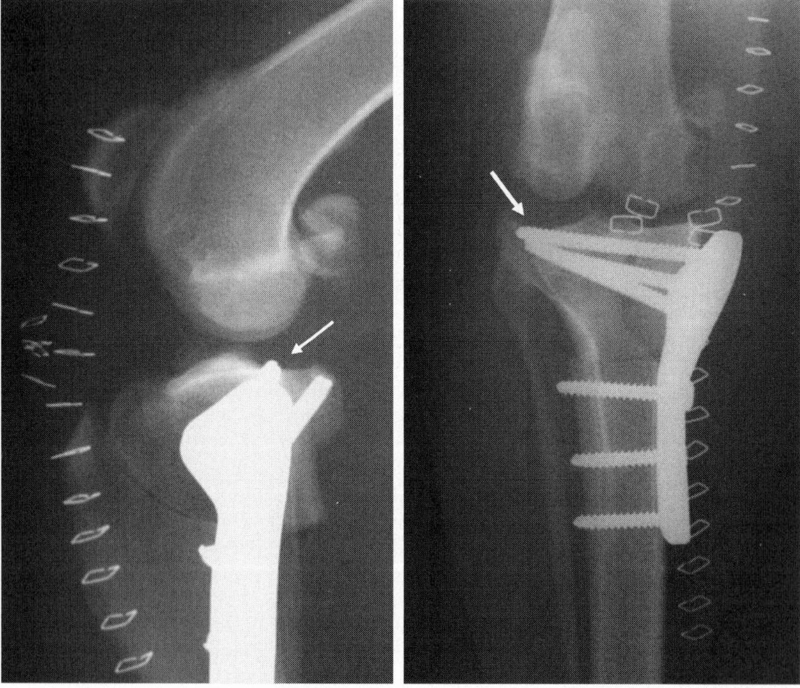

Fig. 16-23 In postoperative radiographs of a tibial plateau leveling procedure, one screw is likely within the joint *(arrows)*. Although this screw is probably not through the articular cartilage, removal and replacement with a shorter screw or redirected screw would be advised.

Loosened orthopedic devices commonly have a radiolucency surrounding the device within the bone (Fig. 16-26). Other than motion (either of the implant or of the fragment), additional causes for a radiolucency around an orthopedic implant are bone necrosis caused by high-speed drills, digital radiographic artifact, or osteomyelitis (Fig. 16-27). A radiolucent zone around a metal implant that is relatively even with a visible sclerotic margin suggests a cause other than infection (Fig. 16-28). Radiolucency surrounding a metal implant that is uneven with ill-defined margins is more likely infectious.[25]

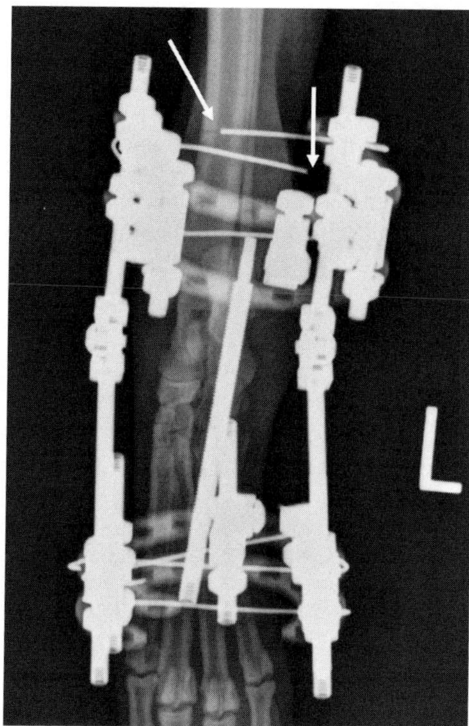

Fig. 16-24 Broken fixation wires *(arrows)* caused by excessive stress on the external fixator.

Some computed radiographic systems produce an artifact seen as a thin radiolucent zone immediately surrounding metallic objects such as pins and screws within bone. This artifact mimics bone lysis from motion or early infection (Fig. 16-29) and must be recognized to avoid an incorrect assessment of loosening or infection.[40,41] Some new direct radiography and computed radiography systems have modified algorithms that do not produce this artifact.

The timing for removal of orthopedic devices varies with the device and with each patient. Methods have been explored to quantify measurement of fracture healing by using ultrasound, CT, or radiography. Most of these efforts attempt to measure the stiffness of the fracture to predict the chance of failure if the fixation device is removed. Direct stiffness measurements of angulation at the fracture site with an applied load correlated more strongly with function outcome than did callus index.[42] However, these techniques are not commonly used with radiographic findings, and clinical assessment remains the most regularly used method to assess union of a fracture. Generally fixation devices may be removed when radiographic evidence of bridging bony callus is present. Fractures stabilized with casts generally have larger periosteal callus. Fractures stabilized with external fixators generally heal with a combination of periosteal and endosteal callus with less periosteal callus when compared with casts. Simple fractures with excellent reduction and stable fixation with external fixators may heal with minimal periosteal and endosteal callus. Comminuted fractures will heal with mainly endosteal callus and bone bridging between fragments if the environment is good and fixation is rigid. Wires used in orthopedic bone repair are usually not removed unless they fragment and cause a problem. Bone plate and screw removal is delayed for 6 to 12 months after surgery to allow adequate time for the

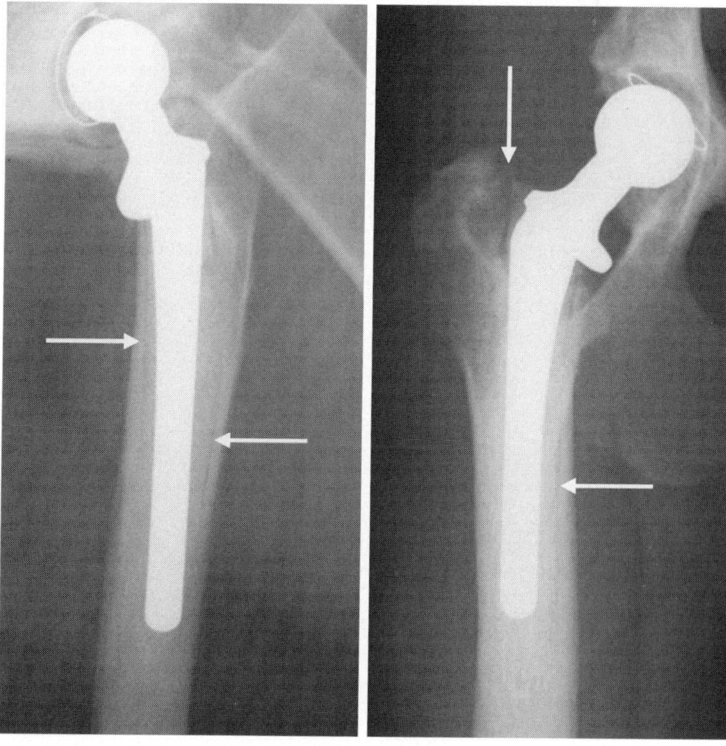

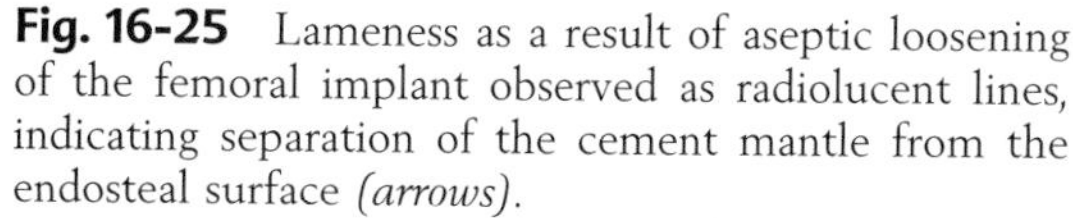
Fig. 16-25 Lameness as a result of aseptic loosening of the femoral implant observed as radiolucent lines, indicating separation of the cement mantle from the endosteal surface *(arrows)*.

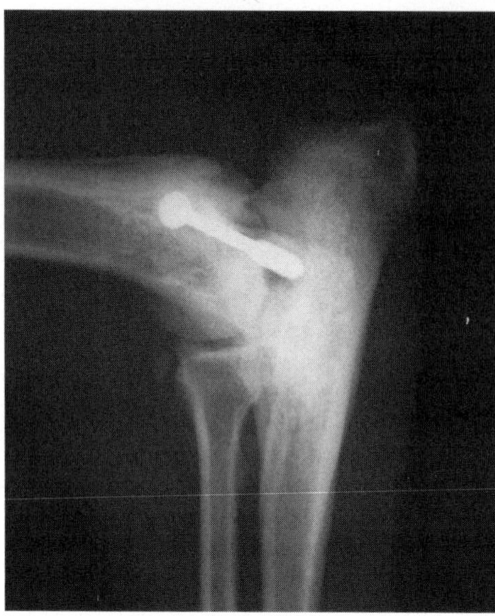
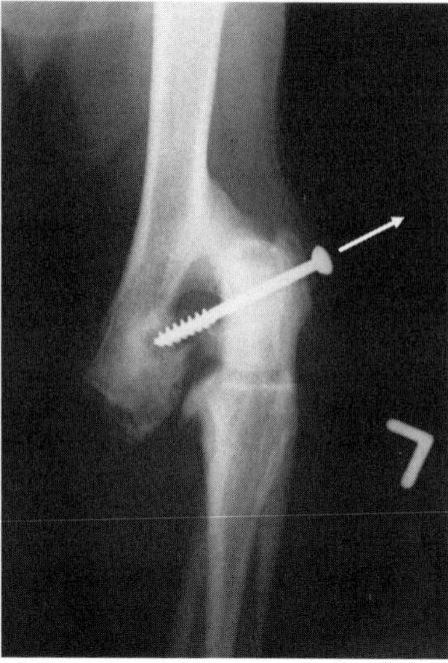

Fig. 16-26 The transcondylar lag screw has loosened and migrated laterally *(arrow)* before bone healing. Consequently, the lateral condylar fracture has formed a malunion and the intercondylar fracture is a nonunion with malarticulation of the medial aspect of the humeral condyle and the medial coronoid process. The radiolucent zone surrounding the screw likely indicates continued motion, most likely caused by interference with the proximal ulna. Remodeling of the medial aspect of the humeral condyle and medial coronoid process is advanced, and repair of the nonunion and malunion will not result in a normal joint.

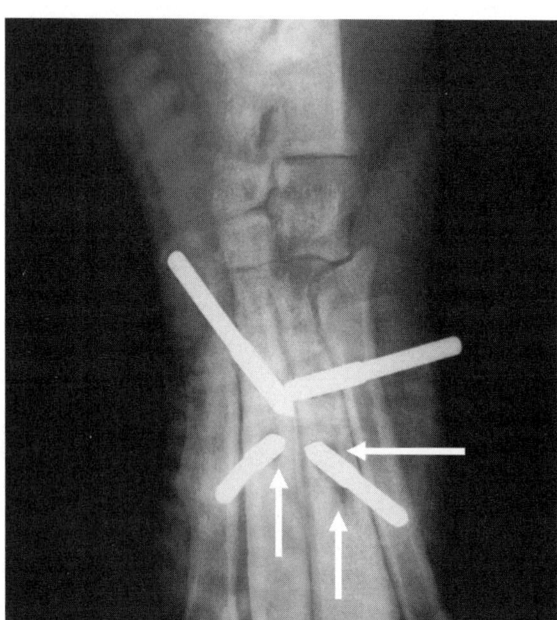

Fig. 16-27 Radiolucencies *(arrows)* surrounding the fixation pins in the metatarsal bones is a result of infection. Purulent discharge was found around the pins. Note the sclerotic reaction within the metatarsal bones.

primary bone healing of the fracture to remodel into dense compact bone.[3]

Soft tissue evaluation completes the radiographic evaluation process. Soft tissue emphysema and swelling is normally seen immediately postoperatively but should resolve in 7 to 10 days. Air pockets that occur after the initial emphysema resolves suggest infection. Soft tissue atrophy is a common sign of disuse and signals significant lameness or disuse of the structure. Mineral opacity in the soft tissues can be seen with dystrophic mineralization caused by previous injury, mineralization of a hematoma associated with the fracture, isolated bone fragment, or cancellous graft material. Mineralization in the soft tissue can also be associated with an aggressive bone lesion such as osteomyelitis or bone tumor. Although rare, fracture and implant-associated sarcomas can occur years after a fracture repair (Fig. 16-30).[43,44]

COMPLICATIONS

Malunion fractures are healed but have abnormal anatomic alignment. These occur from poor initial reduction, shifting of the fragments during the early healing phase, or premature removal of fixation devices before the fracture is stable (Fig. 16-31). Malunion fractures can have a negative effect on function if they are moderate to severe and may require correction (Figs. 16-26 and 16-32). Long bone malunion fractures can be classified as *valgus, varus, antecurvatum, recurvatum, torsional* or *translational* (Fig. 16-33).[3] Torsional (rotational) malunion of less than 10 degrees is difficult to detect on radiographs.[45] A patient can easily compensate for mild shortening of a single bone caused by a malunion. However, if the bone involved is one of a paired system (radius, ulna), the resulting malalignment can lead to dysfunction (Fig. 16-34). Descriptions of malunions can include the terms *functional* and *nonfunctional* to indicate if the malunion is causing dysfunction; however, this is often a clinical finding and not commonly used in a radiographic assessment.[2]

Delayed union is a subjective classification in which a fracture is healing but not as quickly as expected. Generally this indicates a duration longer than typically seen with similar fractures and fixation. A definitive time required for fractures to heal is difficult to define because of the multiple factors that affect the time required for healing, including age, breed, location, type, soft tissue status, defects at the fracture site, and the type of fixation used.[46] Given enough time and no deterioration in stabilization or other complication, a delayed union fracture should eventually heal. If fixation devices are not stable or are migrating, steps may be taken to stabilize the fracture to ensure continued healing.

Nonunion is defined as a fracture that is not healed and has no evidence of progression of the healing process that would result in a bony union. All nonunion fractures first go through a delayed union phase. The key factor in distinguishing a

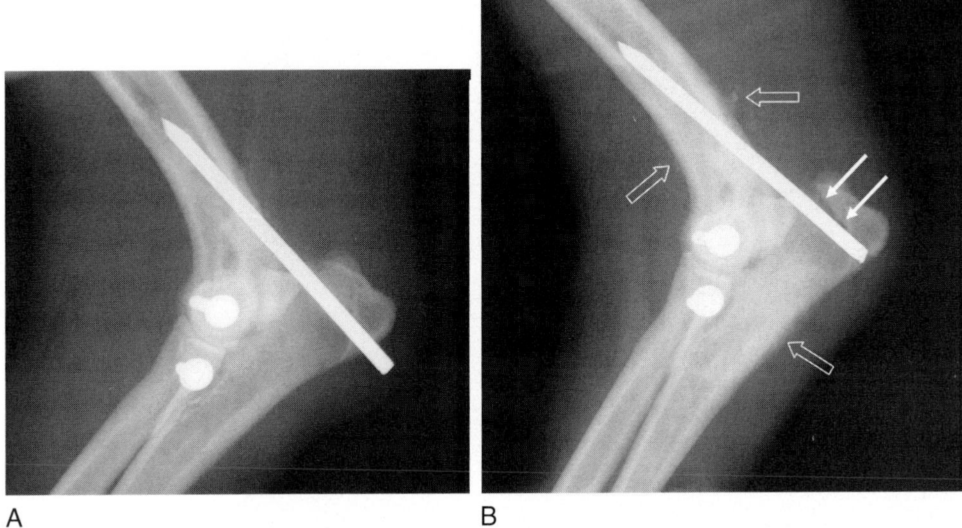

Fig. 16-28 Surgery was performed to repair an elbow luxation. **A,** Postoperative lateral radiographs. **B,** Eleven days later, a smoothly marginated radiolucency *(solid arrows)* surrounding the pin in the proximal ulna is visible, indicating extension and flexion motion of the ulna. The periosteal new bone *(open arrows)* is a result of trauma to the periosteum during surgery and not an indication of infection, although this periosteal appearance could occur as a result of infection.

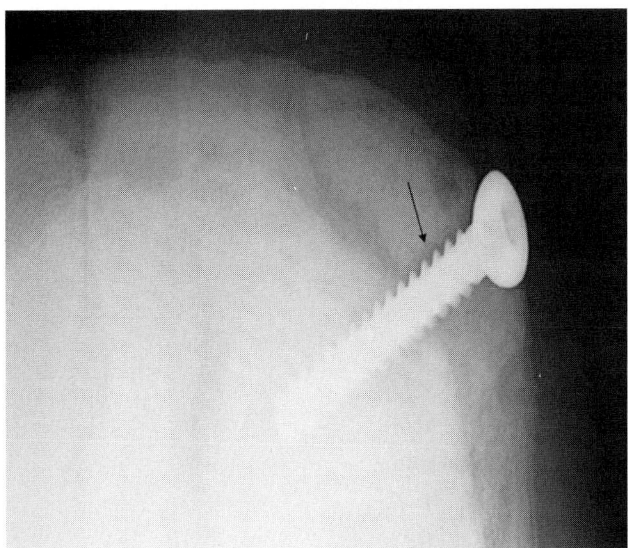

Fig. 16-29 Computed dorsoproximal-dorsodistal radiograph of an equine carpus. A screw has been inserted into the third carpal bone. A radiolucent zone surrounds the screw. This artifact, called the Uberschwinger artifact or rebound effect artifact, occurs when the opacity of adjacent objects is markedly different. It appears as a radiolucent stripe parallel to the interface between the two dissimilar objects. It is caused by the frequency processing algorithm in computed radiography systems in which an "unsharp" (edge enhancement) mask is applied to determine the degree of edge enhancement in the final image.

nonunion from a delayed union is when it can be determined that healing has ceased and will not progress without intervention. Determination of a nonunion is subjective but relies on lack of progression of a healing callus, remodeling of the callus at the fracture ends without bridging, lack of increase in opacity of the fracture line, and duration of the healing process. Some fractures appear to be nonunions that, given enough time, may eventually heal; however, the length of time is much greater than the normal healing time and the outcome is doubtful. Intervention with improved stabilization and possible bone grafts is commonly used to increase the chance of a successful union in a reasonable time.

Some long-term nonunions may develop into a *pseudoarthrosis* as a result of chronic motion at the fracture site (Fig. 16-35). Fibrocartilage fills the fracture gap with a fibrous capsule filled with serum. The patient may have good use of the limb and not have significant pain after formation of the pseudoarthrosis. Many of these are incidental findings and result from previous nondiagnosed and nonrepaired fractures.

In other instances dense, fibrous, and cartilaginous tissue forms that firmly stabilizes a fracture forming a *fibrous union.*[4] In this instance a radiolucent gap or line remains at the fracture site that may or may not opacify over time. A common site for fibrous unions is in fractures of the equine distal phalanx.

Nonunion fractures can be divided into two major classifications, *viable* and *nonviable,* with some defined subclasses.[2]

Viable (reactive, vascular) nonunions are characterized by viable active attempts to heal the fracture with reactive bone and callus formation. Viable nonunions can be divided into three classes.

Hypertrophic ("elephant foot") nonunions are characterized by abundant callus formation and are usually a result of excessive motion in the fracture zone from inadequate fixation, excessive activity by the patient, or premature loosening or removal of the fixation device (Fig. 16-36).

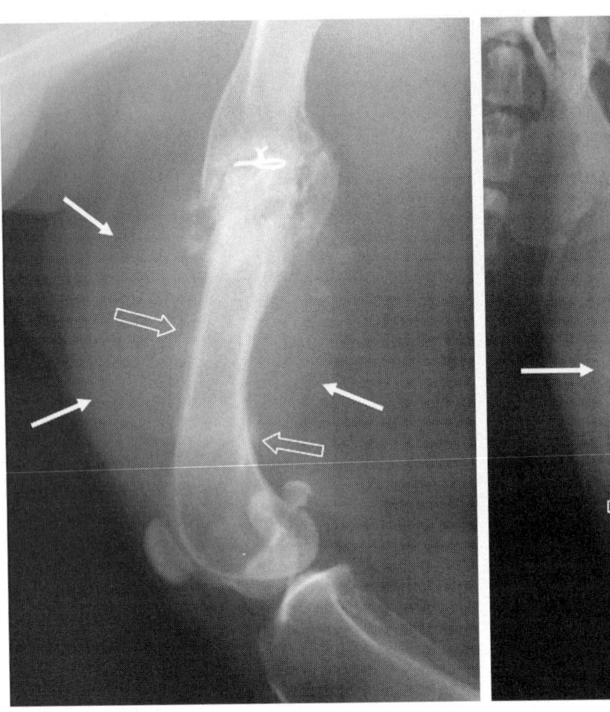

Fig. 16-30 Soft tissue mass *(solid arrows)* and aggressive periosteal new bone *(open arrows)* indicating an aggressive bone lesion at and distal to a malunion fracture.

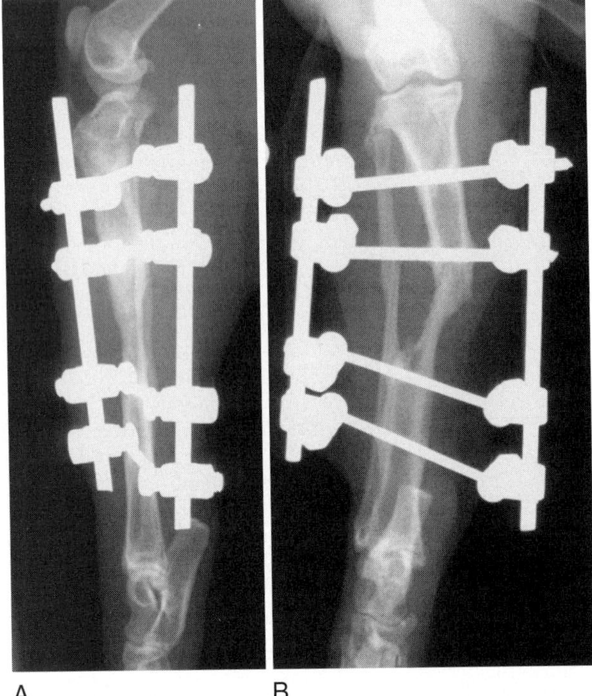

Fig. 16-31 A, Lateral radiograph suggests a healed fracture with good callus. B, Cranial-caudal radiograph shows translational and varus malunion with small amount of callus that will likely fracture when external fixator is removed. Two orthogonal views are required for accurate evaluation.

Moderately hypertrophic ("horse's foot") nonunions are characterized by moderate callus formation that is less than the amount observed with the elephant foot type.

Oligotrophic nonunions have little or no callus with bridging of the fracture fragments by fibrous tissue. These may be difficult to differentiate from nonviable nonunions because of the lack of callus and reaction at the fracture site. Scintigraphy may be used to show blood supply to the fracture gap, indicating viable tissue is present. Generally some bone reaction at the fragment ends will suggest a viable nonunion (Fig. 16-37).

Nonviable nonunions are uncommon and may be easily mistaken for an oligotrophic nonunion, as previously stated. These nonunions occur as a result of severe disruption and lack of adequate blood supply to the fracture site. Nonviable nonunions are further classified into four subgroups.

Dystrophic nonunions occur as a result of poor vascular supply to at least one side of a fragment, preventing bridging callus formation with the opposite fragment. A radiolucent fracture gap will remain with no evidence of callus formation and rounded sclerotic bone edges.

Necrotic nonunions occur as a result of complete loss of vascular supply to the fracture fragment that becomes necrotic and forms a sequestrum at the fracture site. Sepsis may or may not be present. Radiographically the bone fragment retains sharp edges and is sclerotic.

Defect nonunions occur when a large fracture gap is present from the loss or removal of a large fracture fragment. The resulting fracture gap is too large for callus to bridge. The loss may occur at the time of the original injury, during surgery, or later because of sequestra or other complications.

Atrophic nonunions are usually a progression from one of the other types of nonviable nonunion and are characterized by loss of vascularity, resorption, rounding of the fracture ends, and osteoporosis (see Fig. 16-3).

Osteomyelitis associated with a fracture is usually a result of contamination occurring at the time of the fracture, such

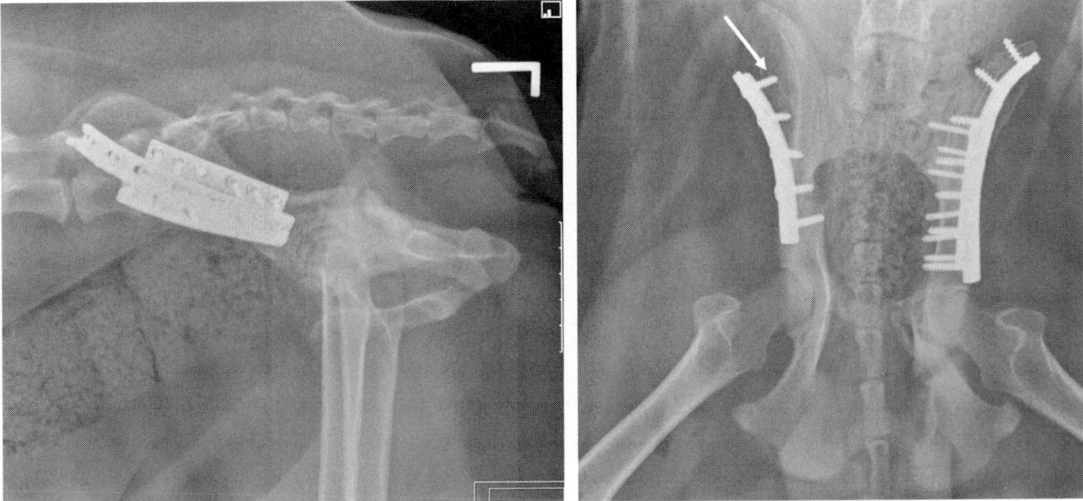

Fig. 16-32 Loosening of the bone plate and screws *(arrow)* from the right ileum, resulting in medial displacement of the acetabulum and malunion. Callus associated with a left acetabular fracture is also present. The significant narrowing of the pelvic canal results in chronic obstipation.

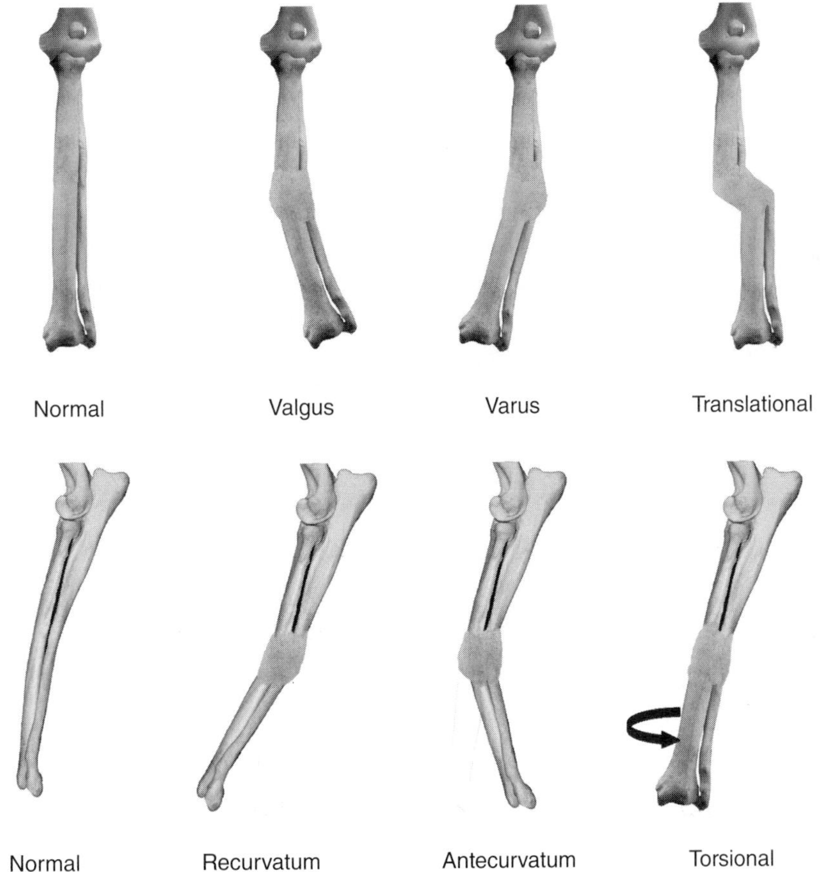

Fig. 16-33 Classification of malunion fractures.

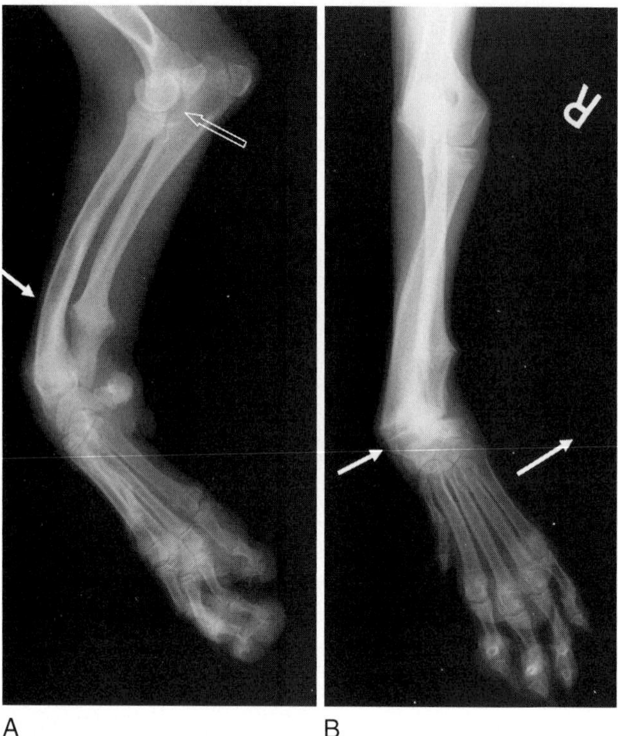

Fig. 16-34 Premature distal physeal closure caused by trauma to the limb. Cessation of longitudinal growth of the ulna results in predictable changes as the radius continues to grow in length. Lateral view (**A**) shows cranial bowing of radius *(solid arrow)* and distal subluxation of the humeroulnar joint *(open arrow)*. Craniocaudal view (**B**) shows valgus angulation of the manus *(arrows)*.

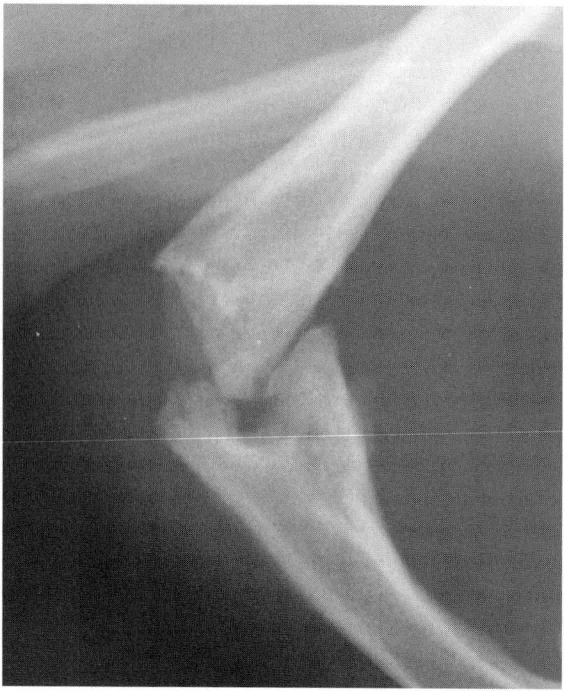

Fig. 16-35 Hypertrophic nonunion of the femoral middiaphysis with pseudoarthrosis. This fracture will not heal without surgical intervention. The dog had an abnormal gate but was not in pain.

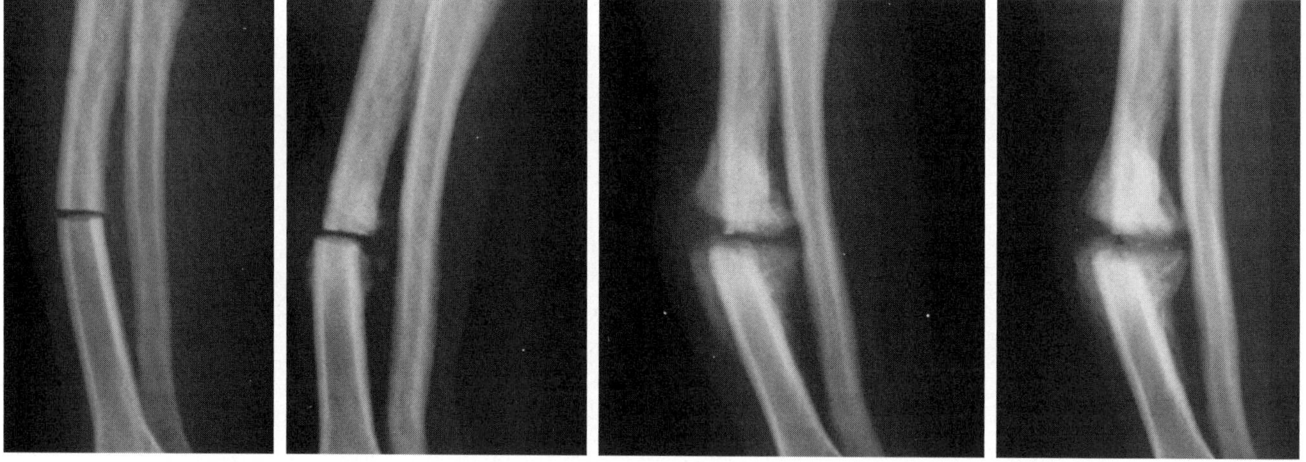

Fig. 16-36 Osteotomy of the radius with lack of fixation develops into a hypertrophic nonunion. Note the exuberant callus around the osteotomy ends with no bridging callus. This appearance is often termed an "elephant foot." (Courtesy Dr. Gregory Daniel, University of Tennessee, Knoxville, Tennessee.)

as an open fracture or contamination during extended surgery. Severe soft tissue damage can also provide a conducive environment for growth of pathogens and predispose the fracture to infection. Early active ossification of a fracture callus can have a fuzzy appearance similar to an early periosteal reaction seen with osteomyelitis, but generally callus is smoother than the periosteal reaction resulting from infection. Also, clinical signs of osteomyelitis should be recognized before radiographic signs are present. The classic clinical signs include, pain, swelling, and heat in the local area with or without a febrile response. In the early stages, soft tissue swelling will be the only radiographic change observed, with rare instances of soft tissue emphysema if a gas-producing organism or draining tract is present. Radiographs made 7 to 10 days after the onset of infection may have early mineralizing periosteal changes. If the infection continues, signs of an aggressive bone

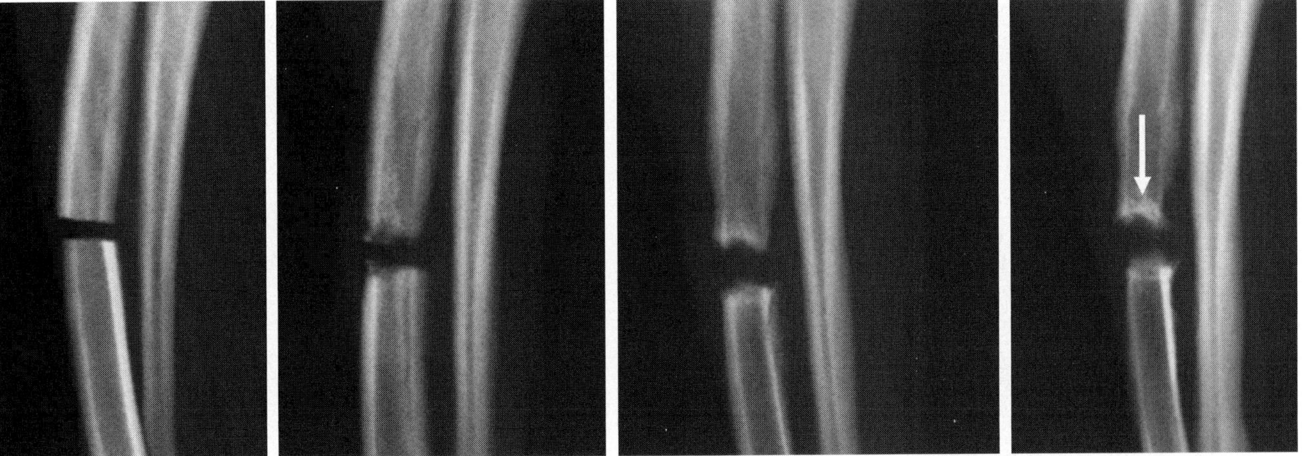

Fig. 16-37 Osteotomy with no fixation develops into an oligotrophic nonunion. Little callus is present at the osteotomy site, with filling in of the ends of the segments seen as a sclerotic band *(arrow)*. (Courtesy Dr. Gregory Daniel, University of Tennessee, Knoxville, Tennessee.)

lesion such as bone lysis may be recognized. Irregular, ill-defined radiolucency surrounding pins or screws with endosteal sclerosis and periosteal reaction at the point of penetration of the device is highly suggestive of osteomyelitis around the pin or screw (Figs. 16-4 and 16-38).

A *bone sequestrum* is a fragment of bone that has lost its blood supply and is no longer viable. The sequestrum may be parosteal, cortical, intramedullary, or a fracture fragment (see Fig. 16-5). Bone sequestra may be *sterile* or *infectious.* A classic sequestrum is recognized as a sharply marginated sclerotic bone fragment (sequestrum) surrounded by or separated from the parent bone by a radiolucent zone that is surrounded by sclerotic bone (involucrum). In some instances a draining tract (cloaca) arises from the radiolucent necrotic area surrounding the sequestrum and extends to the skin surface. Generally less reaction occurs surrounding a sterile sequestrum; however, determining whether the sequestrum is infected or sterile is not always possible.

Angular limb deformities may result from malunion, as previously discussed. However, the most common reference to an angular limb deformity after a fracture is associated with growth disturbances as a result of damage to actively growing (open) physes. Physeal trauma identified as a Salter-Harris type fracture may cause premature closure of part or all of a growth plate, causing cessation of growth in that region of the bone. The most common site for this complication is premature closure of the distal ulnar physis in the dog (see Fig. 16-34). This physis is especially susceptible to injury because of its conical shape, which concentrates forces into the small area of the apex of the physis. This greatly magnifies the force; therefore less force is required to cause significant damage. Other physes distribute the force over a broader area and require more force to cause significant damage. The initial injury results in a Salter-Harris type V fracture that is often not observable radiographically, and the damage is noted only after cessation of growth (closure) causes complications. The radius and ulna are paired bones that must grow in a synchronous manner for normal overall growth of the antebrachium. Premature closure of the distal ulnar physis stops longitudinal growth of the ulna that interferes with the normal linear growth of the radius. As the radius grows longer, the restraint caused by the ulna causes dorsal bowing of the radius, distal subluxation of the humeroulnar joint, distal subluxation of the ulnar carpal joint, and valgus angulation of the manus. The ulnar physis will be "closed" radiographically, as indicated by a lack of the thin radiolucent line normally seen with an open physis. In the antebrachium, closure of the distal radial physis also occurs but is not as common as ulnar closure. Premature closure of the distal radial physis may be partial (Fig. 16-39) or complete compared with premature distal ulnar physis closure, which is usually complete. In premature distal radial physis closure, curvature of the limb is not as common as with premature ulnar closure. More common findings are humeroradial and humeroulnar subluxation,

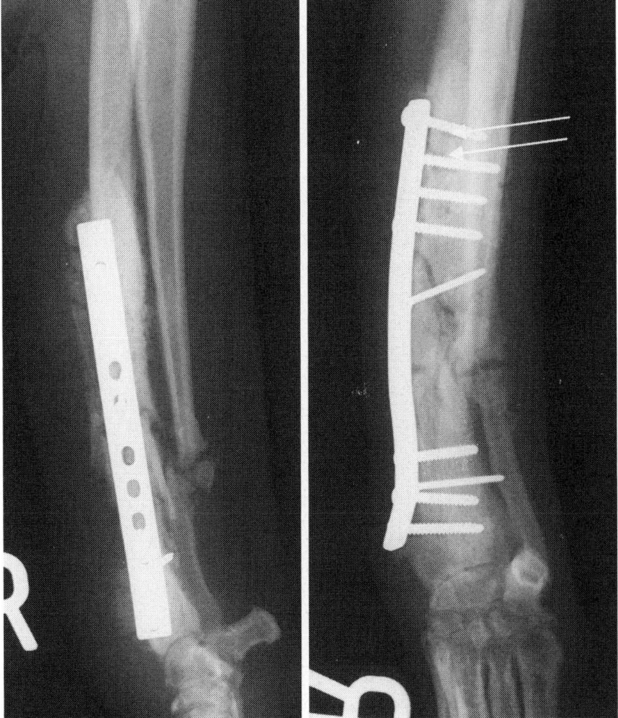

Fig. 16-38 Irregular lytic areas surrounding two plate-associated bone screws caused by infection *(arrows)*. Note the soft tissue swelling visible on the lateral view that is commonly seen with infections and osteomyelitis. Also, the irregular and columnar nature of the periosteal reaction on the craniodistal aspect of the radius is more pronounced than typically seen with callus.

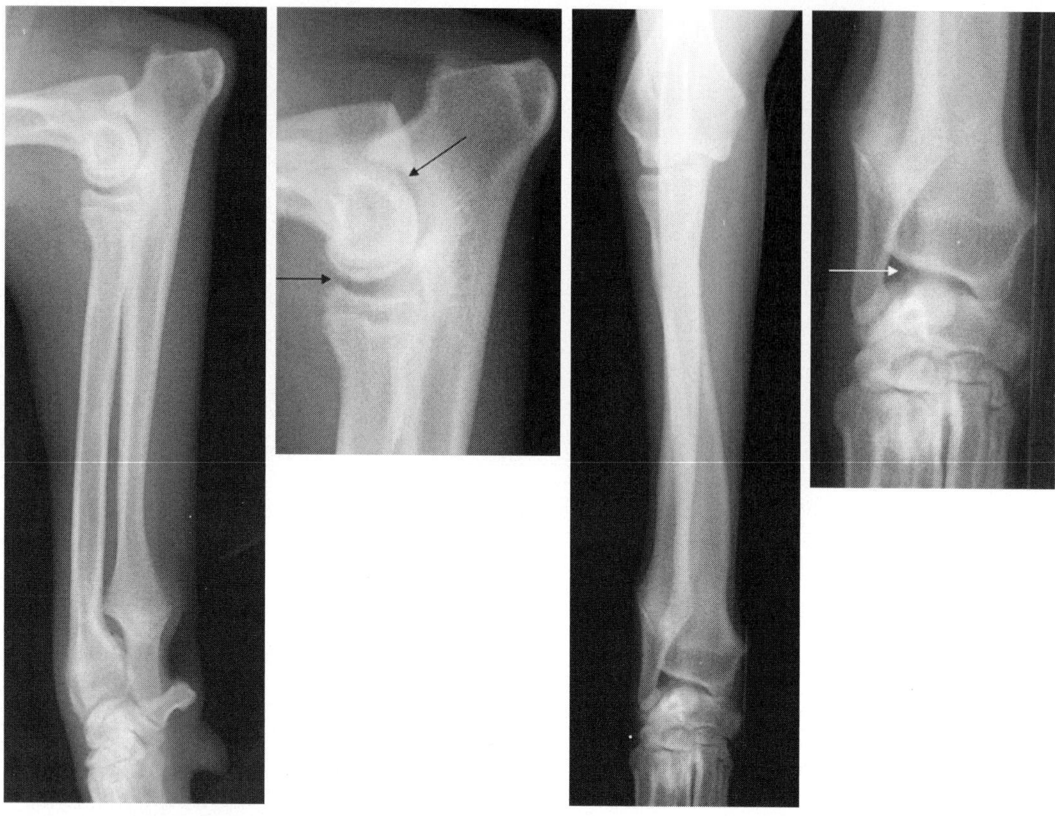

Fig. 16-39 Antebrachial radiographs of a dog with partial closure of the distal radial physis. The physis has closed laterally. The growth retardation has resulted in subluxation of the lateral aspect of the antebrachiocarpal joint *(white arrow)* and humeroradial and humeroulnar subluxation *(black arrows)*. The retarded radial growth results in distal displacement of the radius from the humerus and proximal displacement of the ulna from the humerus. The direction of humeroulnar subluxation with radial closure is opposite from what is observed in ulnar growth retardation (compare to Figure 16-34).

antebrachiocarpal subluxation, and possibly manus deflection, though not as severely valgus as with ulnar closure. In general, the direction and severity of the angular limb deformity depend on factors such as paired versus nonpaired bones, partial or complete physeal closure, and at what age the closure takes place.

REFERENCES

1. Resnick D, Kransdorf MJ: *Bone and joint imaging,* ed 3, Philadelphia, 2005, Elsevier Saunders.
2. Slatter D: *Textbook of small animal surgery, vol 2,* ed 3, Philadelphia, 2003, Saunders.
3. Fossum TW: *Small animal surgery,* ed 2, St. Louis, 2002, Mosby.
4. Rockwood CA, Green DP, Heckman JD et al: *Rockwood and Green's fractures in adults,* ed 5, Philadelphia, 2002, Lippincott Williams & Wilkins.
5. Remedios A: Bone and bone healing, *Vet Clin North Am Small Anim Pract* 29:1029, 1999.
6. Welch RD, Lewis DD: Distraction osteogenesis, *Vet Clin North Am Small Anim Pract* 29:1187, 1999.
7. Nolte DM, Fusco JV, Peterson ME: Incidence of and predisposing factors for nonunion of fractures involving the appendicular skeleton in cats: 18 cases (1998-2002), *J Am Vet Med Assoc* 226:77, 2005.
8. Wheeler P, Batt ME: Do non-steroidal anti-inflammatory drugs adversely affect stress fracture healing? A short review, *Br J Sports Med* 39:65, 2005.
9. Marsh DR, Li G: The biology of fracture healing: optimising outcome, *Br Med Bull* 55:856, 1999.
10. Lienau J, Schell H, Duda GN et al: Initial vascularization and tissue differentiation are influenced by fixation stability, *J Orthop Res* 23:639, 2005.
11. Karladani AH, Granhed H, Karrholm J et al: The influence of fracture etiology and type on fracture healing: a review of 104 consecutive tibial shaft fractures, *Arch Orthop Trauma Surg* 121:325, 2001.
12. Saikku-Backstrom A, Raiha JE, Valimaa T et al: Repair of radial fractures in toy breed dogs with self-reinforced biodegradable bone plates, metal screws, and light-weight external coaptation, *Vet Surg* 34:11, 2005.
13. Welch JA, Boudrieau RJ, DeJardin LM et al: The intraosseous blood supply of the canine radius: implications for healing of distal fractures in small dogs, *Vet Surg* 26:57, 1997.
14. Beale BS: Orthopedic problems in geriatric dogs and cats, *Vet Clin North Am Small Anim Pract* 35:655, 2005.
15. Follak N, Kloting I, Merk H: Influence of diabetic metabolic state on fracture healing in spontaneously diabetic rats, *Diabetes Metab Res Rev* 21:288, 2005.

16. Millis DL: Bone- and non-bone-derived growth factors and effects on bone healing, *Vet Clin North Am Small Anim Pract* 29:1221, 1999.
17. Aaron RK, Ciombor DM, Simon BJ: Treatment of nonunions with electric and electromagnetic fields, *Clin Orthop Relat Res* 419:21, 2004.
18. Barnes GL, Kostenuik PJ, Gerstenfeld LC et al: Growth factor regulation of fracture repair, *J Bone Min Res* 14:1805, 1999.
19. Birnbaum K, Wirtz DC, Siebert CH et al: Use of extracorporeal shock-wave therapy (ESWT) in the treatment of non-unions. A review of the literature, *Arch Orthop Trauma Surg* 122:324, 2002.
20. Goldwirth M, Krasin E: Is it possible to promote fracture repair? Review of biological methods to accelerate fracture repair [Hebrew], *Harefuah* 136:893, 1999.
21. Backstrom KC, Bertone AL, Wisner ER et al: Response of induced bone defects in horses to collagen matrix containing the human parathyroid hormone gene, *Am J Vet Res* 65:1223, 2004.
22. Wilson JW: Vascular supply to normal bone and healing fractures, *Semin Vet Med Surg (Small Anim)* 6:26, 1991.
23. Orsini PG, Rendano VT, Sack WO: Ectopic nutrient foramina in the third metatarsal bone of the horse, *Equine Vet J* 13:132, 1981.
24. Becht JL, Park RD, Kraft SL et al: Radiographic interpretation of normal skeletal variations and pseudolesions in the equine foot, *Vet Clin North Am Equine Pract* 17:1, 2001.
25. Sande R: Radiography of orthopedic trauma and fracture repair, *Vet Clin North Am Small Anim Pract* 29:1247, 1999.
26. Breederveld RS, Tuinebreijer WE: Investigation of computed tomographic scan concurrent criterion validity in doubtful scaphoid fracture of the wrist, *J Trauma* 57:851, 2004.
27. Harris JH, Coupe KJ, Lee JS et al: Acetabular fractures revisited: a new CT-based classification, *Semin Musculoskelet Radiol* 9:150, 2005.
28. Grainger RG, Allison DJ, Adam A et al, editors: *Grainger & Allison's diagnostic radiology: a textbook of medical imaging,* vol 3, ed 4, New York, 2001, Churchill Livingstone.
29. Borrelli J Jr, Ricci WM, Steger-May K et al: Postoperative radiographic assessment of acetabular fractures: a comparison of plain radiographs and CT scans, *J Orthop Trauma* 19:299, 2005.
30. Hoskinson JJ: Equine nuclear scintigraphy. Indications, uses, and techniques, *Vet Clin North Am Equine Pract* 17:63, 2001.
31. Koblik PD, Hornof WJ, Seeherman HJ: Scintigraphic appearance of stress-induced trauma of the dorsal cortex of the third metacarpal bone in racing Thoroughbred horses: 121 cases (1978-1986), *J Am Vet Med Assoc* 192:390, 1988.
32. Berry CR, Daniel GB: *The handbook of veterinary nuclear medicine,* Raleigh, NC, 1996, North Carolina State University College of Veterinary Medicine.
33. Twardock AR: Equine bone scintigraphic uptake patterns related to age, breed, and occupation, *Vet Clin North Am Equine Pract* 17:75, 2001.
34. Tucker RL, Sande RD: Computed tomography and magnetic resonance imaging of the equine musculoskeletal conditions, *Vet Clin North Am Equine Pract* 17:145, 2001.
35. Reef VB: Advances in diagnostic ultrasonography, *Vet Clin North Am Equine Pract* 7:451, 1991.
36. Reef VB: Superficial digital flexor tendon healing: ultrasonographic evaluation of therapies, *Vet Clin North Am Equine Pract* 17:159, 2001.
37. Davidson EJ, Martin BB Jr: Stress fracture of the scapula in two horses, *Vet Radiol Ultrasound* 45:407, 2004.
38. Craig JG, Jacobson JA, Moed BR: Ultrasound of fracture and bone healing, *Radiol Clin North Am* 37:737, 1999.
39. Salter R, Harris W: Injuries involving the epiphyseal plate, *J Bone Joint Surg* 45:587, 1963.
40. Solomon SL, Jost RG, Glazer HS et al: Artifacts in computed radiography, *AJR Am J Roentgenol* 157:181, 1999.
41. Tan TH, Boothroyd AE: Uberschwinger artefact in computed radiographs, *Br J Radiol* 70:431, 1997.
42. Wade R, Richardson J: Outcome in fracture healing: a review, *Injury* 32:109, 2001.
43. Stevenson S, Hohn RB et al: Fracture-associated sarcoma in the dog, *J Am Vet Med Assoc* 180:1189, 1982.
44. Jackson LC, Pacchiana PD: Common complications of fracture repair, *Clin Tech Small Anim Pract* 19:168, 2004.
45. Newton CD, Nunamaker DM: *Textbook of small animal orthopaedics,* Philadelphia, 1985, Lippincott.
46. Piermattei DL, Flo GL, Brinker WO et al: *Brinker, Piermattei, and Flo's handbook of small animal orthopedics and fracture repair,* ed 3, Philadelphia, 1997, WB Saunders.

ELECTRONIC RESOURCES evolve

Additional information related to the content in Chapter 16 can be found on the companion Web site at evolve http://evolve.elsevier.com/Thrall/vetrad/

- Key Points
- Chapter Quiz
- Case Study 16-1
- Case Study 16-2

CHAPTER • 17
Radiographic Features of Bone Tumors and Bone Infections

Donald E. Thrall

Bone tumors and bone infections usually have an aggressive radiographic appearance. The radiographic signs of aggressive bone lesions are discussed in Chapter 12. A definitive distinction between neoplastic and infectious bone lesions is impossible by radiographic means. However, the radiographic features of the bone lesion—such as the number of bones involved and the location of the lesions within the bones–and the signalment, history, and physical and laboratory findings can often be used to prioritize the diagnostic possibilities accurately. Nevertheless, a biopsy with histopathologic evaluation and possibly microbiologic culture is needed for the definitive diagnosis of any aggressive bone lesion.

PRIMARY BONE TUMORS

Primary bone tumors are typically characterized by a single metaphyseal aggressive bone lesion.[1] Such a lesion in a dog or cat should be considered a primary bone tumor until proven otherwise. Although primary bone tumors typically begin in the metaphysis, they may readily involve the epiphysis and diaphysis. The opinion that primary bone tumors do not cross joints or invade adjacent bones is false because both may occur as the tumor enlarges. Such invasion, however, occurs later in the disease process. Additionally, primary bone tumors may metastasize to parenchymal organs and other parts of the skeleton. Subclinical metastasis of osteosarcoma in dogs has usually occurred by the time the primary tumor is diagnosed.

Canine Osteosarcoma

Osteosarcoma is the most common primary bone tumor in dogs; other histologic types are uncommon. Interestingly, in dogs the age distribution of osteosarcoma is bimodal with a small peak in incidence at approximately 2 years of age and then a larger peak in incidence later in adult life.[2]

Osteosarcomas usually originate in the metaphysis of long tubular bones in large and giant breeds. Common forelimb osteosarcoma sites are the proximal humerus and the distal radius (away from the elbow). In the hindlimb, the distal femur and proximal tibia (toward the stifle) are common locations, but tumors in the distal tibia also occur. Osteosarcomas may be primarily lytic (Fig. 17-1), primarily sclerotic (blastic or productive) (Fig. 17-2), or mixed, with both lytic and productive features (Fig. 17-3); the mixed presentation is most common. Of note, the degree of lysis versus sclerosis is not a feature that should be used in deciding whether a lesion is aggressive (see Chapter 12).

Osteosarcomas may also be characterized by a range of periosteal reactions, varying from active (also called irregularly marginated) (Fig. 17-4) to inactive (also called smoothly marginated) (see Figs. 17-1 and 17-2). Although bone infections may have an active periosteal reaction, extremely aggressive and amorphous types of periosteal reactions are more commonly associated with tumors.

Codman's triangle, which is an isolated cuff (triangle) of reactive subperiosteal new bone,[3] is a roentgen sign sometimes considered pathognomonic for a primary bone tumor (Fig. 17-5). However, a Codman's triangle can be present at the boundary of any benign or malignant mass that elevates the periosteum and is not specific for any bone condition.[3]

Feline Osteosarcoma

Osteosarcoma is also the most commonly encountered primary bone tumor in cats, but its prevalence is lower than in dogs.[4-8] Age distribution in cats is not bimodal; mean age at time of diagnosis is approximately 10 years.[5] As in dogs, feline osteosarcomas result in an aggressive bone lesion, but the hindlimbs are affected more often than the forelimbs. The radiographic appearance of osteosarcoma in cats has been reported to be primarily osteolytic,[6] but a spectrum of tumor opacities has also been reported.[4] Thus the radiographic spectrum of feline osteosarcoma appears to not be significantly different from that in dogs (Fig. 17-6). Pulmonary metastasis from feline osteosarcoma is less common than with canine osteosarcoma.[8,9]

Osteosarcoma as a Secondary Event

Situations can occur in which the development of osteosarcoma is secondary to another bone abnormality. For example, dogs developing polyostotic bone infarction are prone to develop osteosarcoma.[10] Bone infarcts may be idiopathic[11] or caused by bone trauma, such as total hip arthroplasty.[12] Idiopathic polyostotic bone infarction is a rare condition characterized by formation of multifocal medullary opacities in both long and short tubular bones (Fig. 17-7). The specific cause-and-effect relation between bone infarction and bone sarcoma is unknown. Dogs developing idiopathic polyostotic bone infarction and subsequent osteosarcoma are occasionally small-breed dogs (Shelties and Terriers) in contrast to the large breeds that typically develop primary osteosarcoma. Bone infarction resulting from physical injury to the bone, such as from internal fixation, may also predispose to development of osteosarcoma (Fig. 17-8).[13]

Rarely, occurrence of a fracture or use of an internal fixation device will lead to the development of a primary bone tumor. Case history reports have been published in both dogs and cats in which the development of osteosarcoma after skeletal trauma has been documented (see Chapter 15).

FUNGAL BONE INFECTIONS

Fungal disease in dogs typically involves large-breed young adults.[14] Fungal osteomyelitis is uncommon in cats. Fungal osteomyelitis is most commonly identified in geographic

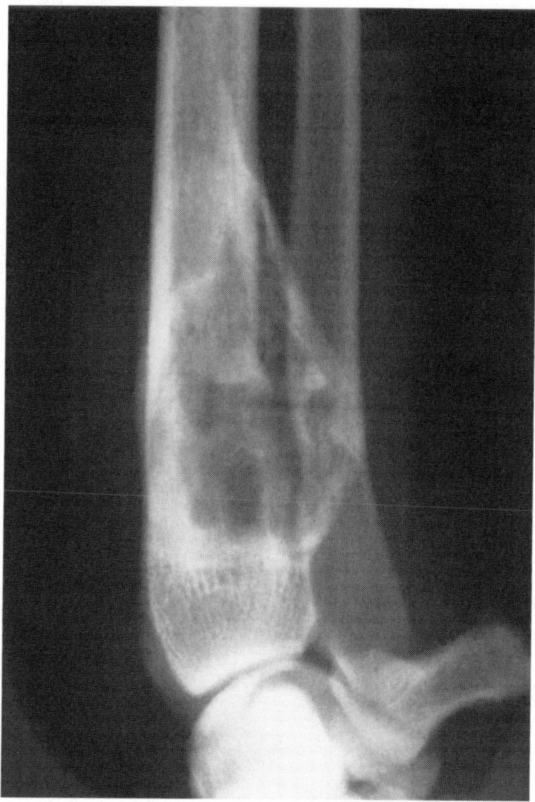

Fig. 17-1 Lateral view of the distal antebrachium. A primarily lytic lesion involves the distal radial metaphysis. The lesion is aggressive because of the lack of a defined transition zone between normal and abnormal bone. The cortex is expanded caudally. Margins of this lesion are relatively smooth. This lesion has not crossed the region of the closed physis, but many osteosarcomas extend into the diaphysis. The diagnosis is osteosarcoma.

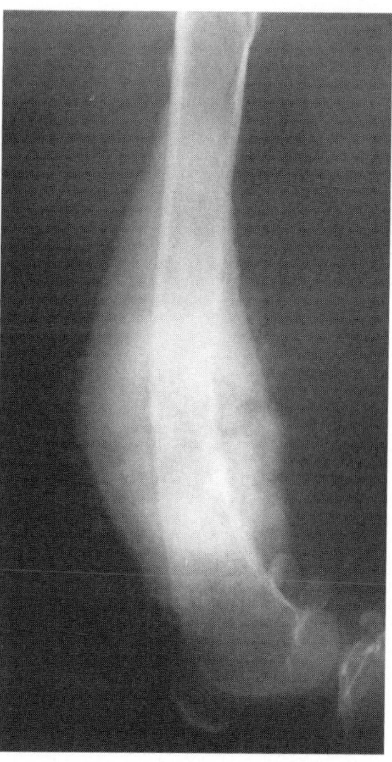

Fig. 17-2 Lateral view of the femur. A predominantly blastic (sclerotic) lesion is present in the distal diaphysis and metaphysis. The periosteal reaction is smooth, and little evidence is present of cortical destruction. However, the lesion is aggressive because of the lack of a sharp transition zone proximally between normal and abnormal bone. The diagnosis is osteosarcoma.

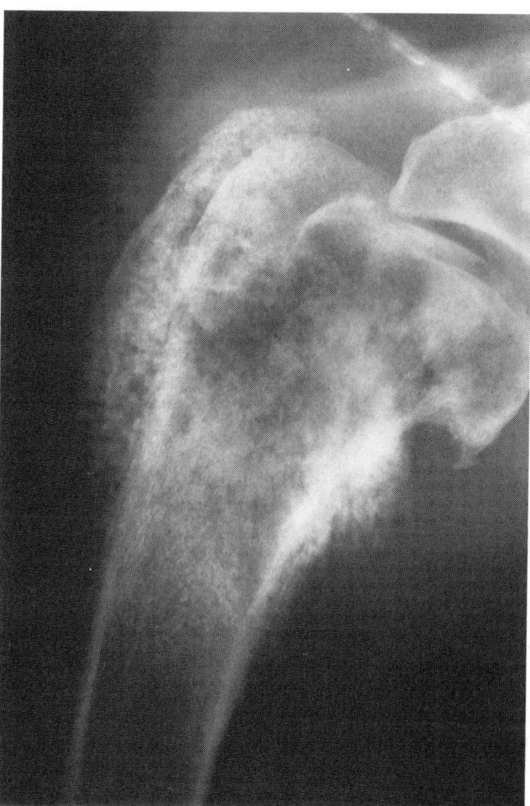

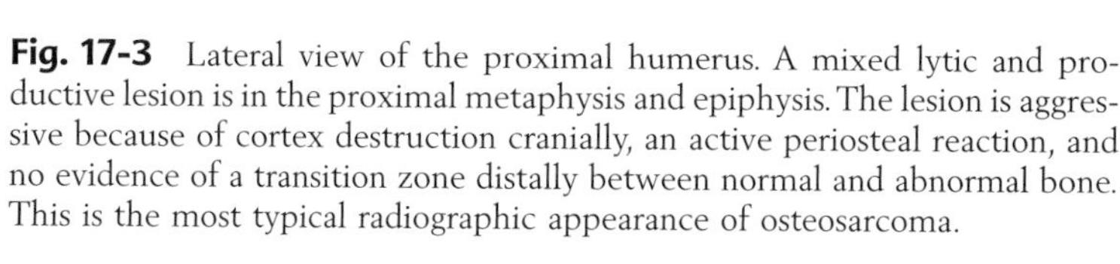

Fig. 17-3 Lateral view of the proximal humerus. A mixed lytic and productive lesion is in the proximal metaphysis and epiphysis. The lesion is aggressive because of cortex destruction cranially, an active periosteal reaction, and no evidence of a transition zone distally between normal and abnormal bone. This is the most typical radiographic appearance of osteosarcoma.

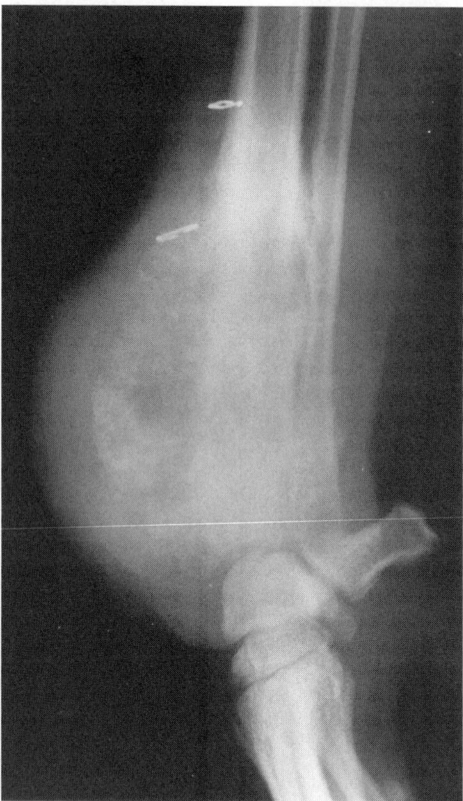

Fig. 17-4 Lateral view of the distal antebrachium. A mixed lytic and productive lesion is present in the distal radius. The lesion is aggressive because the cortex is destroyed cranially and caudally, an active periosteal reaction is present, and an indistinct transition zone is seen proximally between normal and abnormal bone. The metallic wires were inserted after a biopsy. The periosteal reaction is quite irregular. Infections, especially bacterial infections, do not typically result in this extent of periosteal irregularity. The diagnosis is osteosarcoma.

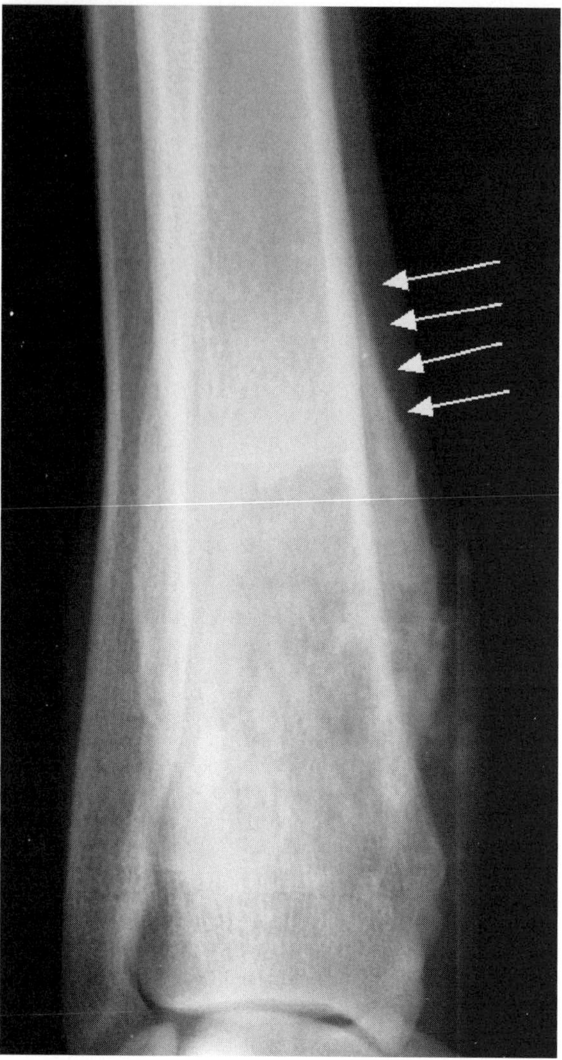

Fig. 17-5 Craniocaudal view of the distal antebrachium of a dog with a distal radial osteosarcoma. The appearance of the triangular periosteal reaction at the proximomedial aspect of the lesion *(arrows)* has been termed a Codman's triangle and is often associated with osteosarcoma to the extent that it is presumed to be pathognomonic. However, this triangle results from periosteal elevation and can be present in neoplastic infections and traumatic lesions. A Codman's triangle can also be seen in Figs. 17-1 and 17-2.

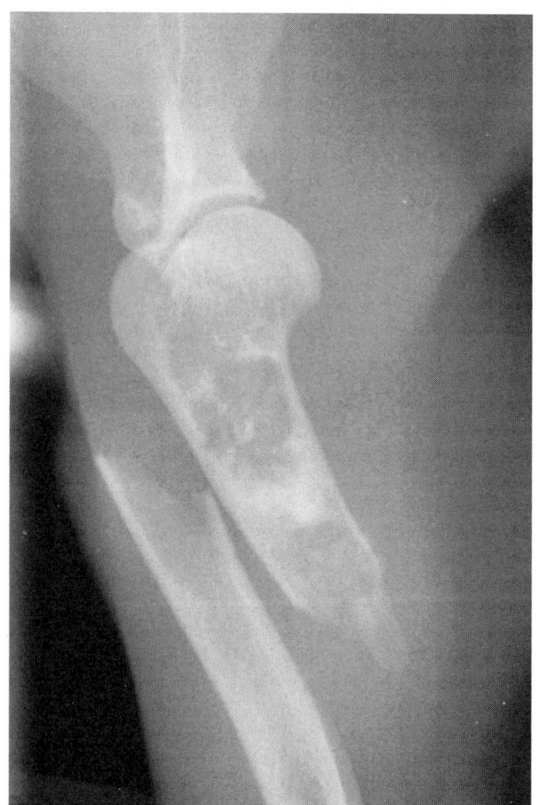

Fig. 17-6 Lateral view of the proximal humerus in a cat. An aggressive lesion is in the proximal humerus. The lesion is primarily lytic but some peripheral sclerosis is present, especially distally. The fracture is likely a pathologic fracture caused by decreased structural integrity of the bone. The diagnosis is osteosarcoma.

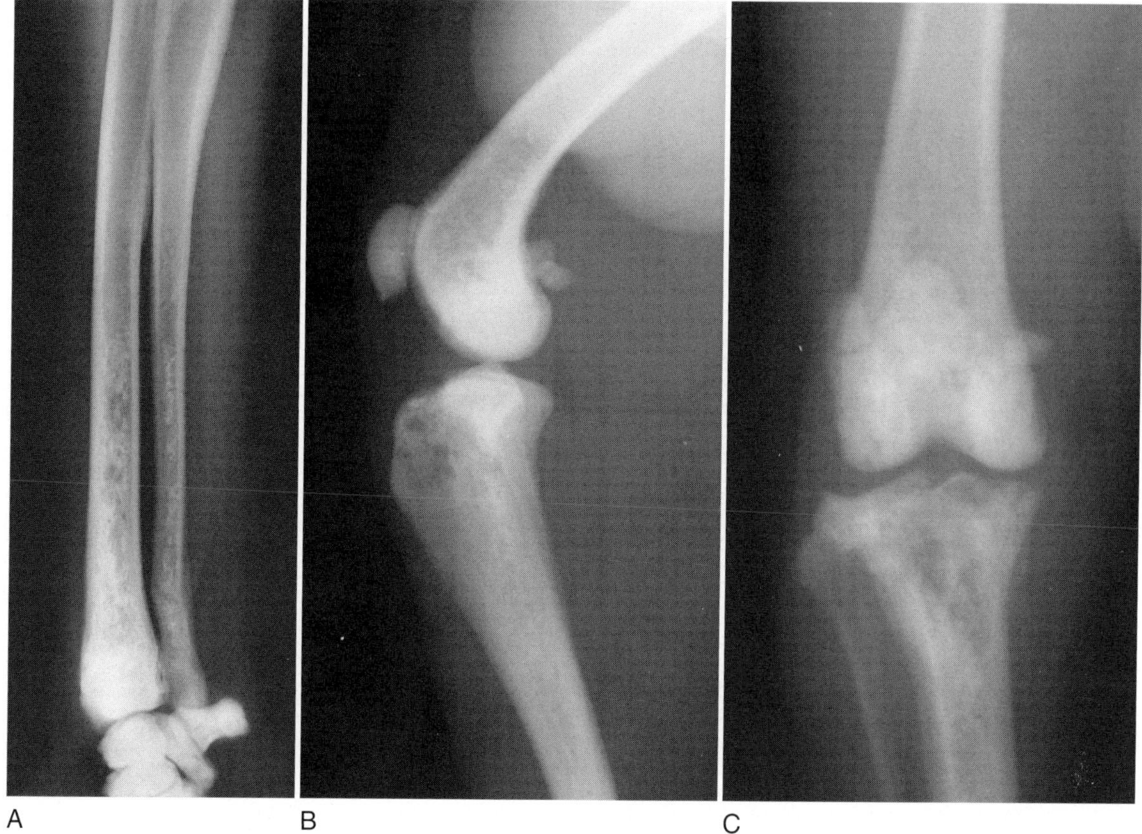

Fig. 17-7 A, Lateral view of the antebrachium. Multifocal regions of opacity are present within the medullary cavity of the distal radius and ulna that are caused by bone infarction. Lateral **(B)** and craniocaudal **(C)** views of the stifle of the same dog. Bone infarcts are again visible. An aggressive, primarily lytic, lesion is also present in the proximal tibia that was diagnosed as osteosarcoma. This tumor developed as a consequence of the uncharacterized bone derangement associated with the infarcts.

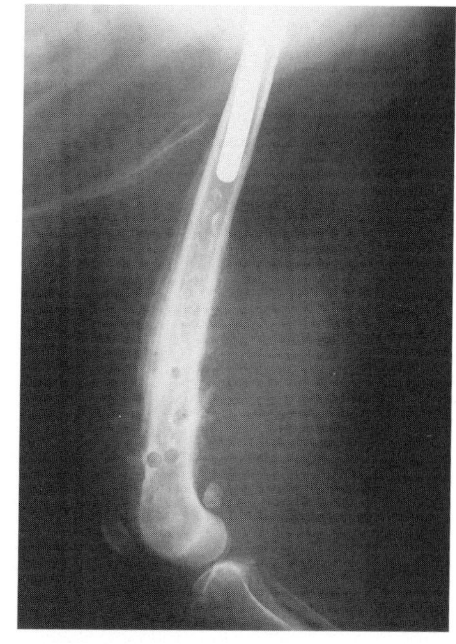

Fig. 17-8 Lateral view of the femur. The stem of the femoral component of a total hip prosthesis is visible. The prosthesis had been present for 5 years. Focal opacities in the medullary cavity of the femur developed shortly after implant insertion and were interpreted as bone infarcts. The dog became acutely lame. This radiograph shows a lamellar periosteal reaction is present cranially but an irregular, active periosteal reaction is present caudally. Also noted is soft tissue swelling, which contains regions of mineralization; distally, no obvious transition between normal and abnormal bone is present. These radiographic signs indicate an aggressive process. Multiple biopsies of the femur were obtained; circular biopsy sites are visible. The histologic diagnosis was osteosarcoma, and the tumor most likely resulted from the longstanding infarcts.

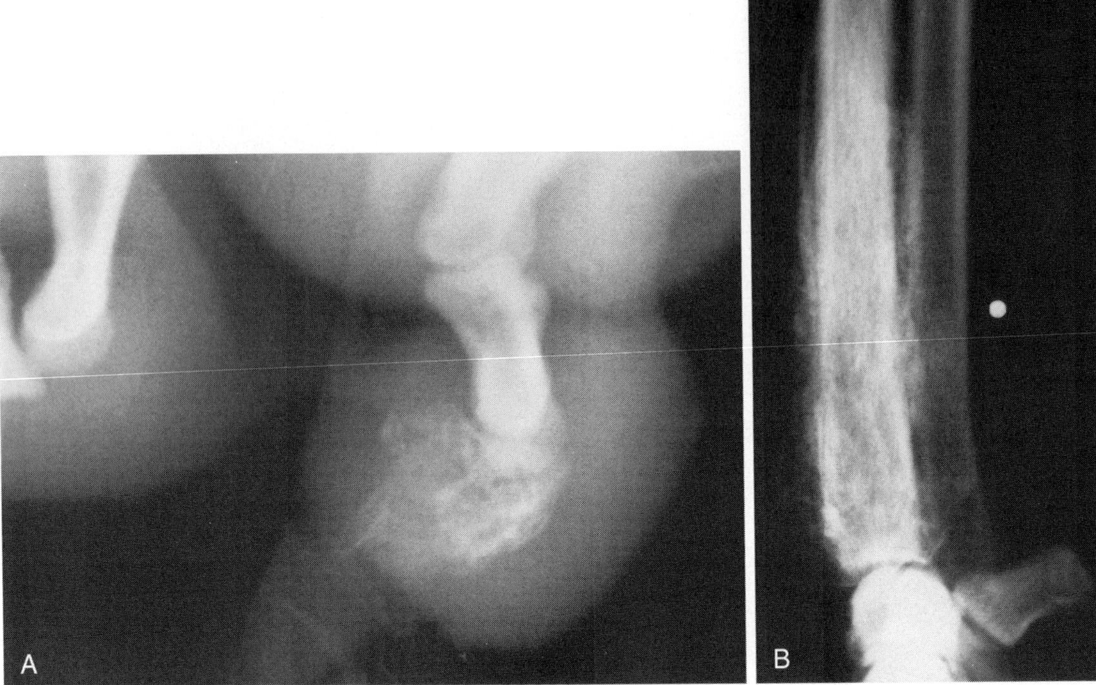

Fig. 17-9 Lateral radiographs of a rear-limb distal phalanx (A) and the distal antebrachium (B) of a 5-year-old, mixed-breed dog with a history of lameness and weight loss. The phalanx is characterized by multifocal regions of lysis, with some evidence of new bone formation. The cortex of the phalanx is destroyed. The distal radius is characterized by mottled regions of increased and decreased bone opacity. The cortex is destroyed cranially and caudally, and an active periosteal reaction is present. No sharp transition zone is present proximally between normal and abnormal bone. The phalanx and radial lesions are both aggressive. Taken alone, each is consistent with primary neoplasia. Taken collectively, a more likely diagnosis is mycotic osteomyelitis or metastatic solid tumor. This dog is relatively young, lives in a blastomycosis-endemic area, and had no identifiable primary tumor. Blastomycosis titers were high, and *Blastomyces* species was isolated from a bone biopsy.

regions where predisposing fungi are endemic, such as the southeast (blastomycosis) and the southwest (coccidioidomycosis) regions of the United States. However, infected dogs may relocate to nonendemic areas where they may be examined by veterinarians who do not have a high index of suspicion for fungal infections.

Fungal osteomyelitis is generally of hematogenous origin, leading to a polyostotic distribution within the skeleton; the appendicular and axial skeleton may be involved. In the appendicular skeleton, hematogenous afflictions typically involve the metaphyseal region of long bones because of the rich capillary network located there. This capillary network acts as a filter and the microenvironment is rich in nutrients, providing fertile ground for colonization. Nevertheless, diaphyseal infections arising from hematogenous dissemination also occur. Bone lesions of fungal osteomyelitis can appear quite aggressive radiographically, leading them to be confused with tumors. Fungal osteomyelitis should be considered in any dog in whom polyostotic aggressive bone lesions are identified (Fig. 17-9).

Rarely, fungal osteomyelitis will be monostotic and metaphyseal-epiphyseal in location (Fig. 17-10). Such lesions are usually impossible to distinguish radiographically from a bone tumor. Thus any monostotic metaphyseal aggressive lesion should be biopsied before a course of therapy is selected. Other radiographic evidence, such as pulmonary infiltrates or mediastinal lymphadenopathy, or clinical signs of systemic debilitation may support the diagnosis of an infectious process, but a biopsy of the bone lesion is necessary for a definitive diagnosis.

BACTERIAL BONE INFECTIONS

Most bone infections in dogs and cats are of bacterial origin.[15] Bacterial bone infections are acquired by (1) direct inoculation, such as from an open fracture, a bite wound, or surgery; (2) extension from soft tissue injury; or (3) hematogenous dissemination.[15] Direct inoculation and extension from the soft tissue are much more common causes of bacterial bone infection in dogs and cats than is hematogenous dissemination.

Direct inoculation or extensions from soft tissue as causes of bacterial bone infection have no predilection for skeletal localization; lesions develop at the site of injury (Fig. 17-11). Therefore bacterial osteomyelitis usually involves only one limb, but more than one bone may be involved. A history of previous trauma or surgery is usually present, and any breed can be affected. Thus little confusion should exist between bacterial osteomyelitis resulting from direct inoculation or extension and a primary bone tumor.

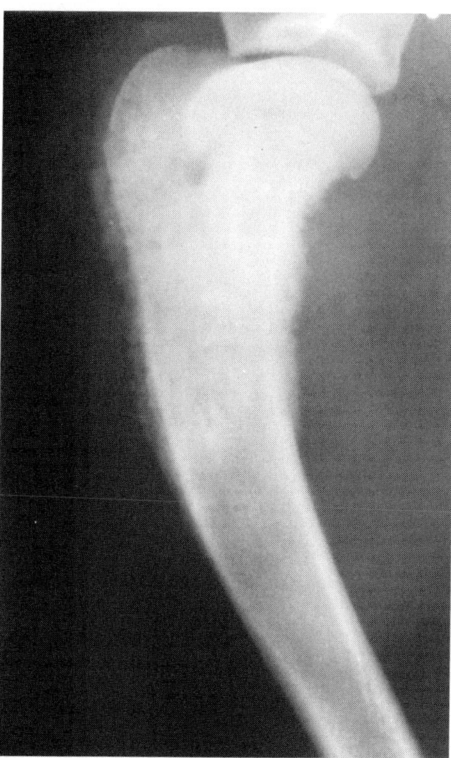

Fig. 17-10 Lateral view of the proximal humerus. A predominantly proliferative lesion is present in the metaphysis and the epiphysis. Cortex destruction, active periosteal reaction, and an indistinct transition zone distally between normal and abnormal bone are visible. Therefore the lesion is aggressive. Other bone lesions were not detected. The appearance of the lesion is consistent with a primary bone tumor. The focal lytic region was produced by a biopsy. *Actinomyces* species was identified. The bone lesion resolved after appropriate drug therapy.

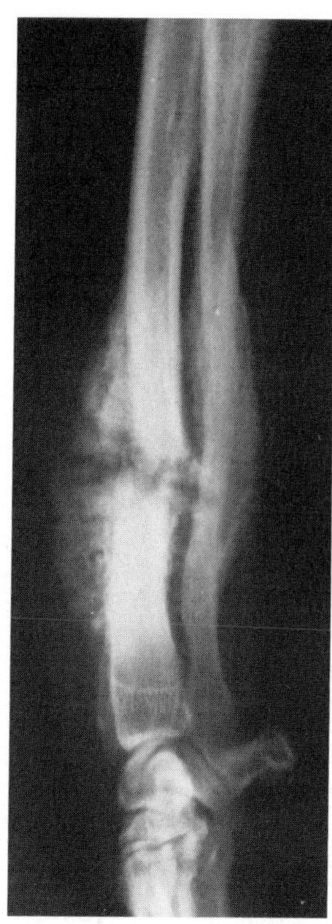

Fig. 17-11 Lateral view of the antebrachium of a 2-year-old dog that was bitten by another dog 2 months previously. The dog was lame and the limb was swollen. The radius is characterized by increased opacity in the distal diaphysis and metaphysis, an active periosteal reaction, and a fracture. The periosteal reaction has a palisade appearance in some areas. A palisading periosteal reaction may be produced by a tumor but seems more commonly associated with bacterial osteomyelitis. The ulna is characterized by a relatively smooth periosteal reaction, increased bone opacity, and apparent bending around the radial lesion. No sharp transition zones are present proximally or distally in either the radius or ulna. Both the radial and the ulnar lesions are aggressive. Although pathologic fractures occasionally develop from primary bone tumors, the history and signalment and the fact that both the radius and the ulna are involved extensively suggest infection as the most likely diagnosis. The final diagnosis is dog bite–induced radial fracture and bacterial osteomyelitis.

Although bacterial bone infections and bone tumors result in aggressive bone lesions, the lesions have little in common. Osteomyelitic bone lesions in dogs and cats are typically not metaphyseal in location and may involve more than one bone and generally are not as aggressive as those resulting from bone tumors. Most bacterial osteomyelitic lesions will have a periosteal reaction. The less-aggressive appearance of osteomyelitic lesions relative to bone tumors particularly applies to the periosteal reaction, where spiculation, commonly found in tumors, is unusual. Osteomyelitic periosteal reactions often have a palisading or columnar appearance to the periosteal reaction, in which vertically oriented columns of new bone are oriented perpendicular to the cortex (Figs. 17-11 through 17-13). Certainly this type of periosteal reaction can be seen in neoplastic bone lesions, but it seems more typical of bacterial bone infections.

Hematogenous bacterial bone infection typically results in polyostotic metaphyseal lesions because of the rich blood supply in this region of the bone; circulating bacteria are able to colonize this rich environment after being filtered by the extensive capillary network. Lesions of hematogenous bacterial osteomyelitis may be either lytic, productive, or mixed depending on the relative virulence of the organism and defense capacity of the bone (Fig. 17-14). Fortunately, bone is relatively resistant to infection. Most dogs and cats with hematogenous bacterial osteomyelitis are skeletally immature, making confusion with neoplasia unlikely.

PROTOZOAN BONE INFECTIONS

Hepatozoonosis is a rare protozoan infection that may cause polyostotic aggressive lesions.[16] *Hepatozoon* infections have been diagnosed in dogs throughout the world; in the United States, most infections occur in the South.[17] The primary vector of *Hepatozoon* infections is the brown dog tick, *Rhipicephalus sanguineus*. Radiographically, findings are primarily limited to the periosteum and range from irregular periosteal

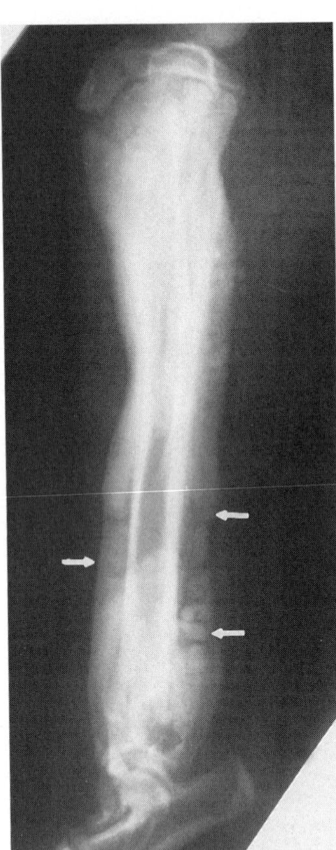

Fig. 17-12 Lateral view of the tibia of a 6-month-old dog made 3 weeks after external fixation of an open distal tibial physeal fracture. The limb is swollen, warm, and painful. Extensive periosteal reaction is present along the bone. In some areas the periosteal reaction has a palisade appearance *(arrows)*. A palisading periosteal reaction may be produced by a tumor but seems more commonly associated with bacterial osteomyelitis. Considering the age of the patient, the history, the extension of the periosteal reaction along the entire shaft of the bone, and the palisade appearance of the periosteal reaction, the most likely diagnosis is bacterial osteomyelitis. Neoplasia is not a likely diagnosis in this patient.

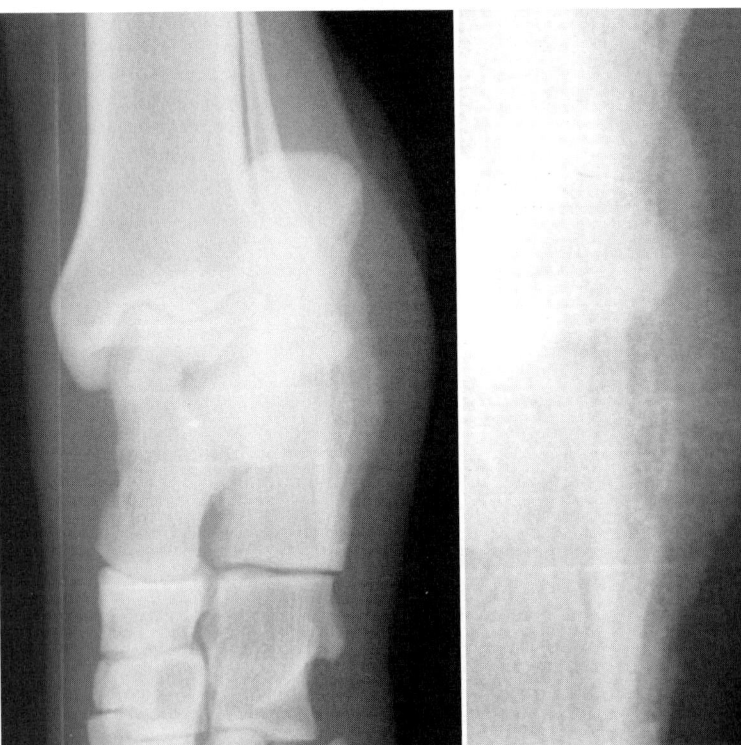

Fig. 17-13 A, Dorsolateral-plantaromedial oblique view of the tarsus of a dog with tarsal swelling. An irregular periosteal reaction is present on the plantarolateral margin of the calcaneus. **B,** Close-up of the periosteal reaction, which has a palisading appearance. The irregularity of the periosteal reaction makes this lesion aggressive, but this is an unusual location for a primary tumor or hematogenous infection. The most likely diagnosis is infection associated with puncture wound.

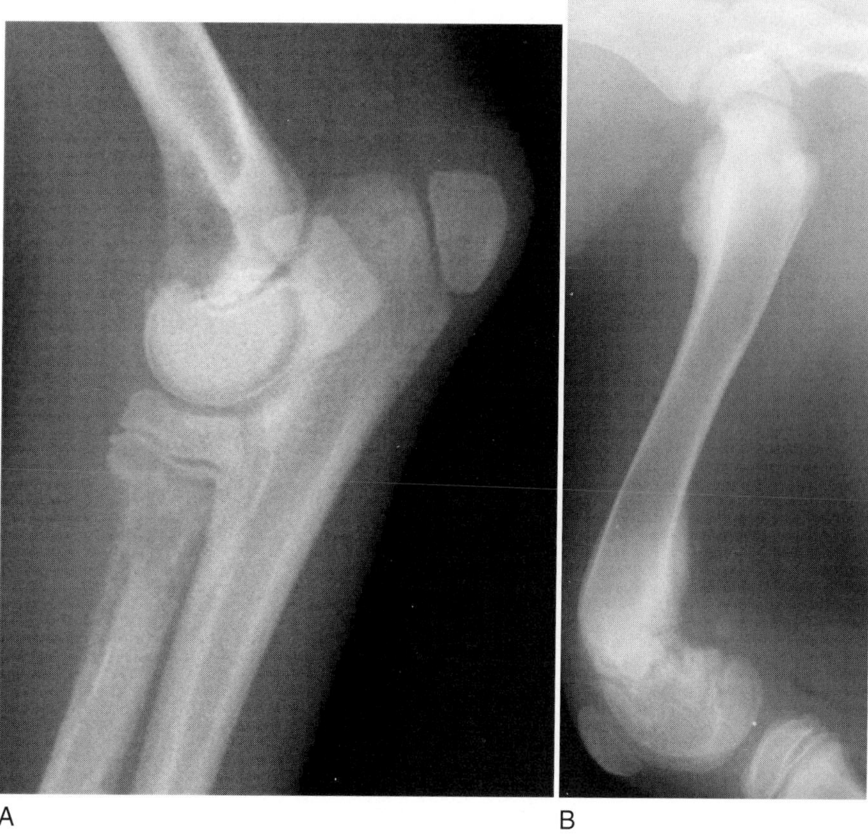

Fig. 17-14 **A,** Lateral radiograph of the elbow of a young dog. Aggressive lytic lesions are present in the distal humerus and proximal radius. Other limbs were also affected. **B,** Lateral view of the femur of a young dog. Aggressive lesions are present in the proximal and distal aspect of the femur; the main abnormality is the presence of an active periosteal reaction. Other limbs were similarly affected. Lesions in these dogs do not have a distribution consistent with primary bone tumor. The young age also makes metastatic neoplasia unlikely. Hematogenous osteomyelitis was documented in both dogs. The primarily lytic appearance in one dog versus the productive appearance in the other depends on the relative virulence of the organism and defense capacity of the infected bone.

proliferation to smooth laminar thickening of the periosteum.[18] Lesions have been described in the axial and the appendicular skeleton.[18] The appearance of the irregular periosteal reaction is consistent with a polyostotic infection or metastasis. The smooth periosteal reaction is misleading because it is not typically associated with disseminated bone infection. Dogs with hepatozoonosis usually have systemic dysfunction. Common clinical signs are fever, weight loss, muscle atrophy, ocular discharge, and generalized pain.[16]

With animal patients with cancer being treated more aggressively and living longer, metastatic bone tumors have become more common than once thought. Any malignant tumor has the potential to metastasize to the skeleton, but in general bone metastasis from epithelial tumors is more common than from mesenchymal tumors.[19,20] In dogs, mammary, lung, liver, thyroid, urinary, and prostate cancers are a common source of bone metastasis.[19,21,22] Metastatic tumor sites in the skeleton arise hematogenously, leading to a polyostotic distribution (Fig. 17-15). The hematogenous origin also suggests that a metaphyseal distribution would be most common, but diaphyseal lesions are not unusual. The most common sites of metastatic bone tumors are in the axial skeleton and the proximal extent of long bones in the appendicular skeleton.[19] Metastatic bone tumors are aggressive radiographic lesions, and, as with primary bone tumors, they may be sclerotic, mixed, or predominantly osteolytic. Patients with metastatic bone tumors are generally older; they also usually have a history of primary tumor, making the index of suspicion higher for tumor than for mycotic infection.

SUBUNGUAL TUMORS VERSUS SUBUNGUAL INFECTIONS

The digit is another location where radiographic differentiation between infectious and neoplastic causes can be difficult. Subungual tumors are relatively common in the dog, with the most common type being squamous cell carcinoma.[23] Most subungual squamous cell carcinomas involve large-breed dogs with black haircoats.[23,24] Melanomas are another common canine subungual tumor.[25] Inflammatory conditions of the digit, such as pododermatitis, also occur; these may be difficult to differentiate radiographically from tumors. Radiographic changes in dogs with pododermatitis and digital tumors have been characterized.[26] Tumors and pododermatitis were fairly evenly distributed between the manus and the pes. Also, the frequency of bone involvement is similar between subungual tumors and pododermatitis: 25 of 48 (52.1%) for pododermatitis and 33 of 52 (63.5%) for digital tumors. Regarding radiographic changes, pododermatitis could not be differentiated from malignant tumors because both conditions resulted in aggressive bone lesions. However, lesions characterized primarily by osteolysis were more likely to be caused by a malignant neoplasm.[26] In another study of dogs with digit masses, digit osteolysis was seen with all types of masses but was more commonly associated with squamous cell carcinoma (Figs. 17-16 and 17-17).[27]

Digital tumors typically involve a single digit, but syndromes of multiple-digit tumors have been described in dogs and cats (Fig. 17-18).[28-33]

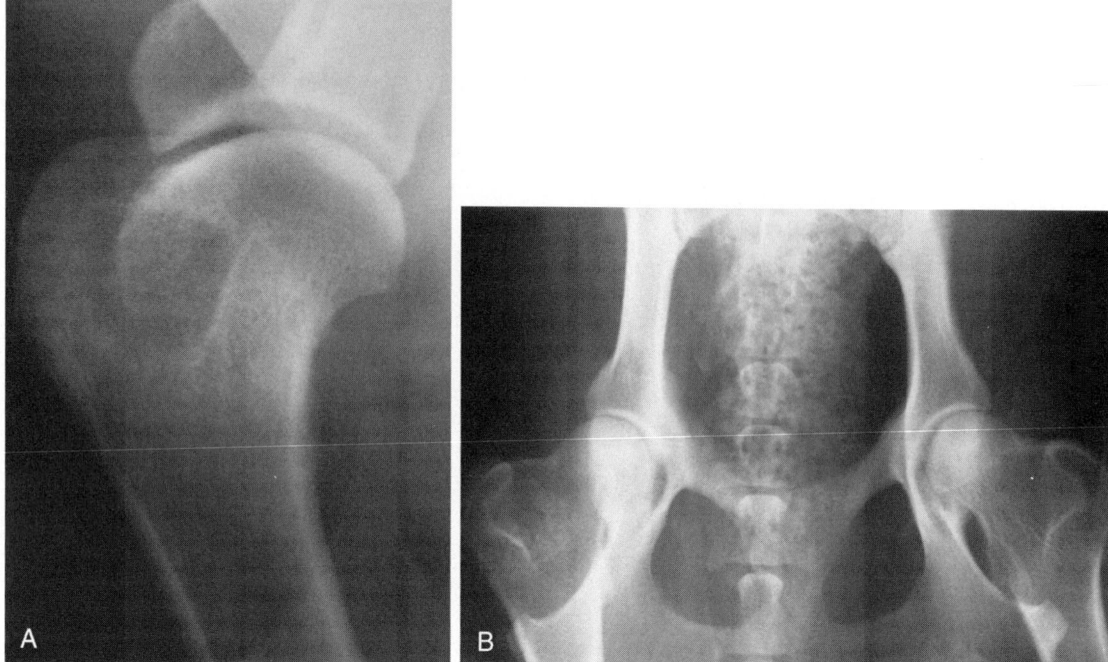

Fig. 17-15 Lateral view of the proximal humerus (A) and ventrodorsal view of the pelvis (B) of a 10-year-old Border Collie with previously irradiated nasal carcinoma and recent onset of lameness. In the humerus is a focal region of decreased bone opacity that has indistinct margins; thus this lesion is aggressive. Active periosteal reaction is also present on the caudal humeral metaphysis. In the pelvis is a region of mixed increased and decreased opacity in the right proximal femur, medial to the greater trochanter. The femoral lesion also has indistinct margins and is therefore aggressive. Polyostotic aggressive lesions in an older dog with a known malignant tumor are most likely caused by metastatic cancer. The diagnosis is metastatic nasal carcinoma.

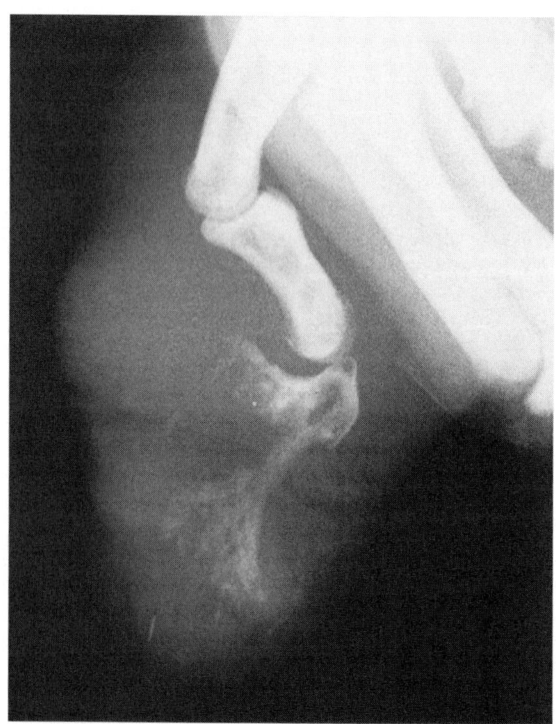

Fig. 17-16 Lateral view of the distal phalanx of the fifth digit of a dog. Extensive lysis of the distal phalanx is present; the lesion is aggressive. This radiographic appearance is more consistent with neoplasia than with pododermatitis, but histopathologic assessment will be needed for a definitive diagnosis. The diagnosis is subungual melanoma. (Reprinted from Voges AK, Neuwirth L, Thompson JP et al: Radiographic changes associated with digital, metacarpal and metatarsal tumors, and pododermatitis in the dog, *Vet Radiol Ultrasound* 37:327, 1996.)

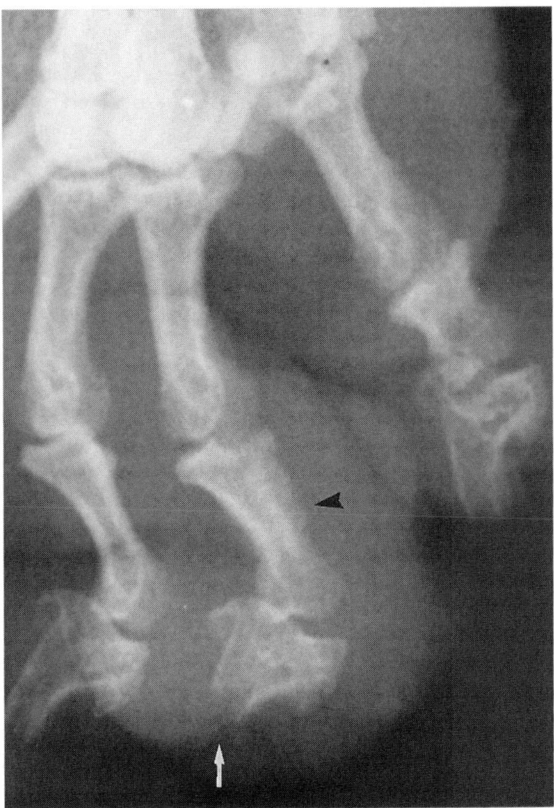

Fig. 17-17 Lateral view of the swollen third digit of a dog. Lysis of the most distal aspect of the distal phalanx is present *(white arrow)*, as is periosteal proliferation on the palmar aspect of the middle phalanx *(black arrowhead)*. The entire digit is swollen. These radiographic changes could result from either a tumor or inflammatory disease, but with the amount of productive new bone an inflammatory lesion is more likely. A biopsy is needed for a definitive diagnosis, which was pododermatitis. (Reprinted from Voges AK, Neuwirth L, Thompson JP et al: Radiographic changes associated with digital, metacarpal and metatarsal tumors, and pododermatitis in the dog, *Vet Radiol Ultrasound* 37:327, 1996.)

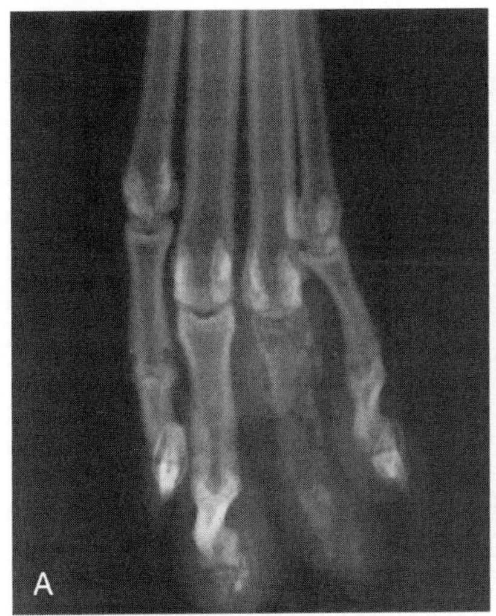

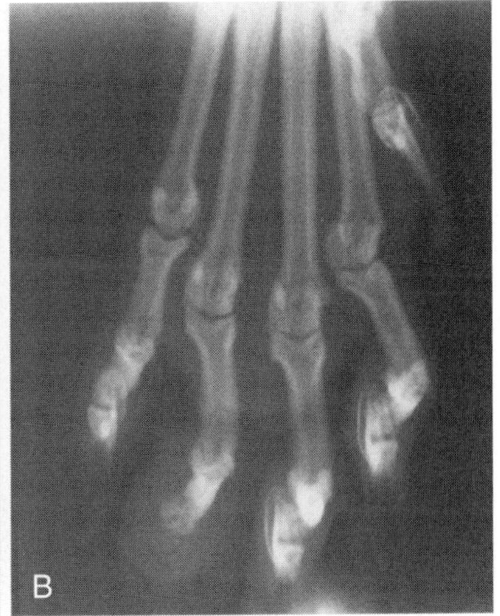

Fig. 17-18 Dorsopalmar radiograph of the manus (A) and dorsoplantar radiograph of the pes (B) of a 14-year-old cat with swollen digits on each manus and pes. The manus shows swelling of the fourth digit with lysis of the distal phalanx of that digit. The pes has lysis of the distal phalanx of the third digit and lysis of the proximal, middle, and distal phalanges of the fourth digit; some reactive bone is present on the proximal phalanx of the fourth digit. In radiographs of the thorax, multiple lung masses were present. Histologic diagnosis of the lung and digital lesions is squamous cell carcinoma. The digital tumors represent metastatic sites.

REFERENCES

1. Alexander J, Patton C: Primary tumors of the skeletal system, *Vet Clin North Am* 13:181, 1983.
2. Misdorp W, Hart A: Some prognostic and epidemiological factors in canine osteosarcoma, *J Natl Cancer Inst* 62:537, 1979.
3. Mirra J, Gold R, Picci P: Osseous tumors of intramedullary origin. In Mirra J, Picci P, Gold R, editors: *Bone tumors: clinical, radiologic and pathologic correlations, vol 1,* Philadelphia, 1989, Lea & Febiger, pp 270-271.
4. Kessler M, Tassani-Prell M, von Bomhard D et al: Osteosarcoma in cats: epidemiological, clinical and radiological findings in 78 animals (1990-1995) [in German], *Tierarztl Prax* 25:275, 1997.
5. Heldmann E, Anderson M, Wagner-Mann C: Feline osteosarcoma: 145 cases (1990-1995), *J Am Anim Hosp Assoc* 36:518, 2000.
6. Turrel J, Pool R: Primary bone tumors in the cat: a retrospective study of 15 cats and a literature review, *Vet Radiol* 23:152, 1982.
7. Quigley P, Leedale A: Tumors involving bone in the domestic cat: a review of 58 cases, *Vet Pathol* 20:670, 1983.
8. Bitetto W, Patnaik A, Schrader S et al: Osteosarcoma in cats: 22 cases (1974-1984), *J Am Vet Med Assoc* 190:91, 1987.
9. Liu S, Dorfman H, Patnaik A: Primary and secondary bone tumors in the cat, *J Sm Anim Pract* 15:141, 1974.
10. Riser W, Brodey R, Biery D: Bone infarctions associated with malignant bone tumors in dogs, *J Am Vet Med Assoc* 160:414, 1972.
11. Dubielzig R, Biery D, Brodey R: Bone sarcomas associated with multifocal medullary bone infarction in dogs, *J Am Vet Med Assoc* 179:64, 1981.
12. Sebastyen P, Marcellin-Little D, DeYoung D: Femoral medullary infarction secondary to canine total hip arthroplasty, *Vet Surg* 29:227, 2000.
13. Marcellin-Little D, DeYoung D, Thrall D et al: Osteosarcoma at the site of bone infarction associated with total hip arthroplasty in a dog, *Vet Surg* 28:54, 1999.
14. Kerl M: Update on canine and feline fungal diseases, *Vet Clin North Am Small Anim Pract* 33:721, 2003.
15. Johnson K: Osteomyelitis in dogs and cats, *J Am Vet Med Assoc* 205:1882, 1994.
16. Macintire D, Vincent-Johnson N, Dillon A et al: Hepatozoonosis in dogs: 22 cases (1989-1994), *J Am Vet Med Assoc* 210:916, 1997.
17. Ewing D, Panciera R: American canine hepatozoonosis. *Clin Microbiol Rev* 16:688, 2003.
18. Drost W, Cummings C, Mathew J et al: Determination of time of onset and location of early skeletal lesions in young dogs experimentally infected with *Hapatozoon americanum* using bone scintigraphy, *Vet Radiol Ultrasound* 44:86, 2003.
19. Cooley D, Waters D: Skeletal metastasis as the initial clinical manifestation of metastatic carcinoma in 19 dogs, *J Vet Intern Med* 12:288, 1998.
20. Russell G, Walker M: Metastatic and invasive tumors of bone in dogs and cats, *Vet Clin North Am* 13:163, 1983.
21. Brodey R, Reid C, Sauer R: Metastatic bone tumors in the dog, *J Am Vet Med Assoc* 148:29, 1966.
22. Geodegebuure S: Secondary bone tumors in the dog, *Vet Pathol* 16:520, 1979.
23. Vail D, Withrow S: Tumors of the skin and subcutaneous tissues. In Withrow S, MacEwen E, editors: *Small animal clinical oncology,* ed 2, Philadelphia, 1996, W.B. Saunders, p 167.
24. O'Brien M, Berg J, Engler S: Treatment by amputation of subungual squamous cell carcinomas in dogs: 21 cases (1987-1988), *J Am Vet Med Assoc* 201:759, 1992.
25. Aronsohn M, Carpenter J: Distal extremity melanocytic nevi and malignant melanomas in dogs, *J Am Anim Hosp Assoc* 26:605, 1990.
26. Voges A, Neuwirth L, Thompson J et al: Radiographic changes associated with digital, metacarpal and metatarsal tumors, and pododermatitis in the dog, *Vet Radiol Ultrasound* 37:327, 1996.
27. Marino D, Matthiesen D, Stefanacci J et al: Evaluation of dogs with digit masses: 117 cases (1981-1991), *J Am Vet Med Assoc* 207:726, 1995.
28. Paradis M, Scott D, Breton L: Squamous cell carcinoma of the nail bed in three related giant schnauzers, *Vet Record* 125:322, 1989.
29. O'Rourke M: Multiple digital squamous cell carcinomas in 2 dogs, *Mod Vet Pract* 66:644, 1985.
30. Gottfried S, Popovitch C, Goldschmidt M et al: Metastatic digital carcinoma in the cat: a retrospective study of 36 cats (1992-1998), *J Am Anim Hosp Assoc* 36:501, 2000.
31. Pollack M, Martin R, Diters R: Metastatic squamous cell carcinoma in multiple digits of a cat: case report, *J Am Anim Hosp Assoc* 20:835, 1984.
32. May C, Newsholme S: Metastasis of feline pulmonary carcinoma presenting as multiple digital swelling, *J Sm Anim Pract* 30:302, 1989.
33. Scott-Moncrief J, Elliott G, Radovsky A et al: Pulmonary squamous cell carcinoma with multiple digital metastases in a cat, *J Sm Anim Pract* 30:696, 1989.

ELECTRONIC RESOURCES evolve

Additional information related to the content in Chapter 17 can be found on the companion Web site at evolve http://evolve.elsevier.com/Thrall/vetrad/.

- Key Points
- Chapter Quiz
- Case Study 17-1
- Case Study 17-2

CHAPTER 18
Radiographic Signs of Joint Disease in Dogs and Cats

Graeme S. Allan

Many radiographic signs of joint disease are nonspecific (Box 18-1, Fig. 18-1). Also, animals with progressive joint diseases may have different signs when examined during different phases of the disease.

The clinician must determine whether lameness is caused by a monoarticular or a polyarticular problem. A hallmark of immune-mediated joint diseases is their polyarticular distribution. The same finding applies to hematogenously disseminated septic arthritis. Most other joint diseases involve one or only a few joints.

Do systemic signs of disease exist? Cats with feline chronic progressive polyarthropathy or *Mycoplasma* arthritis have systemic signs of illness, including transient fever, malaise, and stiffness as well as lameness. Animals with signs of bleeding disorders and concurrent joint pain should be examined for signs of hemarthrosis. Systemic lupus erythematosus (SLE) is a multiorgan disease, of which polyarthropathy may be a mild clinical sign. These points are mentioned only to underscore that sound knowledge of joint pathophysiologic characteristics is as important in the diagnosis of joint disease as is the ability to make and interpret radiographs of joints.

SIGNS OF JOINT DISEASE

Increased Synovial Volume

Any moderate increase in joint capsular or intracapsular soft tissue volume may be detected on good-quality radiographs. The joint cartilage, synovial fluid, synovial membrane, and joint capsule cannot be differentiated on survey radiographs because they are all of soft tissue opacity and therefore silhouette each other. In most joints, any increase in synovial mass appears as periarticular soft tissue swelling, which is identified radiographically by the increased opacity of affected soft tissues.

In the stifle, the infrapatellar fat pad sign may be used to evaluate synovial volume. The normal infrapatellar fat pad is readily identified on lateral stifle radiographs as a triangular radiolucent region immediately caudal to the patellar ligament (Fig. 18-2). When stifle synovial mass increases, either from increased synovial fluid or soft tissue, a combination of inflammatory response and effusion causes the fat pad to become less visible.

If necessary, the joint cartilage and the synovium may be evaluated by contrast arthrography. This technique has been used to help identify chondral flaps and tears in dogs with osteochondritis dissecans and synovial hypertrophy in villonodular synovitis.

Altered Thickness of the Joint Space

The joint space is the region of soft tissue opacity between the subchondral bone of opposing weight-bearing surfaces of a joint. This space consists of two layers of articular cartilage separated by a microfilm of synovial fluid. In early joint disease, synovial effusion may cause widening of the joint space. As joint disease progresses, attrition of articular cartilage results in a thinner appearance of the joint space (Fig. 18-3). Radiographs made while the patient is weight bearing on an affected joint are required if changes in the thickness of the joint space are to be assessed accurately. Radiographs of the recumbent animal are not adequate for this purpose. Exceptions to this rule may be patients in which stress radiography has been used to amplify signs of joint laxity or when muscle contracture is present, thereby compressing the joint space. Contracture of the infraspinatus and quadriceps muscles, for example, reduces the shoulder and stifle joint spaces, respectively.

Decreased Subchondral Bone Opacity

The subchondral bone is separated from the synovial fluid by an intact layer of articular cartilage. Any disease process that changes the character of synovial fluid, causing the articular cartilage to erode, potentially threatens the integrity of subchondral bone. In inflammatory joint disease, inflammatory exudates may cause pronounced subchondral bone loss. Infectious arthritis may extend into subchondral bone. Subchondral bone loss initially appears as a ragged margin of subchondral bone, but it may extend to cause marked destruction of bone. When bone loss affects smaller carpal and tarsal bones, these small cuboidal bones may be dramatically reduced in mass (Fig. 18-4).

Increased Subchondral Bone Opacity

In benign joint disease, such as degenerative joint disease, subchondral bone may be more opaque than normal because of stress remodeling. Increased subchondral bone opacity usually appears as a subchondral zone of increased opacity 1 to 2 mm wide.

Subchondral Bone Cyst Formation

Subchondral bone cysts, a feature of degenerative joint disease in human beings, are occasionally encountered in young dogs with osteochondrosis[1] and in mature dogs with advanced degenerative joint disease.[2]

Altered Perichondral Bone Opacity

At the chondrosynovial junction, articular cartilage merges with the synovial membrane. The highly vascular membrane is sensitive to inflammation. Synovial inflammation, or hypertrophy, may result in erosion of the bone adjacent to the synovium. Early inflammation causes the adjacent bone to appear ragged and spiculated. Longstanding or severe synovial inflammation or hypertrophy may cause pronounced bone erosion. Perichondral bone erosion is characteristic of some immune-mediated joint diseases and villonodular synovitis.

Perichondral Bone Proliferation

In degenerative joint disease, fibrocartilage elements form at the chondrosynovial junction. Gradual ossification of this fibrocartilaginous periarticular collar produces osteophytes. Progressive enlargement of osteophytes may result in their incorporation into the adjacent joint capsule.[2]

Articular Soft Tissue Mineralization

As a consequence of many chronic joint diseases, mineralization may occur within the joint capsule, within the synovial membrane, or free within the synovial fluid. Occasionally,

Box • 18-1

Radiographic Signs of Joint Disease

- Increased synovial volume
  - Compressed infrapatellar fat pad sign
- Altered thickness of the joint space
- Decreased subchondral bone opacity
- Increased subchondral bone opacity
- Subchondral bone cyst formation
- Altered perichondral bone opacity
- Perichondral bony proliferation
- Mineralization of joint soft tissues
- Intraarticular calcified bodies
- Joint displacement or incongruency
- Joint malformation
- Intraarticular gas

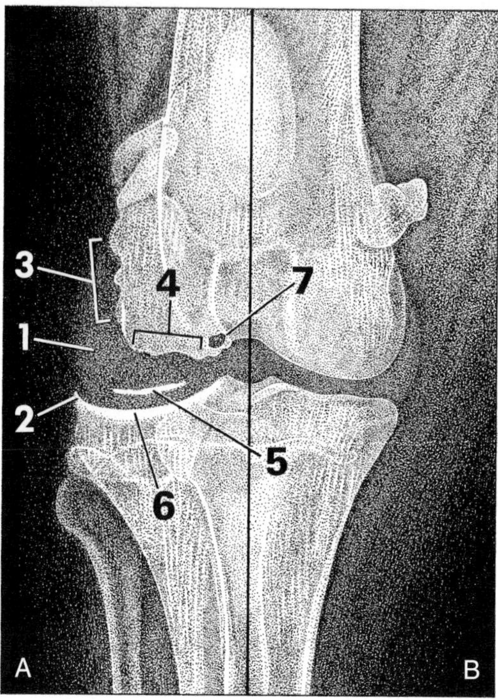

Fig. 18-1 Radiographic signs of joint disease **(A)** compared with a normal joint **(B)**. Increased synovial mass *(1)*, perichondral osteophyte *(2)*, and enthesophyte formation *(3)* are commonly observed radiographic changes. Erosion of the subchondral bone surface *(4)* and joint mice *(5)* are signs seen less often, whereas increased subchondral bone opacity *(6)* and subchondral bone cyst formation *(7)* are signs of chronic joint disease.

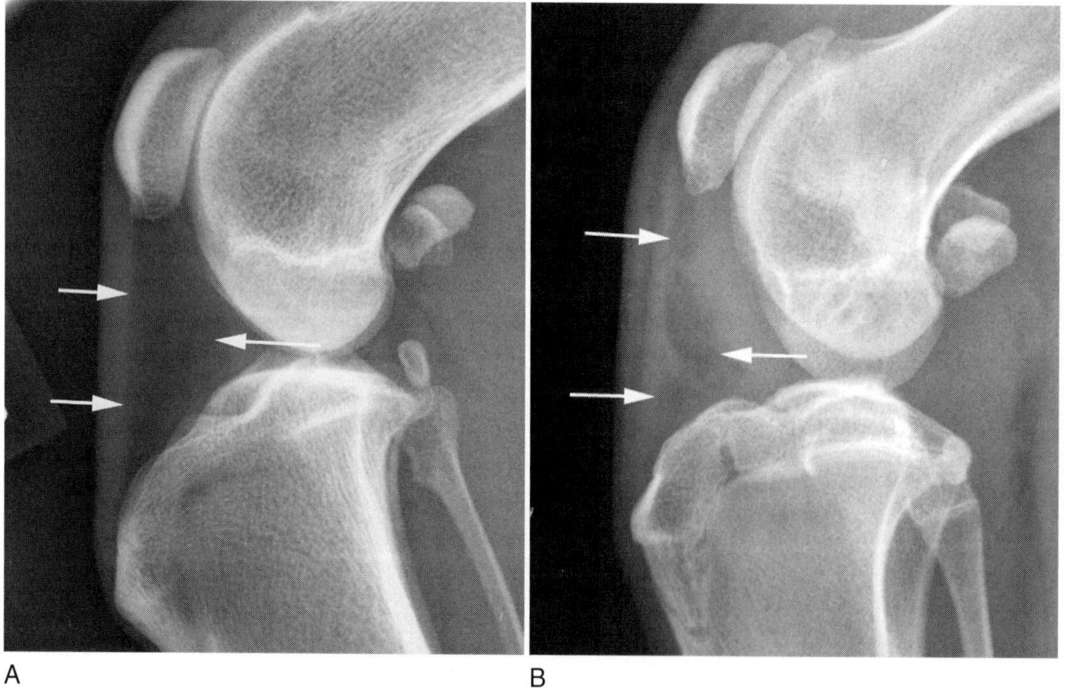

Fig. 18-2 Changes in the infrapatellar fat pad, located between the arrows, is a sensitive indicator of absence **(A)** or presence **(B)** of increased synovial volume in the stifle.

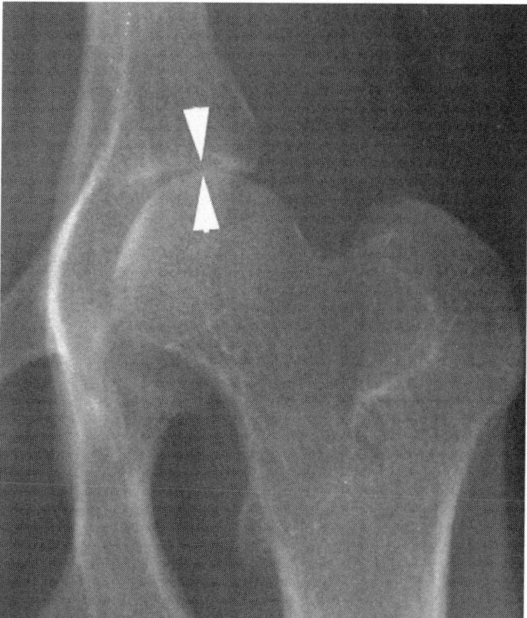

Fig. 18-3 A narrow articulate joint space *(between the arrowheads)* is interpreted as reduction in cartilage thickness.

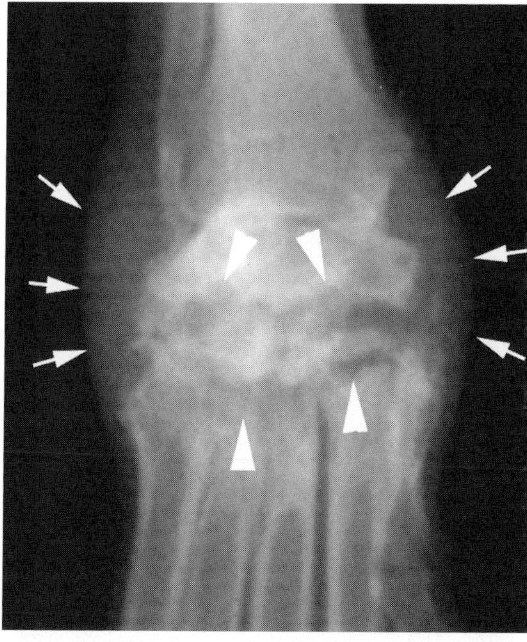

Fig. 18-4 Periarticular soft tissue swelling *(arrows)* and subchondral bone erosion *(arrowheads)* seen in the carpus of a dog with an erosive polyarthropathy.

large accumulations of articular or periarticular calcific material may be observed. Large osteochondromas have been reported within the joints of dogs[3] and cats,[4] and intrameniscal calcification and ossification have been observed in the stifle joints of cats.[5] Pseudogout (or calcium pyrophosphate deposition disease), which also causes mineralization of articular and periarticular soft tissues,[6,7] has been reported in dogs.

Intraarticular Calcified Bodies

Small, well-defined articular and periarticular calcific opacities are occasionally observed in dogs and cats. Such mineralized fragments are sometimes called *joint mice.* Not all such fragments are free within the joint, although they may appear so radiographically. Articular calcified bodies usually fall into three fairly distinct categories: avulsed fragments of articular or periarticular bone, osteochondral components of a disintegrating joint surface, or small synovial osteochondromas (Table 18-1).[8] They must be differentiated from sesamoid bones.[9]

Table • 18-1

Some Common Causes of Calcified Intraarticular Bodies

JOINT	ETIOLOGY
Shoulder	OCD of the head of the humerus
	Mineralization of the bicipital tendon/sheath
	Synovial osteochondroma
	Separate centers of ossification on the glenoid rim
Elbow	Ununited anconeal process
	Fragmented coronoid process
	OCD of the humeral medial condyle
Hip	Avulsion epiphyseal fractures after femoral luxation
	Avascular necrosis of the femoral head
Stifle	OCD of the femoral condyles
	Avulsion fractures of the:
	Origin of the long digital extensor tendon
	Origin or insertion of the cruciate ligaments
	Origin of the Popliteus
	Meniscal calcification
	Synovial osteochondroma
	Fragmented or fractured sesamoid bones
Tarsus	OCD of the talus

In all joints, soft tissue periarticular mineralization may occur as a result of degenerative joint disease.

Joint Displacement or Incongruency

When the normal spatial relation between the adjacent osseous components of a joint is disturbed, some type of displacement has occurred. A good example is the cranial drawer sign in a stifle with a ruptured cranial cruciate ligament. In this condition, clinically detectable displacement is not always easy to demonstrate radiographically but is best seen when stressed mediolateral radiographs of the stifle are made with the tarsal joint held in maximal flexion.[10] Joint displacement is usually a consequence of trauma to fibrous or ligamentous supporting structures. Another example is coxofemoral joint laxity, a feature of canine hip dysplasia. Special stress radiographs are required to assess the extent of laxity in the coxofemoral joints accurately, because laxity is not adequately assessed on standard ventrodorsal extended radiographs of the pelvis.

Radiographic identification of elbow joint incongruency from unbalanced growth of the radius and ulna is subjective, unless the step between the ulna and radial articular surfaces is greater than 2 mm. Accurate detection of elbow incongruency of as little as 2 mm is difficult, however, so the usefulness of survey radiography of the elbow to identify incongruency is questioned.[11] Computed tomography (CT) may be the most preferable imaging modality to increase the sensitivity for detecting this problem (Fig. 18-5).

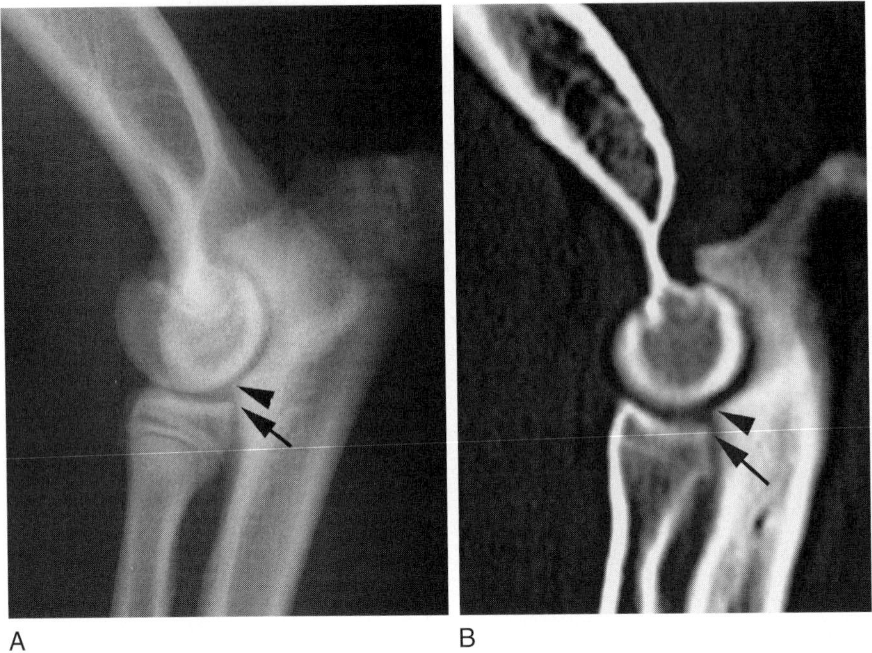

Fig. 18-5 Survey mediolateral radiograph *(left)* and CT image *(right)* of the same elbow, which is characterized by a well defined "step" between the head of the radius *(arrow)* and the distal end of the semilunar articular surface of the ulna *(arrowhead)*. (Courtesy Dr. J. Beck, Brisbane Veterinary Specialist Centre, Brisbane, Australia.)

Joint Malformation

Joint malformation represents the end product of osseous remodeling and is usually the result of malunion of bones of traumatized joints, chronic degenerative joint disease, or congenital joint disease.

OSTEOPHYTES AND ENTHESOPHYTES

Osteophytes

The proposed pathogenesis of osteophyte formation is that abnormal joint cartilage loading leads to cartilage wear, fibrillation, and loss of cartilage. The products of cartilage degradation mediate synovial hyperplasia and subsequent development of osteophytes.[12] Initially, osteophytes consist of cartilage and later become radiographically visible when they are mineralized. They are seen as bony outgrowths of bone, usually at the periphery of articular cartilage. They occur as a component of osteoarthritis.

Entheses and Enthesophytes

An enthesis is the point of insertion of a tendon, ligament, joint capsule, or fascia to bone. During embryogenesis ligaments or tendons are attached to cartilage, but subsequent metaplasia of fibroblasts at their attachment site results in formation of fibrocartilage. This change extends into the tendon or ligament, and enchondral ossification proceeds within the remaining cartilage. Enthesitis is inflammation of the site of tendon or ligament attachment to bone. An enthesophyte is a boney spondylopathy that develops at an enthesis (Fig. 18-6).[13]

Because enthesophytes, osteophytes, and ankylosing spondylopathy appear radiographically similar, confusion in terminology often occurs when referring to these structures on a radiograph. To separate osteophytes around or within joints from enthesophytes, where the common entheses are

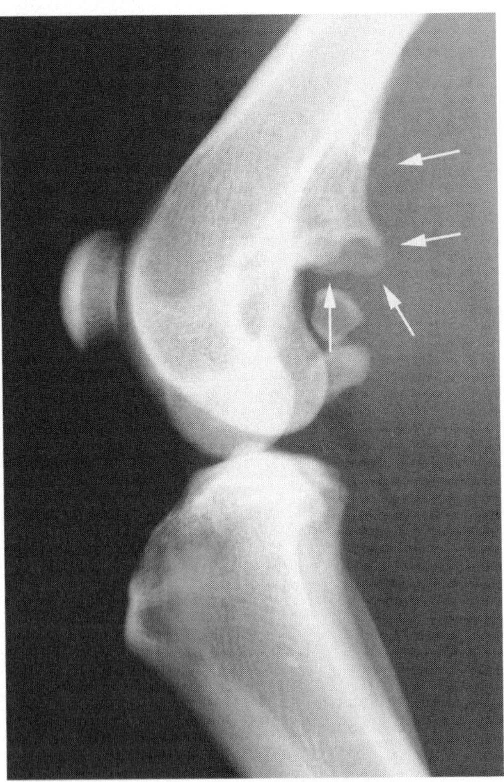

Fig. 18-6 A large enthesophyte arising from the enthesis of origin of the gastrocnemius muscle *(arrows)*.

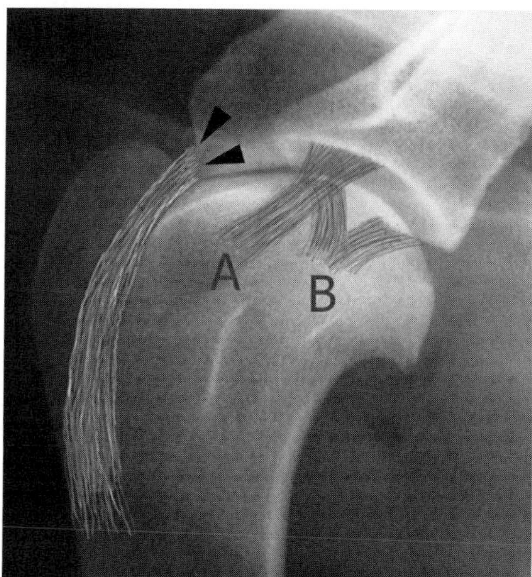

Fig. 18-7 In the scapulohumeral joint the intraarticular tendon of origin of biceps brachii muscle arises from its enthesis *(arrowheads)* on the scapular tuberosity. Other entheses around the shoulder are related to the lateral *(A)* and medial *(B)* glenohumeral ligaments and the joint capsule and tendons of insertion of supraspinatus, infraspinatus, and subscapularis muscles (not depicted).

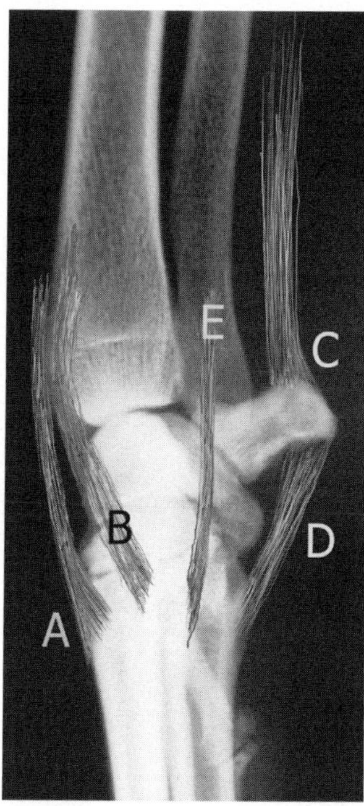

Fig. 18-8 Entheses around the carpus. In addition to the many intraarticular ligaments and the joint capsule (not depicted) are periarticular entheses of extensor carpi radialis and extensor carpi ulnaris *(A)*, abductor pollicis longus *(B)*, flexor carpi ulnaris *(C)*, the check ligaments of the accessory carpal bone *(D)*, and flexor carpi radialis *(E)*.

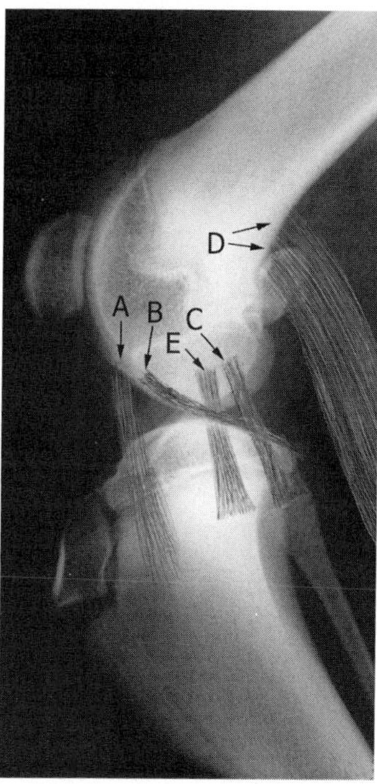

Fig. 18-9 The stifle. Entheses of origin of the long digital extensor *(A)*, popliteus *(B)*, lateral collateral ligament *(C)*, gastrocnemius *(D)*, and medial collateral ligament *(E)*. Not depicted are the cranial and caudal cruciate ligaments.

located is useful information (Figs. 18-7, 18-8, and 18-9). In complex joints such as the carpus and tarsus, a large number of intraarticular ligaments are present. Every diarthrodial joint has a joint capsule, and intraarticular and periarticular ligaments and joint capsules insert onto bone at their respective entheses. New bone formation arising in or around joints where no known entheses are present are usually referred to as osteophytes.

Intraarticular Gas

Spontaneous or induced gas diffusion (vacuum phenomenon) into a joint has been reported in both horses[14] and dogs.[15-19] It has also been observed within the intervertebral disc spaces of dogs that have a prolapsed disc and may be observed after interventional joint procedures. The presence of intraarticular gas is more easily identified during CT examinations than during routine radiography because of the greater contrast enhancement of CT images compared with conventional radiographs.[18]

The prevailing theory is that noniatrogenic intraarticular gas migration represents diffusion of nitrogen from extracellular fluid into an adjacent joint space when negative pressure is present in the joint. This may occur naturally or be induced by applying traction to a joint. The vacuum phenomenon has many causes in dogs and cats (Box 18-2). The phenomenon is observed when excessive distraction is applied to the coxofemoral joints during distraction radiography and has been reported in 20% of a series of shoulder joint radiographs of dogs with osteochondritis dissecans (OCD) of the humeral head.[16,17] Because traction is used during positioning of the shoulder for an OCD examination, gas diffusion is theorized to be induced by traction. Interestingly, gas diffusion was not a feature of normal (non-OCD) contralateral joints of dogs in this series.[16] Positive clinical associations with intraarticular gas include degenerative disc disease, cervical vertebral instability, OCD, and osteoarthritis (Figs 18-10 to 18-13). Intraarticular gas slowly diffuses out of the joint, a process that takes several hours, after normal intraarticular pressure is reestablished.

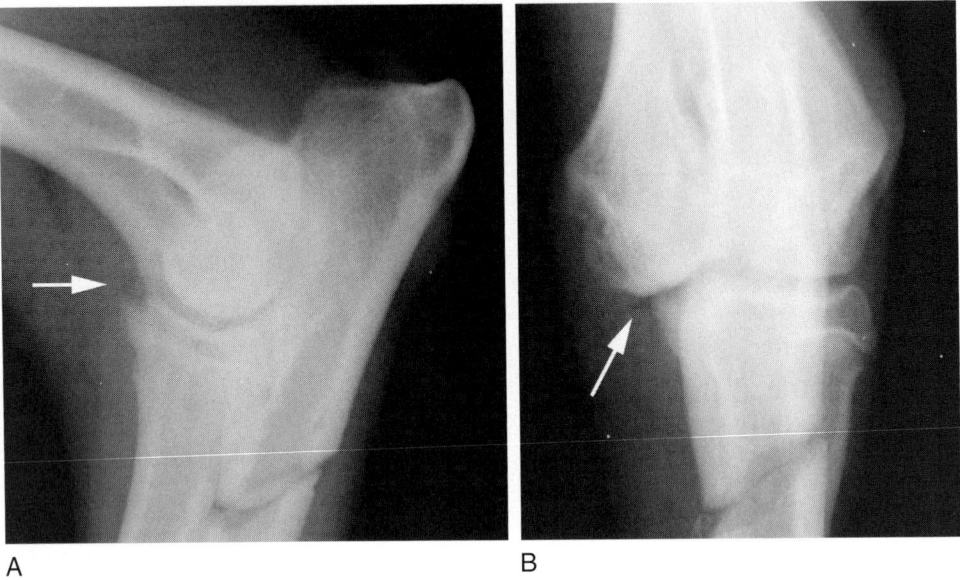

Fig. 18-10 Intraarticular gas *(arrows)* in the humeroradial joint after arthrotomy to treat fragmented medial coronoid process. An ulna osteotomy was part of the same procedure. (Courtesy University Veterinary Centre, Sydney, Australia.)

Box • 18-2

Causes of Intraarticular Gas

Iatrogenic
After arthrotomy/arthroscopy
Negative-contrast arthrography
Arthrocentesis
Tension on joints
  PennHIP distraction radiography
  Positioning shoulders with OCD for radiography

Trauma
Joint luxation
Penetrating injuries

Infection
Gas-producing microorganisms

Spontaneous
Intervertebral disc disease
Osteoarthritis

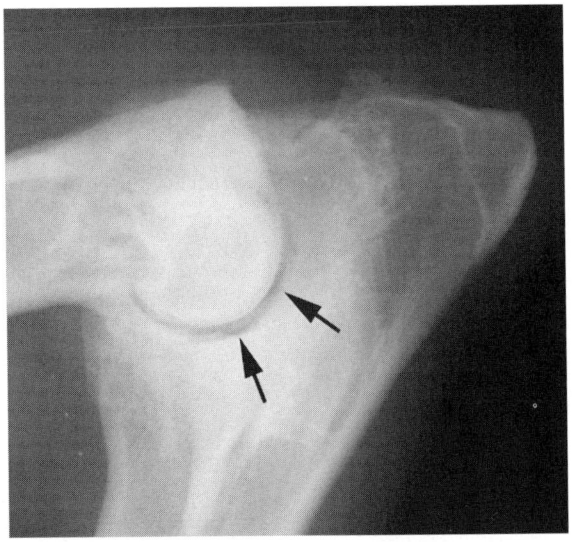

Fig. 18-11 Spontaneous intraarticular gas in the elbow of a dog with osteoarthritis *(arrows)*. (Courtesy Kingston Animal Hospital, Kingston, Australia.)

SESAMOID BONES

Sesamoid bones are commonly present adjacent to the elbow, stifle, tarsus, and the metacarpophalangeal and metatarsophalangeal joints. If sesamoid bones are not visualized on a radiograph, they may be absent or have not ossified at the time of radiography. The clavicle is present in up to 96% of large dogs and in all cats, but the sesamoids in the iliopubic cartilage were identified in only 11% of one group of Greyhounds.[20] In the same group of dogs, the elbow sesamoid, located in the tendon of origin of the supinator, had an incidence of 31%, the lateral plantar tarsometatarsal sesamoid 50%, and the intraarticular tarsometatarsal sesamoid 27%, whereas the popliteal sesamoid is ossified in 84% to 94% of dogs.[9,10] Sesamoid bones are identified by their size, shape, and location (Figs. 18-14 to 18-21, Table 18-2). Occasionally, displaced sesamoids are regarded as a sign of muscular or tendinous injury. Although this may be true, and has been reported in conjunction with ruptured cruciate ligaments[10] and trauma of the tendon of origin of the popliteus[21,22] and gastrocnemius,[23,24] variation in sesamoid location may also occur in the absence of a pathologic condition.[25]

Meniscal Ossicles in Nondomestic Cats

A lunula, or meniscal sesamoid, is commonly present in large nondomestic cats, such as lions, where it is located in the cranial horn of the medial meniscus. A similar intraarticular ossicle in the stifle has been reported in reptiles, amphibians, rabbits, rodents, edentates, lemurs, birds, and nonhuman primates.[28]

CONTRAST RADIOGRAPHY OF JOINTS

Radiographs with added contrast medium enhance visualization of important intraarticular structures, such as the articular cartilage and synovium. Contrast radiography has been most useful in the evaluation of the canine shoulder joint for evidence of OCD. Other applications include evaluation of capsular trauma, documentation of synovial hypertrophy, and identification of radiolucent-joint mice. Interest in methods of evaluating dogs with bicipital tenosynovitis and fragmented coronoid processes has resulted in renewed enthusiasm for contrast arthrography.[29-31] When compared with sonography, arthrography was considered a more sensitive method of identifying abnormalities in the bicipital tendon and intertubercular groove of the humerus.[32]

Either a positive-contrast or negative-contrast medium may be used (Figs. 18-22 and 18-23). A diluted mixture of an isotonic positive-contrast medium such as iohexol is recommended for positive-contrast studies, the concentration being reduced to 100 mg/mL of iodine by the addition of sterile diluent. For average-sized dogs, a volume of 2 to 4 mL is injected into the shoulder joint.[33] This dose can be varied for studies that evaluate the bicipital tendon, in which the objective is to fill the bicipital tendon sheath; 0.4 mL/kg body weight can be used for this application.[29] For elbow arthrography in dogs, the optimal volume was 2 mL in one report; in that study, lower volumes were preferred to higher volumes.[30] Strict adherence to sterile technique is mandatory. When iodine concentrations greater than 100 mg/mL are used, the opaque contrast medium may camouflage underlying articular structures, rendering them invisible.

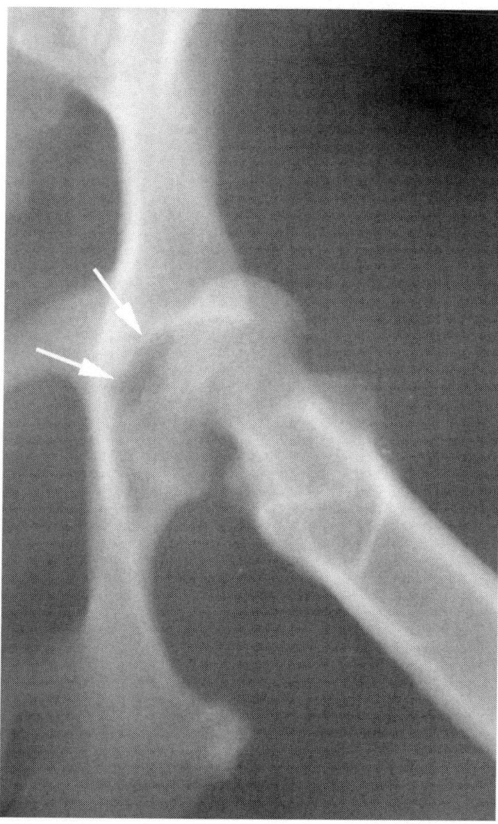

Fig. 18-12 Trauma-related intraarticular gas *(arrows)* in a dog with closed coxofemoral luxation. (Courtesy Sylvania Veterinary Hospital, Sydney, Australia.)

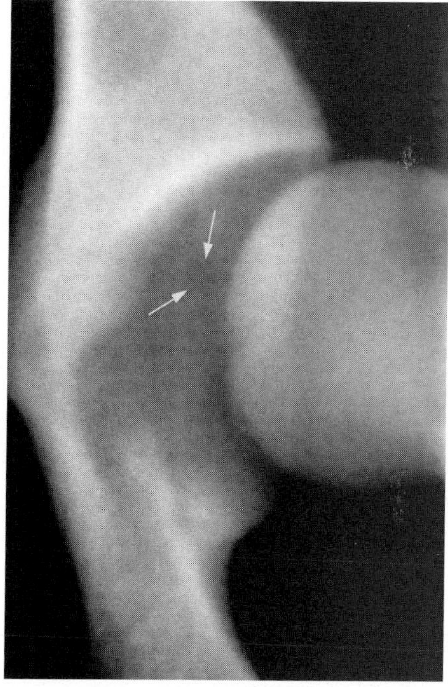

Fig. 18-13 Coxofemoral intraarticular gas *(arrows)* induced by excessive distraction during PennHIP radiography. (Reprinted from *BSAVA manual of canine and feline musculoskeletal imaging*, BSAVA Publications, Quedgeley, Gloucester, England, 2006.)

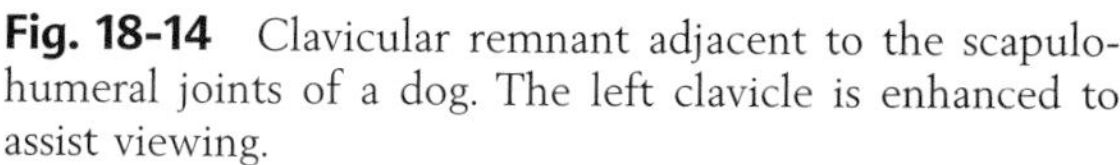

Fig. 18-14 Clavicular remnant adjacent to the scapulohumeral joints of a dog. The left clavicle is enhanced to assist viewing.

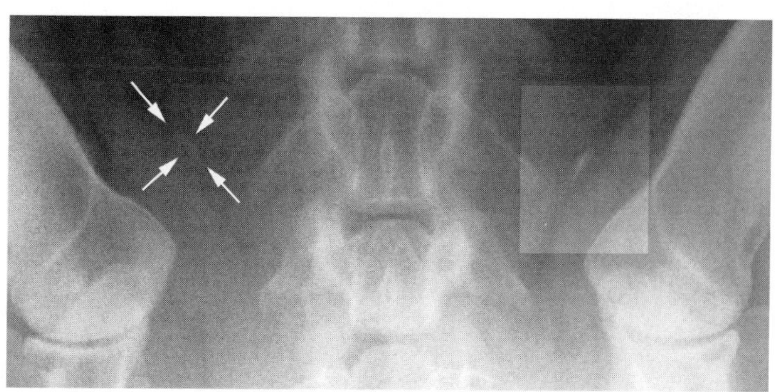

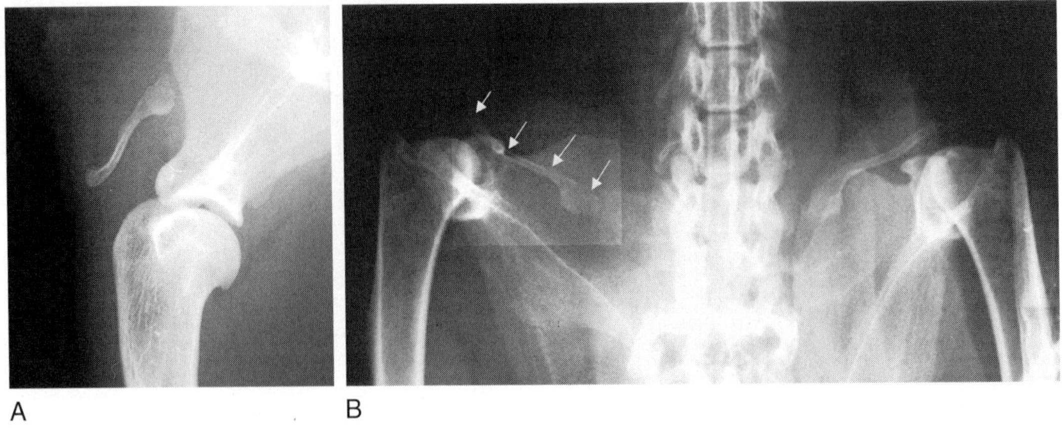

Fig. 18-15 Feline clavicle in lateral (A) and ventrodorsal (B) views. In this cat the clavicle is extensively ossified (*arrows*).

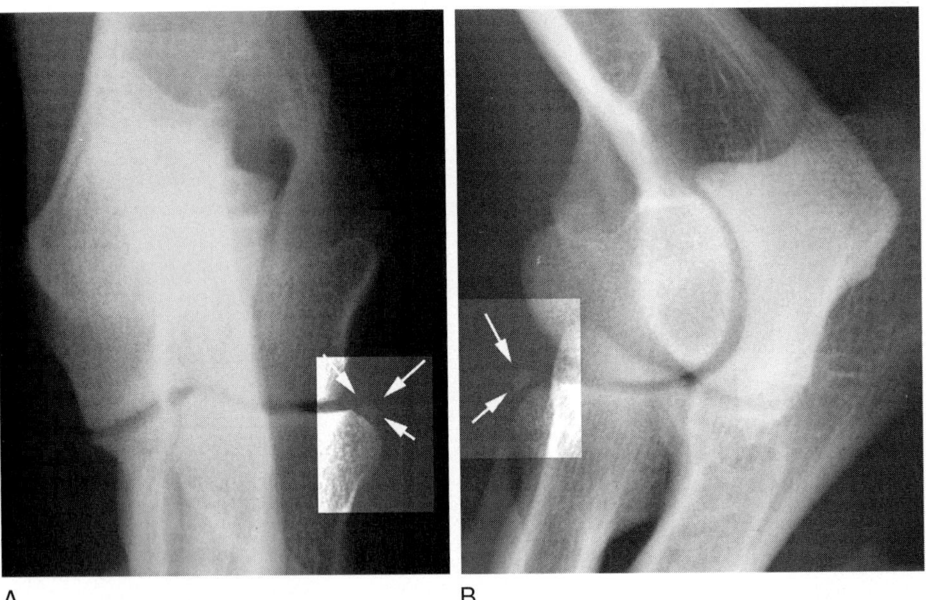

Fig. 18-16 The elbow sesamoid, in the tendon of origin of the supinator, is seen adjacent to the craniolateral surface of the head of the radius *(arrows)*.

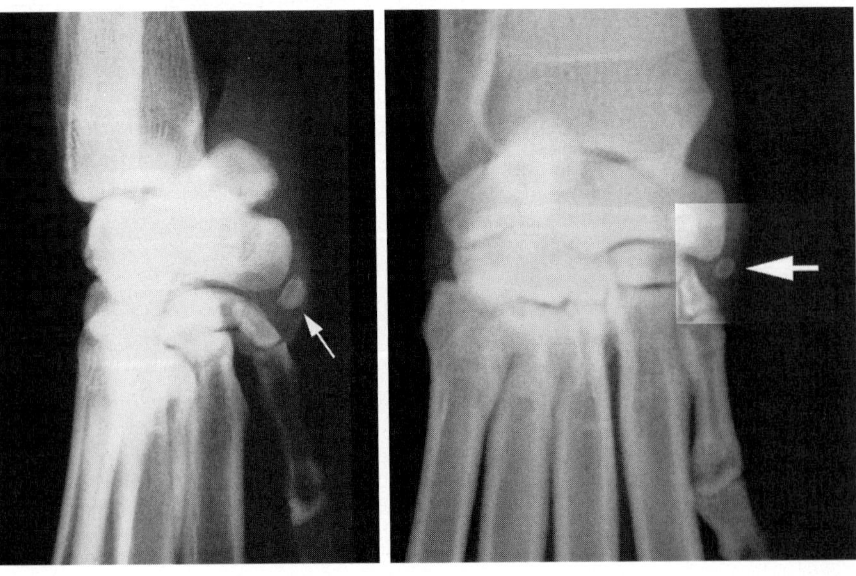

Fig. 18-17 The carpal sesamoid is located in the tendon of the abductor pollicis longus on the medial side of the carpus at the level of the intercarpal articulation *(enhanced box, large arrow)*. The tendon inserts onto the proximal end of the first digit. (Reprinted from BSAVA Manual of Canine and Feline Musculoskeletal Imaging, BSAVA Publications, Quedgeley, Gloucester, England, 2006.)

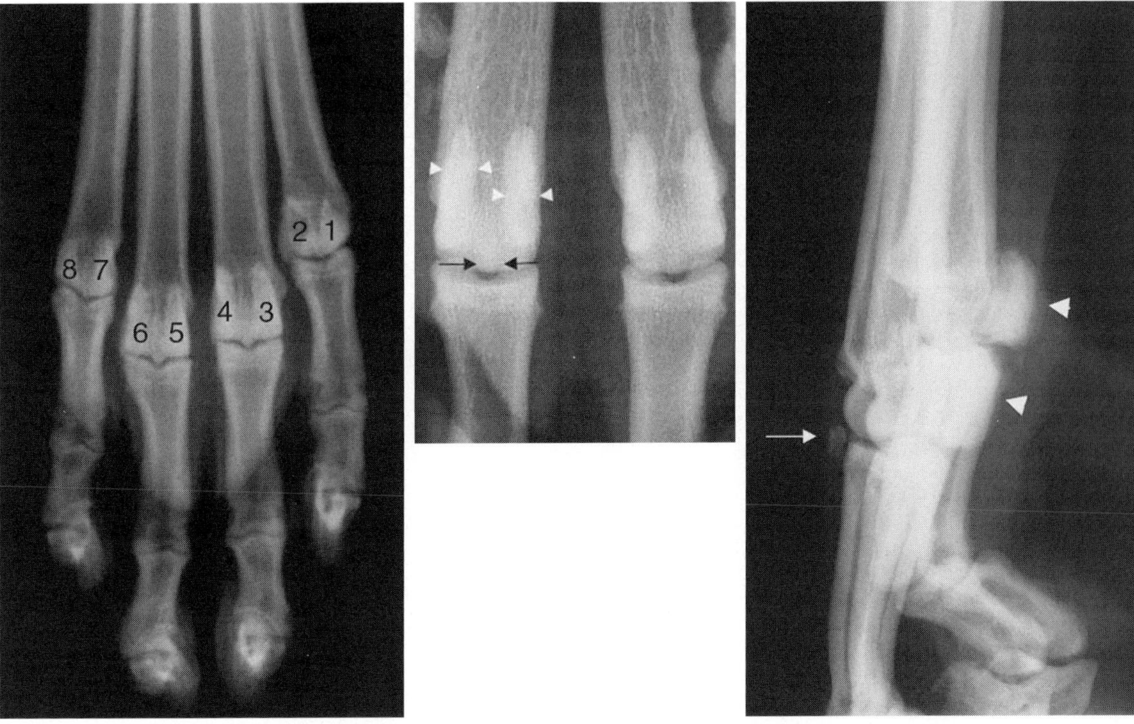

Fig. 18-18 The metacarpophalangeal and metatarsophalangeal sesamoids are paired *(arrowheads)* on the palmar (plantar) surface and single on the dorsal surface *(arrows)*. They are numbered from medial to lateral. (Reprinted from BSAVA manual of canine and feline musculoskeletal imaging, BSAVA Publications, Quedgeley, Gloucester, England, 2006.)

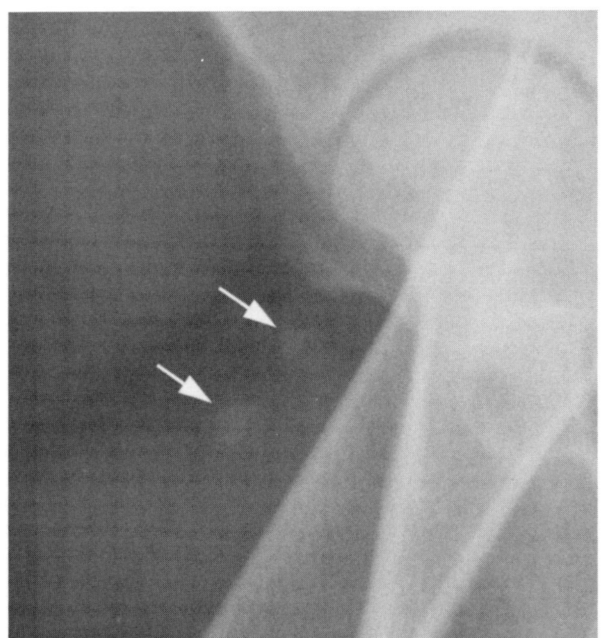

Fig. 18-19 The iliopubic sesamoids are occasionally seen cranial to the pubic eminence on lateral radiographs of the pelvis of large dogs *(arrows)*.

Air or carbon dioxide may be used for negative-contrast arthrography. When gas is used, it should be injected into the joint space through a Millipore filter (Millipore Corporation, Billerica, Mass.) to ensure that it is free of particulate matter or microorganisms.

SESAMOID DISEASE

A syndrome of metacarpophalangeal (MCP) sesamoid bone fragmentation (Fig. 18-24) has been reported in several large breeds of dogs, but it occurs most commonly in Rottweilers.[34] The underlying cause appears to be osteonecrosis[35] of selected sesamoids, although developmental, traumatic, and degenerative conditions have also been cited as possible precipitating causes. Eight palmar/plantar sesamoids are present on the four main digits of each of the forefeet and hindfeet, but sesamoid fragmentation mainly affects the palmar sesamoids numbered two and seven. In an early description of the syndrome, the incidence was 44% in one group of Rottweilers.[36] In a prospective study of 55 Rottweilers, the radiographic incidence of sesamoid disease at 12 months of age was 73%, with an incidence of clinical signs attributable to sesamoid disease in 65% of affected dogs. Sesamoid disease was identified as the cause of forelimb lameness in 50% of young Rottweilers.[37]

Radiographic images obtained with dorsopalmar projections usually allow identification of affected sesamoid bones, but oblique lateral projections with the digits separated by traction may provide additional information. Radiographically, fragmented sesamoid bones appear as a cluster of ossific fragments on the palmar aspect of the joint, adjacent to an unaffected paired sesamoid. The ossicles are usually multiple,

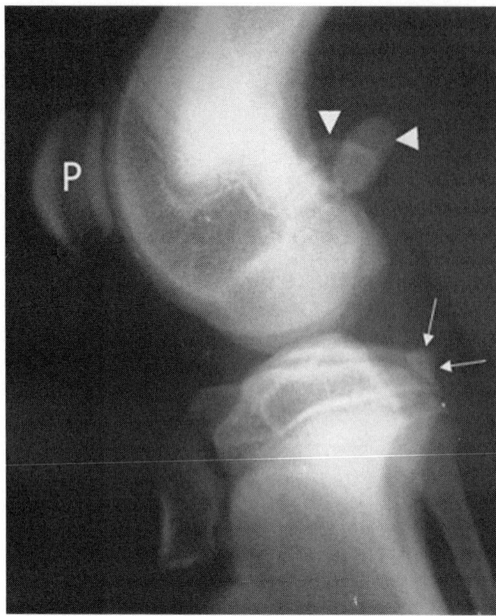

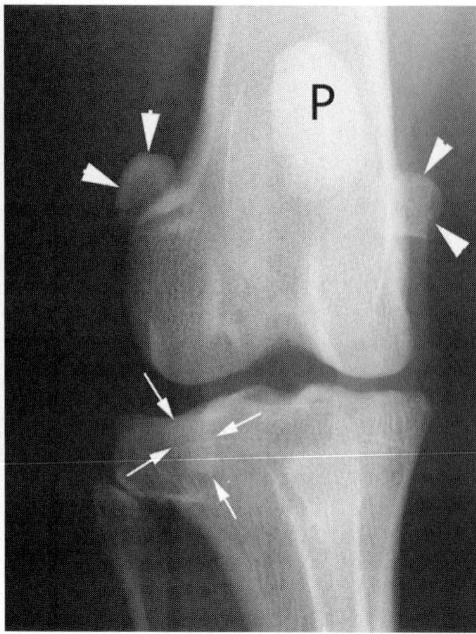

Fig. 18-20 The patella *(P)* is easily identified on the cranial aspect of the femoral condyle. The paired fabellae *(arrowheads)* are seen on the caudal aspect of the femoral condyle, where they lie adjacent to the medial and lateral condyles near the origin of the gastrocnemius. The popliteal sesamoid *(arrows)* is located caudolaterally, adjacent to the head of the tibia.

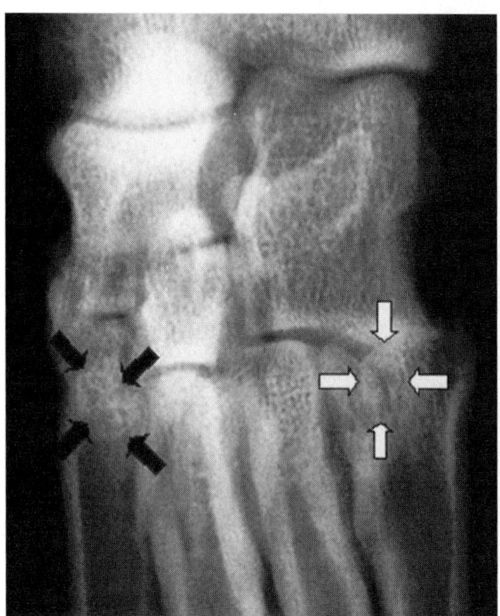

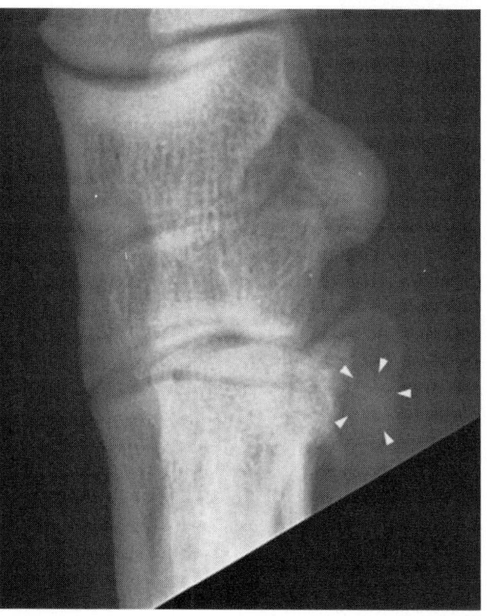

Fig. 18-21 The lateral tarsometatarsal sesamoid *(white arrows)* and the medially located intraarticular tarsometatarsal sesamoid *(black arrows)* are inconsistently present in dogs and can be difficult to locate. On the lateral image *(right panel)* one can be seen *(arrowheads)*. (Reprinted from BSAVA Manual of Canine and Feline Musculoskeletal Imaging, BSAVA Publications, Quedgeley, Gloucester, England, 2006.)

with rounded margins that conform to a variety of shapes and sizes. In racing Greyhounds, clearly defined transverse sesamoid "fractures" have been reported, leading to a belief that trauma is the cause of sesamoid fragmentation in this breed.[38] Although much less frequently than in the metacarpophalangeal sesamoids, the fabellae are also prone to fragmentation (Fig. 18-25).

The most commonly seen example of sesamoid displacement is medial luxation of the patella (Fig. 18-26). Although patella luxation can occur in any animal, it is most frequently seen in toy dogs and also in Devon Rex cats. Some breeds have an inherited predisposition to patella luxation. Other sesamoids are also prone to displacement. Distal displacement of the popliteal sesamoids or the fabellae has been cited as a sign that indicates rupture or trauma to their respective tendons, although this is not always true (Fig. 18-27 and Case Study 18-1 on the Evolve site [http://evolve.elsevier.com/Thrall/vetrad]).

Osteoarthritis

Osteoarthritis is a slowly progressive degenerative joint disease of synovial joints in which synovial effusion and cartilage degradation are key components. It is the most common joint abnormality seen in small animal practice and occurs most frequently in the weight-bearing joints of medium-sized to large dogs, although it may affect any synovial joint of both dogs and cats. The best example of canine osteoarthritis occurs as a result of canine hip dysplasia. The incidence of hip dysplasia varies from breed to breed and in many large breeds exceeds 50%. The next most frequent locations are the canine shoulder and stifle joints. Signs of shoulder osteoarthritis were identified in 33% to 50% of groups of dogs surveyed either at necropsy or radiographically; 20% of dogs in another survey had evidence of stifle osteoarthritis at necropsy.[2,39,40]

Osteoarthritis may be a primary aging change (idiopathic) or as a result of a developmental or acquired disorder. Examples of canine developmental disorders include osteochon-

Table • 18-2

Sesamoid Bones Visible on Radiographs of Joints of the Canine

APPENDICULAR SKELETON	JOINT NAME/LOCATION
Shoulder	Clavicle (medial end of tendinous intersection in the brachiocephalicus) (see Figs. 18-14 and 18-15)
Elbow	Tendon of origin of the supinator (see Fig. 18-16)[26]
Carpus	Tendon of the abductor pollicis longus (see Fig. 18-17)
Metacarpophalangeal	Paired palmar sesamoid bones (located in the tendons of insertion of the interosseous muscles) (see Fig. 18-18) Single dorsal sesamoid (located in the extensor tendons)
Coxofemoral	None* (see Fig. 18-19)
Femorotibial	Patella (tendon of insertion of the quadriceps femoris) (see Fig. 18-20) Sesamoid bones of the gastrocnemius (fabellae) Medial head Lateral head Popliteal sesamoid (tendon of the popliteus)
Tarsus	Lateral plantar tarsometatarsal sesamoid bone (see Fig. 18-21)[27] Intraarticular tarsometatarsal sesamoid bone[27]
Metatarsophalangeal	Paired plantar sesamoid bones (see Fig. 18-18) Single dorsal sesamoid bone

*Sesamoid bone located in the iliopubic cartilage may be seen cranial to the iliopubic eminence.[20]

drosis, fragmented coronoid process, ununited anconeal process, hip dysplasia, patellar luxation, achondroplasia, and conformational disorders such as valgus and varus deformities of the carpus. Acquired disorders capable of causing osteoarthritis in dogs include trauma, joint instability, epiphyseal aseptic necrosis, recurrent hemarthrosis, and acquired postural or conformational defects such as joint malalignment after fracture repair.[41]

Radiographic Signs of Progression of Osteoarthritis in Dogs

The stifle joint is often used to study the progression of osteoarthritis in dogs. The initial stages of osteoarthritis are asymptomatic, and changes are not typically detected radiographically. The first pathologic change is a mild nonsuppurative synovitis, accompanied by a significant increase in the volume of synovial mass. Focal articular cartilage degeneration follows. The joint space may appear widened during this stage.[42] Osteophytosis is the radiographic feature that demonstrates the greatest degree of change over time in the stifle of dogs with naturally occurring joint instability. When grading stifle osteoarthritis, evaluating the changes in the number and size of periarticular osteophytes is more reliable than evaluating subchondral sclerosis, intraarticular mineralization, or synovial effusion, but signs of synovial effusion and compression of the infrapatellar fat pad are identifiable radiographic features that often accompany stifle instability.

Osteophyte formation commences as early as 3 days after cranial cruciate ligament transection and can be seen radiographically at the margins of the femoral trochlea as early as 2 weeks after the onset of stifle instability. Initially, osteophytes consist of cartilage, and they do not become radiographically visible until they are mineralized. The proximal and distal ends of the trochlear ridges are the sites of the earliest osteophyte changes in the stifle joint, but later changes occur on the lateral and medial femoral condylar surfaces and the tibial condyles. Enthesophyte formation at points of origin and insertion of the cruciate and collateral ligaments occurs later than osteophytosis on the trochlear ridges.

Early identification of osteophytes on trochlear ridges is facilitated by using specific radiographic projections, such as flexed mediolateral, craniomedial-caudolateral, and caudomedial-craniolateral oblique radiographs of the stifle. As well as special positioning, fine-detail film-screen combination is recommended as the optimal image receptor.[12,43-45]

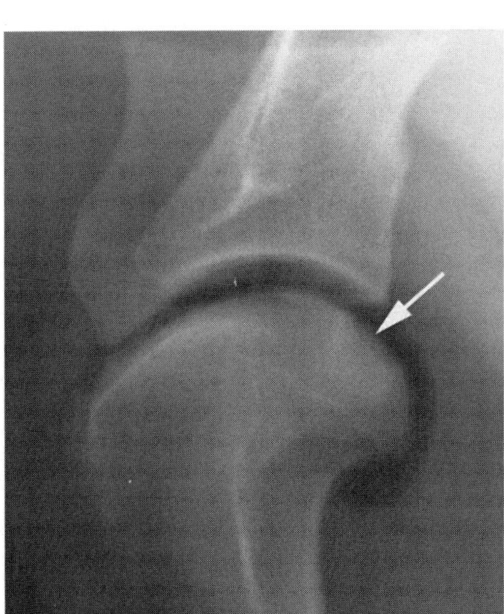
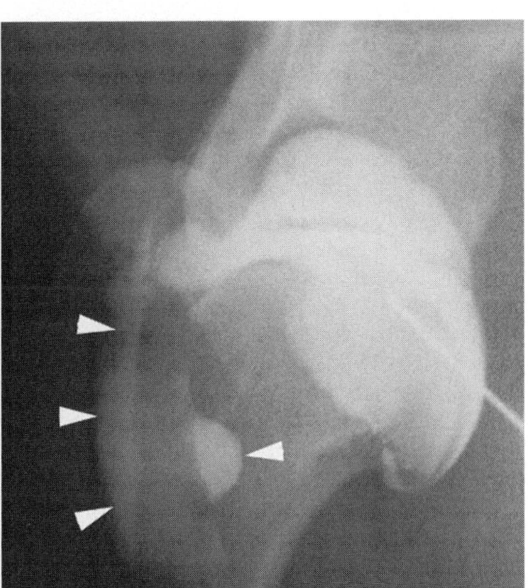

Fig. 18-22 Contrast arthrography of the shoulder. *Left*, Negative-contrast arthrogram highlighting an OCD lesion *(arrow)* on the humeral head was achieved by injecting 10 mL of air. *Right*, A positive-contrast arthrogram of a canine shoulder was achieved by injecting 6 mL iohexol (90 mg/mL of iodine). Note opacification of the biceps tendon bursa *(arrowheads)*.

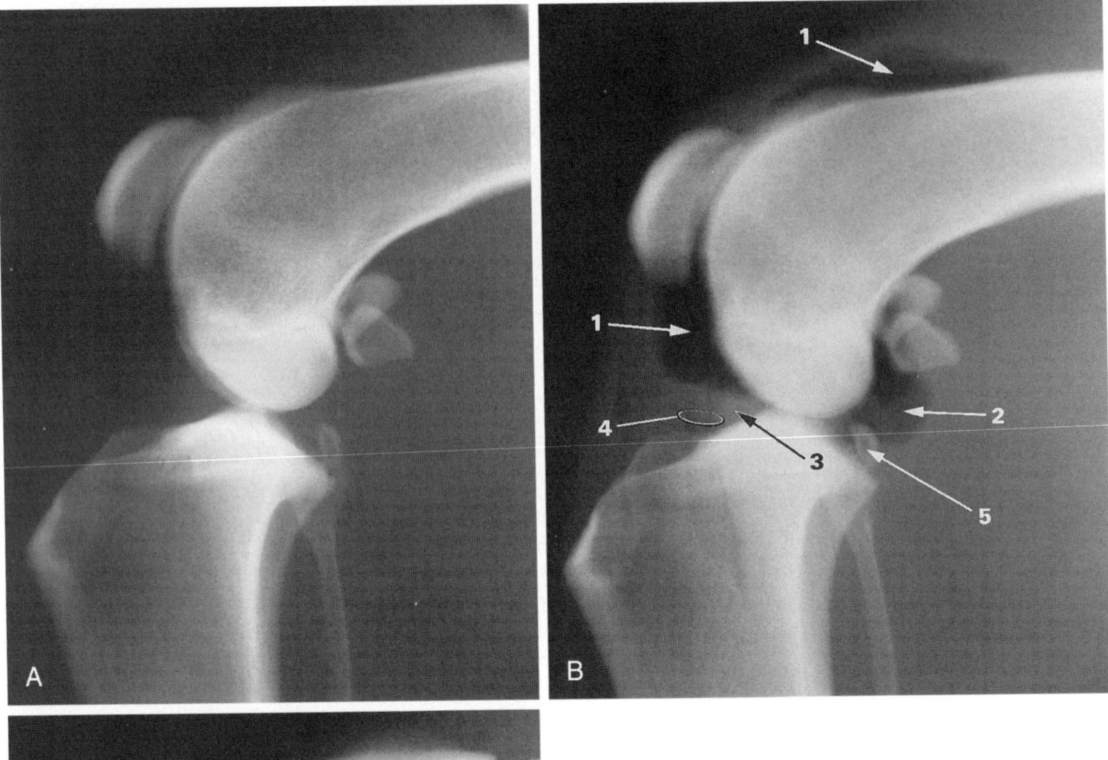

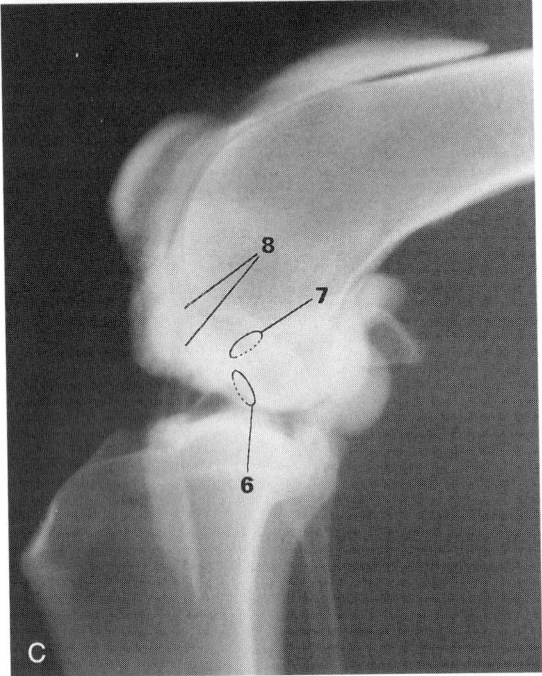

Fig. 18-23 Contrast arthrography of the stifle. **A,** Lateral noncontrast radiograph of a normal stifle. **B,** Negative-contrast arthrography of the stifle illustrated in **A.** Ten milliliters of air was injected into the cranial aspect of the joint space *(1)*. Note the caudal joint sac *(2)*, the menisci *(3)*, and the air in the bursa surrounding the tendon of the extensor digitorum longus muscle *(4)*. Air is also visible in the bursa of the popliteus muscle that is adjacent to the popliteal sesamoid *(5)*. **C,** A positive-contrast arthrogram of the contralateral stifle was achieved by injecting 10 mL iohexol (60 mg/mL of iodine). Additional intraarticular features demonstrated by this technique include the cranial *(6)* and the caudal *(7)* cruciate ligaments (linear filling defects) and the articular cartilage *(8)*.

In the coxofemoral joint, synovial effusion induces joint laxity, which appears radiographically as subluxation. The presence of hip laxity is a powerful indicator of the risk of development of coxofemoral osteoarthritis.[46-49] Workers studying passive coxofemoral joint laxity, as quantified by a unitless distraction index (DI), reported a strong correlation between the DI and subsequent development of degenerative joint disease. In four breeds studied (Borzoi, German Shepherd, Rottweiler, and Labrador Retriever), the likelihood of coxofemoral osteoarthritis varied with the breed and with the DI. Interestingly, the threshold DI, below which coxofemoral osteoarthritis is unlikely to occur, is different for the different breeds. For the German Shepherd, the threshold DI is 0.3; it appears to be higher (0.4) for the Labrador Retriever and Rottweiler.[50,51]

Radiographic changes of degenerative joint disease vary according to the stage of the disease. The most readily recognizable change is enthesophyte and osteophyte formation, which follows neovascularization of the chondrosynovial junction with resultant fibrocartilage formation. This fibrocartilage collar gradually ossifies with the formation of perichondral new bone (Fig. 18-28). Enthesophytes develop on nonweight-bearing surfaces and are eventually incorporated into adjacent ligamentous or capsular attachments.[38,39]

On radiographs obtained during weight bearing, continued attrition of the articular cartilage may be detected as thinning

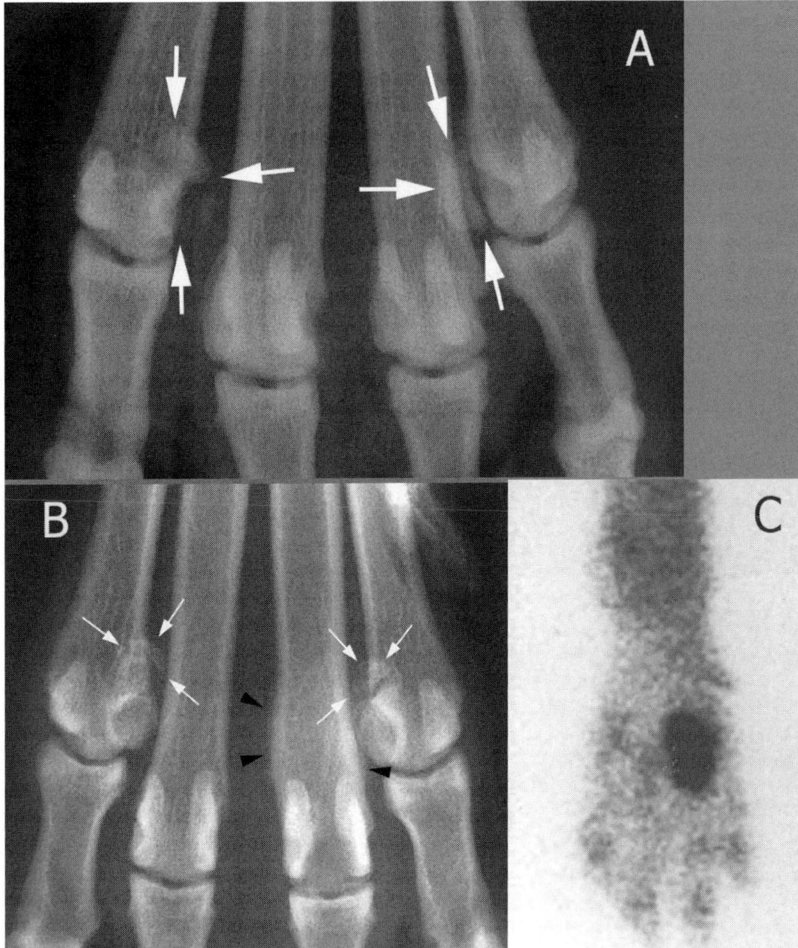

Fig. 18-24 A, Fragmentation of sesamoids 2 and 7 in a Rottweiler *(arrows)*. **B,** A similar Rottweiler *(white arrows)* shows concurrent osteitis of the distal end of a metacarpal bone *(black arrowheads)*. **C,** By using nuclear scintigraphy the osteitis was identified as the active lesion, and the fragmented sesamoids were diagnosed as fragmented but not clinically significant. (**B** and **C** courtesy Dr. R.M. Zuber, Gladesville Veterinary Hospital, Sydney, Australia.)

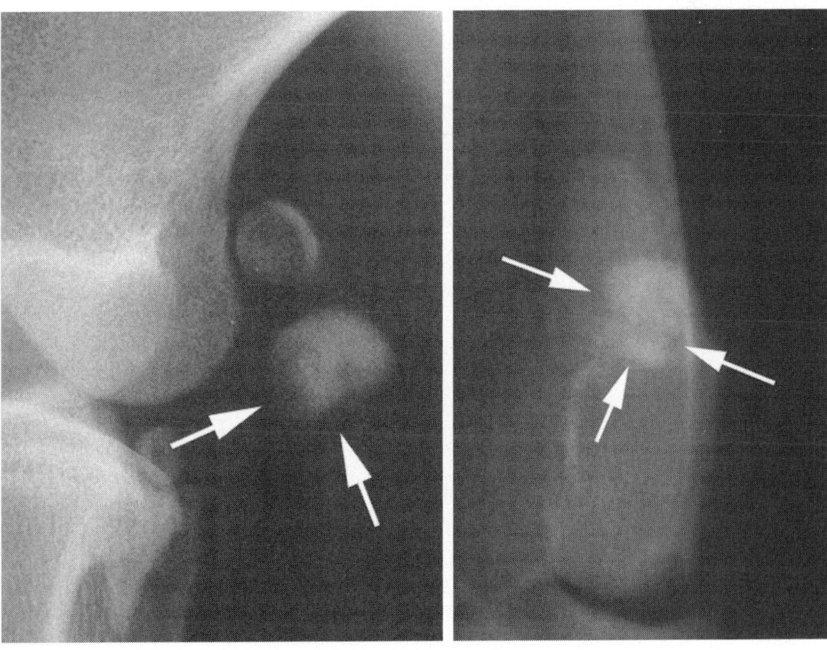

Fig. 18-25 Fragmentation of the lateral fabella *(arrows)* of an adult Staffordshire Bull Terrier. (Courtesy Sylvania Veterinary Hospital, Sydney, Australia.)

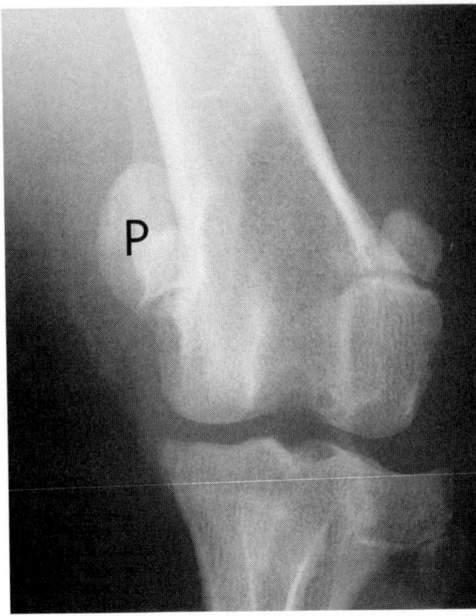

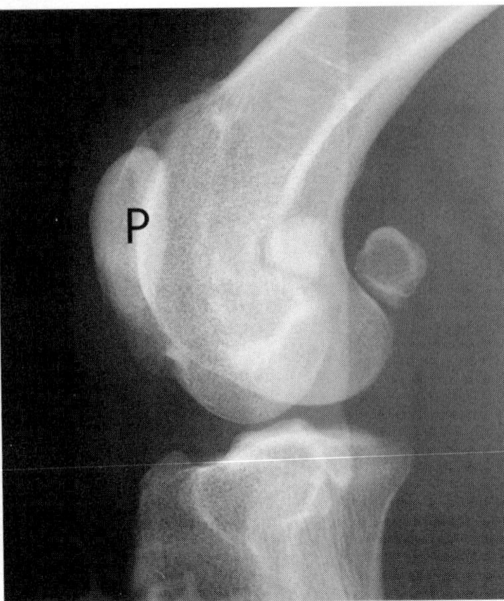

Fig. 18-26 Chronic medial luxation of the patella associated with varus angulation of the femoral condyle. On the lateral image the luxated patella is superimposed on the trochlea of the femoral condyle. (Courtesy Animal Referral Hospital, Sydney, Australia.)

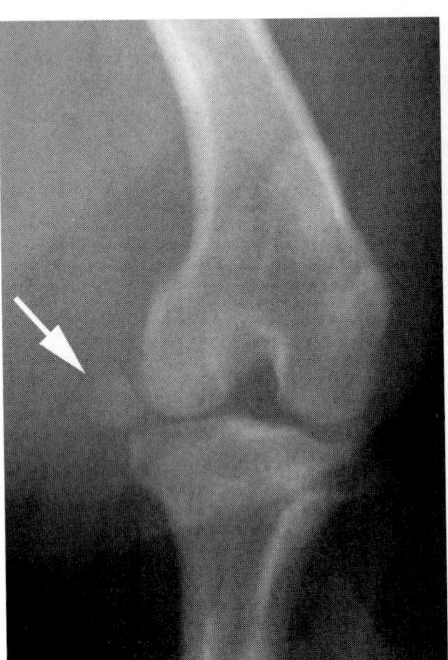

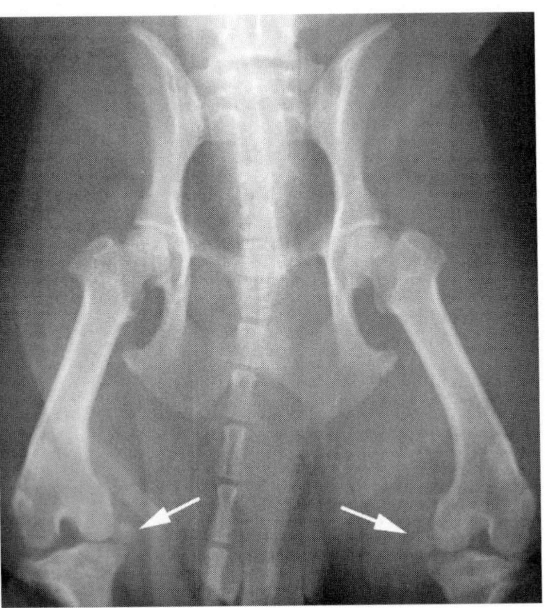

Fig. 18-27 A, Distal displacement of the medial fabella *(arrow)* of the left stifle of a 2-year-old male West Highland White Terrier. This change may be associated with rupture of the medial head of the gastrocnemius muscle, but examination of the contralateral stifle **(B)** revealed that displacement was bilaterally symmetrical *(arrows)*. In this circumstance, distal displacement of the medial fabellae is unlikely to be clinically significant. (Courtesy University Veterinary Centre, Sydney, Australia.)

of the radiolucent joint space. Pathologic alteration of the subchondral bone shelf, including eburnation, compression, and necrosis, may be detected radiographically as increased subchondral opacity of the weight-bearing surface. Subchondral cyst formation, a feature of osteoarthritis of the human femoral head, has also been observed in joints of small animals.[2,51]

Affected joints exhibit decreased range of movement, which results in increased loading of the diminished weight-bearing surface. The combination of increased load, diminished subchondral strength, and loss of shock-absorbing cartilage results in alteration in the shape of the subchondral bone table. This remodeling of subchondral bone is complemented by the addition of peripheral new bone in the form of perichondral osteophytes. Altered shape of the osseous components of affected joints is readily identified radiographically.[51] The gamut of the radiographic changes seen in degenerative joint disease is outlined in Box 18-3.

Osteoarthritis in Cats

Primary causes of articular cartilage degeneration and consequent osteoarthritis in cats include the storage disease mucopolysaccharidosis and osteochondral dysplasia of Scottish Fold cats. Established secondary causes of feline osteoarthritis (Fig. 18-29) include developmental and traumatic conditions that alter joint stability as well as dietary (hypervitaminosis A) and neuropathic causes (diabetes mellitus). Many infectious and immune-based arthropathies alter the integrity of articular cartilage, leading to a cascade of articular changes, with osteoarthritis as the end result.[52] Radio-

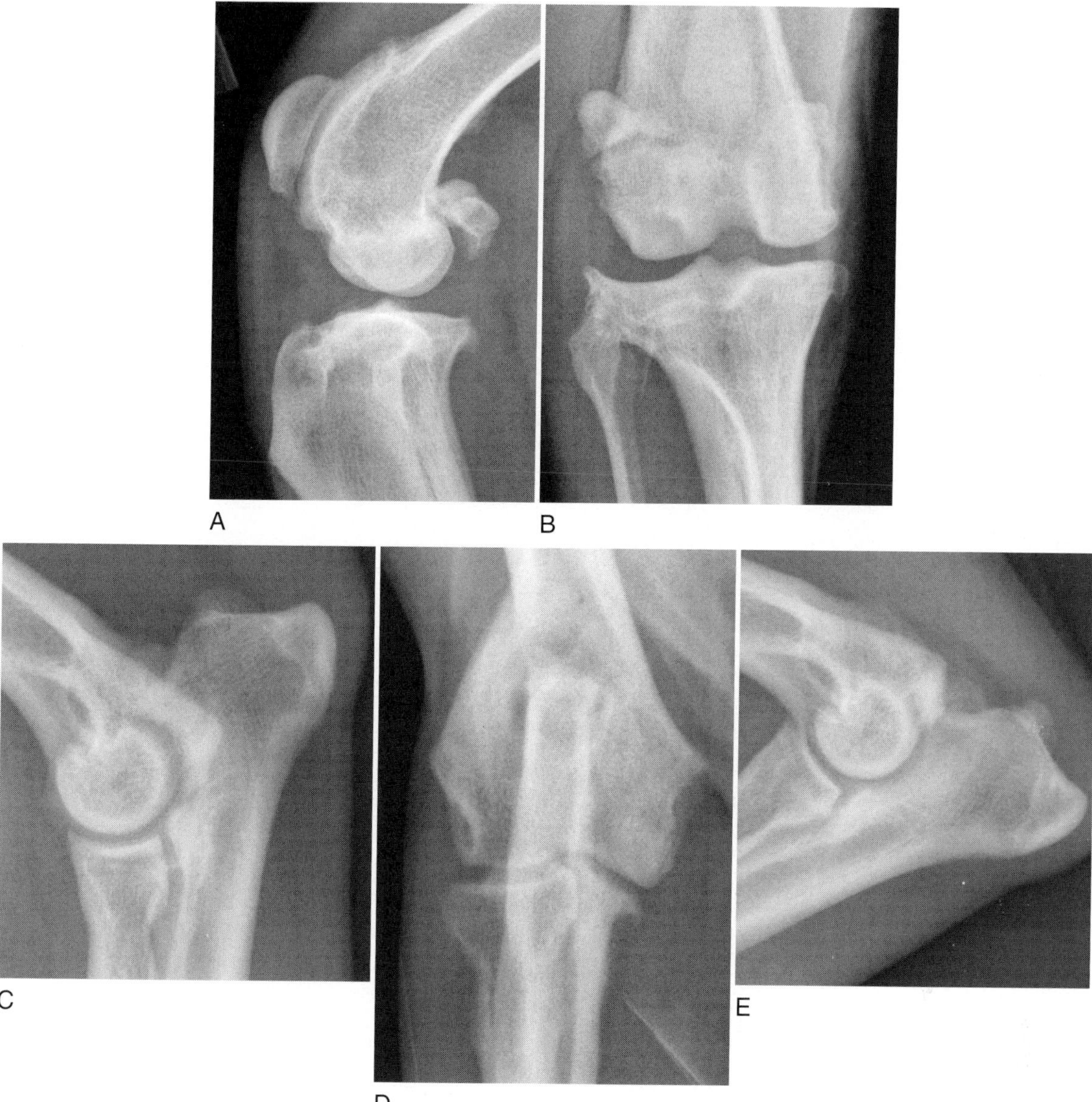

Fig. 18-28 A and B, A 7-year-old German Shepherd had chronic weight-bearing lameness of the right pelvic limb. Perichondral osteophytes and enthesophytes are visible on the distal femur and the proximal tibia. Synovial effusion is also evident. The presence of a prominent enthesophyte at the origin of the cranial cruciate ligament suggests these changes are attributable to chronic joint instability originally caused by cruciate ligament rupture. C to E, Osteoarthritis in the elbow of a 2-year-old German Shepherd. Osteophytes on the cranial aspect of the head of the radius (C) and on the medial edge of the coronoid process of the ulna (D) and enthesophyte formation on the anconeal process (E) are degenerative changes often seen secondary to the fragmented medial coronoid process.

graphic prevalence of signs of osteoarthritis in cats older than 12 years of age is as high as 90%, which is far greater than the incidence of clinical signs of osteoarthritis in older cats.

Cats with uncomplicated osteoarthritis may be free of clinical signs of joint disease, and radiographic signs of this condition are often accidentally discovered, but most of the syndromes listed in Box 18-4 are characterized by recognizable clinical signs that are accompanied by appendicular skeletal pain and lameness.

The radiographic signs of osteoarthritis in cats are similar to those reported in dogs. Periarticular new bone formation as osteophytes or enthesophytes develops around affected joints (see Fig. 18-29). Although the articular cartilage is invisible on survey radiographs, remodeling and increased opacity of subchondral bone add to the changed appearance of joint architecture.[1] Subchondral bone changes usually imply underlying changes in the joint cartilage. Signs of synovial effusion and/or thickened periarticular soft tissue are seen less commonly in cats than in dogs, whereas the incidence of intraarticular soft tissue calcification is seen more commonly in cats. Other changes that accompany feline osteoarthritis include intraarticular and periarticular soft tissue calcification, often ascribed to synovial osteochondromatosis, and prolific periarticular osteophytosis.

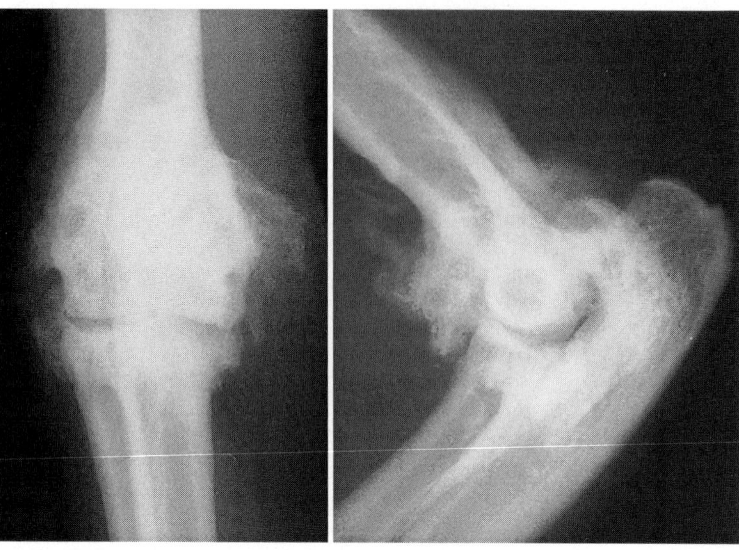

Fig. 18-29 Craniocaudal *(left)* and mediolateral *(right)* projections of a feline elbow with marked degenerative joint disease. Exuberant periarticular new bone formation is present around the elbow. On the lateral projection, an uneven radiolucent joint space indicates poor joint congruity. (Reprinted from Allan GS: Radiographic features of feline joint diseases, *Vet Clin North Am Small Anim Pract* 30:281, 2000.)

Box 18-3

Radiographic Signs of Osteoarthritis

- Synovial effusion
- Initial widening, then thinning, of the radiolucent joint space
- Perichondral enthesophyte formation of non-weight-bearing surfaces
- Increased subchondral bone opacity
- Remodeling of subchondral bone
- Mineralization of intraarticular and periarticular soft tissues
- Subchondral cyst formation (rare)
- Subluxation of the coxofemoral joint

Box 18-4

Causes of Osteoarthritis in Cats

Primary
- SFCOD
- MPS
- Age-related cartilage degeneration

Secondary
- Congenital
- Hip dysplasia
- Trauma
  - Traumatic joint instability
  - Physeal fractures
- Infectious/inflammatory
  - Viral (calicivirus, coronavirus)
  - Bacterial (bacterial L-form, mycoplasma, bite wounds)
  - Fungal (cryptococcosis, histoplasmosis)
- Nutritional
  - Hypervitaminosis A
- Neuropathic
  - Diabetes mellitus
- Immune mediated
  - Rheumatoid arthritis
  - Progressive proliferative polyarthropathy
- SLE
  - Idiopathic polyarthritides

Reprinted from Allan GS: Radiographic features of feline joint diseases, *Vet Clin North Am Small Anim Pract* 30:281, 2000.

HIP DYSPLASIA

Hip dysplasia is abnormal development of the coxofemoral joints. Hip dysplasia principally occurs in large dogs but also affects small dogs and cats. The incidence in males and females is similar. The condition is typically bilateral, but unilateral hip dysplasia has been reported in approximately 11% of dogs radiographed with the conventional extended ventrodorsal projection.

Hip dysplasia is an inherited disorder. Heritability estimates range from 2% to 6%. With the use of more sensitive radiographic interpretation and newer methods of imaging the coxofemoral joints, the estimated heritability in German Shepherds has been raised from 46% to 61%.[53,54] Environmental factors influence the phenotypic expression of hip dysplasia.[55] The role of nutrition has been extensively studied. Overnutrition is regarded as one of the principal nongenetic factors that influence the expression of canine hip dysplasia.[56] Hip dysplasia is a developmental, age-related disorder; it is not present at birth. A variable amount of time must elapse before radiographic changes manifest. Once present, these radiographic changes usually progress as the affected animal ages.

The earliest recognizable changes in the coxofemoral joints are a combination of perifoveal cartilage erosion, hypertrophy of the round ligament of the femoral head, synovial effusion, and synovitis.[57] None of these is recognizable radiographically, but the strongest clue to their presence can be obtained by testing for signs of joint laxity, which appears to be precipitated by synovial effusion. Joint laxity may be palpated (Ortolani's sign, Barden's lift method), visualized radiographically (Figs. 18-30 and 18-31),[42,58,59] or investigated sonographically. Subsequent radiographic changes are those of osteoarthritis (Fig. 18-32). The order of subsequent changes is (1) perichondral osteophyte formation, (2) remodeling of the femoral head and neck, (3) remodeling of the acetabulum, and (4) increased opacity of subchondral bone of the femoral head and acetabulum. An early and sensitive sign of new bone formation has been described.[60] Solitary bony enthesophytes on the caudal aspect of the femoral neck may be visualized as an opaque line (Fig. 18-33) directed distally rather than around the femoral neck; this line has been

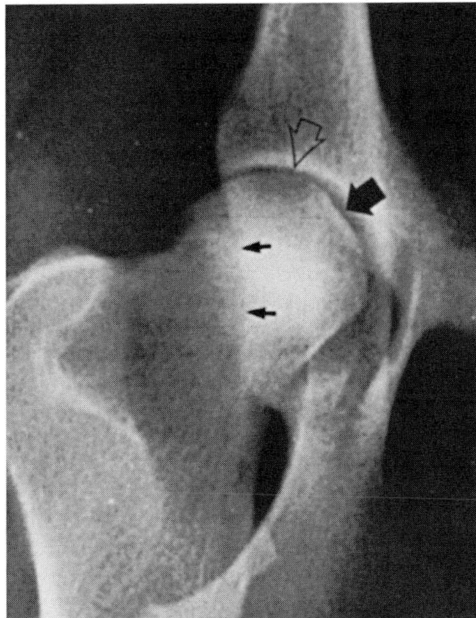

Fig. 18-30 Normal mature coxofemoral joint. Note that two thirds of the femoral head lies medial to the dorsal effective acetabular margin *(small arrows)*. The cranial margin of the femoral head is separated from the adjacent acetabulum by a fine radiolucent line, which represents the radiolucent joint cartilage and a microfilm of synovial fluid *(open arrow)*. The flattened portion of the femoral head is normal and represents the fovea capitis femoris *(solid arrow)*.

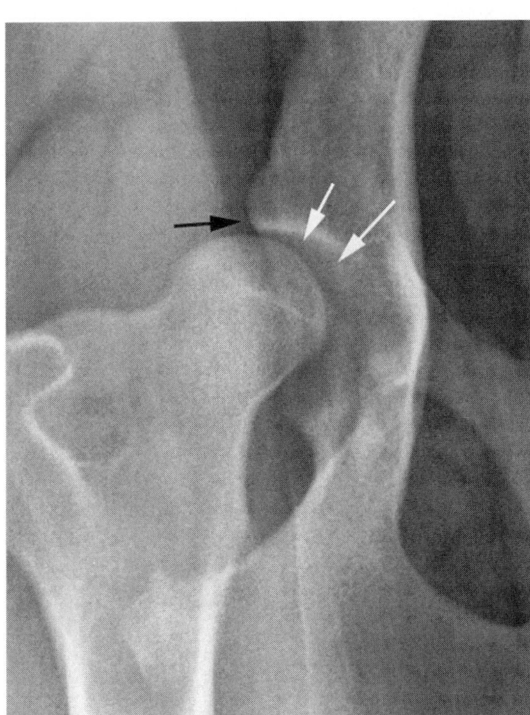

Fig. 18-31 Moderate hip dysplasia. Subluxation of the femoral head is accompanied by remodeling of the acetabulum. The cranial effective acetabular margin is angulated *(black arrow)*, and the acetabulum is shallow. Note the wedge-shaped joint space *(white arrows)*.

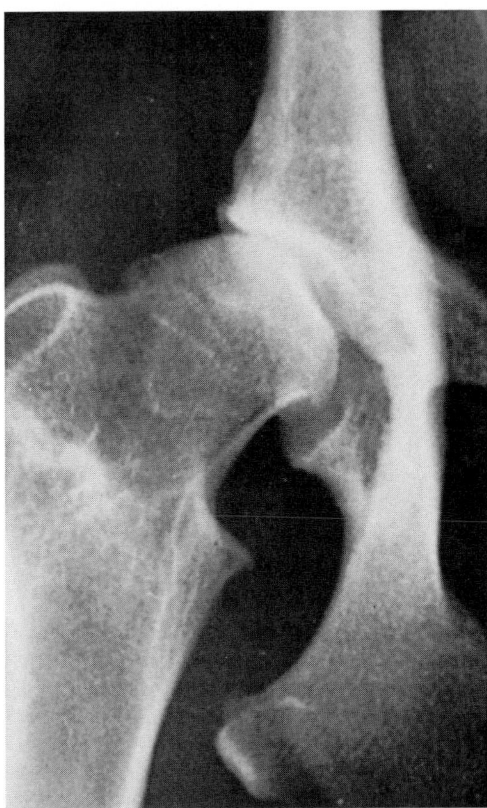

Fig. 18-32 Advanced hip dysplasia. The acetabulum and the femoral head have undergone advanced remodeling. Osteophytes have formed on the femoral neck and head as well as on the cranial effective acetabular margin. New bone formation has filled the acetabular fossa, and the opacity of acetabular subchondral bone is increased. These are easily recognized signs of degenerative joint disease.

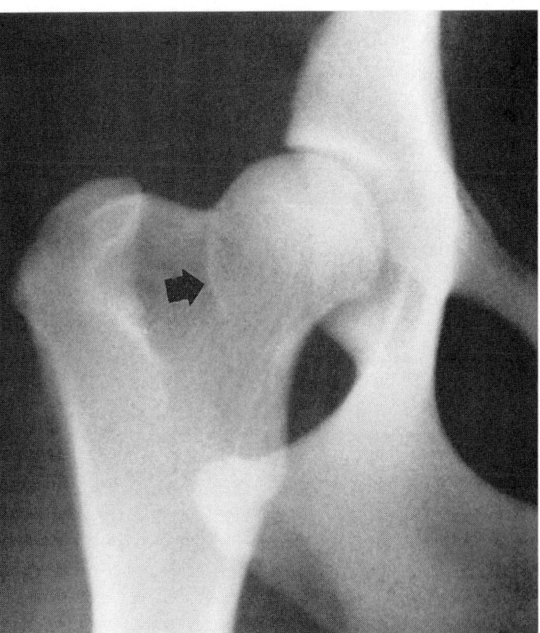

Fig. 18-33 A sentinel sign of early degenerative joint disease is the Morgan line, representing enthesophyte formation on the caudal aspect of the femoral neck, medial to the trochanteric fossa *(arrow)*.

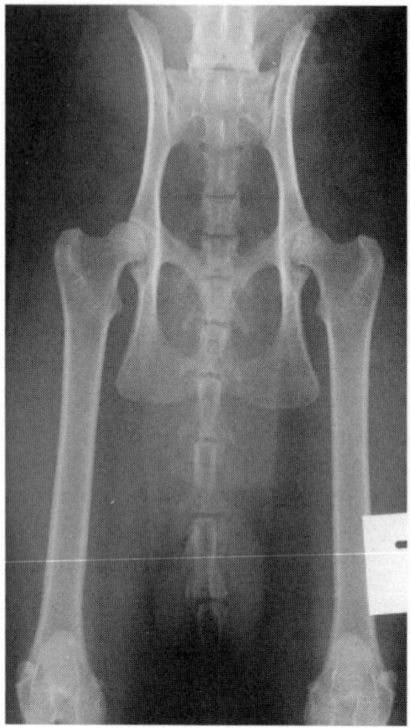

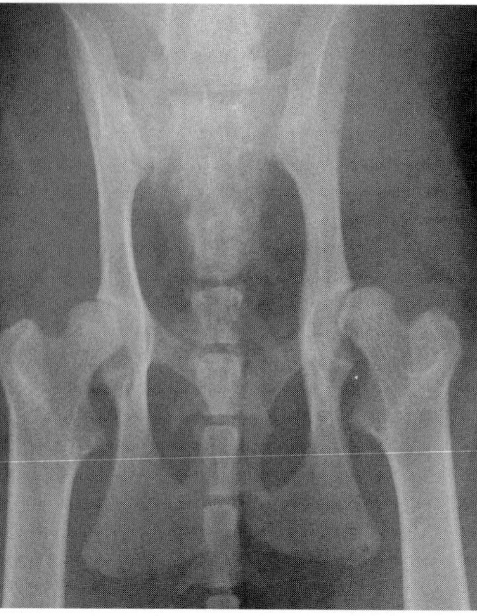

Fig. 18-34 Feline coxofemoral joints. *Left,* Normal hip conformation. *Right,* Abnormal hip conformation demonstrating coxofemoral subluxation. (Right panel courtesy University Veterinary Centre, Sydney, Australia.)

called the Morgan line. Because it is sometimes evident in animals whose coxofemoral joint laxity is camouflaged on the extended view, it should be regarded as an early and significant sign of coxofemoral osteoarthritis. As the degenerative phase advances, the femoral head loses its spheroidal shape and becomes flattened along its articular surface. The femoral neck becomes thickened, and the surface of the neck becomes irregular as a result of the growth of a collar of perichondral osteophytes. The acetabulum loses its cuplike shape and becomes shallow. Increased bone opacity of subchondral articular surfaces represents bone sclerosis, a response to cartilage thinning. A variable degree of coxofemoral subluxation is always present, and coxa valga is common. Subchondral cyst formation is an infrequent manifestation of osteoarthritis in small animals but may occasionally be observed.

The incidence of hip dysplasia in domestic shorthaired cats, based on standard hip radiography, has been estimated at 6.6%.[61] The incidence is higher in purebred cats (12.3%), with some breeds such as the Maine Coon having an incidence of 18% to 21%.[61,62] When passive coxofemoral laxity is evaluated by stress radiography, the overall incidence of feline hip dysplasia may be as high as 32%.[63] The prevalence of feline hip dysplasia is much lower than the prevalence in dogs.

Radiographic criteria for diagnosing feline hip dysplasia include the presence of signs of coxofemoral subluxation (Fig. 18-34), enthesophyte formation on the acetabular margins, and remodeling and degenerative changes of the femoral head and neck (Fig. 18-35). Unlike canine hip dysplasia, most degenerative changes in cats appear on the craniodorsal acetabular margins, with a low incidence of degenerative remodeling reported on the femoral head and neck.

The optimal method of screening canine coxofemoral joints to quantify dysplastic changes is disputable. Methods of evaluating the coxofemoral joints can be divided into those than proactively identify signs of subluxation, or joint laxity, and those that examine for visible radiographic evidence of osteoarthritis. Phenotypic screening programs used internationally fall into the latter group and rely on assessment of the extended ventrodorsal radiographic projection (Fig. 18-36), although this projection has long been recognized as an insensitive indicator of coxofemoral joint laxity. To reliably identify coxofemoral joint laxity, a stressed ventrodorsal projection is used. With the femurs placed in a distracted position (Fig. 18-37), coxofemoral laxity can be quantified and

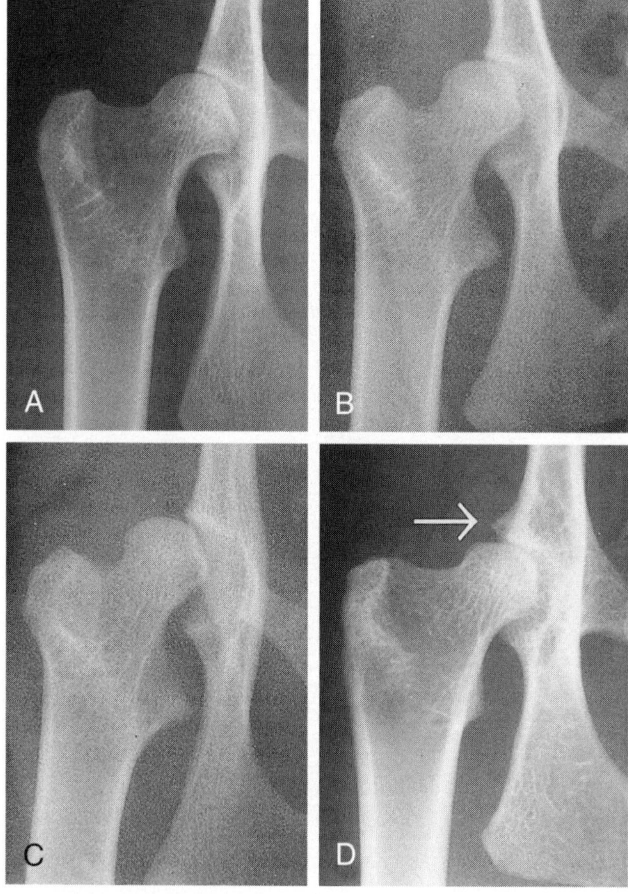

Fig. 18-35 A to D, Feline hip dysplasia. Varying degrees of coxofemoral subluxation (B and C) are compared with a "normal" (A) feline coxofemoral joint. Degenerative changes, with osteophyte formation on the cranial effective acetabular margin *(arrow),* are a typical manifestation of feline coxofemoral osteoarthritis (D). (Reprinted from Allan GS: Radiographic features of feline joint diseases, *Vet Clin North Am Small Anim Pract* 30:281, 2000.)

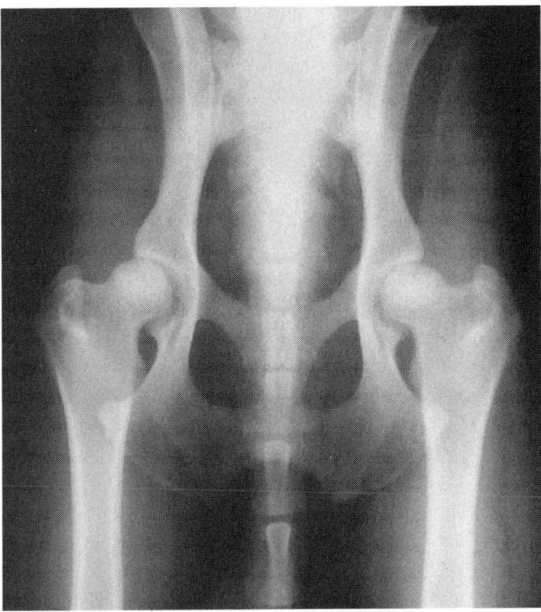

Fig. 18-36 Extended ventrodorsal projection of the coxofemoral joints (OFA preferred view). Note bilateral symmetry of the pelvis and parallel femurs. The coxofemoral joints appear to be normal. (Courtesy Dr. Ian Robertson, North Carolina State University, Raleigh, NC.)

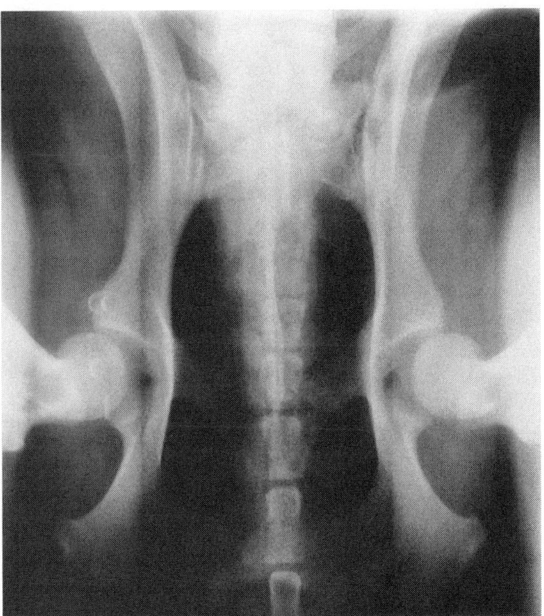

Fig. 18-37 Ventrodorsal distraction projection (PennHIP view). Bilateral coxofemoral subluxation (laxity) is evident. This radiograph is of the same dog shown in Figure 16-11. (Courtesy Dr. Ian Robertson, North Carolina State University, Raleigh, NC.)

the calculated laxity index (DI) used to rank individual dogs within their breed with respect to hip joint tightness/looseness.[64] The DI is also a useful indicator of the likelihood of future coxofemoral degenerative changes. This information can be obtained at a much earlier age by using distraction radiography than with the standard extended ventrodorsal projection. Alternative methods of achieving a similar result look at dorsolateral subluxation, measuring a dorsolateral subluxation score or a subluxation index. Proponents of the dorsolateral subluxation score (DLS) claim that a combination of the DLS

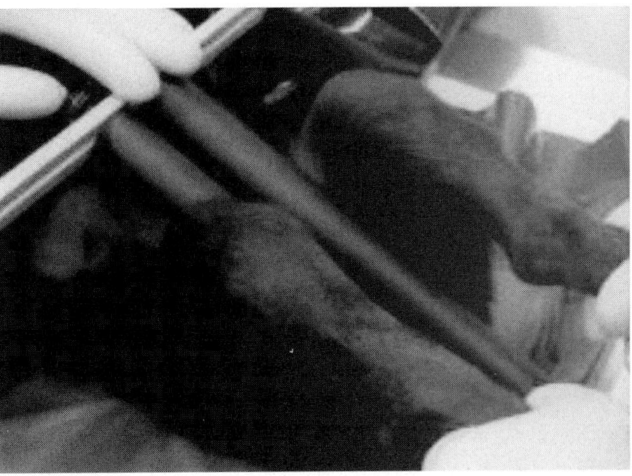

Fig. 18-38 The distracted PennHIP view is achieved by holding a rubberized distraction device between the patient's thighs, with the femurs held at 90 degrees to the pelvis. The femurs are gently pressed against the distractor during the radiographic exposure.

and measurement of Norberg's angle also serves as a useful predictor of future development of the coxofemoral osteoarthritis.[57] All the newer methods of evaluating the coxofemoral joints recognize that assessing coxofemoral laxity is an important component of complete assessment of the coxofemoral joints.

Most current screening programs require that the extended ventrodorsal radiograph of the coxofemoral joints be made and submitted for evaluation. The method of obtaining the projection required by the Orthopedic Foundation for Animals (OFA), which is similar to the projections used by other screening programs internationally, has been described in detail.[65] With the dog in dorsal recumbency, the hindlimbs are extended with the femurs parallel and the stifles rotated inward so that the patellae are located over the middle of the cranial surface of the distal femur. The x-ray beam should be centered over the coxofemoral joints, and the radiograph should include the entire pelvis and the femurs. The pelvis must appear symmetrical in the radiograph, without evidence of pelvic rotation (see Figs. 18-34, *A*, and 18-36). Although satisfactory radiographic quality may be achieved without the assistance of chemical restraint,[66] failure to anesthetize the subject may decrease radiographic sensitivity for signs of coxofemoral joint laxity.[67] Because the extended ventrodorsal projection is an insensitive method of detecting signs of coxofemoral subluxation,[64,68] care must be taken to ensure accurate subject positioning and satisfactory radiographic quality.

The PennHIP method[46,47,64] also requires the dog to be placed in dorsal recumbency. The femurs are placed in a neutral position to duplicate standing. This neutral position avoids spiral tensioning of the joint capsule, a significant disadvantage of the OFA projection. The hindlimbs are held with the femurs neutrally positioned, and a radiograph is made while the coxofemoral joints are compressed to obtain an image of the coxofemoral joints at their most congruent position. A distraction device is then placed between the femurs for the second radiograph (Fig. 18-38). When the femurs are pressed against the bars of the distracter, any coxofemoral laxity that is naturally present is visualized radiographically. The two views of the hips are compared, and any coxofemoral laxity is quantified by a unitless measure, the DI. A third (OFA) projection is made so that secondary signs of hip dysplasia, such as degenerative joint disease, can be evaluated (Fig. 18-39).

The PennHIP method has several inherent advantages over the traditional (OFA) method of evaluating the coxofemoral

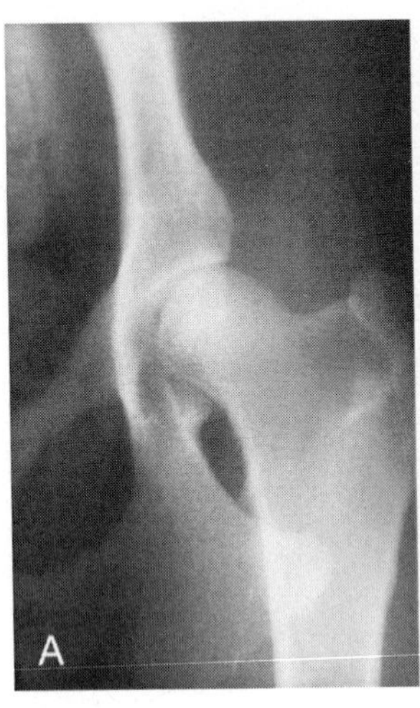

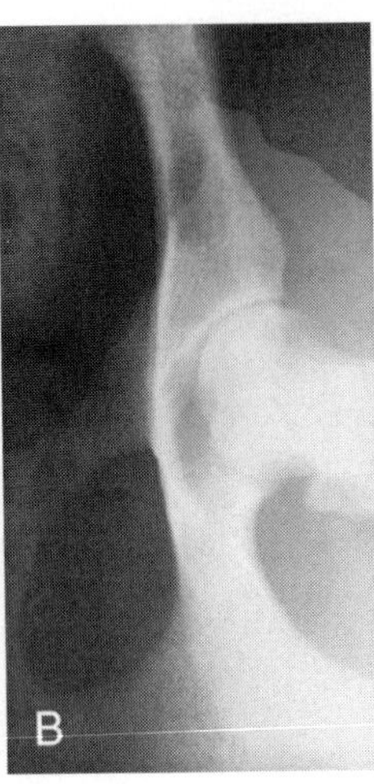

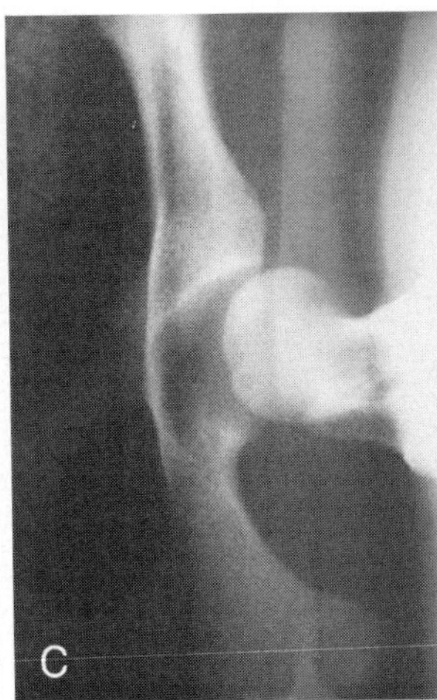

Fig. 18-39 A to C, A completed PennHIP study with the coxofemoral joints in the extended (A), neutral compressed (B), and distracted (C) projections. Note the amount of coxofemoral subluxation revealed in this dog with the distracted projection.

Box • 18-5

Comparison of OFA and PennHIP Methods for Hip Dysplasia Radiography

Extended Ventrodorsal Projection

Advantages

- Currently the most popular screening program internationally
- Does not require special training or accessory equipment
- Only one radiograph required
- Has amassed a large database of information about the coxofemoral phenotype
- Animals can be radiographed without personnel exposure

Disadvantages

- Inaccurate in young animals; accuracy increases with age; optimal time to radiograph is 24 to 36 months
- An insensitive method of identifying coxofemoral joint laxity
- Requires rigid application to achieve beneficial results in breeding programs
- Technique of extending the femurs camouflages signs of joint laxity by spiral tensioning of the joint capsule

PennHIP Distraction Projection

Advantages

- A valuable screening method for breeders before litters are placed in homes (as early as 16 weeks)
- An accurate method of predicting dysplastic changes in young animals from 6 months
- A sensitive method available for identifying joint laxity
- Generates a unitless index (DI) that can be used to predict whether osteoarthritis will develop
- Has a greater heritability than the OFA method

Disadvantages

- Requires special training to certify users
- Requires special equipment
- Multiple radiographic projections required
- Personnel exposure during radiographic exposure is difficult to avoid

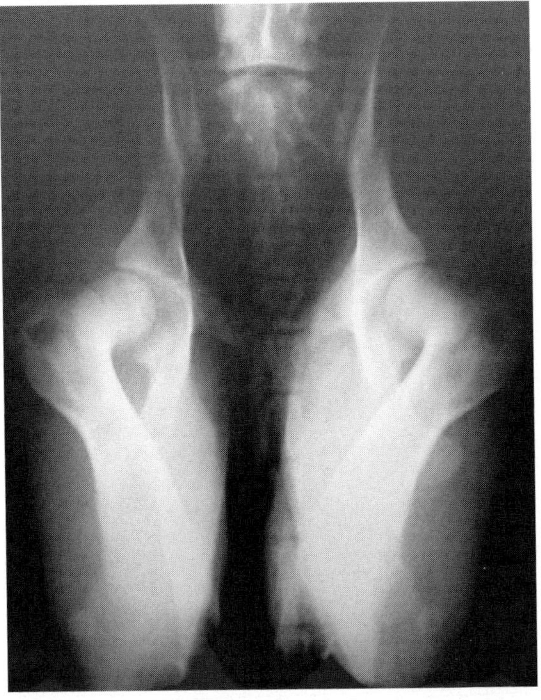

Fig. 18-40 Radiographic image of the pelvis of a dog positioned for the Fluckiger technique. The stifles are adducted and rotated inward. The femurs are held at an angle of approximately 45 degrees to the table top, and the legs are pressed toward the table top to accentuate signs of any joint laxity that may exist in the coxofemoral joints.

joints (Box 18-5). First, it quantifies joint laxity, which is generally accepted as the beginning of a chain of events that culminates in varying degrees of coxofemoral osteoarthritis. Second, the examination can be done on young dogs. The predictive value of the DI is constant after 6 months of age, thereby providing valuable information to breeders at an early age when selecting their stock. Third, the technique predicts a DI below which degenerative changes are unlikely to occur. Conversely, the DI and the subsequent development of osteoarthritis appear to have a direct relation when the DI is greater than 0.3 (for German Shepherds) or 0.4 (for Labrador Retrievers and Rottweilers).

A variant of the PennHIP method has been described (Fluckiger technique) in which the Ortolani maneuver is simulated with the dog in dorsal recumbency (Fig. 18-40).[69] This

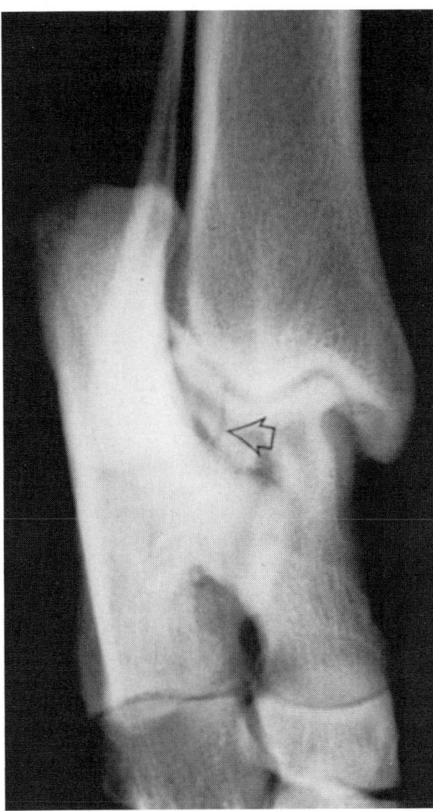

Fig. 18-41 A 3-year-old German Short-Hair Pointer with acute onset of non-weight-bearing lameness of the left pelvic limb. A fracture through the lateral trochlear ridge of the talus is shown *(arrow)*. The diagnosis is articular fracture of the talus. (Courtesy University Veterinary Centre, Sydney, Australia.)

method discloses craniodorsal and lateral coxofemoral laxity, which is defined by a subluxation index (SI). The radiographic image of dogs positioned for the Fluckiger method appear similar to those positioned for the DLS method, except that the femurs are more perpendicular to the pelvis in the latter. These two methods measure "functional laxity" of the coxofemoral joints, compared with the PennHIP method, which measures "passive laxity."

Proponents of the DLS method argue that hip dysplasia is defined by the presence of osteoarthritis, which is debatable.[70] Not all dogs with coxofemoral laxity develop osteoarthritis, but does this mean they are not dysplastic, or just fortunate to have escaped the consequences of having joint laxity? The question of what constitutes phenotypic freedom from hip dysplasia continues to be debated.

TRAUMA INVOLVING THE OSSEOUS COMPONENTS OF JOINTS

Any fracture that communicates with a joint space is an articular fracture (Fig. 18-41). Articular fractures must be diagnosed accurately to ensure appropriate surgical reduction and stabilization Radiographic examinations should include two projections made at right angles to one another (Fig. 18-42). To these should be added oblique views and projections during flexion and stress, when needed. These additional projections are of most value when chip or avulsion fractures are suspected or when the osseous structures of interest are superimposed on other osseous structures.

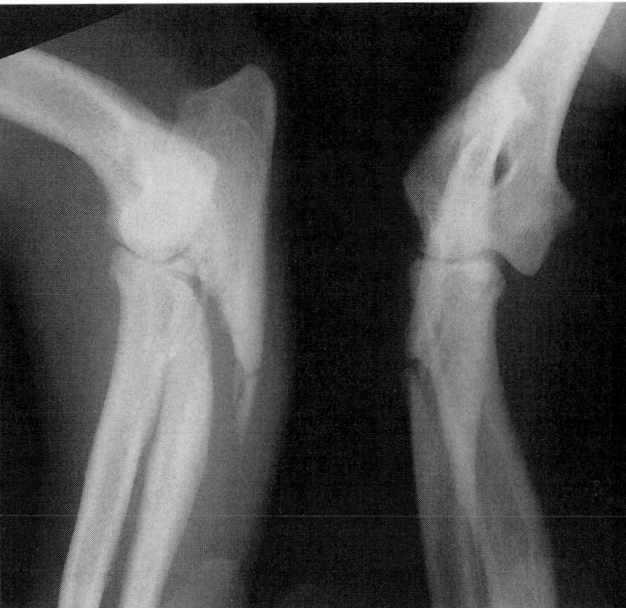

Fig. 18-42 A long, oblique fracture of the ulna penetrates the humeroulnar joint at the medial coronoid process.

Articular fractures frequently occur in immature animals because of the incidence of physeal and epiphyseal trauma in these patients. Because the proximal femoral physis is intracapsular, all femoral capital physeal fractures are intraarticular fractures (Fig. 18-43). In other joints, physeal fractures that involve the joint are usually classified as Salter type III or IV fractures.[71]

Premature physeal closure may follow repair of Salter fractures and is observed within 2 to 3 weeks of surgery. It should be regarded as a potential consequence, regardless of the type of physeal trauma, and periodic radiography is advised to minimize the problems associated with undetected premature physeal closure.

SPRAINS AFFECTING JOINTS

Supporting soft tissue structures of joints appear as soft tissue opacities that silhouette each other and with adjacent soft tissues. Therefore they are not clearly visualized on a radiograph. The radiographic features of severe sprains include (1) periarticular soft tissue swelling; (2) avulsion fractures at points of attachment of ligaments, tendons, and capsules to bone (entheses); (3) joint instability or subluxation; and (4) spatial derangement of the osseous components of a joint.

Sprains must be diagnosed promptly. In many instances, appropriate medical or surgical therapy ensures return to normal joint function after moderate to severe sprain injuries. Many patients with profound sprains, such as carpal hyperextension injuries, may be effectively treated, thus allowing the affected animal to ambulate satisfactorily instead of surviving with a disability.

The clinical assessment (palpation and manipulation) of a sprained joint is usually the best diagnostic tool. Radiographic examination adds information that is useful for treatment planning while documenting the presence and magnitude of the sprain and identifying avulsed osseous fragments. A useful technique for radiographic assessment of a sprained joint is stress radiography (Fig. 18-44 and 18-45). In practice, this technique involves application of force to the joint in question to demonstrate displacement of its osseous components. The forces applied are the same stresses to which the joint

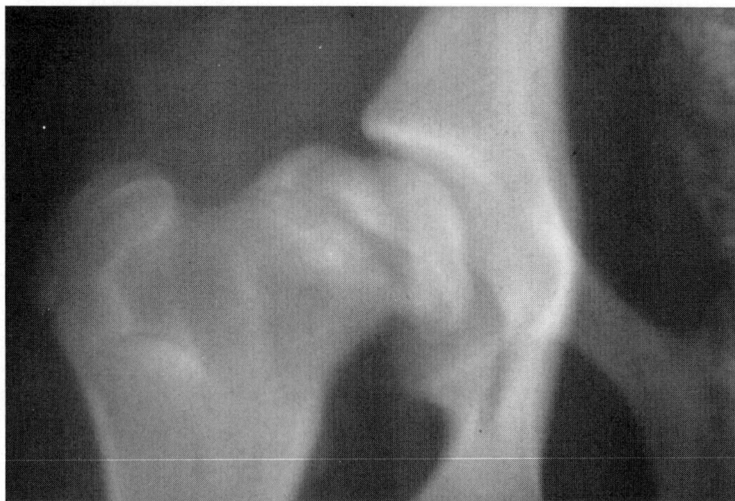

Fig. 18-43 Because the femoral capital epiphysis is entirely intracapsular, any fracture involving the femoral head, as illustrated, is an articular fracture.

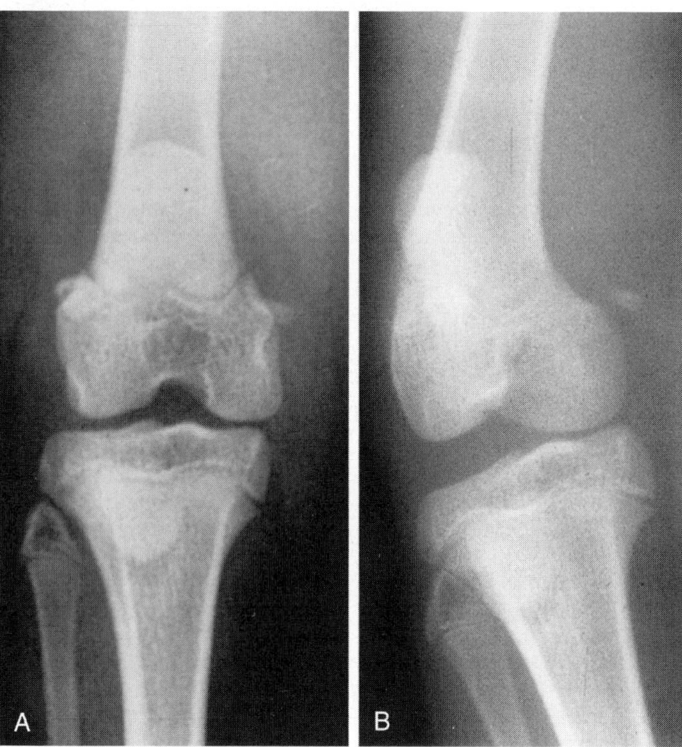

Fig. 18-44 An 8-month-old Burmese cat was lame in the left pelvic limb. A craniocaudal radiograph **(A)** was normal. In a stressed craniocaudal radiograph **(B)**, widening of the lateral aspect of the joint space was apparent. The diagnosis is ruptured lateral collateral ligament.

would be subjected in normal daily activity and are defined as compressive, rotational, traction, shear, and wedge forces (Fig. 18-46).[72]

An excellent example of a compressive stress is a radiograph of a joint during weight bearing. Ligamentous trauma, as in carpal hyperextension injuries, is readily detected by this technique. The cranial drawer sign seen in cranial cruciate ligament trauma is a practical example of a shearing stress. It is stress that is used routinely in clinical examination of the stifle. The same manipulative procedure may be applied to the stifle during radiography. Traction stress involves pulling the osseous components of the joint away from one another. One useful application of traction stress involves capital physeal fractures of the femoral head. When traction is applied to the femur in the extended ventrodorsal position, capital physeal fractures are easy to identify.

A technique using traction stress has been described for identifying medial scapulohumeral joint instability in small dogs. With the patient in lateral recumbency, nontraction and traction radiographs are made of the shoulder joint. A significant increase in the shoulder joint space has been identified as a sign of medial shoulder joint instability.[73] Traction and wedge stresses (see Case Study 18-2 on the Evolve site [http://evolve.elsevier.com/Thrall/vetrad]) are useful for examining joints for small avulsion fractures and intraarticular-joint mice. Unilateral trauma to collateral ligaments of the elbow and stifle may be disclosed with wedge stresses. Because stress radiography requires that personnel hold the patient during x-ray exposure, utmost care must be taken to ensure that such persons wear appropriate protective clothing.

TENDONS, DESMOPATHIES

Injuries to tendons and ligaments are important causes of lameness in dogs and cats and must be distinguished from skeletal and articular causes of lameness. Many tendons and

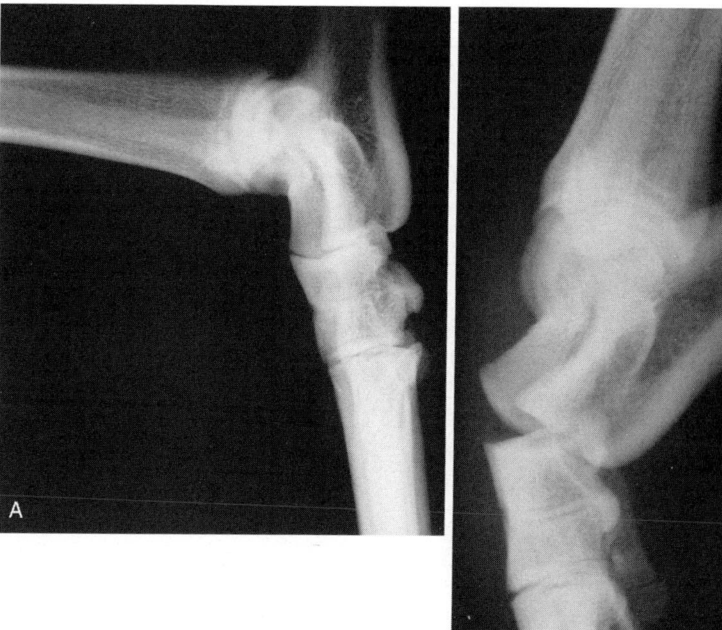

Fig. 18-45 A, A neutral lateral radiograph of a racing Greyhound appears normal. B, Stress radiography was performed, which allowed identification of instability of the proximal intertarsal joint.

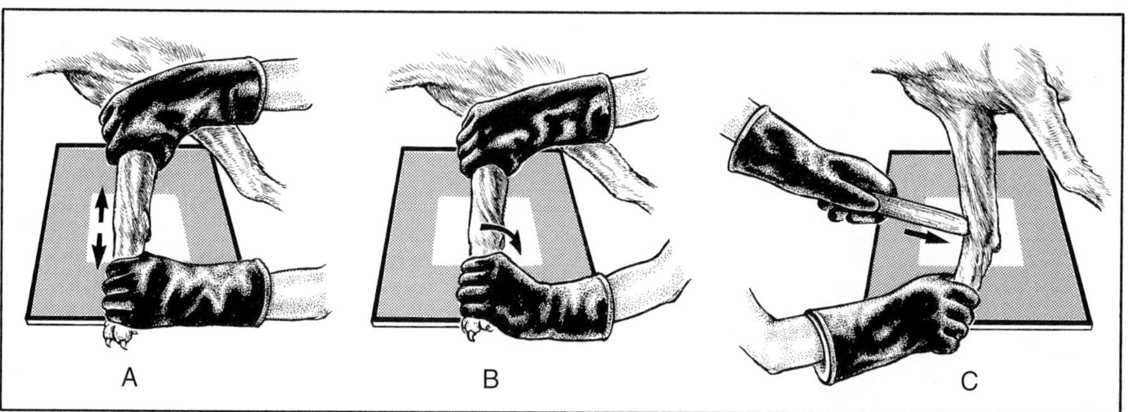

Fig. 18-46 Stress radiography of joints involves the application of traction (A), rotational (B), and wedge (C) forces to demonstrate subluxation that may not be evident on standard radiographic projections. (Modified from Farrow CS: Stress radiography: applications in small animal practice, *J Am Vet Med Assoc* 181:777, 1982.)

ligaments are intimately associated with joints, lying within them (cruciate ligaments), passing through them (bicipital tendon, long digital extensor tendon), or inserting adjacent to a joint (popliteus tendon). This section includes some of the common desmopathies that occur around joints.

SHOULDER

Bicipital Tendon (Biceps Brachii)

Gross changes in dogs with bicipital tenosynovitis include synovial effusion, synovial hyperplasia of the bursa, chondromalacia of the intertubercular (bicipital) groove with osteophyte formation at its edges, and metastatic calcification of the biceps tendon.

The latter two changes can be seen on survey radiographs of the shoulder (Fig. 18-47) when they occur in affected dogs. Occasionally discrete mineralized opacities (joint mice) may be seen superimposed on the tendon within the bicipital groove.[74] In extreme cases, the entire bicipital bursa appears calcified (Fig. 18-48).

Positive contrast arthrography usually demonstrates thickened and irregular synovial margins that diminish the volume of fluid within the synovial bursa, causing irregular margination of the tendon and synovium.

Ruptured Bicipital Tendon

Bicipital tendonopathy and bursitis may also be evaluated sonographically. Sonography may reveal changes in the bicipital tendon or bursa in instances of bursitis and tendonitis. The location of a rupture in the tendon may be identified radiographically and sonographically (Figs. 18-49 and 18-50).

Sonography can also be used to identify the supraspinatus and infraspinatus tendons, the teres minor tendon, and the

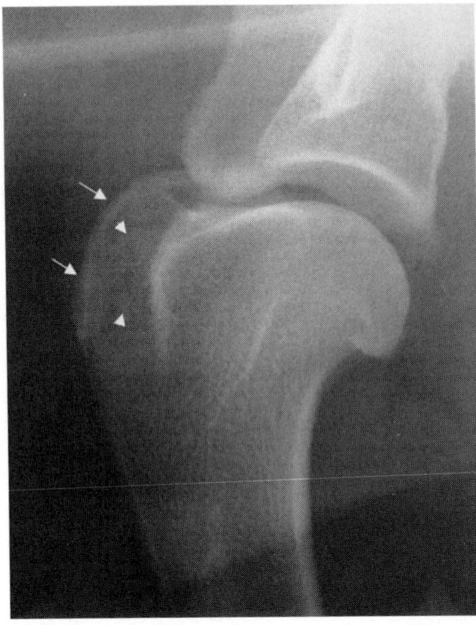
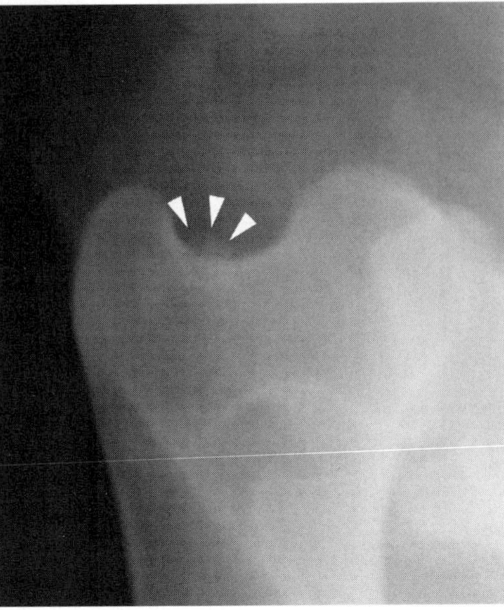

Fig. 18-47 Bicipital tendonitis. *Left,* New bone proliferation superimposed on the bicipital *groove (arrowheads)* and along the margin of the greater tubercle of the humerus seen in a dog with bicipital tendonitis. *Right,* A cranioproximal-craniodistal "skyline" view showing osteophytes in the bicipital groove.

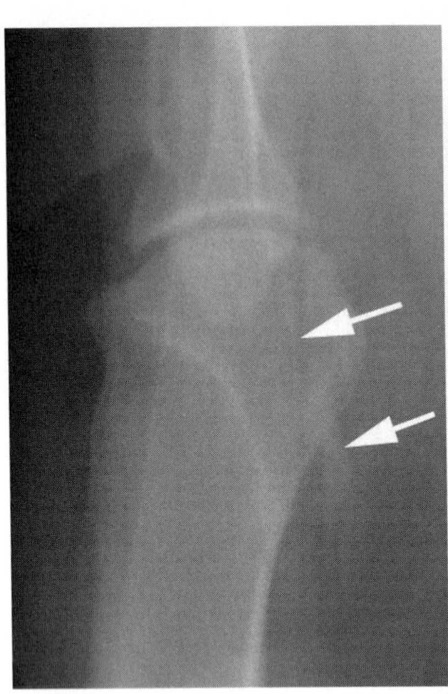
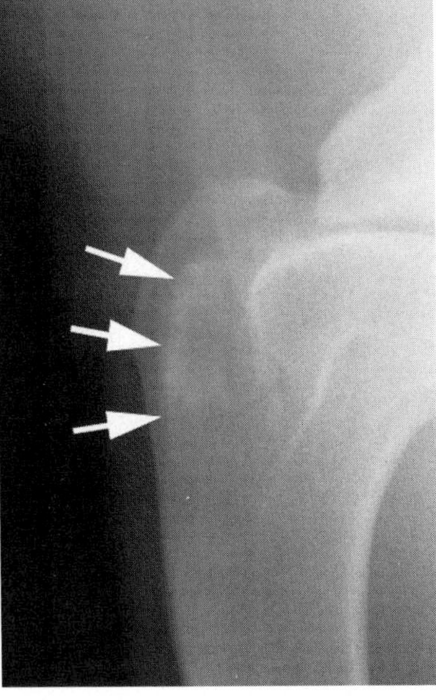

Fig. 18-48 Extensive mineralization surrounding the bicipital tendon was interpreted as calcifying bursitis in a dog with chronic tendonopathy of biceps brachii. (Courtesy Dr. M. Fetterplace, Ingleburn Veterinary Hospital, Ingleburn, Australia.)

caudal aspect of the humeral head. In clinical settings sonography assists in identification of synovial effusion and proliferation within the bicipital bursa, supraspinatus and bicipital tendonitis, dystrophic calcification, and osteochondrosis of the humeral head, but the lateral glenohumeral ligament was not seen in one study of tendons and ligaments around the shoulder joint.[75,76] Advanced imaging modalities such as magnetic resonance imaging (MRI) (Fig. 18-51) have demonstrable advantages when evaluating tendons and ligaments around joints.

THE CARPUS

Several important tendons pass close to the carpus or insert onto bones adjacent to it. Osteophytes arising and extending from the medial sulcus of the distal radius (Fig. 18-52) follow the path of the tendon of abductor pollicis longus and are a response to synovitis where the tendon passes over the sulcus. Osteophytosis has been associated with stenosis of the synovial sheath of the tendon.[77] Extensor carpi radialis inserts on the dorsal surface of the proximal end of metacarpals 2 and 3. An enthesopathy at the points of insertion can result in new bone formation that can be identified on lateral radiographs of the carpometacarpal region. Flexor carpi ulnaris inserts on the proximal surface of the accessory carpal bone, and the check ligaments of the accessory carpal bone originate from the distal surface. Again, an enthesopathy can be identified on the proximal and distal surfaces of the accessory carpal bone when an enthesopathy of these tendons and ligaments is present. The tendons and ligaments around the carpus can be assessed sonographically (Fig. 18-53) as well as by MRI.

Carpal Flexural Deformity

Attributed to asynchronous development of the manus and flexor tendons, carpal flexural deformity is recognized by the

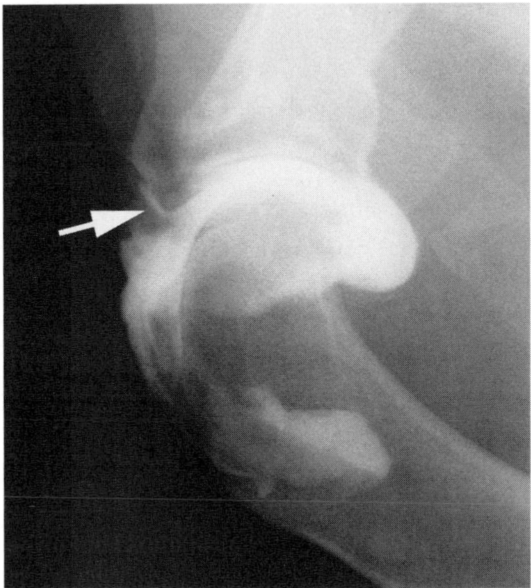

Fig. 18-49 Flexed lateral views of a shoulder arthrogram of a dog with a ruptured tendon or origin of the biceps tendon. The well-defined distal edge of the supraglenoid tubercle *(arrow)* was interpreted as indicating separation of the tendon and its proximal enthesis.

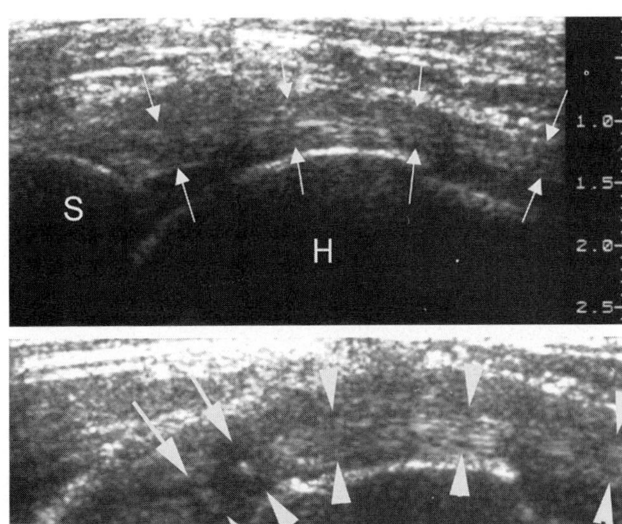

Fig. 18-50 Composite image of the right *(top)* and left *(bottom)* biceps tendon. The normal striated right tendon is visible *(arrows)* in the upper image. The lower image is of the ruptured left biceps tendon. The void *(arrows)* representing the rupture contrasts with the normal striated tendon distally *(arrowheads)*. *S*, Scapular; *H*, humerus. (Courtesy University Veterinary Centre, Sydney, Australia.)

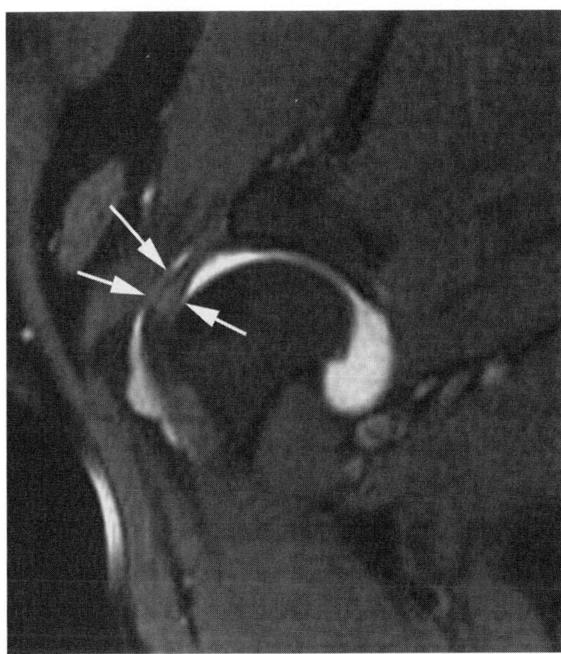

Fig. 18-51 A 2-year-old neutered Labrador Retriever had left forelimb lameness for 2 months. Shoulder radiographs were unremarkable. On a T1-weighted fat-saturated MRI sequence taken after intraarticular gadolinium injection (contrast arthrogram), the biceps tendon was shown to have a heterogeneous signal, with abnormal hyperintensity just proximal to the cranial margin of the humeral head *(arrows)*. The diagnosis, based on this finding, was chronic biceps tenosynovitis. Biceps tenotomy was performed and the lameness improved. (Courtesy Dr. Chess Adams, University of Wisconsin, Madison, Wis.)

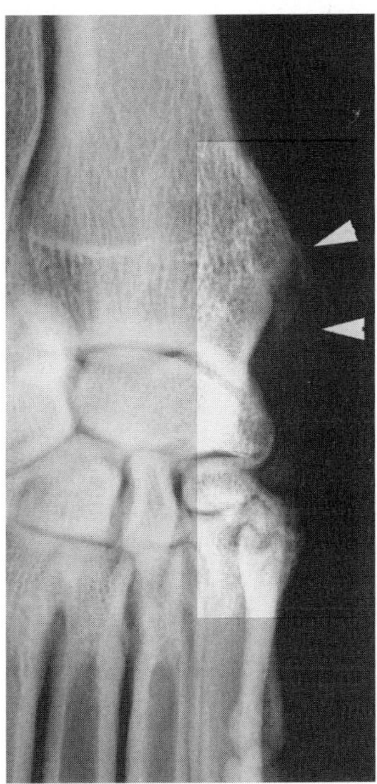

Fig. 18-52 Osteophyte formation arising from the distomedial surface of the radius following the path of the tendon of abductor pollicis longus *(arrowheads)*, which was interpreted as indicating bursitis and tendonopathy where the tendon passes over the medial sulcus. (Courtesy Dr. P. Young, All Pets Veterinary Hospital, Albury, Australia.)

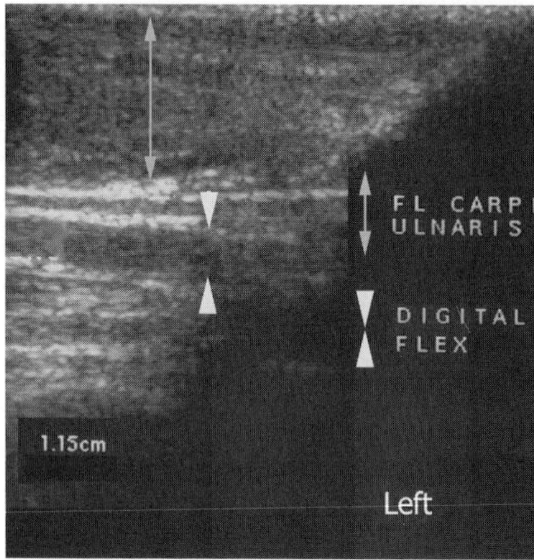

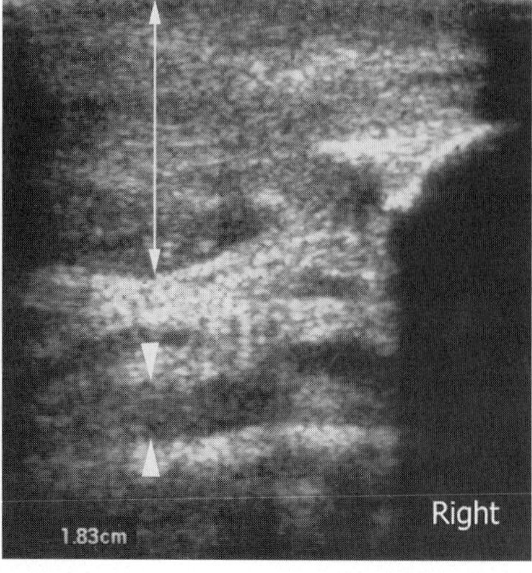

Fig. 18-53 Chronic trauma to the tendon of insertion of flexor carpi ulnaris has resulted in thickening of the affected right tendon, which is easier to comprehend when compared with the left tendon at the same level. (Courtesy Dr. Soo Kuan, Northern Sydney Veterinary Specialist Centre, Sydney, Australia.)

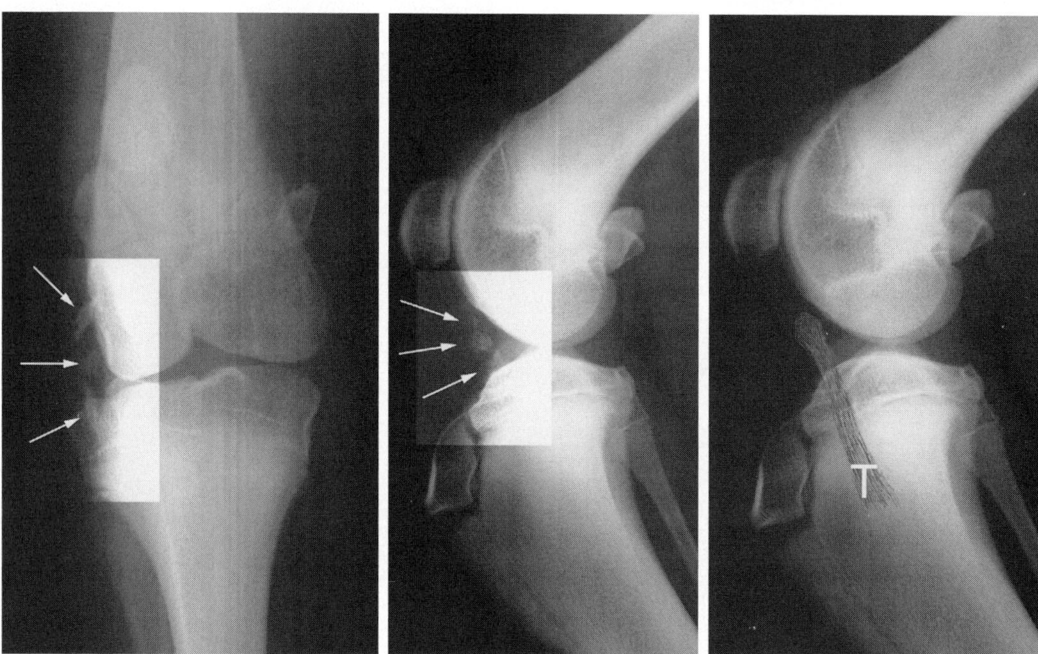

Fig. 18-54 Stifle of an immature Rottweiler. Fragments of bone on the craniolateral aspect of the stifle *(arrows)*, a result of avulsion of the tendon of origin *(T)* of the long digital extensor muscle. (Courtesy Dr. A.P. Black, Northern Sydney Veterinary Specialist Centre, Sydney, Australia.)

curled toes and flexed digits visible in affected animals. The condition affects puppies in the first year of life. From a radiological perspective the manus appears normal.

THE STIFLE

In the stifle sonography is a reliable technique for identification of osteochondrosis lesions in the lateral femoral condyle. The menisci were less reliably imaged in small dogs than in large dogs, but the cranial cruciate ligament and femoral articular cartilage can be seen. The patella ligament and the origin and tendon of the long digital extensor muscle can be reliably imaged, but the collateral ligaments and joint capsule were not seen.[78,79] Sonography identified 20% of ruptured cruciate ligaments in one study of cranial cruciate ligament rupture in dogs. Although not an incisive diagnostic procedure for this condition, it does permit evaluation of soft tissue changes that occur within the stifle as a result of joint instability.[80]

Long Digital Extensor Tendon

Avulsion of the origin of the long digital extensor tendon produces characteristic radiographic changes because the proximal enthesis usually avulses fragments of bone from the extensor fossa. Bone fragments are identified craniolateral to the stifle joint space (Fig. 18-54). Where chronic desmopathies of the tendon and its bursa are present, a tunnel of calcification sometimes develops around the tendon and can be identified radiographically (Fig. 18-55).

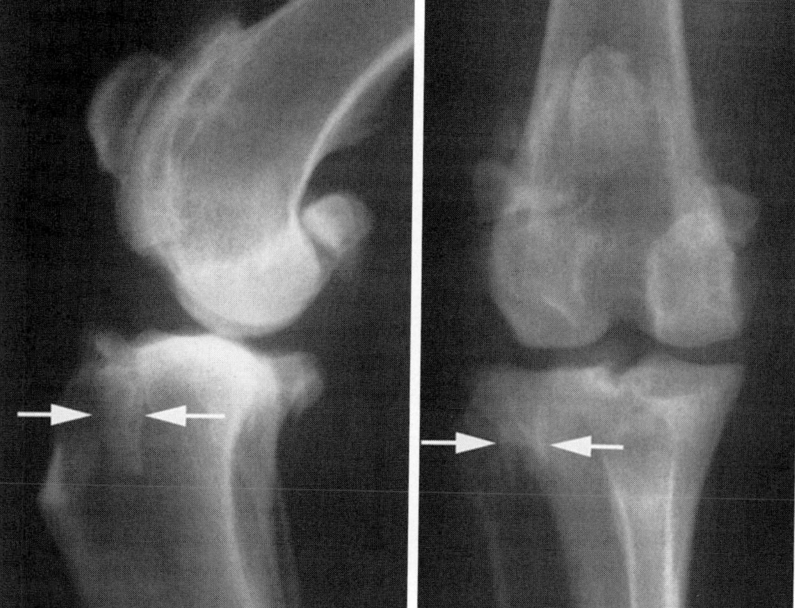

Fig. 18-55 A column of calcified tissue following the path of the long digital extensor tendon *(arrows)* was interpreted as calcifying bursitis and tendonopathy. Osteophytosis, a sign of osteoarthritis, is present around the trochlear ridges of the femoral condyle.

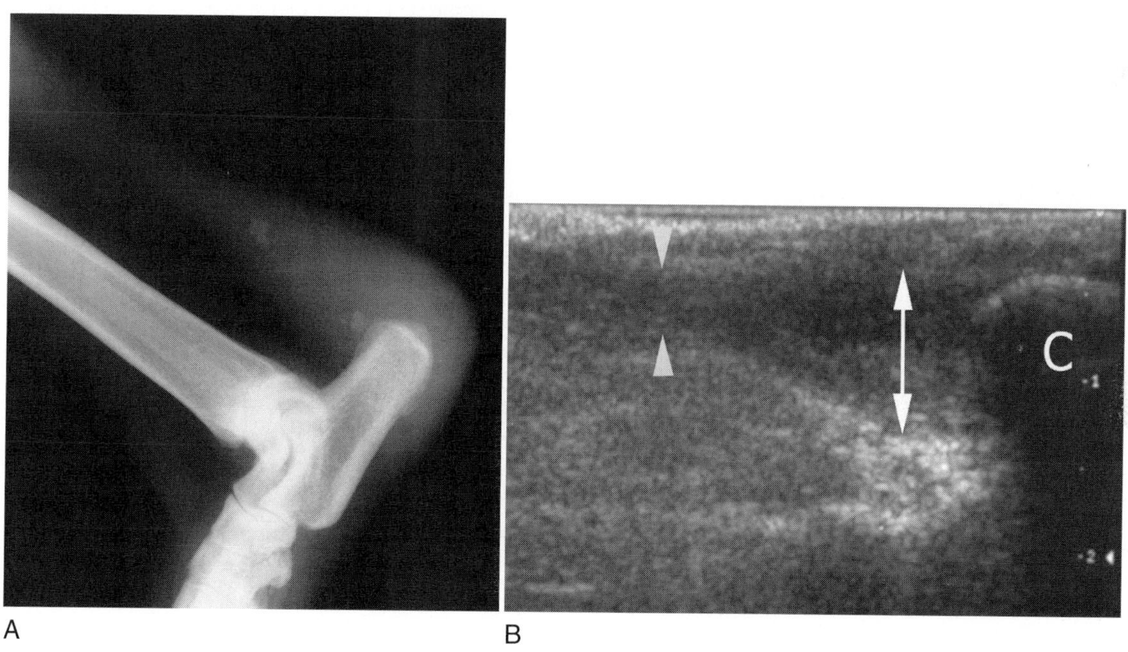

Fig. 18-56 Soft tissue swelling and dystrophic calcification along the path of the Achilles tendon in a dog **(A)**, and sonographic evidence of focal swelling of the distal end to the Achilles tendon in a cat **(B)** adjacent to the calcaneus *(C)*, interpreted in both cases as Achilles tendon injury. (A courtesy Dr. M. McLachlan, Petersham Veterinary Hospital. Reproduced from *BSAVA manual of canine and feline musculoskeletal imaging*, BSAVA Publications, Quedgeley, Gloucester, England, 2006.)

TARSUS

The Achilles tendon is composed mainly of the tendons of flexor digitorum superficialis and gastrocnemius muscles, with contribution of tendons from biceps femoris, semitendinosus, and gracilis muscles. It inserts onto the calcaneal tuberosity. Chronic desmopathies of the Achilles tendon cause soft tissue swelling, occasionally containing dystrophic calcification (Fig. 18-56). Sonography enables identification of partial and total ruptures of the deep and superficial structures comprising the Achilles tendon. Tendinous trauma can be distinguished from muscle trauma.[81]

HYPERVITAMINOSIS A

Excessive dietary vitamin A produces an ankylosing arthropathy and spondylopathy. Although both dogs and cats can be affected, the disorder seems more likely to affect cats. The food mostly associated with hypervitaminosis A is bovine liver, and when fed as an exclusive diet the clinical syndrome of vitamin A excess can be recognized after a few months.

Affected cats become obtunded, apprehensive, reluctant to jump, hypersensitive to neck palpation and lame. The underlying connective tissue disorder causes vertebral ankylosis and an ankylosing osteoarthritis of the forelimbs.

Recognizable radiographic manifestations of hypervitaminosis A may be seen in as little as 10 weeks after introduction of a diet rich in vitamin A. Changes include ankylosing spondylopathy of the cervical and cranial thoracic vertebral column and periarticular enthesopathy and osteoarthritis of the shoulder and elbow joints (Figs. 18-57 and 18-58). In advanced disease the additional bone becomes seamlessly incorporated with existing bone so that the architecture of the original bones is completely remodeled. Other regions of the vertebral column and other joints of the appendicular skeleton may become involved, but the aforementioned bones and joint appear to be the primary site of bony changes in cats.

These ankylosing changes are permanent; they do not resolve once a balanced diet is substituted, but some of the clinical signs of hypervitaminosis A resolve once the dietary imbalance is corrected.

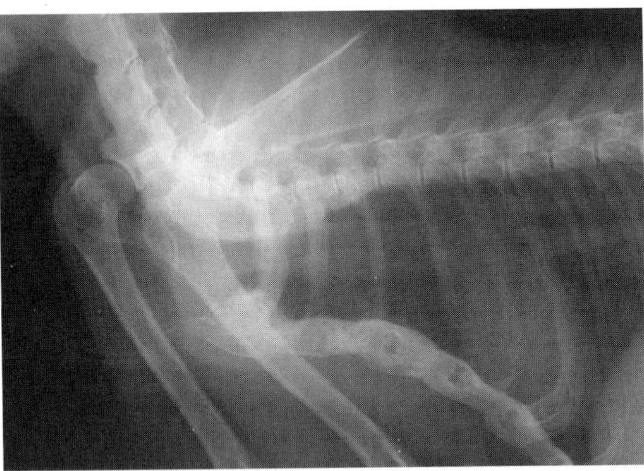

Fig. 18-57 Ankylosing spondylopathy of the cervical and cranial thoracic vertebrae and the sternum of a cat with hypervitaminosis A. (Reprinted from Allan GS: Radiographic features of feline joint diseases, *Vet Clin North Am Small Anim Pract* 30:281, 2000. Courtesy University of Queensland, Australia.)

MUCOPOLYSACCHARIDOSIS

The storage diseases that comprise mucopolysaccharidosis (MPS) are characterized by the accumulation of glycosaminoglycans in tissue. Both dogs and cats are affected by MPS. The best-studied animal form is the feline form of MPS VI. It causes polyarthropathies because of faulty cartilage formation, a result of dermatan sulfate accumulation in connective tissue because of deficiency of the lysosomal enzyme *N*-acetylgalactosamine-4-sulphatase.

The morphologic appearance of affected cats ranges from normal to short-legged dwarfs with facial dysmorphism. Feline MPS VI has two genotypes. The least affected phenotype ranges from being physically and clinically normal to having osteoarthritis of the shoulder and stifle joints. The classic form produces phenotypic features of dwarfism and facial dysmorphia. These cats tend to show lameness and develop hindlimb paresis.

Radiographic abnormalities are from epiphyseal dysplasia and range from signs of osteoarthritis in the shoulder and stifle to gross malformation of the appendicular and axial skeleton (Figs. 18-59 and 18-60). Severely affected animals are osteopenic. The subchondral bone of articular surfaces is distorted, and periarticular soft tissue mineralization is common. Epiphyseal dysplasia results in distortion of the epiphyses of the appendicular skeleton, which reflects high levels of lysosomal storage in chondrocytes, adversely affecting mineralization of the matrix during enchondral ossification.

Vertebral malformation is a recognizable feature of feline MPS VI. The vertebral bodies are short and square, the pedicles elongated, and articular processes malformed. Epiphyseal dysplasia causes distortion of the epiphyses of vertebral bodies. New bone formation around articular facets and ankylosing spondylopathy are common.

SCOTTISH FOLD CHONDRO-OSSEOUS DYSPLASIA

Scottish Fold chondro-osseous dysplasia (SFCOD) is inherited as an autosomal dominant trait that causes defective cartilage maturation. Although folding of the auricular cartilage is a defining visible feature of SFCOD, the cascade of changes

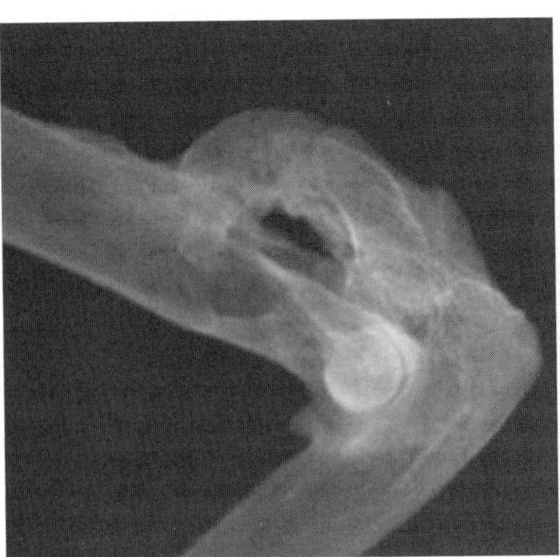

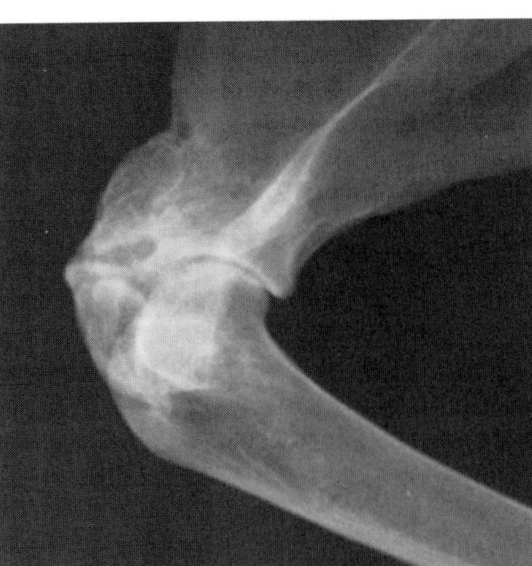

Fig. 18-58 Radiographs of the elbows and a shoulder obtained from the skeleton of a cat that was euthanized because of the crippling ankylosing arthropathy caused by hypervitaminosis A.

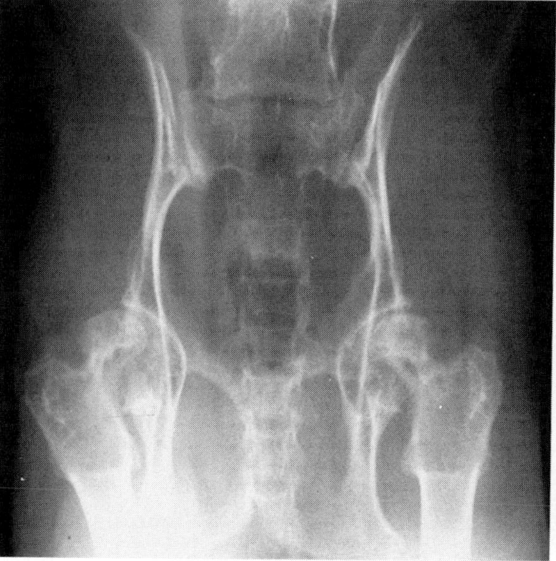
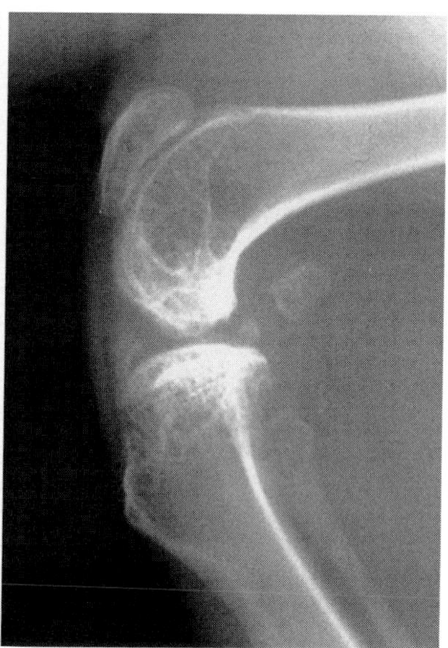

Fig. 18-59 Malformation of the coxofemoral joints, pelvis, and stifle caused by mucopolysaccharidosis type VI in a cat. (Courtesy Dr. A.C. Crawley, Adelaide, South Australia. Reprinted from Allan GS: Radiographic features of feline joint diseases, *Vet Clin North Am Small Anim Pract* 30:281, 2000.)

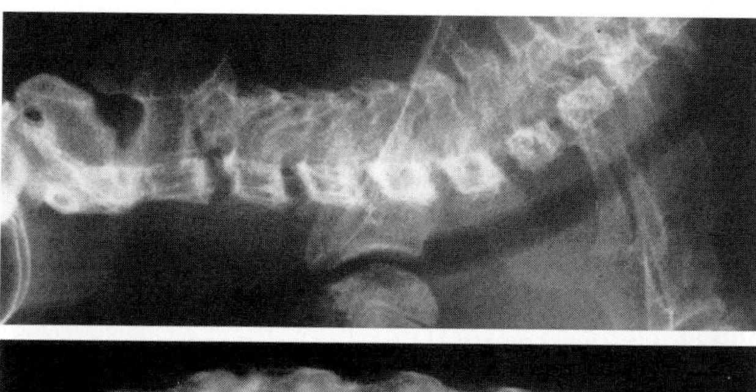
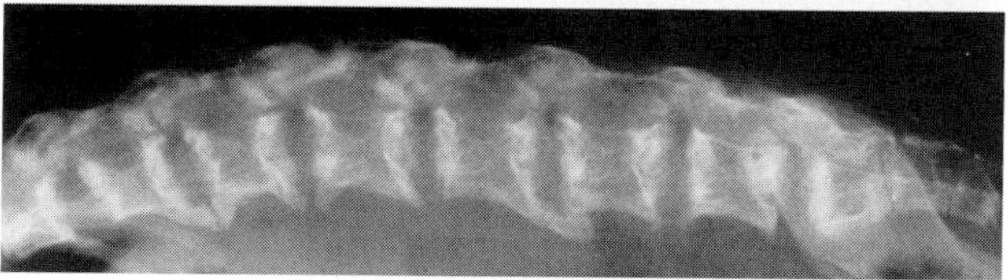

Fig. 18-60 Cervical and lumbar vertebral malformation caused by MPS type VI in a cat. (Courtesy Dr. A.C. Crawley, Adelaide, South Australia. Reprinted from Allan GS: Radiographic features of feline joint diseases, *Vet Clin North Am Small Anim Pract* 30:281, 2000.)

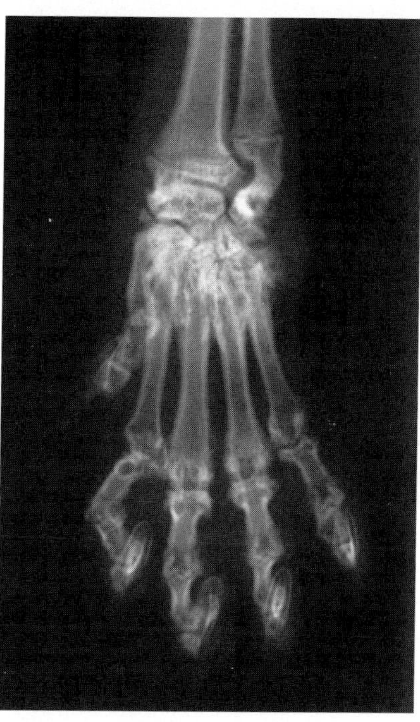

Fig. 18-61 Carpometacarpal ankylosis and metacarpal and phalangeal malformation in a Scottish Fold cat. (Courtesy Sylvania Veterinary Hospital, Sydney, Australia.)

caused by faulty cartilage maturation affecting the skeleton are seen in both homozygotes and heterozygotes of this condition. In extreme forms the polyarthropathy caused by SFCOD can be crippling, and affected animals can be disinclined to ambulate and unable to jump.

Defective cartilage formation manifests skeletal changes that affect joints and entheses. The joints of the distal limbs are most spectacularly affected, but some long bones such as the metacarpi, metatarsi, and the phalanges may also develop abnormally (Fig. 18-61).

Large enthesophytes can form around joints at points of tendinous origin or insertion (entheses). An ankylosing arthropathy frequently results in fusion of the carpi and tarsi (Fig. 18-62) and their articulations with the metacarpi and metatarsi. Malformed bones in the manus and pes may not grow to a normal length, and these bones may appear shorter and fatter than normal. Vertebral malformation can be spectacular in the tail (Fig. 18-63), where the caudal vertebrae may be short and wide. Spondylopathy of the caudal vertebrae may combine to produce a tail that is short and relatively inflexible.[82]

HEMARTHROSIS

Intraarticular hemorrhage may occur in dogs with coagulopathies or after joint trauma. Hemarthrosis was reported in a dog with suspected warfarin toxicosis.[83] Other coagulopathies in the dog that may cause hemarthrosis include hemophilia A and B; von Willebrand's disease; deficiencies in factors VII, X, and XI; and liver disease. Isolated, infrequent

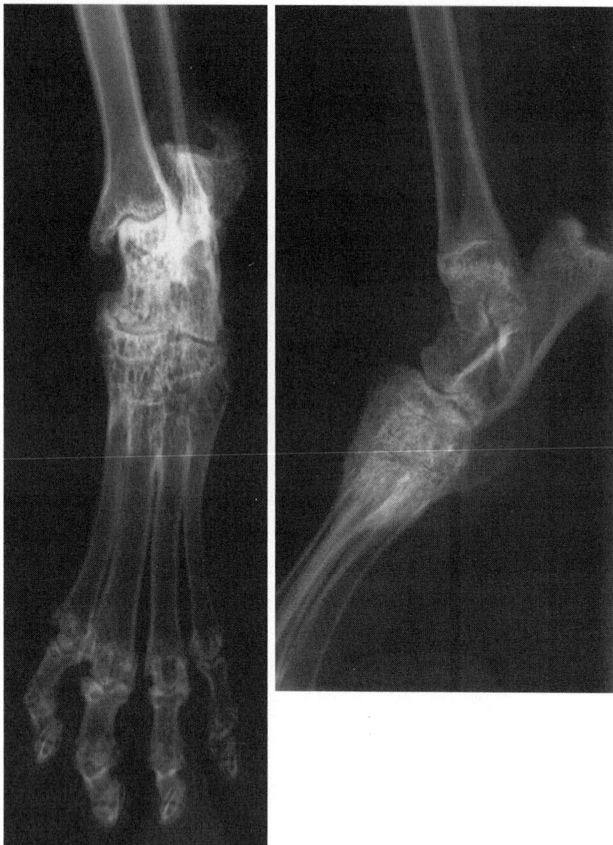

Fig. 18-62 Radiographic examples of tarsal and tarsometatarsal ankylosis and metatarsal malformation in a Scottish Fold cat with SFCOD.

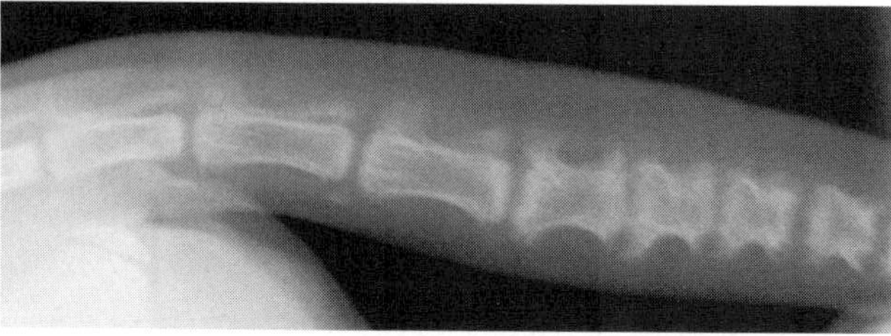

Fig. 18-63 Caudal vertebral malformation and spondylosis in a Scottish Fold cat with SFCOD. (From Allan GS: Radiographic features of feline joint diseases, *Vet Clin North Am Small Anim Pract* 30:281, 2000.)

episodes of intraarticular bleeding do not significantly alter the articular cartilage. Repeated hemorrhage may lead to severe damage to the cartilage as well as the subchondral bone.

Affected animals have severe non-weight-bearing lameness of affected limbs, and affected joints are swollen and painful. Radiographic examination in acute hemarthrosis reveals joint soft tissue swelling, which may be extensive.[83] After chronic intraarticular hemorrhage, the joint cartilage may be eroded and thin. The subchondral bone appears irregular if it is involved in the destructive process. Remodeling of bones adjacent to affected stifles was reported in dogs after repeated intraarticular injections of whole blood.[84] In advanced hemarthrosis, signs similar to osteoarthritis may be present.

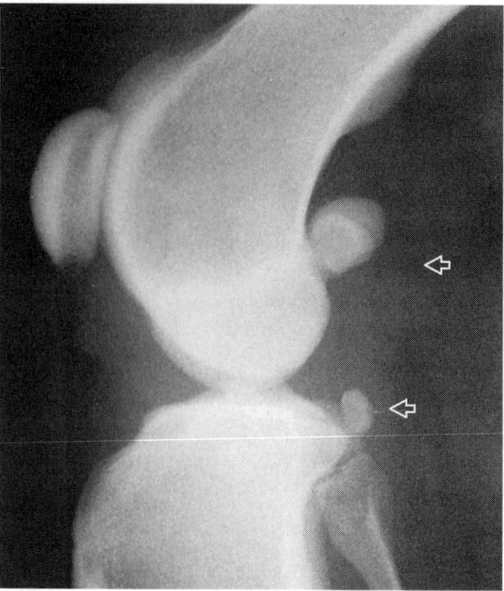

Fig. 18-64 An 8-year-old male Australian cattle dog had neurologic signs related to the hindquarters as well as pain in the right stifle. In the lateral view of the right stifle, the infrapatellar fat pad is compressed by synovial effusion. Note the bulging caudal compartment of the stifle joint *(arrows)*. Discospondylitis was identified in radiographs of the thoracic spine. Laboratory diagnosis was septic arthritis based on isolation of *Staphylococcus aureus* from the synovial fluid.

INFECTIOUS ARTHRITIS

Infectious arthritis is an infrequently diagnosed joint disease in small animals, with the incidence being lower than that of immune-mediated joint disease. Infectious arthritis is difficult to diagnose radiographically. Initial radiographic changes are similar to those seen in any effusive, nonerosive joint disease (Figs. 18-64 and 18-65). Irreversible joint damage has occurred by the time a definitive radiographic diagnosis can be made. Ideally, the arthritis should be diagnosed and successfully treated without definitive radiographic changes becoming apparent.[85]

Polyarticular infectious arthritis may occur as a result of bacteremia associated with an isolated focus of infection (endocarditis, discospondylitis, or omphalophlebitis) or in conjunction with a systemic diseases (as in *Mycoplasma* arthritis, canine leishmaniasis, or feline caliciviral lameness).[86,87] Polyarticular infectious arthritis must be differentiated from immune-mediated joint disease. The former is more likely to affect the larger, more proximal joints of the appendicular skeleton, whereas the latter more commonly affects the joints nearer the distal extremities (Box 18-6).

Monoarticular infectious arthritis most likely results from extension of focal osteomyelitis into an adjacent joint, direct joint trauma, or foreign body penetration (grass seed awns), or it may occur after joint surgery or intraarticular therapy.

Hematogenous dissemination of infection to joints is more common in young animals. Septic arthritis caused by surgery, particularly cruciate ligament repair, is more common in older animals.

The earliest radiographic changes are synovial effusion and increased synovial mass, which represent an inflammatory response of the synovium (see Figs. 18-64 and 18-65). Soft tissue swelling is usually demarcated by the distended joint capsule. Joint capsule distention is more easily identified in carpal, tarsal,

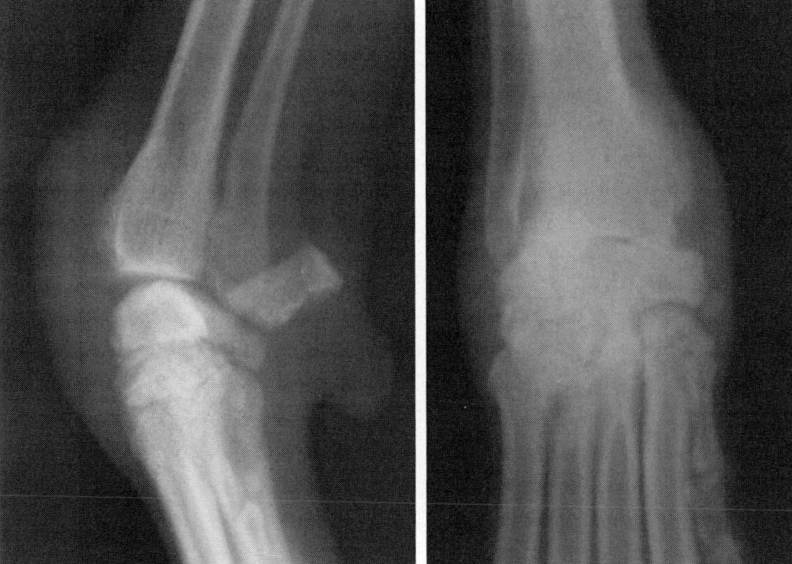

Fig. 18-65 Pericarpal swelling and periosteal new bone proliferation seen in this carpus are characteristics of more advanced septic arthritis. (Compare this image with Fig. 18-66.)

Box • 18-6

Polyarthropathies Affecting the Appendicular Skeleton of Dogs and Cats

- Immune-mediated joint diseases
  - Rheumatoid arthritis
  - SLE
  - Feline periosteal proliferative polyarthritis
  - Feline nonerosive immune-mediated polyarthropathy
- Septic arthritis
  - Hematogenous septic arthritis
    - Bacterial or fungal septic arthritis
- Inflammatory arthritides
  - Leishmaniasis
  - Rocky Mountain spotted fever
    - *Rickettsia rickettsii*
  - Lyme disease
    - *Borrelia burgdorferi*
  - Mycoplasma arthritis
  - Chinese Shar Pei fever syndrome
  - Feline calicivirus, coronavirus
  - Greyhound polyarthritis
- Hemarthrosis
- Chronic, recurrent, caused by blood dyscrasias
- Hypervitaminosis A
- Primary osteoarthritis/osteoarthrosis
- Disseminated idiopathic skeletal hyperostosis syndrome
- Familial or genetic skeletal dysplasias
  - SFCOD
- Feline MPS
  - Canine hip dysplasia
  - Canine elbow dysplasia
  - Heritable polyarthritis in adolescent Japanese Akita
  - Stiff Beagle disease (polyarteritis nodosa)
  - Osteochondrosis
- Drug-induced and vaccine-mediated polyarthritis
- Feline osteochondromatosis

and stifle joints. A useful landmark in the stifle is the infrapatellar fat pad. When the fat pad silhouette is compressed cranially, it becomes smaller or unclear, indicating synovial effusion is present. In untreated infectious arthritis, joint cartilage destruction follows synovial effusion and is followed by subchondral and perichondral bone destruction (Fig. 18-66).

Specific radiographic features of infectious arthritis become conspicuous after the articular cartilage is destroyed and subchondral osteomyelitis is established. Destruction of the femoral head was noted radiographically 4 weeks after the onset of clinical signs of coxofemoral infectious arthritis.[88] The width of the radiolucent joint space is progressively reduced as the articular cartilage is destroyed. Radiographs obtained during weight bearing are needed to detect this change. Destruction of the subchondral bone plate and subsequent subchondral osteomyelitis cause the margins of the joint space to appear uneven or ragged. Continued subchondral bone destruction produces large cystic subchondral radiolucent spaces (Fig. 18-67). Bone sclerosis adjacent to the osteolytic bone appears as increased osseous opacity, a sign of osseous inflammatory response to the infection (Box 18-7). Extensive osteomyelitis around affected joints can develop in severe or advanced cases of osteomyelitis (see Fig. 18-67).

Increasingly, septic arthritis is being identified in joints that have chronic osteoarthritis. Initial radiographs reveal changes consistent with degenerative joint disease, often leading to inappropriate therapy for the infection. Radiographs made 2 to 4 weeks later reveal more aggressive signs of periosteal new bone formation and intraarticular bone destruction.[88] Septic arthritis should be suspected when acute lameness and joint pain are identified in individual animals whose osteoarthritis has previously been well controlled.

The diagnosis of septic arthritis is based on cytologic assessment of synovial fluid and microbiologic examination of synovial fluid and/or synovium and joint capsule. Radiographic assessment alone has low specificity for septic arthritis, but survey radiographs are useful to rule out other conditions as well as to follow the progress of a joint infection once a diagnosis of septic arthritis is confirmed.

Infective Arthropathies in Cats

In cats hematogenously disseminated septic arthritis may be caused by a variety of microorganisms, which include

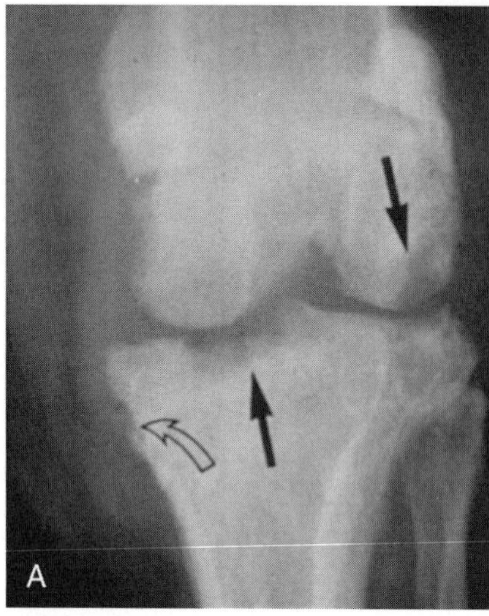

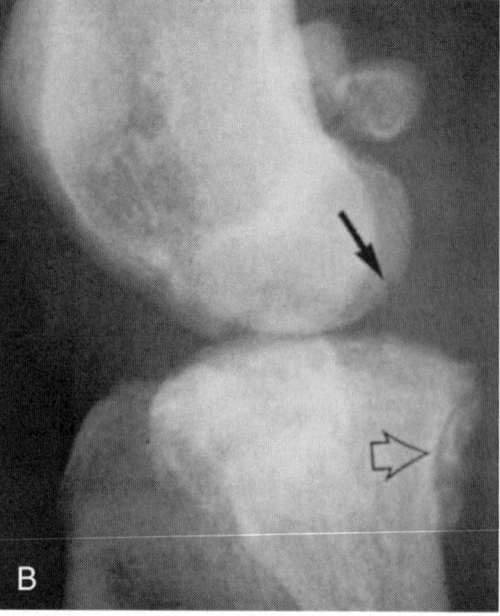

Fig. 18-66 An 8-year-old male Australian cattle dog had stifle swelling and pain that persisted after repair of a ruptured cranial cruciate ligament. **A** and **B**, Subchondral bone erosion involves the medial condyle of the tibia and the femoral condyles *(solid arrows)*. Periarticular new bone formation is also evident *(open arrow)*. Note the concurrent medial patellar luxation. Laboratory diagnosis was septic arthritis based on isolation of *Staphylococcus aureus* from the synovial fluid.

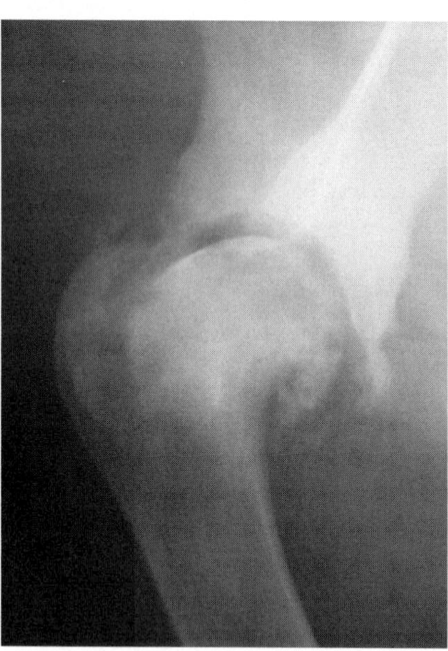

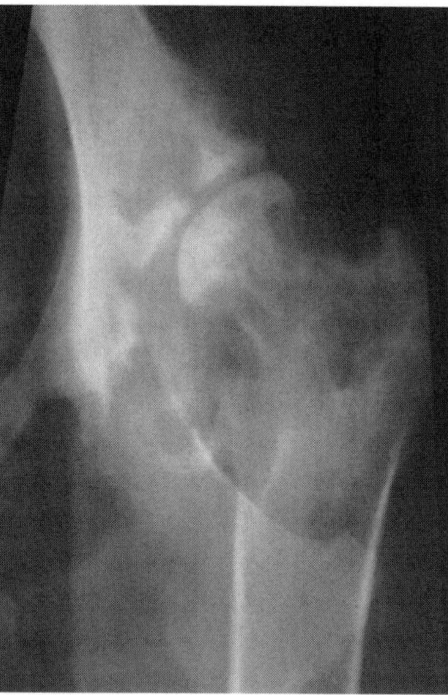

Fig. 18-67 Advanced septic arthritis in two dogs. In each dog extensive bone destruction has extended into the bones surrounding the affected joint, and accompanying calcification of periarticular soft tissues is present. *Staphylococcus intermedius* was cultured from synovial fluid in the dog shown on the right. (Left image courtesy Alice Springs Veterinary Hospital, Alice Springs, Australia.)

Box • 18-7

Progression of Radiographic Signs of Infectious Arthritis

- Increased synovial mass indicating synovial effusion and widened radiolucent joint space
- Diminished radiolucent joint space indicating destruction of articular cartilage
- Loss of the smooth surface of the subchondral bone plate—an early sign of infectious penetration of subchondral bone
- Osteolucent signs of destruction of subchondral and perichondral bone usually highlighted by a peripheral border of increased osseous opacity
- In advanced infectious arthritis, weight-bearing surfaces may collapse, causing distortion of joint architecture

Mycoplasma gateae, Mycoplasma felis, bacterial L-form infection (*Pasteurella* spp.), calicivirus (transient arthritis in kittens), coronavirus (feline infectious peritonitis), and fungi (cryptococcosis, histoplasmosis).

Hematogenously disseminated septic arthritis initially causes a nonerosive polyarthropathy characterized by lameness and joint swelling (synovial effusion and synovial thickening). Affected cats may be unwell, showing signs of systemic illness. Viremic polyarthropathies tend to be transient, whereas bacterial arthritis can have a protracted course.

Direct injection of bacteria from bite wounds can result in mixed infections of microorganisms, which may include anaerobic bacteria.

Bacterial arthritis from penetrating bite wounds causes lameness, which is usually restricted to one joint. Synovial effusion and periarticular soft tissue thickening precede (by weeks or months) secondary changes such as subchondral bone erosion. Joint infections that extend through the synovium and joint capsule into extracapsular tissue stimulate periosteal new bone formation on bone surfaces adjacent to the joint. Septic arthritis can lead to osteomyelitis in the bones on either side of an affected joint.

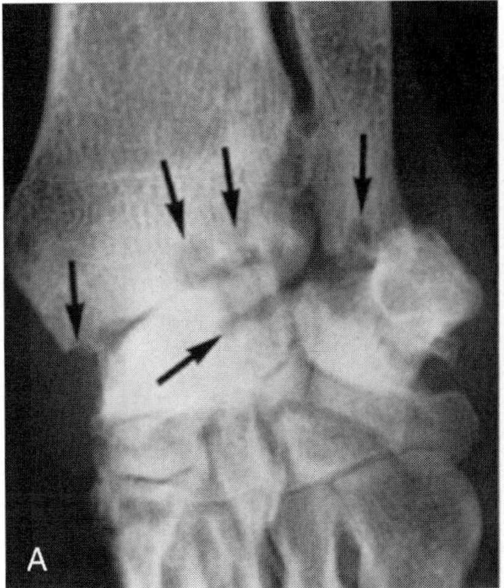

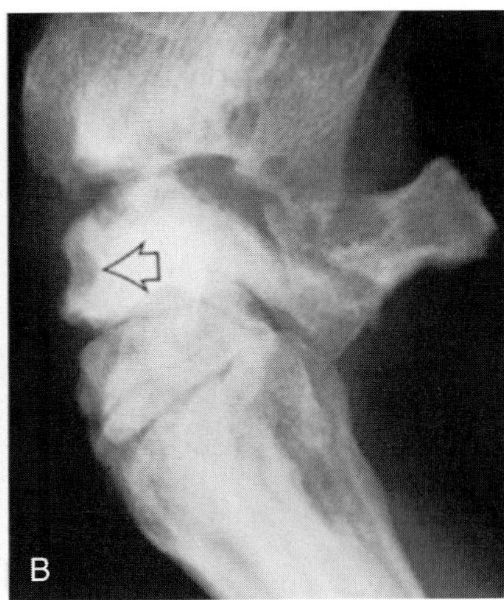

Fig. 18-68 An 8-year-old male (neutered) Corgi cross-breed had non-weight-bearing lameness of the right forelimb, valgus deviation of the left manus, and left carpal joint swelling and crepitus. **A,** Dorsolateral-palmaromedial projection (right carpus). Shown is extensive subchondral erosion of the styloid process of the ulna and the articular surfaces of the distal radius and radial carpal bone *(arrows)*. **B,** Lateral projection during flexion. In addition to the changes seen in **A,** note the erosion of the non-weight-bearing dorsal surface of the radial carpal bone *(arrow)*. Laboratory diagnosis was canine rheumatoid arthritis. (Courtesy University Veterinary Centre, Sydney, Australia.)

IMMUNE-MEDIATED ARTHROPATHIES

Rheumatoid Arthritis

Rheumatoid arthritis is a severe, progressive, erosive polyarthritis that has been reported in dogs.[89] A similar condition has been identified in cats.[90,91]

Radiographic changes usually occur in distal joints of the extremities. The more proximal large joints (stifle and elbow) are occasionally affected. Synovial effusion occurs initially. Radiographs made early in the course of the disease are typically characterized by nonspecific soft tissue swelling around affected joints. The joint capsule may be distended. The first radiographic signs of an osseous pathologic process may be detected several weeks after the onset of clinical signs. Initial changes are mild but, as would be expected in a progressive disease, the magnitude of radiographic abnormalities becomes more obvious as the disease advances.

The progression of radiographic changes includes (1) perichondral decreased bone opacity, (2) subchondral bone destruction and cyst formation, (3) signs of perichondral osteolysis and erosion (Fig. 18-68), (4) narrowing of the joint space, (5) progressive decreased opacity of epiphyses adjacent to affected joints, (6) destruction of subchondral and perichondral bone, (7) mushrooming of the ends of the metacarpi and metatarsi (which occurs in advanced arthritis and represents collapse of subchondral bone), and (8) varying degrees of joint subluxation and luxation (Fig. 18-69). Other changes more characteristic of degenerative joint disease (perichondral osteophytes/enthesophytes, subchondral sclerosis, and calcified periarticular tissues) may also be present.[89]

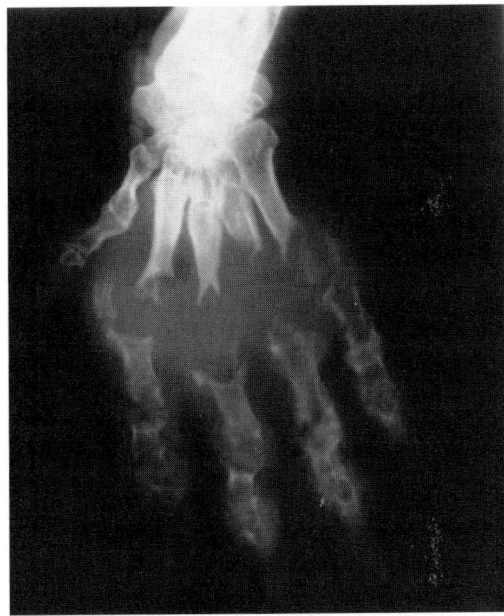

Fig. 18-69 The left manus of a small dog with polyarticular disease resulting in destruction of all the metacarpophalangeal joints. These changes were caused by rheumatoid arthritis. (Courtesy Dr. A. Martin, Hornsby Veterinary Hospital, Sydney, Australia.)

Systemic Lupus Erythematosus

SLE is a multisystemic disease that affects dogs of all breeds as well as cats. The disorder has a variety of clinical manifestations, including polyarthritis, anemia, nephropathy, skin disease, pericarditis, myocarditis, and lymphadenopathy.[92,93] The diagnosis of SLE is complicated and made on the basis of the concurrence of clinical manifestations and serologic evidence of the disease.

The immunopathologic features of SLE should be consistent with the clinical involvement (e.g., if arthritis is present, immune complexes should be demonstrable in tissue biopsy samples).

The relative frequency of the different clinical manifestations seen in SLE varies according to different authors. In one study, 121 patients were reviewed, and joint disease was reported to be the most frequent clinical sign (69%), followed by hematologic (53%), renal (50%), cutaneous (33%), and intrathoracic (17%) manifestations.[92]

Arthritis that occurs in SLE is described as nonerosive and effusive. Polyarthritis (five or more joints affected) is typical, but monoarticular and pauciarticular arthritis have been reported. Clinically, affected animals are reluctant to move because they often have a shifting lameness. Affected joints may be swollen, painful, and warm. The joints most commonly affected are the carpus, tarsus, metatarsus, stifle, and elbow.

Radiographic signs are usually absent or are minimal. In chronic SLE, the joint space of affected joints may be narrowed, and the joint capsule is distended. A mild periosteal response has been reported at the junction of the joint capsule and the bone. Contrast arthrography has been useful in detecting distention of the joint capsule. The synovial margin outlined by arthrography has been reported as being irregular and indistinct.

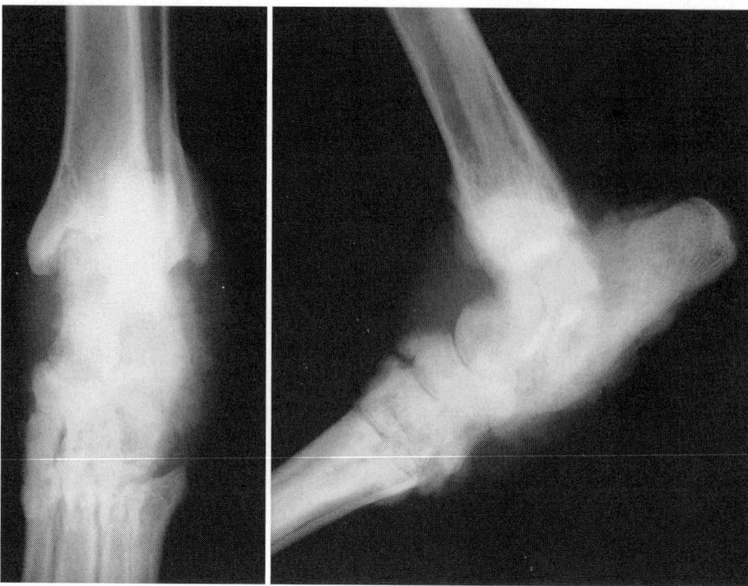

Fig. 18-70 A 2-year-old male domestic cat had progressive, generalized lameness preceded by fever and lassitude. Regional lymph nodes were palpably enlarged. Radiographs made 1 month after onset of clinical illness show periosteal new bone formation on many tarsal bones. Subchondral osteolysis is pronounced in the distal intertarsal articulations. Some tarsal bones have foci of osteolysis. Peritarsal soft tissue swelling is evident. Laboratory diagnosis was feline chronic progressive polyarthritis. (Courtesy University Veterinary Centre, Sydney, Australia. Reprinted from Allan GS: Radiographic features of feline joint diseases, *Vet Clin North Am Small Anim Pract* 30:281, 2000.)

Feline Noninfectious Polyarthritis

Feline noninfectious polyarthritis is a disease of male cats aged 1 to 5 years.[90,91,94] The polyarthritis is categorized as erosive or nonerosive.[95] There are two types of erosive polyarthritis: the periosteal proliferative form and the erosive form. The erosive form is more commonly referred to as *feline rheumatoid arthritis.* A group of nonerosive, effusive polyarthropathies thought to be immune mediated also occur in cats and are associated with a variety of conditions.

Periosteal Proliferative Form

Affected cats display clinical signs characterized by fever, malaise, and stiffness, which are followed by periarticular soft tissue swelling and regional lymphadenopathy. Radiographic changes may be identified in affected joints after a few weeks of clinical illness. The joints most commonly affected are the carpi and tarsi. The stifle, elbow, shoulder, and hip joints are affected to a lesser extent.

During the first month, periarticular soft tissue swelling is the predominant sign. Swelling may be either intracapsular or extracapsular. One to 3 months after the onset of clinical signs, periosteal new bone production at points of joint capsular attachment may be identified. During this phase, the bone adjacent to affected joints may have decreased bone opacity and a coarse trabecular pattern. Perichondral new bone formation is pronounced 2 or 3 months after onset of the disease.

Extensive enthesopathy may bridge smaller joint spaces. More severe radiographic manifestations include perichondral bone erosion and formation of subchondral cysts. Narrowing of affected joint spaces may occur late in the disease.[90] The radiographic signs of the periosteal proliferative form of feline chronic progressive polyarthritis include periarticular soft tissue swelling, periosteal new bone formation, perichondral enthesophyte production, perichondral and subchondral erosion, subchondral cysts, osteopenia of bone adjacent to affected joints, and narrowed joint spaces (Figs. 18-70 and 18-71). Arthrography has been used to detect proliferative synovitis in affected joints.[96]

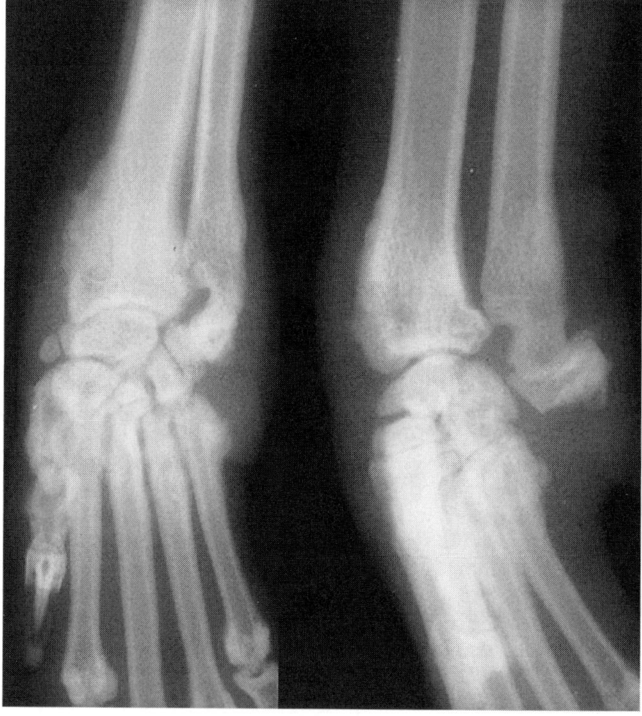

Fig. 18-71 The tarsus of a young cat with feline chronic progressive polyarthritis. (Courtesy University Veterinary Centre, Sydney, Australia. Reprinted from Allan GS: Radiographic features of feline joint diseases, *Vet Clin North Am Small Anim Pract* 30:281, 2000.)

Erosive Form

A second, more erosive form of feline noninfectious polyarthritis has been described; it resembles human rheumatoid arthritis and is seen in older cats.[90,91] This form of the disease is characterized radiographically by severe subchondral bone erosion, perichondral bone erosion, and subchondral cyst formation. Perichondral enthesophyte formation, bone destruction at points of ligamentous insertion to bone, and subluxation of small joints of the extremities also occur.

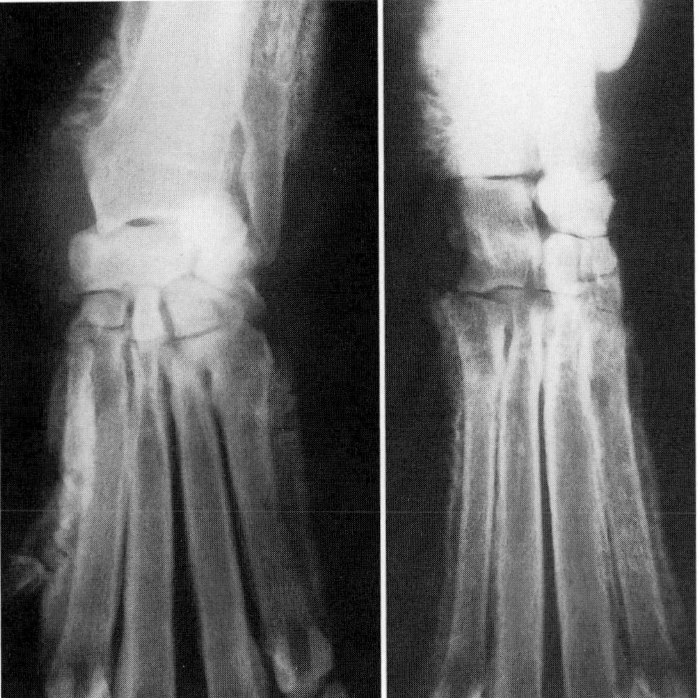

Fig. 18-72 A 6-year-old male Australian cattle dog had swollen paws and progressive lameness for 6 weeks. The forelimb had periosteal new bone formation on the radius, ulna, and metacarpal bones. Periosteal new bone formation was noted on the tarsal and metatarsal bones of the hindlimb. Histologic diagnosis was hypertrophic osteopathy caused by pulmonary neoplasia.

A diagnosis of feline rheumatoid arthritis requires a positive rheumatoid factor test, characteristic histologic changes seen on a synovial biopsy, or both. Both test results are negative in cats with feline proliferative polyarthritis.[95]

Feline Nonerosive Polyarthritis

Two categories of nonerosive polyarthritis have been described in cats.[95] They are feline SLE and idiopathic polyarthritis. Idiopathic polyarthritis has four subtypes: (1) uncomplicated polyarthritis; (2) reactive polyarthritis, associated with a disease process elsewhere in the body; (3) enteropathic polyarthritis, associated with gastrointestinal disease; and (4) malignant-related idiopathic polyarthritis, associated with myeloproliferative disease.

Radiography is used to distinguish the erosive from the nonerosive form of feline polyarthritis. The latter group is identified as having periarticular soft tissue swelling, joint capsule distention, and synovial fluid accumulation.

Hypertrophic Osteopathy

Hypertrophic osteopathy is a generalized osteoproductive disorder of the periosteum that affects the long bones of the extremities (Fig. 18-72). It is usually caused by cardiopulmonary disease or neoplasia. When neoplasia is involved pulmonary (primary or secondary) neoplasms are most likely, but hypertrophic osteopathy is also reported in animals with primary intraabdominal neoplasia without pulmonary involvement. Nonneoplastic causes of hypertrophic osteopathy include inflammatory lung disease (e.g., blastomycosis), intrathoracic foreign bodies, *Dirofilaria immitis* infestation, and spirocercosis.

The pathogenesis of hypertrophic osteopathy is incompletely understood. The most consistent pathologic finding in affected animals is increased blood flow to the extremities. This increased flow results in an overgrowth of vascular connective tissue, with subsequent fibrochondroid metaplasia and subperiosteal new bone formation. New bone formation typically commences on the digits and progressively extends toward the axial skeleton.

Periosteal new bone formation results in cortical thickening. The periosteal surface appears nodular or spiculated when visualized radiographically. When joints are involved, the bone surfaces that are not covered with cartilage are roughened and large perichondral osteophytes form.

THE SYNOVIUM

Synovial Cysts

Synovial cysts present as a pain-free, soft, flocculent swelling, usually around or near a joint in both dogs and cats. In dogs synovial cysts have been identified arising from articular process joints of the vertebral column, the carpus, metacarpus, and hock. Synovial cysts in cats have been located mainly on the medial aspect of the elbow. These cysts are lined by synovium and arise from joints or bursae. Fluid accumulates in the cyst either as one-way flow of synovial fluid through a normal communication with a bursa or by herniation of synovium through the joint capsule. Concurrent osteoarthritis of the elbow has been a common finding in cats. When positive-contrast medium has been used to define the cyst lumen, the cysts have been demonstrated to communicate with a joint space.

Survey radiographs reveal a large, homogenous, soft tissue swelling (Fig. 18-73). Positive contrast cystography identifies the size and shape of the cyst lumen and whether it commu-

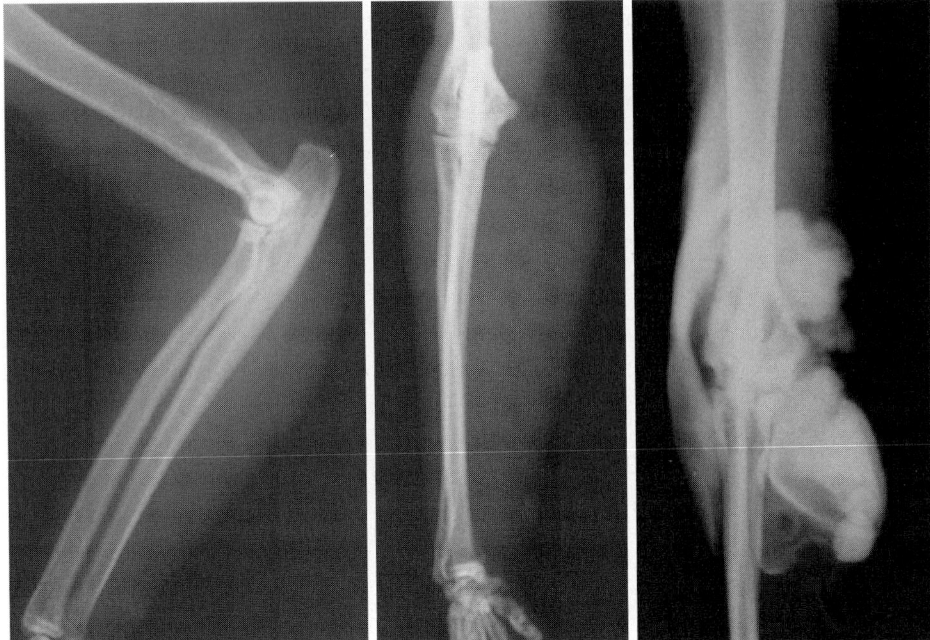

Fig. 18-73 Survey radiographs of a feline antebrachium demonstrate soft tissue swelling, but the extent of the synovial cyst causing this swelling is revealed after an injection of 10 mL Omnipaque (180 mg/mL) into the cyst. (Courtesy Melbourne Veterinary Referral Centre, Melbourne, Australia.)

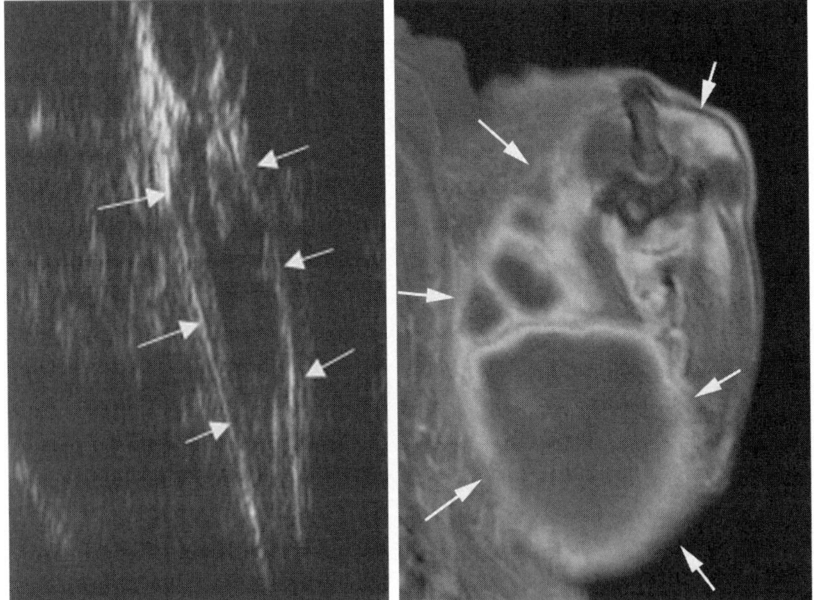

Fig. 18-74 Synovial cysts in different cats depicted by sonography *(left)* and MRI *(right)*. A contrast-enhanced T1-weighted MRI in the transverse plane (right) reveals a multiloculated synovial cyst, which is a usual finding in this condition. (Courtesy Dr. J. White and the University Veterinary Centre, Sydney, Australia.)

nicates with a joint. Sonography can be used to confirm the presence of a cyst lumen (Fig. 18-74) and the nature of the cyst wall. Advanced imaging studies (CT, MRI) should permit greater geographic detail of the extent of the cyst (see Fig. 18-74), particularly where they arise from facet joints.

Villonodular Synovitis

Villonodular synovitis is an intracapsular joint disorder characterized by nodular synovial hyperplasia, which is thought to represent a response of the synovium to trauma. Experimentally, villonodular synovitis has been reproduced in dogs by

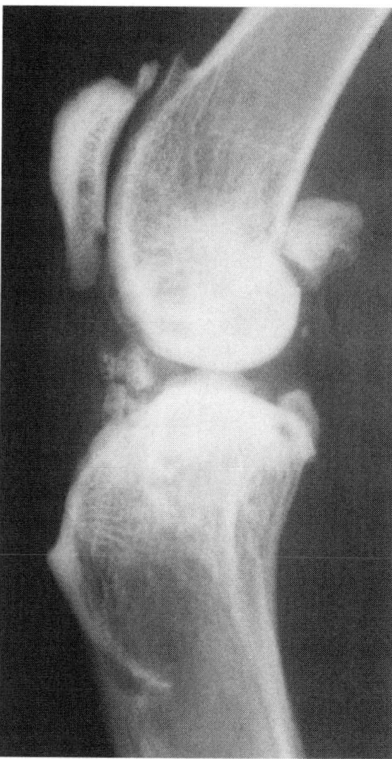

Fig. 18-75 A 5-year-old female (neutered) Burmese cat had bilateral stifle enlargement. Mineralization of the infrapatellar fat pad and within the stifle joint compartment was evident radiographically. Histologic diagnosis was synovial osteochondroma.

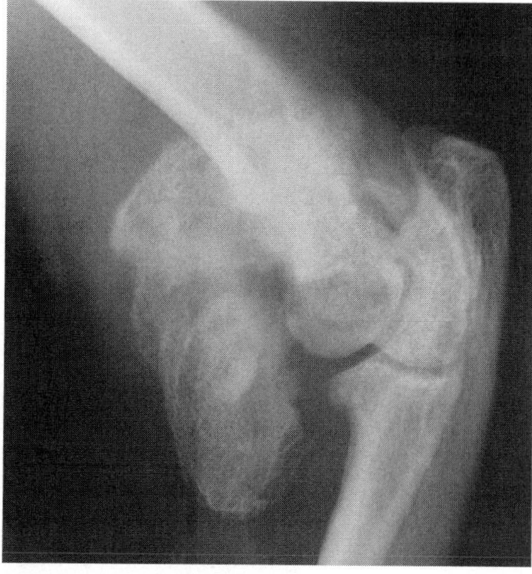

Fig. 18-76 A 6-year-old male (neutered) Burmese cat had progressive lameness of the right forelimb for 6 weeks. Radiographically a large, well-defined, ossified mass was visible on the craniomedial aspect of the right elbow. Histologic diagnosis was extraarticular synovial osteochondroma.

repeated intraarticular injections of whole blood. Villonodular synovitis is an established, although uncommon, disorder of human beings that has also been reported in horses and dogs.[97-100] In dogs the condition has been identified in the carpus, the coxofemoral joint, and the stifle.

The radiographic signs of villonodular synovitis may be nonspecific but include articular soft tissue swelling alone or with erosion of cortical bone at the chondrosynovial junction. These cortical erosions may appear cystlike, with slightly opaque borders. In severe proximal femoral villonodular synovitis in human beings, the femoral neck has been described as looking like an apple core. The articular cartilage and subchondral bone are not involved in the disease process. Arthrography may be used to identify the intracapsular nodular masses of hypertrophied synovium.

The differential diagnosis for perichondral erosive lesions, characteristic of villonodular synovitis, should include synovial osteochondromatosis, rheumatoid arthritis, and joint neoplasia.

Synovial Osteochondromas

Synovial osteochondromas have long been recognized in the joints of human beings. These lesions are described as islands of cartilage produced by the synovial membrane. Foci of cartilage become pedunculated and may become separated from their pedicles to form loose bodies within the joint. Reports of synovial osteochondromatosis in cats suggest that Burmese cats are overrepresented, and that in some cats the condition may be confused with other benign disorders characterized by periarticular ossification, such as meniscal calcification.

The radiographic appearance of mineralized synovial osteochondromas varies. These lesions are usually well-defined, rounded, often multiple intraarticular nodules of calcific opacity (Fig. 18-75). Not all chondromas become calcified; contrast arthrography may be necessary for their diagnosis. Synovial osteochondromas may also arise from extraarticular foci of synovial tissue (Fig. 18-76).

Synovial osteochondromas have been reported in the dog and the cat.[101,102] Their cause is unknown, but the theory of synovial metaplasia is generally accepted. These lesions have been reported to cause severe lameness in some dogs. Surgical removal of synovial osteochondromas relieves clinical signs of joint pain and lameness.[101]

Intrameniscal calcification and ossification have been reported in the stifle joint of cats.[5] Radiographically, these lesions appear similar to the reported appearance of osteochondromas within the feline stifle joint. Other conditions in cats in which intraarticular and periarticular mineralization may be confused with synovial osteochondromatosis are mild forms of MPS VI and hypervitaminosis A.[52,103]

Joint Neoplasia

The primary joint neoplasm, synovial sarcoma, arises from primitive mesenchymal precursor cells of the synovial membrane of joints and bursae.[104] These tumors are uncommon in the dog and are rare in the cat.[105] They occur most frequently in middle-aged, medium-sized to large dogs. The most commonly affected joints are the stifle and the elbow. Synovial sarcomas grow slowly and are first noticeable as a homogeneous soft tissue mass that involves or is near a joint. Initially, radiographs reveal a mass of soft tissue. Portions of the tumor may be calcified, with mineral deposits appearing as hazy and punctate or as linear streaks.

Canine synovial sarcomas are more likely to invade adjacent bone than their counterpart in human beings. Initial bone involvement usually appears as a spiculated periosteal response followed by ragged erosion of the cortical bone adjacent to the tumor. Occasionally the neoplasm initially appears relatively nonaggressive, mimicking a simple cyst, only to change later into a more extensive and destructive disease (Fig. 18-77). Destruction of cancellous bone may be extensive

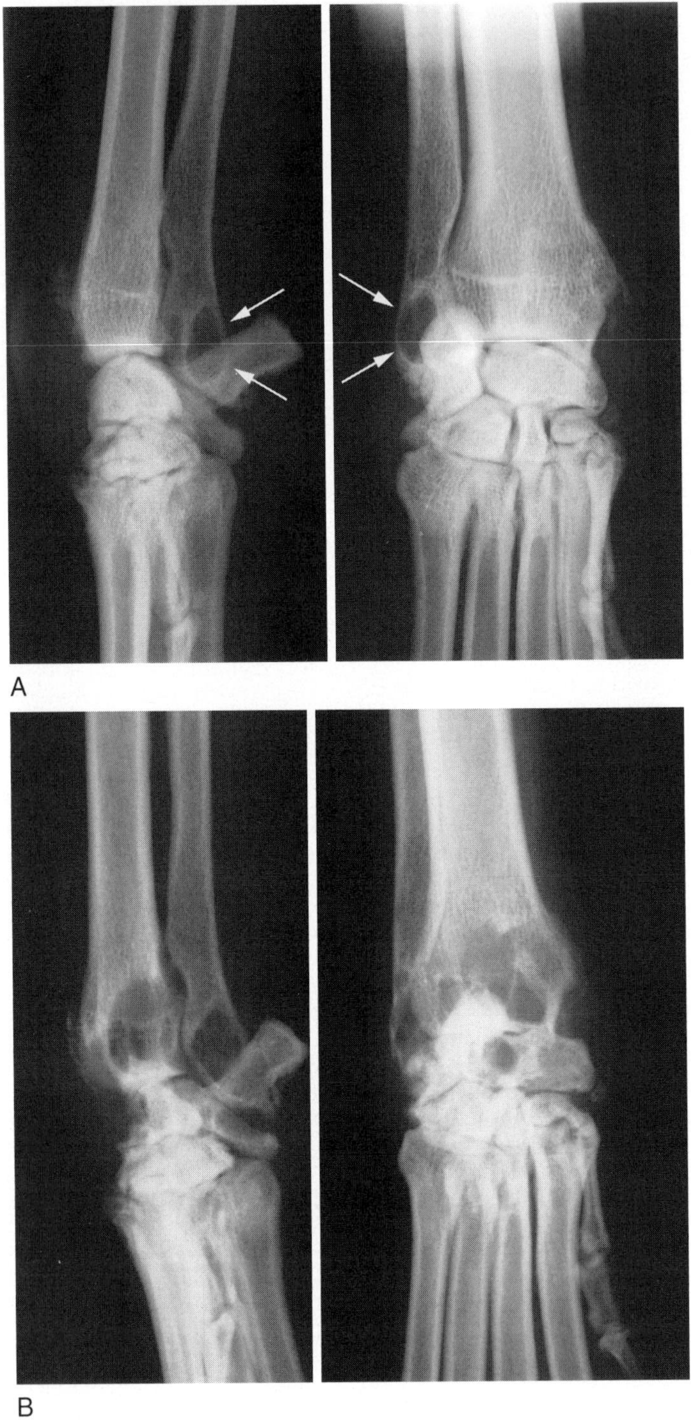

Fig. 18-77 A simple cyst present in the distal end of the left ulna *(arrows)* was identified 6 weeks after the onset of soft tissue swelling around the antebrachiocarpal joint and clinical signs of left forelimb lameness in a dog. The lesion changed dramatically over the succeeding 12 months **(B)**, by which time a multiloculated cystlike change was present in the distal radius, ulna, and the proximal row of carpal bones. Histologic diagnosis was synovial cell carcinoma. (Courtesy Dr. P. Young, All Pets Veterinary Hospital, Albury, Australia.)

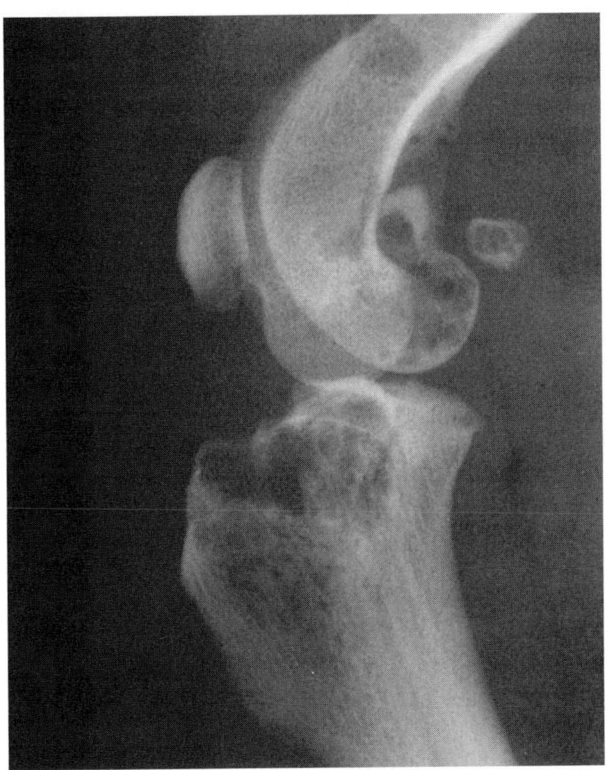

Fig. 18-78 Multiple radiolucent lesions are evident on both sides of this dog's stifle. Histologic diagnosis was synovial sarcoma.

and most commonly occurs on both sides of the joint (Fig. 18-78). The tumor is locally invasive with an unpredictable capacity to metastasize,[106] although distant metastasis, particularly to the lungs, occurs in as many as half of reported patients.[104] Radiographic examination of the thorax is therefore mandatory in patients with suspected synovial sarcoma.

Many neoplasms mimic the radiographic appearance of synovial sarcomas (Fig. 18-79). In a recent study of joint neoplasms, synovial sarcomas were represented in only 27% of cases.[107] The other neoplasms with a radiographic appearance similar to that of synovial sarcomas included fibrosarcoma, rhabdomyosarcoma, fibromyxosarcoma, malignant fibrous histiocytoma, liposarcoma, and undifferentiated sarcoma. The once pathognomonic findings of an intraarticular tumor with osteodestructive potential affecting the bones on either side of the joint cannot be assumed to be caused by a synovial cell sarcoma. Histologic evaluation of the lesion is mandatory to establish its origin.

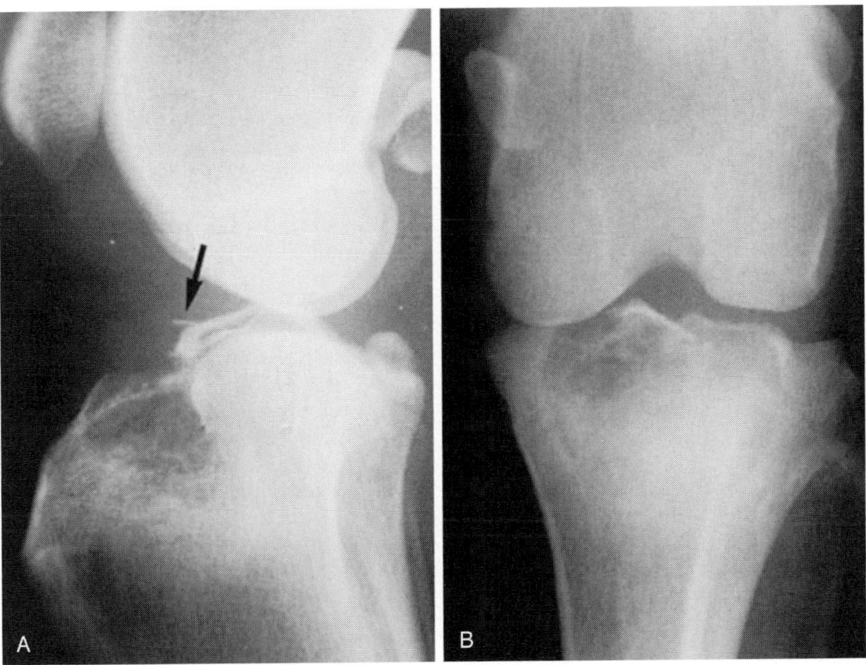

Fig. 18-79 A 2-year-old female Great Dane had gradual enlargement of the proximal left tibia and subsequent acute onset of non-weight-bearing lameness of the left hindlimb. **A** and **B,** A focus of osteolysis within the medial condyle of the proximal tibia extends to involve the joint space. A small bone fragment is free within the joint space *(arrow)*. Histologic diagnosis was hemangiosarcoma. (Courtesy University Veterinary Centre, Sydney, Australia.)

REFERENCES

1. Basher AWP, Doige CE, Presnell KR: Subchondral bone cysts in a dog with osteochondrosis, *J Am Anim Hosp Assoc* 24:321, 1988.
2. Morgan JP, Pool RR, Miyabayashi T: Primary degenerative joint disease of the shoulder in a colony of Beagles, *J Am Vet Med Assoc* 190:531, 1987.
3. Flo GL: Synovial chondrometaplasia in five dogs, *J Am Vet Med Assoc* 200:943, 1992.
4. Kealy JK, McAllister H: *Diagnostic radiology and ultrasonography of the dog and cat*, ed 3, Philadelphia, 2000, W.B. Saunders, p. 282.
5. Whiting PG, Pool RR: Intrameniscal calcification and ossification in the stifle joints of three domestic cats, *J Am Anim Hosp Assoc* 21:579, 1985.
6. de Haan JJ, Anderson CB: Calcium crystal associated arthropathy in a dog, *J Am Vet Med Assoc* 200:943, 1992.
7. Short RP, Jardine JE: Calcium phosphate deposition disease in a Fox Terrier, *J Am Anim Hosp Assoc* 29:363, 1993.
8. Mahoney PN, Lamb CR: Articular, periarticular and juxtaarticular calcified bodies in the dog and cat: a radiologic review, *Vet Radiol Ultrasound* 37:3, 1996.
9. Wood AKW, McCarthy PH: A study of irregularly occurring ectopic and sesamoid bones in the dog, *Vet Radiol* 27:22, 1986.
10. DeRooster H, van Bree H: Popliteal sesamoid displacement associated with cruciate rupture in the dog, *J Small Anim Pract* 40:316, 1999.
11. Mason DR, Schultz KS, Samii VF et al: Sensitivity of radiographic evaluation of radio-ulnar incongruence in the dog in vivo, *Vet Surg* 31:125, 2002.
12. Widmer WR, Buckwalter KA, Braunstein EM et al: Radiographic and magnetic resonance-imaging if the stifle joint in experimental osteoarthritis in dogs, *Vet Radiol Ultrasound* 35:371, 1994.
13. McGonagle D, Benjamin M, Marzo-Ortega H et al: Advances in the understanding of entheseal inflammation, *Curr Rheumatol Rep* 4:500, 2002.
14. Specht TE, Poulos PW, Metcalf MR et al: Vacuum phenomenon in the metatarsophalangeal joint of a horse, *J Am Vet Med Assoc* 197:749, 1990.
15. Morgan JP: *Radiology of skeletal diseases–principles of diagnosis in dogs*, Davis, CA, 1981, Veterinary Radiology Associates, p. 22.
16. van Bree H: Vacuum phenomenon associated with osteochondrosis of the scapulohumeral joint in dogs: 100 cases (1985-1991), *J Am Vet Med Assoc* 201:1916, 1992.
17. *PennHIP Training Manual*, Synbiotics Corp., San Diego, CA, 1998, p. 22.
18. Hathcock JT: Vacuum phenomenon of the canine spine: CT findings in 3 patients, *Vet Radiol Ultrasound* 35: 285, 1994.
19. Weber WJ, Berry CR, Kramer RW: Vacuum phenomenon in 12 dogs, *Vet Radiol Ultrasound* 36:493, 1995.
20. McCarthy PH, Wood AKW: Anatomical and radiological studies of the iliopubic cartilage in adult Greyhounds, *Anat Histol Embryol* 15:73, 1986.
21. Pond MJ, Lasonsky JM: Avulsion of the popliteus muscle in the dog: a case report, *J Am Anim Hosp Assoc* 12:60, 1976.
22. Eaton Wells RD, Plummer GV: Avulsion of the popliteus muscle in an Afghan hound, *J Small Anim Pract* 19:743, 1978.
23. Chaffee VW, Knecht CD: Avulsion of the medial head of the gastrocnemius in the dog, *Vet Med Small Anim Clin* 70:929, 1975.
24. Robinson A: Atraumatic bilateral avulsion of the origins of the gastrocnemius muscle, *J Small Anim Pract* 40:498, 1999.
25. Rendano VT, Dueland R: Variation in location of gastrocnemius sesamoid bones (fabellae) in a dog, *J Am Vet Med Assoc* 173:200, 1978.
26. Wood AKW, McCarthy PH, Howlett CR: Anatomic and radiographic appearance of a sesamoid bone in the tendon of origin of the supinator muscle of dogs, *Am J Vet Res* 46:2043, 1985.
27. Wood AKW, McCarthy PH: Radiologic and anatomic observations of plantar sesamoid bones at the tarsometatarsal articulations of Greyhounds, *Am J Vet Res* 45:2158, 1984.
28. Walker M, Phalan D, Jensen J et al: Meniscal ossicles in large non-domestic cats, *Vet Radiol Ultrasound* 43:249, 2002.
29. Barthez PY, Morgan JP: Bicipital tenosynovitis in the dog—evaluation with positive contrast arthrography, *Vet Radiol Ultrasound* 34:325, 1993.
30. Lowry JE, Carpenter LG, Park RD et al: Radiographic anatomy and technique for arthrography of the cubital joint in clinically normal dogs, *J Am Vet Med Assoc* 203:72, 1993.
31. Muir P, Johnson KA: Supraspinous and biceps brachii tendonopathy in dogs, *J Am Anim Pract* 35:239, 1994.
32. Rivers B, Wallace L, Johnson GR: Biceps tenosynovitis in the dog: radiographic and sonographic findings, *Vet Comp Orthop Traumatol* 5:51, 1992.
33. Muhumnza L, Morgan JP, Miyabayashi T et al: Positive-contrast arthrography: a study of the humeral joints in normal Beagle dogs, *Vet Radiol* 29:157, 1988.
34. Cake MA, Read RA: Canine and human sesamoid disease, *Vet Comp Orthop Traumatol* 8:70, 1995.
35. Robins GM, Read RA: Diseases of the sesamoid bones. In Bojrab MJ, editor: *Disease mechanisms in small animal surgery*, ed 2, Philadelphia, 1993, Lea & Febiger, p. 1094.
36. Vaughan LC, France C: Abnormalities of the volar and plantar sesamoids in Rottweilers, *J Small Anim Pract* 27:551, 1986.
37. Read RA, Black AP, Armstrong SJ et al: Incidence and clinical significance of sesamoid disease in Rottweilers, *Vet Rec* 130:533, 1992.
38. Davis PE, Bellenger CR, Turner DM: Fractures of the sesamoid bones in the Greyhound, *Aust Vet J* 45:15, 1969.
39. Ljunggren G, Olsson S-E: Osteoarthrosis of the shoulder and elbow joints in dogs: a pathologic and radiographic study of necropsy material, *J Am Vet Radiol Soc* 16:33, 1975.
40. Tirgari M, Vaughan LL: Arthritis of the canine stifle joint, *Vet Rec* 96:394, 1975.
41. Marshall JL: Peri-articular osteophytes—initiation and formation in the knees of the dog, *Clin Orthop* 62:37, 1969.
42. Lust G, Summers BA: Early, asymptomatic stage of degenerative joint disease in canine hip joints, *Am J Vet Res* 42:1849, 1981.
43. Gilbertson E: Development of periarticular osteophytes in experimentally induced osteoarthritis in the dog. A study using microradiographic, microangiographic and fluorescent bone-labelling techniques, *Ann Rheum Dis* 34:12, 1975.
44. Marshall J: Periarticular osteophytes: initiation and formation in the knee of the dog, *Clin Orthop* 62: 37, 1969.
45. Innes JF, Costello M, Barr FJ et al: Radiographic progression of osteoarthritis of the canine stifle joint: a prospective study, *Vet Radiol Ultrasound* 45:143, 2004.

46. Smith GK, Popovitch CA, Gregor TP et al: Evaluation of risk factors for degenerative joint disease associated with hip dysplasia in dogs, *J Am Vet Med Assoc* 206:642, 1995.
47. Smith GK, Gregor TP, Rhodes WH et al: Coxofemoral joint laxity from distraction radiography and its contemporaneous and prospective correlation with laxity, subjective score, and evidence of degenerative joint disease from conventional hip-extended radiography in dogs, *Am J Vet Res* 54:1020, 1993.
48. Popovitch CA, Smith GK, Gregor TP, et al: Comparison of susceptibility for hip dysplasia between Rottweilers and German shepherd dogs, *J Am Vet Med Assoc* 206:648, 1995.
49. Lust G, Williams AJ, Burton-Worster N et al: Joint laxity and its association with hip dysplasia in Labrador Retrievers, *Am J Vet Res* 54:1990, 1993.
50. Marshall JL, Olsson S-E: Instability of the knee: a long-term experimental study in dogs, *J Bone Joint Surg (Am)* 53:1561, 1971.
51. Sokoloff L: The pathology of osteoarthritis and the role of ageing. In Nuki J, editor: *The aetiopathogenesis of osteoarthritis*, Tunbridge Wells, England, 1980, Pitman Medical Publishing, pp. 1-15.
52. Allan GS: Radiographic features of feline joint diseases. In Watrous BJ, editor: *Veterinary clinics of North America*, Philadelphia, 2000, W.B. Saunders, pp. 281-302.
53. Hedhammar A, Olsson S-E, Andersson S-A et al: Canine hip dysplasia: study of heritability in 401 litters of German shepherd dogs, *J Am Vet Med Assoc* 174:1012, 1979.
54. Leighton EA, Smith GK, McNeil M et al: *Heritability of the distraction index in German Shepherd dogs and Labrador Retrievers*, Proceedings of the American Kennel Club Conference on Molecular Genetics and Genetic Health, Florham Park, NJ, 1994.
55. Lust G, Rendano VT, Summers BA: Canine hip dysplasia: concepts and diagnosis, *J Am Vet Med Assoc* 187:638, 1985.
56. Hedhammar A, Wu F-M, Krook L et al: Overnutrition and skeletal disease, *Cornell Vet* 64:9, 1974.
57. Todhunter RJ, Grohn YT, Bliss SP et al: Evaluation of multiple radiographic predictors of cartilage lesions in the hip joints of eight-month old dogs, *Am J Vet Res* 64:1472, 2003.
58. Lust G, Beilman WT, Dueland R et al: Intra-articular volume and hip joint instability in dogs with hip dysplasia, *J Bone Joint Surg (Am)* 62:576, 1980.
59. Lust G, Beilman WT, Rendano VT: A relationship between degree of laxity and synovial fluid volume in coxofemoral joints of dogs predisposed for hip dysplasia, *Am J Vet Res* 41:55, 1980.
60. Morgan JP: Canine hip dysplasia: significance of early bony spurring, *Vet Radiol* 28:2, 1987.
61. Keller GG, Reed AL, Lattimer JC et al: Hip dysplasia: a feline population study, *Vet Radiol Ultrasound* 40:460, 1999.
62. Root CR, Sande RD, Pfleuger S et al: *A disease of Maine Coon cats resembling congenital canine hip dysplasia*, Chicago, 1987, Proceedings of the Annual Meeting of the American College of Veterinary Radiologists.
63. Langenbach A, Grigor U, Green P et al: Relationship between degenerative joint disease and hip joint laxity by use of distraction index and Norberg angle measurements in a group of cats, *J Am Vet Med Assoc* 213:1439, 1998.
64. Smith GK, Biery DN, Gregor TP: New concepts of coxofemoral joint stability and the development of a clinical stress radiographic method for quantitating hip joint laxity in the dog, *J Am Vet Med Assoc* 196:59, 1990.
65. Rendano VT, Ryan G: Canine hip dysplasia evaluation, *Vet Radiol* 26:170, 1985.
66. Farrow CS, Back RT: Radiographic evaluation of non-anesthetized and non-sedated dogs for hip dysplasia, *J Am Vet Med Assoc* 194:524, 1989.
67. Aronson E, Kraus KH, Smith J: The effect of anesthesia on the radiographic appearance of the coxofemoral joints, *Vet Radiol* 32:2, 1991.
68. Belkoff SM, Padgett G, Soutas-Little RW: Development of a device to measure canine coxofemoral joint laxity, *Vet Comp Orthop Traumatol* 1:31, 1989.
69. Fluckiger MA, Friedrick GA, Binder H: A Radiographic stress technique for evaluation of coxofemoral joint laxity in dogs, *Vet Surg* 28:1, 1999.
70. Farese JP, Todhunter RJ, Lust G et al: Dorsolateral subluxation of hip joints in dogs measured in a weight-bearing position with radiography and computed tomography, *Vet Surg* 27:393, 1998
71. Salter RB, Harris WR: Injuries involving the epiphyseal plate, *J Bone Joint Surg* 45:587, 1963.
72. Farrow CS: Stress radiography: applications in small animal practice, *J Am Vet Med Assoc* 181:777, 1982.
73. Puglisi TA, Tangner CH, Green RW et al: Stress radiography of the canine humeral joint, *J Am Anim Hosp Assoc* 24:235, 1988.
74. Davidson EB, Griffey SM, Vasseur PB et al: Histopathological, radiographic, and arthrographic comparison of the biceps tendon in normal dogs and dogs with biceps tenosynovitis, *J Am Anim Hosp Assoc* 36:522, 2000.
75. Long CD, Nyland TG: Ultrasonographic evaluation of the canine shoulder, *Vet Radiol Ultrasound* 40:372, 1999.
76. Mitchell RAS, Innes JF: Lateral glenohumeral ligament rupture in three dogs, *J Small Anim Pract* 41:511, 2000.
77. Grundmann S, Montavon PM: Stenosing tenosynovitis of the abductor pollicis longus muscle in dogs, *Vet Comp Orthop Traum* 14:95, 2001.
78. Kramer M, Stengel H, Gerwing M et al: Sonography of the canine stifle, *Vet Radiol Ultrasound* 40:282, 1999.
79. Reed AL, Payne TJ, Constantinescu GM: Ultrasonographic anatomy of the normal canine stifle, *Vet Radiol Ultrasound* 36:315, 1995.
80. Gnudi G, Bertoni G: Echographic examination of the stifle joint affected by cranial cruciate ligament rupture in the dog, *Vet Radiol Ultrasound* 42:266, 2001.
81. Kramer M, Gerwing M, Michele U et al: Ultrasonographic examination of injuries to the Achilles tendon in dogs and cats, *J Small Anim Pract* 42:531, 2001.
82. Malik R, Allan GS, Howlett CR et al: Chondro-osseous dysplasia in Scottish Fold cats, *Aust Vet J* 76:85, 1998.
83. Bellah JR, Weigel JP: Hemarthrosis secondary to suspected warfarin toxicosis in a dog, *J Am Vet Med Assoc* 182:1126, 1983.
84. Hoaglund FT: Experimental haemarthrosis: the response of canine knees to injection of autogenous blood, *J Bone Joint Surg* 49:285, 1967.
85. Bennett D, Taylor DJ: Bacterial infective arthritis in the dog, *J Small Anim Pract* 29:207, 1988.
86. Moise NS, Crissman JW, Fairbrother JF et al: *Mycoplasma gateae* arthritis and tenosynovitis in cats: case report and experimental reproduction of the disease, *Am J Vet Res* 44:10, 1983.
87. Ernst S, Cogin JM: What is your diagnosis? Mycoplasma arthritis, *J Am Vet Med Assoc* 215:19, 1999.
88. Schrader SC: Septic arthritis and osteomyelitis of the hip of six mature dogs, *J Am Vet Med Assoc* 181:894, 1982.
89. Bennett D: Immune-based erosive inflammatory joint disease of the dog: canine rheumatoid arthritis: I. Clini-

cal, radiological and laboratory investigations, *J Small Anim Pract* 28:779, 1987.

90. Pedersen NC, Pool RR, O'Brien T: Feline chronic progressive polyarthritis, *Am J Vet Res* 41:522, 1980.
91. Carro T: Polyarthritis in cats, *Comp Cont Educ Pract Vet* 16:57, 1994.
92. Grindem CB, Johnston KH: Systemic lupus erythematosus: Literature review and report of 42 new canine cases, *J Am Anim Hosp Assoc* 19:489, 1983.
93. Bennett D: Immune-based non-erosive inflammatory joint disease of the dog: I. Canine SLE, *J Small Anim Pract* 28:871, 1987.
94. Moise NS, Crissman JW: Chronic progressive polyarthritis in a cat, *J Am Anim Hosp Assoc* 18:965, 1982.
95. Bennett D, Nash AS: Feline immune-based polyarthritis: a study of thirty-one cases, *J Small Anim Pract* 29:501, 1988.
96. Cantwell HD: Radiographic diagnosis, *Vet Radiol* 27:149, 1986.
97. Kusba JK, Lipowitz AJ, Wize M et al: Suspected villonodular synovitis in a dog, *J Am Vet Med Assoc* 182:390, 1983.
98. Somer T, Sittnikow K, Henriksson K et al: Pigmented villonodular synovitis and plasmacytoid lymphoma in a dog, *J Am Vet Med Assoc* 197:877, 1990.
99. Marti JN: Bilateral pigmented villonodular synovitis in a dog, *J Small Anim Pract* 38:256, 1997.
100. Hanson JA: Radiographic diagnosis—carpal villonodular synovitis, *Vet Radiol Ultrasound* 39:15, 1998.
101. Flo GL, Stickle RL, Dunstan RW: Synovial chondrometaplasia in five dogs, *J Am Vet Med Assoc* 191:1417, 1987.
102. Hubler M, Johnson KA, Burling RT et al: Lesions resembling osteochondromatosis in two cats, *J Small Anim Pract* 27:181, 1986.
103. Crawley AC, Yogalingam G, Muller VJ et al: Two mutations within a feline mucopolysaccharidosis type VI colony cause three different phenotypes, *J Clin Invest* 101:109, 1998.
104. Vail DM, Powers BE, Getzy DM et al: Evaluation of prognostic factors for dogs with synovial sarcoma: 36 cases (1986-1991), *J Am Vet Med Assoc* 205:1300, 1994.
105. Silva-Krott IU: Synovial sarcoma in a cat, *J Am Vet Med Assoc* 203:1430, 1993.
106. McGlennon NJ, Houlton JEF, Gorman NT: Synovial sarcoma in the dog—a review, *J Small Anim Pract* 29:139, 1988.
107. Whitelock RG, Dyce J, Houlton JEF et al: A review of 30 tumours affecting joints, *Vet Comp Orthop Traumatol* 10:146, 1997.

ELECTRONIC RESOURCES evolve

Additional information related to the content in Chapter 18 can be found on the companion Web site at evolve http://evolve.elsevier.com/Thrall/vetrad/.

- Key Points
- Chapter Quiz
- Case Study 18-1
- Case Study 18-2

CHAPTER • 19
The Stifle and Tarsus

Valeria Busoni

THE STIFLE

Radiographic Examination

The lateromedial view is the basic radiographic view of the stifle and can be obtained on the standing horse with a portable or fixed radiographic unit. With good collimation this view does not require the use of a grid because enough contrast is present, even in a large horse. Centring is 5 to 7 cm proximal to the tibial plateau, between the cranial and middle third of the stifle region. The cassette should be vertical to the ground to avoid geometric distortion, and exposure must be sufficient to visualize the femoral condyles; as a result the femoral trochlea may be overexposed, so use of a hot light, or another less-exposed radiograph, may be needed. A lateromedial view of the flexed stifle is used to examine further the cranial and central intercondylar areas of the tibia.

Depending on the equipment used (portable or fixed radiographic unit) and the type of disease suspected, a caudolateral-craniomedial oblique view and/or a caudocranial view are indicated. The caudolateral-craniomedial oblique view allows good visualization of the two most common sites of disease in the young horse: the lateral trochlear ridge (osteochondrosis site) and the medial femoral condyle (subchondral cystlike lesion site). Because the superimposed femoral condyles are often underexposed on the lateromedial view when the radiograph is made with a portable unit, the caudolateral-craniomedial oblique view is a valuable complement for assessment of the stifle in the field. The caudocranial view is mainly aimed at the assessment of the femorotibial joints and the investigation of osteoarthrosis. This view requires the use of a grid for optimal contrast and therefore is difficult to obtain with a portable x-ray unit on a large horse.

The skyline view of the patella (cranioproximal-craniodistal oblique view) is imperative when patellar disease is being investigated. This view can be easily obtained with a portable x-ray unit because a grid is not necessary and the required exposure is relatively low.

With the advent of digital radiography and its inherently greater contrast resolution, radiographic evaluation of the soft tissues of the stifle is possible to a certain extent. Lateromedial radiographs of the stifle allow good visualisation of the patellar ligaments and the cranial fat pad (Fig. 19-1). Localization of soft tissue swelling as being extraarticular or intraarticular is possible by using the silhouette sign and evaluating fat pad displacement (Fig. 19-1).

Ultrasonography for Supplemental Stifle Imaging

Subchondral cystlike lesions and osteophyte formation on the medial tibial or femoral articular margins as a result of osteoarthrosis of the medial femorotibial joint are the most common radiographic signs of femorotibial disease.[1] Bony fragments, new bone formation, or radiolucent areas at ligament insertions, suggesting avulsion fractures or enthesopathy, may also be seen.[1-4] However, because of the high incidence of soft tissue lesions involving menisci and ligaments, femorotibial pain may be present with no or minor radiographic signs.[2,5,6] When clinical signs suggest femorotibial involvement, the radiographic examination may not provide a complete picture of the severity of joint damage because assessment of soft tissue lesions is not possible. The mid-term prognosis for a return to work or the long-term prognosis for development of osteoarthrosis mainly depends on the severity of the soft tissue injuries, in particular meniscal damage.[6] A combination of ultrasonographic examination and radiographic examination is therefore necessary for complete assessment of the stifle. Ultrasonography of the weight-bearing stifle allows easy assessment of the femoropatellar and femorotibial synovial recesses, the femoral trochlea, the patellar ligaments, the menisci, the collateral ligaments, and the medial femorotibial joint margins (Fig. 19-2). In the flexed stifle, ultrasonography allows visualisation of the cranial horns of the menisci, the cranial meniscal ligaments, and a portion of the articular surface of the medial femoral condyle (Fig. 19-2).

Diseases of the Femoropatellar Joint

Osteochondrosis

Although osteochondrosis lesions develop early in life, osteochondrosis of the femoropatellar joint is a common radiographic finding in both young and older horses.[7] Lateromedial or caudolateral-craniomedial oblique views are necessary to evaluate the femoral trochlea in young horses with synovial distension of the femoropatellar joint. Radiographic signs of osteochondrosis include flattening, irregular subchondral surface, heterogeneous opacity of the trochlear ridge, and presence of bony fragments attached by a radiolucent junction to the bone surface at the cranial aspect of the trochlea (Fig. 19-3). The most common site of osteochondrosis lesions is the lateral femoral trochlear ridge, especially the middle third.[1,7,8] The trochlear groove may occasionally be involved or have a lesion without involvement of the trochlear ridge. Lesions of the medial femoral trochlear ridge are less common (see Fig. 19-3).[8,9] Patellar lesions are rare and mainly seen associated with trochlear abnormalities.[8] Taking into account the age of development of permanent osteochondral lesions of the femoral trochlea, radiographic screening of the stifle for osteochondrosis should not be performed before 8 to 12 months of age.[7] Because of possible bilateral involvement, both stifles should always be examined. Because the femoral trochlea cannot be evaluated on the caudocranial view, and lateromedial and caudolateral-craniomedial oblique views do not allow precise estimation of the mediolateral extent of the lesion, ultrasonographic examination of the cranial aspect of the stifle may be helpful before surgery to define better the long-term prognosis (Fig. 19-4).

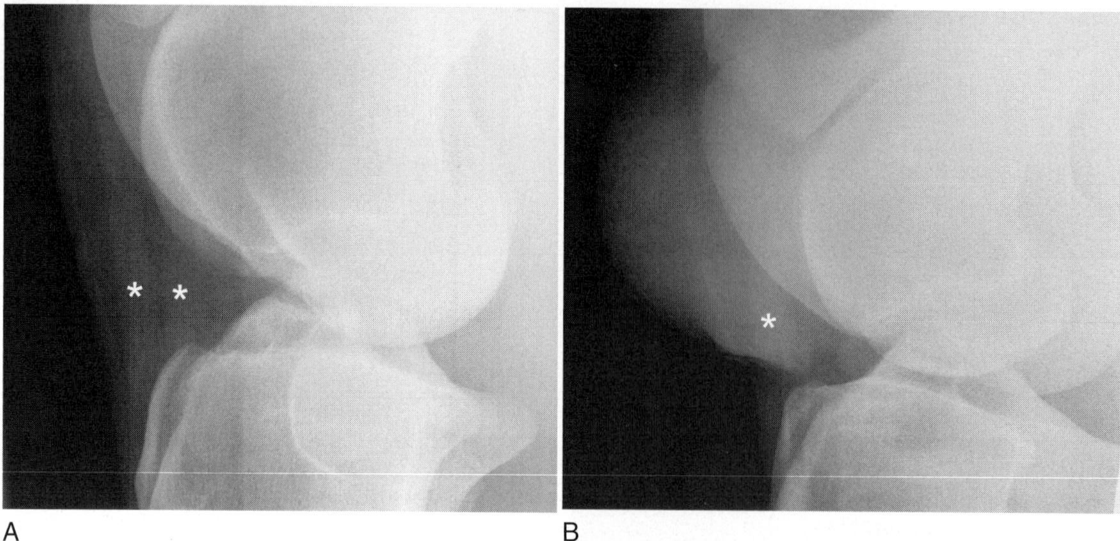

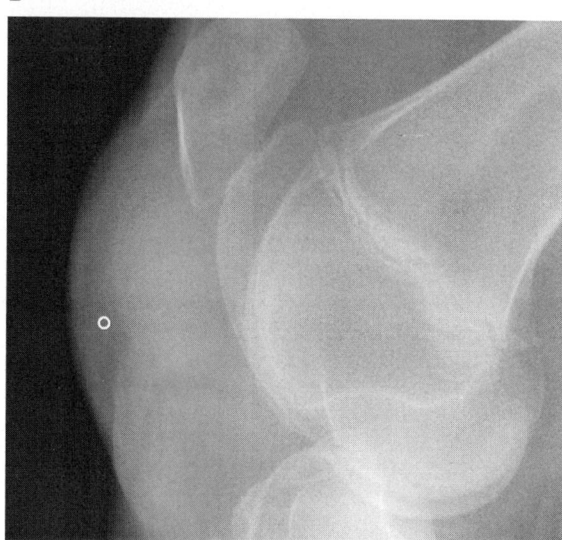

Fig. 19-1 Lateromedial radiographs of three equine stifles. **A,** Normal stifle. The patellar ligaments *(asterisks)* are delineated by the different opacity of the fat pad at the cranial aspect of the joint. **B,** A slightly oblique craniolateral-caudomedial view. A localized extraarticular soft-tissue swelling is visible. The middle patellar ligament is still visible *(asterisk)*. The horse had an extraarticular abscess. **C,** A soft tissue swelling at the cranial aspect of the stifle. The swelling is intraarticular (femoropatellar and femorotibial), and the patellar ligaments are no longer visible. The fat pad *(open circle)* is pushed cranially.

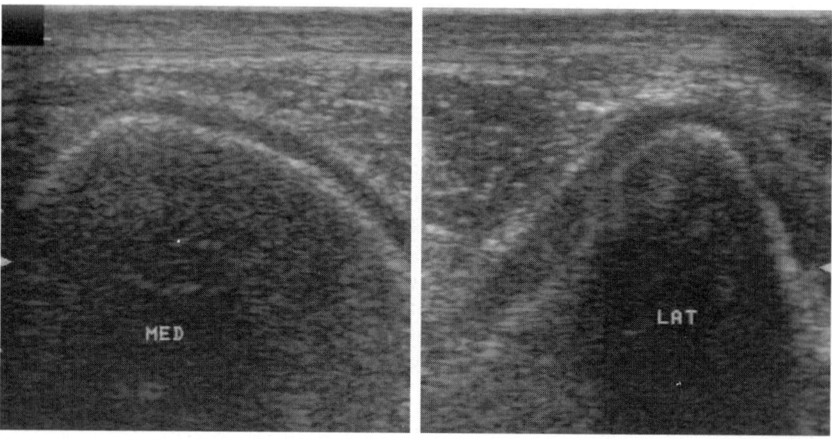

Fig. 19-2 Ultrasound (US) images of the normal equine stifle (**A** to **D**) and meniscal tears (**E**). **A,** Transverse US images of the medial *(med)* and lateral *(lat)* ridges of the femoral trochlea in a normal horse. The hyperechoic line is the subchondral bone surface. The hypoechoic band that covers the bone surface is the articular cartilage.

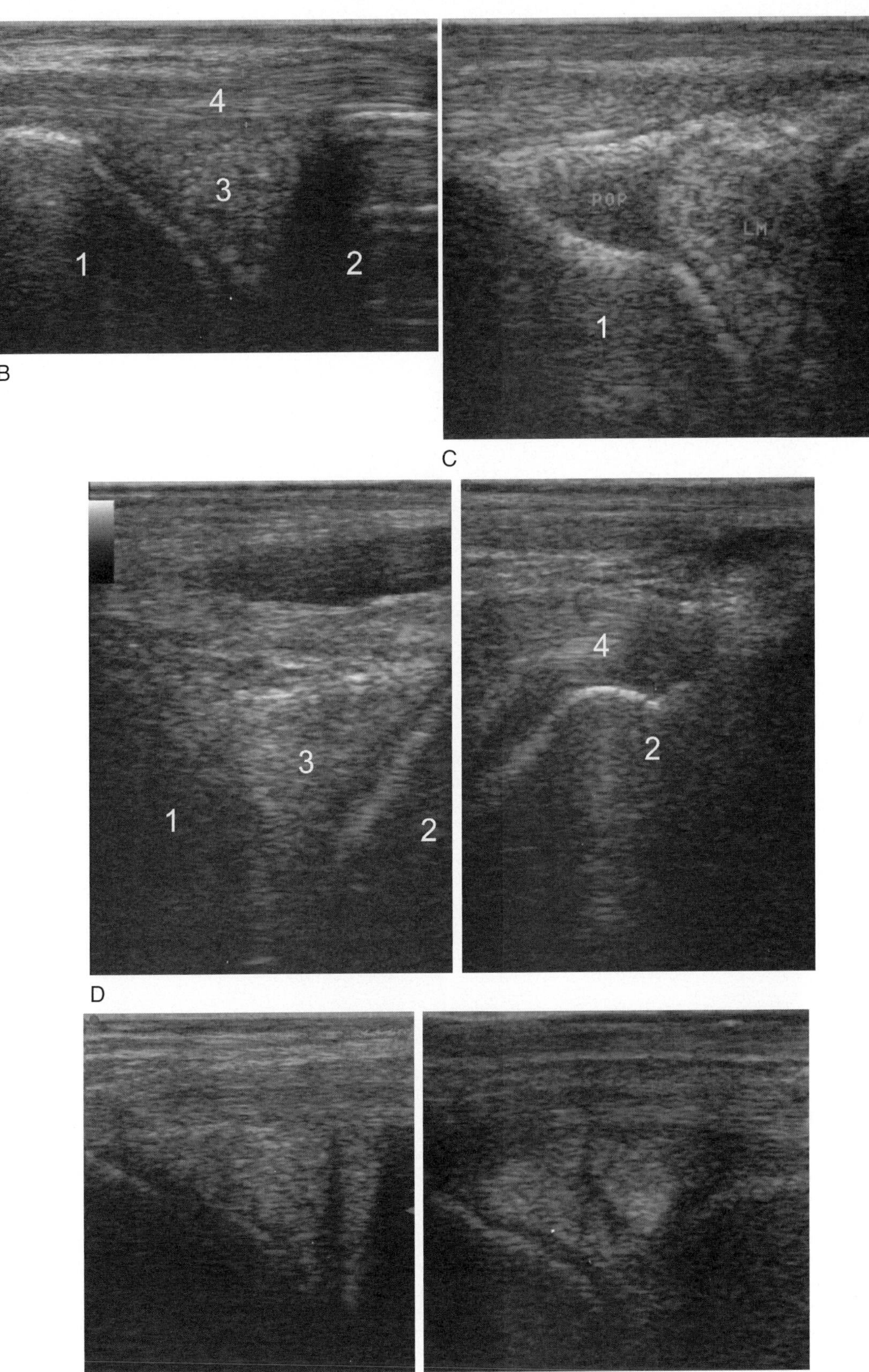

Fig. 19-2, cont'd **B,** Longitudinal US image of the stifle obtained at the medial aspect of the joint in a normal horse. *1,* Femur; *2,* tibia; *3,* medial meniscus; *4,* medial collateral ligament. **C,** Longitudinal US image of the stifle obtained at the lateral aspect of the joint in a normal horse. The hypoechogenicity of the popliteus tendon *(pop)* is caused by the oblique orientation of the fibers in relation to the US beam. *1,* Femur; *2,* tibia; *LM,* lateral meniscus. **D,** Longitudinal *(left)* and transverse *(right)* US images of the flexed stifle obtained at the cranial aspect of the joint in a normal horse. *1,* Femur; *2,* tibia; *3,* cranial horn of the lateral meniscus; *4,* cranial meniscal ligament of the medial meniscus inserting on the proximal tibia. **E,** US images of meniscal tears in two horses with stifle lameness. The hypoechoic linear images that cross the menisci are indicative of meniscal damage. *Left,* Horizontal tear of the medial meniscus. *Right,* Oblique tear of the lateral meniscus.

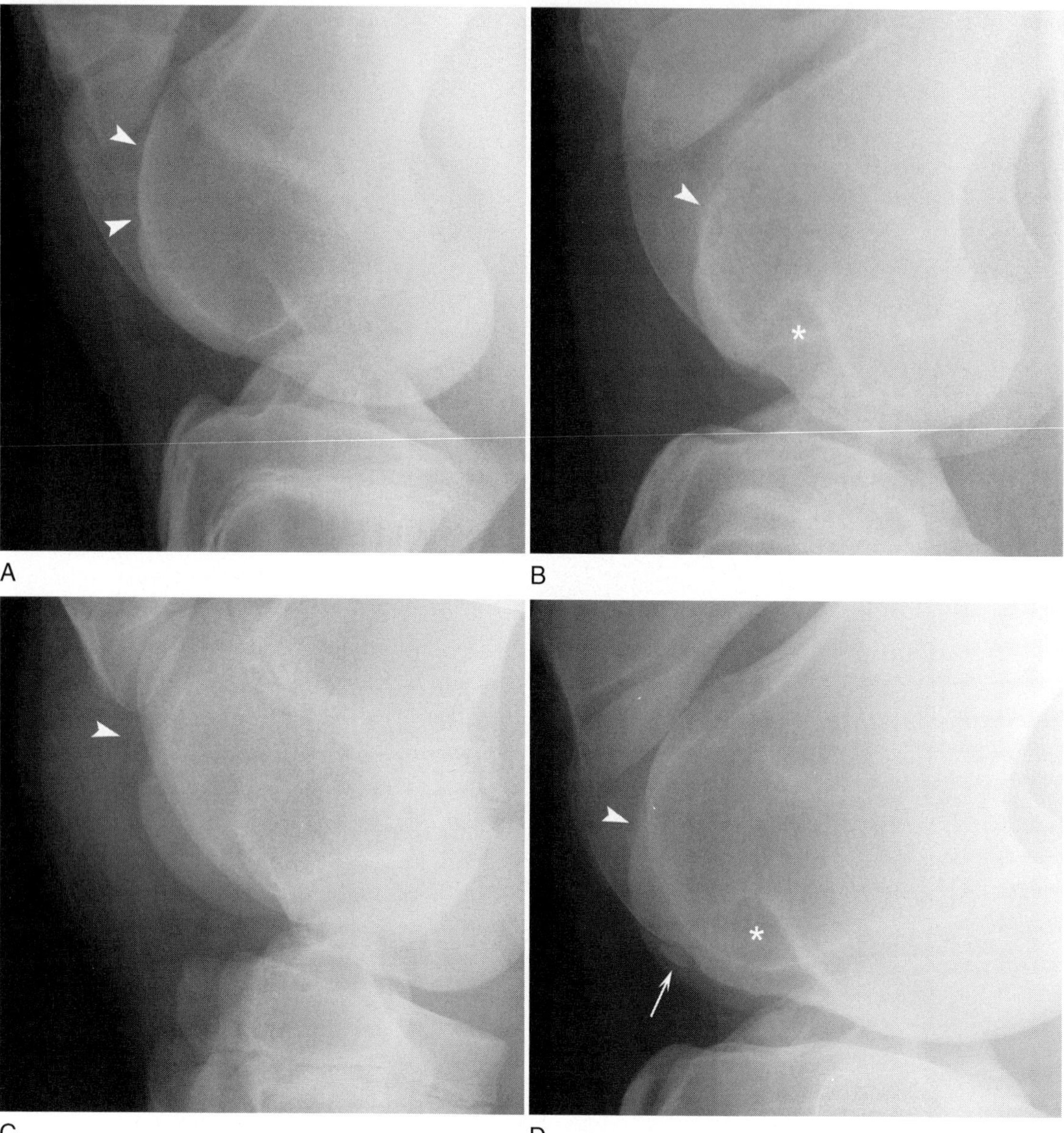

Fig. 19-3 Lateromedial (A, B, D) and caudolateral-craniomedial oblique (C) radiographs of the stifle of four horses with osteochondrosis of the femoral trochlea. **A,** The lateral trochlear ridge is flattened and its subchondral bone surface is irregular *(arrowheads)*. **B,** The view is slightly craniolateral-caudomedial and the lateral trochlear ridge is superimposed on the trochlear groove. The lateral trochlear ridge is flat in its middle third and the subchondral bone has heterogeneous reduced *opacity (arrowhead)*. The extensor fossa of the distal femur *(asterisk)* is abnormally delineated by a cranial sclerotic border. This radiographic finding is seen in horses with chronic synovial distension and is often associated with osteochondrosis. **C,** The middle third of the lateral femoral trochlear ridge has a large radiolucent defect with small radiopaque fragments located cranial to it *(arrowhead)*. The femoropatellar joint is markedly distended. **D,** The lateral trochlear ridge is flat and irregular in its middle third *(arrowhead)*. The medial trochlear ridge has a bony fragment separated by a radiolucent junction from a defect in the subchondral bone *(arrow)*. The extensor fossa *(asterisk)* is more conspicuous than normal.

Patellar Fragmentation

Patellar fragmentation involves the patellar apex and is primarily seen in horses that have undergone medial patellar desmotomy.[10-12] The fragmentation is considered to be the consequence of patellar instability after desmotomy.[11] One or multiple bone fragments may be present (Fig. 19-5). Remodelling of the tibial tuberosity at the insertion of the patellar ligaments and remodelling or enthesopathy of the patella may be seen in association with fragmentation of the apex and help distinguish this condition from osteochondrosis.[10-12]

Upward Patellar Fixation

No radiographic sign can be used to confirm the clinical diagnosis of recurrent upward patellar fixation. Radiographic examination of the stifle is recommended to exclude other

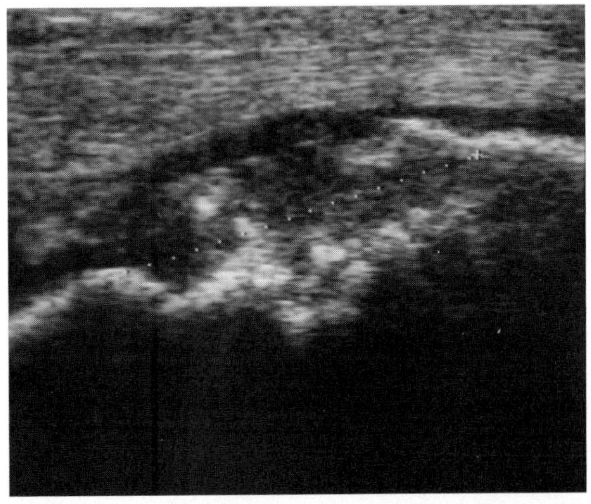

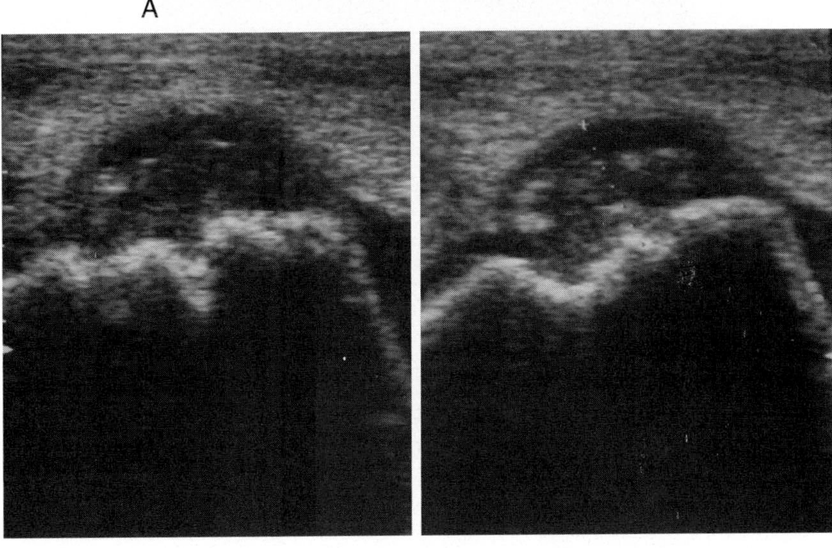

Fig. 19-4 Longitudinal (A) and transverse (B) ultrasonographic images of the lateral trochlear ridge of a horse with osteochondrosis. The cartilage thickness is uneven. The subchondral bone surface does not produce a smooth hyperechoic line at the site of the lesion because it is not ossified. The subchondral bone is hypoechoic and its surface is irregular. Compare this figure to the normal aspect of the femoral trochlear in Figure 19-2, *A*.

concurrent stifle lesions that may affect the choice of treatment and prognosis. Horses with recurrent partial upward patellar fixation may have remodelling of the patellar apex on lateromedial radiographs.[8]

Patellar Luxation and Trochlear Dysplasia

Lateral patellar luxation is an uncommon congenital condition and may be unilateral or bilateral.[13,14] Lateral patellar luxation is often the consequence of femoral trochlear dysplasia with trochlear ridge hypoplasia and a shallow trochlear groove. Lateral patellar luxation may be associated with incomplete ossification of the medial patellar angle.[13,14] Patellar luxation is recognized in horses of all ages as a cause of a nonpainful gait alteration, more commonly in miniature breeds and ponies.[8,15] Radiographically, lateral patellar luxation is seen as a malpositioning of the patella (Fig. 19-6). An increase in the craniocaudal dimension of the patella on the lateromedial view of the stifle is caused by displacement and rotation of the patella compared with the normal axis of the limb.

Osteomyelitis of the Patella

Chronic osteomyelitis of the patella may develop as a consequence of a longstanding abscess at the cranial aspect of the stifle.[8] Radiographic signs are seen on the lateromedial and caudolateral-craniomedial oblique view. A cranioproximal-craniodistal view of the patella is essential to assess the full extent of the bone involvement (Fig. 19-7). Radiographic signs are periosteal reaction on the cranial patellar surface and areas of reduced opacity within the patella, resulting in a patchy heterogeneous appearance of the patella on radiographs (see Fig. 19-7). Ultrasonography can help assess concurrent soft tissue infection, localize the abscess, and confirm bony involvement seen as roughening of the bone surface.

Diseases of the Femorotibial Joints

Subchondral Cystlike Lesions

Subchondral cystlike lesions of the stifle are juvenile osteoarticular abnormalities but may be seen in horses of any age.[4] Their typical radiographic appearance is a round to oval radiolucent area with well-defined margins within the subchondral bone of the femoral (Fig. 19-8) or, less commonly, the tibial condyles. Subchondral bone cysts may have a distal base of variable extent depending on communication and proximity with the joint space; they may also be surrounded by a sclerotic rim. The subchondral surface of the femoral condyle is flattened at the level of the cyst. Small bone cysts may be difficult to see within the thick femoral condyle, especially in large horses. Flattening or indentation of the femoral subchondral surface may be the only radiographic sign visible in some horses.[16] Ultrasonography of the medial femoral condyle surface in the flexed stifle may be used to confirm radiographic suspicion. Radiographic signs of degenerative joint disease may be present in older horses with a cystlike lesion as a result of

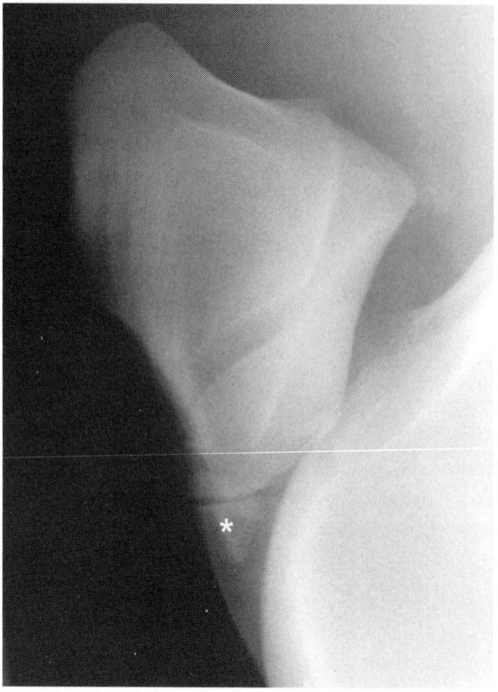

Fig. 19-5 Lateromedial radiograph of the patella of a horse with patellar fragmentation *(asterisk)* after medial patellar desmotomy.

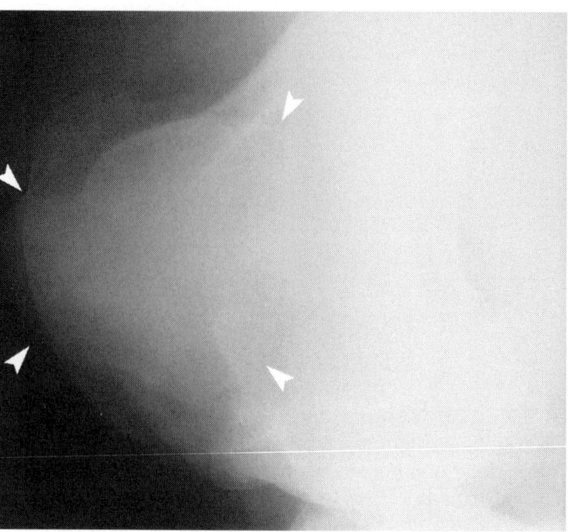

Fig. 19-6 Lateromedial radiograph of the stifle of an adult Appaloosa horse with permanent lateral patellar luxation: the patella *(arrowheads)* is superimposed on the femoral trochlea.

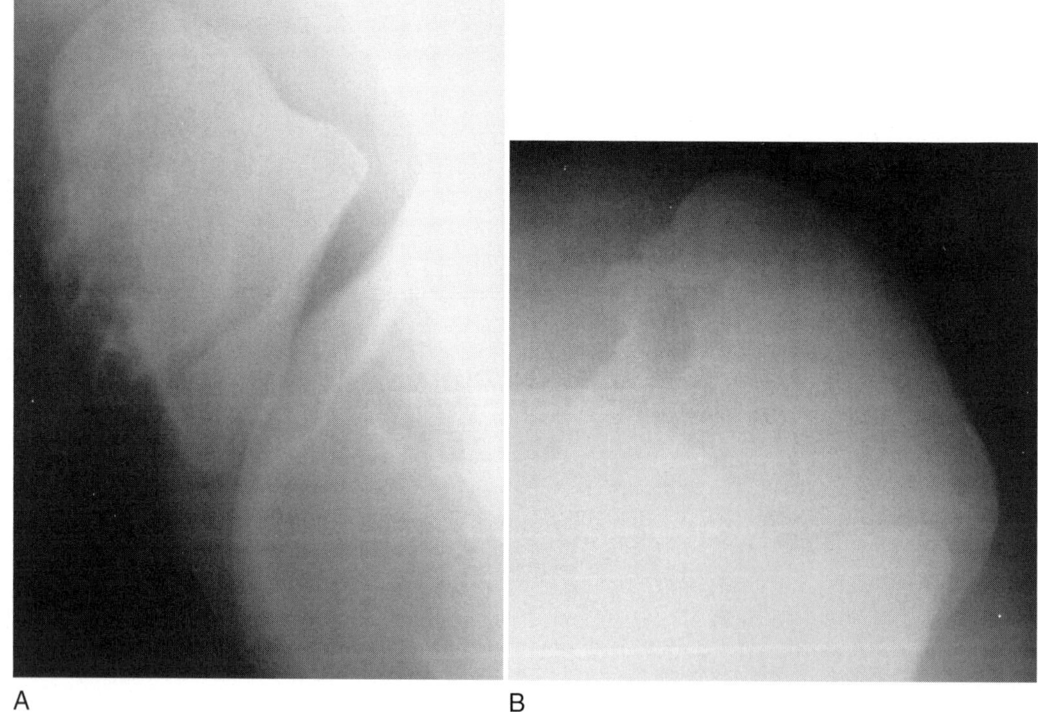

Fig. 19-7 Lateromedial (A) and cranioproximal-craniodistal oblique (B) radiographs of the patella of a horse with an abscess at the cranial aspect of the stifle and subsequent patellar osteomyelitis. The patella is heterogeneous and contains radiolucent areas. The cranial patellar surface is irregular. A large radiolucent defect is seen in the patella in the cranioproximal-craniodistal oblique view.

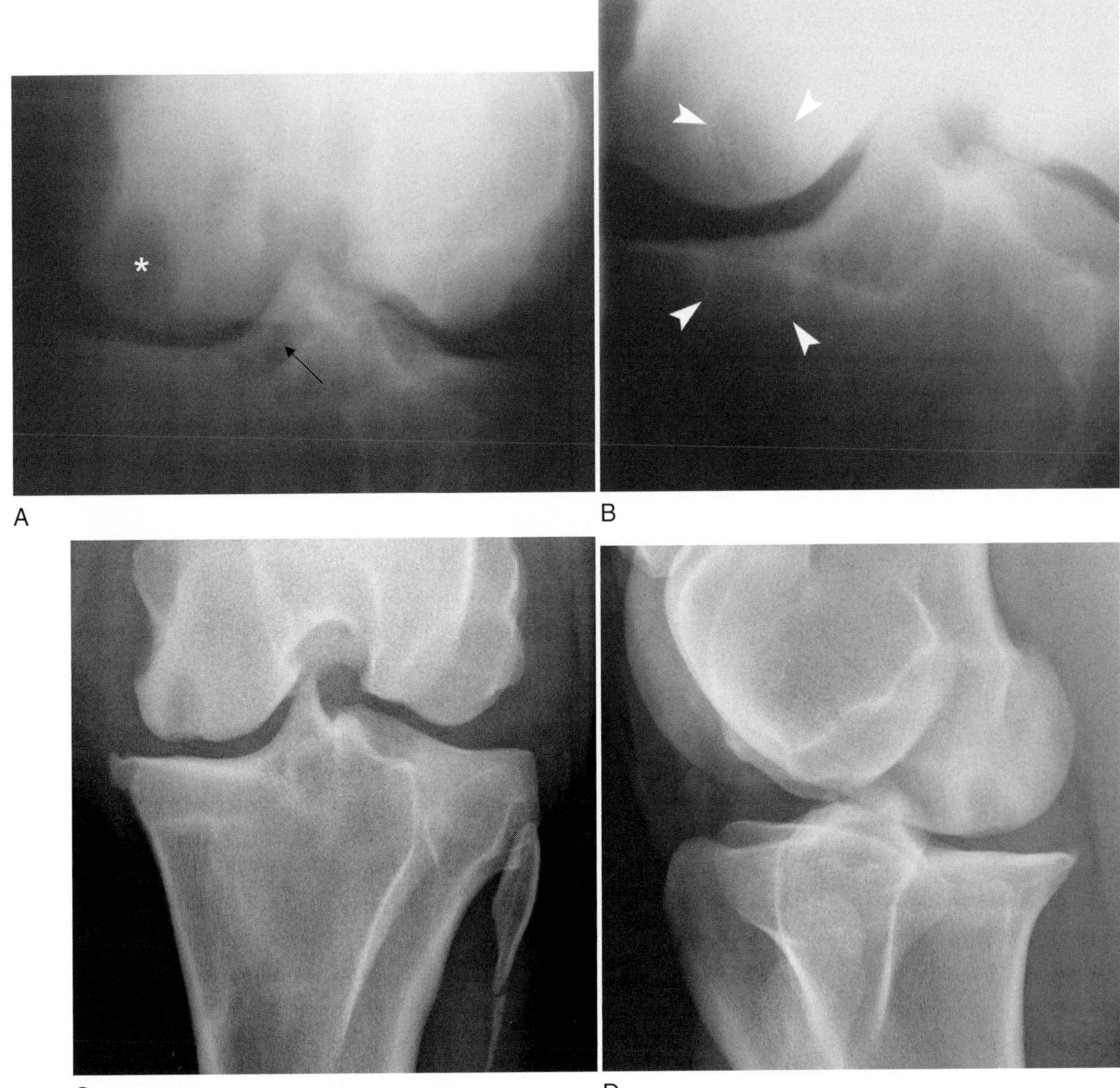

Fig. 19-8 Radiographs of the stifle of three horses with subchondral bone cysts. **A,** A large, oval, well-marginated radiolucent area *(asterisk)* is visible in the medial femoral condyle. Also note the radiolucent region in the tibia just distal to the medial intercondylar eminence *(black arrow)*. This is a normal finding in the equine tibia and should not be confused with a cystlike lesion. **B,** Two round radiolucent areas *(arrowheads)* are surrounded by a thin sclerotic rim located in the medial femoral and tibial condyles. **C** and **D** show craniocaudal and caudolateral-craniomedial views, respectively. A large, oval, subchondral radiolucent region with faint marginal sclerosis is present in the medial femoral condyle. Flattening of the medial femoral condyle is visible. Osteophytes on the medial tibial condyle and medial intercondylar eminence indicate degenerative joint disease. Note the normally segmented fibula in **C.**

chronic synovitis and secondary meniscal damage (see Fig 19-8, *C* and *D*). The most common location for subchondral cystlike lesions is the weight-bearing area of the medial femoral condyle.[8,17] Osseous cystlike lesions have also been reported in the caudal aspect of the femoral condyles in foals.[18] Lateral femoral condyle and proximal tibial cystlike lesions are less common (Fig. 19-8, *B*).[8,19] Subchondral cystlike lesions may be difficult to see on slightly underexposed lateromedial radiographs because of superimposition of the femoral condyles. A caudocranial view of optimal exposure and contrast and/or a caudolateral-craniomedial oblique view are the most useful for confirming and localizing the lesion.

Degenerative Joint Disease

Degenerative joint disease of the femorotibial joint can be a sequel to any stifle injury and is commonly seen in horses with stifle lameness and meniscal damage.[5,6,8] Involvement of the medial femorotibial joint is more common than involvement of the lateral compartment.[5,8] The most common radiographic signs are remodelling of the tibial and femoral joint margins with production of large-based osteophytes (see Figs. 19-8, *C* and *D*, and 19-9). Tibial osteophytes are usually large with smooth margins and tend to grow such that their proximal surface is not in the same plane compared with the tibial plateau. Femoral osteophytes are more commonly seen on the

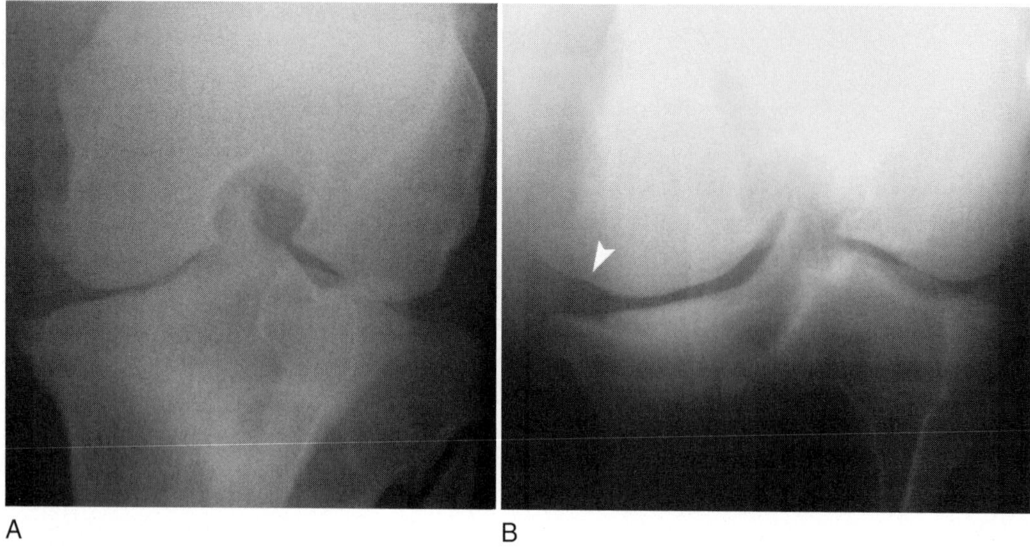

Fig. 19-9 Caudocranial radiographs of the stifle of two horses with meniscal injuries and degenerative joint disease. **A,** Femoral and tibial osteophytes on the medial articular margins and new bone formation on the medial tibial intercondylar eminence are visible. **B,** Femoral and tibial large-based osteophytes are present on the medial articular margins. Note the change in curvature between the condyle surface and the femoral osteophyte *(arrowhead)*.

medial condyle margin. They are usually large-based and, as tibial osteophytes, their distal surface is not in continuity with the arc of the condylar surface (see Fig. 19-9). Narrowing of the femorotibial joint space is less common and is a sign of meniscal prolapse more than a consequence of cartilage thinning in degenerative joint disease (Fig. 19-10). Areas of subchondral bone sclerosis and lucencies are mainly seen in advanced articular damage with meniscal injury and prolapse.

Radiographic Signs of Meniscal and Meniscal Ligament Damage

The menisci, which are of soft tissue opacity, occupy the space between the distal femoral condyles and the proximal tibial plateau; they cannot be seen on radiographs. Therefore meniscal damage can only be suspected on radiographs when calcification is present in the femorotibial joint space or close to it (Fig. 19-11), or on the basis of secondary bony abnormalities (radiolucent areas, new bone formation, avulsion fragments) at the site of insertion of the cranial meniscal ligaments on the proximal tibia (Fig. 19-12). New bone formation cranial to the medial intercondylar eminence of the tibia has been reported as the most frequent radiographic finding in horses with meniscal damage (Fig. 19-13).[20] The imaging technique of choice to evaluate meniscal and meniscal ligaments damage in the horse is ultrasonography (see Fig. 19-2). When the site of pain responsible for the lameness has been proven to be the stifle, or when distension of the femorotibial joint is present, a radiographically normal stifle should not be considered a lesion-free joint because soft tissue injuries, in particular meniscal damage, are a frequent cause of lameness in the horse.[5,6]

Radiographic Signs of Cruciate Ligament and Collateral Ligament Damage

Indirect radiographic signs of cruciate ligament damage are seen as radiolucent areas at the ligament insertion sites on the distal femur or bone remodelling at the tibial insertions.[2,3] Avulsion of bone at the cruciate ligament insertions, mainly of the tibial intercondylar eminence, have also been reported.[2,3,21-23]

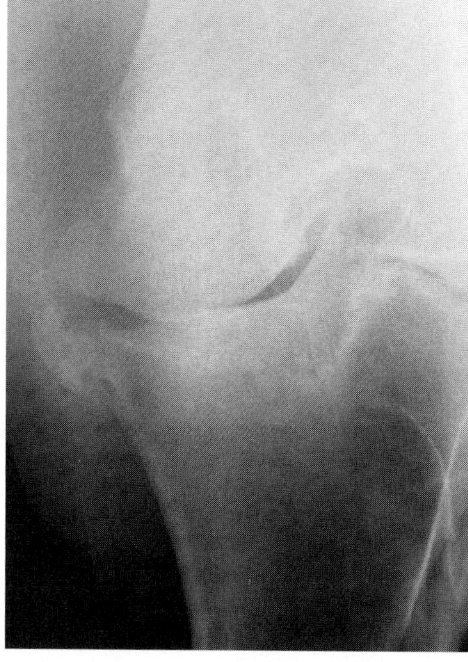

Fig. 19-10 Caudocranial view of the stifle of a horse with severe medial meniscal damage, calcification, and prolapse. The medial femorotibial joint space is narrowed, and the proximal tibial condyle is sclerotic because of a prolapse of the medial meniscus. Calcified meniscal material is present outside the articular space at the medial aspect of the joint. The medial femoral and tibial joint margins have large osteophytes. The cranial intercondylar area of the tibia is heterogeneous and surrounded by a sclerotic rim, suggesting cranial meniscal ligament enthesopathy.

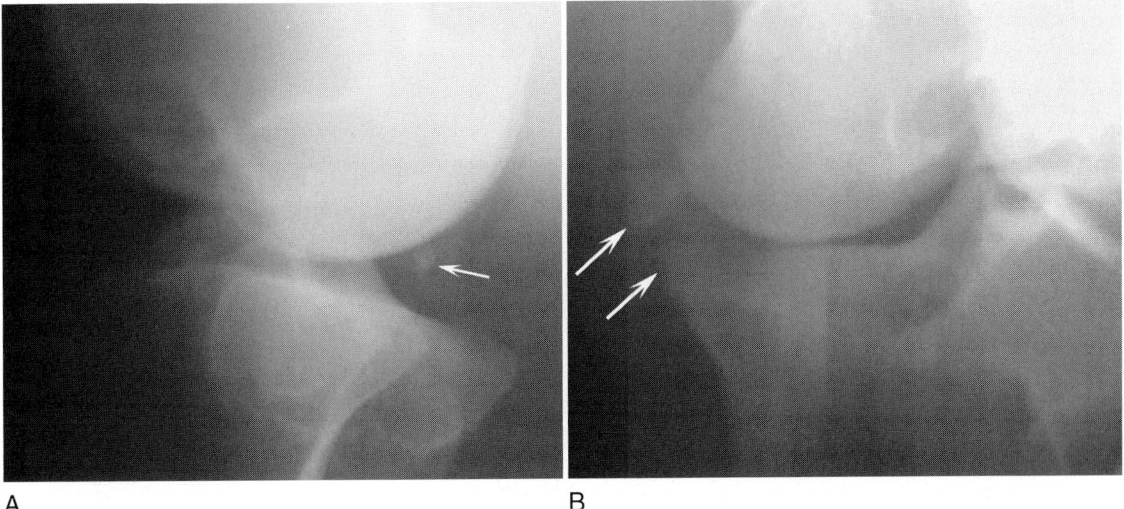

Fig. 19-11 Lateromedial (A) and caudocranial radiograph (B) of the stifle of two horses with meniscal calcification. **A,** A small radiopaque focus *(arrow)* is present between the femoral condyle and the caudal aspect of the tibial plateau compatible with calcification in the caudal horn of the medial meniscus. **B,** Two large radiopaque bodies *(arrows)* at the medial aspect of the medial femorotibial joint correspond to calcified portions of a prolapsed medial meniscus.

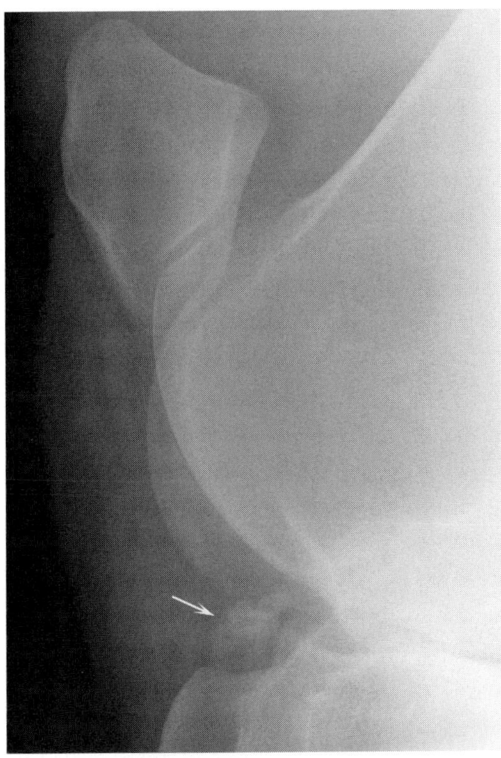

Fig. 19-12 Close-up caudolateral-craniomedial radiograph of the stifle in a horse with severe medial meniscal damage and prolapse. A large bony fragment is at the cranial aspect of the femorotibial joint space *(arrow)* representing an old avulsion fragment at the cranial meniscal ligament attachment.

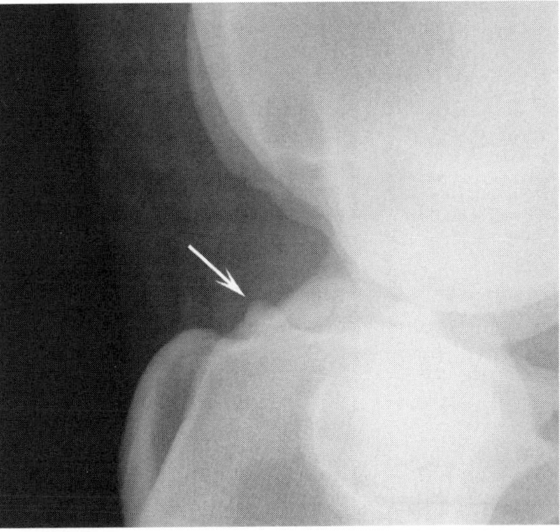

Fig. 19-13 Flexed lateromedial radiograph of an equine stifle. A prominent bony proliferation is present cranial to the tibial intercondylar eminence *(arrow)*. Ultrasound showed a horizontal fissure and a partial prolapse of the medial meniscus and damage to the medial cranial meniscal ligament.

Collateral ligament damage of the stifle as a consequence of acute trauma does not result in any radiographic abnormality except joint swelling. Ultrasonography allows an easy assessment of the medial and lateral collateral ligaments (see Fig. 19-2, *B*). Chronic desmopathy involving the bony insertion (enthesopathy) may be visible on caudocranial views of the stifle as a change in shape or an increased irregularity of the surface of the medial or lateral femoral epicondyles.

Fractures Involving the Stifle

Patellar Fractures

Patellar fractures most commonly involve the medial angle of the patella.[24,25] These fractures occur mainly in steeplechase and eventing horses when the flexed joint hits a fixed fence.[24-26] Fractures of the medial angle may be incidental and not related to lameness at the time of the radiographic examina-

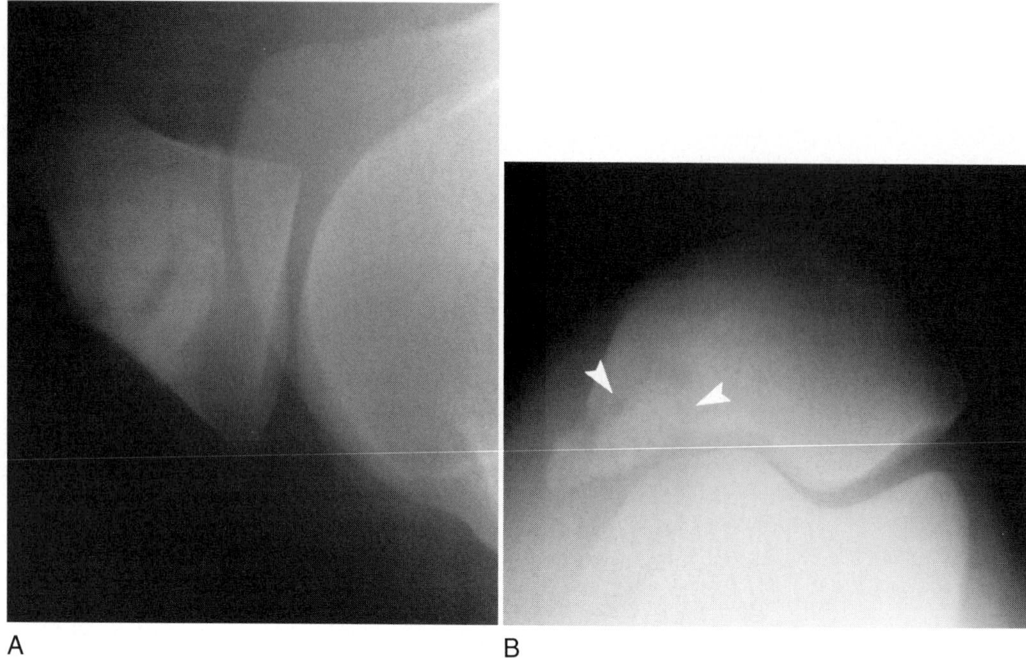

Fig. 19-14 Flexed lateromedial radiograph **(A)** and cranioproximal-craniodistal oblique radiograph **(B)** of the stifle of a horse with an old undisplaced fracture of the medial angle of the patella. **A,** The patella has increased opacity and a radiolucent line at the level of the medial angle. The medial articular surface is irregular and interrupted by the radiolucent line. **B,** The fracture of the medial angle of the patella is seen as an ill-defined radiolucent line *(arrowheads)* separating two bony fragments. The fracture involves the medial articular surface of the patella.

tion. These fractures may be suspected on the lateromedial view because of an area of heterogeneously increased opacity visible in the site of the medial patellar angle (Fig. 19-14). A cranioproximal-craniodistal view of the stifle allows confirmation of the diagnosis and a complete assessment of the extent and morphologic features of the fracture. Complete or comminuted fractures of the patella result from severe trauma.[4] Patellar fracture may be associated with fractures of the trochlear ridges of the femur.[8]

Tibial and Femoral Fractures

Fractures of the tibial tuberosity are the most commonly reported fractures involving the proximal tibia in adult horses.[8,27] Fractures involving the intercondylar eminence or the caudal aspect of the proximal tibia are seen in association with cruciate ligament damage and often involve the ligament insertion sites.[2,3,21-23] The proximal aspect of the tibial diaphysis is the most common site for incomplete fracture of the tibia, which usually begins at the lateral aspect of the bone and spirals distally (Fig. 19-15).[8,28] Radiographic diagnosis of these incomplete fractures may be challenging even if several oblique views are made. Complete rest and repeat radiographs approximately 1 week after the onset of the acute lameness are indicated. At this stage the fracture line becomes more visible because of resorption of the fracture margins.

Fractures of the femur involving the distal epiphysis are uncommon in adult horses. Trochlear ridge fractures are seen as free sharp fragments and a bony defect in the trochlea or as radiolucent lines in the trochlear ridge in incomplete undisplaced fractures. These fractures result from direct external trauma and may be associated with patellar fractures.[4,8] Femoral avulsion fractures of the origin of the common tendon of the peroneus tertius and the extensor digitorum longus are reported in foals.[4,29-31]

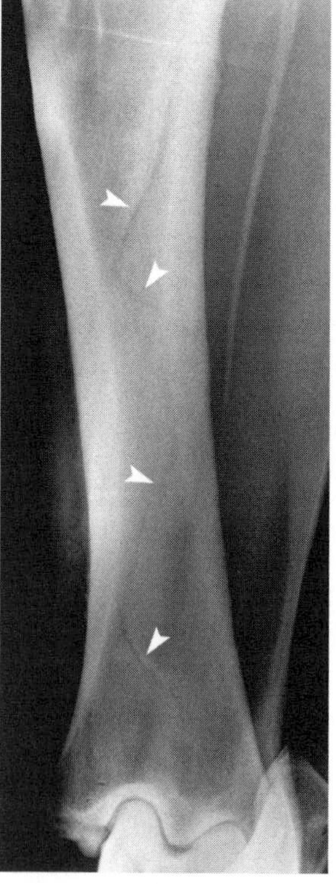

Fig. 19-15 Caudocranial radiograph of the tibial diaphysis of a horse with an incomplete fracture of the tibia. A radiolucent line begins at the lateral aspect of the proximal tibia and spirals distally through the entire tibial diaphysis *(arrowheads)*. This radiograph was made 1 week after the onset of the acute lameness.

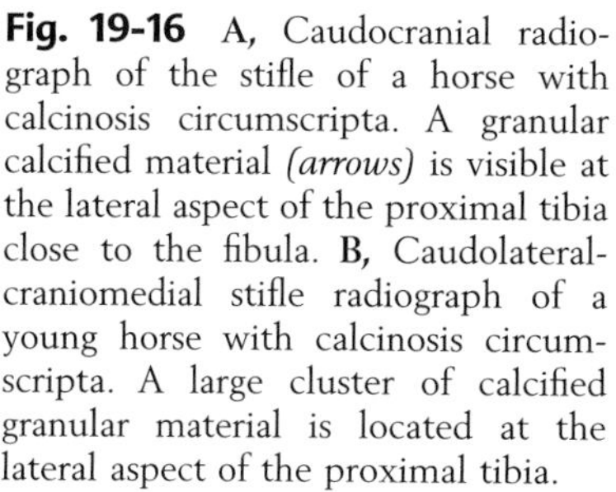

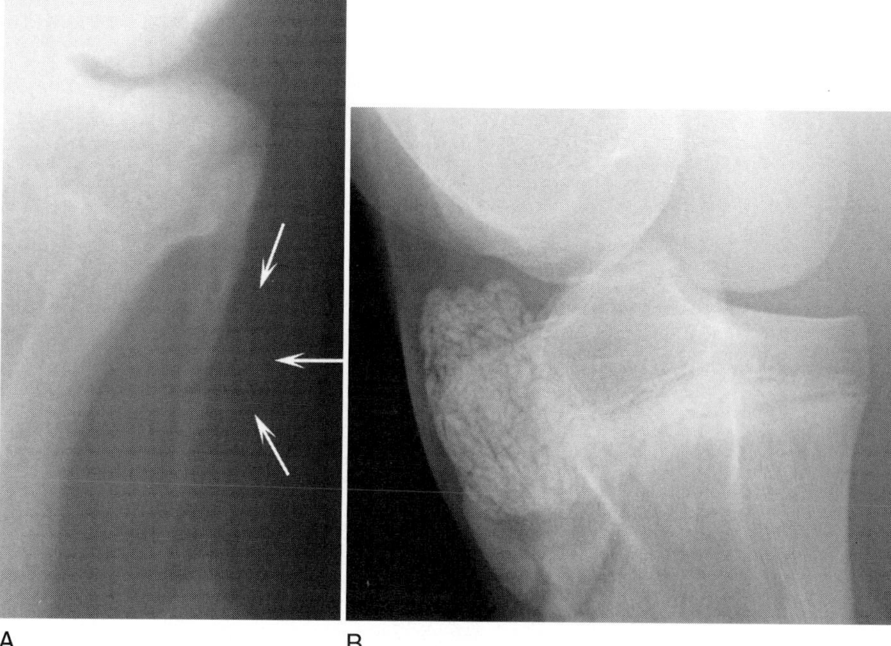

Fig. 19-16 A, Caudocranial radiograph of the stifle of a horse with calcinosis circumscripta. A granular calcified material *(arrows)* is visible at the lateral aspect of the proximal tibia close to the fibula. **B,** Caudolateral-craniomedial stifle radiograph of a young horse with calcinosis circumscripta. A large cluster of calcified granular material is located at the lateral aspect of the proximal tibia.

Fibular Fractures

Fibular fractures have been reported as a cause of lameness.[8] Care should be taken not to confuse the normal radiolucent line traversing the proximal fibula as a result of incomplete ossification with a fracture line (see Fig. 19-8, C). Callus formation is a useful radiographic sign of the presence of a previous fracture.[8]

Miscellaneous Conditions Involving the Stifle

Calcinosis Circumscripta

Calcinosis circumscripta, also called tumoral calcinosis, is defined as localized deposits of calcium salts in the skin and in the subcutaneous tissues.[32] The lesions of calcinosis circumscripta appear grossly as hard, spherical, nonpainful, subcutaneous or periarticular swellings. The etiology of calcinosis circumscripta is unknown. In the horse the predilection site is the lateral aspect of the stifle close to the extensor groove of the tibia.[4,32] The lesion is visible radiographically as a well-circumscribed, roughly oval accumulation of granular mineral opacities at the lateral aspect of the proximal tibia (Fig. 19-16). Calcinosis circumscripta may be an incidental radiographic finding because the lesion rarely causes lameness.[4,8] Most commonly the owner reports a firm, nonpainful swelling that has been slowly increasing in size. The lesions are usually bilateral, and radiographic examination of the contralateral limb is important if surgical removal is considered.

Septic Arthritis and Osteomyelitis

Septic arthritis is inflammation of a joint caused by bacterial invasion and proliferation.[33] Septic arthritis may occur in foals or adult horses. Haematogenous spread is the most common cause of septic arthritis in foals, whereas septic arthritis in adult horses is usually a consequence of penetrating wounds, injection, or surgery.[33]

Infection of the stifle joint in adult horses is rare. Periarticular infection and abscess after trauma and penetrating wounds are more common than bacterial joint invasion.[33] In foals, the femoropatellar joint and the femorotibial joints are common sites of septic arthritis.[8] Bone changes appear late in the condition in adult horses, whereas they are often seen at the beginning of the condition in foals. Bone changes attributable to osteomyelitis are located differently depending on the joint infected. When the femoropatellar joint is affected, osteolysis is mainly seen on the patellar articular surface (Fig. 19-17). Subchondral bone abnormalities on the femoral trochlea may be more difficult to assess because the trochlear ridges normally have an irregular bone surface in young foals during ossification. Femorotibial involvement is often uniaxial (medial or lateral). Bone involvement is seen as ill-defined radiolucent areas in the subchondral bone of the tibial plateau

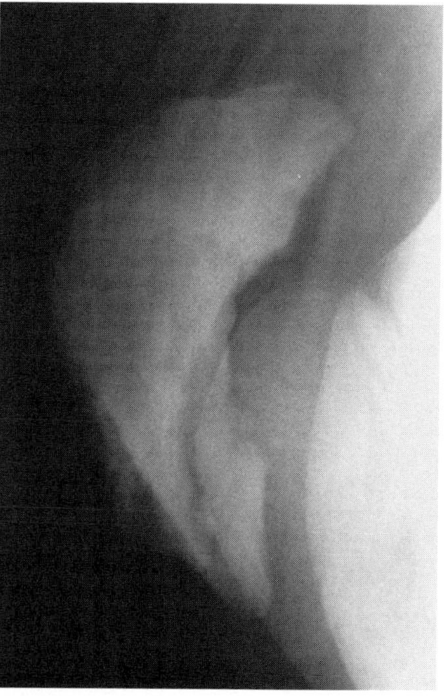

Fig. 19-17 Lateromedial radiograph of the patella of a foal with septic arthritis of the femoropatellar joint. The patella is severely affected; the articular surface is quite irregular, and severe lysis of the subchondral bone is visible.

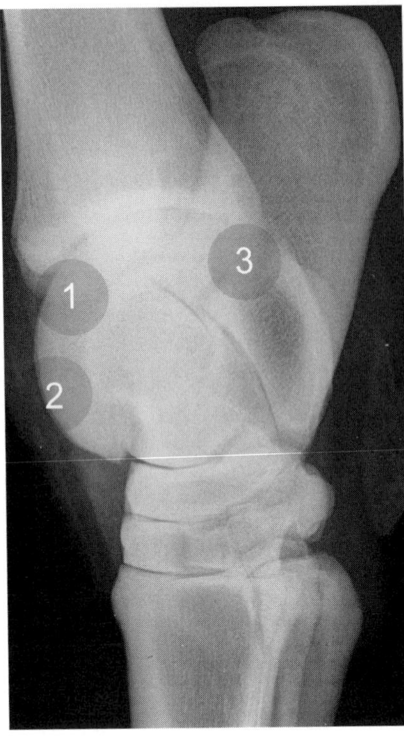

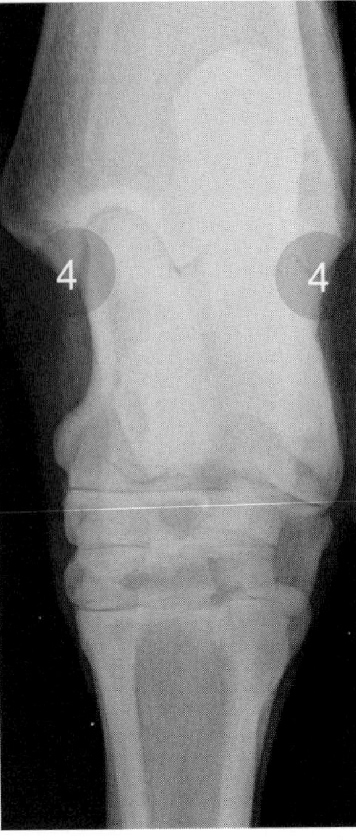

Fig. 19-18 Sites of osteochondrosis in the equine tarsus. *1*, Intermediate ridge of the tibial cochlea; *2*, ridges of the talus; *3*, proximal tubercle of the talus; *4*, tibial malleoli.

and/or the femoral condyles, with the medial femoral condyle being more commonly affected.[8,18] Well-defined radiolucent areas in the subchondral bone remain evident as a sequela of osteomyelitis when infection is eliminated.

Periarticular Soft Tissue Swelling

Localized periarticular soft tissue swelling is common in the stifle region. Main causes are seromas, hematomas, and abscesses, mainly occurring after penetrating injuries, falls, or trauma during jumping. Radiographic examination is used to assess concurrent bone involvement. If lameness is severe, joint involvement should be checked. Ultrasonography is the technique of choice to localize the swelling and establish its relation to the joint cavity. The nature of the content may be confirmed by aseptic centesis of the swelling. The increased contrast resolution of computed radiography allows localization of the soft tissue swelling by using the silhouette sign with the patellar ligaments and meniscal opacity and looking at the position relative to the patellar fat pad (see Fig. 19-1).

THE TARSUS

Radiographic Examination

A standard radiographic series of the tarsus includes dorsoplantar, dorsolateral-plantaromedial oblique, plantarolateral-dorsomedial oblique, and lateromedial views. A flexed lateromedial view may be used to visualize the plantar articular surface of the talus. A plantaroproximal-plantarodistal view of the calcaneus is important for assessing lesions of the sustentaculum tali, proximal talar tubercle, and calcaneus.

Because of the paucity of soft tissues around the tarsal joint, a grid is not needed to obtain good-quality radiographs in terms of contrast. A grid may be used when major soft tissue swelling is present around the joint, especially in draft horses.

Diseases of the Tarsocrural Joint

Osteochondrosis and Subchondral Cystlike Lesions

The tarsus is a common location for osteochondrosis lesions in the horse.[8,9,34-36] Although osteochondral lesions of the tarsocrural joint may be seen after 5 months of age, osteochondrosis is a frequent radiographic finding in horses of any age and in many breeds.[7,9,34,35] Radiographic abnormalities are not always associated with clinical signs.[8,36,37] In the tarsus, osteochondrosis may affect different sites (Fig. 19-18), with the most commonly affected being the intermediate cochlear ridge of the distal tibia.[8,9,35,36] In this location lesions are seen radiographically as bony fragments attached to the distal tibia by a radiolucent junction (Fig. 19-19). Less commonly, fragments become free in the joint and are seen in the distal aspect of the joint pouches at the dorsal or medial aspect of the distal talus and central tarsal bone regions. In some horses with minor involvement of the distal tibia a roughening and a radiolucent concave defect may be the only radiographic signs. Larger radiolucent defects with no adjacent bony fragment are most commonly seen in radiographs of horses in whom the fragment has already been removed (Fig. 19-20). The talar ridges, in particular the lateral talar ridge, are also a site of osteochondrosis (Fig. 19-21).[8,9,36,38] Radiographically the affected ridges have a flattened or irregular contour and may have a heterogeneous opacity. Sometimes bony fragments attached by a radiolucent junction to the talar ridge are seen. Large fragmentations of the distal aspect are more common on the lateral ridge of heavy horses and are usually clinically significant (Fig. 19-22).[36] Central smooth depressions without subchondral bone changes are commonly seen, especially in the medial talar ridge in clinically normal horses (Fig. 19-23). Semicircular subchondral defects in the weight-bearing portion of the talar ridge have been reported in association with severe lameness.[39] Other sites of osteochondrosis of the tarsus are the medial and lateral tibial malleoli and the medial proximal tubercle of the talus.[8] Horses affected by osteochondrosis of the tibial malleoli have osteochondral fragments with smooth contours separated from the malleolus by a radiolucent gap. The fragments may be located axially or distally to the malleolus (Fig. 19-24). Involvement of the medial malleolus is more common.[36] At the medial proximal tubercle of the talus osteochondrosis is seen either as a separate bony fragment or as a large and prominent tubercle (Fig. 19-25).

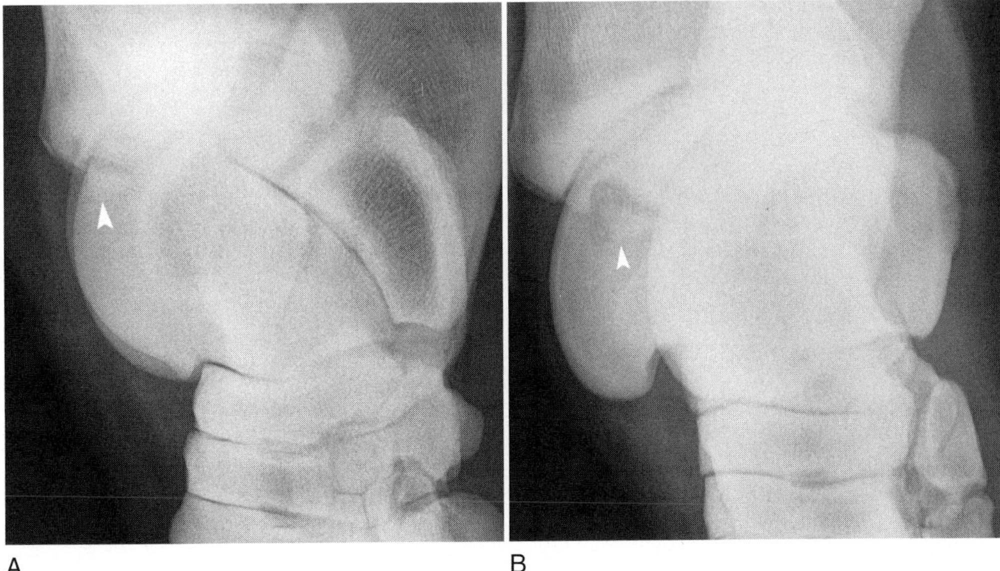

Fig. 19-19 Lateromedial (A) and plantarolateral-dorsomedial oblique (B) radiographs of the tarsus of a horse with osteochondrosis of the intermediate ridge of the tibia. A bony fragment attached by a radiolucent junction is visible distal to a concave defect in the intermediate ridge of the tibial cochlea *(arrowhead)*. The fragment is easier to see on the plantarolateral-dorsomedial oblique view because only the lateral trochlear ridge of the talus is superimposed on it.

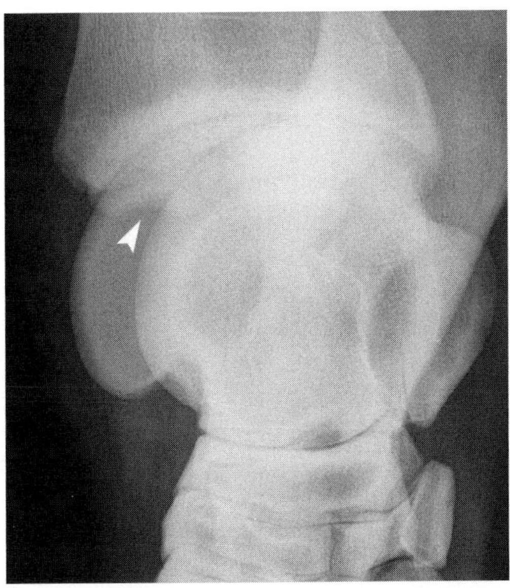

Fig. 19-20 Postoperative plantarolateral-dorsomedial oblique radiograph of the tarsus of a horse with osteochondrosis of the intermediate ridge of the tibia. A concave radiolucent defect *(arrowhead)* is present in the intermediate trochlear ridge of the tibial cochlea. The bony fragment had been removed at arthroscopy.

Subchondral cystlike lesions are considered a juvenile osteoarticular abnormality but may develop in skeletally mature horses after trauma or sepsis.[40] The occurrence of cystlike lesions in the tarsus is lower than in the stifle.[41] In the tarsocrural joint subchondral cystlike lesions are seen radiographically as round, usually small radiolucent areas, often surrounded by a thin sclerotic rim in the distal tibia or talus. In adult horses progressive cystlike radiolucencies may occasionally develop after subchondral trauma, mainly in the distal tibia.[42] Occult subchondral cystlike lesions, not visible on radiographs and possibly of septic origin, are also reported in the tarsocrural joint.[43]

Collateral Ligament Injury

Injuries to the collateral ligaments of the tarsocrural joint are the consequence of a sprain of the tarsus.[8] The horse usually has acute lameness and a severe articular swelling of the tarsocrural joint. Most horses have no radiographic signs except swelling of the tarsocrural joint at the onset of lameness. Avulsion fragments occasionally are seen at the tibial malleoli (Fig. 19-26). The diagnosis of the ligament damage is achieved by ultrasonography (Fig. 19-27). Ultrasonography allows a detailed assessment of the long and short collateral ligaments at the medial and lateral aspect of the joint (Fig. 19-27). Radiographic signs of enthesopathy appear as bony proliferation at the sites of attachment of the collateral ligament and may be seen in chronic sprains or 4 to 6 weeks after trauma.[8,42]

Diseases of the Distal Intertarsal and Tarsometatarsal Joints

Degenerative Joint Disease

Degenerative joint disease of the tarsus is common. The distal intertarsal and tarsometatarsal joints are the most frequently affected, either alone or in combination.[8,42,44,45] Although degenerative joint disease of these joints is considered one of the most common causes of hindlimb lameness, the clinical significance of most of the radiographic signs consistent with degenerative changes varies among horses.[8,43,46] Radiographic signs are changes in shape and opacity of the joint margins, osteophyte formation, thinning of the joint space, ill-defined subchondral bone/cartilage interface, subchondral plate irregularities, subchondral lysis, and trabecular bone sclerosis (Fig. 19-28). The association of several of the cited radiographic

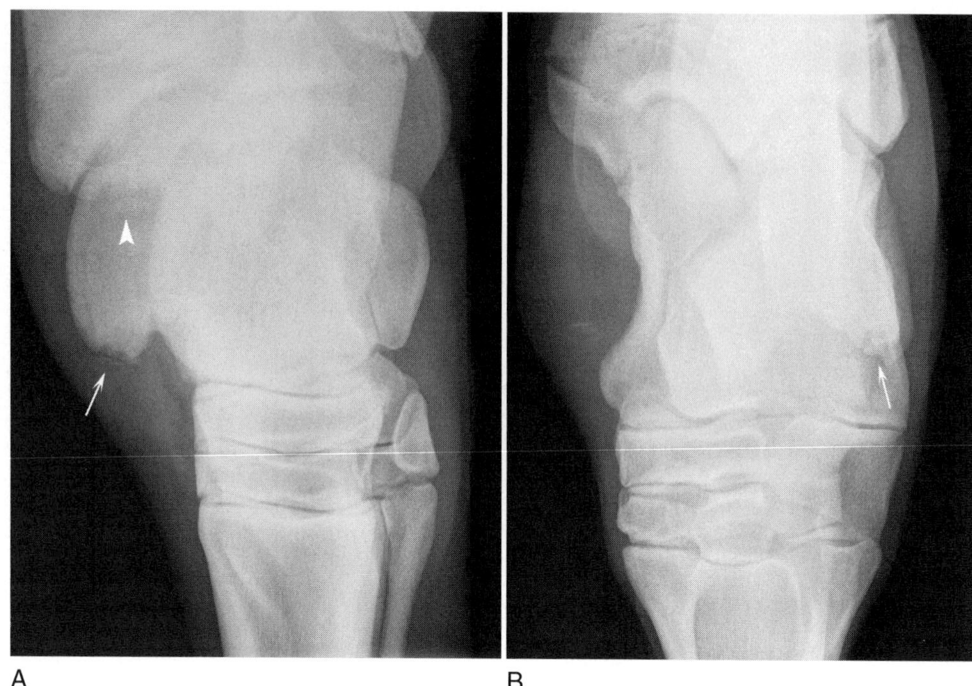

Fig. 19-21 Plantarolateral-dorsomedial oblique (A) and dorsoplantar (B) radiographs of the tarsus of a young horse with osteochondrosis of the intermediate ridge of the tibia and the lateral talar ridge. A bony fragment separated by a radiolucent line from the intermediate ridge of the tibia is visible on the plantarolateral oblique view *(arrowhead)*. A defect in the distal extremity of the lateral trochlear ridge is visible on both views *(arrow)*. At this level the bone surface is irregular, and two thin bony fragments are attached by a radiolucent junction to the edge of the ridge. Tarsocrural joint effusion is evidenced by the soft tissue swelling on the dorsoplantar view. Free bony fragments are also visible at the medial aspect of the distal talus.

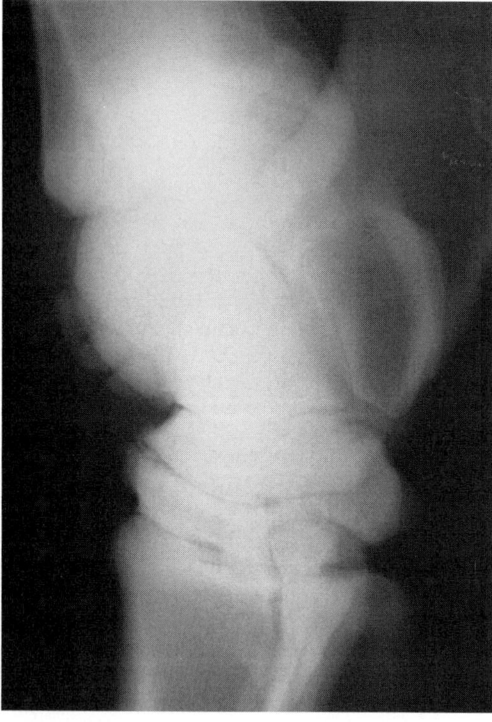

Fig. 19-22 Lateromedial radiograph of the tarsus of a draft horse with osteochondrosis of the lateral talar ridge, tarsal bone collapse, and distal intertarsal degenerative joint disease. Three large fragments are seen on the lateral ridge of the talus attached by a radiolucent junction. The fragmentation involves the dorsal aspect of the entire distal third of the trochlear ridge.

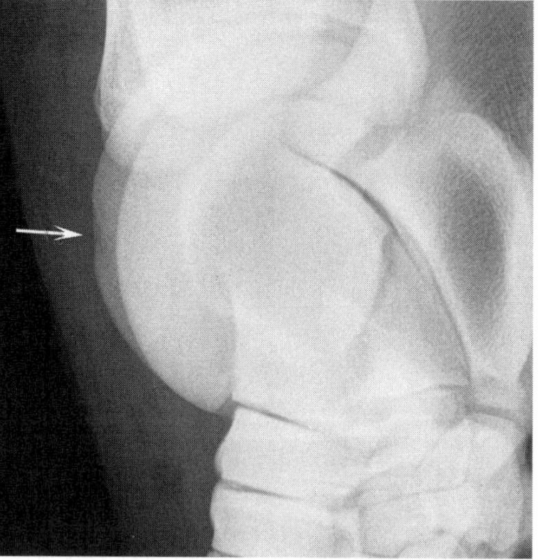

Fig. 19-23 Lateromedial radiograph of the tarsus of a clinically normal horse. A small area of flattening *(arrow)* is visible at the junction between the middle and distal third of the medial trochlear ridge of the talus. This is an incidental radiographic finding without clinical significance.

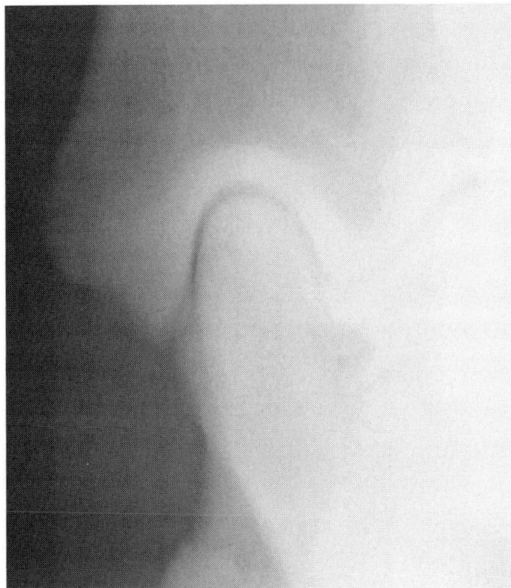

Fig. 19-24 Dorsoplantar radiograph of the tarsus of a horse with osteochondrosis of the medial malleolus. A small osteochondral fragment with smooth margins is visible distal to the medial malleolus.

signs, including changes in opacity at the joint margins, is more likely to be responsible for clinical signs. Remodelling or bony spurs with smooth contours and no change in opacity at the margins of the tarsometatarsal joint are often an incidental finding with no clinical significance (Fig. 19-29). Because subchondral bone plate irregularities are often associated with osteophyte formation at the distal intertarsal joint margins (but not in the tarsometatarsal joint), this radiographic finding is likely to be more significant clinically in the distal intertarsal joint than in the tarsometatarsal joint.[44] Subchondral bone lysis, independently from the location, should always be considered associated to a certain degree with joint pain. The more lytic the changes in the subchondral bone, the more likely that clinical signs will be present.

Degenerative joint disease of the distal intertarsal or tarsometatarsal joints is often bilateral and often begins in the dorsal aspect of the joints. An uneven distribution of biomechanical forces seems to be an important etiologic factor of the disease.[46] Mild dorsal collapse of the tarsal bones is often mainly associated with degenerative joint disease of the distal intertarsal joint. On the lateromedial views of the tarsus of these horses is a mild to moderate bulging of the dorsal profile of the distal tarsal rows, and intertarsal and tarsometatarsal joint spaces converge dorsally. In severely affected horses the entire joint is involved.

Incomplete Ossification of Tarsal Bones and Tarsal Collapse

Incomplete ossification of the tarsal bones is reported in newborn foals.[42,47,48] However, because of lack of recognition of clinical signs or lack of concern for angular deformity by some owners, foals may be seen by the veterinarian later in life. The condition is more common in premature or twin foals and is thought to be a consequence of skeletal immaturity at birth.[8,42] Radiographically, incomplete ossification of the central and/or the third tarsal bone occurs, with the third tarsal bone being more commonly and more severely affected. Dorsal or lateral collapse of the affected bone is common (Fig. 19-30). Collapse leads to dorsal fragmentation of the tarsal bone and the clinical consequences of angular limb deformity

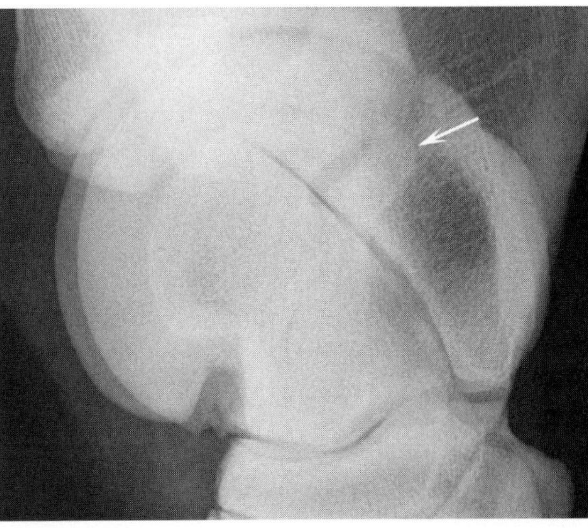

A

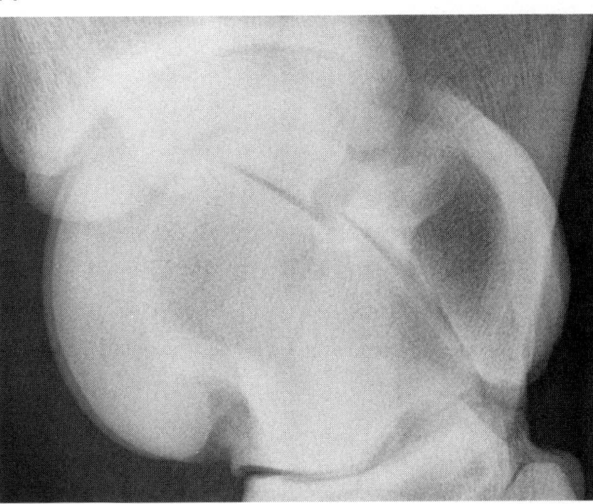

B

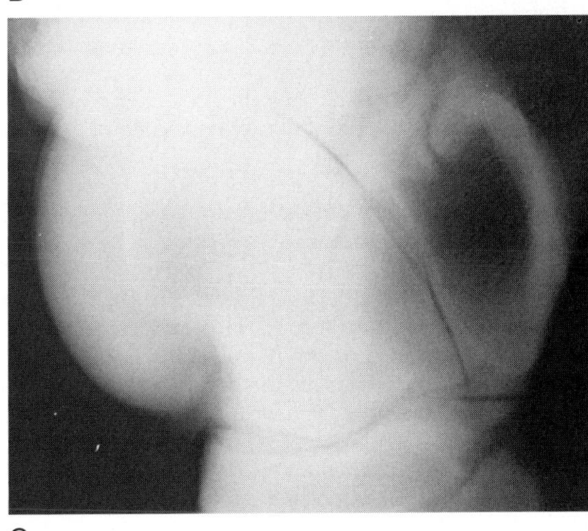

C

Fig. 19-25 Lateromedial radiographs of the tarsus from three horses illustrating different radiographic appearances of the proximal tubercle of the talus. **A,** Normal proximal tubercle of the talus *(arrow)*. **B,** Prominent proximal tubercle of the talus. **C,** Fragmentation of the proximal tubercle of the talus.

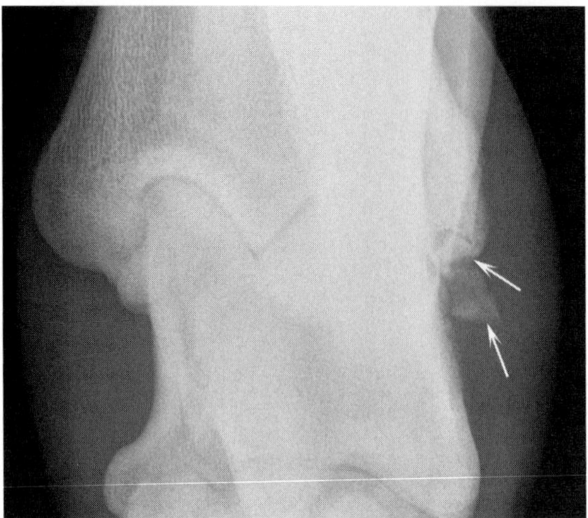

Fig. 19-26 Dorsoplantar radiograph of the tarsus of a horse with an avulsion fracture of the lateral malleolus. Two sharp bony fragments *(arrows)* distal to the lateral malleolus and a concave defect in the malleolus are visible. The tarsocrural joint is severely distended.

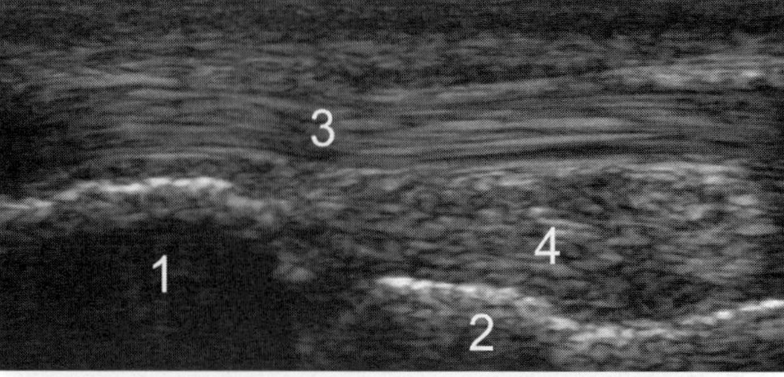

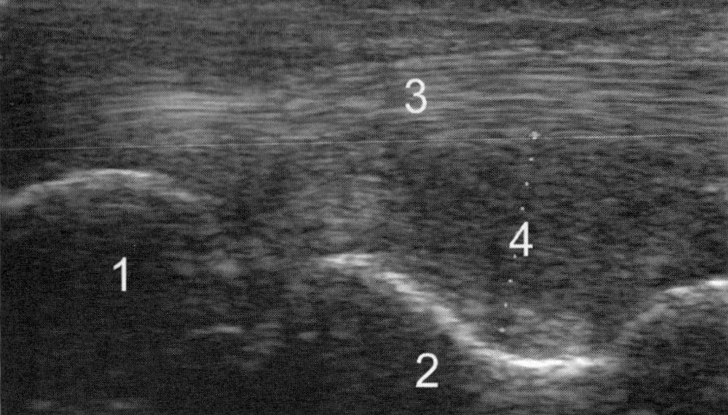

A

B

Fig. 19-27 Ultrasound (US) images of the collateral ligaments of the tarsus. **A,** Longitudinal US images of the tarsus obtained at the lateral aspect of the joint at the level of the lateral digital extensor tendon in a normal horse *(top)* and in a horse with tarsal sprain *(bottom)*. *1,* Tibial malleolus; *2,* talus; *3,* lateral extensor tendon; *4,* short bundle of the lateral collateral ligament. In the bottom image the short bundle of the collateral ligament is thickened and hypoechoic and displaces abaxially the lateral extensor tendon. **B,** Longitudinal US images of the tarsus obtained at the medial aspect of the joint at the level of the medial collateral ligament in a normal horse. *1,* Tibial malleolus; *2,* talus; *3,* long bundle of the medial collateral ligament; *4,* short bundle of the medial collateral ligament.

(tarsus valgus). Foals with incomplete ossification of the tarsal bone may develop degenerative joint disease of the distal intertarsal and tarsometatarsal joints.[42] Prognosis for future athletic soundness seems to be related to the degree of bone collapse (guarded prognosis in foals with more than 30% of collapse of a tarsal bone).[47,48]

Subchondral Cystlike Lesions

Subchondral cystlike lesions in the central and third tarsal bones and in the proximal metatarsus occasionally occur.[8] Subchondral cystlike lesions are radiolucent round to oval areas often surrounded by sclerotic trabecular bone. Because of their small size and the superimposition of the tarsal bones, their diagnosis requires an attentive radiographic reading. In the central and third tarsal bones they are considered a predisposing factor for degenerative joint disease of the distal intertarsal joint.[8,49]

Diseases of the Talocalcaneal and Proximal Intertarsal Joints

Degenerative Joint Disease

Degenerative joint disease of the talocalcaneal and proximal intertarsal joints is uncommon.[50,51] However, because of the high clinical significance of the radiographic findings consistent with degenerative changes in these joints, awareness of this condition is important; it may be responsible for severe hindlimb lameness, with guarded to poor prognosis.[42,50,51] Radiographic signs are subchondral lysis and sclerosis, irregular subchondral surface, and changes in joint space width (Fig. 19-31). Subchondral bone lysis is often the predominant radiographic sign.[51] In the talocalcaneal joint osteophyte formation is difficult to assess because of the anatomy of the joint. The radiographic signs are more evident on the lateromedial view (Fig. 19-32).

Fractures Involving the Tarsus

Fracture of the Distal Tibia and Malleolar Fractures

Tibial stress fractures are common in racehorses and occasionally involve the distal tibia.[28] Intraarticular involvement may follow if the stress fracture spirals distally and becomes comminuted. Severely comminuted intraarticular fractures of the distal tibia are the result of violent traumatic events, including kicks from other horses, dramatic falls, and encounters with vehicles. Physeal Salter-Harris type II fractures are the most frequently encountered tibial fracture in foals.[8]

Sprains of the tarsus result in collateral ligament injury and severe synovial effusion.[8] Avulsion fracture of the malleolus may occur in association with collateral ligament damage.[8,42,52] One or more separated sharp bony fragments are seen at the lateral or medial aspect of the proximal tarsal row close to the fractured malleolus, which has a bony defect (see Fig. 19-26). The lateral malleolus is more commonly involved.[8,42] The size and shape of the fragment, the bony defect, the shape of the

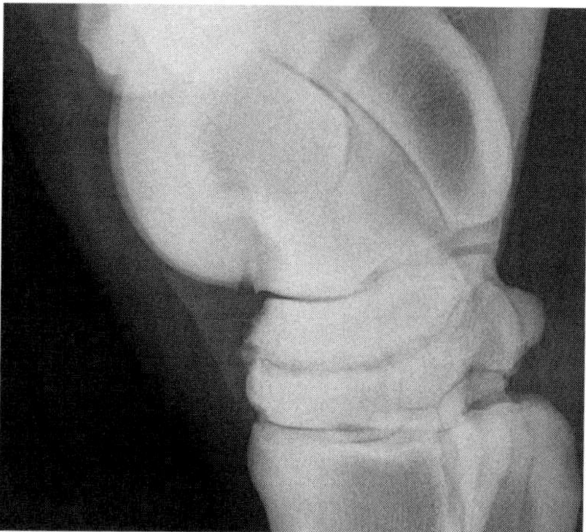

Fig. 19-28 Lateromedial radiograph of the tarsus of a horse with distal intertarsal degenerative joint disease. Osteophyte formation has occurred at the dorsal aspect of the distal intertarsal joint. The joint space is ill defined and seems enlarged because of radiolucency of the lytic subchondral bone. The trabecular bone of the central and third tarsal bone is sclerotic.

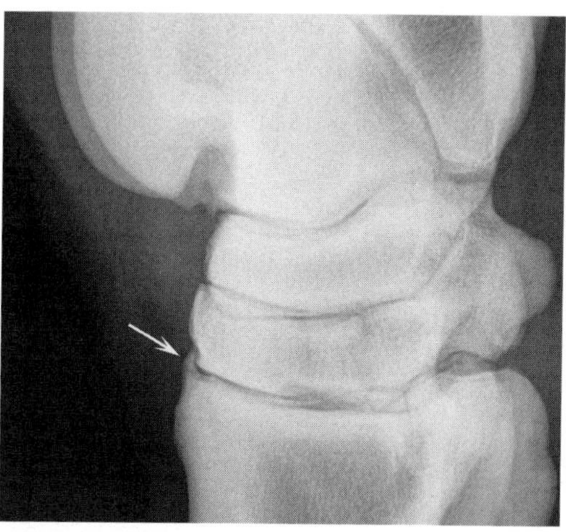

Fig. 19-29 Lateromedial radiograph of the tarsus of a clinically normal horse. A large bony spur with well-defined contour is present at the dorsoproximal margin of the third metatarsal bone *(arrow)*. No changes in opacity are present in the articular margins or in the subchondral bone. The distal margin of the third tarsal bone is smooth and well defined.

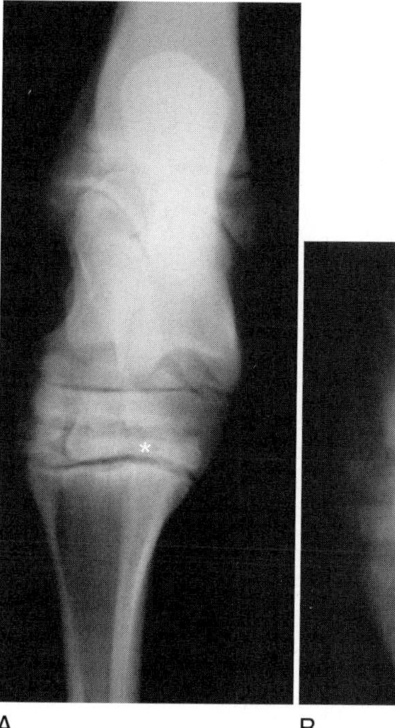

A

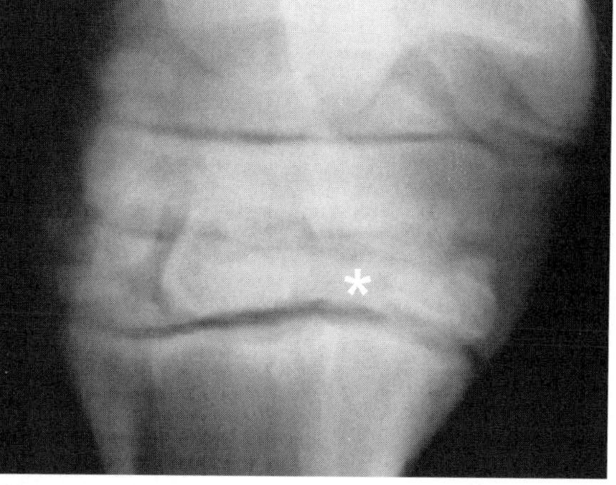

B

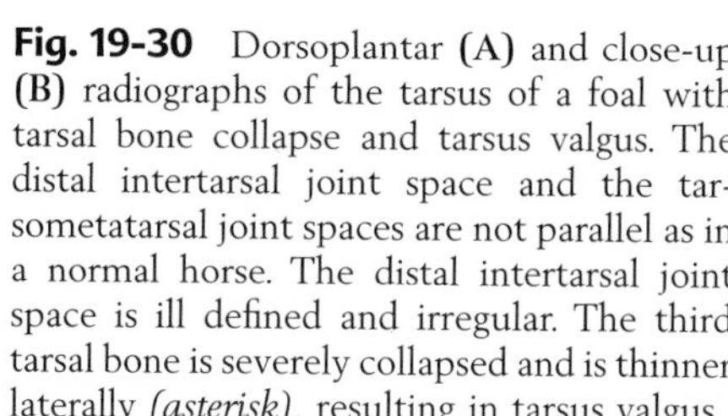

Fig. 19-30 Dorsoplantar (A) and close-up (B) radiographs of the tarsus of a foal with tarsal bone collapse and tarsus valgus. The distal intertarsal joint space and the tarsometatarsal joint spaces are not parallel as in a normal horse. The distal intertarsal joint space is ill defined and irregular. The third tarsal bone is severely collapsed and is thinner laterally *(asterisk)*, resulting in tarsus valgus.

fractured malleolus, and the clinical history and signs should help differentiate this condition from osteochondrosis (see Fig. 19-24).[8,42]

Central and Third Tarsal Bones and Proximal Metatarsal Fractures

Fractures of the central and third tarsal bones and the proximal metatarsus occur in racehorses, mainly Standardbreds.[53,54] Fractures of the central and third tarsal bones are difficult to detect because of the complex anatomy of the tarsus and the superimposition of tarsal bones. Often several oblique views are needed to identify the fracture line. If the fracture line cannot be seen at the first radiographic examination but the clinical history and signs strongly suggest a tarsal fracture, the horse should be rested and radiographs should be repeated 7 to 10 days after the lameness onset.[8,42] Rarefaction of the fracture margins will make the fracture line more obvious. Fractures of the central and third tarsal bones are usually slab fractures.[8] Third tarsal bone fractures are more commonly dorsal or dorsolateral.[42] A significant association between a wedge-shaped conformation of the third tarsal bone and the occurrence of slab fractures of this bone has been demonstrated in racehorses.[55] Intraarticular fractures of the proximal metatarsus involving the dorsal aspect of the bone are reported in racehorses.[54,56] These fractures are more commonly incomplete.[54,56]

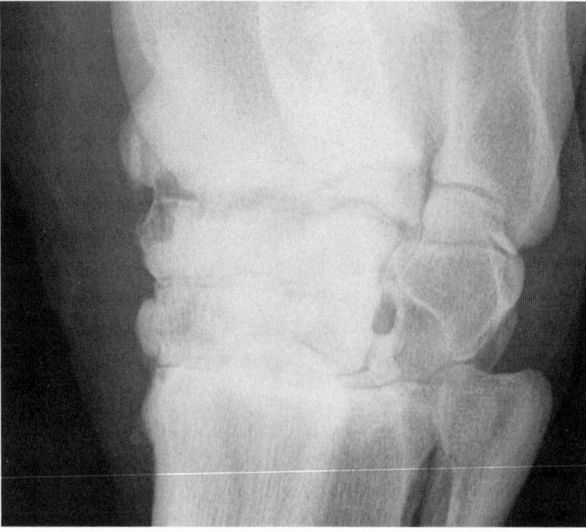

Fig. 19-31 Dorsolateral-plantaromedial oblique radiograph of the tarsus in a horse with severe hindlimb lameness and moderate distension of the tarsocrural joint attributable to degenerative disease of the proximal intertarsal joint. The tarsocrural joint is swollen. Remodeling of the dorsomedial margins of the intertarsal and tarsometatarsal joints has occurred. A severe subchondral lysis and subchondral bone surface irregularity are present in the proximal intertarsal joint. The proximal intertarsal joint space appears wider because of the subchondral lysis. The distal intertarsal and tarsometatarsal joints are also thinner than normal.

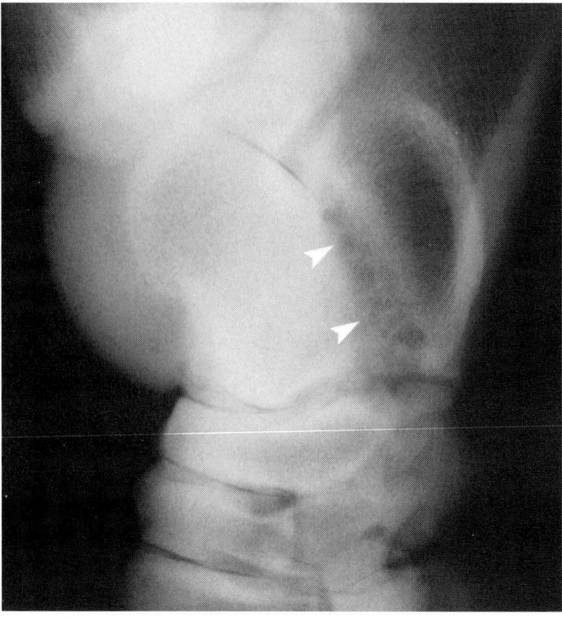

Fig. 19-32 Lateromedial radiograph of a horse with severe hindlimb lameness and moderate distension of the tarsocrural joint. The distal portion of the talocalcaneal joint appears widened *(arrowheads)* because of severe subchondral bone lysis. These findings are indicative of severe degenerative joint disease of the talocalcaneal joint.

Miscellaneous Conditions Involving the Tarsus

Septic Arthritis

Septic arthritis may occur in foals or adult horses.[33] The tarsocrural joint is the most commonly affected, especially in adult horses.[8] Diagnosis of septic arthritis is not a radiographic diagnosis but is based on clinical signs and analysis of the synovial fluid. Radiographic examination is essential to establish bone or physeal involvement, especially in foals. Soft tissue and joint swelling in a non-weight-bearing limb may be the only radiographic signs of septic arthritis. When bone damage occurs, it is seen as ill-defined subchondral radiolucencies. Radiographic changes may be apparent within 7 to 10 days after the onset of clinical sings. In the small bones of the tarsus in foals, radiolucent changes may be delayed because infarction caused by infection may slow bone resorption.[33]

Osteomyelitis of the Calcaneus

Osteomyelitis of the calcaneus involving the tuber calcanei and/or the sustentaculum tali is seen in horses after penetrating injuries of the point of the tarsus.[57,58] Septic calcaneal bursitis and infection of tarsal synovial sheath may be associated with osteomyelitis of the tuber calcanei and osteomyelitis of the sustentaculum tali, respectively.[56,57] Radiographic signs of calcaneal osteomyelitis are only seen after substantial bone loss has occurred, typically 10 to 15 days after injury. Repeated radiographic assessment is therefore always suggested to follow up traumatic wounds of the tarsus. Radiographic abnormalities indicative of calcaneal infection are ill-defined areas of decreased bone opacity indicating osteolysis and irregular bone contour (Fig. 19-33). Mild to moderate bony proliferation is more common in chronic sepsis with proliferative osteitis.[58] Fragmentation and sequestra, seen as bony fragments surrounded by a radiolucent halo, which is then enveloped by sclerotic bone, may develop on the tuber calcanei as a result of the minimal tissue covering the region and the relatively poor blood supply.[58,59]

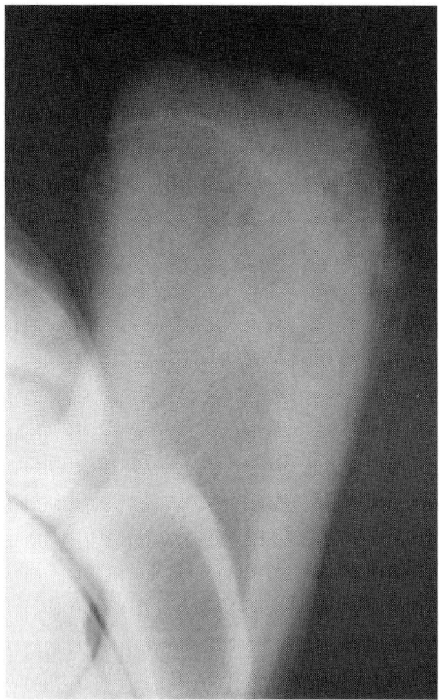

Fig. 19-33 Lateromedial radiograph of the calcaneus of a horse with a penetrating injury of the point of the tarsus. Several ill-defined radiolucent areas are present in the calcaneus, mainly at its plantar aspect. No marked periosteal reaction is visible, but some marginal irregularity of the dorsal and plantar contours of the calcaneus likely represent bony proliferation. No sharp transition zone exists between abnormal and normal bone. Surrounding soft tissues are swollen. These findings categorize the bone lesion as aggressive and suggest calcaneal osteomyelitis after the penetrating injury.

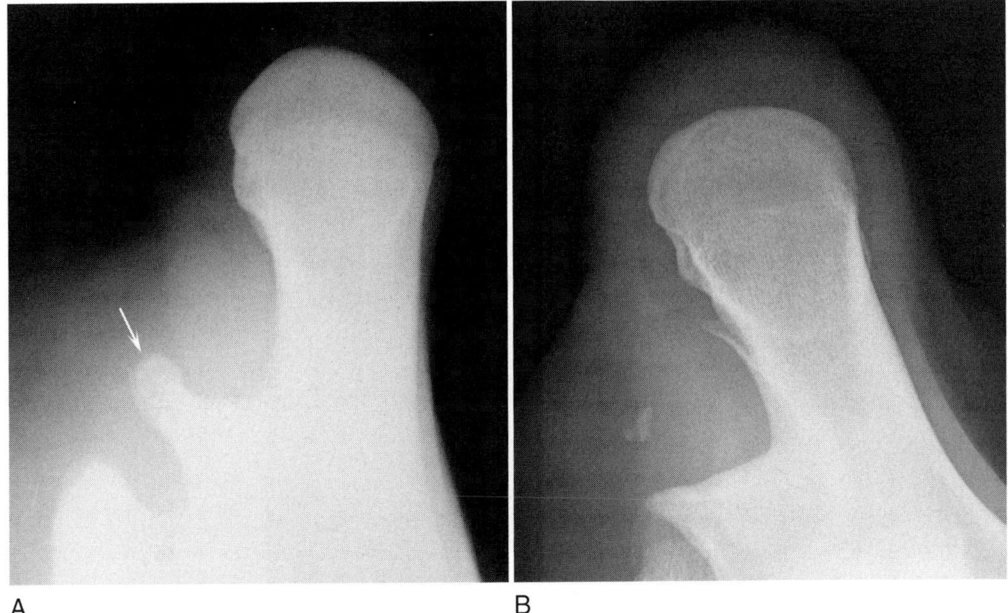

Fig. 19-34 Plantaroproximal-plantarodistal oblique views of the sustentaculum tali of two horses with aseptic chronic tenosynovitis of the tarsal sheath. **A,** A prominent, smooth, bony proliferation is present on the medial margin of the sustentaculum tali *(arrow)*. **B,** The soft tissues plantar to the sustentaculum tali are thickened, and two focal areas of mineralization with smooth margins are visible plantar to the sustentaculum tali. These likely represent dystrophic calcifications in the soft tissues. Mild remodeling of the medial margin of the sustentaculum tali and a bony proliferation on the axial surface of the tuber calcanei are visible.

Abnormalities of the Sustentaculum Tali and Tarsal Sheath Tenosynovitis

The tarsal sheath is the synovial sheath enveloping the lateral digital flexor tendon at the level of the tarsus.[60] The lateral digital flexor tendon joins the medial digital flexor tendon at the plantar aspect of the proximal metatarsus to form the deep digital flexor tendon.[60] The lateral digital flexor tendon passes over the sustentaculum tali, which serves as a gliding groove.[60] Tenosynovitis of the tarsal sheath frequently produces an obvious effusion easily detectable on radiographs as soft tissue swelling at the medial aspect of the tarsus or between the distal tibia and the calcaneus. Radiographic abnormalities of the sustentaculum tali may be seen in horses with chronic aseptic tenosynovitis or when local infection is present as a consequence of a penetrating wound (Figs. 19-34 and 19-35).[8] In chronic tenosynovitis, bony proliferations at the insertion of the flexor retinaculum are a sign of enthesopathy. Calcifications may be seen in the soft tissues (see Fig. 19-34).[8] In horses with proven or suspected infection of the tarsal sheath, an irregular contour of the sustentaculum tali, osteolysis with or without bony proliferation, fragmentation, and sequestra are signs of concurrent bone involvement and osteomyelitis (Fig. 19-35). Dysplasia of the sustentaculum tali has been reported as a cause of tarsal sheath tenosynovitis because of mechanical medial displacement of the lateral digital flexor tendon during movement.[8]

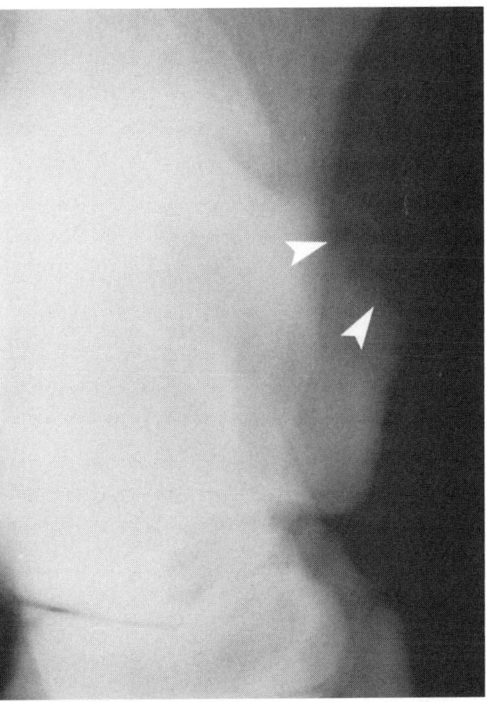

Fig. 19-35 Plantarolateral-dorsomedial oblique radiograph of the tarsus of a horse with a penetrating wound of the tarsus and septic tenosynovitis of the tarsal sheath. A large heterogeneous radiolucent area *(arrowheads)* is visible in the sustentaculum tali, suggesting osteomyelitis.

Proximal Insertion Suspensory Desmopathy and Enthesopathy

Proximal insertion desmopathies of the suspensory ligament are a common cause of lameness in sport horses.[61] Radiographic signs may be visible in chronic insertional desmopathy when the point of tendon insertion onto bone is involved. Lateromedial radiographs of the tarsus and proximal metatarsus are characterized by subcortical sclerosis or thickening of

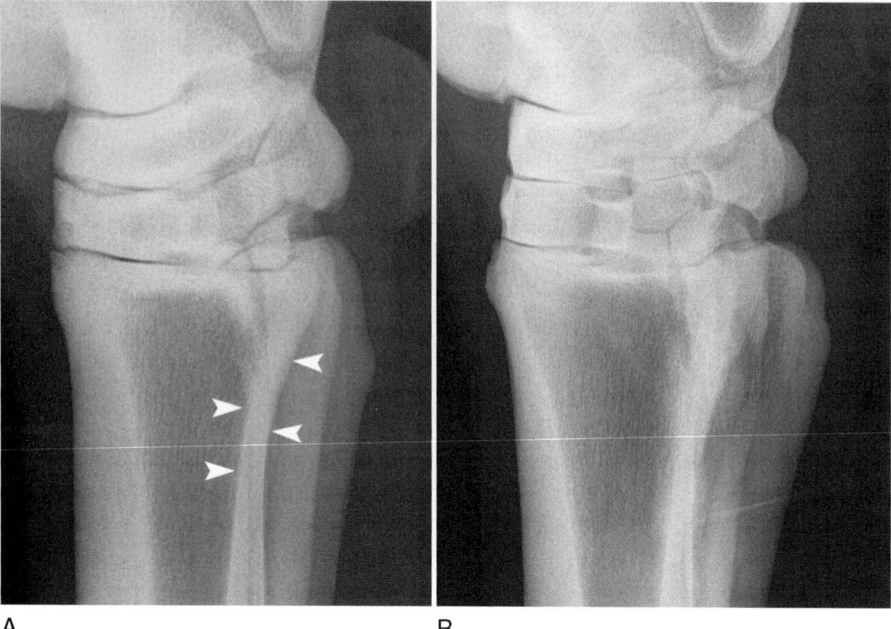

Fig. 19-36 Lateromedial radiographs of the proximal metatarsal region of a normal horse **(A)** and a horse with proximal insertional desmopathy of the suspensory ligament **(B)**. **A,** The plantar cortex of the third metatarsal bone is smooth at the level of the insertion of the proximal suspensory ligament *(arrowheads)*. **B,** The plantar surface of the plantar cortex of the third metatarsal bone is quite irregular, and mild subcortical sclerosis is present (the projection is slightly different compared with **A**). Ultrasonography confirmed proximal suspensory desmopathy with bony involvement at the enthesis.

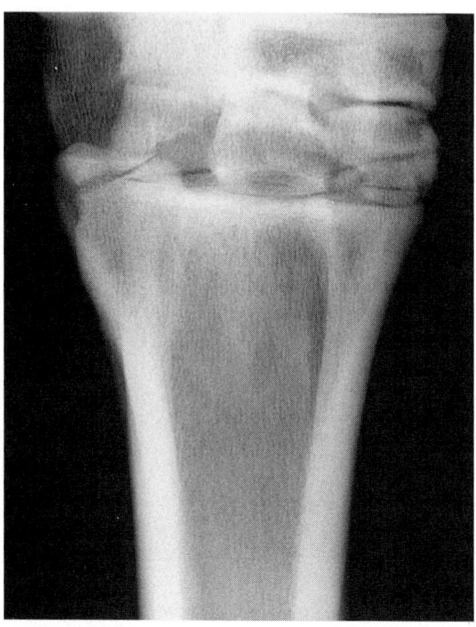

Fig. 19-37 Dorsoplantar radiograph of the proximal aspect of the metatarsus of a horse with proximal insertional desmopathy of the suspensory ligament. Note the ill-defined increased opacity involving the proximolateral aspect of the third metatarsal bone.

the plantar cortex of the third metatarsal bone (Fig. 19-36). The dorsoplantar view of the proximal metatarsus may be characterized by an increased homogeneous or mixed opacity (Fig. 19-37), often visible as proximodistal ill-defined stripes. Radiographic evaluation of the contralateral limb is indicated to either compare radiographic appearance with a normal bone or assess bilateral involvement because this condition is frequently bilateral in the hindlimbs. Avulsion fracture may occur at the site of the proximal insertion of the suspensory ligament on the third metatarsal bone.

REFERENCES

1. Jeffcott LB, Kold SE: Stifle lameness in the horse: a survey of 96 referred cases, *Equine Vet J* 14:31, 1982.
2. Edwards RB, Nixon AJ: Avulsion of the cranial cruciate ligament insertion in a horse, *Equine Vet J* 28:334, 1996.
3. Prades M, Grant BD: Injuries to the cranial cruciate ligament and associated structures: summary of clinical, radiographic, arthroscopic and pathological findings from 10 horses, *Equine Vet J* 21:354, 1989.
4. Walmsley JP: The stifle. In Ross MW, Dyson SJ, editors: *Diagnosis and management of lameness in the horse,* St. Louis, 2003, Saunders.
5. De Busscher V, Busoni V, Bolen G et al: Soft tissue lesions of the equine femoro-tibial joints diagnosed by ultrasonography: 74 cases (2000-2005), *J Equine Vet Sci* 26:434, 2006.
6. Flynn KA, Whitcomb MB: Equine meniscal injuries: a retrospective study of 14 horses, *Proc Am Assoc Equine Pract* 48:249, 2002.
7. Dik KJ, Enzerink E, Van Weeren PR: Radiographic development of osteochondral abnormalities in the hock and stifle of Dutch Warmblood foals, from age 1 to 11 months, *Equine Vet J* 31(suppl):9, 1999.
8. Butler JA, Colles CM, Dyson SJ et al, editors: The stifle and tibia. In *Clinical radiology of the horse,* ed 2, London, 2000, Blackwell.
9. Kane AJ, Park RD, McIlwraith CW et al: Radiographic changes in Thoroughbred yearlings. Part 1: prevalence at the time of the yearling sales, *Equine Vet J* 35:354, 2005.
10. Gibson KE, McIlwraith CV, Park RD et al: Production of patellar lesions by medial patellar desmotomy in horses, *Vet Surg* 18:466, 1989.
11. Labens R, Busoni V, Peters F et al: Ultrasonographic and radiographic diagnosis of patellar fragmentation secondary to bilateral medial patellar ligament desmotomy in a Warmblood gelding, *Equine Vet Educ* 17:201, 2005.
12. McIlwraith CW: Osteochondral fragmentation of the distal aspect of the patella in horses, *Equine Vet J* 22:157, 1990.
13. Engelbert TA, Tate LP, Richardson DC et al: Lateral patellar luxation in miniature horses, *Vet Surg* 22:293, 1993.

14. Hermans WA, Kerjes AW, Van Des Mey GKK et al: Investigation into the heredity of congenital lateral patellar (sub)luxation in the Shetland Pony, *Vet Q* 9:1, 1987.
15. Kobluk CN: Correction of patellar luxation by recession sulcoplasty in three foals, *Vet Surg* 22:298, 1993.
16. Scott GS, Crawford WH, Colahan PT et al: Arthroscopic findings in the horses with subtle radiographic evidence of osteochondral lesions of the medial femoral condyle: 15 cases (1995-2002), *J Am Vet Med Assoc* 224:1823, 2004.
17. Howard RD, McIlwraith CW, Trotter GW: Arthroscopic surgery for subchondral cystic lesions of the medial femoral condyle in horses: 41 cases (1988-1991), *J Am Vet Med Assoc* 206:842, 1995.
18. Hance SR, Schneider RK, Embertson RM et al: Lesions of the caudal aspect of the femoral condyles in foals: 20 cases (1980-1990), *J Am Vet Med Assoc* 202:637, 1993.
19. Textor JA, Nixon AJ, Lumsden J et al: Subchondral cystic lesions of the proximal extremity of the tibia in horses: 12 cases (1983-2000), *J Am Vet Med Assoc* 218:408, 2001.
20. Walmsley JP: Vertical tears of the cranial horn of the meniscus and its cranial ligament in the equine femorotibial joint: 7 cases and their treatment by arthroscopic surgery, *Equine Vet J* 27:20, 1995.
21. Rose PL, Graham JP, Moore I et al: Imaging diagnosis—caudal cruciate ligament avulsion in a horse, *Vet Radiol Ultrasound* 42:414, 2001.
22. Sanders-Shamis M, Bukowiecki CF, Biller DS: Cruciate and collateral ligament failure in the equine stifle: seven cases, *J Am Vet Med Assoc* 193:573, 1988.
23. Mueller PO, Allen D, Watson E et al: Arthroscopic removal of a fragment from an intercondylar eminence fracture of the tibia in a two-year-old horse, *J Am Vet Med Assoc* 204:1794, 1994.
24. Dik KJ, Nemeth F: Traumatic patella fractures in the horse, *Equine Vet J* 15:244, 1983.
25. Dyson S, Wright I, Kold S et al: Clinical and radiographic features, treatment and outcome in 15 horses with fracture of the medial aspect of the patella, *Equine Vet J* 24:264, 1992.
26. Dyson SJ: Stifle trauma in the event horse, *Equine Vet Educ* 6:234, 1994.
27. Arnold CE, Schaer TP, Baird DL et al: Conservative management of 17 horses with nonarticular fractures of the tibial tuberosity, *Equine Vet J* 35:202, 2003.
28. Ross MW: The crus. In Ross MW, Dyson SJ, editors: *Diagnosis and management of lameness in the horse,* St. Louis, 2003, Saunders.
29. Blikslager AT: Avulsion of the origin of the peroneus tertius tendon in a foal, *J Am Vet Med Assoc* 204:1484, 1994.
30. Holcombe SJ, Bertone A: Avulsion fracture of the origin of the extensor digitorum longus muscle in a foal, *J Am Vet Med Assoc* 204:1652, 1994.
31. *The American Heritage Stedman's Medical Dictionary,* 2004, Houghton Mifflin Company: http://medical-dictionary.thefreedictionary.com/calcinosis%20circumscripta. Accessed October 31, 2005.
32. Dodd DC, Raker CW: Tumoral calcinosis (calcinosis circumscripta) in the horse, *J Am Vet Med Assoc* 57:968, 1970.
33. Bertone A: Infectious arthritis. In Ross MW, Dyson SJ, editors: *Diagnosis and management of lameness in the horse,* St. Louis, 2003, Saunders.
34. Sandgren B: Bony fragments in the tarsocrural and metacarpo- or metatarsophalangeal joints in the Standardbred horse—a radiographic survey, *Equine Vet J Suppl* 6:66, 1988.
35. Grondahl AM: The incidence of osteochondrosis in the tibiotarsal joint of Norwegian Standardbred trotters—a radiographic study, *Equine Vet Sci* 11:272, 1991.
36. Richardson DW: Diagnosis and management of osteochondrosis and osseous cyst-like lesions. In Ross MW, Dyson SJ, editors: *Diagnosis and management of lameness in the horse,* St. Louis, 2003, Saunders.
37. Jørgensen HS, Proschowsky H, Falk-Rønne J et al: The significance of routine radiographic findings with respect to subsequent racing performance and longevity in Standardbred trotters, *Equine Vet J* 29:55, 1997.
38. McIlwraith CW, Foerner JJ, Davis DM: Osteochondritis dissecans of tarsocrural joint: results of treatment with arthroscopic surgery, *Equine Vet J* 23:155, 1991.
39. Simpson CM, Lumsden JM: Unusual osteochondral lesions of the talus in a horse, *Aust Vet J* 79:752, 2001.
40. Dyson SJ: Radiography and radiology. In Ross MW, Dyson SJ, editors: *Diagnosis and management of lameness in the horse,* St. Louis, 2003, Saunders.
41. Trotter GW, McIlwraith CW: Osteochondritis dissecans and subchondral cystic lesions and their relationship to osteochondrosis in the horse, *J Equine Vet Sci* 1:157, 1981.
42. Debareiner RM, Carter GK, Dyson SJ: The tarsus. In Ross MW, Dyson SJ, editors: *Diagnosis and management of lameness in the horse,* St. Louis, 2003, Saunders.
43. Garcia-Lopez JM, Kirker-Head CA: Occult subchondral osseous cyst-like lesions of the equine tarsocrural joint, *Vet Surg* 33:557, 2004.
44. Laverty S, Stover SM, Bélanger D et al: Radiographic, high detail radiographic, microangiographic and histological findings of the distal portion of the tarsus in weanlings, young and adult horses, *Equine Vet J* 23:413, 1991.
45. Björnsdóttir S, Axelsson M, Eksell P et al: Radiographic and clinical survey of degenerative joint disease in the distal tarsal joints in Icelandic horses, *Equine Vet J* 32:268, 2000.
46. Björnsdóttir S, Ekman S, Eksell P et al: High detail radiography and histology of the centrodistal tarsal joint of Icelandic horses 6 months to 6 years, *Equine Vet J* 36:5, 2004.
47. Dutton DM, Watkins JP, Walker MA et al: Incomplete ossification of the tarsal bones in foals: 22 cases (1988-1996), *J Am Vet Med Assoc* 213:1590, 1998.
48. Dutton DM, Watkins JP, Honnas CM et al: Treatment response and athletic outcome of foals with tarsal valgus deformities: 39 cases (1988-1997), *J Am Vet Med Assoc* 215:1482, 1999.
49. Watrous BJ, Hultgren BD, Wagner PC: Osteochondrosis and juvenile spavin in equids, *Am J Vet Res* 52:607, 1991.
50. White NA, Turner TA: Hock lameness associated with degeneration of the talocalcaneal articulation: report of two cases in horses, *Vet Med Small Anim Clin* 75:678, 1980.
51. Smith RKW, Dyson SJ, Schramme MC et al: Osteoarthritis of the talocalcaneal joint in 18 horses, *Equine Vet J* 37:166, 2005.
52. Jakovljevic S, Gibbs C, Yeats JJ: Traumatic fractures of the equine hock: a report of 13 cases, *Equine Vet J* 14:62, 1982.
53. Tulamo RM, Bramlage LR, Gabel AA: Fractures of the central and third tarsal bone in horses, *J Am Vet Med Assoc* 182:1234, 1983.
54. Ross MV, Sponseller ML, Gill HE et al: Articular fracture of the dorsoproximolateral aspect of the third metatarsal bone in five Standardbred racehorses, *J Am Vet Med Assoc* 203:698, 1993.
55. Baird DH, Pilsworth RC: Wedge-shaped conformation of the dorsolateral aspect of the third tarsal bone in the Thoroughbred racehorse is associated with development

of slab fractures in this site, *Equine Vet J* 33:617, 2001.
56. Pilsworth RC: Incomplete fracture of the dorsal aspect of the proximal cortex of the third metatarsal bone as a cause of hind limb lameness in the racing Thoroughbred: a review of three cases, *Equine Vet J* 24:147, 1992.
57. Hand DR, Watkins JP, Honnas CM et al: Osteomyelitis of the sustentaculum tali in horses: 10 cases (1992-1998), *J Am Vet Med Assoc* 219:341, 2001.
58. Post EM, Singer ER, Clegg PD et al: Retrospective study of 24 cases of septic calcaneal bursitis in the horse, *Equine Vet J* 35:662, 2003.
59. May KA, Moll HD, Carrig CB et al: What is your diagnosis? *J Am Vet Med Assoc* 214:627, 1999.
60. Barone R: *Anatomie comparée des mammiféres domestiques, tome 2 arthrologie et myologie,* Paris, 1989, Vigot.
61. Dyson SJ, Genovese RL: The suspensory apparatus. In Ross MW, Dyson SJ, editors: *Diagnosis and management of lameness in the horse,* St. Louis, 2003, Saunders.

ELECTRONIC RESOURCES evolve

Additional information related to the content in Chapter 19 can be found on the companion Web site at evolve http://evolve.elsevier.com/Thrall/vetrad/

- Key Points
- Chapter Quiz
- Case Study 19-1
- Case Study 19-2
- Case Study 19-3

CHAPTER • 20
The Equine Carpus

Rachel C. Murray
Sue J. Dyson

ANATOMY

The equine carpus is composed of three main articulations: the antebrachiocarpal or radiocarpal joint; the middle carpal or midcarpal joint, and the carpometacarpal joint. The equine carpus incorporates two rows of cuboidal bones, the carpal bones.[1] The antebrachiocarpal joint is formed by the distal radius proximally and the proximal row of carpal bones (radial, intermediate, ulnar, and accessory carpal bones) distally. The middle carpal joint is the articulation formed between the proximal (radial, intermediate, and ulnar carpal bones) and distal (second, third, and fourth carpal bones) rows of carpal bones. The carpometacarpal joint describes the articulation between the distal row of carpal bones and the second, third, and fourth metacarpal bones. Vertically oriented joints between adjacent carpal bones within each row are referred to as intercarpal joints. The antebrachiocarpal and middle carpal joints provide flexion and extension for the carpus, whereas the carpometacarpal joint is capable of only minimal motion.

Within each row, the carpal bones are connected by two interosseous ligaments, described as intercarpal ligaments, and two transverse dorsal ligaments.[1] Within the middle carpal joint are two palmar ligaments, which attach the proximal and distal row of carpal bones. The medial palmar intercarpal ligament joins the radial with the second and third carpal bones, and the lateral palmar intercarpal ligament joins the ulnar with the third and fourth carpal bones.

When the carpus is flexed, the radial carpal bone moves distally relative to the intermediate and ulnar carpal bones. The accessory carpal bone, situated on the palmar aspect of the carpus, articulates with the distal lateral aspect of the radius and the ulnar carpal bone.[2,3]

The complex anatomy of the carpus makes radiographic interpretation challenging. Comparison with a normal set of radiographs and with bone specimens is helpful.

NORMAL VARIATIONS

The presence of the first and fifth carpal bones is variable, as is their shape and size and proximity to adjacent bones (Figs. 20-1 and 20-2). These bones should not be confused with osteochondral fragments. The first carpal bone occurs in approximately 30% of horses but varies in widely in size and may articulate with one or both of the second carpal and metacarpal bones.[3] The fifth carpal bone occurs only rarely. Lucent zones in the ulnar carpal bone at the site of articulation of the fifth carpal bone, and the second carpal and the proximal aspect of the second metacarpal bones at the site of articulation of the first carpal bone (see Fig. 20-1), are normal features of these articulations and should not be misinterpreted as a lytic lesion. The accessory carpal bone may occasionally develop from more than one center of ossification. Fusion usually subsequently occurs, but radiographic separation may be identified during the first 6 months of age.[3,4]

Incidental findings in the distal aspect of the radius include medial and lateral protrusions of the cortex at the distal radial physis in a mature horse (Fig. 20-3), noted particularly on oblique projections. The caudal aspect of the radius may be slightly irregular immediately proximal to the physis.[5] If fusion of the distal radial and distal ulnar epiphyses is delayed, a radiolucent line or rounded radiolucency may remain in the distal radial epiphysis, possibly with a notch in the articular surface at this location. Vestigial remnants of the ulna may occur in some horses and are visible radiographically when ossification of a fibrous remnant occurs.[3]

Small radiolucent zones may occur within any carpal bone, especially the ulnar and second carpal bones, the majority of which are of no clinical significance.

When interpreting radiographs, articulations between the carpal bones should not be confused with sagittal plane fractures of the third carpal bone.[6] For example, in dorsoproximal-dorsodistal (skyline) views of the distal row of carpal bones, the articulation between the third and fourth carpal bones should not be confused with a parasagittal fracture of the lateral aspect of the third carpal bone. On the dorsomedial-palmarolateral oblique view, the articulation between the second and third carpal bones should not be confused with a parasagittal fracture of the medial aspect of the third carpal bone.

Variations in carpal bone shape and structure can depend on the training history of the horse. For example, in horses that have raced or undergone strenuous galloping training, smooth enlargement or modeling of the dorsal aspect of carpal bones is frequently found, and entheseous new bone on the dorsal surface of the carpal bones as the only radiologic abnormality may be clinically insignificant.[3]

Training also has an effect on subchondral and cancellous bone density and mineralization. Therefore horses worked on a soft surface with low training intensity are likely to have thinner subchondral bone at the carpal articular surfaces and less dense cancellous bone than horses with a history of strenuous galloping exercise.[7] This should be taken into account when evaluating radiographs and be differentiated from the severe subchondral bone sclerosis in the third carpal bone that may be associated with osteochondral and slab fractures.[8] Interpretation of the clinical significance of sclerosis of the radial facet of the third carpal in both Thoroughbred and Standardbred racehorses may require nuclear scintigraphy to distinguish between adaptational and pathologic change.

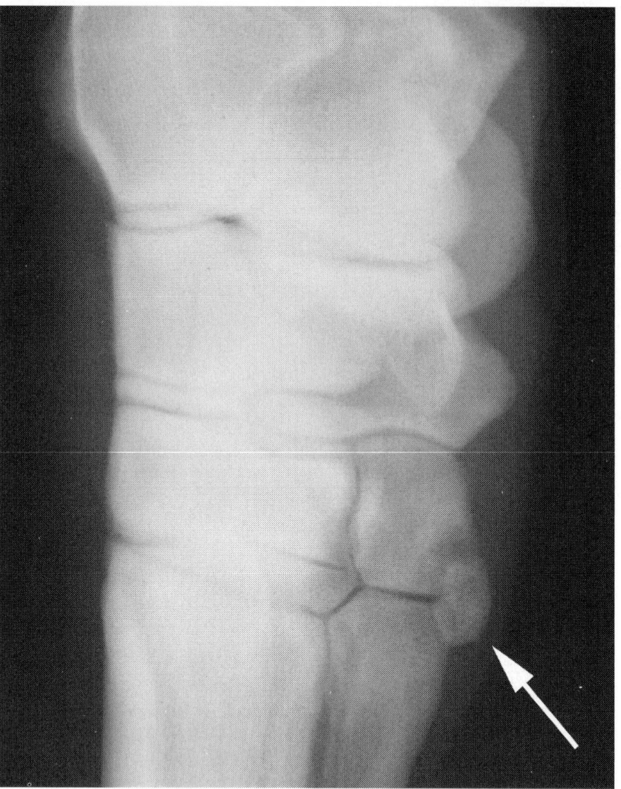

Fig. 20-1 Dorsomedial-palmarolateral view of a carpus. A first carpal bone is present *(arrow)*. Also note the radiolucent zone in the adjacent second carpal bone. These are normal variants.

The presence of small enthesophytes or osteophytes is frequently incidental in mature sports horses but should also be considered as a potential indicator of osteoarthritic change when lameness is isolated to the carpal joints by local analgesia. The significance of these findings may depend on the athletic demands of the horse.

ABNORMALITIES

Developmental

Distal Radial Physitis/Epiphysitis

Distal radial physitis is most commonly seen in horses from 4 to 12 months of age,[9] although the distal radial physis in horses up to 2 years old that have recently entered training may also be affected.[10,11] Physitis occurs when endochondral ossification in the metaphyseal growth cartilage is disrupted.[10]

Standard views are recommended, although the dorsopalmar may be most useful. The physis appears wider with irregular margins as a result of remodeling of the surrounding metaphysis (Fig. 20-4). The physis appears flared at the edges from periosteal new bone formation, with the edges of the physis appearing to protrude from the surface of the cortex on both proximal and distal aspects of the physis.[3,10] Associated soft tissue swelling may be present at the site.

Incomplete Ossification of Carpal Bones

Premature or dysmature foals may have incomplete ossification of the carpal bones at birth (Fig. 20-5). This may lead to secondary angular limb deformity resulting from collapse of the poorly ossified carpal bones that cannot withstand the forces of normal weight bearing.[12,13]

Although a dorsopalmar view is the most useful for assessing the degree of deformity,[12,13] obtaining a full radiographic

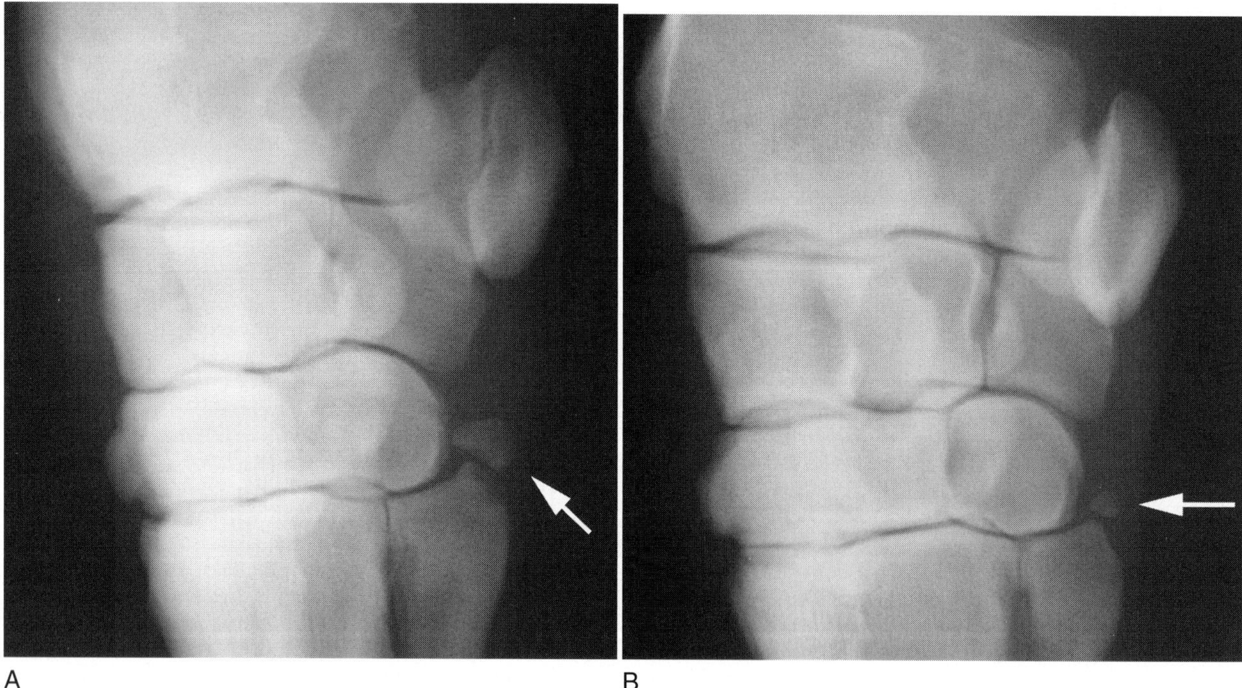

Fig. 20-2 **A,** Dorsolateral-palmaromedial oblique view of a left carpus. A fifth carpal bone is present *(arrow)*. Also note the unusual shape of the base (head) of the fourth metacarpal bone. These are normal variants. **B,** Dorsolateral-palmaromedial oblique view of the right carpus of the same horse as in **A.** A fifth carpal bone is present *(arrow)* but it is smaller and rounder than in the left forelimb. The shape of the base of the fourth metacarpal bone is more normal.

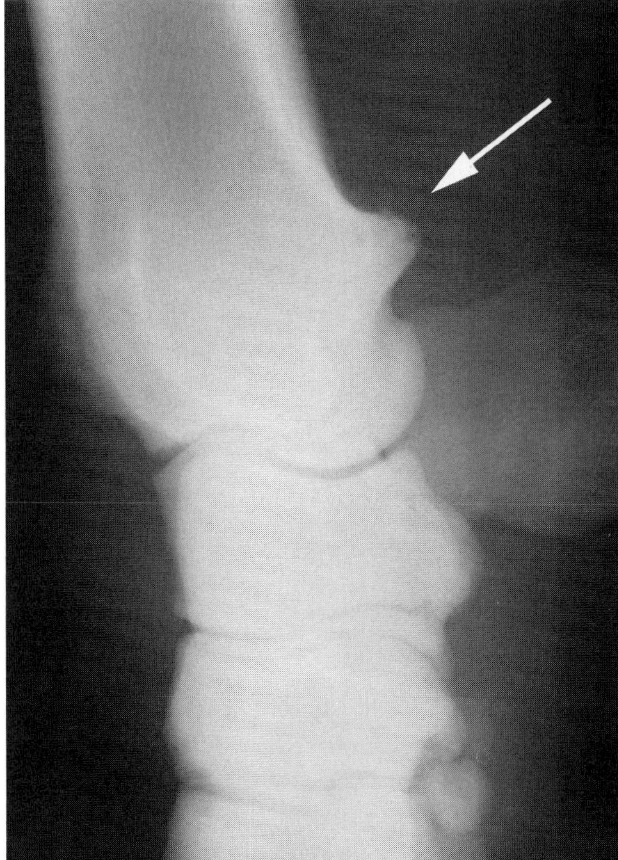

Fig. 20-3 Lateromedial view of a carpus, deliberately underexposed, to demonstrate the prominent medial and lateral protrusions (superimposed) at the caudal aspect of the distal radial physis (*arrow*). This is a normal variant. Also note the presence of both first and fifth carpal bones.

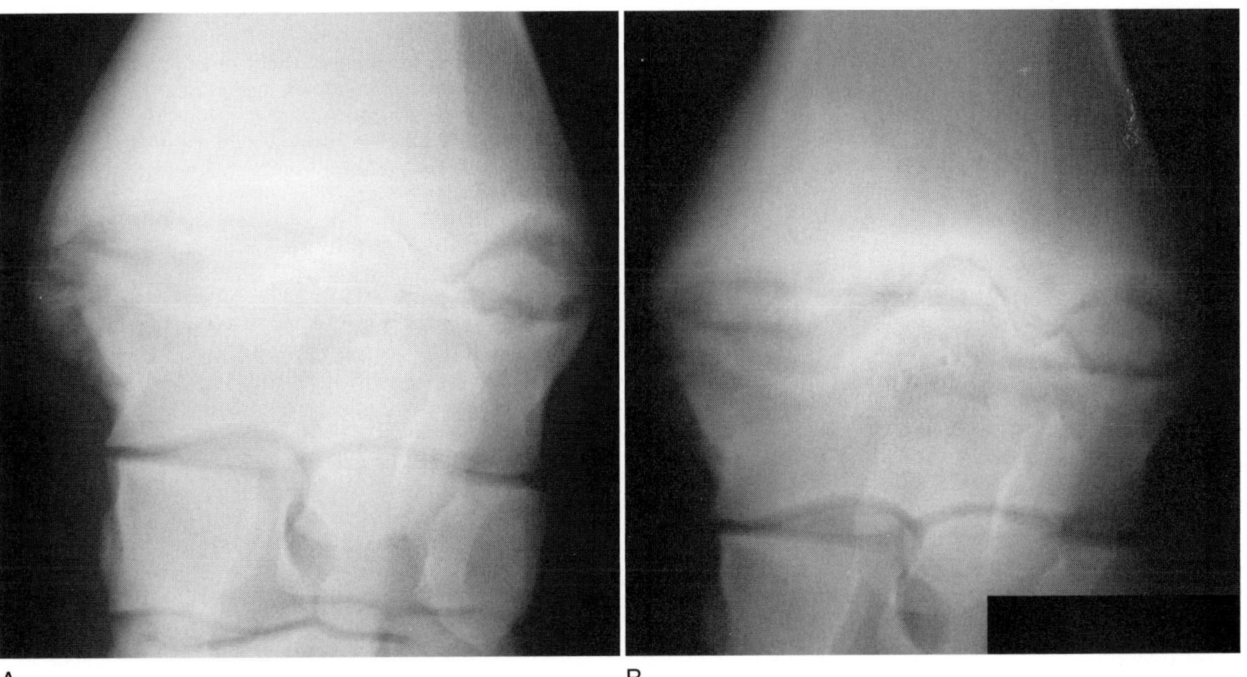

Fig. 20-4 Dorsopalmar views of a carpus of a weanling foal. Medial is to the left. **A** is underexposed to show the flaring of the distal metaphyseal region of the radius, especially notable medially, and the irregular new bone on the medial aspect of the distal radial epiphysis. The distal radial physis is quite irregular, consistent with distal radial physitis. **B** was obtained by using higher exposure. Generalized sclerosis of the distal metaphyseal region of the radius is present medially. Note the irregular widening of the physis.

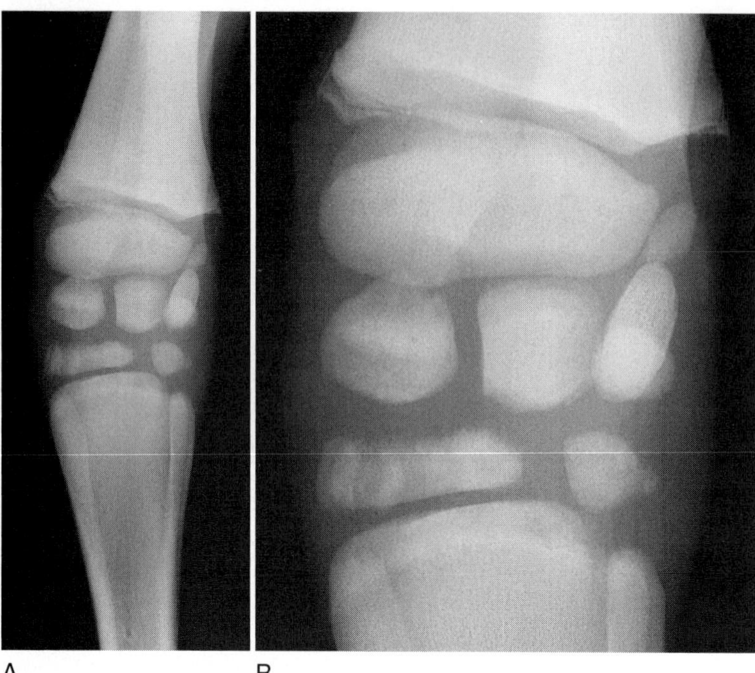

Fig. 20-5 Dorsopalmar view (A) and close-up view (B) of a carpus of a premature foal. Medial is to the left. The carpal bones are small and have irregular margins as a result of incomplete ossification. An angular limb deformity is already present.

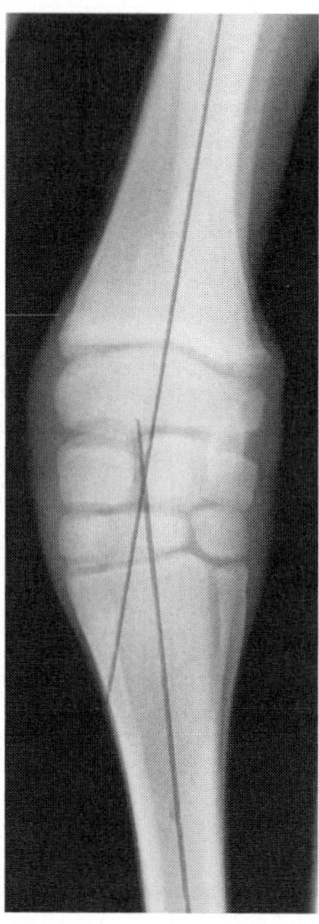

Fig. 20-6 Dorsopalmar view of a carpus of a 6-week-old foal. Medial is to the left. Mild soft tissue swelling is present on the medial aspect of the carpus. The carpal bones are more rounded than normal and the joint spaces are wider as a result of incomplete ossification. A carpal valgus deformity is associated with this incomplete ossification. Lines bisecting the long axes of the radius and third metacarpal bone intersect at the level of the proximal row of carpal bones.

series is recommended because potential exists for carpal bone deformity in a variety of configurations. The carpal bones appear small and rounded, without their normal cuboidal shape (Fig. 20-6).[3,14] Relative enlargement of intercarpal joint spaces is therefore present. Angular limb deformity may be noted on radiographs, with the deformity at the level of the carpal bones and not the distal radial physis.[3,12,13] Collapse and malformation of one or more carpal bones may be observed in severe cases.

Angular Limb Deformities

Angular limb deformities can arise from congenital, developmental, or acquired conditions.[12,13,15-17] Congenital problems relate to in utero factors such as positioning, infective or chemical insult, nutrition, and skeletal maturity at birth. Developmental abnormalities have been attributed to a variety of factors associated with developmental orthopedic disease, including nutrition, exercise, and overloading, although damage to one side of the joint, epiphysis, or physis leading to asymmetric growth will be exaggerated in the developing horse. Acquired deformities may be the result of trauma, including fracture, or infection.

Standard radiographic views are for severe deformity, if onset is acute, or swelling or lameness is present. Extended dorsopalmar views, including as much of the distal radius and proximal metacarpal region as possible, are most useful in the majority of cases (Fig. 20-7).[3,15]

On dorsopalmar views, the long axis of the radius is out of line with the long axis of the third metacarpal bone. At the level of carpus, valgus deformity (lateral deviation of the distal aspect of the limb) is observed most frequently, but varus deformity (medial deviation) does occur. The location of the abnormality is usually at the level at which maximal deviation occurs. By drawing lines bisecting the long axis of radius and the long axis of the third metacarpal bone, the level of deviation can be determined. When no angular limb deformity is present, the lines drawn through the long bones should be continuous. However, when deviation is present, these lines intersect at the level of maximal deviation, giving a guide to the structures involved. This technique can also be useful for measuring the degree of deformity and monitoring response to treatment. No variation in obliquity of sequential radiographs should occur because this can alter the degree of deviation assessed from the intersecting lines. Another guide to normal alignment is the positioning of the joint surfaces. When no abnormality is present, the articular surfaces of the antebrachiocarpal, middle carpal, and carpometacarpal joints

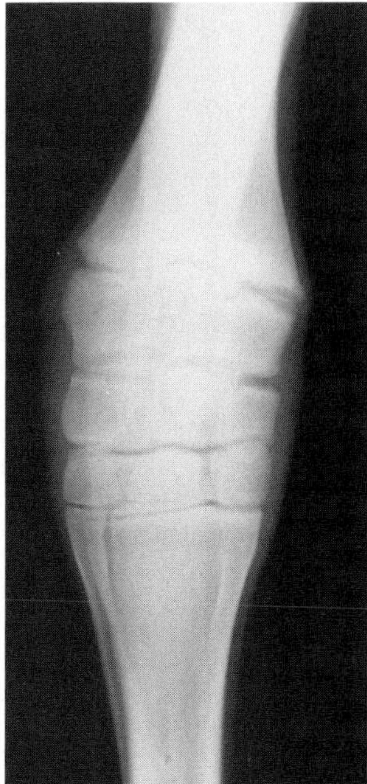

Fig. 20-7 Dorsopalmar view of a carpus of a 4-month-old foal. Medial is to the left. A carpal valgus angular limb deformity is present. The distal radial epiphysis is slightly wedge shaped, being taller medially. The distal radial physis is not parallel with the antebrachiocarpal, middle carpal, or carpometacarpal joints.

should be parallel and perpendicular to the long axis of the limb. With joint-based abnormalities, a loss of articular surface alignment in the affected joint(s) may occur.[3,13,15]

Abnormalities that can be observed include the following, which can be targeted on the basis of the level of maximal deviation.[3,12,13,15-17]

Diaphyseal deformity: This occurs only rarely. The site of maximal deviation is at the level of the diaphysis, making a straight line bisecting the affected long bone impossible to draw.

Distal radial physis abnormality: On dorsopalmar radiographs, the physis may be relatively widened on the medial or lateral aspect and narrow or fused on the opposite side. This is associated with deviation away from the widened side because metaphyseal growth continues on that side but is restricted on the apparently closed aspect of the physis. Location of maximal deviation is at the level of the distal radial physis.

Epiphyseal growth imbalance: The distal radial epiphysis may appear wedge shaped on dorsopalmar radiographs. This may result from dysplasia of the distal radial epiphysis. The lateral styloid process may also be characterized by delayed development. Fusion of the distal radial and distal ulnar epiphyses should occur between 3 and 6 months of age. Altered development of the distal ulnar epiphysis can be seen as lack of growth on the lateral aspect of the distal radius. Location of maximal deviation is at the level of the epiphysis, and the distal radial physis and antebrachiocarpal articular surfaces are no longer parallel.

Incomplete ossification of carpal bones: In severe ossification defects, collapse or deformity of one or more incompletely ossified carpal bones may occur, resulting in angular limb deformity. Location of maximal deviation is at the level of the carpal bones where the collapse or deformity occurs. Lines through the joint spaces may no longer be parallel.

Flaccidity or damage to periarticular structures: Location of maximal deviation may be variable, although it is often at the distal articular surface of the radius. Widening of joint space(s) on one side may occur, although the degree of deformity can vary if medial or lateral stresses are applied.

Osseous or Subchondral Cystlike Lesions

Subchondral or osseous cystlike lesions have been reported in the carpal bones, the proximal aspect of the second or fourth metacarpal bones, and the distal aspect of the radius, with or without an articular component.[3,18] The most commonly reported site is the ulnar carpal bone. Osseous cystlike lesions in the proximal aspect of the second metacarpal bone seem to occur most frequently when a first carpal bone is present (see Fig. 20-1) and may occur in conjunction with a cystlike lesion in the first carpal bone. Osseous cystlike lesions are frequently noted as an incidental finding, but some are associated with lameness.[19] Generally those situated deep in the bone, particularly in the first, second, and ulnar carpal bones, and proximal aspect of the second metacarpal bone, are unlikely to be associated with lameness. However, lesions associated with articular margins and subchondral cystlike lesions in the distal medial aspect of the radius are more likely to be clinically significant (Fig. 20-8).[20] Lameness can vary in severity and progression, and clinical progression may not closely relate to radiographic signs. The use of other diagnostic techniques can give guidance about the current activity of the bone around the cystic lesion; for example, scintigraphic imaging can determine osteoblastic activity at the site.

Osseous cystlike lesions are generally considered developmental abnormalities, but trauma to the articular cartilage and subchondral bone can potentially lead to formation of these cystlike lesions.[21] Osseous cystlike lesions in the ulnar carpal bone with or without an adjacent osseous fragment have been linked to tearing of the attachment of the lateral palmar intercarpal ligament and associated with lameness.[22] If cystlike lesions are observed in a foal, then septic osteomyelitis should be considered and other diagnostic procedures used to investigate the presence of septic foci.

Standard views are recommended. Subchondral or osseous cystlike lesions are seen as well circumscribed circular or semicircular lucent areas within the carpal bones, the distal aspect of the radius, or in the proximal aspect of the second or fourth metacarpal bones. An area of opacity may surround the lucent zone. For articular lesions, clear communication with the articular surface may be present, although more frequently the lesions are adjacent to the articular surface and a clear communication cannot be clearly established. Radiographic evidence of secondary osteoarthritis may be visible (see Fig. 20-8).

Soft Tissue Problems

Periarticular Soft Tissues

Although alterations to periarticular soft tissues may be noted on radiographs, ultrasonographic assessment is frequently more informative than is radiographic evaluation. For synovial structures or with penetrating wounds, contrast medium may be necessary to outline filling defects or define communication with other structures.

Periarticular soft tissue swelling may be either focal or diffuse and generalized. Cellulitis is most commonly observed as diffuse soft tissue swelling that is not purely localized to the region of the carpus and affects the limb circumferentially. However, the presence of a foreign body or wound may lead to more focal enlargement. If a foreign body is radiopaque

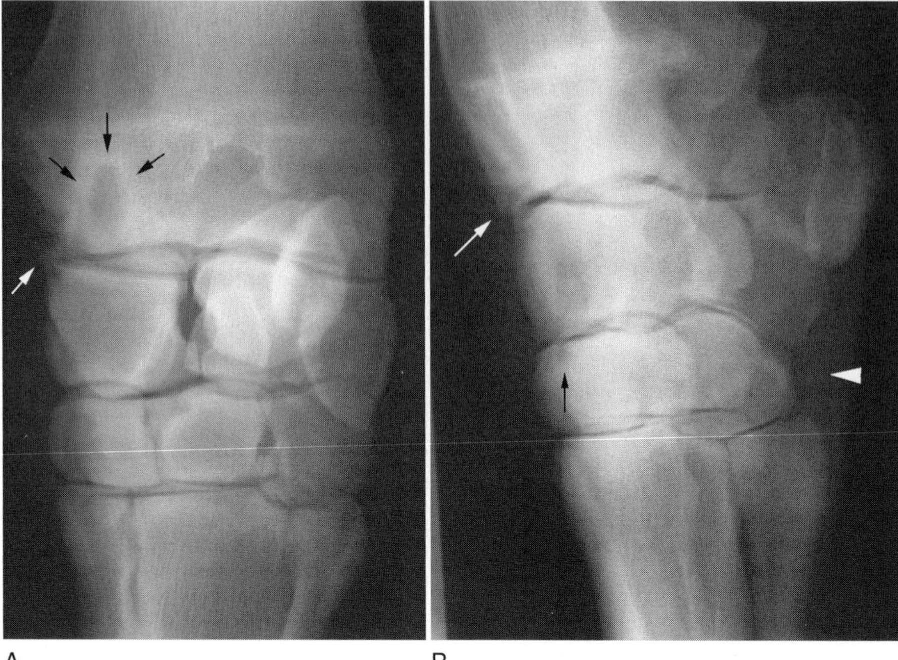

Fig. 20-8 A, Dorsopalmar view of a carpus. Medial is to the left. Periarticular osteophyte formation is visible on the medial aspect of the antebrachiocarpal joint *(white arrow)* in association with an osseous cystlike lesion *(black arrows)* surrounded by a sclerotic rim in the distal medial aspect of the radius. B, Dorsolateral-palmaromedial oblique view of the same carpus as in A. Modeling of the dorsal articular margins of the antebrachiocarpal joint is present *(white arrow)*. A small lucent zone is also present in the proximal aspect of the third carpal bone *(black arrow)*. Note the presence of a fifth carpal bone *(arrowhead)* and the small osseous spur on the proximal aspect of the accessory carpal bone.

then it may be detected radiographically, but ultrasonography is often more useful.

Conditions associated with swelling on the dorsal aspect of the carpal region are presented below.

Carpal hygroma A carpal hygroma is a subcutaneous sac or acquired bursa usually positioned over the dorsal aspect of the carpal region.[6] A hygroma usually occurs as a result of blunt trauma at the site and is generally nonpainful, although it may have been painful at the site when the inciting event occurred. Gait alteration is not generally observed unless the hygroma is so large that carpal flexion is restricted.

Standard radiographic views and direct contrast medium injection into the mass are required for diagnosis, with ultrasonography to evaluate the adjacent soft tissues. Radiographic diagnosis is based on soft tissue swelling over the dorsal aspect and the presence of a defined structure that has no communication with other structures after contrast medium injection.

Distension/synovitis of extensor carpi radialis, common digital extensor, or long digital extensor tendon sheaths In neonatal or young foals with distension of the tendon sheath of extensor carpi radialis, rupture of the extensor carpi radialis tendon should be considered, particularly if flexural deformity is also present.[23] In horses of any age, traumatic or septic damage to an extensor tendon sheath may occur, potentially with coexisting tendon damage. Ultrasonographic examination is often more useful in assessment of these injuries than is radiographic examination, although the use of radiography with contrast medium injection adds information about communication between synovial cavities. To determine if communication exists between the carpal joints and tendon sheath(s), double-contrast techniques may also be useful. Contrast medium injection can also be used to demonstrate filling defects associated with adhesion formation or synovial proliferation.

Radiographs are characterized by soft tissue swelling over the dorsal aspect of the carpus. Swelling may be more defined in the region of the tendon sheath. Chronic synovitis may be associated with periosteal new bone formation on adjacent structures. In particular, extensor carpi radialis synovitis may be associated with periosteal new bone on the cranial distal aspect of the radius.[24]

Herniation of carpal joint synovial membrane Herniation of a joint capsule can occur as a result of trauma. It is likely to be nonpainful and only noted as an incidental finding. On radiographs a focal or slightly generalized soft tissue swelling is visible, most frequently dorsolateral.[3] Contrast medium injection reveals communication between the subcutaneous swelling and the joint of origin.

Synovitis The antebrachiocarpal joint cavity remains separate from the other joints of the carpus in most horses, whereas the middle and carpometacarpal joints usually communicate.[2] Distension of either the antebrachiocarpal or middle carpal joints is associated with swelling on the dorsal aspect, often obscuring the normal dorsal radiolucencies associated with the fat pads.[25] An antebrachiocarpal joint effusion is located as a swelling on the dorsal aspect in the proximal third of the carpal region at the level of the articulation between the radius and proximal row of carpal bones, whereas middle carpal joint distension is located at the mid-carpal level at the level of the articulation between the two rows of carpal bones. Carpometacarpal joint distension is difficult to see, but an effusion in the middle carpal joint may suggest synovitis in this joint. The osseous tissues should be carefully examined for abnormalities that could lead to the detected synovitis. Further examination of the soft tissues may be performed with ultrasonography.

Conditions Associated with Swelling on the Palmar Aspect of the Carpal Region

Generalized swelling may occur circumferentially at the level of the carpus and therefore be seen as swelling on the palmar aspect in addition to other sites in conditions such as cellulitis. Generalized periarticular soft tissue swelling on the dorsal aspect of the carpus may be caused by fractures or severe osteoarthritis. Swelling localized to the palmar aspect may be associated with palmar wounds, foreign body penetration, or trauma.

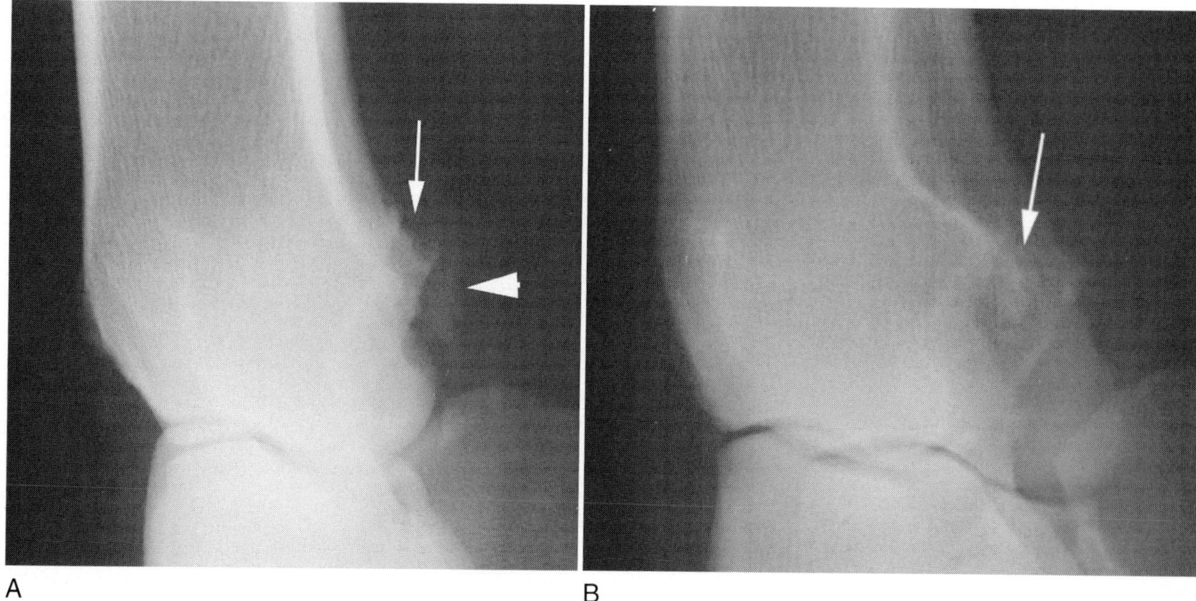

Fig. 20-9 A, Lateromedial view of a carpus. Linear mineralization *(arrowhead)* is present in the soft tissues on the distal caudal aspect of the radius, confirmed ultrasonographically to be within the deep digital flexor tendon. An osseous projection *(arrow)* is present at the level of the transverse ridge of the radius, which was impinging on the deep digital flexor tendon. **B,** Dorsolateral-palmaromedial oblique view of the same carpus as in **A.** Normal bony prominences are on the caudomedial and caudolateral aspects of the radius, but the radiopacity between these *(arrow)* represents the abnormal osseous projection that was impinging on the deep digital flexor tendon.

Distension of the carpal sheath Conditions affecting the carpal sheath lead to swelling on the palmar aspect, which may be detectable radiographically.[26] Radiographic examination is necessary in horses with carpal sheath distension to identify or rule out osseous abnormalities.[27] Ultrasonographic examination is necessary to evaluate the soft tissue structures within the carpal sheath. Primary idiopathic synovitis or hemorrhage appears unremarkable on radiographic examination, apart from the soft tissue swelling caused by the carpal sheath distension. Desmitis of the accessory ligament of the deep digital flexor tendon, superficial digital flexor tendonitis, or deep digital flexor tendonitis within the sheath is associated with carpal sheath distension but is better evaluated by ultrasonography because no abnormalities are generally detected on radiographs.

Radiographic abnormalities are seen with acute or chronic fracture of the accessory carpal bone or palmar fractures of the other carpal bones, which all have the potential to cause carpal sheath distension.[28-30]

Osteochondroma of the distal caudal aspect of the radius and radial physeal exostoses Distension of the carpal sheath can be caused by the presence of an osteochondroma, a cartilage-covered exostoses,[27,31] or an axial exostosis on the caudal aspect of the distal radial physis (Fig. 20-9). Both lesions may result in an impingement lesion on the deep digital flexor tendon and associated secondary synovitis. Horses with an osteochondroma are generally lame, with the lameness being exacerbated by flexion. However, horses with a physeal exostosis may have sporadic severe lameness that may not induce detectable synovitis of the carpal sheath.

An osteochondroma is identified as an exostosis located on the distal caudal aspect of the radius just proximal to the distal radial physis (Fig. 20-10). It appears as a bony outgrowth that

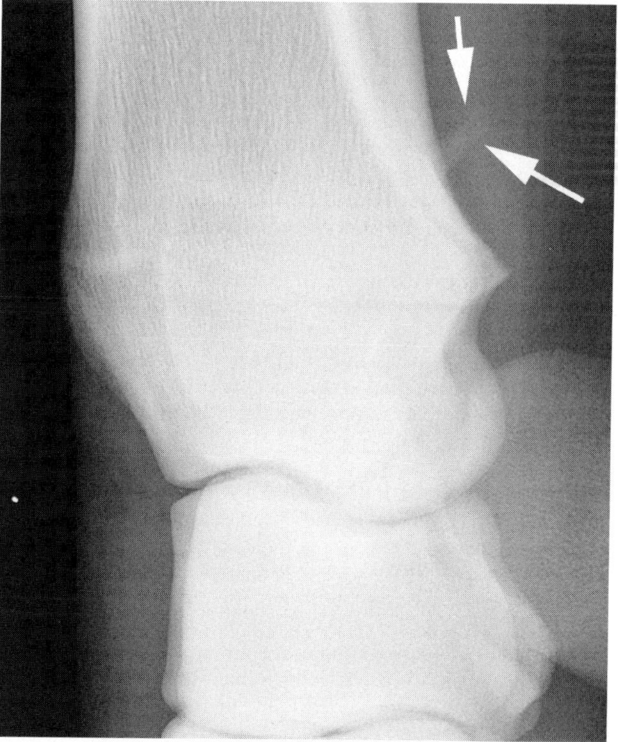

Fig. 20-10 Lateral view of the distal radius of a 4-year-old Clydesdale. A small columnar region of new bone arises from the distocaudal aspect of the radius *(arrows)*. This is a common location and appearance of osteochondroma in the horse.

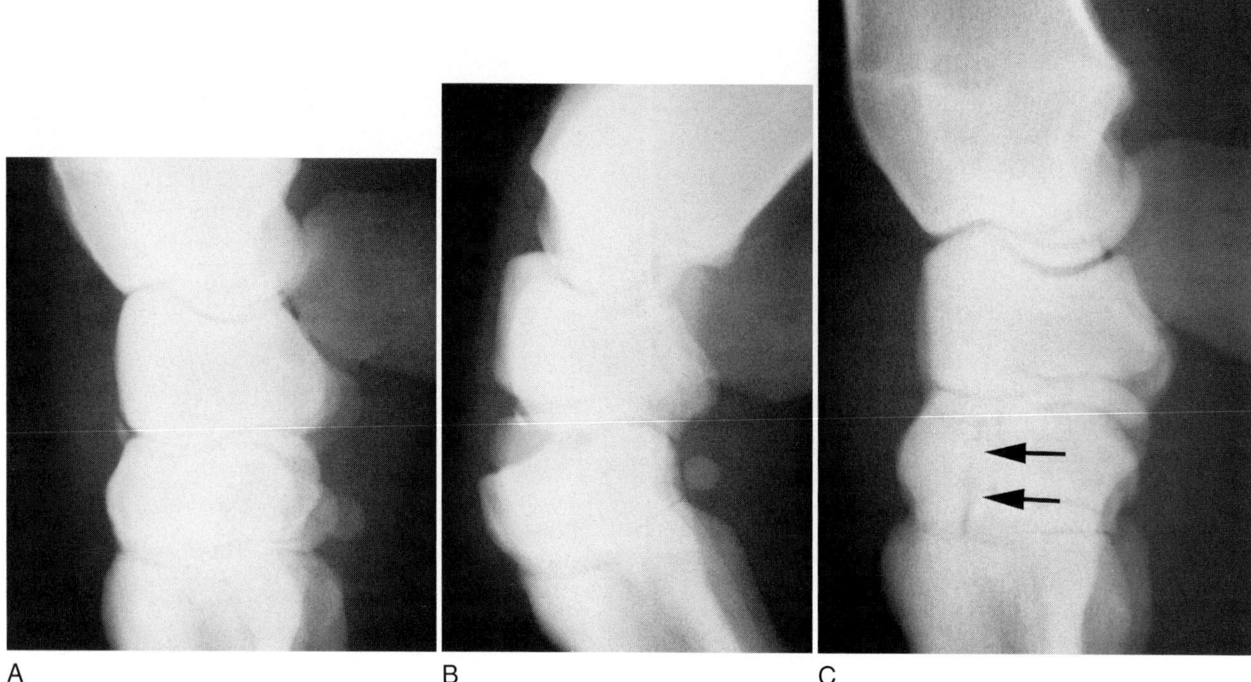

Fig. 20-11 A, Lateromedial view of a carpus. The radiograph is deliberately underexposed to demonstrate soft tissue swelling at the level of the middle carpal joint dorsally and a chip fracture on the dorsal aspect of the joint (distal dorsal radial chip fracture). Also note the presence of a second carpal bone. **B,** Flexed lateromedial view of the same carpus as in **A.** The radial carpal bone has moved distally relative to the intermediate and ulnar carpal bones. A chip fracture is visible on the dorsodistal aspect of the radial carpal bone. Also note the presence of a second carpal bone. **C,** Lateromedial view of a carpus. A very large slab fracture of the third carpal bone is visible *(arrows)*, associated with soft tissue swelling on the dorsal aspect of the carpus. Also note the irregularity of the caudal aspect of the radius at the level of the physis, a normal variant.

is continuous with the cortex. Exostoses at the level of the distal radial physis must be differentiated from the normal medial and lateral protuberances and in some horses may best be detected in oblique views. Concurrent damage of the deep digital flexor tendon often occurs and can be detected by ultrasonographic examination. Treatment is by surgical excision of the osteochondroma or physeal exostosis.

Mineralized opacities within the periarticular soft tissues Dystrophic mineralization may be diffuse or localized and occurs as a result of trauma (see Fig. 20-9) or local corticosteroid injection.

Osseous and Osteochondral Abnormalities

Osteochondral damage of the antebrachiocarpal and middle carpal articular surfaces occurs most frequently in Thoroughbred racehorses,[32] although the incidence is also high in racing quarter horses[33] and Standardbreds.[6,34] Racing on dirt tracks is associated with a higher incidence of carpal lesions than is racing on turf.[35] Carpal injures are uncommon in horses that are not subjected to race training, which may be a function of reduced stresses on the carpal joints or more advanced age at which they undergo athletic training.[35] Nonracehorses also seem more tolerant of radiographic abnormalities consistent with osteoarthritis. In racehorses in the United States, an asymmetry in the incidence of middle carpal joint osteochondral lesions has been noted between the two forelimbs, with an increased incidence of fractures in the right forelimb.[33] This finding has been attributed to the oval shape of the racetrack and uniform direction of the races in the United States.[33-36]

In racehorses, the middle carpal joint is most frequently affected, whereas in nonracehorses the antebrachiocarpal joint has a higher prevalence of injury. Most lesions occur on the dorsal aspect. In Thoroughbred and quarter horses, the most frequent site of osteochondral injuries is the distal, dorsal radial carpal articular surface (Fig. 20-11), followed by the proximal dorsal third carpal articular surface (primarily medially) and then the distal dorsal aspect of the intermediate carpal bone.[33,34,37] Lesions that can be observed may involve articular cartilage erosion, osteochondral chip fractures or slab fractures (see Fig. 20-11). Chip fractures occur near the dorsal margin of a carpal bone, affecting only one articular surface. Slab fractures are primarily observed at a less-marginal location and involve both proximal and distal articular surfaces of the affected carpal bone. In the dorsal medial aspect of the third carpal bone, dorsal plane osteochondral slab fractures tend to occur most commonly, followed by very large osteochondral chip fractures, which are located less close to the dorsal margin.[38] Sagittal plane, incomplete slab fractures are observed less frequently.

Carpal Bone Sclerosis

Osteochondral injuries affecting the middle carpal joint have been suggested to be primarily chronic overload injuries.[35,39] Although a single massive overload of a normal structure can occur, repetitive trauma resulting in microdamage, leading to ultimate overload, is considered a more common etiology for

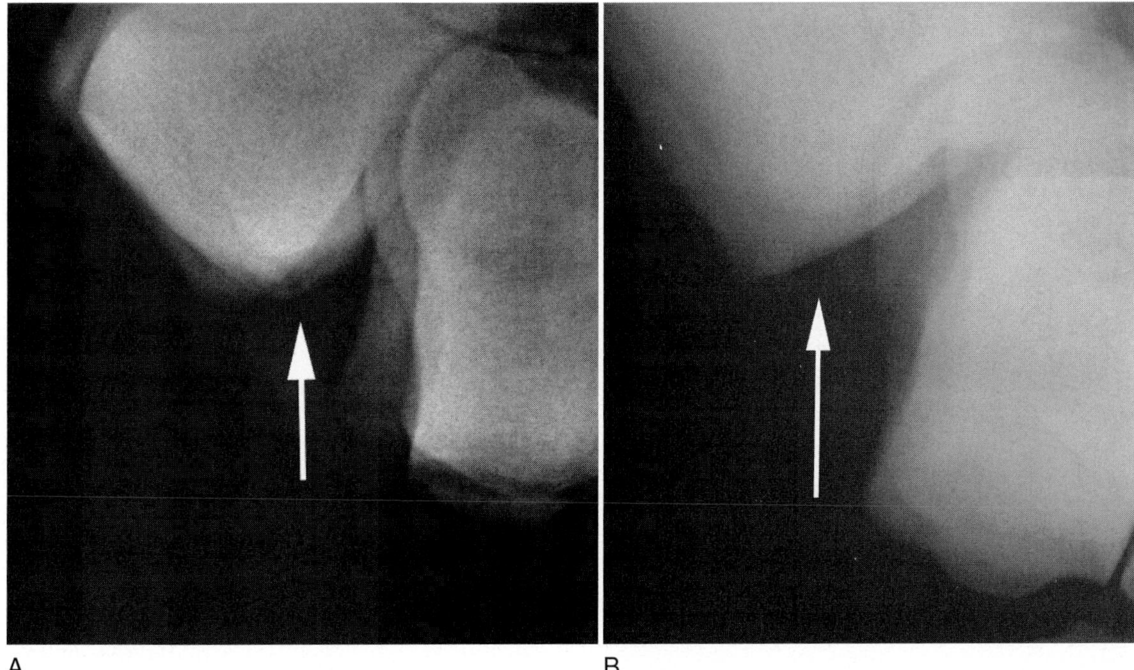

Fig. 20-12 A, Flexed lateromedial view of a carpus. A small subchondral radiolucent area is visible in the distal dorsal aspect of the radial carpal bone *(arrow)*. Arthroscopic examination of the middle carpal joint confirmed the presence of a focal chondro-osseous defect. B, Flexed lateromedial view of a carpus (not the same horse as in A). A small subchondral radiolucent area is visible in the distal dorsal aspect of the radial carpal bone *(arrow)*. Arthroscopic examination of the middle carpal joint confirmed the presence of a focal chondro-osseous defect.

osteochondral injury.[7,35,40] In the radial carpal bone, osteochondral fractures may be preceded by lucency, apparent softening and collapse of the subchondral bone,[35,41] seen as a focal radiolucency on the distal aspect of the bone (Fig. 20-12). This has also been reported to occur at focal sites in the third carpal bone.[35] In the third carpal bone, cartilage erosion and fracture are often associated with bone sclerosis and loss of trabecular pattern, as detected radiographically.[35,42] In pathologic bones, this sclerosis is maximal in the medial facet approximately 10 to 20 mm palmar to the dorsal margin (Fig. 20-13).[42] This sclerosis has been suggested to be associated with decreased absorption of concussive forces by the trabecular bone, followed by increasing demands on the articular cartilage and subchondral bone to attenuate these forces.[7,35,40] This apparent stress concentration in the articular cartilage and subchondral bone has been suggested as the cause of articular cartilage failure and subchondral bone loss.[42]

Subchondral lucency of the third carpal bone has been reported in Standardbred racehorses.[43] Areas of lucency are often surrounded by subchondral sclerosis.[44] These appear to be sites of bone collapse after repetitive trauma. This is seen most clearly in dorsolateral-palmaromedial oblique views.

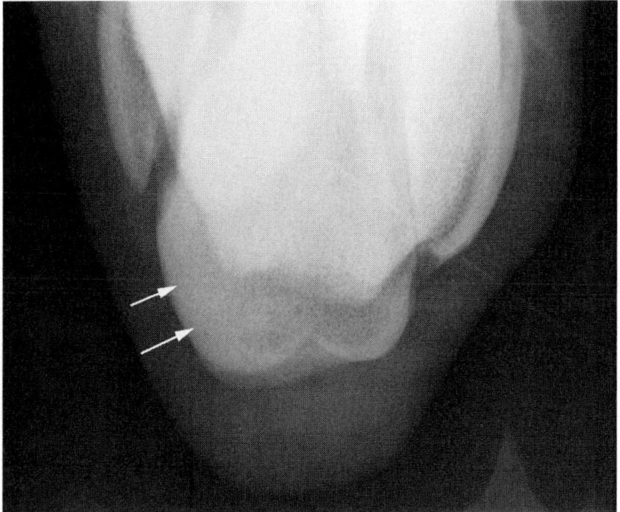

Fig. 20-13 Dorsoproximal-dorsodistal oblique view of the distal row of carpal bones. Medial is to the left. Increased radiopacity (sclerosis) of the radial facet of the third carpal bone is visible *(arrows)*. No significant radiological abnormality was seen in any other radiographic projection.

Carpal Bone Chip Fractures

Dorsal aspect Osteochondral fragmentation or chip fracture formation is most likely to involve the dorsal articular borders of the distal aspect of the radius, proximal and distal aspects of the radial and intermediate carpal bones, and the proximal aspect of the third carpal bone (Figs. 20-11, 20-14, and 20-15).[33,34,38,45] However, the expected lesion distribution differs among breeds, with most lesions occurring on the medial aspect of the middle carpal joints in Standardbred racehorses but affecting both the antebrachiocarpal and middle carpal joints in Thoroughbred and quarter horse racehorses. Although affected horses are usually markedly lame at the time of initial damage, the degree of lameness may reduce to a mild level or progress to become severe. Although effusion and local pain may be present, only very mild signs may be observed in some horses.

All radiographic views should be evaluated, including a dorsopalmar, lateromedial, at least two obliques, a flexed lateromedial, and dorsoproximal-dorsodistal views of each row of carpal bones. The contralateral limb should routinely be evaluated because lesions are commonly found bilaterally.

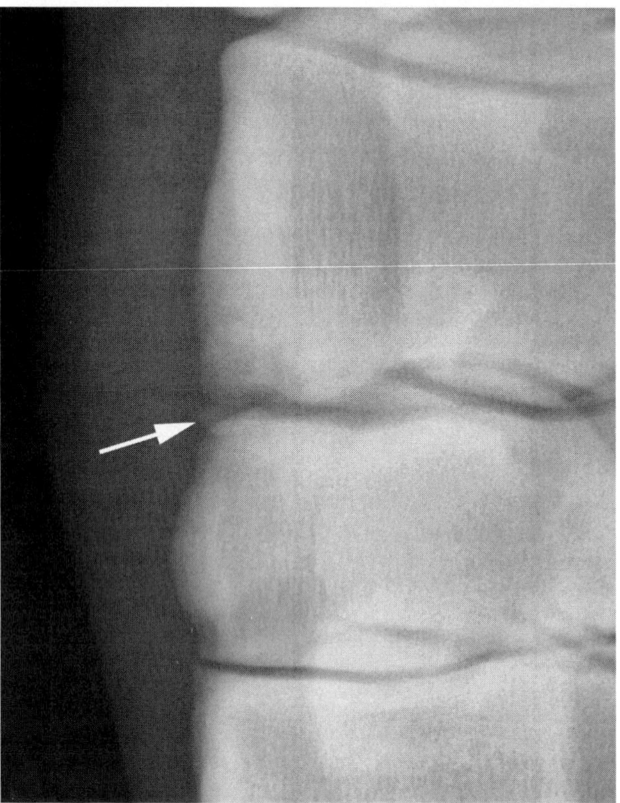

Fig. 20-14 Dorsolateral-palmaromedial oblique view of a carpus. A small chip fracture is present *(arrow)* on the dorsomedial aspect of the middle carpal joint.

When interpreting radiographs in horses with suspected osteochondral fragmentation, all potential lesion sites should be carefully evaluated. The third carpal bone should be assessed for degree of sclerosis, and the radial carpal bone should be assessed for apparent lucency, rounding of the dorsal extent, and collapse of the subchondral bone, all changes that may precede actual fragmentation. Signs of osteoarthritis may also be present with chronic injury to the carpus, including osteophyte and enthesophyte formation (see Fig. 20-15).

Palmar aspect Osteochondral fractures of the palmar aspect of the carpal joints are generally associated with a single traumatic incident, such as during recovery from general anesthesia, including direct impact injuries or hyperextension of the carpus.[46] Horses are at least moderately lame, with a marked response to flexion.

Occasionally migration of osteochondral fragments from the dorsal aspect may result in detection of fragments in the palmar aspect of the antebrachiocarpal or middle carpal joints. Evaluation of the entire joint, not solely focused on the palmar aspect, is therefore important.

Carpal Bone Slab Fractures

Slab fractures extend from one articular surface to another in proximal to distal direction. The third carpal bone is the most frequently affected,[32,47,48] although fractures of the fourth, radial, and intermediate carpal bones have been reported.[49] Racehorses are the most likely to be affected.

Dorsal plane slab fractures are the most likely to occur, particularly affecting the medial facet of the third carpal bone.[32-35,39] They may range in depth from 8 to 25 mm and may be displaced or nondisplaced (Fig. 20-16). Lameness varies in severity from mild to severe. With complete displaced fractures significant effusion, soft tissue swelling, and severe lameness are usually present, but horses with nondisplaced incomplete fractures may also have no localizing clinical signs. Complete radiographic evaluation of the contralateral limb should also be performed because lesions may occur bilaterally.

A complete series of radiographs should be obtained, including dorsoproximal-dorsodistal views. Fractures of the radial facet are best visualized on lateromedial, flexed

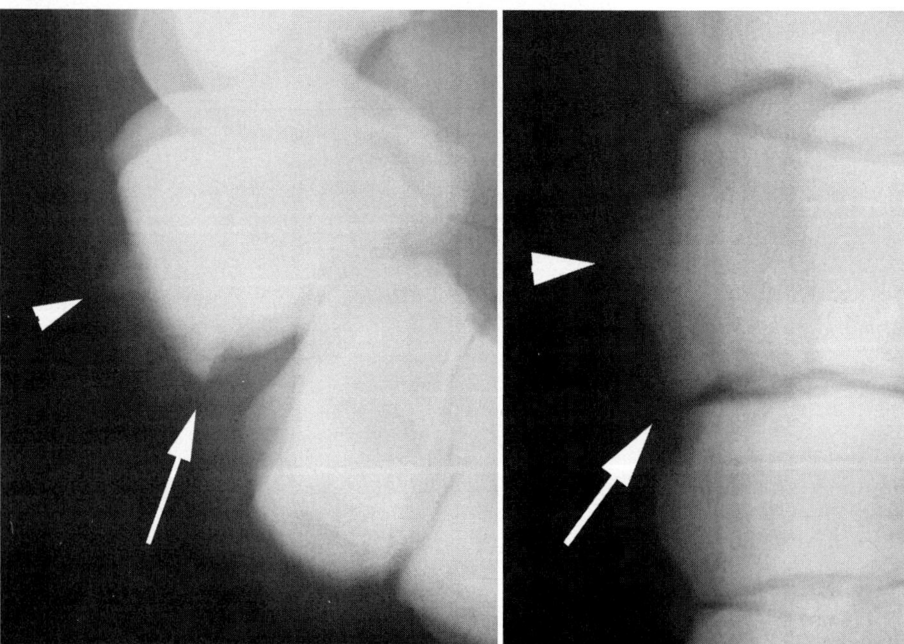

Fig. 20-15 **A,** Flexed lateromedial view of a carpus. A nondisplaced chip fracture of the distal dorsal aspect of the radial carpal bone is visible *(arrow)*. Also note the entheseous nonarticular new bone on the dorsal aspect of the radial carpal bone *(arrowhead)*. The radiograph is deliberately underexposed to demonstrate the new bone. **B,** Dorsolateral-palmaromedial oblique view of the same carpus as in **A.** Modeling of the distal dorsal aspect of the radial carpal bone and a chip fracture are visible *(arrow)*, contiguous with entheseous new bone on the middle of the dorsal aspect of the bone *(arrowhead)*.

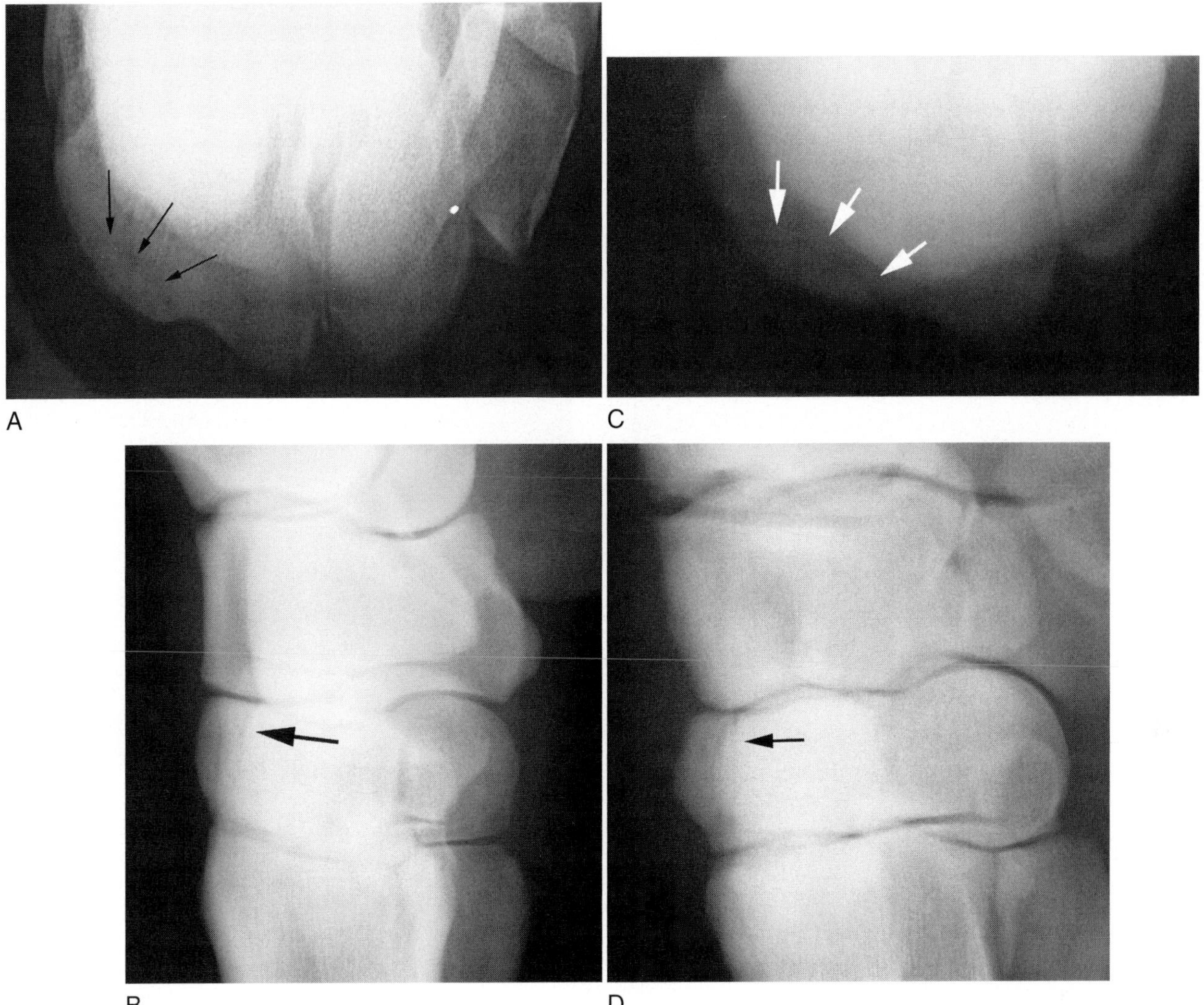

Fig. 20-16 **A,** Dorsoproximal-dorsodistal oblique view of the distal row of carpal bones (slightly obliqued). Mild increased radiopacity of the radial facet of the third carpal bone and a nondisplaced slab fracture are visible *(arrows)*. No significant abnormality was seen in any other radiographic projection. **B,** Dorsomedial-palmarolateral oblique view of a carpus. A faint line in the third carpal bone may represent a fracture *(arrow)*; however, the complexity of this joint prevents making a definitive diagnosis on the basis of this finding. **C,** Dorsoproximal-dorsodistal oblique view of the distal row of carpal bones of the same limb as **B.** Medial is to the left. A nondisplaced slab fracture of the radial facet of the third carpal bone is visible *(arrows)*. This illustrates the value of the dorsoproximal-dorsodistal oblique views to assess potential slab fractures. **D,** Dorsolateral-palmaromedial oblique view of a carpus. A radiographically incomplete slab fracture of the third carpal bone is visible *(arrow)*. Also note the mottled radiopacity of the bone dorsal to the fracture. The distal dorsal aspect of the radial carpal bone is modeled, being more rounded than normal and "cut back," moving the point of impact on the third carpal bone in a palmar direction. This change may predispose to fracture of the third carpal bone. Also note the modeling of the articular margins of the antebrachiocarpal joint and possibly a small osseous fragment on the distal dorsal aspect of the radius.

lateromedial, and dorsolateral-palmaromedial oblique views and a dorsoproximal-dorsodistal view of the distal row of carpal bones.[50] In some horses a fracture can only be seen in the dorsoproximal-dorsodistal projection, especially if the fracture is nondisplaced (see Fig. 20-16). Concurrent damage to the dorsal distal aspect of the radial carpal bone is a frequent occurrence, as is concurrent third carpal bone sclerosis.

Sagittal plane fractures occur less commonly than dorsal plane fractures and may be incomplete.[51-53] They primarily affect the medial facet of the third carpal bone (Fig. 20-17). As with other osteochondral fractures, horses are quite lame at the time of fracture, and the contralateral limb may be involved. Fracture of other carpal bones has been reported but is relatively rare.

Sagittal fractures of the third carpal bone are best seen on dorsoproximal-dorsodistal and dorsomedial palmarolateral oblique views. The lucent fracture line is often located parallel to the articulation between the second and third carpal bones. Radiographs of the entire carpus should be assessed for concurrent osteochondral injury.

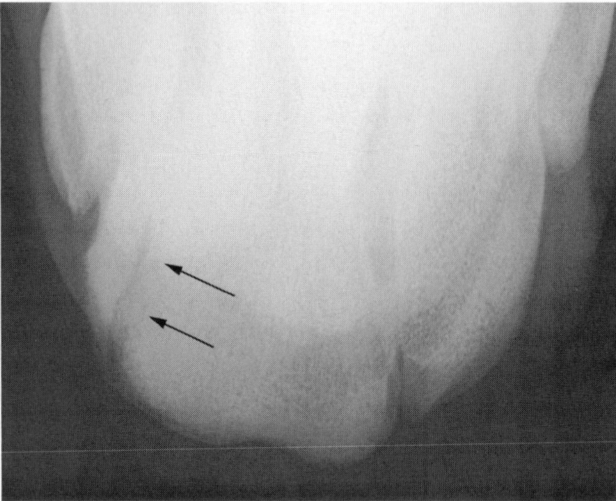

Fig. 20-17 Dorsoproximal-dorsodistal oblique view of the distal row of carpal bones. Medial is to the left. Increased radiopacity (sclerosis) of the radial facet of the third carpal bone and an incomplete parasagittal fracture are visible *(arrows)*. The margins of the fracture line are indistinct, indicating chronicity. No significant radiologic abnormality was seen in any other radiographic projection.

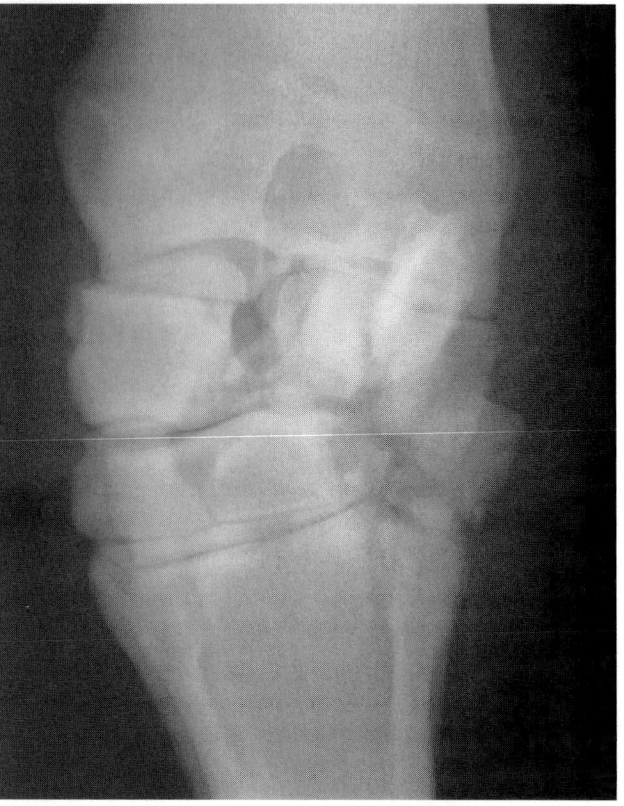

Fig. 20-18 Dorsopalmar view of a carpus. Lateral is to the right. Multiple displaced fractures are on the lateral aspect of the carpus, resulting in partial collapse of the carpus with abaxial displacement of part of the fourth carpal bone. Identifying all fractures, even from a complete radiographic series, will be difficult. Computed tomographic examination of such a fracture will be more precise in localizing all fractures.

Comminuted and Multiple Fractures

Multiple or comminuted fractures are unusual but do occur, especially in racehorses.[6] They may also occur in other types of horses as a result of direct trauma or a single-event injury. Affected horses are generally in severe pain and usually do not bear weight on the limb. Carpal instability is a frequent finding. Prognosis is generally guarded to poor.

Full radiographic examination of the carpus is required to assess the extent and nature of osseous injury. Concurrent joint effusion and soft tissue swelling are usually present (Fig. 20-18).

Fractures of the Accessory Carpal Bone

Accessory carpal bone fractures usually occur as a result of a single incident, such as a fall, that either causes hyperextension of the carpus or results in direct trauma to the accessory carpal bone itself. Soft tissue swelling palmar to the carpus is present. Horses usually have moderate to severe pain and resent flexion of the carpus.[28-30]

Fractures most commonly occur through the lateral groove of the ulnaris lateralis tendon in a dorsal plane (vertical) (Fig. 20-19). Although most fractures are simple, comminuted fractures can occur. Because the flexor muscles provide constant distraction forces and motion, a fibrocartilaginous nonunion frequently occurs at this site. The fibrous union results in a persistent lucent line on radiographs. Bony proliferative changes are also often noted radiographically during the fibrous healing period. However, the prognosis for function is usually favorable.

Less commonly, proximal dorsal chip fractures of the accessory carpal bone occur close to the articular surface. Because standard views may result in superimposition of these fragments over the other carpal bones, further oblique views may be required. A dorsal 80-degree lateral-palmaromedial oblique view has been recommended. Such fractures should be surgically removed, otherwise secondary osteoarthritis will ensue.

Periosteal New Bone on the Dorsal Aspect of the Carpal Bones, the Distal Aspect of the Radius, and the Proximal Aspect of the Metacarpal Bones

Enthesophytes not associated with the articular surface or joint margins are likely to be caused by strain on the intercarpal ligaments. Enthesophytes are often observed in association with osteoarthritis (see Figs. 20-15 and 20-20) but may occur as a result of direct periosteal trauma.[3]

Hypertrophic Osteopathy

Hypertrophic osteopathy is often associated with intrathoracic disease. Enlargement of the proximal carpal region and mild lameness may occur from fibrous and osseous enlargement of the distal radius resulting from hypertrophic osteopathy.[54] Pain is usually felt on palpation of the affected area.

Radiographs are characterized by palisading periosteal new bone perpendicular to the cortex. This palisading bone does not usually affect the carpal joints.

Articular Problems

Luxation/Subluxation

Luxation is the complete loss of contact between articular surfaces, and subluxation is partial loss of contact between the articular surfaces and may be intermittent. Generally luxation and subluxation are caused by disruption of the lateral or medial collateral ligaments, with or without damage of the adjacent soft tissues. Although alterations in joint congruency may be noted on radiographs, more direct visualization of

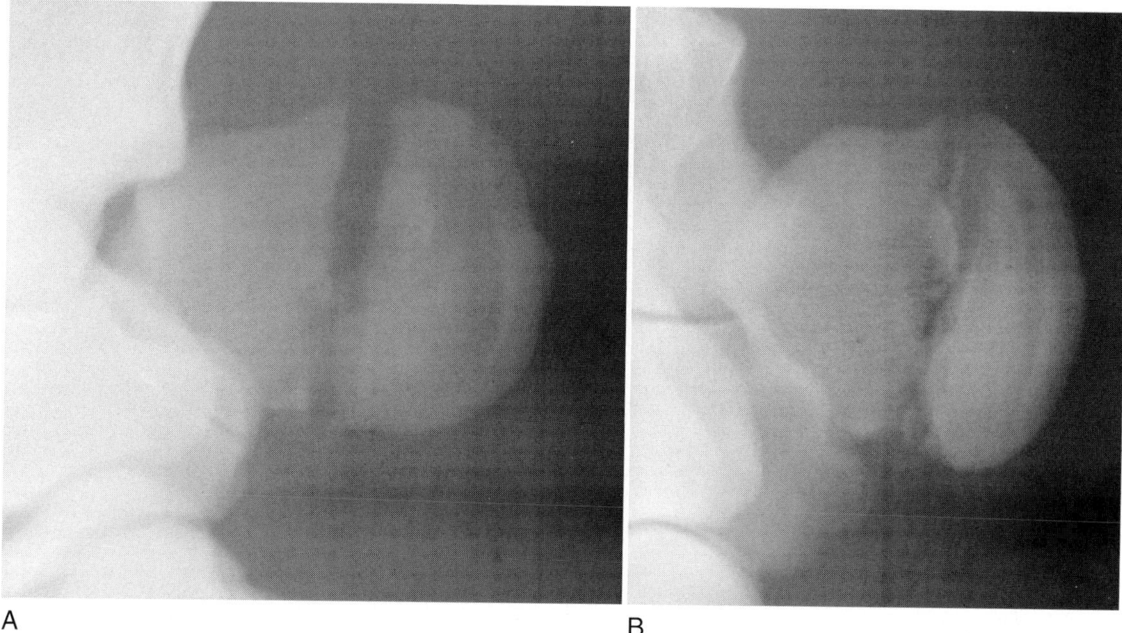

Fig. 20-19 A, Flexed lateromedial view. A slightly displaced fracture of the accessory carpal bone is visible. B, Dorsolateral-palmaromedial oblique view of the same carpus as in A. A complete fracture of the accessory carpal bone is present.

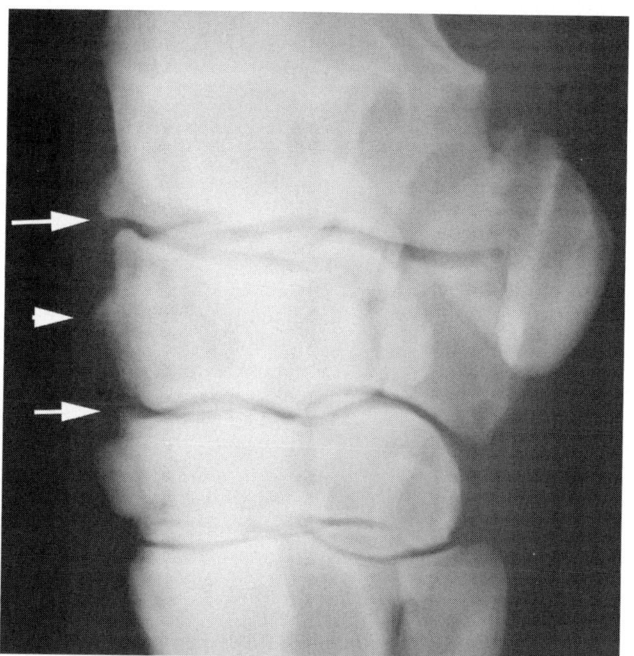

Fig. 20-20 Dorsolateral-palmaromedial oblique view of a carpus. Extensive periarticular osteophyte formation involving the dorsomedial aspects of the antebrachiocarpal and middle carpal joints is visible *(arrows)*, consistent with advanced osteoarthritis. Entheseous new bone on the dorsal aspect of the intermediate carpal bone is also present *(arrowhead)*. Also note the new bone on the proximodorsal aspect of the accessory carpal bone. A small radiolucent zone in the distal palmar aspect of the ulnar carpal bone is visible but is an incidental finding.

collateral ligament structure is possible with ultrasonographic evaluation. Luxation or subluxation of individual carpal joints or all the joints of the carpus may be seen depending on the extent of injury to the soft tissue structures.

In addition to standard views, stressed dorsopalmar and/or stressed lateromedial radiographs should be used to assess joint stability. The presence of asymmetric joint spaces and altered proximal-distal alignment of carpal bones on either dorsopalmar or lateromedial views indicate subluxation, although they may not always be detected without stressed views. In complete luxation, complete loss of alignment of the articular surface in the affected joint is observed.

Radiographs should be examined to detect avulsion fractures at the origin or insertion of collateral ligaments, seen as a discontinuity of the cortex or presence of radiopaque fragments. Enthesophytes at the origin or insertion of collateral ligament may signify chronic damage. Severe luxations may be associated carpal bone fractures, which may result in radiopaque intercarpal ligament avulsion fragments within the joint space. In the case of an open luxation, gas can be present within the joint and local soft tissues.

Osteoarthritis

Osteoarthritis is generally characterized by periarticular osteophyte formation, narrowing of the joint space, subchondral lucent zones, subchondral bone sclerosis or thickening, and joint capsule distension. The degree of radiographic change is not always correlated with the degree of pain or lameness, and radiographic changes may sometimes be quite advanced at the time of lameness onset, so predicting onset and degree of lameness from radiographic examination is difficult.[3,6]

Antebrachiocarpal joint Osteoarthritis in the antebrachiocarpal joint is most commonly observed in flat racehorses and is usually caused by repetitive overloading injury of the articular osteochondral structure.[35,39] Stress-related subchondral bone injury is present with overlying cartilage damage and cartilage wear lines, which are not visible radiographically.

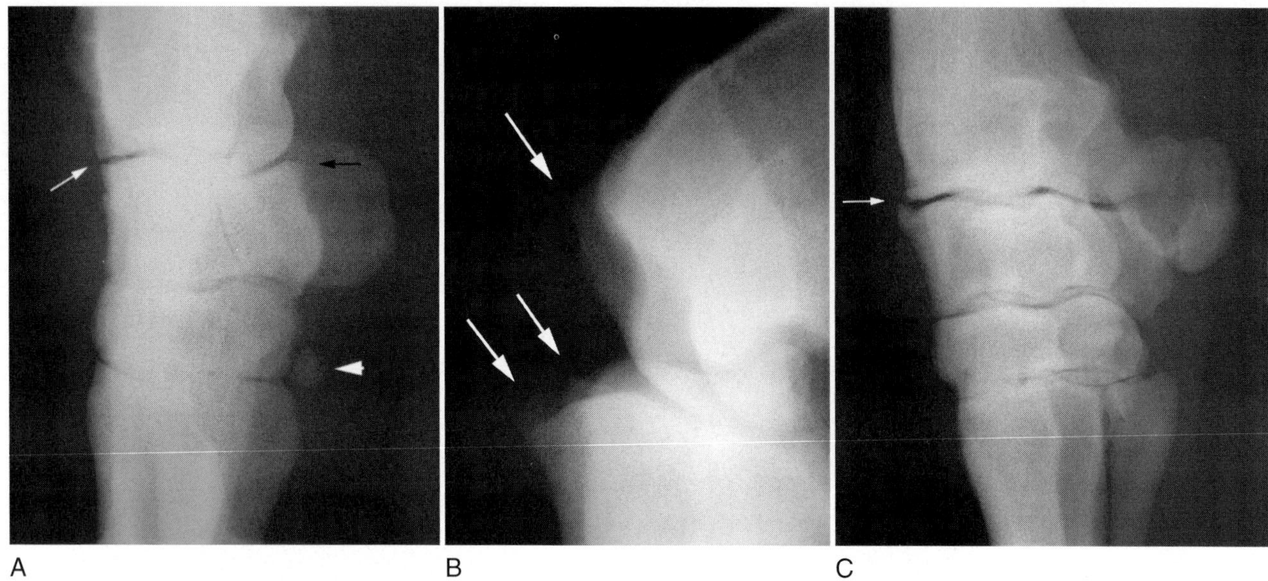

Fig. 20-21 A, Dorsomedial-palmarolateral oblique view of a carpus. Soft tissue swelling is present on the dorsolateral aspect of the carpus centered around the antebrachiocarpal joint. Modeling of the dorsal articular margins of the antebrachiocarpal joint is visible *(white arrow)*, as is an osteophyte on the palmaroproximal aspect of the ulnar carpal bone *(black arrow)*, consistent with osteoarthritis of the antebrachiocarpal joint. Note also the presence of a second carpal bone *(arrowhead)*. **B,** Flexed lateromedial view of the same carpus as in **A.** Periarticular osteophyte formation on the distal dorsal aspect of the radius and the proximodorsal aspects of the radial and intermediate carpal bones is visible *(arrows)*, consistent with osteoarthritis of the antebrachiocarpal joint. **C,** Dorsolateral-palmaromedial oblique view of the same carpus as **A** and **B.** A large osteophyte on the proximodorsal aspect of the radial carpal bone and modeling of the distal dorsal aspect of the radius are visible *(arrow)*.

Osteochondral fragments are frequently present in these horses.[33,34] For nonracehorses, osteoarthritis is more likely to occur in older horses, with osteochondral fragments being unusual unless the horse has a prior racing history.[3,6] Although small periarticular osteophytes are sometimes observed in horses without clinically detectable lameness, their presence can indicate osteoarthritic change. When severe changes are present, including loss of joint space and ankylosis, they are likely to be associated with lameness no matter the horse's athletic requirements, with the horse severely resenting flexion and abducting the limb to avoid flexion during movement. However, when mild changes are present, the breed and use of the horse can influence the prognosis and potential significance of mild osteoarthritic change, suggesting a significant effect on performance in a racehorse but having little significance for a pleasure or show horse.

Periarticular osteophytes are most commonly detected on the dorsal aspect, particularly of the radial and intermediate carpal bones, but may also be observed on the palmar aspect of the joint (Figs. 20-21 and 20-22).[3] Joint capsule distension is sometimes present, particularly when intercarpal ligament, chronic synovitis, or joint capsule damage is present in association with the osteochondral changes. Osteochondral fragments are observed as radiopacities within the joint space or at the joint margins.

Middle carpal joint Osteoarthritis in the middle carpal joint occurs in a similar manner to the antebrachiocarpal joint.[7,40] Periarticular osteophytes are most frequently observed on the dorsal aspects of the radial and third carpal bones, although palmar osteophytes may be observed. Modeling of the dorsal articular margins of the radial and third carpal bones may also be seen. The dorsal distal aspect of the radial carpal bone should be well defined, with a clear subchondral margin and corner to the bone. With repetitive overloading, damage may be seen as radiolucency of the dorsodistal corner (see Fig. 20-12, *A*) and eventually either loss in the form of a clearly defined osteochondral fragment (see Fig. 20-14) or gradual rounding of the corner.[41] This results in decreased dorsal loading of the medial aspect of the third carpal bone, moving the site of maximal loading on the third carpal bone, and increasing risk of osteochondral damage to the radial facet of the third carpal bone articular surface, potentially leading to sclerosis (seen as marked increase in radiopacity), slab fracture (observed as a radiolucent line, with or without a defect in the articular surface), osteochondral collapse (see as a defect in the articular surface), or more generalized osteoarthritis.[35]

Carpometacarpal joint Osteoarthritis of the carpometacarpal joint occurs much less commonly than does osteoarthritis of the two proximal articulations and occurs largely in older horses.[6] No specific type of work history appears to predispose to the condition. Onset is generally insidious, progressing to severe lameness.

Osteoarthritic change is generally characterized by narrowing or collapse of the joint space, frequently focal or confined to either the medial or lateral side only, involving the articulation with either the second or fourth metacarpal bones (Fig. 20-23).[3] Unlike the high-motion joints of the carpus, changes are likely to include subchondral lucency as well as subchondral sclerosis and often periosteal new bone extending along the proximal metaphysis and diaphysis of the affected metacarpal bone.

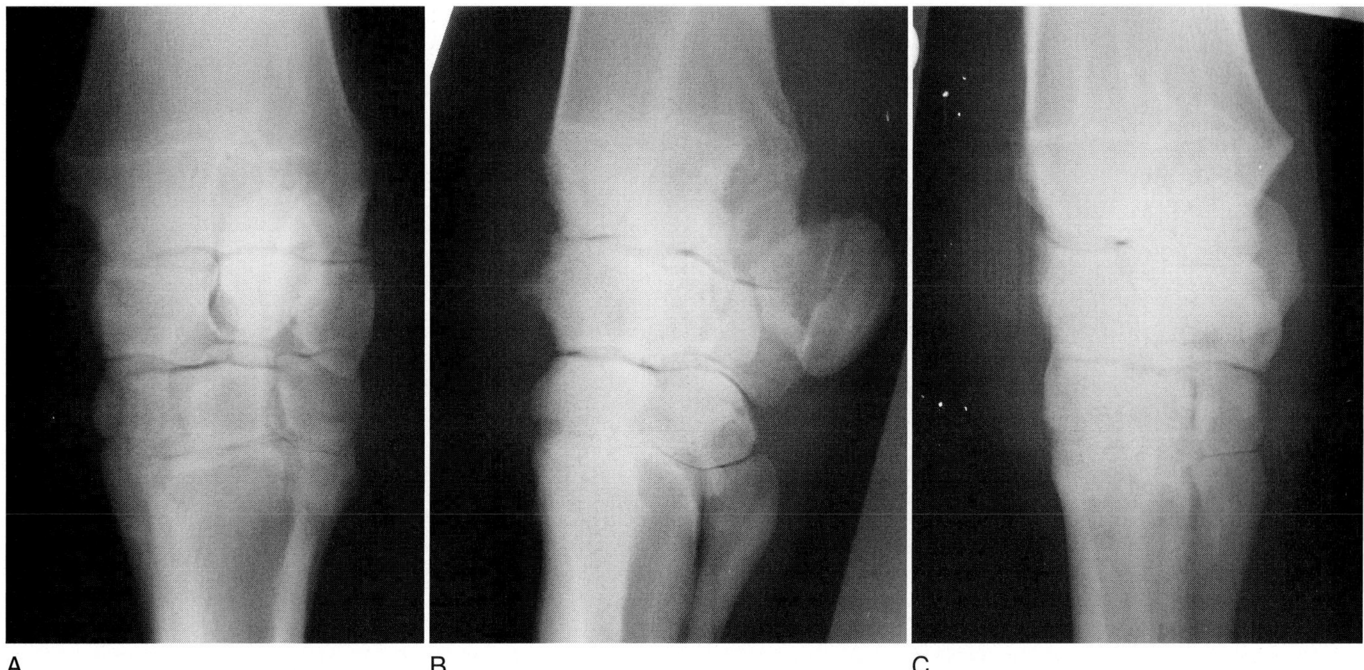

Fig. 20-22 A, Dorsopalmar view of a carpus. Lateral is to the right. Narrowing of the antebrachiocarpal joint medially and of the entire carpometacarpal joint is visible, consistent with advanced osteoarthritis. The horse was an international-level event horse that had received multiple intraarticular injections of corticosteroids. **B,** Dorsolateral-palmaromedial oblique view of the same carpus as in **A.** Extensive soft tissue swelling on the dorsal aspect of the carpus and modeling of the dorsal distal aspect of the radius are present. Prominent entheseous new bone is visible on the dorsal aspect of the radial carpal bone. **C,** Dorsomedial-palmarolateral oblique view of the same carpus as **A** and **B.** Extensive soft tissue swelling is present on the dorsal aspect of the carpus, narrowing of the antebrachiocarpal, middle carpal, and carpometacarpal joint spaces, as is modeling of the articular margins of the antebrachiocarpal joint and entheseous new bone on the dorsal aspect of the intermediate carpal bone.

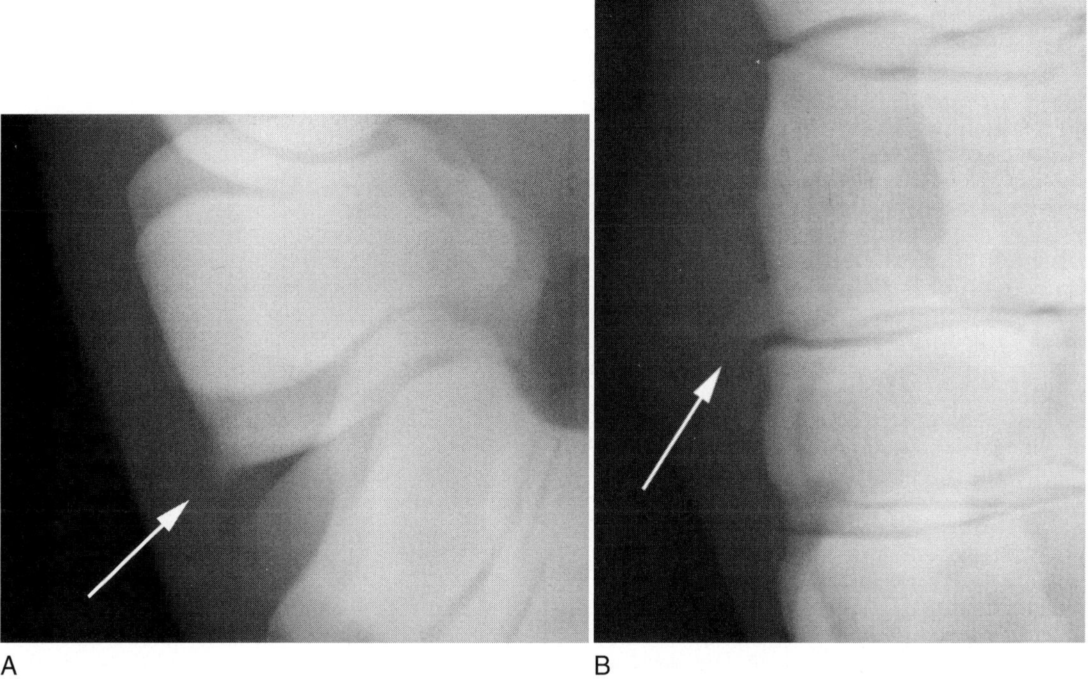

Fig. 20-23 A, Flexed lateromedial view of a carpus. A large osteophyte is present on the distal dorsal aspect of the radial carpal bone *(arrow)*, consistent with osteoarthritis of the middle carpal joint. The radiograph is deliberately underexposed. **B,** Dorsolateral-palmaromedial oblique view of the same carpus as in **A.** Periarticular soft tissue swelling is centered at the middle carpal joint, and a large osteophyte *(arrow)* is present on the distal dorsal aspect of the radial carpal bone.

Sepsis

Septic arthritis and osteomyelitis Horses with septic arthritis usually become severely lame within 24 hours of infection, with heat and swelling of the carpal region. If septic arthritis is suspected, diagnosis and treatment should be instigated as an emergency because early treatment is linked to improved prognosis.[55] Once articular cartilage damage and osteomyelitis are present, prognosis for a positive outcome reduces dramatically, with the horse being unlikely to return to athletic function. Septic arthritis can occur as a result of a penetrating wound, hematogenous infection, or spread from adjacent tissues in conditions such as septic tenosynovitis or osteomyelitis.[56] Although rare, iatrogenic infection caused by intraarticular injection or arthroscopy can occur.[56,57]

Septic arthritis of the carpal joints occurs not uncommonly in foals with failure of passive transfer of immunity, high sepsis score, or multisystemic disease.[58] These foals may be relatively less lame than older horses with septic arthritis.[56] However, the prognosis in foals is more guarded than that for adult horses, even if treatment is instigated at the onset of clinical signs.[56,57] A significant proportion of foals with septic arthritis have concurrent osteomyelitis.[58] Radiolucent changes in the bone may rapidly occur after the onset of clinical signs but can be more difficult to visualize in the carpal bones than in the distal radius. Infarction can also occur and can delay recognition of bone involvement because radiolucency is less apparent.[55]

Radiographic signs include distension of the affected joint and sometimes generalized soft tissue swelling. Widening of the joint space may be present in the early stages, particularly when the limb is not bearing weight. In the more chronic phase, damage to the articular surfaces may be visible. Articular cartilage loss leads to joint space narrowing, and subchondral bone destruction is observed as irregular subchondral lucency or decreased opacity. Areas of sclerosis may also be observed. Reactive new bone on the periarticular aspects is seen as a disorganized, low-opacity irregularity on the joint margins. Increasing bridging of the antebrachiocarpal, middle carpal, or carpometacarpal joints occurs, with accompanying new bone within the intercarpal joints, progressing toward ankylosis.[3]

Further diagnosis needs to be made on the basis of synoviocentesis and synovial analysis with Gram stain and culture. Hematologic examination and blood culture are also recommended in foals. Management of septic arthritis usually requires joint lavage, intraarticular and systemic antimicrobial therapy, and antiinflammatory use at a minimum. Open drainage and synovial debridement and use of antimicrobial-impregnated methylmethacrylate or regional antimicrobial infusion have all been used as additional options for management.[55]

REFERENCES

1. Sisson S: Equine syndesmology. In Getty R, editor: *The anatomy of the domestic animals,* Ed 5, Philadelphia, 1975, WB Saunders, pp 349-375.
2. Smallwood JE, Shiveley M: Radiographic and xeroradiographic anatomy of the equine carpus, *Equine Pract* 1:22, 1979.
3. Butler JA, Colles CM, Dyson SJ et al: *Clinical radiology of the horse,* ed 2, Oxford, 2003, Blackwell Science Ltd.
4. Auer J, Smallwood J, Morris E et al: The developing equine carpus from birth to 6 months. A radiographic study, *Equine Pract* 4:35, 1982.
5. Myers VS: Confusing radiological variation at the distal end of the radius of the horse, *J Am Vet Med Assoc* 147:1310, 1986.
6. Ross M: Carpus. In Ross MW, Dyson SJ, editors: *Diagnosis and management of lameness in the horse,* St. Louis, 2003, Elsevier Science, pp 376-394.
7. Murray RC, Vedi S, Birch HL et al: Subchondral bone thickness, hardness and remodeling are influenced by short term exercise in a site specific manner, *J Orthop Res* 19:1035, 2001.
8. Young A, O'Brien T, Pool R: Exercise related sclerosis in the third carpal bone of the racing thoroughbred, *Proc Am Assoc Equine Pract* 34:339, 1988.
9. O'Donohue DD, Smith FH, Strickland DL: The incidence of abnormal limb development in the Irish Thoroughbred from birth to 18 months, *Equine Vet J* 24:305, 1992.
10. Watkins JP: Osteochondrosis. In Auer JA, editor: *Equine surgery,* Philadelphia, 1992, W.B. Saunders, pp 971-984.
11. Ellis DR: Physitis. In Ross MW, Dyson SJ, editors: *Diagnosis and management of lameness in the horse,* St. Louis, 2003, Elsevier Science, pp 554-556.
12. Auer JA: Angular limb deformities. In Auer JA, editor: *Equine surgery,* Philadelphia, 1992, W.B. Saunders, pp 940-956.
13. Auer JA, Marten RJ, Morris EL: Angular limb deformities in foals: congenital factors, *Compend Contin Educ Pract Vet* 4:13, 1983.
14. Adams R, Poulos P: A skeletal ossification index for neonatal foals, *Vet Radiol* 29:217, 1988.
15. Parente EJ: Angular limb deformities. In Ross MW, Dyson SJ, editors: *Diagnosis and management of lameness in the horse,* St. Louis, 2003, Elsevier Science, pp 557-561.
16. Caron JP: Angular limb deformities in foals, *Equine Vet J* 20:225, 1988.
17. Gaughan EM: Angular limb deformities in horses, *Compend Contin Educ Pract Vet* 20:944, 1998.
18. Ellis D: Some observations on bone cysts in the carpal bones of young thoroughbreds, *Equine Vet J* 17:63, 1985.
19. McIlwraith CW: Subchondral cystic lesions (osteochondrosis) in the horse, *Comp Contin Ed Pract Vet* 4:S396, 1982.
20. Specht TE, Nixon AJ, Colahan PT: Subchondral cyst-like lesions in the distal portion of the radius of four horses, *J Am Vet Med Assoc* 193:949, 1988.
21. Walmsley JP: Diagnosis and management of osteochondrosis and osseous cyst-like lesions. In Ross MW, Dyson SJ, editors: *Diagnosis and management of lameness in the horse,* St. Louis, 2003, Elsevier Science, pp 455-470.
22. Adams SB, Santschi EM: Management of flexural deformities in young horses, *Equine Pract* 21:9, 1999.
23. Platt D, Wright I: Chronic tenosynovitis of the carpal extensor tendon sheaths in 15 horses, *Equine Vet J* 29:11, 1997.
24. Dietze A, Rendano V: Fat opacities dorsal to the equine antebrachiocarpal joint, *Vet Radiol* 25:205, 1984.
25. Mackey-Smith MP, Cushing LS, Leslie JA: Carpal canal syndrome in horses, *J Am Vet Med Assoc* 160:993, 1972.
26. Dyson SJ: The carpal canal and carpal synovial sheath. In Ross MW, Dyson SJ, editors: Diagnosis and management of lameness in the horse, St. Louis, 2003, Elsevier Science, pp 685-687.
27. Dyson S: Fractures of the accessory carpal bone, *Equine Vet Educ* 2:188, 1990.
28. Barr ARS, Sinnott MJA, Denny HR: Fractures of the accessory carpal bone in the horse, *Equine Vet J* 126:432, 1990.
29. Barr A, Sinnott M, Denny H: Fractures of the accessory carpal bone in the horse, *Vet Rec* 127:432, 1990.
30. Held JP, Patton CDS, Shores M: Solitary osteochondroma of the radius in three horses, *J Am Vet Med Assoc* 193:563, 1988.

31. Wyburn RS, Goulden BE: Fractures of the equine carpus: a report on 57 cases, *NZ Vet J* 22:133, 1974.
32. Park RD, Morgan JP, O'Brien T: Chip fractures in the carpus of the horse; a radiographic study of their incidence and location, *J Am Vet Med Assoc* 157:1305, 1970.
33. Palmer SE: Prevalence of carpal fractures in Thoroughbred and Standardbred racehorses, *J Am Vet Med Assoc* 188:1172, 1986.
34. Bramlage L, Schneider R, Gabel A: A clinical perspective on lameness originating in the carpus, *Equine Vet J* 6(suppl):12, 1988.
35. Auer JA, Fackelman GE: Treatment of degenerative joint disease of the horse: a review of and commentary, *Vet Surg* 10:80, 1981.
36. McIlwraith CW, Yovich JV, Martin GS: Arthroscopic surgery for the treatment of osteochondral chip fractures in the equine carpus, *J Am Vet Med Assoc* 191:531, 1987.
37. Schneider RK, Bramlage LR, Gabel AA et al: Incidence, location and classification of 371 third carpal bone fractures in 313 horses, *Equine Vet J* 6(suppl):33, 1988.
38. Bramlage LR: Surgical diseases of the carpus, *Vet Clin North Am (Large Anim Pract)* 5:261, 1983.
39. Murray RC, Zhu CF, Goodship AE et al: Exercise affects the mechanical properties and histological appearance of equine articular cartilage, *J Orthop Res* 17:725, 1999.
40. Dabareiner RM, White NA, Sullins KE: Radiographic and arthroscopic findings associated with subchondral lucency of the distal radial carpal bone in 71 horses, *Equine Vet J* 28:93, 1996.
41. Young DR, Richardson DW, Markel MD et al: Mechanical and morphometric analysis of the third carpal bone of Thoroughbreds, *Am J Vet Res* 52:402, 1991.
42. Uhlhorn H, Carlsten J: Retrospective study of subchondral sclerosis and lucency in the third carpal bone of Standardbred trotters, *Equine Vet J* 31:500, 1999.
43. Ross MW, Richardson DW, Beroza GA: Subchondral lucency of the third carpal bone in Standardbred racehorses: 13 cases (1982-1988), *J Am Vet Med Assoc* 195:789, 1989.
44. Thrall DE, Lebel JL, O'Brien TR: A five year survey of the incidence and location of equine carpal chip fractures, *J Am Med Assoc* 158:1366, 1971.
45. Dabareiner RM, Sulins KE, Bardley W: Removal of a fracture fragment from the palmar aspect of the intermedial carpal bone in a horse, *J Am Vet Med Assoc* 203:553, 1993.
46. De Hann CE, O'Brien TR, Koblik PD: A radiographic investigation of third carpal injury in 42 racing Thoroughbreds, *Vet Radiol* 28:88, 1987.
47. Stephens PR, Richardson DW, Spencer PA: Slab fractures of the third carpal bone in Standardbreds and Thoroughbreds: 155 cases (1977-1984), *J Am Vet Med Assoc* 193:353, 1988.
48. Auer JA, Watkins JP, White NA et al: Slab fractures of the four and intermediate carpal bones in five horses, *J Am Vet Med Assoc* 188:595, 1986.
49. Uhlhorn H, Ekman S, Haglund A et al: The accuracy of the dorsoproximal-dorsodistal projection in assessing third carpal bone sclerosis in Standardbred trotters, *Vet Radiol Ultrasound* 39:412, 1988.
50. Fischer AT, Stover SM: Sagittal fractures of the third carpal bone in horses: 12 cases (1977-1985), *J Am Vet Med Assoc* 192:106, 1987.
51. Gertsen KE, Dawson HA: Sagittal fracture of the third carpal bone in a horse, *J Am Vet Med Assoc* 169:633, 1976.
52. Palmer SE: Lag screw fixation of a sagittal fracture of the third carpal bone in a horse, *Vet Surg* 12:54, 1986.
53. Mair T, Dyson S, Fraser J et al: Hypertrophic osteopathy (Marie's disease) in Equidae: a review of twenty-four cases, *Equine Vet J* 28:256, 1996.
54. Beinlich CP, Nixon AJ: Radiographic and pathologic characterization of lateral palmar intercarpal ligament avulsion fractures in the horse, *Vet Radiol Ultrasound* 45:532, 2004.
55. Bertone AL: Infectious arthritis. In Ross MW, Dyson SJ, editors: *Diagnosis and management of lameness in the horse*, St. Louis, 2003, Elsevier Science, pp 685-687.
56. Schneider RK, Bramlage LR, Moore RM et al: A retrospective study of 192 horses affected with septic arthritis/tenosynovitis, *Equine Vet J* 24:436, 1992.
57. Meijer MC, van Weeren PR, Rijkenhuizen AB: Clinical experiences of treating septic arthritis in the equine by repeated joint lavage: a series of 39 cases, *J Vet Med A Physiol Pathol Clin Med* 47:351, 2000.
58. Steel CM, Hunte AR, Adams PLE et al: Factors associated with prognosis for survival and athletic use in foals with septic arthritis: 93 cases (1987-1994), *J Am Vet Med Assoc* 215:973, 1999.

ELECTRONIC RESOURCES evolve

Additional information related to the content in Chapter 20 can be found on the companion Web site at
evolve http://evolve.elsevier.com/Thrall/vetrad/
- Key Points
- Chapter Quiz
- Case Study 20-1

CHAPTER • 21
The Metacarpus and Metatarsus

Stephen K. Kneller

ANATOMIC CONSIDERATIONS

Third Metacarpus and Third Metatarsus: The Cannon Bone

Radiographically, the third metacarpus and metatarsus (MC III and MT III) are nearly the same (Fig. 21-1). The midportion of the dorsal cortex is thicker than the remaining cortex, and it thins gradually toward the ends of the bone. This variable cortical thickness is often mistaken for abnormal bone remodeling or periosteal response. The palmar/plantar cortex is more uniform in thickness and is interrupted at the junction of the proximal and middle third by the nutrient foramen. Unlike the nutrient foramina of smaller bones, those in MC III and MT III are channels, which may be mistaken for a fracture on lateral and oblique views, especially in the rear limb (Fig. 21-2).

The proximal physis has fused by the time of birth. The distal epiphysis is within the metacarpophalangeal (metatarsophalangeal) joint and is one of the first sites to become abnormal in metabolic bone disease, although its appearance varies in the normal animal at different ages.

On the lateral view, the metacarpus and metatarsus differ at the distal end (see Fig. 21-1). The metacarpus is relatively straight, whereas the distal end of the metatarsus usually curves slightly, giving the dorsal border a slightly convex appearance.

Interest exists in quantifying the thickness, shape, and symmetry of the metacarpus in racing horses for assessment of racing and training potential. The significance and utility of this process appears unclear at this point.[1,2]

Second and Fourth Metacarpi and Metatarsi: The Splint Bones

These small bones articulate with the carpus or tarsus and taper distally. The size and shape vary among animals and limbs.[3] The degree of natural outward curvature also varies. The distal end is usually in the form of a slight bulbous enlargement of variable size and shape, but the margins are smooth and distinct.

In the forelimb, the medial splint bone (MC II) is usually longer than the lateral (MC IV), although MC IV may be the same length or longer than MC II. In the rear limb, when compared with MT II, MT IV is relatively massive and irregular at the proximal aspect, often extending proximal to MT III.

The proximal epiphysis of the splint bones, apparently present in the fetus, is fused and therefore not visible at birth. The distal epiphysis is cartilaginous and therefore is not visible radiographically at birth. As it ossifies, the distal epiphysis is separated from the body of the bone by cartilage until fusion occurs. Care should be taken to avoid mistaking the normal epiphysis as a fracture (Fig. 21-3).

Mach Bands: False Fracture Lines

A visual phenomenon in radiography that causes some confusion is edge enhancement, or mach bands.[4] This phenomenon is especially evident in radiographs of equine metacarpi and metatarsi. Simply stated, as one bone edge crosses another on a radiograph, a radiolucent line may appear. This line may often be seen on the palmar or plantar aspect of the equine metacarpus and metatarsus, resulting in erroneous diagnoses of cortical fracture of MC III or MT III, as well as fractures of the smaller metacarpal and metatarsal bones (Fig. 21-4). To guard against erroneous diagnoses, the anatomic contour of each bone must be followed carefully, with additional radiographs obtained for clarification as needed.

CHARACTERIZATION OF LESIONS

Soft Tissue Enlargement and Mineralization

Abnormal size and shape of the soft tissues in the metacarpal and metatarsal areas may be evident on radiographs as enlargements over the dorsal surface, with early metacarpal periostitis; generalized enlargements along the palmaroplantar surface, with suspensory desmitis and flexor tendon abnormalities; and localized areas along the small metacarpal or metatarsal bones, usually proximally, with interosseous ligament damage.[3-5] Because minimal soft tissue is present in these areas, such soft tissue abnormalities should also be evident on visual inspection and palpation of the horse.

The purpose of radiographically evaluating the soft tissues is threefold. First, in a busy practice, performing a quick physical examination and proceeding with radiographic examination is a common temptation. Finding soft tissue enlargements radiographically should stimulate a more thorough physical examination of the area in question. Second, although thorough study of the radiographs is paramount, finding a soft tissue abnormality should lead to an in-depth review of the underlying bony structures to evaluate the extent of the lesion and to further characterize it. The third purpose is correlation of abnormalities, that is, evaluating the association or lack of association of bony lesions with soft tissue enlargements in size, shape, and proximity as well as relative activity. For example, in many horses tendons and ligaments may be delineated because of the loose, fat-laden adventitia interposed between them. In such horses, a low degree of inflammation may result in loss of visualization of these margins on high-quality radiographs.

Soft tissue mineralization may be identified, especially in the suspensory ligament and flexor tendon areas. Surface debris and medication should be removed to avoid confusion. Mineralization within the soft tissues is usually dystrophic as a result of injury of some duration. The injury may be from

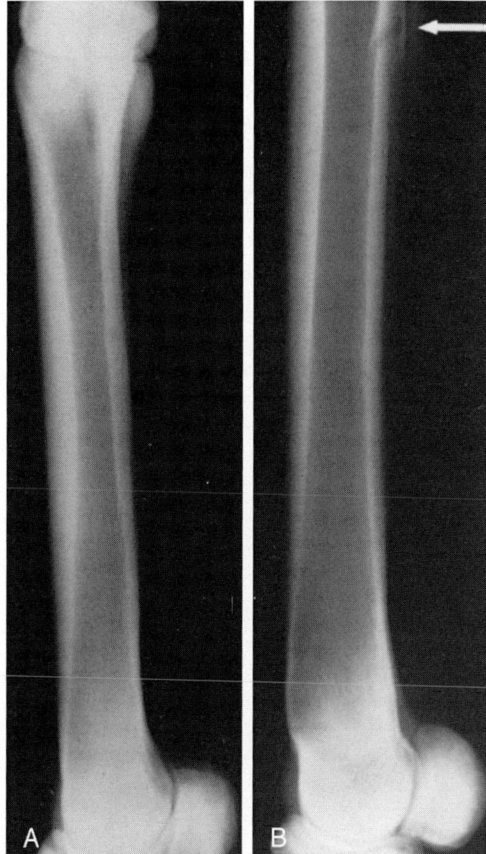

Fig. 21-1 Normal lateral radiographs of the metacarpus (A) and the metatarsus (B). Note that the metacarpus is straight, whereas the metatarsus curves slightly at the distal end. The dorsal cortex in both bones is thicker, especially at the midportion. The large nutrient foramen is evident in the metatarsus *(arrow)*.

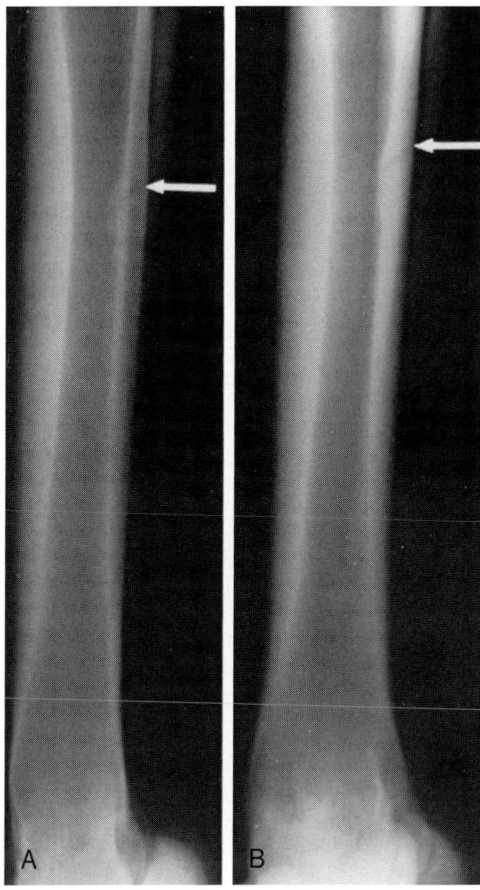

Fig. 21-2 Lateral (A) and dorsomedial-plantarolateral (B) views of the left metatarsus of a 1-year-old Thoroughbred colt. The nutrient foramen appears as a channel through the plantar cortex of MT III *(arrows)*.

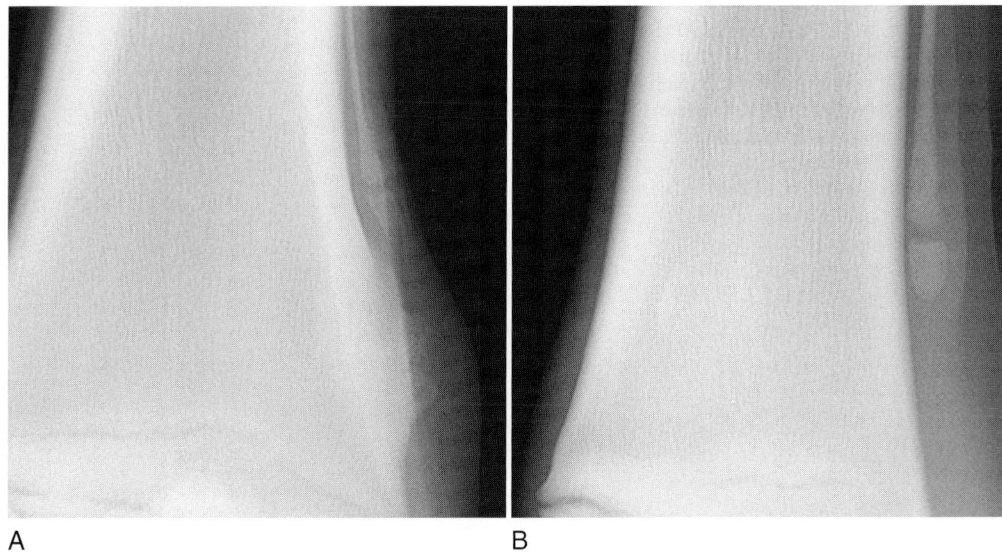

Fig. 21-3 Dorsolateral-plantaromedial (A) and dorsomedial-plantarolateral (B) radiographs of the distal aspect of the left metacarpus of a 2-month-old Quarter horse. The distal epiphyses of MT IV (A) and II (B) have not fused to the diaphyses; this appearance should not be confused with a fracture. A region of smooth, periosteal, trauma-induced reaction is visible on the distolateral aspect of the third metacarpal metaphysis.

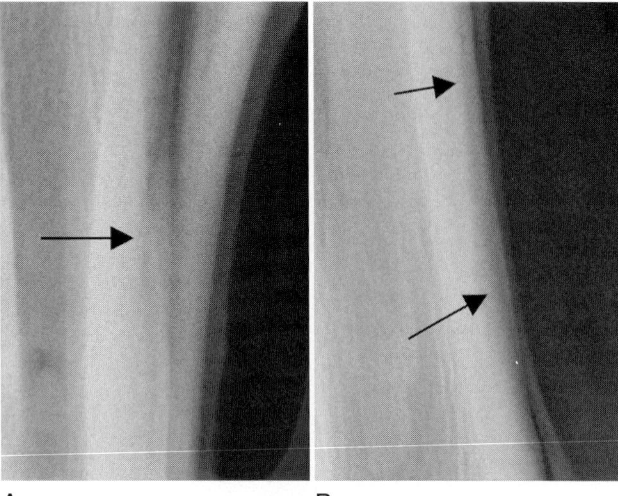

Fig. 21-4 Dorsomedial-palmarolateral radiographs of the proximal (A) and distal (B) aspect of the metacarpal region of two different horses. In each, a black line *(arrows)* is created when the cortex of MC IV overlaps the cortex of MT II. This line is caused by the mach effect and should not be misinterpreted as a fracture.

work-related stress, resulting in damaged or torn structures, or it may be caused by drug injections.

Penetrating foreign objects may also be present in soft tissues. Therefore familiarity with the normal appearance of soft tissue is important to recognize foreign objects that have an opacity similar to adjacent soft tissue. These foreign objects result in a disturbance of the normal size, shape, or opacity relationships.

Mineralization in the skin and subcutaneous tissues may result from surface injuries and must be differentiated from deeper mineralization. In the rear limb, the chestnut may contain mineral and be mistaken for disease.

Mineral opacity between the small metacarpal or metatarsal bones and MC or MT III is a common finding as a result of trauma to the interosseous ligament (splint disease) (Fig. 21-5). This opacity may represent actual mineralization of the interosseous ligament or an associated periosteal reaction. As in any dystrophic mineralization, this radiographic sign is not evident until some time after the injury. Accurate positioning is imperative when assessing for mineralization of the interosseous ligament because overlap of the bones may produce a similar appearance (Fig. 21-6). In some horses, because of the bone contour, multiple views at slightly different angles must be made to separate the bones completely throughout the length of overlap. When this mineralization is evident, previous injury has occurred in the interosseous ligament. Splint disease is discussed more thoroughly in the following section.

Periosteal Response

On high-quality radiographs, periosteal surfaces of the metacarpus and metatarsus should be smooth and well defined. Because of the geometry of the bones, the dorsal surface of MC III or MT III may appear indistinct on radiographs unless a high-intensity illuminator (hot light) is used. If using digital images, the brightness should intentionally be increased substantially to look for regions of periosteal response. Periosteal response is a healing response, and the appearance depends on the stage of healing. If the inciting cause is removed, the periosteal response becomes mature and organized over time.

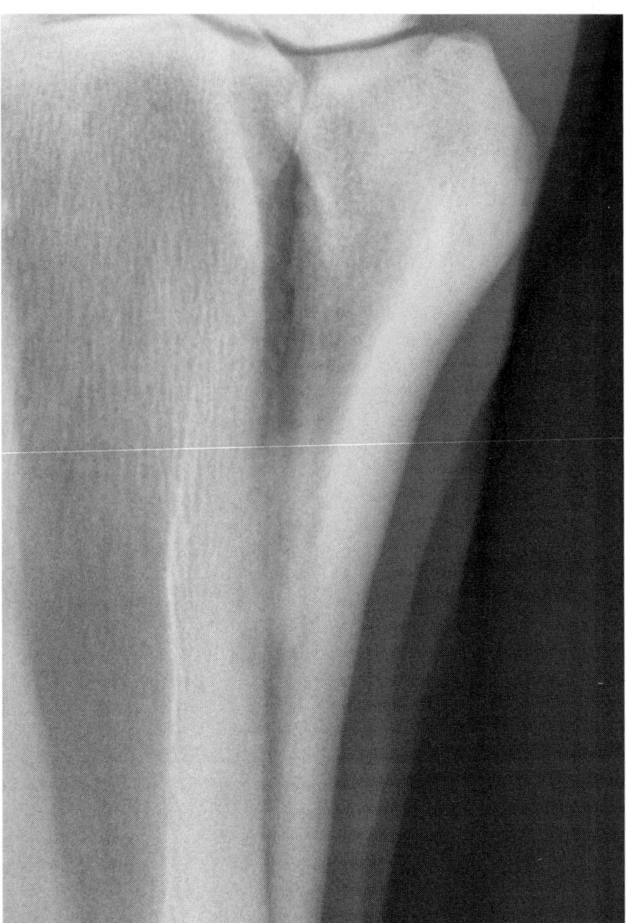

Fig. 21-5 Dorsolateral-palmaromedial radiograph of the proximal aspect of the metacarpus of a 13-year-old Percheron. An irregular margin and amorphous hyperostosis are visible between MC III and MC IV consistent with enthesophytosis from interosseous ligament pulling.

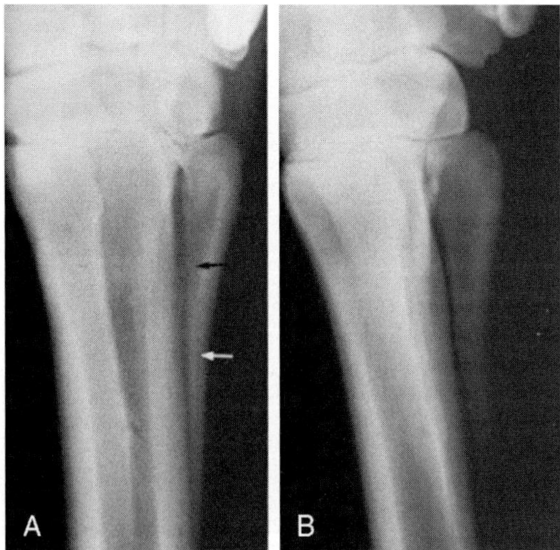

Fig. 21-6 A, Dorsolateral-palmaromedial radiograph of the metacarpal region of an 11-year-old Morgan mare in which MC IV can be seen. The space between MC III and MC IV is not clearly visible, suggesting mineralization of the interosseous ligament *(arrows)*. B, Same view at a different angle. A clear separation of MC III and MC IV is visible, with no abnormal mineralization.

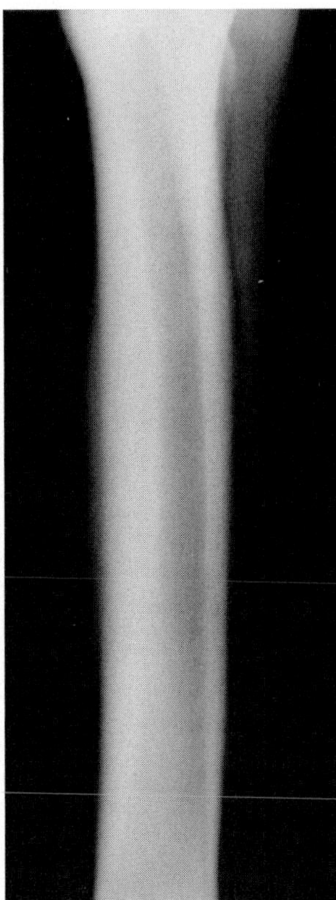

Fig. 21-7 Lateral view of the left metacarpus of a 2-year-old racing Quarter horse. A layer of periosteal new bone is present on the dorsal aspect of the midportion of MC III. The right MC III had similar changes.

The dorsal surface of the MC III may develop a periosteal response because of microfractures; this is commonly referred to as *metacarpal periostitis* or *bucked shins* (Fig. 21-7). Care should be taken to evaluate the cortex for fracture lines.

Another relatively common location for periosteal response is between MC/MT II and III, with lesions between MC/MT III and IV occurring less frequently. Lesions between MC/MT II and III are usually associated with the proximal half of the splint bones and are caused by interosseous ligament damage (splint disease) (Fig. 21-8). The periosteal response is variable in size; the response initially is ill defined and irregular, but it gradually becomes smooth, opaque, and smaller as it matures, fusing the small bones to the larger bones. A large, irregular periosteal response may mimic a fracture, yet a fracture may be masked by the callus formation.

Cortical Bone Abnormalities

Cortical lysis in the metacarpal and metatarsal bones is usually associated with localized trauma. Injury to the periosteum of MC III or MT III may cause death of the outer third of the bone, with a resulting sequestrum (Fig. 21-9). This is related to the thick cortex of these bones and the inability of the endosteal blood supply to maintain viability of the dorsal cortex after periosteal disruption.

Metacarpal and metatarsal fractures are common, especially in racing horses. The most common fracture site in these regions is the distal half of MC II and IV and MT II and IV. As previously mentioned, care must be taken to avoid mistaking cartilaginous plates and mach bands for fractures. Fractures may also occur in the proximal half of MC II and IV and MT II and IV, and these fractures may be mistaken clinically for typical splints.

Aside from complete fractures of MC III and MT III, which are obvious, incomplete fractures may be difficult to diagnose (Fig. 21-10). They do, however, occur in specific locations. These incomplete stress fractures are usually seen in racing horses. The lesion most readily diagnosed is the sagittal distal condylar fracture (Fig. 21-11). This fracture frequently affects MC III, extending proximally from the metacarpophalangeal joint; it may be displaced significantly. Often this fracture may be seen only on the dorsopalmar or slightly oblique view, and it may be easily missed on underexposed radiographs. Evidence exists that distal condylar fractures are often predisposed from previous stress injury in thoroughbred racing horses.[6]

Stress fractures may also be found in the dorsal cortex, especially associated with metacarpal periostitis (Fig. 21-12). These fractures occur most often on the dorsomedial aspect near the junction of the middle and distal third of the bone. Because of their shape, these lesions have been called *saucer fractures.*

Fractures also occur in the palmar or plantar cortex. The most common site is approximately 2 to 3 cm from the proximal articular surface, although they may occur in the midportion of the bone. Associated lesions have been reported as avulsion fractures, stress fractures, and stress response, sometimes linked with disease of the suspensory ligament.[5,7-9] Some appear radiographically only on the dorsopalmar or dorsoplantar view as a thin crescent- or linear-shaped region of decreased opacity (Fig. 21-13). Other appearances associated with proximal suspensory desmitis include an irregular trabecular pattern or slightly increased opacity in the proximal portion of MT or MC III; horses with these radiographic changes are usually characterized by marked increased radiopharmaceutical uptake in the region, as seen in a radionuclide bone scan (Fig. 21-14). Typically these abnormalities are medial to the midsagittal plane, although they may also be lateral. To assess the radiographic opacity of the medullary cavity of MT or MC III if a proximal suspensory ligament is suspected, excellent-quality radiographs are needed because overexposure or underexposure may lead to misinterpretation. Lesions of the proximal aspect of the suspensory ligament are more accurately characterized by bone scintigraphy, ultrasound examination, or magnetic resonance imaging than by radiography.

Abnormal shape of MC and MT III results from growth disturbance and is most often seen at the distal end of the bone. This shape change may be seen as a single, localized problem, or it may be seen in conjunction with more proximal limb abnormalities.

Although the size and shape of the small metacarpal and metatarsal bones vary considerably, abaxial deviation of the distal end of the splint bones is often associated with suspensory desmitis, presumably from outward pressure exerted by the enlarged ligaments (Fig. 21-15). If this outward curving is noted, the suspensory ligaments should be evaluated for inflammation and enlargement, but apparent deviation should not be considered diagnostic for suspensory desmitis.

ULTRASOUND: METACARPAL/METATARSAL REGION

Radiographic evaluation of the soft tissues on the palmar/plantar aspect of the equine limb is severely limited because of the lack of contrast resolution between soft tissue structures. But because of differences in tissue character, diagnostic ultrasound has been found useful to assess anatomic structure and disease conditions in this area.[10,11] The superficial digital flexor tendon (SDF) and the deep digital flexor tendon (DDF), as well as the suspensory and the "check"

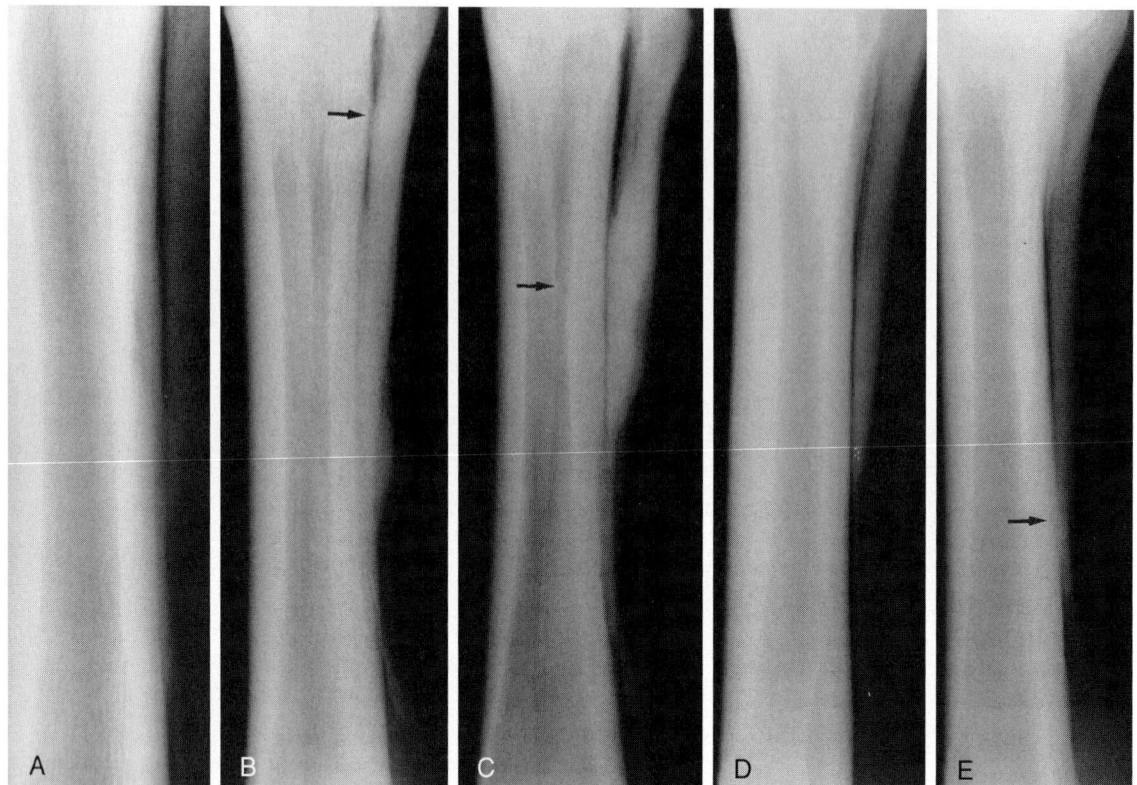

Fig. 21-8 Dorsomedial-palmarolateral radiographs of the metacarpal region of several horses with different appearances of damaged interosseous ligaments (splint lesions). **A,** A 13-year-old Thoroughbred gelding (hunter-jumper) with a recent interosseous injury. A slight periosteal response and a small amount of cortical bone lysis are evident. This is the typical appearance of a 2- to 3-week-old lesion. **B,** A 3-year-old Standardbred gelding. The periosteal response is more organized but still active. It involves most of the attachment area of the interosseous ligament with a separate site of reaction proximally *(arrow)*. **C,** A 2-year-old Standardbred gelding. As in **B,** this lesion is chronic but appears active and is most likely at least 6 weeks old. The periosteal reaction is large and opaque over a localized area, but it has not become smooth. The large mass may produce abnormal pressure on surrounding soft tissues. The nutrient foramen *(arrow)* should not be confused with a lesion. **D,** A 2-year-old Thoroughbred filly. The lesion on the midportion of MC II is inactive. This is typical of a 3- to 6-week-old lesion that has been protected with rest. Such a lesion would be expected to become solid with no enlargement. **E,** A 5-year-old Standardbred gelding. The lesion is near the distal end of MC II *(arrow)*. It is opaque and smooth, blending together with the cortex of MC II and MC III as a chronic inactive lesion. Lameness may result from concussion of MC II and the interosseous ligament, exaggerated by the distal fusion of MC II to MC III. The appearance of the proximal end is caused by overlap of MC II, MC III, and MC IV.

(accessory) ligament, are composed of dense linear fibers that are more echogenic than is surrounding loose tissue (Fig. 21-16). Because these structures are uniform in echotexture, defects such as hemorrhage, fiber disruption, and inflammatory lesions appear as hypoechoic areas within the structure. Also, fluid within tendon sheaths is visible adjacent to structures and tendon sheaths. In addition, the cross-sectional size of these structures is uniform. Calipers found on most ultrasound machines allow relatively precise measurement of structures.

Sonographic anatomy of the metacarpal/metatarsal region has been described.[12-16] Variation has been reported, however, regarding the normal size and appearance of these structures relative to the type and degree of activity and the age of the patient.[17-22] Understanding variations between front limbs and hindlimbs, as well as the effect of the use of the patient, is necessary to avoid erroneous diagnoses and assessments.

Along with variation within patients, technical factors and errors in performance of the examination can severely affect the appearance of the image.[23-25] The quality of ultrasound machines is extremely variable. Equipment that is satisfactory for one purpose is not necessarily satisfactory for another. Image clarity and definition are important when examining structures that are typically 1 cm or less in thickness. Most probes scanning at less than 7 MHz are not satisfactory for accurate evaluation of equine tendons. The ultrasound beam must also be powerful enough to penetrate to the palmar aspect of the limb. For full evaluation, the ability to change the depth of interest to allow adequate assessment of the suspensory ligament as well as the very near SDF is helpful. Probe design is important to allow an adequate area of contact between the probe surface and the limb. The smaller the radius of the probe surface arc, the more difficult it is to use. Even with excellent equipment, the examination technique

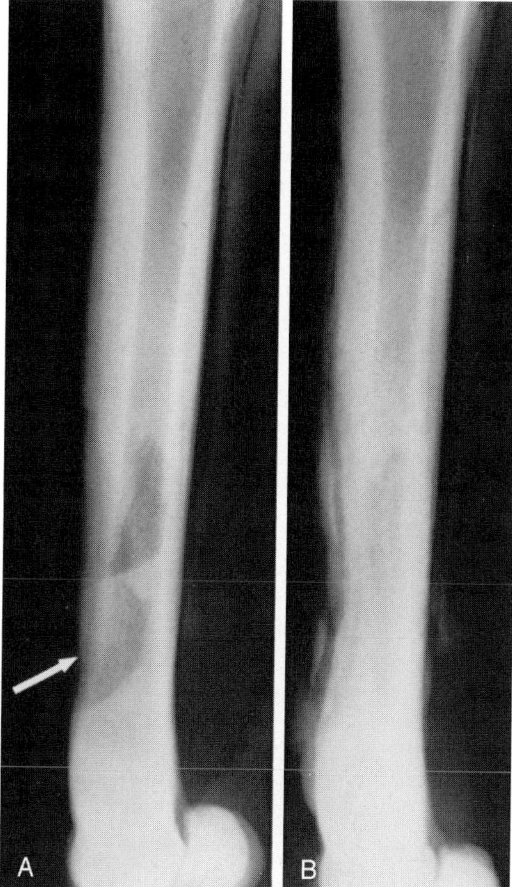

Fig. 21-9 A, Lateral view of the right metatarsal region of a 3-year-old Quarter horse mare 10 days after the limb was severely injured, exposing a large portion of MT III. The large radiolucent areas overlying MT III are caused by missing soft tissue. A faint, dark line is present within the dorsal cortex of MT III *(arrow)*, indicative of fracture or impending sequestration. B, A lateral view 3 weeks later. The sequestered bone can now be seen to extend proximally.

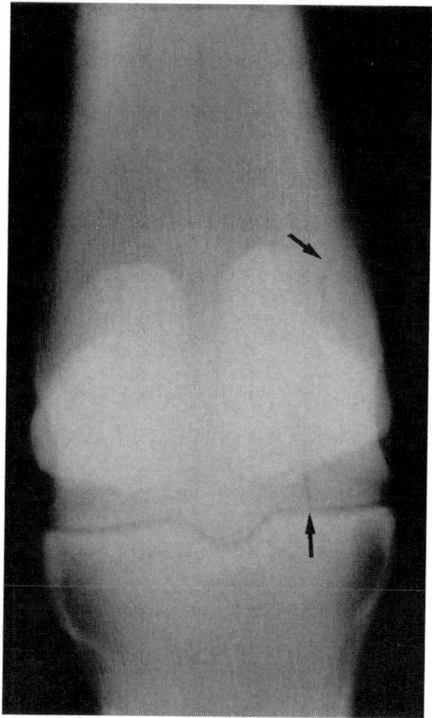

Fig. 21-11 Dorsopalmar radiograph of the left front limb of a 4-year-old Thoroughbred stallion. A sagittal fracture is present in the lateral distal condyle of MC III *(arrows)*. This lesion was not visible on lateral or oblique views.

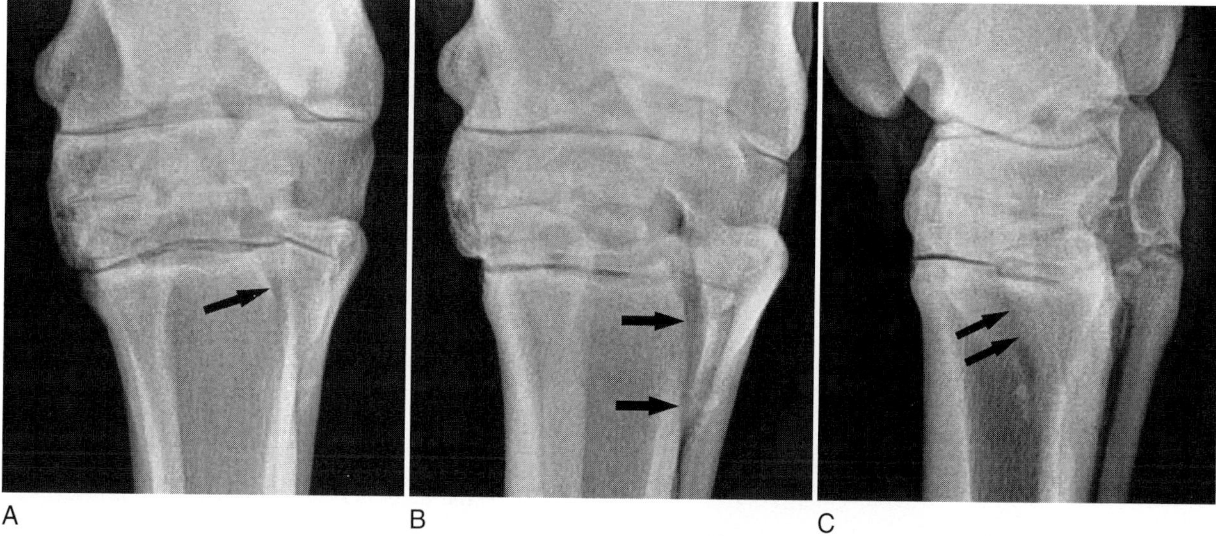

Fig. 21-10 Dorsoplantar (A), dorsomedial-plantarolateral (B), and dorsomedial-plantarolateral (C) radiographs of the right tarsus and proximal metatarsus of a 7-year-old Quarter horse gelding with history of right hindlimb lameness for several months. The owner reported the patient fell in the pasture when the problem began, but no swelling could be palpated at the time of examination. The horse was sound at a walk, but mild lameness was present when trotting and jogging. An oblique fracture of the proximal plantarolateral aspect of MT III is visible *(arrows)*. The cortical disruption at the distal end of the fracture is evident on the dorsolateral-plantaromedial view (A). The distal intertarsal joint space is not visible because of fusion of the joint. (Radiographs courtesy Dr. Susan Bontkowski, private practice, Cary, Ill.)

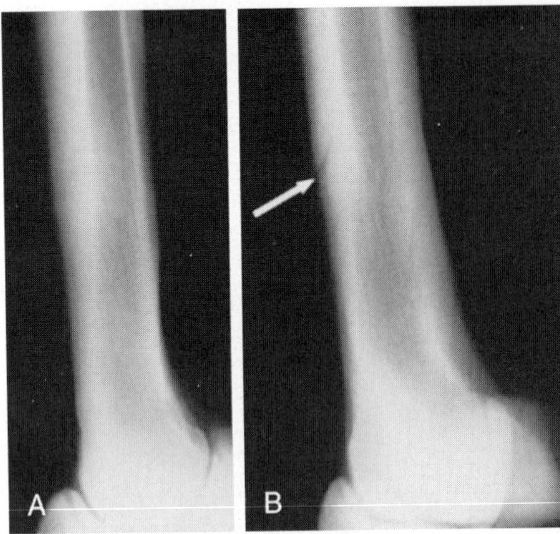

Fig. 21-12 Lateral (A) and dorsolateral-palmaromedial (B) views of the left metacarpal region of a 6-year-old Thoroughbred gelding that became lame immediately after a race 2 weeks before the radiographs were made. The stress fracture *(arrow)* evident in **B** is barely visible in **A**.

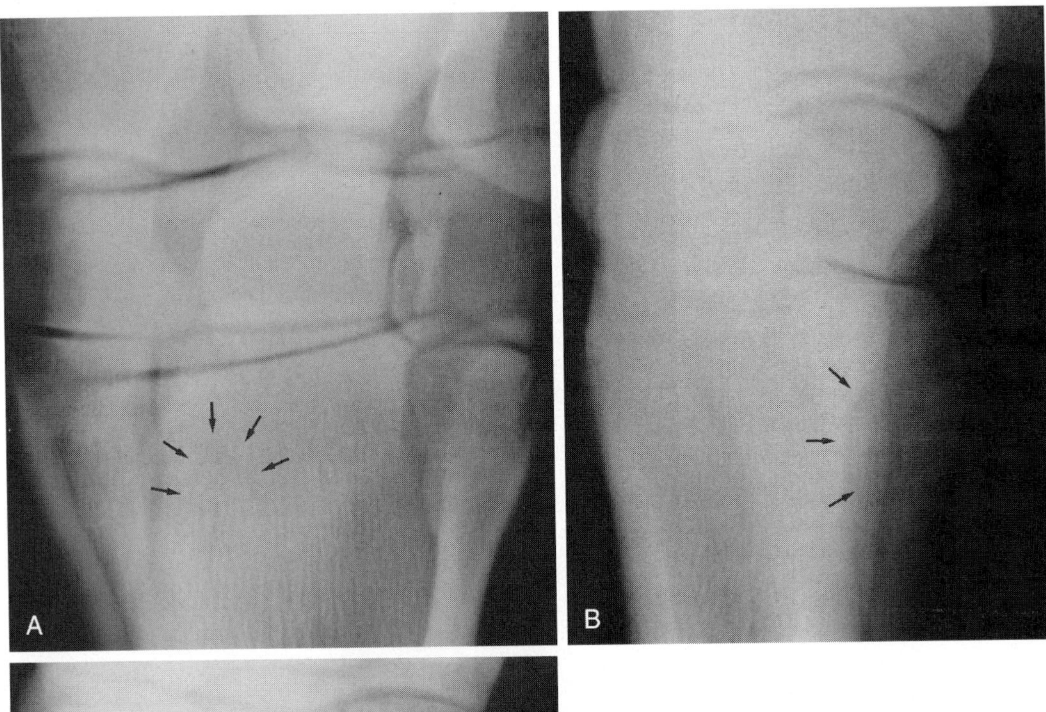

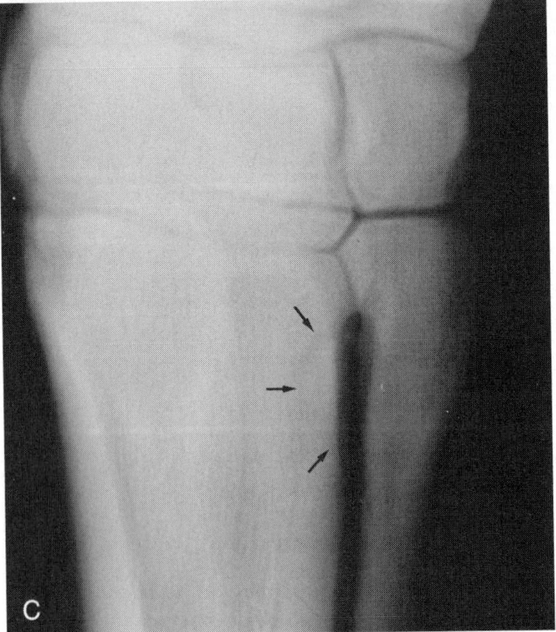

Fig. 21-13 Dorsopalmar (A), lateral (B), and dorsomedial-palmarolateral (C) radiographs of the right proximal metacarpus of a 2-year-old Standardbred colt with acute lameness in the right forelimb. A fracture is evident on all three views *(arrows)* in the medial aspect of the palmar cortex. On the dorsopalmar view, the fracture is identified as radiolucent lines that do not conform to the normal trabecular pattern. Although the fracture in this horse is best seen on the lateral and dorsomedial-palmarolateral views, such fractures are often only seen on the dorsopalmar view.

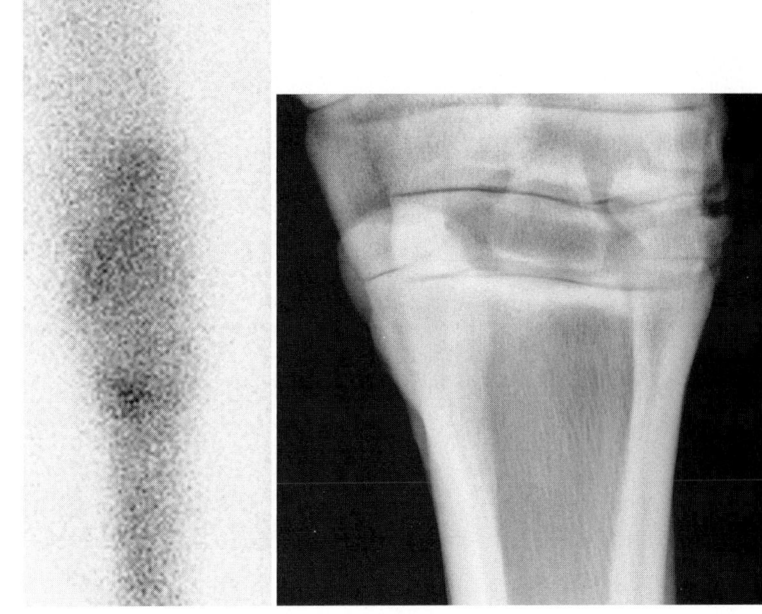

Fig. 21-14 A, Plantar bone scintigram of the tarsus of a 10-year-old Irish Sport horse with lameness localized to the proximal left metatarsal region. A focal region of increased radiopharmaceutical uptake is visible in the proximolateral aspect of the metatarsal area. B, Dorsoplantar radiograph of the region characterized by the increased radiopharmaceutical uptake seen in A. Increased medullary bone opacity is present.

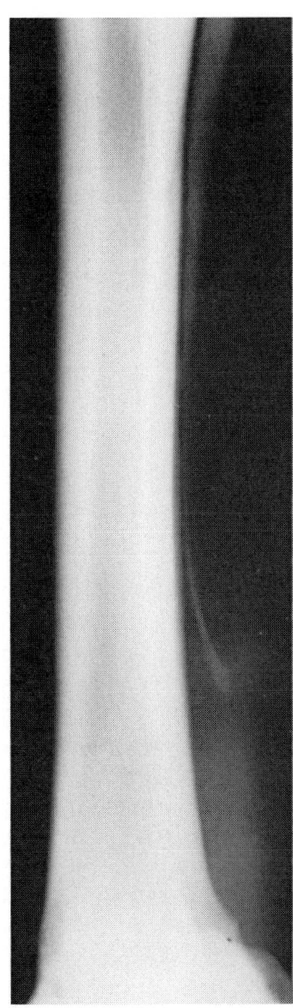

Fig. 21-15 Dorsomedial-plantarolateral view of MT II in an 8-year-old Standardbred gelding. Soft tissue enlargement is present on the plantar surface of the metatarsal area. MT II is deviated sharply at the distal end, which is consistent with suspensory desmitis.

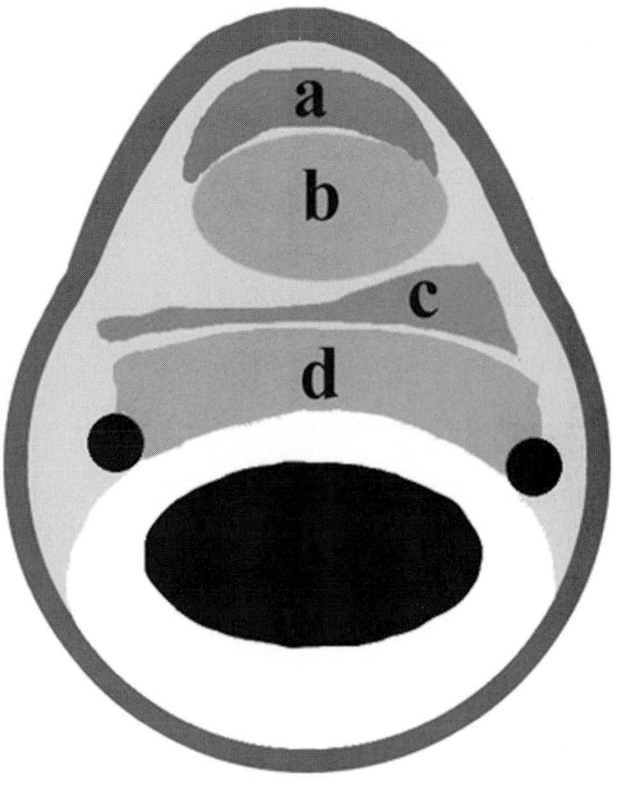

Fig. 21-16 Cross-sectional anatomy. *a*, SDF; *b*, DDF; *c*, accessory (check); *d*, suspensory ligament.

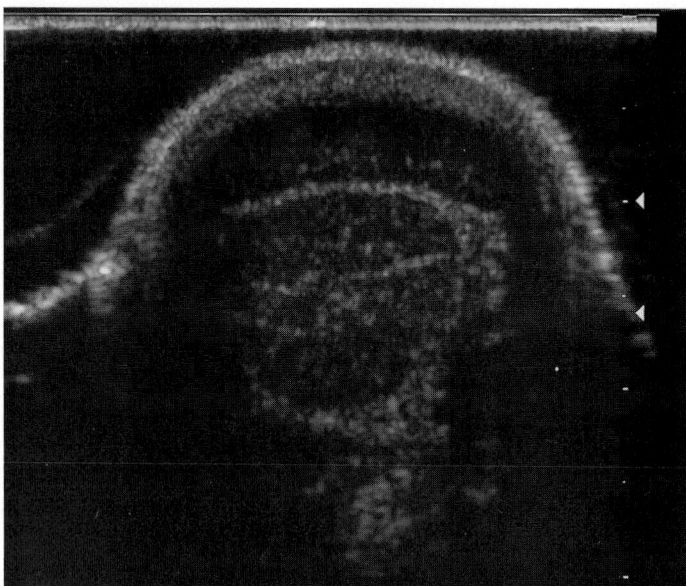

Fig. 21-17 Sonogram of equine tendons. A "stand-off" device was used; however, the probe angle was not correct. Notice the difference in the appearance of the tendons compared with Figure 21-18.

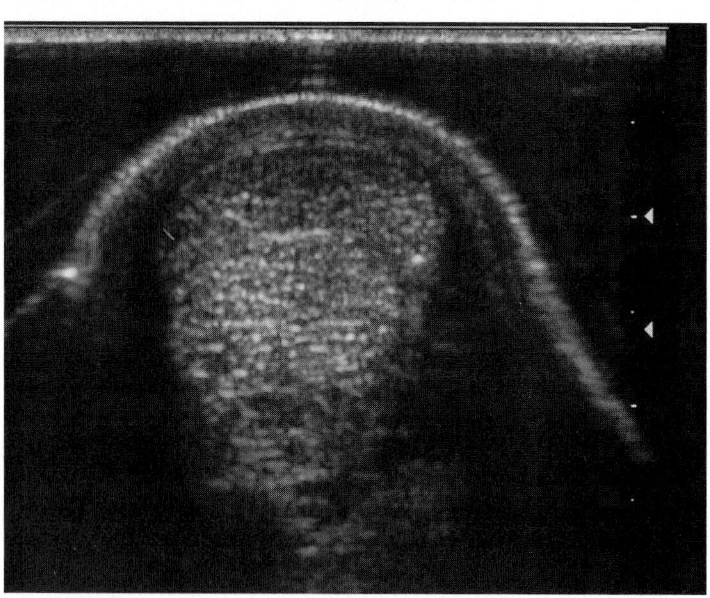

Fig. 21-18 Sonogram of equine tendons. A "stand-off" device was interposed between the probe and the skin to allow better visualization of near-field structures. The probe angle is correct. Notice the clarity of the SDF tendon compared with Figure 21-17.

must be exacting. Incorrect alignment of the probe with the limb may lead to incorrect interpretation. Proximal-distal malalignment can cause echogenicity of structures to appear different. Compare the appearance of tendons in Figure 21-17 with the appearance in Figure 21-18. The only difference between these images is a slight difference in the proximal-distal angle of the probe with the limb.

Many methods are used to prepare the surface of the skin to create optimal interface with the probe surface. Shaving the hair over the examination area is most desirable. Some clients are adverse to shaving or clipping the hair. Dermally applied therapeutic agents may produce scabs and blisters on the surface, preventing preparation of a smooth skin surface, which leads to poor contact between the transducer and the patient. Procedures such as covering the surface with mineral oil is sometimes used in lieu of clipping the hair. If allowable, actual shaving of a thin strip along the tendon surface creates an excellent interface when wiped with alcohol before use of ultrasound coupling gel. Nearly all ultrasound examinations of this region are performed with the transducer perpendicular to the structures (in cross section) from the palmar-plantar aspect of the limb. Depending on the probe design, the anatomy of the tendons and ligaments may be demonstrated nicely in longitudinal section; however, because the image is produced from a thin "slice" of tissue, examination of these structures in this fashion alone can result in considerable misinformation. Probe design is also a factor in the production of images in cross section. Unless the tendons are rather large or considerable soft-tissue enlargement is present from fluid accumulation, the surface at the point of probe contact may be small because of the contour of the tendons. This may produce a very narrow window through which clear images may be seen. With the curved design of many probes, the echoes are concentrated in the near field, making superficial structures such as the SDF difficult to demonstrate. To counter this problem, materials of uniform echogenicity may be used between the probe and the limb as a "stand-off" device (see Fig. 21-18).[26,27]

To aid in communication and for follow-up comparison, the regions of the limb are typically divided into six zones (Fig. 21-19). Other methods have been proposed such as the use of measurements from palpable structures.[28]

Sonographic examination of the metacarpal-metatarsal region is used to add information to the examination procedure. Sonography can be helpful for evaluating the extent of lesions and monitoring healing processes. It should not replace a thorough lameness examination. Sonography is used to identify hypoechoic lesions in the tendons and ligaments caused by hemorrhage, edema, and fiber disruption. These lesions may be large central pockets (core lesions) (Fig. 21-20), or they may appear as diffuse disruption (Fig. 21-21). Healed lesions tend to appear isoechoic or hyperechoic to the surrounding structure. Depending on the time of sonography relative to an injury, a lesion will vary in appearance relative to the stage and degree of healing. As with any modality, improper use may lead to erroneous diagnoses and conclusions. In addition to general consideration of the major tendons and ligaments, specific diagnoses are also possible.[29-31] A word of caution is necessary at this point. A number of parameters that may lead to misinterpretation have been previously mentioned, including suitability of equipment, understanding of imaging physics, and patient variation. In addition to patient variation, vascular structures and previous injuries may cause confusion. Thorough knowledge of the local anatomy is imperative. The clinician must fully understand the modality and its use through training and experience before depending on it with client-owned animals. Excellent texts are available that deal specifically with sonography.[32,33]

Ultrasound has been documented as a reliable method to evaluate lesion healing over time by comparison of images made at different dates.[34] However, magnetic resonance (MR)

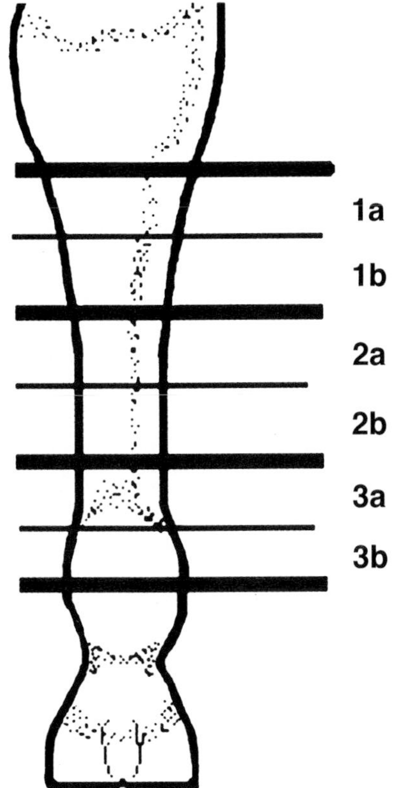

Fig. 21-19 Identification of the six zones typically used to identify location of lesions in an equine tendon ultrasound.

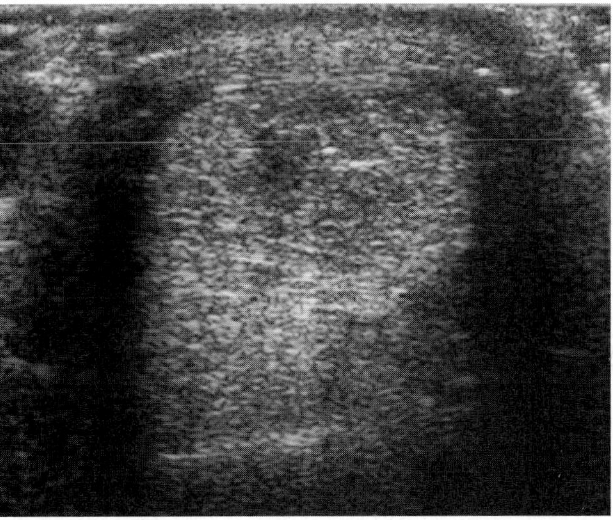

Fig. 21-20 Sonographic image of an equine tendon ultrasound image. A large hypoechoic lesion is present in the SDF; such a lesion is often referred to as a core lesion.

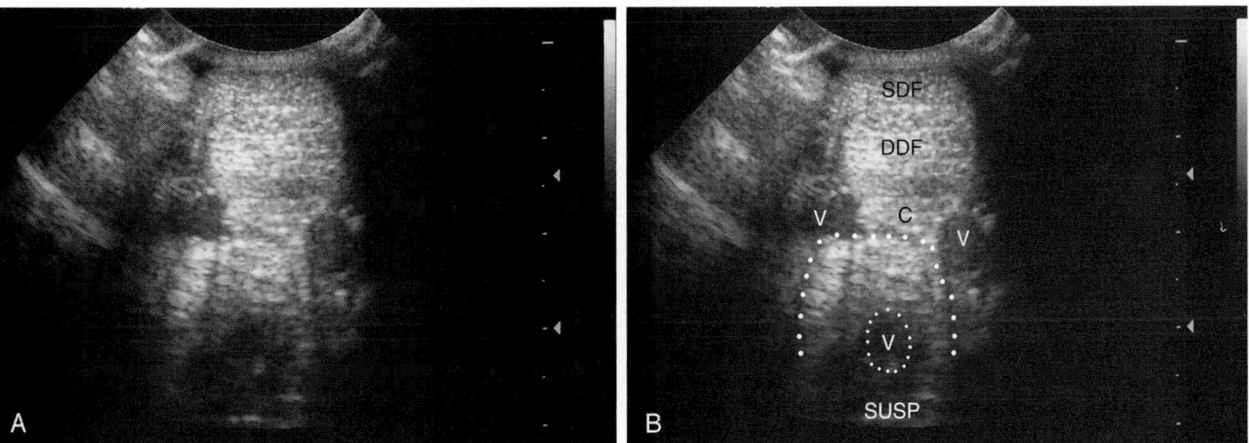

Fig. 21-21 A, Equine tendon sonographic image. Normal tendons are visualized. A hypoechoic lesion is present near the bifurcation of the suspensory ligament. In addition, blood vessels appear as hypoechoic to anechoic round structures. Notice acoustic enhancement as well as edge refraction related to the vessels. B, The same image as in A, with structures labeled. The suspensory ligament *(SUSP)*, containing the hypoechoic lesion, is outlined in *white dots.* C, Inferior check ligament (accessory ligament of the DDF); *V,* vessels.

imaging has shown to be more effective in demonstrating chronic tendon lesions than has diagnostic ultrasound.[35] In addition, MR imaging has been used to demonstrate lesions in the tissues associated with the metacarpal/metatarsal region that have been inaccessible with other imaging modalities.[36]

REFERENCES

1. Walter LJ, Davies HM: Analysis of a radiographic technique for measurement of equine metacarpal bone shape, *Equine Vet J* April(suppl):141, 2001.
2. Davies HM, Watson KM: Third metacarpal bone laterality asymmetry and midshaft dimensions in Thoroughbred racehorses, *Aust Vet J* April:224, 2005.
3. Getty R: *Sisson and Grossman's the anatomy of the domestic animals,* ed 5, Philadelphia, 1975, WB Saunders.
4. Lane EJ, Proto AV, Phillips TW: Mach bands and density perception, *Radiology* 121:9, 1976.
5. Bramlage LE, Gabel AA, Hackett RP: Avulsion of the origin of the suspensory ligament in the horse, *J Am Vet Med Assoc* 176:1004, 1980.
6. Radtke CL, Danova NA, Scollay MC et al: Macroscopic changes in the distal ends of the third metacarpal and metatarsal bones of Thoroughbred racehorses with condylar fractures, *Am J Vet Res* Sept:1110, 2003.
7. Lloyd KCK, Koblik P, Reagle C et al: Incomplete palmar fracture of the proximal extremity of the third metacarpal bone in horses: ten cases (1981-1986), *J Am Vet Med Assoc* 192:798, 1988.
8. Dyson S: Proximal suspensory desmitis: clinical, ultrasonographic, and radiographic features, *Equine Vet J* 23:25, 1991.
9. Pleasant RS, Baker GH, Muhlbauer MC et al: Stress reactions and stress fractures of the proximal palmar aspect of the third metacarpal bone in horses: 58 cases (1980-1990), *J Am Vet Med Assoc* 201:1918, 1992.
10. Spaulding K: Ultrasonic anatomy of the tendons and ligaments in the distal metacarpal-metatarsal region of the equine limb, *Vet Radiol* 25:155, 1984.
11. Nicholl RG, Wood AK, Martin IC: Ultrasonographic observation of the flexor tendons and ligaments of the metacarpal region of horses, *Am J Vet Res* 54:502, 1993.
12. Cauvin ER, Munroe GA, Boswell J et al: Gross and ultrasonographic anatomy of the carpal flexor tendon sheath in horses, *Vet Rec* 141:489, 1997.
13. Smith RK, Jones R, Webbon PM: The cross-sectional areas of normal equine digital flexor tendons determined ultrasonographically, *Equine Vet J* 26:460, 1994.
14. Wood AK, Sehgal CM, Polansky M: Sonographic brightness of the flexor tendons and ligaments in the metacarpal region of horses, *Am J Vet Res* 54:1969, 1993.
15. Cuesta I, Ribar C, Pinedo M et al: Ultrasonographic measurement of palmar metacarpal tendon and ligament structures in the horse, *Vet Radiol Ultrasound* 36:131, 1995.
16. Denoix JM, Busoni V: Ultrasonographic anatomy of the accessory ligament of the superficial digital flexor tendon in horses, *Equine Vet J* 31:186, 1999.
17. Gillis CL, Meagher DM, Pool RR et al: Ultrasonographically detected changes in equine superficial digital flexor tendons during the first months of racing, *Am J Vet Res* 54:1797, 1993.
18. Gillis CL, Meagher DM, Cloninger A et al: Ultrasonographic cross-sectional area and mean echogenicity of the superficial and deep digital flexor tendons in 50 trained thoroughbred racing horses, *Am J Vet Res* 56:1265, 1995.
19. Gillis CL, Poole RR, Meagher DM et al: Effect of maturation and aging on the histomorphometric and biochemical characteristics of equine superficial digital flexor tendon, *Am J Vet Res* 58:425, 1997.
20. Riemersma DJ, De Bruyn P: Variations in cross-sectional area and composition of equine tendons with regard to their mechanical function, *Res Vet Sci* 41:7, 1986.
21. Birch HL, McLaughlin L, Smith RK et al: Treadmill exercise-induced tendon hypertrophy: assessment of tendons with different mechanical functions, *Equine Vet J* 30(suppl):222, 1999.
22. Wilson DA, Baker GJ, Pijanowski GJ et al: Composition and morphologic features of the interosseous muscle in Standardbreds and Thoroughbreds, *Am J Vet Res* 52:133, 1991.
23. Miles CA: Ultrasonic properties of tendon: velocity, attenuation, and backscattering in equine digital flexor tendons, *J Acoust Soc Am* 99:3225, 1996.
24. Miles CA, Fursey GA, Birch HL et al: Factors affecting the ultrasonic properties of equine digital flexor tendons, *Ultrasound Med Biol* 22:907, 1996.
25. van Schie JT, Bakker EM, van Weeren PR: Ultrasonographic evaluation of equine tendons: a quantitative in vitro study of the effects of amplifier gain level, transducer-tilt and transducer-displacement, *Vet Radiol Ultrasound* 40:151, 1999.
26. Biller DS, Myer W: Ultrasound scanning of superficial structures using an ultrasound standoff pad, *Vet Radiol* 29:138, 1988.
27. Wood AK, Newell WH, Borg RP: An ultrasonographic offset system for examination of equine tendons and ligaments, *Am J Vet Res* 52:1945, 1991.
28. Pugh CR: A simple method to document the location of ultrasonographically detected equine tendon lesions, *Vet Radiol Ultrasound* 34:211, 1993.
29. Dyson SJ, Arthur RM, Palmar SE et al: Suspensory ligament desmitis, *Vet Clin North Am Equine Pract* 11:177, 1995.
30. Wright IM, McMahon PJ: Tenosynovitis associated with longitudinal tears of the digital flexor tendons in horses: a report of 20 cases, *Equine Vet J* 31:12, 1999.
31. Lepage OM, Leveille R, Breton L et al: Congenital dislocation of the deep digital flexor tendon associated with hypoplasia of the sustentaculum tali in a thoroughbred colt, *Vet Radiol Ultrasound* 36:384, 1995.
32. Nyland TG, Mattoon JS: *Veterinary diagnostic ultrasound,* Philadelphia, 1995, WB Saunders.
33. Reef VB: *Equine diagnostic ultrasound,* Philadelphia, 1998, WB Saunders.
34. Wilderjans H, Boussauw B, Madder K et al: Tenosynovitis of the digital flexor tendon sheath and annular ligament constriction syndrome caused by longitudinal tears in the deep digital flexor tendon: a clinical and surgical report of 17 cases in warmblood horses, *Equine Vet J* 35:270, 2003.
35. Kasashima Y, Kuwano A, Katayama Y et al: Magnetic resonance imaging application to live horse for diagnosis of tendonitis, *J Vet Med Sci* 64:577, 2002.
36. Zobrod CJ, Schneider RK, Tucker RL: Use of magnetic resonance imaging to identify suspensory desmitis and adhesions between exostoses of the second metacarpal bone and the suspensory ligament in four horses, *J Am Vet Med Assoc* 224:1815, 2004.

ELECTRONIC RESOURCES evolve

Additional information related to the content in Chapter 21 can be found on the companion Web site at evolve http://evolve.elsevier.com/Thrall/vetrad/

- Key Points
- Chapter Quiz
- Case Study 21-1

CHAPTER • 22
Metacarpophalangeal/Metatarsophalangeal Articulation

Lisa G. Britt
Russell L. Tucker

ANATOMY

The anatomic structures of the metacarpophalangeal (MCP) and metatarsophalangeal (MTP) articulations are so similar that differentiating the right from the left or the front limb from the hindlimb on unlabeled radiographs is inaccurate. The MCP or MTP articulations are hinge joints, formed by the distal end of the metacarpal (or metatarsal) bone and the proximal end of the proximal phalanx. The articular surface of the proximal phalanx is concave and has a sagittal groove opposing the sagittal ridge at the distal end of the third metacarpal (MC III) or the third metatarsal (MT III) bone. This ridge and groove divide the weight-bearing surface into two unequal parts. The largest surface is on the medial (or axial) side, where loading is greatest. The sagittal ridge of MC III or MT III is received into a depression at the palmar* surface that is created by the proximal sesamoid bones and the intersesamoidean ligament. The joint has two radii of articulation. The dorsal radius serves the weight-bearing portion, and the palmar radius conforms to the articulation with the proximal sesamoid bones.[1] The junction of these radii of articulation often appears flat and may be confused with a lesion of the articular surface.

The joint capsule attachments at the proximal end of the proximal phalanx are immediately periarticular, with no redundant capsule or recesses. The capsule attaches to the distal end of MC III or MT III at the periarticular margins. Dorsally, a large recess extends proximally and forms a pouch that allows full extension of the joint. A bursa is interposed between the extensor tendons and the dorsal joint pouch. The palmar joint capsule extends proximal to the sesamoid bones between the suspensory ligament and MC III or MT III.[1] Ligaments associated with the MCP and MTP articulations have been described and are illustrated in Chapter 23.[2]

RADIOGRAPHIC EXAMINATION

The intent of the radiographic examination is to visualize adequately the articular and periarticular skeletal structures and the adjoining soft tissues. The examination should include the proximal interphalangeal joint and the distal ends of the metacarpal or metatarsal bones. Identification markers recorded in the emulsion are essential in radiographic examination of the MCP or MTP articulation; right versus left and front versus hind should be clearly designated. If oblique views are obtained, the direction of x-ray beam travel (i.e., name of the projection) must be designated. Markers should be placed to the lateral surface of all views, with the exception of the lateromedial view, for which markers should be placed dorsally.[3]

Survey radiographic examination of the joint should include a lateromedial, a dorsopalmar, and two oblique projections (dorsal 45-degree lateral-palmaromedial and dorsal 45-degree medial-palmarolateral), with the limb bearing weight if possible. The survey examination should precede any special radiographic projections or contrast studies of the joint. The lateromedial projection should be made with the primary beam centered at the articulation and directed parallel to an imaginary line connecting the collateral fossae at the distal end of MC III or MT III. A true lateromedial projection is essential for proper assessment of the sagittal ridge of distal MC III or MT III.[4] The dorsopalmar projection warrants thoughtful positioning. Because the plane of the joint is at an angle to the solar surface of the hoof, the primary beam is directed from dorsoproximal to palmarodistal at approximately 30 to 40 degrees (dorsal 35-degree proximal-palmarodistal view). This should result in the projection of the proximal sesamoid bones over the distal MC III or MT III and the joint space projected with maximal width.[5,6] The dorsal 45-degree lateral-palmaromedial and dorsal 45-degree medial-palmarolateral oblique projections should be a routine part of the survey examination. These oblique views are necessary to view the abaxial aspects of the articular surfaces, the periarticular margins, and the proximal sesamoid bones. Oblique views made in a dorsal 60-degree lateral-palmaromedial or dorsal 60-degree medial-palmarolateral direction allow the best visualization of the dorsal eminence of the proximal phalanx, which is located near midline, and the axial aspect of the proximal sesamoid bones. Some prefer using the 60-degree oblique view as the routine oblique view rather than the oblique views made at 45 degrees because axial lesions may be common (Fig. 22-1).[7]

Additional projections of the joint may be indicated according to the information gained from survey radiographs.[4] The lateromedial projection during flexion is performed while the foot is held off the ground as if the sole of the hoof were being visually inspected. Alternate positions include variations in the degree of flexion and flexed oblique views. These projections may provide better visualization of subarticular surfaces at the dorsal aspect of distal MC III or MT III, the proximal part of the proximal phalanx, and the articular margins of the proximal sesamoid bones.[6]

The dorsodistal-palmaroproximal projection is made while the limb is not bearing weight. In this study, a tangential view of the articular margin of the distal MC III or MT III bone is created. The foot is elevated on a block and the limb is extended. The primary beam direction is approximately 125

*"Palmar(o)" is used throughout this chapter with the understanding that "plantar(o)" should be substituted if reference is being made to the hindlimb.

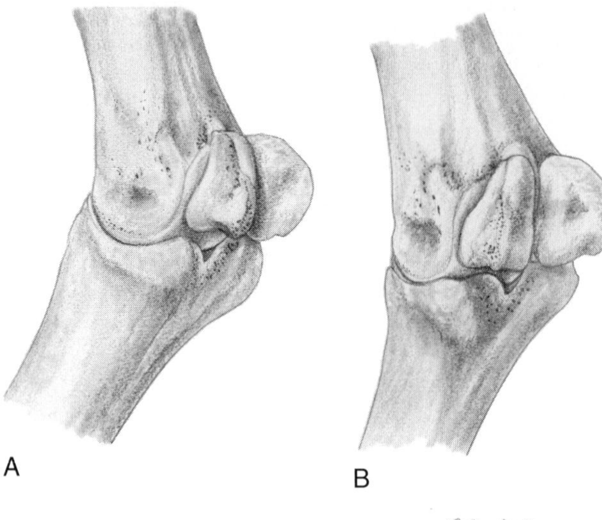

Fig. 22-1 The effect of angle of obliquity on the different aspects of the proximal sesamoid bones that can be projected. **A,** The dorsal 30-degree proximal, 45-degree medial (or lateral)-palmarodistolateral (or medial) oblique view of the MCP joint best demonstrates the abaxial aspect of the sesamoid bones where the branches of the suspensory ligament attach. **B,** Dorsal 30-degree proximal, 60-degree medial (or lateral)-palmarodistolateral (or medial) oblique view of the fetlock joint maximizes the evaluation of the dorsal eminence of P1. (Drawing by Gheorghe M. Constantinescu, DVM, University of Missouri, Columbia.)

degrees to the axis of the metacarpal or metatarsal bone.[8] The degree of flexion and the angle of the primary beam determine the tangent of the joint surface that is visualized.

The palmaroproximal-palmarodistal projection is used to visualize the palmar articular surface of MC III or MT III and the proximal sesamoid bones. Positioning of the patient requires that the x-ray tube be placed close to the horse's body. The limb should be positioned as far caudal as possible, and the foot is placed on a supporting tunnel containing a cassette.[6] Some magnification results from the use of this projection because of the distance between the proximal sesamoid bones and the film cassette.

The abaxial surfaces of the proximal sesamoids may be further examined by placing a cassette medial or lateral to the joint on the affected side. The x-ray beam is then directed in a dorsal 50-degree proximal, 45-degree lateral-distopalmaromedial or dorsal 50-degree proximal, 45-degree medial-distopalmarolateral direction, respectively, and creates a tangential view of the proximal sesamoid bones.[9] The described positioning results in the x-ray beam being directed downward at the sesamoid bones at an angle of 50 degrees from horizontal. This tangential projection is beneficial in assessing if articular involvement is present with sesamoid lesions and thus directs the surgical approach (Fig. 22-2, *A* and *C*).

Contrast arthrography of the MCP or MTP joint is sometimes useful. Five to 10 mL of water-soluble contrast medium containing 300 to 400 mg/mL of iodine is adequate. Injection of contrast medium should follow arthrocentesis and withdrawal of an equal volume of synovial fluid. Injection is made into the lateral pouch of the joint, proximal to the lateral

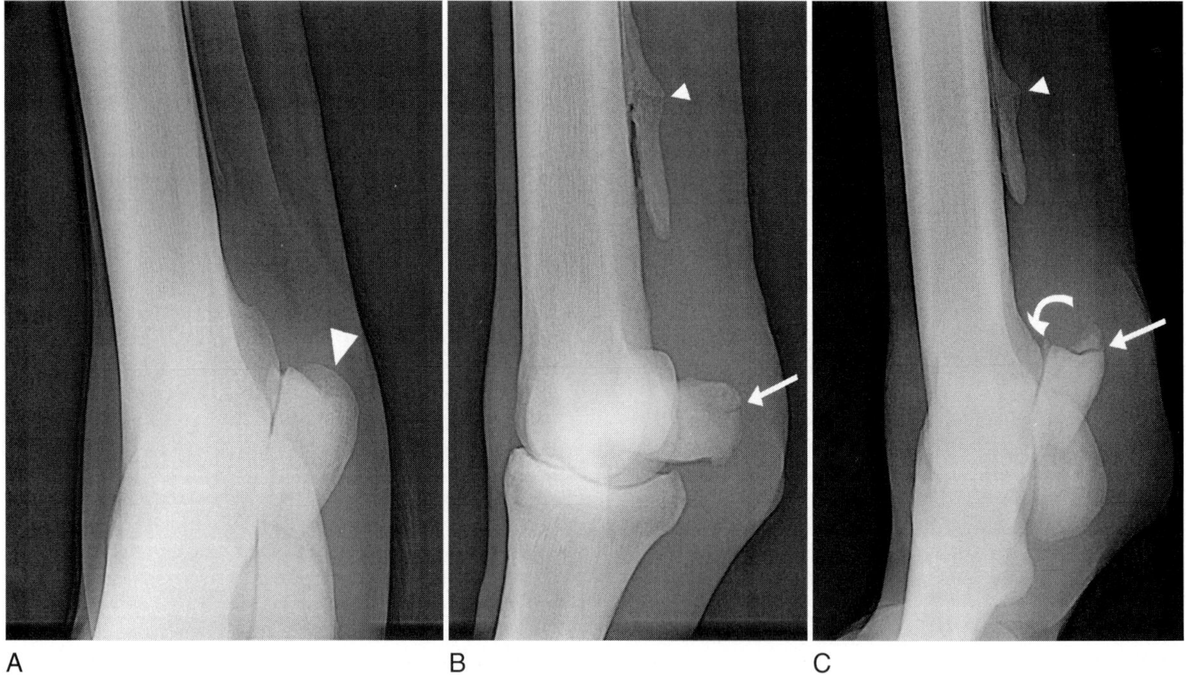

Fig. 22-2 **A,** A dorsal 50-degree proximal, 45-degree medial-distopalmarolateral view demonstrating the normal appearance of the proximal abaxial sesamoid on this tangential view *(arrowhead)*. **B** and **C,** Oblique views of an apical sesamoid fracture. **B,** A dorsal 30-degree proximal, 60-degree lateral-palmarodistomedial oblique view. An incomplete fracture of the lateral sesamoid bone is visible *(arrow)*. A chronic fracture of the distal MC IV is also present *(arrowhead)*. **C,** A dorsal 50-degree proximal, 45-degree medial-distopalmarolateral view of the same horse. This view demonstrates that the sesamoid fracture is complete and articular *(straight arrow)* with a small articular fragment *(curved arrow)*. (Courtesy Scott E. Palmer, VMD, Dipl. ABVP-Equine, New Jersey Equine Clinic, Clarksburg, New Jersey.)

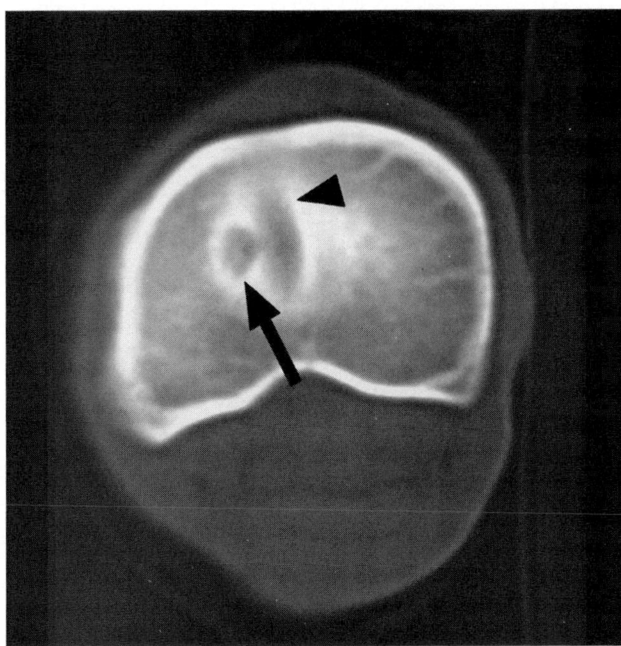

Fig. 22-3 A transverse 1.5-mm thick CT image of the proximal aspect of P1. A small, oval, hypoattenuating cystic lesion *(arrow)* is surrounded by hyperattenuating sclerotic bone just lateral to and communicating with the fossa for the median sagittal ridge *(arrowhead)*.

sesamoid bones and dorsal to the suspensory ligament. The joint should be vigorously flexed, extended, and massaged before radiography to distribute the contrast medium throughout the joint.

ALTERNATIVE IMAGING MODALITIES

Ultrasound offers many advantages in the evaluation of the soft tissues surrounding the MCP or MTP joint and is frequently used to complement the radiographic examination. Portable ultrasound machines can be used to image the extensor and flexor tendons, the suspensory and distal sesamoidean ligaments, the synovial lining and joint recesses, and cortical margins. The normal sonographic features of the MCP and MTP joints have been described.[10]

In addition to conventional radiography, computed tomography (CT) may be useful in selected patients to image the MCP or MTP joint. Like radiography, CT is based on x-ray absorption by tissues; however, the system is much more sensitive to attenuation differences and has excellent contrast resolution. The CT information is displayed in tomographic slices that have superb radiographic detail and eliminate superimposition of overlying structures. CT excels in the evaluation of bones and is useful in imaging complex fractures and subchondral lesions in the MCP and MTP joints (Fig. 22-3).

Recently, magnetic resonance (MR) imaging has been used to evaluate the distal limbs in horses, including the MCP or MTP joints.[11-13] A distinct advantage of MR is the exceptional contrast resolution (Fig. 22-4). Additionally, MR imaging is multiplanar. MR examinations are commonly performed by using several types of acquisition sequences to demonstrate different anatomic and pathologic features. MR systems usually require that horses be under general anesthesia. However, some MR systems are available for imaging the limbs of standing horses. Motion artifact remains a limitation, especially proximal to the distal phalanx, although work is being done to improve motion correction techniques.[14]

RADIOGRAPHIC INTERPRETATION OF DISEASES OF THE METACARPOPHALANGEAL/ METATARSOPHALANGEAL ARTICULATION

Joint disease in the horse is often associated with repeated trauma and, as with any species, the pathologic changes may be characteristic of the joint and of the function required of the horse. A study of racetrack injuries in horses has provided an overview of pathologic findings and pathogenesis of MCP or MTP joint disease.[15] Lameness and distension of a joint are the initial clinical signs that typically precede the request for radiographic examination. The earliest signs of joint disease may remain obscure on radiographs because wear lines in the articular cartilage or synovial hypertrophy are usually not recognized. Radiographs of the contralateral joint may be obtained for comparison. Although pathologic change is often bilateral, it is usually in different stages of development.

Joint Effusion

Joint effusion is usually a result of trauma, with degenerative changes in the articular surfaces and joint capsule. Radiographic signs include soft tissue swelling and joint distention. With chronic insults, dystrophic calcification of the periarticular soft tissues may also be present.[16]

Villonodular Synovitis

Villonodular synovitis is characterized by a firm, nonfluctuating swelling at the dorsal aspect of the joint. The villonodular masses arise from enlargement of the synovial villi of the joint capsule and are associated with repetitive trauma. The condition is usually diagnosed by clinical signs, history, palpation, and ultrasound. With time, the radiographic signs will include mild to severe erosion of distal MC III or MT III at the region just distal to the dorsal joint capsule attachment.[17-19] Periarticular bony proliferation may be present (Fig. 22-5). With arthrography, radiolucent, space-occupying masses of the synovial villus hypertrophy can usually be identified in the dorsal recess of the joint (Fig. 22-6).

Supracondylar Lysis

In MC III or MT III, the radiographic features of supracondylar lysis are similar to those seen in villonodular synovitis, except that the former occurs at the palmar surface of the bone. Changes are caused by chronic proliferative synovitis. Radiographic signs are joint distention and lysis of bone at the palmar cortex of MC III or MT III, distal to the joint capsule attachment (see Fig. 22-5, *B*). Arthrography may be difficult to perform because of the presence of hypertrophied synovium and diminished synovial joint space. Contrast medium permeates an undulating, irregular-mass filling defect. The erosive concavity formed in the bone is usually readily apparent (see Fig. 22-6).

Degenerative Joint Disease

Degenerative joint disease is a nonspecific term describing deterioration of articular and periarticular structures. The pathologic events culminate in degenerative hypertrophic osteoarthritis/osteoarthrosis, regardless of the initiating causes or biochemical alterations. It is a chronic disorder characterized by progressive deterioration of articular cartilage that results in a radiographic loss in joint space and reactive changes in the joint margin and capsule.[15]

The first stages include cartilage degeneration and formation of wear lines characteristic of hinge joints. These wear lines are grooves in the articular surface that are oriented par-

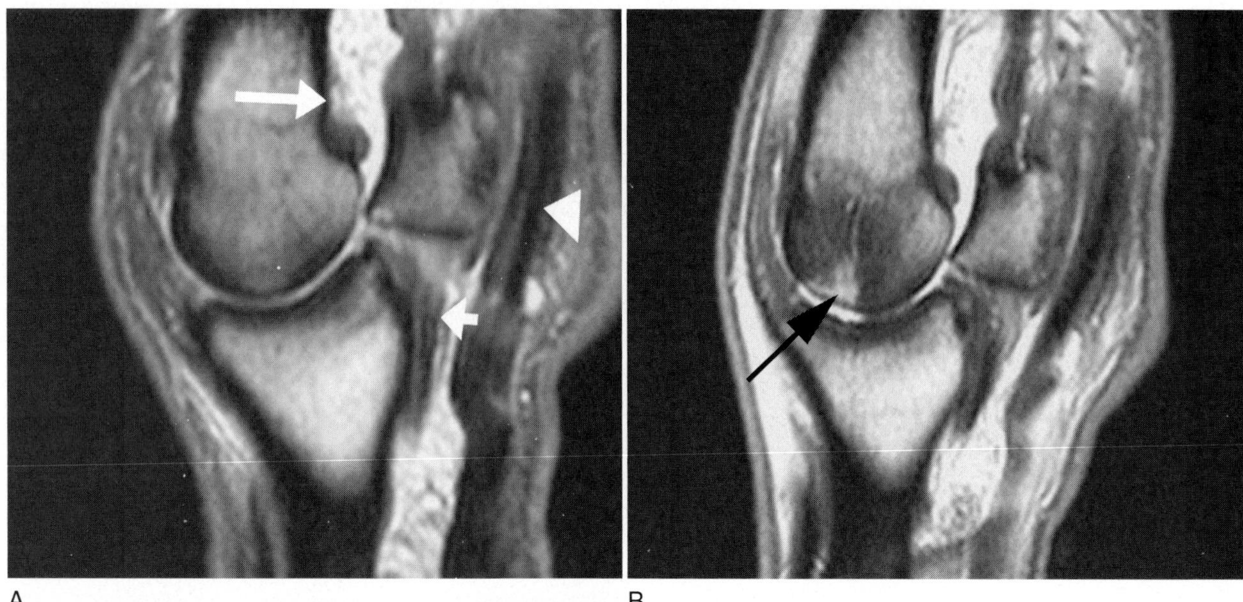

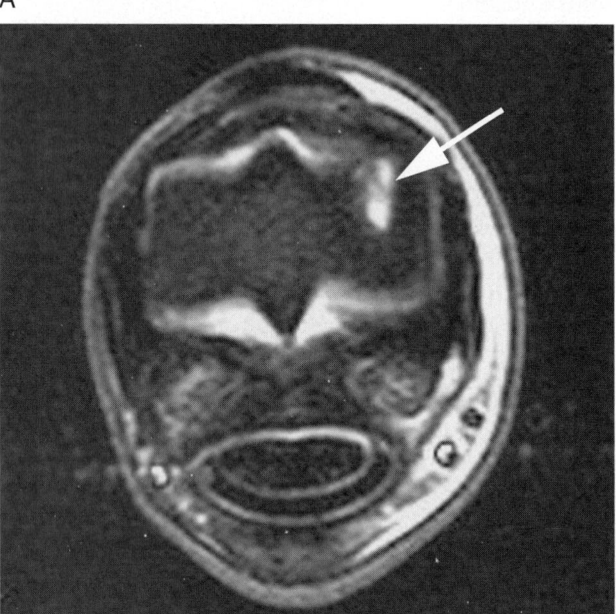

Fig. 22-4 MR images of right and left distal MC III. **A,** A sagittal proton density–weighted MR image of the MCP joint. The deep digital flexor tendon can be seen coursing along the palmar aspect *(arrowhead)* and the distal sesamoidean ligaments originating on the distal margin of the proximal sesamoid bone *(short arrow)*. The synovial fluid in the caudal palmar pouch can be clearly visualized on this image *(long arrow)*. **B,** A sagittal proton density–weighted MR image of the contralateral MCP joint. A distal MC III medial condyle hyperintensity extends into the joint *(arrow)*, causing an associated articular cartilage defect. **C,** A transverse spectral presaturation with inversion recovery weighted image that removes signal derived from fat. This increases the visibility of the MC III medial condyle lesion *(arrow)*.

allel to the direction of joint motion. Cartilaginous fibrillation and erosions form in the surface, and subsequent wear results in narrowing of the joint space. If reduction in the width of a joint space is confirmed on two radiographic views, cartilage thinning is likely. Progressive loss of joint width is a subjective finding and must be carefully assessed with clinical signs to determine its significance (Fig. 22-7).

Radiographic signs of degenerative joint disease are soft tissue swelling, narrowed joint space, and bone remodeling with lysis and proliferation. These findings may occur in any combination. Joint capsule thickening may be suspected but is rarely visualized, even on high-detail radiographs. Soft tissue swelling results from hypertrophy and proliferation of other periarticular tissues.

Chronic arthritis is characterized by sclerosis or eburnation of subchondral bone, with loss of trabecular architecture as a result of erosion of the overlying articular cartilage. Repetitive stress or trauma at the joint capsule attachments results in enthesophyte formation (Fig. 22-8). Similar, but not identical, are periarticular bony osteophytes that form at the joint margins in response to damage to the articular surface (see Fig. 22-7). Of note, many joint disorders can progress to a common end point having the stereotypic features of chronic degenerative joint disease.[15] The initiating factors of degenerative joint disease may be difficult or impossible to determine in the late stages of the disease process.

Cortisone Arthropathy

The changes associated with cortisone arthropathy may involve articular and periarticular structures and have variable degrees of degeneration and proliferation. Repeated steroid injections result in localized demineralization of bone and decreased trabecular detail. Long-term changes include mineralization in the periarticular soft tissues associated with deposition of steroid within those structures. A differential diagnosis of steroid-induced arthritis should be considered in the presence of degenerative change or collapse of subchondral bone with mineralization in periarticular soft tissue (Fig. 22-9).

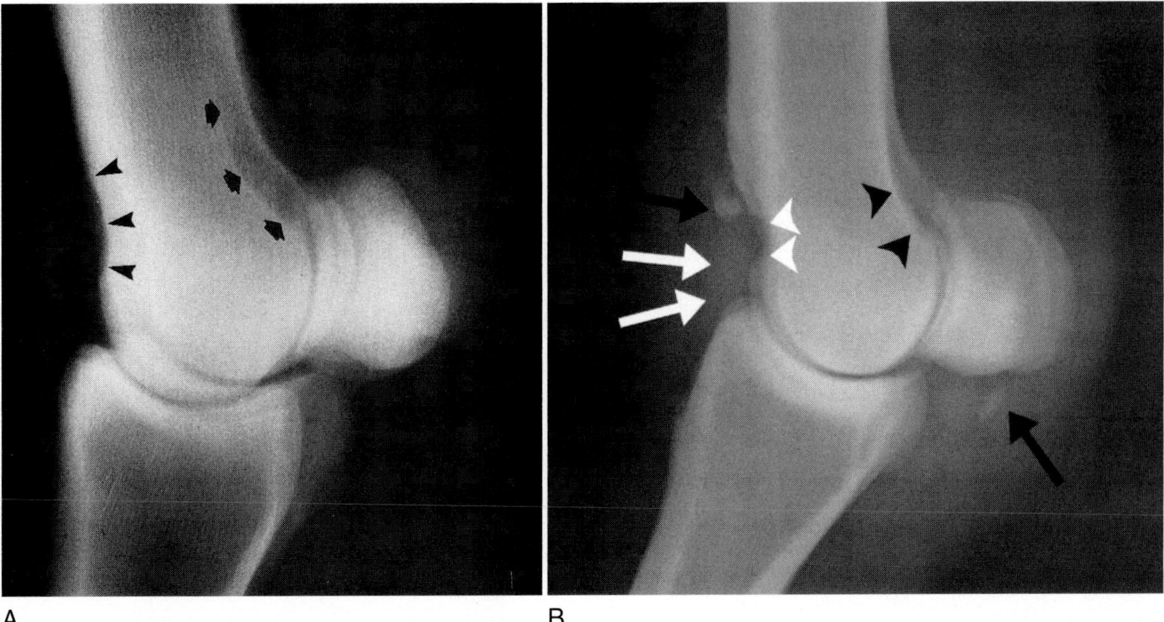

Fig. 22-5 Lateromedial radiograph of an MCP joint with changes of mild (A) and severe (B) villonodular synovitis. A, Swelling dorsal to the joint, erosion of bone at the dorsoproximal joint capsule attachment *(arrowheads)*, and early evidence of supracondylar lysis at the palmar cortex *(arrows)* are all visible. Bony proliferation is visible at the proximodorsal periarticular border of the proximal phalanx. B, This joint has more chronic changes with severe joint effusion *(white arrows)*, bone erosion at the dorsoproximal joint capsule attachment *(white arrowheads)*, supracondylar lysis *(black arrowheads)*, and periarticular bone fragments *(black arrows)*. Bone remodeling is also present at the proximodorsal aspect of the proximal phalanx as well as along the palmar border of the sesamoid bones.

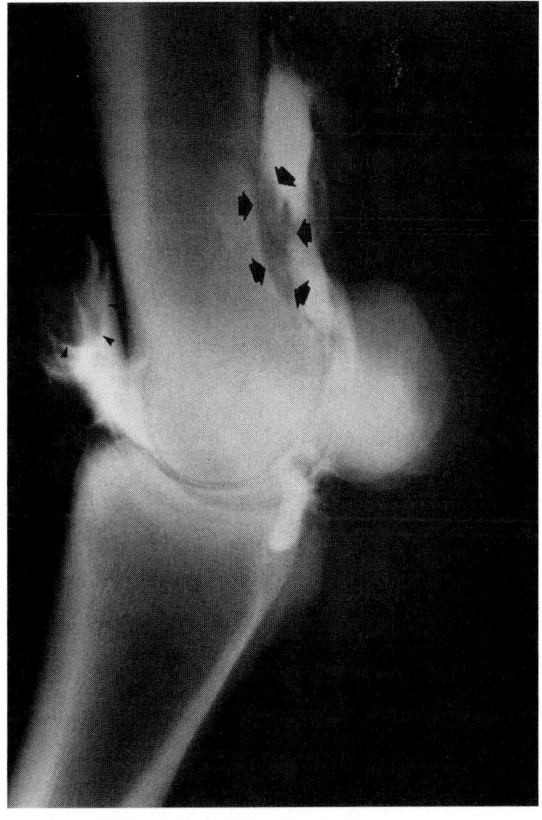

Fig. 22-6 Positive-contrast arthrogram (same horse as in Fig. 22-5, *A*). Two radiolucent, space-occupying masses are present in the dorsoproximal joint space *(arrowheads)*. A space-occupying mass at the palmar surface fills the area of supracondylar lysis *(arrows)*.

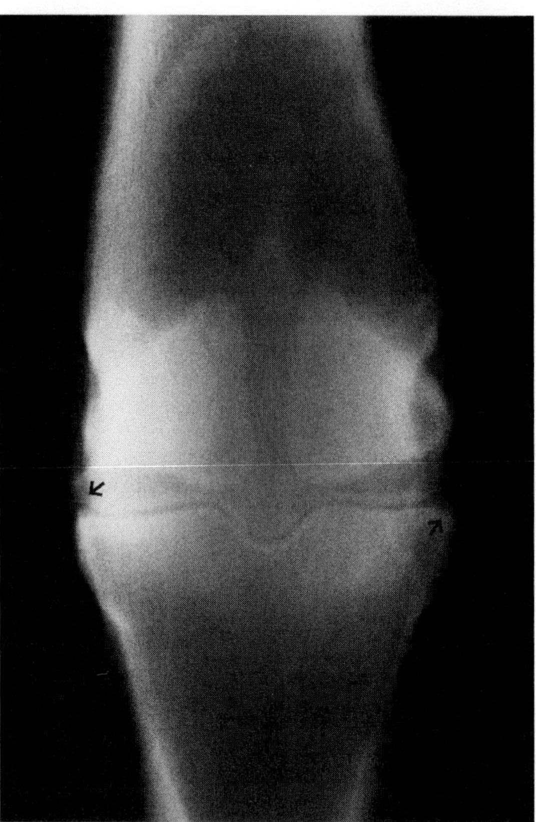

Fig. 22-7 Dorsopalmar radiograph with changes of chronic degenerative joint disease. Narrowing of the joint space and formation of osteophytes at the joint margins are visible *(arrows)*.

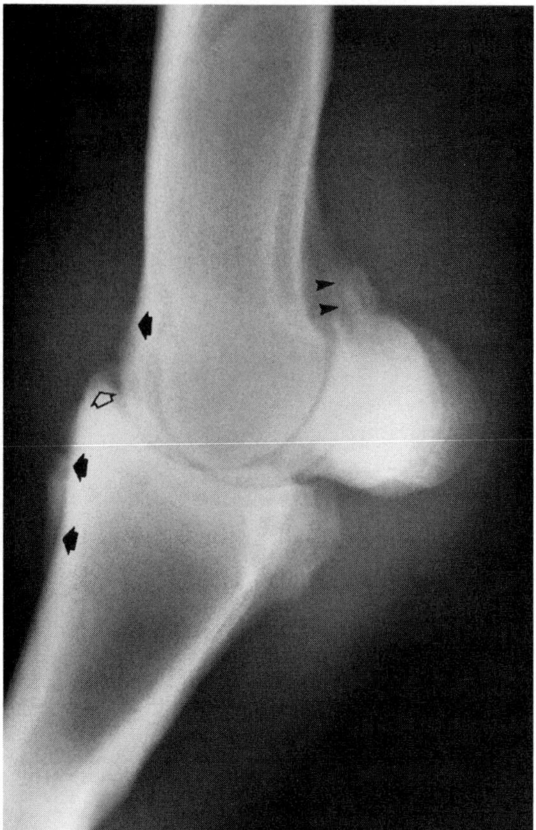

Fig. 22-8 Lateromedial radiograph of a horse with chronic degenerative joint disease, sesamoiditis, and desmitis. Generalized soft tissue swelling and joint distention are present. Chronic osteochondral fractures are present at the apexes of the proximal sesamoid bones *(arrowheads)*. Degenerative bone proliferation (enthesophyte) is present at the dorsoproximal surface of the proximal phalanx and at the joint capsule attachment on the dorsodistal surface of MC III *(solid arrows)*. A periarticular osteophyte is evident on the dorsal rim of the proximal phalanx *(open arrow)*. Other changes include supracondylar lysis, remodeling of bony trabeculae in the proximal sesamoid bones, and bone proliferation at the attachments of the deep sesamoidean ligaments at the proximal palmar aspect of the proximal phalanx.

Osteochondrosis

Osteochondrosis may be found in the distal aspect of MC III or MT III.[20-23] The radiographic findings are well-demarcated radiolucencies that may extend several centimeters deep to the articular margin. A lateromedial radiograph of the joint may best demonstrate the depth of the lesion in the condyle. The shape of the defect may be a shallow concavity, a deep concavity, crescentic, oval, or circular.[23] The changes are found at the junction of the radii of articulation between the MCP or the MTP joint and the metacarposesamoidean or metatarsosesamoidean articular surface (Fig. 22-10). These lesions have been called *traumatic osteochondrosis*—an indication of the controversy regarding their etiology.[15] Arthrographically, cavitation of the joint surface may exist, although advanced degenerative subchondral bone changes can also be found with the overlying cartilage intact at the articular surface.

Osteochondral fragments of the palmar aspect of the joint have been given three classifications.[24] Type I fragments occur at the proximal end of the proximal phalanx, just medial or lateral to the sagittal groove; type II fragments have an origin from the wing of the proximal phalanx. Type III fractures originate from the basilar margin of the sesamoid bones and are discussed under the section on sesamoid basilar fractures (Figs. 22-11 and 22-12). Type I or II fragments have the highest incidence in Standardbreds and were originally reported as avulsion fractures.[25,26] Because of the anatomic origins, symmetry of the lesions and breed predilection, these fragments have been reported to be the result of osteochondrosis. These fragments are the subject of much controversy. Studies have focused on radiography,[27-29] etiology,[30] heritability,[31,32] the effect of patient size,[33] epidemiology[34,35] surgical treatment,[36,37] and prognosis.[29] Subchondral bone cysts can also be seen at the proximal end of the first phalanx and are often difficult to see radiographically (see Fig. 22-3).

Osteochondrosis of the sagittal ridge of MC III or MT III is usually diagnosed in young horses and occurs with variable radiographic expression (Fig. 22-13). Radiographic signs may vary from small flattening to large excavations of subchondral bone of the sagittal ridge. Lesions are usually best visualized on flexed lateral projections of the MCP or MTP joint. Detached osteochondral fragments may be found in close association to the bone defect or may be nestled in distant recesses of the joint.[38]

Septic Arthritis

Septic arthritis may be associated with hematogenous spread of microorganisms, such as occurs with omphalophlebitis, or by direct contamination as a result of trauma or nonsterile invasive techniques. Radiographic signs of early septic arthritis are periarticular soft tissue swelling and distention of the joint. Progression of the disease results in malalignment, subluxation, or collapse of the joint (Fig. 22-14) and bony changes of subchondral bone lysis and periosteal proliferation

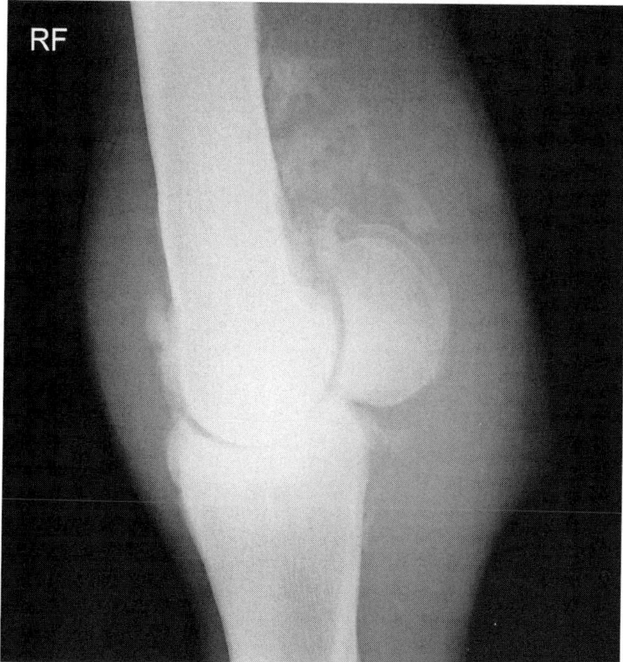

Fig. 22-9 Lateromedial radiograph of a horse with cortisone arthropathy. There is narrowing of the joint space and severe periarticular bone remodeling of the dorsal and palmar aspects of the distal metacarpal, proximal aspect of P1, and the apical margins of the proximal sesamoid bones. Mineralization in periarticular soft tissues is typical of cortisone arthropathy. (Courtesy Stephanie Nykamp, DVM, D.ACVR, Ontario Veterinary College, Guelph, Ontario, Canada.)

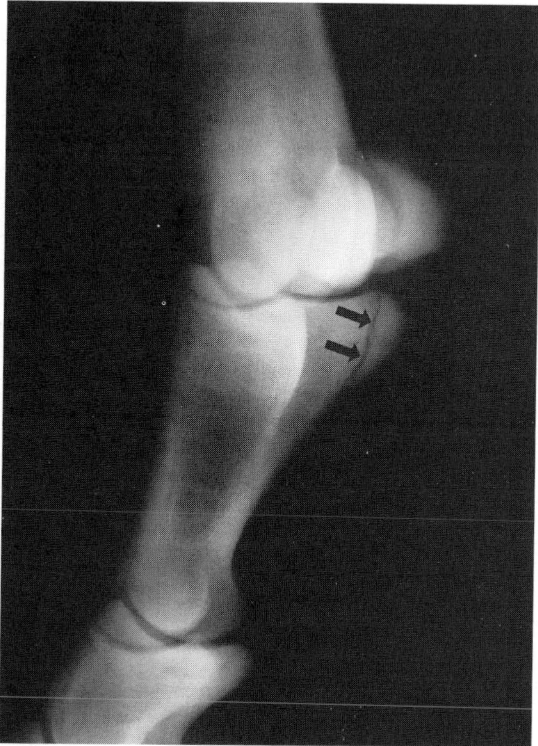

Fig. 22-11 Dorsal 45-degree medial-palmarolateral radiograph of the MCP joint with a type II fragment *(arrows)* originating from the medial palmar eminence of the proximal phalanx.

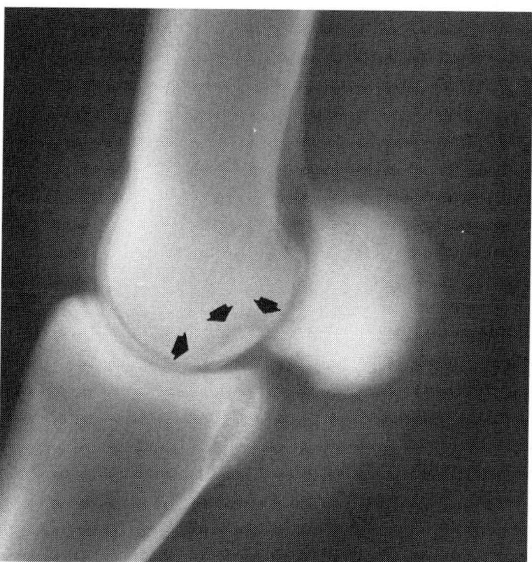

Fig. 22-10 Lateromedial radiograph of a horse with distal metacarpal osteochondrosis. An opaque osteochondral fragment is visible within a deep concavity of radiolucency *(arrows)*.

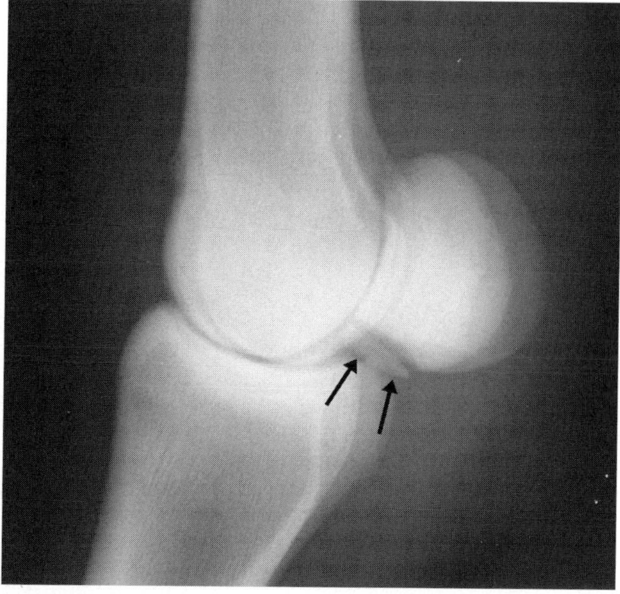

Fig. 22-12 Lateromedial radiograph of an MCP joint with a type III fracture *(arrows)* originating from the basilar margin of a proximal sesamoid.

at the joint margins (Fig. 22-15). The cartilage space may appear increased at areas of subchondral bone lysis. Diminished joint space is evidence of the loss of articular cartilage that typically precedes subchondral bony change.

The radiographic sign of an increase in the apparent joint space must be critically analyzed. Incomplete ossification of the cartilage model is normally present in young, developing animals. The large soft tissue space at articular margins progressively diminishes with skeletal maturity. Furthermore, radiographs made in non-weight-bearing horses will cause joint spaces to be widened compared with weight-bearing projections. Whenever possible, the horse should bear normal weight on the joint at the time of radiography. Increased thickness of the articular cartilage has not been documented in animals. Excessive fluid or soft tissue in the joint space, as

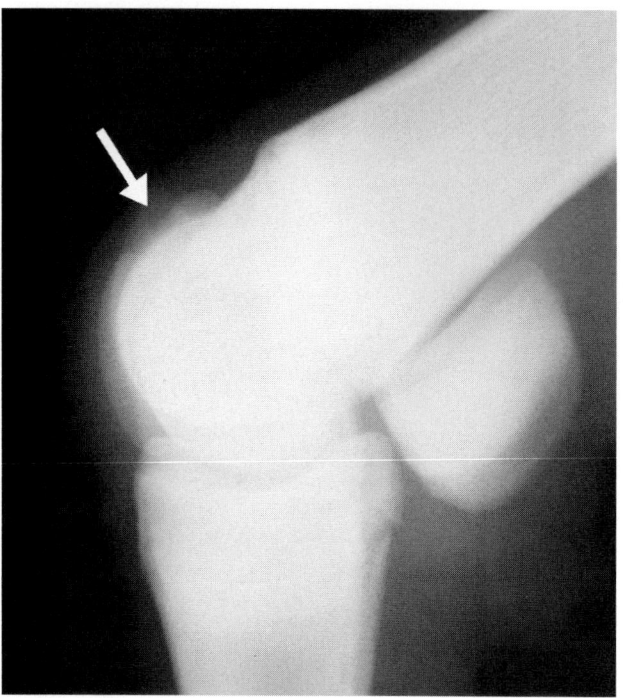

Fig. 22-13 Lateromedial radiograph of a flexed MCP joint with osteochondrosis of the sagittal ridge of MC III. There is excavation of subchondral bone *(arrow)*.

occurs with immune-mediated arthritis, results in a wider joint space. However, such diseases have not been documented in the horse.

Nonseptic inflammatory joint diseases have varied causes and may be difficult to classify. Radiographic signs are distention of the joint and displacement of periarticular soft tissues. If the condition is chronic, bone production at the joint margins or periarticular osteophytes may be found.

Condylar Fractures

Fractures in the distal condyle of MC III or MT III can be difficult to visualize radiographically. The radiographic signs include uneven joint surface, interruption of the metaphyseal cortex, and the presence of a radiolucent fracture line extending from the joint surface to the cortex. The dorsodistal-palmaroproximal projection, angled at 125 degrees in a non-weight-bearing position, has been useful to identify condylar fractures of the distal MC III or MC III that were not apparent on standard radiographic series.[8] These fractures usually occur at the lateral side of the joint (see Figs. 22-4 and 22-16) and may be completely displaced, completely nondisplaced, or incomplete.[39,40] Prognosis after surgical treatment varies.[40,41]

Fractures of the proximal phalanx often communicate with the articular surface. Fracture location and severity must be considered relative to surgical repair and prognosis.[42]

Periarticular Chip Fractures

Chip fractures are more common in racehorses and occur equally in the front limbs. They commonly arise from the medial or lateral periarticular eminences at the proximal dorsal rim of the proximal phalanx.[43] Acute chip fractures may have sharp borders and angular configurations. Chronic chip fractures undergo remodeling and have smooth, rounded

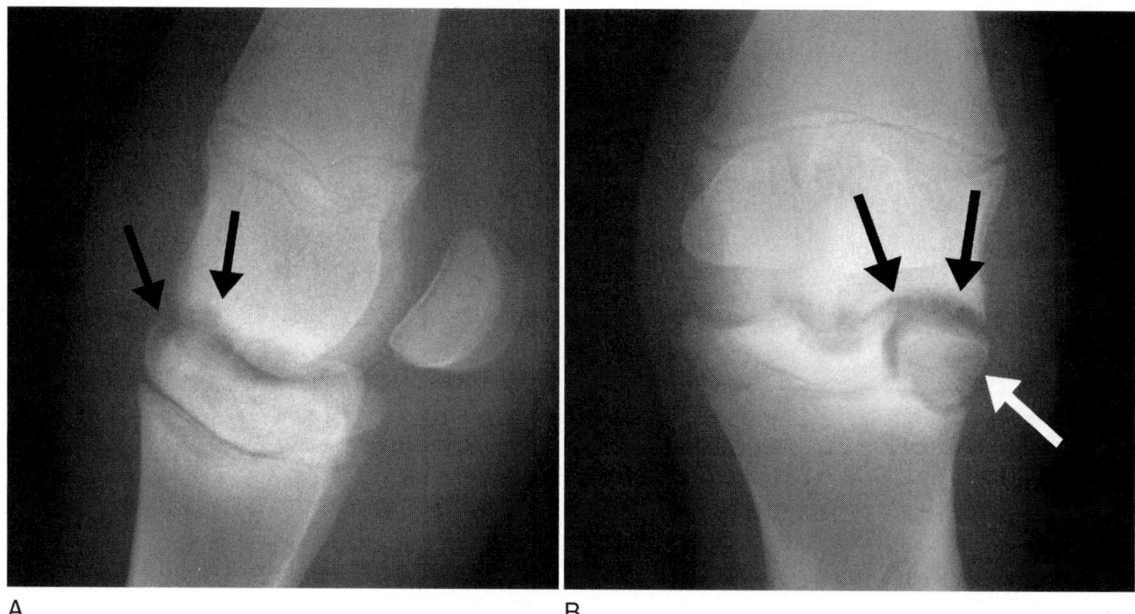

Fig. 22-14 Lateromedial and dorsopalmar views of a 1-month-old filly with soft tissue swelling, septic arthritis, and osteomyelitis. **A,** There is severe osteolysis of the subchondral bone of the distal aspect of the third metatarsal bone and the proximal epiphysis of the proximal phalanx *(arrows)*. **B,** Not only is severe erosion of the subchondral bone of the distal aspect of the third metatarsal bone visible *(black arrows)*, but so is a large osteolytic fragment involving the medial side of the proximal epiphysis of the proximal phalanx *(white arrow)*. These changes are consistent with advanced septic arthritis and septic epiphysitis with a pathologic Salter III fracture of the epiphysis.

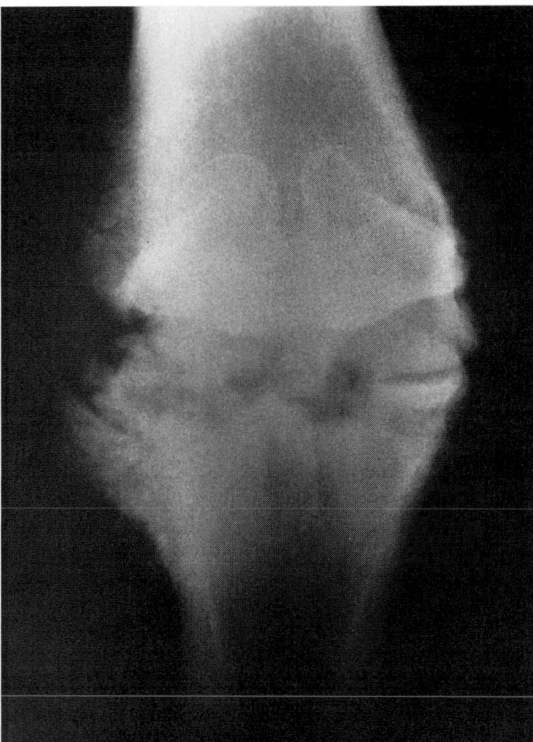

Fig. 22-15 Dorsopalmar radiograph of a horse with chronic septic arthritis. Generalized soft tissue swelling is visible. The joint space has collapsed, and severe erosion of subchondral bone of the opposing joint surfaces has occurred. Bone proliferation is evident on all periarticular surfaces.

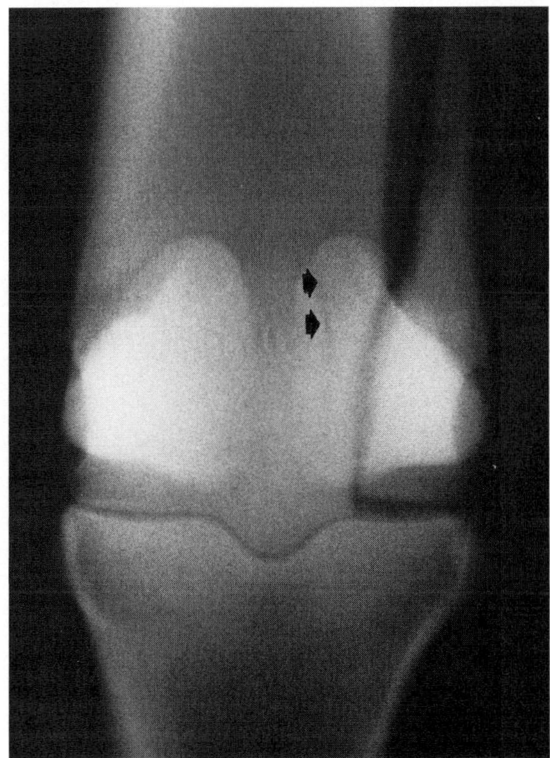

Fig. 22-16 Dorsopalmar radiograph of a horse with a slab fracture of the lateral condyle of MC III. Some fracture lines may be difficult to visualize *(arrows)*. Marked displacement of a fragment such as this is often not present.

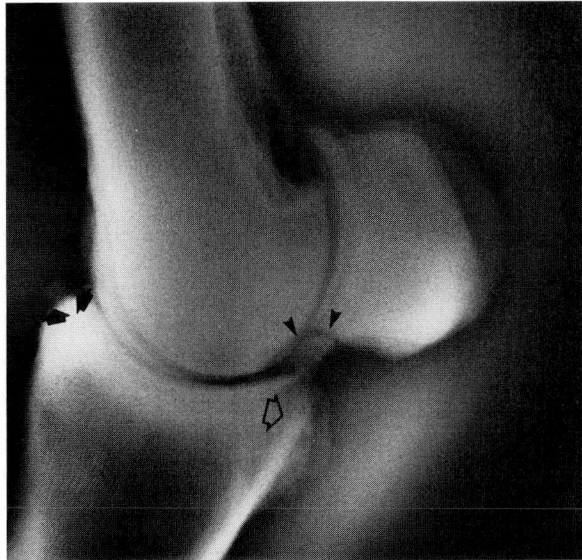

Fig. 22-17 Lateromedial radiograph of a horse with chronic degenerative joint disease. An osteochondral (chip) fracture is present at the dorsal periarticular rim of the proximal phalanx *(solid arrows)*. A basilar osteochondral fracture of the proximal sesamoid is evident *(arrowheads)*. Bone proliferation is present at the attachment of the deep sesamoidean ligaments at the palmaroproximal border of the proximal phalanx *(open arrow)*. Villonodular erosion of bone and supracondylar lysis are also apparent.

borders. The latter are usually attached to the joint capsule or to the joint margin as an exostosis (Fig. 22-17). Free joint bodies may displace or move about within the joint.

Osteochondral fragments arising from the plantarolateral eminences of the proximal phalanx (see Fig. 22-17) have been reported as fractures[15,25,26,30,44] and are considered by some to be manifestations of osteochondrosis.[24,27-36,45,46]

Fractures of the Proximal Sesamoids

Proximal sesamoid fractures are consistently of three types: apical, mid-body, or basilar.[37] Some may be found as osteochondral fragments separated from the sesamoid apex (apical fractures; see Figs. 22-2 and 22-8) or base (basilar fractures, see Figs. 22-12 and 22-17). Fractures through the body of a sesamoid may have a narrow cleavage line, indicating that the suspensory apparatus remains intact (Fig. 22-18, *A*). Wide separation of sesamoid fragments usually indicates bilateral sesamoid fractures and disruption of the fibers of the suspensory ligament (see Fig. 22-18, *B*). Hyperextension of the MCP or MTP joint is apparent if stress is applied to the joint or if the limb is bearing weight with disruption of the suspensory ligament.

Abaxial fractures are detected by using special radiographic projections. These fractures result from avulsion of bone by a portion of the attachment of the branches of the suspensory ligament on the medial or lateral abaxial aspects of the respective proximal sesamoid (Fig. 22-2, *A* and *C*, and Fig. 22-19).

The prognosis of sesamoid fractures is correlated to the type of fracture and damage to the associated structures. Reviews of the clinical aspects of apical[47] and basilar[48] sesamoid fractures are available.

Sesamoiditis

Sesamoiditis is indicated radiographically by bony proliferation on nonarticular surfaces of the proximal sesamoid bones.[49] Linear or cystic lysis may appear to penetrate the sesamoid from the abaxial surface (Fig. 22-20). Sesamoiditis

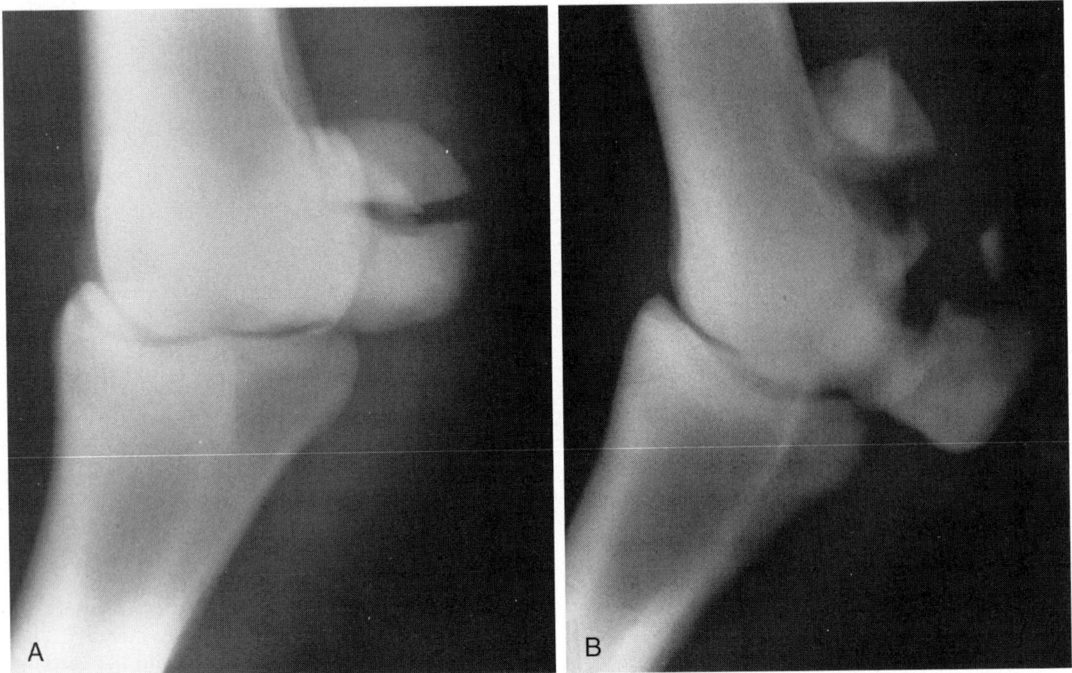

Fig. 22-18 A, A dorsal 45-degree medial-palmarolateral radiograph. Fractures through the medial sesamoid bone are apparent. The joint is extended, but separation of the fragments is minimal. The suspensory ligament remains intact. **B,** Lateral radiograph of a horse with fractures of the medial and lateral proximal sesamoid bones. The joint is hyperextended, and marked separation of the fragments is visible. The suspensory ligament has separated.

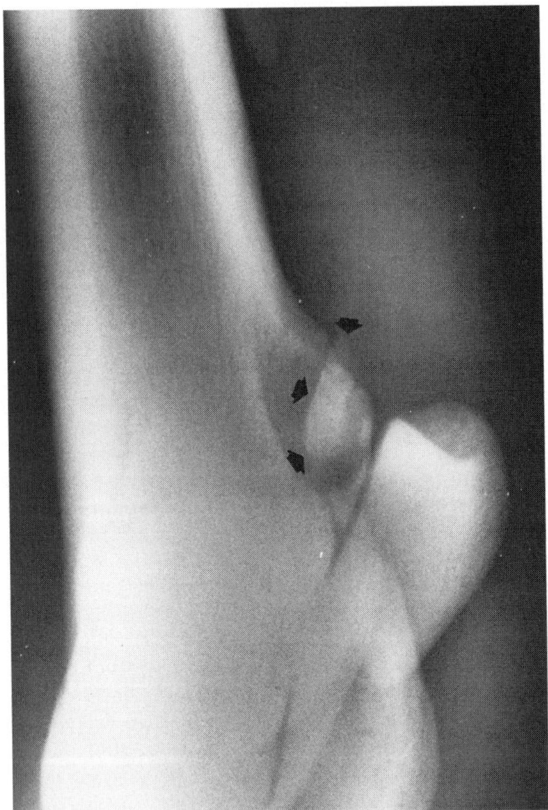

Fig. 22-19 Dorsal 50-degree proximal, 45-degree medial-palmarodistolateral view radiograph of a horse with a periarticular fracture of the medial proximal sesamoid *(arrows)*. The fracture originates at an articular surface and emerges at the abaxial surface of the sesamoid.

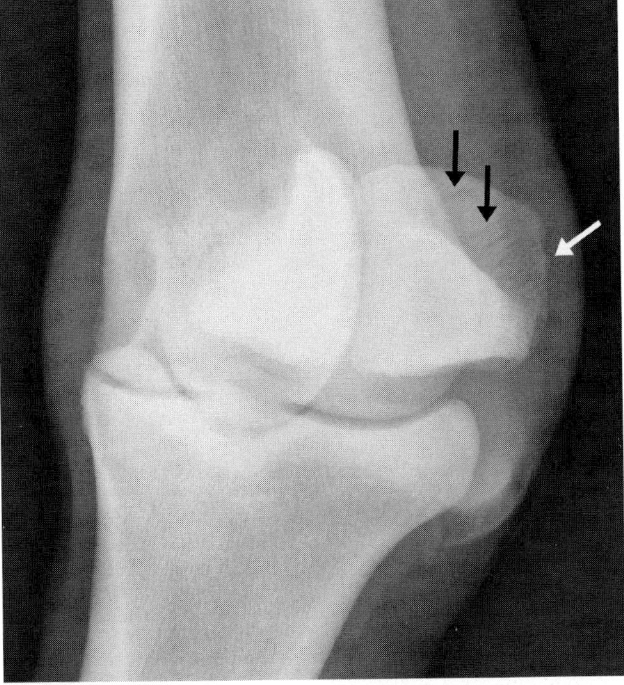

Fig. 22-20 Dorsal 45-degree medial-palmarolateral oblique view of a horse with sesamoiditis of the medial proximal sesamoid, which is projected. Degenerative remodeling is present with increased size of vascular channels within the sesamoid bone *(black arrows)* and bone remodeling of its palmar surface *(white arrow)*. Soft tissue swelling surrounds the MCP joint.

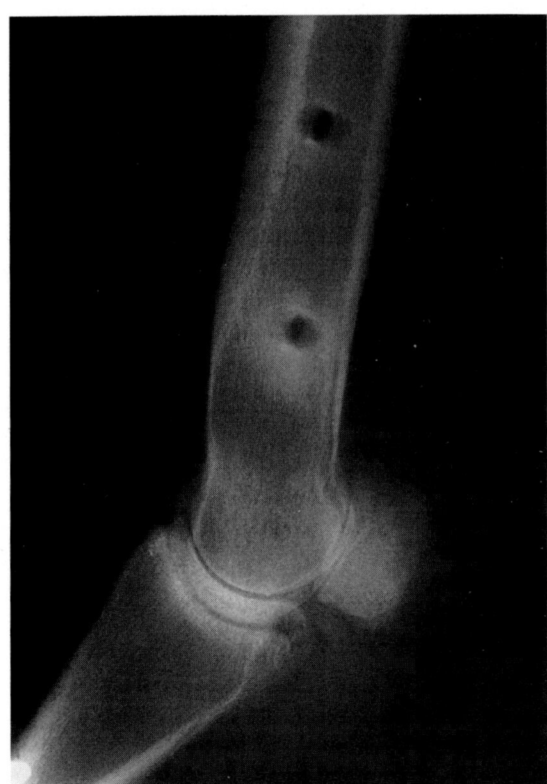

Fig. 22-21 Lateromedial radiograph of the distal metacarpal/metacarpophalangeal III, the MCP joint, and the proximal phalanx of a horse recently having external support removed from the leg. Bone sclerosis is present around transverse pin tracts, but the remaining bone has advanced osteopenia. Generalized remodeling of bone has occurred, and the cortices are thin. Osseous trabeculae are coarse and irregular, with no organized pattern. The sesamoid bones have a spongelike appearance, and avulsion of bone has occurred along the basilar margins.

is usually associated with degenerative change in the suspensory ligament and degenerative remodeling or fracture at the distal ends of MC II or MT IV.

Disuse Atrophy of Bone

Disuse atrophy occurs most rapidly in the proximal sesamoid bones but may also be recognized in the tubular bones as a reduction in bone opacity. Trabeculae within the bone become large and coarse. This change occurs as a result of altered stress or axial weight bearing and may not signify primary pathologic change in the joint (Fig. 22-21).

REFERENCES

1. Getty R: *Sisson and Grossman's the anatomy of the domestic animals,* ed 5, Philadelphia, 1975, W.B. Saunders, pp 357-360.
2. Weaver JC, Stover SM, O'Brien TR: Radiographic anatomy of soft tissue attachments in the equine metacarpophalangeal and proximal phalangeal region, *Equine Vet J* 24:310, 1992.
3. Rendano VT: Equine radiology: the fetlock, *Mod Vet Pract* 58:871, 1977.
4. Butler JA, Colles CM, Dyson SJ et al: *Clinical radiology of the horse,* London, 1993, Blackwell, pp 83-99.
5. Allan GS: Radiography of the equine fetlock, *Equine Pract* 1:40, 1979.
6. Morgan JP: *Techniques of veterinary radiography,* ed 5, Ames, IA, 1993, Iowa State University.
7. O'Brien: T. *Radiography for the ambulatory equine practitioner,* Jackson, WY, 2005, Teton.
8. Hornof WJ, O'Brien TR: Radiographic evaluation of the palmar aspect of the equine metacarpal condyles: a new projection, *Vet Radiol* 21:161, 1980.
9. Palmer SE: Radiography of the abaxial surface of the proximal sesamoid bones of the horse, *J Am Vet Med Assoc* 181:264, 1982.
10. Denoix JM, Jacot S, Perrot P: Ultrasonographic anatomy of the dorsal and abaxial aspects of the equine fetlock, *Equine Vet J* 28:54, 1996.
11. Martinelli MJ, Baker GJ, Clarkson RB et al: Magnetic resonance imaging of degenerative joint disease in a horse: a comparison to other diagnostic techniques, *Equine Vet J* 28:410, 1996.
12. Martinelli MJ, Kuriashkin IV, Carragher BO et al: Magnetic resonance imaging of the equine metacarpophalangeal joint: three dimensional reconstruction and anatomic analysis, *Vet Radiol Ultrasound* 38:193, 1997.
13. Tucker RL, Sande RD: Magnetic resonance imaging and computed tomography: Evaluation of equine musculoskeletal conditions, *Vet Clin North Am [Eq Prac]* 17:145, 2001.
14. McKnight AL, Manduca A, Felmlee JP et al: Motion correction techniques for standing equine MRI, *Vet Radiol Ultrasound* 45:513, 2004.
15. Pool RR, Meagher DM: Pathologic findings and pathogenesis of racetrack injuries, *Vet Clin North Am [Eq Prac]* 6:1, 1990.
16. Gillette EL, Thrall DE, Lebel JL: *Carlson's veterinary radiology,* ed 3, Philadelphia, 1977, Lea & Febiger, p 435.
17. Barclay WP, White KK, Williams A: Equine villonodular synovitis: a case survey, *Cornell Vet* 70:72, 1979.
18. Nickels FA, Grant BD, Lincoln SD: Villonodular synovitis of the equine metacarpophalangeal joint, *J Am Vet Med Assoc* 168:1043, 1976.
19. van Veenendaal JC, Moffat RE: Soft-tissue masses in the fetlock joint of horses, *Aus Vet J* 56:533, 1980.
20. Petterson H, Reiland S: Periarticular subchondral "bone cysts" in horses, *Clin Orthop* 62:95, 1969.
21. Hornof WJ, O'Brien TR, Pool RR: Osteochondritis dissecans of the distal metacarpus in the adult racing thoroughbred horse, *Vet Radiol* 22:98, 1981.
22. Edwards GB: Interpreting radiographs. 2: The fetlock joint and pastern, *Equine Vet J* 16:4, 1984.
23. O'Brien TR, Hornof WJ, Meagher DM: Radiographic detection and characterization of palmar lesions in the equine fetlock joint, *J Am Vet Med Assoc* 178:231, 1981.
24. Foerner JJ, Barclay WP, Phillips TN et al: Osteochondral fragments of the palmar/plantar aspect of the fetlock joint. *Proceedings of the 33rd Annual Meeting of the American Association of Equine Practitioners,* 1987, p 739.
25. Birkeland R: Chip fractures of the first phalanx in the metatarsal phalangeal joint of the horse, *Acta Radiol* 319(suppl):73, 1972.
26. Petterson H, Ryden G: Avulsion fractures of the caudoproximal extremity of the first phalanx, *Equine Vet J* 14:333, 1982.
27. Sandgren B: Bony fragments in the tarsocrural and metacarpo- or metatarsophalangeal joints in the Standardbred horse: a radiographic survey, *Equine Vet J* 6(suppl):66, 1988.
28. Carlsten J, Sandgren B, Dalin G: Development of osteochondrosis in the tarsocrural joint and osteochondral fragments in the fetlock joints of Standardbred trotters. I. A radiological survey, *Equine Vet J* 16(suppl):42, 1993.

29. Grøndahl AM, Engeland A: Influence of radiographically detectable orthopedic changes on racing performance in Standardbred trotters, *J Am Vet Med Assoc* 206:1013, 1995.
30. Dalin G, Sandgren B, Carlsten J: Plantar osteochondral fragments in the fetlock joints of Standardbreds: result of osteochondrosis or trauma? *Equine Vet J* 16(suppl):62, 1993.
31. Grøndahl AM, Dolvik NI: Heritability estimations of osteochondrosis in the tibiotarsal joint and of bony fragments in the palmar/plantar portion of the metacarpo- and metatarsophalangeal joints of horses, *J Am Vet Med Assoc* 203:101, 1993.
32. Philipsson J, Andréasson E, Sandgren B et al: Osteochondrosis in the tarsocrural joint and osteochondral fragments in the fetlock joints in Standardbred trotters. II. Heritability, *Equine Vet J* 16(suppl):38, 1993.
33. Sandgren B, Dalin G, Carlsten J et al: Development of osteochondrosis in the tarsocrural joint and osteochondral fragments in the fetlock joints of Standardbred trotters. II. Body measurements and clinical findings, *Equine Vet J* 16(suppl):48, 1993.
34. Grøndahl AM: The incidence of bony fragments and osteochondrosis in the metacarpo- and metatarsophalangeal joints of Standardbred trotters: a radiographic study, *Equine Vet Sci* 12:81, 1992.
35. Sandgren B, Dalin G, Carlsten J: Osteochondrosis in the tarsocrural joint and osteochondral fragments in the fetlock joints in Standardbred trotters. I. Epidemiology, *Equine Vet J* 16(suppl):31, 1993.
36. Fortier LA, Foerner JJ, Nixon AJ: Arthroscopic removal of axial osteochondral fragments of the plantar/palmar proximal aspect of the proximal phalanx in horses: 119 cases (1988-1992), *J Am Vet Med Assoc* 206:71, 1995.
37. Copelan RW, Bramlage LR: Surgery of the fetlock joint, *Vet Clin North Am [Large Anim Pract]* 5:221, 1983.
38. Yovich JV, McIlwraith CW, Stashak TS: Osteochondritis dissecans of the sagittal ridge of the third metacarpal and metatarsal bones in horses, *J Am Vet Med Assoc* 186:1186, 1985.
39. Zekas LJ, Bramlage LR, Embertson RM et al: Characterization of the type and location of fractures of the third metacarpal/metatarsal condyles in 135 horses in central Kentucky (1986-1994), *Equine Vet J* 31:304, 1999.
40. Rick MC, O'Brien TR, Pool RR et al: Condylar fractures of the third metacarpal bone and third metatarsal bone in 75 horses: radiographic features, treatments, and outcome, *J Am Vet Med Assoc* 183:287, 1983.
41. Zekas LJ, Bramlage LR, Embertson RM et al: Results of treatment of 145 fractures of the third metacarpal/metatarsal condyles in 135 horses (1986-1994), *Equine Vet J* 31:309, 1999.
42. Holcombe SJ, Schneider RK, Bramlage LR et al: Lag screw fixation of noncomminuted sagittal fractures of the proximal phalanx in racehorses: 59 cases (1973-1991), *J Am Vet Med Assoc* 206:1195, 1995.
43. Yovich JV, McIlwraith CW: Arthroscopic surgery for osteochondral fractures of the proximal phalanx of the metacarpophalangeal and metatarsophalangeal (fetlock) joints in horses, *J Am Vet Med Assoc* 188:273, 1986.
44. Nixon AJ, Pool RR: Histologic appearance of axial osteochondral fragments from the proximoplantar/proximopalmar aspect of the proximal phalanx in horses, *J Am Vet Med Assoc* 207:1076, 1995.
45. Barclay WP, Foerner JJ, Phillips TN: Lameness attributable to osteochondral fragmentation of the plantar aspect of the proximal phalanx in horses: 19 cases (1981-1985), *J Am Vet Med Assoc* 191:855, 1987.
46. Grøndhal AM: Incidence and development of ununited proximoplantar tuberosity of the proximal phalanx in Standardbred trotters, *Vet Radiol Ultrasound* 33:18, 1992.
47. Spurlock GH, Gabel AA: Apical fractures of the proximal sesamoid bones in 109 Standardbred horses, *J Am Vet Med Assoc* 183:76, 1983.
48. Parente EJ, Richardson DW, Spencer P: Basal sesamoidean fractures in horses: 57 cases (1980-1991), *J Am Vet Med Assoc* 202:1293, 1993.
49. Blevins WE, Widmer WR: Radiology in racetrack practice, *Vet Clin North Am [Eq Prac]* 6:31, 1990.

ELECTRONIC RESOURCES evolve

Additional information related to the content in Chapter 22 can be found on the companion Web site at evolve http://evolve.elsevier.com/Thrall/vetrad/

- Key Points
- Chapter Quiz
- Case Study 22-1

CHAPTER • 23
The Phalanges

Elizabeth A. Riedesel

TECHNICAL FACTORS

Patient Preparation

Diagnostic nerve blocks are helpful to localize the origin of pain, especially in the horse with multiple abnormalities.[1] The significance of many radiographic abnormalities of the equine phalanges is difficult to ascertain unless pertinent facts obtained from the history and physical examination are correlated with the radiographic findings. Dirt, skin lesions, and iodine-containing medications can all produce opacities that complicate radiographic interpretation. All such material should be removed from the haircoat and hoof wall. Shoes and any additional pads should be removed so that optimal radiographs of the distal phalanx can be obtained. The sole and sulci of the frog should be thoroughly cleaned. The sulci may then be filled with a material of soft tissue opacity (such as Play-Doh, Hasbro, Pawtucket, RI) to the level of the solar surface (Fig. 23-1, *A*). Packing the central and collateral sulci eliminates radiolucent linear regions created when the air-filled sulci are superimposed on the distal phalanx in the dorsal 65-degree proximal palmarodistal* oblique view (see Fig. 23-1, *B*).

Recommended Views

The equine foot is structured such that certain anatomic areas can be imaged as a group (Table 23-1). Excellent descriptions of positioning are available for additional information.[2,3]

NORMAL RADIOGRAPHIC ANATOMY (INCLUDING VARIATIONS)

Osseous Structures

Normal radiographic anatomy of the digit is illustrated in Chapter 14 and other published sources.[4-6] However, several anatomic variations that are frequently misinterpreted as abnormal are worthy of mention.[7] A nutrient foramen occurs in the proximal phalanx of approximately 87% of Thoroughbreds and Standardbreds that are at least 1 year of age.[8,9] When present, these foramina are sometimes bilaterally symmetric and can be located in either the palmar or dorsal cortex. No horses were identified in those surveys to have both a dorsal and a palmar nutrient foramen; however, the author has noted both to be present occasionally in foals. When present in the dorsal cortex, the foramen is typically seen in a lateromedial view as a radiolucent line running obliquely proximal to distal through the mid-diaphyseal cortex (Fig. 23-2). In a dorsopalmar view, it appears as a thin lucent line within the medullary region. When in the palmar cortex, the foramen is located in the distal third and courses in a shorter oblique-to-transverse direction. Of greatest importance is that these foramina should not be mistaken for fractures. Variability in the location of the nutrient foramen of the hindlimb proximal phalanx has not been reported. Variations have not been reported in other breeds, but they likely occur.

Variations may also occur in the appearance of trabeculae in the medullary cavity of the proximal phalanx (Fig. 23-3). A prominent radiolucent center in the medullary cavity surrounded by a ringlike radiopacity is a normal variation and does not indicate cyst formation (Fig. 23-3, *B*).

If the lateromedial view is slightly oblique, two normal structures become more conspicuous and can be misinterpreted as abnormal. The first is the ridge for the V-shaped attachment of the oblique sesamoidean ligament along the palmar cortex of the proximal phalanx. The second is the eminence for attachment of the collateral ligaments of the distal interphalangeal joint along the dorsal aspect of the middle phalanx.

The radiographic appearance of the normal distal phalanx in the dorsal 65-degree proximal-palmarodistal oblique view varies in several respects.[10-12] The most obvious difference is the number and distribution of vascular channels (Fig. 23-4). The number of vascular channels is typically greater in the rear distal phalanx than in the front distal phalanx (ranges of 9 to 19 and 5 to 16, respectively).[10] All vascular channels radiate from the solar canal to the solar border. On their path to the periphery, some give rise to secondary branches that reach the solar border. Although this branching pattern is unique to individual animals, the major channels identified at the solar margin should communicate with the solar canal.

A smoothly rounded concavity in the toe of the distal phalanx may be seen in the normal horse. This notch is referred to as the *crena margins solaris* or, more commonly, the *crena* or toe notch. In a radiographic study of the foredigit of the developing quarter horse, a crena was identified in foals between 4 and 22 weeks of age in 83% of the distal phalanges evaluated.[13] The depth of this notch usually does not exceed 1.5 cm.[11] The crena is more conspicuous in front than in hind feet.[10] Ninety percent of sound racing Thoroughbreds have bilateral symmetry in the presence of the crena in the front feet, 5% asymmetry in the front feet, and 5% in neither front foot.[12]

The shape of the extensor process of the distal phalanx may also differ among individual animals (Fig. 23-5).[10] The margin of the normal process, however, should be smooth regardless of its shape.

The palmar processes of the distal phalanx become more extensively ossified with age. The morphologic development of the palmar process has been described in the foal (3

*Palmar(o) is used throughout this chapter with the understanding that plantar(o) should be substituted if reference is being made to the rear digit.

Table • 23-1

Views for Equine Phalanx Evaluation

EXAMINATION	STRUCTURES EVALUATED	VIEWS
Pastern	P1	Dorsal 45-degree proximal- palmarodistal oblique
	Proximal interphalangeal joint	Lateromedial
	P2	Dorsal 35-degree lateral-palmaromedial oblique
		Dorsal 35-degree medial-palmarolateral oblique
Digit	P3	Dorsopalmar with horizontal beam and dorsal 45-degree proximal- palmarodistal oblique
	Distal interphalangeal joint	Dorsal 65-degree proximal-palmarodistal oblique with horse standing on cassette
		Lateromedial, with foot on block to include solar margin of P3 and soft tissues of sole on the radiograph
		Two oblique views: dorsal 65-degree proximal, 45-degree lateral-palmarodistomedial and dorsal 65-degree proximal, 45-degree medial-palmarodistolateral (both with horse standing on cassette); obliques are especially useful when P3 fracture is suspected

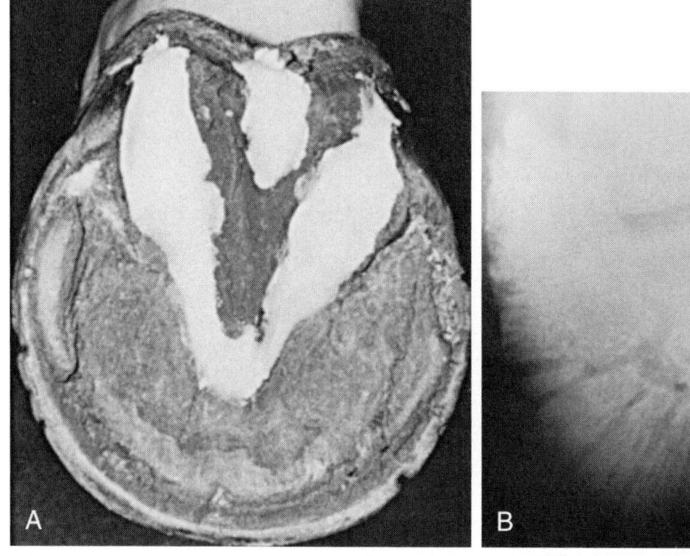

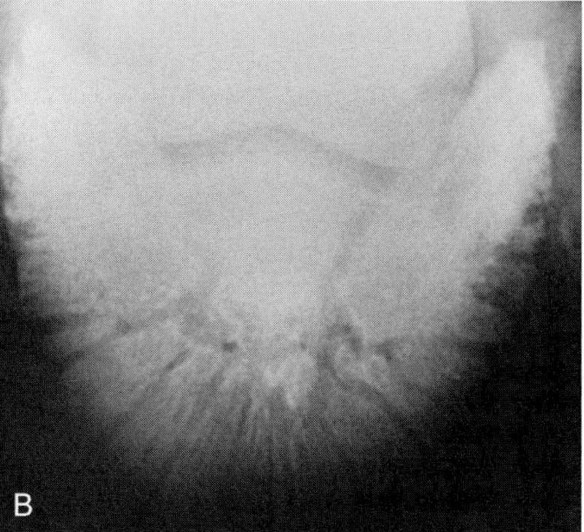

Fig. 23-1 A, The central and collateral sulci of the foot have been packed with a pliable material of similar radiopacity as the sole (Play-Doh). B, Dorsal 65-degree proximal-palmarodistal view of a normal P3 with the sulci packed. Note the good definition of vascular channels without superimposed air artifacts.

to 32 weeks of age).[14] Compare the palmar processes of the three horses (5 months old, 8 years old, and 15 years old) in Figure 23-6.

Soft Tissue

No muscle exists in the phalangeal region of the foot. Many tendons and supporting ligaments, however, are present in addition to joint capsules. Minimal amounts of fat are present in the phalangeal region. Knowledge of the attachment sites of the joint capsules, tendons, and ligaments of the foot is imperative for accurate interpretation of the osseous changes seen in radiographs of the phalanges. Figures 23-7 and 23-8 illustrate the attachment sites of these major structures. Additional information on soft tissue attachments is available.[6,15] Most of these soft tissues do not create independently distinct shadows. However, the deep digital flexor tendon can often be seen in the lateromedial view as a slightly more opaque soft tissue band as it passes between the level of the proximal aspect of the middle phalanx and the proximal margin of the navicular bone.[10] The hoof capsule generally is considered to produce a uniform soft tissue opacity. However, the junction between the stratum medium and the stratum internum of the dorsal hoof wall can frequently be seen in a properly exposed lateromedial view.[12] The junction of the coronary band and the most proximal extent of the hoof wall is not always clearly distinct in lateromedial and dorsopalmar views.

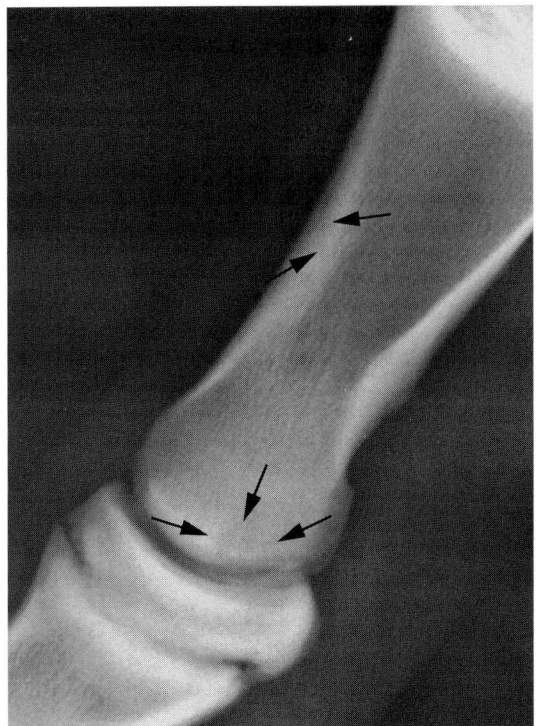

Fig. 23-2 Radiolucent lines are visible in both the dorsal *(long arrows)* and palmar cortices of P1 of this foal. These are normal small nutrient foramina. A circular radiolucency is also present in the distal palmar subchondral bone of P1 *(short arrows)*. This is a cystlike osteochondrosis lesion.

The ergot may create a radiopacity when superimposed on the proximal phalanx in the dorsopalmar view (see Fig. 23-3, *B*). In the lateromedial view, the ergot opacity can be seen along the palmar surface of the skin.

Articular Cartilage and Collateral Cartilages

The properly positioned dorsal 45-degree proximal palmarodistal view is the best view for evaluation of the width of the metacarpophalangeal, proximal interphalangeal, and distal interphalangeal joints. In the normal foot, the metacarpophalangeal joint is usually the narrowest of these articulations, the proximal interphalangeal joint is slightly wider, and the distal interphalangeal joint is the widest (see Fig. 23-3, *A*). If the horse is not bearing weight evenly on the leg, the asymmetrical loading forces can cause the appearance of narrowing of the loaded side and widening of the nonloaded side of the joint (see Fig. 23-12, *B*). This artifact can be recognized because it similarly affects all three joints. The collateral cartilages are not visible in the normal foot.

Alternate Imaging of the Foot

Increased access to computed and digital radiography, ultrasound, nuclear scintigraphy, magnetic resonance imaging (MRI), and computed tomography is enhancing the anatomic and physiologic assessment of foot lameness. The development of an open MRI system for use in the sedated standing horse is in use clinically and has the potential to improve evaluation of soft tissues of the digit.[16,17] Although this chapter cannot fully discuss the contributions of these modalities, specific notation will be made regarding major alternate imaging findings where applicable.

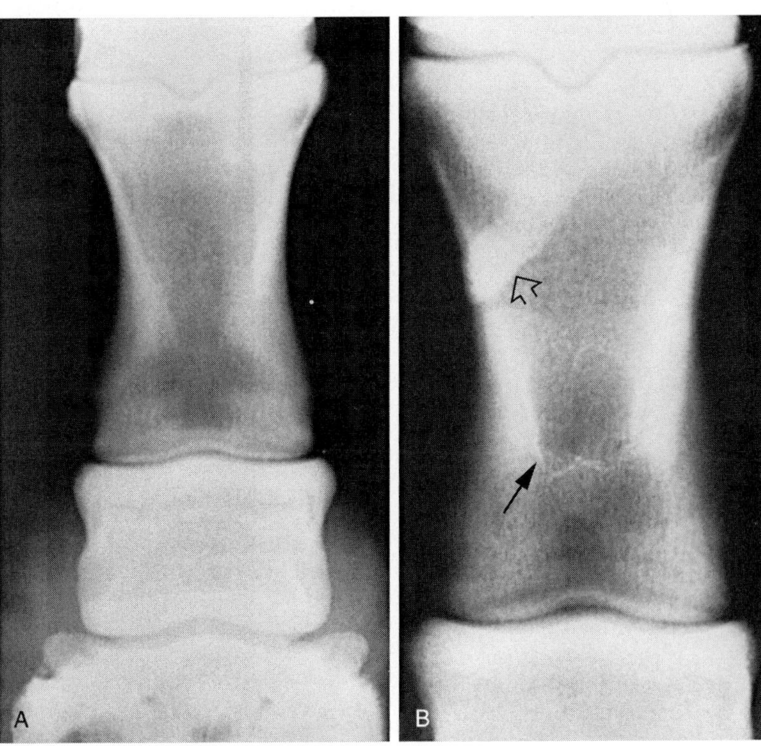

Fig. 23-3 Dorsopalmar view of two normal equine proximal phalanges. **A,** Note the normal thickness of the lateral and medial cortices of P1 at the junction of the middle and distal third of the bone. The radiolucent medullary cavity is seen between the thickest parts of the cortex. The widest joint space is usually the distal interphalangeal joint, with the joint spaces becoming progressively narrower toward the metacarpophalangeal joint. **B,** A thin rim of opaque trabeculation surrounds the central medullary cavity of P1 *(solid arrow)*. The ergot is elongated in this animal and is seen because of its summation with P1 *(open arrow)*.

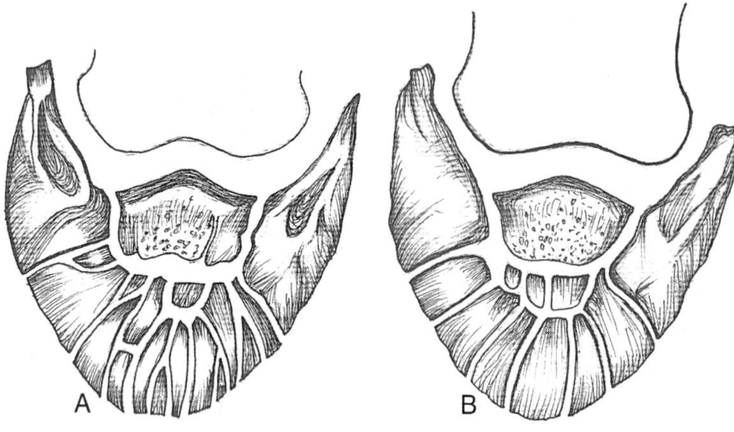

Fig. 23-4 A and B, Two variations in the pattern of vascular channel formation in the normal P3.

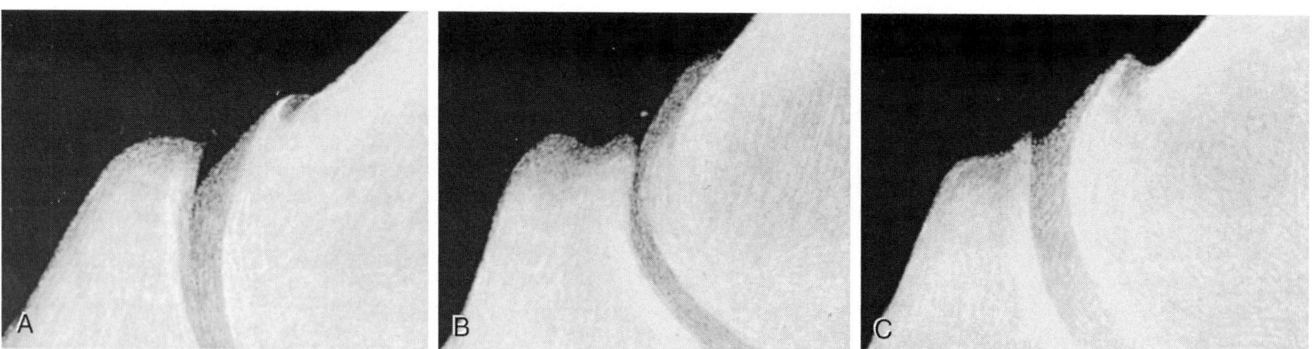

Fig. 23-5 A to C, Normal variations in the shape of the extensor process of P3, as might be seen on the lateromedial view. (Illustration by Richard M. Shook, DVM.)

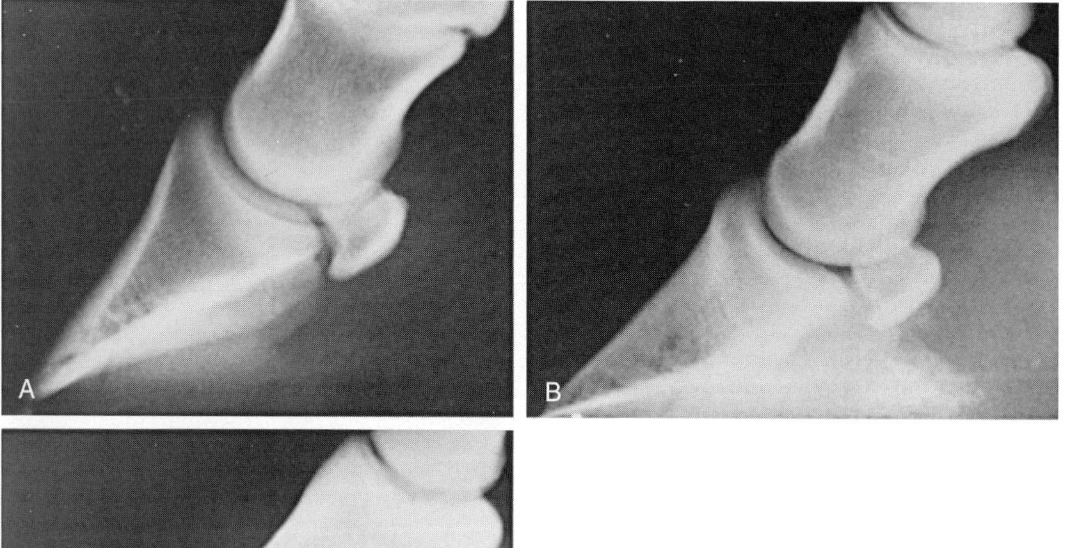

Fig. 23-6 Palmar processes of the normal P3 in the horse become more extensively ossified with age. Lateromedial views of **A,** a 5-month-old foal; **B,** an 8-year-old Standardbred; and **C,** a 15-year-old Arabian crossbreed.

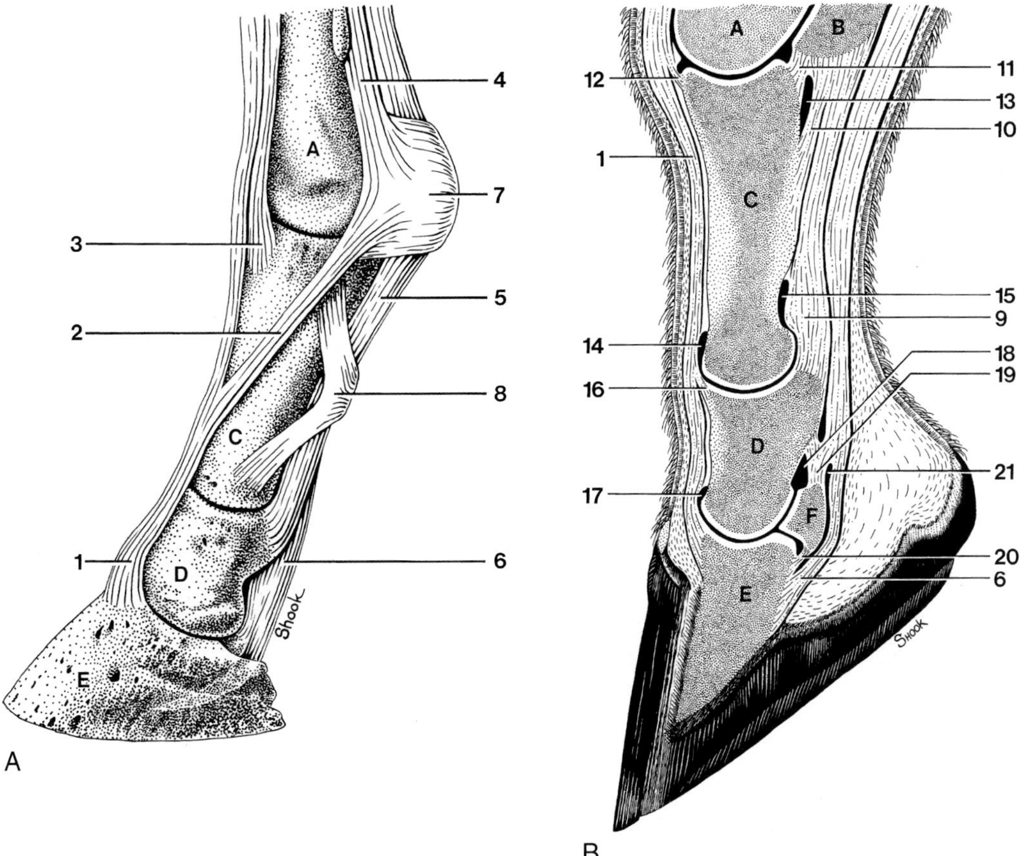

Fig. 23-7 Lateral views of the tendon and ligament attachments of the digit. **A,** Superficial tissues; **B,** Sagittal section. (Illustration by Richard A. Shook, DVM.)

The following anatomic key is for Figures 23-7 and 23-8.

A. Third metacarpal bone
B. Proximal sesamoid bone
C. P1
D. P2
E. P3
F. Distal sesamoid (navicular) bone

1. Common digital extensor tendon
2. Extensor branch of the interosseous (suspensory) ligament
3. Lateral digital extensor tendon
4. Interosseous (suspensory) ligament
5. Superficial digital flexor tendon
6. Deep digital flexor tendon
7. Superficial transverse metacarpal ligament (palmar annular ligament)
8. Proximal digital annular ligament
9. Superficial (straight) sesamoidean ligament
10. Middle (oblique) sesamoidean ligament
11. Deep (cruciate) sesamoidean ligament
12. Metacarpophalangeal joint capsule (blended with fibers from the common digital extensor tendon)
13. Distal palmar recess of the metacarpophalangeal joint
14. Dorsal recess of the proximal interphalangeal joint capsule
15. Palmar recess of the proximal interphalangeal joint
16. Proximal interphalangeal joint capsule (blended with fibers from the common digital extensor tendon)
17. Dorsal recess of the distal interphalangeal joint
18. Palmar recess of the distal interphalangeal joint
19. Collateral sesamoidean ligament
20. Distal sesamoidean impar ligament
21. Podotrochlear bursa
22. Medial collateral ligament of the metacarpophalangeal joint
23. Lateral collateral ligament of the proximal interphalangeal joint
24. Medial collateral ligament of the distal interphalangeal joint

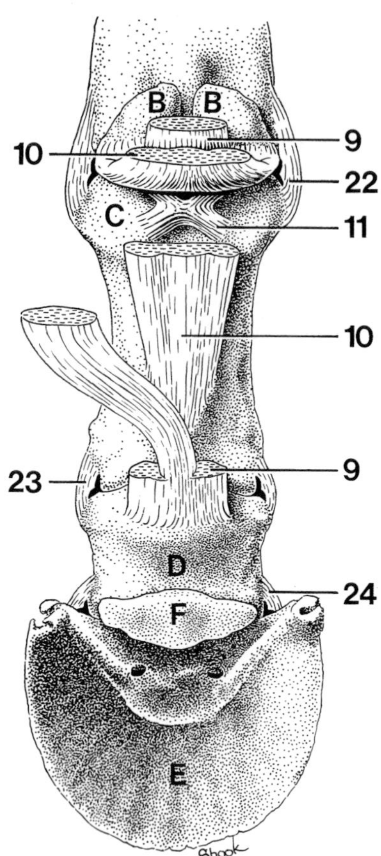

Fig. 23-8 Palmar view of the sesamoidean and collateral ligament attachments of the digit. (See Anatomic Key in legend for Fig. 23-7.) (Illustration by Richard A. Shook, DVM.)

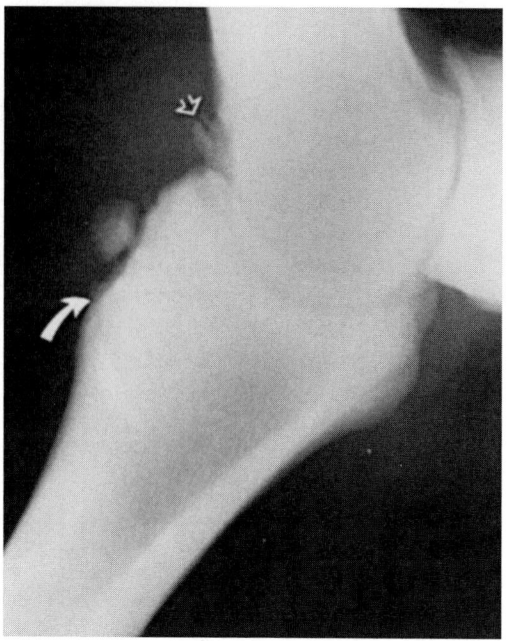

Fig. 23-9 Lateromedial view of the metacarpophalangeal joint. Small chip fragments from the dorsoproximal edge of P1 are evident *(open arrow)*. Periosteal proliferation, cortical sclerosis *(curved arrow)*, and avulsion fragmentation or dystrophic calcification of the insertion of the lateral digital extensor tendon are also visible.

RADIOGRAPHIC CHANGES CAUSED BY DISEASES OF THE PHALANGES

General Comments

Common diseases affecting the digit are acute trauma leading to fracture; chronic repetitive trauma leading to desmitis, tendonitis, enthesopathy, and degenerative joint disease; and infection. Inflammation of the laminae of the hoof wall (laminitis), leading to a disturbance of the mechanical support of the foot, is the only common effect initiated by metabolic disease. Neoplasia of the digit is extremely rare.

Because the digit has little soft tissue, standard x-ray exposure technique is typically selected to best define the bony structures. Still, soft tissue abnormalities do occur. Either the soft tissues must be evaluated by a high-intensity light, or additional images must be made to optimize soft tissue evaluation. Use of a relatively higher kilovoltage peak and lower milliampere seconds produces a radiograph with a longer scale of contrast and better resolution of soft tissues. The postcapture image manipulation offered by computed and digital radiography allows evaluation of osseous and soft tissue structures with one exposure per view.

The radiographic signs of abnormal soft tissue include alteration of thickness, contour, or opacity. Increased pericapsular soft tissue thickness may be seen with intracapsular fluid accumulation, synovial tissue thickening, extracapsular inflammation (cellulitis), or fibrosis. If radiographic signs of soft tissue enlargement are strictly confined to the region of the joint, intracapsular fluid accumulation with or without synovial tissue thickening is the likely cause. If the enlargement extends proximally and distally beyond the sites of joint capsule attachment, an extracapsular process (fluid and cellular) is likely present, which obscures evaluation of intracapsular changes. Isolated enlargement, away from the joint, is most likely related to direct local trauma with or without infection. An irregular surface contour suggests acute laceration or chronic granulation tissue. Large areas of periosteal new bone may persist for a long time after resolution of the inciting cause. The soft tissue contour bulges over such an area of periosteal new bone but may not be actually thickened.

Increased opacity within pericapsular soft tissue is usually caused by dystrophic mineralization. Lesions that commonly become mineralized include chronic sprain or strain of supporting ligaments and tendons (Fig. 23-9), pericapsular deposition of corticosteroids, and focal necrosis attributable to neurectomy (Fig. 23-10). Ossification of the collateral cartilages of the distal phalanx should not be mistaken for dystrophic mineralization of soft tissue.

Decreased opacity within the soft tissues is caused by air or gas in the subcutis or the fascial planes of the tendons and ligaments. Soft tissue gas pockets commonly follow diagnostic nerve block and open skin wounds but rarely are caused by a gas-producing organism.

The radiographic signs of abnormal bone include alteration of contour, margination, and opacity. These signs are caused by a combination of new bone formation and bone removal. Repeated patterns of bone change tend to be associated with specific injury to the phalanges and associated joints. Figures 23-11 and 23-12 depict the variable appearances of the periosteal surface, joint space, and subchondral bone that occur in the more common diseases of the phalanges.

Strain and Sprain Injuries

Regions of new bone formation are commonly seen on the cortical surfaces of the phalanges, especially in the proximal and middle phalanx. Many of these are caused by strain and sprain injuries. Strain injury (tendonitis) results from damage to muscle or tendon induced by overuse or overstress.[3] In its

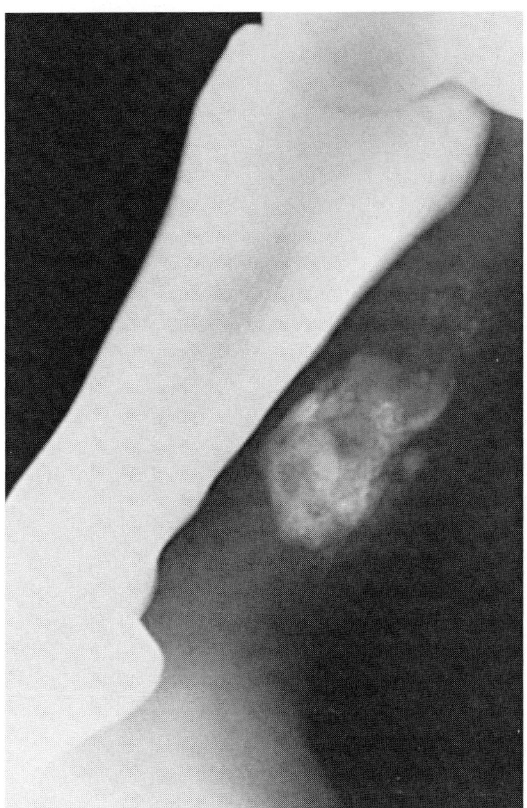

Fig. 23-10 Dystrophic calcification in the palmar soft tissues caused by previous neurectomy.

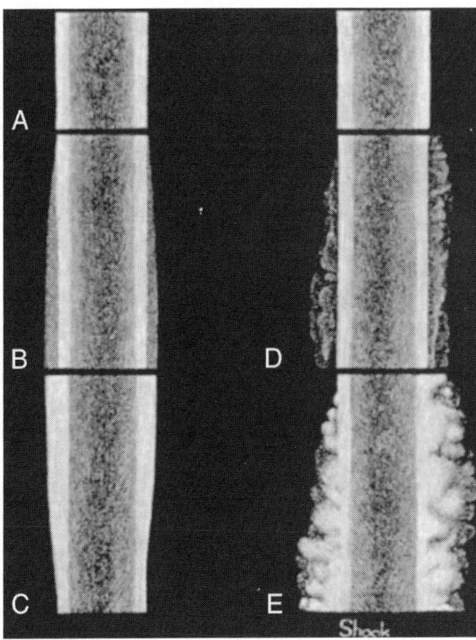

Fig. 23-11 Variable appearance of contour and opacity of periosteal bone proliferation and likely causes. *A*, Normal cortex. *B*, Smooth margin, mildly opaque; recent subperiosteal hemorrhage from direct trauma or exudate of infection. C, Smooth margin, opaque; inactive, remodeled trauma. *D*, Irregular margin, mildly opaque; recent or active response to direct traumatic injury including sprain/strain or infective periostitis. *E*, Irregular margin, opaque; chronic sprain/strain or infection. Note the loss of distinction between periosteal new bone and original cortex in C and *E*. (Illustration by Richard A. Shook, DVM.)

mildest form, strain causes only inflammation. With chronic repeated strain or more severe acute strain, disruption within the soft tissue unit or avulsion from its bone attachment occurs. Radiographically, the swelling or inflammation in the tendon may not be evident. Soft tissue changes are best imaged by ultrasound, vascular and soft tissue pool phase scintigraphy, and MRI. The latter has been shown to be sensitive to lesions of the deep digital flexor tendon throughout the foot region (Fig. 23-13).[18] Although uncommon, dystrophic mineralization can develop in a chronically inflamed tendon.

Radiography is useful for assessing the bony attachment sites of the tendons. Knowledge of the attachment sites of the flexor and extensor tendons on the phalanges is therefore needed (see Figs. 23-7 and 23-8). Avulsion fracture at the attachment site can occur and will be evident as a bone fragment displaced in the direction of traction of the tendon. New bone formation at a tendon or ligament attachment site is called an enthesophyte. When seen early it will likely be minimal in volume and have a mildly irregular surface. If the strain injury continues, the enthesopathy enlarges and continues to have a fuzzy, irregular margin. Such a change is occasionally seen at the insertion of the lateral digital extensor tendon on the dorsolateral proximal surface of the proximal phalanx (see Fig. 23-9). With further progression, the enthesopathy takes on a smooth, hooklike, or spurlike shape, projecting in the direction of tension or traction. Radiographically aging or determining the activity of these bone changes is difficult. Periosteal new bone formation is typically not visible until 5 to 7 days (in the foal) or 10 to 14 days (in the adult) after stimulation. When a prominent smooth enthesophyte is seen on a first radiographic evaluation of a horse, it should be taken as a signal of strain injury that occurred at least 5 to 6 weeks previously.

Sprain injury (desmitis) results from damage to the supporting ligaments of joints induced by movement of the bony components beyond their normal range.[3] Similar to strain injury, the mild sprain injury causes inflammation that is not likely to cause visible changes radiographically. Greater degrees of injury result in loss of stability to the joint, allowing complete or partial luxation.

Stress views may be needed to detect subluxation. Laxity in a subluxated joint is often more apparent at physical examination than at radiography, especially if the horse is unwilling to bear full weight on the leg. Conversely, complete luxation is typically evident and may be accompanied by avulsion fractures at the ligament insertion sites. Non-weight-bearing flexed dorsal 45-degree lateral-palmaromedial oblique and flexed dorsal 45-degree medial-palmarolateral oblique views may improve the visualization of the origin and insertion sites for the collateral ligaments of the distal interphalangeal joint.[19] Larger fractures of the phalanges may also be associated with joint luxation. This is commonly seen with comminuted fractures of the middle phalanx and associated loss of congruency of the proximal interphalangeal joint (see Fig. 23-18). Secondary changes expected with subluxation are enthesophyte formation at the ligament insertion sites and some degree of degenerative joint disease. The range of change will depend on the severity of the initial injury and the frequency of recurring subluxation. Although not the result of overt joint instability, a common site of enthesophyte formation associated with ligament insertion is on the palmar or plantar margin of the proximal phalanx at the insertion of the middle (oblique) sesamoidean ligament (Fig. 23-14). Most enthesophytes do not regress after healing of the soft tissues involved in the inciting sprain or strain injury.

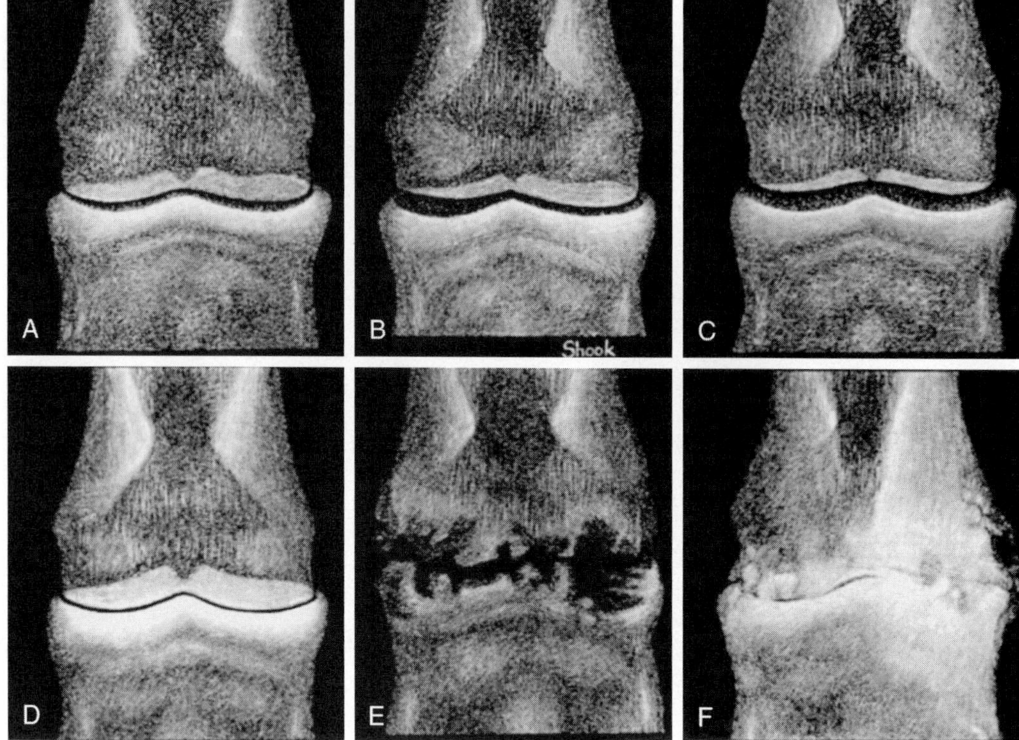

Fig. 23-12 Changes in joint space width, subchondral bone opacity, or both, as seen in the dorsopalmar view of the proximal interphalangeal joint, and likely causes. **A,** Normal joint space and subchondral bone. **B,** Widened joint space on the lateral or medial side, no subchondral bone changes. Artifact is caused by asymmetric weight distribution on the foot or unbalanced hoof trimming. **C,** Widened joint space, no subchondral bone changes; not weight bearing at time of radiography or increased intraarticular fluid volume. **D,** Uniformly narrowed joint space, no subchondral bone changes. Artifact caused by x-ray beam angulation or uniform degenerative wearing and loss of articular cartilage. **E,** Widened joint space, lysis of the subchondral bone; active septic arthritis. **F,** Narrowed joint space, irregular opacity, and contour of subchondral bone; chronic low-grade septic arthritis or chronic osteoarthritis caused by trauma-related instability or poor conformation. (Illustration by Richard A. Shook, DVM.)

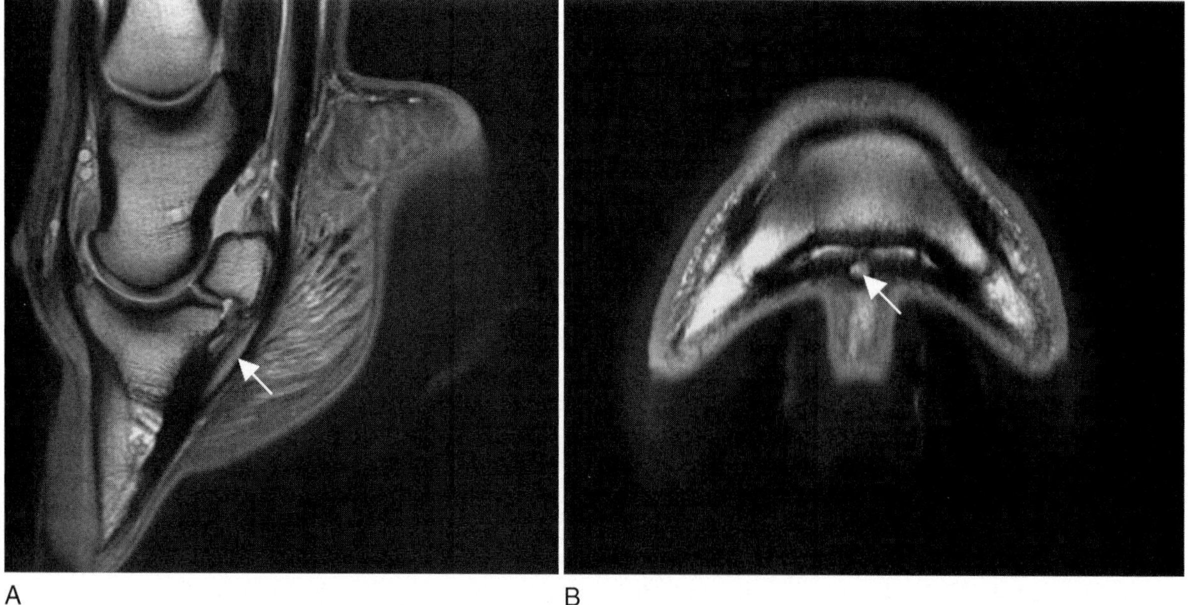

Fig. 23-13 Sagittal (**A**) and transverse (**B**) proton density-weighted MRIs of an equine digit. A large hyperintense core lesion in the deep digital flexor tendon *(arrows)* is visible. This lesion would not be visible on radiographs, CT, or nuclear medicine images. The lesion might be visible by ultrasound, but examining this region of the digit with ultrasound is difficult because of the poor acoustic characteristics of the overlying tissues.

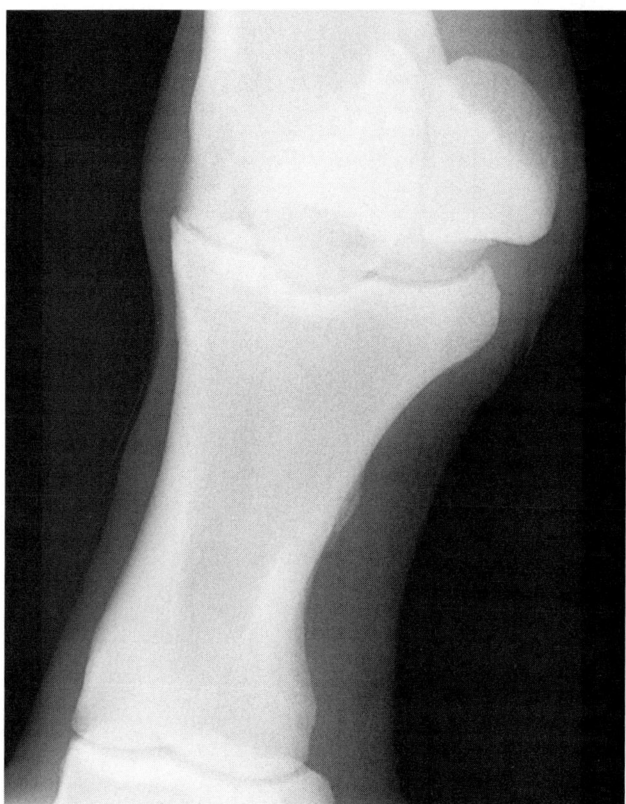

Fig. 23-14 Dorsal 45-degree lateral-palmaromedial view of P1. Note the enthesopathy on the palmarolateral aspect of P1 caused by pulling of the attachment of the middle sesamoidean ligament.

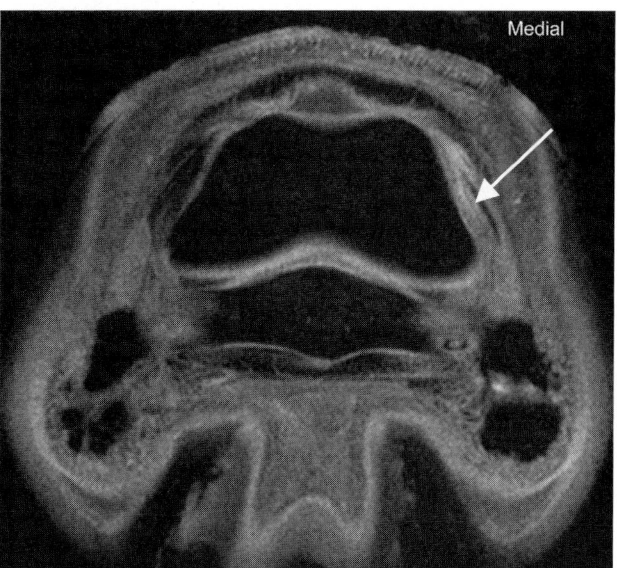

Fig. 23-15 Transverse gradient-echo image of the P3 region of a horse with interphalangeal collateral desmitis. Note the increased signal within and adjacent to the medial collateral interphalangeal ligament *(arrow)* compared with the normal lateral side.

Collateral ligament desmitis of the distal interphalangeal joint has been found to be a significant cause of foot lameness in the absence of radiographic changes. MRI has been found to be the most useful diagnostic imaging modality to define the changes in these ligaments (Fig. 23-15).[20-22]

FRACTURE DISEASE

Proximal Phalanx

The location of fractures of the proximal phalanx (P1) depends on the type of stress applied. The common fracture types are osteochondral edge (chip) fractures at the proximal dorsal periarticular margin and the palmar or plantar proximal tuberosity and longitudinal fractures of the body (diaphysis).[23,24] By far, the most common fracture involving P1 is the osteochondral fracture of the proximal dorsal edge, either at the medial or at the lateral eminence (see Fig. 23-9). This occurs as an overextension injury of the metacarpophalangeal joint in racehorses. This fracture and those of the palmar eminence are described in Chapter 21.

Various classification schemes have been applied to all other fractures of P1.[25-28] By general classification, the fractures are noncomminuted or comminuted, incomplete or complete, monoarticular or biarticular, and in a primarily sagittal or dorsal plane to the long axis of P1. Figure 23-16 illustrates these fractures of P1. Several retrospective surveys of Thoroughbred and Standardbred racehorses with these types of fractures have been reported with an attempt to correlate fracture configuration to prognosis.[25,26,28-31] The most frequently reported fracture configuration in these breeds is the noncomminuted, incomplete, monoarticular sagittal fracture (see Fig. 23-16, *A*). This fracture is common in 2- and 3-year-olds in race training or active racing. It occurs in both front limbs and hindlimbs of these breeds. However, reported fractures are somewhat more common in the front limbs of Thoroughbreds and the hindlimbs of Standardbreds. This fracture typically originates at the proximal articular surface just lateral to or within the midline plane of the sagittal groove (Figs. 23-17, *A;* also see Fig. 23-16, *A*). Few originate medial to the midline plane.

Two variations of the noncomminuted, incomplete, monoarticular sagittal fracture occur. The short (less than 30-mm extension into the diaphysis) variation is slightly more common than the long (more than 30-mm extension into the diaphysis) variation. Both fractures may course in a slightly spiral or oblique manner. This effect is depicted as two parallel or "offset" radiolucent lines representing the fracture plane in the dorsal and palmar cortices. The short fracture may be more difficult to identify on an initial radiographic evaluation. Both variations of fracture are seen only on dorsopalmar views. Because the fracture plane typically has very little gap, the x-ray beam must pass parallel to the fracture line for the fracture gap to be detected. Repeat radiographs in 7 to 10 days should allow identification of the fracture more readily, after lysis of bone along the fracture edges has occurred during the first stages of healing. When imaging occurs several weeks after the onset of lameness, periosteal new bone will likely be present on the dorsal or palmar surface, indicating callus. At this stage, the new bone is visible on the lateromedial view, the fracture line on the dorsopalmar view may be less visible, and sclerosis in the adjoining bone should be seen.

Horses with either the short or the long variation of the noncomminuted, incomplete, monoarticular sagittal fracture have a good prognosis for survival and return to athletic performance. However, in a survey of Standardbreds, these horses had slower racing times and decreased performance indexes (order of finish times purse) regardless of fracture length or medical versus surgical treatment.[31] This type of fracture is not mentioned in a report of diagnosis and treatment of quarter horse racehorses.[32]

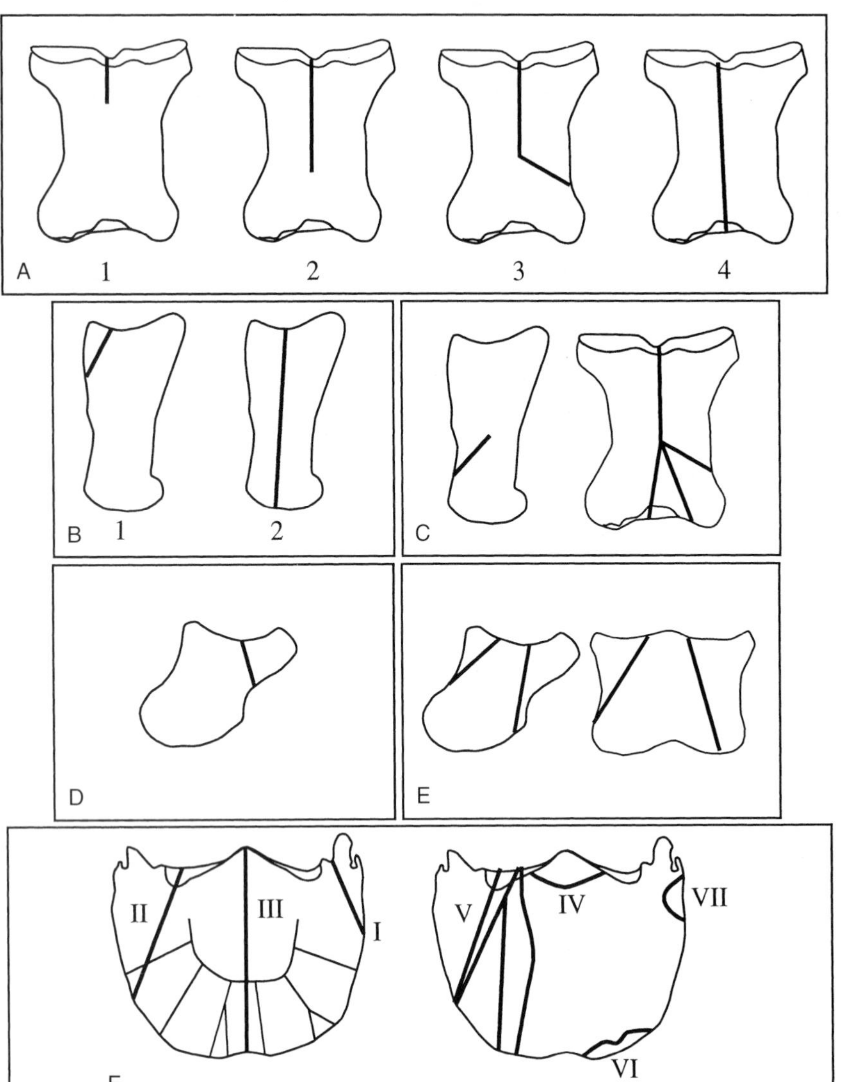

Fig. 23-16 Common fractures of the phalanges. P1: **A,** Sagittal plane fractures, noncomminuted. *1,* Incomplete, monoarticular (short, less than 30-mm variation); *2,* incomplete, monoarticular (long, more than 30-mm variation); *3,* complete, monoarticular; *4,* complete, biarticular. **B,** Dorsal plane fractures, noncomminuted. *1,* Complete, monoarticular; *2,* complete, biarticular. **C,** Comminuted, complete, biarticular, dorsal, and/or sagittal plane. P2: **D,** Palmar/plantar eminence (monoarticular, complete). **E,** Comminuted, complete, biarticular. P3: **F,** *I,* Nonarticular, palmar/plantar process; *II,* articular, extending from distal interphalangeal joint to solar margin; *III,* articular, mid-sagittal, divides into equal parts; *IV,* articular, extensor process; *V,* articular, comminuted body fracture (not of types II, III, or IV); *VI,* solar margin; *VII,* solar border of palmar/plantar process in foals.

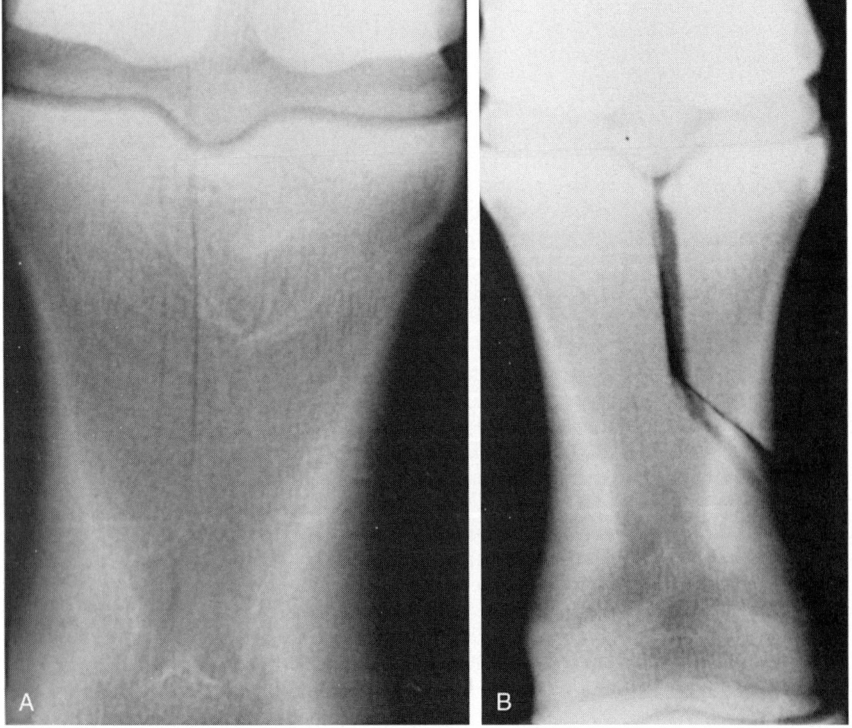

Fig. 23-17 Incomplete (**A**) and complete (**B**) sagittal fracture of P1. The plane of the primary x-ray beam must be parallel to the fracture plane to identify this lesion when no fragment displacement is present.

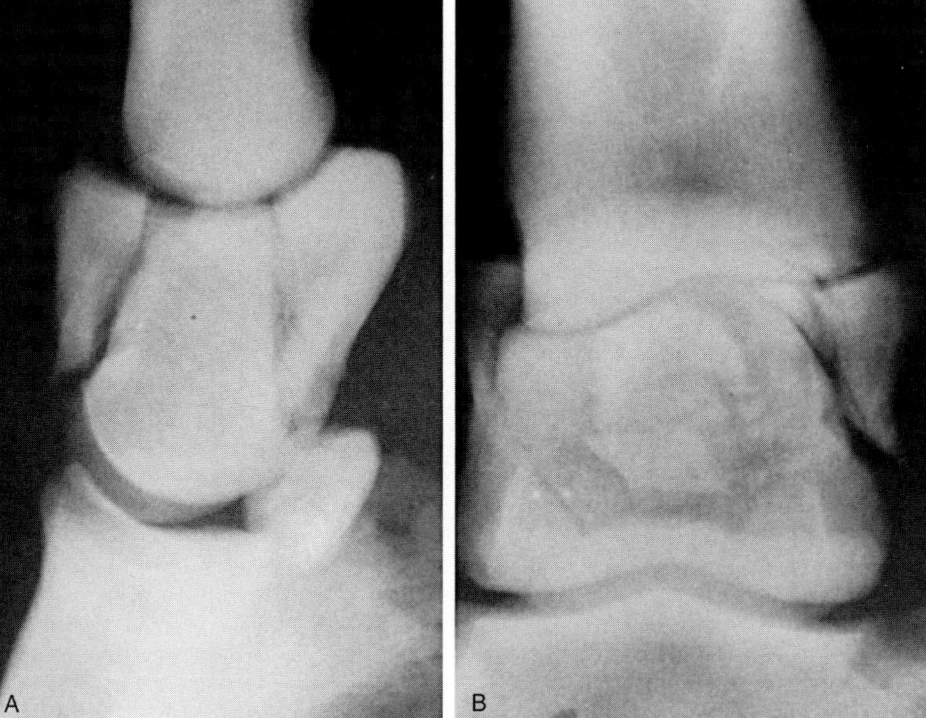

Fig. 23-18 Comminuted, multiple fractures of P2. In the lateromedial view (A) the palmar fracture extends into the distal interphalangeal joint in the area of the navicular bone.

Noncomminuted, complete sagittal fractures of P1 occur with considerably less frequency than do incomplete fractures in racehorses. This type of fracture is, however, reported to be more common in the Western performance horse.[3] Two variations of this fracture occur: one is biarticular involving origin at the metacarpophalangeal joint and exit at the proximal interphalangeal joint; the other is monoarticular and typically exits through the lateral distal palmar or plantar cortex (see Figs. 23-16, *A* and 23-17, *B*). These fractures are most readily seen in the dorsopalmar view. Although these horses have a good prognosis for survival with conservative or surgical treatment, prognosis for return to an equal level of performance is more guarded than with the noncomminuted, incomplete, monoarticular sagittal fracture. Significantly fewer racehorses with fracture into the proximal interphalangeal joint have returned to racing.[28]

Comminuted fractures of P1 (see Fig. 23-16, C) accounted for approximately 30% and 16% of P1 fractures, excluding dorsal proximal chip fractures, in two large surveys, respectively.[26,30] The majority of Thoroughbreds in one survey were 2 years old.[26] The average age of horses in another survey was 8.3 years (range, 2 to 23 years).[30] Variations of this type include comminution throughout the phalanx, only in the proximal portion, or only in the distal portion. These fractures frequently have one exit through the lateral rather than the medial cortex. These fractures typically are biarticular and are more likely to be complicated by being open. The multiple fracture planes of the comminuted fracture are visible in both lateromedial and dorsopalmar views. Oblique views should also be made to obtain a more thorough depiction of the fracture configuration. Comminuted fractures have the most guarded prognosis for survival and very poor prognosis for return to athletic performance.

Much less commonly reported are incomplete or complete dorsal plane fractures that originate at the proximal articular surface (see Fig. 23-16, *B*).[26,29,33] These fractures may be detected only on lateromedial views. The incomplete fracture typically courses distally toward the dorsal cortex. The complete variation either breaks through the dorsal cortex or extends the entire length of the phalanx to exit in the proximal interphalangeal joint. The latter variation typically splits P1 into roughly equal dorsal and palmar or plantar halves. Other sporadically reported fractures of P1 include physeal fractures (typically Salter-Harris II) and incomplete distal articular fractures.[26]

Middle Phalanx

Fractures of the middle phalanx (P2) include comminuted fracture (most common), fracture of the plantar or palmar proximal eminence (fracture of both medial and lateral eminences is more common than a single eminence fracture), and osteochondral chip fracture (rare) (Fig. 23-18; see also Figs. 23-16, *D* and *E*). Physeal fracture can occur in the skeletally immature horse but is infrequently reported. The comminuted (complete and typically biarticular) and eminence fractures (complete monoarticular) are most common in horses whose activity subjects P2 to extreme simultaneous compression and torsion forces while the foot is fixed to the ground.[34] Thus these types of fractures are most common in working or performing Western horses, polo ponies, and jumpers. For both common fractures, the hindlimbs are reported to be involved approximately twice as frequently as the front limbs.[34-38] However, the front limb is more equally affected by comminuted fracture. The hindlimb is considerably more frequently reported to have a plantar eminence fracture without other comminution. Neither type of fracture is difficult to identify radiographically. When the eminence is fractured without comminution, the fragments are variably displaced in a plantar direction. In the most severe instances, the proximal interphalangeal joint is simultaneously luxated, allowing the distal end of P1 to descend distally and override P2. Because the proximal articular surface of P2 is involved in this fracture, successful repair typically includes arthrodesis of the proximal interphalangeal joint. Prognosis for survival with such repair is good, and prognosis for return to usable soundness is fair to good.[36-37] Comminuted fractures can involve only the proximal portion of P2 but, more commonly, the fracture planes extend into the distal interphalangeal joint. Decision to treat and the type of treatment of the comminuted P2 fracture depend on many factors; however, one of the most important is the degree of involvement of the distal interphalangeal joint. Additional oblique views at different angles compared with the standard (see Table 23-1) may be needed to fully identify the planes of comminution. Computed tomography has been used to improve assessment of the degree and configuration of comminution.[34] With computed tomography, the number of fracture planes was found to decrease toward the distal end of P2. Of the reported horses having P2 fractures, those with comminuted fractures were most likely to be euthanatized at the time of diagnosis or euthanatized during the course of postsurgical healing because of continued lameness.[34,35,38] Yet many of the horses successfully recover to reach breeding or athletic soundness. Secondary degenerative joint disease in the distal interphalangeal joint may significantly complicate long-term recovery for return to athletic performance.

Distal Phalanx

A fracture classification system (types I through VII) describes the fractures of the distal phalanx (P3).[39,40] This classification system is illustrated in Figure 23-16, *F.* Fractures are typed on the basis of region of the bone affected, articular or nonarticular involvement, and anatomic plane of the fracture, as follows:

- I Nonarticular fracture of palmar or plantar process
- II Articular fracture, extending from distal interphalangeal joint to solar margin
- III Articular fracture, midsagittal, divides into equal parts
- IV Articular fracture, extensor process
- V Articular fracture, comminuted body fracture (not of type II, III, or IV)
- VI Solar margin fracture
- VII Palmar process fracture

Trauma is the most common cause of P3 fractures; however, they also occur as pathologic fractures secondary to infective pedal osteitis and laminitis. Because the hoof wall restricts displacement of bone fragments, diagnosis of the P3 fracture depends on visualization of the fracture line. If the plane of the primary x-ray beam is not parallel to the fracture plane, the superimposed parts of the bone obscure the fracture line, and the diagnosis is missed. Therefore four views of P3 are recommended when a fracture is suspected: (1) lateromedial; (2) dorsal 65-degree proximal-palmarodistal oblique; (3) dorsal 65-degree proximal, 45-degree lateral-palmarodistal oblique; and (4) dorsal 65-degree proximal, 45-degree medial-palmarodistal oblique. Views 2 through 4 are done with the horse standing on the reinforced cassette or cassette tunnel. Type VI fracture requires careful assessment of the solar margin. Overexposure of the image makes this fracture difficult to see.

A wide variety of horses sustain fractures of the P3. Quarter horses were most common in a review of a large number of horses.[40] Type II fractures were found most often in a report of 65 horses.[41] Lesions usually involved the lateral aspect of the left front limb or the medial aspect of the right front limb (Fig. 23-19).[41,42] In the racehorses of that series, the forelimb that bore the most weight in turns was at greatest risk (horses were raced counterclockwise). In another report of 274 horses, type VI was the most frequently identified type of fracture.[40] The type VI fracture was found in association with radiographic signs of laminitis in 42 feet (32% of type VI fractures) (see Fig. 23-28, *B*).[40]

The progression of healing of a P3 fracture is difficult to determine radiographically because of the minimal amount of external (periosteal) osseous callus produced by this bone. Fractures of the extensor process tend to produce the greatest amount of new bone (Fig. 23-20). The periosteum of P3 is poorly developed and does not respond with abundant proliferation to the stimulation of direct trauma. Treatment by corrective shoeing and stall rest has led to healing in 3 to 19 months, with young horses and nonarticular fractures showing the most rapid and complete progression to bone union. Prognosis for return to athletic activity is good for type I and guarded for types II and IV.[40,43] Solar margin (type VI) fractures have a good prognosis if not associated with laminitis or severe pedal osteitis.

Palmar process ossicles have been identified radiographically in the forelimbs of foals aged 3 to 32 weeks.[44] Although these ossicles have been suggested to be separate centers of ossification, the microradiographic and histologic appearance in the majority of foals studied was consistent with fracture healing.[14,44] Radiographically, these are seen as a triangular fragment at the palmar aspect of the distal angle of the palmar process, or as an oblong fragment separated by a radiolucent line extending from the incisure of the palmar process to the

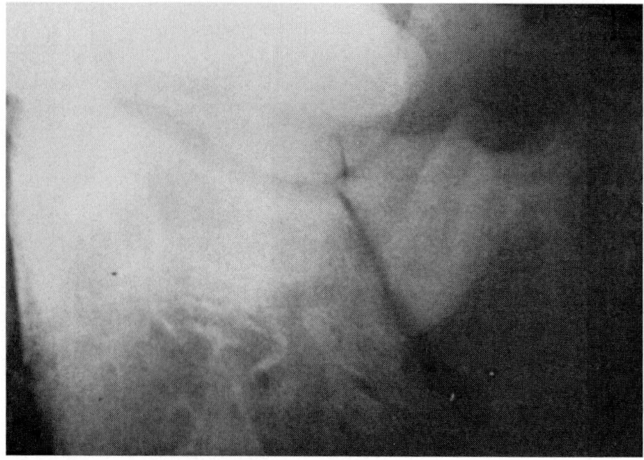

Fig. 23-19 Type II fracture of P3. Dorsal 65-degree proximal, 45-degree lateral-palmarodistomedial oblique view. An oblique projection such as this is often necessary to determine whether the fracture extends into the distal interphalangeal joint, as it does in this horse.

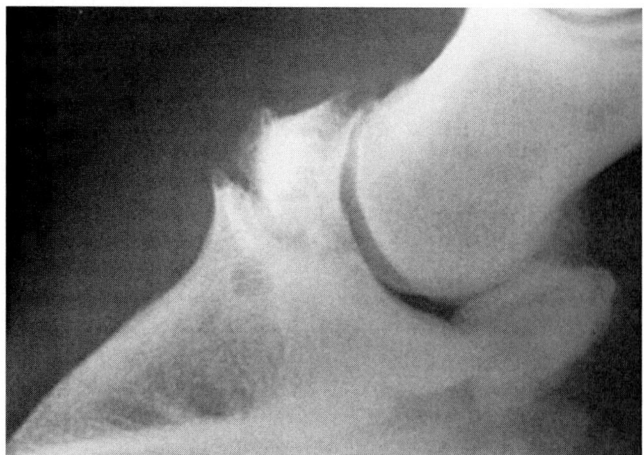

Fig. 23-20 Chronic fracture of the extensor process of P3. The fracture extends into the distal interphalangeal joint and has led to degenerative osteoarthrosis. Note that periarticular changes are not prominent on the distal end of P2.

solar margin (VII—solar border of palmar/plantar process in foals in Figs. 23-16, *F* and 23-21).[44] Fractures have been identified at either or both medial and lateral palmar borders. Radiography is an insensitive method for identifying all foals affected with these fractures. An investigation regarding a cause for these fractures found no significant relation to extensive trimming of the heels.[45] Mild, short-duration lameness was attributed to these fractures in this group of foals. Healing was radiographically complete in an average of 8 weeks, and foals were sound. Foals through 12 weeks of age have a lucent line between the proximal and distal angles of the palmar process. This line is normal and should not be mistaken for a fracture (Fig. 23-22).

INFECTION

Osteomyelitis and Septic Osteitis

Infection of the phalanges results most commonly from trauma or as a complication of surgical treatment and less commonly as the result of hematogenous dissemination of bacteria. Lacerations and puncture wounds by foreign objects carry a high risk of secondary infection of the soft tissue and bone. Sequestrum formation associated with bacterial infection is likely associated with a currently or periodically draining soft tissue lesion. Sequestra vary widely in length and thickness. Oblique views may be necessary to profile the sequestrum. The periosteal new bone associated with a sequestrum may be smooth or mildly irregular (Fig. 23-23).

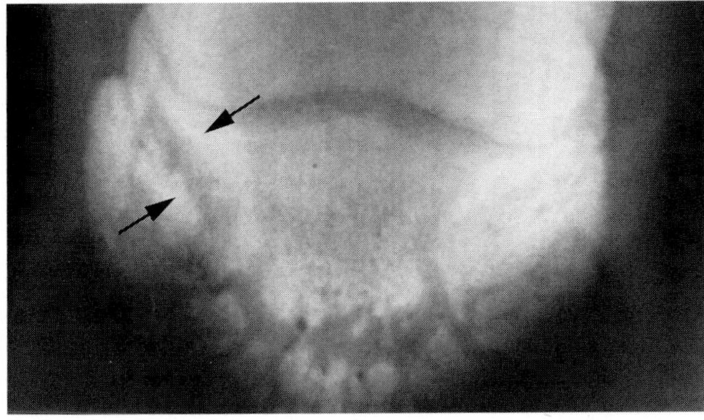

Fig. 23-21 A palmar process fracture in the P3 of a foal (type VII in Fig. 23-16, *F*). *Arrows* indicate a radiolucent line extending from the incisure of the palmar process to the solar margin.

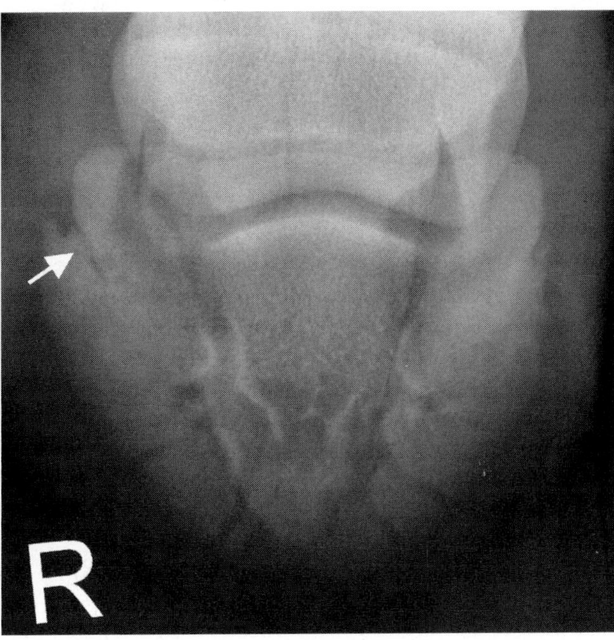

Fig. 23-22 Dorsal 65-degree proximal-palmarodistal view of the P3 of a normal foal. Note the normal radiolucent line in the palmar process *(arrow)*, which should not be confused with a fracture.

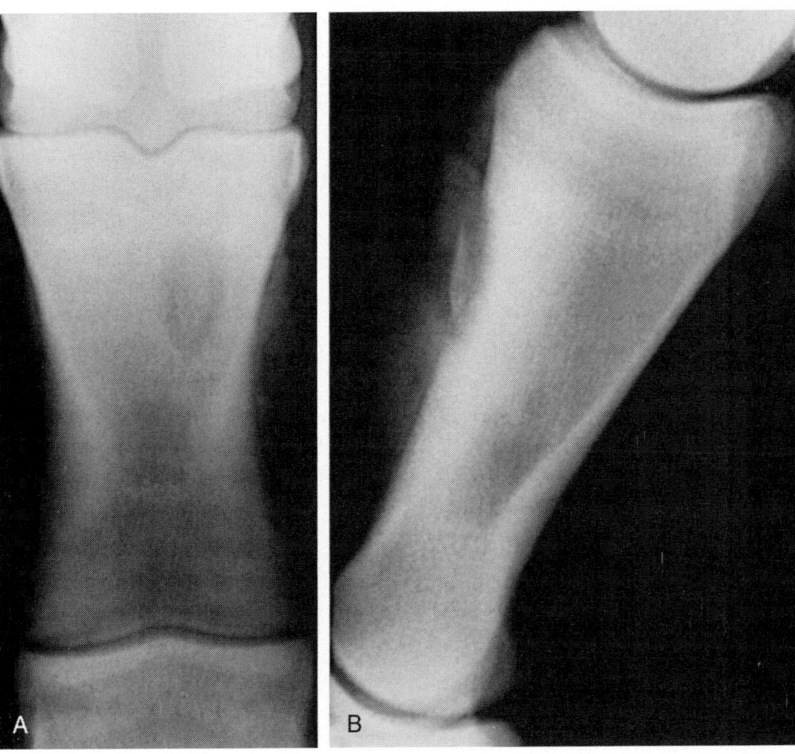

Fig. 23-23 Sequestrum formation involving the dorsal cortex of P1. **A,** The dorsopalmar view shows an ovoid radiolucent defect in the proximal part of the phalanx that surrounds a smaller oval opacity. Active periosteal new bone formation is also evident. **B,** The lateromedial view shows the cortical sequestrum, the defect in the underlying cortex, and the adjacent periosteal proliferation. Sequestration of bone may be caused by trauma-induced avascular necrosis or by bacterial infection.

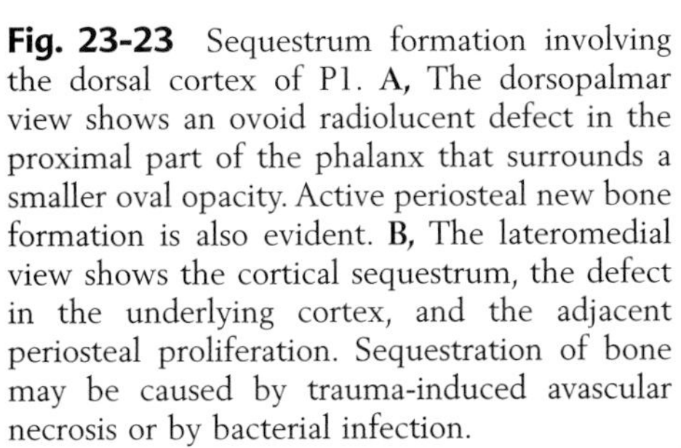

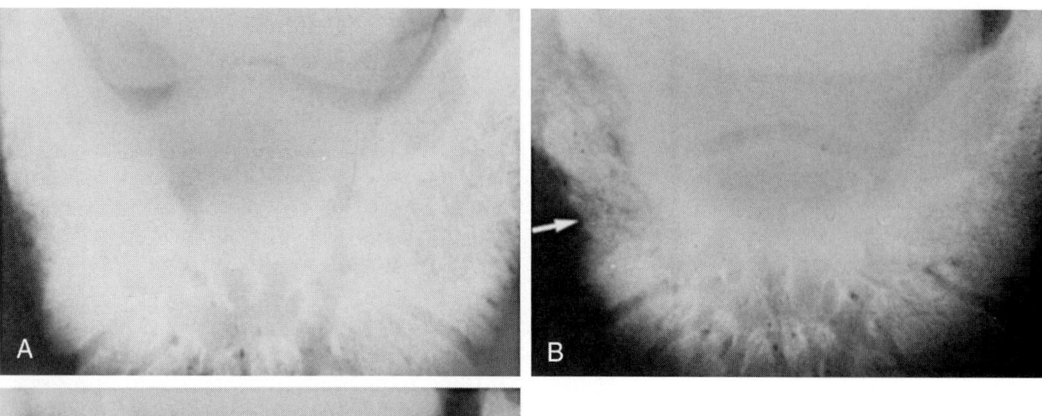

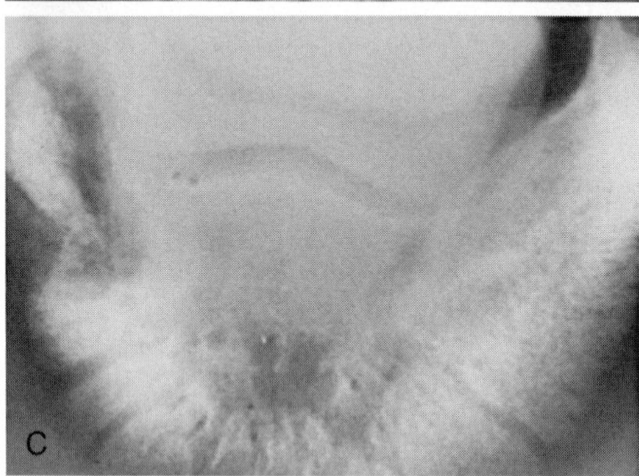

Fig. 23-24 Serial dorsal 65-degree proximal-palmarodistal projections of the palmar processes of the P3 of an acutely lame 5-year-old Thoroughbred. **A,** Initial examination shows minimal radiographic abnormality. **B,** Six days later, a radiolucent defect *(arrow)* is evident in the medial palmar process with loss of trabecular bone detail (compare with lateral palmar process). **C,** Nine days later, more extensive lysis of bone has occurred, with separation of a sequestered fragment. The radiographic diagnosis is septic osteitis with sequestrum formation.

Septic (infective) pedal osteitis refers to infection of P3. Common radiographic changes are discrete areas of lysis, irregular margin, and decreased opacity of P3 typical of chronic inflammation. Gas may be present in the soft tissue adjacent to the surface of P3. A pathologic fracture is uncommon. Separation of a piece of P3 may represent a pathologic fracture or sequestrum (Fig. 23-24).[46] Clinically, a draining tract at the sole or coronary band may be found. Contrast sinography or images made with a metallic stylet in the tract are useful to confirm association with a bone lesion or to detect communication with the distal interphalangeal joint or navicular bursa. To avoid iatrogenic introduction of infection into the joint or bursa, an arthrogram to detect leakage out of the joint cavity should be considered in those horses with draining tracts at the coronary band. Extension of infection to these synovial cavities necessitates aggressive treatment.[47] If a metallic foreign body is evident at physical examination, radiographs should be made before removal to determine the depth of its penetration and its relation to the regional bone.

Septic Arthritis

Infective agents are introduced into the joint by penetrating wounds, iatrogenic injections, or hematogenous introduction. The latter occurs most commonly in foals. However, neither the proximal nor the distal interphalangeal joints are typically involved in the septic polyarthritis syndrome of foals.[48] Any laceration near a joint that is associated with significant and persistent lameness warrants concern for extension to the joint and infection.

The joint pouches of the distal interphalangeal joint are large. During the initial stage of infection, no radiographic changes may be visible. Inflammation of the synovium and effusion may create a focal enlargement or a bulge in the contour at the joint level. If the distal interphalangeal joint is infected, a bulge at or just proximal to the coronary band should be evident. Rarely is widening of the joint space detected, especially if the horse is still bearing weight.[49] Lameness caused by infected joints is usually quite painful and the horse is reluctant to fully bear weight. This further complicates critical assessment of the width of the joint space.

Positive-contrast arthrography was used in horses suspected to have joint infection but no bone changes.[49] This was successful for identification of communication of the contrast medium from the joint to the external wound. One of the earliest bone reaction signs is fuzziness at the joint capsule insertion or chondro-osseous junction on the perimeter of the joint surfaces. As cartilage begins to deteriorate, thinning of the joint space is seen. As the infection invades the deeper regions of the cartilage and reaches the subchondral bone, the subchondral bone margin becomes irregular because of lysis (see Figs. 23-12, *E* and *F*, and 23-25). Lysis of the subchondral bone causes the joint to be widened unevenly.[49] At this stage, periosteal new bone should be evident at the joint margins. Septic arthritis always has a guarded prognosis.

DEGENERATIVE JOINT DISEASE

Degenerative joint disease is a chronic disorder of synovial joints characterized by progressive deterioration of articular cartilage and reactive changes in the joint margin and joint capsule.[50] Among the multiple causes of degenerative joint disease are acute trauma, infection, poor limb conformation, developmental orthopedic disease, and chronic repetitive trauma associated with athletic activity such as racing and other styles of competitive performance. These causes typically produce what is thought of as secondary degenerative joint disease. Primary degenerative joint disease, in comparison, is considered an age-related disease of slow onset, resulting in gradual degradation of normal joint structure and function. The proximal and distal interphalangeal joints can be affected by any of these causes. The general changes expressed radiographically are new bone formation (osteophytes) at the periarticular (chondro-osseous) margin, enthe-

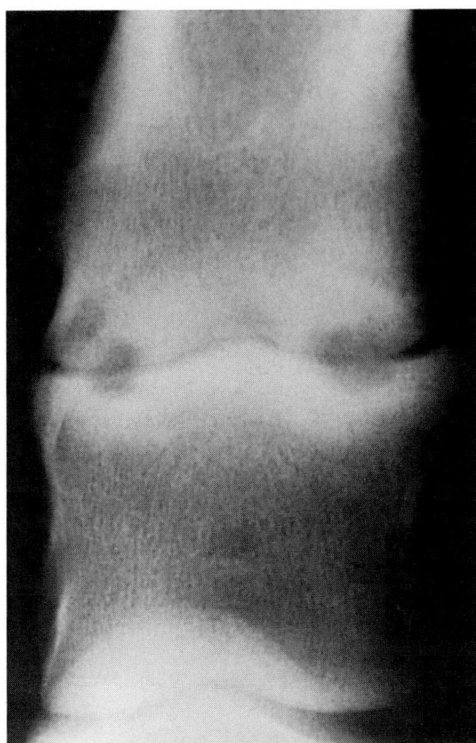

Fig. 23-25 Decreased width of the proximal interphalangeal joint space with large, multiple indistinctly margined subchondral bone defects. The radiographic signs in this foal are attributable to septic arthritis with erosion of articular cartilage leading to osteomyelitis of the subchondral epiphyseal bone. The absence of the periosteal reaction, which usually accompanies lysis caused by osteomyelitis, suggests a fulminating infection.

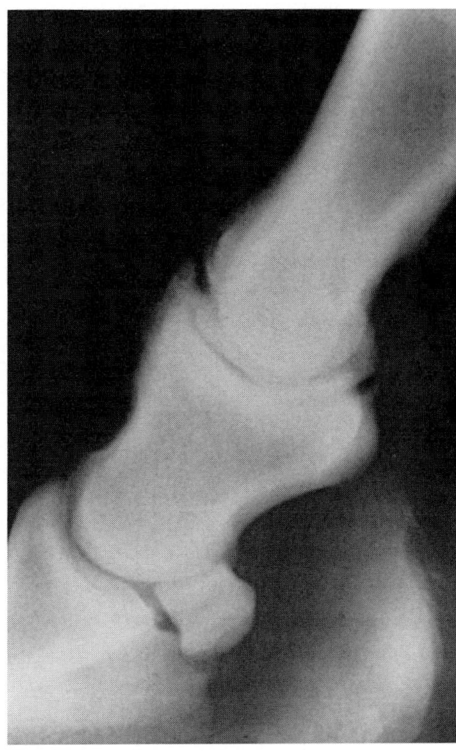

Fig. 23-26 Osteoarthrosis of the proximal interphalangeal joint. The contours of the opposing surfaces of P1 and P2 are flattened. The articular surfaces are also broader as a result of remodeling and new bone formation at the periarticular margins. These periarticular osteophytes are often sharply spiculated in the mildly unstable joint.

sophytes at the sites of supporting ligaments and joint capsule, sclerosis and lucency in the subchondral bone, and changes in the joint space width (Figs. 23-26 and 23-27). A wide spectrum of combination and degree of the above changes is seen (see Fig. 23-12). In the situation of secondary degenerative joint disease, radiographic changes unique enough to reveal the primary insult may be present. However, in many horses the primary insult is not evident.

The proximal interphalangeal joint is a high-load, low-motion joint, meaning that a large range of movement does not occur during the stride motion of the limb. As a consequence, a smaller region of the joint surface sustains a more constant weight-bearing load for a longer period in the athletic horse.[50] This relation is the basis of an explanation for the characteristic features of progressive proximal interphalangeal degenerative joint disease seen in athletic horses, especially those active in Western-style events.[51] The movements of athletic activity are proposed to concentrate the load on the articular cartilage excessively and initiate fibrous thickening of the supporting soft tissues to restrict joint motion further. Continued compression leads to full-thickness necrosis of the cartilage. Simultaneously, remodeling of the underlying bone occurs in the forms of sclerosis and resorption. The natural attempts to heal the cartilage lesions are not successful, and gaps are left in the articular cartilage surface. Osteogenic granulation tissue from the exposed subchondral bone bridges these joint gaps, initiating the process of ankylosis.

Radiographically, typical periarticular osteophytes and enthesophytes develop. Fibrous thickening of the joint capsule and collateral ligaments, along with compression remodeling of the articular cartilage and subchondral bone, occurs but can be subtle radiographically. Focal regions of subchondral bone resorption may be large enough to be seen as lysis. The osteogenic granulation tissue in the subchondral sites of bone resorption becomes visible as bone-to-bone contact.[50] This is the start of ankylosis of the joint (see Fig. 23-12, *F*).

If these initial ankylosis sites are sufficiently stable, additional ankylosis progresses to complete the union of the bone surfaces. However, if activity is continued, the initial ankylosis sites can break down and generate more periarticular new bone (see Fig. 23-27). During the ankylosis process, lameness is likely to persist. In these horses, the natural ankylosis must be replaced by surgical arthrodesis so that the lameness can be resolved.

In the standard images of the proximal interphalangeal joint, the new bone changes are readily seen in all views. The subchondral bone sclerosis and resorption changes are most easily seen on the dorsopalmar or oblique views. Adequate x-ray beam penetration and careful scrutiny of the subchondral bone margin are necessary to confirm that subchondral bone resorption is truly present. The increased opacity of irregularly deposited new bone formation adjacent to unaffected bone can simulate decreased bone opacity, which may then be misinterpreted as bone lysis. Correlating the location of new bone in all views helps avoid this misinterpretation.

Osteoarthritis from causes other than infection or articular fracture is much less frequently reported with specific reference to the distal interphalangeal joint. It is also not as radiographically obvious. When present, the radiographic signs of osteoarthritis are small periarticular osteophytes on the dorsal edges of P2 and P3 (see Fig. 23-20), enthesophytes

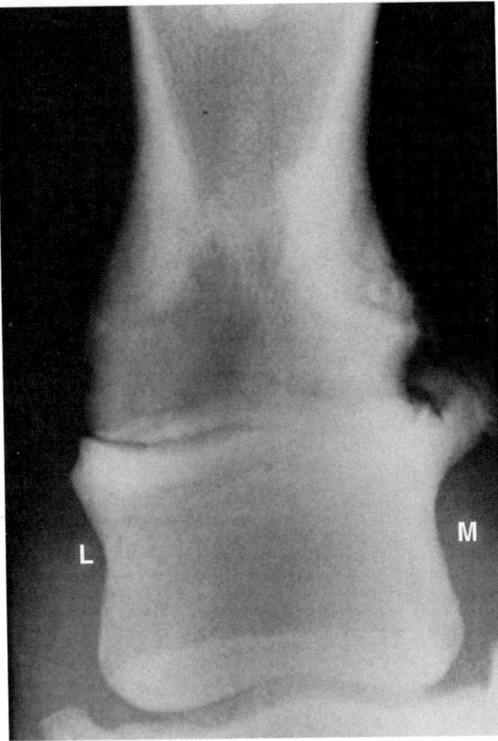

Fig. 23-27 Dorsopalmar view showing large enthesophytes at the attachments of the medial collateral ligaments. In addition, collapse of the medial portion of the proximal interphalangeal joint with subchondral sclerosis of the opposed surfaces of P1 and P2 is seen. Osteoarthritis is caused by trauma. *L*, Lateral; *M*, medial.

on the eminences for the collateral ligaments on P2, and narrowing of the distal interphalangeal joint. If asymmetric narrowing of the joint is noted on the dorsopalmar view (see Fig. 23-12, *B*), this may be attributable to true asymmetric cartilage degeneration, asymmetrical weight bearing, or unbalanced compressive forces caused by unbalanced trimming or wear of the hoof.

MRI will likely play a larger diagnostic and research role in the earlier recognition of changes that eventually lead to degenerative joint disease. In a series of 11 lame horses evaluated with MRI, subchondral trabecular bone damage was found that was not radiographically evident.[52] These changes consisted of subchondral bone fluid signals with and without cyst formation. Determining whether the subchondral changes, particularly the cysts, were initiated by trauma, prior osteochondrosis lesion, or some other bone insult was not possible because of insufficient histologic assessment.

LAMINITIS

The normal orientation of P3 to the hoof is maintained by the interdigitating leaves of the laminar corium and the hornlike lamellae of the hoof wall. The laminar corium is attached to the dorsal surface of P3 by a modified periosteum, which contains a tightly meshed network of blood vessels.[53,54] Insult to this unique anatomic structure can result in the loss of mechanical support of P3 within the hoof capsule. Laminitis is the general clinical term used to refer to the complex of signs expressed by the horse and its effects on the structural relations of the hoof wall, P3, and sole from a variety of insults. Most horses that develop clinical laminitis do so as a result of a systemic illness. Concussion trauma to the feet is a less well-defined cause of laminitis. Horses with protracted, severe, unilateral limb lameness have been considered to be at risk for developing contralateral limb laminitis.[55]

Although differences of opinion exist regarding the terminology and categorization of this complex condition, several clinical phases or stages of laminitis are recognized: developmental, acute, and chronic.[56] Developmental laminitis is defined as the period between the initial insult to the first expression of lameness. It may be as short as 24 hours or as long as 60 hours.[56] This is likely an imperceptible stage to the owner unless access to excessive grain is known to have occurred or a systemic disease or other condition is present that warrants concern for initiation of laminitis. This period is a prevention phase for mechanical failure of the foot complex.[56] Acute laminitis represents the phase from the first expression of lameness through 72 hours without evidence of mechanical collapse or at any time that signs of mechanical collapse occur.[56] Radiographs may be indicated in either the developmental or the acute phase to serve as a baseline for future comparison. Horses may fully recover from either developmental or acute laminitis. If, however, radiographic or clinical signs of P3 displacement are seen, the phase of chronic laminitis has been entered.[56]

Radiographic Evaluation of Laminitis

Radiographic evaluation of any horse with a clinical impression of pain and lameness caused by laminitis is justified. The goals of radiography are to detect changes indicative of mechanical failure and observe changes that contribute to the formulation of prognosis and therapy. All four feet should be evaluated initially. Although lameness may be expressed in only one leg, structural changes may be radiographically present in several feet. Front feet are most commonly affected. Optimal lateromedial, dorsopalmar, and dorsal 65-degree proximal-dorsodistal oblique views are recommended. Placement of radiopaque markers on the hoof wall has been advocated to help identify soft tissue landmarks.[57-59] One marker is placed on the midsagittal plane at the junction of the hoof wall and the coronary band. The second, a linear marker preferably of known length, is placed on the midsagittal plane of the dorsal hoof wall (Fig. 23-28, C). This should be of sufficient length to extend approximately half to two thirds the length of the dorsal hoof wall. The third is placed at the point of the frog of the sole. Occasionally a fourth marker is placed on the white line junction of the hoof wall and heel bulb (angle of the wall). These markers assist in initial radiographic assessment and the measurement or identification of landmarks needed for planning corrective shoeing.

The radiographic signs of P3 displacement are definitive evidence of chronic laminitis. The sign seen is either palmar deviation (rotation) of P3 from the hoof wall, distal (vertical or sinking) displacement of P3, or a combination. A spectrum of severity is found. In the normal foot the dorsal cortex of P3 should be parallel to the dorsal margin of the hoof wall in the lateromedial view. Divergence of these surfaces, with the toe region of P3 deviating or rotating in a palmar direction, is an indication of mechanical separation of the dermal and epidermal laminae (see Fig. 23-28, *A*). This is the easiest of the P3 displacements to detect radiographically. When a straight edge is used to mark the comparative lines of the hoof wall and dorsal cortex (Fig. 23-29, *A*), these lines should be parallel in the normal foot. In the horse with palmar deviation of P3, these lines diverge at the toe region and converge proximally. The angle at the point of convergence can be measured and is referred to as the degree of rotation (see Fig. 23-29, C).

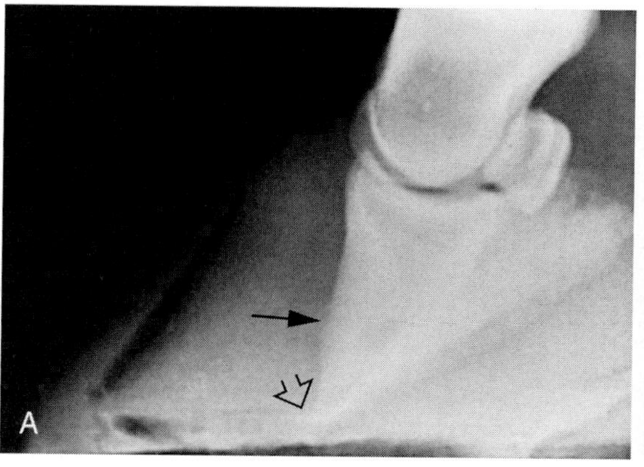

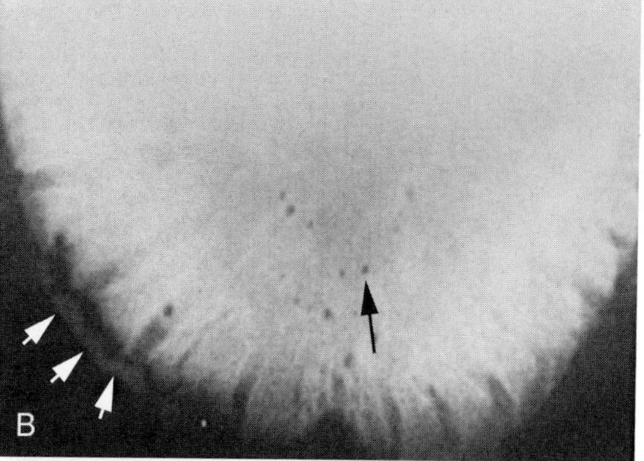

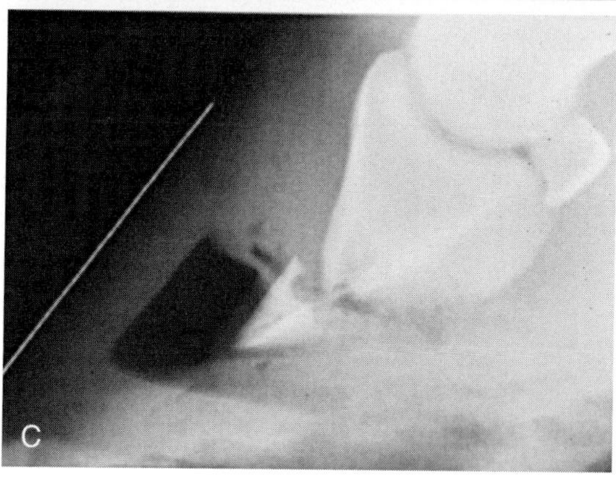

Fig. 23-28 A, Severe palmar deviation-rotation of P3 resulting from chronic laminitis. Gas is seen between the hoof wall and the soft tissues of the corium. Indistinct dorsal surface *(solid arrow)* and dorsal angulation ("ski tip" appearance) of the toe of P3 *(open arrow)* are additional changes seen in chronic laminitis. **B,** Pathologic type VI fracture of P3 caused by laminitis. A thin bone fragment is separated from the solar margin *(white arrows)*. Punctate radiolucent defects *(black arrow)* are enlarged vascular channels viewed end-on. **C,** Larger fracture of the toe with concurrent palmar deviation-rotation. The large accumulation of gas between the hoof wall and the laminar corium is most likely caused by a concurrent subsolar abscess and septic osteitis.

Vertical displacement of P3 can be more difficult to detect and is often overlooked.[60] In the normal foot, the proximal edge of the extensor process of P3 is positioned roughly at the same plane or just proximal to the junction of the hoof wall and coronary band.[54,61] The vertical distance between the proximal limit of the dorsal hoof wall and the proximal limit of the extensor process of P3 has been measured to generate a "founder" distance (see Fig. 23-29, *B*).[58] When corrected for magnification, this distance in 25 normal horses was an average of 4 mm (range, −2 to 11 mm) in the front feet and an average of 4.6 mm (range, −2 to 9 mm) in the hind feet.[58]

An increase in the thickness of the dorsal soft tissues has been suggested to be an early sign of laminar inflammation or edema and thus a sign of acute laminitis. The thickness of the dorsal soft tissues has been measured on radiographs of clinically normal horses.[12,55,58,59] A statistical difference was found in thickness among normal ponies, Hanoverians, and Thoroughbreds.[58] The average thickness of the front feet for all horses, when corrected for magnification, was 16.3 mm (range, 11.1 to 20.2 mm).[58] When only Thoroughbreds were compared between two studies,[12,58] the average thickness was 16.3 mm (range, 13.9 to 19.7 mm) compared with 14.6 mm, respectively (both values corrected for magnification). For other specified breeds, from one study the measurements (corrected for magnification) were found for the front feet ranges of ponies (11.1 to 16.1 mm) and Hanoverians (17 to 19.1 mm) and for the hind feet ranges of ponies (11.7 to 16.1 mm), Hanoverians (15.9 to 20.4 mm), and Thoroughbreds (14.3 to 17.9 mm).[58] A marker of known length must be in the image to correct for magnification. If this is not available, an alternative is to calculate the dorsal soft tissue thickness as a percentage of the palmar cortex length. In 41 sound Thoroughbreds the average was 24.2%; a measurement greater than 28.1% should be considered abnormal for the Thoroughbred (see Fig. 23-29, *B* and *D*).[12] When not corrected for magnification, a dorsal soft tissue thickness greater than 20 mm has been suggested to be abnormal for any breed.[62]

Other radiographic changes that can be seen with chronic and progressive laminitis include a very thin sole. The change in the position of the toe of P3 may cause a convex bulge in the sole's contour, or the toe may penetrate through the sole. Radiolucency at the laminar junction can be seen as a single linear lucency in the lateral view (see Fig. 23-28, *A*) and as a series of parallel linear lucencies in the dorsal 65-degree proximal palmarodistal oblique view. This linear radiolucency could be caused by air dissecting between the hoof wall and the laminar corium when necrosis has eroded through to the coronary band or white zone of the sole or to a vacuum phenomenon that causes nitrogen to diffuse from the blood. Larger regions of radiolucency are more likely to be associated with secondary infection of the soft tissue (see Fig. 23-28, *C*). An increase in small circular lucencies is often seen in the central region of P3 in the dorsal 65-degree proximal palmarodistal oblique view (see Fig. 23-28, *B*). These lucencies represent an increased number of and wider vascular channels extending from the solar canal to the dorsal cortex. This is typically seen in combination with new bone along the dorsal cortex. The new bone also creates a prominent domed shape to the dorsal surface of P3. The toe of P3 frequently develops a "lipping" shape from either new bone, resorption of the palmar cortex, or an angular orientation of a solar margin fracture (type VI) (see Fig. 23-28, *A* and *B*). Osteitis of variable severity usually develops. Additionally, disuse of the limbs can further decrease the bone's opacity. Infectious osteitis can occur in the most severely affected horses. A break in the pastern angle (rotation of P3 about the distal interphalangeal joint) can occur if contraction of the deep digital flexor tendon occurs or if the more rapid growth of the hoof wall at the heel is improperly managed.

Because of the severe morbidity and protracted treatment required for chronic laminitis, indicators of prognosis for

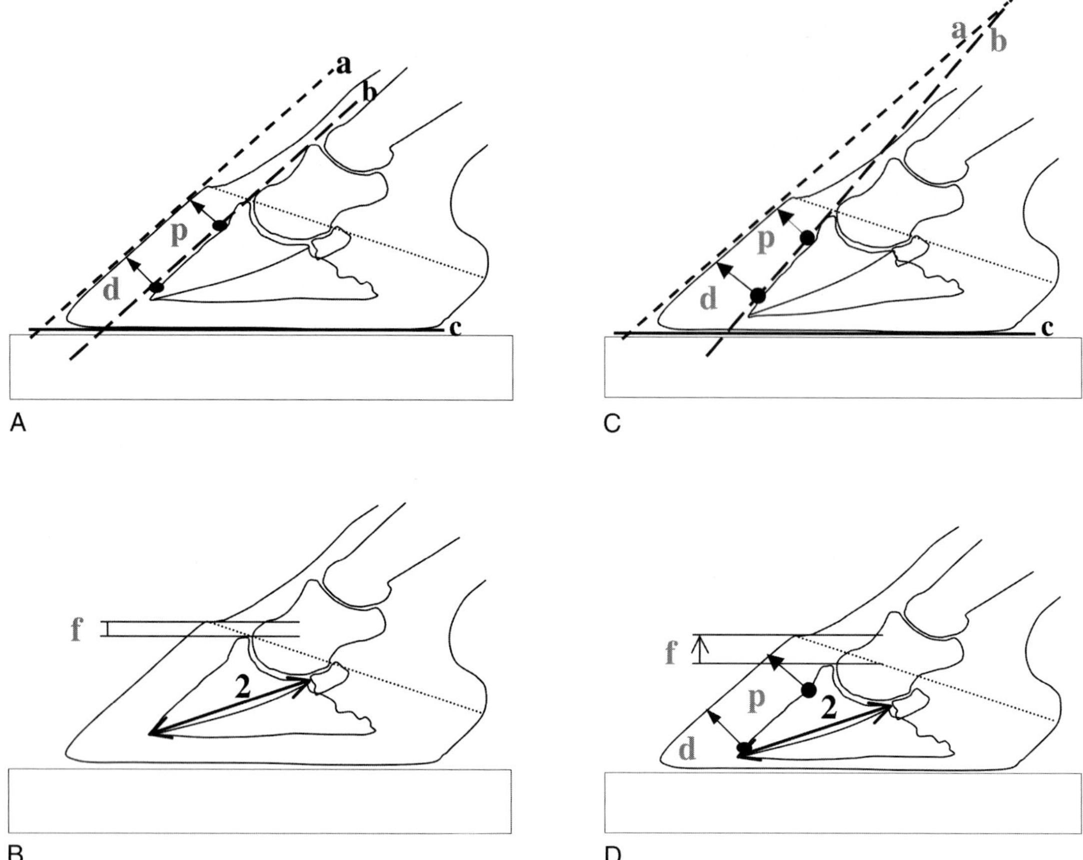

Fig. 23-29 A and B, Radiographic measurements of the normal foot. **A,** Line *a* is parallel to the hoof wall. Line *b* is parallel to the dorsal cortex of P3. Line *c* is parallel to the weight-bearing surface of the hoof wall. Angle *ac* is the hoof axis. Angle *bc* is the foot axis. Distance *p* is the thickness of the dorsal soft tissues measured 5 mm distal to the junction of the extensor process with the dorsal cortex. Distance *d* is the thickness of the dorsal soft tissues measured 6 mm proximal to the most distal point of the dorsal cortex. **B,** Line *2* is the length of the palmar cortex measured from the solar margin at the distal toe to the palmar articular edge between P3 and the distal sesamoid bone. Distance *f* is the vertical distance or "founder" distance measured between coronary band and proximal edge of the extensor process. **C** and **D.** Radiographic measurements of the foot with chronic laminitis. **C,** Foot with chronic laminitis exhibiting P3 displacement as rotation only. Lines *a* and *b* are no longer parallel and converge proximally forming angle *ab* or the rotation angle. Distance *d* is greater than distance *p*. **D,** Foot with chronic laminitis exhibiting P3 displacement as vertical displacement (sinking) only. Founder distance *f'* is increased. Distance *p* equals *d*, but both are greater than normal. The percentage that *d* is of line *2* will be greater than normal. (See text for normal and abnormal values.) (Reprinted from Lindford RL, O'Brien TR, Trout DR: Qualitative and morphometric radiographic findings in the distal phalanx and digital soft tissues of sound Thoroughbred racehorses, *Am J Vet Res* 54:38, 1993; and Cripps PJ, Eustace RA: Radiological measurements from the feet of normal horses with relevance to laminitis, *Equine Vet J* 31:427, 1999.)

success or failure of treatment are desired. Various radiographic measurements have been retrospectively assessed in an effort to define reliable predictors of outcome for horses with chronic laminitis.[59,63,64] Figure 23-29 illustrates several of these measurements. Even though none has been completely reliable when used as the only indicator, trends have been identified. In general, the more deviant from normal, the more guarded to worse the prognosis. In a series of 91 horses, the degree of P3 rotation was inversely correlated with return to athletic performance. Horses with less than 5.5 degrees of deviation had a favorable prognosis for return to athletic work, horses with 6.8 to 11.5 degrees had a guarded prognosis, and horses with more than 11.5 degrees of deviation were not useful as performance animals but some could be salvaged for breeding.[63] In another study, neither the degree of P3 rotation nor distal displacement correlated with outcome, and lameness severity was a more accurate predictor.[64] In a recent study of horses with severe clinical features of chronic laminitis, 54% with a rotation angle greater than 20 degrees and 88% with a rotation angle less than 2 degrees were successfully treated and returned to riding soundness.[59] As a predictor of outcome to riding soundness, founder distance was useful when it was either in the low range of normal or well beyond the upper limit. In horses with severe chronic laminitis, no animal with a founder distance less than 7.9 mm failed to respond to treatment, and only one horse with a founder distance greater than 15.2 mm was a success.[59] However, some horses with physical evidence of a sinking P3 had founder distances within the normal range.[59] With the measurement of dorsal soft tissue thickness (measured at the distal point) calculated as a percentage of the palmar cortex length, a measurement of greater than 28.1% should be considered abnormal for the fore foot of Thoroughbreds.[12] Dorsal wall thickness was not found to be an isolated predictor of outcome with treatment.[59] Even so, increased dorsal soft tissue thickness was found to be a risk factor for development of clinical laminitis in the contralateral limb of horses with unilateral limb lameness.[55] In that series of horses, increased dorsal wall thickness and sinking were more common than palmar deviation of P3. Some cautions regarding the use of radiographic measurements deserve mention. Measurements probably are most valuable when used for serial assessment of an individual horse. Strict attention to detail must be maintained in the production of images. Positioning of both the horse's foot and the x-ray beam is critical. An oblique projection angle can significantly alter measurement. Likewise, placement of any markers should be standardized. Failure to adhere to strict standardization renders comparative measurements unreliable.

A recent cadaver limb study found a greater number of overall changes with MRI than were radiographically evident.[65] Laminar disruption, focal laminar gas, laminar fluid, signal changes in the cancellous bone consistent with bone fluid, increased size and number of P3 dorsal cortical vascular channels, alteration in the corium coronae, and distension of the distal interphalangeal joint were identified. MRI evaluation may help determine a set of findings of clinical and investigative importance.

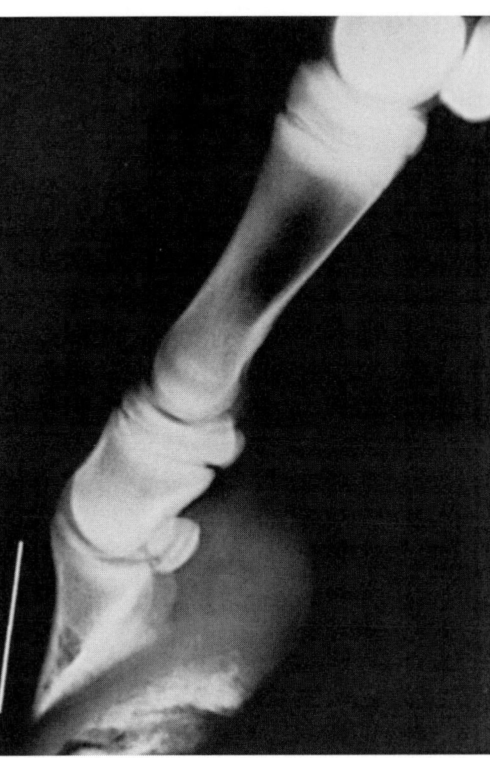

Fig. 23-30 Flexural deformity of the distal interphalangeal joint in a 4-month-old foal. The dorsal surface of P3 remains parallel to the dorsal hoof wall *(white line)*, but both of these structures assume an abnormally vertical position.

FLEXURAL DEFORMITY OF THE INTERPHALANGEAL JOINTS

Distal Interphalangeal Joint

This is the most common joint location of the flexural deformities of the phalanges. The clinical appearance of this is an almost vertical orientation of the hoof wall to the ground (Fig. 23-30). Flexural deformity may be either congenital or acquired. Genetic influences and teratogenic insults during embryonic developmental are factors that may lead to congenital deformities.[3,66] The acquired form is most common in rapidly growing foals and has been related to pain that initiates a persisting flexion withdrawal response, lack of exercise, or poor nutritional management in the growing foal. Both overfeeding and unbalanced diets have been cited as potentiating factors.[67] The exact manner in which these various influences interact to produce flexural deformities is unknown, but several theories suggest a difference in the rate of bone growth versus tendon and ligament lengthening.[67,68] All theories imply a faster rate of lengthening of metacarpal III or metatarsal III than for the deep digital flexor tendon-check ligament unit. Increasing tension on this tendon-ligament unit leads to flexion of the distal interphalangeal joint, with the foal assuming a "toe dancer" stance. Changes seen in P3 of these foals range from none to varying irregularity of the solar margin centered at the toe. The irregularity is caused by widened vascular channels and bone resorption at the solar margin.[69] If the deformity is corrected early, the bone changes can resolve to a normal appearance.

Proximal Interphalangeal Joint

Abnormal flexion alignment is uncommon and may be either congenital or acquired (Fig. 23-31). Visually, a bulge in the dorsal pastern contour has been referred to as *dorsal subluxation;* this represents the position of distal P1 relative to the normal pastern axis.[70,71] The proximal interphalangeal joint is, however, flexed. Thoroughbred racehorses have developed this malalignment after injury to the soft tissue support struc-

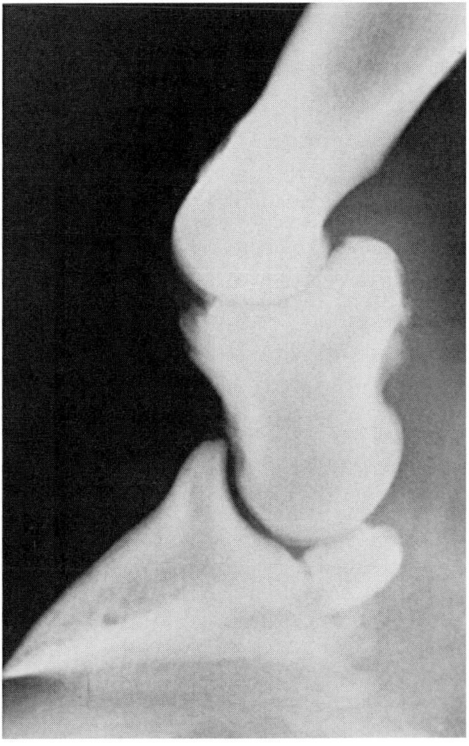

Fig. 23-31 Flexural deformity (dorsal subluxation) of the proximal interphalangeal joint. Enthesophytes of the dorsal joint capsule and superficial digital flexor tendon insertion sites of P2 indicate the chronicity of this injury.

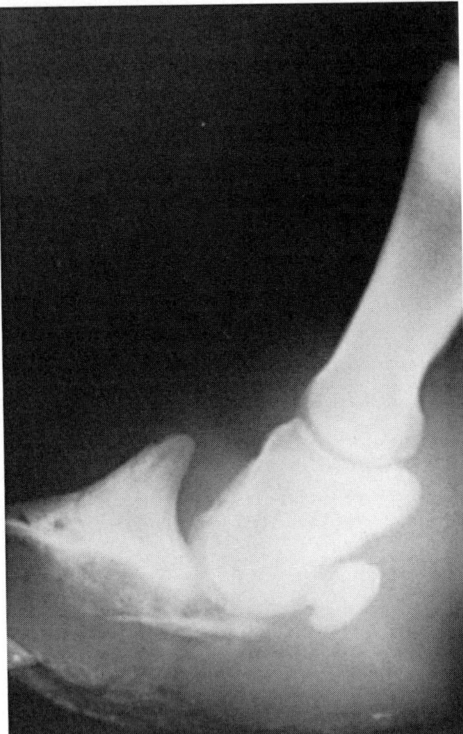

Fig. 23-32 Luxation of the distal interphalangeal joint as a result of osteomyelitis and pathologic fracture of the flexor surface of P3. Dorsal displacement of P3 is caused by avulsion of the deep digital flexor tendon insertion and the subsequent unreciprocated traction of the common digital extensor tendon. The distal sesamoidean impar ligament is also ruptured, allowing proximal displacement of the navicular bone.

tures of the metacarpophalangeal joint.[70] Dorsal subluxation has also occurred after corrective desmotomy of the suspensory ligament for treatment of flexural deformities of the metacarpophalangeal joint.[70] A number of young horses have been observed with this deformity in the hindlimb. The flexion is prominent when the horse is not bearing weight, but with full weight the alignment is reduced, often accompanied by a clicking sound.[71,72] A combination of deep digital flexor tendon contracture and concomitant superficial digital flexor tendon laxity has been postulated as the cause for this hindlimb deformity.[71] No specific bone changes other than joint alignment are expected.

Hyperextension Alignment of the Interphalangeal Joints

Hyperextension of the proximal interphalangeal joint is an unusual appearance that occurs with rupture of both the straight (superficial) sesamoidean ligament and the superficial digital flexor tendon. It may also be seen in combination with overextension of the distal interphalangeal and metacarpophalangeal joints as a congenital deformity in foals. No additional bone changes are typically present.[73]

Hyperextension of the distal interphalangeal joint may occur in newborn foals as a congenital abnormality affecting all three joints of the foot. Weakened flexor tendons may also be seen as a result of poor nutrition, slow or incomplete recovery from a systemic disease, or after prolonged periods of external support (splinting or casting) of the leg.[3] Acquired hyperextension is also caused by rupture of the deep digital flexor tendon or avulsion of its insertion (Fig. 23-32). This lesion occurs with traumatic laceration of the tendon or extension of infection from a deep sole abscess to the palmar surface of P3.

OSTEOCHONDROSIS (SUBCHONDRAL CYSTLIKE LESIONS)

The phalanges are not affected by classical osteochondritis dissecans, meaning that osteochondral fragments associated with subchondral bone defects are not reported. Single, oval to circular, radiolucent lesions surrounded by a thin or variably thick sclerotic rim are sporadically reported in the distal end of P1, the proximal and distal ends of P2, and the base of the extensor process or body of P3.[74] These have been called subchondral cysts, osseous cysts, or subchondral cystlike osteochondrosis. Considerable question still exists regarding whether any of these lesions in the phalanges represents true defective growth of the articular-epiphyseal complex (abnormal endochondral ossification process).[75] Figure 23-33 illustrates two examples of the subchondral cystlike lesion.

Clinical expression of lameness is suggested to relate to the extent of articular surface involvement. Some lesions have no visible connection to the articular cartilage or joint space lucency. Others have a thin neck or a broader base of connection to the articular cartilage or joint space lucency. The latter two have a greater chance of being associated with pain and lameness. These lesions are generally associated with joint effusion or lameness in horses of training age, that is, younger than 3 years. A higher incidence of occurrence has been reported in the pelvic limb in a group of quarter horses, although either the thoracic or the pelvic limb may be affected.[76] Some lesions have been found in clinically sound older horses presented for prepurchase evaluation.[74] The subchondral cystlike defects in the distal part of P1 frequently lead to extensive degenerative joint disease in the proximal interphalangeal joint (see Fig. 23-33, *B*). In such instances, surgical arthrodesis may be needed to allow return to useful function.[23,77,78] In one series of 13 horses in which solitary phalangeal subchondral cystlike lesions were treated by conservative management, lameness disappeared in seven horses over a period of 1 month to 2.5 years.[79] In four of these animals the defect could not be identified radiographically 1.5 to 2.5 years after the initial diagnosis.

PEDAL OSTEITIS

Diffuse roughening of the solar border of P3, creating a ragged, lacy appearance when viewed in the lateromedial or dorsal 65-degree proximal palmarodistal oblique projection, may be an indication of pedal osteitis (Fig. 23-34).[11] Pedal osteitis is the response of P3 to inflammation and is manifested by demineralization, either focal or more diffuse. The change is most commonly seen as a result of chronic bruising, sole abscess without extension of infection in the bone, flexural deformities, and other conditions.[80] Once the primary insult and pedal osteitis become inactive, little change in the appearance of the roughened contour of the solar margin is seen. Also, because the normal appearance of the solar surface of P3 varies considerably, a mild degree of irregularity may be misleading. A positive response to hoof testers, an increased number and diameter of vascular channels seen concomitantly with demineralization of the bone, and thinning of the sole of the foot increase the probability of pedal osteitis as a current cause of lameness. Thus clinical signs must be considered in the determination of whether a radiographically irregular margin of P3 is an indicator of current or previous pathologic condition.

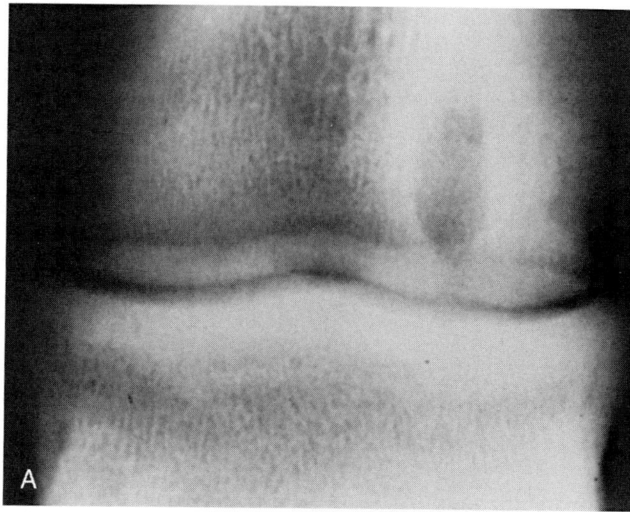

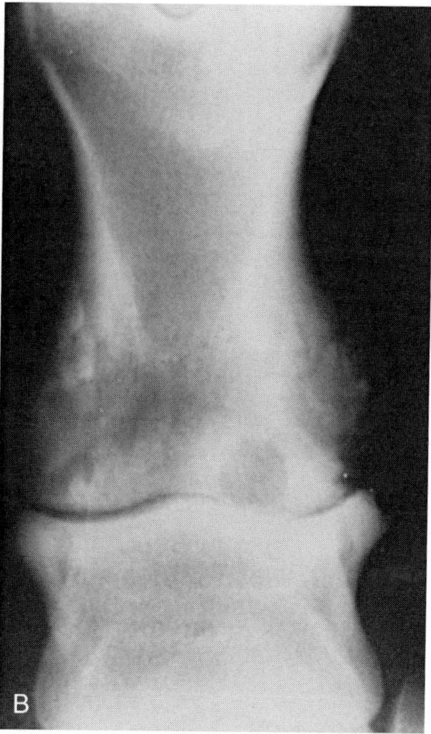

Fig. 23-33 Dorsopalmar views of solitary, radiolucent subchondral cystlike bone defects (osteochondrosis) of P1. **A,** Elliptic defect with narrow necklike connection to articular cartilage/joint space and surrounding zone of sclerosis. Osteoarthrosis is not evident in this 1-year-old Thoroughbred. **B,** Spherical defect surrounded by sclerotic subchondral bone. Collapse of contiguous joint space and periarticular osteophyte formation indicate the presence of osteoarthrosis in a 6-year-old quarter horse that had been lame for 1 month.

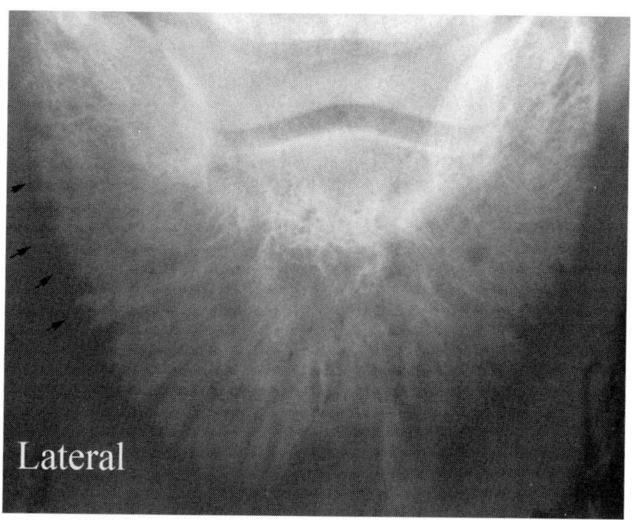

Fig. 23-34 Dorsal 65-degree proximal-palmarodistal view of the P3 of a horse with pedal osteitis. Note the irregular margin of the lateral aspect of P3 *(arrows)*.

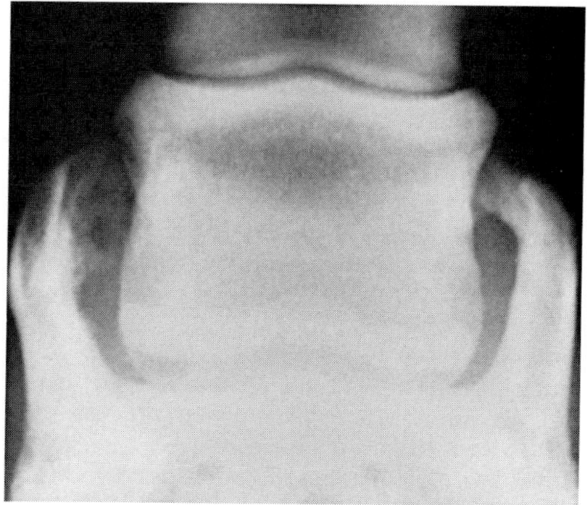

Fig. 23-35 Ossification of the collateral cartilage of P3. Uniform ossification is seen in both the lateral and the medial collateral cartilage. Such advanced changes usually do not cause lameness if the foot is broad at the heel.

COLLATERAL CARTILAGES

Ossification/Calcification (Sidebones)

This is a common finding in radiographs of the distal part of the digit, especially in draft breed horses. When the proximal edge of the ossified collateral cartilage extends beyond the proximal margin of the navicular bone, sidebone formation is considered present (Fig. 23-35).[11] Even an extensive degree of ossification may not be clinically significant, especially in older horses, horses with a broad foot, and horses that have no pain on manipulation of the heel area.

Asymmetric mineralization of the collateral cartilages may indicate increased stress on the ossified portion (Fig. 23-36).

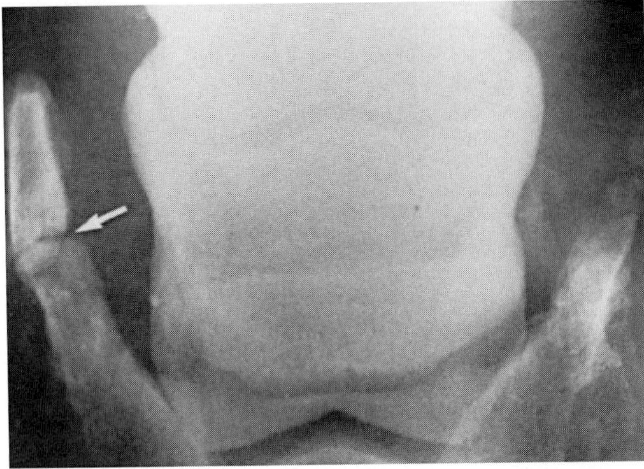

Fig. 23-36 Asymmetric ossification of the collateral cartilage of P3 may indicate abnormal stress on the affected side of the foot and warrants close examination of the heel and navicular bone for additional abnormalities. In this horse, the radiolucent defect *(arrow)* is a cartilage remnant between two separate centers of ossification, not a fracture.

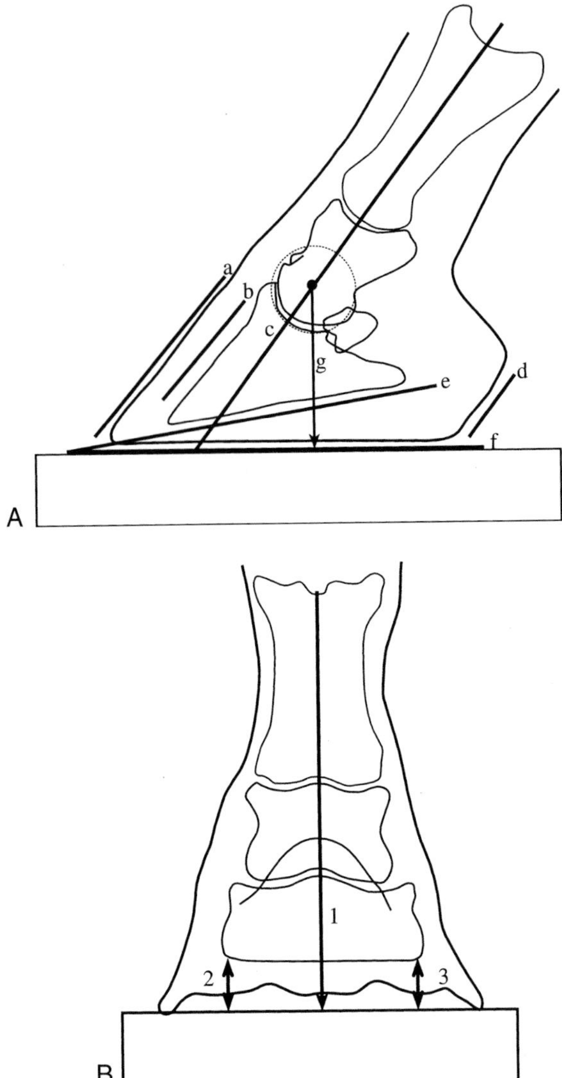

Fig. 23-37 Radiographic measurements for foot balance. **A,** Assessment from lateromedial view of normal foot. *a,* Line parallel to dorsal hoof wall; *b,* line parallel to dorsal cortex of P3; *c,* line that bisects P2 into equal dorsal and palmar halves; *d,* line drawn parallel to the bulbs of the heel; *e,* line drawn parallel to the solar surface of P3; *f,* line drawn parallel to the bearing surface of the hoof wall; *g,* line from center of best-fit circle for the distal interphalangeal joint drawn perpendicular to the bearing surface of the hoof wall. Line *a* should be parallel to lines *b, c,* and *d.* Line *g* should intersect at the mid-point of the bearing surface of the hoof wall. Angle *af,* 45 to 55 degrees in a front foot; 50 to 55 degrees in a hind foot; Angle *ef,* 5 to 10 degrees. **B,** Assessment from dorsopalmar view of the normal foot. *1,* Line bisecting the phalanges; *2* and *3,* lines from respective lateral and medial solar margins of P3 to bearing surface of the hoof wall. These lines should be parallel to line *1.* Distance *2* = *3.*

Careful physical examination is warranted in this instance to determine if localized disease is present within the foot. The navicular bone should also be closely evaluated in the previous example because collateral cartilage ossification may accompany a more significant degenerative lesion in the navicular bone.[81]

A radiolucent linear defect or gap in the ossified cartilage usually indicates the junction between a separate, peripheral ossification center and the part of the cartilage that is ossifying from the palmar process of the phalanx (see Fig. 23-36). In a study of Finnish trotters, almost all radiolucent gaps between separate ossification centers were located in the middle or distal part of the ossified cartilage.[82] Fracture of the ossified collateral cartilage is unusual. Response to digital pressure applied to the coronary band, in the area of suspected fracture, helps differentiate a fracture from an incomplete pattern of ossification. Occasionally a fracture at the base or attachment of the cartilage to the palmar process can extend to involve the palmar process and the distal interphalangeal joint.

Infection (Quittor)

Penetrating wounds or lacerations in the coronary band region can introduce infection into the collateral cartilages. Necrosis associated with infection of this cartilage is called quittor. In acute infections, radiography should be considered to rule out a metallic foreign body or deeper lesion in the adjacent bones. In chronic infections, a draining tract is typical. Extension to the distal interphalangeal joint is uncommon unless it occurs iatrogenically during aggressive establishment of drainage or debridement of the necrotic cartilage.

HOOF BALANCE

Unbalanced trimming and improper shoeing of the foot can result in lameness in horses.[83] They have also been suggested as causes for development of navicular syndrome and degenerative joint disease of the interphalangeal joints. Lateromedial and dorsopalmar radiographic views of the foot can be used in conjunction with direct measurements on the foot to assess foot balance.[11,84-88] When radiographic views are used in this manner, particular attention must be paid to positioning of the foot, the center of the x-ray beam, and degree of weight bearing on the limb being assessed. The measurements used to assess foot balance radiographically are shown in Figure 23-37. In the lateromedial view, the dorsal hoof wall should be parallel to the wall at the heel. The pastern axis, as seen in the lateromedial view, is a line that divides P2 into equal dorsal and palmar halves. Ideally, this line similarly bisects P1 and is parallel to the dorsal cortex of P3. When this line is carried through to intercept with a line on the bearing surface of the hoof wall, it should create an angle of 45 to 55 degrees (front foot) or 50 to 55 degrees (hind foot) with the bony solar margin.[3,84] Significant differences were induced in the angles of the interphalangeal joints when the hoof angle was altered.[84] The greatest difference in angle occurred in the distal interphalangeal joint. Clinically, such a change in the angle of the distal interphalangeal joint may have an effect on the strain on the deep digital flexor tendon.[84] The angle of intercept of a line parallel to the solar margin of P3 and the line of the weight-bearing surface of the hoof wall should be 5 to 10 degrees.[11] The length of the toe region compared with the heel region of the bearing surface of the hoof wall is judged by comparison with the distal interphalangeal joint. A line from the center of the best-fit circle of curvature of the joint space, when drawn perpendicular to the weight-bearing surface, should be at the middle of the weight-bearing surface.[11,86] The lateral and medial portions of the hoof wall should be of equal length. An elaborate set of measurements has been made on the dorsopalmar view to assess the effects of uneven mediolateral hoof wall trimming.[85,86] This method was used to assess the effects of using the corrective full rolling shoe in horses that were lame as a result of interphalangeal degenerative joint disease.[88]

MISCELLANEOUS DISEASES AFFECTING THE PHALANGES

Keratoma is an abnormal mass of squamous epithelial cells with abundant keratin and granulation tissue. These develop within the hoof wall or in the sole and are rare. They are considered to be caused by traumatic or infectious insult to the hoof.[89] Horses in that report had been lame for relatively long periods as a result of prior hoof injuries.

Visible deformity of the hoof wall or sole is clinically evident. The mass effect can cause localized osteolysis of an adjacent area of P3. The lytic region typically involves the surface of P3. An oblique projection angle may be needed to demonstrate this feature. The margins of the lytic area are smooth, and the shape is typically round because the process of bone change is slow. Differential diagnoses for this type of bone lesion are septic pedal osteitis (margin should be more irregular); bone cyst (typically more centralized in the body of P3); and squamous cell carcinoma, fibrosarcoma, or mast cell tumors of the hoof wall or sole tissues.[11,89,90] Histologic evaluation of soft tissue masses of the sole and hoof is needed for definitive diagnosis.

Hypertrophic osteopathy is rare in the horse. The lesions in the limbs are characterized by fairly diffuse soft tissue swelling of all four limbs and periosteal new bone formation in the diaphyseal regions of the long bones, including the phalanges. The amount of new bone is variable. Most of the reported examples had palisade-like new bone formation. Articular margins or surfaces are usually not altered. Of horses and donkeys described with hypertrophic osteopathy, the phalanges were affected in 12 (approximately half).[91-93] The majority of animals had intrathoracic disease associated with the limb lesions. The bilateral symmetry, multilimb involvement, and character of the periosteal new bone are characteristic of this disease.

Mastocytosis is a tumorous swelling of the skin that can sometimes involve the subcutis and adjacent muscle. A report summarized the findings in six horses; three had the lesion in the distal limb that created radiographic abnormalities.[94] The common radiographic lesion was localized soft tissue swelling several centimeters in size, with granular mineralization. A poorly defined periosteal new bone response was found in one horse with a pastern region lesion. However, this horse had been unsuccessfully treated, and the periosteal response may have been a consequence of treatment rather than a result of the mastocytosis. Although several lesions were close to a joint, no architectural lesions in the joint were identified. The Arab breed was overrepresented in this series.

REFERENCES

1. Nyrop KA, Coffman JR, DeBowes RM et al: The role of diagnostic nerve blocks in the equine lameness examination, *Comp Contin Educ Vet Pract* 5:S669, 1983.
2. Morgan JP, Neves J, Baker T: *Equine radiography*, Ames, IA, 1991, Iowa State University.
3. Stashak TS: *Adams' lameness in horses*, Philadelphia, 1987, Lea & Febiger.
4. Schebitz H, Wilkens H: *Atlas of radiographic anatomy of the horse*, Philadelphia, 1978, WB Saunders.
5. Smallwood JE, Holliday SD: Xeroradiographic anatomy of the equine digit and metacarpophalangeal region, *Vet Radiol* 28:166, 1987.
6. Denoix JM: *The equine distal limb atlas of clinical anatomy and comparative imaging*, Ames, IA, 2002, Iowa State University.
7. Becht JL, Park RD, Kraft SL et al: Radiographic interpretation of normal skeletal variations and pseudolesions in the equine foot, *Vet Clin North Am Equine Pract* 17:1, 2001.
8. Kneller SK, Losonsky JM: Variable locations of nutrient foramina of the proximal phalanx in the forelimbs of Thoroughbreds, *J Am Vet Med Assoc* 197:736, 1990.
9. Losonsky JM, Kneller SK: Variable location of nutrient foramina of the proximal phalanx in the forelimbs of Standardbreds, *J Am Vet Med Assoc* 193:671, 1988.
10. Rendano VT, Grant B: The equine third phalanx: its radiographic appearance, *J Am Vet Radiol Soc* 19:125, 1978.
11. Butler FA, Colles CM, Dyson SJ et al: *Clinical radiology of the horse*, London, 1993, Blackwell Scientific.
12. Linford RL, O'Brien TR, Trout DR: Qualitative and morphometric radiographic findings in the distal phalanx and digital soft tissues of sound Thoroughbred racehorses, *Am J Vet Res* 54:38, 1993.
13. Smallwood JE, Albright SM, Metcalf MR et al: A xeroradiographic study of the developing equine foredigit and metacarpophalangeal region from birth to six months of age, *Vet Radiol* 30:98, 1989.
14. Kaneps AJ, Stover SM, O'Brien TR: Radiographic characteristics of the forelimb distal phalanx and microscopic morphology of the lateral palmar process in foals 3-32 weeks old, *Vet Radiol Ultrasound* 36:179, 1995.
15. Weaver JCB, Stover SM, O'Brien TR: Radiographic anatomy of soft tissue attachments in the equine metacarpophalangeal and proximal phalangeal region, *Equine Vet J* 24:310, 1992.
16. Werpy NM: Magnetic resonance imaging for diagnosis of soft tissue and osseous injuries in the horse, *Clin Tech Equine Pract* 3:389, 2004.
17. Mair TS, Kinns J, Jones RD et al: Magnetic resonance imaging of the distal limb of the standing horse, *Equine Vet Educ* 17:74, 2005.
18. Dyson S, Murray R, Schramme M et al: Lameness in 46 horses associated with deep digital flexor tendonitis in the digit: diagnosis confirmed with magnetic resonance imaging, Equine Vet J 35:681, 2003.
19. Butler JA, Colles CM, Dyson SJ et al: *Clinical radiology of the horse*, ed 2, London, 2000, Blackwell Scientific.
20. Dyson SJ, Murray R, Schramme M et al: Collateral desmitis of the distal interphalangeal joint in 18 horses (2001-2002), *Equine Vet J* 36:160, 2004.

21. Zubrod CJ, Farnsworth KD, Tucker RL et al: Injury of the collateral ligaments of the distal interphalangeal joint diagnosed by magnetic resonance, *Vet Radiol Ultrasound* 46:11, 2005.
22. Dyson SJ, Murray P, and Schramme MC: Lameness associated with foot pain: results of magnetic resonance imaging in 199 horses (January 2001-December 2003) and response to treatment, *Equine Vet J* 37:113, 2005.
23. McIlwraith CW, Goodman NL: Conditions of the interphalangeal joints, *Vet Clin North Am Equine Pract* 5:161, 1989.
24. Kawcak CE, McIlwraith CW: Proximodorsal proximal phalanx osteochondral chip fragmentation in 336 horses, *Equine Vet J* 26:392, 1994.
25. Markel MD, Richardson DW: Noncomminuted fractures of the proximal phalanx in 69 horses, *J Am Vet Med Assoc* 186:573, 1985.
26. Ellis DR, Simpson DJ, Greenwood RES et al: Observations and management of fractures of the proximal phalanx in young Thoroughbreds, *Equine Vet J* 19:43, 1987.
27. Fackleman GE, Peutz IP, Norris JC et al: The development of an equine fracture documentation system, *Vet Comp Orthop Trauma* 6:47, 1993.
28. Holcombe SJ, Schnieder RK, Bramlage LR et al: Lag screw fixation of noncomminuted sagittal fractures of the proximal phalanx in racehorses: 59 cases (1973-1991), *J Am Vet Med Assoc* 206:1195, 1995.
29. Markel MD, Martin BB, Richardson DW: Dorsal frontal fractures of the proximal phalanx in the horse, *Vet Surg* 14:36, 1985.
30. Markel MD, Richardson DW, Nunamaker DM: Comminuted proximal phalanx fractures in 30 horses, surgical vs. nonsurgical treatments, *Vet Surg* 14:135, 1985.
31. Tetens J, Ross MW, Lloyd JW: Comparison of racing performance before and after treatment of incomplete, midsagittal fractures of the proximal phalanx in Standardbreds: 49 cases (1986-1992), *J Am Vet Med Assoc* 210:82, 1997.
32. Goodman NL, Baker BK: Lameness diagnosis and treatment in the Quarterhorse racehorse, *Vet Clin North Am Equine Pract* 6:85, 1990.
33. Dechant JE, MacDonald DG, Crawford WH: Repair of complete dorsal fracture of the proximal phalanx in two horses, *Vet Surg* 27:445, 1998.
34. Rose PL, Seeherman H, O'Callaghan MO: Computed tomographic evaluation of comminuted middle phalangeal fractures in the horse, *Vet Radiol Ultrasound* 38:424, 1997.
35. Colahan PT, Wheat JD, Meagher DM: Treatment of middle phalangeal fractures in the horse, *J Am Vet Med Assoc* 178:1182, 1981.
36. Martin GS, McIlwraith CW, Turner AS et al: Long-term results and complications of proximal interphalangeal arthrodesis in horses, *J Am Vet Med Assoc* 184:1136, 1984.
37. Doran RE, White NA, Allen D: Use of a bone plate for treatment of middle phalangeal fractures in horses: seven cases (1979-1984), *J Am Vet Med Assoc* 191:575, 1987.
38. Crabill MR, Watkins JP, Schneider RK et al: Double-plate fixation of comminuted fractures of the second phalanx in horses: 10 cases (1985-1993), *J Am Vet Med Assoc* 207:1458, 1995.
39. Gabel AA, Bukowiecki CF: Fractures of the phalanges, *Vet Clin North Am Large Anim Pract* 5:233, 1983.
40. Honnas CH, O'Brien TR, Linford RL: Distal phalanx fractures in horses: a survey of 274 horses with radiographic assessment of healing in 36 horses, *Vet Radiol* 29:98, 1989.
41. Scott EQ, McDole M, Shires MH et al: A review of third phalanx fractures in the horse: 65 cases, *J Am Vet Med Assoc* 174:1337, 1979.
42. Scott EQ, McDole M, Shires MH et al: Fractures of the third phalanx (P3) in the horse at Michigan State University, 1964-1979. In *Proceedings of the 25th Annual Convention of the American Association of Equine Practitioners*, Miami, 1979, p 439.
43. O'Sullivan CB, Dart AJ, Malikides N et al: Nonsurgical management of type II fractures of the distal phalanx in 48 Standardbred horses, *Aust Vet J* 77:501, 1999.
44. Kaneps AJ, O'Brien TR, Redden RF et al: Characterization of osseous bodies of the distal phalanx of foals, *Equine Vet J* 25:285, 1993.
45. Kaneps AJ, O'Brien TR, Willits NH et al: Effect of hoof trimming on the occurrence of distal phalangeal palmar process fractures in foals, *Eq Vet J* 26(suppl):36, 1998.
46. Baird AN, Seahorn TL, Morris EL: Equine distal phalangeal sequestration, *Vet Radiol* 31:210, 1990.
47. Cauvin ERJ, Munroe GA: Septic osteitis of the distal phalanx: findings and surgical treatment in 18 horses, *Equine Vet J* 30:512, 1998.
48. Steel CM, Hunt AR, Adams PL et al: Factors associated with prognosis for survival and athletic use in foals with septic arthritis: 93 cases (1987-1994), *J Am Vet Med Assoc* 215:973, 1999.
49. Honnas CM, Vacek JR, Schumacher J: Diagnostic and therapeutic protocols for septic arthritis of the distal interphalangeal joint, *Vet Med* Dec:1215, 1992.
50. Pool RR, Meagher DM: Pathologic findings and pathogenesis of racetrack injuries, *Vet Clin North Am Equine Pract* 6:1, 1990.
51. Pool RR: Pathologic manifestations of joint disease in the athletic horse. In McIlwraith CW, Trotter GW, editors: *Joint disease in the horse,* Philadelphia, 1996, W.B. Saunders.
52. Zubrod CH, Schneider RK, Tucker RL et al: Use of magnetic resonance imaging for identifying subchondral bone damage in horses: 11 cases (1999-2003), *J Am Vet Med Assoc* 224:411, 2004.
53. Kainer RA: Clinical anatomy of the equine foot, *Vet Clin North Am Equine Pract* 5:1, 1989.
54. Goetz TE: Anatomic, hoof and shoeing considerations for the treatment of laminitis in horses, *J Am Vet Med Assoc* 190:1323, 1987.
55. Peloso JG, Cohen ND, Walker MA et al: Case-control study of risk factors for the development of laminitis in the contralateral limb of Equidae with unilateral lameness, *J Am Vet Med Assoc* 209:1746, 1996.
56. Hood DM: Laminitis in the horse, *Vet Clin North Am Equine Pract* 15:287, 1999.
57. Curtis S, Ferguson DW, Luikart R et al: Trimming and shoeing the chronically affected horse, *Vet Clin North Am Equine Pract* 15:463, 1999.
58. Cripps PJ, Eustace RA: Radiological measurements from the feet of normal horses with relevance to laminitis, *Equine Vet J* 31:427, 1999.
59. Cripps PJ, Eustace RA: Factors involved in the prognosis of equine laminitis in the UK, *Equine Vet J* 31:433, 1999.
60. Baxter GM: Acute laminitis, *Vet Clin North Am Equine Pract* 10:627, 1994.
61. Herthel D, Hood DM: Clinical presentation, diagnosis, and prognosis of chronic laminitis, *Vet Clin North Am Equine Pract* 15:375, 1999.
62. O'Brien TR, Baker TW: Distal extremity examination: How to perform the radiographic examination and interpret the radiographs. In *Proceedings of the 32nd Annual Convention of the American Association of Equine Practitioners,* Nashville, 1986, p 553.

63. Stick JA, Hann HW, Scott EA et al: Pedal bone rotation as a prognostic sign in laminitis of horses, *J Am Vet Med Assoc* 180:251, 1982.
64. Hunt RJ: A retrospective evaluation of laminitis in horses, *Equine Vet J* 25:61, 1993.
65. Murray RC, Dyson SJ, Schramme MC et al: Magnetic resonance imaging of the equine digit with chronic laminitis, *Vet Radiol Ultrasound* 44:609, 2004.
66. McIlwraith CW, James LR: Limb deformities in foals associated with ingestion of locoweed by mares, *J Am Vet Med Assoc* 181:255, 1982.
67. Owen JM: Abnormal flexion of the corono-pedal joint or "contracted tendons" in unweaned foals, *Equine Vet J* 7:40, 1975.
68. Fackelman GE: Equine flexural deformities of developmental origin. In *Proceedings of the 26th Annual Convention of the American Association of Equine Practitioners*, Anaheim, CA, 1980, p 97.
69. Arnbjerg J: Changes in the distal phalanx in foals with deep digital flexor tendon contraction, *Vet Radiol* 29:65, 1988.
70. Grant BD: The pastern joint. In Mansmann RA, McAllister EG, editors: *Equine medicine and surgery*, ed 3, Santa Barbara, CA, 1982, American Veterinary Publications.
71. Shiroma JT, Engel HN, Wagner PC et al: Dorsal subluxation of the proximal interphalangeal joint in the pelvic limb of three horses, *J Am Vet Med Assoc* 195:777, 1989.
72. Wagner PC, Watrous BJ: *Equine pediatric orthopedics: a practitioner monograph*, Santa Barbara, CA, 1991, Veterinary Practice Publishing.
73. Wagner PC, von Matthiessen P: Treating congenital limb deformities in the foal, *Vet Med* 1993, p 989.
74. Dowling BA, Dart AJ, Hodgson DR: Subchondral cystic lesions involving the second phalanx in two horses, *Aust Vet J* 76:328, 1998.
75. Hurtig MB, Pool RR: Pathogenesis of equine osteochondrosis. In McIlwraith CW, Trotter GW, editors: *Joint disease in the horse*, Philadelphia, 1996, W.B. Saunders.
76. Trotter GW, McIlwraith CW, Norrdin RW et al: Degenerative joint disease with osteochondrosis of the proximal interphalangeal joint in young horses, *J Am Vet Med Assoc* 180:1312, 1982.
77. Trotter GW, McIlwraith CW: Osteochondritis dissecans and subchondral cystic lesions and their relationship to osteochondrosis in the horse, *Equine Vet Sci* 5:157, 1981.
78. Trotter GW, McIlwraith CW: Osteochondrosis in horses: pathogenesis and clinical syndromes. In *Proceedings of the 27th Annual Convention of the American Association of Equine Practitioners*, New Orleans, 1981, p 141.
79. Pettersson H, Reiland S: Periarticular subchondral bone cysts in horses, *Clin Orthop* 62:95, 1969.
80. Reeves MJ, Yovich JV, Turner AS: Miscellaneous conditions of the equine foot, *Vet Clin North Am Equine Pract* 5:221, 1989.
81. Reid CF: Radiography and the purchase examination in the horse, *Vet Clin North Am Large Anim Pract* 2:151, 1980.
82. Ruohoniemi M, Tulamo R-M, Hackzell M: Radiographic evaluation of ossification of the collateral cartilages of the third phalanx in Finnhorses, *Equine Vet J* 25:453, 1993.
83. Moyer W, Anderson JP: Sheared heels: diagnosis and treatment, *J Am Vet Med Assoc* 166:53, 1975.
84. Bushe T, Turner TA, Poulos P et al: The effect of hoof angle on coffin, pastern, and fetlock joint angles, *Proc Am Assoc Equine Pract* 33:729, 1987.
85. Caudron I, Grulke S, Farnir F et al: Radiographic assessment of equine interphalangeal joints asymmetry: articular impact of phalangeal rotations (part I), *J Vet Med* 45:319, 1998.
86. Caudron I, Grulke S, Farnir F et al: Radiographic assessment of equine interphalangeal joints asymmetry: articular impact of asymmetric bearings (part II), *J Vet Med* 45:319, 1998.
87. Colles CM: Interpreting radiographs 1: the foot, *Equine Vet J* 15:297, 1983.
88. Caudron I, Miesen M, Grulke S et al: Radiological assessment of the effects of a full rolling motion shoe during asymmetrical bearing, *Equine Vet J* 23(suppl):20, 1997.
89. Lloyd KCK, Peterson PR, Wheat JD et al: Keratomas in horses: seven cases (1975-1986), *J Am Vet Med Assoc* 193:967, 1988.
90. Ritmeester AM, Denicola DB, Blevins WE et al: Primary intraosseous mast cell tumor of the third phalanx in a Quarter horse, *Equine Vet J* 29:151, 1997.
91. Messer NT, Powers BE: Hypertrophic osteopathy associated with pulmonary infarction in a horse, *Comp Contin Educ Vet Pract* 5:S636, 1983.
92. Sweeney CR, Stebbins KE, Schelling CG et al: Hypertrophic osteopathy in a pony with a pituitary adenoma, *J Am Vet Med Assoc* 195:103, 1989.
93. Mair TS, Dyson SJ, Frasser JA et al: Hypertrophic osteopathy (Marie's disease) in Equidae: a review of twenty-four cases, *Equine Vet J* 28:256, 1996.
94. Samii VF, O'Brien TR, Stannard AA: Radiographic features of mastocytosis in the equine limb, *Equine Vet J* 29:63, 1997.

ELECTRONIC RESOURCES evolve

Additional information related to the content in Chapter 23 can be found on the companion Web site at evolve http://evolve.elsevier.com/Thrall/vetrad/

- Key Points
- Chapter Quiz
- Case Study 23-1

CHAPTER • 24
The Navicular Bone

Federica Morandi
Barbara J. Watrous
Robert L. Toal

ANATOMY

The normal radiographic anatomy of the navicular bone (distal sesamoid bone) is shown in Chapter 13. The navicular bone has two surfaces (flexor and articular), two borders (proximal and distal), and two extremities (medial and lateral). The navicular bone typically ossifies from a single center (Fig. 24-1).[1] It has two separate hyaline cartilage–covered articular surfaces. The larger proximal articular surface conforms to the condyles of the middle phalanx. A smaller distal articular surface, associated with the distal navicular border, is essentially a narrow facet that articulates with the distal phalanx. The distal articular surface of the navicular bone and the articular surface of the distal phalanx are usually parallel but can be convergent.[2] The flexor surface has a prominent central ridge—termed the central eminence. The deep digital flexor tendon and adjacent bursa make contact with the fibrocartilage-covered flexor surface. The navicular bone is held in position by three strong ligaments. The paired suspensory navicular ligaments originate from the dorsolateral and dorsomedial aspects of the proximal phalanx and attach to the proximal navicular border and both extremities. The distal sesamoidean, or impar, ligament originates from a projection on the distal navicular border just caudal to the articular surface. The impar ligament inserts on the distal phalanx deep to the deep digital flexor tendon. Blood vessels and sensory nerves traverse these ligaments and ramify into the navicular bone and synovial membrane by way of both borders.[3] No evidence exists for an anatomic communication between the distal interphalangeal joint and the navicular bursa.[4]

INDICATIONS FOR RADIOGRAPHY

Indications for navicular radiography include the assessment of bony changes in navicular syndrome, the identification of significant bone abnormalities during prepurchase examination, the assessment of bone or bursal involvement in foot wounds or abscesses, the evaluation of suspected trauma, and the collection of information about the morphologic progression or remission of navicular bone abnormalities.

PREPARATION FOR RADIOGRAPHIC EVALUATION

Accurate radiographic evaluation of the navicular bone depends on a radiograph that is properly positioned and exposed and on a foot that is free of distracting artifacts. Proper preparation for navicular radiography is similar to that for the distal phalanx discussed in Chapter 22.

Positioning aids, such as a reinforced cassette, grooved wooden blocks, and a cassette tunnel, assist in radiographic evaluation of the navicular bone (Fig. 24-2). Use of a grid for angular dorsoproximal-palmarodistal views is optional. A grid improves radiographic detail by reducing film fog from scatter radiation. Because the grid is fragile, its use is limited to techniques during which the foot does not bear weight directly on the grid, such as with a cassette tunnel.

RADIOGRAPHIC VIEWS

The location of the navicular bone and its complex shape require that at least three different views be made for complete radiographic evaluation. These views include the angular dorsoproximal-palmarodistal views, the lateromedial view, and the palmaroproximal-palmarodistal oblique view (Box 24-1).[2] The horizontal beam dorsopalmar view is an additional view that is helpful for evaluating the extremities of the navicular bone. In addition, dorsoproximolateral-palmarodistomedial and dorsoproximomedial-palmarodistolateral oblique views project the extremities of the navicular bone without superimposition on the middle phalanx.

Dorsoproximal-Palmarodistal Views

Angular dorsoproximal-palmarodistal views of the navicular bone may be made by two different hoof-positioning techniques.[5-7] These methods include (1) the high coronary stand-on route, in which the foot stands directly on a reinforced cassette, cassette tunnel, or grooved wooden block. The x-ray beam is centered just proximal to the coronary band and angled 45 or 65 degrees proximally from horizontal; and (2) the upright pedal route, in which the hoof rests on the toe in tiptoe fashion, with the dorsal hoof wall positioned either 80 or 90 degrees from horizontal; the x-ray beam is directed horizontally (Fig. 24-3).

By varying the x-ray beam angulation incident on the navicular bone in the high coronary route or by altering the position of the hoof in the upright pedal route, an accurate projection of either the proximal or distal navicular border can be obtained. This is because the proximal and distal navicular borders are not parallel (they diverge in a palmar direction), and thus a true geometric projection of both borders cannot be obtained in a single dorsoproximal-palmarodistal radiograph.

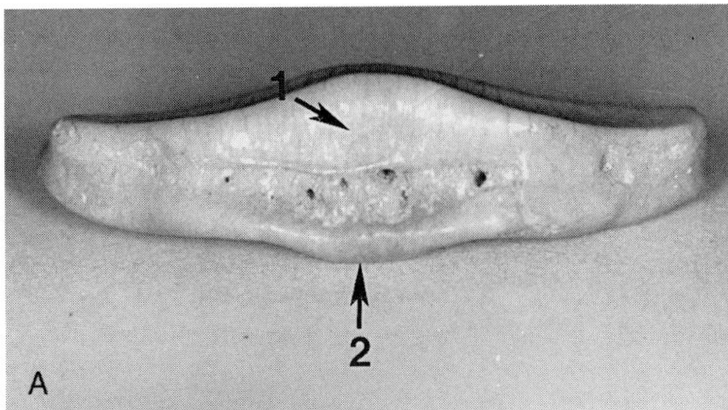

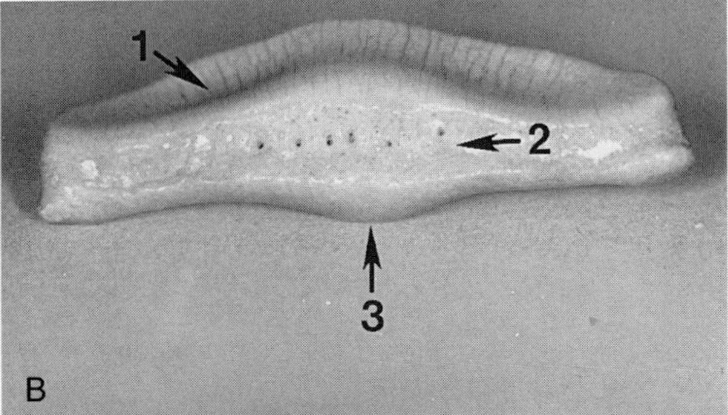

Fig. 24-1 The navicular bone. **A,** En face view of the distal border. *1,* The small articular surface with the distal phalanx; *2,* the projection off the distal border where the impar ligament attaches. **B,** En face view of the proximal border. *1,* The articular surface with the middle phalanx; *2,* the proximal border itself where the suspensory navicular ligament attaches; *3,* the central eminence. The view in **B** is analogous to that obtained in a palmaroproximal-palmarodistal radiograph.

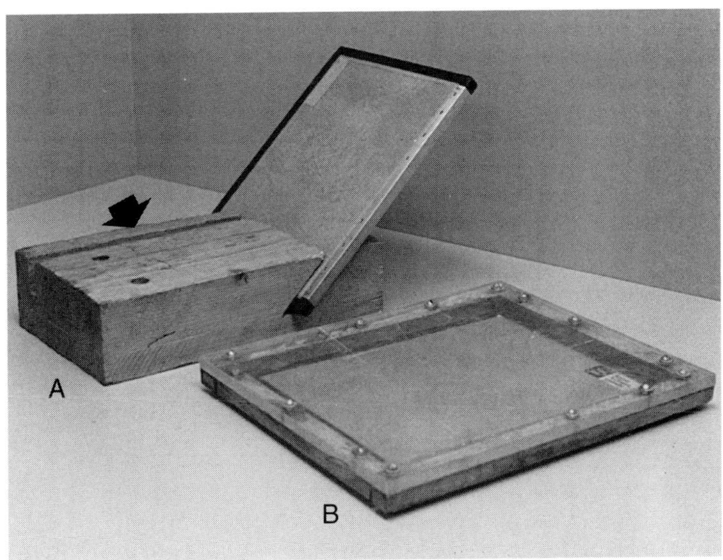

Fig. 24-2 Types of positioning aids for navicular radiography. *A,* A wooden block for angular dorsoproximal-palmarodistal views. The longitudinally oriented slot *(arrow)* is used for lateral views. The grooves are of sufficient width to allow combined insertion of a grid and cassette. *B,* A cassette tunnel covered with Plexiglas protects the cassette (and grid) during dorsoproximal-palmarodistal views.

An undistorted projection of the proximal navicular border is achieved by using the 45-degree high coronary stand-on route or the 90-degree upright pedal route. The distal navicular border is obscured by these routes because it is projected below the level of the distal interphalangeal joint. Because only the proximal navicular border can be accurately evaluated in these two projections, they are used as supplemental views (see Fig. 24-3, *A* and *C*).

A 65-degree high coronary stand-on route or an 80-degree upright pedal route projects the distal navicular border proximal to the distal interphalangeal joint and superimposes the entire navicular bone behind the middle phalanx. The distal navicular border is well visualized, and although the proximal border is slightly distorted, it is readily identified. Either one of these two positioning methods is recommended for the angular dorsoproximal-palmarodistal projection because when they are done properly, the entire navicular bone is projected through the middle phalanx (see Fig. 24-3, *B* and *D*).

Stand-on techniques are technically easier but result in slightly more magnification of the navicular bone when compared with the upright pedal route.[6] Magnification can be minimized on the high coronary stand-on route by using a grooved wooden block. A cassette and grid are placed in a precut groove behind the hoof as it rests on the block. Because of the position of the cassette, less magnification of the navicular bone occurs when compared with other stand-on techniques (see Fig. 24-3, *B*).

Lateromedial View

In the lateral view, both navicular extremities should be projected superimposed. If some degree of angulation occurs, this factor must be recognized and taken into account during interpretation or an incorrect assessment of navicular bone remodeling will be made. The foot is placed on a wooden block so that the x-ray tube can be positioned low enough to center the beam on the lateral (transverse) axis of the navicular bone. A wooden block also elevates the hoof, allowing the cassette to straddle it proximally and distally. The entire hoof should be included on the radiograph.

Palmaroproximal-Palmarodistal View

The palmaroproximal-palmarodistal view (Fig. 24-4) projects the flexor cortex, medulla, and central eminence. The concept is to isolate most of the bone between the palmar processes of the distal phalanx. The horse stands on a reinforced cassette or cassette tunnel. The foot is positioned as far caudal as

Box • 24-1

Radiographic Views of the Navicular Bone

Dorsoproximal-Palmarodistal Views

High coronary stand-on route
- 45 degrees: Projects proximal border and extremities
- 65 degrees: Projects both borders and extremities

Upright pedal route
- 90 degrees: Projects proximal border and extremities
- 80 degrees: Projects both borders and extremities

Lateromedial View

Foreshortened projection along the axis of the bone
- Projects both borders and both surfaces in profile
- Extremities are superimposed

Palmaroproximal-Palmarodistal Oblique View

Beam is angled tangential to the flexor surface
- Projects the flexor cortex, medulla, and central eminence
- Extremities are obscured by palmar processes of distal phalanx

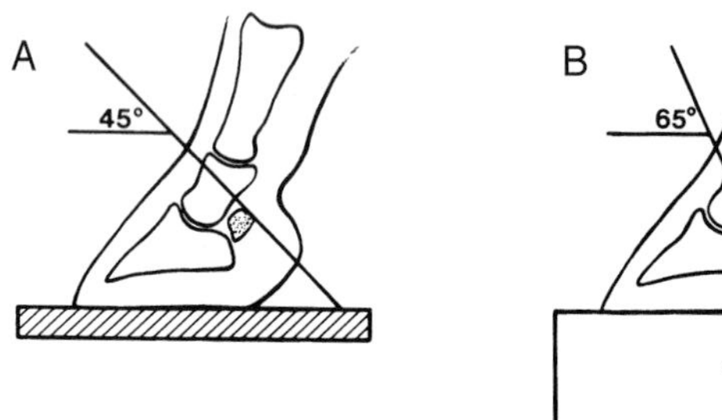

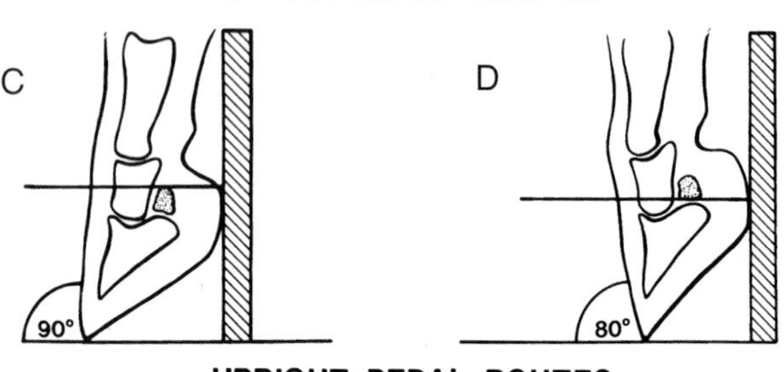

Fig. 24-3 Angular dorsoproximal-palmarodistal views. High coronary routes: **A,** Direct stand-on method. **B,** Wooden block technique. **C** and **D,** Upright pedal routes illustrated showing beam or hoof angulation relative to the horizontal plane. Only the proximal navicular border is well visualized in **A** and **C,** whereas both proximal and distal borders are clearly projected in **B** and **D.**

possible while still bearing weight.[8] Local analgesia may be required to obtain ideal foot positioning. Paradoxically, some prefer that the foot be more slightly forward than in the normal standing position.[8,9] Regardless of foot location, the primary beam is positioned tangential to the estimated plane of the flexor cortex and is centered between the bulbs of the heel. Too steep of a beam angle with the foot may result in superimposition of the ergot over the navicular bone. Reduced angulation alters the apparent width of the flexor cortex and results in an indistinct interface between cortical and trabecular bone.[8] Excessive superimposition of the palmar processes of the distal phalanx on the navicular bone can also occur. Oblique palmaroproximal-palmarodistal projections distort the navicular shape and superimpose it behind the palmar processes of the distal phalanx.

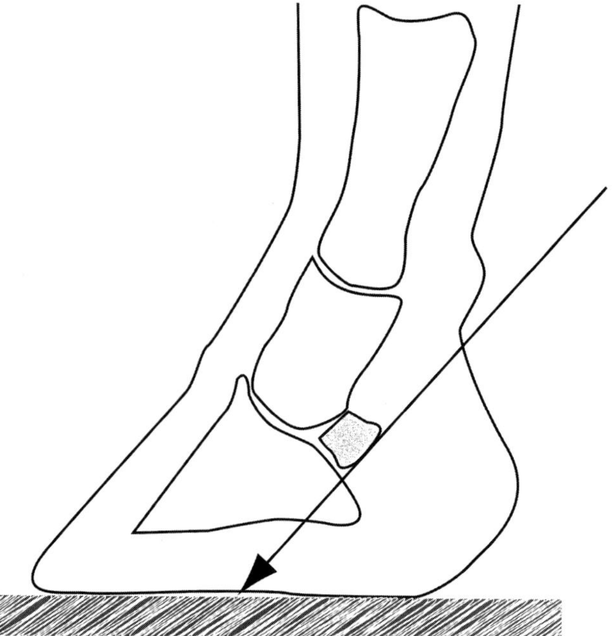

Fig. 24-4 Setup to acquire a palmaroproximal-palmarodistal view of the navicular bone. The distal interphalangeal joint is positioned in extension, with the x-ray beam angled tangentially to the flexor surface of the navicular bone.

Dorsopalmar View

In the dorsopalmar view, the x-ray beam is directed horizontally toward the hoof, which is in a normal weight-bearing position. The foot should be placed on a wooden block to allow the cassette to straddle the hoof and the navicular bone. This view is useful in evaluating the extremities of the navicular bone, particularly when subtle abnormalities are suspected.

NORMAL RADIOGRAPHIC APPEARANCE

In the angular dorsoproximal-palmarodistal views, the navicular bone is of uniform radiopacity. Its spindle shape varies somewhat from horse to horse. The extremities are fairly symmetric and are bluntly pointed. The proximal border is smoothly marginated. The shape of the proximal border has been classified variously as concave, undulating, straight, or convex.[10] The distal border has a variable number (usually no more than seven) of cone-shaped radiolucencies representing synovial invaginations. Their size is variable, with the height being approximately 1.5 times the width of the cone at the base. Size is related to degree of work, although their shape should remain somewhat triangular.

The lateral view offers a clear, unobstructed view of the navicular bone but presents a foreshortened image. Both extremities should be superimposed; a well-defined medullary cavity is visualized. The flexor surface is convex palmarly and is smoothly marginated. In some normal horses, a smoothly marginated dimple of variable depth is seen in the mid-portion of the central eminence. The proximal and distal borders are smooth, as are the articular surfaces. Some horses may have a mild elongation of the proximal or distal border, or both.[2] The joint space between the navicular bone and the distal phalanx is usually parallel, but a convergent joint is sometimes present.

In the palmaroproximal-palmarodistal view, a well-defined medullary cavity of uniform trabecular pattern with four or five small radiolucent foramina may be seen. The cortex is of homogeneous opacity and is of uniform thickness centrally, with some thinning peripherally. The width of the flexor cortex varies from 2.0 to 3.6 mm because of breed differences and geometric magnification.[2,8] The flexor surface is smoothly marginated with a prominent central eminence. The central eminence is usually rounded and prominent, but in some horses it may appear flattened normally. A small crescent-shaped radiolucency may be seen within the cortex of the central eminence, representing a normal midsagittal synovial fossa. This fossa is occasionally seen as a dimple on the flexor surface on the lateral view. In some horses, a lucent crescent is seen within the central eminence, even in bones without a dimple. This is caused by a trabecular bone island interposed between two parallel cortical bone plates of the central eminence.[11,12] The ends of both extremities are rounded, being variably superimposed over the palmar processes of the distal phalanx. The articular surface is occasionally seen in this view.

NAVICULAR DISEASE

The term *navicular disease* is used in this discussion to denote a chronic progressive syndrome involving the navicular bone, its fibrocartilaginous flexor surface, its ligaments and capsular attachments, the deep digital flexor tendon, and the navicular bursa. The distal interphalangeal joint may be involved to a lesser degree but its role in this syndrome is controversial. The precise source of pain in navicular lameness remains obscure. Variable response to local analgesia of the medial and lateral palmar digital nerves, the distal interphalangeal joint space, and the navicular bursa is noted. This variable response suggests that sensory nerves innervating the synovial membranes of the collateral sesamoidean ligament, the distal sesamoidean impar ligament, and the navicular bone itself play a separate or combined role in mediating pain in navicular disease.[4,13] In addition, pain arising from the dorsal margin of the sole has been shown to be attenuated by analgesia of the distal interphalangeal joint or palmar digital nerve block.[14] This further complicates the interpretation of nerve block results in horses suspected of having navicular origin pain.

Navicular disease is primarily a slowly developing, intermittent, bilateral forelimb lameness.[15,16] It is also occasionally recognized in the hindlimb.[17] In general, navicular disease is most common between 3 and 18 years of age, with a peak incidence of 9 years of age at presentation. Males have involvement more often than do females, geldings have a greater risk than stallions, and the breed prevalence varies according to the population characteristics of the reporting institutions.[18,19]

No pathognomonic clinical test is available for navicular disease. The diagnosis is based on a characteristic gait, localization of pain to the palmar part of the heel, identification of radiographic signs of navicular degeneration, and elimination of other causes of lameness.[15,20] When navicular lameness is suspected, both feet should be radiographed because radiographic changes are often bilateral even if clinical signs are not.

The pathophysiology of navicular syndrome is multifactorial. Classically, it has been characterized as navicular fibrocartilaginous degeneration with secondary tendon fibrillation. Palmar cortex bone erosions can develop later.[5,15,20,21] Other bony changes involving the distal border synovial invaginations (enlargement) have also been noted.[21-23] Abnormalities such as dilated vessels, vascular thrombosis, granulation tissue, and empty synovium-lined invaginations have been observed histologically to a variable degree.[3,20-29] Whether these findings represent a continuum of events or are separate, isolated abnormalities is unknown. Enthesopathy involving the ligaments of the proximal and distal borders can occur with or without distal border foramina changes. Many of the gross and histologic features of navicular syndrome support the concept of a degenerative arthrosis.[23,27,29-31] Some evidence shows that chronic passive venous congestion of the foot is related to navicular changes of elevated subchondral bone pressure and arterial hyperemia.[27,32,33]

Similar confusion exists regarding the significance of radiographic changes in the navicular bone in horses with lameness attributed to navicular disease. Poor correlation of pathologic and radiographic findings with clinical signs and prognosis has been demonstrated.[18,24,26,28,34] Horses without radiographic abnormalities may have clinical navicular lameness, and horses with pathologic and radiographic changes may be sound.[28,35] This paradox is explained in part by the fact that horses have different pain thresholds, are subjected to wide ranges of physical exercise, and are evaluated in variable stages of disease.[8] Additionally, some pathologic changes may represent insignificant wear lesions or may be located in tissues of soft tissue opacity and thus are not radiographically discernible.[20,26] Several authors agree that radiographic signs of navicular disease in an otherwise clinically normal horse are significant and may warrant a cautious prognosis for future soundness.[8,36] However, no universal agreement exists regarding the clinical significance of all radiographic signs seen in navicular disease.

Radiographic Signs of Navicular Degeneration

Radiographic abnormalities associated with navicular degeneration are varied. Bony abnormalities may occur separately but usually occur in combination, unilaterally or bilaterally. Their clinical relevance regarding presence, absence, or degree of lameness in a given animal is varied.[34] Additionally, no clear association exists between changes in the radiographic appearance of navicular bones and clinical outcome after treatment.[37] Thus radiographic changes of navicular degeneration must be interpreted in context with the presenting clinical signs. This is similar for other musculoskeletal conditions.

The major radiographic signs of navicular degeneration are shown in Box 24-2. A diagram depicting various radiographic

Box • 24-2

Roentgen Signs of Navicular Degeneration

Proximal Border and Extremities
Enthesophytes (spurs) on the extremities
Remodeling

Distal Border Changes
Synovial invaginations
Small osseous fragments

Flexor Cortex Changes
Cortical erosions
Mineralization of deep digital flexor tendon

Medullary Cavity Changes
Radiolucent cysts
Sclerosis

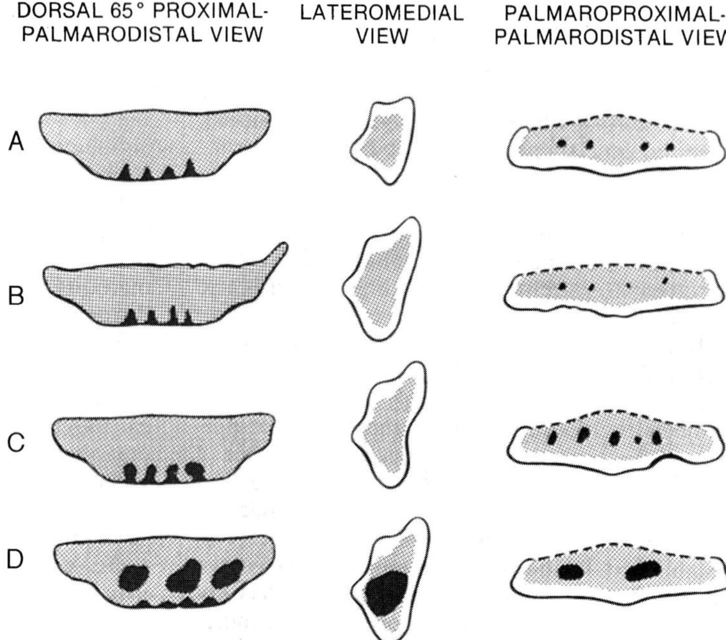

Fig. 24-5 Radiographic changes seen in navicular degeneration. Dorsal 65-degree proximal-palmarodistal view: *A*, normal; *B*, remodeling enthesophyte on extremity and irregular proximal border; *C*, lollipop-shaped invaginations on distal border; *D*, cystlike lesion formation. Lateromedial view: *A*, normal; *B*, elongated navicular profile from remodeling (enthesophyte formation); *C*, flexor cortical erosion; *D*, cystlike lesion formation. Palmaroproximal-palmarodistal view: *A*, normal; *B*, flexor cortical erosions; *C*, enlarged fossae and flexor cortical erosions; *D*, cystlike lesion formation. (Modified with permission from Richard Park, Fort Collins, Colo.)

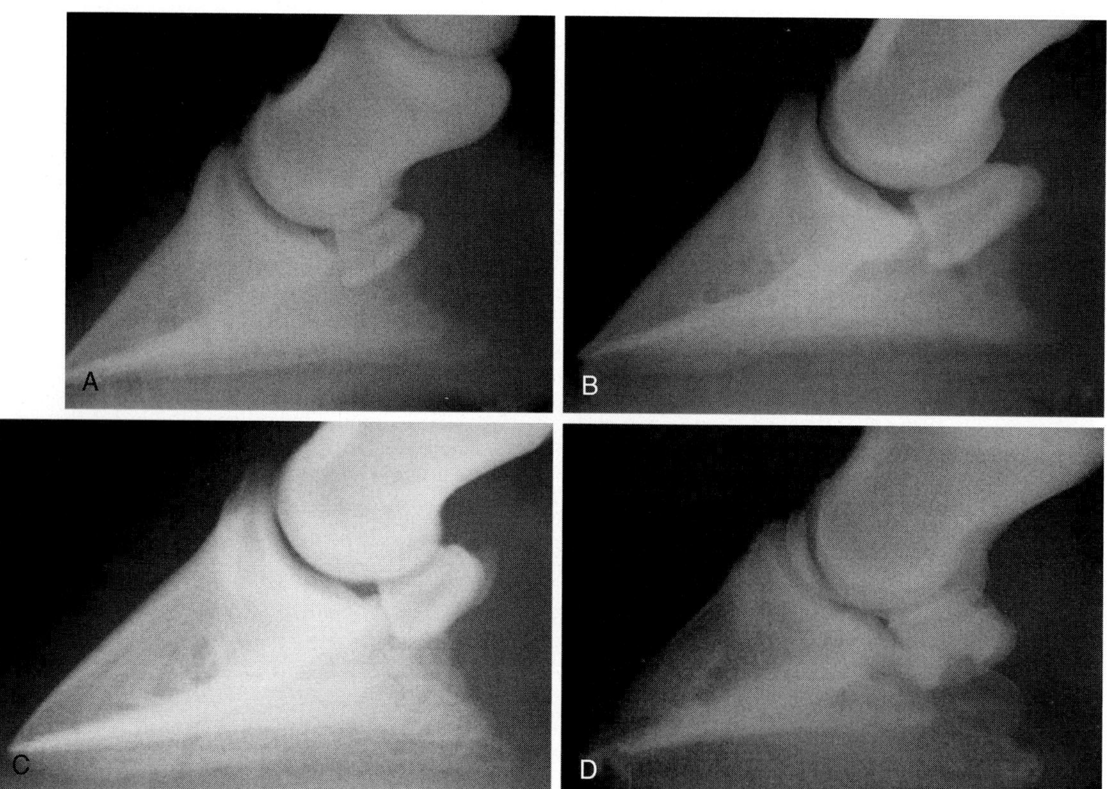

Fig. 24-6 Lateral views of the navicular bone. **A,** Normal navicular bone. **B,** Proximal elongation caused by remodeling. **C,** Enthesophyte (spur) on proximal border. **D,** Flexor cortex lysis.

signs of navicular degeneration is shown in Figure 24-5. Radiographic manifestations of navicular degeneration and normal variants are shown in Figures 24-6 through 24-9.

Proximal Border and Navicular Bone Extremities

The heredity aspects of the shape of the proximal navicular border and its relation to risk for navicular syndrome have been studied in Warmbloods.[10] The conclusion was that horses with a convex-shaped proximal border had the least risk for development of severe navicular disease.

Dystrophic mineralization at sites of ligamentous or tendon attachment is termed enthesophytosis.[29,38] Mineralization of the suspensory navicular ligament along the proximal border results in a roughened or undulating appearance of the

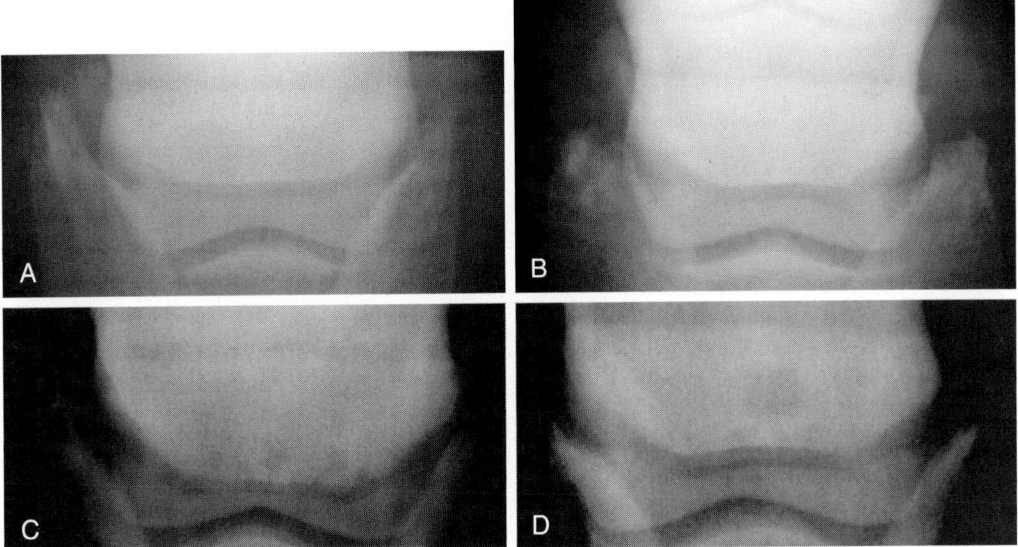

Fig. 24-7 Dorsoproximal-palmarodistal views of the navicular bone. **A,** Normal navicular bone. **B,** Remodeling of lateral extremity. **C,** Lollipop-shaped synovial invaginations of the distal navicular border. **D,** Cystlike cavitation over the plane of the navicular medullary cavity. Remember that flexor cortical erosions often falsely mimic medullary cavity cysts on angled dorsoproximal-palmarodistal views. Thus the palmaroproximal-palmarodistal and/or lateral view would be needed in this situation to determine the location of the lesion accurately.

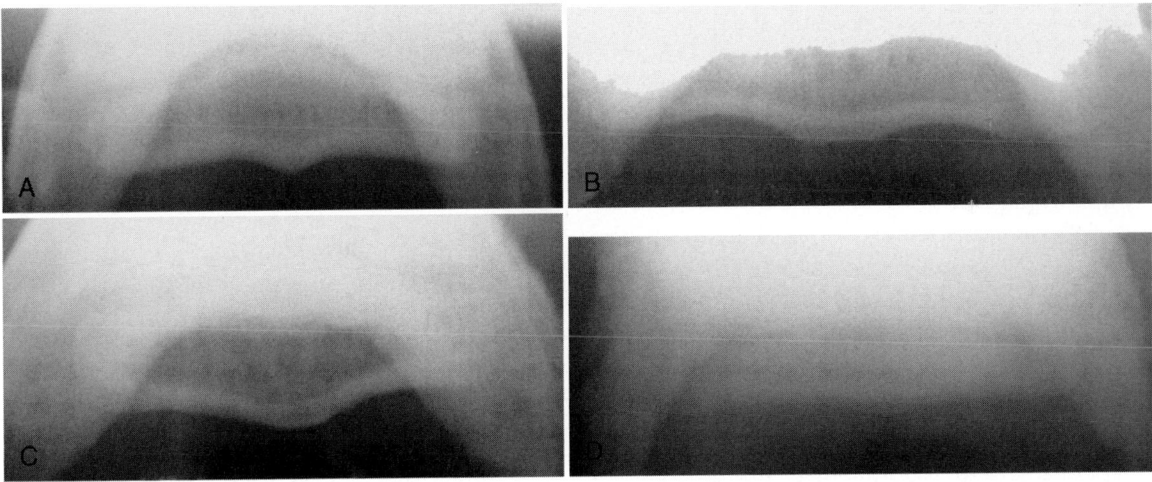

Fig. 24-8 Normal variations in the appearance of the navicular flexor cortex are shown. The flexor cortex should be smoothly marginated and have an abrupt demarcation from the less-opaque medullary spongiosa. **A,** Prominent central eminence. **B,** Blunted central eminence. **C,** Crescent-shaped radiolucency in central eminence. **D,** Either altered beam angulation or patient motion may result in indistinct interface between the cortex and the medullary spongiosa, falsely suggesting navicular sclerosis. The lateral view in this horse was normal, and a repeat palmaroproximal-palmarodistal projection with better beam angulation showed normal corticomedullary distinction.

bone margin. Pronounced enthesophytes on the extremities of the navicular bone have been termed spurs. When enthesophytosis is excessive, the overall shape of the bone is altered. This is called remodeling (see Figs. 24-6, *B* and *C*, and Fig. 24-7, *B*).

In general, enthesophytes are manifestations of a degenerative process.[5,15,38,39] They are occasionally seen in nonlame animals, particularly in older, heavily worked animals.[18,24,26] Enthesophytes in younger horses and extensive enthesophytes in others should be considered significant, particularly if accompanied by lameness.

Enthesophytes are best seen in angular dorsoproximal-palmarodistal views as new bone formation on the extremities or as bone proliferations along the proximal border

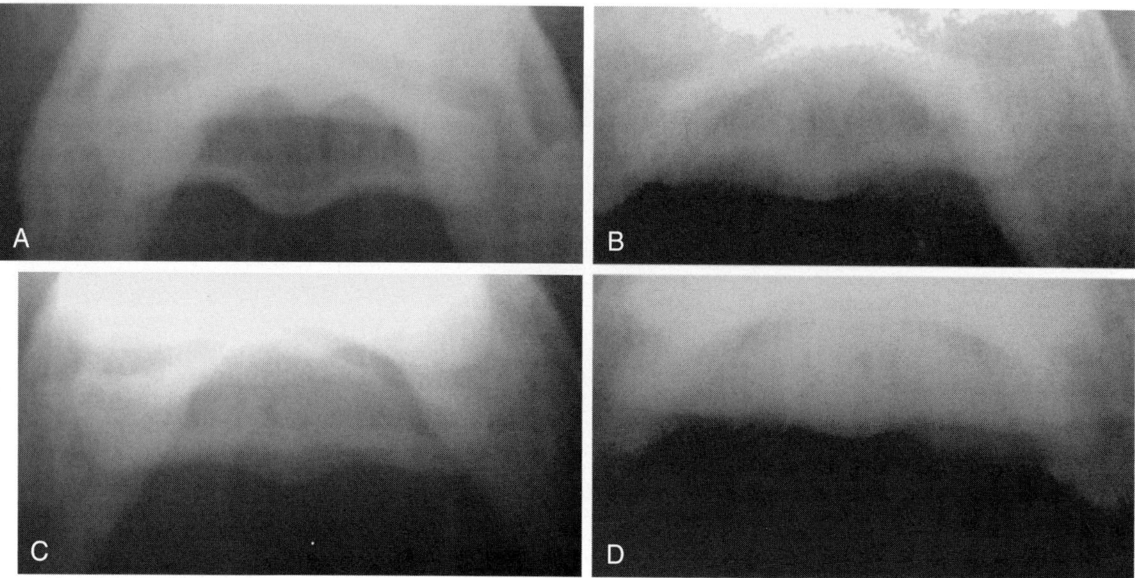

Fig. 24-9 Palmaroproximal-palmarodistal views of the navicular flexor cortex and medulla showing various abnormalities. **A,** En face view of enlarged distal border synovial invaginations. Note the crescent lucency in the central eminence. **B,** Flexor cortex erosions result in a loss of the normal smooth flexor contour. **C,** Large focal cortical lysis causing disruption of the flexor cortex over the central eminence. **D,** Extensive subchondral bone sclerosis. This was also seen on the lateral view.

(irregular border) (see Fig. 24-7, *B*). In the lateral view, excessive remodeling gives the bone an elongated appearance (see Fig. 24-6, *B* and *C*). Caution should be exercised because improperly positioned lateral views may artifactually distort the bone profile. Similarly, normal variants exist that resemble remodeling laterally when angular dorsoproximal-palmarodistal images are normal.[29]

Distal Border Changes

The radiolucent invaginations along the distal border of the navicular bone are called synovial invaginations or synovial fossae (previously referred to as "vascular channels"). These are best seen in the dorsal 65-degree proximal-palmarodistal view. They are normally inverted cone to columnar in shape. Increased size and number are physiologic changes related to type and frequency of work.[2,3] A change in shape to a lollipop or mushroom is considered a signal of abnormal degenerative change (see Fig. 24-7, *C*).[29,30,40] These abnormal synovial invaginations may be a sign of arthrosis of the distal interphalangeal joint, albeit a navicular manifestation. The presence of synovial invaginations in the extremities of the navicular bone has been considered abnormal by some, but they do not correlate with lameness.[34]

Horses with clinical navicular disease have a high incidence of abnormal synovial invaginations, but their clinical specificity remains uncertain. This is because lollipop-shaped synovial invaginations have been reported in 11% of normal horses, and no correlation exists with degree of lameness in confirmed navicular lameness.[34]

Radiolucent changes of the distal border cannot be seen well in lateromedial views. The palmaroproximal-palmarodistal view, however, projects them end-on within the trabecular portion of the bone. Increases in size of visible fossae in this view are abnormal (see Fig. 24-8).[8,9] The range of normal shape variation of fossae for this view, however, has not been established.

Mineralization associated with the distal sesamoidean impar ligament is another degenerative change. The significance of this is similar to that of enthesophytes involving the proximal border. Occasionally, osseous bodies can be seen associated with the distal border. These can be seen in normal and lame horses alike. Small osseous fragments occasionally indicate chip fractures of the distal border and are discussed in the section on navicular fractures. Small osseous fragments of the distal border are best seen in the angular dorsoproximal-palmarodistal views.

Flexor Cortex Changes

Gross pathologic involvement of the navicular flexor fibrocartilage is varied. Lesions include yellowish discoloration, cartilage thinning, focal erosions, and cartilage ulcerations, with or without subchondral bone involvement.[5,26,30] Some of the abnormalities may be age-related phenomena, but all have been seen in navicular disease to varying degrees.[24,26]

Bursa, tendon, and cartilage changes are not usually seen radiographically; only subchondral bone defects are routinely detectable. Early osseous lesions are best seen on the palmaroproximal-palmarodistal view, whereas severe defects may be recognized in other views as well. A reliable radiographic sign consists of focal or diffuse subchondral bone cortical lysis (see Fig. 24-9).[8] Flexor cortex erosions are rarely seen in sound horses and have a significant correlation to the presence and degree of lameness.[2,23,34] Large, discrete flexor cortical erosions may simulate medullary cystlike lesions in the dorsopalmar view. Localization of such cystlike lesions radiographically is vital. Flexor cortical erosions are often associated with tendinous adhesions, whereas medullary cysts are not.[30,38] This added information may be important in the overall management of the animal. Navicular variants of a flat central eminence and a crescent lucency within the cortex of the central eminence exist (see Fig. 24-8). These are normal variations and should not be misdiagnosed as navicular degeneration. Well-positioned lateral radiographs depict the flexor cortex in profile axially. Minor dimpling of the central eminence in this view may be a normal variant or may be the result of geometric distortion. Abrupt irregular cavitations are

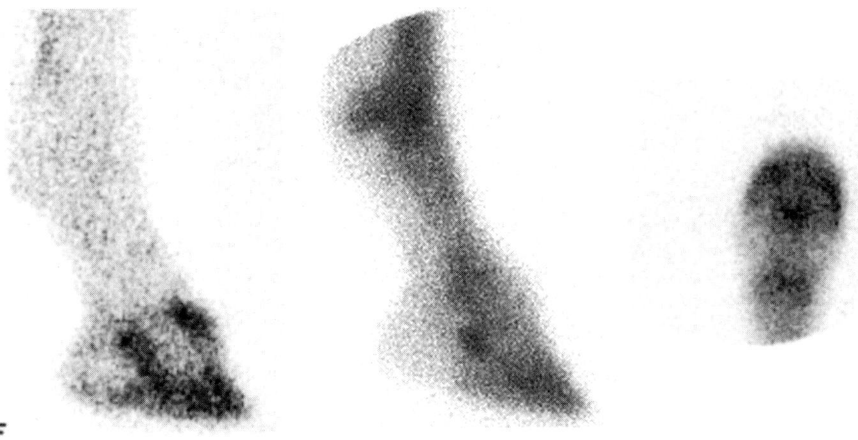

Fig. 24-10 Static images of the right front foot of a horse presented for evaluation of foot pain. The image at *left* is a soft tissue phase lateral view of the distal limb obtained within 5 minutes of the injection of approximately 120 mCi of technetium-99m hydroxyethylene diphosphonate. The images at *center* and *right* are lateral and solar views of the same foot, obtained approximately 1 hour later. Notice the increased focal uptake in the region of the navicular bone, apparent on all views. The uptake at the level of the coronary band on the soft tissue image is normal.

abnormal (see Fig. 24-6, *D*). Abnormalities of the flexor cortex observed on a lateral radiograph should be further evaluated by the palmaroproximal-palmarodistal view.

Dystrophic mineralization of the deep digital flexor tendon may be seen in conjunction with flexor erosions. This finding is reported rarely and indicates severe tendon degeneration, rendering a poor prognosis.[37,41] Faint visualization of the deep digital flexor tendon on the lateral view is a frequent normal finding. Diseased tendons that are sufficiently mineralized may be seen in both lateral and palmaroproximal-palmarodistal views.

Medullary Cavity Changes

Medullary trabecular disruption in the form of trabecular lysis or cystlike cavitations is abnormal. This is rarely seen in sound horses (see Fig. 24-7, *D*). These radiolucencies may be seen on the angular dorsoproximal-palmarodistal, palmaroproximal-palmarodistal, and occasionally lateral views. They range in size from 0.5 to 1.5 cm and are round to oval. They usually are single but may be multiple. Marginal sclerosis is variable, ranging from complete to none at all.

Lytic lesions located within the middle or distal phalanx may be superimposed over the navicular bone. By evaluating other views or repeating the dorsoproximal-palmarodistal view at a different angle, whether the suspect lesion changes in position or remains associated with the navicular bone may possibly be seen. Similarly, lucent artifacts that result from air trapped in the frog by packing material, or from focal gas in the hoof wall or sole from a surface defect or abscess, may be misinterpreted as radiolucent bone lesions. Air pockets usually present as linear radiolucent shadows. When doubt exists, the frog should be repacked.

Extensive erosions of the flexor cortex can falsely mimic medullary cavity cysts on angular dorsoproximal-palmarodistal views. On a palmaroproximal-palmarodistal view, the suspect lesion can be localized regarding whether it originates from the flexor cortex or the medullary cavity (see Fig. 24-9, *B* and *C*). Localization of such lesions is also possible on a lateral projection (see Fig. 24-6, *D*).

Sclerosis of the medullary spongiosa is said to be an early finding in horses lame because of navicular disease.[2,8,34] This is seen as a fine trabecular pattern that blends with the flexor cortex, resulting in an indistinct interface between the flexor cortex and the medullary spongiosa (see Fig. 24-9, *D*).[2,8] This finding is not reliable because it can often be seen in normal horses as a result of a poorly positioned radiograph (see Fig. 24-8, *D*).[2,34,42,43] When present, it is observed on both the lateral and palmaroproximal-palmarodistal views; therefore these views should always be examined in conjunction.[44]

Normal Radiographic Findings

Many horses with clinical navicular lameness have normal radiographs.[19] These animals may have disease that better falls into the category of navicular bursitis or other nonosseous causes of heel pain. Before this conclusion is reached, however, an adequate number of high-quality radiographs should be obtained.

Technetium-99m bone scintigraphy is an extremely valuable adjunct when radiographic findings are equivocal or when the bone is normal but disease of the navicular soft tissues is suspected. This is true because nuclear scintigraphy is more sensitive than radiography in identifying early soft tissue and bone abnormalities, although a scintigram provides primarily physiologic as opposed to anatomic information. Because physiologic alterations associated with navicular degeneration are likely to precede gross anatomic changes, scintigraphy of the navicular bone should be done when clinical signs are compatible with navicular lameness but radiographs are normal (Fig. 24-10).[45]

FRACTURES

Navicular fractures are infrequently reported; therefore data are not available from which to draw firm conclusions about their incidence and pathophysiology. Most navicular fractures are traumatic or pathologic in origin. Both chip and complete fracture types have been described. A diagram of navicular fractures is shown in Figure 24-11.

Care should be taken to avoid misinterpreting artifacts as navicular fractures. The sulci of the frog may cast overlying linear radiolucent shadows in the dorsoproximal-palmarodistal projection that simulate complete navicular fracture. This situation occurs when the foot is unpacked or when air is trapped in the sulcus by packing material. Sulcal lines typically extend beyond the periphery of the navicular bone. Complete fractures are confined to the bone and are seen on dorsoproximal-palmarodistal and palmaroproximal-palmarodistal views. Gravel or debris in the foot or a foot with scaly horn may simulate chip fractures. With proper hoof preparation (cleaning, paring, and packing), these artifacts can be eliminated. Lateral views or dorsoproximal-palmarodistal radiographs made at different angles help localize a suspect opacity. When in doubt about navicular fractures, the hoof should be cleaned and repacked before more radiographs are made.

Osseous Fragments of the Distal Border

Small osseous fragments associated with the distal border of the navicular bone and impar ligament are occasionally seen. They

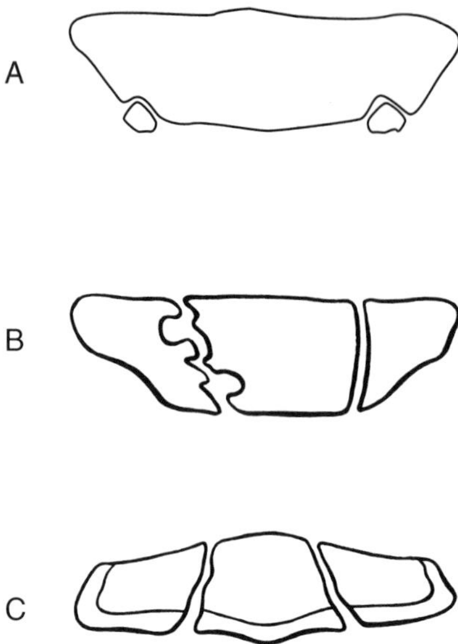

Fig. 24-11 Types of navicular fractures. **A,** Chip fractures of the distal navicular border, dorsal 65-degree proximal-palmarodistal projection. **B** and **C,** Complete navicular fractures: dorsal 65-degree proximal-palmarodistal and palmaroproximal-palmarodistal projections, respectively.

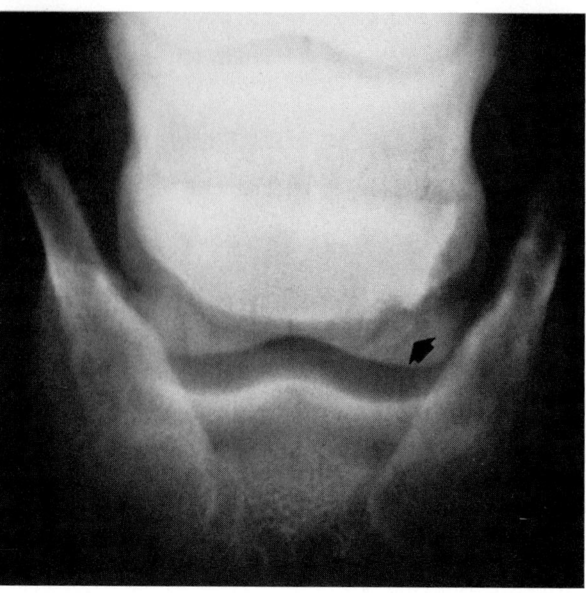

Fig. 24-12 Chip fracture at the distal navicular border. The small fragment *(arrow)* and the underlying fracture bed can be seen.

are usually identified on the dorsoproximal-palmarodistal view but may also be seen superimposed over the medullary cavity of the navicular bone on the palmaroproximal-palmarodistal projection. These osseous bodies have more than one pathogenesis. They may be caused by chip fractures, damage to the impar ligament with secondary mineralization, separate centers of ossification within the impar ligament, or synovial osseous metaplasia.[31,38] When present, osseous bodies may be unilateral or bilateral, involve both the medial and lateral aspects of the bone, or involve only one side of the bone. Larger fragments are most often found on the medial side of the bone.

Osseous bodies that are true chip fractures may appear as small (0.2 to 1.2 cm), rectangular bone fragments separated from the distal border by a radiolucent zone. A fracture bed within the navicular bone corresponding in size and shape to the fragment is often seen.[46] Dystrophic mineralization of the impar ligament may have a similar appearance, but a fracture bed is not seen.

The presence of osseous bodies does not always indicate navicular disease, but an association has been noted by some investigators.[23] These bodies have not been shown to influence clinical signs or prognosis of navicular disease (Fig. 24-12).

Complete Fractures

Complete navicular fractures may occur in normal or diseased navicular bones.[13,47-53] They are most frequently seen in the forelimb, but hindlimb fractures have been reported.[52] Initiating causes include direct navicular trauma and repeated concussive forces on a pathologic navicular bone in a neurectomized patient. Lameness associated with complete fracture is usually acute, but may be chronic, and is moderate to severe. In general, the long-term prognosis for competitive performance is poor.[46] Postmortem studies of limited numbers of fractured navicular bones show fibrous unions between the fragments.[48] Variable instability is inherent because of the hingelike motion allowed by the fibrous component.

Usually, one or two vertical or oblique fracture lines may be seen within the body or at the body-extremity junction of the navicular bone. A prominent fracture line is usually present. Fracture fragments have irregular to smooth margins and are minimally displaced. Occasionally, fragments have mild degenerative changes of bony resorption and sclerosis adjacent to the fracture line (Fig. 24-13). Healing is thought to occur from a noncalcified fibrous union because bony union is not observed radiographically, regardless of fracture duration. Absence of periosteum and progenitor cells, constant fragment motion, and influx of regional synovial fluid are all thought to play a role in navicular fracture healing with fibrous rather than bony union.[54]

Multipartite Navicular Bone

What appear to be bilaterally symmetric fractures are occasionally seen in minimally lame animals with otherwise normal navicular bones. This finding has fostered the belief that the lines represent multiple navicular bone ossification centers that have not fused. Congenital multipartite sesamoids are occasional, incidental findings in other species. Although the navicular bone develops from a single ossification center, aberrant formation is theoretically possible.[1] Radiographic differentiation between a congenitally multipartite navicular bone and a chronic fracture is impossible. Radiographically, multipartite (bipartite or tripartite) sesamoid bones are often bilateral. Individual fragments have smooth, rounded margins with wide radiolucent gaps between. In addition, multiple ossification centers initially cause no to minimal lameness. If instability is present, however, degenerative changes resulting in lameness may occur (see Fig. 24-13).

In some lame horses, a multipartite navicular bone also undergoes changes that are compatible with advanced navicular degeneration. This circumstance has two plausible explanations. One is that a pathologic fracture of a primarily diseased bone has occurred. Another is that fracture or multiple ossification centers are present initially. The resultant instability causes chronic secondary degenerative changes. Thus, when a multipartite sesamoid navicular bone is seen in conjunction with severe degenerative navicular changes, determining whether the navicular bone is fractured or multipartite is difficult (see Fig. 24-13). When marked distortion of the individual fragments is present or when multiple navicular bones are involved, a multipartite development is likely. A case of bipartite navicular bone has also been reported in association with bipartite distal phalanx.[55]

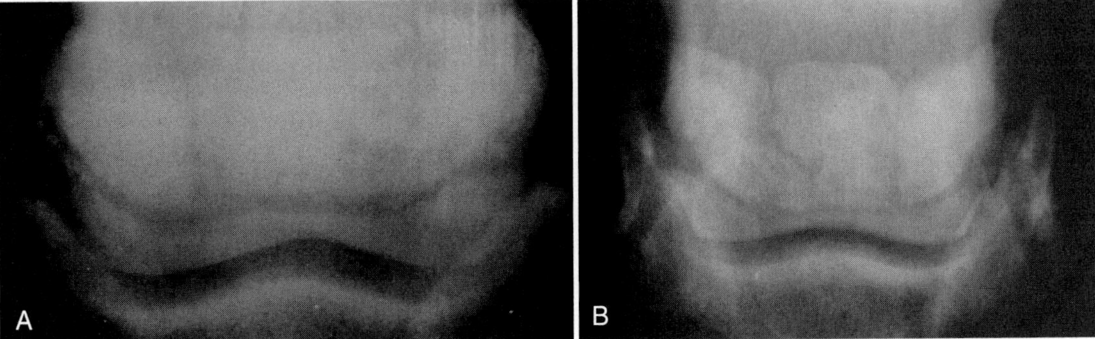

Fig. 24-13 A, Complete navicular bone fractures. The left fracture line is seen as a discrete linear lucent defect; the right fracture is seen as a broad lucent zone separating the right eminence from the body of the navicular bone. **B,** Tripartite navicular bone; notice the smooth margins of the navicular fragments. This was a mature horse with tripartite naviculars in both front feet and minimal lameness. (Courtesy of Dr. Robert J. Bahr, Oklahoma State University, Stillwater, Okla.)

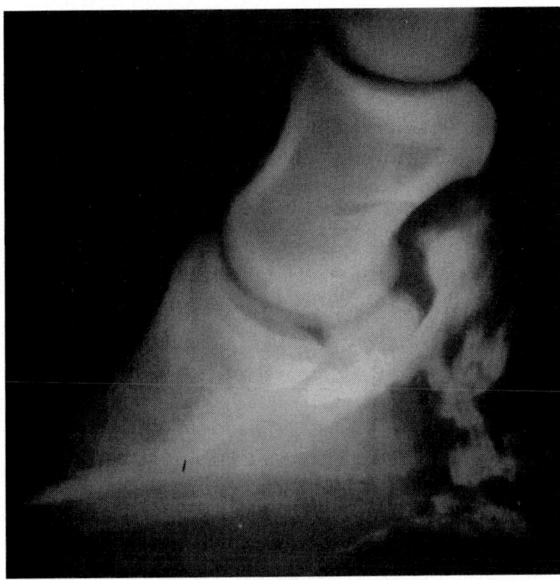

Fig. 24-14 Fistulogram after a nail puncture wound. The tract communicates with the navicular bursa.

NAVICULAR SEPSIS

Navicular sepsis may result from penetrating puncture wounds or deep lacerations that involve the bursa or the bone itself. Radiographic signs relative to the navicular bone occurring after a puncture wound to the navicular bursa vary. The length of time between the initial injury and the first radiographic evaluation influences the findings.[56]

If a horse presents within 3 weeks of injury and initial radiographs are negative, a fistulogram or radiograph made after insertion of a blunt probe should be considered. This examination helps establish if the puncture wound involves the navicular bursa or bone (Fig. 24-14). This is important because a puncture wound that involves the bone or bursa warrants a more cautious prognosis and more vigorous therapy because osteomyelitis may result. A negative fistulogram does not eliminate the possibility that the navicular bone or bursa was involved in the initial injury because partial tract healing in the deeper areas of the wound could prevent passage of contrast medium during fistulography, resulting in a falsely negative study.

Regardless of whether a fistulogram is performed during the initial evaluation, follow-up radiographs should be made within the subsequent 3 to 12 weeks because radiographic evidence of navicular infection may take 6 weeks or longer to become apparent. Also, an estimated 50% of horses with navicular sepsis that have initially negative radiographs subsequently develop radiographic signs of bone infection. Once present, navicular osteomyelitis may progress and result in serious complications, leading to chronic lameness that may eventually necessitate euthanasia.

Of the standard projections to evaluate the navicular bone, the lateral and palmaroproximal-palmarodistal views are more valuable than the angled dorsoproximal-palmarodistal views in detecting and staging osteomyelitis of the navicular bone.

Initial radiographic signs of navicular bone infection appear as focal areas of decreased opacity in the flexor cortical bone with disruption and irregularity of the flexor surface. These lesions are often initially located abaxial to the central eminence. The greater the duration of the injury without treatment, the more extensive the disease will be in terms of depth of the irregularity into the navicular bone and its abaxial extent.

More severe long-term findings associated with puncture wounds and navicular osteomyelitis include septic arthritis of the distal interphalangeal joint (Fig. 24-15), secondary joint disease, pathologic fracture of the navicular bone, and subluxation of the distal interphalangeal joint. Rupture of the deep digital flexor tendon or navicular impar ligament causes subluxation of the distal interphalangeal joint, which may only be observed during weight bearing. In some horses, degenerative changes similar to those seen in navicular disease have been observed as long-term sequelae.

MISCELLANEOUS CONDITIONS

Another condition that affects the navicular bone is degenerative arthritis. The navicular bone participates in forming the distal interphalangeal joint. The articular border of the navicular bone adjacent to the middle phalanx is normally rounded. Periarticular osteophytes can be seen that result in subtle, pointed, spurlike projections. These have been seen in sound horses as well as in horses lame from navicular disease; thus their significance is uncertain. Reports of significant pathologic processes involving the articular cartilage in navicular disease are rare.[26] However, some changes seen in navicular degeneration are believed to be a form of distal interphalangeal joint arthrosis.[26,27,29]

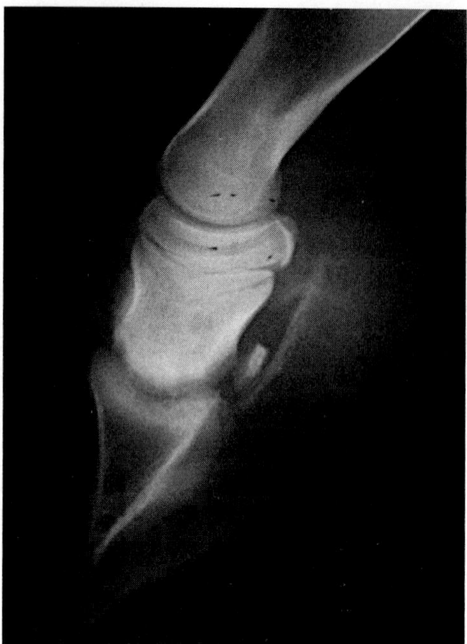

Fig. 24-15 Lateral forefoot of a young horse 4 weeks after a nail puncture of the navicular bursa. Septic arthritis of the distal interphalangeal joint, osteolysis and displacement of the navicular bone, and dystrophic mineralization of the deep digital flexor tendon are present.

Congenital absence of the navicular bone (agenesis) has been reported.[57,58]

ULTRASONOGRAPHIC EVALUATION OF THE NAVICULAR BONE AND ASSOCIATED SOFT TISSUE STRUCTURES

Sonography of the navicular bone and associated soft tissue structures has been of limited use because of the inability to penetrate the hoof wall with conventional ultrasound imaging equipment. The proximal aspect of the navicular bone can be visualized by way of the palmar aspect of the middle phalanx just proximal to the bulbs of the heels, but it provides information limited to the paired proximal suspensory ligaments, proximal margin of the navicular bone, and proximal portion of the tendon of insertion of the deep digital flexor muscle. Approach to the podotrochlear apparatus (navicular bone, collateral and impar ligaments of the navicular bone, distal deep digital flexor tendon, and podotrochlear bursa) through the frog (referred to as the transcuneal approach) has been recently described. The procedure requires trimming the dry superficial layers of the frog to moist pliable tissue, producing a wide central cuneal sulcus. The foot is then soaked in warm water for 10 to 15 minutes up to 12 hours to hydrate the frog, creating an acoustic window to the navicular bone and its distal attachments. Mechanical, fixed curvilinear, linear, or phased-array transducers may be used with a frequency range of 6 to 10 MHz.[59,60] Sagittal, parasagittal, and transverse scans are performed. Structures visible on the longitudinal views include the palmar surfaces of the distal phalanx and fibrocartilage of the navicular bone, distal palmar recess of the distal interphalangeal joint, impar ligament, bursa, deep digital flexor tendon, and digital cushion. Transverse scans provide visualization of the palmar fibrocartilage of the navicular bone, navicular bursa, the fibrocartilaginous and fibrous parts of the deep digital flexor tendon, distal digital annular ligament, and digital cushion (Figs. 24-16 and 24-17).[59]

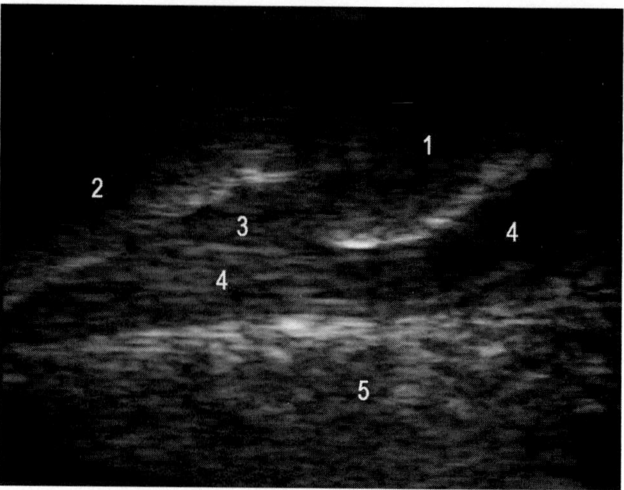

Fig. 24-16 Sagittal ultrasonographic image of the podotrochlear apparatus obtained with a linear probe by the transcuneal approach. *1*, Navicular bone; *2*, distal phalanx; *3*, distal impair sesamoidean ligament; *4*, deep digital flexor tendon; *5*, digital cushion. (Courtesy of Dr. Valeria Busoni, Université de Liège, Liège, Belgium.)

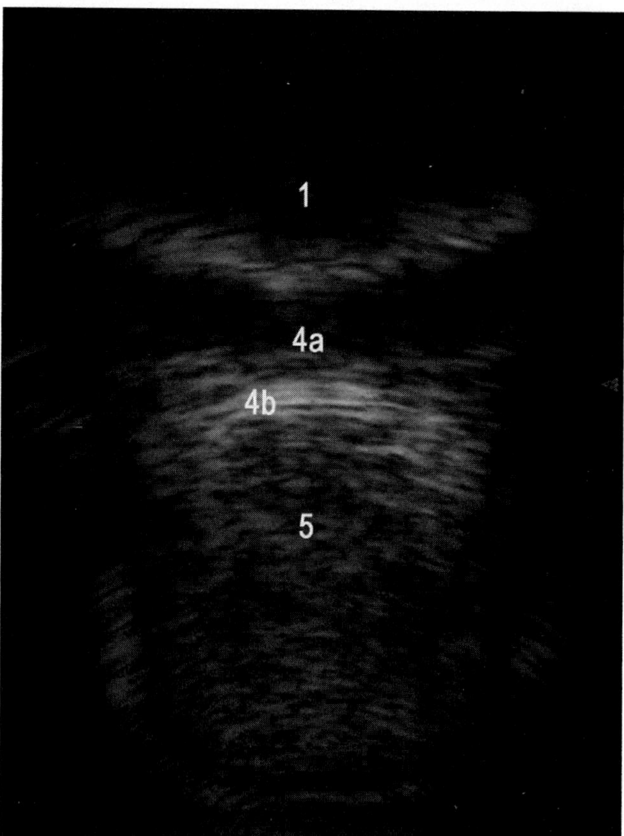

Fig. 24-17 Transverse ultrasonographic image of the podotrochlear apparatus obtained with a microconvex probe using the transcuneal approach at the level of the navicular bone. *1*, Navicular bone; *4a*, fibrocartilaginous portion of the deep digital flexor tendon; *4b*, fibrous portion of the deep digital flexor tendon; *5*, digital cushion. (Courtesy of Dr. Valeria Busoni, Université de Liège, Liège, Belgium.)

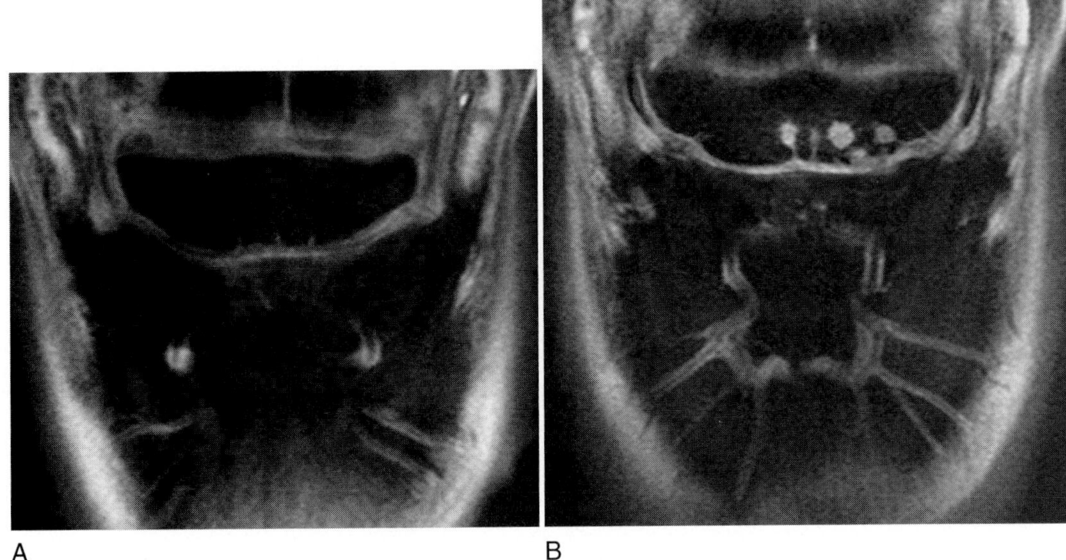

Fig. 24-18 A, Dorsal plane STIR image of a normal navicular bone; notice the small, conical hyperintense synovial invaginations. **B,** Dorsal plane gradient echo image of the navicular bone showing enlarged lollipop-shaped synovial invaginations and irregular margination of the medial aspect of the distal border of the navicular bone. (Courtesy of Dr. Russell L. Tucker, Washington State University, Pullman, Wash.)

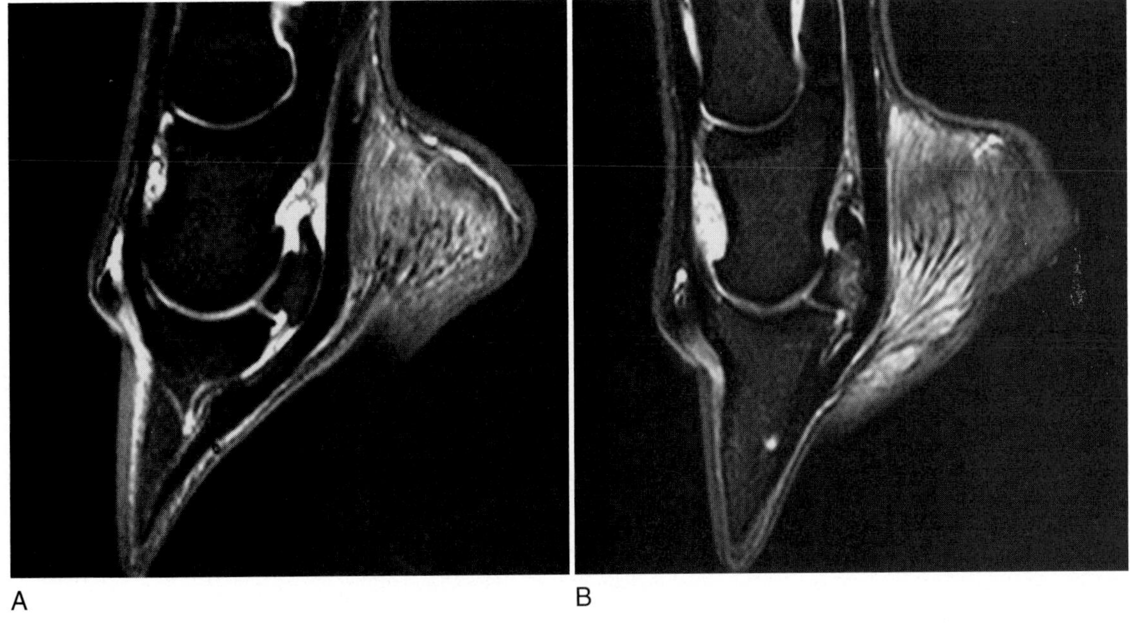

Fig. 24-19 Sagittal plane STIR images of the foot and navicular bone. **A,** Normal navicular bone. **B,** Increased fluid signal within the navicular bone, indicating marrow edema. Notice the thickening of the suspensory navicular ligament. (Courtesy of Dr. Russell L. Tucker, Washington State University, Pullman, Wash.)

MAGNETIC RESONANCE AND COMPUTED TOMOGRAPHIC EVALUATION OF THE NAVICULAR BONE

In recent years, computed tomographic (CT) imaging and magnetic resonance (MR) imaging have become more available in equine medicine. In addition, the development of open magnets that allow imaging of the standing horse, without the need for general anesthesia, has made MR imaging especially popular for the investigation of foot pain. MR and CT imaging have been shown to allow visualization of the size, shape, and position of the synovial invaginations better than radiography (Fig. 24-18).[61] Osseous changes and changes in surface contour (lateral wings, articular and flexor surface) are better seen with CT,[43,61,62] and in one study CT was speculated to be more reliable than conventional radiography in assessing the flexor surface of the navicular bone.[42] Deep digital flexor tendon lesions associated with navicular changes have been identified with both CT and MR imaging but are best seen by MR imaging.[61] In general, MR imaging is a more powerful modality for the depiction of soft tissue lesions, including loss of signal of fibrocartilage, distension of the navicular bursa and/or of the distal interphalangeal joint (with or without chronic inflammation), distension of the digital tendon sheath, and surface and core defects of the deep digital flexor tendon and impair ligament.[43,61,63,64] In addition, MR imaging can allow detection of abnormal signal within the navicular bone marrow (Fig. 24-19), navicular enthesophytes, and evidence of mineralized fragments within the impair ligament.[63,64] Sequences used for navicular imaging in clinical patients include three-dimensional (3D) T1-weighted spoiled gradient echo (SPGR) imaging, 3D T2* gradient echo (GRE) imaging, and short tau inversion recovery (STIR) or fat-saturated 3D T2* GRE in the sagittal, dorsal, and transverse planes.[63,65] GRE and SPGR have the advantages of allowing 3D acquisition and a sufficiently short acquisition time for practical clinical scanning compared with spin echo or fast spin echo sequences. Fat suppression techniques are used to reduce interference from fat signal and are especially useful in detecting bone medullary fluid (see Figs. 24-18, *A*, and 24-19).

MR and CT imaging are superior to conventional radiography for navicular imaging, facilitating earlier and more accurate diagnosis.[43,61] However, the relative merits of CT and MR imaging in the evaluation of foot pain in the horse have yet to be fully determined.[63]

REFERENCES

1. Getty R: *Sisson and Grossman's the anatomy of the domestic animals*, Philadelphia, 1975, W.B. Saunders.
2. Kaser-Hotz B, Ueltschi G: Radiographic appearance of the navicular bone in sound horses, *Vet Radiol Ultrasound* 33:9, 1992.
3. Colles CM, Hickman J: The arterial supply of the navicular bone and its variations in navicular disease, *Equine Vet J* 9:150, 1977.
4. Bowker RM, Ruckershouser SJ, Kelly BV et al: Immunocytochemical and dye distribution studies of nerves potentially desensitized by injections into the distal interphalangeal joint of the navicular bursa of horses, *J Am Vet Med Assoc* 203:1708, 1993.
5. Oxspring GE: The radiology of navicular disease with observations on its pathology, *Vet Rec* 15:1434, 1935.
6. Campbell JR, Lee R: Radiological techniques in the diagnosis of navicular disease, *Equine Vet J* 4:135, 1972.
7. Watrous BJ: *A guide to equine field radiography*, Trenton, NJ, 1995, Veterinary Learning Systems, p 13.
8. O'Brien TR, Millman TM, Pool RR et al: Navicular disease in the Thoroughbred horse: a morphologic investigation relative to a new radiographic projection, *J Am Vet Radiol Soc* 16:39, 1975.
9. Rose RJ, Taylor BJ, Steel JD: Navicular disease in the horse: an analysis of seventy cases and assessment of a special radiographic view, *J Equine Med Surg* 2:492, 1978.
10. Dik K, van den Broek J: Role of navicular bone shape in the pathogenesis of navicular disease: a radiological study, *Equine Vet J* 27:390, 1995.
11. Poulos P, Brown A: On navicular disease in the horse: a roentgenological and patho-anatomic study: I. Evaluation of the flexor central eminence, *Vet Radiol* 30:50, 1989.
12. Berry C, Pool R, Stover S et al: A radiographic/morphologic investigation of a radiolucent crescent within the flexor central eminence of the navicular bone in the Thoroughbred. In *Proceedings of the American College of Veterinary Radiology Annual Meeting,* Nov 29-Dec 1, 1990, Chicago.
13. Dyson SJ, Kidd L: A comparison of responses to analgesia of the navicular bursa and intra-articular analgesia of the distal interphalangeal joint in 59 horses, *Equine Vet J* 25:93, 1993.
14. Schumacher J, Steiger R, Schumacher J et al: Effects of analgesia of the distal interphalangeal joint of palmar digital nerves on lameness caused by solar pain in horses, *Vet Surg* 29:54, 2000.
15. Stashak TS, editor: *Adam's lameness in horses*, ed 4, Philadelphia, 1987, Lea and Febiger, p 499.
16. Rose RJ: *The treatment of navicular disease—a review and current concepts.* Presented at the 29th Annual Convention of the American Association of Equine Practitioners, December 1983, Las Vegas, NV.
17. Valdez H, Adams OR, Peyton LC: Navicular disease in the hindlimbs of the horse, *J Am Vet Med Assoc* 172:291, 1978.
18. Ackerman N, Johnson JH, Dorn CR: Navicular disease in the horse: risk factors, radiographic changes, and response to therapy, *J Am Vet Med Assoc* 170:183, 1977.
19. Wright IM: A study of 118 cases of navicular disease: clinical features, *Equine Vet J* 25:488, 1993.
20. Pool RR, Meagher DM, Stover SM: Pathophysiology of navicular syndrome, *Vet Clin North Am Equine Pract* 5:109, 1989.
21. Wilkinson GT: The pathology of navicular disease, *Br Vet J* 109:38, 1953.
22. Smith F: The pathology of navicular disease, *Vet J* 23:72, 1886.
23. Wright IM, Kidd J, Thorp BH: Gross histological, histomorphometric features of the navicular bone and related structures in the horse, *Equine Vet J* 30:220, 1998.
24. Colles CM: Ischaemic necrosis of the navicular bone and its treatment, *Vet Rec* 104:133, 1979.
25. Fricker CH, Riek W, Hugelshofer J: Occlusion of the digital arteries: a model for pathogenesis of navicular disease, *Equine Vet J* 14:203, 1982.
26. Doige CE, Hoffer MA: Pathologic changes in the navicular bone and associated structures of the horse, *Can J Comp Med* 47:387, 1983.
27. Svalastoga E: Navicular disease in the horse: a microangiographic investigation, *Nord Vet Med* 35:131, 1983.
28. Ostblom L, Lund C, Melsen F: Histologic study of navicular bone disease, *Equine Vet J* 14:199, 1982.
29. Poulos PW, Smith MF: The nature of enlarged "vascular channels" in the navicular bone of the horse, *Vet Radiol* 2:60, 1988.
30. Svalastoga E, Reimann I, Nielsen K: Changes of the fibrocartilage in navicular disease in horses, *Nord Vet Med* 35:373, 1983.
31. Svalastoga E, Neilsen K: Navicular disease in the horse: the synovial membrane of bursa podotrochlearis, *Nord Vet Med* 35:28, 1983.
32. Svalastoga E, Smith M: Navicular disease in the horse: the subchondral bone pressure, *Nord Vet Med* 35:31, 1983.
33. Colles CM: *Concepts of blood flow in the aetiology and treatment of navicular disease.* Presented at the 29th Annual Convention of the American Association of Equine Practitioners, December 1983, Las Vegas, NV.
34. Wright IM: A study of 118 cases of navicular disease: radiological features, *Equine Vet J* 25:493, 1993.
35. Turner T, Kneller S, Badertscher R et al: Radiographic changes in the navicular bones of normal horses. In *Proceedings of the 32nd Annual Meeting of the American Association of Equine Practitioners,* Nashville, TN, 1986, p 309.

36. Huskamp B, Becker M: Diagnose und prognose der röntgenologischen Veranderungen an den Strahl-beinen der Vordergliedma Ben der Pferde unter besonderer Berucksichtigung der Ankau fsuntersuchung: Ein Versuch zur Schematisierung der Befunde, *Praktische Tierarzt* 61:858, 1980.
37. Wright IM: A study of 118 cases of navicular disease: treatment by navicular suspensory desmotomy, *Equine Vet J* 25:501, 1993.
38. Poulos P, Brown A, Brown E et al: On navicular disease in the horse: a roentgenological and patho-anatomic study: II. Osseous bodies associated with the impar ligament, *Vet Radiol* 30:54, 1989.
39. Turner TA: The anatomic, pathologic, and radiographic aspects of navicular disease, *Comp Contin Educ Pract Vet* 4:350, 1982.
40. MacGregor C: Radiographic assessment of navicular bones based on changes in the distal nutrient foramina, *Equine Vet J* 18:203, 1986.
41. Turner TA: Dystrophic calcification of the deep digital flexor tendons resulting from navicular disease, *Vet Med Small Anim Clin* 77:571, 1982.
42. Ruohoniemi M, Teruahartiala P: Computed tomographic evaluation of Finnhorse cadaver forefeet with radiographic problematic findings on the flexor aspect of the navicular bone, *Vet Radiol Ultrasound* 40:275, 1999.
43. Widmer W, Buckwalter K, Fessler J et al: Use of radiography, computed tomography and magnetic resonance imaging for evaluation of navicular syndrome in the horse, *Vet Radiol Ultrasound* 41:108, 2000.
44. De Clercq T, Vershooten F, Ysebaert M: A comparison of the palmaroproximal-palmarodistal view of the isolated navicular bone to other views, *Vet Radiol Ultrasound* 41:525, 2000.
45. Trout DR, Hornof WJ, O'Brien TR: Soft-tissue and bone-phase scintigraphy for diagnosis of navicular disease in horses, *J Am Vet Med Assoc* 198:73, 1991.
46. van De Watering CC, Morgan JP: Chip fractures as a radiologic finding in navicular disease of the horse, *J Am Vet Radiol Soc* 16:206, 1975.
47. Lillich JD, Ruggles AJ, Gabel AA et al: Fracture of the distal sesamoid bone in horses: 17 cases (1982-1992), *J Am Vet Med Assoc* 207:924, 1995.
48. Vaughan LC: Fracture of the navicular bone in the horse, *Vet Rec* 73:895, 1961.
49. Arnbjerg J: Spontaneous fracture of the navicular bone in the horse, *Nord Vet Med* 31:429, 1979.
50. Reeves MJ: Miscellaneous conditions of the equine foot, *Vet Clin North Am Equine Pract* 5:221, 1989.
51. Smythe RH: Fracture of the navicular bone in the horse—comment, *Vet Rec* 73:1009, 1961.
52. Kaser-Hotz B, Ueltshci G, Hess N et al: Navicular bone fractures in the pelvic limb in two horses, *Vet Radiol Ultrasound* 32:283, 1991.
53. Rick MC: Navicular bone fractures. In White NA, Moore JN, editors: *Current practice of equine surgery*, Philadelphia, 1990, J.B. Lippincott, pp 602-605.
54. Vaughn LC: Fractures of the navicular bone, *Vet Rec* 73:95, 1961.
55. Benninger MI, Deiss E, Ueltschi G: Bipartite distal phalanx and navicular bone in an Andalusian stallion, *Vet Radiol Ultrasound* 46:69, 2005.
56. Richardson GL, O'Brien T: Puncture wounds into the navicular bursa of the horse: role of radiographic evaluation, *Vet Radiol* 26:203, 1985.
57. Reid CF: Radiology panel-film interpretation session notes. In *Proceedings of the 22nd Annual Convention of the American Association of Equine Practitioners*, 1976, Dallas, TX.
58. Modransky C, Thatcher C, Welker F et al: Unilateral phalangeal dysgenesis and navicular bone agenesis in a foal, *Equine Vet J* 19:347, 1987.
59. Busoni V, Denoix JM: Ultrasonography of the podotrochlear apparatus in the horse using a transcuneal approach: technique and reference images, *Vet Radiol Ultrasound* 42:534, 2001.
60. Grewal JS, McClure SR, Booth LC et al: Assessment of the ultrasonographic characteristics of the podotrochlear apparatus in clinically normal horses and horses with navicular syndrome, *J Am Vet Med Assoc* 225:1881, 2004.
61. Whitton RC, Buckley C, Donovan T et al: The diagnosis of lameness associated with distal limb pathology in a horse: a comparison of radiography, computed tomography and magnetic resonance imaging, *Vet J* 155:223, 1998.
62. Tietje S: Computed tomography of the navicular bone region in a horse: a comparison with radiographic documentation, *Pferdeheilkunde* 11:51, 1995.
63. Dyson S, Murray R, Schramme M et al: magnetic resonance imaging of the equine foot: 15 horses, *Equine Vet J* 35:18, 2003.
64. Busoni V, Heirmann M, Trenteseaux J et al: Magnetic resonance imaging findings in the equine deep digital flexor tendon and distal sesamoid bone in advanced navicular disease—an ex vivo study, *Vet Radiol Ultrasound* 46:279, 2005.
65. Dyson SJ, Murray R, Schramme MC: Lameness associated with foot pain: results of magnetic resonance imaging in 199 horses (January 2001-December 2003) and response to treatment, *Equine Vet J* 37:113, 2005.

ELECTRONIC RESOURCES evolve

Additional information related to the content in Chapter 24 can be found on the companion Web site at evolve http://evolve.elsevier.com/Thrall/vetrad/

- Key Points
- Chapter Quiz
- Case Study 24-1

SECTION IV

Neck and Thorax

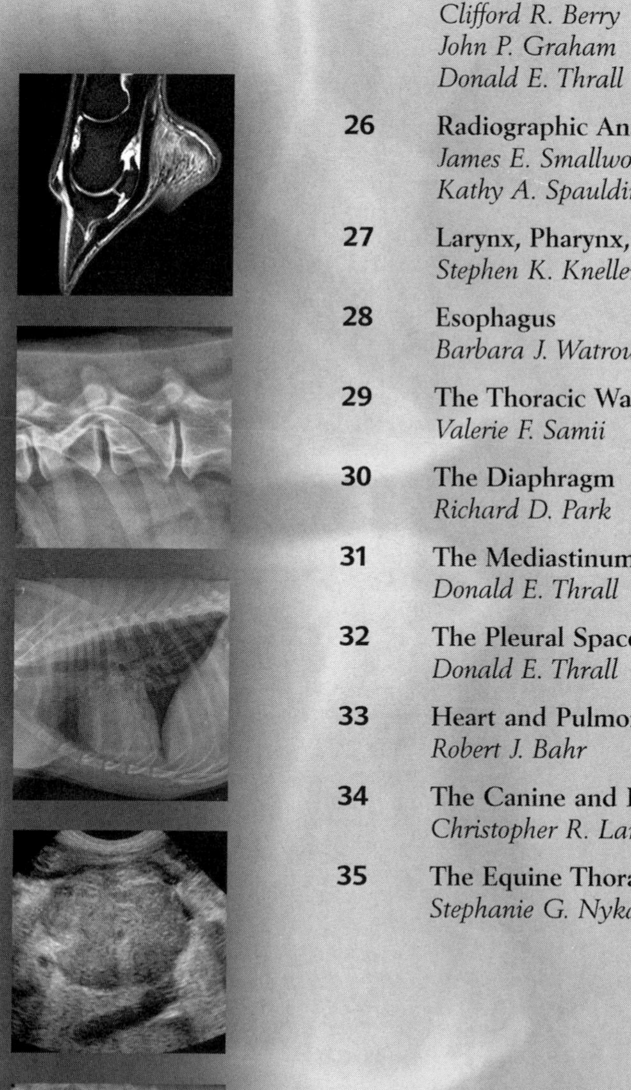

CHAPTER • 25
Interpretation Paradigms for the Small Animal Thorax

Clifford R. Berry
John P. Graham
Donald E. Thrall

RADIOGRAPHIC INTERPRETATION OF THE SMALL ANIMAL THORAX

Overview

This chapter provides a framework for beginning interpreters of radiographs of the thorax. Basic information on how to produce a diagnostic radiograph, recommend views, and a structure for interpretation are presented. This chapter is not intended to be a standalone resource for thoracic radiographic interpretation. Rather, it is an overview of some important principles that will assist the reader in the evaluation of the more detailed chapters that focus on individual regions and diseases.

Thoracic radiographs are one of the most commonly performed radiographic examinations in small animal practice.[1-3] Important information about major medical problems, such as heart disease and cancer, is often obtained from thoracic radiographs. Follow-up radiographs can be used to evaluate clinical response to therapy or progression of disease. Thoracic radiography can also be frustrating in that the technical aspects of obtaining high-quality radiographs are demanding and patient positioning is critical. Also, many radiographic abnormalities are nonspecific. Evaluation of the lung can be frustrating because of low confidence in discerning normal from abnormal and discrimination between various abnormal lung patterns. With experience and an organized approach to interpretation, all these challenges can be overcome.

This chapter presents a review of normal anatomy and pertinent physiology; however, the reader is challenged to think in terms of a radiographic/pathologic correlation. Understanding why certain abnormalities appear as they do will aid in interpretation.

Technique and Positioning

Thoracic radiographic examination must consist of a minimum of two orthogonal radiographs, although a three-view examination (right and left lateral and ventrodorsal [VD] or dorsoventral [DV] radiographs) is becoming the routine standard of care in small animal practice.[4,5] When describing a right versus a left lateral radiograph, the terminology refers to the recumbency of the patient during radiography. In actuality, the correct term for a lateral radiograph made with the patient in right recumbency, a so-called right lateral, based on the "point of entrance to point of exit" principle, is left-right lateral; in practice, however, lateral views are typically named according to the recumbency of the patient.[6] On the other hand, for VD and DV radiographs, the name does describe the actual point of entrance to point of exit path of the x-ray beam and not the recumbency of the patient. For example, a VD radiograph is made with the patient in dorsal recumbency and the point of entrance to exit of the primary x-ray beam is ventral to dorsal through the patient.[7,8]

With film-screen systems, thoracic radiographs should be made with a high kilovoltage peak and low milliampere seconds technique. This will lead to a long contrast scale in a body region having inherent short-scale contrast because of the air in the lung.[1] Using a low kilovoltage peak, high milliampere seconds technique for the thorax will result in excessive image contrast and lesions being overlooked. Once milliampere seconds value has been determined, the highest milliampere and the fastest time should be used to minimize respiratory motion artifact. Radiographs should be obtained on peak inspiration.[9]

In technically adequate radiographs, the thoracic inlet to the caudal most extent of the caudodorsal lung field should be included in the field of view. Occasionally, a 14-inch by 17-inch cassette may not allow inclusion of the entire thorax of a giant breed dog in one image, and each lateral and VD or DV view may have to be divided into cranial and caudal sections to obtain complete coverage. On the lateral radiograph, the thoracic limbs should be pulled as far forward as possible so that the soft tissues of the brachium are not superimposed over the cranial aspect of the thorax. If properly exposed, evaluation of the caudodorsal lung field on the lateral view and the peripheral lung field on the VD/DV view should be possible without the aid of a hot light. Overexposure will give the false impression of a pneumothorax and prevent subtle lung lesions from being seen. A common digital radiographic artifact is oversaturation of the lungs with complete blackening in areas of the right cranial, accessory, and peripheral lung fields.

Making thoracic radiographs on peak inspiration maximizes lung contrast.[9] In panting dogs timing the exposure to respiration may be difficult. Holding the mouth shut for several seconds, bringing the anode to full speed rotation, and then allowing the dog to take a deep inspiration may help synchronize the exposure with inspiration. In a radiograph made at peak inspiration, the caudodorsal aspect of the caudal lung lobes will be caudal to T12, and increased aeration of the accessory lung lobe will be present. This will result in separation of the cardiac silhouette from the diaphragm. The cranial margin of the left cranial lung lobe should extend to the level of the first rib. On the VD/DV radiograph, indicators of inspiration include increased thoracic cavity width and thoracic cavity length, the diaphragmatic cupola (dome) will be caudal to mid-T8 vertebral body and the caudolateral aspect of the caudal lung lobes will be caudal to T10.

The effect of patient positioning on thoracic radiographic appearance must be understood.[6-8] In right lateral radiographs,

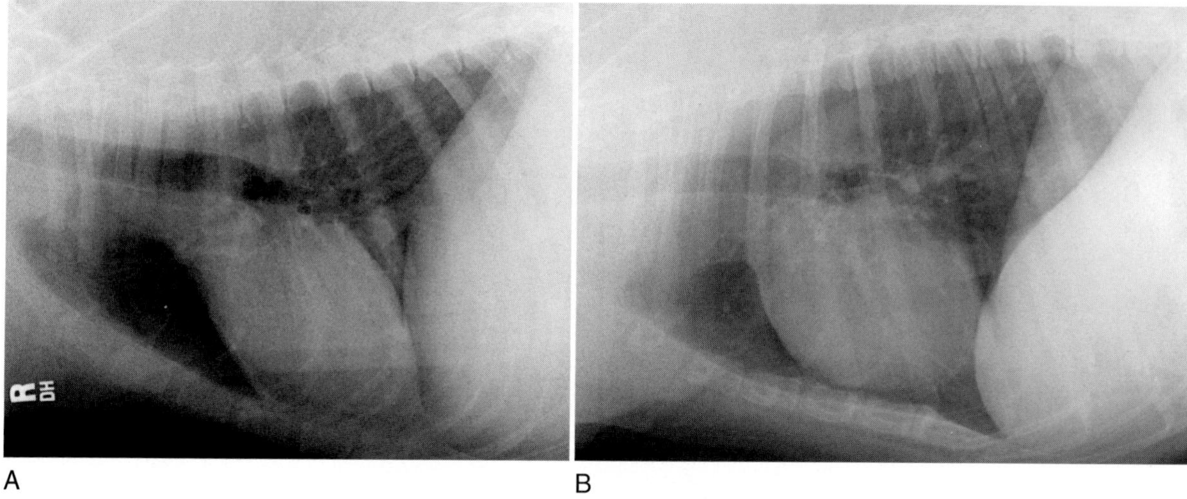

Fig. 25-1 Comparison of right and left lateral thoracic radiographs from an adult dog (Golden Retriever). On the right lateral **(A)** view the diaphragmatic crura are parallel and the right crus is cranial to the left. The heart is oval in shape, and the caudal vena cava insertion is confluent with the most cranial crus (right one). A lesion in the left lung would be better visualized. On the left lateral radiograph **(B)** the diaphragmatic crura diverge as they course dorsally, with the left crus being cranial to the right. The caudal vena cava inserts into the caudal crus. A lesion in the right lung would be better visualized.

the cardiac silhouette is oval or egg shaped (Fig. 25-1). The diaphragmatic crura are usually parallel to each other, with the right crus being more cranial than the left. The right diaphragmatic crus can usually be identified by tracing the dorsal border of the caudal vena cava to the point where it becomes confluent with the right crus at the caval hiatus. Air within the fundus of the stomach may be visible behind the left diaphragmatic crus. Overlap between the right and left cranial lobe pulmonary arteries and veins is common on right lateral radiographs, which will make assessment of the relative size of the pulmonary arteries and veins difficult in this view compared with the left lateral.

In the left lateral radiograph the left diaphragmatic crus in usually more cranial than the right (see Fig. 25-1). The right and left crura diverge from each other as the diaphragm is traced from a ventral to dorsal position. The caudal vena cava can be traced to silhouette with the right crus, usually at a point caudal to the left crus. Food or air within the fundic portion of the stomach can be identified caudal to the left crus. The apex of the cardiac silhouette tends to become displaced from the sternum, giving a circular appearance to the overall cardiac shape. This should not be mistaken as a sign of either right ventricular hypertrophy, in which the cardiac apex may rotate dorsally from the sternum, or pneumothorax, in which the cardiac silhouette is elevated away from the sternum. Distinguishing the right from left cranial lobe pulmonary vessels and pulmonary arteries from pulmonary veins is typically easier in a left lateral than a right lateral radiograph, and relative vessel size is easier to evaluate.

The right and left diaphragmatic crura have a convex appearance (thoracic surface) and are superimposed over the larger convex cupola of the diaphragm (Fig. 25-2) on a VD radiograph.[7,8] The cardiac silhouette tends to be more elongated than in a DV radiograph. Changes in the descending aorta and great vessels are more conspicuous on the VD view, and the accessory lung lobe region between the cardiac silhouette and diaphragm is elongated.

On a DV radiograph the cardiac shape is more oval because of its upright position, and the apex is often displaced to the left by cranial excursion of the diaphragm pushing the heart to the left (see Fig. 25-2).[10] Better visualization of the caudal lobar pulmonary vessels and bronchi can be achieved in the DV view because they are magnified and are more perpendicular to the primary x-ray beam (Fig. 25-3). The accessory lobe region is less aerated in a DV view because of cranial displacement of the diaphragm. These differences between right versus left lateral views and VD versus DV views are more pronounced in medium-size and large dogs and may not be apparent in small dogs and cats.

Other helpful radiographic views of the thorax include oblique radiographs to evaluate rib and pleural abnormalities. Radiographs made with a horizontally directed x-ray beam in which the patient is placed in lateral recumbency or is held in a standing position can take advantage of gravity to move pleural fluid away from areas of interest, such as possible lung masses. The use of a horizontal x-ray beam requires an adjustable x-ray tube head. A common application of horizontal beam radiography is in evaluating cats with severe pleural effusion to determine whether a cranial mediastinal mass is also present. Another useful radiograph is what has been termed the "humanoid" radiograph (Fig. 25-4). This is a VD radiograph in which the thoracic limbs are pulled caudally rather than cranially. This allows the scapula and associated musculature to rotate away from the cranial thorax, providing better visualization of the cranial lung lobes.

One important effect of recumbency is the difference in conspicuity of a lung lesion (mass or infiltrate) depending on whether the lesion is in the dependent or nondependent lung.[11] The dependent lung rapidly becomes less aerated; thus its radiographic opacity increases. The increased opacity of the dependent lung causes the lung to silhouette with any lung lesion that is of soft tissue opacity (Fig. 25-5). Large lesions (4 to 6 cm) in the dependent lung may be invisible radiographically. When the opposite view is obtained, the previously dependent lung quickly becomes aerated, providing contrast for the lesion and allowing it to be visualized.

INTERPRETATION PARADIGM OVERVIEW

The thorax can be divided into four basic anatomic regions: the extrathoracic region, the pleural space, the pulmonary

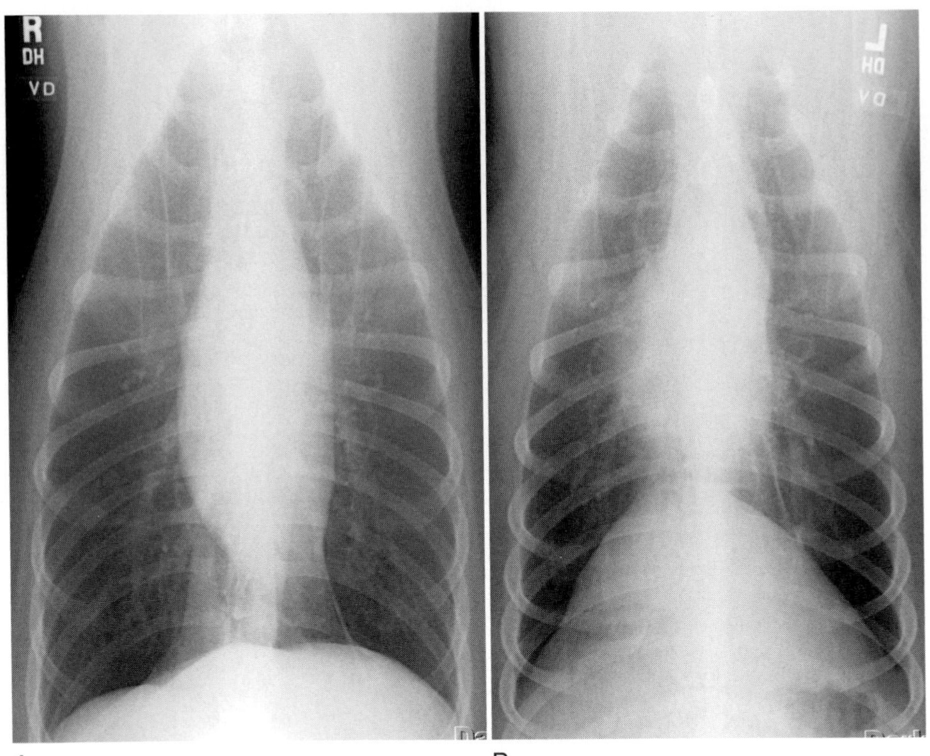

Fig. 25-2 Comparison of VD and DV radiographs from an adult dog. On the VD radiograph **(A)** the cardiac silhouette is more elongated and oval in shape. On the DV radiograph **(B)** the cardiac silhouette is more upright and shorter in the cranial to caudal direction. In **B,** the dome of the diaphragm has moved cranially compared with **A,** and this leads to a lower volume of aerated lung in the DV view. Occasionally in a DV view, the diaphragm will move sufficiently cranial to displace the heart into the left hemithorax.

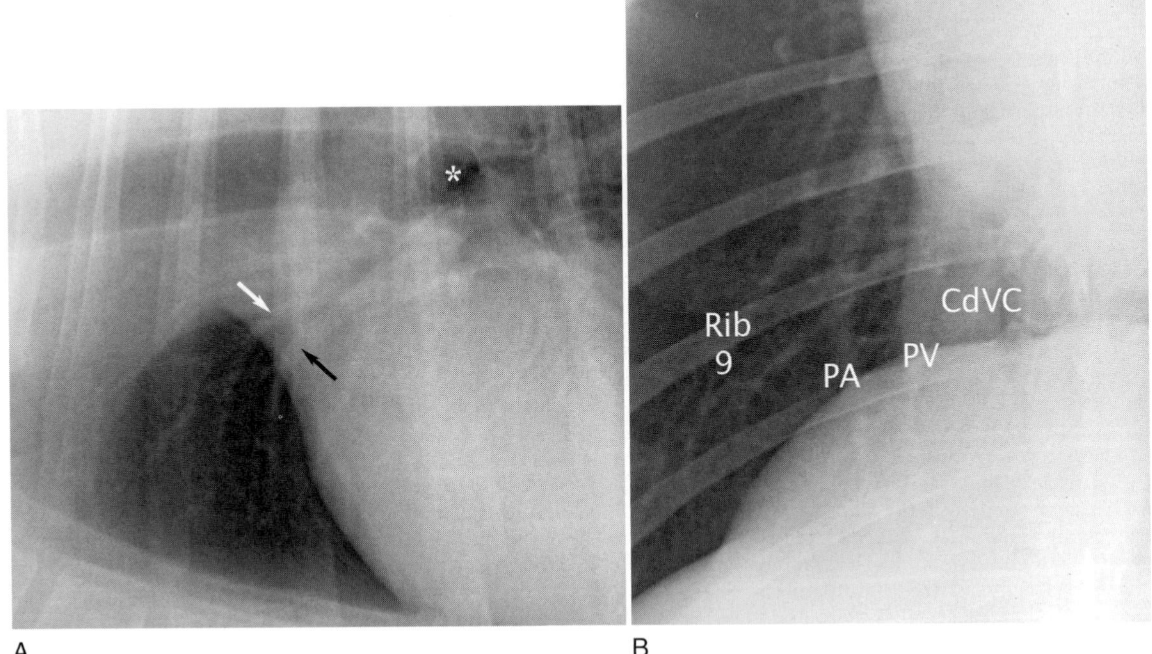

Fig. 25-3 Close-up evaluation of right lateral **(A)** and VD **(B)** radiographs of the thorax from an adult dog. In **A,** the *white arrow* points to the pulmonary artery of the right cranial lung lobe and the *black arrow* points to the pulmonary vein of the right cranial lung lobe. *Asterisk,* Bronchus origin of the right cranial lobe. In **B,** the caudal lobar pulmonary artery (*PA,* lateral), bronchus, and pulmonary vein (*PV,* medial) are clearly visualized. Notice that the vessels form a summation shadow that is the shape of a square as they cross the ninth rib. *CdVC,* Caudal vena cava.

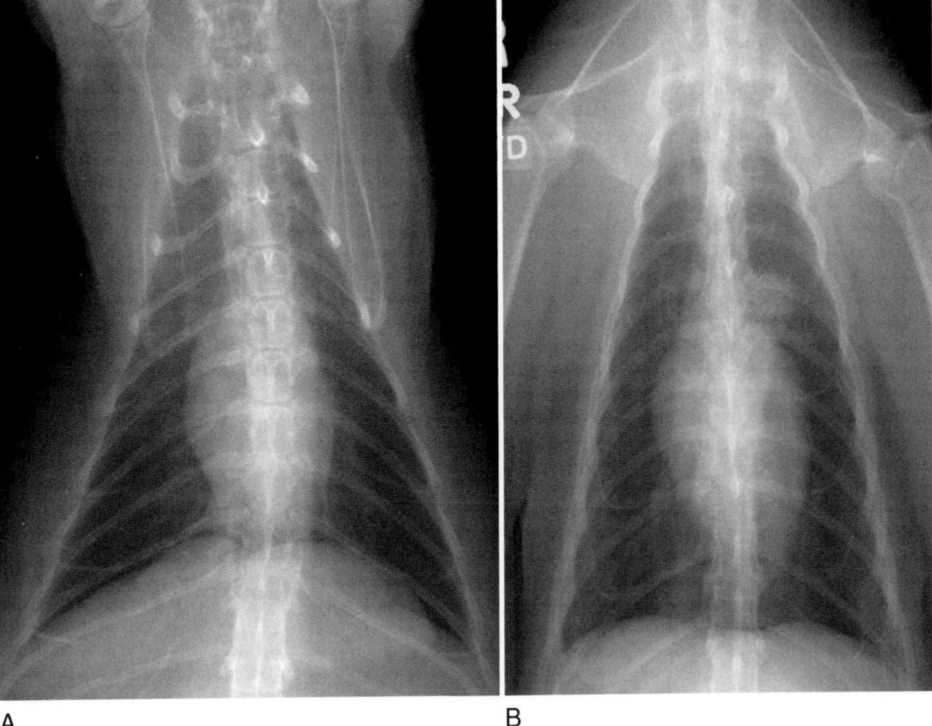

Fig. 25-4 VD radiographs of a feline thorax. **A,** The scapulae are superimposed over the cranial thoracic lung fields, adding opacity to the cranial lobes. **B,** A humanoid radiograph in which the thoracic limbs have been pulled caudally, rotating the scapulae for clear visualization of the cranial lung lobes.

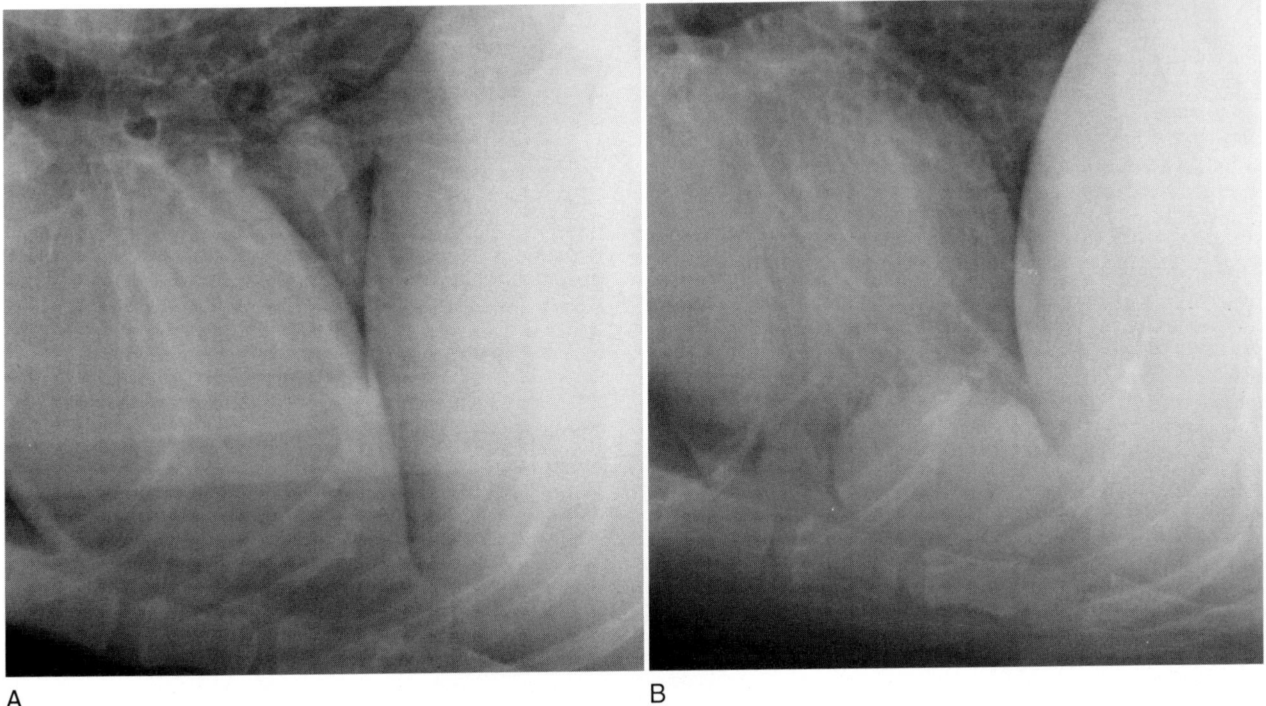

Fig. 25-5 Right lateral **(A)** and left lateral **(B)** radiographs of a dog with a right middle lung lobe mass. The right middle lung lobe mass is peripheral and ventral and is seen only in **B.** This mass could not be identified on the VD radiograph. This affirms the need for routinely obtaining each lateral and either a VD or DV view of the thorax.

parenchyma, and the mediastinum (including the heart and great vessels). Evaluation of each of these four areas is the basis for interpreting thoracic radiographs because expected structures and opacities typify each region. Memorization of basic anatomic boundaries and borders of each region and a basic understanding of the physiology relating to structures within a given region are important for interpretation.

The Normal Thoracic Radiograph

Recognition of radiographic abnormalities is based on a thorough understanding of normal radiographic appearance. Every anatomic structure present on a radiograph has a characteristic size, shape, opacity, margin, contour, number, and location. This interpretation paradigm overview progresses in a systematic fashion from the extrathoracic to intrathoracic structures. For the most part, common thoracic diseases may involve only one of the four regions noted. When two or more of these regions are involved, the radiographs become more complicated, so it is important to have an understanding of the basic pathophysiologic mechanisms involved in various thoracic diseases. For example, in dogs with right heart failure (passive congestion and backward failure), pleural effusion, enlargement of the caudal vena cava, hepatic venous congestion, and ascites would be expected. These areas are secondarily involved. Therefore, two of the main anatomic regions (mediastinum and the pleural space) are involved even though a single disease is responsible for the radiographic abnormalities. Again, recognizing the connection between the two regions on the basis of the underlying pathophysiologic characteristics of the disease is important.

When interpreting thoracic radiographs, several key factors should be kept in mind. The first is that the thoracic radiograph represents an instantaneous snapshot of the thorax and a particular stage of a specific disease process. This is like making a photograph of a marathon race at mile 5 and assuming that the marathoners will look the same at the end of the race or that the outcome of the marathon will always be the same based on the appearance of the race at that moment. The disease may be more advanced than the radiographic abnormalities suggest, or certain changes characteristic of the disease may not yet be present. In actuality, radiographic changes typically lag behind the pathophysiologic stage of the disease; this is true for most imaging examinations, not just radiographs of the thorax.

The second factor to consider is that radiographic abnormalities are visualized only after the normal radiographic anatomy of a particular structure has undergone change. These anatomic alterations may be a direct result of the disease (e.g., true anatomic abnormality) or a secondary change (e.g., as that described for right heart failure). In either instance, an understanding of normal anatomy, the anticipated radiographic anatomic variations, and possible radiographic abnormalities based on the underlying pathophysiologic characteristics is imperative. Finally, although the interpretation of images involves looking for changes in anatomy, these anatomic changes may not be related to the patient's clinical signs or disease. This relates to basic interpretive principles (see Chapter 5) and the concept of each abnormality representing a window (past event), mirror (current disease), or picture (current disease with possible future prognostic information). For example, an unstructured interstitial pattern in a patient who has lived in an urban environment may be unrelated to the clinical signs of a cough.

Extrathoracic Structures

The extrathoracic region includes the thoracic skeleton and soft tissue of the thoracic wall and diaphragm. These boundaries include the sternum ventrally, the vertebral bodies and ribs dorsally, the ribs, intercostal soft tissues, subcutaneous structures and forelimbs laterally, and the diaphragm caudally. Starting ventrally and working in a clockwise direction on the lateral radiograph, the sternum consists of eight sternebrae and the intersternebral disc spaces. The first sternebral segment is the manubrium and is elongated compared with other sternebrae. The last sternebral segment is the xiphoid process that extends caudoventral to the level of the falciform fat. The intersternebral discs are fibrocartilaginous joints similar to the intervertebral discs. Costal cartilages from the first eight ribs insert at the intersternebral disc space. The remaining costal cartilages insert near the xyphoid process or on the preceding rib's costal cartilage. Degenerative changes of the sternebrae and intersternebral disc spaces are common. New bone, similar in appearance to the osteophytes forming as a result of spondylosis deformans, as well as intersternebral disc space collapse with end plate sclerosis, can be seen. These changes are more common in older dogs and, to a lesser extent, in older cats.

The ribs generally course in a craniodorsal to caudoventral direction. Costal cartilages may mineralize early in the life in both dogs and cats and generally course in a caudodorsal to a cranioventral direction from the costochondral junction to the sternum.

The costochondral junction between the body of the rib and the costal cartilage can undergo extensive degenerative change with heterogeneous amorphous mineralization patterns. These are degenerative changes and should not be confused for intrapulmonary masses, pleural lesions, or aggressive rib lesions (Fig. 25-6).

The cranial aspect of the thorax is bounded by soft tissue structures within the ventral neck at the thoracic inlet. This

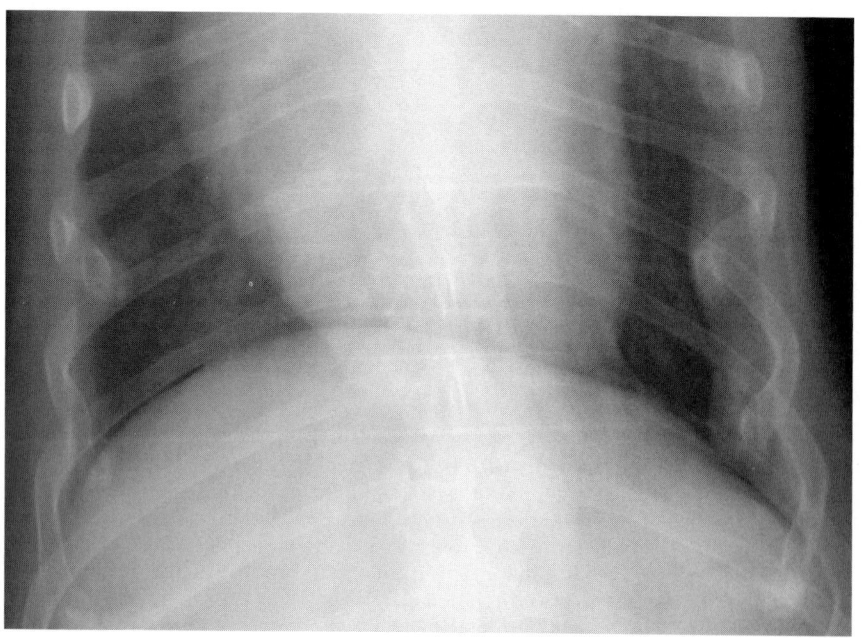

Fig. 25-6 Close-up VD radiograph of a Bassett Hound with extrapleural indentations (the "extrapleural sign") from degenerative changes associated with the costochondral junctions. This pushes the parietal pleural into the thorax, creating an additional soft tissue opacity superimposed over the lateral lung field.

includes the cervical trachea and caudal cervical vertebrae. The shoulder joints should be evaluated for degenerative changes. Abnormalities within the humerus and scapula should be noted. Dorsally the vertebral bodies should be evaluated along with the scapula for any change. The diaphragm should be assessed for the normal lung-diaphragm interface and positioning. The crura and dome or cupula of the diaphragm are evaluated for changes in contour or position relative to each other. Tracing each of the ribs should be a priority on every radiographic projection to ensure the absence of rib lesions. Individuals interpreting thoracic radiographs may treat the ribs as background "noise" and not examine them completely. This occurs because so few rib lesions occur compared with cardiopulmonary lesions. To overcome this, some have advocated temporarily rotating thoracic radiographs out of their normal orientation; this new position (Fig. 25-7) can make the ribs more conspicuous to the eye (or brain). This exercise may be useful to those learning to interpret thoracic radiographs, but skilled radiologists rarely use this maneuver.

On the basis of the lateral radiograph, the soft tissues ventral to the sternum, such as soft tissue, fatty mass(es), or nipples, may result in superimposed lung opacity. Nipple shadows typically are bilateral and within one intercostal space of each other in opposite lung fields on the VD or DV radiograph and will not appear within the pulmonary parenchyma on the lateral radiograph. If the interpreter cannot decide if the apparent pulmonary nodule is caused by superimposition of a nipple, a small amount of barium can be applied to the nipple and the radiograph repeated (Fig. 25-8).

The cranial abdomen should be assessed for hepatic changes and the positioning of the stomach. The diaphragm position within the thorax should also be assessed. Ascites or abdominal masses may not allow the patient to take a deep breath, thereby obviating an inspiratory radiograph. Also, peritoneal gas will collect along the peritoneal side of the diaphragm between the diaphragm and the liver. Any of these changes described above warrant further evaluation. This is especially true for a dog or cat with an apparent pneumoperitoneum without a history of recent (within the past 4 weeks) abdominal surgery.

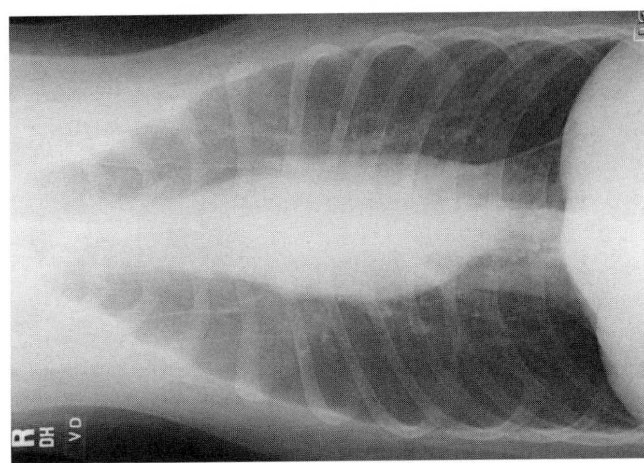

Fig. 25-7 VD radiograph from a dog in which the radiograph has been rotated 90 degrees from its normal orientation. This maneuver may make the ribs more conspicuous to beginning interpreters, but skilled radiologists rarely use this maneuver.

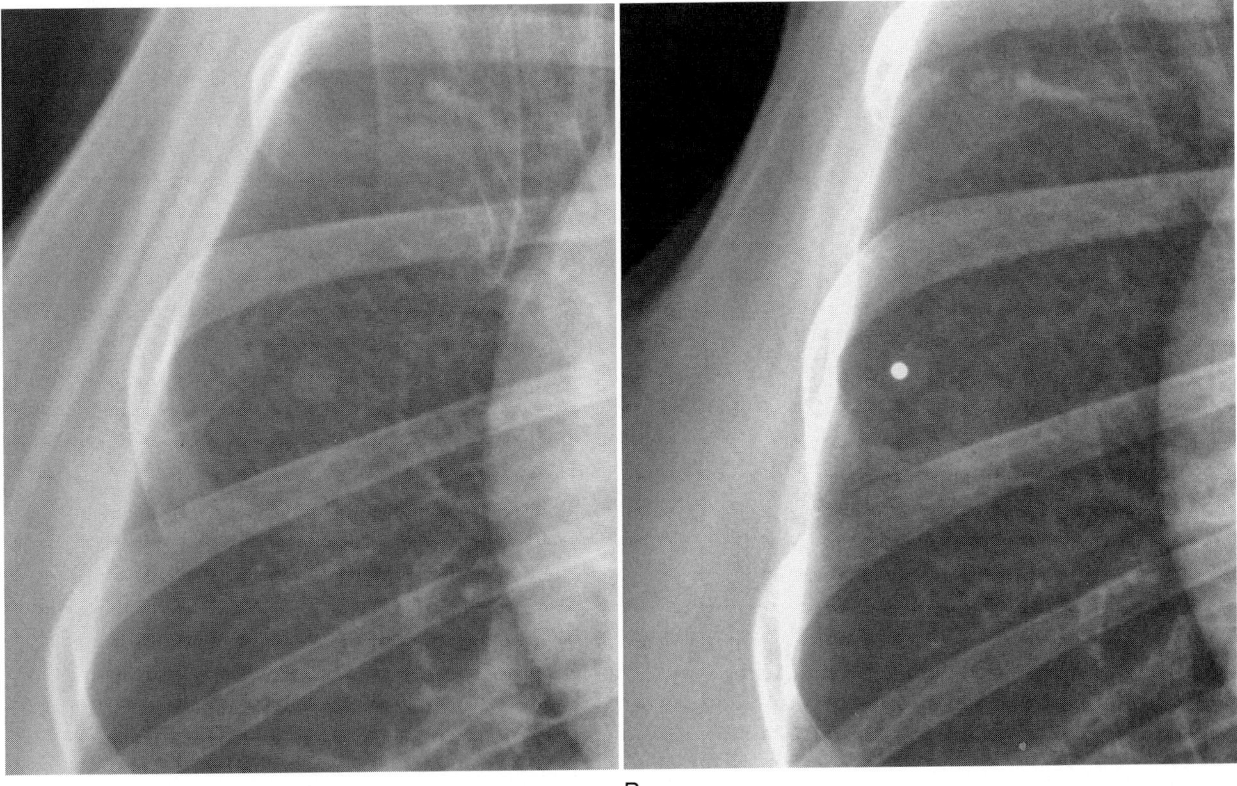

Fig. 25-8 A, Close-up VD radiograph in which an apparent lung nodule is seen. B, The same dog after a marker was taped to the right cranial thoracic nipple. The marker is superimposed on the presumed nodule, indicating it is caused by the nipple and is not in the lung.

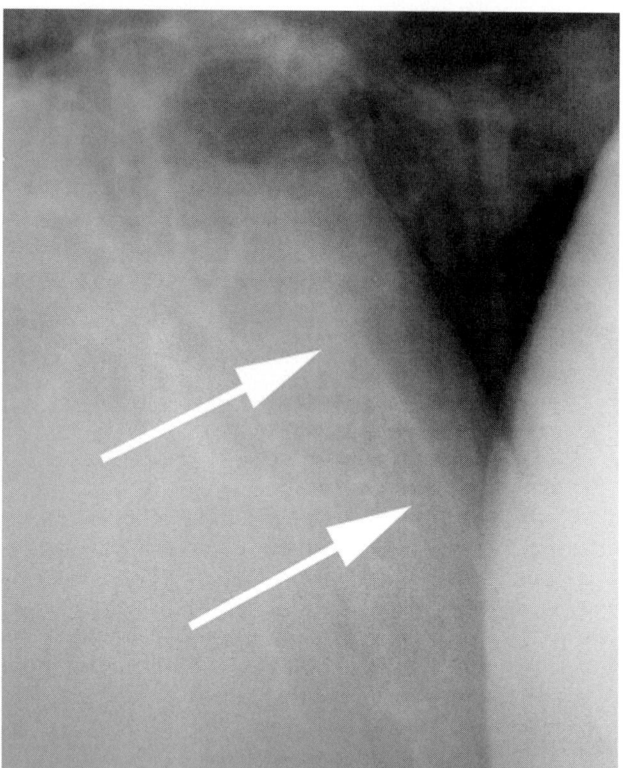

Fig. 25-9 Left lateral radiograph of a dog. An area of pleural thickening is noted between the right middle and right caudal lung lobes *(arrows)*. This is a common finding in older dogs and is not significant.

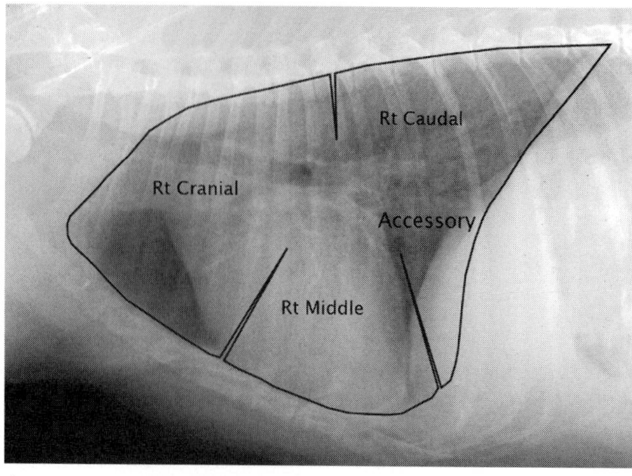

A

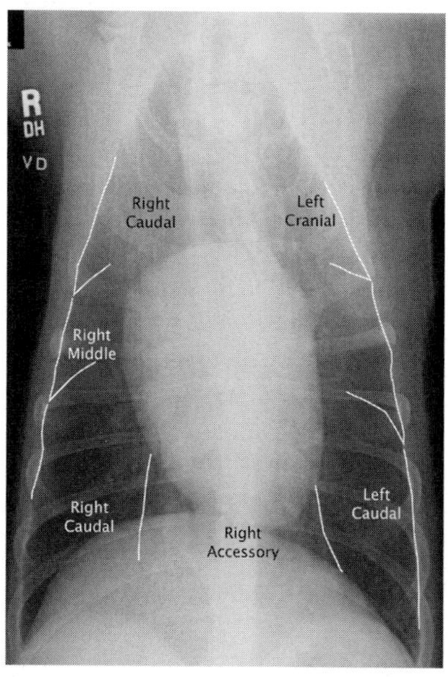

B

Fig. 25-10 Right lateral view **(A)**, VD view **(B)**, and illustration **(C)** documenting the position of the expected pleural fissures between the different lung lobes. The illustration **(C)** shows that if the lung lobe is retracted away from the parietal margin and replaced by air, it will appear black (true pneumothorax) and no vascular markings will be present beyond the lung lobe margin. This may require a hot light for complete evaluation. If the lung lobe is retracted from the parietal margin by fluid, the intervening space will have a soft tissue opacity.

Pleural Space

The pleural space is the next region to be evaluated. The pleural space is composed of two mesothelial layers called the parietal and visceral pleura. The parietal pleura lines the thoracic cavity and is fused with the thoracic wall (intercostal spaces and ribs) and diaphragm. Medially, the parietal pleura reflects dorsally at the level of the sternum and ventrally at the level of the vertebrae to form the mediastinal pleura. At the pulmonary hilum the parietal pleura also reflects onto the outer pulmonary surface, becoming the visceral pleura. Normally, the pleural space contains a very small amount of fluid that is not radiographically visible. Even though production of pleural fluid is continuous, the fluid is also continually absorbed and a net accumulation of fluid does not occur. In older patients, pleural thickening may be present, particularly between the right middle and right caudal lung lobe, seen best on a left lateral radiograph (Fig. 25-9); however, this is not considered a significant radiographic abnormality. The anatomic localization of the normal pulmonary fissures is important because these are sites of fluid or air accumulation and also represent boundaries and borders for lung disease. These potential pleural fissures are illustrated in Figure 25-10.

Pleural space abnormalities are space occupying and can be divided into abnormal accumulations of air (pneumothorax) or fluid (pleural effusion), pleural mass(es) (including herniation of abdominal contents after traumatic tears of the diaphragm), and extrapleural lesions with thoracic invasion (rib tumor). In abnormal accumulation of air and fluid, the lung lobes retract away from the thoracic wall, with air (appearing black on the radiograph) or fluid (appearing gray or white on the radiograph) in the pleural space between the parietal and visceral pleura. Pleural masses can be difficult to identify if concomitant pleural effusion is present. An extrapleural sign is the indentation of the pulmonary parenchyma by a normal or abnormal extrathoracic structure. In Bassett Hounds and other chondrodystrophic breeds, normal extrathoracic indentations are present at the level of the costochondral junctions (see Fig. 25-6).

Pulmonary Parenchyma

The pulmonary parenchyma consists of three structures that are normally visualized on routine thoracic radiographs: (1) the walls of the airways to the level of the secondary divisions of the bronchi (normal), (2) the pulmonary arteries and the pulmonary veins, and (3) the lung interstitium, or the con-

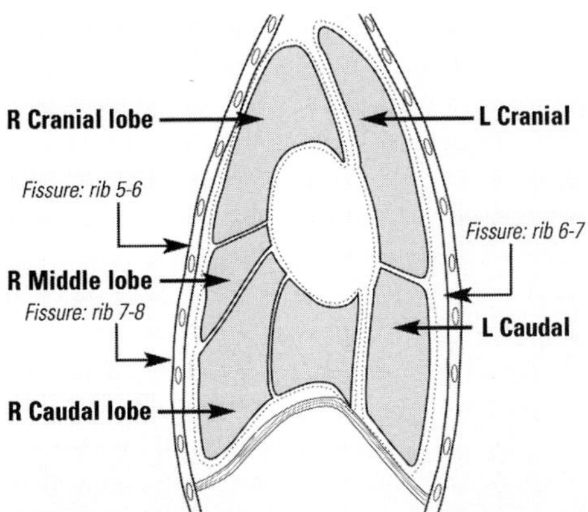

Fissure lines - thickest lateral and get thinner medially. They go from caudolateral to craniomedial direction and have a cranial curve.

Pulmonary vessels - greatest diameter of vessel is medial (toward heart) and tapers laterally.

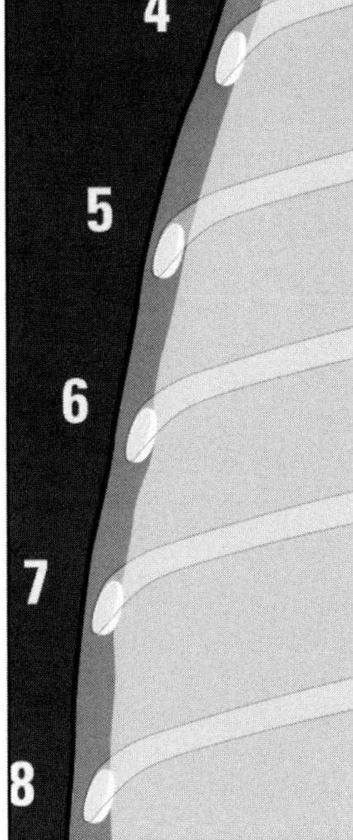

Normal
Lack of visualization of fissures and pleural space.

4
5
6
7
8

Pleural fluid
Soft tissue opacity in fissures
Radiolucent lung
Soft tissue opacity separating lung from rib crescent (thoracic wall)

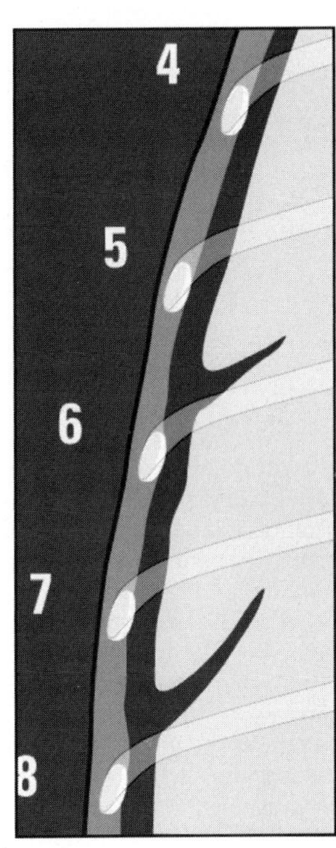

Pneumothorax
Air in fissures
Radiopaque lung
Air opacity separating the lung from rib crescent (thoracic wall)

C

Fig. 25-10, cont'd For legend see opposite page.

nective tissue framework of the lung. If the radiograph is obtained on inspiration versus expiration, a dramatic difference will occur in the ability to visualize each of these structures (Fig. 25-11).

On lateral radiographs, pulmonary arteries are dorsal to the corresponding bronchus, which in turn is dorsal to the corresponding pulmonary vein. This is apparent only in the cranial aspect of the thorax. The pulmonary vessels (arteries versus veins) cannot be differentiated in the caudal aspect of the thorax on the lateral radiograph. On the VD or DV radiograph, the pulmonary artery to a given lung lobe is lateral to the primary or principle lobar bronchus, whereas the pulmonary vein is medial and ventral. These relations are vital and should be memorized.

On an adequately exposed normal radiograph, the branching pulmonary vessels should be traceable to the periphery of the lung field. On overexposed radiographs or images obtained with digital radiographic systems, where the imaging plate is oversaturated, the lung field will appear black and can be mistaken for a pneumothorax. More importantly, normally obvious radiographic pulmonary lesions are not seen. The veterinarian has to take responsibility for the diagnostic quality and repeat the radiographs until appropriately exposed and positioned thoracic radiographs are obtained. This should not be at the expense of compromising the patient's health, however. The pulmonary vessels have the largest overall diameter closest to the heart and taper and branch toward the periphery. The branching is linear in the normal dog and cat and should not be curved, irregular, or blunted. The vessels are normally of soft tissue opacity. In general, the size of any pulmonary artery should match the size of the corresponding pulmonary vein at the same level.

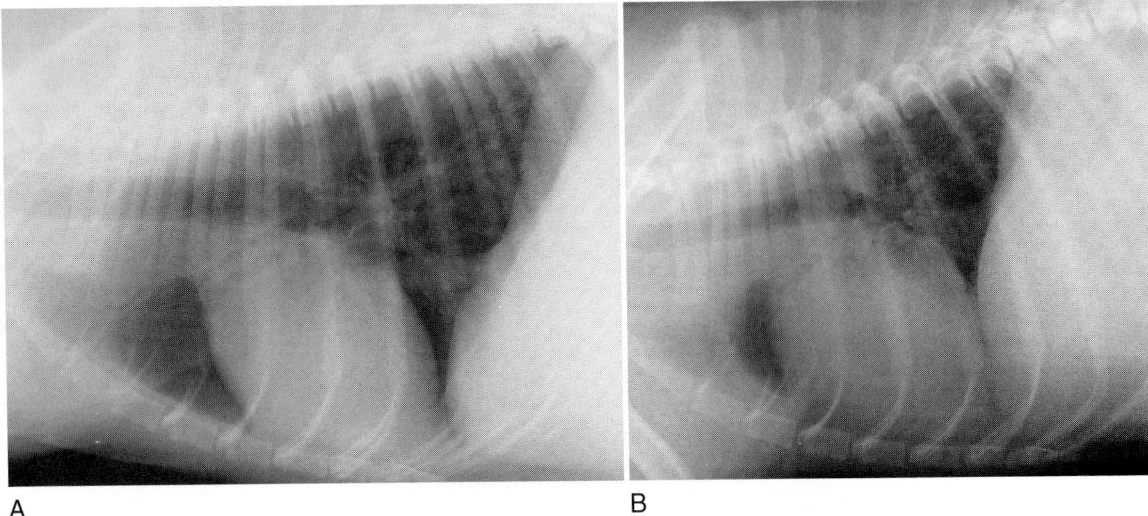

Fig. 25-11 Right lateral radiographs of the same dog obtained during peak inspiration **(A)** and peak expiration **(B)** with normal tidal volume excursions. Note the increased distance between the heart and diaphragm, the decreased interstitial lung opacity, and the overall increase in lung size (volume) on the inspiratory radiograph compared with the expiratory radiograph.

Although the relative size of pulmonary arteries and veins is usually sufficient to assess whether either vessel is abnormal, absolute size can be quantified. For example, the pulmonary artery and vein supplying the right cranial lung lobe should not have a diameter greater than the proximal aspect of the fourth rib. Also, the diameter of the caudal lobe pulmonary artery and vein should equal the thickness of the ninth rib at the point where the vessels cross the rib. In other words, the summation shadow of the intersecting vessel and ninth rib should be a square. If the vessel is enlarged the summation shadow will be rectangular, with the largest dimension being horizontal, whereas if the vessel is small the summation shadow will be rectangular, with the largest dimension being vertical. Relations, such as the relative size of the caudal lobe vessels and the ninth rib, are only guidelines and are not always accurate.

The interstitium is the non-air-containing part of the lung where the pulmonary vessels, bronchi, lymphatics, and pulmonary parenchyma/connective tissue (alveolar septum, interlobar septum) are located. The interstitium is the source of the lacy soft tissue opacity between vessels and airways that are discerned on close inspection of normal thoracic radiographs. Varying degrees of pulmonary connective tissue exist among species. As a result, the lungs of animals with more connective tissue normally appear more opaque (white). In order of increasing amounts of pulmonary connective tissue are the dog and cat, the horse, cattle, and then pigs.

Two lungs, with each occupying approximately 50% of the thoracic cavity, are present. The right lung is divided into cranial, middle, caudal, and accessory lobes. The left lung is divided into cranial (further subdivided into the cranial and caudal subsegments) and caudal lobes. These lobes occupy specific areas of the thoracic cavity. Even though interlobar fissures are not identifiable on routine thoracic radiographs, the expected anatomic location of these fissures should be understood and memorized.

On the VD or DV radiograph, interlobar fissures curve in a cranial and medial direction toward the pulmonary hilum (trachea) and away from the thoracic wall, with the convex side of the curve located cranially (Fig. 25-12). The position

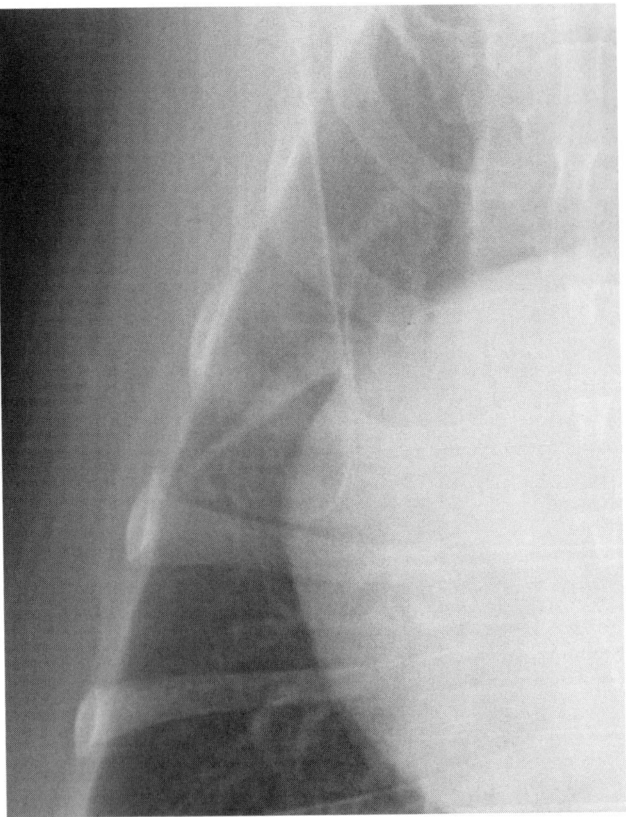

Fig. 25-12 VD radiograph of a dog wherein fat has been deposited between the right cranial and the right middle lung lobe in a central location. In this dog the fissure between these two lung lobes is widest centrally (not peripherally, as would be expected with pleural fluid or a pneumothorax).

of lung lobes can be inferred from the known location of interlobar fissures, as seen in Fig. 25-10. One important consideration is that on the lateral radiograph, the dorsal extent of the accessory lung lobe is dorsal to the caudal vena cava, whereas the lateral most extent on the VD or DV radiograph is demarcated by the caudal ventral mediastinal reflection.

Interpretation Paradigm(s) for the Pulmonary Parenchyma

One method for assessing radiographic alterations of the lung is based on a description of the predominant abnormal radiographic pulmonary pattern.[11-14] This is based on the hypothesis that diseases affecting the alveoli have a different appearance than do diseases affecting only the bronchi. These appearances will then be different from a disease that affects only the interstitium, or the pulmonary vasculature. This type of descriptive hypothesis, termed the pattern recognition approach, is flawed from several aspects. First, a given disease often affects multiple regions of the lung and thereby does not result in just one pulmonary pattern. Second, a lung pattern does not equate to a disease; for example, all alveolar patterns are not caused by pneumonia. Third, beginning interpreters are so anxious to categorize the lung pattern they forget to consider that the radiograph may be normal. Fourth, the pattern recognition system does not automatically lead the interpreter to consider which test to use to determine the underlying cause of the abnormal pattern. Despite the problems associated with the pattern recognition approach, a basic understanding of the classic lung patterns is necessary before considering any other interpretive paradigm.

Regardless of the interpretation paradigm, the first decision to be made is to determine whether the lung is normal. This is often more difficult than identifying which lung pattern is present because of the many nondisease factors that affect the radiographic appearance of lung. Some of the more common factors that influence lung appearance are the following:

- Radiographic technique. An incorrect diagnosis of increased interstitial opacification will be made in underexposed radiographs.
- Body condition. Overweight patients will often have poor ventilation, leading to an incorrect assessment of an alveolar or interstitial pattern. The superimposed adipose tissue will also lead to increased background opacity to the lung, contributing to the false sense of an interstitial pattern (Fig. 25-13).
- Sedation. Sedated patients often do not ventilate as fully as nonsedated patients, and the resultant decreased amount of air within the lung will be misinterpreted as either an alveolar pattern, an interstitial pattern, or both. The effect of aeration on lung opacity was previously illustrated (see Fig. 25-11).
- Patient position. In lateral recumbency the dependent lung rapidly loses air and has an increased opacity. In lateral radiographs, this will contribute to an overall increase in lung opacity that may be misinterpreted as an alveolar or interstitial pattern. This phenomenon is not as pronounced in VD or DV views. Thus as a general rule of thumb, lungs will always look more opaque (abnormal) in lateral views than in the VD or DV view (Fig. 25-14).
- Interpretive bias. Patients that are being radiographed for lung assessment typically have a clinical sign or condition that suggests intrathoracic disease. This will bias the interpreter because the goal is to find something wrong in the radiograph that explains the clinical signs. This will lead to misinterpretation of normal lung appearance, or lung altered by one of the above phenomena, as abnormal.

Once the lung has been determined to be abnormal, in the classic pulmonary pattern approach the interpreter attempts to categorize the abnormality according to one of the classic patterns: alveolar, bronchial, interstitial, or vascular. A complicating issue is that a combination of patterns can occur. In the classic pattern recognition system, the predominant pattern should be classified first.

Some jargon terms used in pulmonary patterns do not have satisfactory definitions and should be avoided. The first term is *infiltrate.* The definition of infiltrate, according to Webster's Dictionary, is "to cause (a liquid, for example) to permeate a substance by passing through its interstices or pores." This definition has nothing to do with most of the pathologic processes seen in the lungs. This definition could be used to describe cardiogenic pulmonary edema, in which increased hydrostatic pressure within the left ventricle (elevated end-diastolic left ventricular pressure) causes elevations in left atrial pressure and thereby pulmonary venous pressure. Even in this pathologic state the reality is that, according to Starling forces at the capillary, the elevated hydrostatic pressure prevents the normal interstitial lung fluid from moving back into the capillaries at the venule side. For physicians interpreting thoracic radiographs of human beings, no agreement has been reached for what the term *infiltrate* is to mean, and the same confusion exists in veterinary medicine.

The second term is *consolidation.* The definition of consolidation, according to Webster's Dictionary, is "the act or process of consolidating; the state of being consolidated; the merger of two or more commercial interests or corporations." Again, consolidation is a term that has little meaning regarding a pulmonary pattern and does not provide any help toward reaching an accurate prioritized differential diagnosis list.

Most veterinary radiologists use infiltrate and consolidation to mean an increased lung opacity without giving a specific pattern. Some may argue that consolidation is another term for an alveolar pattern, but to keep it simple, an alveolar pattern can be defined and consolidation ignored. In either instance, a differential list is not available for either pulmonary infiltrate or pulmonary consolidation.

Paradigm Using a Classic Pattern Approach

From a simplistic standpoint, thoracic radiographic abnormalities can be considered to cause either added pulmonary opacity or decreased pulmonary opacity. More commonly, radiographic opacity changes of the pulmonary parenchyma will be increased instead of decreased in appearance (radiolucency).

Decreased opacity of the pulmonary parenchyma can be generalized or focal. Decreased opacity superimposed over the lungs could still be caused by subcutaneous emphysema or pneumomediastinum, so evaluation of both orthogonal radiographs is critical. The most common cause of a generalized decrease in pulmonary opacity is a generalized decrease in pulmonary vessel size, such as that resulting from hypovolemia, or hyperinflation attributable to feline asthma. Focal causes of decreased pulmonary opacity include pulmonary lobar emphysema, cavitated pulmonary lesions (tumors or abscess), or pulmonary bulla/blebs such as pneumatoceles or hematoceles. These focal abnormalities do not have an anatomic or lobar predisposition.

Superimposed air over the lungs decreases the expected normal opacity of a lateral thoracic radiograph. Without the orthogonal radiograph, placement of the abnormality within one of the four spaces for evaluation (extrathoracic, pleural space, pulmonary parenchyma, or mediastinum) may not be accurate. The same is true for added thoracic opacity. The causes could include an extrathoracic mass, pleural fluid, alveolar lung disease, or fluid within the esophagus. Again, in each instance the specific area or region of disease must be

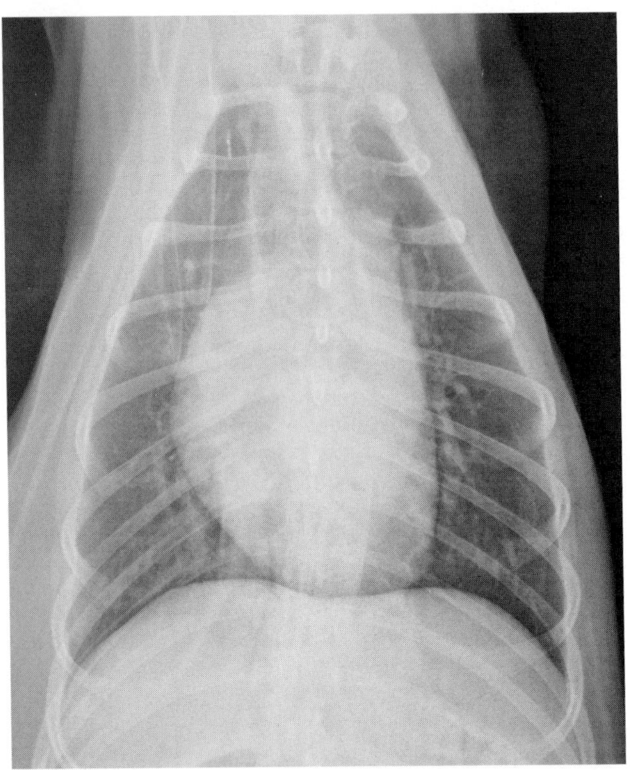

A

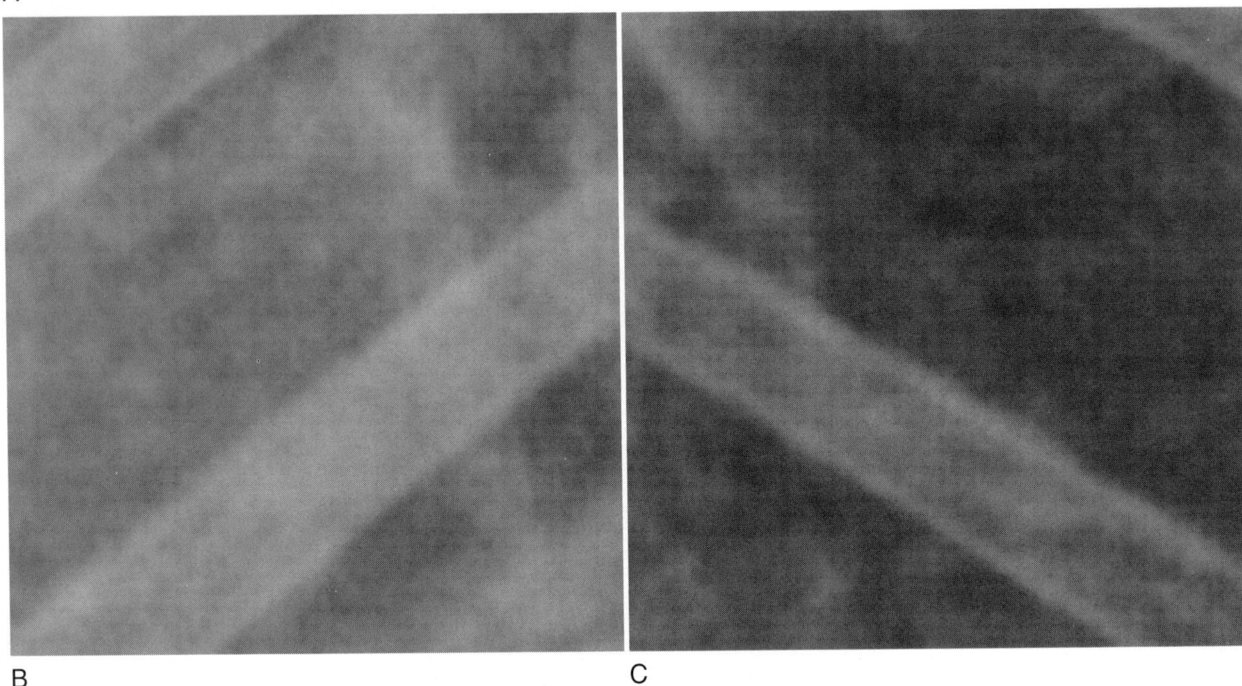

B C

Fig. 25-13 VD thoracic radiograph of a dog where the left forelimb had been removed surgically because of a tumor. Note the difference in thickness of thoracic wall soft tissues on the left versus the right; the decrease on the left is a consequence of surgical removal and disuse atrophy. Note also the increased lung opacity on the right side caused by the greater thickness of thoracic wall tissue on that side. In close-up views from the right (**B**) and left (**C**) caudal lobes, the lung opacity appears increased on the right side. This illustrates how the amount of thoracic wall soft tissue can influence the radiographic opacity of the lung. The lung in **B** would almost certainly be misdiagnosed as having an interstitial pattern by many observers.

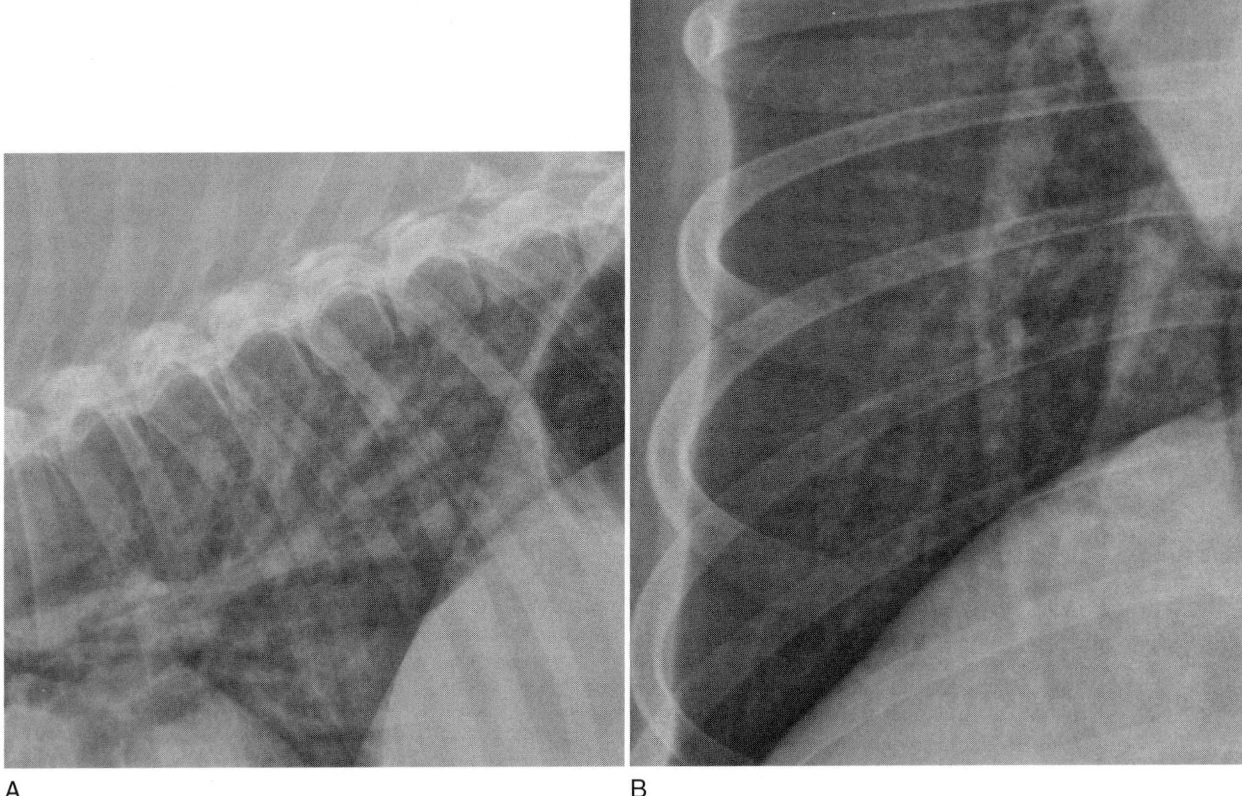

Fig. 25-14 Close-up thoracic radiographs of a moderately obese dog made in lateral (**A**) and VD (**B**) recumbency. Note the increased opacity of the lungs in **A** compared with **B.** This is caused by greater recumbency-associated atelectasis occurring in lateral recumbency. Any suspicious lung opacity seen in a lateral view should be confirmed on the VD or DV view to ensure that it is not caused by atelectasis.

determined. The following discussion is based on the assumption that the practitioner has accurately localized the disease process to the pulmonary parenchyma.

Classical Pulmonary Pattern Recognition

The interpretation paradigm for the pulmonary parenchyma follows a question approach (as is used for evaluating dogs and cats with cardiovascular disease). These questions are summarized in Box 25-1.

If the lungs have increased opacity, describing the location of the abnormality first is easiest. Is the abnormality generalized (equally involves all aspects of all lung lobes)? Or which areas of the thorax are abnormal based on anatomic position and lung lobe position? Is the abnormality located cranioventrally or caudodorsally? If focal or multifocal, what parts of specific lung lobes are involved? If the lobe is not generally abnormal, then each lobe can be subjectively divided into thirds called the peripheral, mid-zone, or hilar thirds extending from the pleural space to the pulmonary hilum.

Second, the severity of the pattern should be noted as mild, moderate, or severe. Even though this is subjective, a peripheral alveolar pattern is not as severe or striking as an alveolar pulmonary pattern that involves the entire lobe. This is important for follow-up radiographs so that the pattern can be determined to be resolving or getting worse.

Third, is a mediastinal shift seen on the VD radiograph? If present, is the shift is away from a space-occupying lesion (contralateral) or toward a lesion, typically implying volume loss within a given lung lobe (ipsilateral)? The pathophysiologic characteristics of lung lobe elasticity, recoil, and collateral ventilation are beyond the scope of this text.[15] Suffice it to say that a contralateral or ipsilateral mediastinal shift can help the interpreter focus on a specific lung lobe where a specific disease process is present.

Once the anatomic location (position, severity, and shift) has been described, the type of pulmonary pattern should be considered. A process of elimination is used, starting with the easiest pattern to recognize to the hardest pattern to recognize. The pulmonary patterns include (1) alveolar, (2) bronchial, (3) vascular, and (4) interstitial. A combination of patterns can also occur. The predominant pattern should be classified first. Because many diseases can involve multiple areas of the lung (bronchi, alveoli, or interstitium), the dominant pattern and location should be used to help formulate the differential list.

After pattern identification, a differential diagnosis list can be formulated on the basis of the position, severity, and shift of the abnormality and the dominant pulmonary pattern. Now other roentgen abnormalities, the signalment of the patient, the clinical history, and clinical signs can be used to formulate a prioritized differential list. Prioritization is key because a definitive diagnosis is usually not possible because of the lack of sensitivity and specificity of each of the pulmonary patterns.

Alveolar Pattern

An alveolar pattern results from abnormal cells or fluid within the terminal air spaces of the lung. Determining the character of the material in the alveolus is impossible radiographi-

Box • 25-1

Interpretation Paradigm for Evaluating the Pulmonary Parenchyma

1. Are the lungs more *opaque* or more *lucent* then expected? Remember, the most common abnormality seen will be increased pulmonary opacity. If the lungs are more radiolucent than expected, then see the text.
2. If the lungs are more opaque, then, what is the *position* of the increased opacity? In other words, anatomically, where are the abnormalities located? Be specific to (1) location within the thorax (cranioventral versus caudodorsal versus generalized); (2) within a given lung lobe by using anatomically correct lobar names; and (3) the part within the lung lobe named (hilar, mid-zone, or peripheral; or the entire lobe is affected). How *severe* are the changes (mild, moderate, or severe)?
3. Is the cardiac silhouette *shifted* toward the affected lung (ipsilateral shift) or away from the lesion (contralateral shift)?
4. What is the predominant pulmonary *pattern* noted, and what is the severity of the pulmonary pattern? Remember that the pulmonary vessels, if enlarged, add opacity to the lung fields.
5. What are all the possible *differential diagnoses* based on the anatomic location of the affected lung and the described pulmonary pattern?

Tie all the radiographic information together along with the signalment, clinical history, and signs to formulate an appropriate prioritized differential diagnosis list.

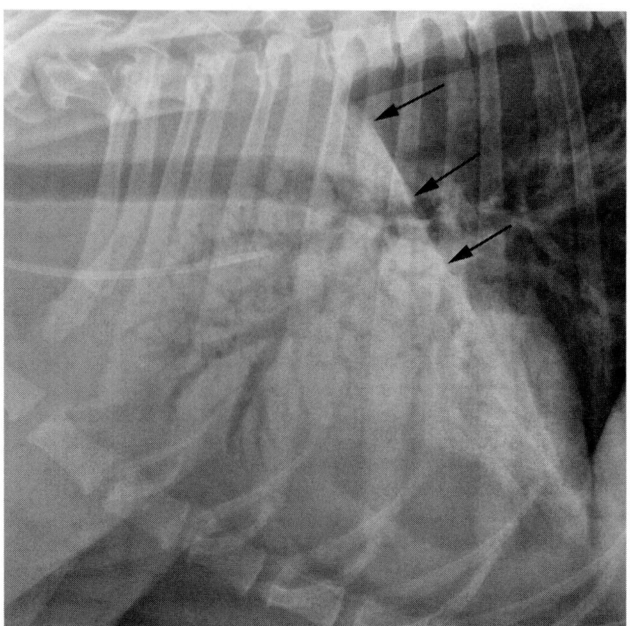

Fig. 25-15 Relatively uniform opacification of the cranioventral aspect of the thorax is visible in this left lateral radiograph. Radiolucent branching tubes are noted in this soft tissue opacity. These are air bronchograms and are present because the dog has alveolar lung disease. Border effacement of the pulmonary vessels and outer bronchial walls is present in the affected lung. Because the radiograph is a left lateral, these changes are more likely to be within the right cranial lung lobe. The surrounding normal pulmonary tissue contrasts with the alveolar lung disease. The *arrows* signify another sign of an alveolar pattern, the lobar sign. The lobar sign results from alveolar disease extending to the edge of the lung lobe where it contrasts against more normally aerated adjacent lung, creating a sharp border.

cally. The features of an alveolar pattern include relatively intense soft tissue opacity per unit area of abnormal lung, air bronchograms, lobar sign, indiscrete margins of the abnormal opacity (unless a lobar sign is present), border effacement of the pulmonary vessels and bronchial walls (intralobar structures), and border effacement with the heart or diaphragm (extralobar structures). Any of these signs can characterize a lung abnormality as alveolar.

The hallmark radiographic sign of the alveolar pattern is the air bronchogram (Fig. 25-15).[1] An air bronchogram has two general causes. An air bronchogram may be created by air in the bronchial lumen with filling of surrounding alveoli with fluid or cells. The fluid or cells replace the air within the alveoli and the lung assumes increased soft tissue opacity. Another cause of air bronchogram formation is collapse of the alveolar air space. The loss of air within the alveoli results in a uniform soft tissue opacity surrounding the radiolucent bronchus. When volume loss is present, a mediastinal shift toward the collapsed lung lobe usually occurs. This is termed atelectasis.[11] Atelectasis is not a pulmonary pattern; it is a differential for an alveolar pattern with an ipsilateral mediastinal shift. It does not imply a specific etiology. Atelectatic lung lobes are often associated with anesthesia, prolonged recumbency, pneumothorax, or pleural effusion.

Diseases resulting in cellular or fluid collection in the alveoli typically result in a relatively intense region of lung opacity compared to other lung patterns. Alveolar disease and a lung mass are the two most intense patterns encountered, per unit area. The intensity from an alveolar pattern results from involvement of the majority of a given volume of lung rather than just a portion of a volume, as would occur with abnormalities affecting the bronchial tree or the interstitium (other than a mass).

The air bronchogram is such a classic sign of an alveolar pattern that beginning interpreters are hesitant to diagnose an alveolar pattern unless an air bronchogram is seen. This is problematic because many patients with cells or fluid in the alveoli do not have an air bronchogram; this is especially true in cats. This results from the alveolar material not being extensive enough to surround an airway sufficiently for it to be seen. Thus air bronchograms are easy to see if extensive alveolar disease is present, but they may not be visible if the alveolar disease is multifocal and not lobar in distribution (Fig. 25-16).

Also, interpreters are so intent on finding an air bronchogram that they often misinterpret normal lung appearance as an air bronchogram. The most common example of this is misinterpretation of a bronchus between two adjacent vessels as an air bronchogram (Fig. 25-17). This can be avoided by noticing that the presumed abnormal lung adjacent to the bronchus does not extend into the periphery of the affected lobe or does not involve the entire lobe.

The lobar sign results from alveolar disease extending to the border of the lung lobe where it contrasts against more normally aerated adjacent lung, creating a sharp border (see Fig. 25-15). Other than the lobar sign, however, the borders of an alveolar pattern are often indistinct because the abnormal region blends to a more normal region within an affected lobe.

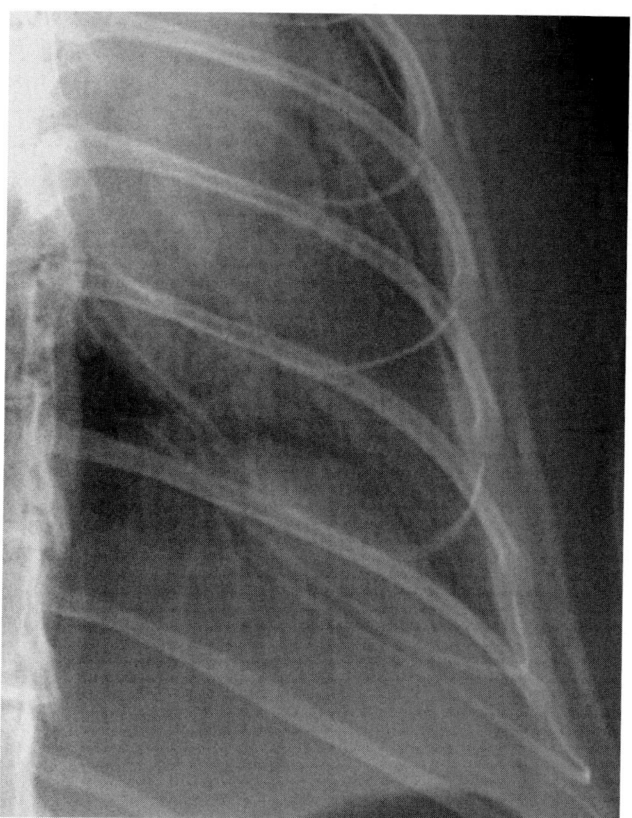

Fig. 25-16 Close-up of the left caudal lung field of a cat with cardiogenic pulmonary edema. Note the ill-defined increase in opacity of the left caudal lobe. The accessory lobe region is more normally aerated. The opacity is severe enough to cause border effacement with the heart, but no air bronchograms are present. The intensity of this opacity per unit area is too great to be an unstructured interstitial pattern; thus it best fits an alveolar pattern, yet without air bronchograms. Care must be taken not to misinterpret an alveolar pattern as interstitial on the basis of a lack of air bronchograms. The concept of intensity per unit area is helpful in this differentiation. Pleural effusion is also present.

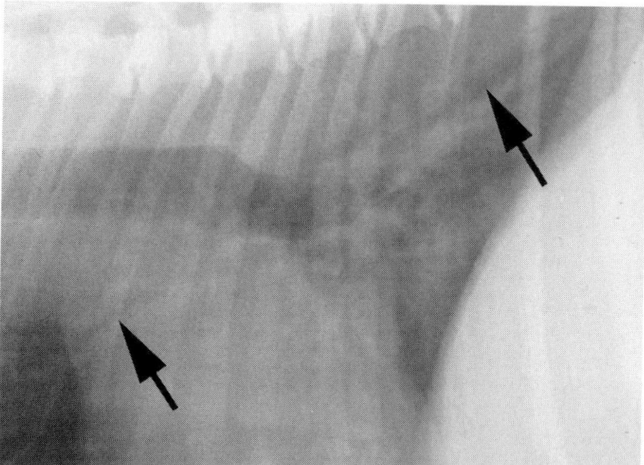

Fig. 25-17 Lateral thoracic radiograph. The region between adjacent vessels *(arrows)* is often misdiagnosed as an air bronchogram. The regions indicated by the *arrows* cannot be air bronchograms because the opacity next to the presumed bronchus does not extend far enough peripheral to the bronchus as it would if it were caused by material displacing air from the lung.

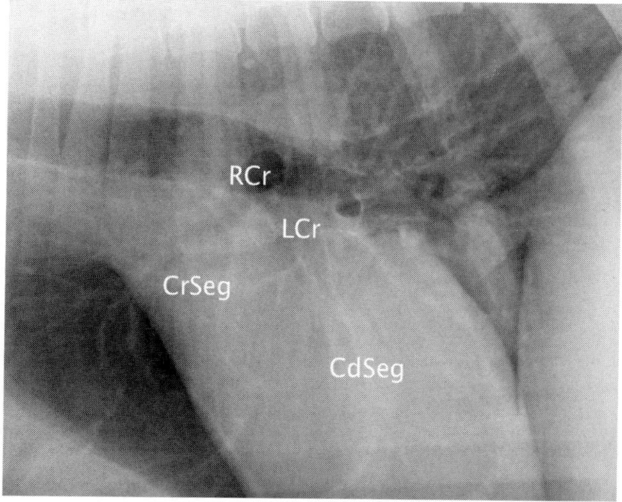

Fig. 25-18 Close-up of the major airways from a right lateral radiograph. If the trachea is traced from the thoracic inlet toward the carina, the circle superimposed over the trachea over the heart base is the right cranial lobar bronchus *(RCr)* and points straight out (the reason for the radiolucent circle) and then takes a 90-degree turn into the right cranial lung lobe. If the ventral margin of the trachea is traced to the level of the carina, an opening enters a tube pointing straight down *(LCr)*. This is the common bronchus into the left cranial lung lobe. It then divides into cranial *(CrSeg)* and caudal *(CdSeg)* subsegments with several millimeters to centimeters from the origin along the ventrolateral aspect of the trachea. The right middle and accessory bronchi originate from the right caudal lobe main stem bronchus caudal to the carina. The right and left caudal lobar bronchi then course in a dorsocaudal direction. Each bronchus should be seen to taper in a normal fashion.

With an alveolar pattern, the pulmonary vessels and outer margins of the bronchial walls are not seen because they are border effaced by the material in the alveoli. An alveolar pattern is not specific for any disease, but the distribution of the alveolar pattern will influence the differential considerations. For example, a cranioventral or ventral alveolar pattern is a common consequence of aspiration pneumonia. A caudodorsal alveolar pattern is a common consequence of noncardiogenic (or neurogenic) pulmonary edema.

Bronchial Pattern

In assessing the bronchi, all the primary bronchi should be traced as they leave the trachea. The right cranial lung lobe bronchus is the first bronchus originating from the trachea at the level of the fifth intercostal space (Fig. 25-18). This is seen as a radiolucent hole on the right lateral radiograph because the bronchus is seen en face. The left cranial lung lobe bronchus can be identified as the next branch of the terminal trachea just before the carina. If the ventral aspect of the trachea is traced past the origin of the right cranial lobe bronchus, a bronchus will be seen in longitudinal orientation coursing ventrally. Within several millimeters to a centimeter (depending on the size of the dog or cat), the bronchus bifurcates into the segmental bronchi (cranial and caudal subsegments) of the left cranial lung lobe. The trachea then terminates into the right and left caudal lobar or primary bronchi (called the carina). The right middle bronchus originates from the ventrolateral aspect of the right caudal lung lobe bronchus within several millimeters of the carina. The

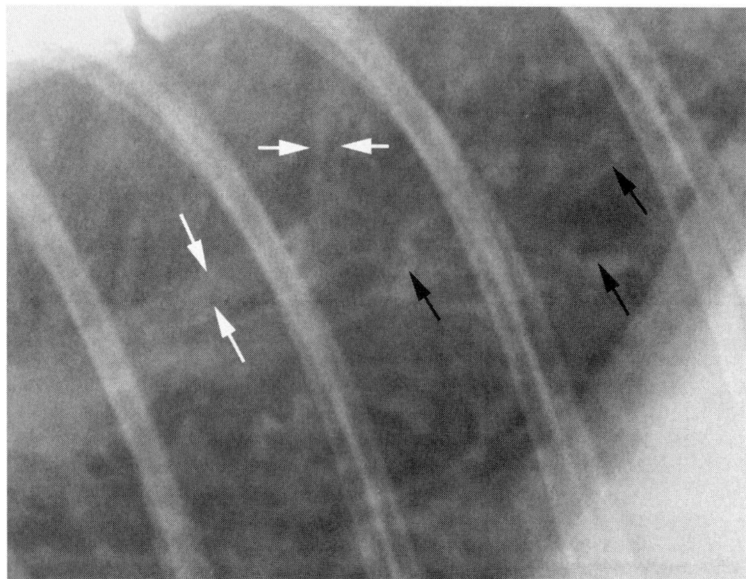

Fig. 25-19 Close-up lateral radiograph of a cat with a bronchial pattern caused by allergic airway disease. Note the conspicuous ring shadows *(black arrows)* and parallel lines *(white arrows)* that result from the airway inflammation.

accessory lung lobe bronchus originates from the ventromedial aspect of the right caudal lung lobe bronchus several centimeters from the carina.

A bronchial pattern consists of abnormal lung opacity caused by thickened bronchi or abnormal cells and/or fluid immediately adjacent to the bronchi. Radiographically, this will appear as an excessive number of opaque rings and lines (Fig. 25-19). The rings represent the abnormal airway region projected end-on, whereas the lines represent the abnormal airway region projected from the side. A bronchial pattern will not be intense per unit area of affected lung because the adjacent alveoli usually remain air filled.

Bronchial mineralization seen in geriatric dogs (Fig. 25-20) and the conspicuity of the airways at the level of the hilar third of the bronchus are often misinterpreted as abnormal airways. Typically bronchial patterns are generalized and, as such, the lung fields should be evaluated in the periphery for the characteristic rings and lines seen in bronchial disease (Fig. 25-21). A magnifying glass may be useful.

Patients with a bronchial pattern may also cause the interpreter to question whether a coexisting unstructured interstitial pattern is present. Diagnosing a bronchointerstitial pattern is tempting for beginning interpreters because it reduces the pressure to fit the abnormalities nicely into one tight niche or pulmonary pattern. This tendency is one of the major pitfalls associated with strict use of the pattern recognition approach. Indeed, coexisting interstitial disease may be present because, as noted above, few diseases actually involve only one anatomic compartment of the lung. In addition, many factors also mentioned above create a false impression of diffuse lung disease when that condition does not actually exist. A solution to this dilemma is discussed below in an alternative paradigm.

Vascular Pattern

Although not considered a pulmonary pattern by some, the pulmonary vessels have an impact on the relative opacity and structure of the lungs. For example, a dog with a left-to-right shunt will have increased lung opacity simply because of pulmonary overcirculation and not necessarily as a result of cardiogenic edema (Fig. 25-22). A dog with severe heartworm disease with severe enlargement of the pulmonary arteries will have curvilinear, tortuous, or even nodular multiple soft tissue opacities (Fig. 25-23).

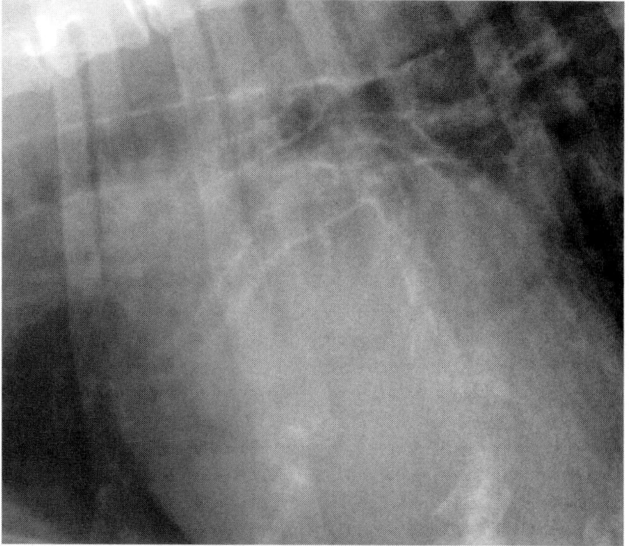

Fig. 25-20 Right lateral radiograph from a geriatric Dachshund. Tracheal and central bronchial mineralization are noted, making the bronchi quite conspicuous. Bronchial mineralization has been described in dogs with Cushing's disease and in geriatric dogs, as well as an incidental finding.

Interstitial Pattern

An interstitial pattern is categorized as either structured (or nodular) or unstructured.[11] A structured pattern is produced by pulmonary nodules (Fig. 25-24) or a pulmonary mass. Nodules and masses are relatively intense per unit area of affected lung and are relatively easy to identify because of discrete margins created by their interface with aerated lung. The easiest place to evaluate for pulmonary nodules is in the periphery of the lung or over the heart or diaphragm.

Pulmonary vessels projected end-on may be confused with a pulmonary nodule. Distinguishing between an end-on vessel and a pulmonary nodule is important for obvious reasons. Pulmonary vessels often are situated adjacent to a bronchus and

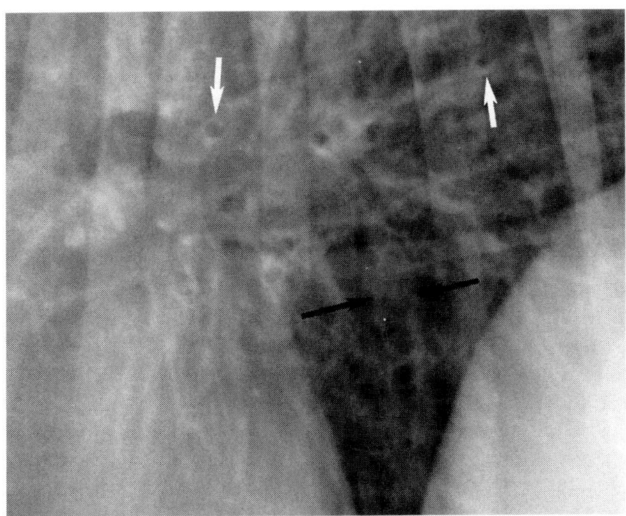

Fig. 25-21 Close-up right lateral radiograph over the area of the caudal heart and accessory lung lobe. This dog has a severe, generalized bronchial pulmonary pattern that is adding opacity to the lung fields. Multiple rings are visible *(white arrows)*. These rings represent end-on airways. The lines *(black arrows)* represent airways in long axis coursing into the pulmonary parenchyma from the pulmonary hilum.

may also have a connected "tail" because part of the vessel is projected laterally (Fig. 25-25). Superficial thoracic wall masses, such as ectoparasites or nipples, may be also be misinterpreted as a pulmonary nodule (see Fig. 25-8).

Pulmonary osteomas are small (2 to 4 mm in size), well-defined nodules (Fig. 25-26) that are sometimes confused with metastasis.[10] These areas of osseous metaplasia are found just beneath the visceral pleura, within the interstitium, in older dogs. They appear as well-defined (mineralized) focal nodules with a ventral predilection but can be found throughout the lung. Pulmonary osteomas are recognized by their small size, being smaller than the minimal size of 5 to 10 mm needed for detection of an isolated soft tissue nodule. Osteomas are visible at such a small size because of their mineralization; pathologic lung nodules rarely mineralize. Shelties and Collies appear to be prone to development of pulmonary osteomas, although specific scientific studies confirming this are not available.

An unstructured interstitial pattern is the most difficult pattern for beginning interpreters to identify because of the many factors previously mentioned that create a false impression of a diffuse pulmonary abnormality. An unstructured interstitial pattern is caused by a collection of fluid, cells, or fibrin within the connective tissue framework of the lung, between alveoli, and around vessels and airways. This will result in a generalized increase in lung opacity that is not intense per unit area of involved lung, but in a pattern that

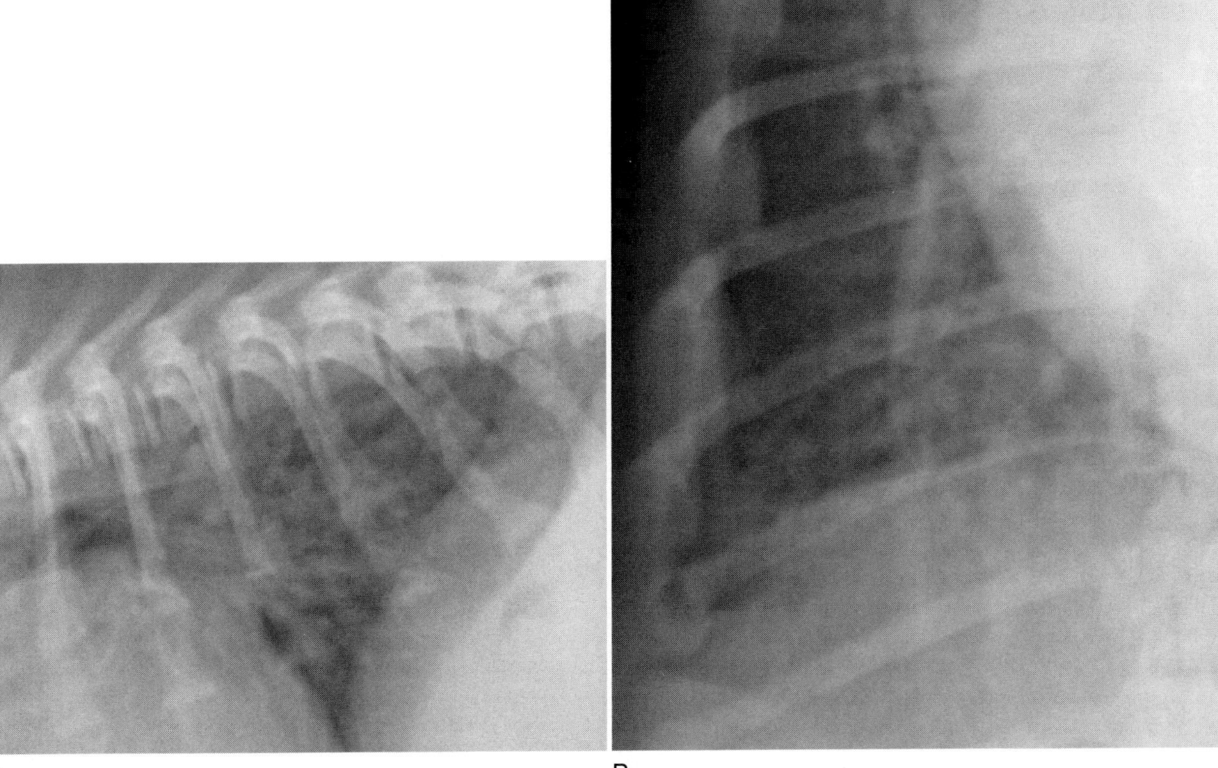

Fig. 25-22 Close-up right lateral (A) and VD (B) radiographs from dog with a left-to-right patent ductus arteriosus. The pulmonary arteries and veins are enlarged, consistent with left-to-right shunting and pulmonary overcirculation. The enlarged pulmonary vasculature causes an overall increase in lung opacity.

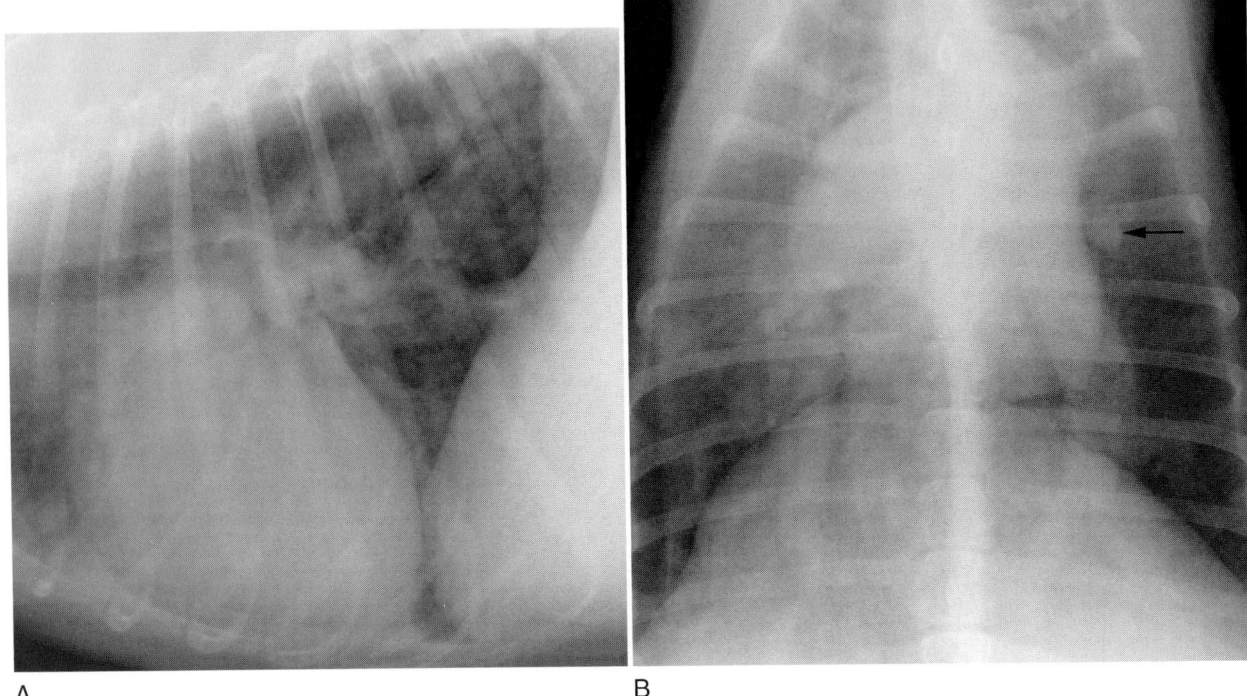

Fig. 25-23 Right lateral (A) and VD radiographs from a dog with severe heartworm disease. The pulmonary arteries are enlarged, blunted, and tortuous. End-on blunted pulmonary arteries can give the impression of pulmonary nodules (*arrow* in B). Eosinophilic granulomas and diffuse interstitial and/or alveolar pulmonary changes are possible in combination with the pulmonary artery changes. All these changes add opacity to the lung. With pulmonary thromboembolism caused by heartworm disease, the affected lung lobe could be radiolucent (a result of regional oligemia) or radiopaque (a result of inflammatory changes associated with verminous thrombosis).

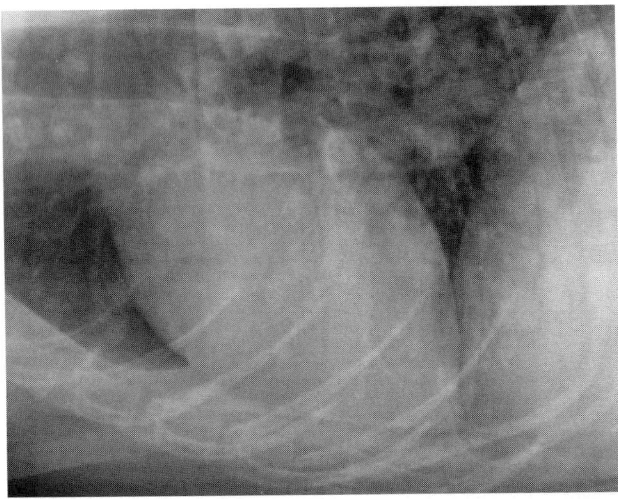

Fig. 25-24 Close-up right lateral radiograph of the mid-ventral thorax. Multiple, variably-sized pulmonary nodules are present. Some of the smallest of these nodules are seen best over a thin section of lung such as the ventral peripheral lung over the heart and diaphragm.

lacks the rings and lines typical of a bronchial pattern (Fig. 25-27). An unstructured interstitial pattern typically is generalized, although not always. An interstitial pattern also causes a loss in vessel definition, but this is difficult for beginning interpreters to appreciate. Fortunately, most clinically significant lung diseases do not lead to an unstructured interstitial pattern as their only radiographic manifestation. The time spent by beginning interpreters trying to decide if a mild, generalized interstitial pattern is present far outweighs the clinical significance of such a finding.

Second Paradigm Alternative to Strict Pattern Recognition

Rather than going through the mental gyrations of trying to fit an abnormal lung appearance into one of the previously defined lung patterns, an alternative approach can be taken. The alternative approach given here may benefit beginning interpreters because it is simpler and interpreters will feel less pressured to find and characterize an abnormal lung pattern. The reader can relax and spend more time initially deciding whether the lungs are truly normal.

Once the lungs are determined to be abnormal (too opaque), the basic decision is whether the airways (alveolar or bronchi) are affected by the disease process. This simplified approach is based on the fact that a definitive diagnosis of a lung disease cannot be made from a radiograph. Radiographs of the lung are most valuable for helping decide how to achieve a diagnosis. If the airways are deemed to be abnormal, then airway sampling with a transtracheal wash or bronchoalveolar lavage may be useful, whereas if the airways are not involved then these techniques have less value in reaching the definitive diagnosis.

Therefore the initial categorization could be aimed at looking for signs of an alveolar *or* bronchial pattern. The signs of these patterns are the same as previously defined. Clearly, if a classic alveolar pattern or bronchial pattern is identified,

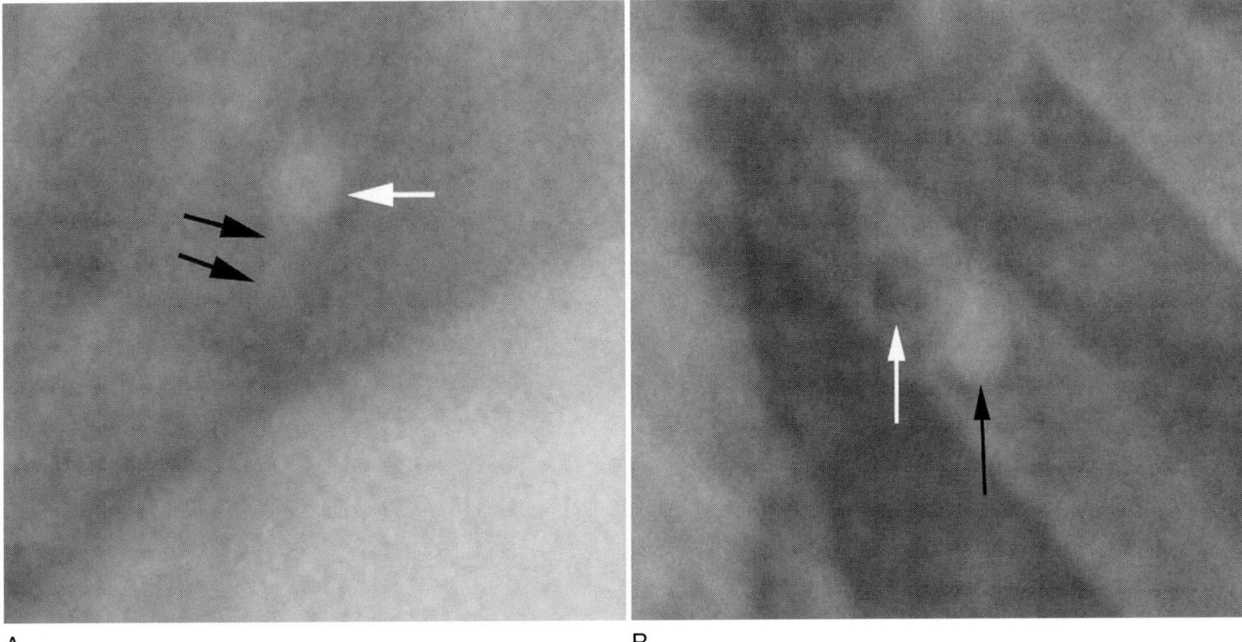

Fig. 25-25 A, Close-up of the right cranial lobe in a VD radiograph. An end-on pulmonary vessel is seen *(white arrow)*. It has an adjacent "tail" *(black arrows)*. B, Close-up of the left caudal lobe in a VD radiograph. An end-on pulmonary vessel is seen *(black arrow)*. It is next to a bronchus *(white arrow)*. End-on pulmonary vessels are quite radiopaque because of their cylindrical nature; that is, the overall thickness struck by the x-ray beam is greater than if the structure were a small sphere.

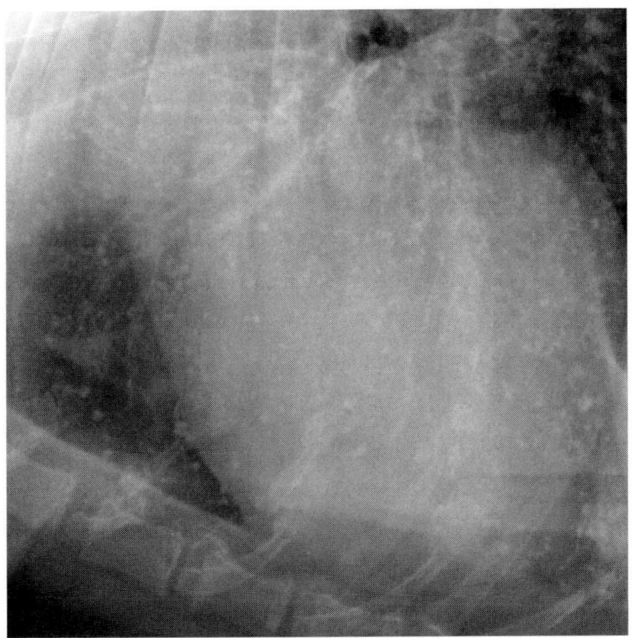

Fig. 25-26 Close-up right lateral radiograph of the cranial thorax. Multiple small, irregularly marginated mineralized opacities are present throughout the lungs, predominantly in a ventral location. These measure 2 to 3 mm in diameter and are mineral opaque. These are consistent with osseous metaplasia and are also called pulmonary osteomas.

then diagnostic considerations based on signalment, breed, history, and lesion distribution can be used, and airway sampling may be quite helpful. However, many patients with abnormal lungs do not have a classic lung pattern, and if the abnormal pattern cannot be determined as alveolar or bronchial, such as might occur in a heterogeneous alveolar pattern, the airways can still be assessed, and, if determined to be abnormal, airway sampling may be beneficial. On the other hand, if no signs of alveolar or bronchial involvement are present, and the intensity of the abnormality per unit area is not great, the likelihood of the abnormality representing an unstructured, interstitial pulmonary pattern increases. With unstructured interstitial disease, the value of airway sampling is diminished and other alternatives must be used to reach the final diagnosis. In fact, the presumed unstructured interstitial pulmonary pattern may be within normal limits, and invasive methods to reach the final diagnosis are not warranted at this time. However, if the unstructured pattern is pronounced, then consideration of methods to identify the final diagnosis, such as lung biopsy, is warranted. This latter paradigm of airway versus no airway involvement also eliminates the confusion associated with the bronchointerstitial pattern because identification of the bronchial component justifies the value of airway sampling as a means to reach the final diagnosis, regardless of whether the interstitium is involved.

Granted, airway sampling is not indicated in every patient with airway involvement, such as in patients with cardiogenic pulmonary edema, but grouping patients by airway versus no airway involvement at least separates them into groups in which the potential value of airway sampling is more clearly defined.

Regardless of the method used to assess the lung, the beginning interpreter will find this to be one of the more difficult concepts to grasp. Only with a consistent approach and expe-

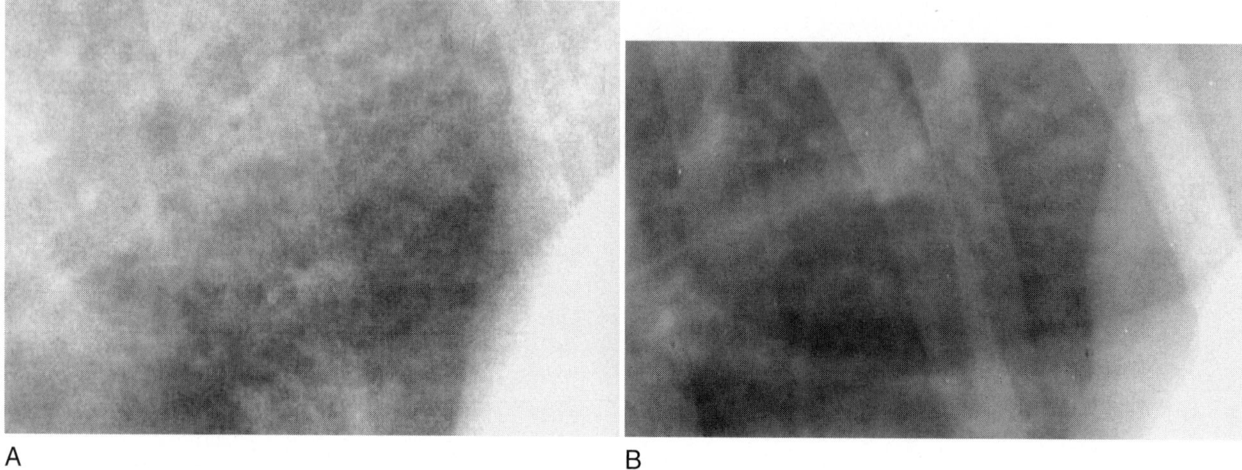

Fig. 25-27 Close-up lateral radiographs of the dorsal caudal aspect of the thorax of a dog with pulmonary lymphoma **(A)** and a normal dog **(B)**. Note the generalized increase in lung opacity in A that has no structure. This is an unstructured interstitial pattern; it is not intense enough per unit area to be confused with an alveolar pattern. It may be tempting to say too many ring shadows are visible, which is true, thus suggesting a bronchial pattern. However, there are not this many bronchi in this region of the lung; these apparent rings are summation shadows from the overlapping interstitial pattern. Note how the vessels are more difficult to identify in **A.** Lymphoma and deep mycoses are the most common cause of an unstructured interstitial pattern, but both conditions are rare.

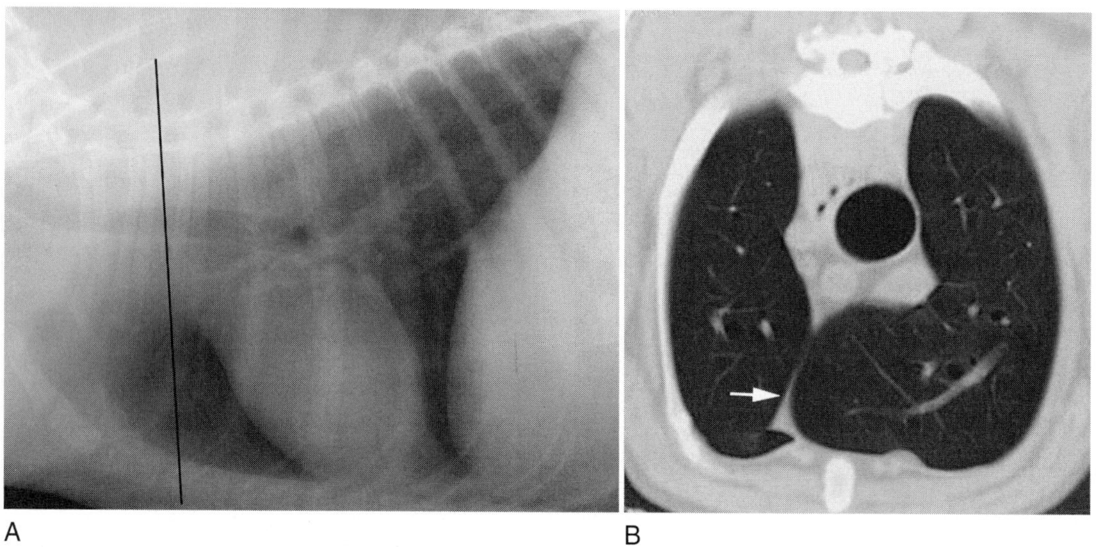

Fig. 25-28 Right lateral radiograph (A) and a single computed tomographic image (B) of the cranial thorax. On the lateral radiograph a *black line* has been placed where the CT study was obtained. On the CT image the right cranial lung lobe (reader's right) passes in front of the heart (out of plane) ventrally toward the left. The soft tissue line *(arrow)* that separates the right cranial and left cranial (reader's left) lung lobes is the cranioventral mediastinal reflection. A mediastinal reflection is an area where a right- or left-sided lung lobe courses across mid-line and then takes on a contralateral location.

rience looking at large numbers of images will proficiency in lung interpretation improve.

The Mediastinum

The mediastinum is the potential space between the right and left pleural sacs. The mediastinum in the dog and cat is incomplete, meaning nonviscid pleural effusions (e.g., transudates) tend to be bilateral. Exudative effusions (e.g., pyothorax or hemothorax) tend to be unilateral because of the plugging of the fenestrated, incomplete mediastinum.

The mediastinum, when viewed from a ventral or dorsal perspective, is characterized by reflections in which certain structures push the mediastinum away from its normal midline location. These mediastinal reflections develop as the lungs grow and cross the ventral aspect of midline. Two primary mediastinal reflections are described (Fig. 25-28). The cranioventral mediastinal reflection forms when the lingula portion of the left cranial lung lobe extends across midline from the left to the right at the thoracic inlet and as the right cranial lung lobe develops and pushes the mediastinum across midline from a right-to-left direction in front of the cardiac silhouette.

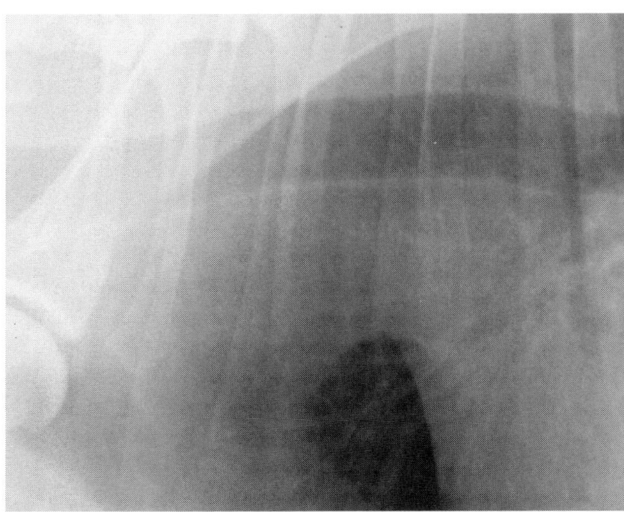

Fig. 25-29 Close-up lateral radiograph. The soft tissue opacity ventral to the trachea is the cranial mediastinum, which contains a large number of structures. These structures are not visible because they are in contact with insufficient interposed fat, leading to border effacement. With pneumomediastinum some structures in this part of the mediastinum can typically be identified.

The caudoventral mediastinal reflection is a result of the growth of the accessory lung lobe as it develops and pushes the mediastinum from the right to the left. The caval mediastinal reflection, or plica vena cava, is not visible as a distinct structure but represents the mediastinum wrapped around the caudal vena cava in the right hemithorax. These reflections are important anatomic landmarks. For example, the caudal ventral mediastinal reflection forms the left lateral–most extent of the accessory lung lobe on the VD or DV radiograph. Within the middle mediastinum, the cardiac silhouette also pushes the mediastinum apart ventrally. The right convexity of the cardiac silhouette displaces the right lung lobe in a rightward direction, and the left convexity of the cardiac silhouette displaces the ventral portion of the left lung lobe in a leftward direction. Dorsally, the mediastinum is a midline structure.

The mediastinum can be divided into cranial, middle, and caudal parts, with each having an imaginary ventral and dorsal compartment. In the cranial mediastinum the trachea is the most conspicuous structure, entering at the thoracic inlet and coursing in a caudal direction to the level of the bronchial bifurcation at the carina. Surrounding the trachea on the lateral radiograph is a confluence of soft tissue structures that cannot be distinguished because of silhouetting with each other (Fig. 25-29). These structures include the brachiocephalic trunk, esophagus, cranial mediastinal lymph nodes, azygous vein, internal thoracic arteries and veins, cranial vena cava, nerves, lymphatics, cardiac silhouette, common carotid arteries, and subclavian vessels. This list is not inclusive but is a reminder of the large number structures present in the dorsal cranial mediastinum.

Occasionally a small amount of gas may be present in the cranial thoracic esophagus or over the heart base area. This finding is more common on the left lateral radiograph compared with the right. In the ventral aspect of the cranial mediastinum, the left cranial lung lobe lingula and the cranial mediastinal reflection is seen. The sternal lymph node is not seen unless enlarged. In a young animal the thymus can occasionally be identified between the right cranial lung lobe and the cardiac silhouette (Fig. 25-30). More commonly, the thymus can be seen on the VD or DV radiograph extending in the cranial mediastinum reflection between the left cranial and right cranial lung lobes. The thymus creates an opacity that is usually curved and triangular in shape and extends from the midline in a convex fashion following the medial border of the left cranial lung lobe into the left hemithorax (see Fig. 25-30). On the VD and DV radiograph, the trachea is normally located to the right of midline. The right lateral margin of the cranial mediastinum on the VD or DV radiograph is usually formed by the lateral margin of the cranial vena cava. The trachea typically enters the thoracic inlet in a midline or just to the right of midline position on the VD or DV radiograph.

Dorsally in the middle mediastinum, the trachea terminates at the carina into the caudal main stem bronchi. The descending aorta is visualized because of its position along the medial border of the left and right caudal lung lobes. The esophagus is usually not visible on the lateral or VD/DV radiograph in this portion of the mediastinum. The dorsal portion of the middle mediastinum also contains the tracheobronchial lymph nodes, phrenic nerve, and vagosympathetic trunk. These structures are not visualized on normal thoracic radiographs.

The most conspicuous opacity in the middle mediastinum is the cardiac silhouette, which is composed of the pericardium, great vessels (ascending aorta, aortic arch, main pulmonary artery), heart, and blood within the heart. The cardiac silhouette occupies two thirds of the middle mediastinum on the lateral radiograph, has an oval appearance, and is located between the fourth and sixth intercostal spaces.[2,3,12,13] Evaluation of the cardiac silhouette should be based on established objective criteria. However, evaluation of the cardiac silhouette can be imprecise because breed variation accounts for a large difference in apparent size. Thoracic conformation must be considered when evaluating cardiac silhouette size in dogs. With a deep, narrow chest such as in Doberman Pinschers, the heart has an upright appearance and is relatively small compared with the overall thoracic volume. On the VD/DV radiograph the heart may appear more rounded rather than oval because of the upright orientation of the heart.

In a medium-size dog with average thoracic confirmation (Golden Retriever or mixed-breed dog) the cardiac base is inclined in a more cranial direction and the cranial heart margin appears to lie along the sternum. On the VD/DV view the cardiac silhouette appears more oval. In small chondrodystrophic dogs, or dogs with a barrel-shaped thorax, the cardiac silhouette typically appears large on the lateral radiograph relative to the overall thoracic volume. The cardiac base has marked cranial inclination, and the heart may appear to occupy 60% to 70% of the thoracic volume. On a VD or DV radiograph, however, the cardiac silhouette will have a more normal size relative to the thoracic volume, which illustrates the importance of obtaining orthogonal radiographs. In addition to breed-related factors, the degree of inspiration can influence the radiographic appearance of the cardiac silhouette.

In general, the heart in dogs should be 3 to 3.5 times the width of an intercostal space on the lateral radiograph (measured in the largest diameter of the cardiac silhouette). In the cat, the maximum diameter of the cardiac silhouette (usually the heart base) should be 2 to 3 times the width of an intercostal space. The basilar to apical length of the cardiac silhouette is usually 60% of the DV height of the thoracic cavity on the lateral radiograph. On the VD or DV radiograph the cardiac silhouette size should not exceed 50% of the pleural to pleural diameter at the ninth intercostal space. These are rules of thumb and should help in the initial assessment of cardiac size.[16,17]

Recently a cardiac measurement technique called the vertebral heart score has been described in which the heart length

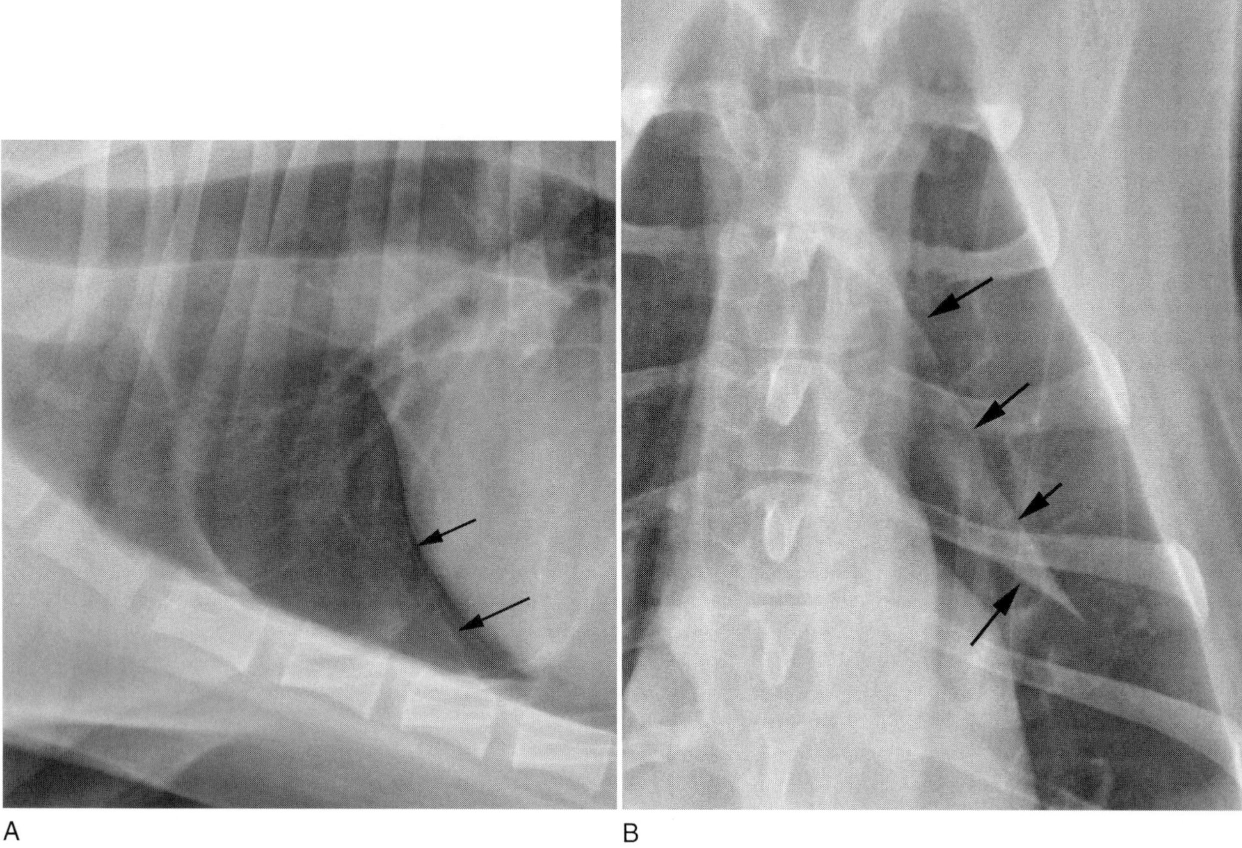

Fig. 25-30 Right lateral (A) and VD (B) radiographs from a young dog with a thymic remnant. The thymus is found in the cranioventral mediastinal reflection identified in Figure 25-28. The *arrows* delineate the thymus on both the right lateral (infrequently seen) and the VD radiographs (most commonly seen and referred to as the "sail sign").

and width on the lateral radiograph is normalized to vertebral length.[18,19] This technique can provide objective criteria for evaluating the heart. The vertebral heart score should not replace subjective radiographic evaluation of cardiac size and shape. Increased accuracy of the vertebral heart score versus subjective evaluation for assessing cardiac abnormalities has not yet been proven.[20] The vertebral heart score may be most useful in assessing the change in size of the heart in an individual patient over time.

The heart tends to be primarily located in the left hemithorax on the VD or DV radiographs and much more so on DV radiographs because of cranial excursion of the diaphragm that displaces the heart to the left. The apex points toward the left costodiaphragmatic angle. The shape of the cardiac silhouette tends to be rounder on the left lateral view because of rotation of the apex from the sternum. The descending aorta and main pulmonary artery extend leftward of the vertebral bodies on the VD/DV radiograph.

The opacity of all the structures of the cardiac silhouette are soft tissue; therefore differentiation of the various chambers, valves, blood, surfaces, and vessels cannot be done without echocardiography or administration of contrast medium.

In actuality, the accuracy of identifying specific cardiac abnormalities in survey radiographs is poor. However, contour, size, and shape changes specific to intracardiac enlargement patterns have been described. These changes are described in Chapter 33. One system that helps familiarize students with evaluation of cardiac abnormalities is the analogy of the cardiac silhouette as a clock face. Specific changes within a given region of the clock face can be correlated with specific chamber or great vessel enlargement (Fig. 25-31). Importantly, cardiac disease cannot be excluded if these changes are absent based solely on survey thoracic radiographs.

When evaluating the heart, great vessels, pulmonary vessels, and parenchyma, certain rules specific to an interpretation paradigm should be followed. These following rules are answers to five questions related to the radiographic abnormalities present:

- Is any roentgen abnormality of the cardiac silhouette present (change in size, shape, opacity, location, margination, and number)? What is the expected normal appearance of the heart based on the breed of the patient?
- If cardiomegaly is present, are the changes consistent with right-sided cardiomegaly, left-sided cardiomegaly, or both (generalized cardiomegaly)?
- Are alterations of the pulmonary arteries and veins present within the peripheral lung field (e.g., undercirculated, overcirculated, pulmonary artery larger than the vein, or pulmonary vein larger than the corresponding artery)?
- Does evidence exist for left heart failure (pulmonary edema), right heart failure, (hepatomegaly, pleural effusion), or both?
- Are the descending aorta, heart base region, main pulmonary artery segment, or the caudal vena cava enlarged? (This question requires evaluation of a

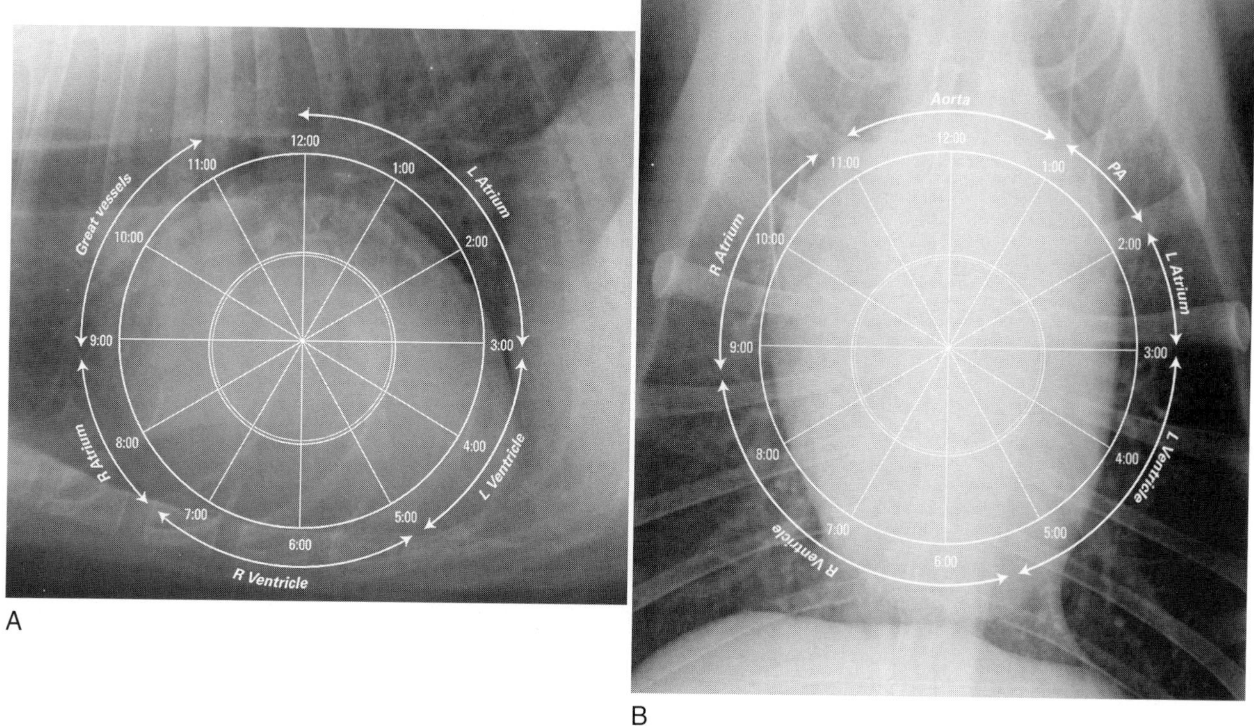

Fig. 25-31 A, Right lateral radiograph with a superimposed clock face. The heart is subdivided into different locations that approximate certain areas of the great vessels and chambers of the heart. *R*, Right; *L*, left. **B,** VD radiograph with a superimposed clock face. The heart is subdivided into different locations that approximate certain areas of the great vessels and chambers of the heart. *R*, Right; *L*, left; *PA*, main pulmonary artery segment.

well-positioned VD/DV radiograph and is critical for evaluating the great vessels for radiographic evidence of poststenotic dilation related to congenital heart defects.)

Notice that these questions integrate several general categories of abnormalities (mediastinum, great vessels, heart, pleural space, and pulmonary parenchyma), and the reader must be familiar with all potential aspects of cardiac-related disease before answering these five questions. Do the answers make sense? Endocardiosis of the mitral valve and valvular insufficiency in a dog would lead to left heart failure (pulmonary edema), but the animal would not be expected to have an enlarged caudal vena or a ductus diverticulum (focal enlargement of the descending aortic arch). Within the context of these answers, the radiographs would need to be reevaluated to ensure that the correct interpretation has been made. This does not mean that multiple abnormalities may not be present; however, an attempt to relate all the radiographic abnormalities into one disease should be made within the known context of expected anatomic and pathophysiologic changes.

The prominent structures of the caudal mediastinum include the caudal vena cava ventrally and the descending aorta dorsally. Normally the esophagus and the other structures of the dorsal middle mediastinum are not seen on either the lateral or the VD/DV radiograph. Occasionally fluid or air may be present in the caudal esophagus on the lateral radiograph. This could be caused by swallowing or gastroesophageal reflux. A repeat radiograph should be obtained. If gas or fluid persist, an esophagram may be indicated to rule out esophageal abnormalities. On the VD or DV radiograph the caudal vena cava will be superimposed over the right caudal lobar pulmonary bronchus and vein, and the descending aorta usually is essentially on the midline just before entering the diaphragm. The caudal ventral mediastinal reflection can also be identified.

In summary, a checklist for the interpretation paradigm for the thorax can be found at http://evolve.elsevier.com/Thrall/vetrad/. The reader is encouraged to download the checklist, print it, and post it next to the view box or viewing station so that radiographs can be reviewed in a systematic fashion.

Anatomic Variants

Individual conformational variation between various dog breeds is quite common. In young animals (younger than 1 year), the thymus is expected to be in the cranial mediastinum. If the animal is older than 1 year, the thymus has usually involuted to the point of not being radiographically detectable. Occasionally, a remnant of the thymus may still be present. Thymomas or other mass lesions of the thymus will have a rounded appearance with enlargement.

Chondrodystrophic breeds have pleural indentations as a result of their typical costochondral deformities. These deformities result in extrapleural opacities visible on the lateral and VD/DV radiographs (see Fig. 25-6). A related finding is the skin fold. Skin folds, however, are characterized by radiolucency lateral to the skin fold margin on the VD/DV radiograph and should not be mistaken for pneumothorax. Skin folds also often extend beyond the margin of the pleural cavity (see Chapter 32).

Dorsal deviation of the trachea in the cranial mediastinum can be caused by flexion of the head and neck at the time of radiographic exposure. If a soft tissue mass is not seen ventral to the trachea or within the cranial mediastinum, then the

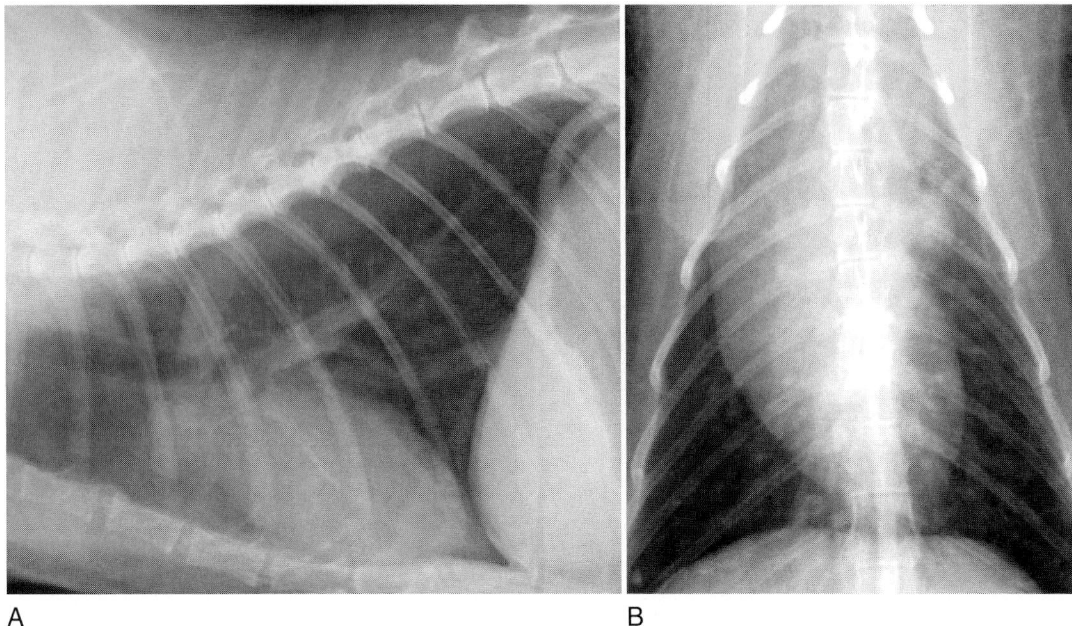

Fig. 25-32 Right lateral (A) and VD (B) radiograph from an 11-year-old cat with a malpositioned heart and tortuous aorta noted on the lateral view and a redundant aortic knob noted on the VD radiograph in the 12 to 1 o'clock position.

most likely cause of tracheal displacement is malpositioning (see Chapter 27).

A redundant tracheal membrane is another tracheal variant. The esophagus and trachealis muscle overlying the trachea will cause a soft tissue opacity superimposed over the dorsal lumen of the trachea in the thoracic inlet extending into the cranial thorax. The degree of soft tissue opacity is related to the degree of laxity of the trachealis muscle. This is called redundant dorsal tracheal membrane and should not be confused with the pathologic condition of tracheal collapse (see Chapter 27). Inspiratory versus expiratory or right versus left lateral radiographs help distinguish tracheal collapse from redundant tracheal membrane. In a dog with a redundant dorsal tracheal membrane, the dorsal border of the trachea can typically be seen above the ventral, luminal soft tissue margin of the trachealis muscle.

As previously mentioned, air can be seen in the esophagus, particularly on the left lateral radiograph at the level of the heart base. This should not be confused with segmental megaesophagus or a foreign body. Repeat radiographs may be obtained to rule out luminal obstruction. In Bulldog and Shar Pei dogs, the esophagus at the thoracic inlet can have a focal redundancy that is normal for the breed.

In obese small animals the cranial and caudal mediastinal reflections are widened because of fat accumulation. Fat will also accumulate along the ventral aspect of the cardiac silhouette, adjacent to the pericardium.[21] Fat along the lateral thoracic wall can also cause an extrapleural sign if the accumulation is sufficiently extensive to displace the parietal pleura medially.

The cardiac silhouette in cats becomes more horizontal in position with age. The normal apicobasilar angle, relative to the sternum, is approximately 45 degrees. In aged cats, this angle may decrease to less than 25 degrees. The aortic arch in older cats is also commonly characterized by a bulge, called a redundant aorta (Fig. 25-32).[20] Excessive accumulation of fat around the heart can result in a double silhouette on the lateral and VD or DV radiograph where the true cardiac silhouette is found within the fat-expanded silhouette.[22] Also, pericardial fat can alter the normal oval appearance of the cardiac silhouette so that a prominent square corner is identified along the right cranial margin of the cardiac silhouette on the VD or DV radiograph. This can be seen in obese dogs as well.

REFERENCES

1. Suter PF: *Thoracic radiograph: a text atlas of thoracic diseases of the dog and cat*, Wettswii, Switzerland, 1984, Peter F. Suter.
2. Suter PF: The radiographic diagnosis of canine and feline heart disease, *Compend Contin Ed Small Anim Pract* 3:441, 1981.
3. Toombs JP, Ogburn PN: Evaluating canine cardiovascular silhouettes: radiographic methods and normal radiographic anatomy, *Compend Contin Ed Small Anim Pract* 7:579, 1985.
4. Forrest LJ: Radiology corner—advantages of the three view thoracic radiographic examination in instances other than metastasis, *Vet Radiol* 33:340, 1992.
5. Barthez PY, Hornof WJ, Theon AP et al: Sensitivity of radiographic protocols when screening dogs for pulmonary metastasis, *J Am Vet Med Assoc* 204:237, 1994.
6. Spencer CP, Ackerman N, Burt JK: The canine lateral thoracic radiograph, *Vet Radiol* 22:262, 1981.
7. Carlisle CH, Thrall DE: A comparison of normal feline thoracic radiographs made in dorsal versus ventral recumbency, *Vet Radiol* 23:3, 1982.
8. Ruehl WW, Thrall DE: The effect of dorsal versus ventral recumbency on the radiographic appearance of the canine thorax, *Vet Radiol* 22:10, 1981.
9. Silverman S, Suter PF: Influence of inspiration and expiration on canine thoracic radiographs, *J Am Vet Med Assoc* 166:502, 1975.
10. Holmes RA, Smith FG, Lewis RE et al: The effects of rotation on the radiographic appearance of the canine cardiac silhouette in dorsal recumbency, *Vet Radiol* 26:98, 1985.

11. Myer CW: Radiography review: the interstitial pattern of pulmonary disease, *Vet Radiol* 21:18, 1980.
12. Myer CW: Radiography review: the vascular and bronchial patterns of pulmonary disease, *Vet Radiol* 21:156, 1980.
13. Silverman S, Poulos PW, Suter PF: Cavitary pulmonary lesions in animals, *J Am Vet Radiol Soc* XVII:134, 1976.
14. Reif JS, Rhodes WH: The lungs of aged dogs: a radiographic-morphologic correlation, *J Am Vet Radiol Soc* 7:5, 1966.
15. Lord PF, Gomez JA: Lung lobe collapse: pathophysiology and radiologic significance, *Vet Radiol* 26:187, 1985.
16. Vanden Broek AM, Darke PG: Cardiac measurements on thoracic radiographs of cats, *J Small Anim Prac* 28:125, 1987.
17. Toal RL, Losonsky JM, Coulter DB et al: Influence of cardiac cycle on the radiographic appearance of the feline heart, *Vet Radiol* 26:63, 1985.
18. Buchanan JW, Bücheler H: Vertebral scale system to measure canine heart size in radiographs, *J Am Vet Med Assoc* 206:194, 1995.
19. Litster AL, Buchanan JW: Measurement of the normal feline cardiac silhouette on thoracic radiographs, *J Am Vet Med Assoc* 216:210, 2000.
20. Lamb CR, Tyler M, Boswood A et al: Assessment of the value of the vertebral heart score in the radiographic diagnosis in dogs, *Vet Rec* 146:687, 2000.
21. Litster AL, Buchanan JW: Radiographic and echocardiographic measurement of the heart in obese cats, *Vet Radiol Ultrasound* 41:320, 2000.
22. Moon M, Keene BW, Lessard P et al: Age related changes in the feline cardiac silhouette, *Vet Radiol Ultrasound* 24:315, 1993.

ELECTRONIC RESOURCES evolve

Additional information related to the content in Chapter 25 can be found on the companion Web site at
evolve http://evolve.elsevier.com/Thrall/vetrad/

- Key Points
- Chapter Quiz
- Paradigm for Interpretation

CHAPTER • 26
Radiographic Anatomy of the Cardiopulmonary System

James E. Smallwood
Kathy A. Spaulding

To use the roentgen-sign method of recognizing abnormal radiographic findings effectively, an understanding of normal radiographic anatomy is required for the specific area of interest. This chapter provides a limited reference for the radiographic anatomy of the cardiopulmonary system. For more detailed information, the reader is referred to a comprehensive text on radiographic anatomy.[1] The radiographic nomenclature used in this chapter is that approved by the American College of Veterinary Radiology in 1983.[2]

REFERENCES

1. Schebitz H, Wilkens H: *Atlas of radiographic anatomy of the dog,* Stuttgart, Germany, 2005, Parey Verlag.
2. Smallwood JE, Shively MJ, Rendano VT, et al: A standardized nomenclature for radiographic projections used in veterinary medicine, *Vet Radiol* 26:2, 1985.

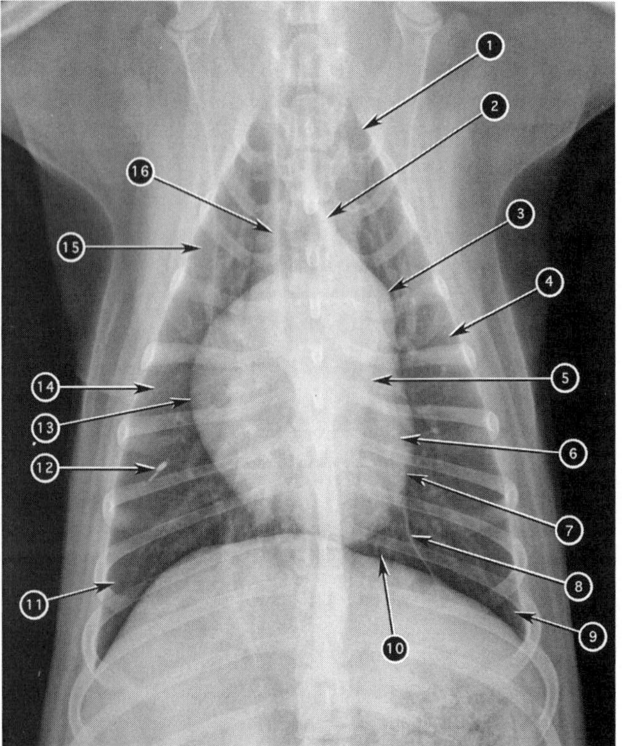

Fig. 26-1 Ventrodorsal Radiograph of Canine Thorax.
1. Cranial part of cranial lobe of left lung
2. Cranial mediastinum (thymus?)
3. Pulmonary trunk
4. Caudal part of cranial lobe of left lung
5. Descending aorta
6. Caudal lobar branch of left pulmonary artery
7. Left ventricle of heart
8. Caudoventral reflection of mediastinum
9. Caudal lobe of left lung
10. Accessory lobe of right lung
11. Caudal lobe of right lung
12. Microchip embedded in subcutis
13. Right ventricle of heart
14. Middle lobe of right lung
15. Cranial lobe of right lung
16. Trachea

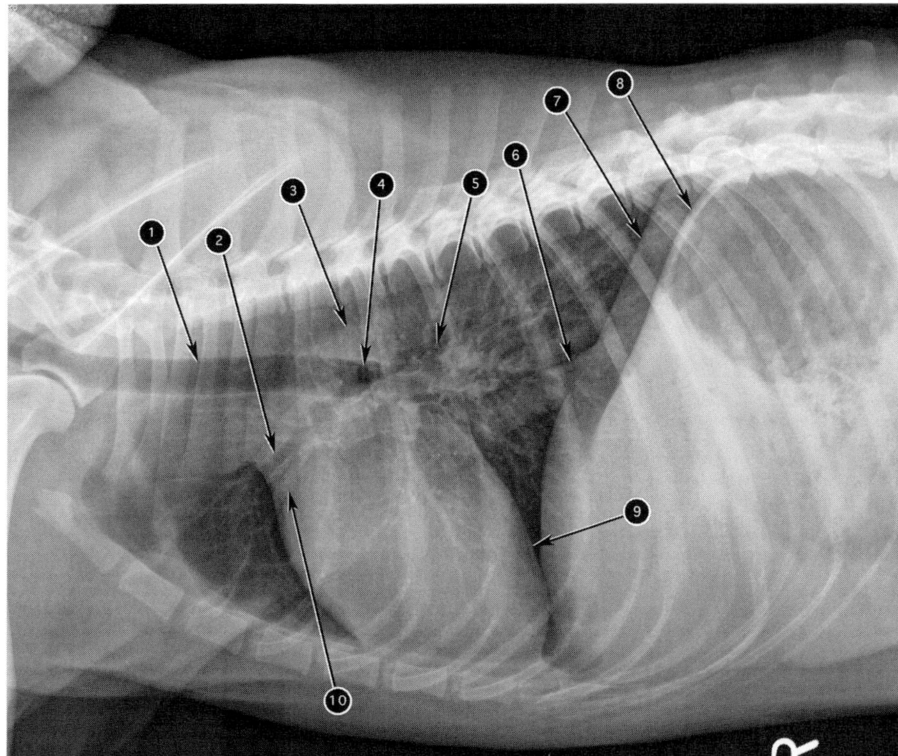

Fig. 26-2 Left-Right Lateral Radiograph of Canine Thorax.
1. Trachea
2. Right cranial lobar bronchus
3. Descending aorta
4. Tracheal bifurcation
5. End-on view of pulmonary vessel
6. Caudal vena cava
7. Right crus of diaphragm
8. Left crus of diaphragm
9. Left ventricle of heart
10. Right cranial lobar pulmonary vein

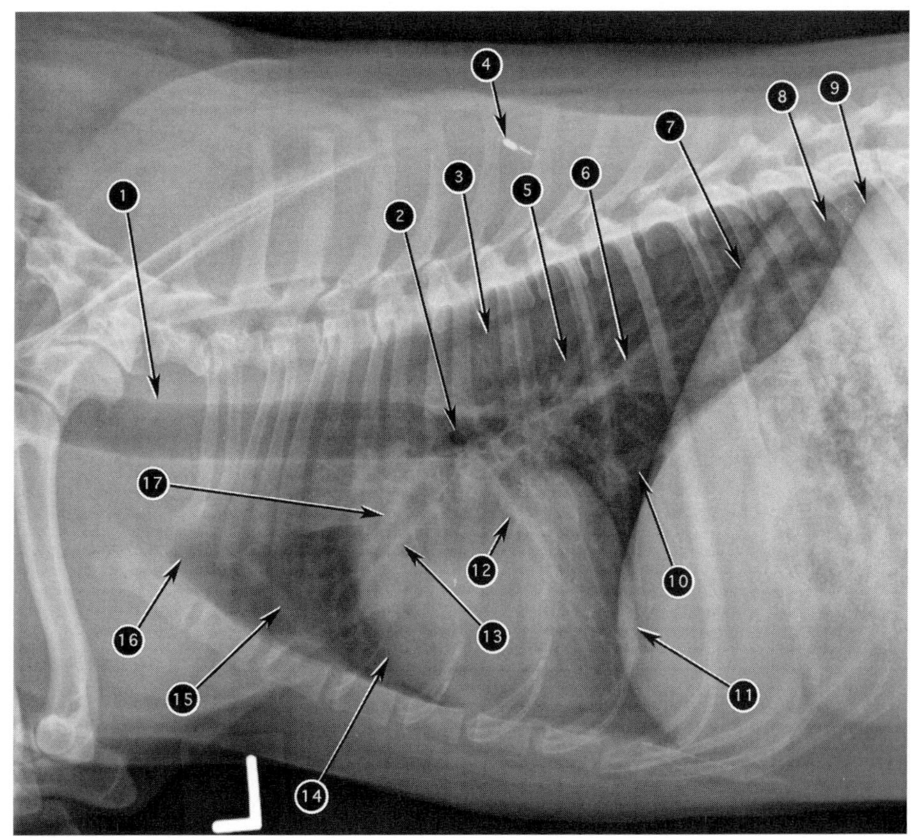

Fig. 26-3 Right-Left Lateral Radiograph of Canine Thorax.
1. Trachea
2. Right cranial lobar bronchus
3. Descending aorta
4. Microchip embedded in subcutis
5. Caudal lobar branch of left pulmonary artery
6. Caudal lobar branch of right pulmonary artery
7. Left crus of diaphragm
8. Gas in fundus of stomach
9. Right crus of diaphragm
10. Caudal vena cava
11. Left ventricle of heart
12. Middle lobar branch of right pulmonary artery
13. Right cranial lobar pulmonary vein
14. Right ventricle of heart
15. Cranioventral mediastinal reflection
16. Apex of left lung
17. Cranial lobar branch of right pulmonary artery

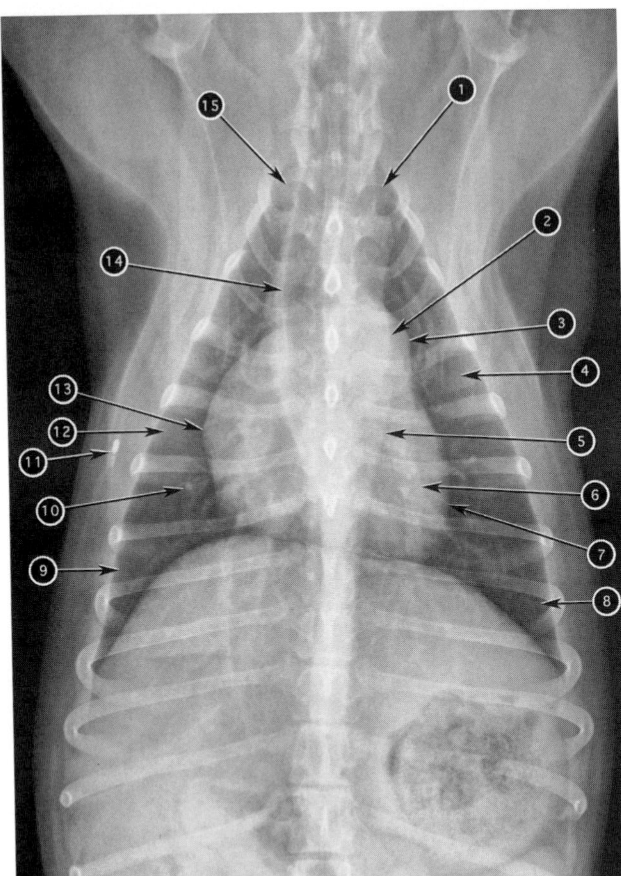

Fig. 26-4 Dorsoventral Radiograph of Canine Thorax.
1. Cranial part of cranial lobe of left lung
2. Aortic arch
3. Pulmonary trunk
4. Caudal part of cranial lobe of left lung
5. Descending aorta
6. Caudal lobar branch of left pulmonary artery
7. Left ventricle of heart
8. Caudal lobe of left lung
9. Caudal lobe of right lung
10. End-on image of pulmonary vessel
11. Microchip embedded in subcutis
12. Middle lobe of right lung
13. Right ventricle of heart
14. Trachea
15. Cranial lobe of right lung

ELECTRONIC RESOURCES evolve

Chapter 26 can also be found on the companion Web site at evolve http://evolve.elsevier.com/Thrall/vetrad/

CHAPTER • 27
Larynx, Pharynx, and Trachea

Stephen K. Kneller

LARYNX AND PHARYNX

Anatomic Considerations

The pharynx, bordered by the base of the tongue and the retropharyngeal wall, is divided into the oropharynx and nasopharynx by the soft palate, which extends to the level of the epiglottis. On high-quality lateral radiographs, many laryngeal structures can be identified (Fig. 27-1).[1]

Laryngeal structures are difficult to see on ventrodorsal views because of overlying structures. In lateral radiographs, the transverse basihyoid bone is usually obvious because it is projected on end and may be mistaken for a foreign object. Radiographs of brachycephalic dogs, as well as those of obese animals, are more difficult to interpret because of the larger amount of soft tissue and fat. This results in a lower air/tissue ratio, providing less contrast as well as opacities that are more irregular.

In very young animals (2 to 3 months of age), laryngeal structures may not be well defined because they are not sufficiently mineralized. Mineralization in laryngeal cartilaginous structures, including the epiglottis, is a normal change of aging. Mineralization may be seen in animals as young as 2 to 3 years and is expected to occur earlier in large and chondrodystrophic dogs. In one study, 96 of 99 clinically normal dogs of random breeds and random age older than 1 year had radiographic laryngeal mineralization.[2] The cricoid cartilage is usually the first laryngeal cartilage to become mineralized.

Depending on the phase and depth of respiration during radiography, the tip of the epiglottis may be just dorsal or ventral to the soft palate, or it may be on the ventral floor of the pharynx. This variation may be seen in normal animals; however, in the presence of swallowing disorders, radiographic and fluoroscopic examination should be performed during swallowing to determine if the epiglottis moves normally.

Hyoid bones have been mistakenly diagnosed as foreign objects. The configuration and relative position of the hyoid bones are rather uniform among small animals; however, the position of the head, tongue, and larynx during radiography causes variation in the angles between hyoid bones. Oblique views may cause significant distortion, leading to erroneous diagnosis.

Radiographic Signs of Disease

Hyoid Bones

Few radiographic abnormalities are evident in the hyoid bones. The most common of these abnormalities are fractures and dislocations.

Space-Occupying Lesions

Mass lesions of the larynx, pharynx, and trachea are also uncommon. When small, these lesions appear as variants in the normal shape of structures, and when large, they may obliterate air-filled cavities. Depending on the shape, physical density, and architecture, foreign objects lodged in the airway may be identified, or they may appear as space-occupying tissue masses.

Space-occupying masses outside the larynx/pharynx are more difficult to identify because they are not surrounded by gas. These lesions are identified through recognition of displacement or encroachment of the air-tissue interfaces. Although masses may develop at any site, enlargement of specific structures, such as a lymph node or the thyroid gland, should be considered as possible causes of such radiographic abnormalities (Fig. 27-2). Swelling in the pharyngeal/laryngeal soft tissues has been reported as a result of rodenticide ingestion.[3,4]

Functional Abnormalities

Functional abnormalities of the larynx are best evaluated by direct visual inspection. Neurogenic disorders result in mild or equivocal radiographic signs.[5] Consistent misplacement of the epiglottis seen on radiographs should prompt visual examination. In the panting dog, the epiglottis lies on the ventral floor of the pharynx.[2] Otherwise, it is in a semierect position, usually with the tip just dorsal or ventral to the soft palate.

TRACHEA

Anatomic Considerations

The trachea is easiest to evaluate on the lateral view; however, its appearance on the ventrodorsal view is useful for assessment of displacement. The trachea is normally found slightly to the right in the cranial mediastinum. This deviation is more exaggerated in brachycephalic breeds and obese dogs; this normal deviation should not be mistaken for displacement from a mass. On the lateral view, the trachea is nearly parallel to the cervical spine, but it is slightly closer to the spine in the caudal cervical region than in the cranial region. Because the thoracic vertebrae angle dorsally, a slight divergence of the trachea from the thoracic spine is present. The trachea angles slightly ventrally at the point of bifurcation into the principal bronchi. The diameter of the trachea is relatively uniform and is slightly smaller than that of the larynx. In normal animals, the trachea does not vary significantly between phases of respiration and remains uniform in diameter.

The trachea is a semirigid tube attached at the larynx and the carina. It is less constrained by surrounding tissues in the cranial mediastinum than in the cervical region. During radiographic examination in the lateral view, the head and neck should be placed in an erect, but not overextended, position. Extreme extension of the neck may cause compression and narrowing of the trachea at the thoracic inlet. Conversely, if the neck is flexed, the trachea is likely to bend in the cranial

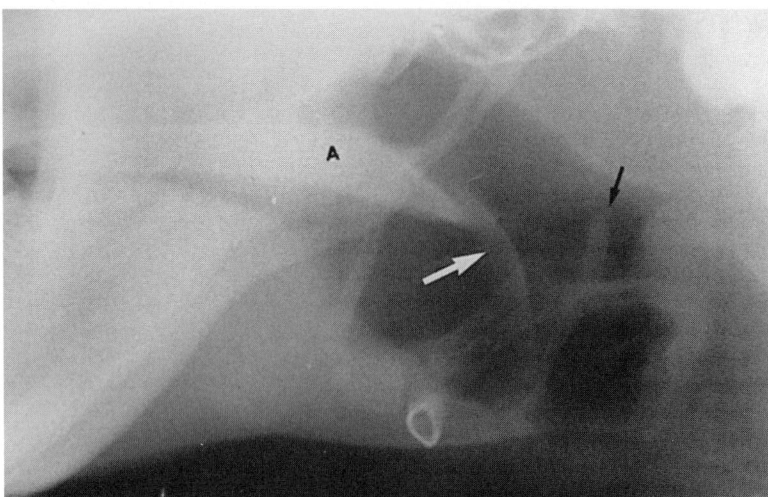

Fig. 27-1 Normal lateral radiograph of the laryngeal region of a 6-month-old mixed-breed dog. The soft palate *(A)* separates the nasopharynx from the oropharynx. The epiglottis *(white arrow)* extends from the larynx to the tip of the soft palate. The cranial cornua of the thyroid cartilage *(black arrow)* should not be mistaken for a foreign object. Note the end-on view of the basihyoid bone.

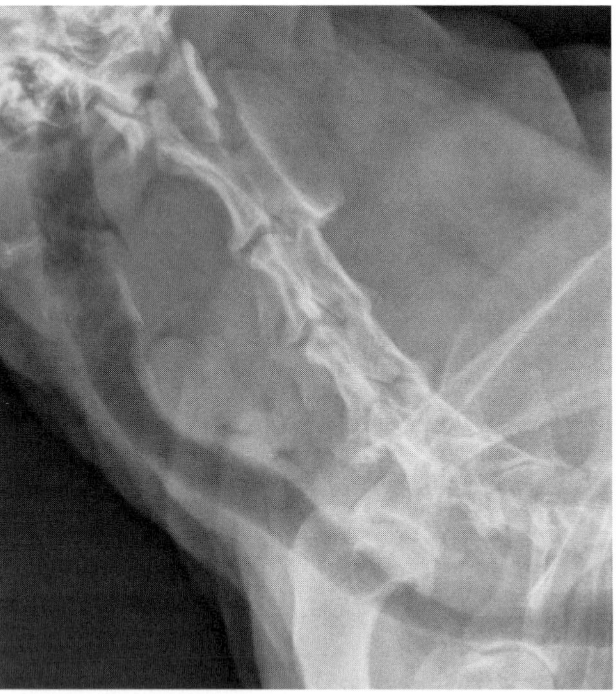

Fig. 27-2 Lateral view of the neck of a dog with a thyroid tumor. Note the ventral displacement of the trachea. Thyroid masses are a common cause of ventral displacement of the trachea in the cervical region. An esophageal mass would be another consideration. In this dog the mass appears lobulated and also surrounded by regions of decreased opacity. These regions may be interpreted as gas, such as might occur with an esophageal mass, but in this dog they were caused by cervical fat surrounding the thyroid mass.

mediastinum, simulating displacement by a cranial mediastinal mass (Fig. 27-3).

Mineralization of the tracheal rings may be seen as part of the aging process, especially in large and chondrodystrophic dogs; however, it is also seen in younger dogs, apparently with no significance. Diseases that stimulate metastatic mineralization may stimulate increased mineralization of the trachea along with other soft tissues.

Tracheal Displacement

Displacement of the trachea can be the first clue to the presence of a mass in the surrounding soft tissue after positioning artifacts and breed variation have been considered. When tracheal displacement is recognized, the immediate area should be scrutinized carefully for the presence of a mass. Occasionally other modalities, such as ultrasound and computed tomography, are needed to identify a mass responsible for tracheal displacement, especially in the heart base region. In the cervical region, mass lesions must be relatively large to cause tracheal displacement. Common causes for tracheal displacement are listed in Table 27-1.

Most masses that displace the trachea rarely compress it unless the mass is massive. Except for tracheobronchial lymphomegaly and gross heart enlargement, masses that narrow the tracheal lumen usually originate within the trachea itself.

Tracheal/Laryngeal Masses

Primary tumors of the larynx or trachea are uncommon. In the canine and feline trachea, osteochondroma and carcinoma, respectively, are the most common types. Carcinoma is the most common tumor of the canine larynx, whereas lymphosarcoma is the most common feline laryngeal tumor. Tracheal and laryngeal tumors often produce clinical signs consistent with airway obstruction. Most laryngeal and tracheal tumors appear as masses within the lumen of the airway. Neoplastic lesions must be differentiated from foreign objects, polyps, or abscesses within the upper airway because these may appear radiographically identical to primary tumors.[6]

Oslerus osleri, found throughout the world, is reportedly the most common respiratory nematode of wild and domestic dogs, but is not commonly diagnosed in the United States.[7] Infection causes single or multiple tracheal mucosal masses (Fig. 27-4). Identification of multiple masses is more consistent with inflammatory disease, but if the parasite causes only a single mass, then other conditions, such as primary tracheal tumor, should be considered.

Tracheal Hypoplasia

Tracheal diameter varies slightly from breed to breed; however, this variation is minimal relative to the size of the animal. English bulldogs have a smaller tracheal diameter than do other breeds but are also more likely to have congenital tracheal hypoplasia (Fig. 27-5).[8] Although subjective assessment is a relatively accurate way of evaluating tracheal size, the ratio of tracheal diameter to thoracic inlet diameter can

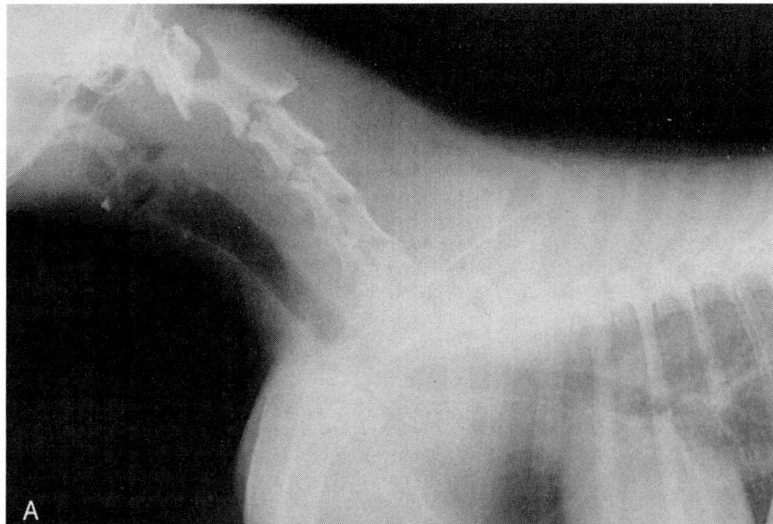

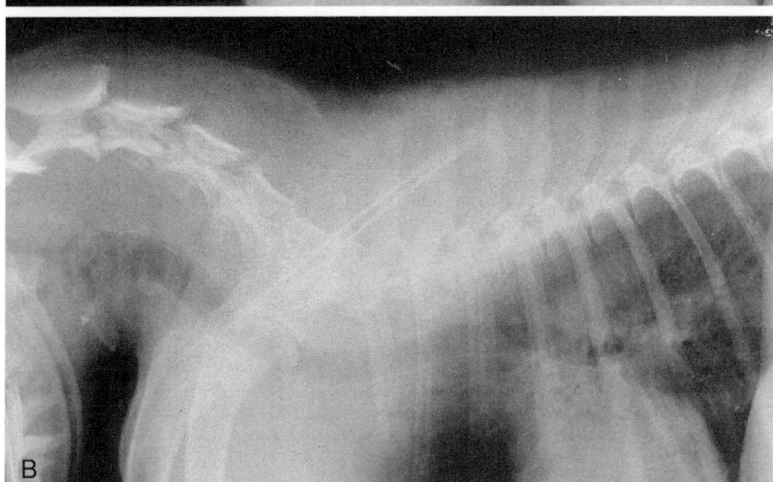

Fig. 27-3 A, Lateral radiograph of a dog with the head and neck correctly positioned. B, Lateral radiograph of the same dog with the neck flexed. Notice the variation in tracheal position. This normal variation may be dramatic, leading to misdiagnosis of a mediastinal mass.

Table • 27-1

Considerations for Radiographically Detectable Deviation of the Trachea in the Lateral Projection

LOCATION OF DEVIATION	DIRECTION OF DEVIATION	CONSIDERATIONS
Cervical	Ventral	Thyroid mass Retropharyngeal lymphomegaly Vertebral/paravertebral mass
Cranial mediastinum	Dorsal	Cranial mediastinal lymphomegaly Thymoma Esophageal enlargement (unusual for tracheal displacement to be dorsal but can occur) Neck position during radiography
Cranial mediastinum	Ventral	Neurogenic tumor Esophageal enlargement/mass
Heart base	Dorsal	Heart base tumor Pulmonary artery enlargement Right atrial enlargement
Tracheal bifurcation	Dorsal	Left atrial enlargement Hilar lymphomegaly (usually ventral but can be dorsal) Generalized cardiomegaly
Tracheal bifurcation	Ventral	Hilar lymphomegaly

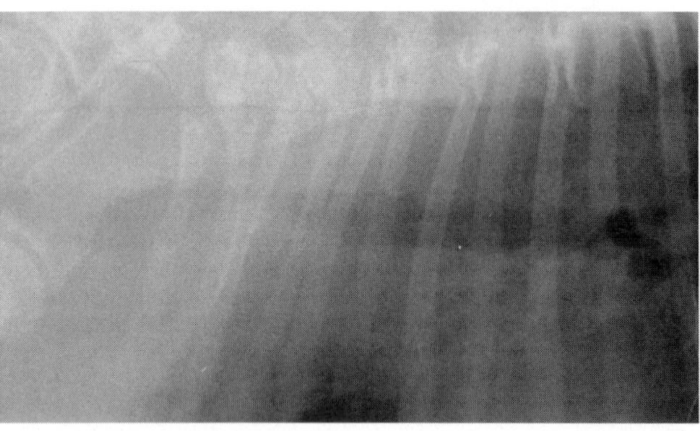

Fig. 27-4 Lateral view of the trachea in a dog with *Oslerus osleri* infection. A relatively large mass arises from the ventral margin of the tracheal mucosa at the level of ribs 1 and 2, and multiple masses are visible from the dorsal aspect of the tracheal mucosa just cranial to the bifurcation.

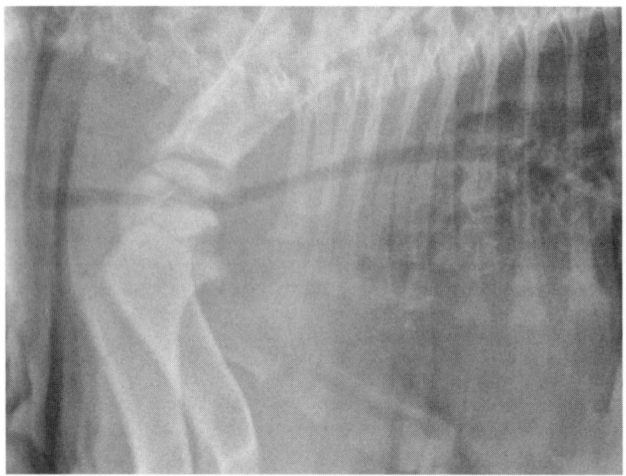

Fig. 27-5 Lateral thoracic radiograph of a 2-month-old English bulldog. This dog became cyanotic on exertion. Note the relatively small size of the trachea consistent with tracheal hypoplasia.

be an objective assessment tool.[9] In nonbrachycephalic dogs, the mean ratio of tracheal diameter to thoracic inlet diameter was 0.20 ± 0.03 compared with 0.16 ± 0.03 in non-Bulldog brachycephalic breeds and 0.13 ± 0.38 in Bulldogs. The range in Bulldogs was 0.07 to 0.21. The smallest ratio in Bulldogs with no clinical signs of respiratory disease was 0.09. The ratio for dogs younger than 1 year was slightly smaller than for older dogs. Accurate lateral positioning is necessary for accurate measurements.

Tracheitis

Airway infections do not usually result in detectable thickening of the tracheal wall or narrowing of the lumen. Rarely, acute dyspnea may occur as the result of inflammatory tracheal disease, with significant decrease in diameter of the tracheal lumen and thickening of the tracheal wall. If the cranial thoracic esophagus contains gas, the esophageal wall will cause border effacement of the dorsal tracheal wall (tracheoesophageal stripe sign), which can be misinterpreted as tracheal wall thickening (Fig. 27-6).

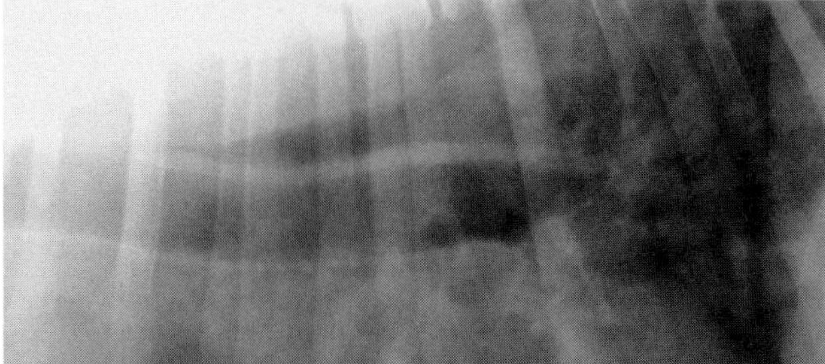

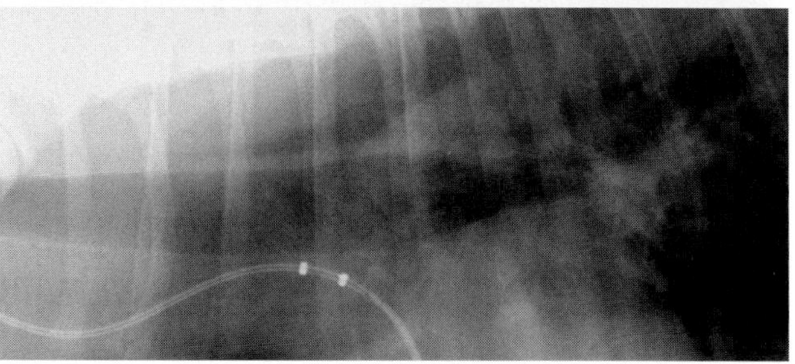

Fig. 27-6 Lateral radiographs of two dogs in which gas can be seen in the esophagus, creating a "tracheoesophageal stripe" sign. This false appearance of tracheal wall thickening can be misinterpreted as abnormal.

Tracheal Collapse

A structurally deficient trachea will result in variation in tracheal size related to the phase of the respiratory cycle, that is, tracheal collapse.[10] This variation is most often seen in toy dog breeds because of weakness in the structural rigidity of the trachea, but tracheal collapse has also been reported in large-breed dogs.[11] Tracheal collapse, because of its dynamic nature, requires special attention for radiographic documentation.

Dynamic narrowing of the tracheal lumen from tracheal instability occurs in the cervical trachea (especially at the thoracic inlet) during inspiration (Fig. 27-7) and in the thoracic trachea (especially at the carina) during expiration (Fig. 27-8). Rarely, with severe loss of rigidity, the site of collapse may not correlate with the phase of respiration; for example, intrathoracic collapse may occur on inspiration. Also, the area that collapses may actually balloon during the opposite respiratory phase.

Occasionally the cervical tracheal lumen appears narrow in dogs with no signs of respiratory disease (Fig. 27-9). Although some believe this is caused by overlying structures such as the esophagus, tracheography (with injection of contrast medium into the trachea) has proved narrowing of the tracheal lumen in some instances. An explanation for this appearance is the redundancy of the trachealis muscle as it folds into the dorsal trachea, thereby narrowing the actual air space. During fluoroscopic examination, the soft tissue trachealis muscle sometimes moves in and out of the lumen during respiration. This radiographic pattern may be seen in large dogs with no evidence of respiratory distress.

For full evaluation of suspected tracheal collapse, lateral radiographs should be made during both inspiration and expiration. Abnormalities in the thoracic trachea are exaggerated during coughing. Fluoroscopic examination may be necessary to demonstrate the dynamic signs. Video clips from fluoroscopic examination of the trachea are available at http://evolve.elsevier.com/Thrall/vetrad/. These include studies of a normal dog as well as patients with tracheal collapse and invagination of the trachealis muscle.

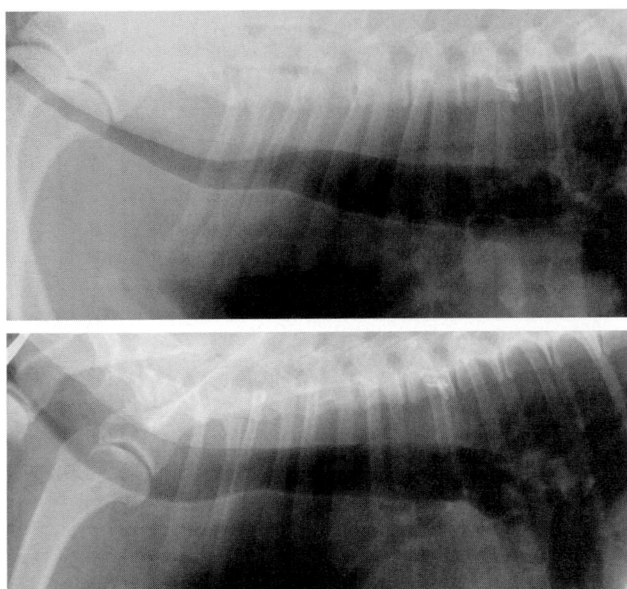

Fig. 27-7 Inspiration *(top)* and expiration *(bottom)* radiographs of a 12-year-old poodle. The cervical trachea is narrowed on inspiration and is larger than the thoracic trachea on expiration. This finding indicates that the weak trachealis muscle is migrating into the lumen by negative intraluminal pressure during inspiration, compromising air flow, and is being forced outward by positive pressure during expiration.

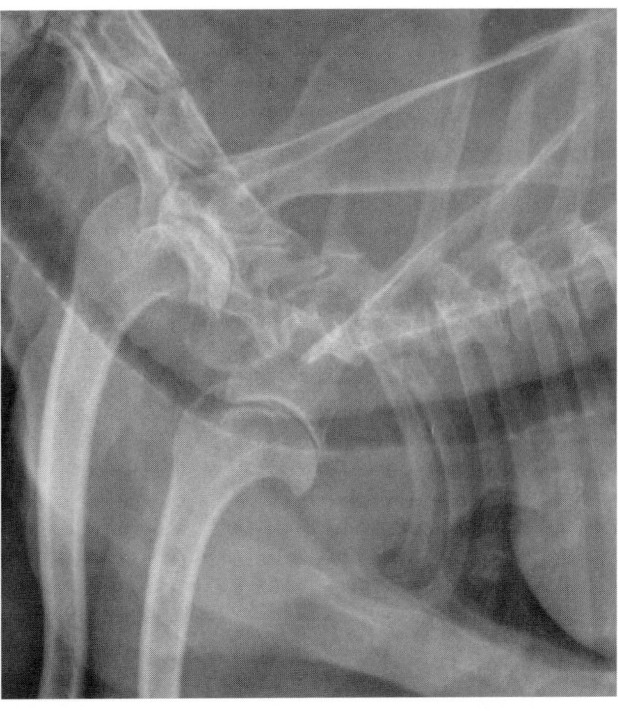

Fig. 27-9 Lateral radiograph of a dog with no clinical signs of respiratory disease.

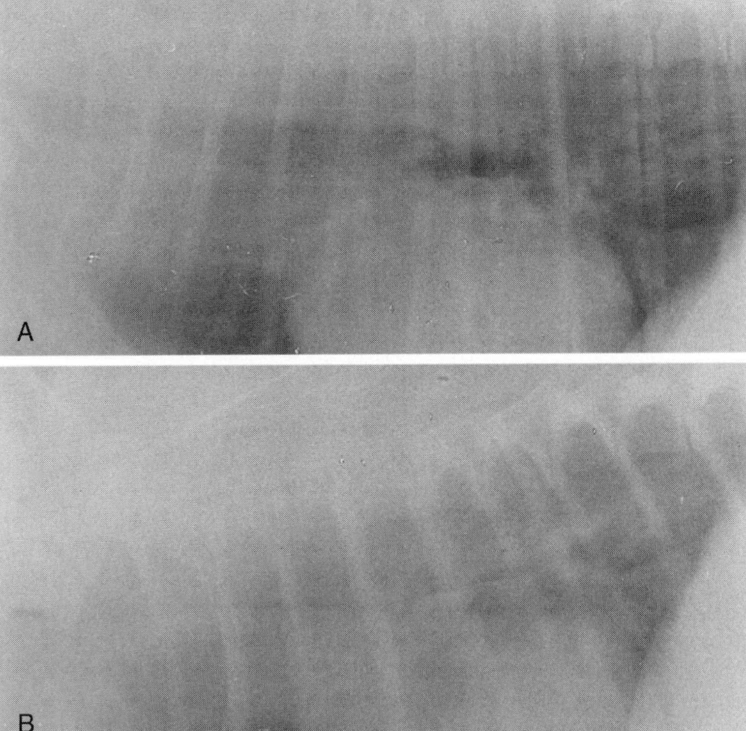

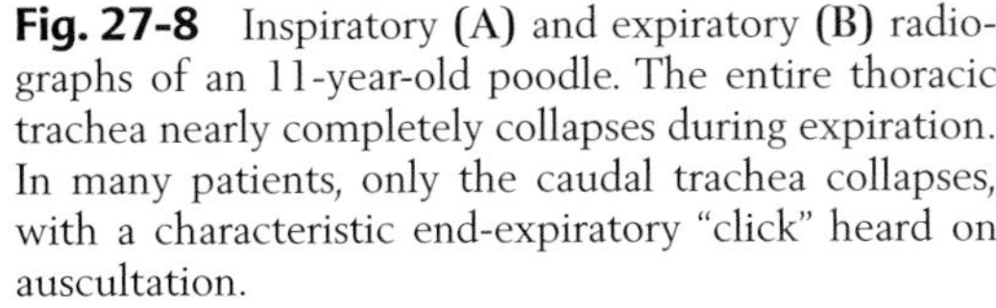

Fig. 27-8 Inspiratory (A) and expiratory (B) radiographs of an 11-year-old poodle. The entire thoracic trachea nearly completely collapses during expiration. In many patients, only the caudal trachea collapses, with a characteristic end-expiratory "click" heard on auscultation.

Tracheal rupture from overdistention of the endotracheal tube cuff is easy to induce in cats. This leads to soft tissue emphysema in the neck and pneumomediastinum, but more importantly can lead to fatal pneumothorax (see Chapter 31). Rupture of the intrathoracic trachea from external trauma has also been reported in cats, with the radiograph having the appearance of a discontinuous trachea, sometimes with a gas-filled diverticulum between the damaged ends.[12]

Alternate Imaging

As previously noted, ultrasound or computed tomographic imaging is helpful for characterization of mass lesions that result in tracheal displacement. Diagnostic ultrasound is not commonly used for assessing the trachea or larynx, but in experienced hands this modality may be useful.[13–17]

REFERENCES

1. O'Brien JH, Harvey CE, Tucker JA: The larynx of the dog: its normal radiographic anatomy, *J Am Vet Radiol Soc* 10:38, 1969.
2. Gaskell CJ: The radiographic anatomy of the pharynx and larynx of the dog, *J Small Anim Pract* 14:89, 1974.
3. Berry CR, Gallaway A, Thrall DE, et al: Thoracic radiographic features of anticoagulant rodenticide toxicity in 14 dogs, *Vet Radiol Ultrasound* 34:391, 1993.
4. Peterson J, Streeter V: Laryngeal obstruction secondary to brodifacoum toxicosis in a dog, *J Am Vet Med Assoc* 208:352, 1996.
5. Reinke JD, Suter PF: Laryngeal paralysis in a dog, *J Am Vet Med Assoc* 172:714, 1978.
6. Carlisle CH, Biery DN, Thrall DE: Tracheal and laryngeal tumors in the dog and cat: literature review and 13 additional patients, *Vet Radiol* 32:229, 1991.
7. Levitan DM, Matz ME, Findlen CS, et al: Treatment of *Oslerus osleri* infestation in a dog: case report and literature review, *J Am Anim Hosp Assoc* 32:435, 1996.
8. Suter PF, Colgrove DJ, Ewing GO: Congenital hypoplasia of the canine trachea, *J Am Anim Hosp Assoc* 8:120, 1972.
9. Harvey CE, Fink EA: Tracheal diameter: analysis of radiographic measurements in brachycephalic and nonbrachycephalic dogs, *J Am Anim Hosp Assoc* 18:570, 1982.
10. Johnson LR, McKiernan BC: Diagnosis and medical management of tracheal collapse, *Semin Vet Med Surg (Small Anim)* 10:101, 1995.
11. Spodnick GJ, Nwadike BS: Surgical management of extrathoracic tracheal collapse in two large-breed dogs, *J Am Vet Med Assoc* 211:12, 1997.
12. Lawrence DT, Lang J, Culvenor J, et al: Intrathoracic tracheal rupture, *J Feline Med Surg* 1:43, 1999.
13. Rudorf H: Ultrasonographic imaging of the tongue and larynx in normal dogs, *J Small Anim Pract* 38:439, 1997.
14. Rudorf H, Herrtage XM, White RA: Use of ultrasonography in the diagnosis of tracheal collapse, *J Small Anim Pract* 38:513, 1997.
15. Rudorf H, Brown P: Ultrasonography of laryngeal masses in six cats and one dog, *Vet Radiol Ultrasound* 39:430, 1998.
16. Bray JP, Lipscombe VJ, White RA, et al: Ultrasonographic examination of the pharynx and larynx of the normal dog, *Vet Radiol Ultrasound* 39:566, 1998.
17. Rudorf H, Lane JG, Wotton PR: Everted laryngeal saccules: ultrasonographic findings in a young Lakeland terrier, *J Small Anim Pract* 40:338, 1999.

ELECTRONIC RESOURCES evolve

Additional information related to the content in Chapter 27 can be found on the companion Web site at evolve http://evolve.elsevier.com/Thrall/vetrad/.

- Key Points
- Chapter Quiz
- Case Study 27–1
- Video 27-1: Dynamic fluoroscopic image of a normal trachea during normal breathing
- Video 27-2: Dynamic fluoroscopic image of a normal trachea during coughing
- Video 27-3: Dynamic fluoroscopic image of a mildly to moderately collapsing trachea
- Video 27-4: Dynamic fluoroscopic image of a severely collapsing trachea
- Video 27-5: Dynamic fluoroscopic image of a life-threatening collapsing trachea
- Video 27-6: Dynamic fluoroscopic image of the trachealis muscle encroaching on the tracheal lumen during inspiration

CHAPTER • 28
Esophagus

Barbara J. Watrous

Disorders of the pharynx and esophagus result in a variety of clinical signs, including regurgitation, dysphagia, abnormal swallowing, and gagging or retching. Secondary signs include weight loss, failure to gain weight or grow normally, and chronic or recurrent respiratory problems. Aspiration pneumonia, tracheitis, and nasal discharge are frequent complications of esophageal dysfunction. In some systemic neuromuscular diseases, the oropharynx, the esophagus, or both may become dysfunctional.

ESOPHAGEAL ANATOMY

The esophagus is a musculomembranous tube bounded at each end by a sphincter. The four layers include the mucosa, a keratinized stratified squamous epithelium with infrequent pigmentation in some canine breeds (e.g., Chow Chows); the submucosa, a loose network of fibrous connective tissue with varying quantities of smooth muscle and mucous glands; the muscularis, which is composed of striated muscle in the dog (the terminal third is smooth muscle in the cat, with its corresponding mucosa thrown into obliquely directed folds); and the adventitia.

The cranial esophageal, or cricopharyngeal, sphincter is composed of paired cricopharyngeus muscles and paired thyropharyngeus muscles. These form an annular band attached to the dorsal aspect of the larynx.

The caudal esophageal sphincter is a complex structure composed of (1) focal thickening of the inner circular layer of esophageal smooth muscle from the muscularis (2) a confluence of gastric rugal folds that lie transverse to the junction (3) and a muscular sling created by the right crus of the diaphragm on the right and the deep oblique smooth muscle layer of the lesser curvature of the stomach on the left. The complexity of this sphincter can be attributed to the effect of the oblique orientation of the esophagus as it attaches to the stomach as well as to the relatively positive intraabdominal pressure that compresses the short intraabdominal segment of the terminal esophagus. In some dogs this intraabdominal segment is not present, but the abdominal pressure should have similar compressive influence on the gastroesophageal junction.[1]

NORMAL RADIOGRAPHIC APPEARANCE

The normal esophagus is difficult to see radiographically (Table 28-1). The cervical esophagus silhouettes with surrounding soft tissues, and the thoracic esophagus is enveloped by the dorsal mediastinum, fascia, and connective tissue.[2] Accumulation of intraluminal gas usually indicates esophageal disease, though small amounts of swallowed air can be seen in the normal esophagus. Common sites for this on the lateral view include the area immediately caudal to the cranial esophageal sphincter, at the thoracic inlet, and dorsal to the heart base (Fig. 28-1). In the region of contact between luminal gas of the trachea and esophagus, an apparent thick soft tissue band is created. This band results from the combined thickness of the tracheal and esophageal walls silhouetting each other. This appearance is called the tracheal stripe sign and is a reliable indicator of the presence of esophageal gas.

Swallowing of air, or aerophagia, occurs most often in apprehensive, sedated, and dyspneic animals. In subsequent radiographs, this focal air accumulation is transient (see Fig. 28-1). In the dorsoventral or ventrodorsal view, this gas is often hidden because of superimposition. General anesthesia may cause marked dilation of a normal esophagus, mimicking megaesophagus. The associated pulmonary atelectasis may also mimic aspiration pneumonia. For this and other reasons, use of anesthesia for thoracic radiography should be avoided.[3]

Fluid occasionally will collect in the caudal aspect of the normal esophagus when dogs are in left recumbency. This fluid creates an oblong region of soft tissue opacity in the caudal aspect of the thorax that should not be confused with a mass or pulmonary disease (Fig. 28-2). This appearance is not typically present in radiographs made with the animal in right recumbency.

The absence of abnormal esophageal radiographic findings does not preclude the presence of esophageal disease; such is often the situation with acute esophageal disease. In addition, the presence of indirect signs of esophageal disease should be anticipated. For example, focal or generalized esophageal dilation may be less apparent when the lumen is fluid filled, creating a positive silhouette sign with the surrounding mediastinum.

ESOPHAGEAL CONTRAST STUDIES

Contrast radiographic examination is often necessary for accurate identification of lesions or further characterization of survey radiographic findings. Differentiation of functional from morphologic causes of dysphagia may be possible with static contrast studies. Specific evaluation of functional abnormalities, however, may be possible only with dynamic fluoroscopic studies. The emphasis in this chapter is on information provided by static survey and contrast radiographic findings.

Contrast Media

Many contrast media are available for esophagography, and selection of a specific one should be made on the basis of suspected disease.[2] Barium sulfate cream and paste have been formulated for extreme radiopacity and to enable good adherence to esophageal mucosa, though mucosal adherence is not achieved in every patient. Suspected mucosal irregular-

Table • 28-1

Survey Radiographic Findings

RADIOGRAPHIC FINDINGS	ESOPHAGEAL STATUS	ETIOLOGIES
Normal	Normal	
	Abnormal	Neuromuscular disease
		Hiatal hernia
		Foreign body (nonradiopaque)
		Esophagitis
		Early strictures
		Fistulas
Radiolucency		
Regional intraluminal	Normal	Aerophagia
	Abnormal	Foreign bodies (nonradiopaque)
		Gastroesophageal intussusception
		Extraluminal masses
		Esophagitis
		Strictures
		Vascular ring anomalies
		Neoplasia
		Segmental hypomotility
Generalized intraluminal	Normal	General anesthesia
		Central nervous system depression
	Abnormal	Megaesophagus
		Neuromuscular hypomotility
		Hypoadrenocorticism
		Autoimmune myositis
		Autoimmune neuritis
		Myasthenia gravis
		Toxicities
		Neoplasia
		Hypothyroidism
		Trauma
Periesophageal	Normal	Subcutaneous emphysema
	Abnormal	Perforation
Radiopacity		
Regional intraluminal	Abnormal	Vascular ring anomalies
		Foreign bodies (radiopaque)
		Spirocerca lupi
		Neoplasia
		Gastroesophageal intussusception
		Diverticula
		Periesophageal masses
Generalized intraluminal	Abnormal	Megaesophagus

ities (e.g., esophagitis, neoplastic infiltrates) and strictures should be initially evaluated with barium paste or cream. Because of their viscosity, however, they tend to maintain a bolus, failing to disperse well or flow around intraluminal lesions. Admixture with liquid barium suspensions is also poor, resulting in clumping in the stomach when an upper gastrointestinal examination with liquid barium sulfate suspension follows an esophagram in which paste was used. Aspiration of paste may lead to asphyxiation; therefore use of paste is not advised when aspiration is a concern.

Liquid barium sulfate suspensions do not adhere well to the mucosa; however, a high-density contrast medium (45% to 85% weight) can be used for esophagography because it is relatively safe when aspirated, mixes well with fluid contents, and readily flows around obstructions. Motility problems in the oropharyngeal and esophageal regions should first be evaluated with liquid barium.

Either barium liquid or barium paste mixed with canned food or kibble is valuable for fully characterizing the volume of a distended esophagus and in animals with problems in swallowing solids but not liquids. Barium-coated food may also be the best choice for identification of strictures or regional motility disorders (see Videos 28-1 and 28-2 available at http://evolve.elsevier.com/Thrall/vetrad/).

Oral aqueous iodine solutions designed for oral administration are relatively nontoxic in body cavities. Therefore their use is indicated when esophageal perforation is suspected. These agents are hypertonic; thus if aspirated they will induce pulmonary edema. They will also cause fluid influx into the gastrointestinal tract, and a volume-depleted animal may be further compromised by fluid loss. If leakage of an aqueous iodine solution occurs into a fluid-filled pleural space or if the leak is minimal, the resulting dilution of the contrast medium may make detection of the extravasated contrast medium or the site of leakage difficult.

Nonionic organic iodine agents are isosmolar and not associated with the complications encountered with ionic contrast media, but they are considerably more expensive. The use of liquid barium if a perforation is suspected is controversial because of the tendency of barium to stimulate a granulomatous reaction on pleural surfaces. The use of barium sulfate can be considered, however, when oral aqueous iodinated contrast medium fails to define a leak. Aqueous iodine contrast media are not recommended for routine esophagography because of their poor coating ability.

Technique

Survey radiographs should always be made immediately before any contrast examination is performed. This provides selection of a suitable radiographic technique and assessment of the status of the esophagus and surrounding tissues. Superimposition of the spine readily obscures even a barium-coated esophageal lumen. Therefore, in addition to the lateral view, an oblique view such as a ventroleft-dorsoright or ventroright-dorsoleft view is recommended to rotate the esophagus into a more visible location. On the lateral view, the opacity over the thoracic inlet from the musculature of the brachium can be reduced by moving one thoracic limb cranially and the other caudally. Survey radiographs should include the cranial esophageal sphincter, the cervical and thoracic esophagus, and caudal esophageal sphincter within the cranial abdomen.

A fractious animal may be given a low dose of a phenothiazine tranquilizer. However, the esophagus is affected by most central nervous system depressant drugs; therefore their use is disadvantageous when motility is being evaluated. Approximately 5 to 20 mL of contrast medium is given to induce several complete swallows for coating the pharynx and esophagus.

Oropharyngeal problems are best evaluated by a series of radiographs made in the midst of a swallow and during a pause after the swallow is completed. The esophageal phase can be evaluated by an additional radiograph made after a sufficient pause to ensure complete transport of the last bolus to the stomach.

The normal appearance of the oropharyngeal region after a swallow of contrast medium reveals coating of the mucosa

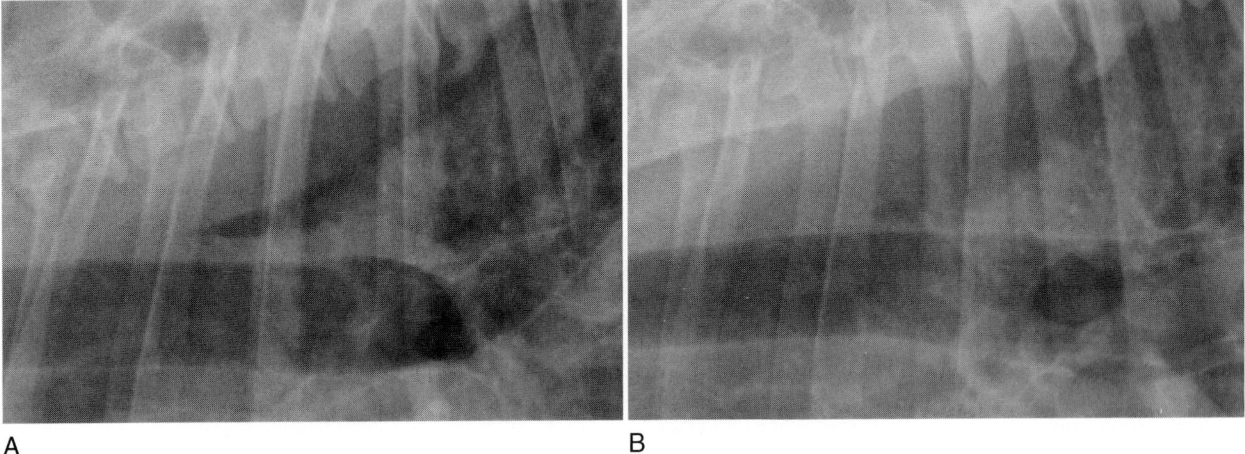

Fig. 28-1 Left (A) and right (B) lateral thoracic radiographs of a normal dog. In A there is a collection of gas in the esophagus dorsal to the terminal aspect of the trachea. Note the apparent thick wall of the trachea in this region. This is not the tracheal wall but an opacity created by silhouetting of the tracheal and esophageal walls, each outlined by the gas in the lumen. This appearance is called the tracheal stripe sign and is a reliable sign of the presence of esophageal gas. B shows the amount of gas is decreased. Swallowed gas typically is transient and will appear different in subsequent radiographs.

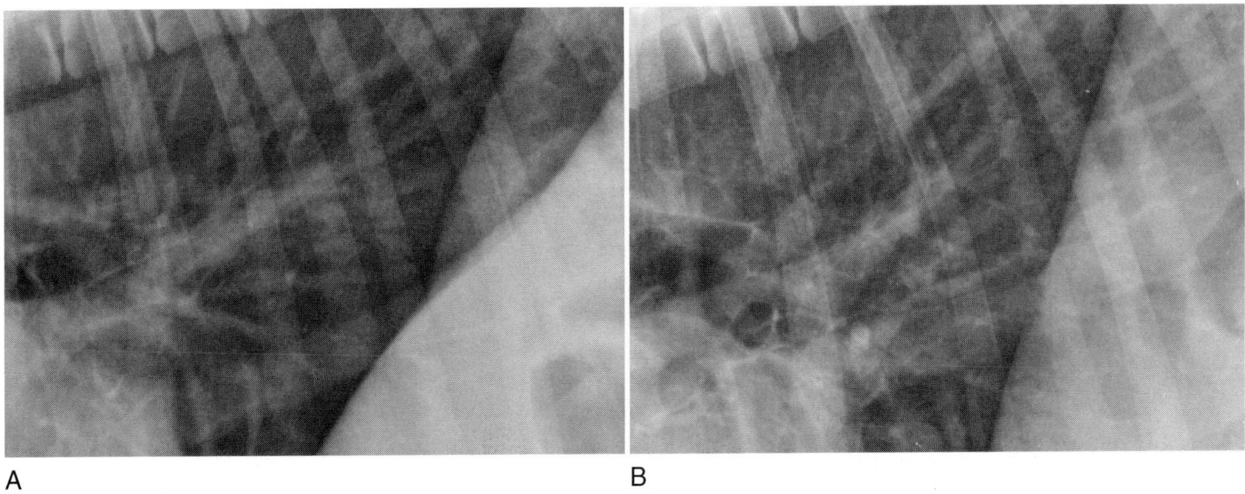

Fig. 28-2 Left (A) and right (B) lateral thoracic radiographs of a normal dog. In A there is a horizontally oriented oblong region of increased opacity between the aorta and caudal vena cava. This is caused by fluid collecting in the caudal thoracic esophagus. This is not seen in B. The appearance illustrated in A is a common finding in canine thoracic radiographs and should not be misinterpreted as disease of the esophagus or other thoracic structure.

without significant retention of the contrast medium (Fig. 28-3). A small amount of contrast medium may occasionally remain in the esophageal lumen immediately caudal to the cranial esophageal sphincter. No contrast medium should persist in the piriform recesses, nasopharynx, or larynx or be present in the trachea unless laryngotracheal aspiration inadvertently occurs.

The normal canine esophageal mucosa appears as a series of longitudinal folds. The lines are close together through most of its length but may separate slightly at the thoracic inlet as the esophagus passes along the left lateral side of the trachea (Fig. 28-4). The feline esophagus has a similar appearance to the level of the heart base, but the caudal esophagus has obliquely directed folds that correspond to the smooth muscle segment (Fig. 28-5). Oblique views eliminate superimposition of the spine and sternum for better visualization of the esophagus (Fig. 28-6).[2,4,5]

OROPHARYNGEAL DYSPHAGIA

Swallowing disorders related to the oropharyngeal phase may be attributable to abnormalities of the tongue, pharynx, or cranial esophageal sphincter. Identification of the underlying disorder, when functional, is difficult, but indirect evidence is often inferred when oral or pharyngeal retention of contrast medium occurs. Mechanical causes of oropharyngeal dysphagia are uncommon but may include foreign bodies, such as fishhooks, perforations of the oral cavity or pharynx, such as by sticks, and infiltrative lesions. These mechanical causes are

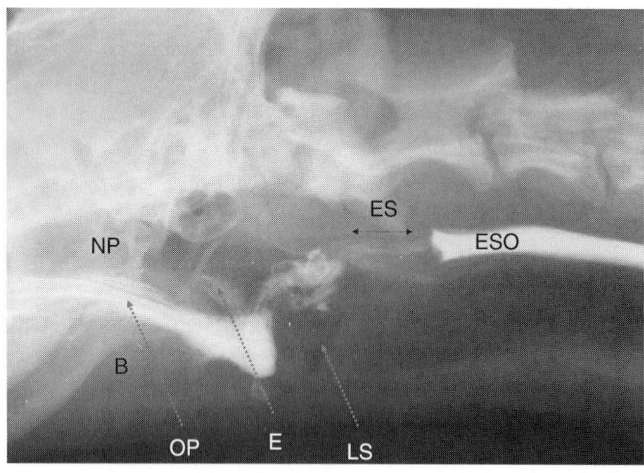

Fig. 28-3 Normal oropharyngeal contrast medium examination of a mature dog (lateral view). *NP,* Nasopharynx; *B,* base of tongue; *OP,* oropharynx; *E,* epiglottis; *LS,* laryngeal saccules filled with air; *ES,* cranial esophageal sphincter; *ESO,* esophagus.

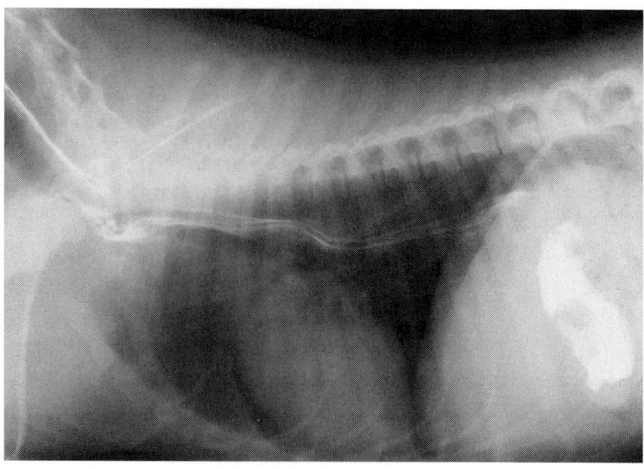

Fig. 28-4 Normal esophagram (lateral view) of a mature dog with barium sulfate cream. The longitudinal folds often separate at the thoracic inlet. A slight ventral deviation of the course of the esophagus at the thoracic inlet is also normal.

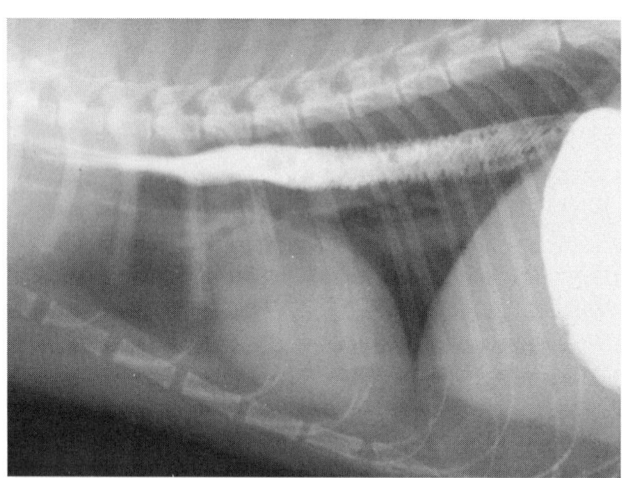

Fig. 28-5 Normal thoracic esophagram in a mature cat. Note the herringbone mucosal pattern in the caudal aspect of the esophagus.

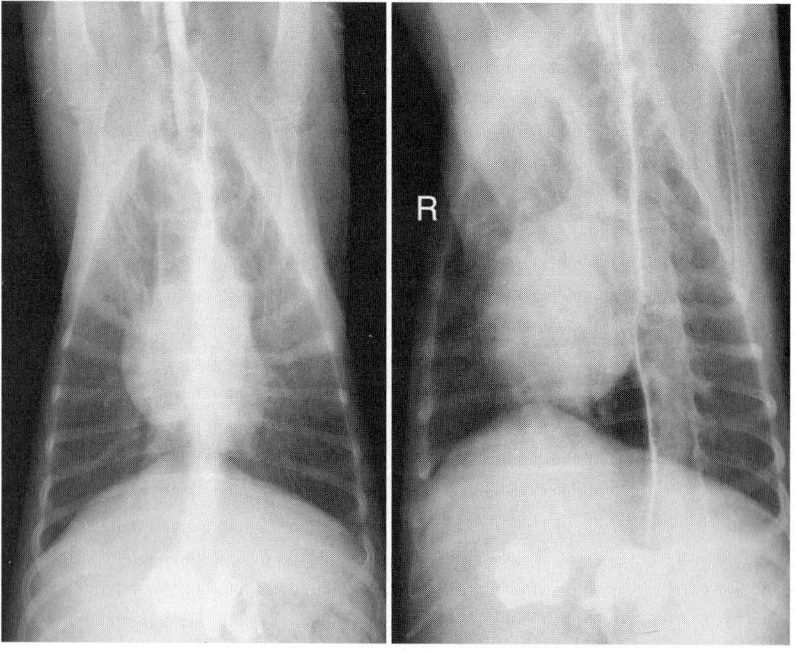

Fig. 28-6 Normal canine esophagram. In the ventrodorsal view **(A),** the esophagus is not well visualized because it is superimposed on the spine. When the sternum is rotated to the dog's right **(B),** the esophagus is much more conspicuously positioned on the right edge of the spine. The correct name of the view seen in B, based on point of entrance to point of exit of the x-ray beam, is ventroleft-dorsoright.

often best identified by a thorough visual examination. With functional abnormalities, survey radiographs are usually unremarkable.

Diseases of the oral stage of swallowing usually involve the tongue. If an abnormality of the oral stage is present, the problem may be noted on prehension, during caudal transport through the oral cavity, or by organization of a bolus in the oropharynx by the tongue. Retention of contrast medium in the oral cavity and oropharynx should not occur (Fig. 28-7). The subsequent pharyngeal and cricopharyngeal stages are normal. The conclusion that contrast medium is retained in the pharynx must be made in delayed radiographs after administration of contrast medium.

Pharyngeal-stage dysphagia can result from neuromuscular disease, adjacent inflammation (Fig. 28-8), or trauma from perforation (Fig. 28-9) or from hyoid injury (Fig. 28-10). The oral stage is normal, but inadequate pharyngeal peristalsis leads to retention of much of the bolus of contrast medium. Inadequate closure of the pharyngeal egresses (nasopharynx, oral cavity, and larynx) may lead to reflux of contrast medium into these regions.

Cricopharyngeal dysphagia may be caused by inappropriate opening or nonopening of the cranial esophageal sphincter (cricopharyngeal asynchrony or achalasia) or failure of that sphincter to close (chalasia). Chalasia is recognized by the persistence of a patent passage between the pharynx and esophagus (Fig. 28-11). Reflux of esophageal contrast medium results in its presence in the pharynx. Pharyngeal paresis, which is an additional cause for pharyngeal retention of contrast medium, often accompanies cricopharyngeal chalasia.

Dysfunction of the cranial esophageal sphincter because of asynchrony or achalasia results in interference with transport

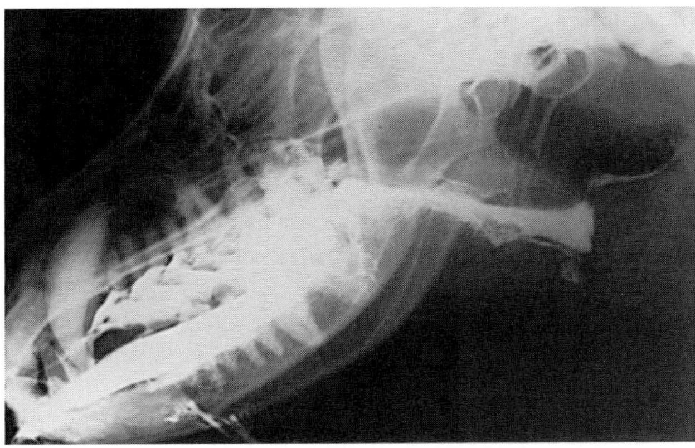

Fig. 28-7 Lateral view of a mature dog with oral dysphagia from hypoglossal neuropathy. Inadequate stripping action of the tongue against the hard and soft palate prevents caudal transport of ingesta, and contrast medium accumulates in the pharynx. A small amount of contrast medium has been swallowed, signifying normal pharyngeal and cricopharyngeal function. (Courtesy New York State College of Veterinary Medicine, Ithaca, NY.)

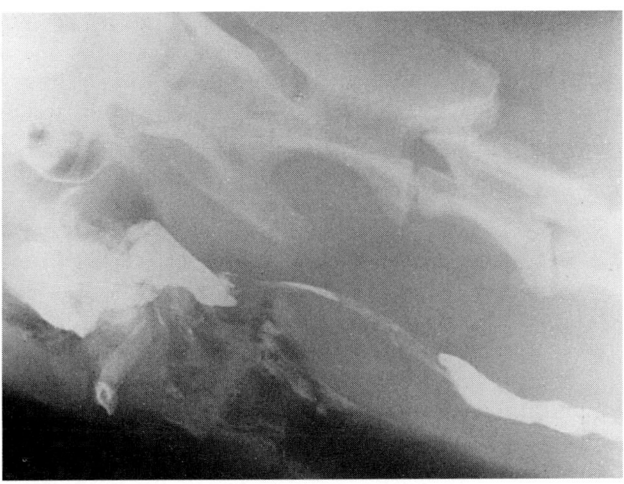

Fig. 28-8 Pharyngeal-stage dysphagia is a result of inadequate sequential cranial-to-caudal contraction by the pharyngeal muscles. Thus transport of a bolus through the cranial esophageal sphincter is usually incomplete. Contrast medium is retained in the pharynx and piriform recesses. This dog with chronic laryngitis and pharyngitis has retropharyngeal swelling and inflammation in addition to scarring of the larynx. In the esophagram there is pharyngeal retention of contrast medium and laryngotracheal aspiration because of disturbed motility.

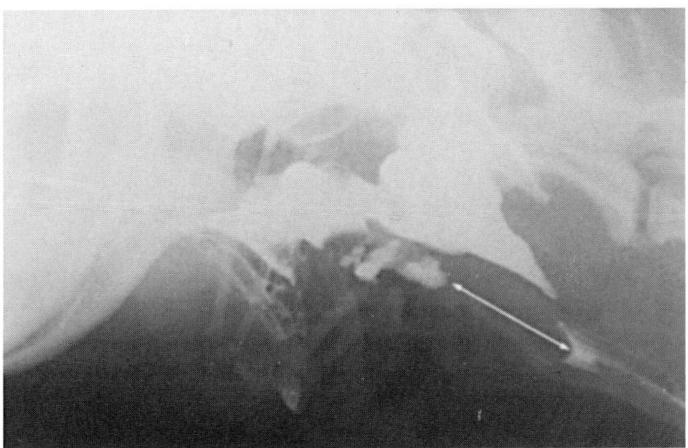

Fig. 28-9 Pharyngeal laceration caused by a stick resulted in a retropharyngeal fistula and pharyngeal paresis. Contrast medium has accumulated in the pharynx and the retropharyngeal abscess. The *arrow* denotes the cranial esophageal sphincter. (Courtesy New York State College of Veterinary Medicine, Ithaca, NY.)

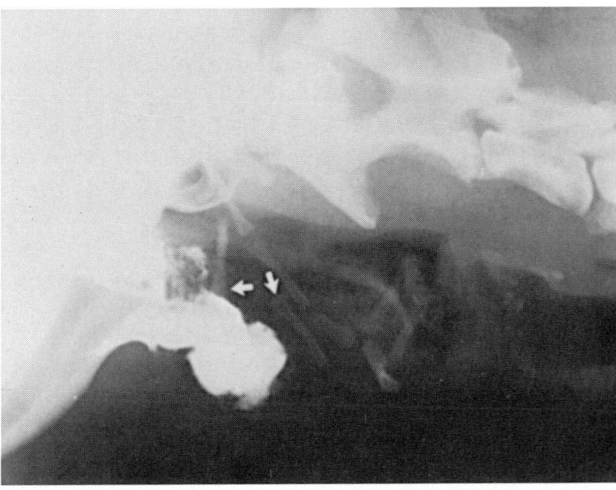

Fig. 28-10 Lateral view of the pharyngeal region of a mature dog. The hyoid apparatus plays an integral role in coordinating laryngeal closure during swallowing. Fracture *(arrows)* or dislocation of the hyoid apparatus may disrupt this process, as in this dog. Contrast medium has collected in the oropharynx but cannot be propelled caudally by the pharynx. (Courtesy New York State College of Veterinary Medicine, Ithaca, NY.)

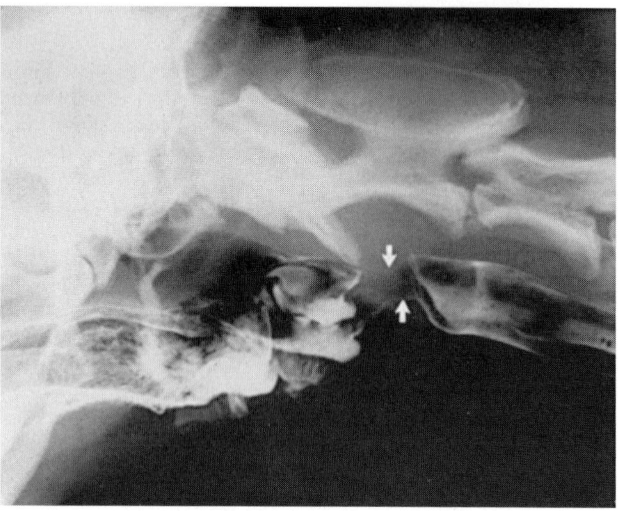

Fig. 28-11 Lateral view of the pharyngeal region of a mature dog with autoimmune polymyositis. Chalasia *(arrows)* and megaesophagus are present. The nonfunctional cranial esophageal sphincter, along with pharyngeal paresis and esophageal hypomotility, results in contrast medium passing freely between the pharynx and esophagus. (Courtesy New York State College of Veterinary Medicine, Ithaca, NY.)

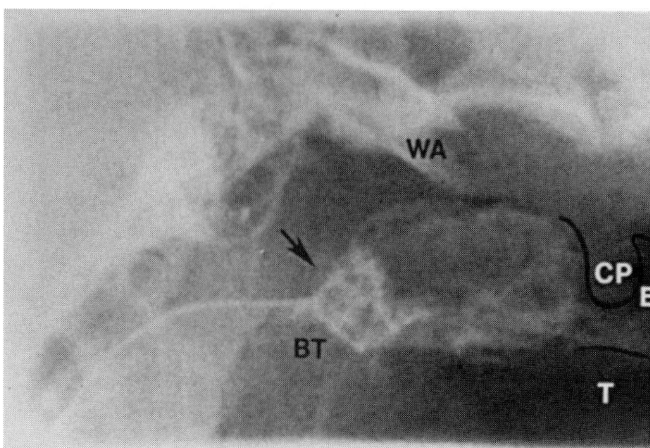

Fig. 28-12 Lateral esophagram of the pharyngeal region of a dog. During the pharyngeal and cricopharyngeal stages of swallowing, the pharynx is in vigorous contraction *(arrow)* against a closing cranial esophageal sphincter *(CP)*. The floor of this passage is open, allowing air and contrast medium to outline the distorted sphincter. Asynchrony between the pharyngeal and the cricopharyngeal stages occurs more commonly than does true cricopharyngeal achalasia. *BT,* Base of tongue; *E,* esophagus; *T,* trachea; *WA,* wings of atlas. (Reprinted from Ettinger SJ, editor: *Textbook of veterinary internal medicine,* ed 2, Philadelphia, 1983, W.B. Saunders.)

Table • 28-2

Summary of Location of Retained Contrast Medium Relative to Type of Oropharyngeal Dysphagia

	DYSPHAGIA			
SITE	NORMAL	ORAL	PHARYNGEAL	CRICOPHARYNGEAL
Oral cavity	±	+	–	–
Nasopharynx	–	–	±	±
Oropharynx	–	+	±	±
Pharynx	–	–	+	+
Valleculae	±	±	+	+
Piriform recesses	–	–	+	+
Esophagus	–	–	±	±
Larynx/trachea	–	–	+	+

+, Present; –, absent.

of the contrast medium into the esophagus. The passage may be visibly distorted, although the pattern of distribution of retained contrast medium is similar to the pattern found in pharyngeal dysphagia (Fig. 28-12). If viewed dynamically, vigorous pharyngeal contractions are seen attempting to force food through the dysfunctional cricopharyngeal sphincter; which increases the probability of aspiration. (See Video 28-3 available at http://evolve.elsevier.com/Thrall/vetrad/. Note the vigorous pharyngeal contractions that are ineffective in propelling ingesta into the esophagus. Persistent ingesta in the pharynx increase the probability of aspiration, which can also be seen.)

Table 28-2 provides a summary of the static contrast radiographic findings in the various forms of oropharyngeal dysphagia.[6]

MEGAESOPHAGUS

Segmental Megaesophagus

Segmental megaesophagus may be congenital or acquired and either functional or mechanical. Segmental megaesophagus frequently is identified on survey radiographs by focal air accumulation. Abnormal regional air accumulation may occur anywhere along the esophagus just cranial to or at the site of localized disease. Air is often noted at the site of acute entrapment of intraluminal foreign bodies, esophagitis, and segmental esophageal hypomotility. Obstruction of the esophageal lumen by vascular ring anomalies (Fig. 28-13), acquired strictures (Fig. 28-14), extraluminal and intrinsic masses, and chronic foreign bodies may or may not result in air accumulation. In chronic disease, fluid, a mixture of fluid

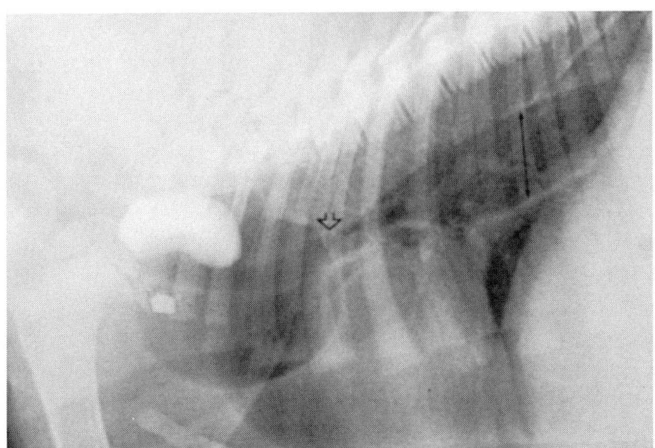

Fig. 28-13 Lateral view of the thorax of a young dog with a persistent right-fourth aortic arch. The characteristic site of esophageal obstruction with persistent right-fourth aortic arch is just cranial to the tracheal bifurcation *(open arrow)*. This animal also had underlying generalized hypomotility and dilation *(arrow)*; the possibility of this also being present must be assessed in patients with vascular ring disease because it influences the prognosis for recovery after surgery. The radiopacities are foreign bodies (stones) within the prestenotic dilated esophageal lumen. Thoracic tracheal depression is evident. Less-common vascular ring anomalies include double aortic arch, aberrant right subclavian artery, and dextroaorta with left subclavian artery. (Courtesy New York State College of Veterinary Medicine, Ithaca, NY.)

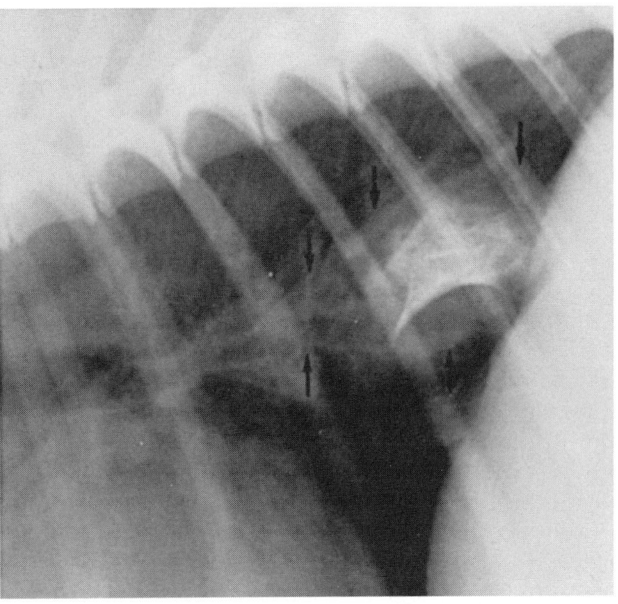

Fig. 28-15 Lateral view of the dorsocaudal thorax of a dog. A radiopaque foreign body is present cranial to the esophageal hiatus. The sharp projection is characteristic of esophageal foreign bodies. A prominent zone of soft tissue *(arrows)* around the bone may be caused by nonmineralized portions of the foreign object but could also reflect esophageal wall thickening. (Courtesy New York State College of Veterinary Medicine, Ithaca, NY.)

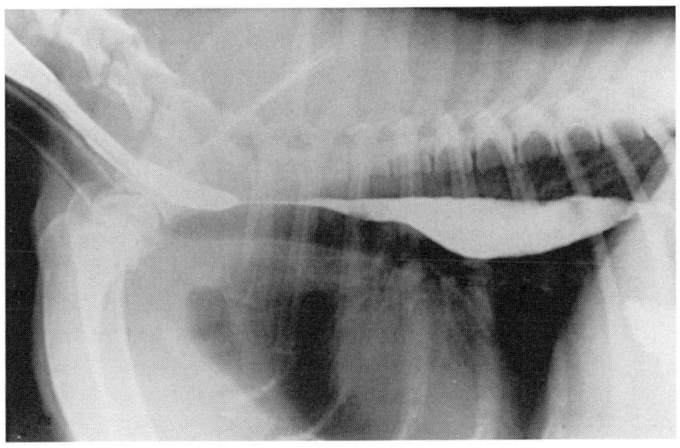

Fig. 28-14 Lateral esophagram of a young adult dog with a cranial thoracic esophageal stricture. The extent of the luminal involvement was best demonstrated by placing an esophageal tube while the dog was anesthetized and gradually administering contrast medium to fill the distensible portions of the esophagus. (Courtesy New York State College of Veterinary Medicine, Ithaca, NY.)

and air, or a heterogeneous pattern of food accumulation may be seen.[7,8]

Foreign Bodies

Entrapment of foreign bodies within the esophageal lumen is a common cause of esophageal dysphagia. Typical features of obstructing foreign objects include a firm or rigid consistency; a sharp, angular, or spiculated shape (Fig. 28-15); or large size relative to the least distensible regions of the esophagus. Bones, fishhooks, and needles are common esophageal foreign objects. Less common foreign objects include linear foreign bodies and trichobezoars, which may be less apparent on survey radiographs. The usual entrapment sites are the cranial cervical region, thoracic inlet, heart base, and caudal thoracic esophagus just cranial to the esophageal hiatus.

Survey radiographs may be satisfactory for identification of radiopaque foreign bodies. The survey radiographic examination should include views of the entire esophagus, including the caudal pharynx and cranial abdomen. Exposure appropriate for evaluation of the lung and pleura is important to rule out sequelae of esophageal disease, including aspiration pneumonia, perforation of the esophagus and secondary pleuritis, mediastinitis, or pulmonary fistula. When suspicion of a foreign body cannot be confirmed by survey radiography, an esophagram is often helpful. Typically, evidence of esophageal dilation with a filling defect caused by the foreign body is apparent in the esophagram (Fig. 28-16). Foreign bodies can cause complete, partial, or no obstruction, with obstruction occurring most often at sites of limited esophageal distention. They may induce esophageal laceration when they are sharp or spiculated or when chronic, leading to mural necrosis. In the cervical esophagus, a tear leads to leakage of luminal contents, which may cause a regional mass effect or facilitate the escape of air into tissues. Secondary abscess may develop. If the tear is intrathoracic a pneumomediastinum (Fig. 28-17) may be seen, but this does not always occur depending on the size of the defect in the esophageal wall. Perforation may lead to mediastinitis, mediastinal abscess, and pleuritis with effusion.

Esophageal and Periesophageal Masses (Neoplastic/Inflammatory)

Intrinsic masses of the esophagus are uncommon. They may be benign or malignant neoplasms or inflammatory masses. The incidence is greater in certain geographic regions, specifically areas endemic for *Spirocerca lupi*. Branchiomas, branchial cleft cysts, papillomas, metastatic tonsillar carcinomas, squamous cell carcinomas, and leiomyosarcomas rarely occur; they cannot be differentiated radiographically. Mass lesions of the thoracic esophagus usually appear as an

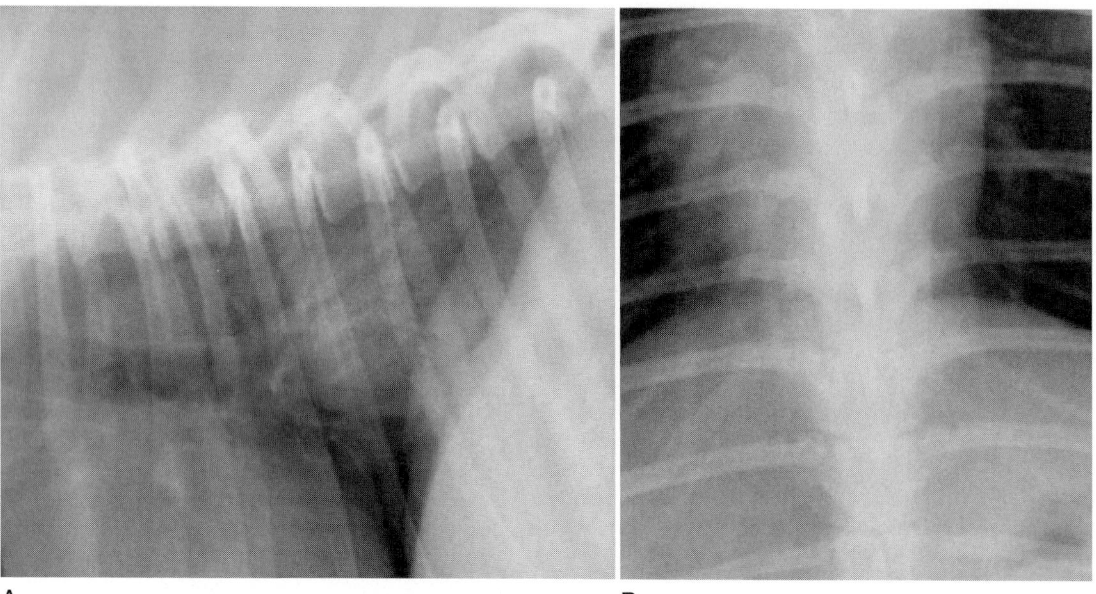

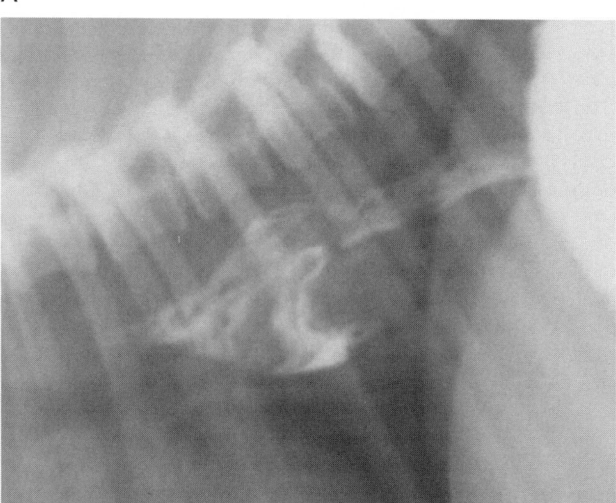

Fig. 28-16 Lateral **(A)** and ventrodorsal **(B)** radiographs of a dog with a history of regurgitation. An ill-defined mass effect is present in the caudal thorax, located on midline. The history and radiographic findings are suggestive of a foreign body, but this is not conclusive. An esophagram was performed **(C)**. Focal dilation of the esophagus and filling defects are created by the foreign body.

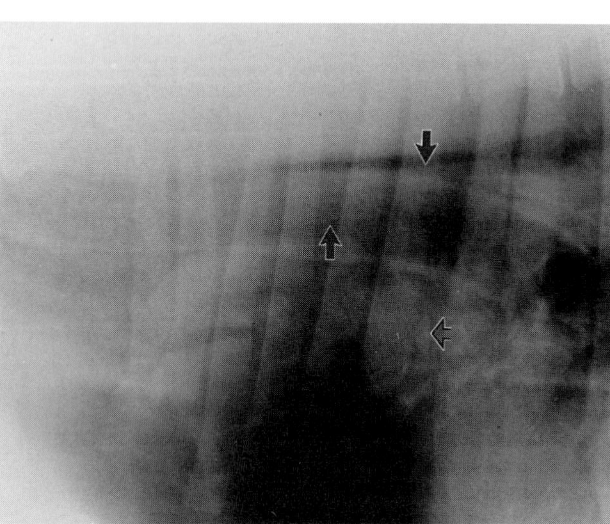

Fig. 28-17 Lateral view of the dorsocranial thorax of a mature dog. Esophageal perforation by a bone has resulted in pneumomediastinum. The outer margins of the esophagus can be seen superimposed on the tracheal lumen *(solid arrows)* next to the brachiocephalic artery. A small bone fragment is visible *(open arrow)* and was present in the mediastinum. (Courtesy New York State College of Veterinary Medicine, Ithaca, NY.)

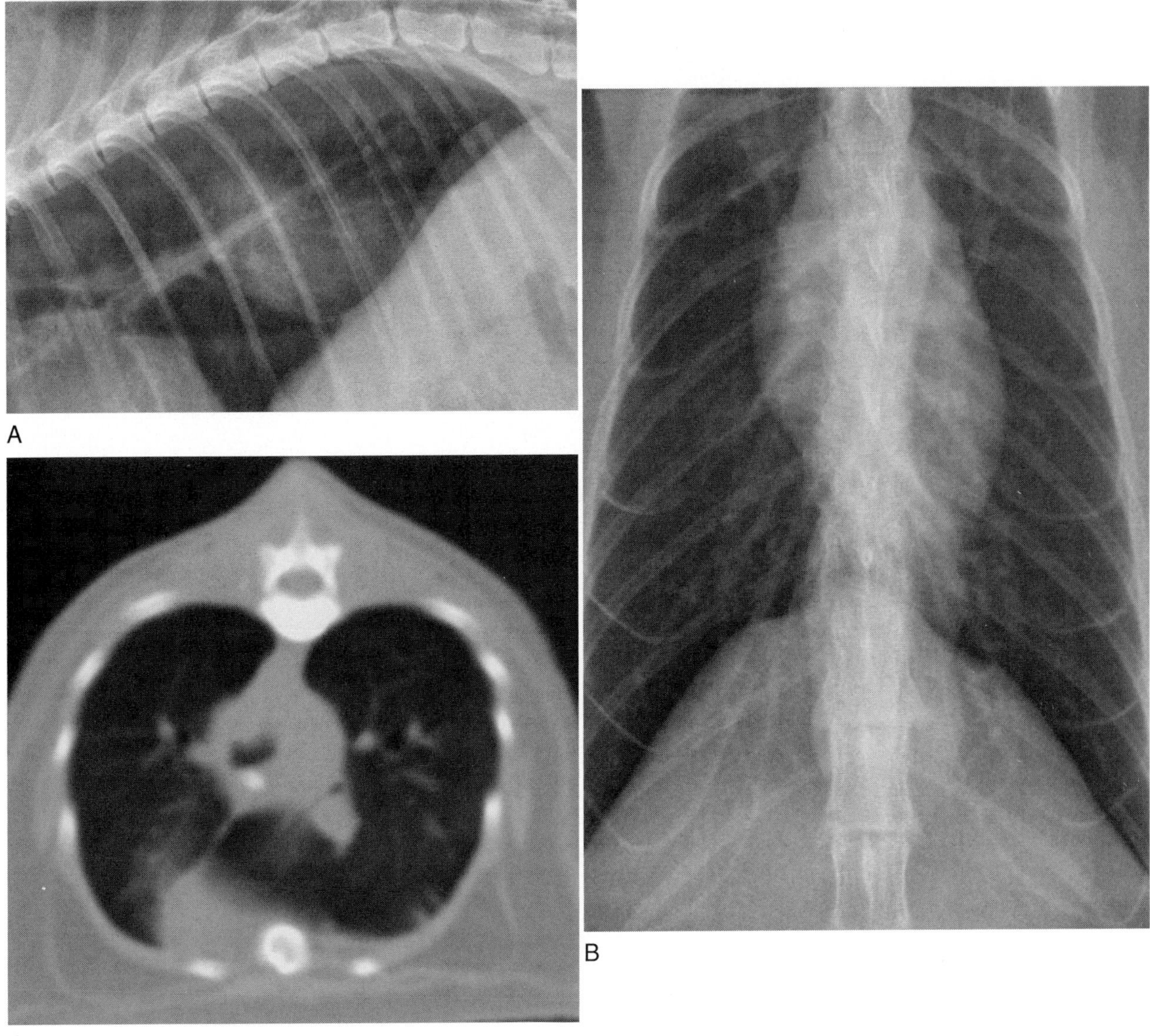

Fig. 28-18 Lateral **(A)** and ventrodorsal **(B)** thoracic radiographs of an elderly cat with a history of regurgitation. In **A** there is an oval undulating mass in the caudal thorax between the aorta and caudal vena cava. In **B** this mass is located on the midline. This mass is consistent with an esophageal mass, but a lung mass cannot be completely ruled out. Accessory lobe masses commonly reside on the midline, but this is an unlikely origin because the caudal vena cava is visible in the lateral view. A computed tomography study of the thorax was acquired **(C)**. The mass is seen as a mural thickening surrounding the gas-filled esophageal lumen; histologic diagnosis was esophageal adenocarcinoma. The evidence of mineralization in the computed tomography image can be seen in the lateral thoracic radiograph but is not as conspicuous.

intrathoracic mass in a position consistent with the esophagus. Differentiation from a nonesophageal mediastinal mass or an accessory lobe mass may be difficult radiographically; an esophagram, a computed tomography, or an endoscopy may be needed to make this distinction (Fig. 28-18).

Mineralization of esophageal masses is rare, although possible (Fig. 28-19). Causes for esophageal mass mineralization include tumor necrosis, osteogenic tumors such as occur with *Spirocerca* infection, and dystrophic mineralization of the esophageal wall. A mineral opacity associated with the esophageal wall may also be seen because of coating of an eroded esophageal mucosa by an orally administered antacid or enteric-coating agent. These medications contain bismuth and other high-atomic-number elements that are radiopaque.[3]

Extrinsic masses may cause displacement and partial to total obstruction of the esophagus, depending on location. Cervical masses that may impinge on the esophagus include thyroid tumors, lymphadenopathy, and cervical abscesses (Fig. 28-20). Invasion of the esophagus by extension may occur, leading to luminal narrowing or wall stiffness and secondary dysfunction. Intrathoracic masses may cause significant esophageal narrowing because of the restriction of space by the spine, sternum, and larger mediastinal structures (e.g., the heart). Accumulation of intraluminal air may be seen cranial to the impinging mass. Oral administration of contrast

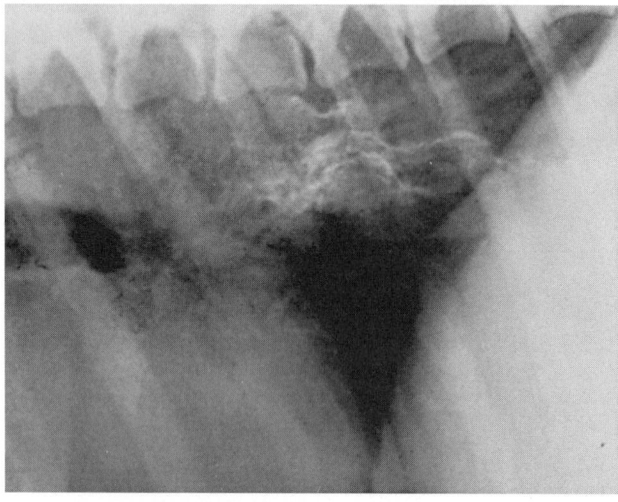

Fig. 28-19 Survey radiograph of the caudodorsal thorax of a mature dog. Abnormal linear to amorphous mineral opacities are present in the dorsal thorax. Differential diagnoses include dystrophic mineralization of the esophagus associated with chronic inflammation or granuloma *(Spirocerca lupi)*, neoplasia with mineralization, chronic radiolucent foreign body, and coating of an eroded mucosa by an antacid or enteric-coating agent. (Courtesy New York State College of Veterinary Medicine, Ithaca, NY.)

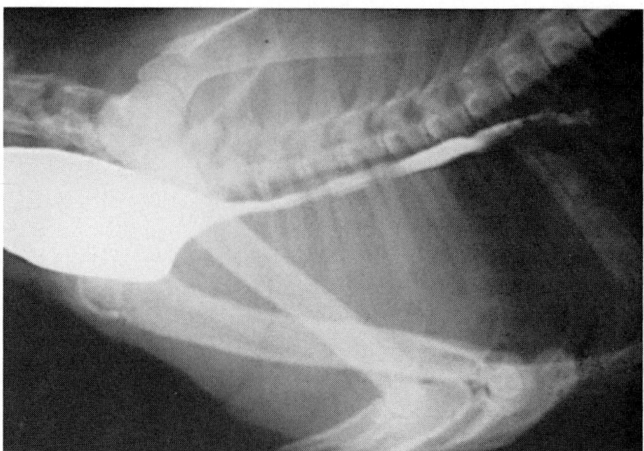

Fig. 28-20 Lateral esophagram of an immature cat with cranial mediastinal lymphosarcoma. The mass is causing elevation of the esophagus and obstruction from restricted expansion capabilities at the thoracic inlet and cranial thorax. (From Ettinger SJ, editor: *Textbook of veterinary internal medicine,* ed 2, Philadelphia, 1983, WB Saunders.)

medium will fill the segmentally dilated esophagus and may demonstrate deviation of the lumen away from the origin of the mass (see Fig. 28-20). Ultrasonography is useful in diagnosing compressive stricture by an extramural mass. Periesophageal lesions may be aspirated or biopsied with ultrasound guidance when visualized on ultrasonography. Cervical masses may be visualized transcutaneously. Intrathoracic periesophageal or mural masses may be examined by way of endoscopic ultrasonography.

Acquired Esophageal Stricture

Esophageal trauma or inflammation may lead to scarring and contracture of the wall. Also, gastric reflux during anesthesia may induce focal esophagitis anywhere along the esophagus, with secondary scarring and luminal narrowing. Subsequent stenosis produces partial and potentially complete obstruction with gradual progression of clinical signs. Depending on the speed of onset and the severity of scarring, prestenotic dilation may not be visible on survey radiographs. The diagnosis is usually made or confirmed by an esophagram (see Fig. 28-14). When liquid barium is used, persistent segmental narrowing on sequential radiographs differentiates the stricture from esophageal spasm. A barium/solid food mixture is important in assessing the distensibility of the narrowed area. See Videos 28-1 and 28-2 at http://evolve.elsevier.com/Thrall/vetrad/ for an example of an esophagram in a dog with an esophageal stricture where liquid and solid food were used. Note the inability to characterize the stricture when liquid barium is used.

Segmental Motor Disease

Segmental esophageal dysfunction is uncommonly recognized. Segmental motility disturbances may affect any portion of the esophagus. Reflux esophagitis is probably the most common form of segmental dysfunction. It usually involves the caudal esophagus and may be associated with hiatal herniation (discussed below). Diffuse esophagitis may produce generalized dilation, but it usually causes intermittent esophageal spasm, which mimics stricture, and focal dilation (Fig. 28-21).

Congenital Causes of Segmental Megaesophagus

Vascular Ring Anomalies

During fetal development of intrathoracic vascular structures, the embryologic arch system is initially duplicated on the right and left sides. Some segments persist after birth and some are transient, with eventual regression of select duplicate parts during cardiovascular development. The aorta is normally derived from the left fourth arch and portions of the left dorsal aorta. The brachycephalic and right subclavian arteries originate from the right fourth aortic arch and portions of the right dorsal aorta.

The most common malformation leading to entrapment of the esophagus is persistence of the right fourth aortic arch; this connects to the main or left pulmonary artery (derived from the ventral root of the right sixth aortic arch) by way of the ductus arteriosus (or ligamentum arteriosus after birth), which forms from the left sixth arch. Constriction occurs with the esophagus, bounded by the heart base ventrally, the aorta on the right, and the pulmonary artery on the left, which is compressed by the ligamentum arteriosum connecting the aorta and pulmonary artery (Fig. 28-22). Dilation of the esophagus occurs cranial to the constriction, with abrupt tapering seen just cranial to the tracheal bifurcation. Luminal contents may include air, fluid, and food (Fig. 28-23). Foreign debris occasionally may be retained (see Fig. 28-13). Radiographic signs on the lateral view usually include ventral deviation of the thoracic trachea (caused by draping of the dilated esophagus over the dorsum of the trachea) and a distinct interface of the dorsal wall of the esophagus silhouetting the cranial thoracic hypaxial muscles when intraluminal air is present. On the ventrodorsal or dorsoventral view, the mediastinum cranial to the heart is widened and either relatively lucent because of air in the esophagus, soft-tissue opaque from fluid accumulation, or heterogeneously opaque from retained food mixed with air. The trachea is deviated to the left near the cranial border of the heart. Tracheal narrowing may also be seen on the ventrodorsal or dorsoventral view.[9] The leftward margin of the descending aortic arch is usually absent. In an esophagram, the segmental dilation of the esophagus with constriction of the lumen just cranial to the tracheal bifurcation is apparent. A shallow indentation created by the contiguous left subclavian artery may be visible cranial to the constriction on the ventrodorsal view (see Video 28-4 of an esophagram in a

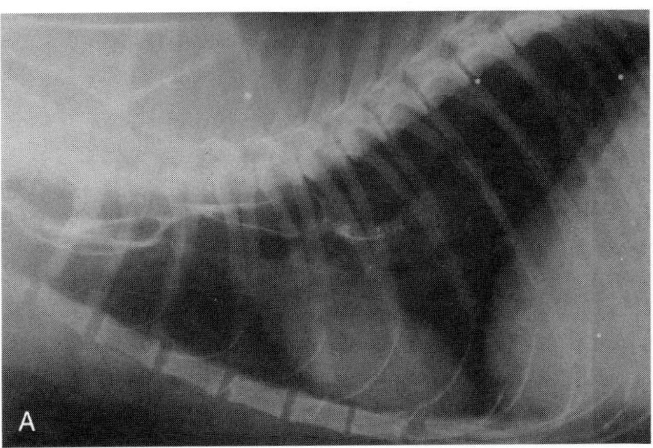

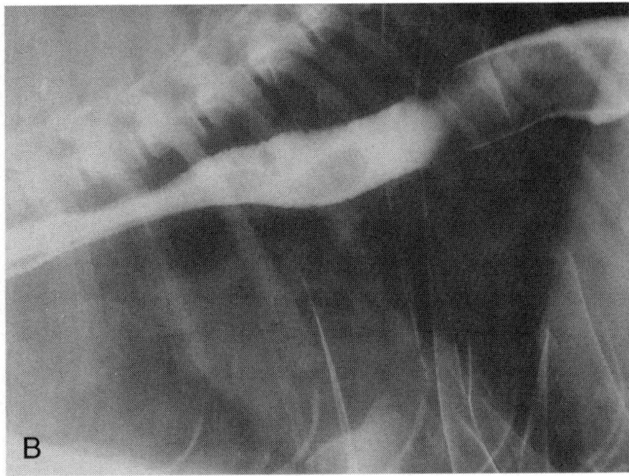

Fig. 28-21 Radiographs of an adult cat with acute regurgitation during meals. **A,** In the initial radiograph, the presence of an esophageal stricture dorsal to the heart base was suspected. The esophagus appeared dilated cranial to this site. **B,** In a subsequent examination, intermittent relaxation of the esophagus was detected at the narrowed site with normal bolus transport during these periods. Focal esophageal spasm was the diagnosis. (Note the mucosal serration of the caudal esophagus, which is typical of the feline esophagus.)

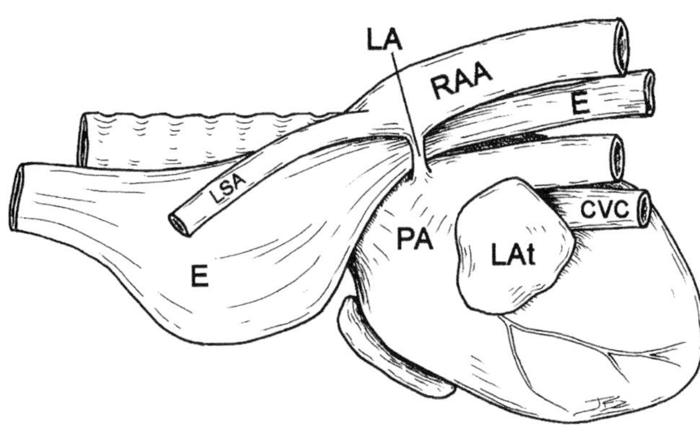

Fig. 28-22 Schematic of persistent right aortic arch. This view, from the left, shows the ligamentum arteriosum *(LA)* connecting the descending right aortic arch *(RAA)* to the main or left pulmonary artery *(PA)* causing constriction of the esophagus *(E)* between these structures and the heart base. *CVC,* Caudal vena cava; *LAt,* left atrium; *LSA,* left subclavian artery.

cat with vascular ring anomaly available at http://evolve.elsevier.com/Thrall/vetrad). Note the area of constriction. Note also that once barium enters the esophagus caudal to the site of compression that contractility is normal. This is an important distinction because generalized esophageal dysfunction may occasionally be concurrent; if this complication is present, esophageal dysfunction will persist even though the vascular ring is corrected.

Less-common vascular ring anomalies include duplication of the aortic arch (Fig. 28-24) and aberrant right subclavian artery (Fig. 28-25). A double aortic arch traps the esophagus between the arches and the heart base. The trachea occasionally may also be constricted, resulting in dyspnea. An aberrant right subclavian artery with a normal aorta traps the esophagus below the artery. The right subclavian artery, normally branching rightward off the brachycephalic trunk, may instead arise directly from the aorta just distal to the left subclavian artery; it then crosses over the top of the esophagus from left to right, constricting the esophagus. A left descending aorta with an aberrant right ligamentum or ductus arteriosus may also encircle the esophagus. If a well-defined normal left descending aortic margin is visible on the ventrodorsal/dorsoventral thoracic radiograph of a patient with dilation of the esophagus cranial to the heart base, one of the less-common vascular ring anomalies should be considered. Ultrasound examination or angiography is needed to characterize these anomalies fully.

Frequently, additional cardiac or vascular anomalies, such as persistent left cranial vena cava, are present but may not be of physiologic significance. The importance of persistent left cranial vena cava in patients with right aortic arch is that it will be an unexpected finding at surgery and may obstruct the normal surgical approach to ligate the ligamentum arteriosus. Rarely, with persistent right aortic arch, the ductus arteriosus may remain patent rather than regress to form the ligamentum arteriosum. If patent, a murmur can usually be auscultated, and extra care will be required when surgically ligating the structure. A vascular ring anomaly occasionally may be accompanied by generalized esophageal dysfunction, leading to generalized megaesophagus (see Fig. 28-13). This will worsen the prognosis for response to surgical correction of the vascular ring anomaly. For this reason, contrast examination of the entire esophagus, not just the portion cranial to the compression, is recommended for complete evaluation of vascular ring anomalies before surgical correction.

Redundant Esophagus

Esophageal redundancy is a rare incidental finding; it may be problematic in young brachycephalic breeds, especially English bulldogs and Shar Peis. Regional dilation may be present at the site of esophageal deviation in the thoracic inlet (Fig. 28-26). In survey radiographs, focal gas accumulation may occur in the caudal cervical and cranial thoracic esophagus, or the radiographs may be normal. Contrast examination highlights a tortuous esophageal path, usually at or just caudal to the thoracic inlet. If the radiograph is exposed in the midst of bolus transport, the peristaltic contraction of the esophagus may mask the redundancy or mimic a focal diverticulum.

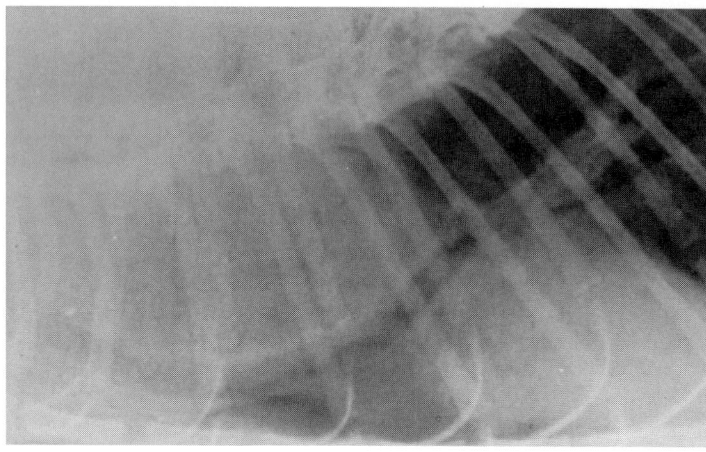

Fig. 28-23 Lateral view of the cranial thorax of a young cat with a persistent right-fourth aortic arch. Food has accumulated in the dilated segment of the esophagus cranial to the obstruction. The trachea deviates ventrally. (Courtesy New York State College of Veterinary Medicine, Ithaca, NY.)

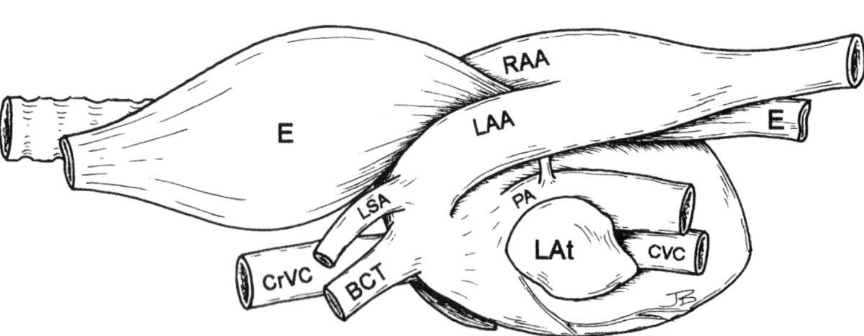

Fig. 28-24 Schematic of double aortic arch. This view, from the left dorsolateral side, shows persistence of both right *(RAA)* and left *(LAA)* aortic arches, which wrap around the dorsal aspect of the esophagus *(E)* and the trachea, leading to constriction. *BCT,* Brachiocephalic trunk; *CrVC,* cranial vena cava; *CVC,* caudal vena cava; *LSA,* left subclavian artery; *PA,* main pulmonary artery; *LAt,* left atrium.

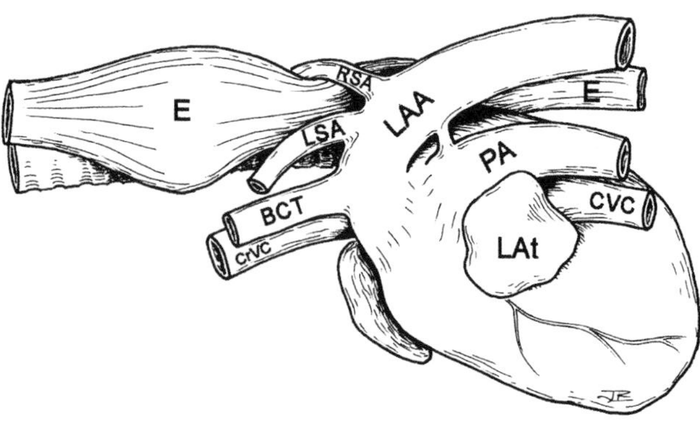

Fig. 28-25 Schematic of aberrant right subclavian artery. This view, from the left side, shows the right subclavian artery *(RSA)* arising leftward from the aortic arch *(LAA)* and coursing over the top of the esophagus *(E)*, causing constriction of the esophagus. *BCT,* Brachiocephalic trunk; *CrVC,* cranial vena cava; *CVC,* caudal vena cava; *LAt,* left atrium; *LSA,* left subclavian artery; *PA,* pulmonary artery.

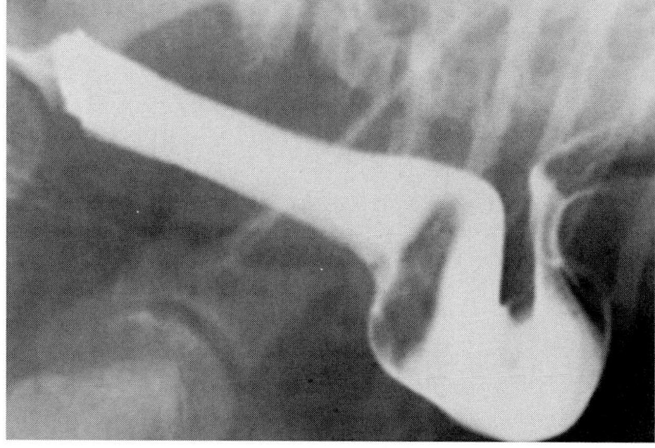

Fig. 28-26 The cranial thoracic esophagus in this immature Bulldog is redundant. The tortuous path, which may be in a transverse or, as in this case, saggital plane, may hamper peristalsis. (Courtesy New York State College of Veterinary Medicine, Ithaca, NY.)

Generalized Megaesophagus

Both congenital and acquired megaesophagus occurs in the cat and dog. The congenital form may be hereditary in both the dog (miniature Schnauzer and Fox Terrier breeds) and the cat. The underlying cause of acquired megaesophagus is often unidentified (idiopathic), although it may be a result of one of many possible causes, including chest trauma, tetanus, organophosphate toxicity, lead toxicity, myasthenia gravis, polymyositis/polymyopathy, autoimmune disease (systemic lupus erythematosus), hypoadrenocorticism, dermatomyositis, thymoma, dysautonomia (cats), gastrointestinal disease (gastric dilation/volvulus, pyloric obstruction, hiatal hernia, esophagitis), central nervous system disease (meningitis, neoplasia, trauma), dyspnea usually caused by upper airway obstruction, and possibly hypothyroidism. A defect in the afferent innervation may be present in both congenital and acquired forms of idiopathic megaesophagus.

Generalized megaesophagus with a gas-filled lumen may be visualized along all or part of its length on survey radiographs. In the lateral view, the cervical portion is apparent beginning just caudal to the cranial esophageal sphincter. In the thorax, the esophagus drapes around the trachea and

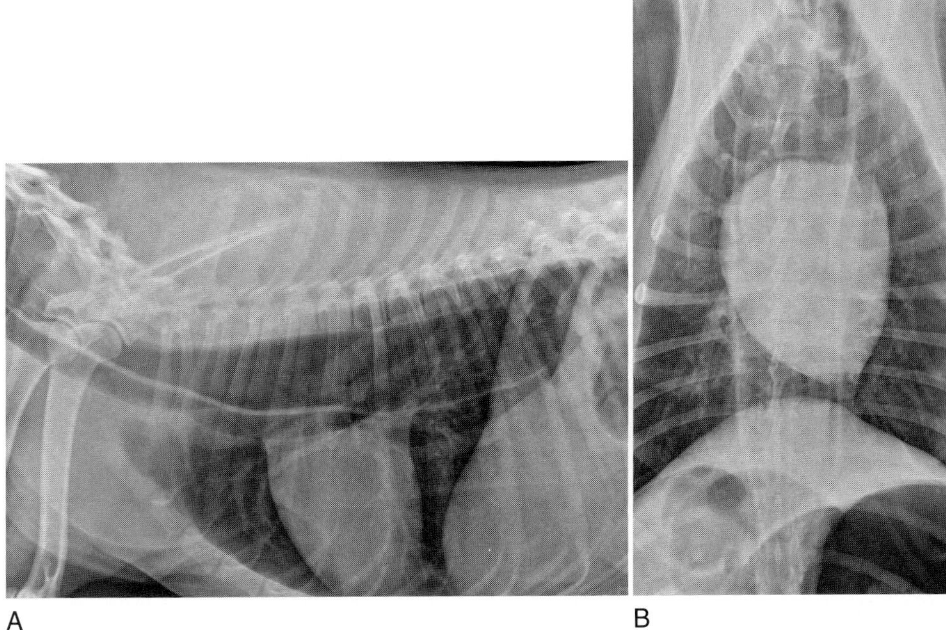

Fig. 28-27 Lateral (A) and ventrodorsal (B) radiographs of a dog with generalized megaesophagus; the esophagus is filled with gas. **A,** Note the sharp demarcation between the esophagus and longus coli muscles, the ventral depression of the trachea, the long tracheal stripe sign, and the visibility of the esophageal walls in the caudal aspect of the thorax. A dilated esophagus is more difficult to see in the ventrodorsal view, but in this patient note the radiopaque lines paralleling the spine on each side of the thorax and how these lines converge caudally as they approach the stomach **(B).**

depresses it ventrally (Fig. 28-27). The thoracic esophagus, when gas filled, may be inadvertently overlooked because of the relative radiolucency of the adjacent lung field. Close scrutiny, however, provides several hallmark findings characteristic of its presence. If the esophagus is fluid filled, the lumen may not be visible because of silhouetting of the soft tissue and fluid (Fig. 28-28).

When the cranial thoracic esophagus dilates, the dorsal wall abuts the paired longus colli muscles, which may be seen as a sharp interface from the thoracic inlet to the ventral aspect of T5 or T6. The ventral wall projects lateral and often ventral to the trachea (see Fig. 28-27, *A*). The draping of the ventral wall over the dorsal tracheal wall results in summation (silhouetting) of the two walls, which creates the tracheal stripe sign. When gas distended, the caudal thoracic esophagus is seen as a pair of thin, soft tissue stripes that converge to a point overlying the diaphragm and cranial abdomen. On the dorsoventral or ventrodorsal view, the dilated, gas-filled cervical esophagus may be hidden by the spine and trachea (Fig. 28-28, *B*). The gas-filled cranial thoracic esophagus produces a wide cranial mediastinum that is relatively radiolucent. The lateral margins may be indented on the left by the descending aorta and on the right by the azygous vein. The caudal thoracic esophagus converges to a **V** at the hiatus of the diaphragm.

ESOPHAGEAL PERFORATION AND FISTULAS

Cervical esophageal perforations result in leakage with sepsis and secondary inflammation. Gradually, an abscess may form or cellulitis may extend along fascial planes through the thoracic inlet to involve the mediastinum and pleural cavity.

Thoracic esophageal perforations result in contamination of the mediastinum and potentially the pleural cavity. Radiographic findings of esophageal perforation may include variable amounts of intraluminal esophageal gas or fluid, cervical gas, cervical swelling, a widened mediastinum or mediastinal mass, pneumomediastinum (see Fig. 28-17), pneumothorax, and/or pleural effusion.

When radiographic interpretation is ambiguous, esophagography is recommended. A water-soluble, organic iodine contrast medium is recommended to minimize contamination of the mediastinum and pleural cavity with a potentially irritating substance. If barium sulfate is inadvertently used and leaks from the esophageal perforation, adequate thoracic lavage will help prevent the granulomatous response caused by the contrast medium and esophageal contents. Occasionally, water-soluble contrast medium will fail to detect a perforation because the contrast medium did not pass through the hole or because of marked dilution in the thoracic effusion. In negative studies, barium sulfate can then be considered.

A fistula between the esophageal lumen and the respiratory tract is uncommon. The site of communication may be esophagotracheal, esophagobronchial, or esophagopulmonary in nature. Foreign bodies have been recognized as a cause of fistula, which can be induced by gradual local esophageal necrosis leading to perforation and by adhesion formation between the esophagus and the adjacent respiratory tract tissue. Potential causes also include malignant esophageal disease, penetrating trauma to the esophagus, infectious or neoplastic pulmonary disease, preexisting esophageal diverticula, and periesophageal lymphadenopathy. In survey radiographs, bronchopneumonia may be noted. The location of the pulmonary infiltrate depends on the site of communication, which may vary. If the animal has a history of coughing

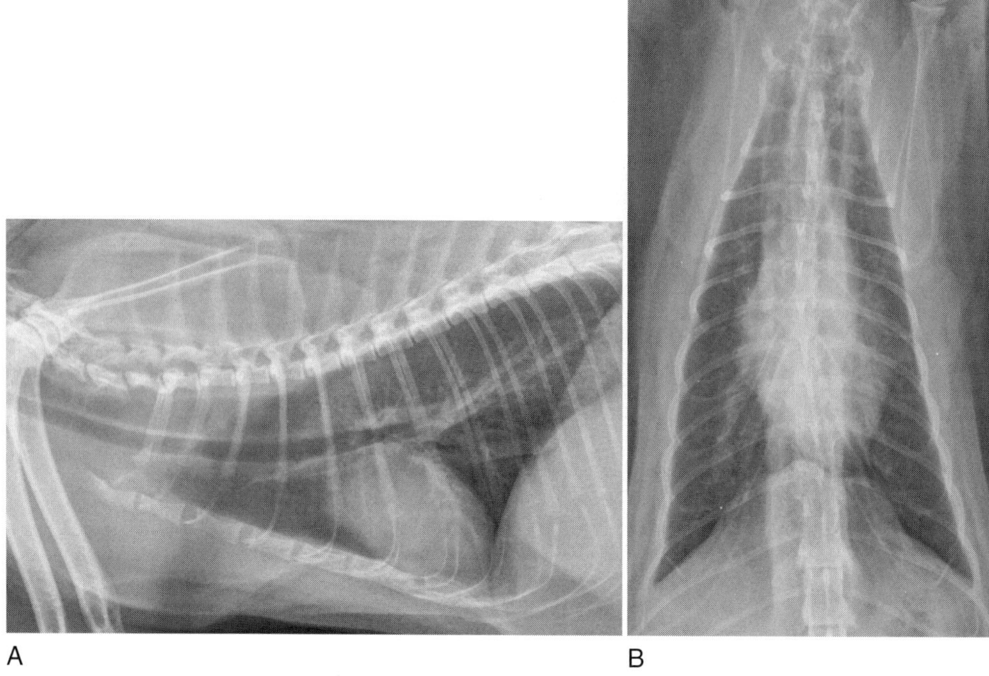

Fig. 28-28 Lateral (A) and ventrodorsal (B) radiographs of a cat with megaesophagus; the esophagus is mainly filled with fluid and air. The dilated esophagus in this cat is not as conspicuous as it would be if filled only with air. In **A,** gas in the cranial portion of the esophagus results in the tracheal stripe sign, and fluid in the esophagus caudally has produced an ill-defined opacity in the caudal aspect of the thorax between the aorta and caudal vena cava. In **B,** the esophagus is also not as conspicuous as if gas filled. The esophagus in the cranial aspect of the thorax is difficult to identify, but in the caudal aspect of the thorax the esophageal wall can be seen.

or choking that is exacerbated by ingestion of fluids, a barium contrast swallow is indicated to locate the fistula (Fig. 28-29). If pleural involvement is noted on the survey radiographs, an isosmotic organic iodide compound is recommended for the esophagram to minimize possible contamination of the pleural space by barium. An ionic organic iodide contrast medium may induce pulmonary edema if communication with the lung parenchyma is present. Inadvertent tracheal aspiration and subsequent alveolarization of contrast medium during a routine swallow should not be misinterpreted as an esophageal fistula.

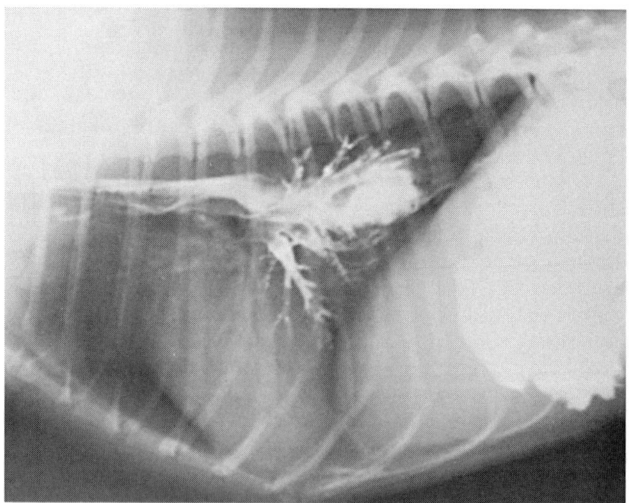

Fig. 28-29 Lateral esophagram of a young dog. Simultaneous filling of the right caudal lobe bronchus and the esophagus is present, indicating a bronchoesophageal fistula. (From Ettinger SJ, editor: *Textbook of veterinary internal medicine,* ed 2, Philadelphia, 1983, WB Saunders.)

DISEASES OF THE HIATUS

The esophagus is tethered to the hiatus of the diaphragm by a phrenoesophageal membrane that normally allows only minor cranial movement of the abdominal segment. A congenital or acquired abnormality of the hiatus may allow for reduced caudal esophageal sphincter tone and reflux, resulting in the development of a sliding hiatal hernia, a periesophageal hiatal hernia, a diaphragmatic hernia, or a gastroesophageal intussusception (see Chapter 29). The differentiation of these disorders may be difficult because of the similarity of clinical signs and survey radiographic findings. In survey radiographs, a variably sized mass effect in the dorsocaudal aspect of the thorax may appear continuous with the diaphragm. The cranial thoracic esophagus may be partly or completely dilated and gas filled cranial to the mass, or it may be normal. Size and visibility of the fundic gas bubble are variable, but the bubble is often not seen with herniation or intussusception. A barium contrast study is required to locate the gastroesophageal junction and the gastric fundus.

Gastroesophageal Reflux

Reflux esophagitis occurs when acidic gastric contents inflame the esophageal mucosa. Reflux may be a normal consequence

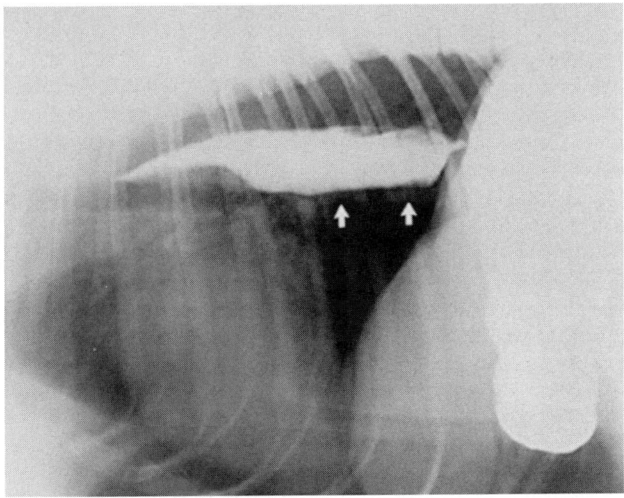

Fig. 28-30 Gastroesophageal reflux is characterized by contrast medium in the caudal esophagus after clearing of this area subsequent to the initial administration of contrast medium. The ventral wall of the esophagus in this dog is thickened *(arrows)* by chronic inflammation, which impairs rapid clearing and further compounds the problem. (Courtesy New York State College of Veterinary Medicine, Ithaca, NY.)

of swallowing, but the retrograde flow of gastric acid should be rapidly cleared by the esophagus. Diagnosis of clinically significant gastroesophageal reflux may be difficult by survey radiography. Survey radiographs may be normal or an esophageal opacity may be present that varies from subtle in the caudal mediastinum, to visible from luminal fluid retention, to dilated and air or fluid filled when the esophagitis is extensive (see Fig. 28-21). Most often, the survey findings are negative or minimal, and they may be overlooked. Contrast examination with static imaging may also be negative. If esophagitis is severe, retention of contrast medium with esophageal mucosal irregularity or ulceration, as well as thickening or diffuse, nonuniform dilation may be seen (Fig. 28-30). Infiltration by inflammatory or granulation tissue usually distorts the mucosal surface, obliterating the longitudinal or oblique folds. Most often, during a gastrointestinal contrast examination, intermittent reflux is seen as recurrence of the appearance of contrast medium within the caudal esophagus as barium gradually transits the stomach. Fluoroscopy is a more accurate means of assessing gastroesophageal reflux.

Hiatal Hernias

With hiatal herniation, a soft tissue mass effect is often present in the dorsocaudal aspect of the thoracic cavity in the lateral view and a mass effect in the caudal thorax, slightly to the left of midline, is present in the ventrodorsal view. Other than hiatal hernia, considerations for such a mass include esophageal mass and pulmonary mass. Hiatal hernias are often dynamic and may appear different, or not even be present, in subsequent radiographs. To determine whether a mass lesion is caused by a hiatal hernia, barium can be administered (Fig. 28-31). Barium will typically allow the misplaced fundus to be identified and the caudal esophageal sphincter, recognized as a focal narrowing of the barium contrast column, is cranially displaced. Variable amounts of rugae-lined gastric fundus are seen as an extension of the caudal esophagus in the thoracic cavity (see Fig. 28-31).

A periesophageal hernia is less common than a hiatal hernia. They cause partial obstruction and displacement of the terminal esophagus laterally away from the herniated gastric fundus. On the ventrodorsal or dorsoventral contrast radiograph, the gastric rugae are seen lateral to the esophagus within the caudal mediastinum.

Gastroesophageal Intussusception

Gastroesophageal intussusception is rare, usually affecting puppies. The stomach, sometimes accompanied by other abdominal viscera (spleen, duodenum, pancreas, and omentum), invaginates into the caudal esophageal lumen. Preexisting congenital or idiopathic megaesophagus may predispose to this intussusception. A large soft tissue or heterogeneous mass is usually present in the caudal mediastinum (Fig. 28-32). Commonly a gas-filled, dilated esophagus is present cranial to the herniation, and the intussuscepted portion of stomach appears as a mass within the esophageal lumen. Rugal folds are often recognized on the surface of the mass, especially when barium is present in the esophagus, because of the invaginated nature of the stomach. A stomach silhouette may be absent from the cranial abdomen or, when gas distended, the stomach lumen may present with a defined communication with the caudal mediastinal mass. Contrast examination in these patients confirms obstruction of the caudal esophagus by the mass with failure of contrast medium to fill the abdominal gastric lumen.

Conclusion

Esophageal disease may be characterized by focal or diffuse involvement. Diffuse disease usually results in megaesophagus characterized by generalized dysfunction, but megaesophagus may also occur with obstruction of the terminal esophagus from a few focal causes. Alternatively, focal or segmental disease may have numerous causes. The common locations of various focal esophageal lesions are listed in Box 28-1. The absence of abnormal esophageal radiographic findings does not preclude the presence of esophageal disease; such findings are often encountered with acute esophageal disease. In addition, the presence of indirect signs of esophageal disease should be anticipated. Focal or generalized esophageal dilation may be less apparent when the lumen is fluid

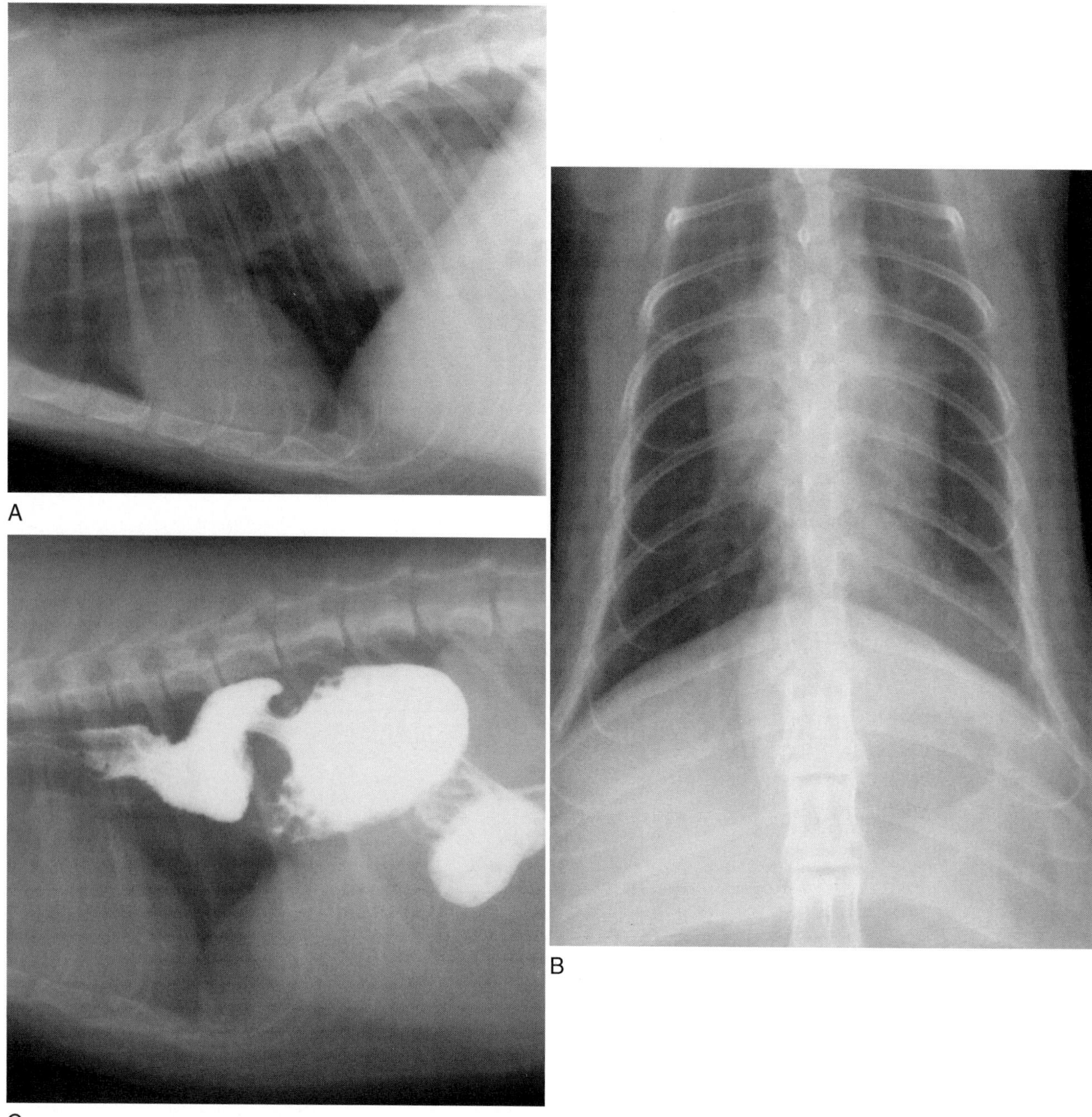

Fig. 28-31 Lateral (A) and ventrodorsal (B) radiographs of a cat with a hiatal hernia. **A,** A mass effect is present in the dorsocaudal aspect of the thoracic cavity. The cranial thoracic esophagus contains more gas than considered normal for a cat. **B,** The mass effect is near the midline but is displaced slightly to the left. Barium was administered. **C,** The fundus is recognized by its rugal folds and is displaced into the thoracic cavity. The caudal esophageal sphincter is apparent.

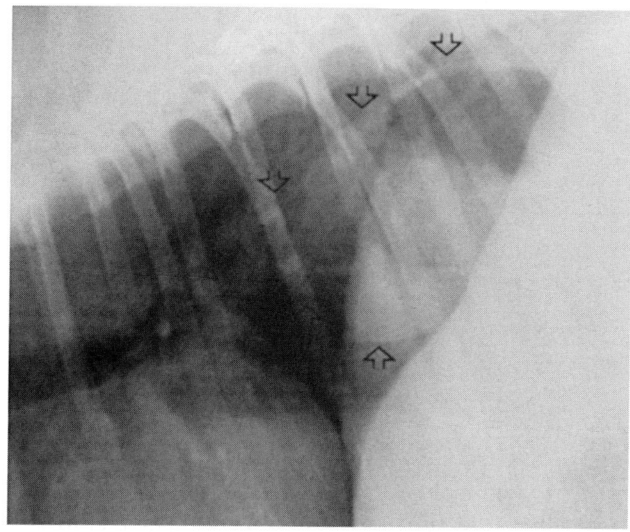

Fig. 28-32 Lateral view of the caudodorsal thorax of a mature dog with a gastroesophageal intussusception. The radiopacity of the gastric contents may be seen in the caudal thorax superimposed over the left diaphragmatic crus and dorsocaudal lung field *(arrows)*. (Courtesy New York State College of Veterinary Medicine, Ithaca, NY.)

filled, thereby creating a positive silhouette sign with the mediastinum. The enlarged lumen, however, affects adjacent visible structures. The weight of the dilated esophagus may cause ventral and right lateral tracheal displacement in the cervical and cranial thoracic regions. The cranial and caudal mediastinum widens around the dilated esophagus. Pulmonary interstitial or alveolar infiltrates occur as a result of aspiration or, less commonly, esophageal fistulation. Pleural effusion, pneumothorax, or pneumomediastinum, as well as lobar consolidation, are occasionally present as a result of esophageal disease.

Box • 28-1

Characteristic Site of Focal Esophageal Disease

Cervical Region

Cricopharyngeal achalasia
Asynchrony
Chalasia
Foreign body
Esophagitis (caustic)
Extension of neoplasia
Perforation
Segmental hypomotility

Cranial Thoracic Region

Vascular ring anomaly
Esophagitis (reflux)
Stricture
Periesophageal mass
Redundancy
Diverticula
Foreign body
Neoplasia
Perforation

Caudal Thoracic Region

Esophagitis (reflux) (patulent caudal esophageal sphincter)
Foreign body
Perforation
Leiomyoma
Gastroesophageal intussusception
Hiatal hernia
Esophageal fistula

REFERENCES

1. Pratschke KM, Fitzpatrick E, Campion D, et al: Topography of the gastro-oesophageal junction in the dog revisited: possible clinical implications, *Res Vet Sci* 76:171, 2004.
2. O'Brien TR: Esophagus. In O'Brien TR, editor: *Radiographic diagnosis of abdominal disorders in the dog and cat: radiographic interpretation, clinical signs, pathophysiology,* Philadelphia, 1978, W.B. Saunders, p. 141.
3. Hall JA, Watrous BJ: Effect of pharmaceuticals on radiographic appearance of selected examinations of the abdomen and thorax, *Vet Clin North Am Small Anim Pract* 30:349, 2000.
4. Kealy JK: The abdomen. In *Diagnostic radiology of the dog and cat,* ed 2, Philadelphia, 1987, W.B. Saunders, p. 41.
5. Brawner WR Jr, Bartels JE: Contrast radiography of the digestive tract. Indications, techniques and complications, *Vet Clin North Am Small Anim Pract* 13:599, 1983.
6. Watrous BJ: Clinical presentation and diagnosis of dysphagia, *Vet Clin North Am Small Anim Pract* 13:437, 1983.
7. Watrous BJ: Esophageal disease. In Ettinger SJ, editor: *Textbook of veterinary internal medicine: diseases of the dog and cat,* ed 2, Philadelphia, 1983, W.B. Saunders, p. 1191.
8. Jones BD, Jergens AE, Guilford WG: Disease of the esophagus. In Ettinger SJ, editor: *Textbook of veterinary internal medicine: diseases of the dog and cat,* ed 3, Philadelphia, 1989, W.B. Saunders.
9. Buchanan JW: Tracheal signs and associated vascular anomalies in dogs with persistent right aortic arch, *J Vet Intern Med* 18:510, 2004.

ELECTRONIC RESOURCES evolve

Additional information related to the content in Chapter 28 can be found on the companion Web site at evolve http://evolve.elsevier.com/Thrall/vetrad/.

- Key Points
- Chapter Quiz
- Case Study 28-1
- Video 28-1: Dynamic fluoroscopic image of a patient with an esophageal stricture being fed liquid barium
- Video 28-2: Dynamic fluoroscopic image of a patient with an esophageal stricture being fed barium-coated kibble
- Video 28-3: Dynamic fluoroscopic image of a patient with cricopharyngeal sphincter dysfunction being fed liquid barium
- Video 28-4: Dynamic fluoroscopic image of a patient with a persistent right fourth aortic arch being fed liquid barium

CHAPTER • 29
The Thoracic Wall

Valerie F. Samii

The thoracic wall is composed of skin, fat, subcutaneous and intercostal musculature, parietal pleura, blood vessels, nerves, and lymphatics. The spine, ribs, costal cartilages, and sternum provide rigid support for the thoracic wall soft tissues. Thoracic wall abnormalities are often overlooked on initial appraisal of thoracic radiographs. Careful inspection of the extrathoracic soft tissue and bony structures is always warranted and can provide information critical to the appropriate diagnosis and treatment.

NORMAL RADIOGRAPHIC APPEARANCE

The soft tissues of the thoracic wall are normally homogeneous in opacity. In particularly obese animals, curvilinear soft tissue opacities, representing extracostal musculature outlined by fat, may be seen paralleling the lateral curvature of the ribs on the dorsoventral (DV) and ventrodorsal (VD) projections (Fig. 29-1). Thirteen pairs of ribs and eight sternebral segments are normal. On the lateral projection, the first few ribs are oriented vertically but become progressively more caudoventral in orientation, from rib head to costochondral junction, in the mid to caudal thoracic spine (Fig. 29-2). On the DV or VD projection, the first few ribs are oriented perpendicular to the spine. In the mid to caudal thoracic spine, ribs curve in a caudolateral direction from their respective vertebrae to their most lateral extent, then continue caudomedially (Fig. 29-3). Slight differences in thoracic wall conformation are common among the various breeds of dog (Fig. 29-4). Breed-associated costochondral conformation leading to a misdiagnosis of pneumothorax or pleural effusion is discussed in Chapter 31.

Mineralization of the costal cartilages may be seen in young dogs and cats and is nearly always present in older animals (Fig. 29-5). Movement at the costochondral and costosternal joints increases as the costal cartilages stiffen from mineralization. This in turn results in osseous proliferation at the costochondral and costosternal joints. The opacities resulting from enlargement of these joints may be confused with lung nodules on DV or VD radiographs. Excessive costochondral or costosternal mineralization may also be confused with aggressive processes such as infection or neoplasia.

Pedunculated soft tissue opacities on the thoracic wall, such as nipples, papillomas, or engorged ticks, may summate with the pulmonary parenchyma and be misdiagnosed as pulmonary nodules. Thorough palpation of the thoracic wall surface usually clarifies the significance of this finding. The inability to identify the presumed pulmonary nodule in the lung on an orthogonal radiograph decreases the likelihood of its presence. Application of positive contrast medium, such as barium paste, on the thoracic wall nodule followed by repeat radiographs can be performed if localization is still in question (Fig. 29-6).

CONGENITAL AND DEVELOPMENTAL ABNORMALITIES

Anomalies of the ribs and sternum are fairly common. Rudimentary ribs are sometimes present on the seventh cervical vertebra (Fig. 29-7) or the first lumbar vertebra (Fig. 29-8). Ribs may be hypoplastic or absent on the thirteenth thoracic vertebral segment (Fig. 29-9). These anomalies may be unilateral or bilateral (Fig. 29-10).

Congenital sternal deformities, such as too few in number, fusion of neighboring segments (Fig. 29-11), pectus carinatum (external protrusion of the sternum), and pectus excavatum (funnel chest or chondrosternal depression) may be incidental findings but have also been reported in animals with peritoneopericardial diaphragmatic hernia (Fig. 29-12).[1,2] Peritoneopericardial diaphragmatic hernias are discussed in Chapter 29.

Pectus excavatum (Fig. 29-13) results in dorsal to ventral narrowing of the thorax and is often associated with respiratory and cardiovascular anomalies. Although pectus excavatum may be congenital or acquired in human beings, all reports in animals describe malformations.[3] The etiology is unknown; however, in a report involving two Welsh terrier littermates, a hereditary component was suggested.[4] Various surgical procedures have been recommended for repair of congenital thoracic wall defects.

THORACIC WALL TRAUMA

Thoracic wall trauma is common in small animals. Soft tissue trauma often goes unnoticed but may be manifested by focal soft tissue swelling or subcutaneous emphysema (Figs. 29-14 and 29-15). Tears of the intercostal musculature can result in separation of ribs and are a common sequela to dog fights, resulting in uneven spacing between ribs.[5] Rib fractures may be identified if fracture fragment displacement is evident (Figs. 29-16 and 29-17). Rib and sternal fractures may be missed if fracture fragments remain in alignment. Many rib fractures are diagnosed retrospectively after callus formation has developed. Multiple rib fractures, particularly segmental fractures, involving the dorsal and ventral aspects of at least two adjacent ribs may create thoracic wall instability, resulting in flail chest.[5,6] The flailing portion of the destabilized thoracic wall moves paradoxically to the normal thoracic wall and is characterized by inward displacement during inspiration and outward displacement during expiration (Fig. 29-18).[5,6] Healing rib fractures may exhibit rounded fracture margins and focal periosteal reaction followed by bridging callus. Over time, the fracture margins and associated osseous callus will remodel, often creating an expansile appearance to the rib once healed (Fig. 29-19). Discrimination of the subtle differences between a healing rib fracture and an aggressive rib

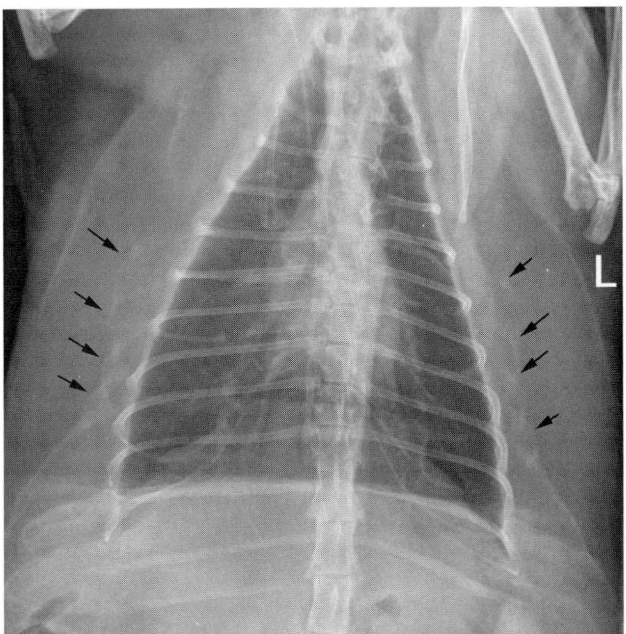

Fig. 29-1 DV thoracic radiograph of an obese cat. Note the bilateral, curvilinear, soft tissue opacities (extracostal musculature) in the fat peripheral to the lateral rib margins *(arrows)*.

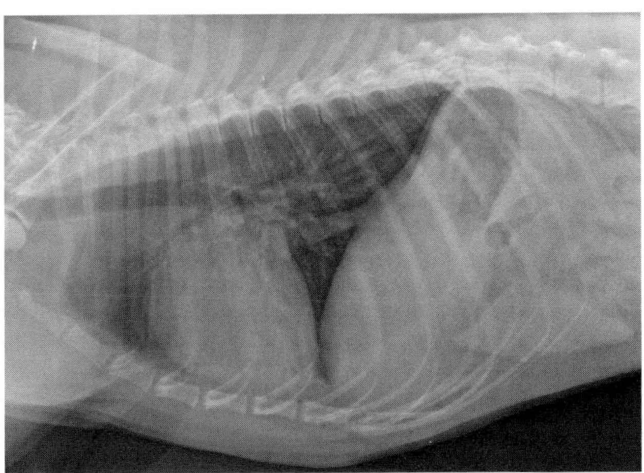

Fig. 29-2 Right lateral thoracic radiograph of a normal adult dog. The first few ribs are oriented vertically but become progressively more caudoventral in orientation, from rib head to costochondral junction, in the mid to caudal thoracic spine.

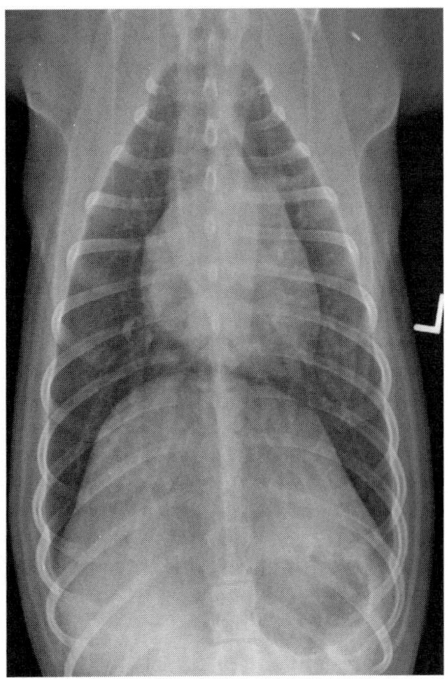

Fig. 29-3 DV thoracic radiograph of a normal adult dog. The first few ribs are oriented perpendicular to the spine. In the mid to caudal thoracic spine, ribs curve in a caudolateral direction from their respective vertebrae to their most lateral extent, then continue caudomedially.

lesion is important. A history of trauma, overriding rib margins, or involvement of multiple adjacent ribs is supportive of a nonneoplastic etiology. When question persists, needle aspiration or biopsy of the rib lesion is indicated. A repeat radiographic evaluation in 2 weeks may also clarify etiology. Progressive lysis and bone proliferation would be expected in an aggressive bone lesion caused by neoplasia.

RIB TUMORS AND INFECTION

A thoracic wall mass that invades the thoracic cavity, regardless of etiology, may create an extrapleural sign.[7,8] An extrapleural sign is characterized by an intrathoracic mass with a well-circumscribed, convex margin facing the lung. The cranial and caudal edges taper along the thoracic wall, giving the mass a broad-based appearance (Fig. 29-20). Extrapleural lesions arise peripheral to the parietal pleura and preferentially extend into the thoracic cavity rather than grow external to the thoracic cavity. They most often originate from ribs but may also arise from connective tissue, nerves, vessels, and muscles. If the convex margin of the extrapleural mass is not sharply delineated, invasion of the pleura overlying the lung should be considered. This occurs more commonly in neoplastic and infectious processes. Occasionally benign extrapleural fat accumulations may be confused with extrapleural neoplastic or infectious processes.[9] Differentiation of fat and soft tissue opacities is important. When in doubt, a needle aspirate of the lesion may clarify its tissue type. The extrapleural sign is best seen when the x-ray beam strikes the lesion tangentially. Oblique radiographs are often necessary to visualize the extrapleural sign.

The characteristic imaging features of the extrapleural sign are helpful in differentiating thoracic wall masses from pulmonary masses. If a lung mass is in contact with the thoracic wall, the junction between the mass and the thoracic wall forms an angle less than 90 degrees (Fig. 29-21, *A*). If a mass originates from the thoracic wall and extends into the thoracic cavity, the junction of the mass and the wall forms an angle greater than 90 degrees (Fig. 29-21, *B*).

Rib infection is uncommon in the dog and cat and usually is the result of trauma caused by a penetrating wound. Occasionally a severe pyothorax may result in rib periostitis. Mycotic rib osteomyelitis may be seen as a result of septicemia. Differentiation of rib osteomyelitis from neoplasia is not possible radiographically. Both processes may illicit mixed productive and lytic, primarily lytic, or primarily productive response. Biopsy is necessary to confirm the pathologic process involved.

Text continued on p. 518

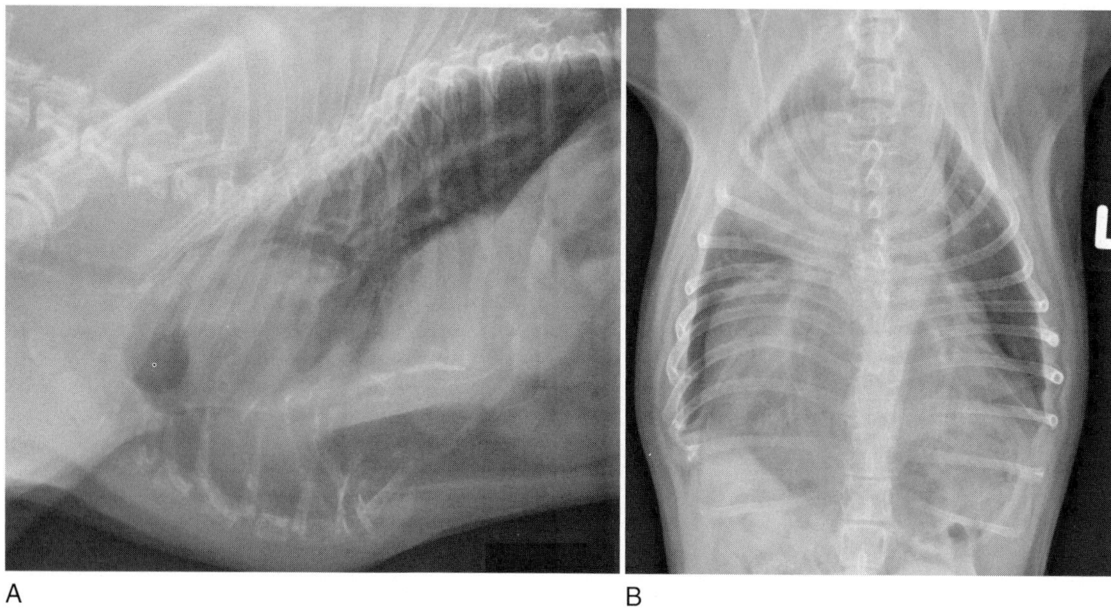

Fig. 29-4 Right lateral (A) and DV (B) thoracic radiographs of an adult Boston Terrier with multiple wedge-shaped vertebrae and hemivertebrae in the mid-thoracic spine. The congenital vertebral anomalies in this dog have resulted in cranioventral angulations of the ribs on the lateral radiograph and a radiating appearance to the rib cage on the DV projection. Scoliosis of the mid-thoracic spine is evident. Extensive mineralization of the costal cartilages is present; this is a normal finding commonly seen in young and old dogs.

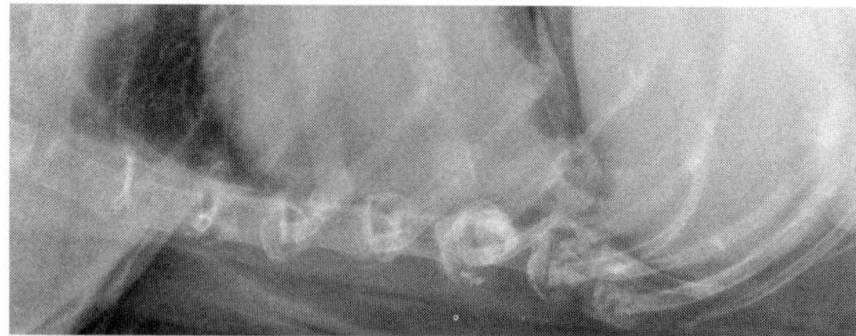

Fig. 29-5 Right lateral radiograph of a middle-aged German Shepherd with extensive costal cartilage mineralization and sternebral and costochondral degeneration.

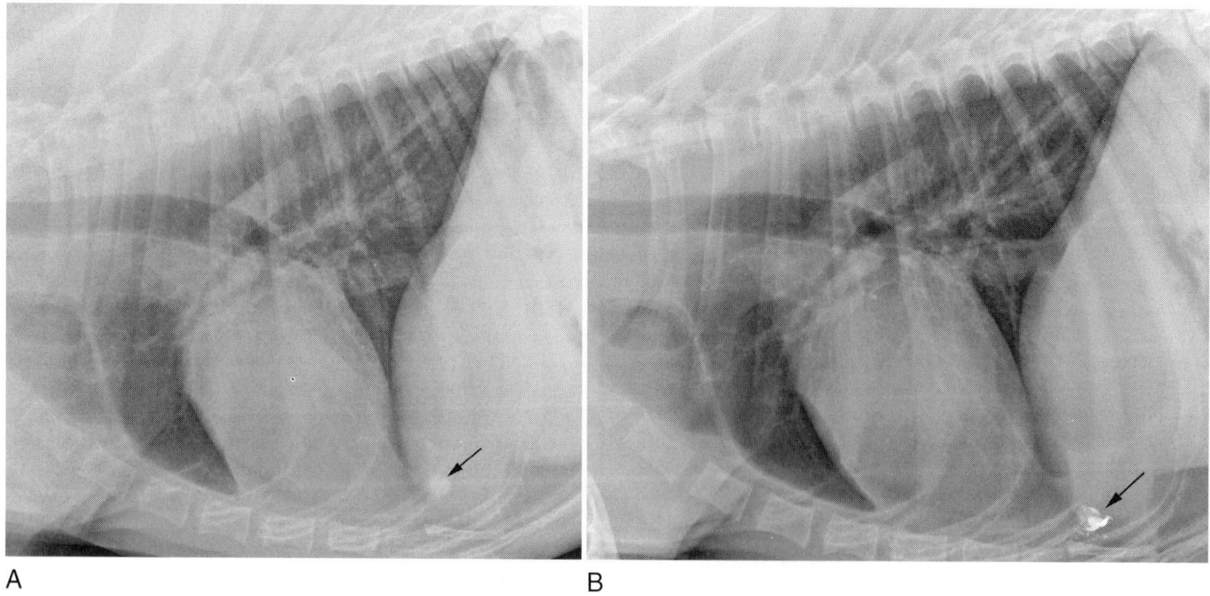

Fig. 29-6 Right lateral thoracic radiographs before (A) and after (B) application of barium paste to a nipple. In **A**, a nodular soft tissue opacity summates with the seventh costal cartilages *(arrow)*. In **B**, barium paste was applied to a palpable nipple on the skin, confirming that the nodule was indeed the nipple *(arrow)*.

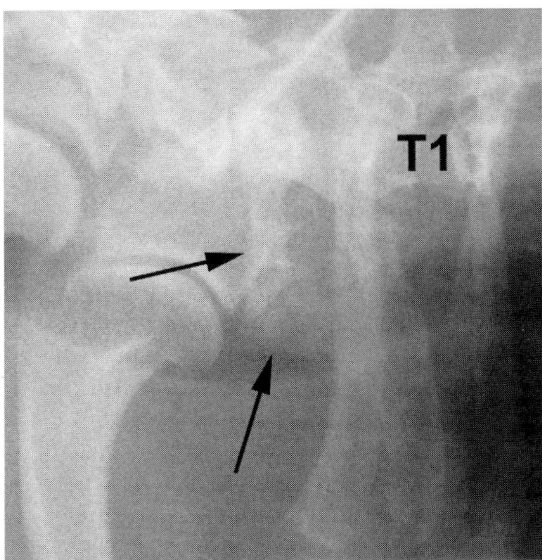

Fig. 29-7 Right lateral cervicothoracic radiograph of a Pekinese dog with a left-sided rudimentary rib on the seventh cervical vertebra, forming a pseudoarthrosis with the first thoracic rib *(arrows)*.

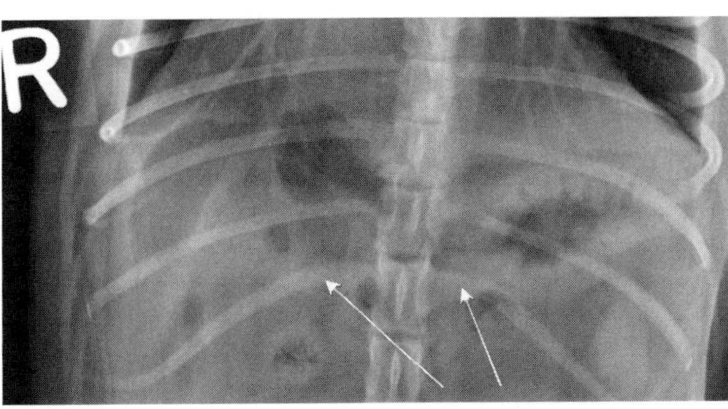

Fig. 29-8 DV caudal thoracic radiograph of a dog with a transitional thoracolumbar vertebral segment. Note the broad-based, thick appearance to the proximal extent of the thirteenth ribs *(arrows)* as compared to ribs 10 to 12. The thirteenth ribs are taking on the characteristics of transverse vertebral processes. This dog only had six lumbar vertebral segments.

Fig. 29-9 DV caudal thoracic radiograph of a dog with a transitional thoracolumbar vertebral segment. The right thirteenth rib is hypoplastic *(arrows)* and only partially mineralized.

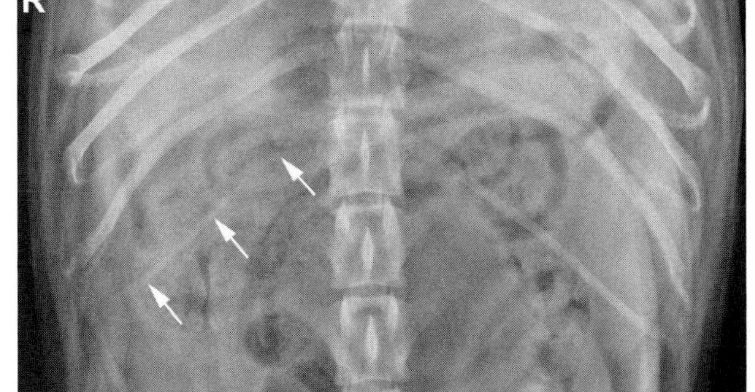

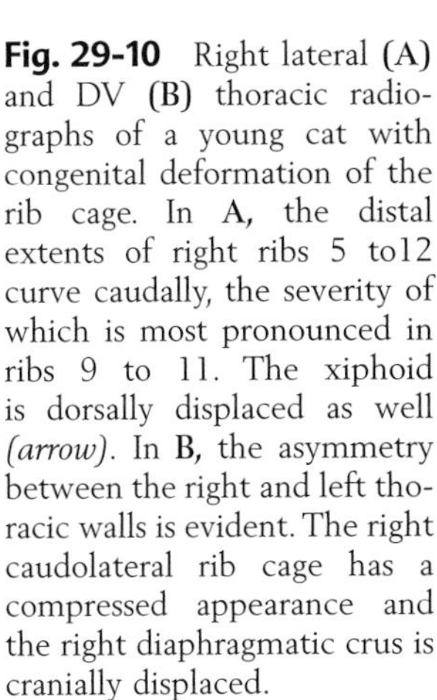

Fig. 29-10 Right lateral (A) and DV (B) thoracic radiographs of a young cat with congenital deformation of the rib cage. In **A**, the distal extents of right ribs 5 to12 curve caudally, the severity of which is most pronounced in ribs 9 to 11. The xiphoid is dorsally displaced as well *(arrow)*. In **B**, the asymmetry between the right and left thoracic walls is evident. The right caudolateral rib cage has a compressed appearance and the right diaphragmatic crus is cranially displaced.

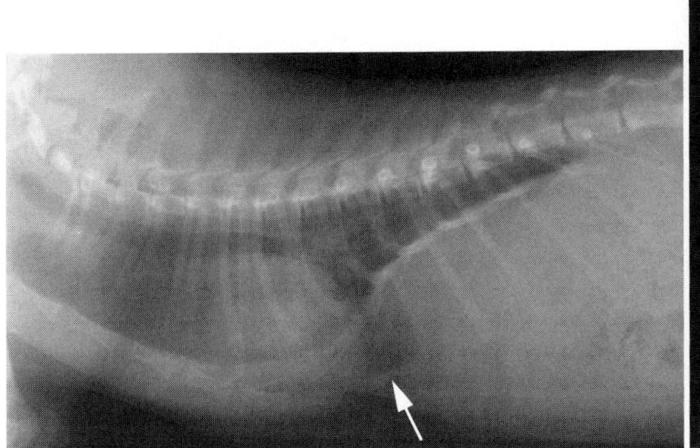

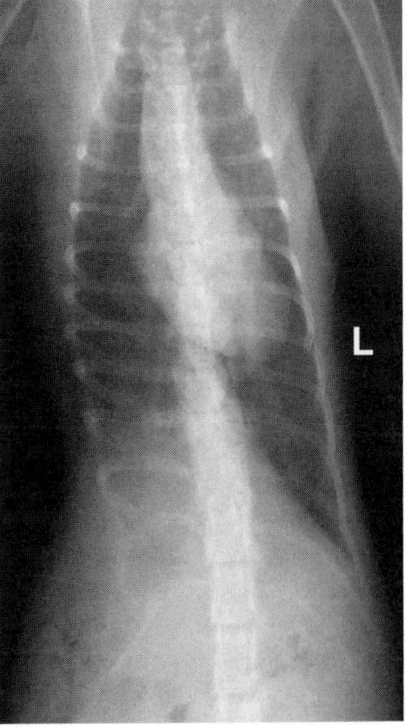

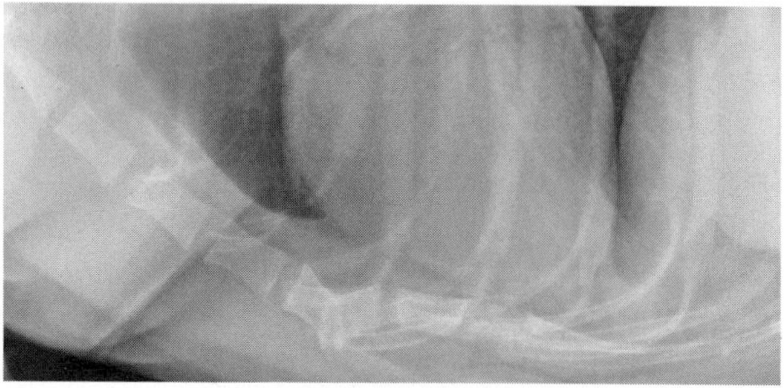

Fig. 29-11 Right lateral radiograph of a young dog's sternum. Fusion of the fourth and fifth sternebral segments is visible, likely a congenital malformation. The dorsal concave margin of the fused segments is smooth, and no evidence of degenerative disease is present that might be consistent with trauma.

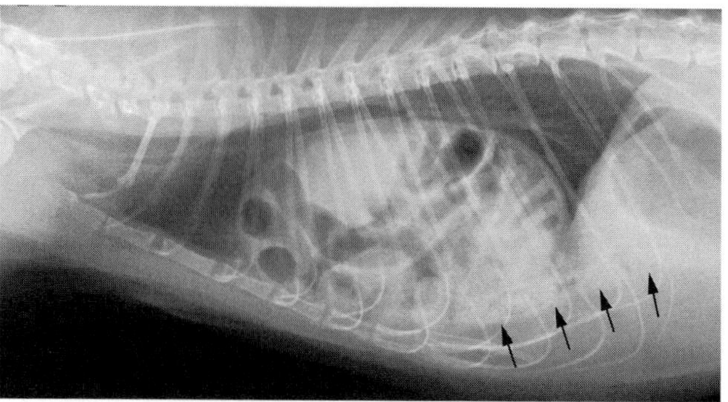

Fig. 29-12 Right lateral thoracic radiograph of a cat with a peritoneopericardial diaphragmatic hernia. The cardiac silhouette is enlarged and oval in shape, causing dorsal deviation of the trachea. Multiple loops of small intestine are present within the thorax summating with the cardiac silhouette. The caudal margin of the cardiac silhouette is confluent with the cranioventral margin of the diaphragm. A dorsal peritoneopericardial mesothelial remnant is not identified. A segment of probable large intestine containing granular material is identified crossing the peritoneopericardial junction *(arrows)*. The liver is probably herniated into the pericardial sac given the lack of liver seen caudal to the diaphragm.

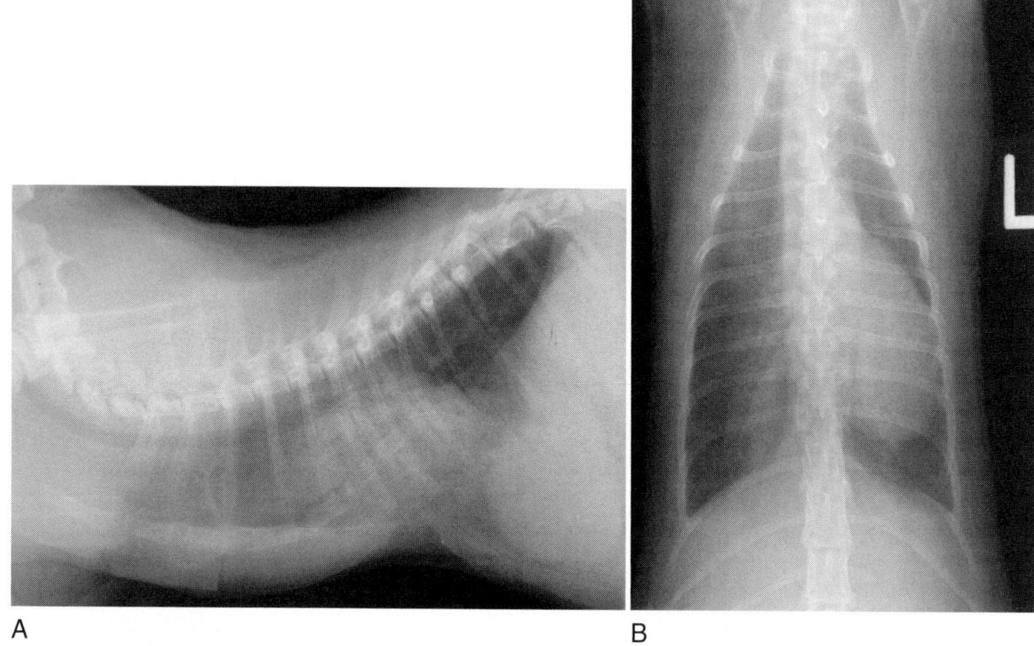

Fig. 29-13 Right lateral (A) and VD (B) thoracic radiographs of an 8-week-old kitten with pectus excavatum (funnel chest or chondrosternal depression). Severe dorsal to ventral narrowing of the thorax is present. The cardiac silhouette and trachea are compressed dorsally against the thoracic spine, and deviation of the cardiac silhouette to the left hemithorax is visible.

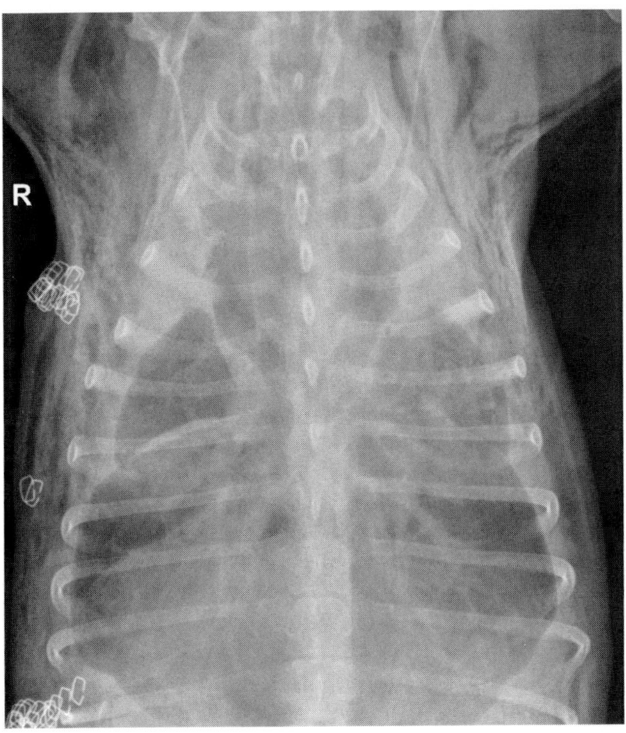

Fig. 29-14 DV thoracic radiographs of a dog with severe subcutaneous emphysema and pneumomediastinum that developed postoperatively. Tracheal trauma/perforation caused by an overinflated endotracheal tube cuff was the suspected cause.

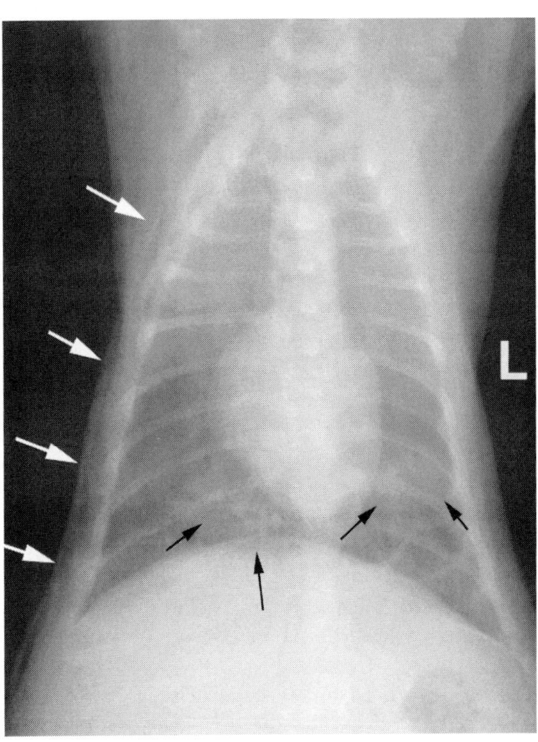

Fig. 29-15 DV thoracic radiograph of a kitten with subcutaneous emphysema along the right thoracic body wall caused by bite wound trauma *(white arrows)*. Ill-defined opacities in the caudal lung lobes represent pulmonary contusions *(black arrows)*.

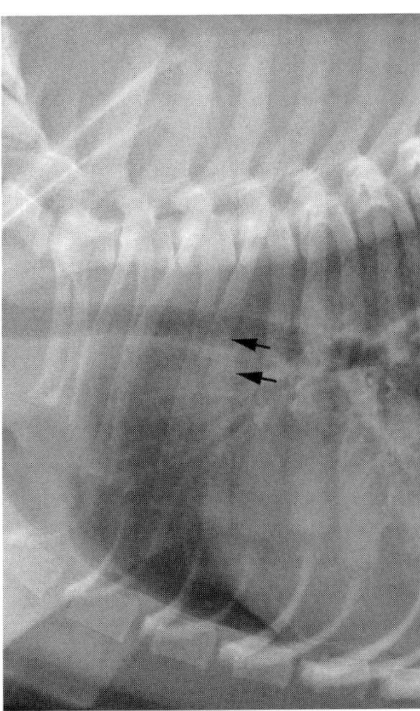

Fig. 29-16 Right lateral cranial thoracic radiograph of a dog. A mid-body, caudally displaced fracture of the right fourth rib is present *(arrows)*. Fracture margins are sharp, and no evidence of bony callus consistent with acute trauma exists.

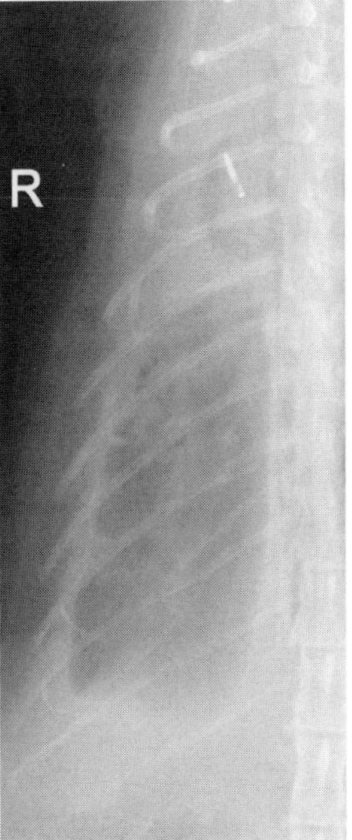

Fig. 29-17 DV radiograph of the right hemithorax of a cat. Right ribs 6 through 10 are fractured at their distolateral extents, the result of being hit by a car. Also present are retraction of the lung lobes from the pleural surface and increased soft tissue opacity within the pleural space caused by traumatic hemothorax.

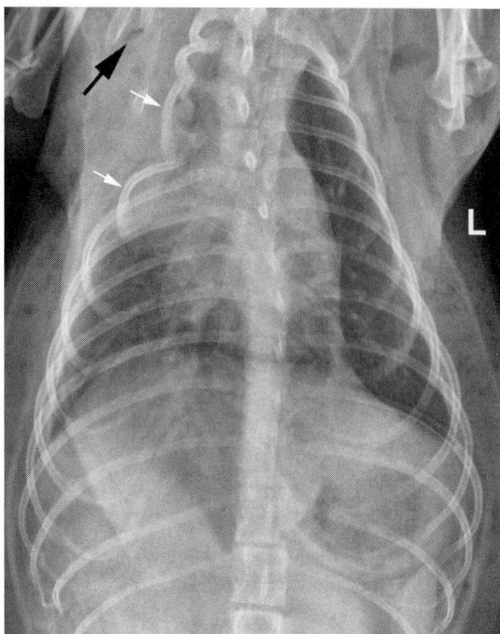

Fig. 29-18 DV thoracic radiograph of a dog with flail chest. Segmental fractures of the right third and fourth ribs *(white arrows)* with resultant collapse of the cranial thoracic wall on this inspiratory radiograph are noted. Partial collapse of the right cranial lung lobe and probable pulmonary contusions at the level of the flail component are present. A comminuted fracture of the distal right scapula *(black arrow)* and subcutaneous emphysema are both present as a result of known trauma (hit by car).

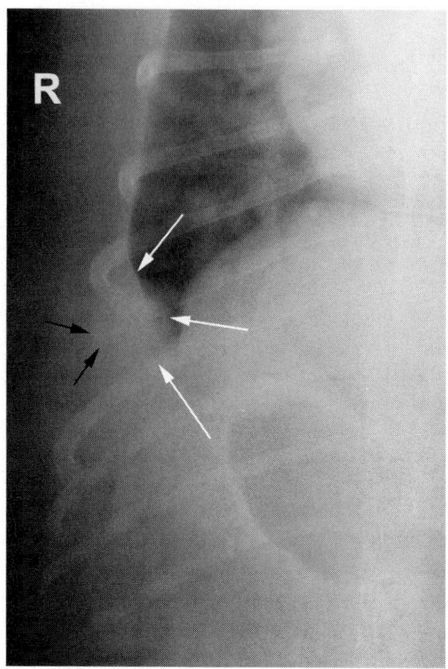

Fig. 29-20 DV caudal thoracic radiograph of a dog. Lysis of the distal aspect of the ninth right rib *(black arrows)* is present, as is an adjacent soft tissue mass. The soft tissue mass is broad based along the intrathoracic wall surface and has a convex margin, displacing the adjacent lung lobe medially *(white arrows)*. These radiographic findings are characteristic of an extrapleural sign. Multiple soft tissue nodules are identified in the caudal right lung lobe consistent with metastatic neoplasia. Histopathologic examination confirmed osteosarcoma of the right ninth rib with pulmonary metastasis.

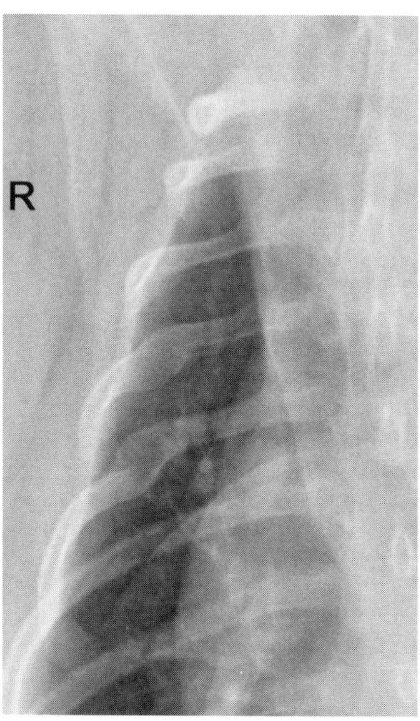

Fig. 29-19 DV cranial thoracic radiograph of a dog with healed right fourth and fifth rib fractures. Note the smooth bony margins and expansile appearance to these malunion fractures.

Rib neoplasia is more common than infection. Primary rib tumors are typically of mesenchymal origin (e.g., chondrosarcoma, osteosarcoma).[10,11] As a result of intrathoracic extension occurring to a greater extent than peripheral extension, most rib tumors are diagnosed late in the course of disease. Pleural effusion is a common result of advanced rib neoplasia. Excessive pleural effusion may summate with the rib lesion, compromising its detection. Positional radiography may be helpful in removing effusion from portions of the thoracic wall where a primary rib lesion is suspected. Carcinomas of urogenital or mammary origin commonly metastasize to ribs. These lesions are often lytic, with varying degrees of periosteal/cortical response (Fig. 29-22). Rib metastases are often overlooked on survey radiographs, where an emphasis is often placed on the detection of pulmonary metastases. Most rib metastases are the result of hematogenous spread and usually are seen in the later stages of disease.

STERNEBRAL TUMORS AND INFECTION

Primary and metastatic sternebral tumors are uncommon. As with ribs, primary sternebral tumors are typically of mesenchymal origin. Most neoplasms causing alteration of sternebral architecture are the result of local invasion by adjacent soft tissue tumors of the thoracic wall.

Sternal infections may result from external trauma, such as bite wounds. Migrating grass awns may lodge against a sternebral segment and result in local osteomyelitis with or without a draining tract. Hematogenous infection may lodge in an

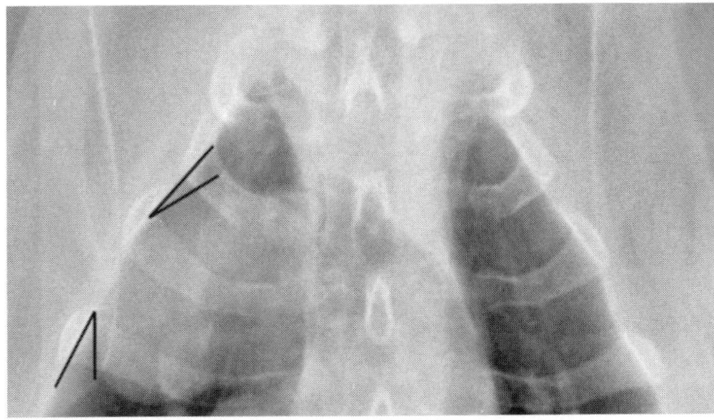
A

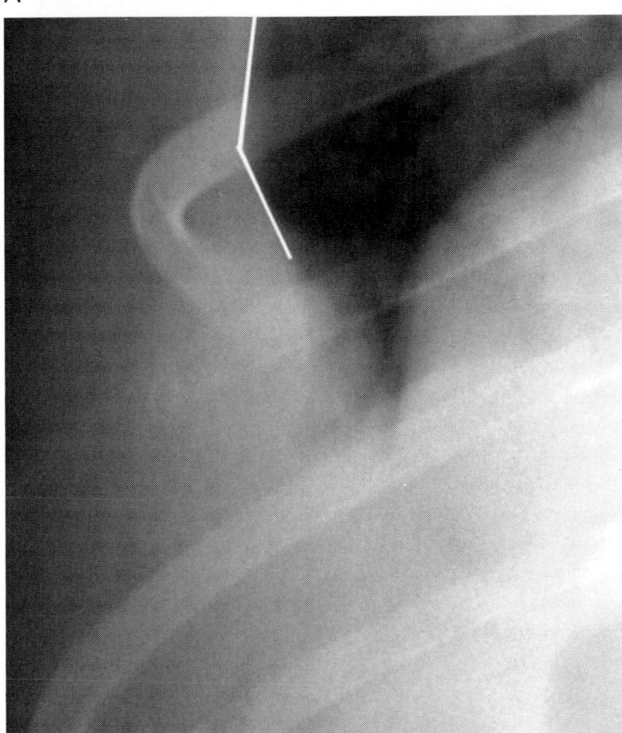
B

Fig. 29-21 DV cranial thoracic radiograph of a dog with a right cranial pulmonary mass **(A)**. The junction of the mass and the thoracic wall forms an angle less than 90 degrees. DV caudal thoracic radiograph of a dog with an intrathoracic wall mass **(B)**. The junction of the mass and the wall forms an angle greater than 90 degrees.

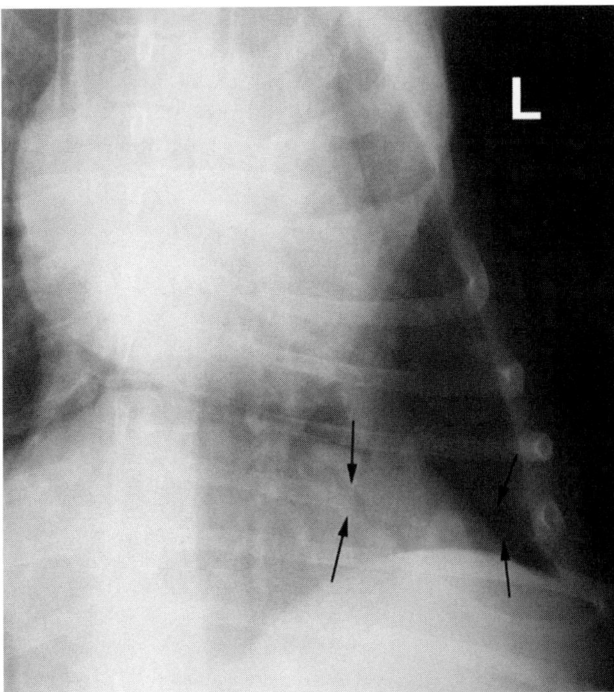

Fig. 29-22 DV thoracic radiograph of a dog with lysis of the distal aspect of the left ninth rib *(arrows)*. Multiple soft tissue nodules are identified in the caudal left lung lobe consistent with metastatic neoplasia. Metastatic carcinoma of left ninth rib and several other bones, as well as the lungs, was confirmed histopathologically. The primary tumor was prostatic carcinoma.

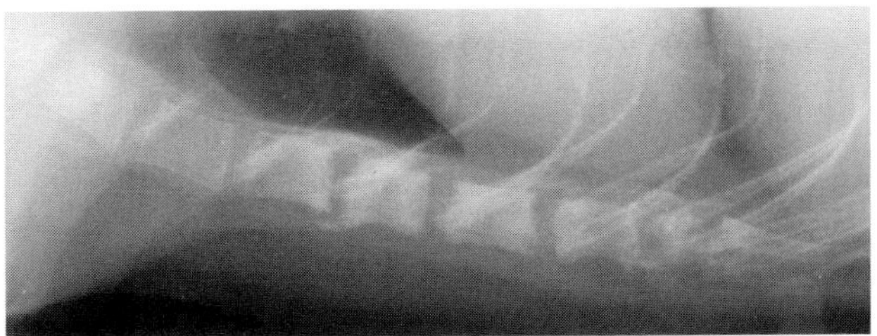

Fig. 29-23 Right lateral radiograph of the ventral aspect of the thorax of a dog. Sternebral endplate lysis and subchondral sclerosis are identified from the caudal endplate of segment 4 through the cranial aspect of segment 8. The intersternebral spaces are subjectively widened, and mild soft tissue swelling is identified ventral to the sternum. A radiographic diagnosis of sternal osteomyelitis was made, supported by clinical signs of swelling, heat, and redness of the sternum and pain on palpation. The dog's urine cultured positive for *Staphylococcus aureus,* and hematogenous spread to the sternum was suspected.

intersternal space, resulting in a endplate lysis and subchondral, reactive osseous proliferation similar in appearance to that seen with discospondylitis (Fig. 29-23).[12]

SOFT TISSUE TUMORS AND INFECTION

Soft tissue tumors of the thoracic wall are fairly common. Benign lipomas are among the most recognized (Fig. 29-24). Most are subcutaneous, though some may infiltrate muscle and fibrous tissues.[13] Interscapular fibrosarcomas at sites of known vaccination may be identified radiographically as a convexly margined soft tissue swelling dorsal to the cranial thoracic spinous processes. Other sarcomas (e.g., hemangiosarcoma, lymphosarcoma) or carcinomas (e.g., mammary adenocarcinoma, squamous cell carcinoma) of soft tissue origin may arise anywhere on the thoracic wall.

Trauma and migrating grass awns are the most common causes of cellulitis and infection of thoracic wall soft tissues. Calcinosis circumscripta of the thoracic wall has been reported in a German Shepherd dog after surgical repair of a patent ductus arteriosus.[14] The exact cause of calcinosis circumscripta is unknown but may be seen after soft tissue injury attributable to inflammatory or neoplastic causes.[14]

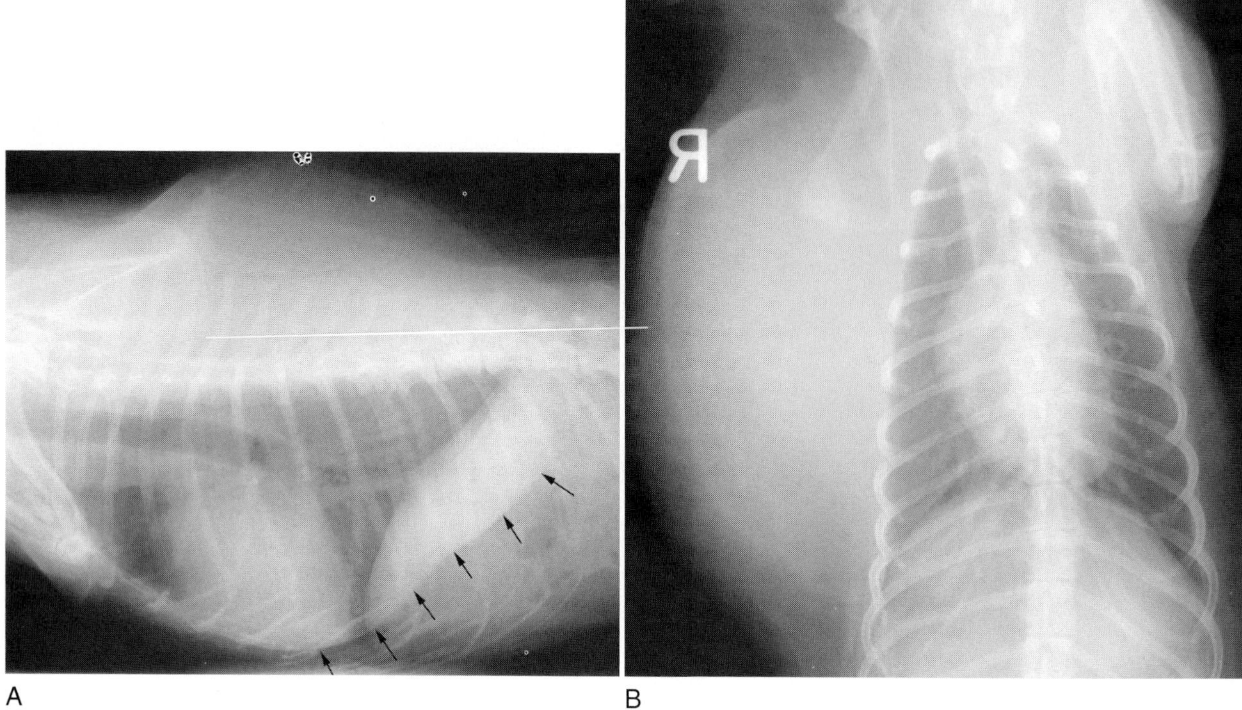

Fig. 29-24 Right lateral (A) and DV (B) thoracic radiographs of a dog. A large, fat opacity mass (lipoma) is identified along the right lateral and dorsal thoracic wall. An overall increase in opacity to the caudal thorax is present on A and right hemithorax compared with left on the DV view (B) because of the summation effect of this mass with the intrathoracic structures. Recognition that this increased opacity is not caused by a pulmonary interstitial pattern is important. The caudoventral aspect of the mass has a distinct border because it is surrounded by room air as the mass is compressed laterally against the radiographic table *(arrows)*.

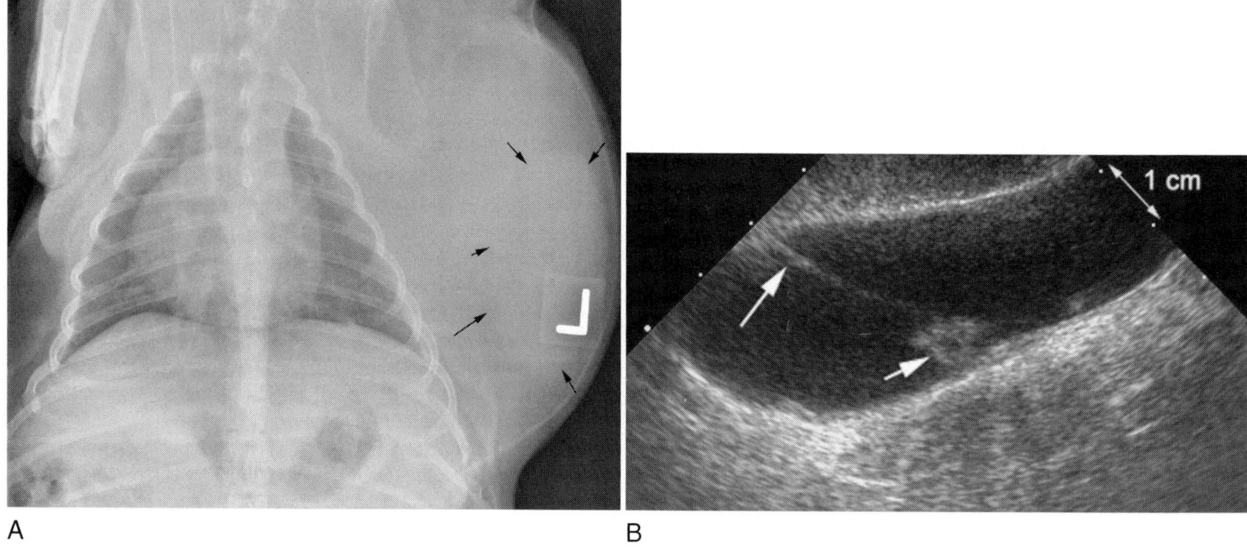

Fig. 29-25 DV thoracic radiograph (A) and left lateral thoracic wall ultrasound image (B) of a dog. In A a large fat opacity mass (lipoma) is identified along the left lateral thoracic wall. An oval, soft tissue mass *(black arrows)* is identified within the larger fat mass. An ultrasound examination (B) was performed to determine the tissue characteristics of the soft tissue region. The soft tissue opacity seen radiographically corresponded to a well-margined, anechoic (black) cystlike structure within a mass of fat on ultrasound. Echogenic strands or septa with frondlike areas of attachment to the cyst wall were identified *(white arrows)*. Ultrasound-guided needle aspirates of the fat mass and cystic structure were performed, and a brown watery fluid was obtained. Cytology was consistent with mature adipocytes (lipoma) and cyst formation lined by hemosiderophages with foci of hematoidin (blood breakdown product) and granulation tissue.

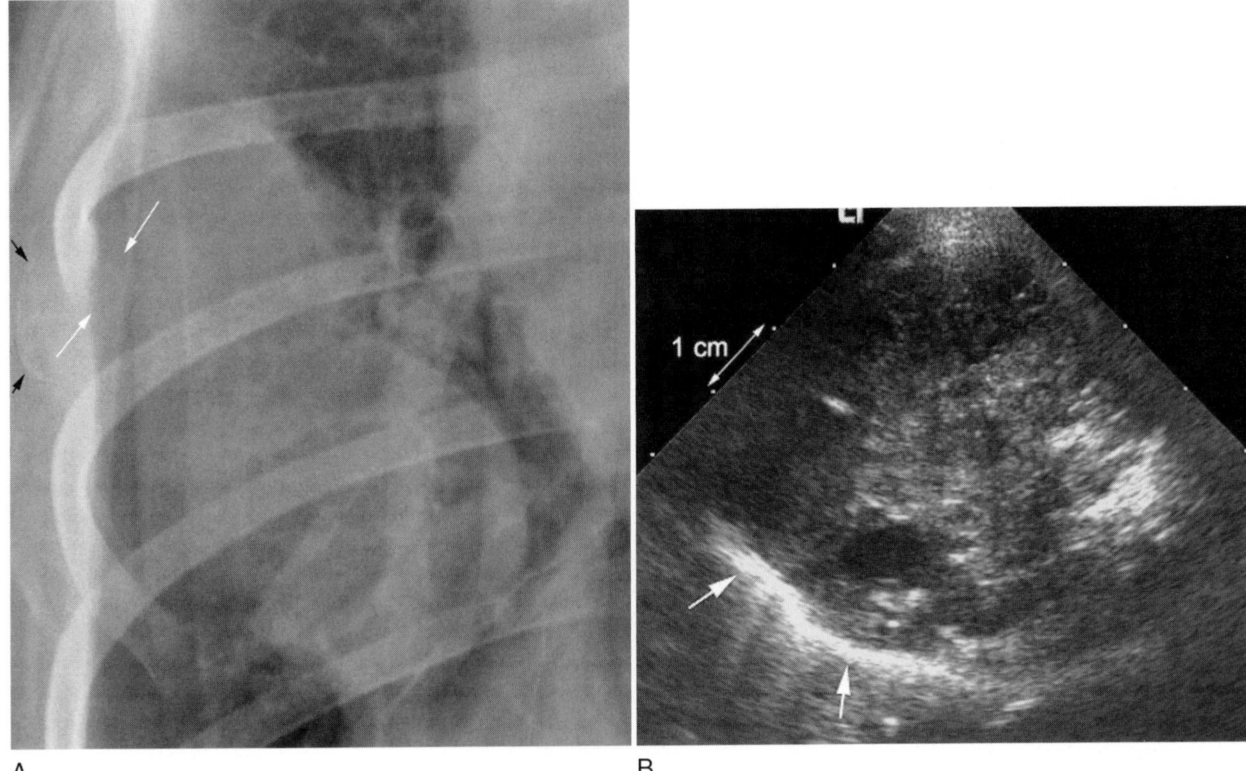

Fig. 29-26 DV caudal thoracic radiograph (A) and right lateral thoracic wall ultrasound image (B) of a dog. In A there is osteolysis of the distal aspect of the right eighth rib *(white arrows)*. A thin rim of mineral with an outer convex margin is identified in the extrathoracic soft tissues lateral to the osteolytic rib *(black arrows)*. This likely represents displaced bone from an expansile rib tumor. No evidence of a productive osseous response is present. A large, lobular soft tissue mass is identified in the caudal right thorax. This mass originates from the eighth right rib. An ultrasound examination was performed to determine the tissue characteristics of the soft tissue mass (B). A heterechoic mass interspersed with hyperechoic, shadowing foci (mineral debris) was identified within the right lateral thoracic cavity at the level of the eighth rib. The distal extent of the remaining rib was irregular and lacked a smooth cortical surface. Anechoic cavitations of varying size were also identified within the mass. These areas lacked evidence of vascularity on Doppler interrogation and likely represented areas of tissue necrosis. The lung surface is identified deep to the mass as a curvilinear hyperechoic interface impeding sound transmission deep to its surface *(white arrows)*. In real time imaging, the lung slid cranially and caudally over the thoracic wall mass during expiration and inspiration, respectively. The histopathologic diagnosis of the rib lesion was chondrosarcoma.

ALTERNATE IMAGING OF THE THORACIC WALL

Ultrasound

Sonography can be used to characterize thoracic wall lesion texture and vascularity further (Fig. 29-25).[15] When distinguishing between a thoracic wall and pulmonary mass is compromised by the presence of pleural effusion, ultrasound may be of help in classifying lesion origin. Sound readily propagates through fluid. Pleural fluid acts as an excellent window for visualization of pleural surfaces. If the mass in question is of pulmonary origin, it will move in conjunction with inspiration and expiration of the lung. If the mass is of thoracic wall origin, the mass will stay fixed to the thoracic wall. Cortical bone discontinuity caused by lysis and remodeling of rib or sternal lesions may also be identified sonographically (Fig. 29-26). Ultrasound-guided needle aspirate or biopsy may be performed for cytologic or histopathologic diagnosis, respectively.

Computed Tomography

Computed tomography (CT) is helpful for evaluating and defining lesion margination, particularly in large lesions that extend well beyond an ultrasound beam's field of view. Vascularity and further depiction of lesion margination can be assessed after intravenous iodinated contrast medium administration (Fig. 29-27). CT has proven to be helpful in surgical planning of vaccine-associated fibrosarcomas in cats (Fig. 29-28).[16] Postcontrast images often depict tendrils of inflammatory or neoplastic tissue dissecting through otherwise normal-appearing soft tissues. CT is also able to differentiate simple lipomas from infiltrative lipomas.[13]

As helical multislice technology becomes more available for use in veterinary patients, CT is likely to be more widely used in practice settings. This newer technology enables scanning of the entire thorax to be accomplished in awake, sedated animals in less than 30 seconds.

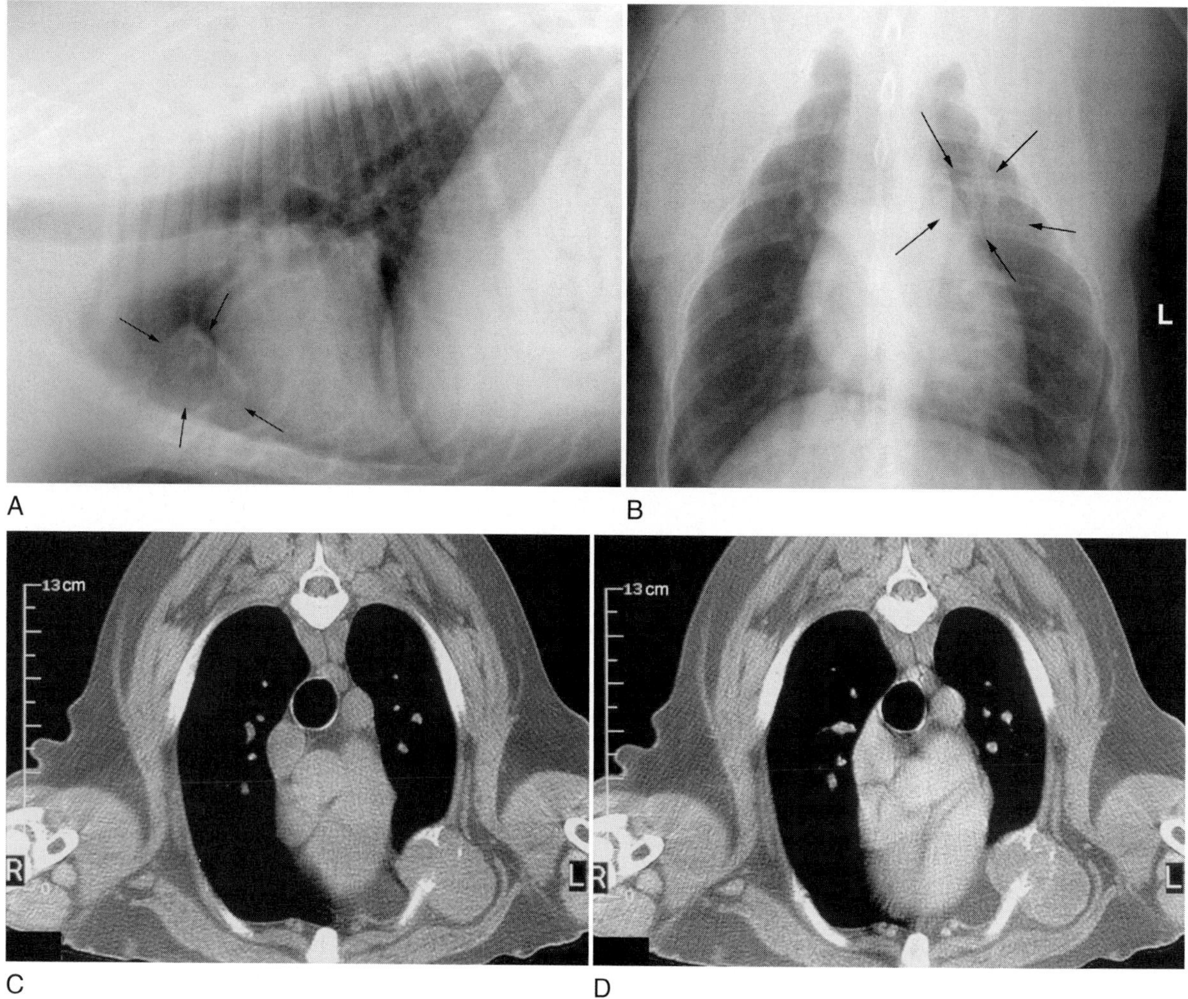

Fig. 29-27 Right lateral **(A)** and DV **(B)** thoracic radiographs of a dog. A poorly margined, mineral opaque mass is present at the level of the left third costochondral junction *(arrows)*. On the DV radiograph, the mass could be mistaken for a pulmonary lesion. Oblique radiographs of the area would be indicated to evaluate for an extrapleural sign. The extrapleural sign is best seen when the x-ray beam strikes the lesion tangentially. Transverse CT images at the level of the third ribs before **(C)** and after **(D)** administration of iodinated intravenous contrast confirm the lesion to be of rib origin. A soft tissue mass is identified associated with the rib lysis in the ventral left thorax creating an extrapleural sign. After contrast medium administration **(D)**, slight enhancement of the soft tissue mass (as well as the cranial heat base, great vessels, and pulmonary vessels) is seen. The histopathologic diagnosis of the rib lesion was osteosarcoma.

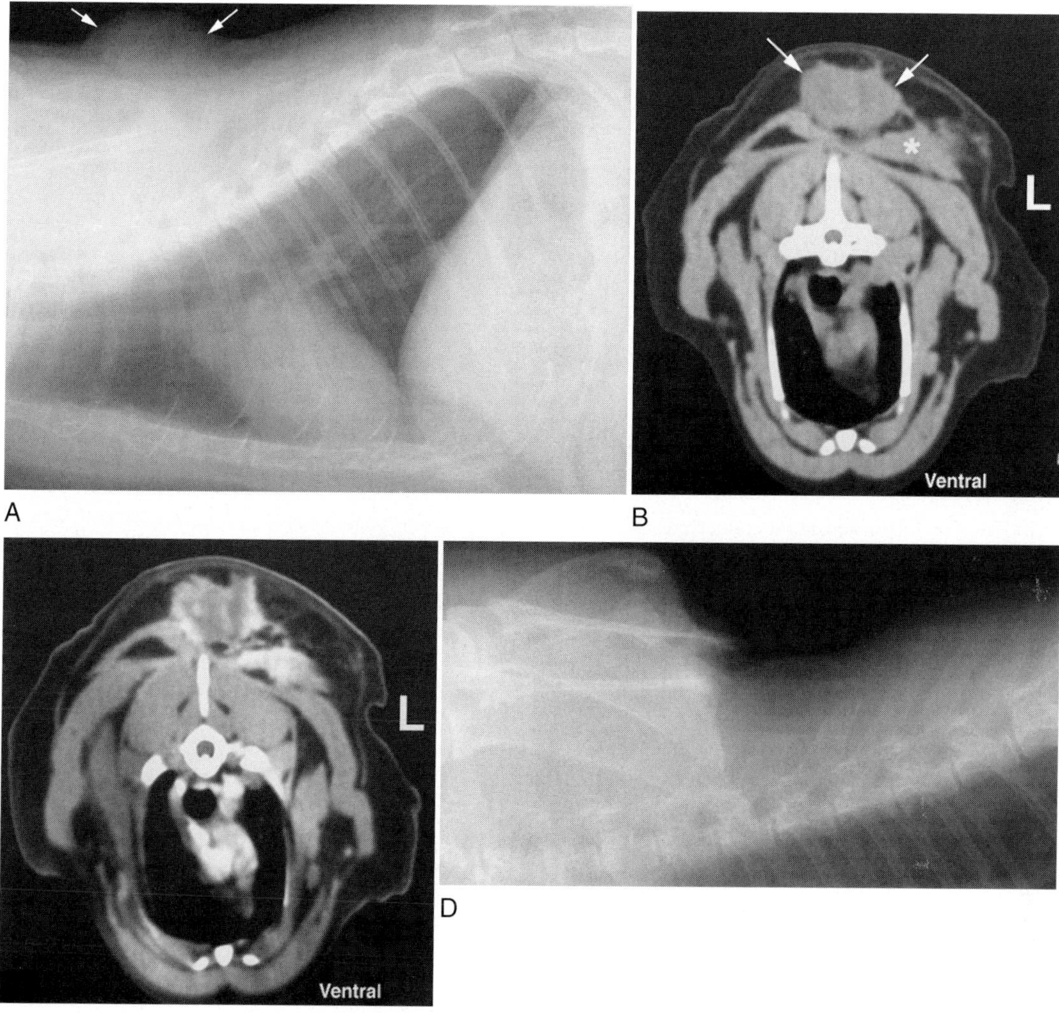

Fig. 29-28 Right lateral thoracic radiograph (A) and precontrast (B) and postcontrast (C) CT images of a cat with a vaccine-associated interscapular fibrosarcoma. A soft tissue mass with a dorsal convex margin is identified in the subcutaneous tissues dorsal to the proximal margin of the scapulae *(white arrows)* on the thoracic radiograph (A). On the precontrast CT image (B) made just caudal to the scapulae, the irregularly margined mass is clearly seen in the fat just dorsal to a thoracic spinous process *(white arrow)*. In addition, soft tissue opaque stranding is identified in the fat surrounding the mass and just lateral to the left trapezius muscle *(asterisk)* that is also thickened and irregular in contour. After intravenous administration of iodinated contrast medium, heterogeneous enhancement of the dorsal subcutaneous mass, left trapezius muscle, and soft tissue stranding within the regional fat are present, consistent with neoplastic infiltration and associated inflammation. Contrast medium opacification of the great vessels cranial to the heart is also seen. Although lysis and remodeling of osseous structures was not identified, soft tissue contrast opacification was observed along the peripheral surfaces of the caudal scapulae and multiple spinous processes. In the interest of obtaining a complete surgical excision, large portions of the scapulae and thoracic spinous processes 2 through 6 were removed (D).

REFERENCES

1. Evans SK, Biery DN: Congenital peritoneopericardial diaphragmatic hernia in the dog and cat: a literature review and 17 additional case histories, *Vet Radiol* 21:108, 1980.
2. Berry CR, Koblik PD, Ticer JW: Dorsal peritoneopericardial mesothelial remnant as an aid to the diagnosis of feline congenital peritoneopericardial diaphragmatic hernia, *Vet Radiol* 31:239, 1990.
3. Fossum TW, Boudrieau RJ, Hobson HP: Pectus excavatum in 8 dogs and 6 cats, *J Am Anim Hosp Assoc* 25:595, 1989.
4. Ellison G, Halling KB: Atypical pectus excavatum in two Welsh terrier littermates, *J Small Anim Pract* 45:311, 2004.
5. Suter PF: Injuries to thoracic wall and sternum. In Suter PF, editor: *Thoracic radiography,* Wettswil, Switzerland, 1984, Peter F. Suter, Zurich, Switzerland.
6. Olsen D, Renberg W, Perrett J et al: Clinical management of flail chest in dogs and cats: a retrospective study of 24 cases (1989-1999), *J Am Anim Hosp Assoc* 38:315, 2002.
7. Myer W: Radiography review: the extrapleural space, *J Am Vet Radiol Soc* 19:157, 1978.
8. Suter PF: The extrapleural sign. In Suter PF, editor: *Thoracic radiography,* Wettswil, Switzerland, 1984, Peter F. Suter, Zurich, Switzerland.
9. Fisher E, Godwin JD: Extrapleural fat collections: pseudotumors and other confusing manifestations, *Am J Roentgenol* 161:47, 1993.
10. Feeney DA, Johnston GR, Grindem CB et al: Malignant neoplasia of the canine ribs: clinical, radiographic, and pathologic findings, *J Am Vet Med Assoc* 180:928, 1982.
11. Baines SJ, Lewis S, White RA: Primary thoracic wall tumours of mesenchymal origin in dogs: a retrospective study of 46 cases, *Vet Rec* 150:335, 2002.
12. Gilding T, Guilliard MJ: What was your diagnosis? Osteomyelitis of the fourth sternebra, *J Small Anim Pract* 44:335, 2003.
13. McEntee MC, Thrall DE: Computed tomographic imaging of infiltrative lipoma in 22 dogs, *Vet Radiol Ultrasound* 42:221, 2001.
14. Davidson EB, Schulz KS, Wisner ER et al: Calcinosis circumscripta of the thoracic wall in a German shepherd dog, *J Am Anim Hosp Assoc* 34:153, 1998.
15. Stowater JL, Lamb CR: Ultrasonography of noncardiac thoracic diseases in small animals, *J Am Vet Med Assoc* 195:514, 1989.
16. Samii VF, McEntee MC: Utility of contrast enhanced computed tomographic imaging of soft tissue sarcomas: overview and case presentations, *Veterinary Cancer Society Newsletter* 22:1, 1998.

ELECTRONIC RESOURCES evolve

Additional information related to the content in Chapter 29 can be found on the companion Web site at evolve http://evolve.elsevier.com/Thrall/vetrad/.

- Key Points
- Chapter Quiz
- Case Study 29-1, includes Video 29-1

CHAPTER • 30
The Diaphragm

Richard D. Park

The diaphragm is the musculocutaneous partition between the thoracic and abdominal cavities. Embryologically, the diaphragm is formed by the septum transversum ventrally and by the mesentery of the foregut and two pleuroperitoneal folds dorsally.

The diaphragm provides approximately 50% of the mechanical respiratory force required for inspiration.[1] The diaphragm also acts as a mechanical partition between the thorax and the abdomen. Lymph vessels from the abdomen penetrate the diaphragm and drain into the thoracic lymph nodes and vessels. Thus inflammatory or neoplastic abdominal disease may spread to the mediastinum and pleural space. Lymph flow from the thorax to the abdomen does not occur.[2]

The diaphragm consists of a tendinous center and three thin peripheral muscles: the pars lumbalis, the pars costalis, and the pars sternalis. The pars lumbalis consists of the right and left crura, which attach to the cranial ventral border of L4 and the body of L3. The attachment area on these vertebrae occasionally has a concave indistinct ventral margin that may be mistaken for bone lysis (Fig. 30-1). The pars costalis attaches in an oblique direction to the thirteenth through eighth ribs, and the pars sternalis attaches to the xiphoid cartilage.[3] The diaphragm is convex and extends into the thorax from its attachments, creating the phrenicocostalis and phrenicolumbalis recesses.

There are three openings through the diaphragm: (1) the dorsally located aortic hiatus encloses the aorta, azygos and hemiazygos veins, and the lumbar cistern of the thoracic duct; (2) the centrally located esophageal hiatus encloses the esophagus and vagus nerve trunks; and (3) the caudal vena cava foramen is located at the junction of the muscular and tendinous portions of the diaphragm.

NORMAL RADIOGRAPHIC ANATOMY

Radiographically, only a small portion of the diaphragm can be seen on any one view. It appears as a thin, convex structure of soft tissue opacity extending in a cranial and ventral direction. Radiographic visualization of the diaphragm depends on adjacent structures being of different opacity. Most of the thoracic surface is visible because of the adjacent gas-filled lungs. Parts of the thoracic surface are not visualized where the lungs are not in contact with the diaphragm—the phrenicocostalis and phrenicolumbalis recesses. A large portion of the abdominal diaphragmatic surface is not seen because it silhouettes the adjacent liver. The ventral abdominal diaphragmatic surface is visible on the lateral view when fat is present within the falciform ligament. The dorsal aspect of the left diaphragmatic crus and the gastric wall appear as one linear structure when gas is present in the gastric cardia.

Diaphragmatic structures that may be distinctly visualized radiographically are the right and left crura, the intercrural cleft, and the cupula (body) (Figs. 30-2 to 30-5). Associated structures that may also be seen are the caudal vena cava and the caudal ventral mediastinum. On the lateral view, the right crus of the diaphragm blends with the caudal vena caval border, and the gastric fundus may be seen adjacent to the abdominal surface of the left crus. The intercrural cleft is a shorter, convex, opaque line caudal and ventral to the crura (see Figs. 30-2 and 30-3). The cupula is the most cranial convex portion of the diaphragm on both the lateral and the dorsoventral or ventrodorsal views. Also on these views, the thoracic surface of the diaphragm may be visualized as one, two, or three convex projections into the thoracic cavity (see Figs. 30-4 and 30-5).

Several normal variations of diaphragmatic position and shape may be seen radiographically. Factors that cause this variable appearance are real and apparent. Real factors consist of breed, age, obesity, respiration, and gravity. Apparent factors are x-ray beam centering and animal positioning during radiographic examination. When all permutations of these variables are considered, more than 51,000 combinations are possible.[4] Most of these variables are not radiographically significant; however, some must be recognized and understood. Changes most apparent radiographically are the position, shape, and visualization of the cupula and crura. The relative position of the crura depends mostly on position and size of the animal and primary x-ray beam centering.

The most dependent crus is usually displaced cranially when an animal is in lateral recumbency. In right lateral recumbency, the crura appear to be parallel (see Fig. 30-3); in left lateral recumbency, they sometimes appear to cross. The crura also appear to be more extensively separated—by up to 2.5 vertebral lengths—if the animal is slightly rotated or if the x-ray beam is centered over the mid- or cranial thorax.[4]

The radiographic appearance of the diaphragm in ventrodorsal or dorsoventral projections varies with x-ray beam centering. The diaphragm may appear as two or three separate domed-shaped structures (see Fig. 30-4) or as a single dome-shaped structure (see Fig. 30-5). The three structures represent the cupula and two crura. A single domed diaphragm may be seen on a ventrodorsal view when the x-ray beam is centered on the mid-abdomen or on a dorsoventral view when the x-ray beam is centered mid-thorax. Two or three separate domed structures are seen when the animal is in the ventrodorsal position and the x-ray beam is centered mid-thorax or on a dorsoventral view with the x-ray beam is centered mid-abdomen.[4]

The diaphragmatic position and shape vary with inspiration, expiration, and intraabdominal pressure. The normal intersection point of the diaphragm and spine is between T11

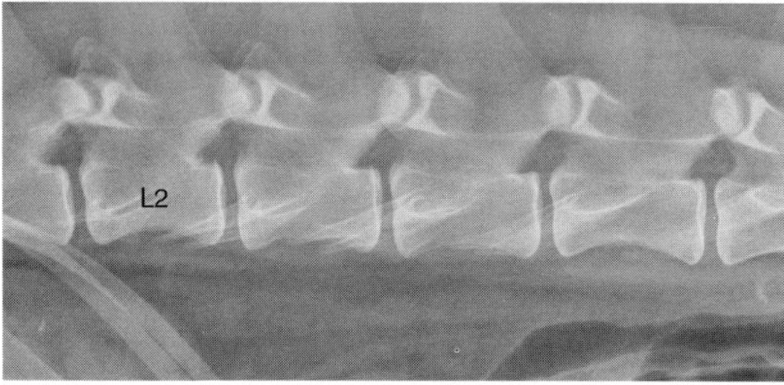

Fig. 30-1 Lateral view of the lumbar spine of a normal dog. Compared with L2 and L5, note the indistinct ventral cortex of L3 and L4 caused by the diaphragm attachment site. This can be misinterpreted as lysis if this normal appearance is not understood.

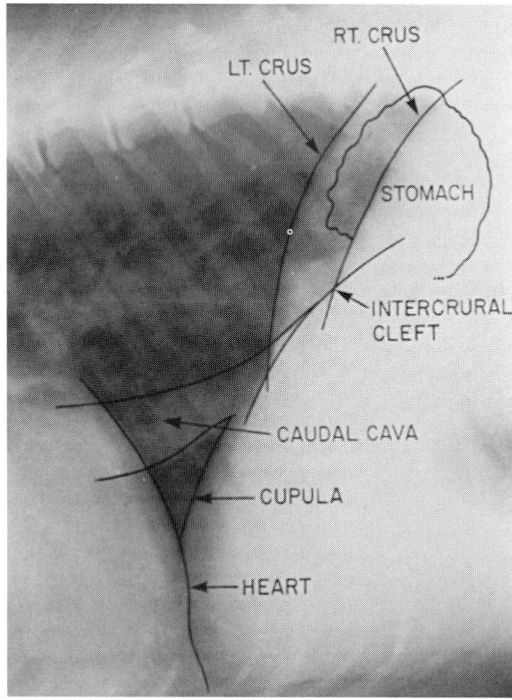

Fig. 30-2 Left lateral recumbent radiograph of the diaphragmatic region of a normal dog. *LT,* Left; *RT,* right.

and T13 but may vary between T9 and L1. The diaphragm changes position with normal respiration from one-half to two vertebral lengths. On extreme inspiration, the diaphragm changes position and shape. On a lateral thoracic view made in extreme inspiration, the diaphragm is oriented more vertically; the shape changes from convex to straight. The diaphragm is displaced cranially by increased intraabdominal pressure, which may be caused by obesity, ascites, gastric or intestinal distention, abdominal pain, or abdominal masses.

Separate diaphragmatic structures are not seen as distinctly in the cat, probably because of the relatively small thoracic size (Fig. 30-6). On extreme inspiration, particularly if the animal is in respiratory distress, small symmetrical muscle projections are noted from the thoracic diaphragmatic surface in the ventrodorsal or dorsoventral view (Fig. 30-7).

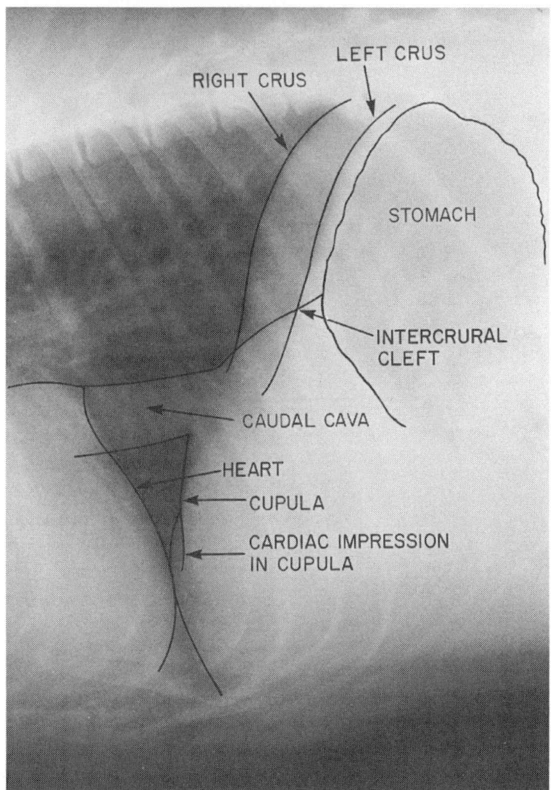

Fig. 30-3 Right lateral recumbent view of the diaphragmatic region of a normal dog.

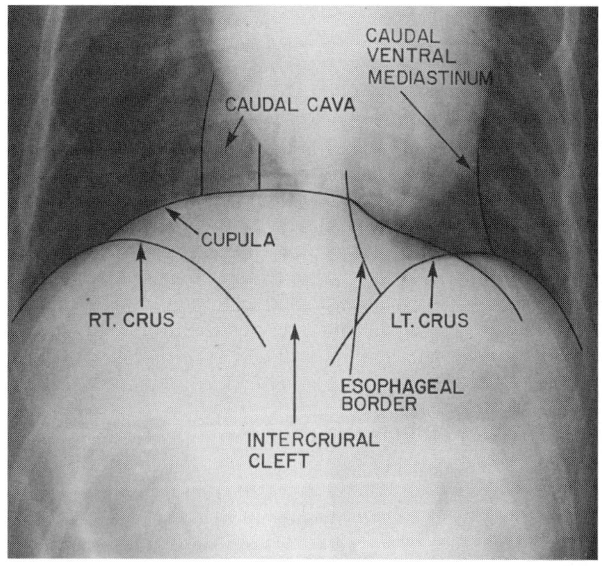

Fig. 30-4 Ventrodorsal view of the diaphragmatic region of a normal dog with the cupula and both crura projecting into the thorax. *LT,* Left; *RT,* right.

RADIOGRAPHIC SIGNS OF DIAPHRAGMATIC DISEASE

The signs directly associated with the diaphragm are not as numerous and specific as those found in many other organs. Radiographic changes observed most frequently with

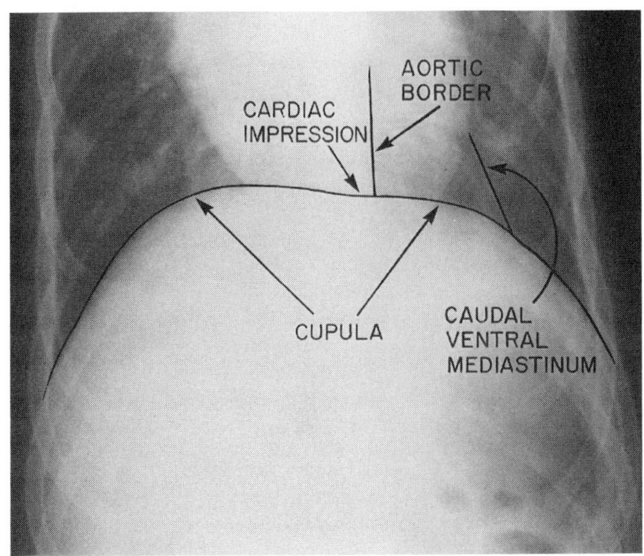

Fig. 30-5 Dorsoventral view of the diaphragmatic region of a normal dog with only one convex shape projecting into the thorax.

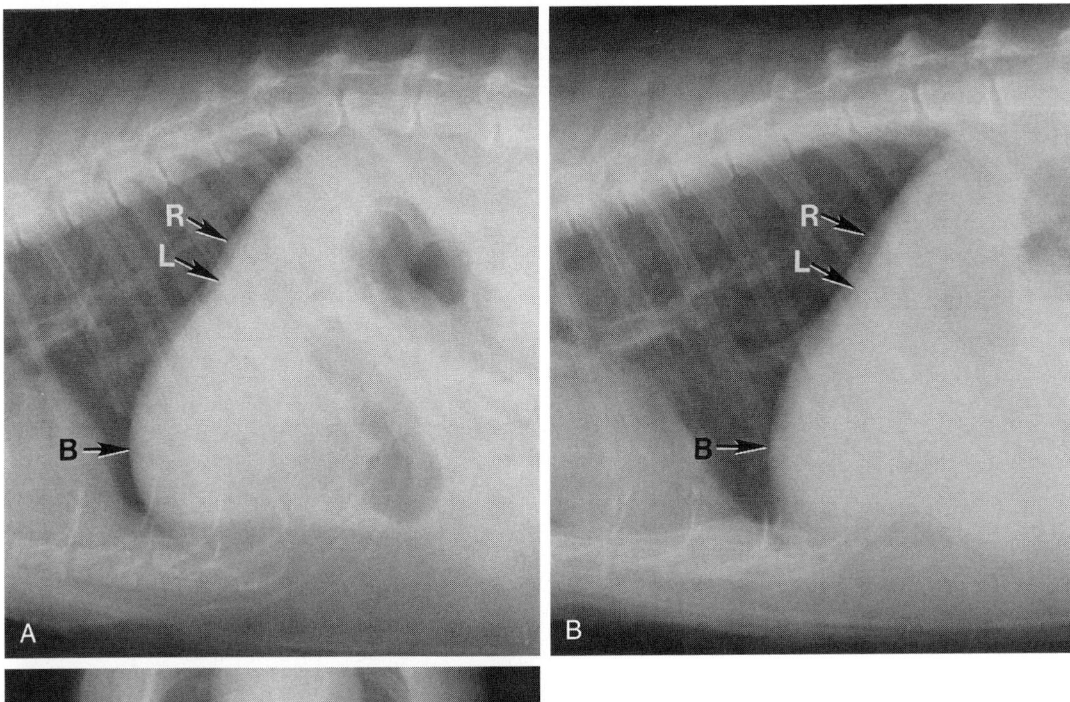

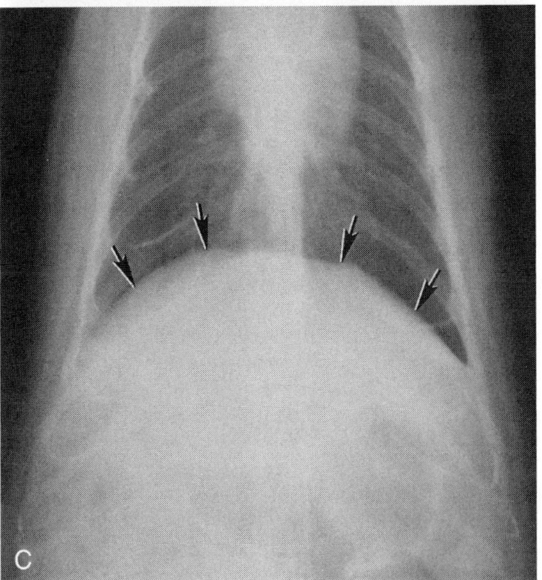

Fig. 30-6 Radiographs of the diaphragmatic region of a normal cat. **A**, Left lateral recumbent view. **B**, Right lateral recumbent view. **C**, Ventrodorsal view. The right *(R)* and left *(L)* diaphragmatic crura are almost superimposed on both recumbent views with little change in position. The body **(B)** has a convex shape projecting into the thorax. In **C**, the diaphragm projects as a single convex opacity into the caudal thorax *(arrows)*.

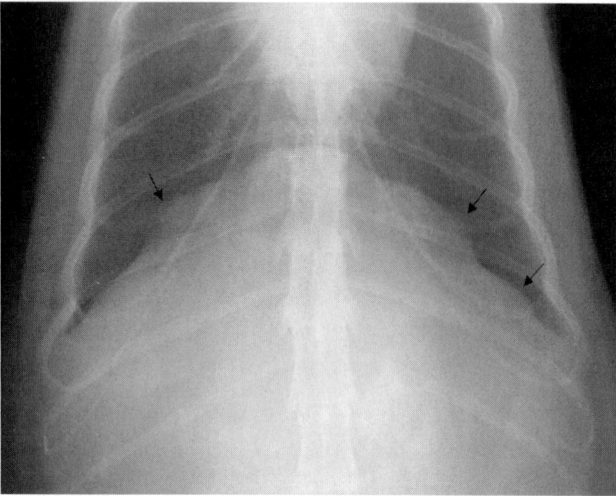

Fig. 30-7 Ventrodorsal view of the diaphragmatic region of a normal cat on deep inspiration. Small, regularly spaced projections *(arrows)* are evident along the thoracic diaphragmatic surface. This so-called "tenting" reflects the pulling of the diaphragm against its costal attachments.

Table • 30-1

Radiographic Signs of Diaphragmatic Disease

RADIOGRAPHIC SIGNS	CAUSES
General loss of diaphragmatic thoracic surface outline	Bilateral pleural fluid Generalized pulmonary disease in caudal lung lobes
Localized or partial loss of the thoracic surface outline	Thoracic masses adjacent to the diaphragm Diaphragmatic hernias Focal pulmonary disease in caudal lung lobes
Shape changes	Thoracic masses adjacent to the diaphragm Hiatal hernias Small diaphragmatic hernias Pleural reaction on the diaphragmatic surface Neoplasia arising from the diaphragm Hemiparalysis of the diaphragm Unilateral tension pneumothorax
Position Changes	
Cranial displacement	Obesity Peritoneal fluid Abdominal pain Abdominal masses or organ enlargement; liver enlargement and masses frequently cause cranial displacement Generalized diaphragmatic paralysis Cranial displacement of the cupula caused by a diaphragmatic defect with the peritoneum and pleura intact
Caudal displacement	Severe respiratory distress—ventilation or perfusion problems Tension pneumothorax Caudal displacement of the cupula caused by contact with the heart

diaphragmatic disease include general or focal loss of the thoracic diaphragmatic surface outline and changes in diaphragmatic shape and position (Table 30-1).

The thoracic diaphragmatic surface outline will not be visualized radiographically if anything of the same opacity, such as soft tissue organs or fluid, is adjacent to the surface. Changes in the diaphragm shape occur most frequently on the cupula; they are often normal and are frequently caused by contact with the heart (Fig. 30-8) or position of the animal during radiographic examination. The shape and position may also appear altered in some large-breed dogs, with the body appearing more convex and extending to a more cranial position in the thorax. This may be the result of a flaccid tendinous membrane, or it may be associated with a peritoneopleural hernia, which often produces no clinical signs.

Thoracic masses or lung disease adjacent to the diaphragm, hiatal and small traumatic diaphragmatic hernias, masses originating from the diaphragm, and chronic pleural inflammatory reactions are the most frequent pathologic causes associated with diaphragmatic shape changes. An asymmetric diaphragmatic shape may occur with unilateral tension pneumothorax or hemiparalysis. Suspected hemiparalysis should be confirmed by observing diaphragmatic movement during fluoroscopy.

Positional changes consist of cranial and caudal displacement. Because the position of the diaphragm changes during the respiratory cycle, minor changes are difficult to diagnose and in most instances are not clinically significant. Severe positional changes may be significant and indicative of thoracic or abdominal disease. Cranial diaphragmatic displacement is usually associated with abdominal disease (see Table 30-1) or generalized diaphragmatic paralysis, which should be confirmed by fluoroscopic observation. Caudal diaphragmatic displacement is usually associated with severe respiratory disease (Fig. 30-9). The caudally positioned diaphragm is an attempt by the animal to increase the level of systemic oxygenation, which may be low because of ventilation or perfusion deficiencies in the lungs. Bilateral tension pneumothorax may also cause a caudally displaced diaphragm from increased pleural pressure. In most instances of pneumothorax, however, the caudally displaced diaphragm is probably an attempt to increase respiratory ventilation.

Although many of the radiographic signs of diaphragmatic disease are not specific, their cause should be determined. In some instances, ultrasonography or additional radiographic studies, such as positional views with a horizontally directed x-ray beam and contrast medium studies, may be indicated to determine the cause of the radiographic signs.

DIAPHRAGMATIC DISEASES

The most frequently observed diaphragmatic diseases in the dog and cat are hernias, which may be traumatic and

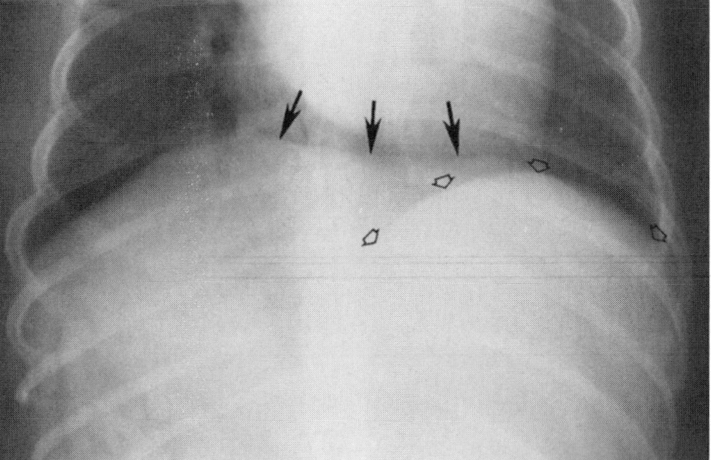

Fig. 30-8 Ventrodorsal view of the diaphragmatic region of a normal dog. A cardiac impression *(arrows)* is present on the diaphragmatic body (cupula). The left diaphragmatic crus *(open arrowheads)* is distinctly visible. The right crus cannot be visualized as a separate structure.

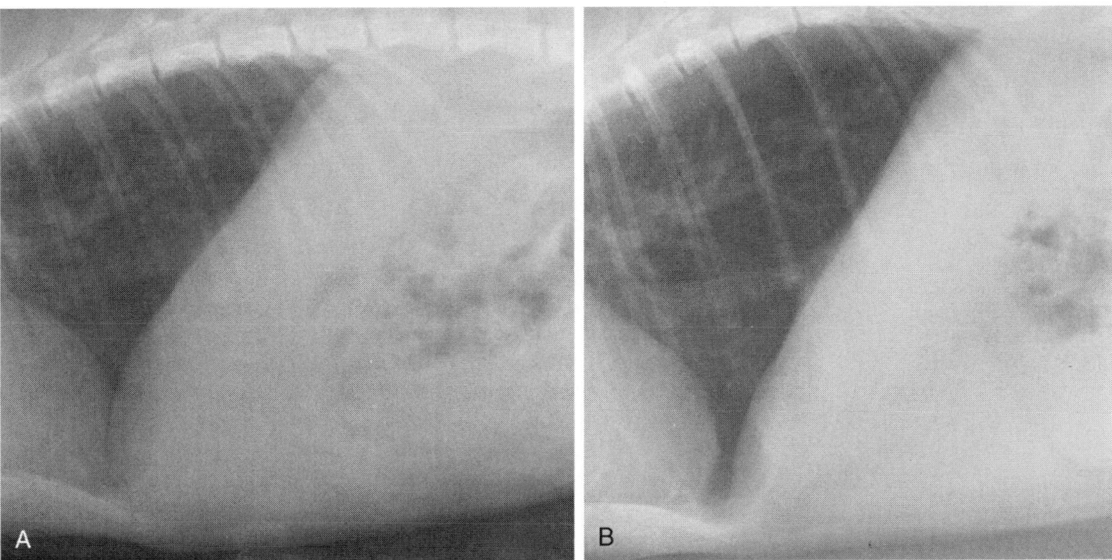

Fig. 30-9 Lateral views of the diaphragmatic region of a normal cat on expiration **(A)** and on extreme inspiration **(B)**. The entire diaphragm is displaced caudally with inspiration and has a flatter contour compared with the expiratory radiograph.

congenitally predisposed. Motor or innervation disturbances occur less frequently.

Diaphragmatic Hernias

A diaphragmatic hernia is a protrusion of abdominal viscera through the diaphragm into the thorax. Diaphragmatic hernias that may be recognized radiographically include traumatic, peritoneopericardial, hiatal, peritoneopleural, and those secondary to congenital diaphragmatic defects.

Abdominal trauma is the most common cause of diaphragmatic hernia. A high momentary increase in abdominal pressure when the glottis is open produces a high pleuroperitoneal pressure gradient that may result in a diaphragmatic hernia. The high pleuroperitoneal gradient may produce a rent in the muscular portion of the diaphragm, or it may force abdominal viscera through congenitally weak or defective areas. Clinical signs that may be observed with diaphragmatic hernias include dyspnea, pain, vomiting, regurgitation, muffled heart sounds, and a weak femoral pulse.[5,6] Some diaphragmatic hernias may not cause clinical signs and are detected incidentally.

Radiography plays an important role in confirming a diagnosis of diaphragmatic hernia and may provide information about location, extent, contents, and secondary complications associated with the hernia.[7-11] If a diagnosis cannot be confirmed from survey radiographs (Box 30-1), ultrasonography and/or other imaging procedures may be performed to provide additional diagnostic information. Other radiographic procedures consist of administration of oral barium sulfate, positional radiographic views, removal of pleural fluid and repeat radiography of the thorax, and positive contrast medium peritoneography.

To ascertain the position of the stomach and proximal small bowel, a small amount (20 to 40 mL) of barium sulfate (30% w/v) can be given orally and radiographs obtained after 15 to 20 minutes (Fig. 30-10). Radiographs made with a horizontal x-ray beam help differentiate solid abdominal organs in the thorax from pleural fluid (Fig. 30-11). Thoracocentesis

Box 30-1

Radiographic Signs Associated with Traumatic Diaphragmatic Hernia

Abdominal Viscera Within the Thorax

Gas- or ingesta-filled bowel
Gas- or ingesta-filled stomach
Identifiable parenchymal organs, such as the liver and spleen

Displacement of Abdominal Structures—Cranial

Liver
Small bowel
Stomach
Spleen

Displacement of Thoracic Structures—Generally Displaced Cranially and Laterally Away from an Abnormal Opaque Area in the Thorax

Heart
Mediastinum
Lungs

Partial or Complete Loss of the Thoracic Diaphragmatic Surface Outline

Pleural fluid or mass
Lung fluid or mass

Divergence of Diaphragmatic Crura or Cranial Angulation of Diaphragm

Pleural fluid

and pleural fluid removal followed by another radiographic examination provide better radiographic visualization of structures within the thorax.

Positive-contrast peritoneography can be performed by injecting 2 mL/kg body weight of an iodinated, preferably nonionic, contrast medium into the peritoneal cavity. The animal should then be positioned such that gravity facilitates contrast medium accumulation around the liver and the diaphragm. Contrast medium within the thorax and an interrupted outline of the abdominal diaphragmatic surface are the most consistent positive-contrast peritoneographic signs of a diaphragmatic hernia (Fig. 30-12).[12,13] Any or all of these procedures may be used, but the most simple should be used first. Peritoneography should be used after other diagnostic procedures have failed to provide the needed information.

Other procedures, including positive-contrast pleurography, portography, cholecystography, angiocardiography, angiography, and nonselective cardiography, have been reported as useful in diagnosing diaphragmatic hernias.[14] These techniques are more difficult and are rarely used.

Ultrasonographic examination of the diaphragm may add diagnostic information, particularly for patients in whom pleural fluid is present and obliterates soft tissue. The examination is best done transhepatically.[15] Ultrasonographic signs of a diaphragmatic hernia include identification of abdominal structures within the thorax, particularly the liver, and an interruption in the diaphragmatic outline.[15-17] An interruption in the diaphragmatic outline may not be consistently seen with diaphragmatic hernias.[18]

Traumatic Diaphragmatic Hernias

In one study, only half of the animals with a trauma-induced diaphragmatic hernia had a history of known trauma.[6] Traumatic diaphragmatic hernias usually involve the muscular portion of the diaphragm.[6,19] It has been suggested that right and left incidence distribution is equal,[15] but a higher inci-

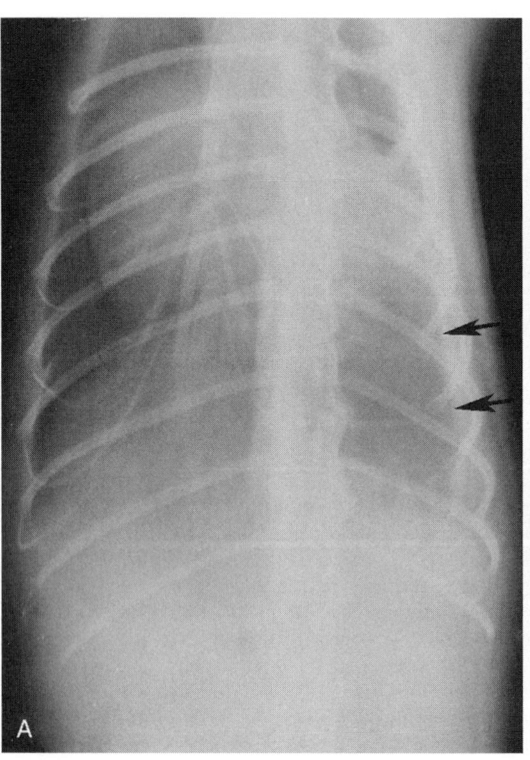

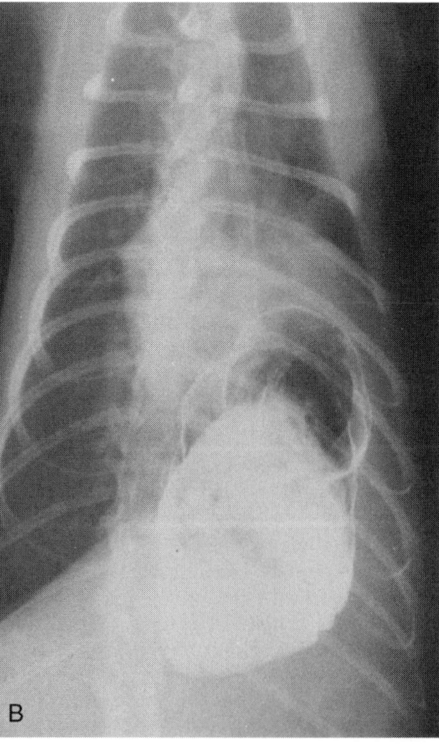

Fig. 30-10 Confirmation of a traumatic diaphragmatic hernia with a barium gastrogram. **A,** Ventrodorsal view of the thorax of a cat. An ill-defined gas opacity is present in the left caudal thorax *(arrows)*. The identity of this opacity is not certain. The heart is displaced toward the right thoracic wall, which is likely accentuated by the slightly oblique position of the animal. **B,** After administration of barium sulfate, the stomach is identified in the left caudal thorax, thus confirming a left-sided diaphragmatic hernia.

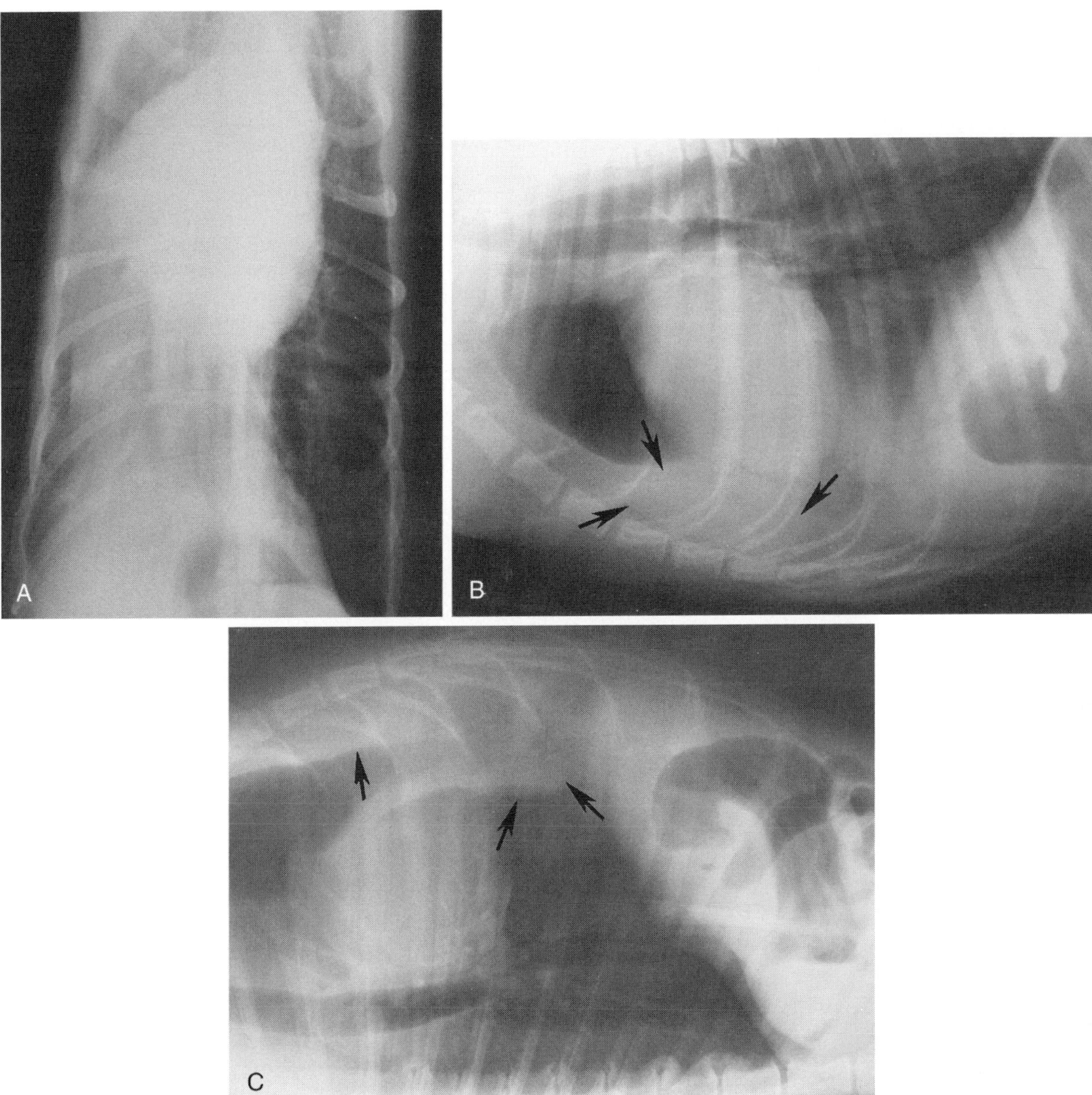

Fig. 30-11 Ventrodorsal (A), lateral (B), and dorsal recumbent, horizontal-beam lateral (C) views of a dog with a traumatic diaphragmatic hernia. **A,** An increased soft tissue opacity in the caudal right thorax with loss of the thoracic diaphragmatic surface outline over the cupula is apparent. **B,** The heart is displaced dorsally, and a soft tissue opacity can be seen between the heart and the sternum *(arrows)*. The thoracic diaphragmatic outline is indistinct over the cupula. **C,** The soft tissue opacity *(arrows)* remains in the same position, which indicates that the opacity is a solid structure and not free pleural fluid. This finding is compatible with a diaphragmatic hernia.

dence on the right side has been reported in the dog.[6] The organs that most frequently herniate are, in order of prevalence, the liver, small bowel, stomach, spleen, and omentum.[6,9,19-21]

The most consistent radiographic signs of traumatic diaphragmatic hernia are abdominal viscera within the thorax; displacement of abdominal or thoracic organs, or both; partial or complete loss of the thoracic diaphragmatic surface outline; asymmetry or altered slope to the diaphragm on the lateral projection[11]; and the presence of pleural fluid (Fig. 30-13).

Identification of abdominal structures in the thorax is a conclusive sign of diaphragmatic hernia. Small bowel is easily identified when it is gas filled; when fluid filled, it appears as a tubular structure. The stomach may be filled with gas, fluid, or ingested material. In addition, gastric rugal folds may provide a marker for identifying the stomach within the thorax. A herniated, gas-distended stomach may appear as a unilateral left pneumothorax, and the stomach should be decompressed and repositioned immediately by surgical intervention (Fig. 30-14).[6] Such instances are life threatening because of potential or actual cardiovascular tamponade.

Herniated solid abdominal parenchymal organs are difficult to distinguish from localized pleural fluid, pulmonary opacity, or both. Omentum is the most difficult to detect

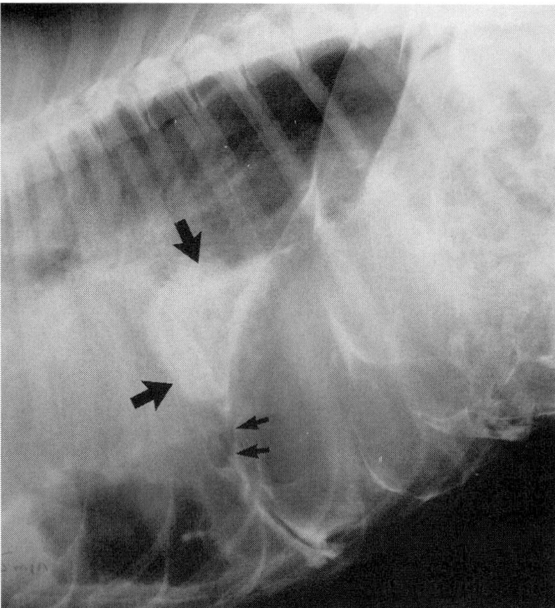

Fig. 30-12 A lateral abdominal radiograph of a positive-contrast peritoneogram. The abdominal surface of the diaphragm has an indistinct outline *(small arrows)*, with contrast medium present within the pleural cavity *(large arrows)*. These are reliable radiographic signs of a diaphragmatic defect and a diaphragmatic hernia.

unless it is herniated in association with other abdominal organs. In such instances, it provides a fat opacity and helps outline other abdominal visceral organs.

In the absence of finding abdominal organs in the thorax, cranial abdominal organ displacement or absence of abdominal organs from their normal location is an indirect sign of diaphragmatic hernia. The liver, spleen, small bowel, and stomach must be assessed most closely for displacement. Including the cranial abdomen on the thoracic radiograph when diaphragmatic hernia is suspected is helpful to evaluate abdominal organ displacement. Barium sulfate may also be administered to identify the stomach and help detect mild to moderate gastric displacement not observed on survey radiographs.

The heart, mediastinum, and lungs may also be displaced, depending on the size and position of abdominal organs within the thorax. The heart and lungs are usually displaced cranially and either medially or laterally by herniated abdominal viscera, and the mediastinum is usually shifted from its midline position. A localized diaphragmatic surface outline loss usually indicates the area through which the diaphragmatic hernia has occurred. Abdominal viscera and/or pleural fluid adjacent to the thoracic diaphragmatic surface cause the outline loss. This occurrence must be distinguished from the many other thoracic conditions that produce soft tissue opacity adjacent to the diaphragm. Pleural fluid is consistently present with chronic diaphragmatic hernias, or if a herniated abdominal organ, most usually the liver, is strangulated through a small diaphragmatic opening.[21] Pleural fluid is a nonspecific sign of diaphragmatic hernia and often masks

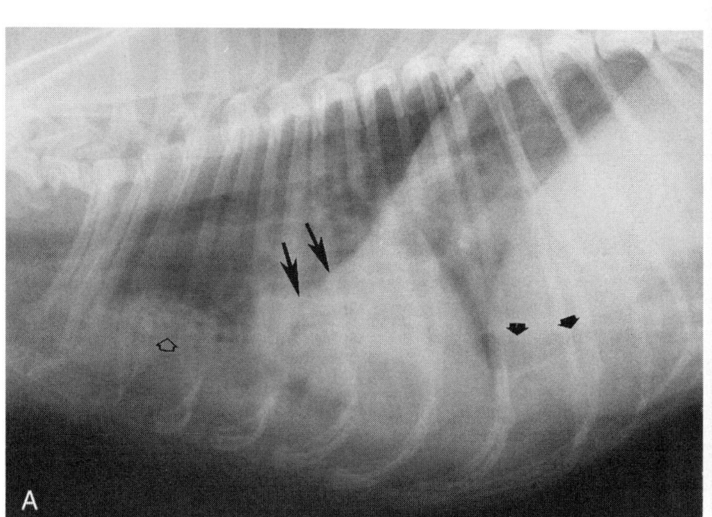

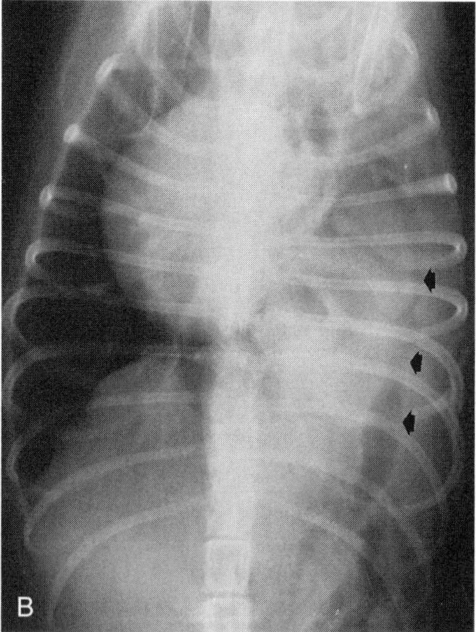

Fig. 30-13 Lateral **(A)** and ventrodorsal **(B)** views of the thorax of a dog with a traumatic diaphragmatic hernia. Radiographic signs of a diaphragmatic hernia in **A** are gas- and ingesta-filled bowel *(open arrow)* within the thorax; cranial displacement of abdominal structures (small bowel *[small solid arrows]*); and a cranially displaced diaphragmatic segment *(large solid arrows)*. Radiographic signs in **B** are the heart displaced from the herniated viscera; gas-filled small bowel within the thorax *(arrows)*; cranially displaced abdominal structures (small bowel, stomach, and liver); and loss of the left diaphragmatic surface outline.

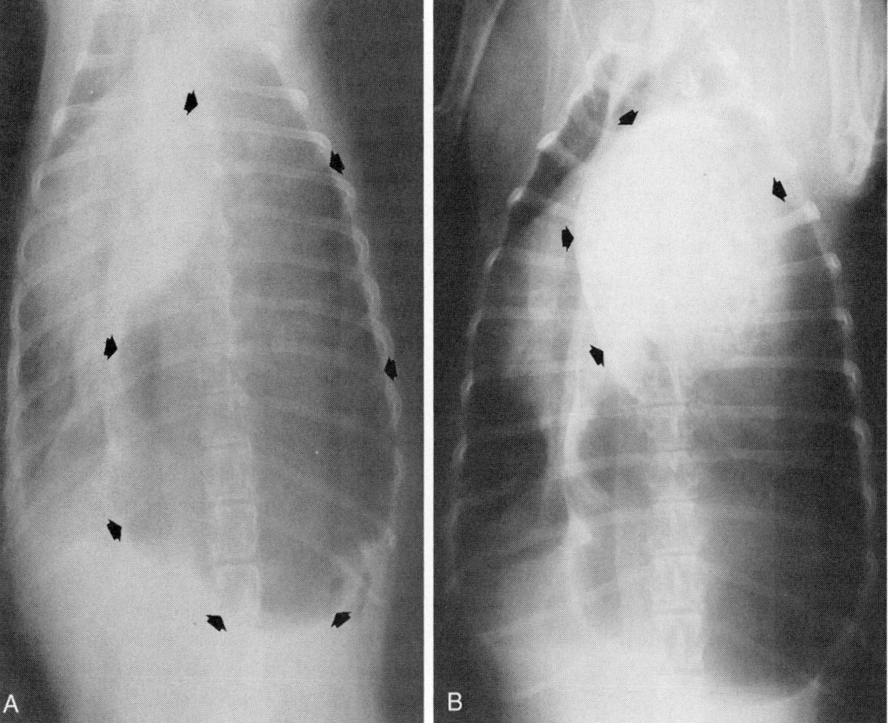

Fig. 30-14 Ventrodorsal views of the thorax of a dog with a traumatic diaphragmatic hernia without **(A)** and with **(B)** barium in the stomach. **A,** The gas-filled stomach *(arrows)* is herniated into the left hemithorax, displacing the heart and lungs to the right. The normal gastric and left diaphragmatic outlines are not present. **B,** Barium is present in the cranial part of the stomach *(arrows)*, and severe gaseous gastric distention is present.

other more important radiographic signs. Thoracocentesis and aspiration of the pleural fluid are often necessary before the hernia can be detected radiographically.

Congenitally Predisposed Diaphragmatic Hernias

Approximately 15% of all diaphragmatic hernias are congenitally predisposed.[9] Included in this group are peritoneopericardial diaphragmatic hernias, hiatal hernias, and peritoneopleural hernias. Herniation in association with congenital diaphragmatic defects may occur in an animal of any age after abdominal trauma or transitory increase in intraabdominal pressure. Defects in diaphragmatic development may be present and never result in a hernia.

Peritoneopericardial Diaphragmatic Hernias

A peritoneopericardial diaphragmatic hernia occurs when abdominal viscera herniates into the pericardial sac through a congenital hiatus formed between the tendinous portion of the diaphragm and the pericardial sac. This has been reported to occur in littermates,[22] and a predisposing trait may be carried on a simple autosomal recessive gene in cats, with a 1:500 to 1:1500 rate of incidence.[23] The hernia may have been present from birth or acquired. Mild increases in intraabdominal pressure may cause abdominal organs to herniate through a congenital hiatus.

Peritoneopericardial hernias may produce clinical signs, or they may be an incidental radiographic finding. These hernias may be present in old or young animals.[5,24-28] The liver is most frequently herniated; the stomach, omentum, and small bowel have a less frequent occurrence of herniation.[29] Hepatic cysts have also been reported to be associated with liver herniation into the pericardial sac.[30]

Radiographic signs associated with peritoneopericardial hernias are listed in Box 30-2. Herniated abdominal organs in the pericardial sac are usually caudal, or caudal and lateral, to the heart. Gas- or ingesta-filled hollow visceral organs are not difficult to identify within the pericardial sac, but the conspicuity of the gas-containing viscus may be a function of left versus right recumbency (Fig. 30-15). Radiographically, gas within the bowel is in abrupt contrast to the adjacent structures of soft tissue opacity. Solid parenchymal organs, unless surrounded by omentum, are difficult to distinguish as separate structures within the pericardium. When abdominal organs are herniated into the pericardial sac, cranial and ventral organ displacement within the abdomen may be seen; but this displacement is usually not as pronounced as that noted with traumatic diaphragmatic hernias.

A large, round cardiac silhouette and a cardiac silhouette with an abnormal convex projection on the caudal border are signs consistent with peritoneopericardial diaphragmatic hernias. These two signs depend on the amount of abdominal viscera within the pericardial sac. Large amounts of viscera produce a large, round cardiac silhouette, whereas smaller

Box • 30-2

Radiographic Signs Associated with Peritoneopericardial Diaphragmatic Hernias

- Abdominal organs identified in the pericardial sac; gas, ingested material, or structures of soft tissue opacity may be present
- Large, round cardiac silhouette
- Convex projection of the caudal cardiac silhouette
- Indistinguishable border of the ventral thoracic diaphragmatic surface and the caudal ventral cardiac silhouette
- Confluent silhouette between the diaphragm and the heart
- Dorsal peritoneopericardial mesothelial remnant between the heart and diaphragm on the lateral view in cats

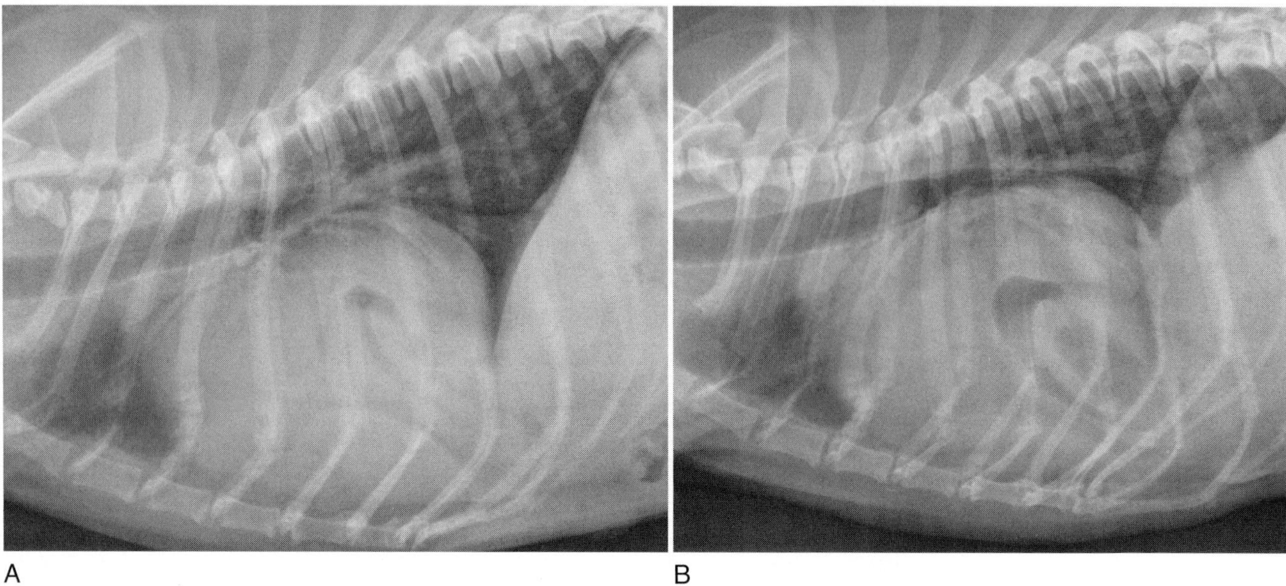

Fig. 30-15 Right (A) and left (B) lateral radiographs of a dog with a peritoneopericardial diaphragmatic hernia. Gas-containing structures are visible in the thorax. Note the larger volume of gas seen in the left lateral view. The amount of gas within organs in the pericardial sac will change depending on the position of the patient; no gas may be visible in some positions.

amounts, such as a portion of the liver or stomach, may only produce an abnormal convex caudal cardiac border. A large, round silhouette must be differentiated from pericardial effusion, generalized heart enlargement, or both. An abnormally convex caudal cardiac border must be differentiated from neoplasia, pleural granulomas, or localized pleural fluid.

An indistinguishable outline to the ventral diaphragmatic surface and the caudal ventral cardiac silhouette is produced by the communication between the two structures. This finding must be differentiated from normal contact between the heart and diaphragm, pleural fluid, localized pleuritis, and pleural granulomas.

An apparently confluent silhouette between the heart and diaphragm may appear as a wide caudal mediastinum; depending on the size of the communication, it may or may not be seen radiographically. This confluent silhouette must also be differentiated from other pathologic conditions listed. On the lateral view, identification of the dorsal peritoneopericardial mesothelial remnant between the heart and diaphragm is a consistent radiographic sign of peritoneopericardial hernia in cats (Fig. 30-16).[31] Additional radiographic studies that may be performed to confirm a diagnosis include oral administration of barium sulfate, nonselective angiography,[32] and peritoneography. Barium sulfate may be used to demonstrate gastrointestinal structures within the pericardial sac or cranial ventral displacement of abdominal structures (Fig. 30-17).

Ultrasonography has been successfully used to diagnose peritoneopericardial diaphragmatic hernias.[15-18] Ultrasonography is a reliable imaging modality to use for documentation of a peritoneopericardial hernia in cases where soft tissue opaque abdominal structures are in the pericardial sac and difficult to differentiate from the heart on radiographs. If available, an ultrasound examination should be considered before contrast examinations are performed to assist in the diagnosis of peritoneopericardial diaphragmatic hernia.

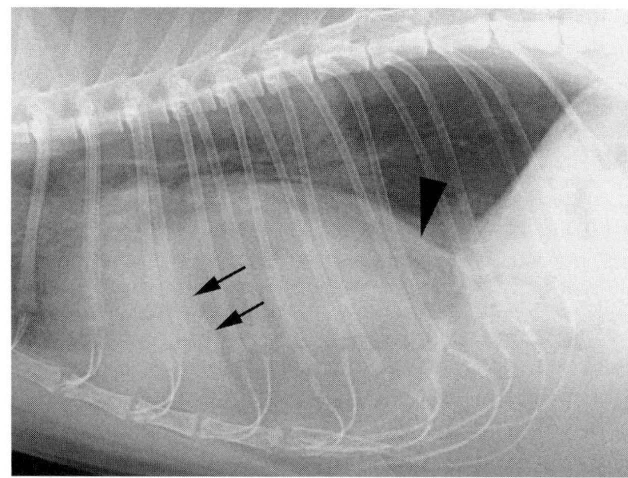

Fig. 30-16 Lateral view of a feline thorax. The cat has a peritoneopericardial diaphragmatic hernia. The outline of a dorsal peritoneopericardial mesothelial remnant is cranial to the diaphragm *(black arrowhead)*. The liver, omentum, and spleen are herniated into the pericardial sac. The caudal border of the heart is visible *(black arrows)* because of fat in the adjacent omentum.

Hiatal Hernias

Hiatal hernias are produced when a portion of stomach enters the thorax through the esophageal hiatus. These hernias are reported to occur through a congenitally or traumatically enlarged esophageal hiatus; they also may result from contraction of the longitudinal esophageal muscle.[33,34]

Two recognized types of hiatal hernias exist: sliding and paraesophageal.[35] The gastroesophageal sphincter and a portion of the stomach, usually the cardia, are herniated into

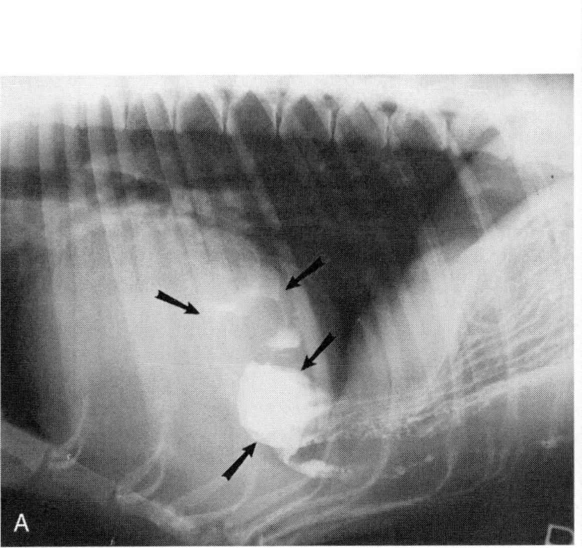

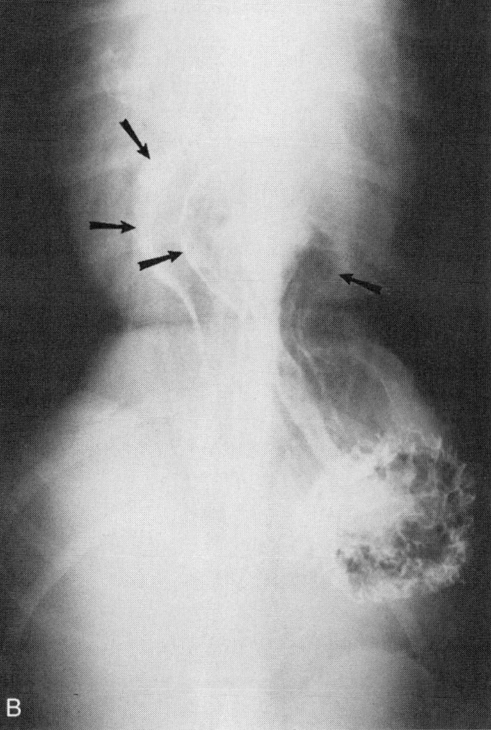

Fig. 30-17 Lateral (A) and ventrodorsal (B) views of the thorax of a dog with a peritoneopericardial diaphragmatic hernia. **A,** The pyloric antrum and proximal duodenum are herniated into the caudal aspect of the pericardial sac and are filled with barium *(arrows)*. The stomach is angled in an abnormal cranial direction, and a convex soft-tissue protrusion is visible on the caudal heart border. **B,** The barium-filled pyloric antrum and proximal duodenum *(arrows)* are within the caudal aspect of the pericardial sac. The pyloric antrum and fundus of the stomach are displaced cranially.

the thorax with sliding hiatal hernias.[36] Sliding hiatal hernias are usually congenital and seen in younger animals.[35] They are often associated with esophagitis from gastroesophageal reflux. As the name implies, the caudal esophagus and the cardia slide intermittently from the abdomen into the thorax. Because the hernia is dynamic, it may not be seen on any one radiograph; fluoroscopic examination is often necessary to make a diagnosis. Patients with nonsliding hiatal hernias have been reported, with the gastroesophageal sphincter and the gastric cardia displaced through the esophageal hiatus and fixed within the thorax.[36] Only a few sliding hiatal hernias have been reported in animals.[37-45] The low incidence may be a reflection of the subtle clinical signs and intermittent manifestations on survey radiographs.

A paraesophageal hiatal hernia is produced when the cardia or cardia and fundus of the stomach or other soft tissue structures herniate through, or alongside, the esophageal hiatus and become positioned adjacent to the esophagus. They are usually static and do not slide between the thorax and abdomen, and the gastroesophageal sphincter is in a normal position.[34,36,46] The herniated stomach may cause esophageal obstruction from external pressure on the caudal esophagus.

Hiatal hernias have been reported in both the dog and the cat.[38,40,42-45] They have been reported associated with other esophageal conditions in Shar Pei dogs.[45] Clinical signs reported with hiatal hernias include vomiting, regurgitation, excessive salivation, dysphagia, and dyspnea.[38,44,45] Hiatal hernia may be suspected from the clinical signs and survey radiographic findings but must be confirmed by an esophagram.

Box • 30-3

Radiographic Signs Associated with Sliding Hiatal Hernias

Survey Radiographs

Soft tissue mass adjacent to the left diaphragmatic crus
Loss of thoracic surface outline on the left diaphragmatic crus
Cranial displacement of the gastric cardia producing an abnormal gastric shape
Dilated esophagus
Pneumonia

Esophagram

Dilated esophagus
Hypomotile esophagus
Gastroesophageal sphincter within the thorax represented by a circumferentially narrowed area of the esophagus
Gastric cardia within the thorax
Gastroesophageal reflux

Radiographic signs of a sliding hiatal hernia are listed in Box 30-3. The most consistent survey radiographic sign is stomach displacement. The cardia appears to be stretched toward the diaphragm or may extend into the thorax. This displacement produces an abnormal shape to the cardia and fundus remaining in the abdomen. The caudal esophagus may or may not be distended, and a soft tissue opacity (mass) may be seen adjacent to the left diaphragmatic crus (Fig. 30-18). The size and visibility of this mass depend on the amount of stomach that has herniated into the thorax. The soft-tissue mass associated with a hiatal hernia must be differentiated from pulmonary masses or a masses originating from the diaphragm. Diaphragmatic neoplastic masses have been reported but are rare.[47]

A dilated caudal esophagus is usually best detected and evaluated with an esophagram. An esophagram is also helpful for differentiating the type of hiatal hernia. The caudal esophageal sphincter and a portion of the cardia are seen cranial to the diaphragm with a sliding hiatal hernia.[48] The caudal esophageal sphincter can be identified as a concentric, smooth, 1- to 2-cm narrowing in the caudal esophagus (Fig. 30-19). Displacement and narrowing of the caudal esophagus by the cardia and fundus can be seen with paraesophageal hiatal hernias. Barium outlining the caudal esophagus can also be seen superimposed over the herniated paraesophageal soft tissue (Fig. 30-20).

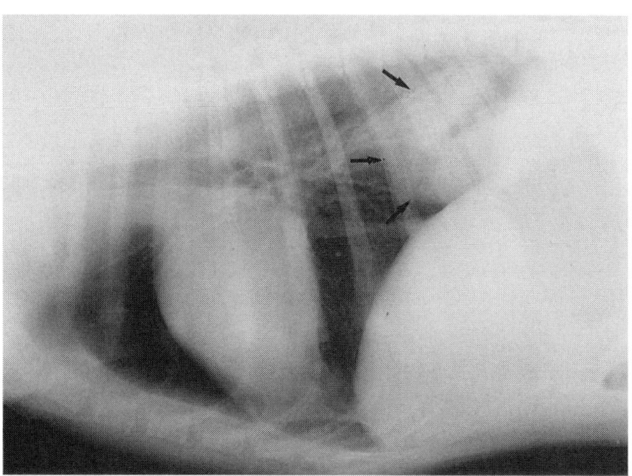

Fig. 30-18 Lateral thoracic view with a soft tissue opacity in the caudodorsal thorax *(arrows)*. The soft tissue opacity has gas within the center and is suspect for a hiatal hernia.

Gastroesophageal Intussusception

Gastroesophageal intussusceptions occur when the stomach, with or without the spleen, duodenum, pancreas, and omentum, invaginates through the esophageal hiatus into the caudal esophagus.[34,36,49,50] They occur most frequently in male and German Shepherd dogs and in animals with a preexisting dilated esophagus.[50] Gastroesophageal intussusceptions usually produce an esophageal obstruction, which results in rapid deterioration of the animal's condition with a high mortality rate; a timely diagnosis is therefore essential.[50]

On survey radiographs, a large soft tissue mass is seen adjacent to the diaphragm, usually accompanied by a dilated esophagus. With an esophagram, gastroesophageal intussusceptions produce a large intraluminal filling defect within the caudal esophagus, rugal folds may be outlined with barium, and barium usually does not usually enter the stomach (Box 30-4 and Fig. 30-21).

Peritonopleural Hernias

Congenital diaphragmatic defects resulting in peritoneopleural hernias have been reported rarely in the dog and cat[51-55] and have been confused with pulmonary masses.[56] The defects are created when the septum transversum or the pleural peritoneal folds do not develop and fuse to form a complete diaphragm. The diaphragmatic defect allows abdominal viscera to enter the thoracic cavity, producing a pleuroperitoneal hernia.

In human beings, diaphragmatic defects have a familial incidence with a multifactorial mode of inheritance.[57] Congenital defects in dogs have been reported in the muscular diaphragm, dorsolateral in position,[58] and in the membranous diaphragm associated with umbilical hernias.[52-54]

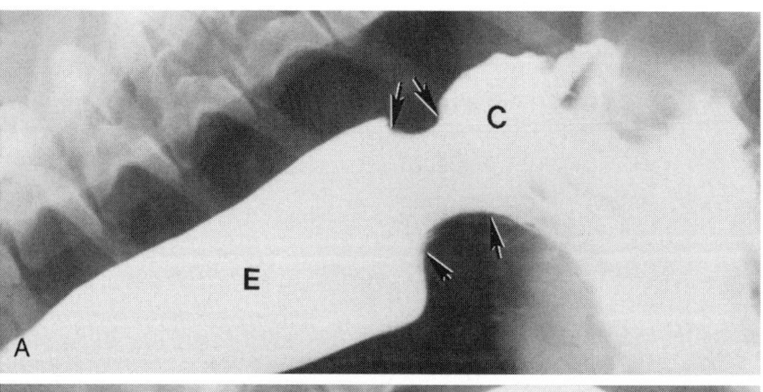

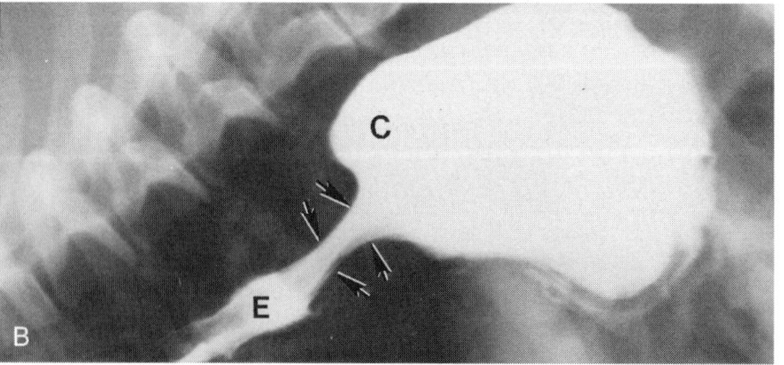

Fig. 30-19 Lateral views of barium esophagram in a patient with a sliding hiatal hernia. **A,** Contrast medium distends the caudal esophagus *(E)*, the gastroesophageal sphincter *(arrows)*, and the cardia *(C)*. The gastroesophageal sphincter and gastric cardia are displaced cranial to the diaphragm through the esophageal hiatus. **B,** The esophagus *(E)* and gastroesophageal sphincter *(arrows)* are outlined but are not distended with barium; most of the barium has passed into the stomach. The gastroesophageal sphincter and gastric cardia are herniated through the esophageal hiatus and are cranial to the diaphragm.

The radiographic signs of peritoneopleural hernias associated with diaphragmatic defects are the same as for traumatic diaphragmatic hernias. With membranous defects, however, the liver (in dogs) or the falciform fat (in cats) is displaced cranially, while remaining in the caudal ventral thorax, and is often confined to the mediastinum because the peritoneal membrane and pleura are intact (Fig. 30-22).[58]

Motor Disturbances of the Diaphragm

The diaphragm is the principal muscle of respiration and is innervated by the phrenic nerve. Most motor disturbances are clinically asymptomatic and have not been well documented in animals.

Motor disturbances of the diaphragm consist of unilateral paralysis, bilateral paralysis, and diaphragmatic flutter.[1] Diaphragmatic paralysis may result from pneumonia, trauma, myopathies, and neuropathies, or the cause may be unidentified.[1] Transient posttraumatic hemidiaphragmatic paralysis has been reported in cats.[59] Diaphragmatic paralysis should be suspected when one or both diaphragmatic crura are displaced cranially (Fig. 30-23). Confirmation of paralysis is best achieved with fluoroscopy. Unequal movement between the crura is seen with unilateral paralysis. With bilateral paralysis, minimal or no diaphragmatic movement or a paradoxic cranial displacement of the flaccid diaphragm may occur during inspiration.[60] Bilateral paralysis may be more difficult to confirm with fluoroscopy because diaphragmatic movement is sometimes produced by compensatory abdominal muscle contraction during respiration.

Diaphragmatic flutter is most often associated with contractions of the diaphragm synchronous with the heartbeat. It is usually transient in nature and can be easily diagnosed with fluoroscopy by observing contractions of the diaphragm in synchrony with the heartbeat.[61]

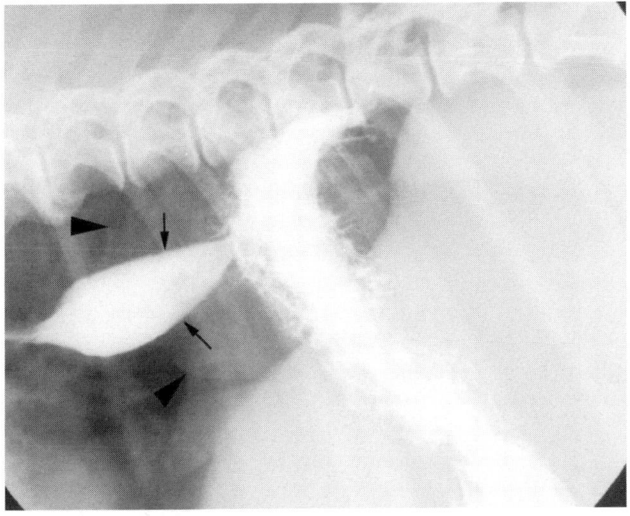

Fig. 30-20 Lateral view of the thorax. Barium is filling and outlining the caudal esophagus *(arrows)*. The barium-filled caudal esophagus is superimposed over a soft tissue opacity organ *(arrowheads)* cranial to the diaphragm and adjacent to one side of the esophagus.

Muscular Dystrophy

Muscular dystrophy caused by dystrophin deficiency has been reported in dogs[62] and cats.[63,64] In cats an irregular, scalloped appearance of the diaphragm, particularly along the ventral margin, was a consistent finding observed on radiographs after 7 months of age.[60] The scalloped margin noted best on the lateral view should not be confused with the normal scalloping observed on the ventrodorsal view in cats on maximal inspiration (see Fig. 30-7). Muscular hypertrophy produced with feline muscular dystrophy has also been reported to cause megaesophagus from extraluminal hiatal obstruction. Definitive laboratory tests, such as immunofluorescence or immunoblot tests, are necessary to establish the diagnosis of muscular dystrophy.

Box • 30-4

Radiographic Signs Associated with Gastroesophageal Intussusception

Survey Radiographs

Soft tissue mass adjacent to the diaphragm
Cranial displacement of the stomach with or without the spleen or duodenum
Dilated esophagus

Esophagram

Intraluminal filling defect in the caudal esophagus
Barium outline of rugal folds
No barium within the stomach

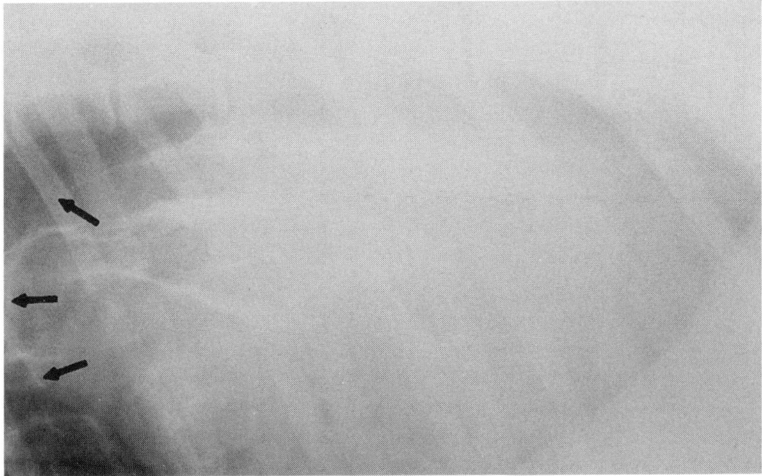

Fig. 30-21 Lateral radiograph of the caudodorsal aspect of the thorax of a dog with a gastroesophageal intussusception. Barium outlines its cranial aspect *(arrows)*. The large soft tissue mass in the caudal dorsal thorax is the stomach intussuscepted into the caudal esophageal lumen. Note the barium coating of the gastric rugae, making them appear as filling defects; this feature is characteristic of gastroesophageal intussusception.

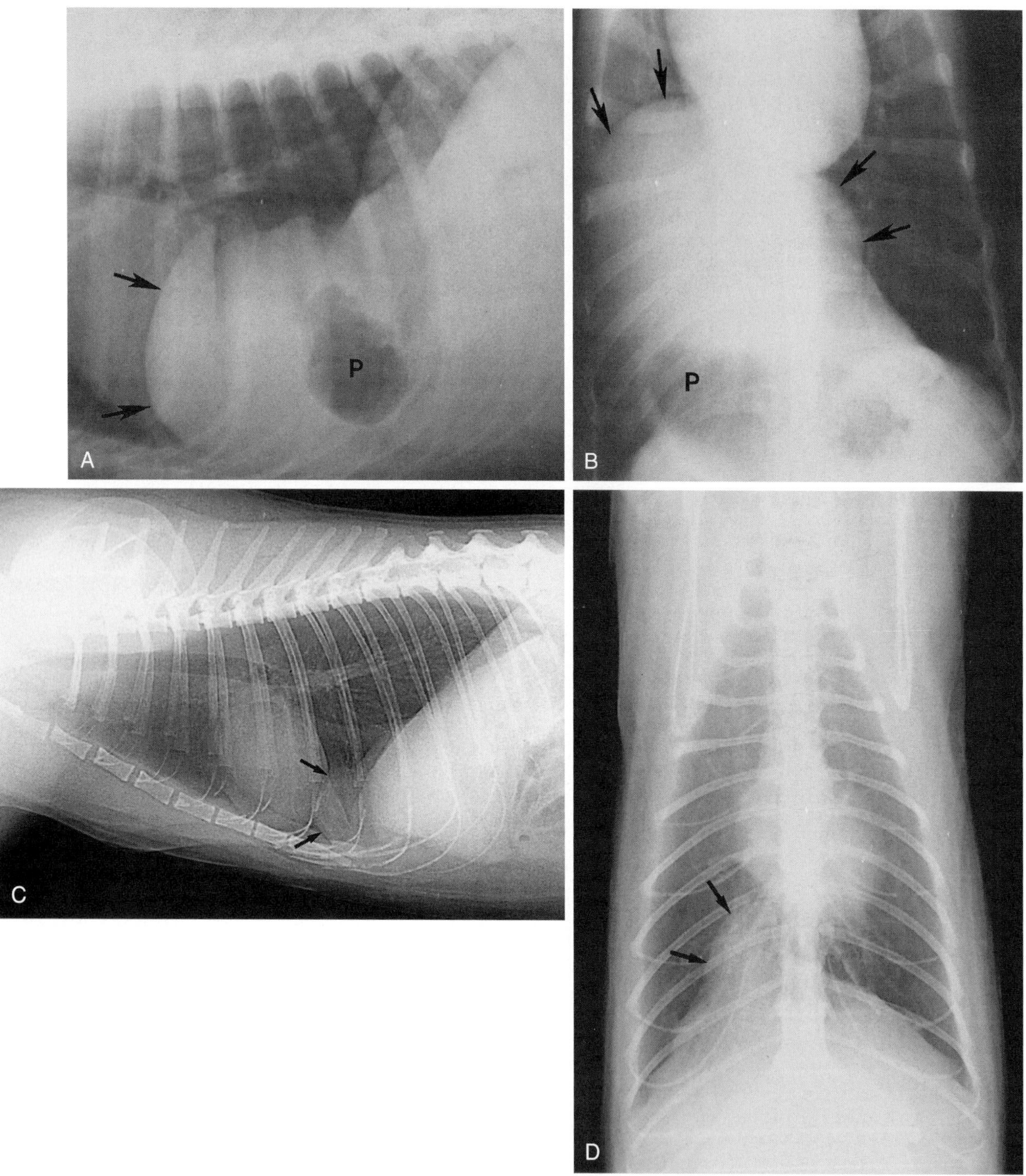

Fig. 30-22 Recumbent lateral and ventrodorsal views of a dog (A and B) and a cat (C and D) thorax. A defect in the membranous portion of the diaphragm is present in both the dog and cat. In the dog (A and B) the liver *(arrows)* and gas-filled pyloric antrum *(P)* are within the thorax, and the stomach and liver are displaced cranially. In the cat (C and D) the falciform ligament and fat are displaced cranially to the diaphragm *(arrows)* and surrounded with intact parietal pleura.

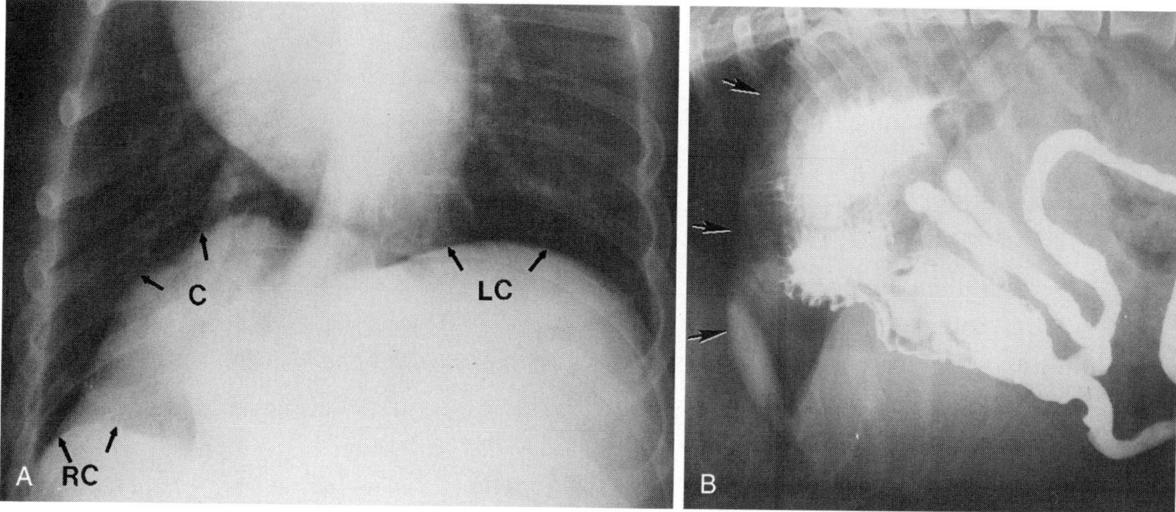

Fig. 30-23 Ventrodorsal (A) and lateral (B) radiographs of the cranial abdomen. Hemiparalysis of the left diaphragm is present. **A,** The left diaphragmatic crus *(LC)* is cranial to the right crus *(RC)*. The cupula *(C)* and right crus *(RC)* are in a normal inspiratory position. **B,** The cranial position of the left diaphragmatic crus *(arrows)* causes the gastric cardia and fundus to be displaced cranially.

REFERENCES

1. Shim C: Motor disturbances of the diaphragm, *Clin Chest Med* 1:125, 1980.
2. Rivero O, del Castillo H: Lymphatics of the diaphragm in the dog, *Acta Radiol (Diagn) (Stockh)* 17:663, 1976.
3. Evans HE: *Miller's anatomy of the dog,* ed 3, Philadelphia, 1993, W.B. Saunders, p. 304.
4. Grandage J: The radiology of the dog's diaphragm, *J Small Anim Pract* 15:1, 1974.
5. Schulman J: Peritoneopericardial diaphragmatic hernia in a dog, *Mod Vet Pract* 60:306, 1979.
6. Garson HL, Dodman NH, Baker GJ: Diaphragmatic hernia: analysis of fifty-six cases in dogs and cats, *J Small Anim Pract* 21:469, 1980.
7. Farrow CS: Radiographic diagnosis of diaphragmatic hernia, *Mod Vet Pract* 64:979, 1983.
8. Silverman S, Ackerman N: Radiographic evaluation of abdominal hernias, *Mod Vet Pract* 58:781, 1977.
9. Wilson GP III, Hayes HM Jr: Diaphragmatic hernia in the dog and cat: a 25-year overview, *Semin Vet Med Surg* 1:318, 1986.
10. Levine SH: Diaphragmatic hernia, *Vet Clin North Am Small Anim Pract* 17:411, 1987.
11. Stokhof AA, Wolvekamp WTC, Hellebrekers LJ et al: Traumatic diaphragmatic hernia in the dog and cat, *Tijdschr Diergeneeskd* 111(suppl 1):62S, 1986.
12. Rendano VT: Positive contrast peritoneography: an aid in the radiographic diagnosis of diaphragmatic hernia, *J Am Vet Radiol Soc* 20:67, 1979.
13. Stickle RL: Positive-contrast celiography (peritoneography) for the diagnosis of diaphragmatic hernia in dogs and cats, *J Am Vet Med Assoc* 185:295, 1984.
14. Williams J, Leveille R, Myer CW: Imaging modalities used to confirm diaphragmatic hernia in small animals, *Compend Small Anim* 20:1199, 1998.
15. Lamb CR, Mason GD, Wallace MK: Ultrasonographic diagnosis of peritoneopericardial diaphragmatic hernia in a Persian cat, *Vet Record* 125:186, 1989.
16. Hay WH, Woodfield JA, Moon MA: Clinical, echocardiographic, and radiographic findings of peritoneopericardial diaphragmatic hernia in two dogs, *J Am Vet Med Assoc* 195:1245, 1989.
17. Hashimoto A, Kudo T, Sawashima I: Diagnostic ultrasonography of noncardiac intrathoracic disorders in small animals, *Res Bull* 55:235, 1990.
18. Hodges RD, Tucker RL, Brace JJ: Radiographic diagnosis (peritoneopericardial diaphragmatic herniation in a dog), *Vet Radiol Ultrasound* 34:249, 1993.
19. Carb A: Diaphragmatic hernia in the dog and cat, *Vet Clin North Am Small Anim Pract* 5:477, 1975.
20. Wilson GP, Newton CD, Burt JK: A review of 116 diaphragmatic hernias in dogs and cats, *J Am Vet Med Assoc* 159:1142, 1971.
21. Boudrieau RJ, Muir WW: Pathophysiology of traumatic diaphragmatic hernia in dogs, *Compend Contin Educ Pract Vet* 9:379, 1987.
22. Feldman DB, Bree MM, Cohen BJ: Congenital diaphragmatic hernia in neonatal dogs, *J Am Vet Med Assoc* 153:942, 1968.
23. Saperstein G, Harris S, Leipold HW: Congenital defects in domestic cats, *Feline Pract* 6:18, 1976.
24. Bjorck GR, Tigerschiold A: Peritoneopericardial diaphragmatic hernia in a dog, *J Small Anim Pract* 11:585, 1970.
25. Gourley IM, Popp JA, Park RD: Myelolipomas of the liver in a domestic cat, *J Am Vet Med Assoc* 158:2053, 1971.
26. Rendano VT, Parker RB: Polycystic kidneys and peritoneopericardial diaphragmatic hernia in the cat: a case report, *J Small Anim Pract* 17:479, 1976.
27. Weitz J, Tilley LP, Moldoff D: Pericardiodiaphragmatic hernia in a dog, *J Am Vet Med Assoc* 173:1336, 1978.
28. Evans SM, Biery DN: Congenital peritoneopericardial diaphragmatic hernia in the dog and cat, *Vet Radiol* 21:108, 1980.
29. Neiger R: Peritoneopericardial diaphragmatic hernia in cats, *Compend Contin Educ Pract Vet* 18:461, 1996.

30. Liptak JM, Bissett SA, Allan GS et al: Hepatic cysts incarcerated in a peritoneopericardial diaphragmatic hernia, *J Feline Med Surg* 4:123, 2002.
31. Berry CR, Koblik PD, Ticer JW: Dorsal peritoneopericardial mesothelial remnant as an aid to the diagnosis of feline congenital peritoneopericardial diaphragmatic hernia, *Vet Radiol* 31:239, 1990.
32. Willard MD, Aronson E: Peritoneopericardial diaphragmatic hernia in a cat, *J Am Vet Med Assoc* 178:481, 1981.
33. Edwards MH: Selective vagotomy of the canine oesophagus: a model for the treatment of hiatal hernia, *Thorax* 31:185, 1976.
34. Teunissen GHB, Happ RP, Van Toorenburg J et al: Esophageal hiatal hernia: case report of a dog and a cheetah, *Tijdschr Diergeneeskd* 103:742, 1978.
35. Ellison GW, Lewis DD, Phillips L et al: Esophageal hiatal hernia in small animals: literature review, *J Am Anim Hosp Assoc* 20:783, 1984.
36. Ellis FH Jr: Controversies regarding the management of hiatus hernia, *Am J Surg* 139:782, 1980.
37. Rogers WA, Donovan EF: Peptic esophagitis in a dog, *J Am Vet Med Assoc* 163:462, 1973.
38. Prymak C, Saunders HM, Washabau RJ: Hiatal hernia repair by restoration and stabilization of normal anatomy. An evaluation in four dogs and one cat, *Vet Surg* 18:386, 1989.
39. Gaskell CJ, Gibbs C, Pearson H: Sliding hiatus hernia with reflex oesophagitis in two dogs, *J Small Anim Pract* 15:503, 1974.
40. Alexander JW, Hoffer RE, MacDonald JM et al: Hiatal hernia in the dog: a case report and review of the literature, *J Am Anim Hosp Assoc* 11:793, 1975.
41. Iwasaki M, DeMartin BW, DeAlvarenga J et al: Congenital hiatal hernia in a dog, *Mod Vet Pract* 58:1018, 1977.
42. Robotham GR: Congenital hiatal hernia in a cat, *Feline Pract* 9:37, 1979.
43. Peterson SL: Esophageal hiatal hernia in a cat, *J Am Vet Med Assoc* 183:325, 1983.
44. Bright RM, Sackman JE, NeNovo D et al: Hiatal hernia in the dog and cat: a retrospective study of 16 cases, *J Small Anim Pract* 31:244, 1990.
45. Stickle R, Sparschu G, Love N et al: Radiographic evaluation of esophageal function in Chinese Shar Pei pups, *J Am Vet Med Assoc* 201:81, 1992.
46. Miles KG, Pope ER, Jergens AE: Paraesophageal hiatal hernia and pyloric obstruction in a dog, *J Am Vet Med Assoc* 193:1437, 1988.
47. Anderson GM, Miller DA, Miller SW: Peripheral nerve sheath tumor of the diaphragm with osseous differentiation in a one-year-old dog, *J Am Anim Hosp Assoc* 35:319, 1999.
48. Steiner GM: Gastro-oesophageal reflux, hiatus hernia, and the radiologist with special reference to children, *Br J Radiol* 50:164, 1977.
49. Pollock S, Rhodes WH: Gastroesophageal intussusception in an Afghan hound, *J Am Vet Radiol Soc* 11:5, 1970.
50. Leib MS, Blass CE: Gastroesophageal intussusception in the dog: a review of the literature and a case report, *J Am Anim Hosp Assoc* 20:783, 1984.
51. Bath GF: Congenital diaphragmatic hiatus in a dog: case report, *J S Afr Vet Assoc* 47:55, 1976.
52. Nicholson C: Defective diaphragm associated with umbilical hernia, *Vet Rec* 98:433, 1976.
53. Sawyer SL: Defective diaphragm associated with umbilical hernia, *Vet Rec* 98:490, 1976.
54. Swift BJ: Defective diaphragm associated with umbilical hernia, *Vet Rec* 98:511, 1976.
55. Valentine BA, Dietze CB, Noden AE: Canine congenital diaphragmatic hernia, *J Vet Intern Med* 2:109, 1988.
56. White JD, Tisdall PLC, Norris JM, Malik R: Diaphragmatic hernia in a cat mimicking a pulmonary mass, *J Feline Med Surg* 5:197, 2003.
57. Wolff G: Familial congenital diaphragmatic defect: review and conclusions, *Hum Genet* 54:1, 1980.
58. Voges AK, Hill RC, Neuwirth L et al: True diaphragmatic hernia in a cat, *Vet Radiol Ultrasound* 38:116, 1997.
59. Vignoli AM, Toniato M, Rossi F et al: Transient port-traumatic hemidiaphragmatic paralysis in two cats, *J Small Anim Pract* 43:312, 2002.
60. Greene CE, Basinger RR, Whitfield JB: Surgical management of bilateral diaphragmatic paralysis in a dog, *J Am Vet Med Assoc* 193:1542, 1988.
61. Mainwaring CJ: Post-traumatic contraction of the diaphragm synchronous with the heartbeat in a dog, *J Small Anim Pract* 29:299, 1988.
62. Cooper BJ, Winand NJ, Stedman H et al: The homologue of the Duchenne locus is defective in X-linked muscular dystrophy of dogs, *Nature* 334:154, 1988.
63. Berry CR, Gaschen FP, Ackerman H: Radiographic and ultrasonographic features of hypertrophic feline muscular dystrophy in two cats, *Vet Radiol Ultrasound* 33:357, 1992.
64. Gaschen FP, Swendrowske MA: Hypertrophic feline muscular dystrophy. A unique clinical expression of dystrophin deficiency, *Feline Pract* 22:23, 1994.

ELECTRONIC RESOURCES evolve

Additional information related to the content in Chapter 30 can be found on the companion Web site at evolve http://evolve.elsevier.com/Thrall/vetrad/.

- Key Points
- Chapter Quiz
- Case Study 30-1

CHAPTER • 31
The Mediastinum

Donald E. Thrall

NORMAL ANATOMY

The mediastinum is the space between the lungs. This space is bounded on each side by a layer of mediastinal pleura, which is a component of the pleural sac. Each right and left pleural sac is composed of mediastinal, diaphragmatic, costal, and pulmonary pleurae (Fig. 31-1). These pleural components within each sac are continuous. The term mediastinal disease usually refers to an abnormality involving the space between the two layers of mediastinal pleura rather than an abnormality of a mediastinal pleural layer.

The mediastinum extends from the thoracic inlet to the diaphragm and is primarily positioned in the median plane of the thorax, essentially dividing the thoracic cavity into right and left halves (Fig. 31-2). The mediastinum may be subdivided into a cranial portion cranial to the heart, a middle portion at the level of and containing the heart, and a caudal portion caudal to the heart. The mediastinum may also be divided into dorsal and ventral portions by a dorsal plane through the tracheal bifurcation. Organs included in the mediastinum are listed in Table 31-1.

Controversy exists regarding whether the mediastinal pleural layers serve as an anatomic separation between the left and right pleural cavities. Some sources suggest that the mediastinal pleura is normally fenestrated[1] and others do not.[2] Regardless, the mediastinal pleura is fragile, and pleural effusion or pneumothorax is commonly bilateral (i.e., not contained to one pleural cavity by the mediastinum). For example, in one study of induced pneumothorax in dogs, 22 of 24 dogs having air injected into one pleural space quickly developed bilateral pneumothorax.[3] Unilateral or asymmetric pleural effusion or pneumothorax may occur if (1) the mediastinal pleura is not fenestrated and the mediastinal pleura remains intact, (2) existing fenestrations have been closed as a result of inflammation, or (3) the pleural fluid is too viscid to pass through existing fenestrations.

The mediastinum, in contrast to the pleural space, is not a closed cavity. The mediastinum communicates cranially with the fascial planes of the neck by way of the thoracic inlet and caudally with the retroperitoneal space through the aortic hiatus. These communications provide the means for the spread of mediastinal disease to the neck and abdomen, and vice versa.

Of the mediastinal organs listed in Table 31-1, only the heart, trachea, caudal vena cava, aorta and, in young animals, thymus are normally visible. Occasionally a portion of the normal esophagus may be seen (see Chapter 27). The other mediastinal organs are not seen either because (1) they are too small to absorb a sufficient number of x-rays, (2) insufficient fat is interposed to provide contrast, or (3) they are in contact with other mediastinal structures of the same radiopacity, leading to border effacement. An example of border effacement of mediastinal structures is the appearance of the cranial mediastinum in a lateral thoracic radiograph. A distinct opacity is created by the cranial mediastinum ventral to the trachea, but individual organs in that portion of the mediastinum cannot be discerned (Fig. 31-3). This opacity is caused by the absorption of x-rays by the left subclavian artery, brachiocephalic trunk, cranial vena cava, mediastinal lymph nodes, and possibly thymus. These organs are not seen individually because they are in contact with each other and insufficient interposed fat is present. Thus the border of these structures is effaced. On the lateral projection, the cranial mediastinum is more radiopaque just ventral to the trachea than just dorsal to the sternum because of the greater thickness of the mediastinum dorsally (Fig. 31-4; see also Fig. 31-3).

In ventrodorsal or dorsoventral thoracic radiographs, most of the cranial mediastinum is superimposed on the spine. The normal width of the mediastinum in this view is usually less than approximately twice the width of the vertebrae (Fig. 31-5). In obese patients, the cranial mediastinum may be widened by fat accumulation and confused with a mediastinal mass (Fig. 31-6). Other imaging techniques, such as ultrasound or computed tomographic imaging, may be necessary to make the final assessment in this situation.

The mediastinum deviates from midline in three normal reflections: the cranioventral mediastinal reflection, the caudoventral mediastinal reflection, and the vena caval mediastinal reflection, or the plica vena cava. The first two are visible in thoracic radiographs of many patients but not universally; the third is not seen.

The cranioventral mediastinal reflection appears in ventrodorsal or dorsoventral radiographs as a curving radiopaque line, on the patient's left, extending from approximately T1 or T2 to the region of the main pulmonary artery. The concave side of the line is to the patient's right (see Figs. 31-4 and 31-5). This reflection is caused by extension of the right cranial lobe across the midline, pushing the mediastinum to the left (see Fig. 31-4). The thickness of the cranioventral mediastinal reflection is affected by the amount of fat it contains. On the lateral view, the cranioventral mediastinal reflection and the margin of the right cranial lobe are frequently identified immediately cranial to the heart (see Fig. 31-3). The cranioventral mediastinal reflection is not visible in every thoracic radiograph. The thymus lies in the cranioventral mediastinal reflection, and sometimes it can be identified in ventrodorsal or dorsoventral radiographs of young animals. The thymus is not as readily seen in lateral thoracic radiographs (Fig. 31-7). In lateral projections of the thorax made before the thymus involutes, however, the thymus may obscure the cranial margin of the heart because of border effacement.

The caudoventral mediastinal reflection is seen only on ventrodorsal or dorsoventral radiographs; it is not seen in lateral projections. It is created by extension of the accessory lobe of the right lung across the midline, thereby pushing the

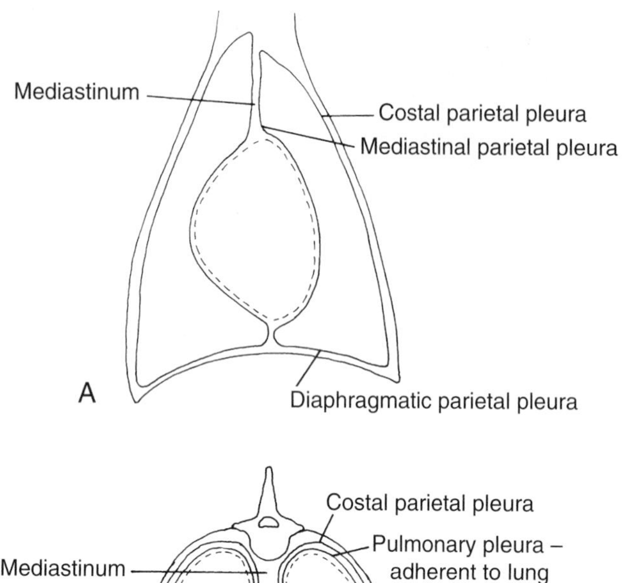

Fig. 31-1 The thorax in dorsal (**A**) and transverse (**B**) planes illustrating the relation of the pleural layers. Two distinct pleural sacs are visible. **A,** Note the continuity of the costal, mediastinal, and diaphragmatic parts of each parietal sac. (Lungs have not been included in **A**.) **B,** Note how the mediastinal pleura is reflected onto the lung as pulmonary pleura. In **B** the lung is depicted by the *dotted line.* Also note that the pleural space is not continuous with the mediastinum. *H,* Heart; *L,* lung; *T,* trachea.

mediastinum to the left. The caudoventral mediastinal reflection appears as a relatively straight radiopaque line in the caudal left hemithorax, extending from the region of the cardiac apex in a caudolateral direction toward the gastric fundus (Fig. 31-8). The caudoventral mediastinal reflection has been incorrectly identified as the sternopericardiac ligament (also called the *cardiophrenic* or *phrenicopericardial ligament*), but the sternopericardiac ligament, which is a continuation of the apex of the fibrous pericardium, is not visible radiographically.[4] The thickness of the caudoventral mediastinal reflection depends on the amount of fat it con-

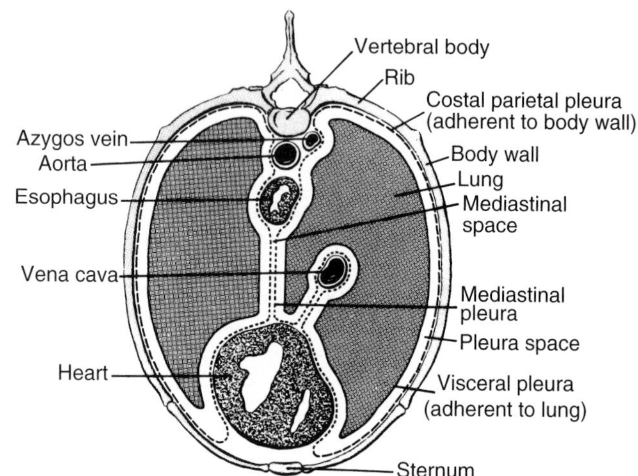

Fig. 31-2 Cross-section of the canine thorax in a transverse plane. The mediastinum divides the thorax into right and left sides. Note the mediastinal space does not communicate with the pleural space. (Reprinted from Thrall DE, Losonsky JM: Dyspnea in the cat: II. Radiographic aspects of intrathoracic causes involving the mediastinum, *Feline Pract* 8:47, 1978.)

Table • 31-1

Mediastinal Organs

ORGAN	CRANIAL MEDIASTINUM	MIDDLE MEDIASTINUM	CAUDAL MEDIASTINUM
Cranial vena cava	x		
Thymus	x		
Sternal lymph nodes	x		
Aortic arch	x		
Brachiocephalic artery	x		
Left subclavian artery	x		
Mediastinal lymph nodes	x		
Trachea	x	x	
Right and left vagosympathetic trunk	x	x	
Dorsal intercostal arteries and veins	x	x	x
Internal thoracic arteries and veins	x	x	x
Esophagus	x	x	x
Thoracic duct	x	x	x
Right and left sympathetic trunks	x	x	x
Right and left phrenic nerves	x	x	x
Descending aorta		x	x
Bronchoesophageal arteries and veins		x	x
Azygous vein		x	x
Heart		x	
Tracheobronchial lymph nodes		x	
Main pulmonary artery		x	
Main pulmonary veins		x	
Principal bronchi		x	
Caudal vena cava			x
Right and left vagus nerves			x

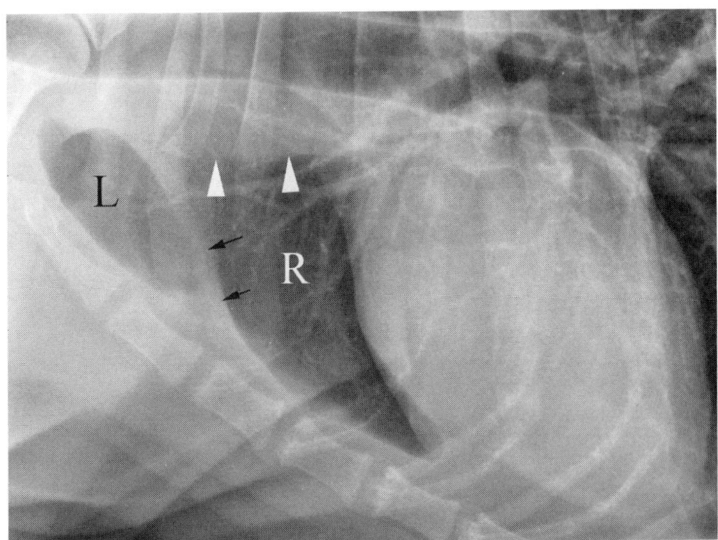

Fig. 31-3 Left lateral radiograph of the thorax of a normal dog. The opacity ventral to the trachea (*white arrowheads* indicate ventral margin of opacity) is part of the cranial mediastinum. Although several different organs are in this part of the mediastinum (e.g., left subclavian artery, brachiocephalic trunk, and cranial vena cava), they cannot be discerned because they are in contact with each other and there is not enough adjacent fat to provide contrast. The mediastinum extends from the vertebrae to the sternebrae, but it is most radiopaque immediately ventral to the trachea because it is thickest at this location (see Fig. 31-4). Also note the cranioventral mediastinal reflection *(black arrows)* between the cranial portion of the left cranial lobe *(L)* and the right cranial lobe *(R)* (see Fig. 31-4).

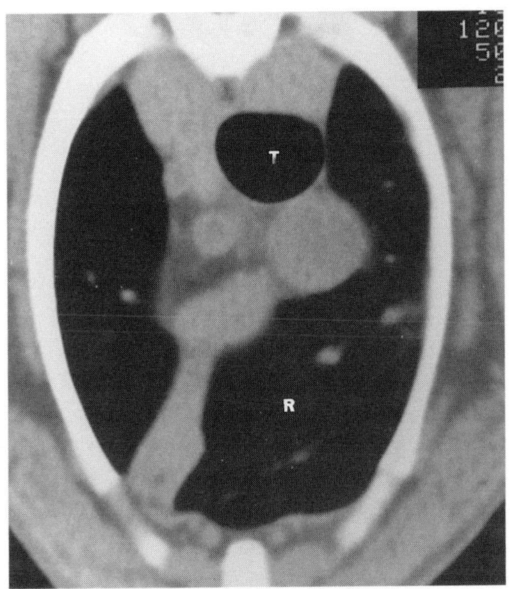

Fig. 31-4 Transverse CT image of the canine thorax at the level of the second thoracic vertebra. Note the greater thickness of the dorsal aspect of the mediastinum. This accounts for the opacity seen ventral to the trachea in lateral thoracic radiographs (see Fig. 31-3). Note the vessels ventral to the trachea *(T)*. Insufficient fat is present for these vessels to be seen in radiographs, but the superior inherent contrast resolution of CT allows them to be identified. Also note the cranioventral mediastinal reflection; the ventral mediastinum is being pushed to the left by the right cranial lung lobe *(R)*.

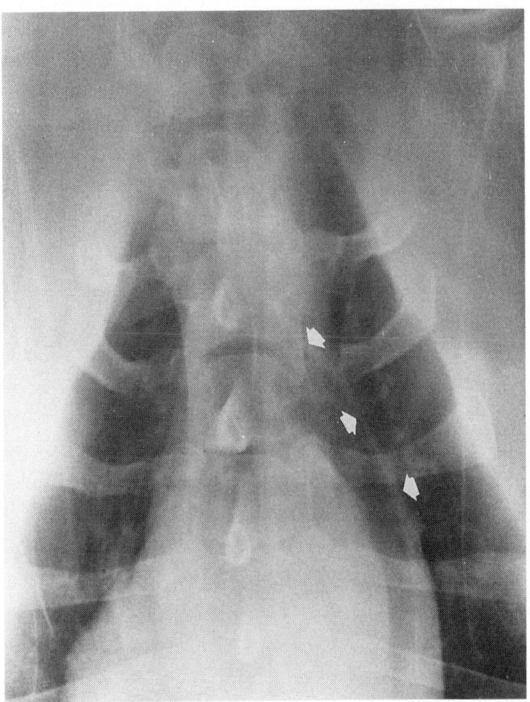

Fig. 31-5 Ventrodorsal radiograph of the cranial aspect of the thorax of a normal dog. The cranial mediastinum is superimposed on the cranial aspect of the thoracic spine; it is relatively indistinct. As an approximation, the width of the normal cranial mediastinum in ventrodorsal or dorsoventral radiographs should not be greater than twice the diameter of the vertebrae. Note the mediastinal reflection between the right cranial lobe and the cranial part of the left cranial lobe *(arrows)*. See Figure 31-3 for the appearance of this reflection in the lateral view and Figure 31-4 for an illustration of the right lung pushing the mediastinum to the left.

tains (Fig. 31-9); in individual animals this may change as body stature changes.

The caudal vena cava mediastinal reflection, or plica vena cava, is not visible as a distinct structure in radiographs of the thorax, but its presence as an extension of the mediastinum to the right should be understood (see Fig. 31-2).

PATHOLOGIC MEDIASTINAL CONDITIONS

Mediastinal abnormalities are divided into four general classifications: mediastinal shift, mediastinal masses, mediastinal fluid, and pneumomediastinum.

Mediastinal Shift

Mediastinal shift occurs as a result of a unilateral decrease in lung volume (ipsilateral shift), a unilateral increase in lung volume (contralateral shift), or the presence of an intrathoracic mass (contralateral shift). A mediastinal shift is not readily apparent on lateral radiographs. Mediastinal position should be evaluated in ventrodorsal or dorsoventral

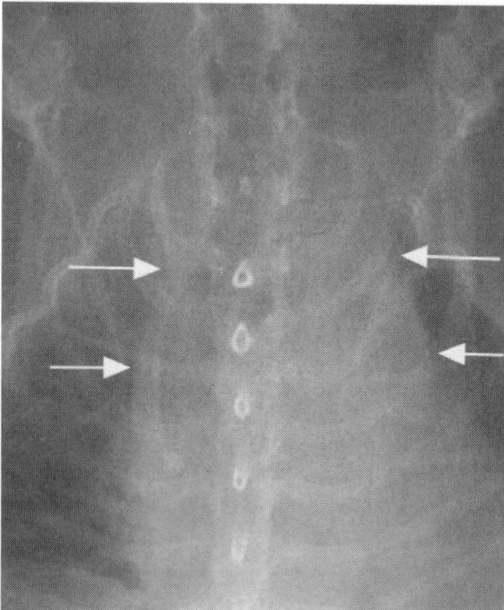

Fig. 31-6 Dorsoventral radiograph of the cranial aspect of the thorax of an obese dog. The cranial mediastinum contains a large amount of fat and appears much wider than twice the diameter of the vertebrae *(arrows)*. Care should be taken to avoid misinterpreting a wide mediastinum in an obese animal as a mediastinal mass. Ultrasound or CT imaging may be necessary to make a final assessment.

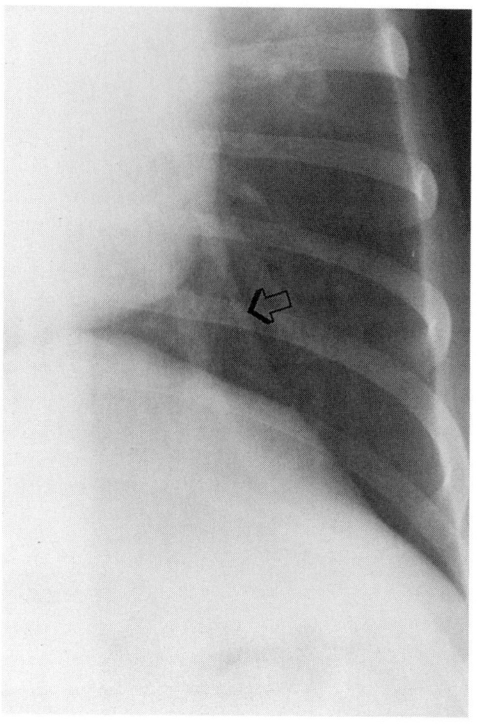

Fig. 31-8 Ventrodorsal radiograph of the caudal thorax of a normal dog. The caudoventral mediastinal reflection is visible *(arrow)*.

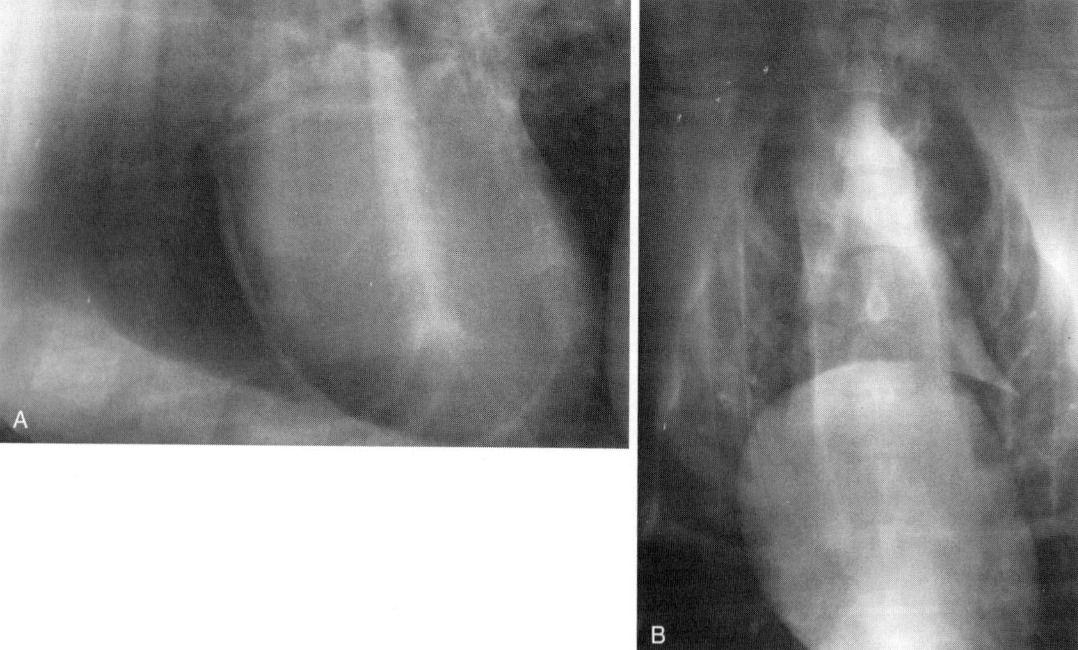

Fig. 31-7 Lateral **(A)** and ventrodorsal **(B)** radiographs of the thorax of a young normal dog. The thymus, located in the cranioventral mediastinal reflection, has not involuted. In the ventrodorsal view **(B)**, the thymus appears as a sail-shaped opacity cranial and to the left of the cardiac base. In the lateral view, the thymus produces a linear region of soft tissue opacity just cranial to the heart. The thymus may be visible in the lateral view in dogs in which it is visible in the ventrodorsal projection.

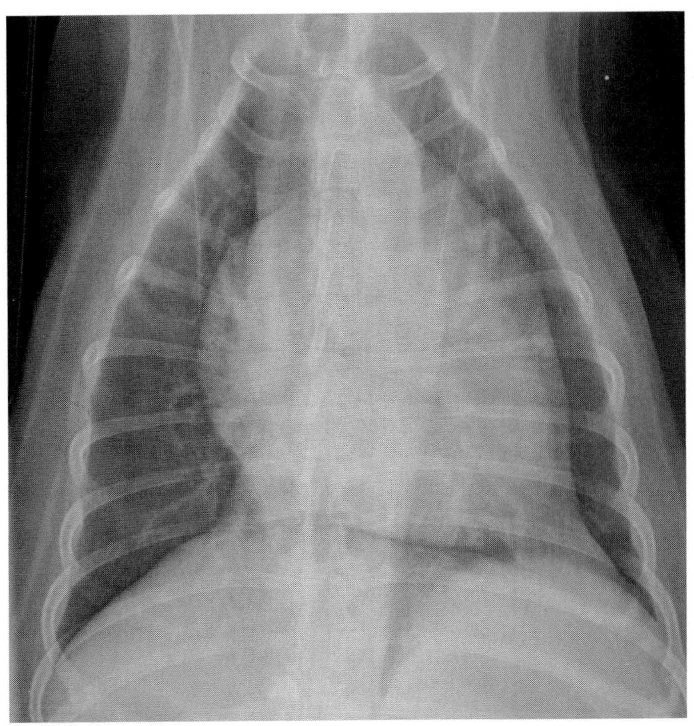

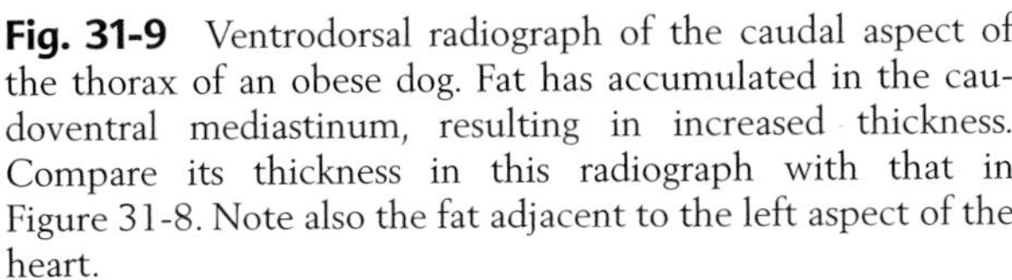

Fig. 31-9 Ventrodorsal radiograph of the caudal aspect of the thorax of an obese dog. Fat has accumulated in the caudoventral mediastinum, resulting in increased thickness. Compare its thickness in this radiograph with that in Figure 31-8. Note also the fat adjacent to the left aspect of the heart.

radiographs by noting the position of visible mediastinal organs, such as the trachea, heart (Fig. 31-10), aorta, and caudal vena cava or by analyzing the cranioventral or caudoventral mediastinal reflections (Fig. 31-11). Improper patient positioning with rotation of the sternum to the right or left will create the false impression of a mediastinal shift. Detection of a mediastinal shift is often the first clue of a thoracic abnormality.

Mediastinal Masses

Mediastinal masses are common, and their radiographic appearance is often similar. The general location of a mass within the mediastinum provides helpful information in formulating a differential diagnosis. Causes of mediastinal masses are listed in Table 31-2. The specific etiology of a mass cannot be determined radiographically; an aspirate or biopsy is usually needed.

Ventrodorsal or dorsoventral projections are usually more useful than the lateral view in deciding whether a thoracic mass is located in the mediastinum versus the lung or elsewhere. Mediastinal location of a thoracic mass should be considered if (1) the mass lies on or adjacent to the midline (Fig. 31-12), (2) the mass is in a position consistent with one of the three previously described mediastinal reflections (see Fig. 31-7), or (3) the mass deviates a mediastinal structure.

Lung masses can often be distinguished from mediastinal masses because they are usually positioned lateral to the mediastinum (Fig. 31-13), and they are more distinctly margined because of the surrounding air-filled lung. In some instances, however, mediastinal masses may protrude laterally and are sharply margined and thus mistaken for a lung mass. On the other hand, lung masses can be positioned quite medially and blend with the mediastinum, making them appear as a mediastinal mass. Radiographically distinguishing lung versus mediastinum as the source of a thoracic mass is not possible in every situation. The correct anatomic location of a thoracic mass be known before a thoracotomy is performed so that the correct surgical approach can be used.

The excellent contrast resolution of computed tomography (CT), the ability to view tomographic slices, and the availability of multiplanar reconstruction techniques, as discussed in Chapter 4, make CT a useful tool to identify the site of mass location correctly (Fig. 31-14).[5] CT is also useful for determining the relations between mediastinal masses and normal mediastinal structures, such as vessels. This latter information is of great value in surgical planning (Fig. 31-15).

The midline location of the accessory lung lobe is also noteworthy. Mass lesions of the accessory lobe will be on the midline and can be easily confused with a mediastinal mass. CT may be needed to differentiate a caudal mediastinal mass from a mass originating in the accessory lung lobe.

Cranial mediastinal masses often cause elevation of the trachea. Elevation of the trachea may also result from a large amount of pleural fluid that results in lung displacement from buoyancy (Fig. 31-16).[6] A small volume of pleural fluid does not result in tracheal elevation unless a mediastinal mass is also present. If pleural fluid is present, definitive identification of a concurrent mediastinal mass is usually not possible. However, if the mass is large enough to compress the trachea, the presence of a mass can be inferred because pleural fluid alone does not cause tracheal compression.

If pleural fluid obscures the mediastinum and a mediastinal mass is being considered, various interventions can be used: (1) The fluid can be removed and the radiographs repeated. (2) The patient can be positioned vertically and a horizontally directed x-ray beam used to obtain a ventrodorsal thoracic radiograph. These horizontal-beam radiographs take advantage of gravity, which causes pleural fluid to migrate away from the area of the suspected mediastinal mass. (3) Ultrasound or CT can be used to search for a mass in the mediastinum.[7,8] The pleural fluid provides an excellent acoustic window for sonographic examination, and ultrasound-guided aspiration or biopsy facilitates making a definitive diagnosis. Ultrasonography of the thorax is technically challenging and is best performed by an experienced sonographer.

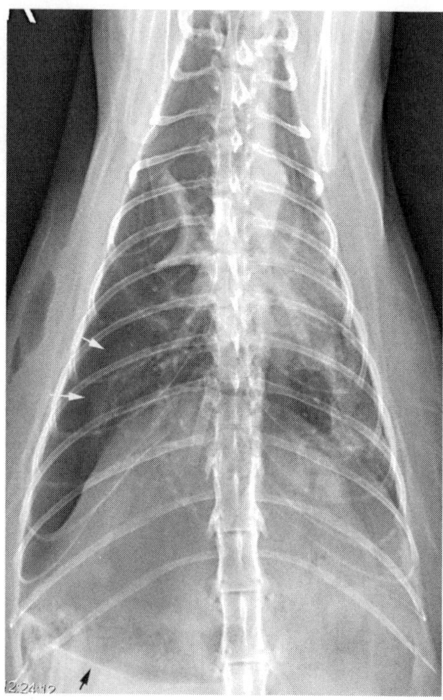

Fig. 31-10 Dorsoventral thoracic radiograph of a cat with a mediastinal shift to the left. The radiograph is acceptably positioned but the heart is displaced to the left. There is an alveolar pattern in the left caudal lobe, and the caudoventral mediastinal reflection, signified by the lobar sign between the left caudal lobe and the accessory lobe, is shifted to the left. The cardiac displacement and abnormal location of the caudoventral mediastinal reflection signify a mediastinal shift, likely due in part to atelectasis of the left caudal lobe. There is also a right-sided pneumothorax. The lung is displaced from the thoracic wall *(white arrows)* and the right side of the diaphragm is caudally displaced *(black arrow)*. The caudal diaphragm displacement is indicative of a right-sided tension pneumothorax, which is also contributing to the mediastinal shift. The mediastinal displacement away from the side of a pneumothorax is an important sign and suggests that the pneumothorax is a tension pneumothorax. The curving opacity to the right of the cranial aspect of the heart is another region of atelectasis and is not related to the mediastinal shift.

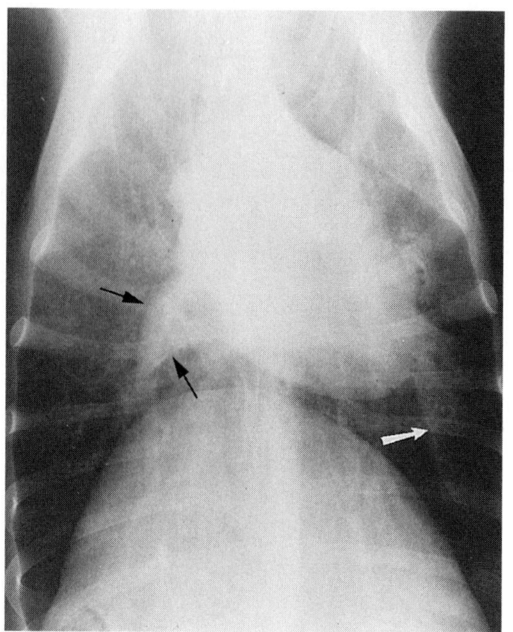

Fig. 31-11 Ventrodorsal radiograph of a dog with mediastinal shift signified by malpositioning of the caudoventral mediastinal reflection *(solid white arrow)* and heart to the left because of decreased volume of the left caudal lung lobe. The right middle lobe is collapsed *(black arrows)*, and alveolar disease is present in the left caudal lobe. The caudoventral mediastinal reflection does not appear as a distinct line, as seen in Figure 31-8, because the increased opacity of the left caudal lobe causes border effacement of the fissure itself.

Mediastinal lymph node enlargement is one of the most common causes of a mediastinal mass, and lymph node enlargement can be associated with a variety of diseases (Table 31-3). Alternatively, some neoplastic and inflammatory diseases that would logically have mediastinal lymph node enlargement often do not (Box 31-1). The major groupings of lymph nodes in the mediastinum are the cranial mediastinal lymph nodes, the sternal lymph nodes, and the tracheobronchial lymph nodes.[9,10]

The cranial mediastinal lymph nodes vary in number and size. Most of them lie along the cranial vena cava and brachiocephalic, left subclavian, and costocervical arteries just ventral to the trachea. Afferent lymphatics come from the muscles of the neck, thorax and abdomen, scapula, last six cervical vertebrae, thoracic vertebrae, ribs, trachea, esophagus, thyroid, thymus, mediastinum, costal pleura, heart, and aorta. Clinically, the cranial mediastinal lymph nodes are usually not affected by abdominal disorders. The cranial mediastinal lymph nodes also receive efferent lymphatics from the intercostal, sternal, middle, and caudal deep cervical, tracheo-

Table • 31-2

Causes of Mediastinal Masses

CAUSE OF MASS	MEDIASTINAL LOCATION
Mediastinal lymphadenopathy	Cranial, cranioventral
Sternal lymphadenopathy	Cranioventral
Hilar lymphadenopathy	Perihilar
Vascular ring anomaly (esophagomegaly)	Craniodorsal*
Neurogenic tumor	Craniodorsal or dorsal
Paraspinal tumor	Dorsal
Mediastinal abscess—usually caused by esophageal perforation	Cranioventral, caudoventral, caudal
Generalized megaesophagus	Dorsal
Spirocerca lupi	Caudodorsal
Mediastinal diaphragmatic hernia	Caudoventral
Ectopic thyroid or parathyroid tumor	Cranioventral, perihilar
Thymoma	Cranioventral
Heart base tumor	Mid-dorsal
Hiatal hernia	Caudal to caudodorsal
Diaphragmatic eventration	Caudal to caudodorsal
Hematoma	Variable, but may have a craniodorsal predilection
Mediastinal cyst (branchial cyst)	Cranioventral

*Severe esophagomegaly may appear cranioventrally.

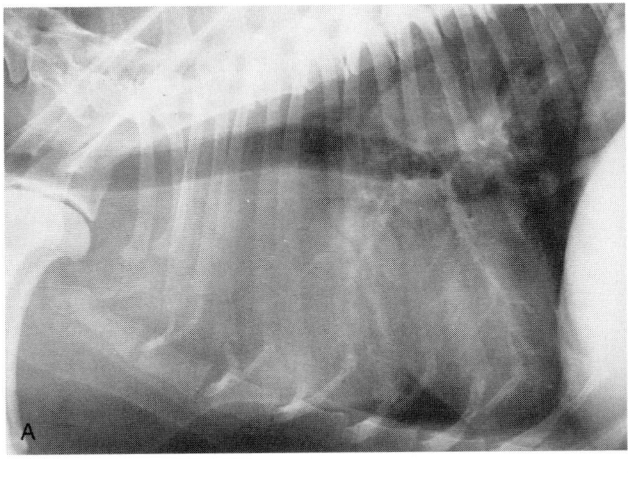

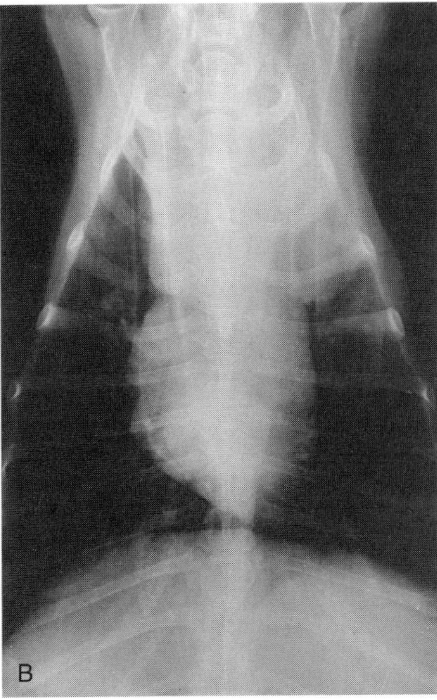

Fig. 31-12 Lateral (A) and ventrodorsal (B) thoracic radiographs of a dog with lymphosarcoma. **A,** A large mass is visible cranial to the heart. Although its position is consistent with mediastinal mass and the trachea is displaced dorsally, the exact position of the mass cannot be determined from the lateral view. **B,** The mass is centered on the midline, suggesting a mediastinal location. The imaging features would be unusual for a lung mass.

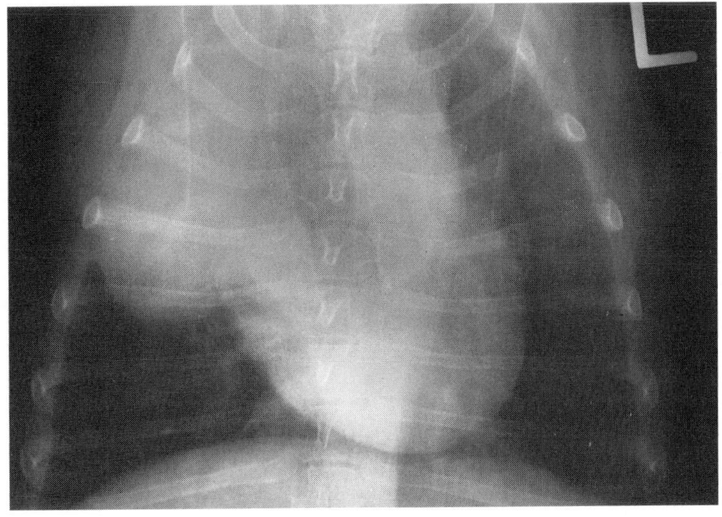

Fig. 31-13 Ventrodorsal radiograph of the thorax of a dog. A large mass is present in the right cranial hemithorax. The probability of such a mass being in the mediastinum is low because (1) the mass is located considerably lateral to the mediastinum, (2) it is not in a position of one of the mediastinal reflections, and (3) no normal mediastinal organs are displaced (the trachea is normally on the right in the cranial thorax). Diagnosis was primary lung tumor in the right cranial lung lobe.

bronchial, and pulmonary lymph nodes. Efferent channels from the tracheobronchial lymph nodes drain into either the thoracic duct or the left tracheal trunk, or both. Enlargement of the cranial mediastinal lymph nodes results in a visible mass in the cranial mediastinum that often creates a mass effect in the cranioventral thorax characterized by elevation of the trachea on the lateral view and widening of the cranial mediastinum on the ventrodorsal view (Fig. 31-17). Radiographic identification of enlarged mediastinal lymph nodes in dogs with lymphosarcoma has been identified as a negative prognostic factor with regard to response to chemotherapy.[11]

The sternal lymph node is usually represented by a single node on each side in the dog and a single node in the cat. The dog occasionally has only a single median node. The sternal node lies in the ventral mediastinum at the level of the second to third sternebra; it is cranioventral to the internal thoracic blood vessels. The afferent lymphatics of the sternal node arise in the abdominal wall and perforate the diaphragm near the middle of the costal arch. Afferent vessels receive tributaries from the ribs, sternum, serous membranes, thymus, adjacent muscles, peritoneal cavity, and mammary glands. Involvement of these nodes secondary to abdominal disease, such as peritonitis or peritoneal tumor seeding, is occasionally noted.[12] Sternal lymph node enlargement appears as an isolated soft tissue opacity dorsal to the region of the second to third sternebra and is best seen on the lateral projection, although

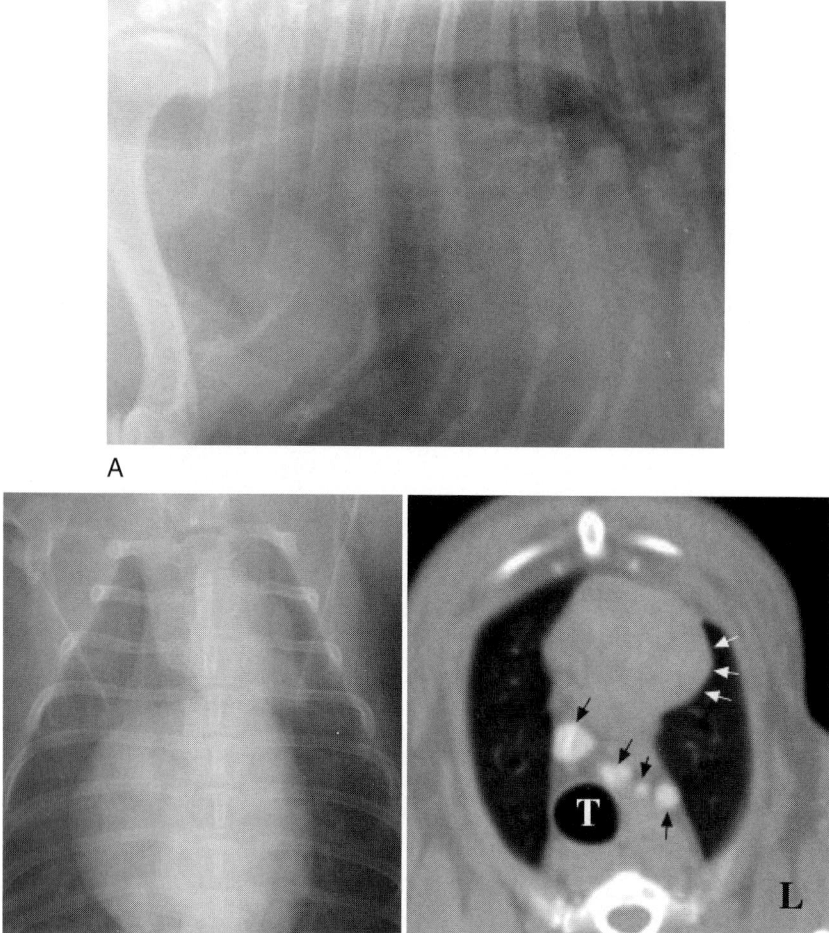

Fig. 31-14 Lateral (A) and ventrodorsal (B) radiographs of the cranial thorax of a dog. A relatively well-marginated mass is visible, signifying it may be pulmonary in origin. The mass is in the region of the medial aspect of the cranial segment of the left cranial lung lobe. However, the proximity of the mass to the midline is also consistent with it being in the mediastinum. The exact location of the mass should be known before a thoracotomy is performed because the approach would be different depending on whether the mass is pulmonary (left thoracotomy) or mediastinal (sternal splitting). **C,** Transverse CT image of the cranial aspect of the thorax (dog is in dorsal recumbency; *L,* left side). Contrast medium has been given intravenously, increasing the opacity of vessels in the mediastinum *(black arrows).* The mass is readily visible and is within the mediastinal space. Note the extension of the mass to the left *(white arrows);* this extension increases the area of the mass surrounded by lung, explaining why it appeared so well marginated in radiographs. This is a good example of a thoracic mass in which mediastinal versus pulmonary location could not be determined from radiographs. *T,* Trachea.

occasionally the mass is sufficiently large enough for the enlargement to be seen on the ventrodorsal view (Figs. 31-18 and 31-19).

The tracheobronchial lymph nodes are subdivided into the right, left, and middle tracheobronchial lymph nodes. The right and left nodes lie on the lateral side of their respective bronchus and also make contact with the trachea. The right node is ventral to the azygous vein and the left is ventral to the aorta. The middle tracheobronchial lymph node is the largest of the group. It is in the form of a V and lies in the angle formed by the origin of the primary bronchi from the trachea. Afferent vessels to the tracheobronchial lymph nodes come from the lungs and bronchi primarily, but they also come from the thoracic parts of the aorta, esophagus, trachea, heart, mediastinum, and diaphragm. Enlargement of the tracheobronchial lymph nodes results in visualization of a soft tissue opacity in the region of the tracheal bifurcation on the lateral view (Fig. 31-20). Enlargement of the tracheobronchial lymph nodes is usually more apparent on the lateral than on the ventrodorsal or dorsoventral projection. Lateral divergence or separation of the principal bronchi may be apparent on the ventrodorsal view (see Figs. 31-18 and 31-20). The conspicuity of enlarged tracheobronchial lymph nodes on the lateral view depends on their size and the amount of adjacent lung opacity. In instances in which the lymph node enlargement exists with lung disease, the lung opacity may hinder visualization of the enlarged tracheobronchial lymph nodes because of border effacement (Fig. 31-21). On the lateral

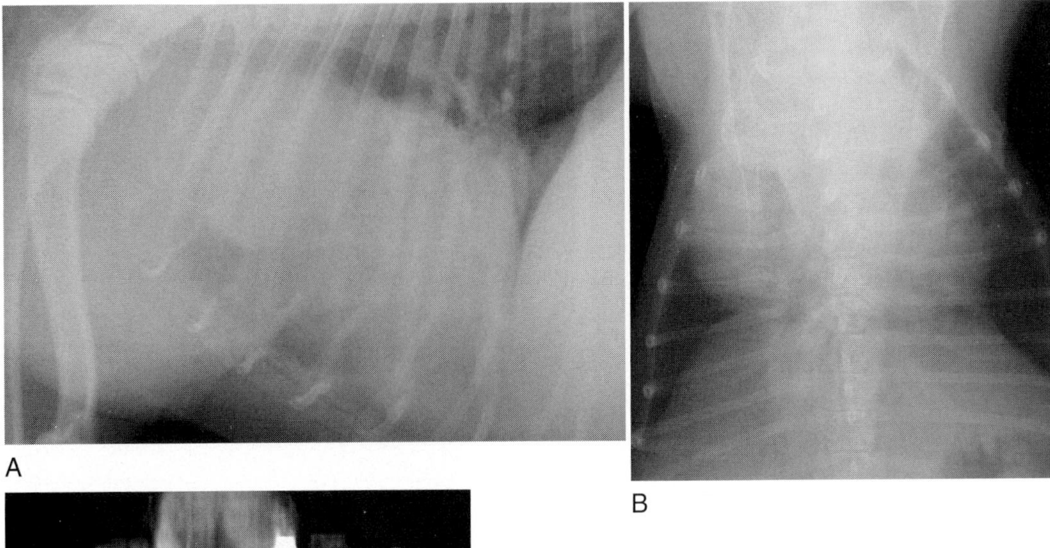

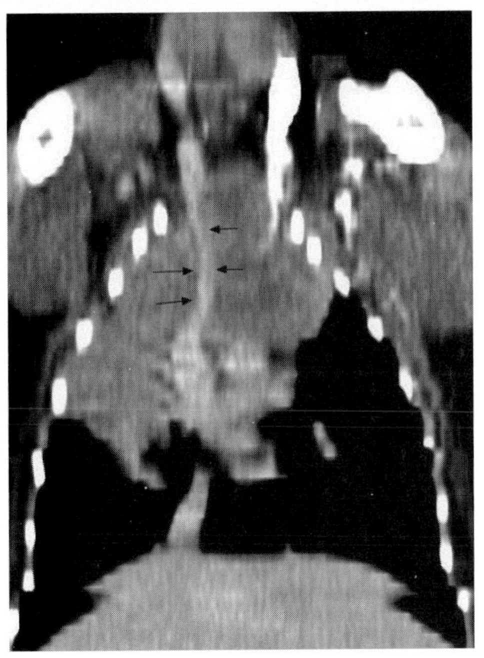

Fig. 31-15 Lateral (A) and ventrodorsal (B) radiographs of the cranial thorax of a dog with a large thoracic mass. In A the mass is causing elevation of the trachea, suggesting it is mediastinal. In B the mass has a midline component but also occupies the right cranial aspect of the thorax. This mass could be either pulmonary or mediastinal in origin, but the tracheal elevation is more consistent with it being mediastinal. From cytologic aspiration a diagnosis of thymoma was made. Surgical resection was planned. A CT study of the thorax was performed to assess the respectability of the mass. Intravenous contrast medium was administered to increase the conspicuity of vessels. In a dorsal plane image of the cranial thorax, computer reconstructed from transverse images (C), the cranial vena cava *(arrows)* is shown to be contained within the mass, indicating that surgical resection will be complicated. This is an excellent example of the value of CT to assess the feasibility of surgical resection of intrathoracic masses.

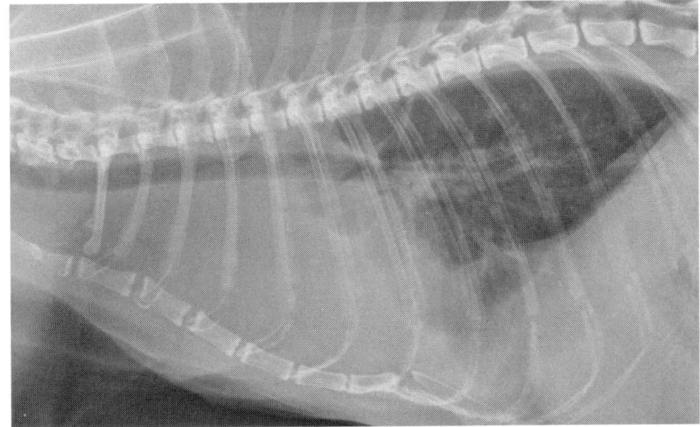

Fig. 31-16 Lateral radiograph of the thorax of a cat with pleural effusion. The trachea is displaced dorsally, but the presence of a mediastinal mass cannot be confirmed radiographically because (1) pleural fluid may be accompanied by tracheal elevation when no mediastinal mass is present because lungs float in the effusion, (2) a mass cannot be seen, and (3) the trachea is not compressed. Radiography after fluid removal, positional radiography with a horizontal x-ray beam, ultrasonography, or CT would be more sensitive for determining whether a mediastinal mass was present in this cat.

Table • 31-3

Causes of Mediastinal Lymphadenopathy

CAUSES OF MEDIASTINAL LYMPHADENOPATHY	NODES TYPICALLY INVOLVED
Lymphosarcoma (feline); lung infiltrates quite uncommon; pleural effusion may be present	Cranial mediastinal, sternal, possibly thymus
Lymphosarcoma (canine); may be accompanied by interstitial lung infiltrate	Cranial mediastinal, sternal, tracheobronchial
Pulmonary mycoses; may be accompanied by mixed lung infiltrates	Tracheobronchial
Lymphomatoid granulomatosis; usually accompanied by mixed lung infiltrates	Cranial mediastinal, sternal, tracheobronchial
Malignant histiocytosis; usually accompanied by mixed lung infiltrates	Cranial mediastinal, sternal, tracheobronchial
Spread of peritoneal inflammation or neoplasia into thorax	Sternal; pleural effusion may be present
Primary lung tumor; pulmonary mass will be present	Tracheobronchial

view, enlarged tracheobronchial lymph nodes may result in elevation, depression, or no positional change of the tracheal bifurcation. Enlarged tracheobronchial lymph nodes that result in elevation of the tracheal bifurcation may be confused radiographically with an enlarged left atrium.

Mediastinal Fluid

Free mediastinal fluid is usually of soft tissue opacity; therefore it may appear radiographically as a mediastinal mass, an enlarged cardiac silhouette if it collects around the heart, or both (Fig. 31-22). If mediastinal fluid is considered, its presence may be detected by horizontal-beam radiography (unless it is trapped or loculated) or ultrasonography. Mediastinal fluid is not commonly recognized. Some causes of mediasti-

Box • 31-1

Diseases Not Typically Associated with Mediastinal Lymphadenopathy

- Mammary adenocarcinoma
- Metastatic lung neoplasia
- Bacterial pneumonia
- Pyothorax
- Thoracic wall tumors (e.g., rib tumors)

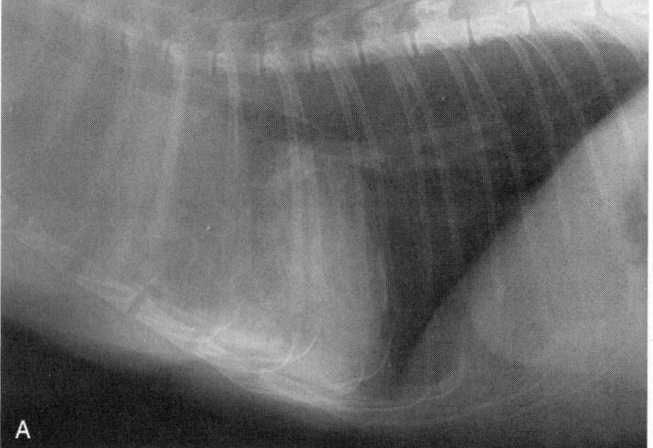

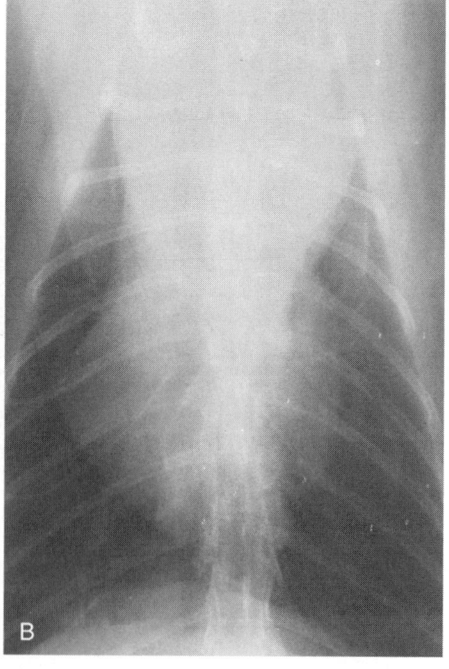

Fig. 31-17 Lateral **(A)** and ventrodorsal **(B)** thoracic radiographs of a cat with enlargement of the cranial mediastinal lymph nodes. A large, homogeneous soft tissue mass in the cranioventral mediastinum is present. The mass is elevating the trachea and displacing the cranial lung lobes laterally and caudally. In cats, distinguishing radiographically between enlargement of the cranial mediastinal lymph nodes and the thymus is nearly impossible. Diagnosis was cranial mediastinal lymphosarcoma.

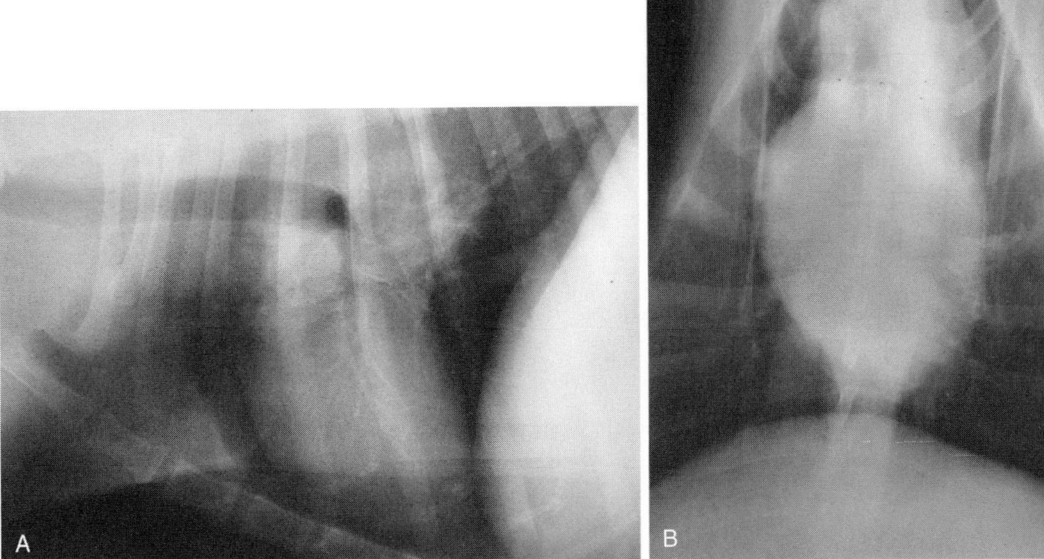

Fig. 31-18 Lateral (A) and ventrodorsal (B) thoracic radiographs of a 9-year-old Dalmatian with a history of generalized peripheral lymphadenopathy. In the lateral radiograph there is a region of soft tissue opacity just dorsal to the second and third sternebrae caused by enlargement of the sternal lymph node. An ill-defined region of increased opacity is also present around the tracheal bifurcation caused by tracheobronchial lymph node enlargement. The enlarged tracheobronchial lymph nodes have also caused elevation of the trachea just cranial to the bifurcation. Also present is a mass effect in the most cranial aspect of the cranial mediastinum that is consistent with cranial mediastinal lymph node enlargement. In the ventrodorsal view, the enlarged sternal and cranial mediastinal lymph nodes have resulted in widening of the cranioventral mediastinum, and the enlarged tracheobronchial nodes have produced lateral displacement of the principal bronchi (see Fig. 31-20). Diagnosis was lymphosarcoma.

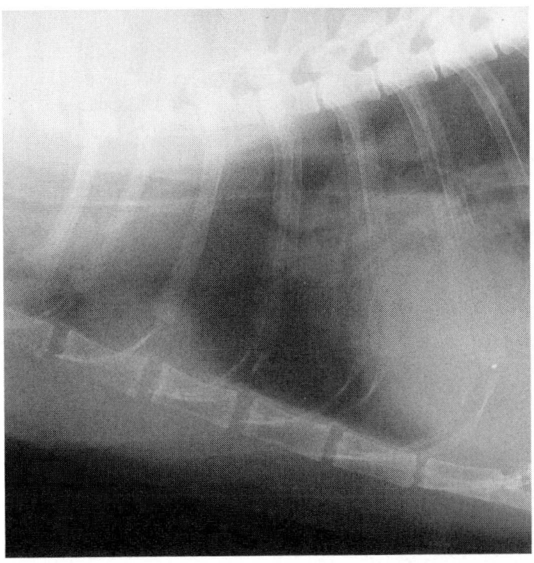

Fig. 31-19 Lateral thoracic radiograph of a cat with lymphosarcoma. A region of increased opacity is present dorsal to the third and fourth sternebrae. This opacity represents an enlarged sternal lymph node. Additionally, a linear gas opacity is present ventral to the trachea, which is consistent with pneumomediastinum. Pneumomediastinum likely occurred as a result of tracheal puncture when blood was being collected from the jugular vein.

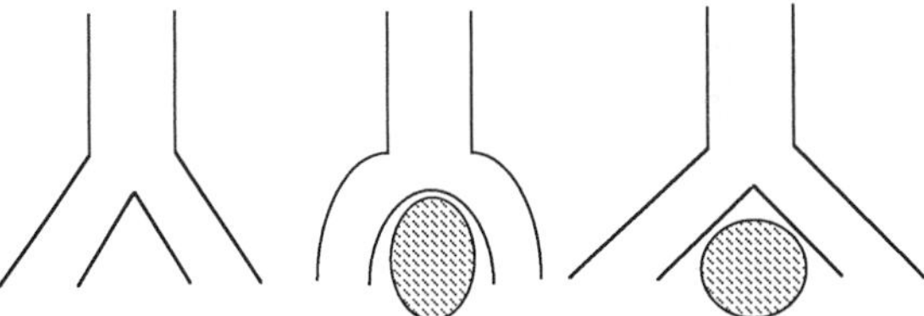

Fig. 31-20 The shape of the principal bronchi in a ventrodorsal radiograph in the normal state *(left)* and when a mass is present between them (*middle* and *right*). An enlarged left atrium or lymph node between the principal bronchi may result in the principal bronchi assuming a curved appearance *(middle)* or being displaced laterally *(right)* or both.

nal fluid are feline infectious peritonitis, trauma, and coagulopathy. Mediastinal fluid may also accumulate as a result of an underlying mass.

Pneumomediastinum

Pneumomediastinum is free gas in the mediastinum. Mediastinal gas provides excellent radiographic contrast, thereby resulting in increased conspicuity of mediastinal organs (Fig. 31-23). If only a small amount of gas is present, the only apparent abnormality may be patchy regions of radiolucency in the cranial mediastinum (see Fig. 31-19). The size of the mediastinum is not greatly increased when pneumomediastinum is present. Therefore pneumomediastinum is not

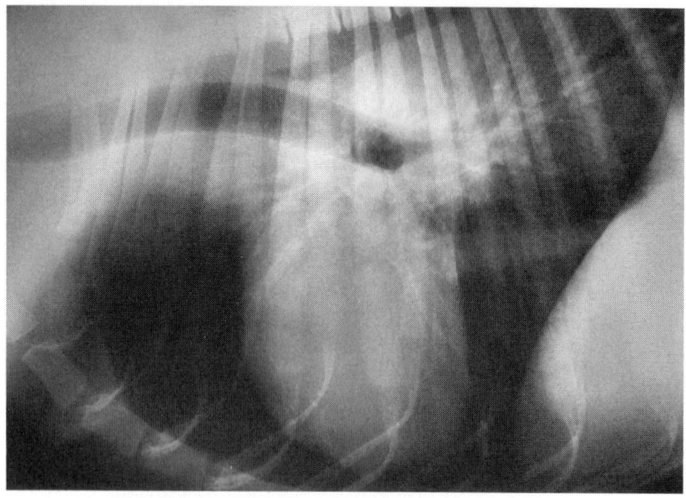

Fig. 31-21 Lateral view of the thorax of a dog with lymphosarcoma. A poorly marginated region of increased opacity is visible around the tracheal bifurcation as a result of tracheobronchial lymph node enlargement. Margins of the enlarged lymph nodes are difficult to identify because lymphoma infiltrate is present in the lung interstitium resulting in border effacement of the enlarged lymph nodes. Definitive identification of enlarged tracheobronchial lymph nodes is more difficult when lung disease is also present.

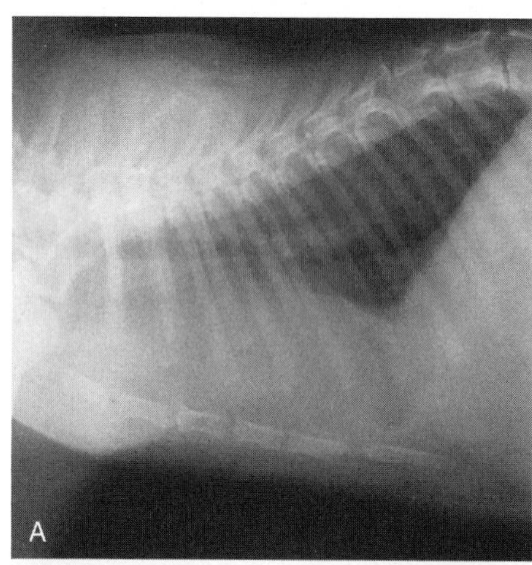

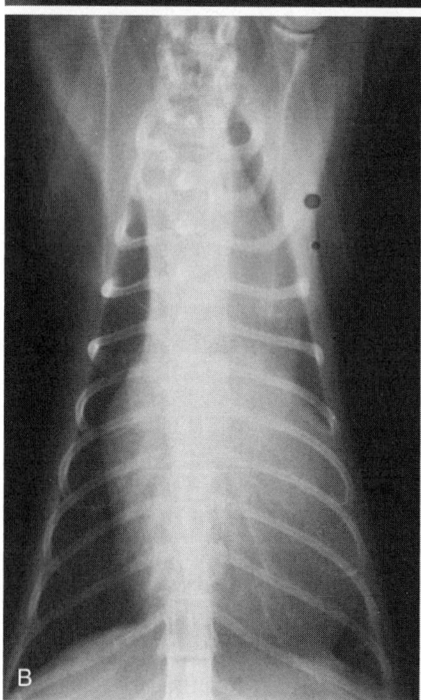

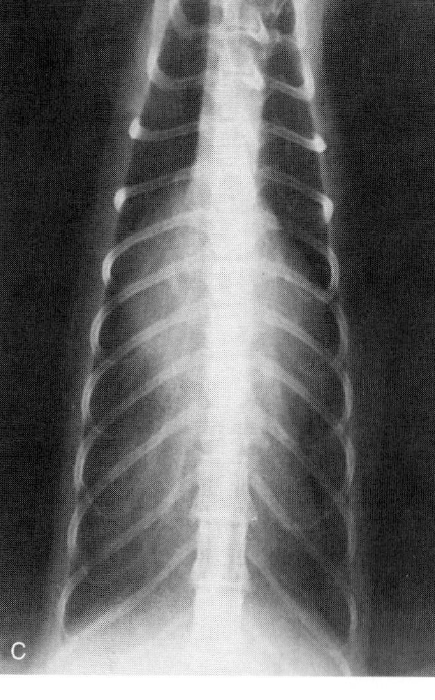

Fig. 31-22 Lateral (A), ventrodorsal (B), and horizontal-beam ventrodorsal (C) views of the thorax of a cat with mediastinal fluid. **A,** The cardiac silhouette is obscured by homogeneous opacification of the ventral thorax. **B,** The cranial mediastinum is wide, and the cardiac silhouette is enlarged with an unusual, rectangular-appearing right margin. **C,** The heart is clearly seen in the middle of the thorax, and the caudal mediastinum is increased in width from caudal gravitation of the free mediastinal fluid. Diagnosis was feline infectious peritonitis. (Reprinted from Thrall DE, Losonsky JM: Dyspnea in the cat: II. Radiographic aspects of intrathoracic causes involving the mediastinum, *Feline Pract* 8:47, 1978.)

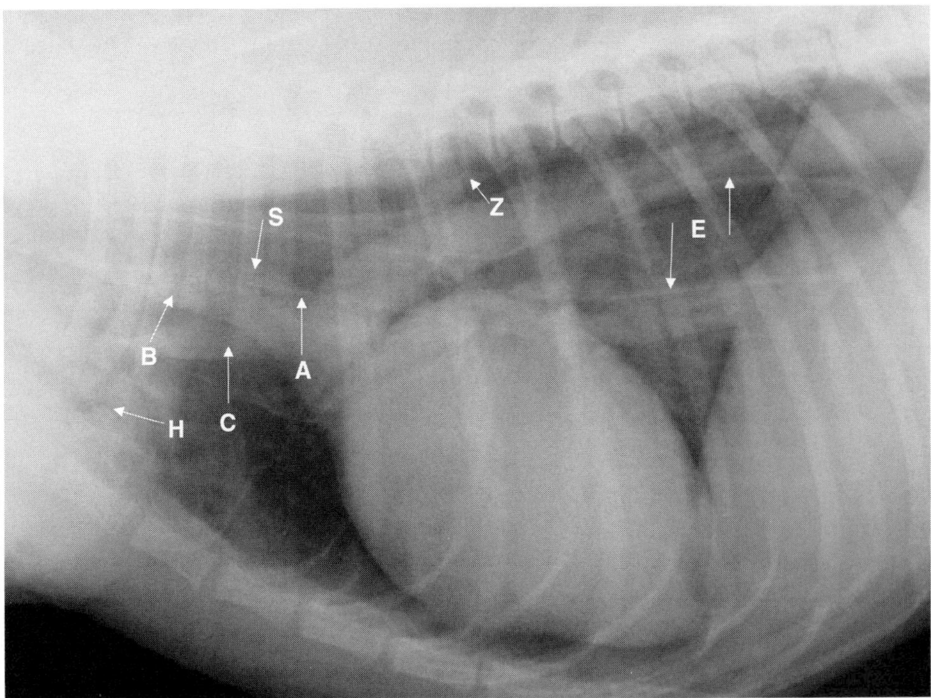

Fig. 31-23 Lateral view of the thorax of a dog with pneumomediastinum. Gas in the mediastinum leads to increased conspicuity of mediastinal organs. Note the adventitial surface of the trachea *(A)*, cranial vena cava *(C)*, brachiocephalic trunk *(B)*, left subclavian artery *(S)*, and azygous vein *(Z)*. None of these structures would be seen without the presence of the mediastinal gas. A gas-filled dilated esophagus is also present *(E)*. Gas in the ventral aspect of the cranial mediastinum creates a heterogeneous appearance *(H)*; no organs reside here to be seen as a result of the increased contrast.

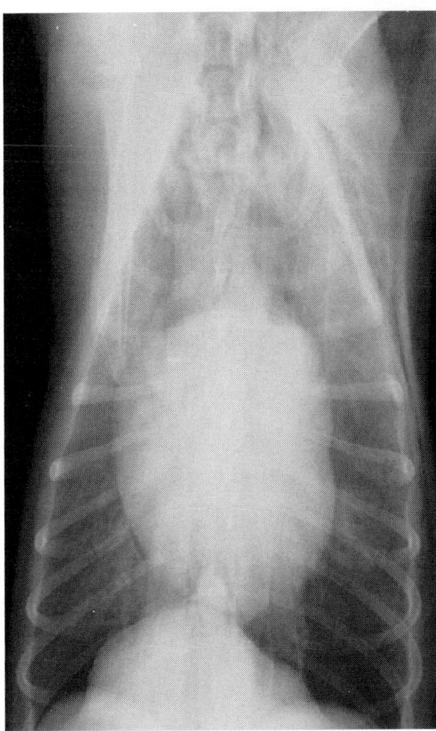

Fig. 31-24 Ventrodorsal view of the thorax of the dog in Figure 31-23. Note how the pneumomediastinum is not as conspicuous as in the lateral view. Some gas is present just to the left of the cranial thoracic spine that is likely in the mediastinum, but the increased conspicuity of mediastinal organs is not present because they are superimposed on each other and on the spine. Subcutaneous emphysema is in the left axilla.

readily seen on ventrodorsal or dorsoventral radiographs (Fig. 31-24).

Pneumomediastinum may progress to pneumothorax if mediastinal pressure results in tearing of mediastinal pleura, thus establishing communication between the mediastinum and the pleural space, or if gas dissects through fenestrations in the mediastinal pleura. On the other hand, pneumothorax does not progress to pneumomediastinum. Dyspnea usually is not seen with pneumomediastinum unless it results in pneumothorax.

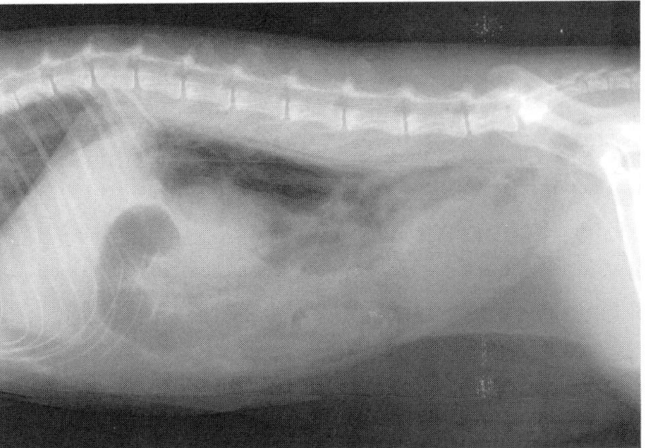

Fig. 31-25 Lateral view of the abdomen of a cat with pneumoretroperitoneum secondary to pneumomediastinum. Gas has dissected through the aortic hiatus into the retroperitoneal space.

Because of the communication of the mediastinum with the neck and retroperitoneal space, pneumomediastinum may result in subcutaneous emphysema or pneumoretroperitoneum (Fig. 31-25). Alternatively, gas in the retroperitoneal space or fascial planes of the neck may diffuse into the mediastinum.

Pneumomediastinum has the following six causes, in decreasing order of likelihood:

1. Air escaping into the lung interstitium from sites of alveolar rupture can diffuse in a retrograde direction in loose connective tissue adjacent to bronchi and vessels into the mediastinum.[13,14] This situation has been called the Macklin effect after its discoverer, and it commonly occurs after blunt thoracic trauma,[15]

such as an automobile accident, and also after iatrogenic pulmonary hyperinflation during anesthesia or resuscitation.[16] Pneumothorax is not present when pneumomediastinum results from the Macklin effect unless the pulmonary pleura becomes torn or the mediastinal air accumulation extends to the pleural space.

2. Caudal extension of gas in neck fascial planes into the mediastinum may occur. Gas in the neck is a common result of neck or oral cavity trauma.
3. A hole in the wall of the trachea may occur as a result of trauma or, less likely, erosion from neoplasia or inflammation. If the hole is intrathoracic, air enters the mediastinum directly. If the hole is in the neck, air may dissect along the trachea through the thoracic inlet into the mediastinum. Pneumomediastinum may occur after jugular venipuncture if the needle inadvertently punctures the trachea. In cattle and horses, pneumomediastinum is frequently seen after transtracheal aspiration procedures. Tracheal rupture in anesthetized cats associated with overdistention of the endotracheal tube cuff is a noteworthy cause of pneumomediastinum.[17,18] Cuff overdistention may be possible during procedures such as dental prophylaxis in which aspiration is considered likely. Cuff overdistention may cause rupture of the trachealis muscle at the point of attachment to the tracheal cartilages. Tracheal rupture may occur at a modest cuff volume and may not be immediately apparent to the anesthetist. Development of subcutaneous emphysema is concurrent with pneumomediastinum and if observed should alert the anesthetist to this potentially fatal complication of anesthesia.

Other less common causes of pneumomediastinum are (4) esophageal perforation as a result of trauma, neoplasia, or inflammation; (5) extension of retroperitoneal gas into the mediastinum; and (6) presence of a gas-producing organism.

REFERENCES

1. Schummer A, Nickel R, Sack W: *The Viscera of the domestic mammals,* ed 2, New York, 1979, Springer-Verlag.
2. Evans H: The respiratory system. In Evans H, editor: *Miller's anatomy of the dog,* ed 3, Philadelphia, 1993, W.B. Saunders.
3. Kern D, Carrig C, Martin R: Radiographic evaluation of induced pneumothorax in the dog, *Vet Radiol Ultrasound* 35:411, 1994.
4. Burk R: Radiographic definition of the phrenicopericardiac ligament, *J Am Vet Radiol Soc* 17:216, 1976.
5. Prather A, Berry C, Thrall D: Use of radiography in combination with computed tomography for the assessment of noncardiac thoracic disease in the dog and cat, *Vet Radiol Ultrasound* 46:114, 2005.
6. Snyder P, Sato T, Atkins C: The utility of thoracic radiographic measurement for the detection of cardiomegaly in cats with pleural effusion, *Vet Radiol* 31:89, 1990.
7. Reichle J, Wisner E: Non-cardiac thoracic ultrasound in 75 feline and canine patients, *Vet Radiol Ultrasound* 41:154, 2000.
8. Konde L, Spaulding K: Sonographic evaluation of the cranial mediastinum in small animals. *Vet Radiol* 32:178, 1991.
9. Bezuidenhout A: The lymphatic system. In Evans H, editor: *Miller's Anatomy of the dog,* ed 3, Philadelphia, 1993, W.B. Saunders.
10. Tompkins M: Lymphoid system. In Hudson L, Hamilton W, editors: *Atlas of Feline anatomy for veterinarians,* Philadelphia, 1993, W.B. Saunders.
11. Starrak G, Berry C, Page R, et al: Correlation between thoracic radiographic changes and remission/survival duration in 270 dogs with lymphosarcoma, *Vet Radiol Ultrasound* 38:411, 1997.
12. Hopper B, Lester N, Irwin P, et al: Imaging diagnosis: pneumothorax and focal peritonitis in a dog due to migration of an inhaled grass awn, *Vet Radiol Ultrasound* 45:136, 2004.
13. Macklin C: Transport of air along sheaths of pulmonic blood vessels from alveoli to mediastinum: clinical implications, *Arch Intern Med* 64:913, 1939.
14. Macklin M, Macklin C: Malignant interstitial emphysema of the lungs and mediastinum as an important occult complication in many respiratory diseases and other conditions: an interpretation of the clinical literature in the light of laboratory experiment, *Medicine* 23:281, 1944.
15. Wintermark M, Schnyder P: The Macklin effect: a frequent etiology for pneumomediastinum in severe blunt chest trauma, *Chest* 120:543, 2001.
16. Brown D, Holt D: Subcutaneous emphysema, pneumothorax, pneumomediastinum and pneumopericardium associated with positive-pressure ventilation in a cat, *J Am Vet Med Assoc* 206:997, 1995.
17. Mitchell S, McCarthy R, Rudloff E, et al: Tracheal rupture associated with intubation in cats: 20 cases (1996-1998), *J Am Vet Med Assoc* 216:1592, 2000.
18. Hardie E, Spodnick G, Gilson S, et al: Tracheal rupture in cats: 16 cases (1983-1998), *J Am Vet Med Assoc* 214:580, 1999.

ELECTRONIC RESOURCES evolve

Additional information related to the content in Chapter 31 can be found on the companion Web site at evolve http://evolve.elsevier.com/Thrall/vetrad/.

- Key Points
- Chapter Quiz
- Case Study 31-1
- Case Study 31-2

CHAPTER • 32
The Pleural Space

Donald E. Thrall

PLEURAL ANATOMY

As described in Chapter 31, there are two pleural sacs in the thoracic cavity, one on the right and one on the left. Each pleural sac is subdivided into mediastinal, diaphragmatic, costal, and pulmonary components. Pulmonary pleura, also called visceral pleura, covers the lung parenchyma. The mediastinal, diaphragmatic, and costal pleurae are parietal pleura. Costal parietal pleura lines the inside of the thoracic cage, diaphragmatic parietal pleura covers the diaphragm, and mediastinal parietal pleura forms the boundaries of the mediastinal space, dividing the thorax into left and right parts.

The left and right pleural sacs are distinct entities (Fig. 32-1). The pleural space is the potential space between parietal and pulmonary pleural layers, between mediastinal and pulmonary pleural layers, and between pulmonary pleural layers in interlobar fissures. The pleural space is thought of as a potential space because it normally contains only a small volume of fluid, which serves as a lubricant, but it can become a real space if it contains fluid, gas, or tissue.

NORMAL RADIOGRAPHIC APPEARANCE OF PLEURA AND PLEURAL THICKENING

Normal pleura is usually not visible radiographically. Visceral pleura outside interlobar fissures cannot be seen because it silhouettes adjacent soft tissue. Visceral pleura within intralobar fissures is surrounded by air in the lung, which provides contrast, but the pleura is so thin that it generally does not absorb a sufficient number of x-rays to produce a detectable radiographic opacity.

Opaque, thin pleural lines are sometimes noted between lobes. Thickened pleura may assume this appearance. Occasionally, however, the x-ray beam strikes normal pleura in an interlobar fissure exactly head on, resulting in absorption of a sufficient number of x-rays for the pleura to be seen (Fig. 32-2). Radiographic determination of whether isolated, thin pleural lines are normal or are due to slight pleural thickening is impossible. In either instance, such a finding is usually of no clinical significance.

When pleural thickening is advanced, wider pleural lines may be seen between lung lobes (Fig. 32-3). In pleural thickening and with pleural effusion, the specific interlobar fissures seen radiographically depend on which fissures are struck tangentially by the x-ray beam. This varies with the position of the patient relative to the x-ray beam.

PLEURAL EFFUSION

Fluid in the pleural space is pleural effusion. This fluid can be an exudate, transudate, or modified transudate (Table 32-1). The nature of the radiographic changes associated with pleural fluid depends on the volume of fluid, the position of the animal in relation to the x-ray beam, the distribution of the fluid, and whether the fluid is free or loculated.

The typical radiographic changes associated with pleural effusion are the same, regardless of fluid type, because neither the distribution of pleural fluid nor its opacity is related to the cause. Pleural fluid distributes itself according to gravity and the ability of the lung to expand, that is, lung compliance. Thus the appearance of pleural effusion in lateral, ventrodorsal, and dorsoventral radiographs made with a vertically directed x-ray beam is different.[1] Radiographic signs of free pleural fluid are listed in Box 32-1.

Interlobar Fissures, Retraction of Lung Margins and Retrosternal Opacification

The thickness and number of interlobar fissures seen with pleural fluid vary according to the amount of fluid and the relative position of the patient and the x-ray beam (Fig. 32-4). Approximately 100 mL of fluid must be present in the pleural space of a medium-sized dog before widened interlobar fissures become visible.[2] Visualization of fluid-containing interlobar fissures results when the x-ray beam strikes the fissure head on. Some fluid-containing fissures may not be seen because their relation to the x-ray beam is not head on.

With small effusions, interlobar fissures are more likely to be seen on ventrodorsal rather than dorsoventral radiographs because when in sternal recumbency, small effusions collect dorsally to the sternum and do not enter interlobar fissures or increase overall thoracic radiopacity to a sufficient degree to be seen.[2] In lateral radiographs, small effusions usually result in visualization of interlobar fissures. As the volume of fluid increases, the number and thickness of interlobar fissures, and the extent of lung retraction from the thoracic wall, increase (Figs. 32-5 and 32-6).

Other differences exist between dorsoventral and ventrodorsal radiographs when pleural fluid is present.[1] In dorsoventral radiographs, the fluid that has gravitated ventrally silhouettes the heart. In ventrodorsal radiographs, pleural fluid does not as readily obscure the heart because the fluid is distributed over a larger area in the dorsal thorax, where it does not make contact with the heart and cause border effacement (Fig. 32-7).

Lung retraction seen with pleural effusion results from fluid located between the visceral and parietal pleura. The magnitude of this separation depends on the volume of fluid present and the compliance of the lung. With normal lungs or with lungs of uniformly decreased compliance, retraction of the lungs away from the thoracic wall is uniform, and the degree of collapse is a function of fluid volume. When only a portion of the total lung volume has decreased compliance, that part of the lung retracts less than normal lung. Thus when

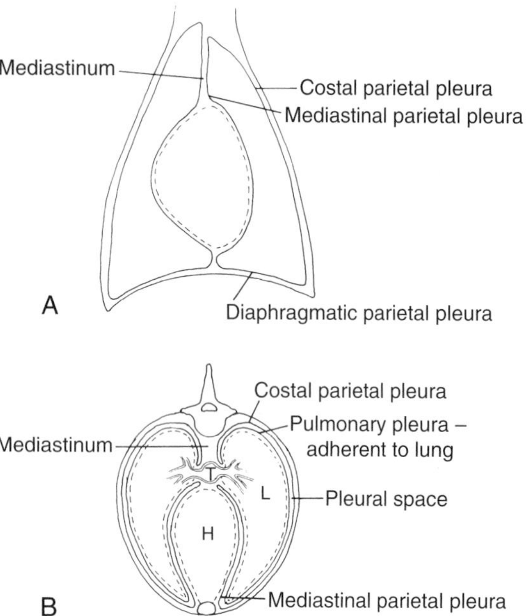

Fig. 32-1 The thorax in dorsal (A) and transverse (B) planes illustrating the relation of the pleural layers. There are two distinct pleural sacs. **A,** Note the continuity of the costal, mediastinal, and diaphragmatic parts of each parietal sac. (Lungs have not been included in **A**.) **B,** Note how the mediastinal pleura is reflected onto the lung as pulmonary pleura. In **B** the lung is depicted by the *dotted line.* Also note that the pleural space is not continuous with the mediastinum. *H,* Heart; *L,* lung; *T,* trachea.

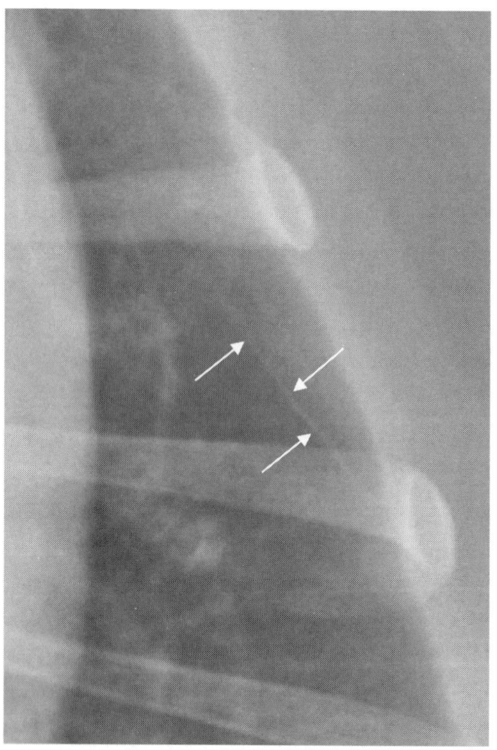

Fig. 32-2 Close-up view of a portion of the left hemithorax of a dog. A thin plural fissure can be seen *(arrows)*. Knowing whether this is caused by x-rays striking a normal fissure or if the pleural layers are slightly thickened is impossible. Clinically, this distinction is not significant.

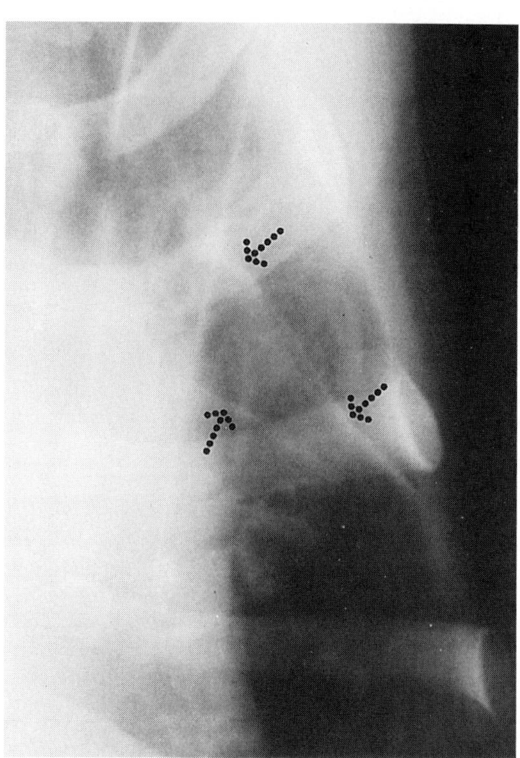

Fig. 32-3 Ventrodorsal thoracic radiograph of a dog in which interlobar fissures *(arrows)* are visible. These fissures are thicker than normal (compare with Fig. 32-2) and may be caused by either pleural thickening or a small pleural effusion. In this dog, pleural effusion was not identified when the thorax was radiographed with a horizontally directed x-ray beam. Thus the most likely cause of these fissure lines is pleural thickening.

Table • 32-1

Causes of Pleural Fluid

CAUSE	FLUID TYPE
Congestive heart failure	M
Pyothorax	E
Malignancy	M
Pneumonia	M, E
Trauma	M
Coagulation defect	M
Hypoproteinemia	T
Mediastinitis	M, E
Chylothorax	M
Diaphragmatic hernia	M

E, Exudate; *M,* modified transudate; *T,* transudate.

nonuniform retraction of lung is seen in patients with pleural effusion, underlying pulmonary disease that has altered lung compliance should be considered.

Retraction of lung from the thoracic wall can be seen on lateral, dorsoventral, and ventrodorsal radiographs (see Figs. 32-5 and 32-6). When fluid is present in the pleural space it surrounds the lung, but the fluid is most apparent radiographically when the x-ray beam strikes the fluid head on (Fig. 32-8). Therefore more pleural fluid is typically present than predicted based on the severity of the radiographic

Box • 32-1

Roentgen Signs of Free Pleural Fluid

Visualization of widened interlobar fissures; fissure is of soft tissue opacity
Retraction of pleural surface of lung away from pleural surface of thoracic wall; space between lung and thoracic wall is of soft tissue opacity
Increased soft tissue opacity dorsal to sternum on lateral radiographs; opacity frequently has scalloped margins
Blunting of costophrenic sulci
Decreased cardiac silhouette visualization in dorsoventral radiographs
Obscured diaphragmatic outline

changes because many large fluid collections are not struck head on by the x-ray beam.

In lateral radiographs pleural fluid often results in a region of homogeneously increased radiopacity dorsal to the sternum (Fig. 32-9; also see Figs. 32-5, C, and 32-6, C). This opacity results from fluid having collected in the ventral aspect of the thorax and layered against the mediastinum in the nondependent hemithorax. If the patient has a unilateral effusion and the fluid is in the dependent hemithorax, this opacity will not be visible because no fluid is layered against the mediastinum. The margin of the retrosternal opacity created by pleural effusion usually appears scalloped because of adjacent, partially collapsed lung, which alters the configuration of the fluid.

Pleural effusion may cause blunting of the costophrenic angle if fluid is present between the dorsocaudal aspect of the lung and diaphragm. In Fig. 32-5, *A*, the costophrenic angles

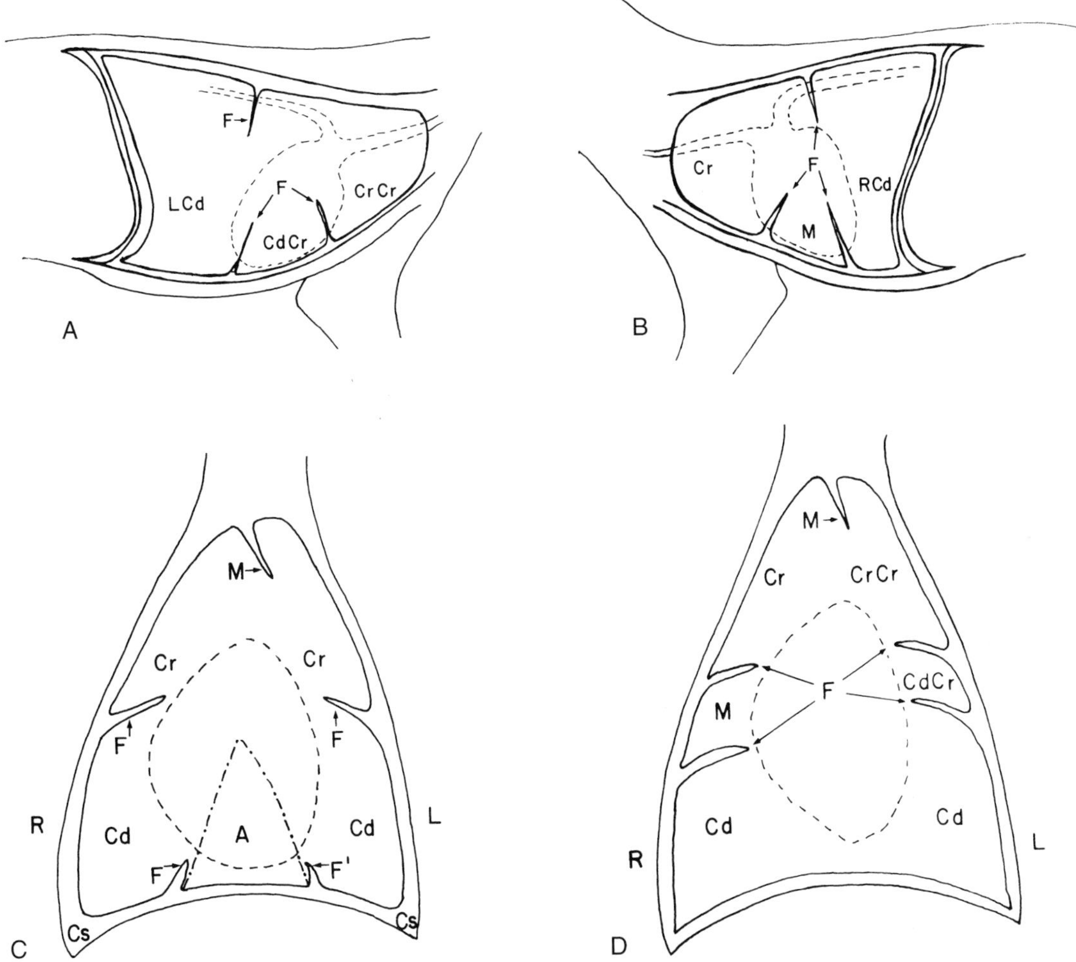

Fig. 32-4 The location of interlobar fissures in the thorax. The exact fissures visible when pleural effusion is present depend on the position of the patient, the volume of fluid, and whether the x-ray beam strikes the fissure tangentially. Only fluid-filled fissures that are struck tangentially are seen. **A,** Fissures of the lateral aspect of the left lung (looking medial to lateral). These fissures are more likely to be seen when the patient is in left recumbency. **B,** Fissures of the lateral aspect of the right lung (looking medial to lateral). These fissures are more likely to be seen when the patient is in right recumbency. **C,** Fissures on the dorsal aspect of the lungs. These fissures are more likely to be seen when the patient is in dorsal recumbency. Note that the costophrenic sulcus becomes rounded when patients with pleural effusion are in dorsal recumbency. **D,** Fissures on the ventral aspect of the lungs. These fissures are more likely to be seen when the patient is in ventral recumbency. *A*, Accessory lobe; *Cd*, caudal lobe; *CdCr*, caudal part of left cranial lobe; *Cr*, right cranial lobe; *CrCr*, cranial part of left cranial lobe; *Cs*, costophrenic sulcus; *F*, interlobar fissure; *F'*, mediastinal reflection between the left caudal lobe and the accessory lobe (pleural fluid may accumulate adjacent to this reflection); *L*, left; *M*, mediastinal reflection; *Md*, right middle lobe; *R*, right.

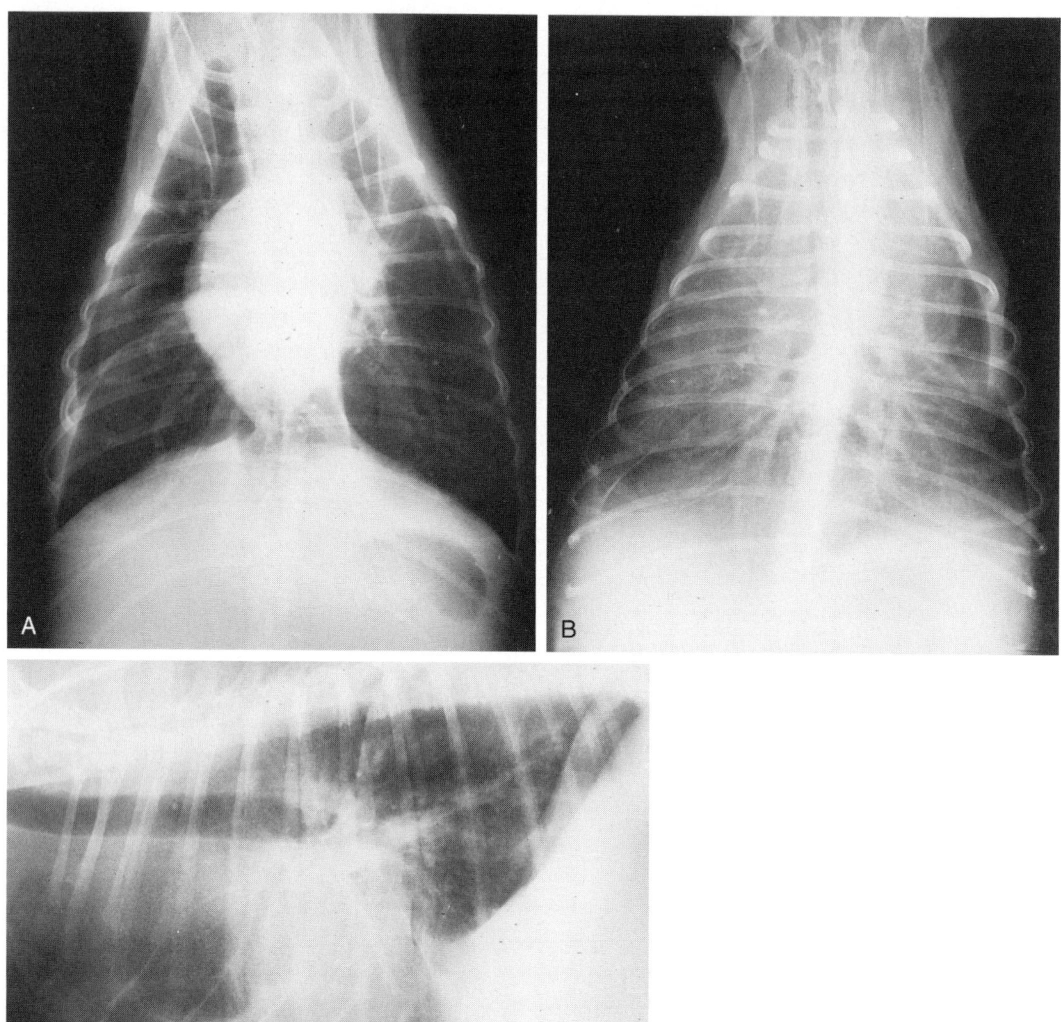

Fig. 32-5 Ventrodorsal (A), dorsoventral (B), and left lateral (C) views of the thorax of a dog with fluid in the pleural space. In the ventrodorsal view (A) there are numerous interlobar fissures, and the right caudal lobe is separated from the thoracic wall by an area of soft tissue opacity. The cardiac silhouette is visible. In the dorsoventral view (B), interlobar fissures and lung displacement away from the thoracic wall are again evident. The cardiac silhouette is not visible, the diaphragm is obscured, and the overall radiopacity of the thorax is increased (see Fig. 32-10). The left lateral view (C) shows interlobar fissures, the cardiac silhouette is partially obscured by surrounding fluid, and the overall radiopacity of the thorax is increased. In addition, an area of radiopacity is just dorsal to the sternum, the margins of which are scalloped because of fluid accumulation in the ventral thorax.

at the caudolateral aspect of the thoracic cavity are sharp, whereas in Figure 32-5, *B*, these angles are round. Rounding of the costophrenic angles will seldom be the only radiographic sign of pleural effusion, and this appearance is rarely used to diagnose pleural effusion.

Asymmetric Distribution of Pleural Fluid

Pleural fluid is usually relatively equally distributed between the right and left pleural spaces. Some patients, however, have asymmetric fluid distribution. Causes of unilateral or asymmetric pleural effusion include a difference in compliance between lung lobes, the closing of mediastinal fenestrations from inflammation or a mass, and an anatomically complete mediastinum. In extensive, unilateral effusion, identification of whether the resultant opacity is caused by a pathologic process in the pleural space, the thoracic wall, or the lung may be difficult, and sonographic or computed tomographic imaging may be necessary to resolve the question.

Pyothorax is a common cause of unilateral or asymmetric pleural effusion because of the viscid nature of the exudate (see Fig. 32-7). Chronic effusions, or inflammatory effusions, often result in extensive fibrosis of the pleura. When the visceral pleura becomes fibrotic, the margin of the retracted lung assumes a rounder shape than normal (Fig. 32-10); this

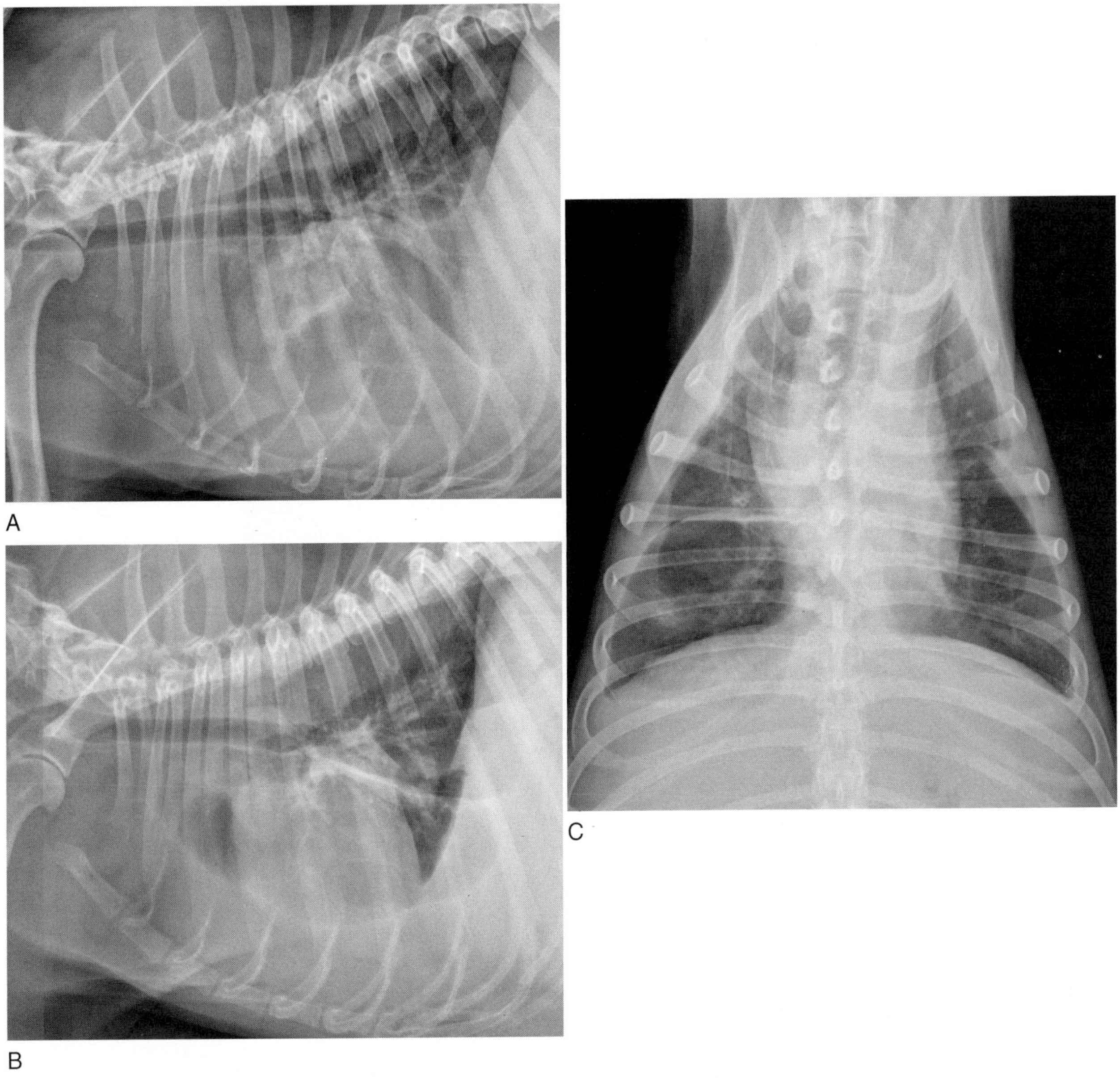

A

B

C

Fig. 32-6 Left lateral (A), right lateral (B), and ventrodorsal (C) radiographs of a dog with a large volume of fluid in the pleural space. In the ventrodorsal view (C), lungs are markedly displaced from the thoracic wall by the fluid. The heart remains visible. In the lateral views the fluid has obscured much of the normal thoracic detail. The pleural fluid makes it unreliable to assess the lungs or mediastinum. This volume of fluid could obscure a large mass in the thorax. The ribs should always be carefully scrutinized in patients with pleural effusion to ensure that the fluid is not the result of a rib tumor. Thoracic ultrasonography or computed tomographic imaging may be helpful in deciding if underlying mass lesions are present.

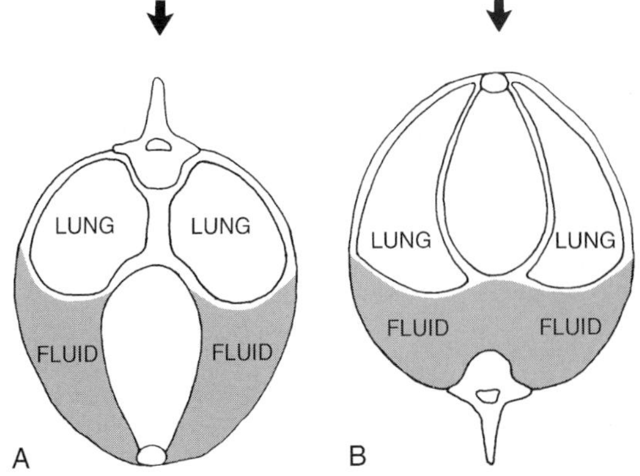

Fig. 32-7 The effect of dorsal versus ventral recumbency on the radiographic appearance of pleural effusion. A, The patient is in ventral recumbency, and fluid gravitates ventrally. The fluid is in contact with the heart, thus obscuring the heart from view. When the patient is placed in dorsal recumbency (B), the fluid gravitates dorsally and is not in contact with the heart; thus the cardiac silhouette is visible. The absolute depth of the fluid is greater when the patient is in ventral recumbency (A) because the ventral part of the thoracic cavity is narrower and the fluid rises to a higher level. Thus overall thoracic radiopacity is greater when the patient is in ventral recumbency.

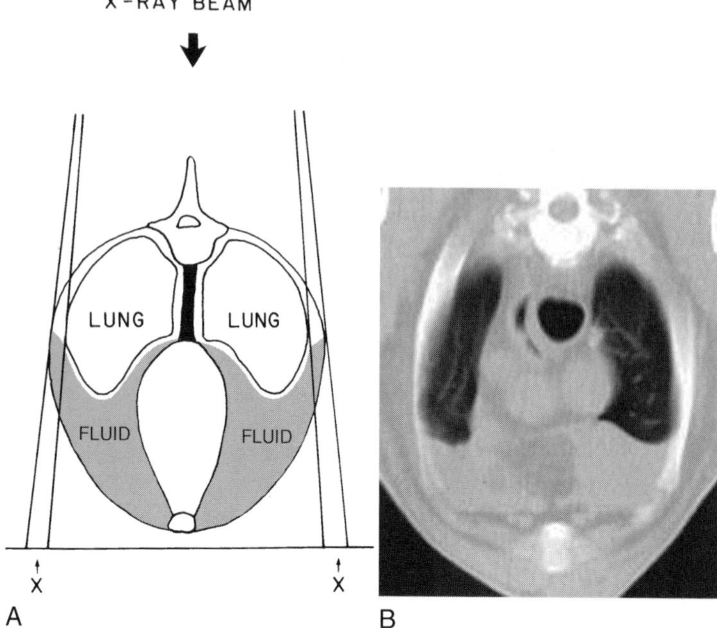

Fig. 32-8 Principle of lung retraction as a result of pleural effusion. **A,** Diagram of a patient with a large amount of pleural fluid being radiographed in ventral recumbency. Fluid has therefore gravitated ventrally, resulting in dorsal displacement of the lung. Extensive dorsal displacement of the ventral aspect of the lung has occurred, but this is not apparent radiographically because the fluid ventral to the lung has not been struck tangentially by the x-ray beam. The only apparent lung retraction is in the regions indicated by *x* because here fluid between the lung and thoracic wall is struck tangentially by the x-ray beam. In the region between the *x*'s, thoracic radiopacity is increased, the heart is obscured, and pulmonary vessels in the partially collapsed lung are visible. (Compare this figure with Fig. 32-5, *B*). **B,** Computed tomographic image of a dog with pleural effusion. This transverse image was acquired at the level of the second thoracic vertebra. Fluid in the ventral aspect of each pleural cavity is causing dorsal displacement of the lung. However, none of the fluid is in a position to be hit "unobstructed" by an oncoming dorsal or ventral x-ray beam. Thus although this fluid may cause some overall increase in opacity in the thoracic radiograph, no interlobar fissures or lung retraction will be seen because the fluid volume is insufficient.

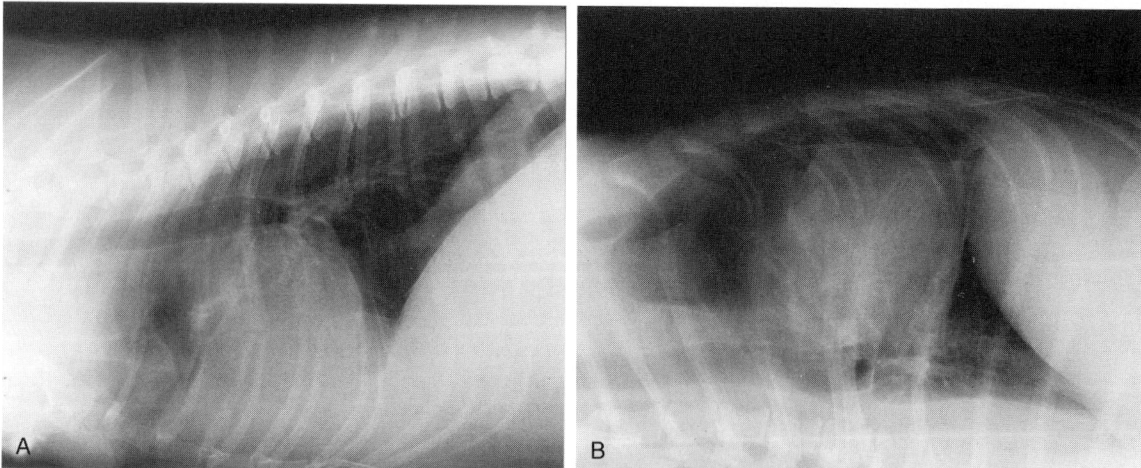

Fig. 32-9 Right lateral (A) and horizontal-beam lateral (dorsal recumbency) (B) radiographs of a dog with pleural effusion. In the right lateral radiograph (A) the opacity is dorsal to the sternum; this finding is consistent with pleural fluid but may also be caused by a mass. In the ventrodorsal view (not shown) there was only minimal evidence of pleural effusion. To clarify the significance of the opacity, the horizontal-beam view was made (**B**). The fluid has gravitated dorsally and is adjacent to the spine, separating the lung from the thoracic wall. An opacity adjacent to the sternum is no longer present. Thus the opacity seen in **A,** dorsal to the sternum, was fluid. Note that no sharp horizontal fluid line is present. Horizontal fluid lines are seen in horizontal-beam radiographs only when there is a free gas-free fluid interface. In **B** the contour of the fluid is conforming to the shape of the partially collapsed lung.

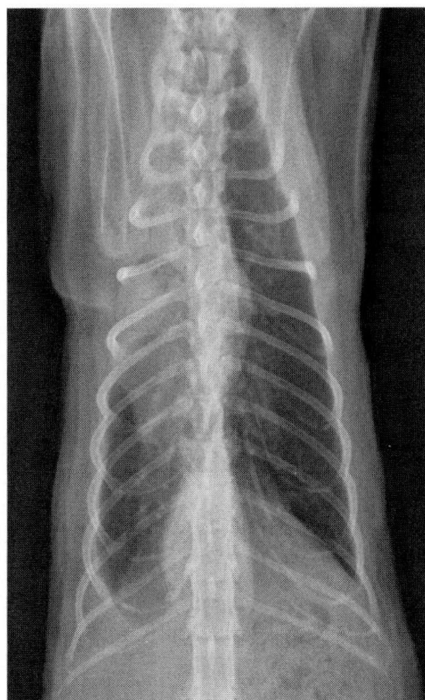

Fig. 32-10 Ventrodorsal thoracic radiograph of a cat with asymmetric pleural fluid. Retraction of the right caudal lobe from the thoracic wall is visible, signifying pleural effusion. Opacification of the cranial aspect of the right hemithorax is visible; whether this represents additional asymmetric fluid, lung opacification, or a mass cannot be ascertained from this radiograph. Additional imaging such as ultrasound or computed tomography would be necessary for this determination. Nevertheless, asymmetric pleural fluid is present, and the margin of the right caudal lung lobe also appears round. These findings are most consistent with pyothorax and pleural thickening. The viscid nature of the exudate in the pleural cavity prevents it from crossing the mediastinum, or perhaps the mediastinal fenestrations are closed because of pleuritis. The rounding of the right caudal lobe is most likely from constrictive visceral pleuritis caused by the pyothorax. Although pyothorax cannot be diagnosed with certainty from radiographs, the findings in this patient are most consistent with this diagnosis.

appearance is highly suggestive of markedly fibrotic pleuritis, as often accompanies pyothorax.

Horizontal-Beam Radiography

Identification of small effusions may not be possible on survey radiographs if the x-ray beam fails to strike a fluid accumulation tangentially (see Fig. 32-8, *B*). To enhance fluid detection, a horizontally directed x-ray beam may be used to ensure a head-on relation between the x-ray beam and the fluid collection. If free pleural fluid is present, it gravitates dependently to the site where the x-ray beam strikes it head on (Fig. 32-11).

A sharply demarcated, straight fluid line is not seen in patients with pleural fluid when radiographed with a horizontal x-ray beam because the configuration of the fluid is altered by the adjacent lung, which retracts because of elastic recoil. Sharp fluid lines are seen in horizontal-beam radiographs only when a free fluid–free gas interface exists. Horizontal-beam radiographs may be useful in distinguishing pleural fluid from an intrathoracic mass as the cause of an intrathoracic opacity (Fig. 32-12; also see Fig. 32-9).

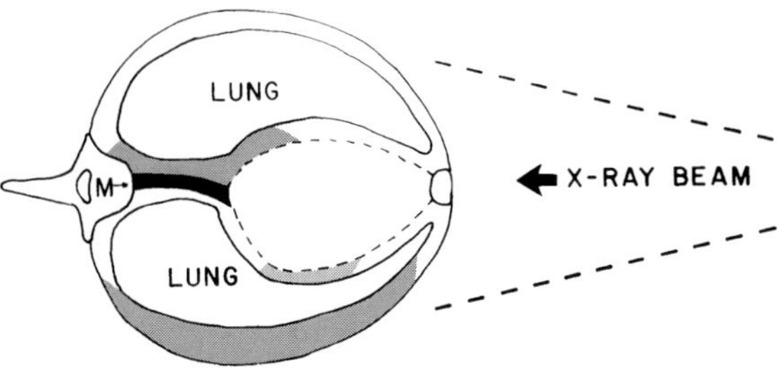

Fig. 32-11 The principle of using a horizontal-beam radiograph to detect pleural effusion. Fluid is represented by *gray stippled areas.* Fluid in the nondependent hemithorax layers against the mediastinum (assuming the mediastinum is complete). This fluid (nondependent side) is not radiographically detectable. Fluid in the dependent hemithorax gravitates to the area between the lung and the thoracic wall, where the horizontally directed x-ray beam strikes it tangentially. *M,* Mediastinum.

Pitfalls in Pleural Fluid Diagnosis

An erroneous radiographic diagnosis of pleural fluid sometimes is made. Thickened pleura may have an appearance identical to pleural fluid (see Fig. 32-3). A distinction may be made by using a horizontally directed x-ray beam.

Mineralized costal cartilage is sometimes confused with pleural effusion. Their position is similar, but the concave surface of costal cartilage is directed cranially, whereas the concave surface of fluid-filled fissures is directed caudally (Fig. 32-13).

Thoracic wall deformities, such as those seen in chondrodystrophoid breeds, may result in increased radiopacity at the margin of the lung field. Without knowledge of this fact, the opacity may be incorrectly misinterpreted as retraction of the lung from the thoracic wall because of pleural fluid (Fig. 32-14).

Significance of Pleural Fluid

Pleural fluid may result from a primary pleural disorder, such as pleural neoplasm, but most often it is a sign of disease elsewhere. Determining the cause of pleural effusion from radiographs is usually impossible. When pleural fluid is present, structures are obscured and extremely large lesions can go unidentified.

When pleural fluid is identified, careful scrutiny of the radiograph is necessary. Subtle radiographic findings such as a rib lesion or asymmetric distribution of the fluid are occasionally noted, which can be of great help in the evaluation of the patient. In patients with a large amount of pleural effusion, the indiscriminate approach of using a horizontally directed x-ray beam with various patient positions to search for other lesions is unrewarding and should not be done. However, making additional radiographs after some of the fluid has been removed may provide important information. Sonographic and computed tomographic imaging of the thorax may also be helpful in elucidating the cause of intractable pleural effusions. Thoracic sonography is technically challenging, and a high skill level is needed for this imaging test to be accurately interpreted.

All pleural effusions are clinically significant, and attempts should be made to reach a definitive diagnosis. Small effusions may not result in abnormal clinical signs, whereas large effusions usually result in dyspnea because of secondary atelectasis. However, small effusions should not be assumed to be less significant than large ones. Thoracocentesis with appropriate fluid analysis should be considered when pleural fluid is identified.[3]

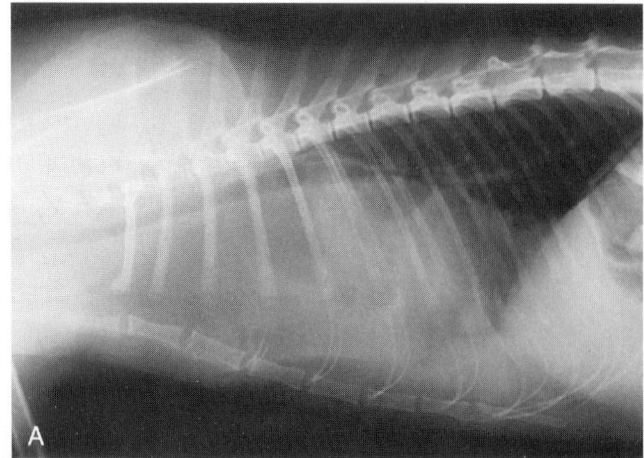

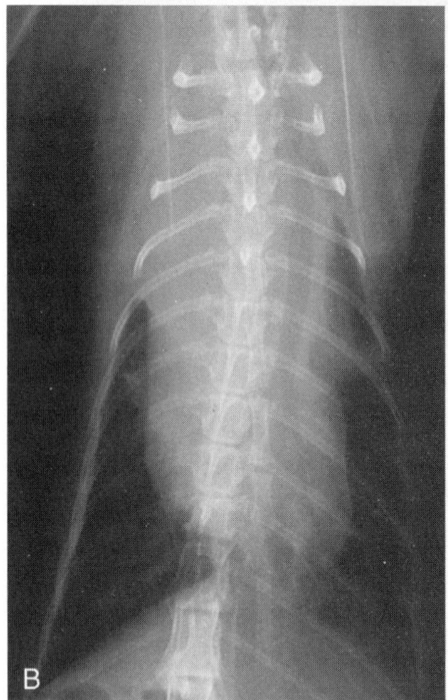

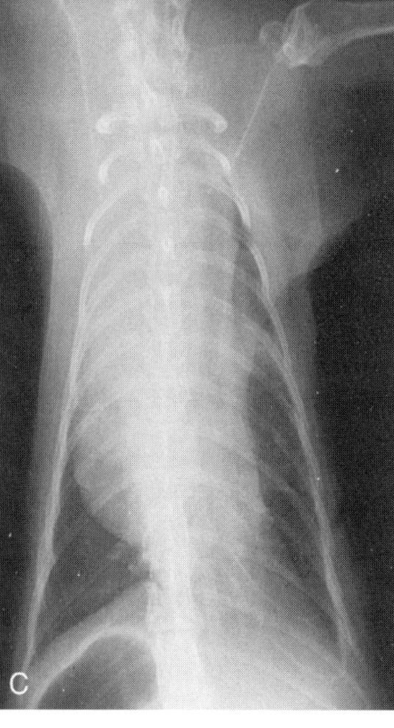

Fig. 32-12 Lateral (A), ventrodorsal (B), and horizontal-beam ventrodorsal (C) (patient supported in upright position) views of the thorax of a cat. In the lateral view (A) there is opacification of the cranial aspect of the thorax. The heart is obscured, suggesting adjacent fluid or a mass. Circular radiolucencies are air bubbles from prior thoracocentesis; a small volume of fluid was removed for cytology. In the ventrodorsal view (B), the cranially located opacity is visible and is on the midline; these findings are consistent with a mediastinal mass. To rule out the possibility that the cranial thoracic opacity was fluid and not a mass, however, a horizontal-beam radiograph (C) was made. The opacity has not moved, suggesting that it is a mass. However, the caudoventral mediastinal reflection has increased in thickness; this is consistent with coexisting mediastinal fluid that has gravitated caudally. No evidence of pleural effusion exists.

Simultaneous Pleural and Peritoneal Effusion

Simultaneous pleural and peritoneal effusions occasionally are detected. In one study, 32 of 48 dogs with simultaneous peritoneal and pleural effusion had either neoplastic or cardiovascular disease. Simultaneous pleural and peritoneal effusion is an indicator of severe disease with poor prognosis.[4]

PNEUMOTHORAX

Gas in the pleural space is termed pneumothorax. Air can enter the pleural space from the outside or from the lung or mediastinum (Box 32-2). The character of the radiographic changes resulting from gas in the pleural space depends on the volume of gas and the relative position of the patient and the x-ray beam. Roentgen signs of pneumothorax are listed in Box 32-3.

Box 32-2

Causes of Pneumothorax

- Trauma
- Tear in lung involving visceral pleura
- Thoracic wall rent
- Extension of pneumomediastinum
- Rupture of cavitary lung mass

Lung Retraction from Pneumothorax

Retraction of the lung from the thoracic wall because of gas in the pleural space can be seen in lateral, ventrodorsal, and dorsoventral radiographs. With a small volume of pleural air, this separation is small and may appear as a fine radiolucent line (Fig. 32-15). As in pleural effusion, air surrounds the lung but is most apparent radiographically when the air is struck head on by the x-ray beam (see Fig. 32-15). Visualization of gas-containing interlobar fissures is not common with pneumothorax because gas usually does enter the fissures of the collapsed lung.

Pneumothorax results in lung collapse because of the elasticity of the lung and the increased pleural space pressure. As lung volume decreases, the lung contains less air and becomes more radiopaque (Fig. 32-16). The degree of increased opacity

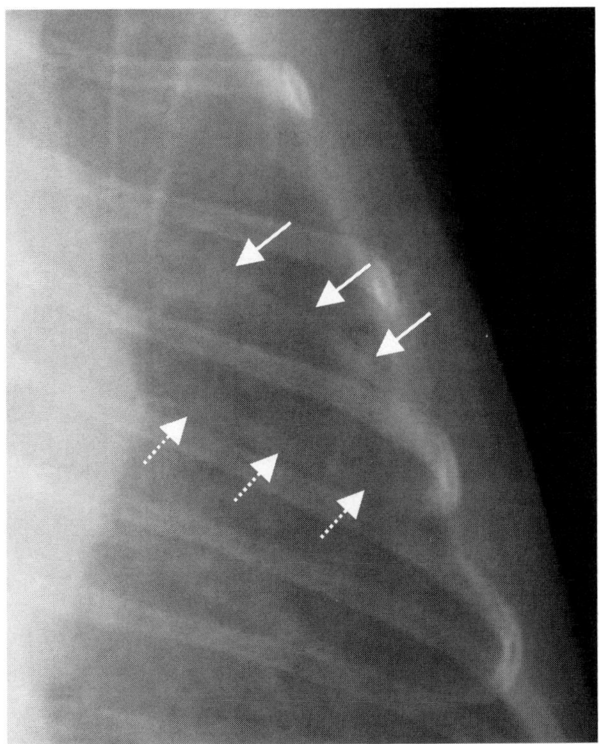

Fig. 32-13 Ventrodorsal radiograph of a dog with pleural effusion. An interlobar fissure is visible *(solid arrows)*. A mineralized costal cartilage is also visible *(dotted arrows)*. Note the similar opacity. For the interlobar fissure, however, the concave surface faces caudally, whereas for the costal cartilage the concave surface faces cranially.

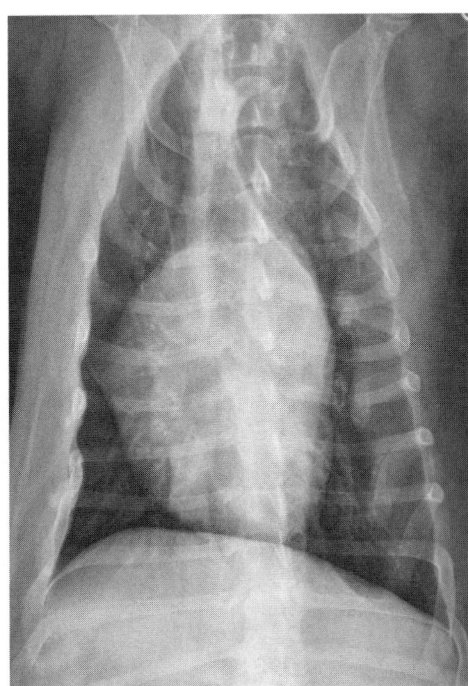

Fig. 32-14 Ventrodorsal view of the thorax of a normal Basset Hound. The sternum is displaced slightly to the left. An area of soft tissue opacity medial to the left thoracic wall is present. This is an artifact created by the irregular thoracic wall configuration in this chondrodystrophic dog. The opacity on the left is caused by the prominent costochondral region; rotation of the patient resulted in its being located at the periphery of the thorax. The location and appearance of this opacity may result in its being confused with pleural effusion; however, interlobar fissures are not seen.

Box • 32-3

Radiographic Signs of Pneumothorax

- Retraction of pleural surface of lung away from pleural surface of thoracic wall; space between lung and thoracic wall is radiolucent
- Lung markings do not extend all the way to thoracic wall
- Lung has increased opacity because of collapse
- Appearance of dorsal displacement of the heart on the lateral view

is directly related to the degree of collapse, and the increased opacity will likely interfere with radiographic evaluation of the lung parenchyma. The pulmonary collapse is also responsible for the lack of visible lung markings extending to the periphery of the thoracic cavity, which is another radiographic sign of pneumothorax.

If the pneumothorax is open, that is, with no valve at the site of gas entrance, gas may continue to enter the pleural space until pleural pressure equals atmospheric pressure. At this point, the lung is maximally collapsed but still maintains roughly the shape of a normal lung because of its elasticity.

"Elevation" of the Heart from the Sternum

Separation of the heart from the sternum is commonly seen in lateral radiographs of patients with pneumothorax (see Fig. 32-15). However, the heart is not actually elevated but displaced into the dependent hemithorax because of a lack of underlying inflated lung to support the heart in its normal midline position. As the heart falls into the dependent hemithorax, it slides dorsally, creating the appearance of elevation when seen on a lateral radiograph (Fig. 32-17). Although pneumothorax is the most common cause of the appearance of elevation of the cardiac silhouette on the lateral view, this radiographic sign has also been seen with decreased heart size, in normal dogs with extremely deep thoracic cavities, and in patients with hyperinflated lungs.

As with pleural effusion, diagnosis of pneumothorax may not be possible from survey radiographs. The likelihood of diagnosing pneumothorax is increased by using a horizontally directed x-ray beam and placing the patient in a position such that the x-ray beam strikes the area of air accumulation head on, such as in lateral recumbency. Decreasing the milliampere seconds by 50% enhances visualization of the air in the horizontal-beam radiograph by rendering the lung more opaque (see Fig. 32-15, C). Justification for use of horizontal-beam radiography to detect pneumothorax should be based on the suspected underlying cause. For example, a pneumothorax resulting from lung disease is a potentially serious event,[5,6] whereas a small pneumothorax occurring after trauma with no associated clinical signs may not be significant.

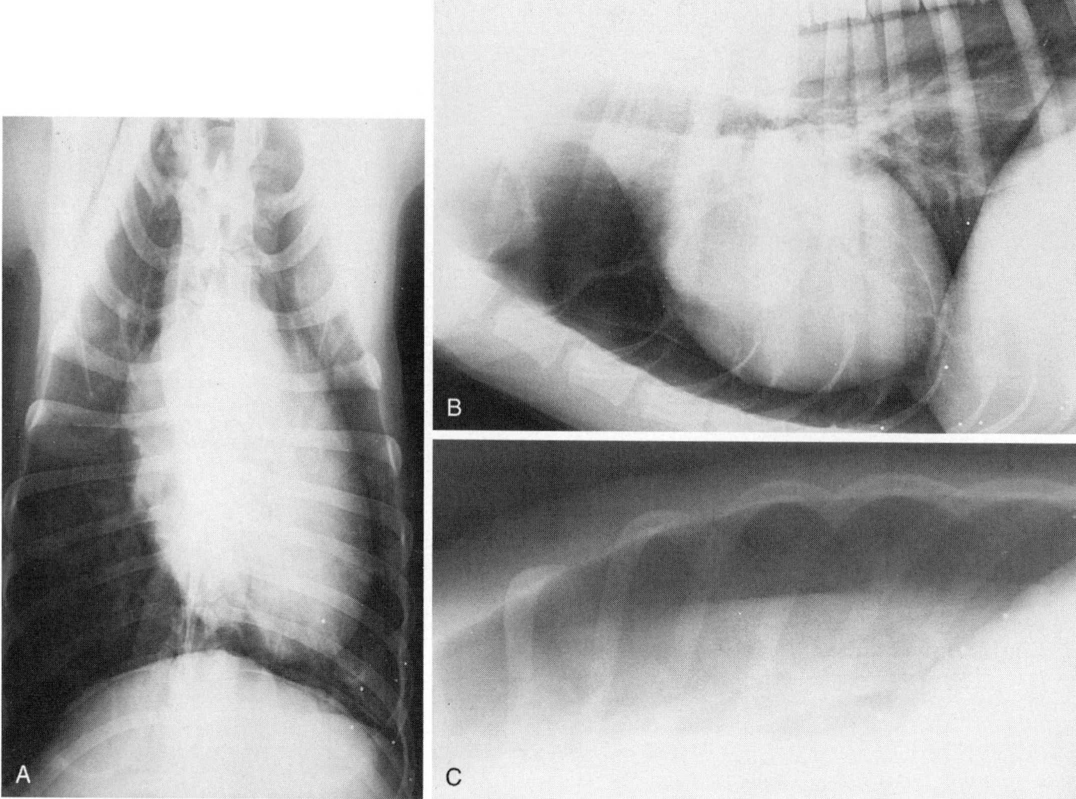

Fig. 32-15 Ventrodorsal (A), left lateral (B), and right lateral recumbent horizontal-beam (C) radiographs of a dog with pneumothorax. In the ventrodorsal view (A) the heart is shifted to the left, but evidence of pneumothorax is not seen because the air has accumulated ventral to the sternum, where it is not struck tangentially by the x-ray beam. A linear region of gas is medial to the right scapula and an area of hemorrhage is in the left caudal lobe. In the right lateral view (B) there is a thin radiolucent line between the diaphragm and a caudal lobe from gas in the pleural space. The heart is separated from the sternum, and a radiolucent area is present between the sternum and the heart. Opaque interlobar fissures extend caudoventrally from the carina and are superimposed on the cardiac apex region because of concurrent pleural effusion. In the horizontal-beam radiograph, the extent of pneumothorax is readily apparent and is larger than would have been predicted from the conventionally positioned radiographs. By placing the patient in right recumbency and using a horizontally directed x-ray beam, air in the left hemithorax was struck tangentially by the x-ray beam. The radiographic mAs was decreased by 50% to facilitate air visualization by rendering the lung more radiopaque.

Some Facts about Pneumothorax

Some attention has been given to identifying the radiographic view with the greatest sensitivity for detection of pneumothorax. In a study of induced pneumothorax, the vertical-beam left lateral recumbent and the horizontal-beam ventrodorsal views had the greatest sensitivity for pneumothorax detection. The right lateral view was most sensitive for assessing differences in the amount of air in the pleural space.[7] Pneumothorax has also been suggested to be easier to detect in dorsoventral radiographs than in ventrodorsal radiographs.[8]

In most animals pneumothorax is bilateral, and this relates either to a bilateral source of pleural air or to movement of air through the mediastinum. Results from a study of induced pneumothorax suggest that air can readily move through the mediastinum because bilateral pneumothorax was observed in 22 of 24 dogs in which a unilateral pleural space injection of air occurred.[7] Unilateral pneumothorax, however, can occur for the same reasons as unilateral pleural effusion.

Some variability regarding the appearance of unilateral pneumothorax exists in lateral radiographs, depending on whether the affected side is dependent or nondependent. Unilateral pleural space air will often be more apparent if the affected side is nondependent because the air collects around the dorsocaudal portion of the caudal lobe. In this situation, the air collection is struck head on by the x-ray beam. If the affected side is dependent, the air may collect against the mediastinum and is not struck head on by the x-ray beam (Fig. 32-18).

Tension Pneumothorax

Tension pneumothorax occurs when pleural space pressure exceeds atmospheric pressure during both phases of respiration. Tension pneumothorax results from a check-valve mechanism at the origin of pleural space gas. In tension pneumothorax, the increased pleural pressure causes the lung to collapse to a greater degree than its maximal collapse in an open pneumothorax. Thus, it may no longer maintain the shape of a lung but may assume the appearance of an amorphous opacity compressed against the midline. With unilateral tension pneumothorax, the increased pleural space pressure tends to cause a contralateral mediastinal shift. Tension pneumothorax may also result in caudal displacement of the

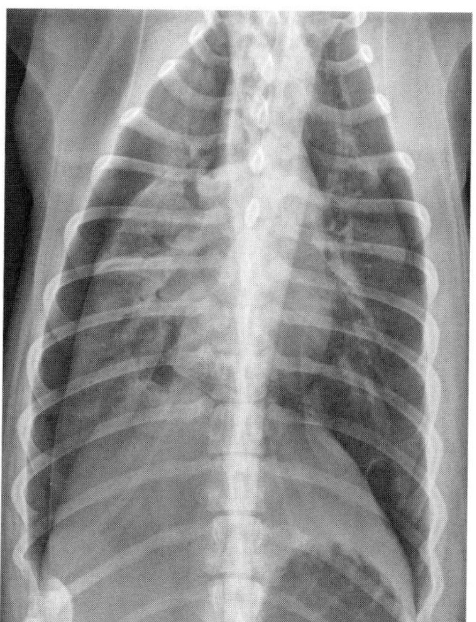

Fig. 32-16 Dorsoventral thoracic radiograph of a dog with a large volume of gas in the pleural cavity. Note the lung retraction and radiolucent region between each lung and the thoracic wall. There is more gas in the right pleural cavity than in the left. The pneumothorax has resulted in atelectasis with a resultant increase in pulmonary opacity. In this situation it is not possible to know whether there is disease in the underlying lung; there was not in this patient. This pneumothorax resulted from a lung bulla in the left caudal lobe that had ruptured spontaneously. There is an extrapleural sign in the right caudal thorax due to a healing rib fracture.

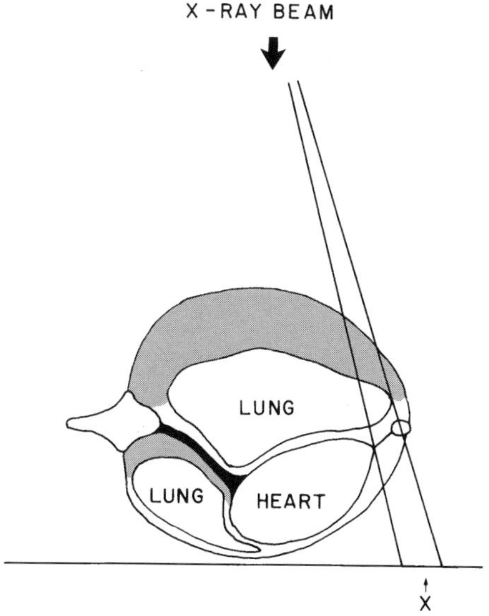

Fig. 32-17 Principle of elevation of the heart from the sternum in lateral radiographs of patients with pneumothorax. When the patient is in lateral recumbency, the lack of a fully inflated lung in the dependent hemithorax allows the heart to gravitate into the dependent hemithorax. As it gravitates, it slides dorsally because of the shape of the thoracic wall, thus creating a space between the heart and the sternum. As x-rays pass through this space, the heart appears elevated from the sternum on the lateral view by the distance *x*.

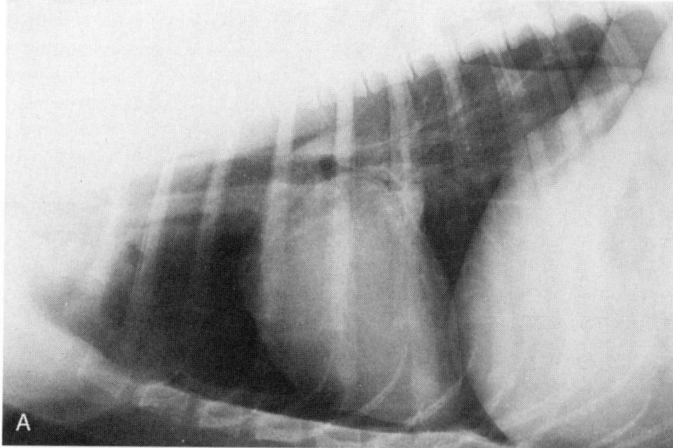

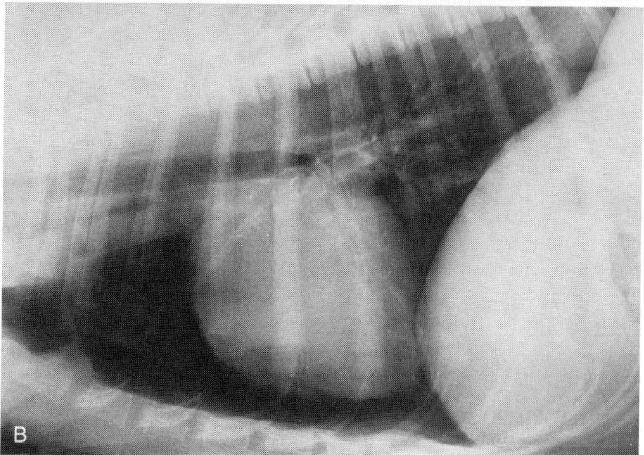

Fig. 32-18 Right (A) and left (B) lateral thoracic radiographs of a dog with a large left and a small right pneumothorax. **A,** The large pneumothorax is nondependent and collects around the left caudal lobe, resulting in clear visualization of collapse of the lobe. A small area of radiolucency is ventral to the heart from a slight shift in cardiac position to the right. Note the lack of heart displacement because of the almost fully inflated dependent right lung, which supports the heart on or near the midline. A traumatic lung bulla is present in the right caudal lobe. Pneumomediastinum is also present. **B,** The large pneumothorax is now dependent. Rather than being located between the lung and the thoracic wall, where it can be struck tangentially by the x-ray beam, air is layered against the dependent side of the mediastinum. Increased separation is present between the heart and the sternum because of atelectasis of the dependent left lung, which permits the heart to fall into the dependent hemithorax. Pneumomediastinum is also present.

diaphragm to the degree that its costal attachments become visible (Fig. 32-19). In a conventional pneumothorax, the heart is usually shifted toward the side of the thorax containing the most air, but in a tension pneumothorax the heart is shifted to the opposite side because of the increased pleural space pressure (Fig. 32-20). Tension pneumothorax is important to recognize because it is a potentially fatal condition requiring immediate thoracocentesis.

Pitfalls in Pneumothorax Diagnosis

Skin folds can result in an extremely radiolucent area superimposed over the lateral aspect of the thorax on ventrodorsal views. In many patients the identification of lung markings in the radiolucent area may not be possible. In these instances the correct diagnosis of skin-fold artifact is usually made by noting that the opacity of the fold extends beyond the limits of the thorax (Fig. 32-21).

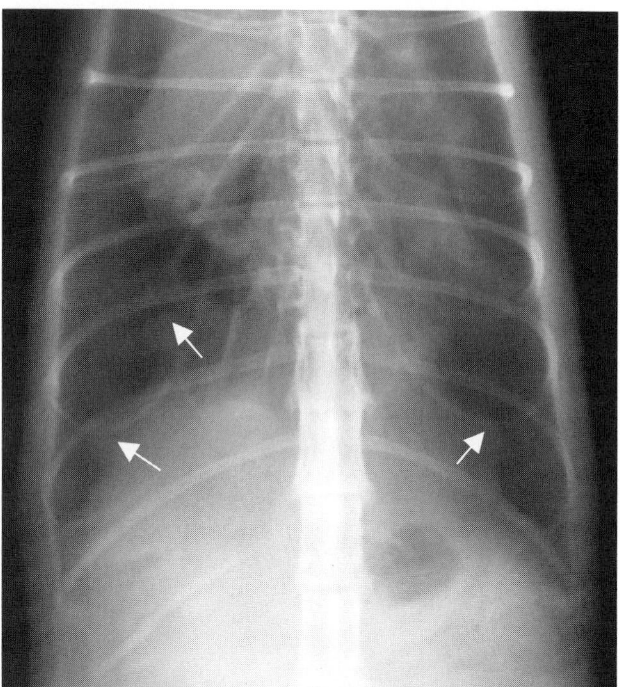

Fig. 32-19 Ventrodorsal radiograph of a cat with tension pneumothorax. The lungs are collapsed and appear as an amorphous opacity adjacent to the midline. Gas is obvious in the pleural space. The diaphragm is being displaced caudally by the increased pleural space pressure, resulting in pulling against its costal attachment sites and creating the tenting appearance *(arrows)*. Tenting can occur with pulmonary hyperinflation, but if seen with pneumothorax it is also a reliable sign of tension pneumothorax.

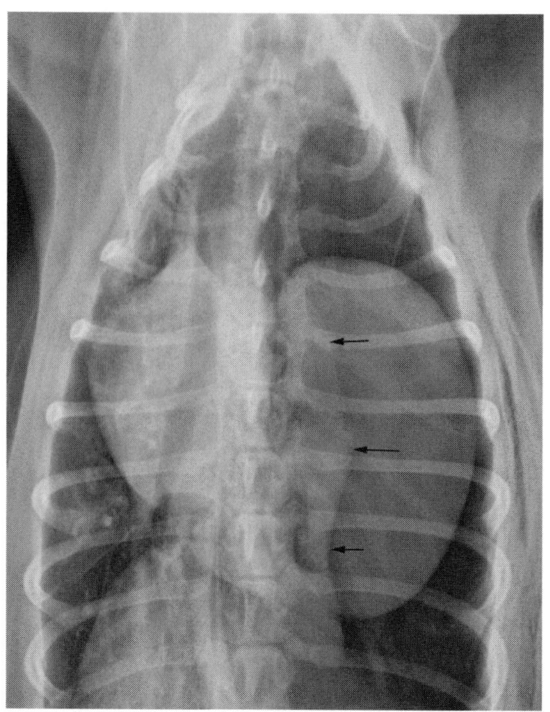

Fig. 32-20 Dorsoventral radiograph of a dog with a left-sided tension pneumothorax. Note the displacement of the heart to the right. The homogeneous mass on the left is a congenital lung cyst. This cyst is not touching the left thoracic wall and is not causing the heart displacement. There is a left-sided pneumothorax and the left lung is collapsed as an amorphous opacity against the midline *(black arrows)*. The left diaphragm is displaced caudally; note the relative radiolucency of the caudal aspect of the left pleural cavity due to the caudal displacement of the diaphragm. The degree of lung collapse, the diaphragm displacement, and the contralateral mediastinal shift (heart shift) are all signs of tension pneumothorax.

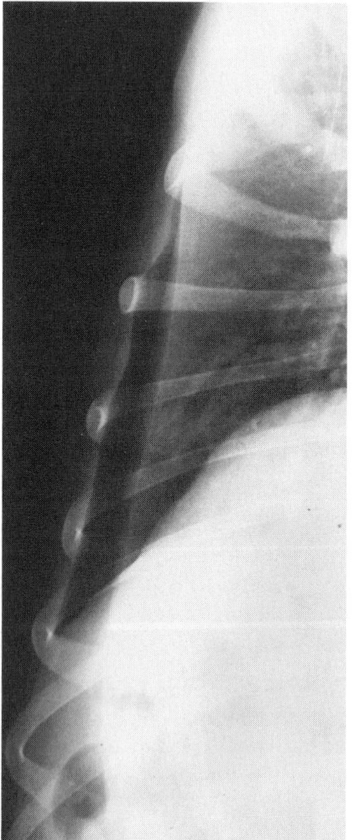

Fig. 32-21 Ventrodorsal view of the thorax of a dog in which a skin fold artifact is visible. These artifacts may easily be confused with pneumothorax. The skin fold itself has the appearance of a lung margin, with adjacent radiolucency that may be caused by gas in the pleural space. No lung markings are visible in the region lateral to the lung. The correct assessment of skin fold artifact is made by noting that the caudal extent of the lung margin extends beyond the limits of the thoracic cavity. Additionally, no air is seen between the lung and the diaphragm.

In chondrodystrophoid breeds, the costochondral region often appears opaque. If the dog's sternum is rotated slightly to one side when making the ventrodorsal or dorsoventral view, the area peripheral to the opacity appears radiolucent; this can be convincing evidence for pneumothorax. Lung markings may be difficult to identify in this radiolucent region, and horizontal-beam radiography may be necessary to conclude pneumothorax is not present (see Fig. 32-14).

REFERENCES

1. Groves TF, Ticer JW: Pleural fluid movement: its effect on appearance of ventrodorsal and dorsoventral radiographic projections, *Vet Radiol* 24:99, 1983.
2. Lord PF, Suter PF, Chan KF, et al: Pleural, extrapleural and pulmonary lesions in small animals: a radiographic approach to differential diagnosis, *J Am Vet Radiol Soc* 13:4, 1972.
3. Bauer T, Woodfield JA: Mediastinal, pleural, and extrapleural diseases. In Ettinger SJ, Feldman EC, editors: *Textbook of veterinary internal medicine*, ed 4, Philadelphia, 1995, WB Saunders.
4. Steyn PF, Wittum TE: Radiographic, epidemiologic, and clinical aspects of simultaneous pleural and peritoneal effusions in dogs and cats: 48 cases (1982-1991), *J Am Vet Med Assoc* 202:307, 1993.
5. Yoshioka M: Management of spontaneous pneumothorax in 12 dogs, *J Am Anim Hosp Assoc* 18:57, 1982.
6. Schaer M, Gamble D, Spencer C: Spontaneous pneumothorax associated with bacterial pneumonia in the dog—two case reports, *J Am Anim Hosp Assoc* 17:783, 1981.
7. Kern DA, Carrig CB, Martin RA: Radiographic evaluation of induced pneumothorax in the dog, *Vet Radiol Ultrasound* 35:411, 1995.
8. Aronson E, Reed AL: Radiology corner-pneumothorax: ventrodorsal or dorsoventral view. Does it make a difference? *Vet Radiol Ultrasound* 36:109, 1995.

ELECTRONIC RESOURCES evolve

Additional information related to the content in Chapter 32 can be found on the companion Web site at evolve http://evolve.elsevier.com/Thrall/vetrad/.

- Key Points
- Chapter Quiz
- Case Study 33-1
- Case Study 33-2

CHAPTER • 33
Heart and Pulmonary Vessels

Robert J. Bahr

Acquired heart disease is relatively common in small animal practice. Congenital anomalies also occur, but much less frequently. Assessing the heart and pulmonary vessels radiographically becomes important when decisions must be made regarding staging a patient with suspected cardiac disease, deciding about therapy protocols, and monitoring response to therapy or progression of disease. This is problematic regarding the heart because it inherently changes its size and shape during each contraction, breed variation exists in heart size and shape,[1,2] and the appearance of the cardiac silhouette is affected by radiographic positioning (see Chapter 25).[3]

With regard to body stature, dogs with a compressed body stature, such as Miniature Schnauzers, and dogs with a muscular frame, such as Rottweilers and Bull Mastiffs, may have a heart that looks larger than otherwise expected. This may be especially true in breeds in which the heart naturally appears round, such as chondrodystrophoid dog breeds and athletic individuals. Conversely, breeds with a laterally compressed but deep thoracic cavity, such as Greyhounds and Collies, may have a heart that, under normal circumstances, could be misinterpreted as small (Fig. 33-1). Thus the breed of the dog should always be considered when the heart is evaluated for size. If any suspicion of a cardiac abnormality exists, either because of radiographic appearance or clinical or historical information, then echocardiography should be the next avenue of investigation.

Radiographic positioning also has an effect on the appearance of the cardiac silhouette in normal dogs (see Chapter 25).[3] Perhaps the most important effect is the difference in cardiac silhouette appearance in ventrodorsal versus dorsoventral radiographs. In dorsoventral radiographs the diaphragm is displaced cranially, which will physically push the heart cranially and into the left hemithorax. The result is a cardiac silhouette that is oriented differently than in a VD view with respect to the primary x-ray beam and a heart that may be displaced into the left hemithorax. These effects are more pronounced in medium and large dogs than in cats or small dogs (Fig. 33-2).

When assessing the heart in radiographs, it should be kept in mind that the cardiac silhouette is composed of tissues other than the heart. The pericardium, any fluid or tissue in the pericardial space, and any tissue or fluid in the mediastinum immediately adjacent to the heart will silhouette with the heart, thereby contributing to the overall size and shape of the cardiac silhouette.[2] This principle is perhaps most important when attempting to assess heart size in obese patients. In such patients the cardiac silhouette is likely larger than the heart because of border effacement caused by fat in the mediastinum. This fat occasionally will be visible as a region of decreased opacity immediately adjacent to the heart (Fig. 33-3).

However, a starting point for radiographic evaluation is necessary, and certain radiographic signs can be used for cardiac assessment. These are discussed according to specific heart chambers. A system of cardiac measurement has been devised to take into account the inherent breed variation in cardiac size. This is called the vertebral heart scale method of evaluation.[4] In this system, the lengths of the long and short axes of the heart are measured and scaled against the length of the vertebral bodies dorsal to the heart, beginning with T4, to quantify heart size. On the basis of such an examination of 100 clinically normal dogs, the normal vertebral heart scale is 9.7 ± 0.5 vertebrae. Because 95% of the normal canine population lies within two standard deviations of the mean, the normal vertebral heart scale ranges from 8.7 to 10.7 vertebral body lengths. This relatively wide range of normal results from inherent breed variation in cardiac size. Although this method may be useful for beginners, it has not proven superior to the subjective heart assessment used by trained radiologists and other specialists.[5,6] Perhaps the best use of the vertebral heart scale is to compare cardiac size on radiographs made on different dates to monitor disease progression or response to treatment.

Importantly, survey radiographic examination is an insensitive and nonspecific modality to use in evaluation of the heart unless cardiac abnormalities are pronounced. Therefore cardiac radiography should be reserved (1) as a screening tool for assessing marked cardiac abnormalities, (2) as a means of evaluating the pulmonary circulation in concert with cardiac function, (3) to gain some insight regarding whether cardiac decompensation has occurred, and (4) to evaluate response to therapy. Any suspected cardiac abnormality must be interpreted in light of signalment and physical findings relative to the cardiovascular system. This chapter provides an understanding of moderate to severe chamber enlargement, describes the features of some of the more common congenital cardiac anomalies as well as the radiographic diagnosis of common acquired cardiac diseases, and provides a description of the radiographic features of heart failure.

For ease of recognition of various parts of cardiac anatomy as well as certain cardiac abnormalities in the dorsoventral or ventrodorsal radiograph, the cardiac silhouette can be visualized in terms of a clock face. The origin of bulges and bumps on the cardiac silhouette, caused by dilation of different parts of the heart or great vessels, can be predicted by using a clock analogy (Fig. 33-4). This system helps note where normal anatomic structures are located.

RADIOGRAPHIC SIGNS

Radiographic Signs of Specific Cardiac Chamber Enlargement

Left Atrium

Enlargement of the left atrium, perhaps the most frequently encountered cardiac enlargement, is essentially always caused by dilation. Left atrial dilation is usually a result of mitral valve

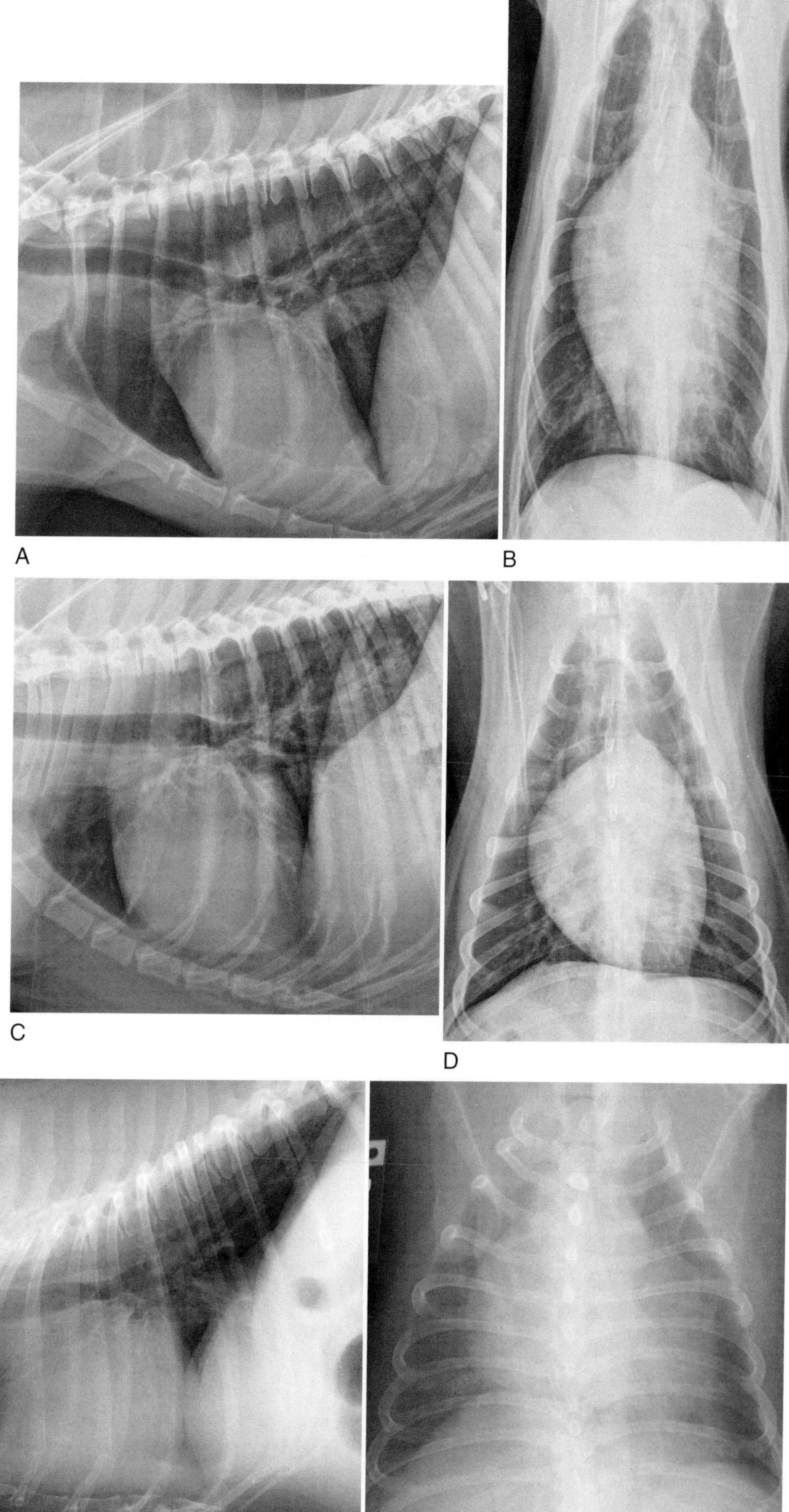

Fig. 33-1 Lateral and ventrodorsal thoracic radiographs from a Borzoi (A and B), Labrador Retriever (C and D), and a Pug (E and F). Each dog is normal. These figures illustrate the effect of breed, or body conformation, on the appearance of the cardiac silhouette. The radiographic appearance of the cardiac silhouette varies widely among breeds.

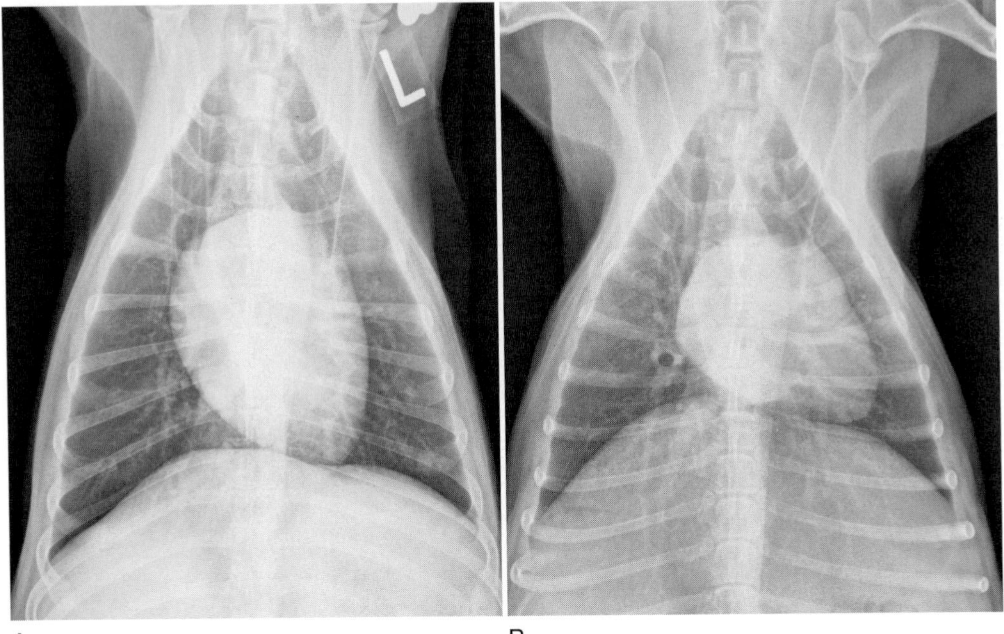

Fig. 33-2 Ventrodorsal (A) and dorsoventral (B) thoracic radiographs of a normal dog. Note the difference in appearance of the cardiac silhouette. In the dorsoventral radiograph the heart appears wider and is displaced into the left hemithorax. Care must be exercised to avoid misinterpreting this displacement as abnormal.

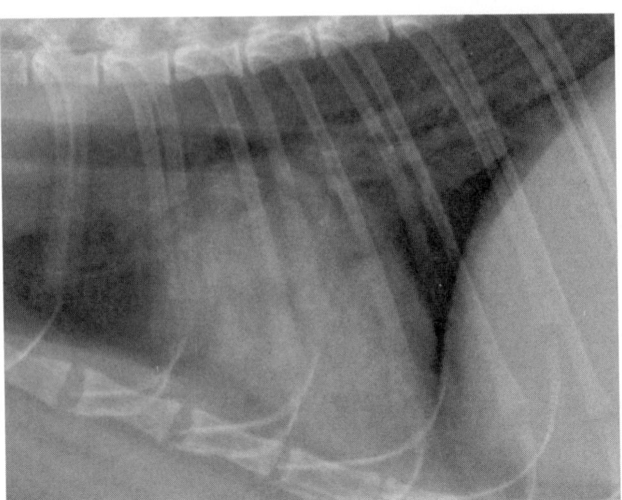

Fig. 33-3 Lateral radiograph of a feline thorax. The heart appears enlarged. However, this is an obese cat and the appearance of the cardiac silhouette is likely being affected by adjacent mediastinal fat. In fact, this cat has regions of slightly decreased opacity cranial and caudal to the heart that support the presence of mediastinal fat adjacent to the heart.

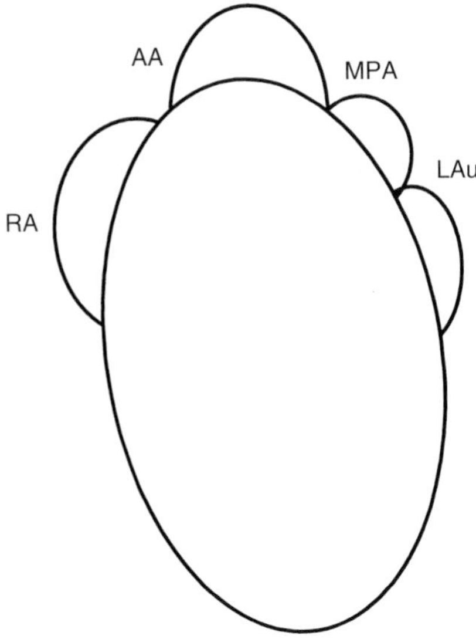

Fig. 33-4 The heart in a ventrodorsal, or dorsoventral, view illustrating the clock face analogy. Locations of dilation of the left auricle *(Lau)*, main pulmonary artery *(MPA)*, aortic arch *(AA)*, and right atrium *(RA)* are shown. Lau, bulge at 2 to 3 o'clock; MPA, bulge at 1 to 2 o'clock; AA, bulge at 11:30 to 12:30 o'clock; RA, bulge at 9:30 to 11:30 o'clock.

disease but can occur with pulmonary overcirculation, as from patent ductus arteriosus. In the lateral view, dilation of the left atrium causes a change in shape of the dorsocaudal aspect of the cardiac silhouette. Rather than the margin of the heart coursing in a dorsal and cranial direction toward the tracheal bifurcation, it tends to course more in a dorsocaudal direction, with the formation of a slight concavity on the caudal margin of the heart. This shape change has been referred to as loss of the caudal waist, but this is a jargon term and should be avoided. Left atrial dilation also causes an increase in height of the caudodorsal heart border and elevation of the tracheal bifurcation (Fig. 33-5).

Because the left atrium lies on midline, severe enlargement causes divergence of the two caudal lobe stem bronchi in the ventrodorsal or dorsoventral view. The normally acute angle (roughly 60 to 90 degrees) between these bronchi appears as a wider angle over the heart base. Also, the enlarged left atrium may create a double opacity in this area (see Fig. 33-5). The left atrium may be enlarged enough to cause selective elevation of the left caudal lobe stem bronchus above the right caudal lobe stem bronchus, as seen in the lateral view. If enough compression of the left caudal lobe stem bronchus has occurred by the enlarged left atrium, it may appear narrower

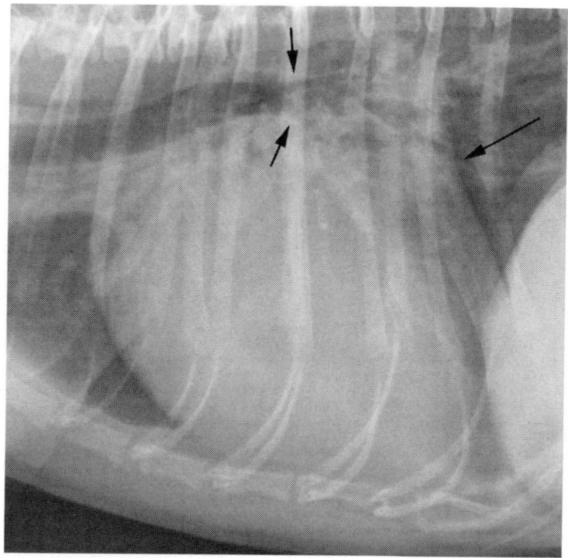

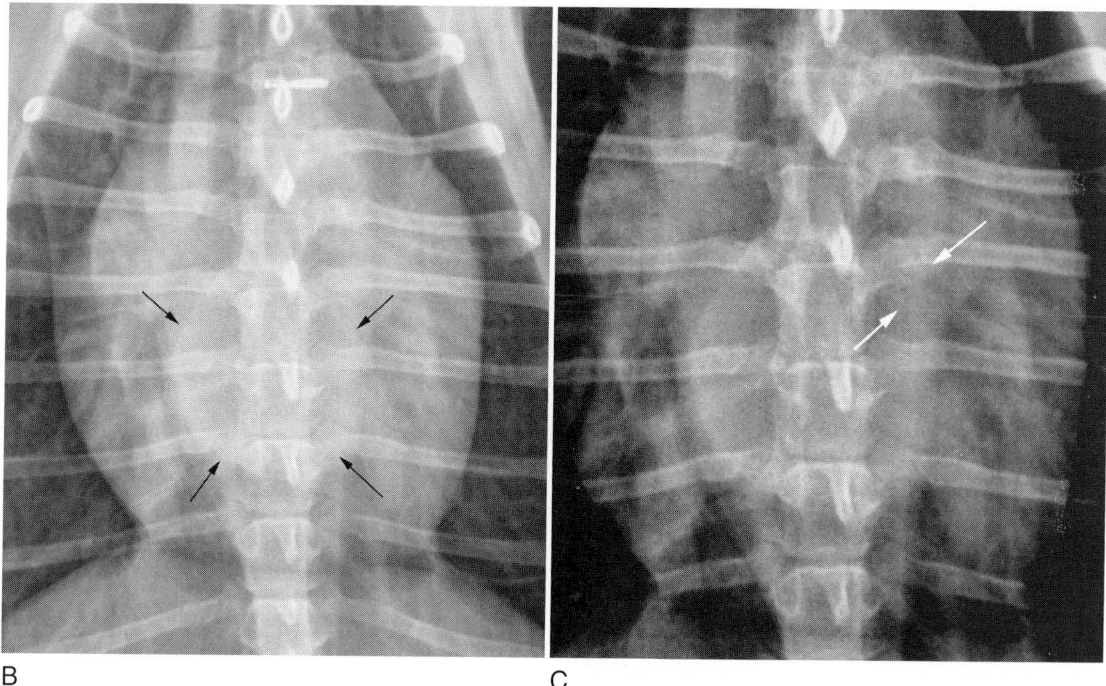

Fig. 33-5 Lateral (A), dorsoventral (B), and close-up dorsoventral (C) radiographs of the tracheal bifurcation region in a dog with marked left atrial dilation. In (A) there is elevation of the trachea and splitting of the main stem bronchi *(short arrows)*. Splitting means the left atrial enlargement has caused dorsal displacement of the left main bronchus. The left atrial dilation has also created a mass effect at the dorsocaudal portion of the cardiac silhouette, leading to a focal concave shape *(long arrow)*. In **B** the dilated left atrium creates a summation effect leading to a region of increased opacity caudal to the tracheal bifurcation *(arrows)*. In **C**, note the poor visualization of the left main stem bronchus *(arrows)* caused by compression by the dilated left atrium.

in the lateral view and nearly invisible in the ventrodorsal or dorsoventral view (see Fig. 33-5). Importantly, dogs with such severe left stem bronchial compression may exhibit a cough that is caused by the bronchial compression and not left heart failure; heart failure medications in such patients are not indicated.

A massively dilated left atrium may also lead to a region of increased opacity superimposed over the cardiac silhouette in the ventrodorsal or dorsoventral view that creates the appearance of a double wall. This is caused by a summation effect of the massively enlarged left atrium being projected superimposed on the remainder of the heart (Fig. 33-6).

Dilation of the left atrial appendage (auricle) occurs less frequently than dilation of the left atrium and when present appears as a focal bulge along the left cardiac border in the 2 to 3 o'clock position according to the clock face

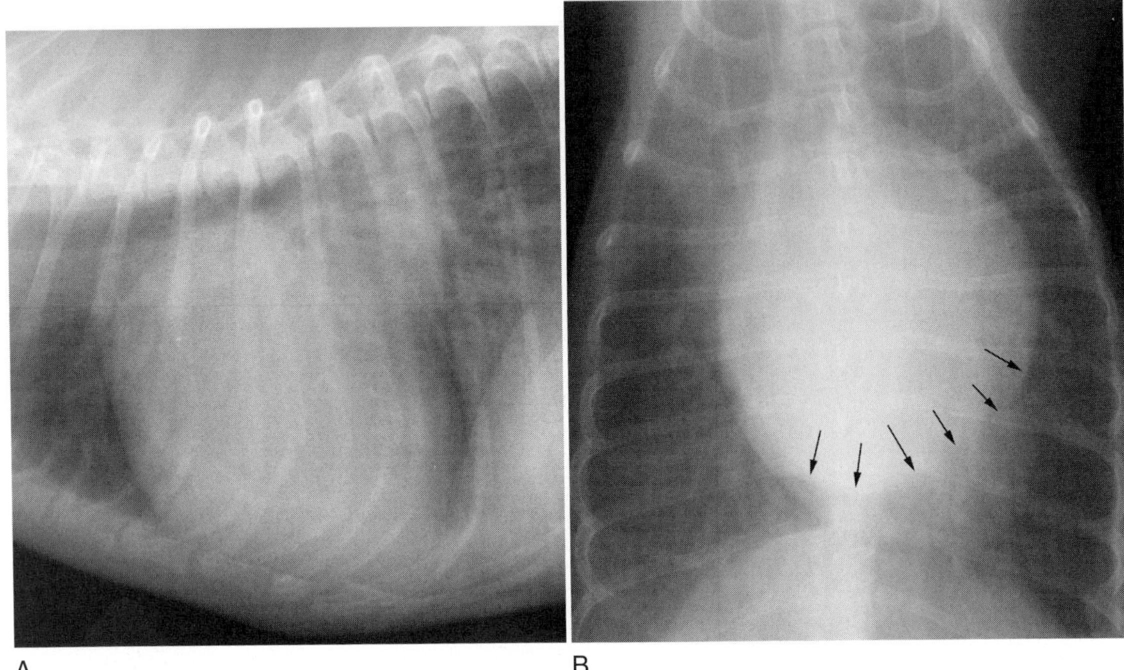

Fig. 33-6 Lateral (A) and ventrodorsal (B) radiographs of a dog with extreme enlargement of the left atrium. In (A) there is a large mass effect in the dorsocaudal region of the cardiac silhouette. When radiographed for the ventrodorsal view, this mass effect becomes superimposed on the remainder of the heart, creating a summation shadow that has been called the "double wall" effect. In **B** the *arrows* depict the margin of the enlarged left atrium.

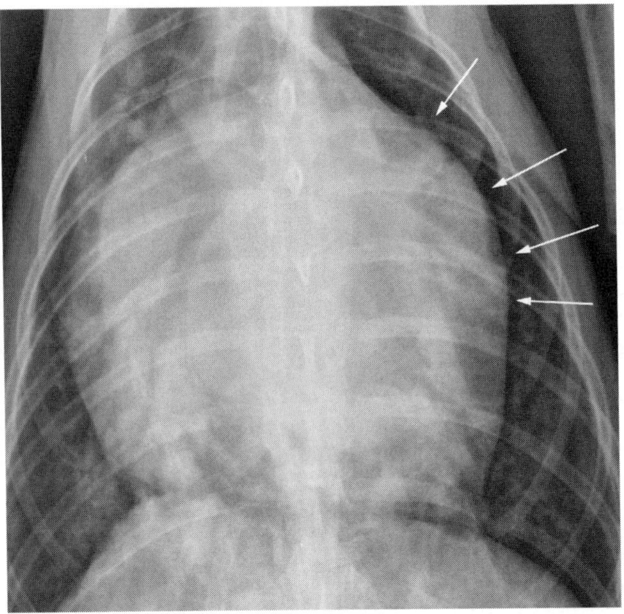

Fig. 33-7 Dorsoventral thoracic radiograph of a dog with a bulge on the cardiac silhouette consistent with either left auricular dilation or displacement.

analogy (Fig. 33-7). An extremely enlarged left atrium can also result in lateral displacement of the left auricle, resulting in its visualization without the auricle actually being dilated.

Left Ventricle

The left ventricle may enlarge as a result of hypertrophy or dilation. Concentric hypertrophy, a likely response to increased afterload such as with aortic stenosis, mainly occurs at the expense of lumen volume and may lead to no, or nonspecific, radiographic signs. Eccentric hypertrophy is a likely response to increased preload, as in patent ductus arteriosus or mitral insufficiency, and can cause visible left ventricular enlargement. Severe, eccentric hypertrophy that results in elongation of the left ventricle can lead to elevation of the entire intrathoracic trachea in the lateral view from the thoracic inlet to the tracheal bifurcation, thus narrowing the angle between the trachea and the thoracic vertebrae. In the ventrodorsal or dorsoventral view, the apex may appear more blunted, and the left heart border may appear to be more rounded than its normally straight appearance.

Dilation of the left ventricle is a likely response to chronically increased preload and is often associated with cardiac failure. Dilation of the left ventricle may either contribute to an overall appearance of "generalized cardiomegaly" or may also result in elongation of the left ventricle, causing tracheal elevation from the thoracic inlet back through the caudal lobe stem bronchi. There is debate, even among experienced radiologists, about the accuracy with which left ventricular hypertrophy or dilation can be diagnosed from survey radiographs.

Right Atrium

Enlargement of the right atrium to the extent that it can be detected radiographically is quite uncommon. Visualization of isolated right atrial enlargement is found in dogs with tricuspid dysplasia. As with the left atrium, enlargement of the right atrium is usually caused by dilation. When visible, right atrial enlargement in the lateral view causes a bulge or mass effect in the craniodorsal aspect of the cardiac silhouette. However, other cardiovascular enlargements, including dilation of the aortic arch and main pulmonary artery, can also cause this

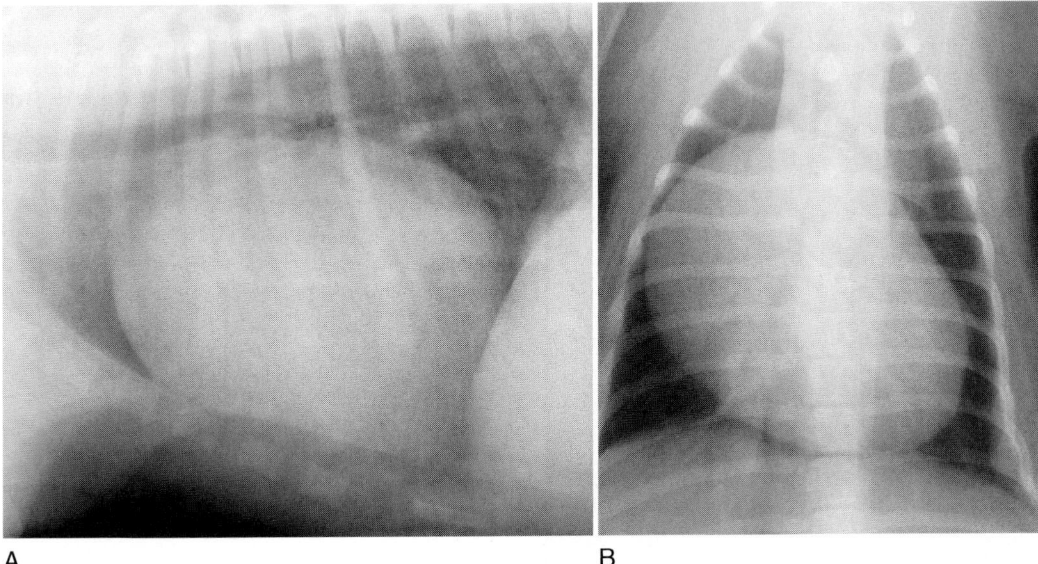

Fig. 33-8 Left lateral (A) and dorsoventral (B) radiographs of a Labrador Retriever with tricuspid dysplasia. A bulge is visible in the region of the right atrium consistent with right atrial enlargement. How far ventral (A) and caudal (B) the enlargement extends on the cardiac silhouette is often surprising.

radiographic appearance. In the ventrodorsal or dorsoventral projection, an increased bulge in the right heart border from the 9 o'clock to 11 o'clock position may be present (Fig. 33-8).

Right Ventricle

As with the left ventricle, the right ventricle may enlarge as a result of hypertrophy or dilation. The most common causes of radiographically detectable right ventricular hypertrophy are heartworm infection and pulmonic stenosis. Hypertrophy mainly occurs at the expense of lumen volume and may lead to no or nonrecognizable radiographic signs. However, the sensitivity of radiographs for detection of right ventricular hypertrophy is greater than for detecting left ventricular hypertrophy; this may be related to the normally thinner wall of the right ventricle, with hypertrophy causing more obvious changes in cardiac size and shape. Because the right ventricle is normally in contact with the sternum, its enlargement, whether from dilation or hypertrophy, often causes an increased sternal contact in the lateral view (Fig. 33-9, *B*). The average dog has an amount of cardiac contact with the sternum ranging from 2.5 to 3 intercostal spaces; thus any sternal contact in excess of 3 intercostal spaces could be abnormal and is consistent with right ventricular enlargement. However, some deep-chested breeds, such as Doberman Pinschers and Irish Wolfhounds, may normally only have approximately 1.5 to 2 intercostal spaces of sternal contact, so 2.5 to 3 spaces would be consistent with right ventricular enlargement for those breeds. Likewise, some barrel-chested breeds, such as the English Bulldog, can normally have more than 3 to 3.5 intercostal spaces of contact.

Ideally, the entire cardiac silhouette should be evaluated in at least two orthogonal views and the right ventricular size estimated in light of its appearance in both views as well as in light of other findings, such as size of the caudal vena cava and right atrium. Severe right ventricular hypertrophy can also lead to the cardiac apex being displaced from the sternum as a result of the change in cardiac shape (Fig. 33-9, C). In ventrodorsal or dorsoventral views, a hypertrophic right ventricle appears more rounded and protrudes further into the right hemithorax than normal, giving the cardiac silhouette a reversed letter D shape (Fig. 33-9, *A*).

Generalized Cardiomegaly

Various combinations of these chamber enlargements may be seen, or all four chambers may be enlarged to the degree that no one chamber enlargement stands out. A common cause for generalized cardiomegaly is myocardial dysfunction. The vertebral heart scale was intended to provide a more accurate assessment tool for overall heart size and can be used here, remembering the inherent problems with this method of size assessment. Generalized cardiomegaly may also be misinterpreted because of underinflation of the lungs, making the thoracic cavity appear smaller than normal. This, in turn, makes the heart appear larger relative to the amount of aerated lung surrounding it (Fig. 33-10).[7]

Radiographic Signs of Major Vessel Enlargement

Caudal Vena Cava

The caudal vena cava is extremely variable in size depending on the phase of respiration and cardiac cycle. It can only be judged to be enlarged if it is consistently larger in diameter than the length of the fifth or sixth thoracic vertebral bodies of the spine as measured in the lateral view.[4] Another measure of caudal vena cava size is that enlargement can only be inferred if the diameter of the caudal vena cava is more than 1.5 times the diameter of the descending aorta.[8] The caudal vena cava can enlarge in response to increased central venous pressure, but the size of the vena cava is not an accurate way to attempt to assess central venous pressure. Valid inferences on cardiovascular disease typically cannot be made on the basis of the size of the caudal vena cava.

Aorta

Widening of the precardiac mediastinum, as seen in the ventrodorsal or dorsoventral views, can indicate widening of the aortic arch. A focal bulge in the descending aorta in ventrodorsal or dorsoventral views is commonly seen in patients

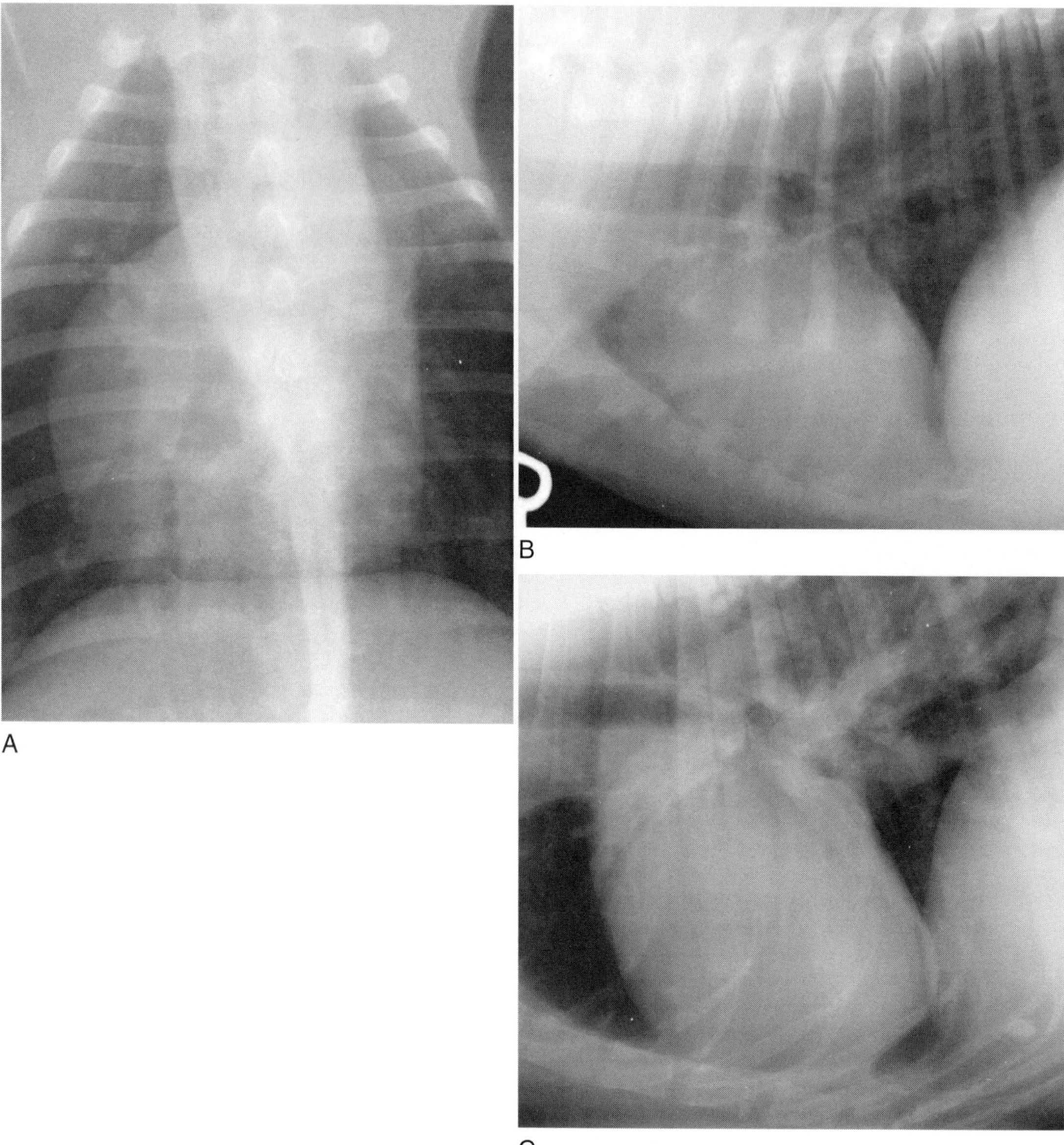

Fig. 33-9 Right ventricular hypertrophy. **A,** Ventrodorsal view of a dog with pulmonic stenosis. Right ventricular hypertrophy has resulted in increased cardiac mass on the right side that creates an appearance of a reverse, or backward, letter D. Enlargement of the main pulmonary artery is also visible. **B,** Right lateral radiograph of a dog with pulmonic stenosis. The increased mass of the right ventricle has resulted in increased contact of the heart with the sternum over a longer distance than normal. **C,** Right lateral radiograph of a dog with heartworms and marked right ventricular hypertrophy. The increased mass on the right side of the heart has caused elevation of the cardiac apex from the sternum. Mild elevation of the cardiac apex from the sternum may be present in normal dogs in a left lateral view, but normal apex displacement should never be this marked or appear in the right lateral view.

with a patent ductus arteriosus (Fig. 33-11). In the lateral views, aortic size is more difficult to assess, but an enlarged aortic arch can create increased mass at the cranial aspect of the cardiac silhouette (see Fig. 33-11). Isolated aortic arch enlargement is rarely seen except with a patent ductus arteriosus or aortic stenosis.

Some older cats will have a more tortuous appearing aorta, as seen in the lateral views, with a more vertical aortic arch orientation; the aortic arch then curves upward and caudally, assuming a serpentine contour as it progresses caudally toward the diaphragm (Fig. 33-12, *A*). In the dorsoventral or ventrodorsal views, this aortic contour can appear unusual in shape and may stand out away from the mediastinum and be misinterpreted as a pulmonary nodule (Fig. 33-12, *B*).[9] This finding in aged cats is considered clinically insignificant.

Main Pulmonary Artery

The main pulmonary artery normally is not seen as a separate structure, but when it enlarges sufficiently in dogs it will appear as a focal bulge in the 1 o'clock position in ventrodorsal or dorsoventral views (see Figs. 33-9, *A*). An enlarged main pulmonary artery is not routinely recognized in lateral views.

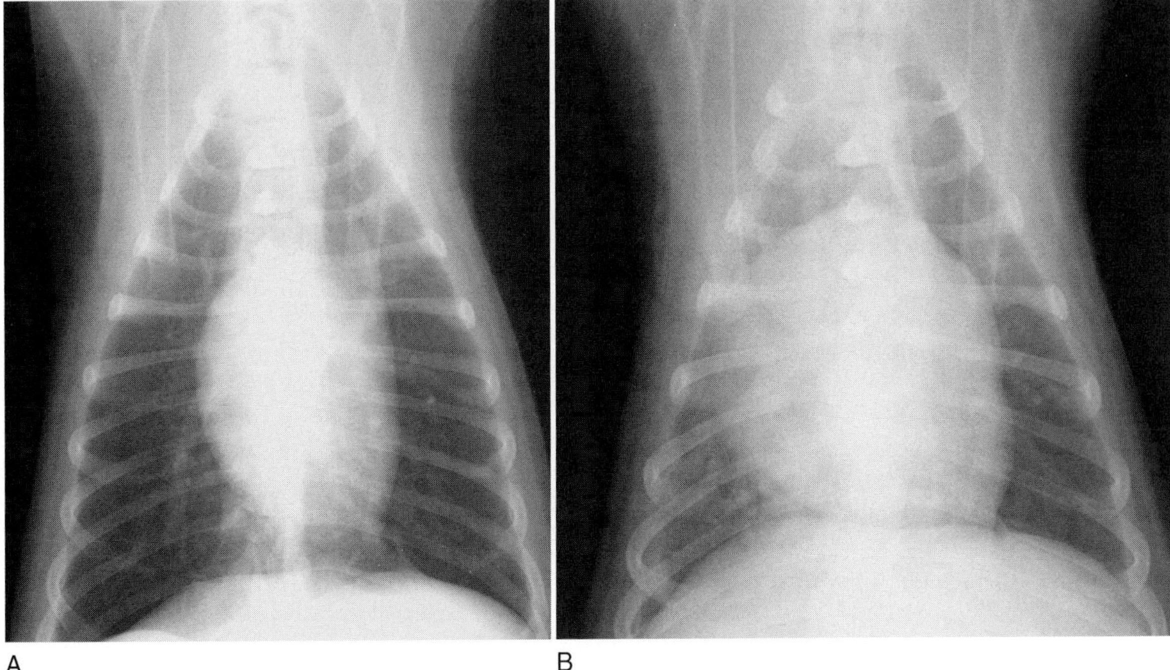

Fig. 33-10 Ventrodorsal thoracic radiographs of the same normal dog made in inspiration (**A**) and expiration (**B**). In **B**, the dog is also sedated, which further reduces tidal volume. Note how the decrease in size of the thoracic cavity in **B** gives the false impression of cardiomegaly. The status of respiration should be noted in every thoracic radiograph before any conclusion is made.

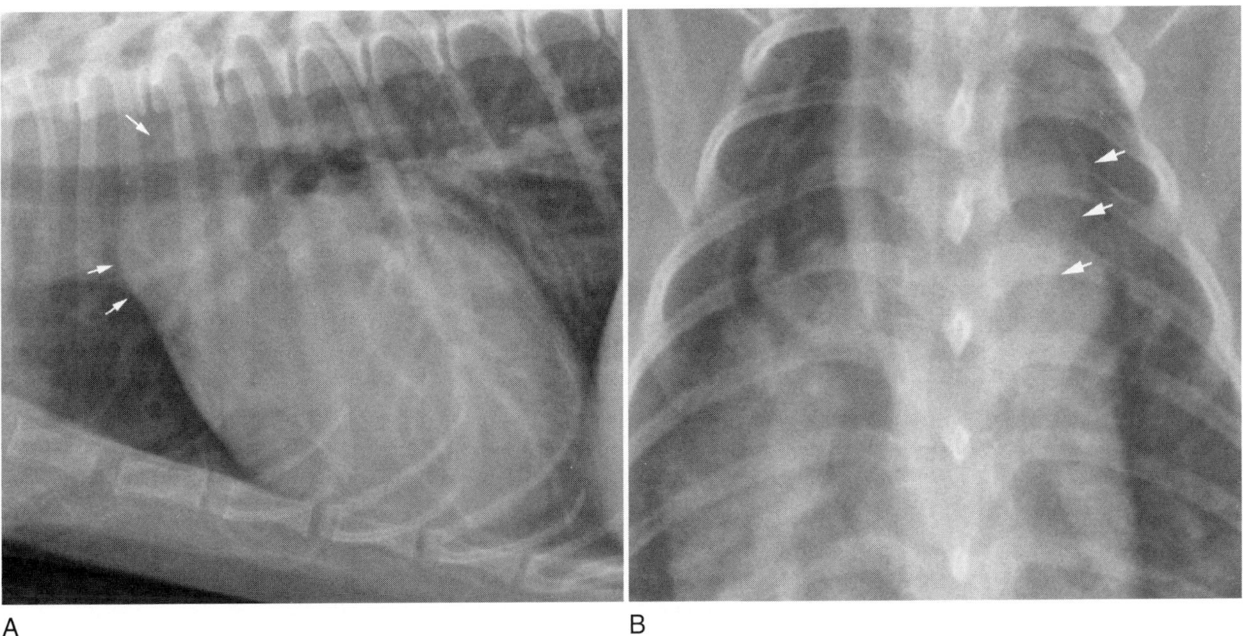

Fig. 33-11 Lateral (**A**) and dorsoventral (**B**) radiograph of a dog with a patent ductus arteriosus. In **A** the left ventricular hypertrophy has resulted in elongation of the cardiac silhouette and secondary elevation of the thoracic trachea. In **B** the enlarged aortic arch appears as an opacity at the cranial, and slightly left, aspect of the cardiac silhouette *(white arrows)*.

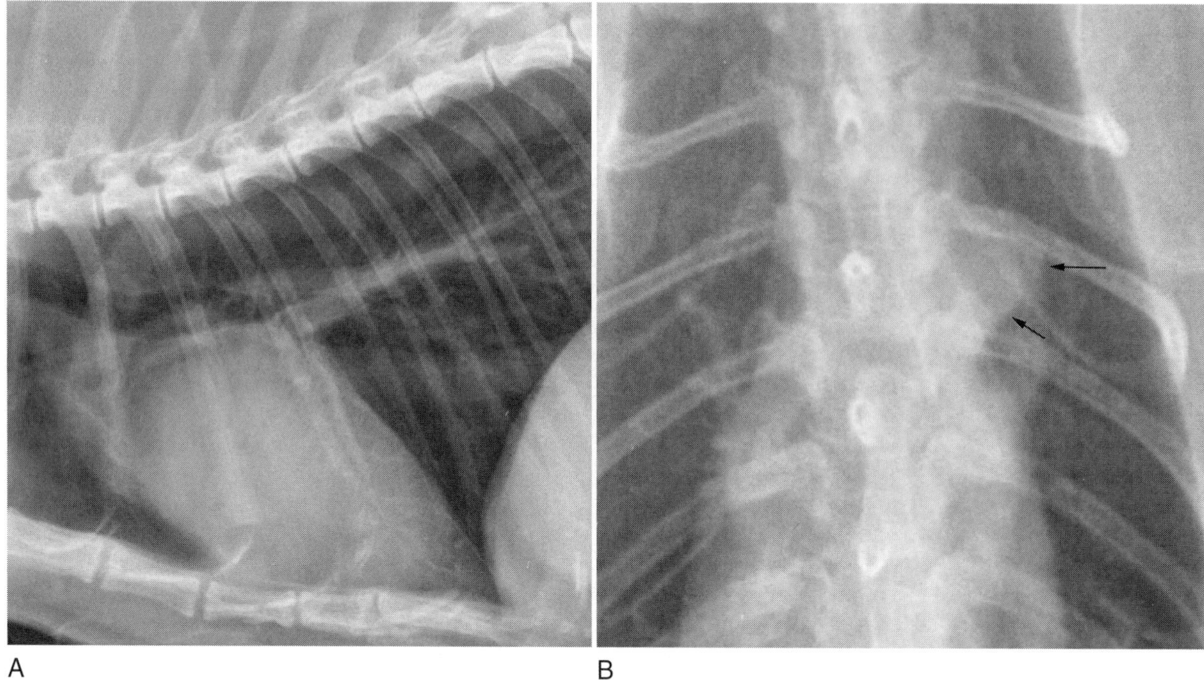

Fig. 33-12 **A,** Lateral radiograph of a cat with a tortuous aorta. This is a commonly encountered appearance in older cats. In **A** the aortic arch is more vertical than normal and the descending aorta is tortuous. In another cat (**B**) with a tortuous aorta, the aortic arch is positioned to the left of midline *(arrows)* and could be misinterpreted as a mediastinal or pulmonary mass.

Common causes of main pulmonary artery enlargement include heartworm disease and pulmonic stenosis.

Radiographic Signs of Pulmonary Vascular Changes

A radiographic assessment of cardiac size or shape is incomplete without also evaluating the main pulmonary artery as well as the peripheral pulmonary arteries and veins. Therefore knowing where to look for and how to differentiate arteries and veins in the lungs is crucial. In the lung, parenchymal vessels and airways are arranged in an organized manner, with the airway always being positioned between the pulmonary artery and pulmonary vein.

In lateral projections, when arteries can be seen as separate structures from veins, the arteries are dorsal and the veins are ventral to an intervening bronchus for any given triad of artery-bronchus-vein.[10] This essentially applies only to the cranial lobe arteries and veins because the caudal lobar arteries and veins are superimposed over each other in the lateral projection and caudal lobe pulmonary arteries cannot be differentiated from veins in a lateral view. The right cranial lobar artery and vein can serve as reference vessels because they are best seen as individual structures when the animal is placed in left lateral recumbency (Fig. 33-13).[3] This is because the right cranial lung lobe is better inflated with the animal in left recumbency, resulting in better definition of these vessels. Although the left cranial lobe will be better inflated in right recumbency, the left and right pairs of cranial lobe vessels will be more superimposed, making their assessment more difficult (Fig. 33-13).

In a ventrodorsal or dorsoventral projection, arteries and veins are most conveniently compared in the caudal lobes. In these views the pulmonary artery is lateral to the pulmonary vein, with the associated bronchus interposed between. The caudal lobe pulmonary vessels are usually better seen in the dorsoventral view than in the ventrodorsal view because of the better lung inflation achieved with the dog in sternal recumbency for a dorsoventral radiograph (Fig. 33-14). In addition to the improved pulmonary inflation in sternal recumbency, the caudal lobar vessels and bronchi are more nearly perpendicular to the x-ray beam than they are with the patient in dorsal recumbency for ventrodorsal radiography. Paired arteries and veins are less well seen in other lobes in either dorsoventral or ventrodorsal views, although occasionally the cranial lobar vessels may be adequately visualized.

Even though a bronchus always lies between a paired artery and vein, the entire distance between these paired vessels is not occupied by the bronchus. The exact position of the bronchus and its actual size can only be seen in survey radiographs if its walls are sufficiently mineralized (see Fig. 33-14, *B*).

Peripheral Pulmonary Arteries

Peripheral pulmonary arteries should essentially be the same size as their associated pulmonary veins.[10] Specifically, cranial lobe arteries should be no larger than the proximal aspect of the fourth rib in a lateral view and caudal lobe arteries no larger than the thickness of the ninth rib in the ventrodorsal or dorsoventral view, where the artery and rib intersect in the image.

A useful method to assess caudal lobe pulmonary artery size in ventrodorsal or dorsoventral radiographs is to assess the shape of the summation shadow created by overlap of a caudal lobe pulmonary artery and the ninth rib. In normal dogs this summation shadow should have sides of equal length. If the artery is enlarged, the long axis of the summation shadow will be in a horizontal direction. If the artery is small, the long axis of the summation shadow will be oriented in a vertical direction (Fig. 33-15).

Peripheral Pulmonary Veins

The peripheral pulmonary veins are similar to pulmonary arteries in that pulmonary veins should be no larger than their corresponding arteries at any given level from the heart; comparisons to the appropriate ribs therefore also apply.

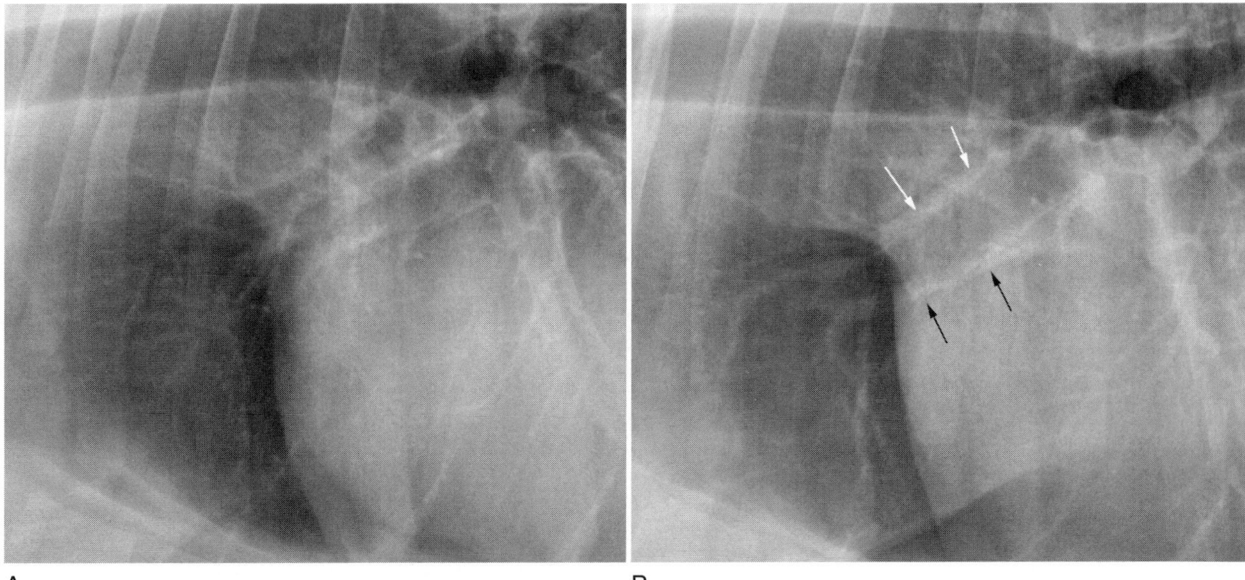

Fig. 33-13 Close-up from right (A) and left (B) lateral radiographs of a normal dog. In A the cranial lobe vessels are superimposed and distinguishing the right cranial lobe artery from the right cranial lobe vein is difficult. In B the artery *(white arrow)* and vein *(black arrow)* for the right cranial lobe are more clearly seen. The ability to distinguish the right cranial artery from the vein is typically easier in a left lateral radiograph. Note the similar size of the artery and vein in **B.**

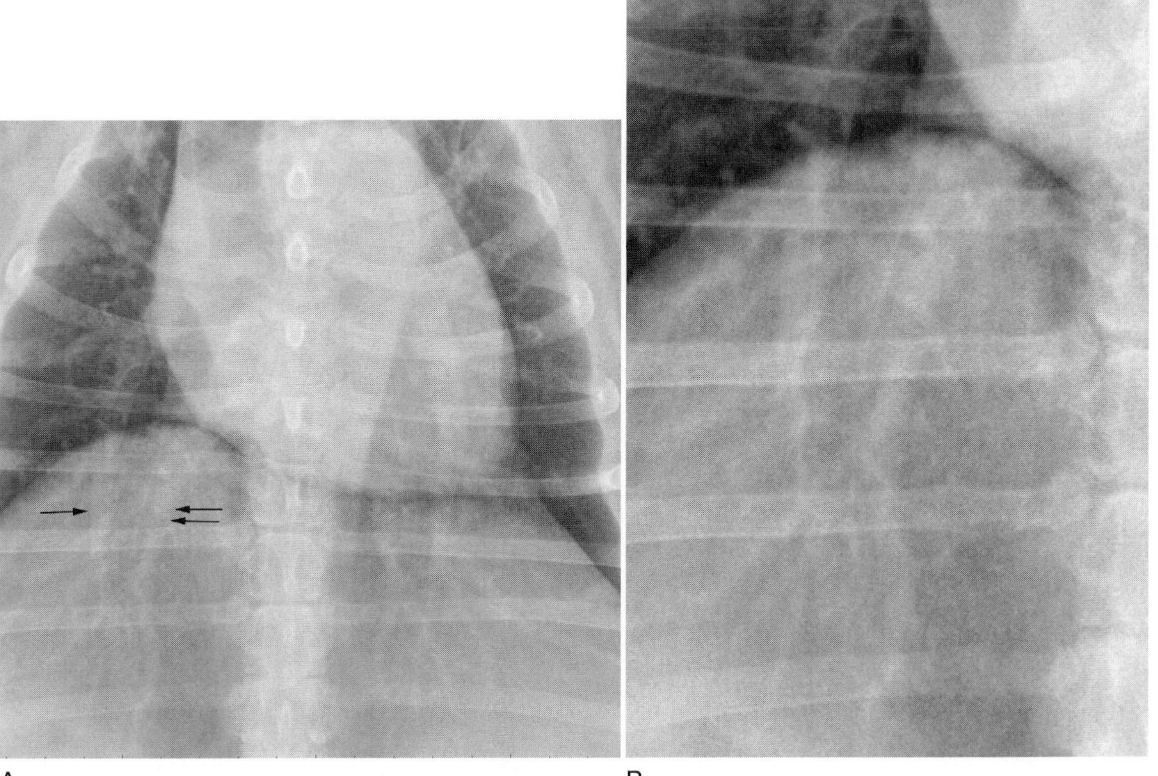

Fig. 33-14 Dorsoventral (A) radiograph of a normal dog. The caudal lobe vessels are conspicuous. The caudal lobe artery *(single arrow)* is lateral to the airway, whereas the vein is medial *(double arrows)*. Close-up view (B) of the right caudal lobe area giving another view of the caudal lobe vessels in this same dog. Upon close inspection, **B** the mineralized wall of the caudal lobe bronchus interposed between the artery and vein can be seen. Note that the bronchus does not occupy the entire space between the artery and vein. When the bronchus is not mineralized, inferring that it occupies the entire distance between its associated artery and vein is inaccurate.

Pulmonary vessels are dynamic; thus their size can change relatively quickly, being a function of intraluminal pressure and volume, which can also change quickly. Situations such as dehydration from diuretic administration or hypervolemia from overzealous intravenous fluid administration can prompt such changes, so interpretation of vessel size must be made with knowledge of any recently administered medications or therapies. More meaningful information is gathered with sequential radiographic examinations, especially if therapies have recently changed.

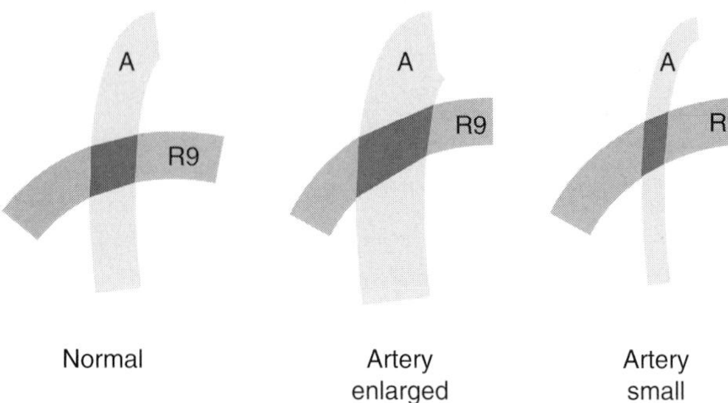

Fig. 33-15 The principle of using the summation shadow created by overlap of a caudal lobe pulmonary artery with the ninth rib *(R9)* to assess artery size. In normal dogs, the summation shadow will have equal sides *(left panel)*. When the artery is enlarged *(center panel)*, the summation shadow will be longer in the horizontal direction than in the vertical direction. When the artery is small *(right panel)*, the summation shadow will be longer in the vertical direction than in the horizontal direction.

Normal size of pulmonary arteries and veins has been described, but certain diseases cause predictable changes in size of either pulmonary arteries alone or pulmonary veins alone or both simultaneously.

Box 33-1 lists common diseases where both pulmonary arteries and veins are expected to be enlarged (Fig. 33-16). The degree of these changes, and therefore how easily they are visualized, depends largely on the severity and duration of the causative disease. Differentiation among these various disease entities depends on evaluating other factors such as the history, physical examination findings, electrocardiography, and echocardiography findings.

Pulmonary artery enlargement without venous enlargement may occur with the diseases listed in Box 33-2. The most common cause of pulmonary arterial enlargement in the dog is heartworm disease (Fig. 33-17). In heartworm disease, arterial

Box • 33-1

Conditions That May Increase the Size of Pulmonary Arteries and Pulmonary Veins

- Left-to-right shunt
  - Patent ductus arteriosus
  - Ventricular septal defect
  - Atrial septal defect
- Peripheral arteriovenous fistula
- Fluid retention due to heart failure
- Iatrogenic intravenous fluid overload

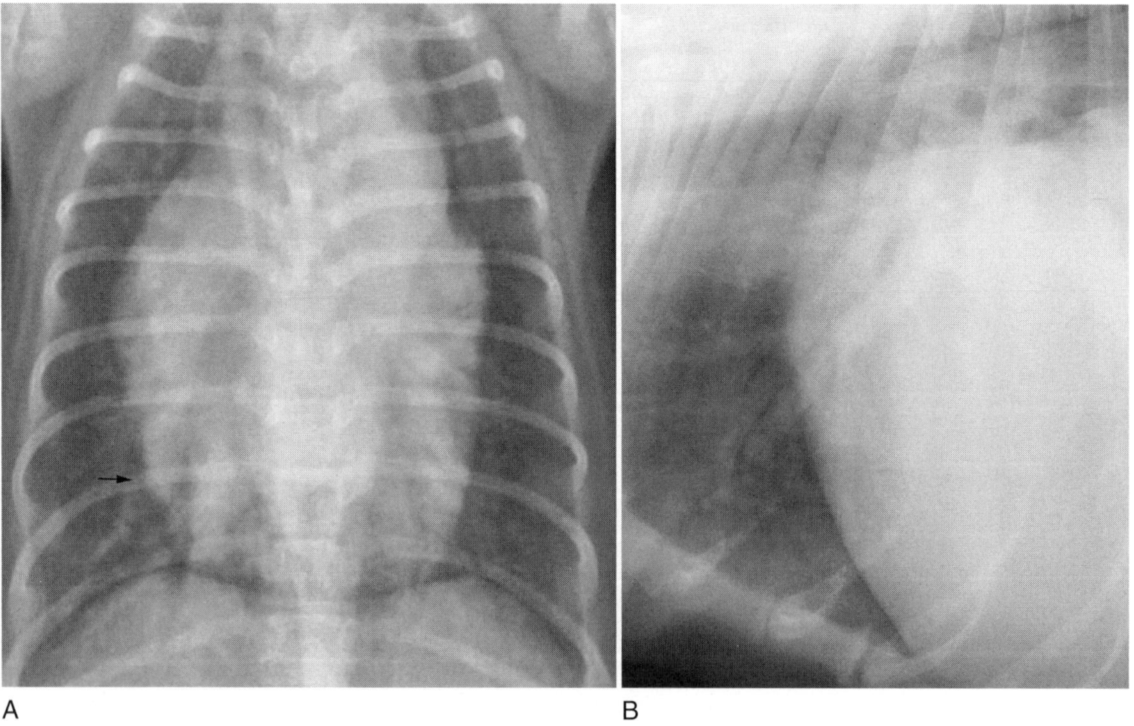

Fig. 33-16 **A,** Dorsoventral radiograph from a dog with a patent ductus arteriosus. The caudal lobe arteries and veins are both enlarged. Note the size of the vessels in the right caudal lobe where they cross the ninth rib *(arrow)*. In a normal dog the caudal lobe vessels should be approximately the same size as the rib. **B,** Lateral thoracic radiograph of another dog with a patent ductus arteriosus where both the artery and vein of the right cranial lobe are enlarged.

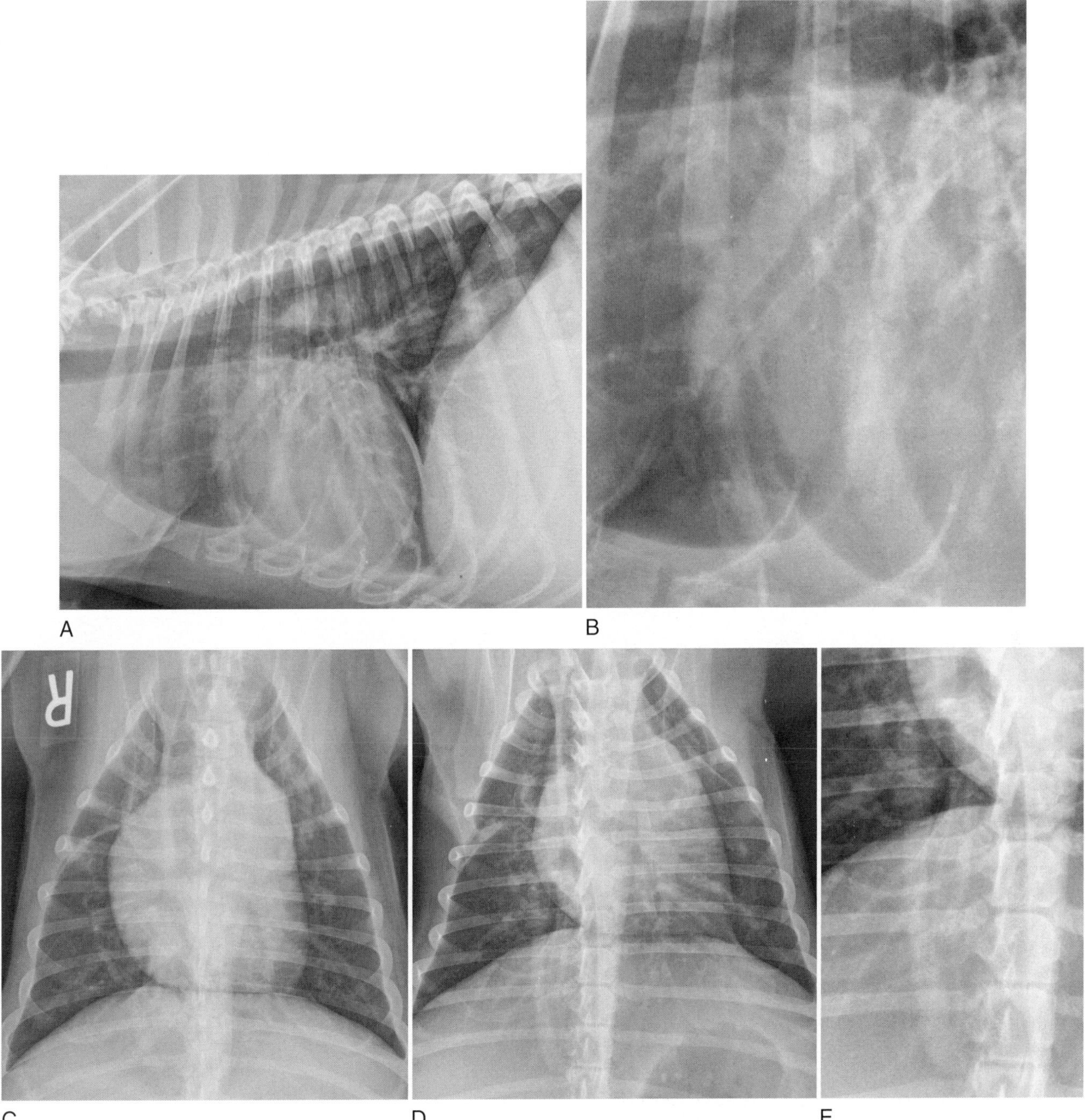

Fig. 33-17 Left lateral (A), close-up left lateral (B), ventrodorsal (C), dorsoventral (D), and close-up dorsoventral (E) radiographs of a dog with heartworm disease. In A and **B,** note the enlargement of the right cranial lobe artery compared with the vein. In C, note the reversed D appearance of the cardiac silhouette, consistent with right ventricular hypertrophy. In D and E note the enlargement of the right caudal lobe artery compared with the vein. These findings are typical of those found in dogs infected with heartworms.

enlargement occurs because of pulmonary hypertension resulting from lesions in the vascular tunica intima or tunica media or because of thromboembolic disease or both. Any or all of the pulmonary arteries may become enlarged, but the pulmonary arteries that enlarge the most frequently in spontaneous heartworm disease are the caudal lobar arteries with a predilection for enlargement of the right more than the left.[11]

In cats with heartworm disease, enlargement of the main pulmonary artery is usually not visualized on survey radiographs.[12-14] This is not because the main pulmonary artery is not enlarged; unlike in dogs, the main pulmonary artery in cats is not positioned so that its border is visible on survey radiographic images. However, with angiography, the main pulmonary artery can be seen when enlarged in most cats with heartworm disease. The peripheral pulmonary arteries do become visibly enlarged in cats with heartworm disease, as in dogs (Fig. 33-18). Enlargement of the central and peripheral portions of the caudal lobar arteries on the ventrodorsal view, with normal-sized caudal pulmonary veins, has been reported to represent the earliest radiographic change seen in sponta-

Box 33-2

Conditions That May Increase the Size of Pulmonary Arteries without Associated Vein Enlargement

- Tunica intima proliferation or tunica media hypertrophy
  - Dirofilariasis
  - Angiostrongyliasis
  - Aelurostrongylus (feline)
- Pulmonary thromboembolism
  - Dirofilariasis
  - Disseminated intravascular coagulation
  - Trauma
  - Angiostrongyliasis
  - Renal disease: amyloidosis, glomerulonephritis
  - Septicemia
  - Pancreatitis
  - Hyperadrenocorticism
- Severe chronic lung disease with pulmonary hypertension

Box 33-3

Conditions That May Increase the Size of Pulmonary Veins without Associated Artery Enlargement

- Cardiac
  - Volume overload
    - Mitral insufficiency
    - Early left-to-right shunts (thinner walls of veins dilate more easily)
    - Patent ductus arteriosus
  - Primary myocardial disease
    - Dilatory cardiomyopathy
    - Hypertrophic cardiomyopathy
    - Restrictive cardiomyopathy
- Noncardiac dysfunction
  - Left atrial obstruction
    - Mass (neoplastic or inflammatory) at heart base
    - Thrombosis within left atrium

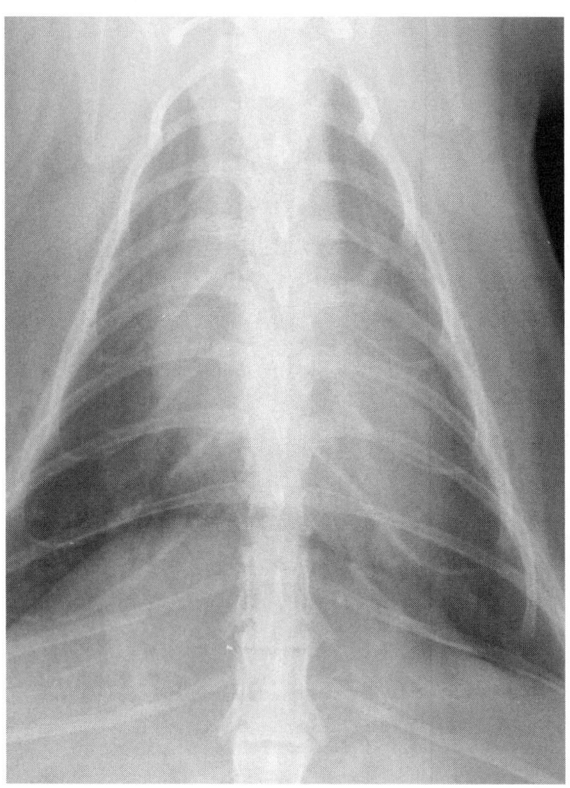

Fig. 33-18 Dorsoventral radiograph of a cat infected with heartworms. Note the enlargement of both caudal lobe pulmonary arteries compared with their respective veins. Enlargement of the main pulmonary artery is not seen, although it is likely present; this is common in cats with heartworm disease.

Box 33-4

Conditions That May Decrease the Size of Pulmonary Arteries and Veins

- Right-to-left shunts
  - Tetralogy of Fallot
  - Ventricular septal defect with pulmonic stenosis
- Severe pulmonic stenosis
- Hypovolemia
- Shock

neous feline heartworm disease. Because feline pulmonary lobar arterial enlargement was shown to resolve and reappear over a span of 4 to 5 months in experimental heartworm infection, vascular changes cannot entirely be relied on when evaluating thoracic radiographs of cats for heartworm disease. A persistent bronchointerstitial pulmonary pattern also occurred in approximately 50% of experimentally infected cats, appearing similar to feline allergic lung disease even after the vascular changes had resolved. Thus cats with radiographic evidence of bronchointerstitial lung opacities should be considered suspects for heartworm disease even in the absence of classic vascular changes. On the basis of the sometimes inconspicuous radiographic signs of feline heartworm disease, echocardiography has been proposed as an alternate screening modality.[15]

Heartworm disease is also the most common cause of pulmonary thromboembolism, caused by arterial occlusion by dying worm emboli or blood clots. This results in an increase in pulmonary opacities that at first appear as a mixed pattern of unstructured interstitial and alveolar opacities but in the later stages, or when an associated host allergic response to the worms occurs, this pulmonary opacity will be predominantly alveolar (Fig. 33-19). Although overt pulmonary infarction is possible with heartworm disease, it is rare.

The differential diagnosis for pulmonary vein enlargement occurring without pulmonary arterial enlargement is listed in Box 33-3. Pulmonary vein enlargement is most commonly seen in dogs with mitral insufficiency (Figs. 33-20 and 33-21).

Diseases associated with decreased size of both the pulmonary arteries and veins are listed in Box 33-4 (Fig. 33-22).

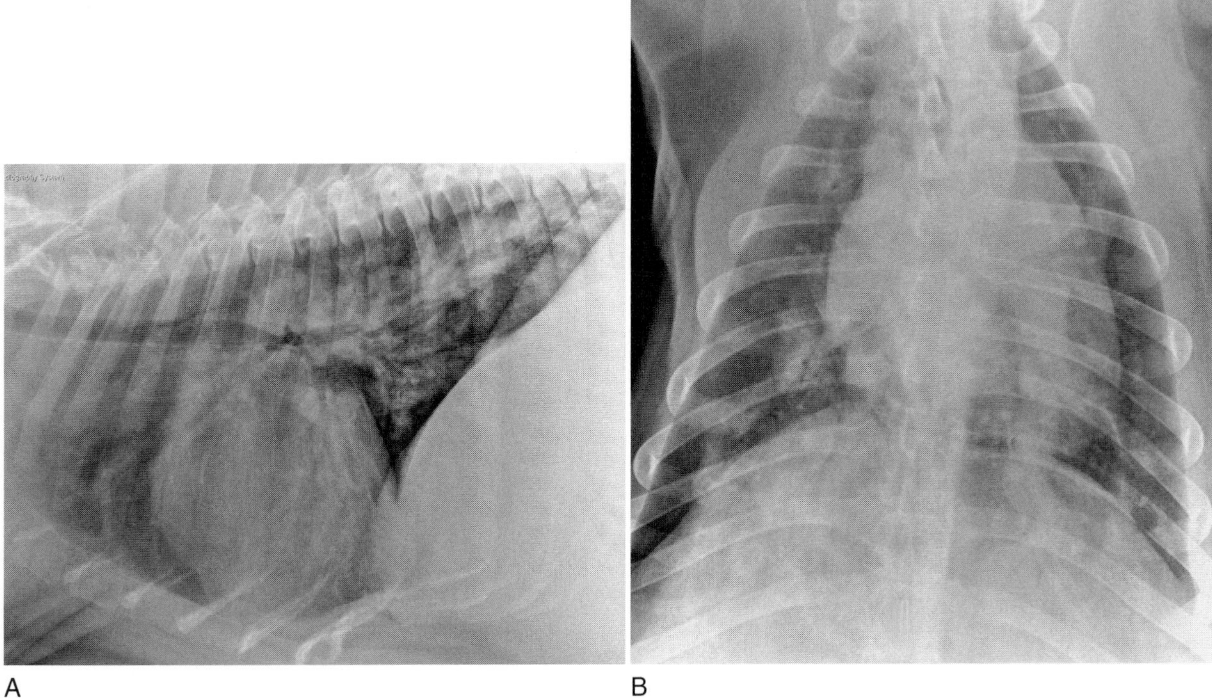

Fig. 33-19 Lateral (A) and dorsoventral (B) radiographs of the thorax of a dog with heartworm disease. Parenchymal pulmonary arteries are enlarged and tortuous. Additionally, a widespread pulmonary pattern is present that is consistent with secondary thromboembolism or allergic pneumonitis.

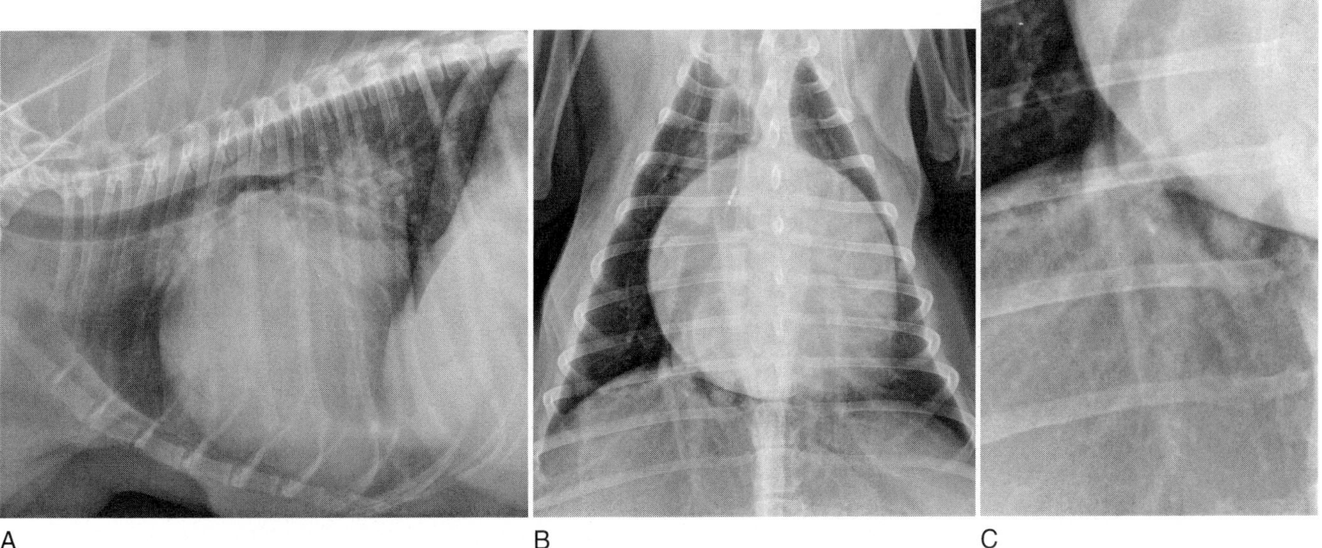

Fig. 33-20 Lateral (A), dorsoventral (B), and close-up dorsoventral (C) views of a dog with compensated mitral insufficiency. In **A** the heart is generally enlarged and the left atrium is dilated. In **B** the heart also appears enlarged and the right caudal pulmonary vein is enlarged compared with the artery. This can also be seen in a close-up (**C**). This is an example of compensated mitral insufficiency. Pulmonary venous hypertension is likely present, evidenced by the pulmonary vein enlargement, but no evidence of pulmonary edema exists to signify left heart failure.

Regardless of cause, the lung fields in these diseases appear hyperlucent because of a lesser contribution by the pulmonary arteries and veins to the overall soft tissue opacity of the lungs. Therefore few x-rays are attenuated on their passage through the aerated lung fields.

Up to this point only a change in size of pulmonary vessels has been considered; shape changes can also occur. A change in shape of pulmonary vessels is most commonly seen in dogs with heartworm disease. In addition to an increase in the size of pulmonary arteries with heartworm disease, vascular tortuosity is possible (see Fig. 33-19), as is nonuniform tapering from the mid-point of the artery distally. Smaller arterial branches may also be dilated. Although rapid peripheral arterial tapering (pruning) from the mid-point of the artery distally, having blunted, squared-off ends (truncation) and focal, saccular dilations of smaller arterial branches, may occur with any disease that causes pulmonary arterial thrombosis or thromboembolism, the incidence of these vascular changes is much greater in heartworm disease.

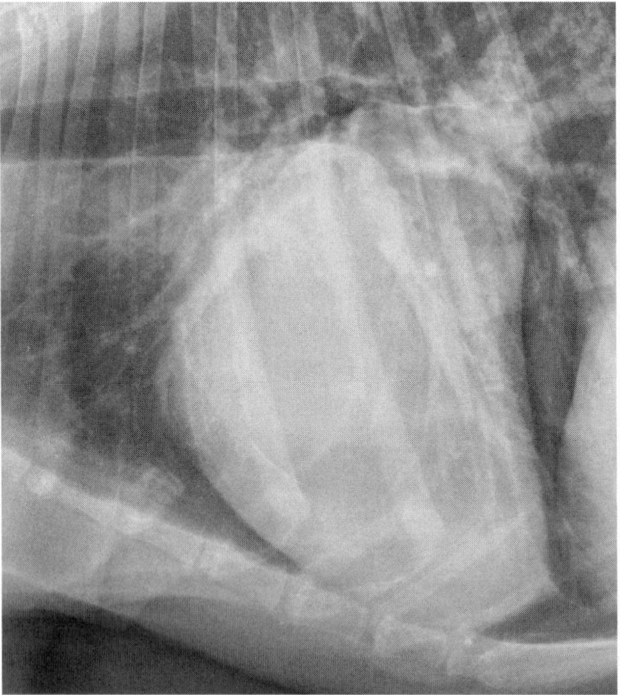

Fig. 33-21 Lateral radiograph of a dog with compensated mitral insufficiency. The left atrium and the right cranial lobe vein are enlarged compared with the artery, a sign consistent with pulmonary venous hypertension.

The margin of pulmonary vessels may also undergo alterations. Pulmonary vascular margination should be relatively sharp and well seen. However, one of the signs of perivascular disease in adjacent lung is either partial or complete loss of visible margins of the outer walls of pulmonary arteries and/or veins. This is usually caused by an accumulation of soft tissue opaque material (fluid, cellular infiltrates, necrotic debris) in either the interstitium or in the alveoli immediately adjacent to the vessel wall, causing border effacement with the vessel and obscuring its margins (Fig. 33-23).

Congestive Heart Failure

Backward left-sided heart failure begins when increased end-diastolic filling pressure in the left ventricle leads to pulmonary venous hypertension. This may progress, if untreated or inappropriately treated, to transudation of fluid from the capillaries into the lung interstitium, causing a hazy, unstructured interstitial pulmonary pattern (pulmonary edema). Pulmonary venous hypertension is recognizable when pulmonary veins are larger than the corresponding lobar artery (see Figs. 33-20 and 33-21).

Cardiogenic pulmonary edema has been described as having a predilection for the perihilar area. This is an association taken from the radiographic appearance of cardiogenic pulmonary edema in human beings. In small animals the finding of a distinct perihilar distribution of cardiogenic pulmonary edema is much less common. The perihilar opacity that occurs because of the summation of the multitude of structures in the perihilar region, coupled with poor aeration from recumbent atelectasis, is often misinterpreted as a real perihilar distribution of disease, especially in patients being assessed for heart failure.

Radiographic visualization of interstitial cardiogenic pulmonary edema is not common because it is short lived, and it

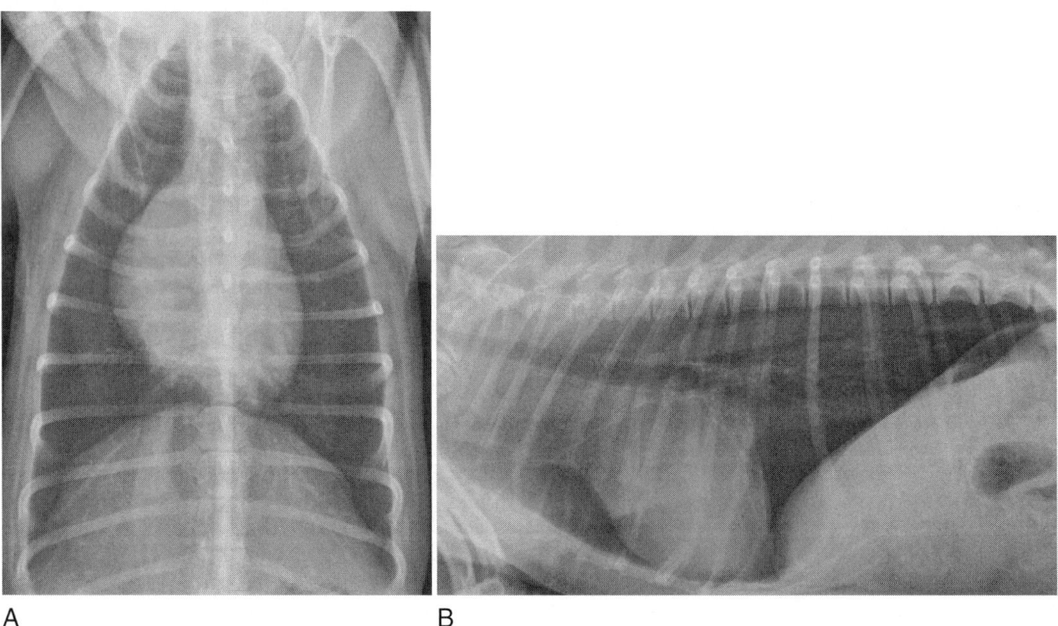

Fig. 33-22 Lateral (A) and ventrodorsal (B) thoracic radiographs of a dog with pulmonary undercirculation from multiple congenital cardiac anomalies. Note the small, inconspicuous pulmonary vessels. The appearance of hypovolemia would be similar.

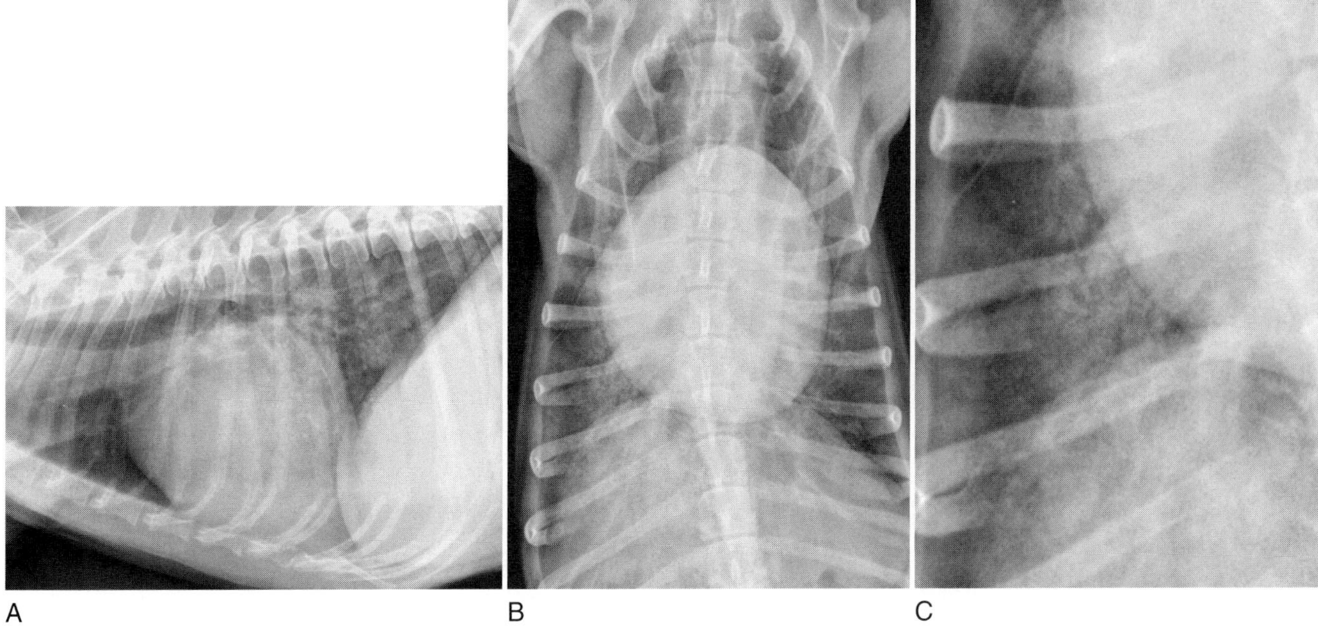

Fig. 33-23 Left lateral (A), dorsoventral (B), and close-up dorsoventral (C) radiographs of a dog with left heart failure attributable to mitral insufficiency. In **A** the heart and left atrium are enlarged. Pulmonary vessels are difficult to identify because of border effacement created by edema in adjacent lung. Increased lung opacity is suggested in the caudal lung lobes, but this may be caused by poor ventilation; any suspicious lung opacity identified in the lateral view must be confirmed in the dorsoventral or ventrodorsal view. In **B,** there is an alveolar pattern in the right middle and caudal lobes. This can be seen in the close-up (**C**). Note the poor visualization of pulmonary vessels in these lobes because of border effacement from the pulmonary edema. This patchy alveolar pattern, without visualization of air bronchograms, is commonly encountered in patients with left heart failure.

also does not create a marked increase in lung opacity. Interstitial pulmonary edema typically progresses to multifocal areas of alveolar pulmonary opacity, obscuring pulmonary vascular structures in the perihilar and middle lung zones. In dogs, pulmonary edema is usually most obvious radiographically in the caudal lobes. Cardiogenic pulmonary edema could be expected to result in generalized homogeneous lung involvement, but this is not common; cardiogenic pulmonary edema is more often patchy, especially in cats (see Fig. 33-23). Some cats also have a component of pleural effusion in addition to pulmonary edema (Fig. 33-24).

Right-sided heart failure usually includes some or all of the following radiographic signs: bilateral pleural effusion with varying degrees of secondary pulmonary atelectasis, ascites, and hepatosplenomegaly. The radiographic appearance of these changes is covered elsewhere in this text.

Acquired Cardiovascular Lesions

Acquired cardiovascular lesions are much more commonly encountered in clinical practice than are congenital lesions. The most common acquired lesions are mitral insufficiency, heartworm disease, and cardiomyopathy.

Mitral Insufficiency

Mitral insufficiency is the most common cause of acquired heart disease in small animal practice, primarily occurring in small breed dogs. Radiographic signs may include various degrees of the following (see Figs. 33-5 to 33-7 and Figs. 33-20 to 33-23):

- Left atrial enlargement, attributable to dilation caused by volume overload from mitral valve regurgitation
- Left ventricular enlargement, from dilation caused by volume overload because not as much blood is ejected from the left ventricle with each systole
- Distended pulmonary veins if venous hypertension has developed
- Pulmonary edema (left heart failure)

Heartworm Disease

Despite the availability of highly effective preventative drugs, heartworm disease is still common in certain parts of the United States. The radiographic changes vary depending on the duration of the infection, the number of worms present, the location of the worms (right heart and/or pulmonary arteries), the rate and degree of cardiac compensation, and the possible die-off of adult worms naturally or in response to antihelmintic medications. Therefore radiographic changes can vary from no abnormal findings or only a mildly affected cardiovascular system to severe involvement (see Figs. 33-17 to 33-19). Common findings are:

- Right ventricular hypertrophy in response to pulmonary hypertension
- Dilation of the main pulmonary artery caused by turbulent blood flow and pulmonary hypertension and possibly the physical presence of heartworms
- Parenchymal pulmonary artery enlargement, truncation, and/or tortuosity from pulmonary hypertension and/or loss in laminar blood flow

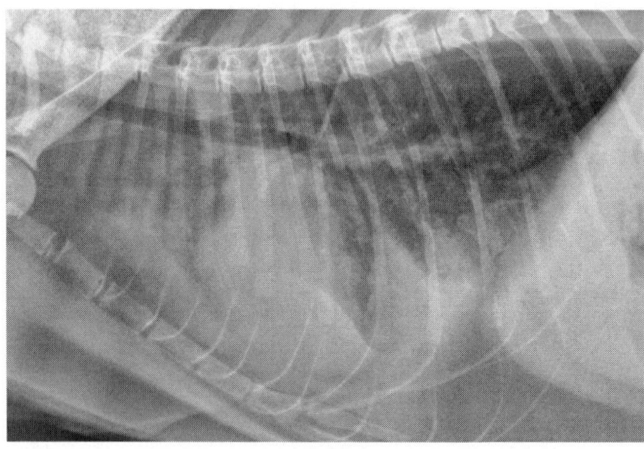

A

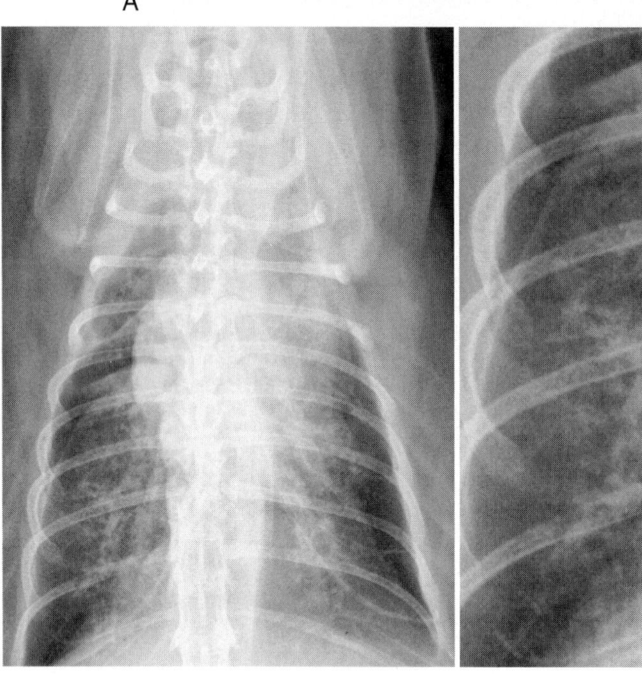

B C

Fig. 33-24 Left lateral (A), ventrodorsal (B), and close-up ventrodorsal (C) radiographs of a cat with left heart failure caused by hypertrophic cardiomyopathy. In **A** interlobar fissures caused by pleural effusion are obvious. The heart cannot be clearly seen in this cat, but it may not appear markedly abnormal in some cats with hypertrophic cardiomyopathy. Increased pulmonary opacity is also suggested in the caudal lung lobes, but this must be confirmed on another view to rule out recumbent atelectasis as a cause. In **B**, there again is evidence of pleural effusion. The caudal lobe pulmonary arteries and veins both appear enlarged; this is often seen in cats in heart failure from cardiomyopathy as a result of fluid retention. A heterogeneous, relatively unstructured pulmonary pattern is present in the caudal lobes that is consistent with pulmonary edema; see close-up in **C**. This heterogeneous pattern is typical of pulmonary edema in cats.

- Peripheral focal or multifocal alveolar pulmonary pattern from pulmonary thromboembolism caused by dead adult worm fragments or secondary eosinophilic pneumonitis
- Hepatomegaly, ascites, and occasionally pleural effusion caused by right-sided heart failure

Cardiomyopathy

Dilated cardiomyopathy occurs from weakened and dysfunctional myocardial contractility. It is most commonly encountered in Doberman Pinschers and Boxers. In dogs, any or all of the following radiographic signs may be seen (Figs 33-25 and 33-26):

- The radiographs may be normal in some dogs with dilated cardiomyopathy
- Generalized cardiomegaly caused by volume overload
- Left atrial dilation may be present because of volume overload or mitral dysfunction from a change in shape of the mitral annulus as a result of the cardiac dilation
- Possible pulmonary vein dilation from mitral valve dysfunction and regurgitation or from fluid retention
- Parenchymal pulmonary artery dilation from fluid retention stimulated by decreased renal perfusion, leading to activation of the renin-angiotensin-aldosterone system
- Possible pleural effusion, hepatomegaly, and/or ascites from right heart failure
- Mixed interstitial and bronchial pattern caused by atypical pulmonary edema; strictly on the basis of radiographic appearance, this distribution of pulmonary edema is unusual and the radiographic pattern is more typical of an allergic airway disease

Hypertrophic cardiomyopathy occasionally occurs in dogs but is more common in cats. Feline hypertrophic cardiomyopathy is characterized by development of a hypertrophied, nondilated left ventricle in the absence of other cardiac diseases. The poor left ventricular diastolic filling leads to reduced cardiac output with secondary increased mitral valve pressure and dilation. Radiographic signs of feline hypertrophic cardiomyopathy include the following (Figs. 33-24 and 33-27):

- Moderate to extreme left atrial dilation. In cats, left atrial dilation with hypertrophic cardiomyopathy can become so large that it extends to the right, giving

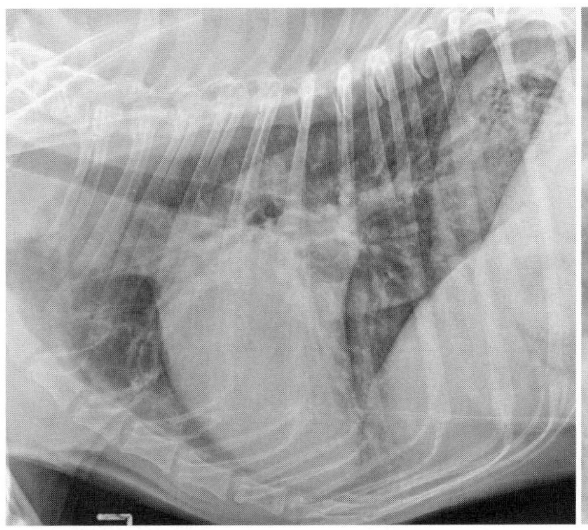
A

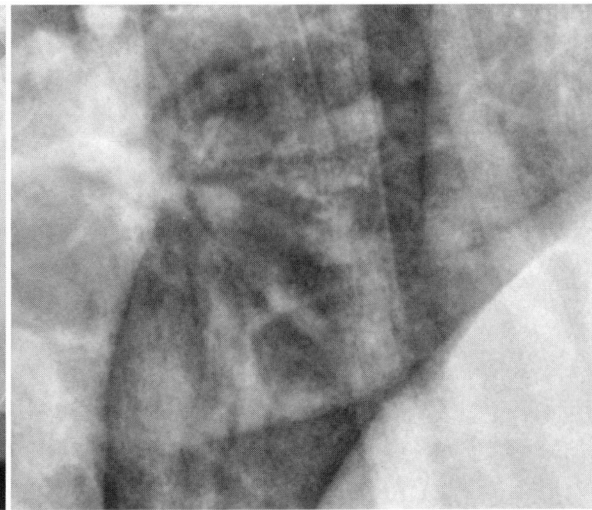
B

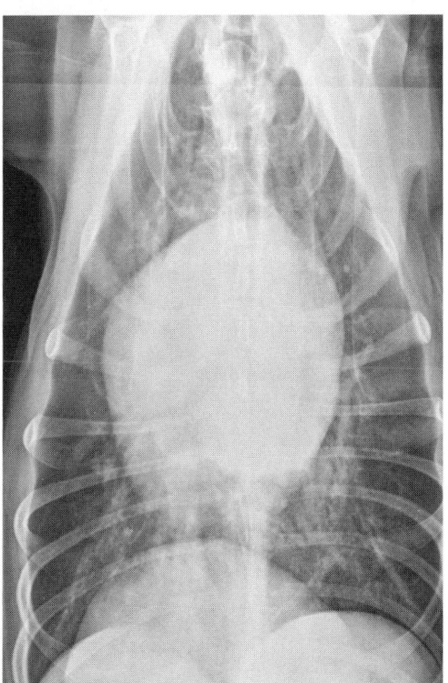
C

Fig. 33-25 Lateral (A), close-up lateral (B), and ventrodorsal (C) radiographs of a dog with dilated cardiomyopathy and left heart failure. The heart in patients with dilated cardiomyopathy may appear normal. In this dog there is enlargement of the left atrium and the right cranial lobe pulmonary vein (A), likely from mitral valve dysfunction with secondary pulmonary venous hypertension. **A** and **C** have the appearance of increased lung opacity. In **B** this opacity can be seen to have a bronchial and unstructured interstitial pattern. This lung pattern is more typical of an inflammatory etiology than cardiogenic pulmonary edema, except in dogs with dilated cardiomyopathy, where it is a typical manifestation of cardiogenic pulmonary edema.

the appearance of biatrial enlargement. Extreme left atrial dilation results in the characteristic "valentine" heart shape in the ventrodorsal or dorsoventral view. Left atrial dilation may be caused by a reduced ability of atrial blood to pass into the restricted size of the left ventricular chamber as a result of the left ventricular myocardial inward hypertrophy, systolic dysfunction, or abnormal systolic anterior motion caused by left ventricular outflow obstruction.

- The left ventricle does not appear enlarged because the hypertrophy is constrictive, or inward, so the myocardium thickens at the expense of the left ventricular chamber size but does not increase its exterior dimensions.
- Enlarged pulmonary veins may appear in early left ventricular decompensation, but visualization of pulmonary venous enlargement is not common in cats with hypertrophic cardiomyopathy.
    - Pulmonary edema will develop as left heart failure progresses if not controlled by medication.
    - Pleural effusion is a late development.

Pericardial Effusion

Although not actually an acquired myocardial or valve problem, pericardial effusion is acquired and can certainly alter the shape and size of the cardiac silhouette. Radiographic signs include the following (Fig. 33-28):

- Large round cardiac silhouette in both lateral and ventrodorsal or dorsoventral views if the effusion is severe enough
- In severely affected patients, the margins of the hugely enlarged cardiac silhouette may touch the thoracic wall bilaterally
- Signs of right heart failure (enlarged caudal vena cava, hepatomegaly, ascites, and occasionally pleural

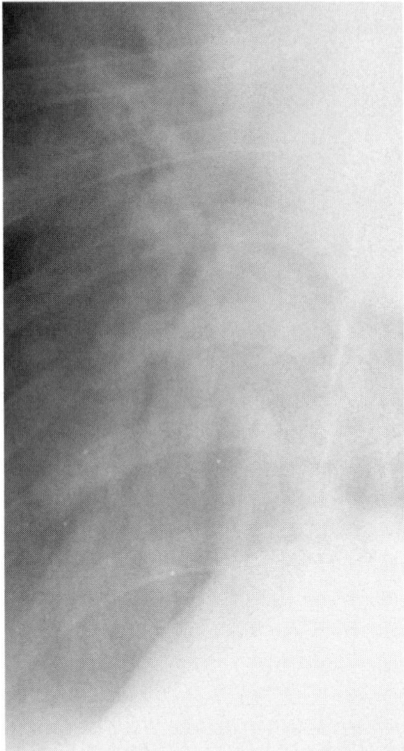

Fig. 33-26 Close-up dorsoventral thoracic radiograph of a dog with dilated cardiomyopathy and heart failure. Both the artery and vein in the right caudal lung lobe are enlarged. This is sometimes seen in dogs with heart failure and is caused by fluid retention. Decreased cardiac output results in activation of the renin-angiotensin-aldosterone pathway with secondary fluid retention.

effusion) may be present if pericardial tamponade is severe enough to prevent diastolic filling of the right atrium and ventricle

- Small to moderate volumes of pericardial effusion often do not have the above-described radiographic signs and can go undetected radiographically.

Congenital Cardiovascular Lesions

Congenital cardiac anomalies are much less commonly encountered than are acquired defects, so only a brief summary is presented.

Patent Ductus Arteriosus

In patent ductus arteriosus, the ductus fails to close normally after birth. This results in an abnormal communication between the descending aorta and the main pulmonary artery. Because of the marked pressure difference between these vessels, a continuous shunting of blood from the aorta into the pulmonary artery occurs during both systole and diastole. This results in pressure and volume overload of the pulmonary circulation and altered myocardial workload. Radiographic signs include the following (Figs. 33-11 and 33-29):

- Segmental enlargement of the proximal aspect of the descending aorta caused by turbulent blood flow and the ductus diverticulum
- Enlargement of the main pulmonary artery from increased pressure and flow
- Enlargement of the left atrium, and possibly the left auricle, from increased blood flow
- Enlarged left ventricle, initially caused by dilation followed by hypertrophy
- Enlarged pulmonary arteries and veins caused by volume and pressure overload

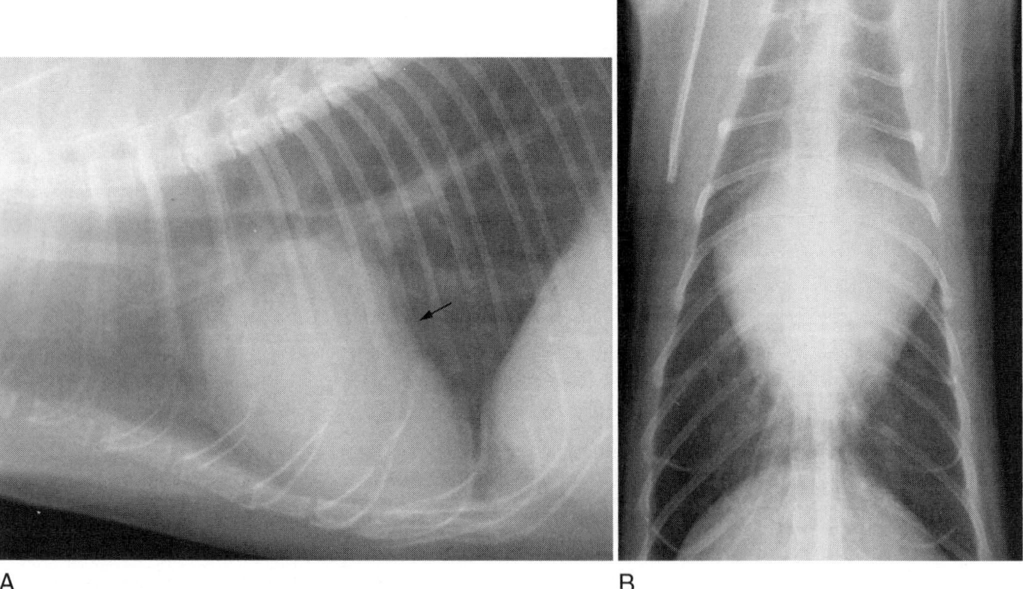

Fig. 33-27 Lateral (**A**) and ventrodorsal (**B**) radiographs of a cat with hypertrophic cardiomyopathy. In **B** the left atrial enlargement is marked and extends to the right side of the patient, creating the so-called "valentine" appearance to the cardiac silhouette. In **A** the left atrium is not as obvious because it is primarily superimposed on the cardiac silhouette; this is dissimilar to the dog, in which an enlarged left atrium causes a mass effect in the region of the tracheal bifurcation. The enlarged left atrium does create a focal concave defect in the shape of the cardiac silhouette in many cats (*arrow* in **A**).

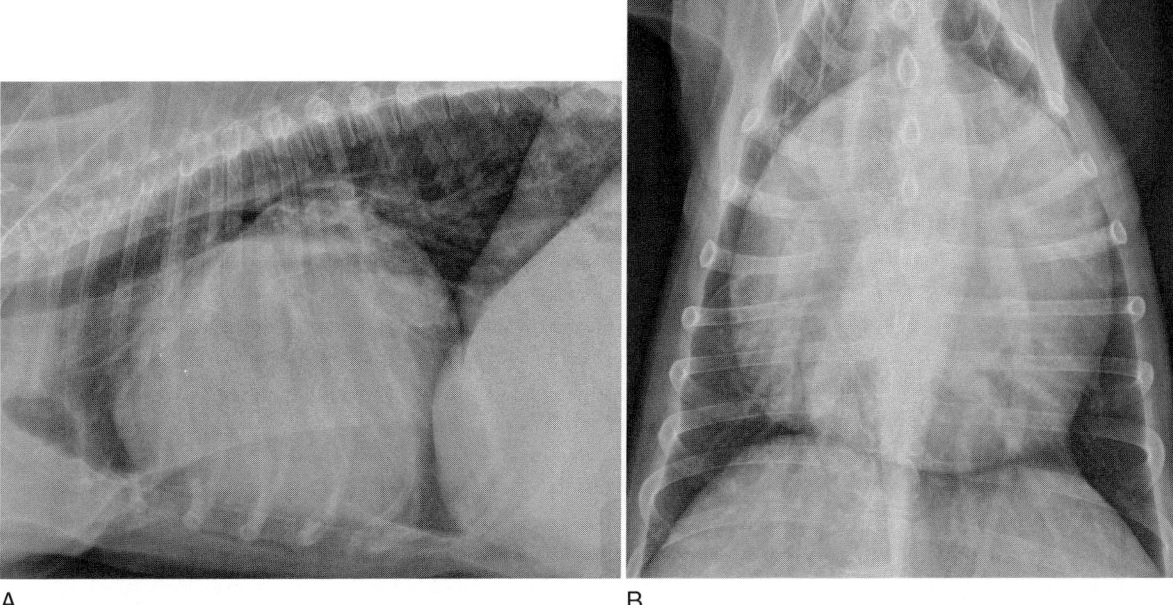

Fig. 33-28 Left lateral (A) and dorsoventral (B) radiographs of a dog with a globoid-appearing cardiac silhouette. This appearance is consistent with pericardial effusion, but based on the radiographs, a peritoneal-pericardial hernia or cardiomegaly cannot be eliminated. This dog had pericardial effusion.

Pulmonic Stenosis

Pulmonic stenosis leads to restriction of flow from the right ventricle into the pulmonary artery. It is typically caused by an abnormal pulmonic valve but can also be associated with narrowing of the pulmonary outflow tract, that is, subvalvular pulmonic stenosis. Radiographic signs include the following (see Fig. 33-9, *A* and *B*):

- Dilated main pulmonary artery caused by turbulence
- Enlarged right ventricle caused by hypertrophy related to increased resistance associated with ejection
- Parenchymal pulmonary vessels are usually normal in size, but if right-sided heart failure develops the pulmonary vessels may be small because of reduced cardiac output

Aortic Stenosis

Narrowing of the subvalvular region of the left ventricle is more common than primary valvular stenosis. As in pulmonic stenosis, the narrowing results in increased resistance to left ventricular ejection. Mitral valve dysfunction and regurgitation may occur as a result of the mitral annulus becoming misshapen. Radiographic signs include the following (Fig. 33-30):

- Enlargement of the aortic arch from turbulent flow, appearing as widening of the precardiac mediastinum
- Elongation of the left ventricle from hypertrophy
- Left atrial dilation if secondary mitral valve dysfunction develops
- Normal pulmonary vessels unless secondary mitral valve dysfunction develops, leading to pulmonary venous hypertension

Ventricular Septal Defect

Abnormal development results in a communication between the left and right ventricle, usually located dorsally in the septum just ventral to the aortic valve. Because systolic pressure is higher in the left ventricle, blood flows into the right ventricle during systole. Little flow is present during diastole because of the similar diastolic pressure in the two ventricles. Because of the upper location of the defect, most shunted blood immediately enters the pulmonary artery and not the right ventricle. The volume of blood shunted with each contraction depends on the size of the defect, but the magnitude of shunting is typically less than with patent ductus arteriosus. The magnitude of radiographic signs depends on the amount of blood shunting through the defect and can include the following (Fig. 33-31):

- Possible mild right ventricular hypertrophy from volume and pressure overload
- Pulmonary arteries and veins may be normal or mildly increased in size because of a mild to moderate increase in pulmonary blood flow; enlargement is typically less than that seen with patent ductus arteriosus

Tricuspid Dysplasia

Tricuspid dysplasia is a congenital malformation of the tricuspid valve. Radiographic signs include the following (see Fig. 33-8):

- Right atrial enlargement from pressure and volume overload
- Pulmonary vessels are usually normal but may become small if cardiac output decreases from the right ventricle.

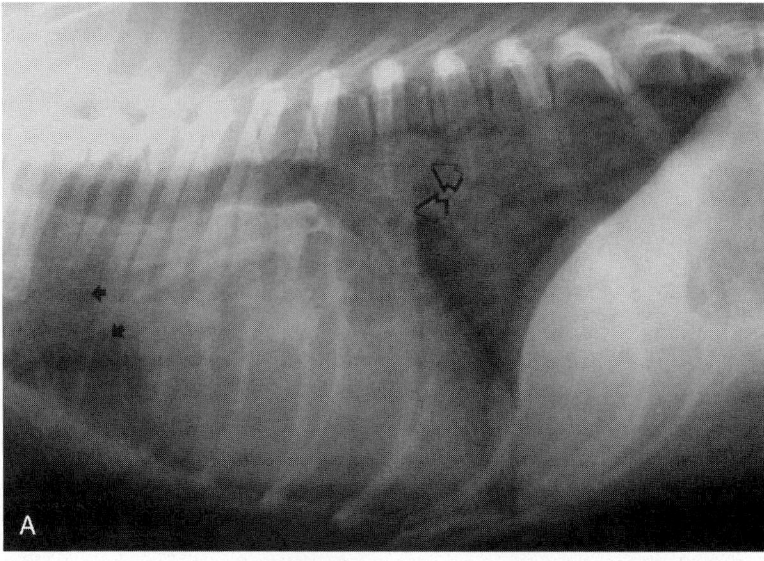

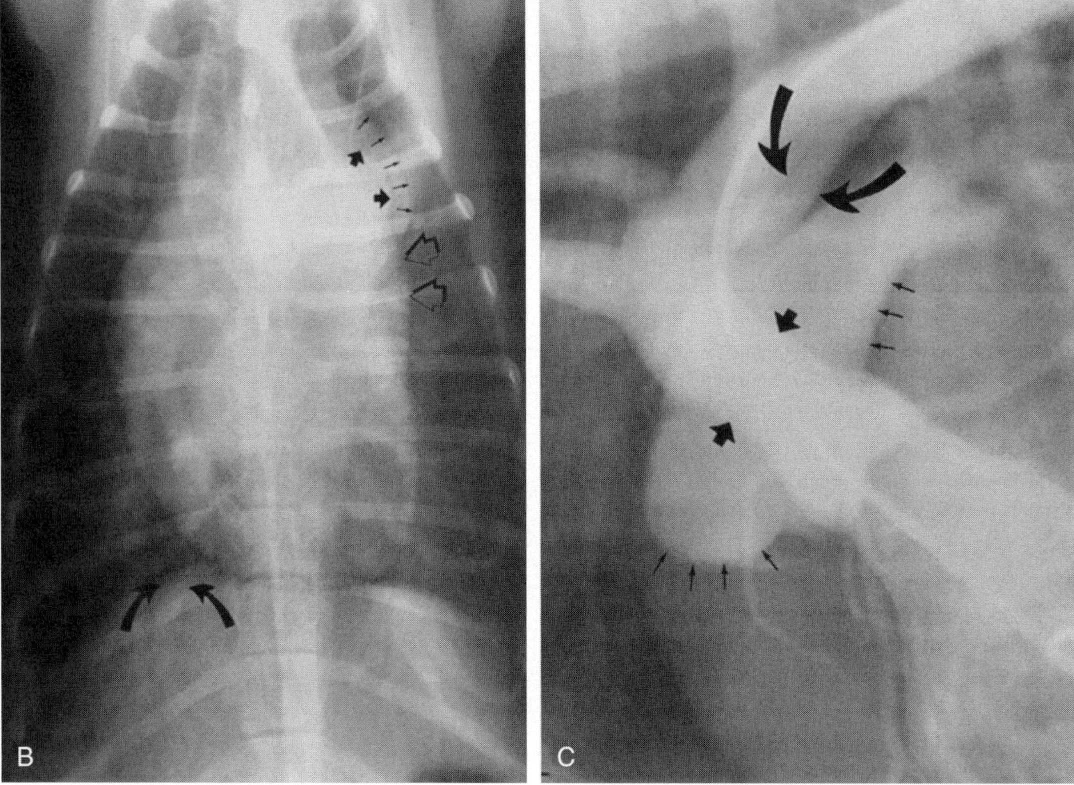

Fig. 33-29 Right lateral (A) and dorsoventral (B) thoracic radiographs of an 8-month-old female Miniature Longhair Dachshund with patent ductus arteriosus. In the dorsoventral projection (B), dilation of the proximal descending aorta *(large solid arrows)* is making the cardiac silhouette appear elongated and creates a distinct bulge. A second distinct bulge *(small thin arrows)* just craniolateral to the descending aorta is caused by dilation of the main pulmonary artery segment. A third distinct bulge *(large open arrows)* along the left cardiac border is caused by dilation and protrusion of the left auricle. Note the enlarged right caudal lobe pulmonary vein *(curved arrows)* and its adjacent artery, caused by pulmonary overcirculation. In the lateral projection (A), the hugely dilated left atrium *(large open arrows)* and the filling of the region of the junction of the right ventricle and the cranial vena cava *(small solid arrows)* caused by aortic and main pulmonary artery segment dilation make the heart base appear wider and the entire cardiac silhouette appear elongated. In a selective left ventricular angiocardiogram (C) (different patient), the dilated main pulmonary artery segment *(small thin arrows)* and the ascending aorta *(solid arrowheads)* are accentuated by positive-contrast medium, and the patent ductus arteriosus *(curved arrows)* lies between the descending aorta and the main pulmonary artery segment and is opacified because of the left-to-right shunting of blood.

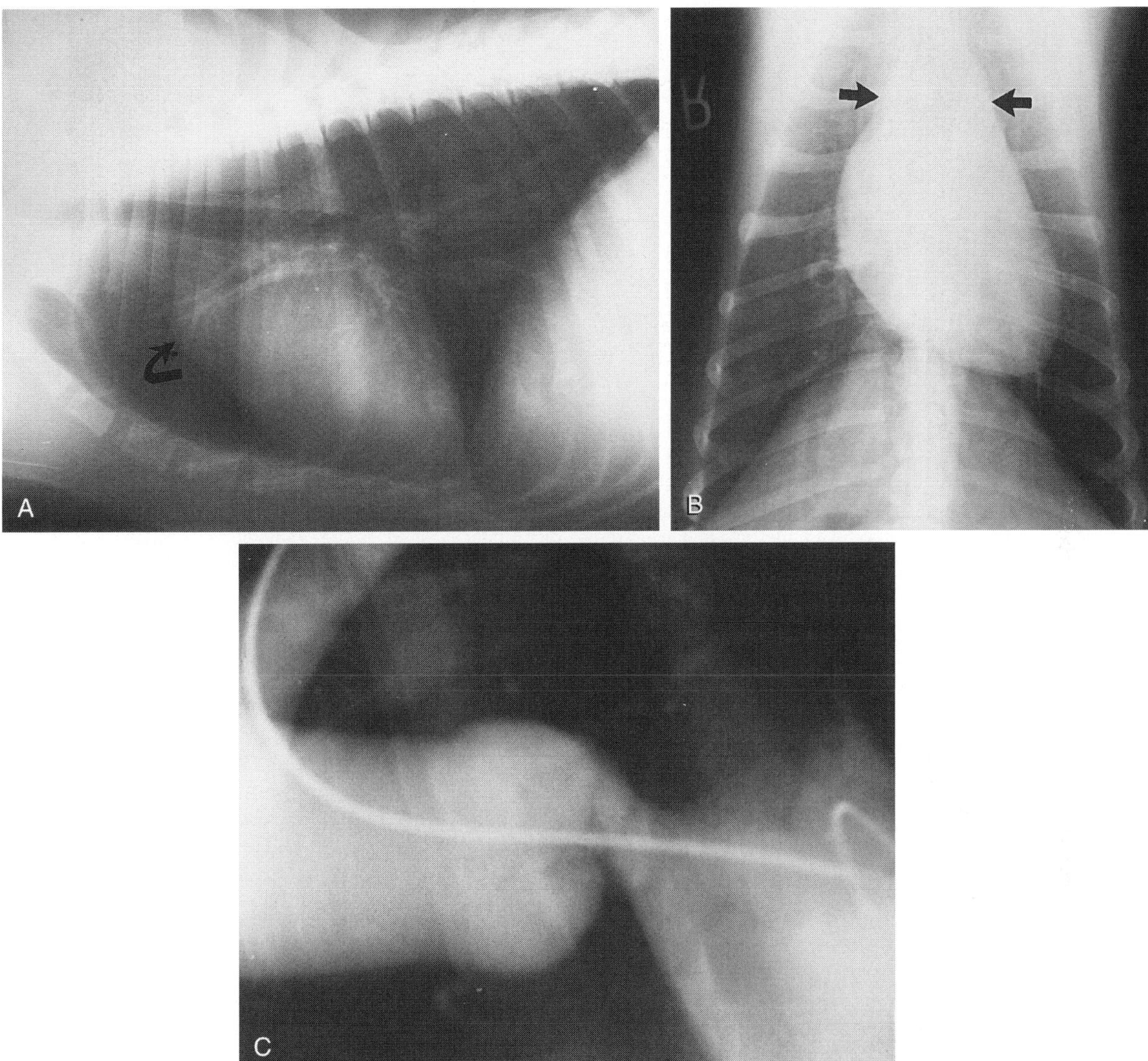

Fig. 33-30 Right lateral (A) and dorsoventral (B) thoracic radiographs of an 11-month-old female Rottweiler with aortic stenosis. The left ventricle is not enlarged in either projection compared with some other patients with this defect. Note the shift of the cardiac apex to the left in B; this is caused by the patient being in sternal recumbency, with cranial displacement of the diaphragm pushing the apex to the left. This is a common source of misdiagnosis of cardiomegaly. The caudal portion of the cranial mediastinum is widened in the dorsoventral projection *(arrows)*, and a bulge is present in the region of the junction of the right ventricle with the cranial vena cava in the lateral view *(curved arrow)*. These radiographic signs are produced by poststenotic dilation of the root of the aorta. In **C** note the narrow subvalvular region and dilation of the aorta distal to the aortic sinus in the angiocardiogram. The aorta should be no wider than the sinus; enlargement of the aorta distal to the sinus is caused by turbulent flow.

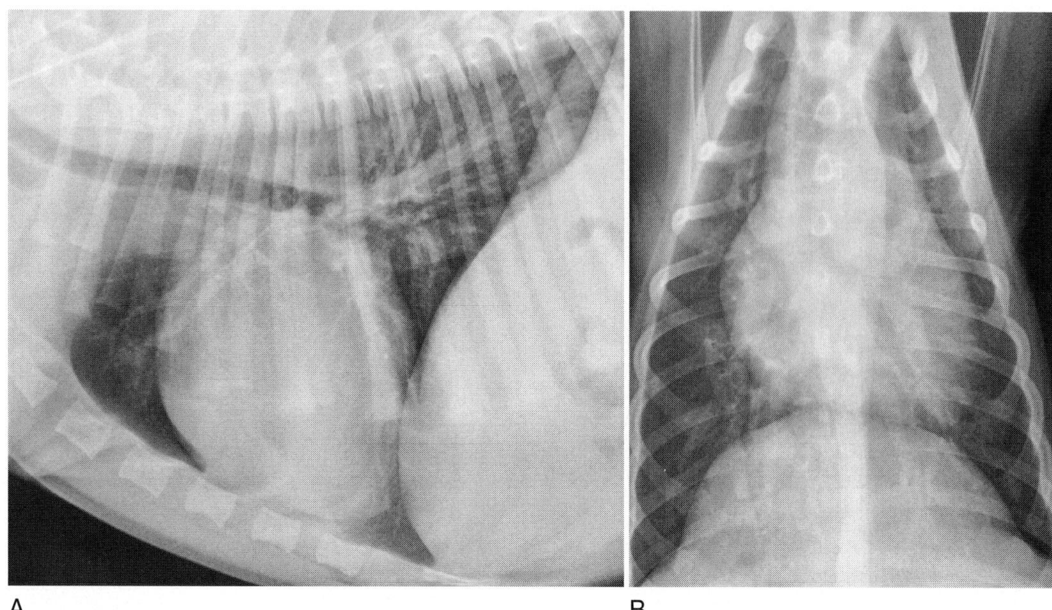

Fig. 33-31 Lateral (**A**) and dorsoventral (**B**) radiographs of a dog with a ventricular septal defect. In **A** there is excessive elevation of the cardiac apex from the sternum consistent with right ventricular hypertrophy, mild dilation of the left atrium, and slight enlargement of the left cranial lobe pulmonary artery and vein, consistent with mild overcirculation. In **B** the apex is displaced to the left as a result of the dog being in sternal recumbency. Slight enlargement of the caudal lobe pulmonary arteries and veins is present, consistent with mild overcirculation. These findings are typical, but not conclusive proof, of a ventricular septal defect.

REFERENCES

1. Kittleson MD: Radiology. In Kittleson MD, Kienle RD, editors: *Small animal cardiovascular medicine,* St. Louis: Mosby, 1998, p 47-71.
2. Lord PF, Suter PF: Radiology. In Fox PR, Sisson D, Moise S, editors: *Textbook of feline and canine cardiology,* Philadelphia: WB Saunders, 1999, p 107-129.
3. Ruehl WW, Thrall DE: The effect of dorsal versus ventral recumbency on the radiographic appearance of the canine thorax, *Vet Radiol* 22:10, 1981.
4. Buchanan JW, Bucheler J: Vertebral scale system to measure canine heart size in radiographs, *J Am Vet Med Assoc* 206:194, 1995.
5. Lamb CR, Tyler M, Boswood A et al: Assessment of the value of the vertebral heart scale in the radiographic diagnosis of cardiac disease in dogs, *Vet Rec* 146: 687, 2000.
6. Lamb CR, Wikeley H, Boswood A et al: Use of breed-specific ranges for vertebral heart scale in the radiographic diagnosis of cardiac disease in dogs, *Vet Rec* 148:707, 2001.
7. Silverman S, Suter PF: Influence of inspiration and expiration on canine thoracic radiographs, *J Am Vet Med Assoc* 166:502, 1975.
8. Lehmukhl L, Bonagura JD, Biller DS et al: Radiographic evaluation of caudal vena cava size in dogs, *Vet Radiol Ultrasound* 38:94, 1997.
9. Moon ML, Keene BW, Lessard P et al: Age related changes in the feline cardiac silhouette, *Vet Radiol Ultrasound* 34:315, 1993.
10. Thrall DE, Losonsky JM: A method for evaluating canine pulmonary circulatory dynamics from survey radiographs, *J Am Anim Hosp Assoc* 12:457, 1976.
11. Losonsky JM, Thrall DE, Lewis RE: Thoracic radiographic abnormalities in 200 dogs with spontaneous heartworm disease, *Vet Radiol* 24:120, 1983.
12. Atkins CE, DeFrancesco TC, Coats JR et al: Heartworm infection in cats: 50 cases (1985-1997), *J Am Vet Med Assoc* 217:355, 1997.
13. Selcer BA, Newell SM, Mansour AE et al: Radiographic and 2-D echocardiographic findings in 18 cats experimentally exposed to *D. immitis* via mosquito bites, *Vet Radiol Ultrasound* 37:37, 1997.
14. Schafer M, Berry CR: Cardiac and pulmonary mensuration in feline heartworm disease, *Vet Radiol Ultrasound* 1996:499, 1995.
15. DeFrancesco TC, Atkins CE, Miller MW et al: Use of echocardiography for the diagnosis of heartworm disease in cats: 43 cases (1985-1997), *J Am Vet Med Assoc* 218:66, 2001.

ELECTRONIC RESOURCES evolve

Additional information related to the content in Chapter 33 can be found on the companion Web site at evolve http://evolve.elsevier.com/Thrall/vetrad/.

- Key Points
- Chapter Quiz
- Case Study 33-1
- Case Study 33-2

CHAPTER • 34
The Canine and Feline Lung

Christopher R. Lamb

The radiology of pulmonary disease is described in four sections: diseases that cause increased opacity, hyperlucency, pulmonary mass lesions, and calcified pulmonary lesions.

INCREASED OPACITY

The radiographic signs of pulmonary diseases that cause increased opacity are customarily described in terms of the anatomic divisions of the lung. The three categories of radiographic signs (patterns) described are bronchial, interstitial, and alveolar. The radiographic aspects of each of these appearances are described in detail in Chapter 25.

Bronchial Pattern

Calcification of the bronchial wall causes an increase in bronchial wall opacity but not thickness (Fig. 34-1). It is common in middle-aged and old dogs and is not significant. In cats with bronchial disease, multifocal pulmonary calcification may be observed as a result of calcification of the peribronchial mucus glands or broncholithiasis (Fig. 34-2).[1] Opaque foci compatible with calcification of peribronchial mucus glands may also be observed in cats without respiratory signs; hence, this can also be an incidental finding.

Thickening of the bronchial wall is most often the result of chronic inflammation; therefore the principal differential diagnoses for a diffuse bronchial pattern are chronic bronchitis (Fig. 34-3),[3,4] pulmonary eosinophilic infiltrates,[5,6] and parasitic infestation, such as aelurostrongylosis.[7] In some instances infiltration of the peribronchial tissues by edema[8] or inflammatory cells may produce the appearance of bronchial thickening on radiographs; therefore bronchopneumonia and peribronchial edema, for example, as a result of cardiac insufficiency (especially heart failure in large-breed dogs with dilated cardiomyopathy), lymphatic dilatation, and acute allergic or inflammatory pulmonary conditions must also be considered as differential diagnoses of the bronchial pattern (Box 34-1). Sampling the lung by a transtracheal aspirate or bronchoalveolar lavage is often helpful in narrowing the list of considerations for a bronchial pattern.

Bronchial dilation and loss of the normal tapering between bronchial walls are signs of bronchiectasis (Fig. 34-4).[9-11] The diameter of a bronchiectatic airway may fluctuate with respiration, being largest on inspiration. Thus the phase of respiration at the time the image is acquired may affect recognition of bronchiectasis. Recognition of bronchiectasis is important because affected patients are more prone to chronic respiratory infections.

Interstitial Patterns

The interstitium is the name given to the non-air-containing elements of the lung, excluding the macroscopic blood vessels. The interstitium includes the alveolar septum, the interlobular septum, and microscopic blood vessels. Accumulation of cells or fluid in the interstitium leads to an increase in the opacity of the lung without obliteration of the air spaces; hence structures outlined by air, such as the cardiac silhouette, caudal vena cava, and the pulmonary vessels, remain visible, although they may be partially obscured.[12] Interstitial disease can be thought of as either nodular or unstructured and localized or diffuse (Boxes 34-2 and 34-3).[12] Obtaining the definitive diagnosis for an interstitial pattern may require direct cytologic sampling, such as from needle aspiration or biopsy. Because many diseases causing an interstitial pattern do not involve the airway per se, sampling by transtracheal aspiration or bronchoalveolar lavage may not be helpful.

Interstitial Nodules

Pulmonary nodules may be first recognized radiographically when they reach 4 to 5 mm in diameter; even at this size, excellent-quality radiographs are needed for their detection. Nodules smaller than 5 mm in diameter must overlap and thereby summate with each other to be visible radiographically. Nodules in the dependent lung may not be seen radiographically because of the partial collapse and increased radiographic opacity of that lung.[13] Focal opacities in the lung could be pulmonary nodules, normal pulmonary vessels seen end on, or foci of heterotopic bone (which occur frequently in the lungs of older, usually large-breed, dogs).[14] These possibilities may be differentiated by the following criteria (Fig. 34-5). Pulmonary vessels seen end on:

- Usually occur close to vessels seen side on
- Are less numerous in the periphery of the lung
- Are never larger in diameter than the nearest side-on vessel but are more opaque because, as a result of their orientation, they represent a greater thickness of tissue.

In contrast, pulmonary nodules:

- Are not consistently associated with vessels
- Have a similar opacity to a side-on vessel of the same diameter
- May be small or large regardless of their location within the lung; hence pulmonary nodules may be recognized with certainty when they are larger than adjacent blood vessels

Foci of pulmonary heterotopic bone:

- Are usually small with a speckled opacity
- Are irregularly shaped on close inspection

Pulmonary nodules may be solitary or multiple, solid or cavitary (see Box 34-2). The cavity of a pulmonary nodule will be visible radiographically only if it contains gas, which may occur if it communicates with an airway or has a necrotic center. Pulmonary nodules may have distinct, smooth margins or may have indistinct margins and tend to coalesce, which makes individual nodules more difficult to recognize. The

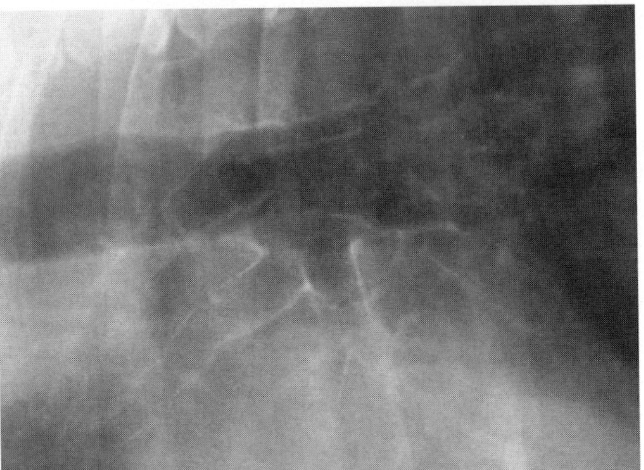

Fig. 34-1 Bronchial calcification. Close-up of a lateral radiograph of an aged dog in which the walls of the principal bronchi are distinctly opaque as a result of calcification.

Box • 34-1

Differential Diagnosis of the Bronchial Pattern

Bronchial calcification
Chronic bronchitis
- Allergic
- Irritant, such as smoke
- Parasitic, such as aelurostrongylosis
- Drug-related, such as bromide in cats

Peribronchial cuffing
- Edema
- Pulmonary eosinophilic infiltrates
- Bronchopneumonia

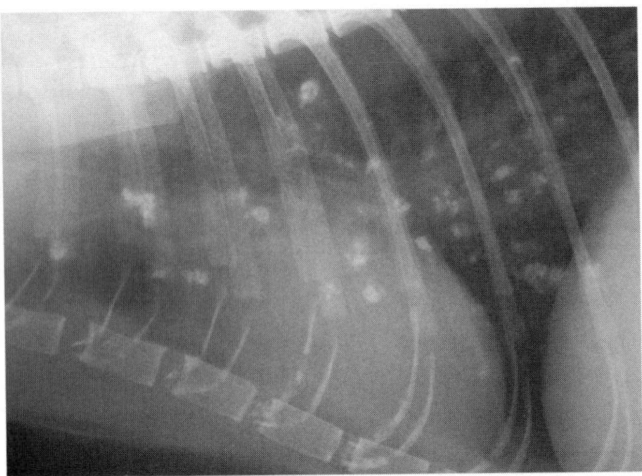

Fig. 34-2 Lateral thoracic radiograph of a cat in which there are multiple small, irregular, opaque foci throughout the lung. This is compatible with calcification of the peribronchial glands.

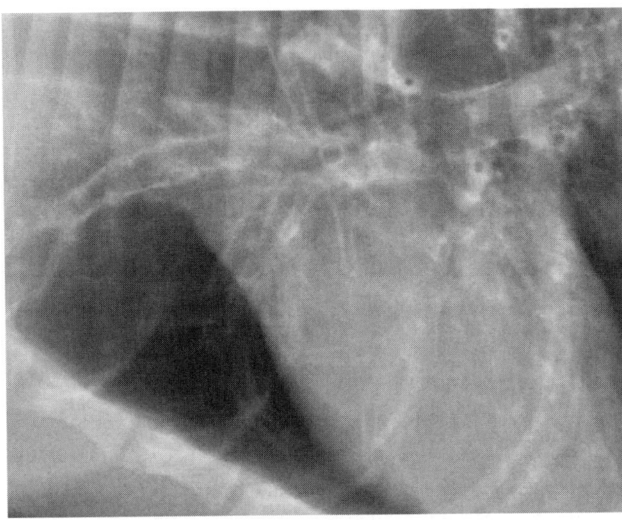

Fig. 34-3 Lateral thoracic radiograph of a middle-aged dog with chronic cough attributable to bronchitis. A striking bronchial pattern well seen overlying the heart is present as a result of thickened bronchial walls.

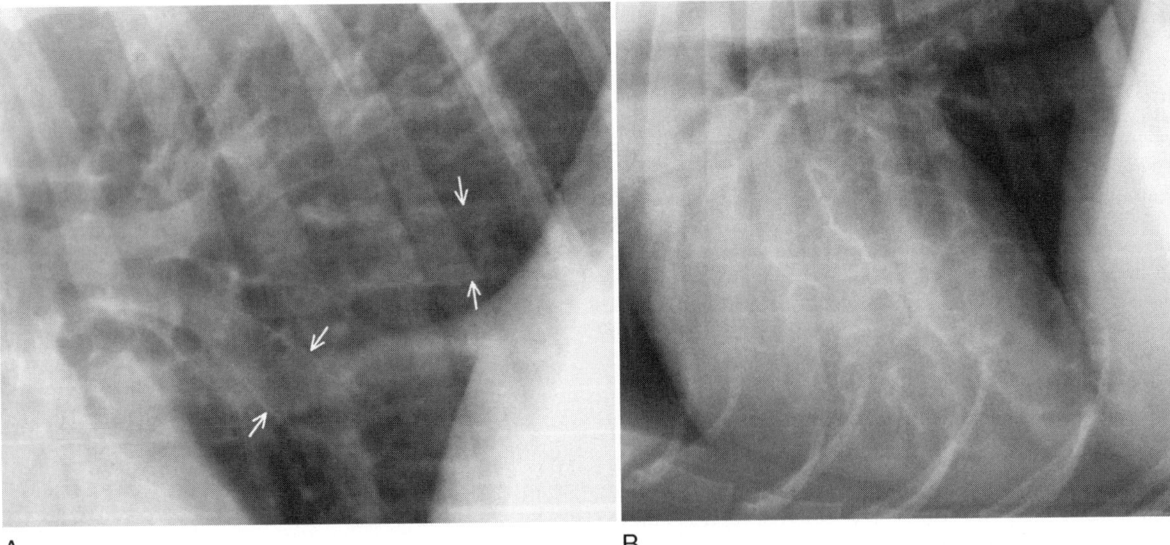

Fig. 34-4 A, Close-up of a lateral thoracic radiograph of a Husky with a history of chronic cough that improved when antibiotics were administered but recurred when medication was discontinued. Endoscopically, excessive mucus and evidence of bronchiectasis were found in the bronchi. Bronchiectasis is visible radiographically as loss of the normal tapering of the bronchial walls *(arrows)*. **B,** Marked saccular bronchiectasis in another dog in which the bronchial walls are markedly thickened and misshapen, producing a bubbly, branching structure superimposed on the cardiac silhouette.

Box • 34-2

Differential Diagnosis of Nodular Interstitial Patterns

- Noncavitary nodule
  - Thoracic wall structure, such as nipple, tick
    - Primary lung tumor
    - Pulmonary metastasis
    - Granuloma
    - Mycotic
    - Heartworm associated
    - Foreign body
    - Eosinophilic (idiopathic)
  - Fluid-filled bulla
  - Hematoma
  - Abscess
  - Cyst
  - Mucus-filled bronchus
- Cavitary nodule
  - Primary lung tumor
  - Pulmonary metastasis
  - Mycotic granuloma, such as blastomycosis
  - Paragonimiasis
  - Abscess
  - Partially fluid-filled bulla
  - Cyst
  - Bronchiectasis

most common solitary nodules in dogs are primary pulmonary tumors, and the most common multiple nodules are pulmonary metastases. The sensitivity of radiography for pulmonary metastasis detection has been estimated to be 65% to 97%.[15-20]

Distinguishing the various causes of pulmonary nodules radiographically is virtually impossible because of the similar appearance of tumors (Fig. 34-6),[15,17-19,21-26] granulomas (Fig. 34-7),[27-29] and abscesses (Fig. 34-8).[26] Also, a fluid- or mucus-filled bronchus could be confused with a nodule in some instances (Fig. 34-9). The pulmonary lesions of acute paragonimiasis appear radiographically as multiple, poorly circumscribed nodules that range from 1 to 4 cm in diameter; subpleural air-filled cavities and bullae (often septated) develop in animals with chronic infection.[30]

Unstructured Interstitial Patterns

A wide variety of causes must be considered when an unstructured interstitial pattern is observed (see Box 34-3). Pathologic and nonpathologic conditions that produce unstructured interstitial patterns can be difficult to distinguish radiographically. Nonpathologic factors include an underexposed radiograph; a radiograph made during expiration rather than peak inspiration; lack of adequate lung inflation associated with obesity, sedation, or abdominal distension; and superimposition of the lung by pleural fluid. Abnormal causes of unstructured interstitial patterns include pulmonary edema, inflammatory or neoplastic cellular infiltrates (Fig. 34-10), and fibrosis. Various systemic diseases may also cause secondary pneumonitis and interstitial patterns, such as uremia (Fig. 34-11).

Some diseases may produce either nodular or unstructured interstitial patterns depending on factors such as etiologic agent, duration, and severity; examples include mycotic

Box • 34-3

Differential Diagnosis of Unstructured (Hazy) Interstitial Patterns

- Diffuse
  - Artifact
    - Underexposed radiograph
    - Underinflated lung, such as end-expiratory exposure, sedation, obesity
    - "Old dog lung"
  - Lymphosarcoma
  - Diffuse pulmonary metastasis
  - Pneumonitis
    - Viral distemper
    - Parasitic, such as dirofilariasis, aelurostrongylosis
    - Metabolic, such as uremia, pancreatitis, septicemia
    - Inhalant, such as allergy, smoke
    - Toxic, such as paraquat
  - Disease in transition
    - Edema
    - Bronchopneumonia
    - Hemorrhage
- Localized
  - Partial lung collapse
  - Hemorrhage
  - Pulmonary embolism
  - Bronchial foreign body
  - Disease in transition
    - Edema
    - Bronchopneumonia
    - Hemorrhage
    - Pulmonary parasites

pneumonia (Fig. 34-12),[27,29,31-33] metastatic neoplasia (Fig. 34-13),[15,17-19,24,34] and dirofilariasis.[35,36]

Alveolar Pattern

The alveolar pattern is a radiographic sign of diseases that displace air from the distal air spaces of the lung (hence it is also referred to as the air space pattern). Lobar collapse and atelectasis, fluid accumulation, and cellular infiltrates (or combinations of these) may produce the alveolar pattern. The radiographic signs of an alveolar pattern are discussed in Chapter 25.

An alveolar pattern may be patchy or diffuse and its appearance may change quickly, particularly when the alveolar pattern is caused by fluid accumulation in the lung. Changes in the severity and distribution of fluid in the lung tend to occur more quickly than movement of cells. When an alveolar pattern is identified radiographically and the differential diagnosis includes pulmonary edema, this possibility may be tested, if clinically acceptable, by repeating the radiographs after 12 hours of treatment with a diuretic. If edema was the cause, a marked decrease in infiltrate will become apparent (Fig. 34-14). Other causes of an alveolar pattern, such as bronchopneumonia (Fig. 34-15) or hemorrhage, are unlikely to change appearance significantly in such a short period. In fact, in these instances a time lag between the onset of clinical signs and the radiographic signs of distal air space disease is often observed, and a similar time lag may occur

Text continued on p. 598

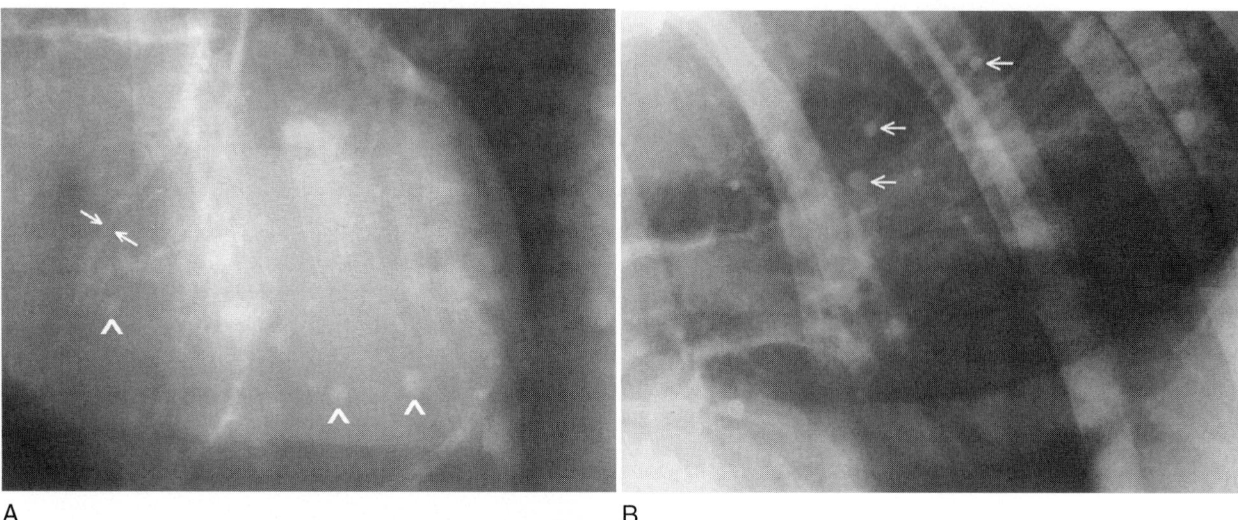

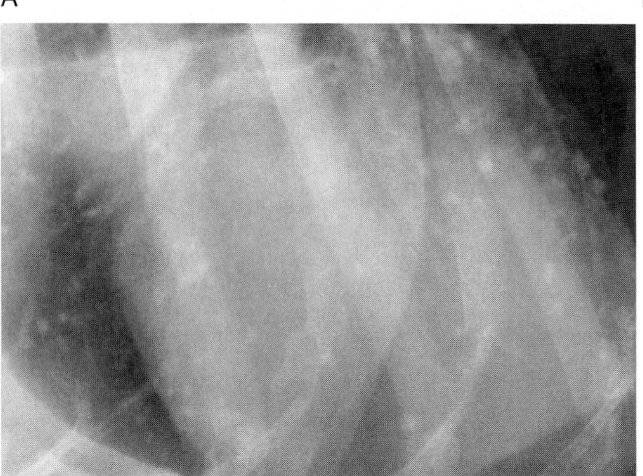

Fig. 34-5 A, Close-up of a lateral thoracic radiograph in which pulmonary nodules are visible. These nodules (some indicated by *arrowheads*) are larger than the adjacent pulmonary vessels *(small arrows)* and occur in peripheral parts of the lung where vessels are normally too small to be seen radiographically. **B,** Pulmonary vessels viewed end on *(small arrows)* are effectively thicker than soft tissue nodules of the same diameter, so they appear more opaque. As in this instance, they are most clearly visible near the pulmonary hilus, where the vessels are largest. **C,** Foci of pulmonary heterotopic bone are distinguished from vessels or soft tissue nodules by their variable shape and speckled opacity.

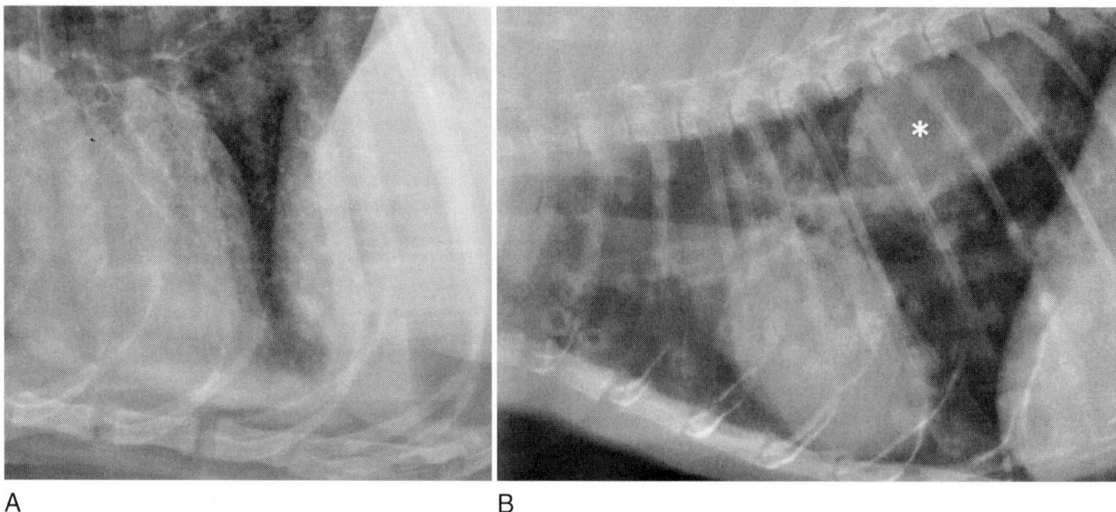

Fig. 34-6 A, Close-up lateral thoracic radiograph of a dog with metastatic hemangiosarcoma. Multiple small nodules are present in the lung. These are easiest to see where the lung is superimposed on the liver. This is often the situation with small military lung nodules. Visualization of such nodules depends highly on radiographic technique, and increasing the image contrast may sometimes be beneficial. **B,** Lateral thoracic radiograph of a cat with primary pulmonary carcinoma *(asterisk)* and pulmonary metastasis. Several of the metastases are cavitary (most clearly visible cranial to the heart).

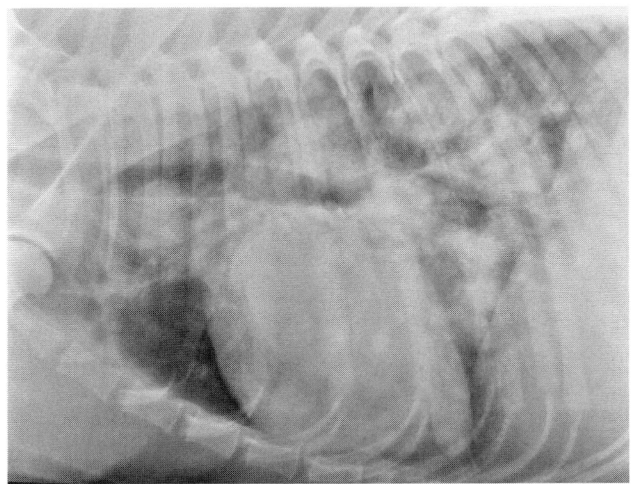

Fig. 34-7 Lateral thoracic radiograph of an 8-month-old Retriever with cough and exercise intolerance. Several large pulmonary nodules are visible. Clinicopathologic tests supported heartworm disease, and the pulmonary lesions resolved after treatment with anthelmintics. Final diagnosis was heartworm-associated eosinophilic pneumonitis.

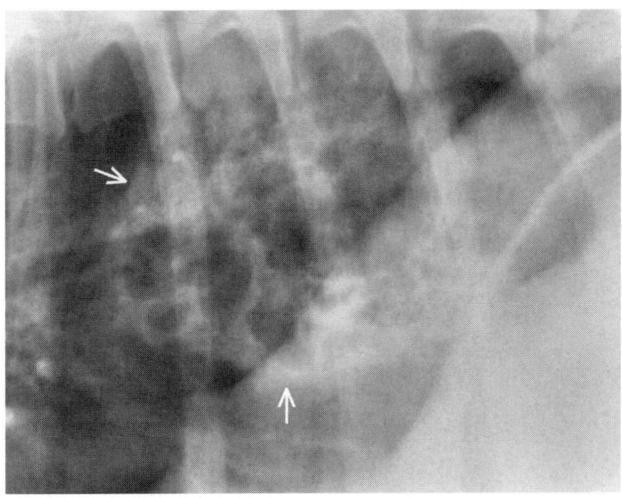

Fig. 34-8 Close-up of the caudodorsal lung field, in which a poorly marginated cavitated lung mass *(arrows)* can be seen. Primary lung tumor was suspected and lobectomy was performed; however, histologic examination indicated abscess caused by septic pulmonary infarction.

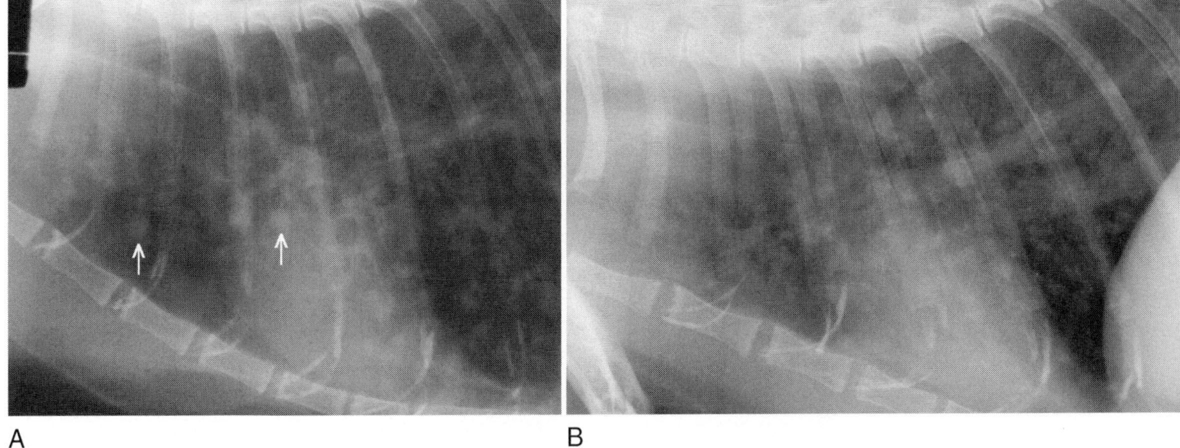

Fig. 34-9 A, Close-up of a lateral thoracic radiograph of a dyspneic cat. Multiple small nodules are visible *(arrows)*. On the basis of examination of the entire radiograph, the lungs were considered hyperlucent, possibly reflecting air trapping. The cat was treated with prednisolone and a mucolytic. In a repeat radiograph 18 days later (**B**), the nodules are no longer evident and the hyperlucency has resolved. Mucus plugging of bronchi in cats or dogs with bronchial disease may mimic pulmonary interstitial nodules of other etiologies. (Courtesy Anita S. Maitra, MRCVS.)

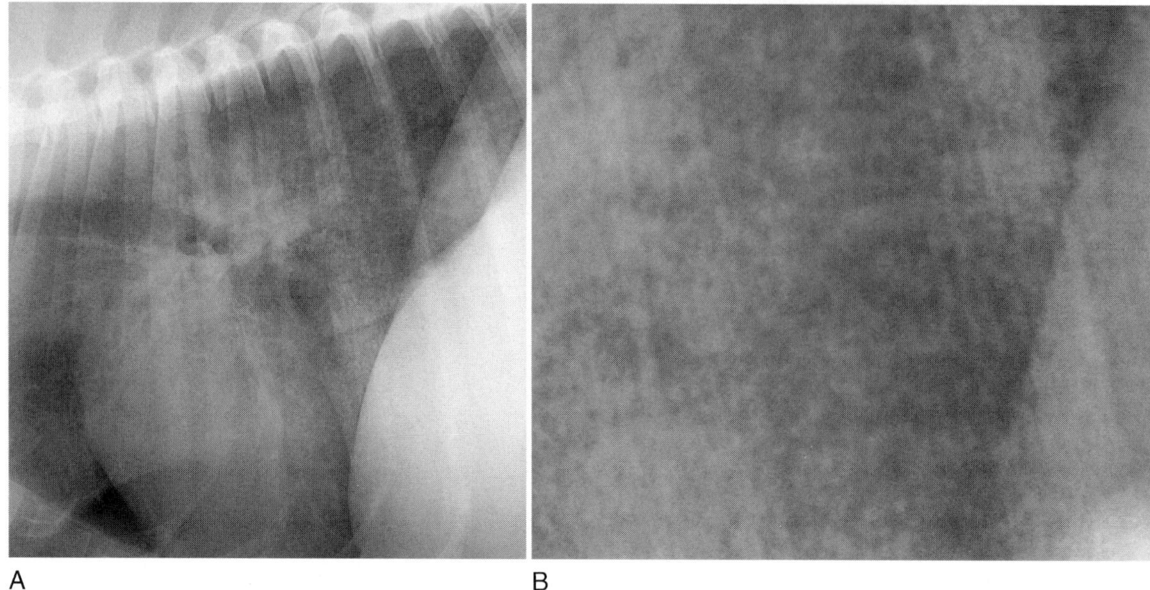

Fig. 34-10 A, Close-up lateral thoracic radiograph of a dog with pulmonary lymphosarcoma. Note the hazy, unstructured, increased lung opacity, most noticeable in the caudal lung lobes. This dog's disease is not more severe in the caudal lobes; it is more conspicuous there because of the greater thickness of lung that is superimposed, creating a more noticeable opacity. Also note the poor visualization of pulmonary vessels because of effacement by the interstitial opacification. B, Magnified view of a portion of the caudal lung of the dog in A. Note the classic lacy, hazy pattern typical of an unstructured lung pattern.

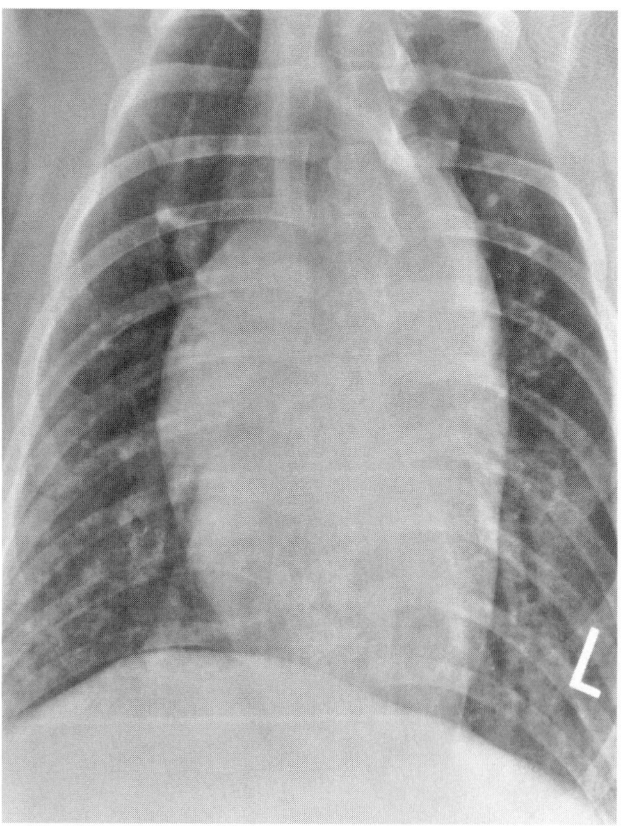

Fig. 34-11 Dorsoventral thoracic radiograph of a dog with chronic renal insufficiency. A bilateral interstitial pattern is most marked in the caudal lung lobes. Histopathologic examination of the lung revealed lesions compatible with uremic pneumonitis.

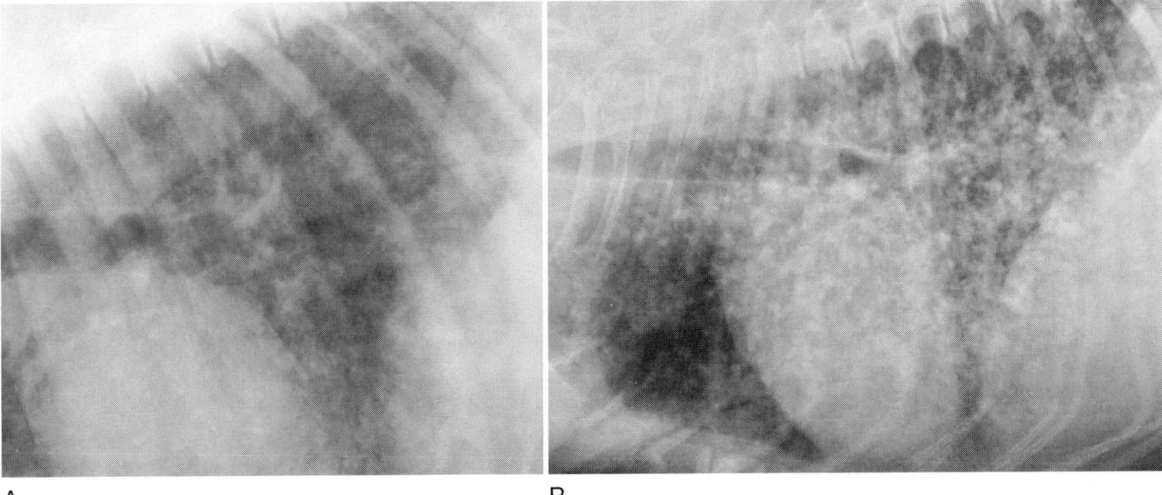

Fig. 34-12 A, Lateral thoracic radiograph of a dog with pulmonary blastomycosis. A disorganized increased opacity is present in the lung. Pulmonary vessels are difficult to see because of effacement. This dog definitely has regions of unstructured lung opacity as well as regions that could be interpreted as a bronchial pattern. In some other areas the pattern has assumed a small, nodular appearance. This variety of pattern appearances may be caused by summation of the interstitial lesions, but it may also actually be caused by the presence of multicompartment involvement or coexistence of multiple lung patterns. Unfortunately, an appearance such as this can be confusing for beginning interpreters. Clearly, though, this is neither an alveolar pattern nor a pure bronchial pattern, supporting its identification as unstructured interstitial. **B,** Micronodular interstitial pattern caused by blastomycosis. When so many small nodules are present, the superimposition leads to coalescence of opacities that obscures underlying pulmonary structures and also makes identification of individual nodules more difficult.

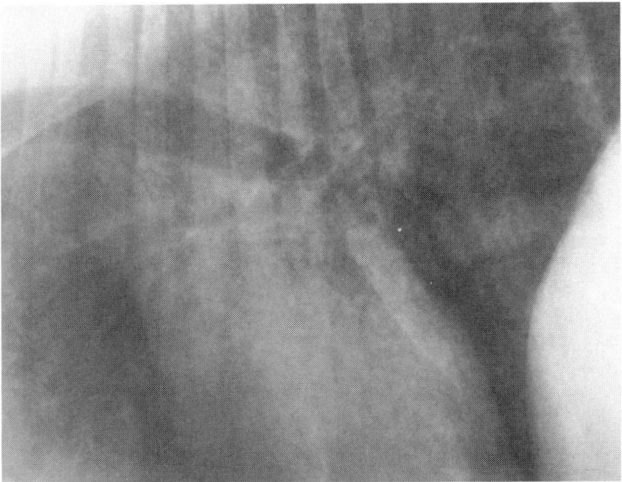

Fig. 34-13 Diffuse interstitial pattern throughout the lung of a dog with metastatic hepatocellular carcinoma. Note that much of the fine detail of the lung (such as the small vessels) is obscured by the metastatic tumor, but the lung remains well aerated and the intensity is not as opaque per unit area of affected lung, which distinguishes this pattern from an alveolar pattern.

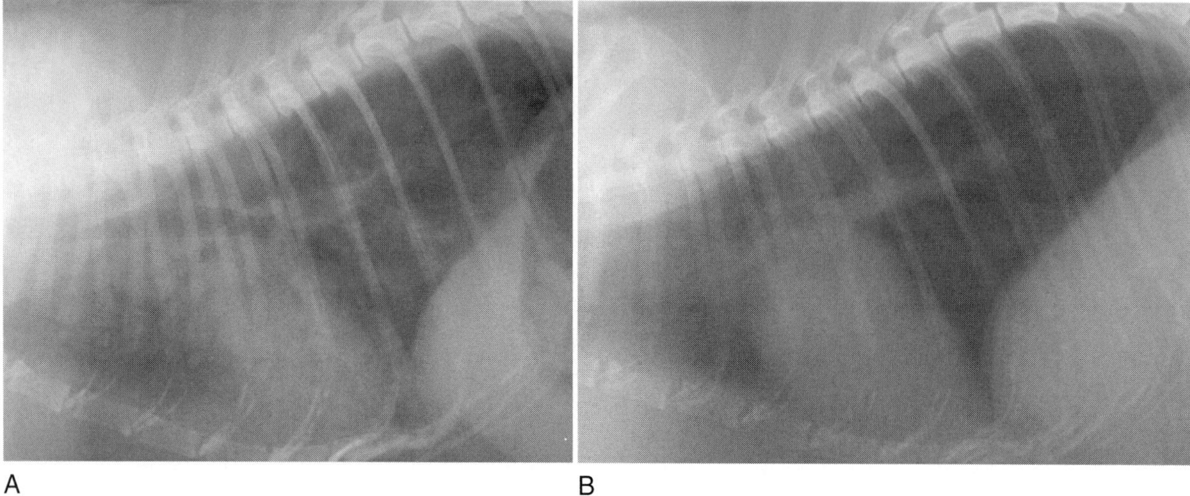

Fig. 34-14 A, Lateral thoracic radiograph of a cat with dyspnea, tachycardia, and murmur. A patchy alveolar pulmonary infiltrate is present, which obscures the cardiac silhouette. This appearance is not specific for any disease; however, the clinical signs suggest the possibility of cardiac disease. Therefore the infiltrate may reflect pulmonary edema. **B,** Repeat lateral radiograph after 12 hours of diuresis shows resolution of the infiltrate and more clearly shows evidence of cardiomegaly. Echocardiography confirmed cardiomyopathy.

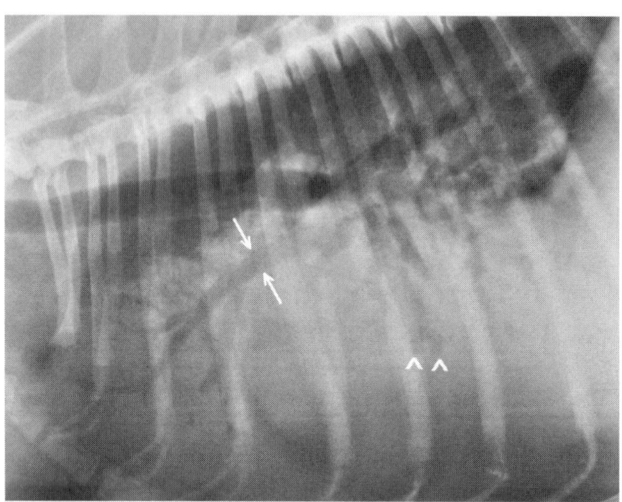

Fig. 34-15 A 5-year-old Standard Poodle had clinical signs and transtracheal aspirate findings consistent with bronchopneumonia. An extensive ventral alveolar pattern and air bronchograms are visible; this appearance is typical of consolidated bronchopneumonia. The left cranial lobar bronchus *(large arrow)* appears to taper and branch normally, but other bronchi appear dilated and blunt ended *(small arrows)*.

Box • 34-4

Differential Diagnosis of Alveolar Patterns

- Localized
  - Bronchopneumonia
  - Edema
    - Cardiac failure
    - Upper respiratory tract obstruction
    - Neurologic disorder, such as seizure, electrocution
    - Transfusion-related acute lung injury
  - Hemorrhage
  - Primary lung tumor
  - Pulmonary metastasis
  - Lobar collapse or atelectasis
    - Airway obstruction, such as by mucus, foreign body
    - Result of pleural effusion
    - Compression by adjacent lesion
  - Dirofilariasis
  - Lobar torsion
  - Pulmonary infarct
- Diffuse
  - Severe bronchopneumonia
  - Severe edema
  - Severe hemorrhage
  - Near drowning
  - Smoke inhalation
  - Terminal paraquat toxicity

during healing. For example, with consolidation as a result of bronchopneumonia, the radiographic lesion may persist for several days despite obvious clinical improvement.

The principal differential diagnoses for an alveolar pattern in dogs are summarized in Box 34-4. Because determining the cause of alveolar pattern is not possible radiographically, sampling the airway by transtracheal aspiration or bronchoalveolar lavage may be helpful, if clinically indicated, in narrowing the considerations for the alveolar pattern. The most common causes are pulmonary edema, bacterial bronchopneumonia, and hemorrhage. Pulmonary edema is most often associated with left-sided cardiac failure, but it can also occur as a sequel to upper airway obstruction,[37] conditions affecting the central nervous system, such as seizures or electrocution,[38,39] and after blood transfusions.[40] Pulmonary edema in dogs often appears most marked in the caudal lung lobes (Fig. 34-16) and is often symmetric in distribution, whereas pulmonary edema in cats has a more variable distribution, often appearing in asym-

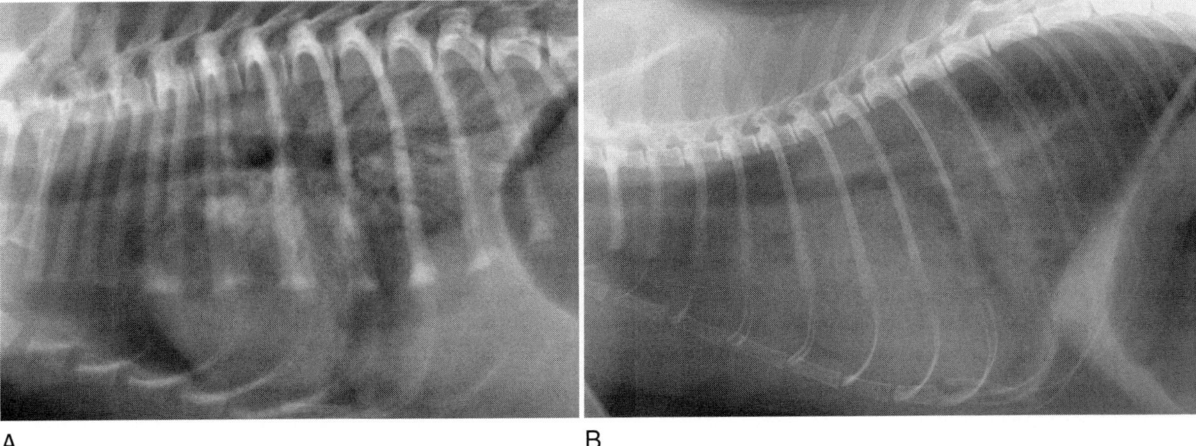

Fig. 34-16 A, Lateral thoracic radiograph of a young dog that bit an electric cord. An alveolar pattern with air bronchograms affecting the caudal lobes can be seen. In these instances, electrical stimulation of the brain causes a burst of sympathetic nerve discharges, which in turn causes acute pulmonary hypertension and pulmonary edema.[46] B, Lateral thoracic radiograph of a cat with pulmonary edema caused by cardiomyopathy. The distribution of the alveolar pattern is mainly in the central and ventral regions of the lung; the caudal lobar tips are not affected. This distribution is typical of pulmonary edema in cats with cardiomyopathy.

metric patches and in the ventral part of the lung, where it may mimic bronchopneumonia (see Fig. 34-16). Air bronchograms are less often seen in cats with pulmonary edema than in dogs with comparable edema.

The distribution of alveolar patterns is variable depending on the cause. Pulmonary disease associated with bacterial bronchopneumonia typically affects the ventral part of the lung and is often asymmetric (see Fig. 34-15). Bronchopneumonia resulting from aspiration (e.g., as with megaesophagus) may be localized to the right middle lobe. Hemorrhage associated with trauma often occurs on the same side of the body as the impact (Fig. 34-17), and thoracic wall lesions, such as rib fractures, may be visible radiographically adjacent to the pulmonary lesion. In contrast, hemorrhage caused by coagulopathy, as from coumarin rodenticide toxicity, may have a patchy or generalized distribution and may be accompanied by signs of pleural and tracheal hemorrhage.[41] Less-common causes of diffuse alveolar patterns include eosinophilic granulomatosis,[28] uremic pneumonitis,[42] acute respiratory distress syndrome,[43] and terminal paraquat toxicity.[44,45]

Replacement of air within a lung lobe may be accompanied by a change in its volume, which usually causes a mediastinal shift (Fig. 34-18). For example, neoplastic infiltration may result in increased lobar volume and a mediastinal shift away from the lesion. Bronchopneumonia or hemorrhage usually results in no recognizable change in volume of the affected lobes. Collapse of a lung lobe usually results in a mediastinal shift toward the affected lobe.[46] In the dog and cat, the right middle lobe is most prone to collapse.[46,47] Approximately 10% of cats with bronchial disease have a collapsed right middle lobe,[4] probably as a result of bronchial obstruction by mucus or exudate (Fig. 34-19). In animals in whom pleural fluid collects around the collapsed lobe, the tendency for a mediastinal shift is reduced, and if sufficient fluid accumulates a mediastinal shift may not be observed.[46]

Lung lobe torsion is another cause of an alveolar pattern, or generalized lobar opacification, in dogs (Fig. 34-20).[48,49] The affected lobe (usually the right middle lobe) may not be visible radiographically because of surrounding pleural fluid. Lung lobe torsion may be difficult to distinguish radiographically from other causes of intense alveolar opacification

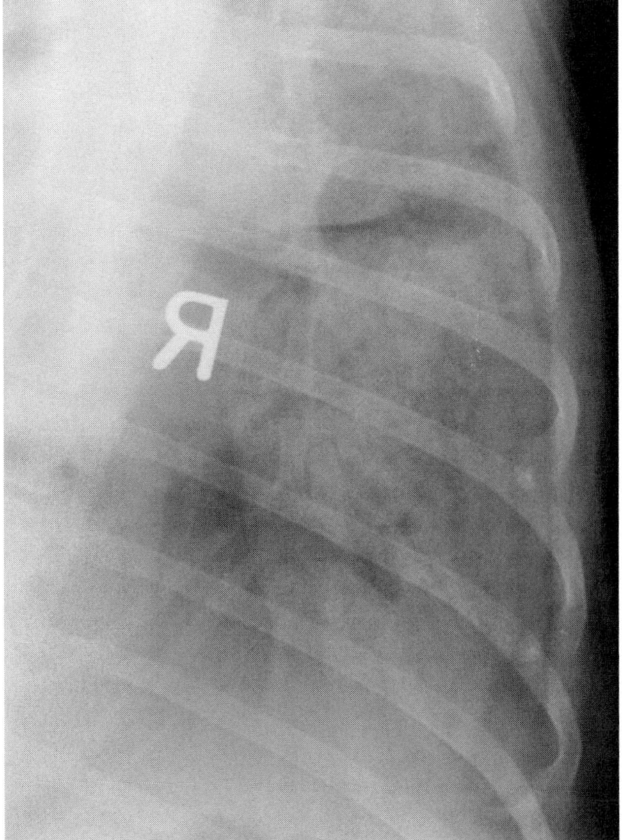

Fig. 34-17 Close-up ventrodorsal thoracic radiograph of a dog struck on the left side by an automobile. The dog was dyspneic and this, unfortunately, influenced the radiographic positioning. The "R" marker is also misplaced. Pneumothorax is present, seen as hyperlucency around the left caudal lobe. An intense alveolar pattern in the left caudal lobe is greater than expected from the amount of secondary atelectasis present. The most likely diagnosis is pulmonary hemorrhage from the road accident.

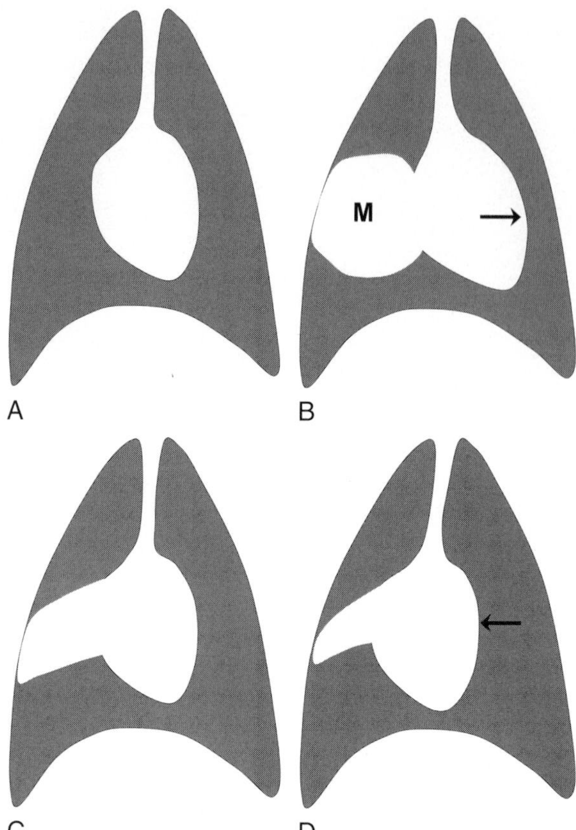

Fig. 34-18 Lesions that result in altered lobar volume are often diagnosed radiographically on the basis of a mediastinal shift. **A,** Normal position of the heart as it appears in a ventrodorsal or dorsoventral radiograph, with apex just to left of midline. **B,** The effect of a unilateral mass *(M)* is a mediastinal shift away from the lesion *(arrow)*. **C,** Some alveolar diseases, such as bronchopneumonia, tend not to change the lung volume. **D,** Collapse of a lobe may produce a mediastinal shift toward the lesion *(arrow)*, although this effect is often reduced by a redistribution of pleural fluid around the collapsed lobe.

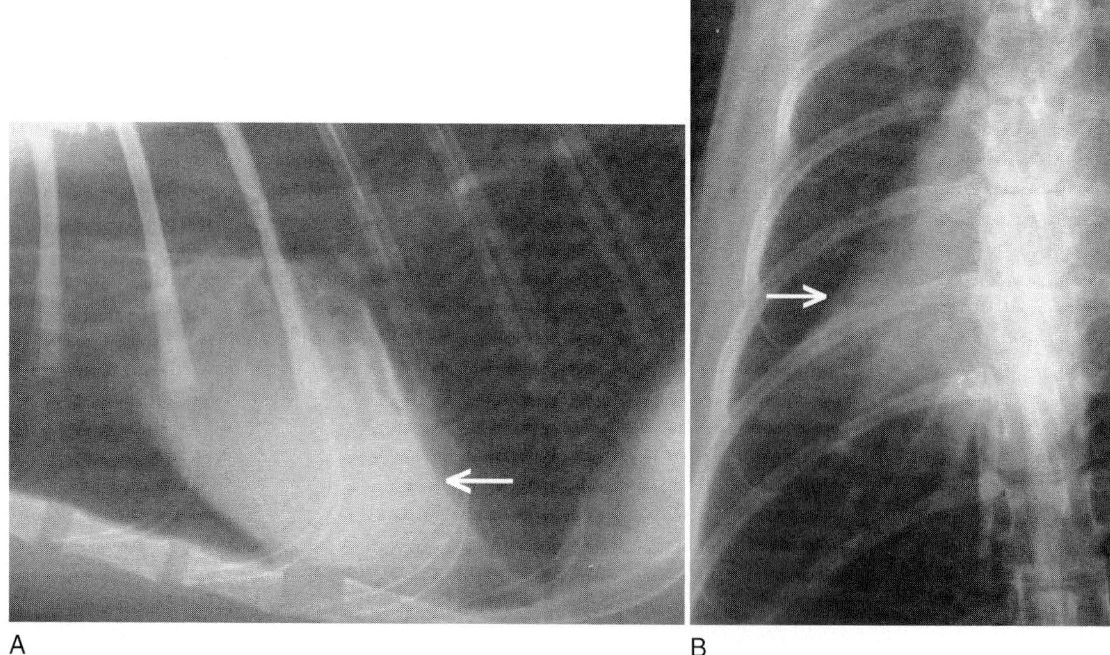

Fig. 34-19 Example of collapse of the right middle lobe in a cat with bronchial disease. In the lateral radiograph (**A**), the collapsed lobe is visible only as a lobar sign *(arrow)* superimposed on the cardiac silhouette. In the ventrodorsal radiograph (**B**), the collapsed lobe appears as a small triangular opacity *(arrow)* adjacent to the cardiac silhouette.

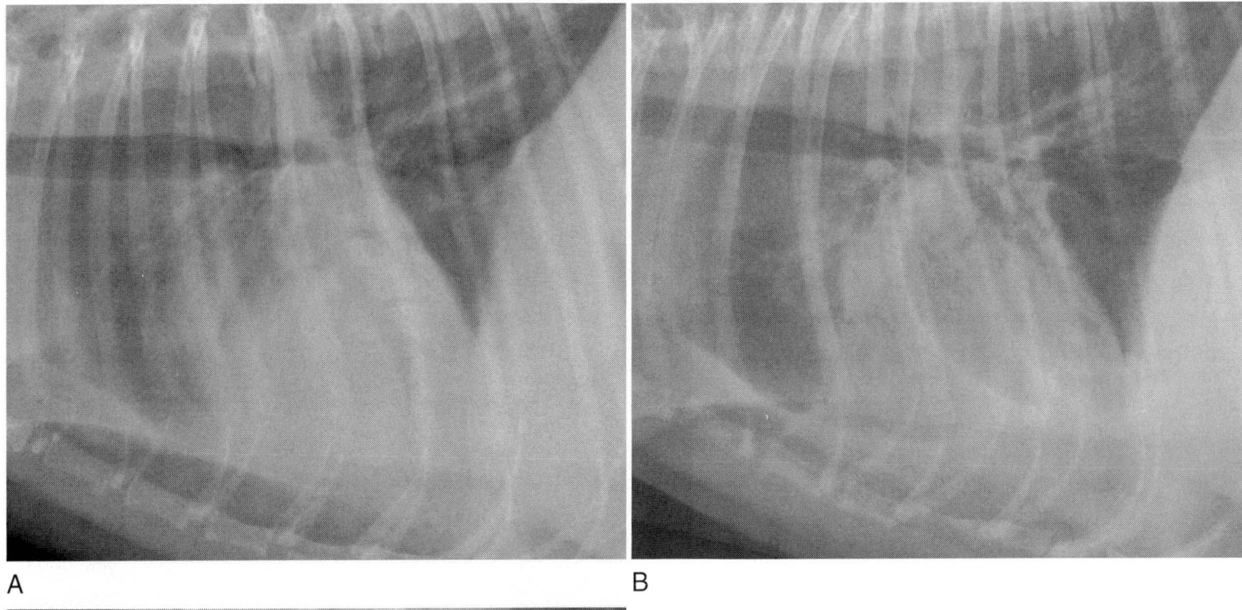

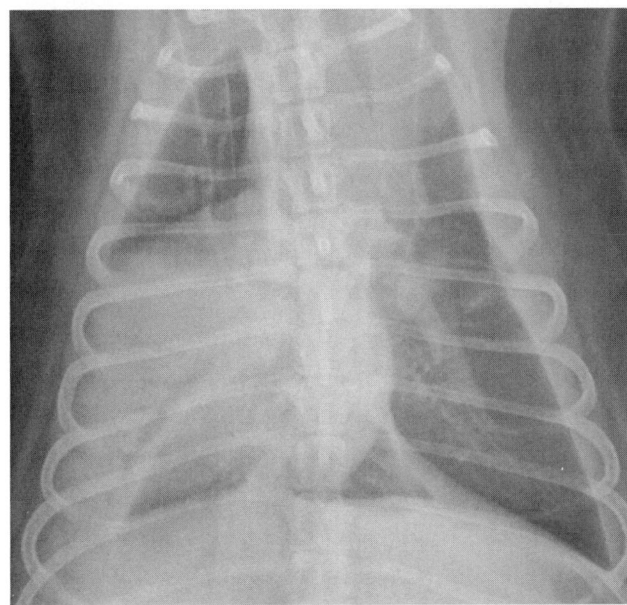

Fig. 34-20 Left lateral (A), right lateral (B), and ventrodorsal (C) thoracic radiographs of a dog with torsion of the right middle lobe. In **A** and **B**, an air bronchogram can be seen superimposed over the cardiac silhouette; this is more conspicuous in the left lateral view (A). In the ventrodorsal view (C) there is evidence of pleural effusion. The right middle lobe is relatively uniformly opacified and its borders merge with the surrounding fluid. The caudal margin of the right middle lobe seems to extend further caudally than normal and the lobar bronchus appears more caudally located in the lobe than normal.

because the twisted bronchus may not be visible. Later in the course of lobe torsion, the affected lobe may take on a mottled appearance as a result of multiple punctuate radiolucencies forming as a consequence of lobar abscessation.

HYPERLUCENCY

Hyperlucency implies that the lung appears less opaque than normal in technically adequate radiographs. In addition to the finding of reduced pulmonary opacity, the cardiac silhouette, aortic shadow, and the ventral aspects of the thoracic vertebrae may be sharply defined. Just as an interstitial infiltrate may be mimicked by underexposure or expiratory exposure, artifactual hyperlucency may be produced by overexposure or iatrogenic overinflation of the lung during anesthesia. Weight loss and hypovolemia also may produce apparent lung hyperlucency by reducing x-ray attenuation in the thoracic wall and lung, respectively. Pathologic causes of diffuse pulmonary hyperlucency, such as feline asthma or emphysema, tend to trap air in the lung and reduce the tidal volume.

Hyperlucency may be classified as diffuse or focal (Box 34-5). Diffuse pulmonary hyperlucency and increased lung volume are observed in some cats as a result of air trapping associated with bronchial asthma[4,50] or emphysema, which can occur as a congenital anomaly (Fig. 34-21)[51,52] or as a result of chronic bronchitis (Fig. 34-22)[4] or aspiration of mineral oil.[53] Other causes of focal pulmonary hyperlucency include congenital bronchogenic cysts, traumatic bullae,[54] pneumatoceles,[26,55] and pulmonary thromboembolism.[56] Bronchial cysts and bullae are usually recognized radiographically as cavitary lesions when they contain gas; however, a fluid-filled cyst or bulla might be mistaken for a solid nodule (Fig. 34-23).

Box 34-5

Differential Diagnosis of Pulmonary Hyperlucency

- Diffuse
  - Nonpulmonary factors
    - Overexposure
    - Hypovolemia
  - Hyperinflation
    - Increased tidal volume, such as metabolic acidosis
    - Iatrogenic (positive-pressure ventilation under anesthesia)
    - Air trapping
    - Emphysema
- Focal
  - Congenital bronchial cyst
  - Localized breakdown of pulmonary parenchyma
    - Emphysema
    - Pneumatocele
    - Bulla
  - Subpleural bleb
  - Bronchiectasis
  - Cavitary soft tissue mass
    - Neoplasm
    - Granuloma
    - Paragonimus cyst
    - Abscess
  - Reduced blood supply
    - Pulmonary thromboembolism

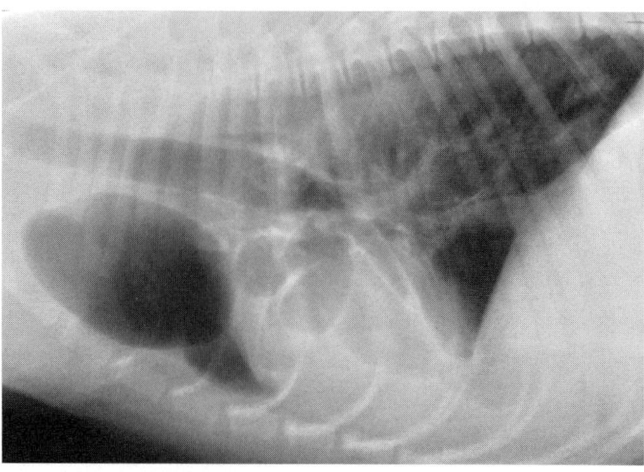

Fig. 34-21 Lateral thoracic radiograph of a 1-year-old retriever with exercise intolerance and slightly increased respiratory effort. Several thin-walled, gas-filled bullae are present in the cranioventral lung field. Final diagnosis was congenital bullous emphysema.

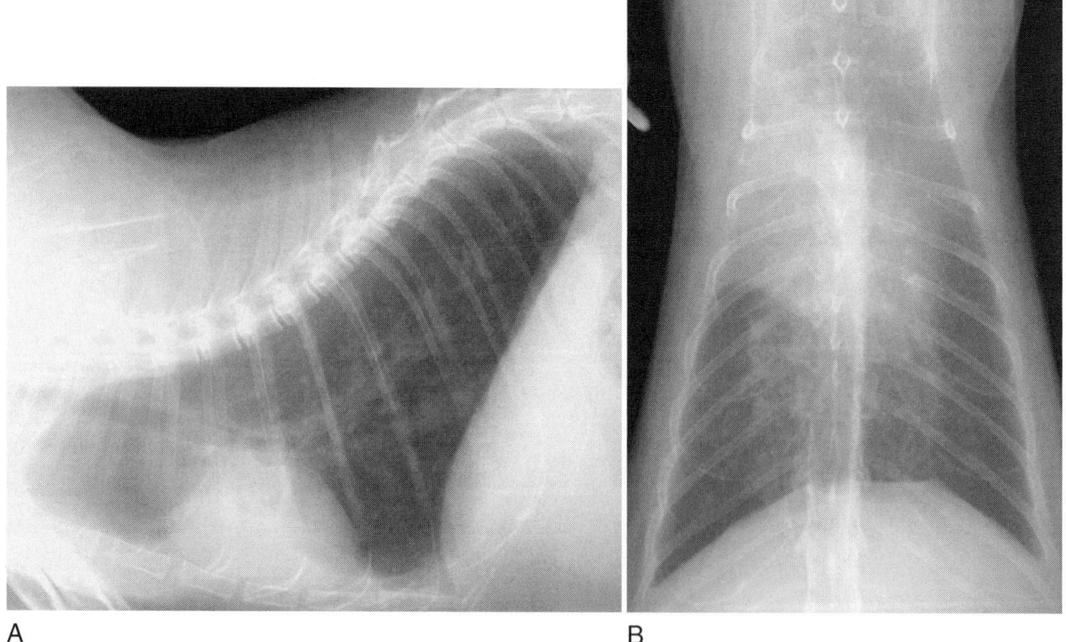

Fig. 34-22 Lateral (A) and ventrodorsal (B) thoracic radiographs of a cat with pulmonary hyperinflation caused by chronic bronchitis. At this time, the bronchial pattern is not as conspicuous in the radiographs. However, the right middle lung lobe is collapsed and the lungs are hyperinflated from air trapping. The lung volume is too great, resulting in caudal extension of the diaphragm and increased distance between the cardiac silhouette and diaphragm in **A.** Slight tenting of the diaphragm is visible in **B.**

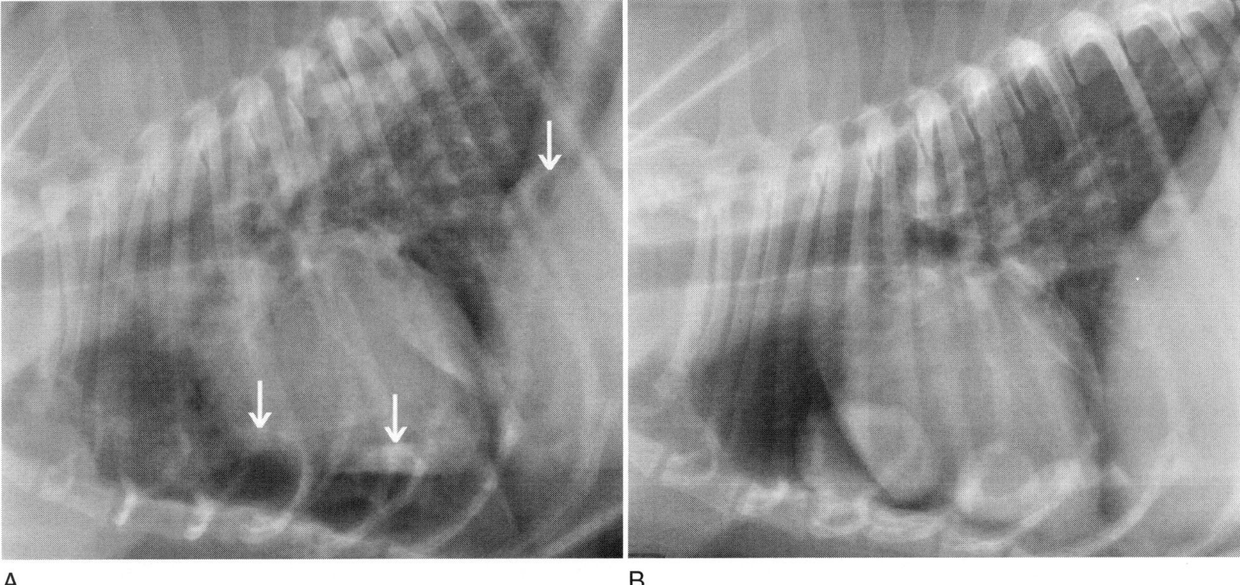

Fig. 34-23 A, Lateral thoracic radiograph of a Terrier-Cross dog hit by a car approximately 1 hour previously. The lucent space between the heart and the sternum indicates pneumothorax. Close inspection also reveals small, gas-filled traumatic lung bullae *(arrows)*. B, Repeat radiograph 24 hours later shows resolution of pneumothorax. The bullae are partially filled with fluid (probably blood) and now appear as sharply defined, round nodules. At this stage they may be misinterpreted as other types of pulmonary nodule; however, the history of recent thoracic trauma, the progression from gas to a gas- and fluid-filled state, and the peripheral location are typical of traumatic lung bullae.

PULMONARY MASS LESIONS

Although pulmonary nodules are described in the section on interstitial patterns, some additional discussion of mass lesions is required. Lesions that are usefully classified as masses are larger than nodules and, because of their size, often cause displacement of adjacent organs. For example, unilateral pulmonary masses often cause a mediastinal shift away from the lesion (see Fig. 34-18). The differential diagnosis of pulmonary masses is as stated for nodules in Box 34-2. Determining the cause of a pulmonary mass lesion often requires direct cytologic sampling, such as from a needle aspirate or biopsy.

Primary neoplasia is the most common cause of a pulmonary mass in the dog or cat. Radiographic diagnosis of a pulmonary mass is usually based on the observation that an intrathoracic mass is surrounded by aerated lung. A pulmonary mass that is in contact with the visceral pleura, or is obscured by concurrent pulmonary lesions or pleural fluid, is more difficult to diagnose radiographically and must be distinguished from a mass arising from the mediastinum, pleural cavity, or thoracic wall.

Box • 34-6

Calcified Pulmonary Lesions

Focal or multifocal
- Bronchial calcification
- Calcified peribronchial mucous glands
- Broncholithiasis
- Heterotopic bone
- Granuloma, such as canine (not feline) histoplasmosis
- Primary lung tumor
- Osteosarcoma metastasis
- Aspirated barium sulfate

Diffuse
- Hyperadrenocorticism
- Hyperparathyroidism
- Chronic uremia
- Idiopathic

CALCIFIED PULMONARY LESIONS

A variety of pulmonary lesions may calcify.[57,58] Calcification is classified as focal or diffuse (Box 34-6). Many instances of focal pulmonary calcification in the dog or cat represent incidental findings; however, calcification is a notable feature of *Histoplasma* granulomas in dogs[31] and is observed in a small number of primary pulmonary neoplasms (Fig. 34-24).[22] Barium sulfate suspension, which may be deposited in the lung during bronchography or when an upper gastrointestinal contrast study is attempted, may be confused with calcification but is more opaque (Fig. 34-25).

Alternative Imaging of Pulmonary Conditions

Radiography is an appropriate first-choice imaging modality for the investigation of most small animals with respiratory

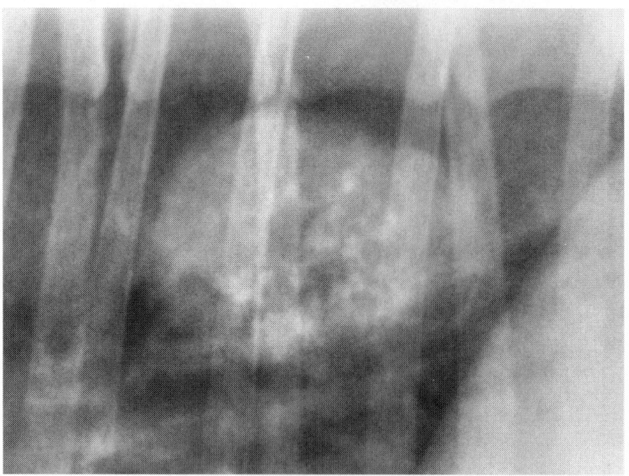

Fig. 34-24 Close-up of a lateral thoracic radiograph of a dog with a partially calcified pulmonary mass. Histologic diagnosis was chondrosarcoma.

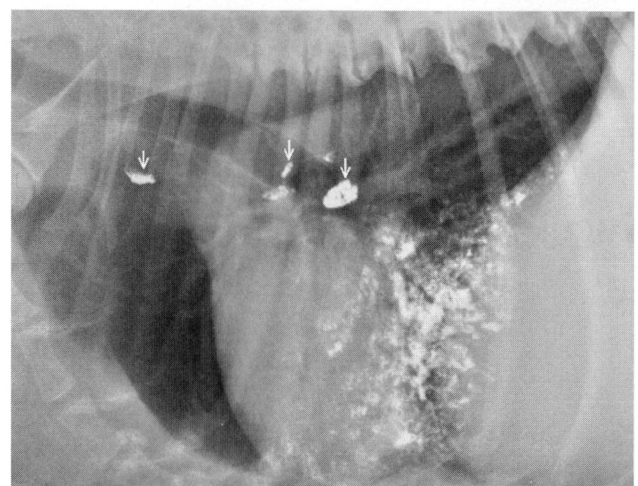

Fig. 34-25 Lateral thoracic radiograph of an old Irish Setter presented for lameness evaluation. This radiograph was made as a routine preanesthetic check and, unexpectedly, barium was seen in the caudoventral lung. The dog had an upper gastrointestinal contrast study several years previously and no history of respiratory signs. The location of the barium in this radiograph is compatible with aspiration and subsequent translocation to the tracheobronchial lymph nodes *(arrows)*. Most aspirated barium is coughed up within a few minutes; barium uptake by macrophages and migration to regional lymph nodes account for a relatively small part of total lung clearance in these patients.

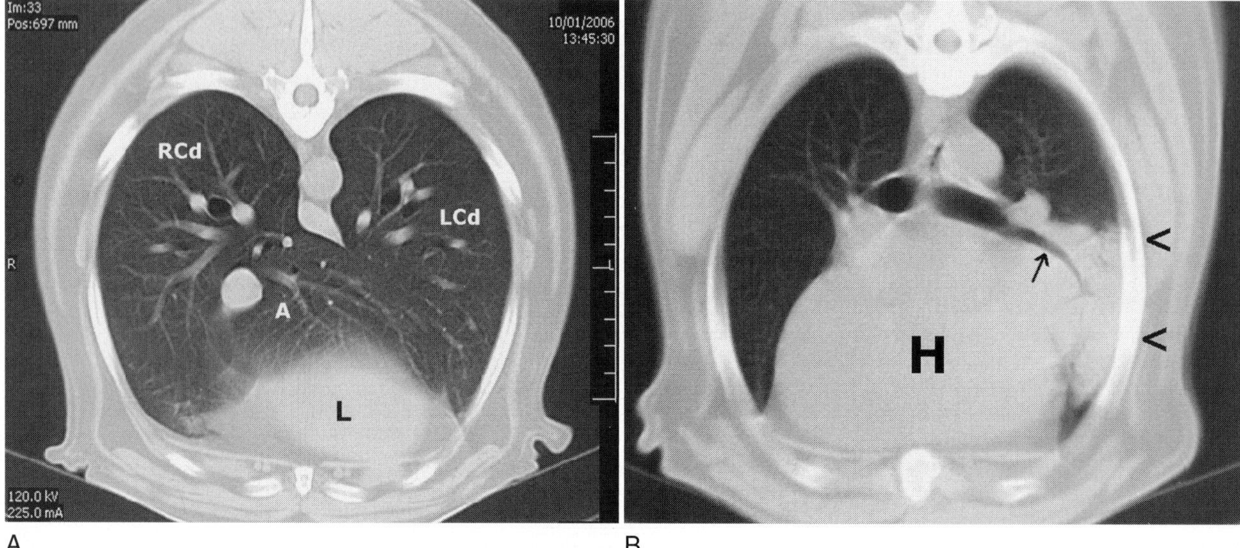

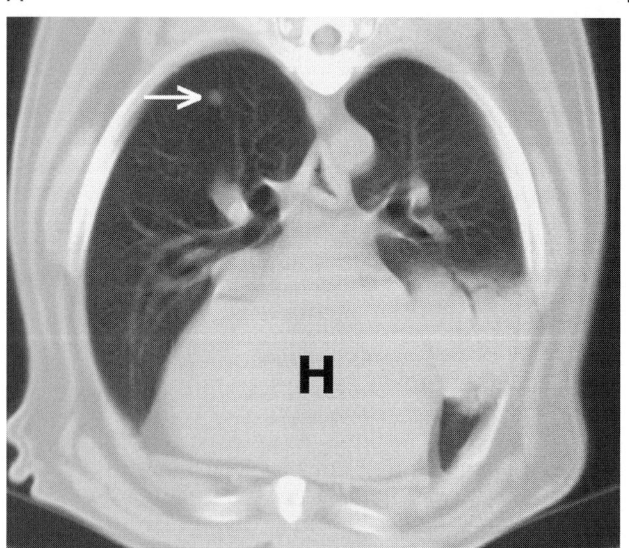

Fig. 34-26 **A,** CT image of the normal canine lung. The pulmonary vessels and bronchi are clearly depicted in this image of the caudal part of the thorax. The soft tissue structure on the ventral aspect of the lung is the liver *(L)*. *RCd,* Right caudal lobe; *LCd,* left caudal lobe; *A,* accessory lobe. **B,** Example of a CT image of a dog with a mass in the left cranial lobe. The anatomic location of the mass is based on identifying the bronchus *(arrow)* that is surrounded by the mass. No sign is present that the mass affects the adjacent rib *(arrowheads)*. *H,* Heart. **C,** Pulmonary nodules were visible *(arrow)* in other CT images of the same dog. This finding suggests that the pulmonary mass has metastasized. Even relatively small, peripheral nodules may be identified using CT when they may not be evident radiographically.

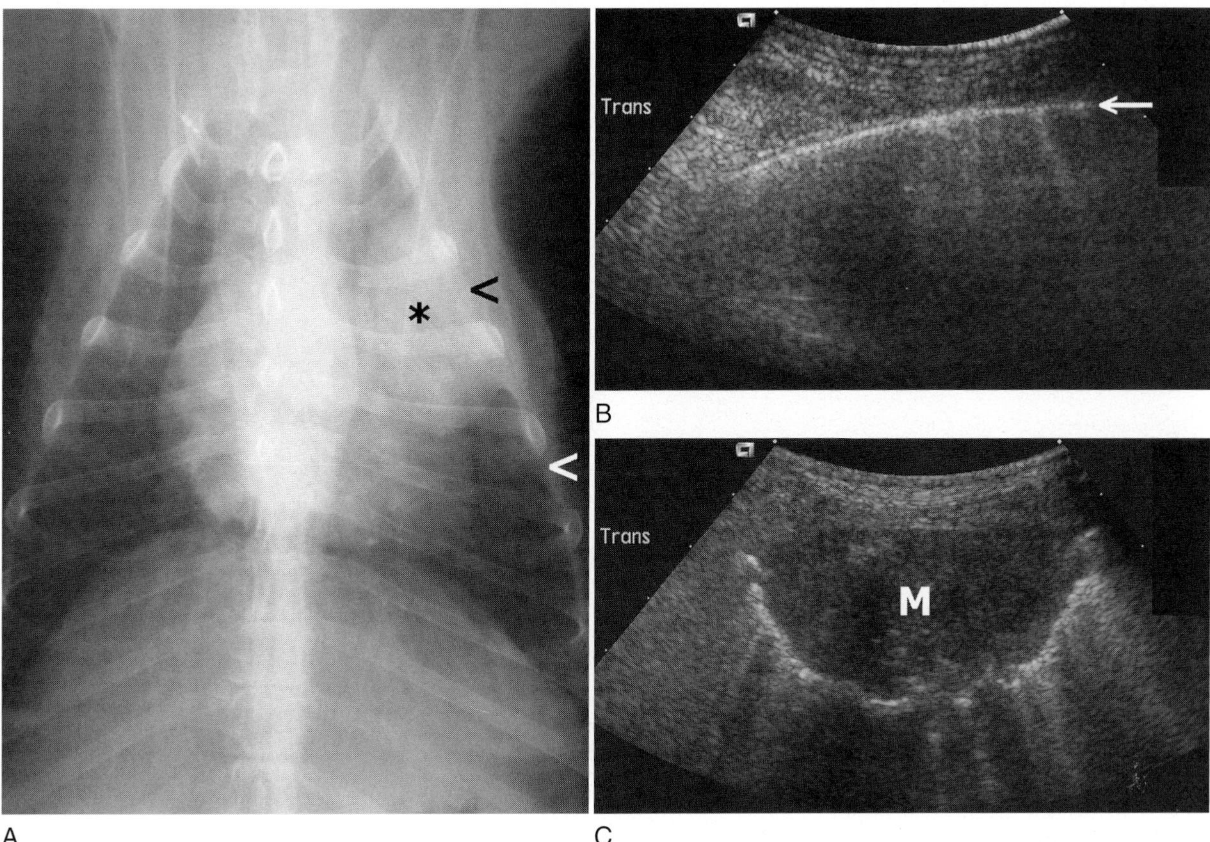

Fig. 34-27 Example of ultrasonography of a pulmonary mass. **A,** Dorsoventral radiograph of a mixed-breed dog with persistent cough in which a mass *(asterisk)* is visible adjacent to the left thoracic wall. **B,** Ultrasound image of the thorax with transducer positioned over the aerated lung (site of *white arrowhead* in **A**) shows the surface of the lung *(arrow)* as a curved, highly echogenic interface with no detail of deeper structures. **C,** In contrast, an ultrasound image of the thorax with the transducer positioned over the mass (site of *black arrowhead* in **A**) shows the internal structures of the mass *(M)* and aerated lung at its lower edge. Cytology based on ultrasound-guided fine-needle aspiration was compatible with carcinoma.

signs, but alternate imaging may be useful in the following circumstances:

- When interpretation is difficult, such as when extensive disease obscures intrathoracic structures
- When more information about the nature and extent of thoracic disease is needed for optimal management, such as delineation of lesion margins as an aid to surgical resection
- When sensitivity for disease must be maximized, such as in a patient with suspected pulmonary metastasis

Computed tomography (CT) and ultrasonography may be useful in these circumstances. Suspected pulmonary metastasis, intrathoracic mass (Fig. 34-26), and nontraumatic (spontaneous) pneumothorax are frequent indications for CT examination of the lung.[59-61]

The inability of ultrasound to penetrate the air-filled lung adequately prevents its use for examination of the normal lung, which reflects virtually all the ultrasound beam, producing a high-amplitude, specular echo and preventing assessment of deeper structures. However, when the lungs are collapsed, consolidated, or displaced by fluid, the ultrasound beam will penetrate.[62,63] Even in the presence of well-aerated lungs, a pulmonary mass will be visible ultrasonographically if it extends to the surface of the lung (visceral pleura) and comes in contact with the thoracic wall or diaphragm (parietal pleura) (Fig. 34-27). The etiology of a pulmonary mass cannot usually be determined from its echogenicity, but ultrasound is a convenient method for guiding fine-needle aspiration or biopsy. Intense pulmonary disease with marked replacement of air (from lobar collapse, bronchopneumonia, or infarction) may be recognized because it produces a liverlike appearance without a mass effect or loss of the normal shape of the lobe. In some cases of consolidation the principal bronchus is visible as an anechoic branching structure known as a fluid bronchogram (Fig. 34-28).

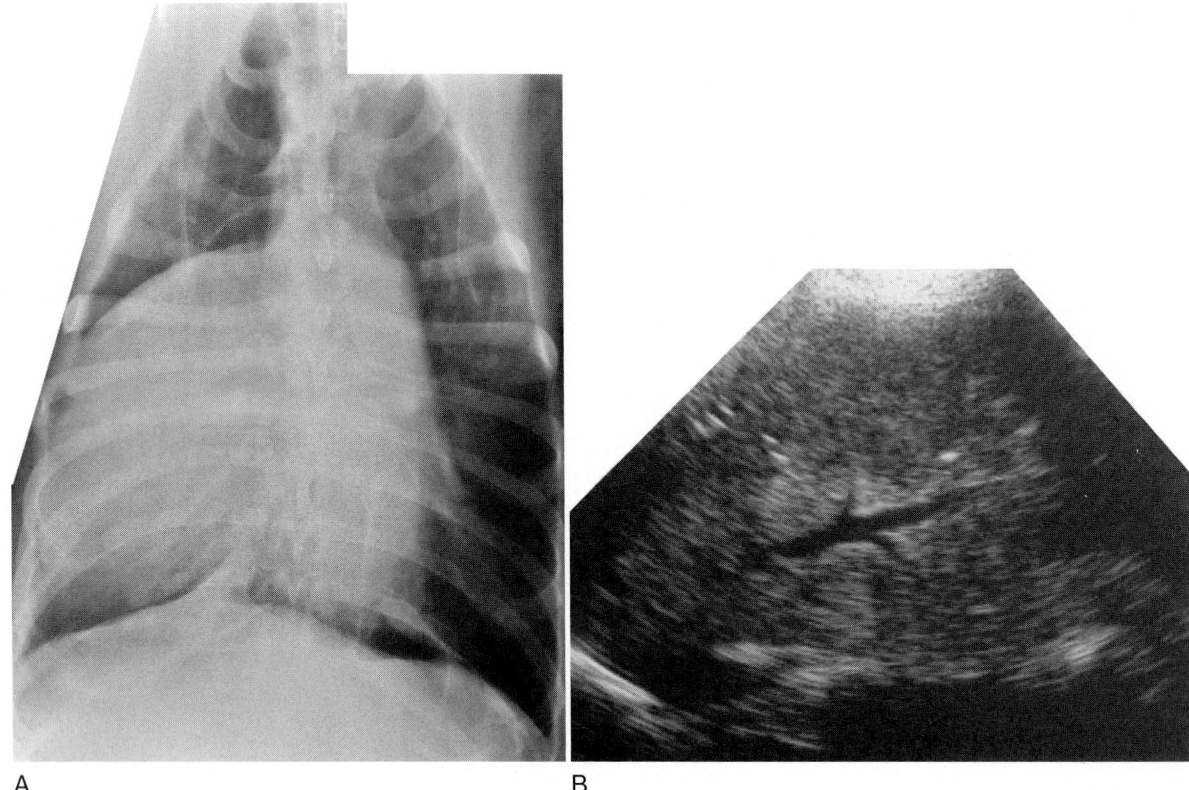

Fig. 34-28 A 3-year-old female Retriever was hit by a car and had a ruptured diaphragm. After surgery to repair this injury, the animal had persistent pneumothorax and intense opacification of the right middle lung lobe. In thoracic radiographs made after referral (ventrodorsal view, **A**), an opaque right middle lobe was visible without apparent loss of volume, and apparent enlargement of the lobe. To define the changes in this lobe better, ultrasonography was performed through an intercostal window (**B**). The primary bronchus was fluid filled, appearing as an anechoic branching structure (so-called fluid bronchogram). Thoracotomy revealed infarction of the right middle lobe. Although torsion was not present at surgery, torsion as a result of the diaphragmatic rupture was considered a likely cause of the infarction. (From Stowater JL, Lamb CR: Ultrasonography of non-cardiac thoracic diseases in small animals, *J Am Vet Med Assoc* 195:514, 1989.)

REFERENCES

1. Allan GS, Howlett CR: Miliary broncholithiasis in a cat, *J Am Vet Med Assoc* 162:214, 1973.
2. Myer CW: Radiography review: the vascular and bronchial patterns of pulmonary disease, *Vet Radiol* 21:156, 1980.
3. Mantis P, Lamb CR, Boswood A: Assessment of the accuracy of thoracic radiography in the diagnosis of canine chronic bronchitis, *J Small Anim Pract* 39:518, 1998.
4. Moise SN, Wiedenkeller D, Yeager AE et al: Clinical radiographic, and bronchial cytologic features of cats with bronchial disease: 65 cases (1980-1986), *J Am Vet Med Assoc* 194:1467, 1989.
5. Corcoran BM, Thoday KL, Henfrey JI, et al: Pulmonary infiltration with eosinophils in 14 dogs, *J Small Anim Pract* 32:494, 1991.
6. Moon M: Pulmonary infiltrates with eosinophilia, *J Small Anim Pract* 33:19, 1992.
7. Losonsky JM, Thrall DE, Prestwood AK: Radiographic evaluation of pulmonary abnormalities after *Aelurostrongylus abstrusus* inoculation in cats, *Am J Vet Res* 44: 478, 1983.
8. Staub NC, Nagano H, Pearce NL: Pulmonary edema in dogs: especially the sequence of fluid accumulation in the lungs, *J Appl Physiol* 22:227, 1967.
9. Myer CW, Burt JK: Bronchiectasis in the dog: its radiographic appearance, *J Am Vet Radiol Soc* 14:3, 1973.
10. Norris CR, Samii VF: Clinical, radiographic, and pathologic features of bronchiectasis in cats: 12 cases (1987-1999), *J Am Vet Med Assoc* 216:530, 2000
11. Hawkins EC, Basseches J, Berry CR et al: Demographic, clinical, and radiographic features of bronchiectasis in dogs: 316 cases (1988-2000), *J Am Vet Med Assoc* 223: 1628, 2003.
12. Myer W: Radiography review: the interstitial pattern of pulmonary disease, *Vet Radiol* 21:18, 1980.
13. Biller DS, Myer CW: Case examples illustrating the clinical utility of obtaining both right and left lateral thoracic radiographs in small animals, *J Am Anim Hosp Assoc* 23:381, 1987.
14. Reif JS, Rhodes WH: The lungs of aged dogs: a radiographic-morphologic correlation, *J Am Vet Radiol Soc* 7:5, 1966.

15. Suter PF, Carrig C, O'Brien TR, et al: Radiographic recognition of primary and metastatic pulmonary neoplasia of dogs and cats, *J Am Vet Radiol Soc* 15:3, 1974.
16. Lang J, Wortman JA, Glickman LT et al: Sensitivity of radiographic detection of lung metastases in the dog, *Vet Radiol* 27:74, 1986.
17. Tiemessen I: Thoracic metastases of canine mammary gland tumors: a radiographic study, *Vet Radiol* 30:249, 1989.
18. Holt D, Van Winkle T, Schelling C et al: Correlation between thoracic radiographs and postmortem findings in dogs with hemangiosarcoma: 77 cases (1984-1989), *J Am Vet Med Assoc* 200:1535, 1992.
19. Hammer AS, Bailey MQ, Sagartz JE: Retrospective assessment of thoracic radiographic findings in metastatic canine hemangiosarcoma, *Vet Radiol Ultrasound* 34:235, 1993.
20. Barthez PY, Hornof WJ, Theon AP et al: Receiver operating characteristic curve analysis of the performance of various radiographic protocols when screening dogs for pulmonary metastasis, *J Am Vet Med Assoc* 204:237, 1994.
21. Barr FJ, Gibbs C, Brown PJ: The radiological features of primary lung tumours in the dog: a review of thirty-six cases, *J Small Anim Pract* 27:493, 1986.
22. Koblik PD: Radiographic appearance of primary lung tumors in cats: a review of 41 cases, *Vet Radiol* 27:66, 1986.
23. Barr F, Gruffydd-Jones TJ, Brown PJ et al: Primary lung tumours in the cat, *J Small Anim Pract* 28:1115, 1987.
24. Miles KG, Lattimer JC, Jergens AE et al: A retrospective evaluation of the radiographic evidence of pulmonary metastatic disease on initial presentation in the dog, *Vet Radiol* 31:79, 1990.
25. Shaiken LC, Evans SM, Goldschmidt MH: Radiographic findings in canine malignant histiocytosis, *Vet Radiol Ultrasound* 32:237, 1991.
26. Silverman S, Poulos PW, Suter PF: Cavitary pulmonary lesions in animals, *J Am Vet Radiol Soc* 17:134, 1976.
27. Ackerman N, Spencer CP: Radiologic aspects of mycotic diseases, *Vet Clin North Am Small Anim Pract* 12:174, 1982.
28. Calvert CA, Mahaffey MB, Lappin MR et al: Pulmonary and disseminated eosinophilic granulomatosis in dogs, *J Am Anim Hosp Assoc* 24:311, 1988.
29. Walker MA: Thoracic blastomycosis: a review of its radiographic manifestations in 40 dogs, *Vet Radiol* 22:22, 1981.
30. Pechman RD: The radiographic features of pulmonary paragonimiasis in the dog and cat, *J Am Vet Radiol Soc* 17:182, 1976.
31. Burk RL, Corley EA, Corwin LA: The radiographic appearance of pulmonary histoplasmosis in the dog and cat: a review of 37 case histories, *J Am Vet Radiol Soc* 19:2, 1978.
32. Wolf AM, Green RW: The radiographic appearance of pulmonary histoplasmosis in the cat, *Vet Radiol* 28:34, 1987.
33. Millman TM, O'Brien TR, Suter PF et al: Coccidioidomycosis in the dog: its radiographic diagnosis, *J Am Vet Radiol Soc* 20:50, 1979.
34. Forrest LJ, Graybush CA: Radiographic patterns of pulmonary metastasis in 25 cats, *Vet Radiol Ultrasound* 39:4, 1998.
35. Ackerman N: Radiographic aspects of heartworm disease, *Semin Vet Med Surg* 2:15, 1987.
36. Carlisle CH: Canine dirofilariasis: its radiographic appearance, *Vet Radiol* 21:123, 1980.
37. Kerr LY: Pulmonary edema secondary to upper airway obstruction in the dog: A review of nine cases, *J Am Anim Hosp Assoc* 25:207, 1989.
38. Lord PF: Neurogenic pulmonary edema in the dog, *J Am Anim Hosp Assoc* 11:778, 1975.
39. Kolata RJ, Burrows CF: The clinical features of injury by chewing electrical cords in dogs and cats, *J Am Anim Hosp Assoc* 17:219, 1981.
40. Looney MR, Gropper MA, Matthay MA: Transfusion-related acute lung injury: a review, *Chest* 126:249, 2004.
41. Berry CR, Gallaway A, Thrall DE et al: Thoracic radiographic features of anticoagulant rodenticide toxicity in fourteen dogs, *Vet Radiol Ultrasound* 34:391, 1993.
42. Moon ML, Greenlee PG, Burk RL: Uremic pneumonitis-like syndrome in ten dogs, *J Am Anim Hosp Assoc* 22:687, 1986.
43. Parent C, King LG, Walker LM et al: Clinical and clinicopathologic findings in dogs with acute respiratory distress syndrome: 19 cases (1985-1993), *J Am Vet Med Assoc* 208:1419, 1996.
44. Darke PGG, Gibbs C, Kelly DF et al: Acute respiratory distress in the dog associated with paraquat poisoning, *Vet Rec* 100:275, 1977.
45. Gee BR, Farrow CS, White RJ et al: Paraquat toxicity resulting in respiratory distress syndrome in a dog, *J Am Anim Hosp Assoc* 14:256, 1978.
46. Lord PF, Gomez JA: Lung lobe collapse: pathophysiology and radiologic significance, *Vet Radiol* 26:187, 1985.
47. Robinson NE, Milar R: Lobar variations in collateral ventilation in excised dog lungs, *Am Rev Respir Dis* 121:827, 1980.
48. Johnston GR, Feeney DA, O'Brien TD et al: Recurring lung lobe torsion in three Afghan Hounds, *J Am Vet Med Assoc* 184:842, 1984.
49. Lord PF, Greiner TP, Greene RW et al: Lung lobe torsion in the dog, *J Am Anim Hosp Assoc* 9:473, 1973.
50. Moise SN, Spaulding GL: Feline bronchial asthma: pathogenesis, pathophysiology, diagnostics, and therapeutic considerations, *Comp Contin Educ Pract Vet* 3:1091, 1981.
51. Herrtage ME, Clarke DD: Congenital lobar emphysema in two dogs, *J Small Anim Pract* 26:453, 1985.
52. Tennant BJ, Haywood S: Congenital bullous emphysema in a dog: a case report, *J Small Anim Pract* 28:109, 1987.
53. Chalifoux A, Morin M, Lemieux R: Lipid pneumonia and severe pulmonary emphysema in a Persian cat, *Fel Pract* 17:6, 1987.
54. Aron DN, Kornegay JN: The clinical significance of traumatic lung cysts and associated pulmonary abnormalities in the dog and cat, *J Am Anim Hosp Assoc* 19:903, 1983.
55. Lamb CR, Neiger R: Differential diagnosis of pulmonary cavitary lesions, *Vet Radiol Ultrasound* 41:340, 2000.
56. Flückiger MA, Gomez JA: Radiographic findings in dogs with spontaneous pulmonary thrombosis or embolism, *Vet Radiol* 25:124, 1984.
57. Thrall DE, Goldschmidt MH, Clement RJ et al: Generalized extensive idiopathic pulmonary ossification in a dog: a case report, *Vet Radiol* 21:104, 1980.
58. Berry CR, Ackerman N, Monce K: Pulmonary mineralization in four dogs with Cushing's syndrome, *Vet Radiol Ultrasound* 35:10, 1994.
59. Prather AB, Berry CR, Thrall DE: Use of radiography in combination with computed tomography for the assessment of noncardiac thoracic disease in the dog and cat, *Vet Radiol Ultrasound* 46:114, 2005.
60. Waters DJ, Coakley FV, Cohen MD et al: The detection of pulmonary metastases by helical CT: a clinicopathologic study in dogs, *J Comput Assist Tomogr* 22:235, 1998.

61. Yoon J, Feeney DA, Cronk DE et al: Computed tomographic evaluation of canine and feline mediastinal masses in 14 patients, *Vet Radiol Ultrasound* 45:542, 2004.
62. Stowater JL, Lamb CR: Ultrasonography of non-cardiac thoracic diseases in small animals, *J Am Vet Med Assoc* 195:514, 1989.
63. Reichle JK, Wisner ER: Non-cardiac thoracic ultrasound in 75 feline and canine patients, *Vet Radiol Ultrasound* 41:154, 2000.

ELECTRONIC RESOURCES evolve

Additional information related to the content in Chapter 34 can be found on the companion Web site at evolve http://evolve.elsevier.com/Thrall/vetrad/.

- Key Points
- Chapter Quiz
- Case Study 34-1

CHAPTER • 35
The Equine Thorax

Stephanie G. Nykamp

RADIOGRAPHIC TECHNIQUE

Radiographing the entire thorax of an adult horse requires a grid and large stationary x-ray tubes that are generally only available at referral centers. Portable radiographic tubes require an excessively long exposure time to penetrate the adult thorax; this results in motion artifact, rendering the images nondiagnostic. Four overlapping 14-inch × 17-inch films are usually required to image the entire thorax. They are positioned in the craniodorsal, caudodorsal, caudoventral, and cranioventral views (Fig. 35-1). In addition to these standard projections, radiographs centered over any specific identified lesions may be useful.

Left and right lateral radiographs of the foal thorax may be made with a single 14-inch × 17-inch cassette and some portable x-ray tubes. Dorsoventral or ventrodorsal radiographs should also be acquired on foals whenever possible.

The horse should be positioned with the thoracic limbs slightly forward to reduce the amount of muscle mass superimposed on the cranial aspect of the thorax. Radiographs should be obtained during peak inspiration. In some instances radiographs should also be obtained during expiration because a comparison of the degree of lung inflation between the inspiratory and expiratory radiographs may be helpful in the diagnosis of air trapping from chronic pulmonary disease.

When thoracic radiographs are obtained with the horse in a standing position, the lung closest to the cassette is seen most clearly. This is opposite to the situation in which thoracic radiographs of small animals are obtained with the patient in lateral recumbency, where the lung farthest from the cassette, the nondependent lung, is seen most clearly. Because of the large width of the equine thorax, the lung farthest from the cassette is magnified and blurred to such an extent that even large lesions can be obscured. Therefore radiographs with the left and right sides of the thorax nearest the cassette are necessary to assess both the left and right lung fields adequately.[1]

Radiographic exposure and degree of inspiration play an important role in the interpretation of thoracic radiographs and must be considered both for initial and serial radiographic examinations. As the quality of the radiograph improves, the amount of perceived interstitial lung pattern decreases.[2] If a radiograph is underexposed or obtained during expiration, the lungs will appear diffusely more opaque than normal, mimicking a mild diffuse interstitial lung pattern often mistaken for disease. If the radiographs are overexposed, small or mild lung lesions may be obscured.

NORMAL ANATOMY

The right and left lungs are not clearly divided by interlobar fissures. The left lung is divided into a cranial and caudal component. The right lung is divided into a cranial and caudal component and the accessory lobe. A prominent cardiac notch is present in the left and right lungs at the level of the third to the sixth ribs.

Craniodorsal Projection

The dorsal portion of the heart, descending aorta, caudal vena cava, hilar pulmonary arteries and veins, trachea, and carina are visible (Fig. 35-2). The hilar portions of the lungs are visible but are difficult to evaluate because of the superimposition of the heart and blood vessels.

Caudodorsal Projection

This view provides the largest unobstructed view of the lungs (Fig. 35-3). The normal equine lung has a mild diffuse bronchointerstitial lung pattern when compared with dogs and cats. The pulmonary blood vessels should be clearly seen tapering toward the periphery of the lung field.

Caudoventral Projection

The caudal borders of the heart, left atrium, caudal vena cava, pulmonary veins, and pulmonary arteries are evident on this view (Fig. 35-4). A small triangle of lung bounded by the caudal vena cava, caudal border of the heart, and cranioventral aspect of the diaphragm is evident. Because of the cardiac notch, the lung is not seen overlying the central portion of the heart. The absence of pulmonary blood vessels in this region should not be mistaken for consolidation of the lung. The diaphragmatic reflection of the pleura follows the costochondral junctions to approximately the ninth rib and then travels dorsally, paralleling the costal arch to the middle of the last rib.[3] This means that the normal lung does not extend ventral to the costochondral junction and, in fact, usually ends approximately 4 inches above the costochondral junction in adult horses at rest. Ventral to the costochondral junction is mediastinal fat that provides contrast between the caudal border of the heart and the diaphragm. This fat opacity should not be mistaken for pleural or pulmonary disease.

Cranioventral Projection

The cranial portions of the lung, cranial mediastinum, aortic arch, and trachea are evident on this projection (Fig. 35-5). The lung is difficult to evaluate in this region because of the superimposition of the thoracic limbs. With the exception of evaluating for a mediastinal mass, this is typically the least helpful of all projections.

Foals

When radiographed immediately after parturition, foals have a mild diffuse interstitial lung pattern because of incomplete expansion of the lungs. In normal foals this opacity should resolve by the time they are 12 to 24 hours old (Fig. 35-6).[4,5] The thymus is large in foals and can sometimes be seen as a soft tissue opacity cranial to the heart. The thymus is largest at approximately 2 months of age and should regress as the foal ages.[5] Atelectasis rapidly occurs when foals are placed in lateral recumbency. This will result in the lungs of recumbent foals appearing more opaque than those of standing foals.[5]

Adults

Age, size, and phase of respiration all affect the radiographic appearance of the lungs. Many adult horses with normal respiratory function and no clinical signs of respiratory disease have a mild, diffuse bronchointerstitial lung pattern as a normal variation.[2,6] This opacity may be caused by the slightly more prominent lobulation and connective tissue seen in horses or by subclinical peribronchial fibrosis.[2,3] The presence of this mild bronchointerstitial lung pattern means that the correlation between radiographic changes and clinical disease is not easily demonstrated, and mild radiographic changes should be interpreted with caution and in relation to the clinical signs (Fig. 35-7).[2,7,8]

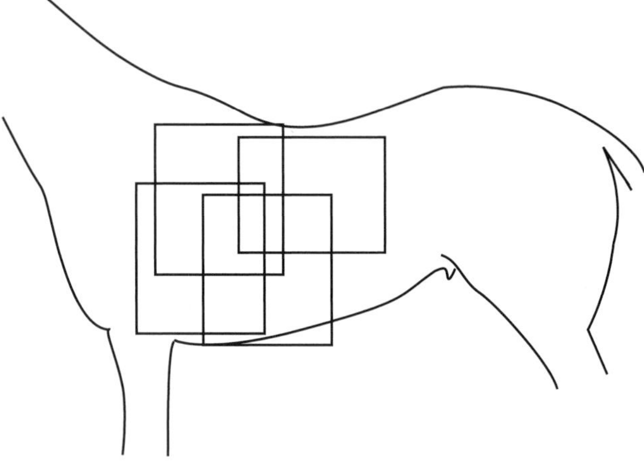

Fig. 35-1 Placement of cassettes for the four radiographic views of the thorax.

Heart

Objective criteria for assessing heart size have not been established in horses.[9] The caudal border of the heart should be straight and should parallel the angle of the ribs. Elevation of the trachea and increased sternal or diaphragmatic contact are indicative of cardiomegaly.[9] Assessment of cardiac size is easiest if the entire cardiac silhouette is on one 14-inch × 17-inch cassette. In foals the cardiac silhouette occupies more of the thoracic cavity than it does in adults.[5] Results from an objective measurement of cardiac size in foals state the height should be 6.6 to 7.8 times the length of a mid-thoracic vertebral body, and the width should be 5.6 to 6.3 times the width of a mid-thoracic vertebral body.[4] Echocardiography is superior to radiography in assessing cardiac size.

ALTERNATIVE IMAGING MODALITIES

Fluoroscopy, the use of real-time radiographic imaging, is useful to evaluate esophageal disease, tracheal collapse, and the motion of thoracic masses.[10] Although this modality is useful, it is not readily available.

The use of ultrasound has become common in equine field practice. Air prevents the transmission of ultrasound waves, so the ultrasound appearance of normal lung is a bright interface

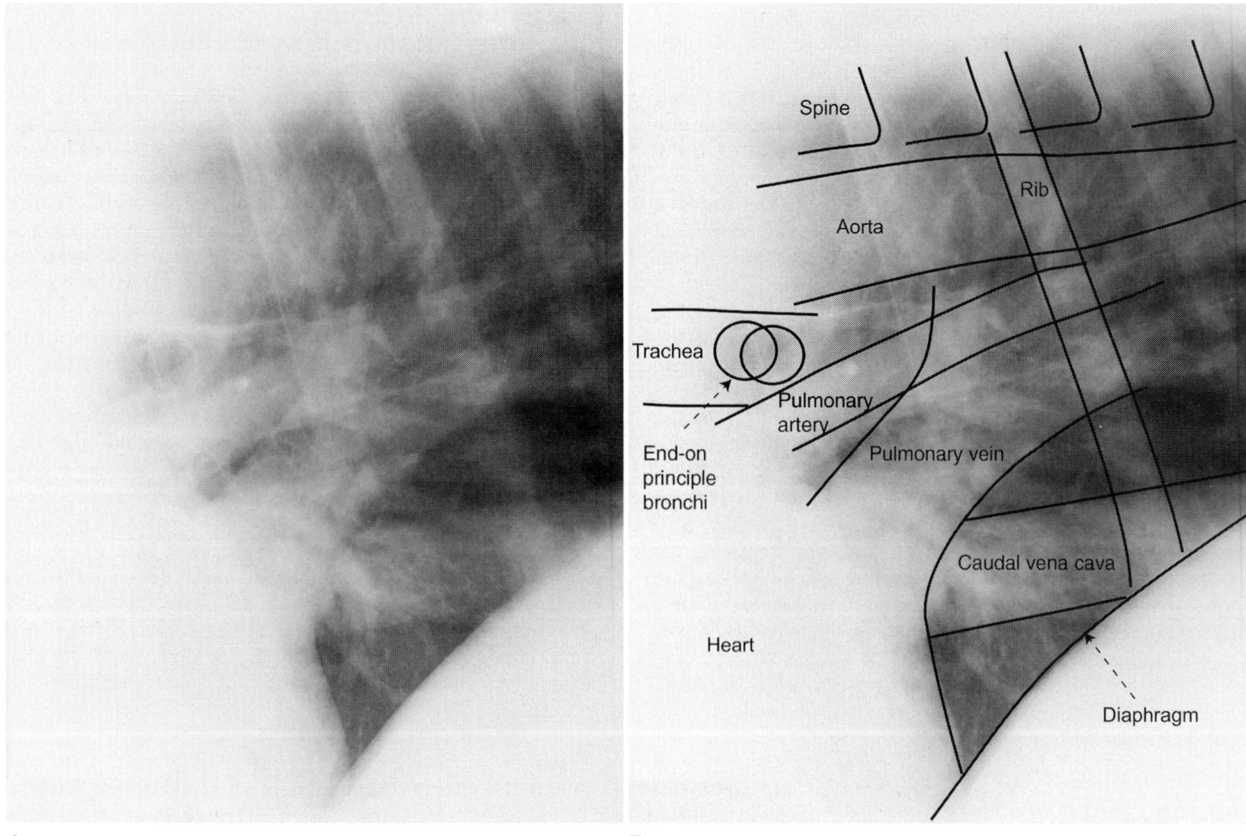

Fig. 35-2 Normal adult thoracic radiograph (**A**), craniodorsal projection, and accompanying line drawing (**B**).

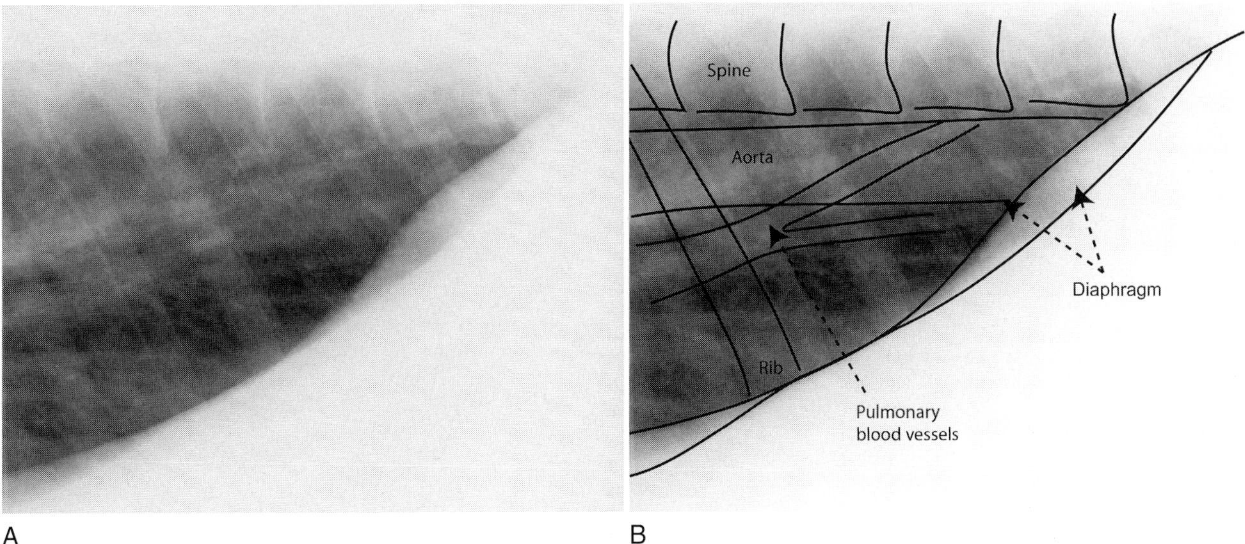

A B

Fig. 35-3 Normal adult thoracic radiograph (A), caudodorsal projection, and accompanying line drawing (B).

A B

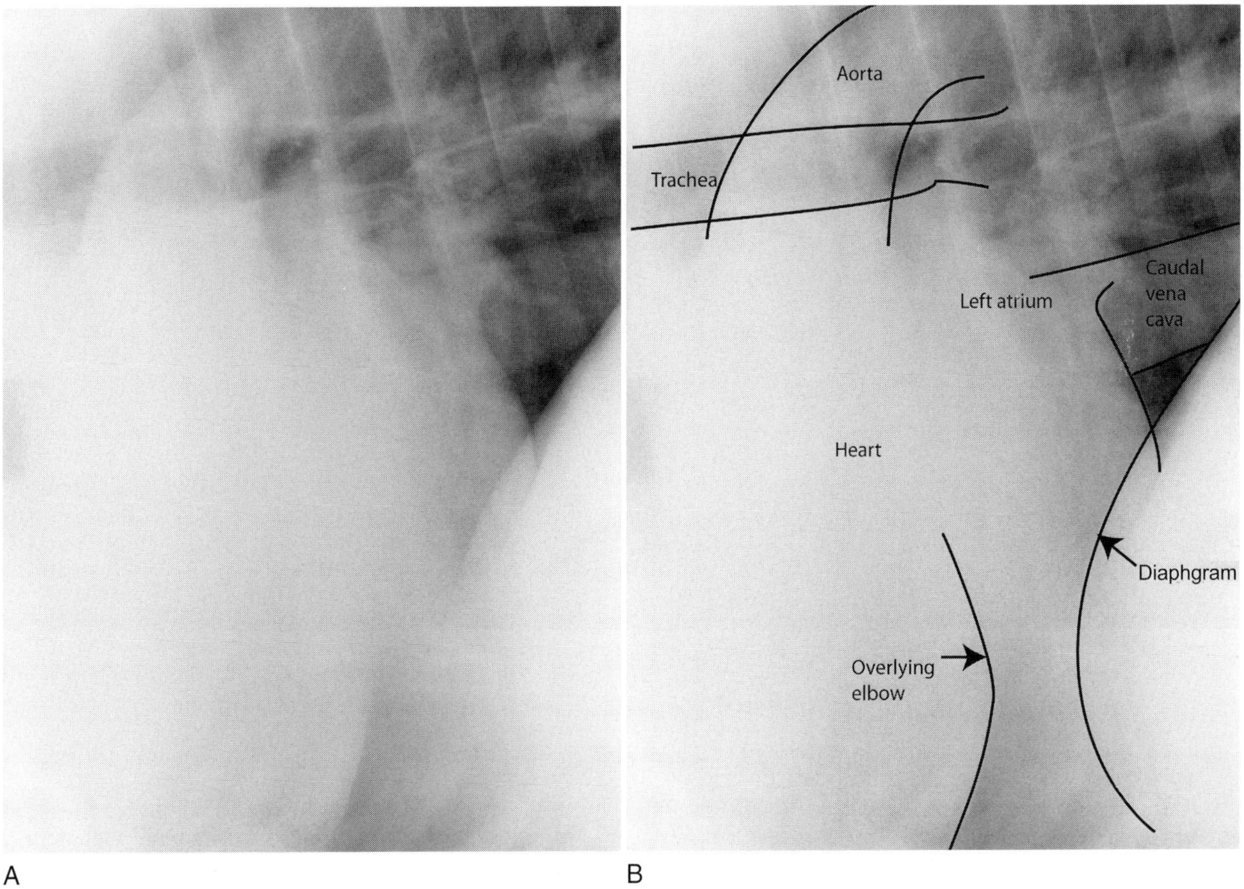

Fig. 35-4 Normal adult thoracic radiograph (A), caudoventral projection, and accompanying line drawing (B).

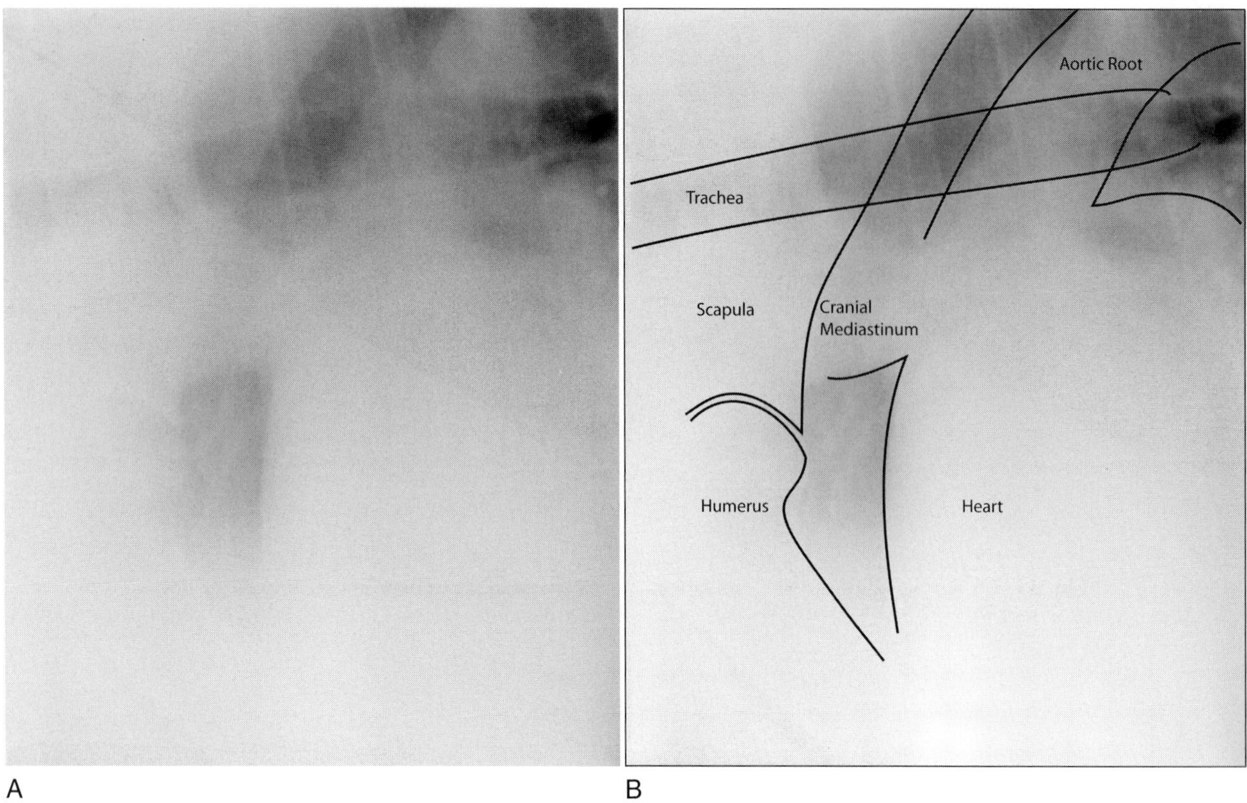

Fig. 35-5 Normal adult thoracic radiograph (A), cranioventral projection, and accompanying line drawing (B).

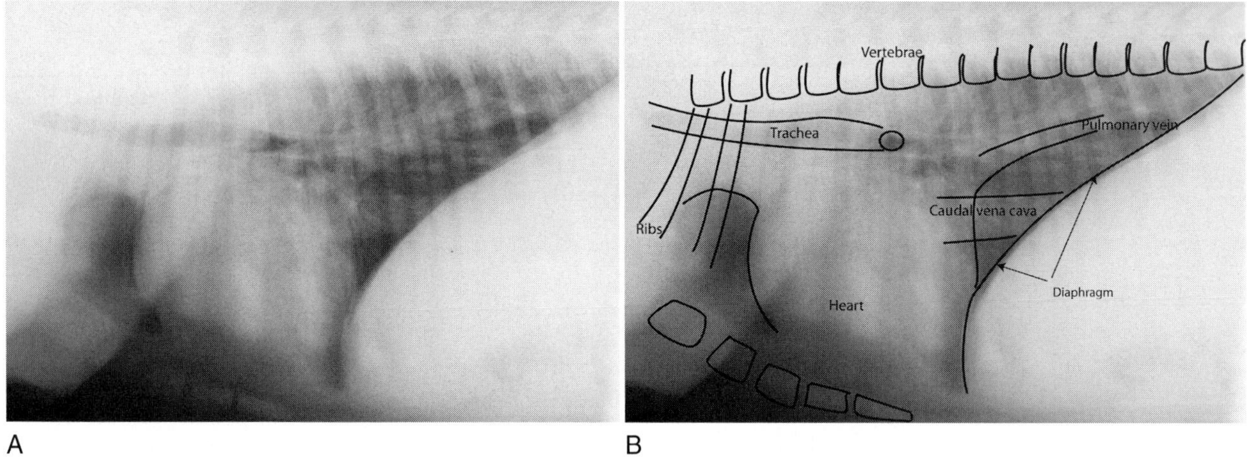

Fig. 35-6 Normal foal thoracic radiograph (A) and accompanying line drawing (B).

with reverberation artifact characterized by equally spaced lines that parallel the surface of the lung (Fig. 35-8).[11] In real time, normal lung can be seen to slide along the body wall during respiration. Ultrasound also allows the detection of consolidation, atelectasis, and abscesses when the lesions extend to the pleural surface. Ultrasound is the diagnostic test of choice for evaluating pleural disease because it is more sensitive to the detection of small amounts of fluid and provides information on the character of the fluid.[10,12,13] Ultrasound can also be used to assess the surface of the lung. A few areas of rough pleural surfaces ("comet tail" artifact) can be seen in the ventral portions of the lung in normal horses, but more extensive lesions will be seen in horses with viral pneumonia and chronic fibrosis (Fig. 35-9).[14,15] Ultrasound is an inexpensive and accessible diagnostic test for serial examinations to assess for resolution or progression of disease.

Nuclear scintigraphy can provide physiologic information about perfusion and ventilation of the lungs. Ventilation studies can be useful in assessing chronic obstructive pulmonary disease and exercise-induced pulmonary hemorrhage.[16,17] The images are characterized by a patchy distribution with hot spots centrally caused by deposition of

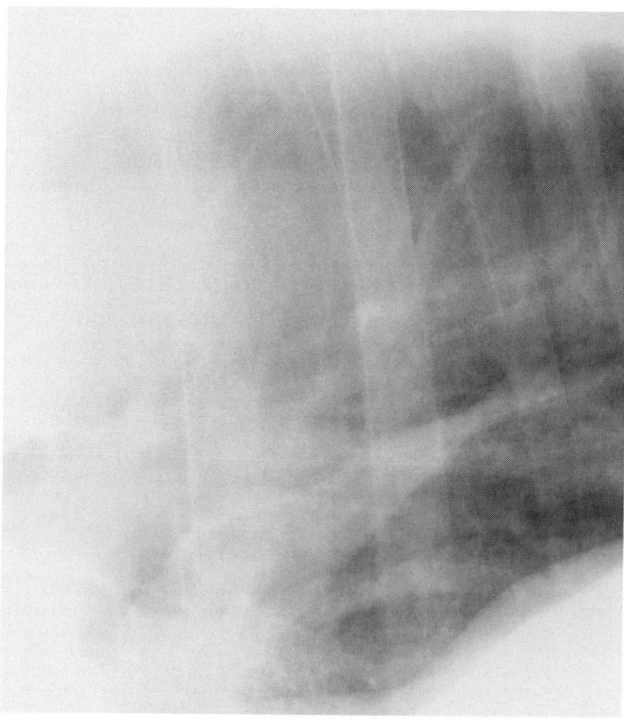

Fig. 35-7 Right lateral radiograph of the caudodorsal thorax in an adult horse with no clinical signs. Note the mild diffuse bronchial lung pattern seen in normal horses.

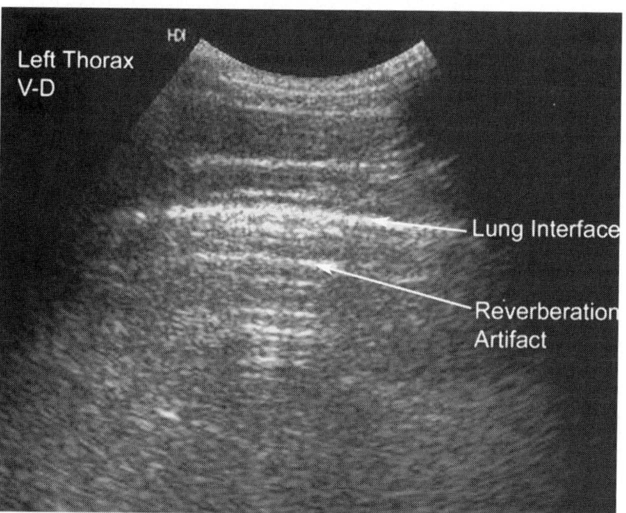

Fig. 35-8 Transverse ultrasound image of the normal left lung (ventrodorsal orientation). Note the equally spaced white lines (reverberation artifact) caused by the sound reflected at the air interface.

the injected isotope in the larger airways and cold spots peripherally from lack of ventilation. Additionally, horses with chronic obstructive pulmonary disease clear the radio pharmaceutical from the lungs faster than do normal horses.[18] Perfusion studies are used to evaluate for pulmonary thromboembolic disease, chronic obstructive pulmonary disease, and other diffuse diseases. In combination with ventilation studies, the patient can be evaluated for ventilation

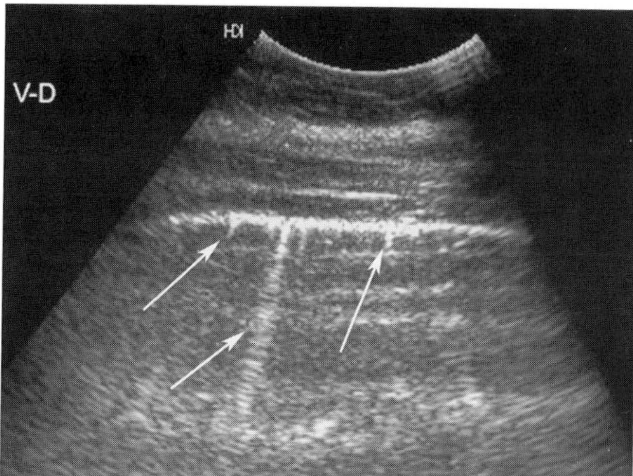

Fig. 35-9 Transverse ultrasound image of the lung. The pleural surface of the lung is rough, which results in a reverberation artifact, otherwise referred to as "comet tail" artifact *(arrows)*. A few comet tails can be seen in normal horses.

and perfusion mismatches. Because of the expensive equipment and need to isolate the patient for approximately 24 hours after the study, these imaging studies are usually limited to referral hospitals.

Computed tomography is an excellent imaging modality for assessment of the thorax, but because of equipment size its use is restricted to small foals and referral institutions.[19]

PULMONARY DISEASE

Radiographs complement a physical examination, they do not replace it. Physical examination can be unremarkable and yet the radiographs be characterized by substantial pulmonary disease. Additionally, the radiographic resolution of disease often lags behind the clinical resolution. This should be considered when evaluating serial studies.[20]

The patterns of pulmonary disease have been discussed elsewhere. The radiographic patterns of pulmonary disease (interstitial, alveolar, bronchial) have a poor correlation with the location of the disease histologically, making the use of these terms confusing. For example, in equine parasitic pneumonia the radiographic pattern seen most often was interstitial, but at necropsy the disease was predominantly in the air spaces (alveolar), and horses with a diffuse interstitial lung pattern had peribronchial disease on histologic examination.[2,21] Radiographic patterns can reflect the severity of the disease, however, with bronchial and interstitial patterns indicating less-severe disease than an alveolar pattern.[20] The distribution of the pulmonary infiltrate provides more insight into the cause of the pulmonary disease.[5,22] Bronchopneumonia and aspiration pneumonia tend to have a cranioventral and caudoventral distribution, whereas pulmonary edema, interstitial pneumonia, and airway disease are more caudodorsal to diffuse in their distribution.

Pneumonia

Inhalation and aspiration pneumonia in the adult horse and foal have a similar radiographic appearance to other species. In adults bronchopneumonia is usually as result of transportation or stress, whereas in foals it is usually caused by sepsis or aspiration.[23,24] In adults and foals, bronchopneumonia can occur as a result of viral pneumonia.[24] Bacterial pneumonia usually occurs in the cranioventral and caudoventral

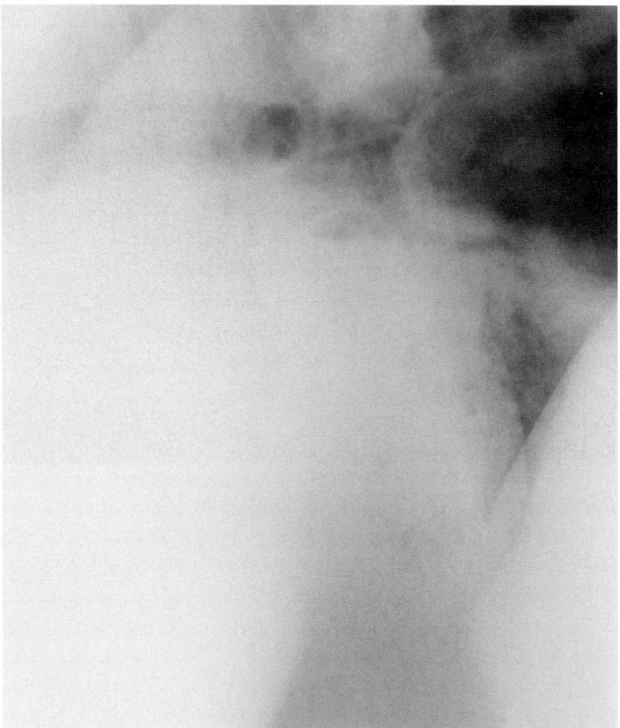

Fig. 35-10 Lateral thoracic radiograph (caudoventral). A fairly intense soft tissue opacity is superimposed on the caudal aspect of the heart that partially silhouettes pulmonary blood vessels, making their margins appear indistinct. This lesion is caused by bronchopneumonia. In the pattern recognition scheme, this lesion is consistent with an interstitial pattern. Dorsal to the carina is a focal, irregularly margined soft tissue nodule. This is a pulmonary abscess.

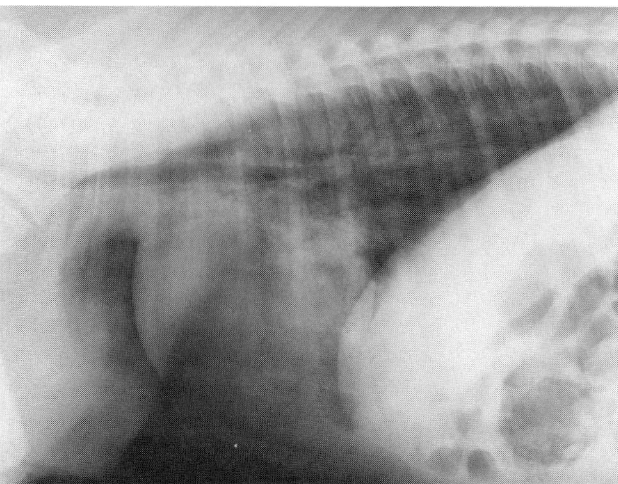

Fig. 35-11 Lateral thoracic radiograph of a foal. A soft tissue opacity is superimposed on the caudal aspect of the heart that obscures the pulmonary blood vessels. In this foal pneumonia developed as a result of aspiration of milk. In the pattern recognition scheme, this lesion is consistent with an alveolar pattern.

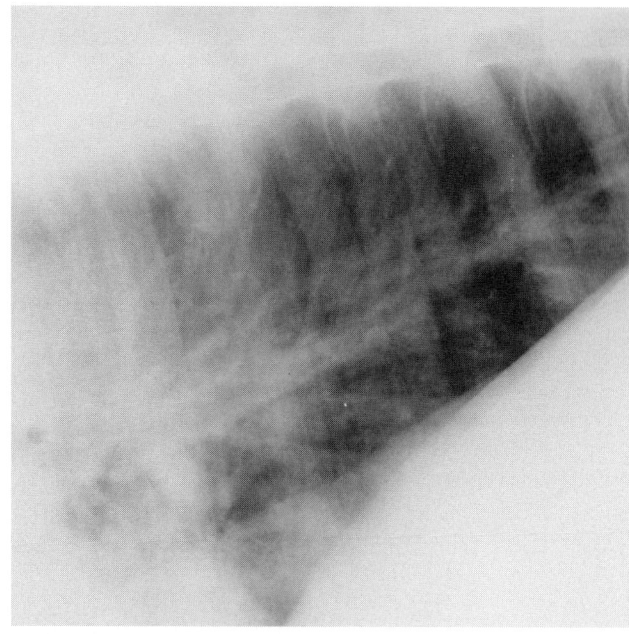

Fig. 35-12 Left lateral radiograph of the caudodorsal thorax in an adult horse with a focal pulmonary abscess. Dorsal to the carina is a circular soft tissue rim that has a gas opacity centrally. In the pattern recognition scheme, this is an interstitial pattern.

portions of the lung.[25] Although it is present in the lung fields cranial to the heart, this region is difficult to image so it is most conspicuous when superimposed on the caudal border of the heart (Fig. 35-10). Bacterial pneumonia can present with an interstitial or alveolar lung pattern depending on the severity (Fig. 35-11).[21] Abscess formation is seen in 10% to 15% of horses with pneumonia (Fig. 35-12).[21]

The ultrasonographic appearance of pneumonic lung is a uniform soft tissue echogenicity that resembles the appearance of liver (Fig. 35-13). Air-filled bronchi will appear as hyperechoic, linear, branching structures that have a reverberation artifact. Fluid-filled bronchi will appear as anechoic branching tubes. Fluid-filled bronchi can be differentiated from blood vessels with Doppler interrogation.

Interstitial pneumonia occurs both in foals and adults and can be acute or chronic.[26,27] The causative agent is usually not identified but may include infectious agents, toxins, systemic inflammatory response syndrome, or allergic factors.[20,23,26-28]

Interstitial pneumonia in foals is usually acute, and affected foals are typically 6 weeks to 6 months of age.[26,29] Chronic interstitial pneumonia has a more favorable prognosis, whereas acute interstitial pneumonia has a high mortality rate.[27,30] Whether the disease is acute or chronic the radiographic changes are the same: a diffuse interstitial lung pattern.[26,29] A mild to moderate bronchial lung pattern may also be present.[27] The disease can result in increased vascular permeability and secondary pulmonary edema.[30] The severity of the changes on the initial radiographs and progression of the changes on subsequent studies are negative prognostic indicators.[20]

Interstitial pneumonia is rare in adults and usually presents as a chronic problem with secondary fibrosis.[31] Because of the fibrosis, affected horses usually respond poorly to treatment.[28] The radiographic appearance is more commonly seen as a diffuse to patchy alveolar lung pattern.[26]

Pneumonia caused by *Rhodococcus equi* in foals is a specific disease entity that frequently has a different radiographic appearance than bronchopneumonia or interstitial pneumonia. *Rhodococcus equi* pneumonia typically has a patchy to diffuse alveolar lung pattern and/or discrete pulmonary nodules (abscesses) (Fig. 35-14).[7,23,32,33] It can also present

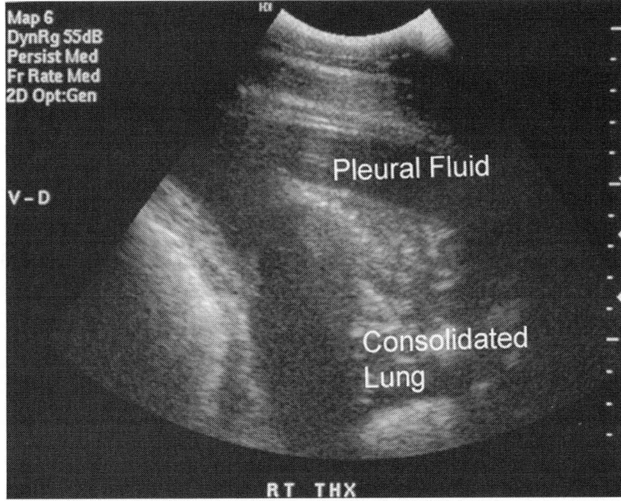

Fig. 35-13 This transverse ultrasound image is characterized by pleural effusion and consolidated lung. Consolidated lung can be recognized by the lack of the normal reverberation artifact seen with aerated lung. The lung has a relatively uniform soft tissue echogenicity similar to the appearance of normal liver and is triangular in shape. The pleural fluid is present between the lung and the body wall.

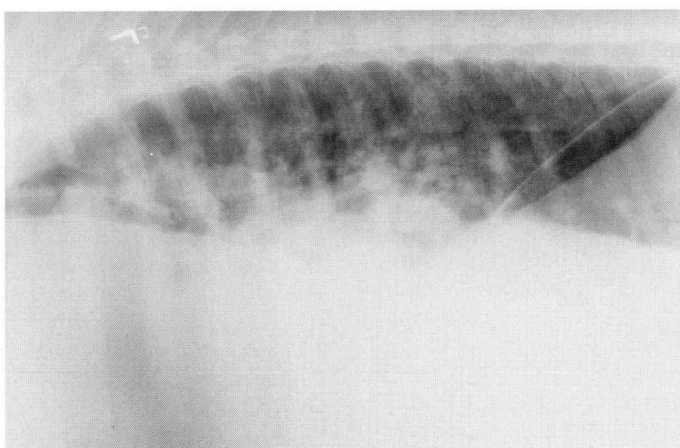

Fig. 35-14 Left lateral radiograph of a 3-month-old foal with pneumonia caused by *Rhodococcus equi* infection. In the ventral portions of the lung is an alveolar lung pattern. In the caudodorsal portions of the lung multiple soft tissue nodules can be seen, the largest of which is cavitated. The nodules are caused by abscess formation.

with consolidation of one lung lobe.[34] Radiographic changes are most apparent at approximately 3 weeks after infection.[34] The severity of the radiographic changes has been negatively associated with prognosis.[35] Foals with an extensive alveolar lung pattern or pulmonary nodules (abscesses) were more likely to die.[33] Tracheobronchial and cranial mediastinal lymphadenopathy can also be detected.[33] In most foals the radiographic signs resolve completely within 3 months of appropriate therapy.[7,34] Ultrasonographic evidence of pneumonia has been highly associated with radiographic abnormalities and may be a useful farm side diagnostic test.[36] Ultrasound may also allow the detection of abscesses within consolidated lung lobes not evident on radiographs (Fig. 35-15).

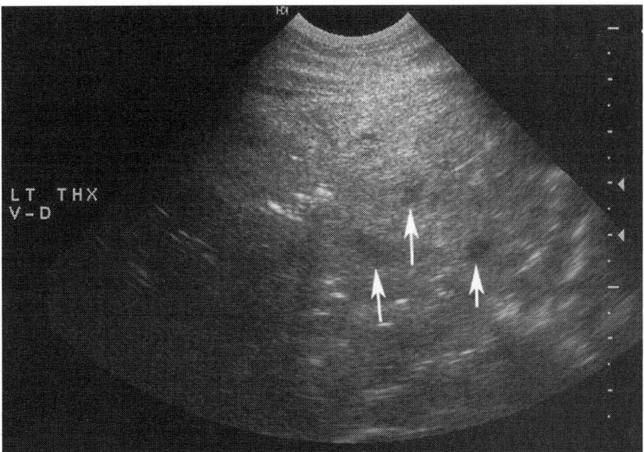

Fig. 35-15 Transverse ultrasound image of the left thorax of the foal in Figure 35-14. The lung is completely consolidated with a heterogenous soft tissue echogenicity. Multiple small, hypoechoic nodules are evident *(arrows)*. These are small abscesses within the consolidated lung.

Fungal pneumonia is rare in horses. It has a wide range of radiographic appearances. Although it cannot be reliably differentiated from bacterial pneumonia on the basis of radiographic appearance, the distribution of fungal pneumonia is usually more diffuse than bacterial pneumonia and typically has an interstitial to indistinct nodular appearance.[21,37-40] Tracheobronchial lymphadenopathy and pleural effusion may also be present.[37,39]

Viral pneumonia itself does not usually result in radiographic changes. However, radiographs can still be indicated to evaluate for concurrent bacterial pneumonia, which is common and results in more severe clinical disease.[14,21,41]

Pulmonary Abscess

Pulmonary abscesses can form as a result of pleuropneumonia or develop independently and predominantly affect foals younger than 6 months of age.[42,43] They can occur anywhere in the lung, but unlike bronchopneumonia, abscesses are most commonly noted in the caudodorsal lung field.[44,45] This may be because they are well contrasted by gas in this region and therefore easier to detect. Abscesses are discrete, focal, soft tissue nodules that may be sharply or poorly margined. If the abscess communicates with a bronchus or contains gas-forming bacteria, a discrete gas-fluid interface will be seen on horizontal-beam radiographs (Fig. 35-16). Well-margined pulmonary consolidation can mimic the appearance of a pulmonary abscess.

By obtaining opposite lateral radiographs centered over the lesion, the abscess can be localized to one side of the thorax. When the abscess is located in the lung closest to the radiographic cassette, it will be smaller and more sharply marginated (Fig. 35-17). If the lesion is located close to midline it will appear approximately the same on both lateral radiographs.[46]

Ultrasound can be used to diagnose pleural-based pulmonary abscesses as well as abscesses that are within consolidated lung and that would not be evident on radiographs. Abscesses are usually hypoechoic to the surrounding pulmonary parenchyma and are defined by the absence of normal pulmonary structures (blood vessels and bronchi) (Fig. 35-18).

Pulmonary Disease in Foals

A caudodorsal and caudoventral interstitial pattern is one of the most common distributions seen in foals.[20] This distribution is nonspecific and can be caused by atelectasis, bacterial pneumonia, viral pneumonia, interstitial pneumonia, prematurity, dysmaturity, or failure of passive transfer, and the causes cannot be differentiated on the basis of radiographs alone (Fig. 35-19).[4,5,27,30,47] Foals with a diffuse distribution of pulmonary disease or a caudodorsal alveolar pattern have a significantly higher mortality rate.[20] Radiographs obtained immediately after parturition often have a diffuse interstitial lung pattern as a result of incomplete expansion of the lungs. This complicates the interpretation of these radiographs because it can mask true pulmonary disease such as sepsis and acute respiratory distress because of a lack of surfactant. If the opacity does not resolve by 12 hours, it is more likely to be caused by underlying disease than by incomplete expansion.[4] Concurrent rib fractures may be present with severe respiratory disease in foals (Fig. 35-20).[4,5,27,30,47] Multiple ribs are usually fractured and can cause myocardial puncture, hemothorax, or pneumothorax.[48]

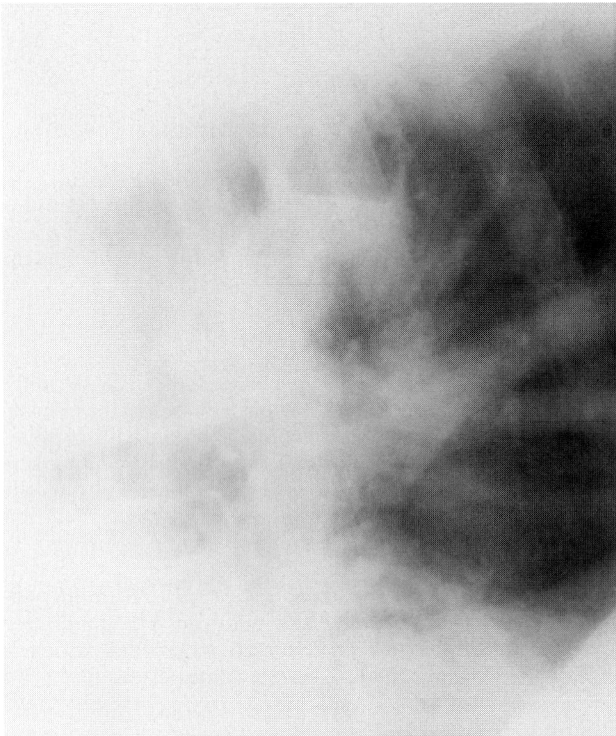

Fig. 35-16 Lateral radiograph of the craniodorsal thorax with a pulmonary abscess. A focal, cavitated pulmonary nodule is present. The dorsal portion of this nodule has a thick rim, and a distinct gas/fluid interface is seen.

Acute respiratory distress syndrome in foals is a respiratory disease with a high mortality rate that can be caused by bacterial or viral infections as well as *Pneumocystis carinii* and coccidiomycosis.[8,29,30,38] Increased vascular permeability leads to pulmonary edema, resulting in a diffuse, interstitial to alveolar lung pattern that cannot be differentiated from other diffuse diseases.[24]

Bronchitis

Only the most severe forms of chronic bronchitis and bronchiolitis result in radiographic changes.[21] Thickening of the bronchi enhance their radiographic visibility, resulting in a pronounced bronchial lung pattern with parallel lines and rings (Fig. 35-21). In end-stage bronchitis tubular to saccular enlargement of the medium bronchi can occur (bronchiectasis).[46]

Recurrent Airway Obstruction (Heaves)

Recurrent airway obstruction (previously known as chronic obstructive pulmonary disease) is a major cause of chronic respiratory disease in horses. The clinical signs are attributed to bronchoconstriction.[49] As such, the majority of horses with recurrent airway obstruction have normal thoracic radiographs. If changes are present they are a diffuse bronchointerstitial lung pattern caused by long-term remodeling of the bronchi.[49] Hyperinflation of the lungs may be present.[50] Hyperinflation of the lungs is characterized by flattening of the diaphragm and no change in lung volume between the inspiratory and expiratory radiographs (i.e., air trapping). Although radiographs are not particularly useful for diagnosing recurrent airway obstruction, they are useful to rule out the presence of a concurrent bronchopneumonia.[49]

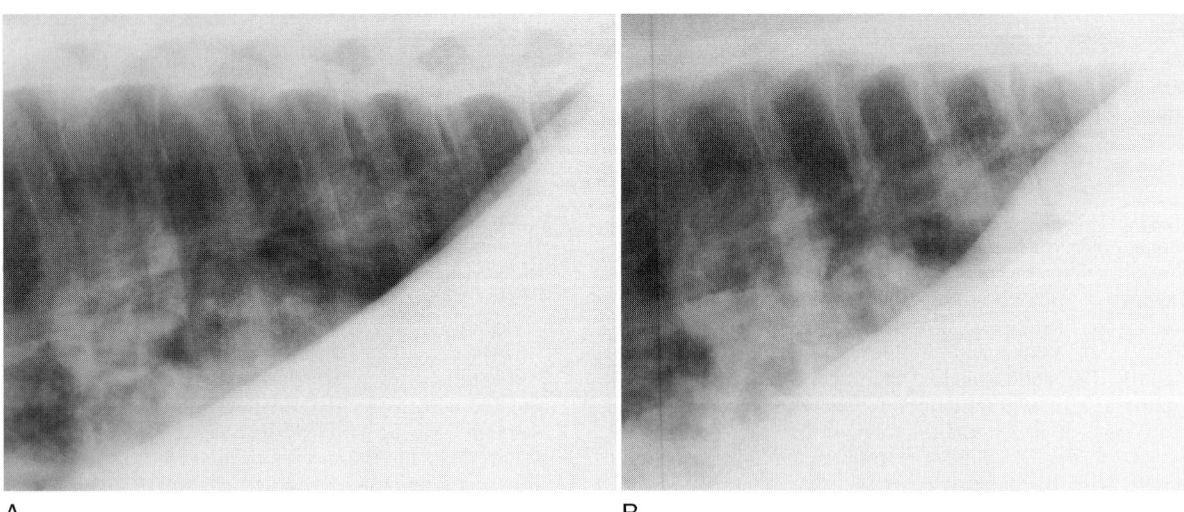

Fig. 35-17 Left (A) and right (B) lateral radiographs of the caudal thorax. The pulmonary nodule is smaller on the left lateral radiograph, which means that the nodule is in the left lung.

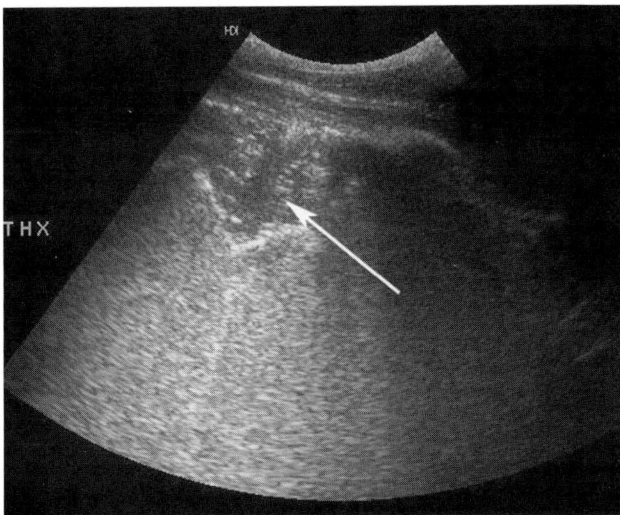

Fig. 35-18 Transverse ultrasound image of the left thorax demonstrates a focal hypoechoic nodule *(arrow)* surrounded by air. This lesion was a pulmonary abscess.

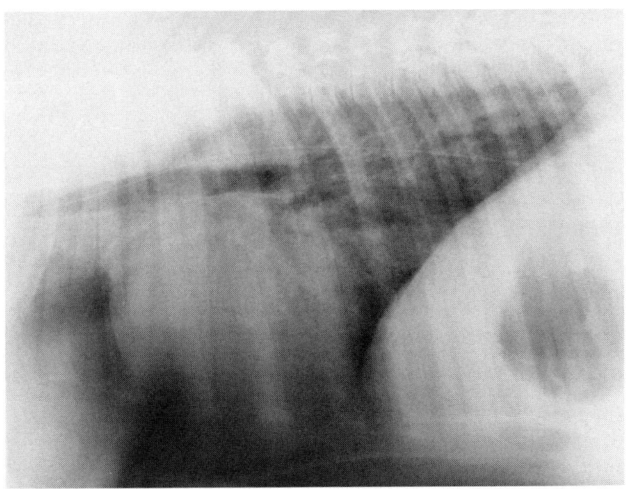

Fig. 35-19 Right lateral radiograph of a premature foal. A diffuse increased soft tissue opacity partially silhouettes the pulmonary blood vessels (interstitial pattern). This diffuse interstitial lung pattern was caused by prematurity and resolved with no treatment. A tube with a radiopaque marker is present in the esophagus.

Exercise-Induced Pulmonary Hemorrhage

Exercise-induced pulmonary hemorrhage is common in racing horses and is characterized by localized or diffuse parenchymal hemorrhage caused by mechanical failure of the walls of the pulmonary capillaries when the internal pressure rises to high levels.[51,52] Many horses with exercise-induced pulmonary hemorrhage have no radiographic abnormalities or a mild, caudodorsal bronchial or interstitial lung pattern that is not distinguishable from airway disease. Therefore radiography is a poor diagnostic tool for exercise-induced pulmonary hemorrhage.[19,56] Repeated episodes of hemorrhage may be necessary for the lesions be become evident radiographically.[57] If a radiographic lesion is present, it is always located in the caudodorsal lung field, superimposed on the diaphragm, and usually presents as a focal area of increased opacity of variable

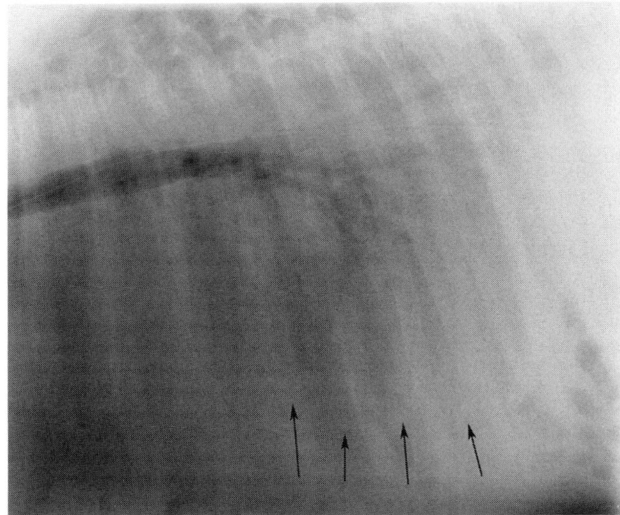

Fig. 35-20 Left lateral radiograph of a foal with severe respiratory distress. A diffuse alveolar pattern is throughout the lungs that silhouettes pulmonary blood vessels. Transverse fractures of the ventral portions of multiple ribs *(arrows)* are present.

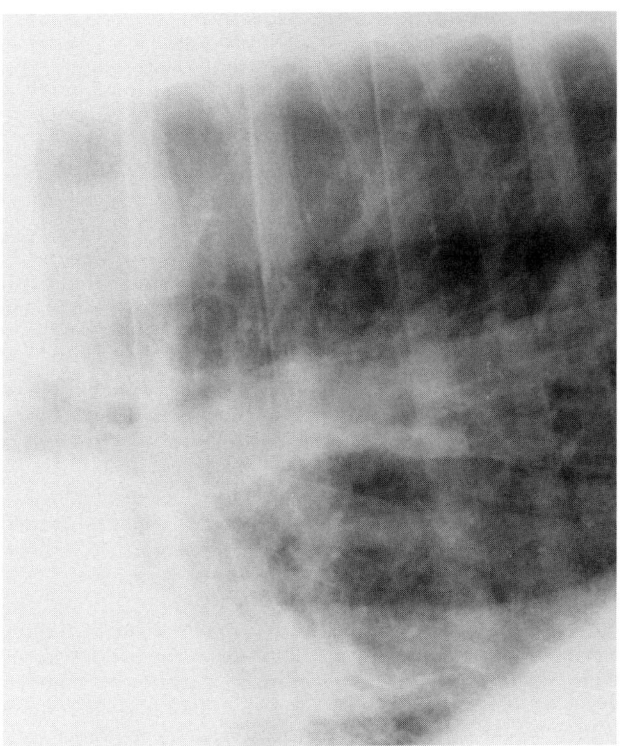

Fig. 35-21 Right lateral radiograph of an adult horse with chronic bronchitis and a bronchial pattern. Note the increased opacity that follows the airways, creating parallel lines and rings.

size (Fig. 35-22).[55-58] The cranial margin of the lesion is round to oval, with indistinct margins. The radiopacity can partially to completely silhouette with the pulmonary blood vessels (interstitial or alveolar pattern).[58] An underlying bronchial lung pattern indicates a chronic lesion.[17] Serial radiographic examinations should provide resolution of the lesion.[58] These lesions occasionally appear cavitated with a distinct gas/fluid

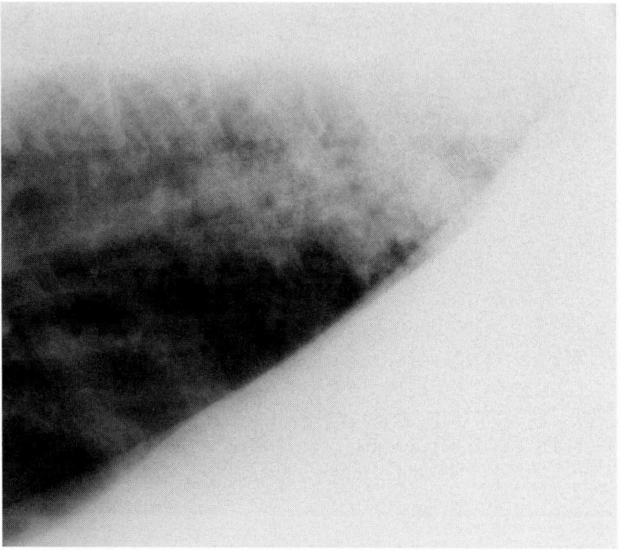

Fig. 35-22 Lateral radiograph of the caudal thorax. A patchy alveolar pattern is superimposed on the dorsal aspect of the diaphragm. This is a common location and appearance of exercise-induced pulmonary hemorrhage.

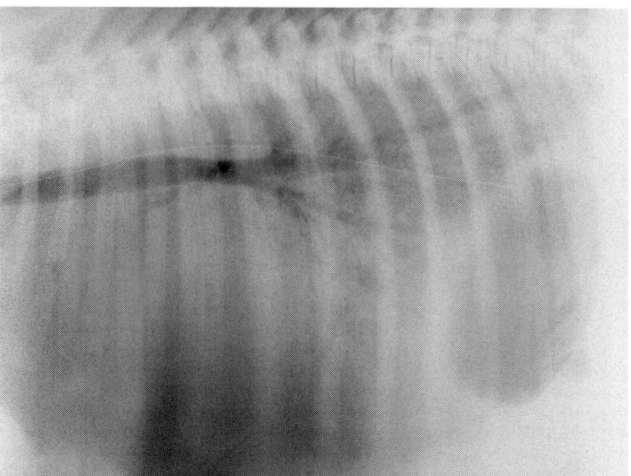

Fig. 35-23 Lateral radiograph of a premature foal with severe pulmonary edema. The lungs are diffusely increased in opacity, and multiple air bronchograms are present (alveolar pattern).

interface, but when this was observed a concurrent infection caused by the hemorrhage was suspected.[58,59] Pleural fluid has also been noted in some horses with exercise-induced pulmonary hemorrhage.[58]

Pulmonary Contusions

Pulmonary contusions can occur as a result of trauma or penetrating wounds. These lesions are seen as poorly marginated areas of increased soft tissue opacity in the lung. The distribution of these lesions corresponds to the location of the trauma.

Pulmonary Edema

Pulmonary edema can result from vasculitis, heart failure, upper airway obstruction, and many other causes.[24,60] The distribution is caudodorsal to diffuse, and the pattern can be interstitial or alveolar (Fig. 35-23).[61] Ultrasonographically, diffuse rough pleural surfaces ("comet tail" artifacts) caused by focal areas of consolidation can be seen.[24]

Neoplasia

Primary and metastatic lung tumors are rare in horses.[62] Lung tumors appear as focal or multifocal soft tissue nodules in the lungs.[48,63-66] These lesions are usually discrete, with no air bronchograms. The presence of pleural fluid is also common with neoplasia.[63,67] The differential diagnoses for these radiographic signs include abscessation and fungal pneumonia. Pulmonary abscesses are the most common cause of multifocal pulmonary nodules and should be considered more likely than neoplasia. If the lesions are pleural based, they can be examined by ultrasound and ultrasound-guided needle aspiration can be performed.[67] Tracheobronchial lymphadenopathy may also be present with primary lung tumors, metastatic tumors, and lymphoma.

Alterations in Pulmonary Vasculature

Assessment of pulmonary vasculature is based on a subjective assessment of the size and number of vessels. The pulmonary veins and arteries generally cannot be distinguished from each other. Diseases that cause overcirculation of the lungs, such as right-to-left shunts, will cause an increase in the size and number of all visible pulmonary blood vessels.[9] Undercirculation of the lungs can be caused by shock or right-to-left shunts.[9]

PLEURAL DISEASE

Pleural Fluid

The most common cause of pleural fluid in the horse is extension of bacterial pneumonia into the pleural space, resulting in pleuropneumonia.[41,42] Other causes of pleural fluid include neoplasia (mesothelioma, metastatic disease, and primary lung tumors), foreign bodies, and trauma (hemorrhage). Pleural fluid is uncommon in foals except as a result of uroperitoneum.[5]

Pleural fluid gravitates to the dependent portion of the thorax and results in a homogenous soft tissue opacity in the ventral thorax (Fig. 35-24). Because horses do not have prominent interlobular fissures, pleural fissure lines are rarely seen. Approximately 1 to 2 L of pleural fluid must be present to be detected radiographically. Therefore normal thoracic radiographs do not eliminate the possibility of pleural fluid.[68] The fluid initially will silhouette the heart and diaphragm, resulting in loss of definition of these structures. As more fluid accumulates, normal lungs will be displaced dorsally. Because of surface tension a discrete, horizontal fluid line is only present if free gas is also present in the pleural space (iatrogenic or traumatic) (Fig. 35-25).

When pleural fluid is present, assessment of the lungs for concurrent disease is difficult to impossible.[21] Consolidated lung lobes are not dorsally displaced by the pleural fluid, so they are obscured. This makes the differentiation of pleural fluid from pneumonia difficult. Fibrin accumulation and inflammation can result in compartmentalization of pleural fluid and unilateral effusions even though the normal mediastinum is not complete. This can add to the difficulty in differentiating pulmonary disease from pleural disease. Repeating the radiographs after thoracocentesis provides more information on the presence and extent of any pulmonary disease.

Ultrasound is superior for evaluating the amount and character of pleural fluid, guiding thoracocentesis, and evaluating

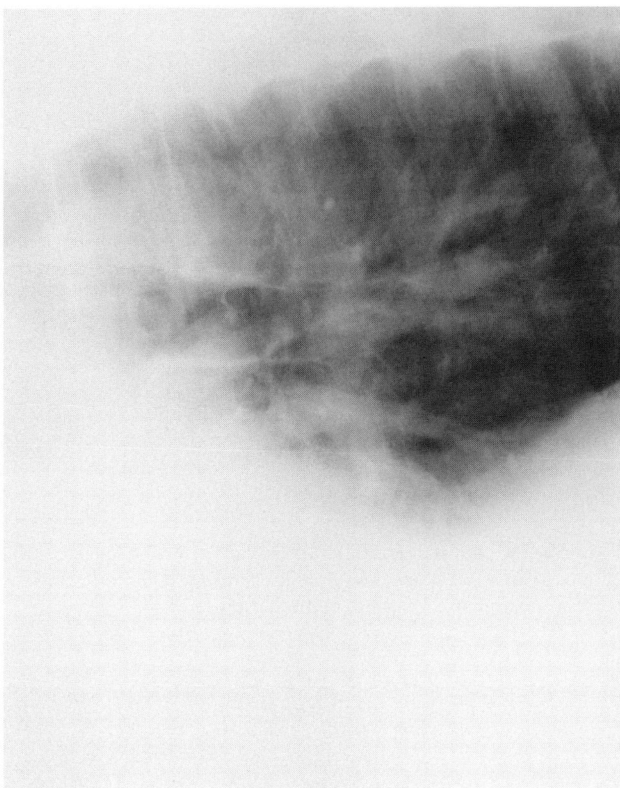

Fig. 35-24 Lateral radiograph of the craniodorsal thorax of a horse with moderate pleural fluid. In the ventral thorax is a uniform soft tissue opacity that silhouettes the heart and diaphragm. A distinct fluid line is not visible because pneumothorax is not present. Differentiation of pleural fluid from consolidated lung can be difficult and often requires ultrasound examination.

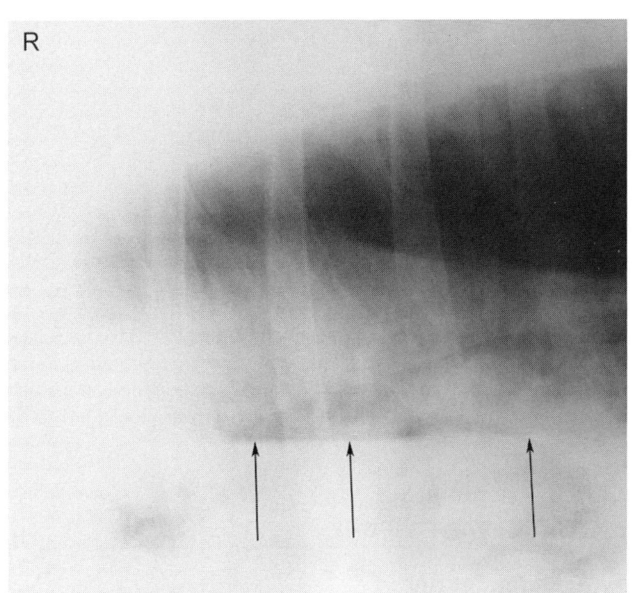

Fig. 35-25 Lateral radiograph of the thorax. In the ventral thorax is a soft tissue opacity that silhouettes the diaphragm. This is caused by pleural fluid. A distinct, horizontal fluid line is evident *(arrows)*. A pleural fluid line is only seen when concurrent pneumothorax is present.

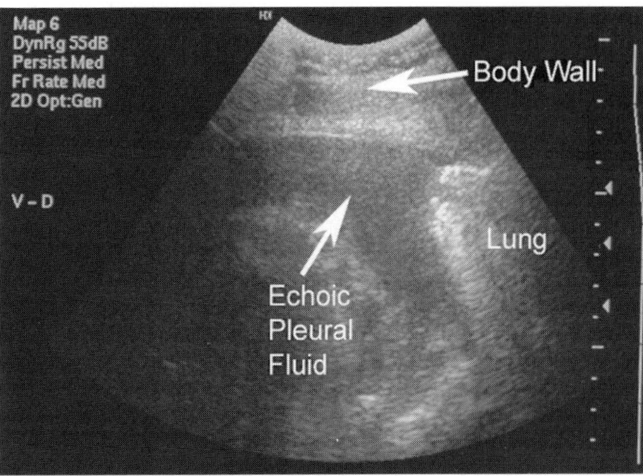

Fig. 35-26 Pleural fluid is seen between the body wall and the lung; the fluid is highly echogenic. The lung is retracted away from the body wall and dorsally.

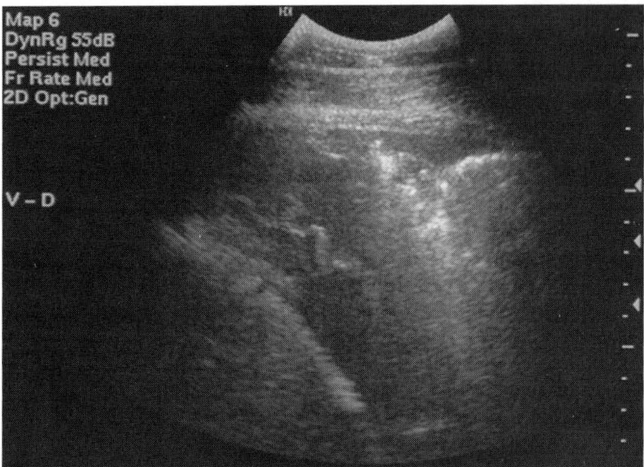

Fig. 35-27 Fibrin tags (adhesions) can be seen as echoic strands in the pleural effusion in this transverse ultrasound image.

for resolution or progression (Fig. 35-26).[69] It also allows the identification of consolidation of the lung and other pleural-based lesions such as abscesses that may be masked by the pleural fluid on the radiographs.[12] The volume of pleural fluid can be estimated with ultrasound based on the level of the fluid relative to various anatomic points. If only a small amount of fluid is present in the ventral thorax, the volume is approximately 0.5 L. If the dorsal extent of the pleural fluid is at the point of the shoulder the volume is approximately 1 to 2.5 L. If the dorsal extent of the pleural fluid is 5 to 7 cm dorsal to the point of the shoulder, the volume is approximately 5 L.[12] The character of the pleural fluid can be inferred by the ultrasound appearance, with more echoic fluids being more cellular, but thoracocentesis is required to diagnose the type of fluid definitively. Ultrasound is also helpful to identify the presence of fibrinous adhesions between the pleural surface of the lung and the body wall (Fig. 35-27).[12] Neither of these changes is able to be identified with radiographs.

Pneumothorax

Pneumothorax in the horse is rare and occurs most commonly as a result of trauma, as a sequela of pleuropneumonia, or from the tearing of pleural adhesions.[70] Iatrogenic causes of pneu-

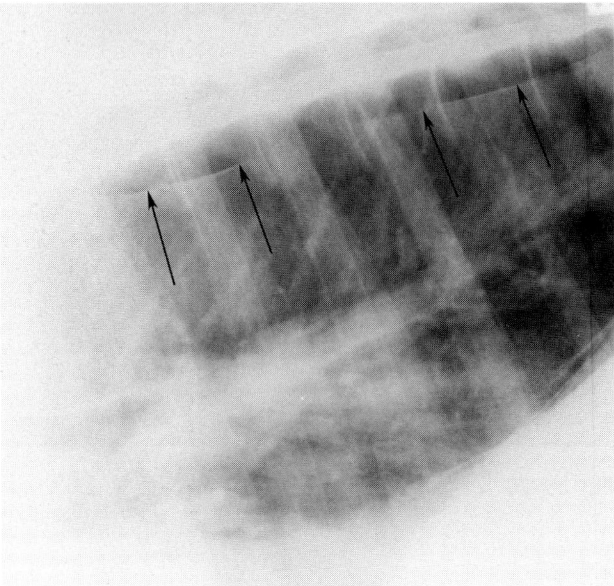

Fig. 35-28 Lateral radiograph of the caudal aspect of the thorax. Pneumothorax results in the lungs being retracted from the dorsal body wall; the edge of the lung can be seen as an opaque white line paralleling the vertebral column *(arrow)*.

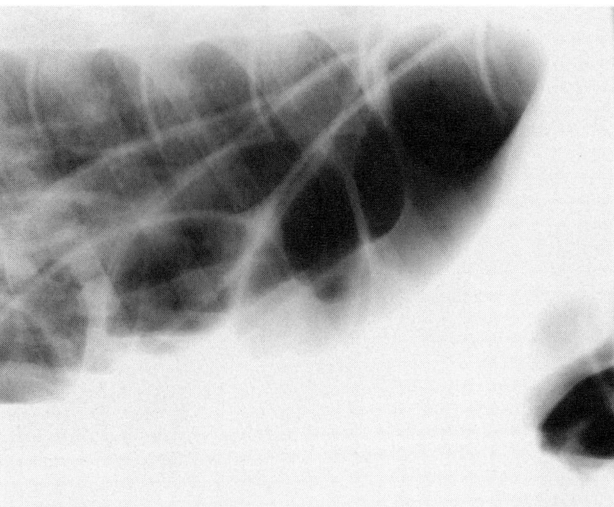

Fig. 35-29 Lateral radiograph of the caudal aspect of the thorax in an adult horse. Multiple loops of gas-filled intestine are seen as a result of a diaphragmatic hernia.

mothorax include complications from thoracocentesis and surgical procedures.

The presence of air in the pleural space results in retraction of the lungs from the body wall, permitting visualization of the dorsal margin of the lung because the air will rise to the dorsal aspect of the thorax. The free gas between the lung and the body wall contrasts with the edge of the lung, making it appear as an opaque white line running roughly parallel to the vertebral column (Fig. 35-28). If pneumothorax is present concurrently with pleural fluid, a distinct horizontal gas-fluid line will be present.

Radiography and ultrasound can both be used to diagnose pneumothorax, although radiography may be slightly more sensitive and is less operator dependent.[70] The ultrasonographic appearance of air is the same whether it is free in the thorax or within the lung (a bright interface with reverberation artifact). The ultrasound diagnosis of pneumothorax requires the operator to identify that the air does not move with respiration (called the "curtain sign").[45] Additionally, if the dorsal portions of the thorax are not evaluated, free air can go undetected.[70] Pneumothorax is easier to detect with ultrasound when pleural fluid is present concurrently.[70]

Diaphragmatic Hernia

Diaphragmatic hernias can occur as a result of trauma, dystocia, strenuous exercise, or laparoscopic surgery. Radiographic identification of a diaphragmatic hernia requires detection of abdominal contents in the thoracic cavity. Most often gas-filled loops of the gastrointestinal tract are detected in the caudodorsal portion of the thorax (Fig. 35-29).[71,72] Pleural fluid may also be present.[72,73] Ultrasound can also be used to diagnose diaphragmatic hernias, particularly when pleural fluid is present. Not all the diaphragm can be visualized with ultrasound, so the actual disruption of the diaphragm may not be identified, but abdominal contents in the thoracic cavity can be seen.[74]

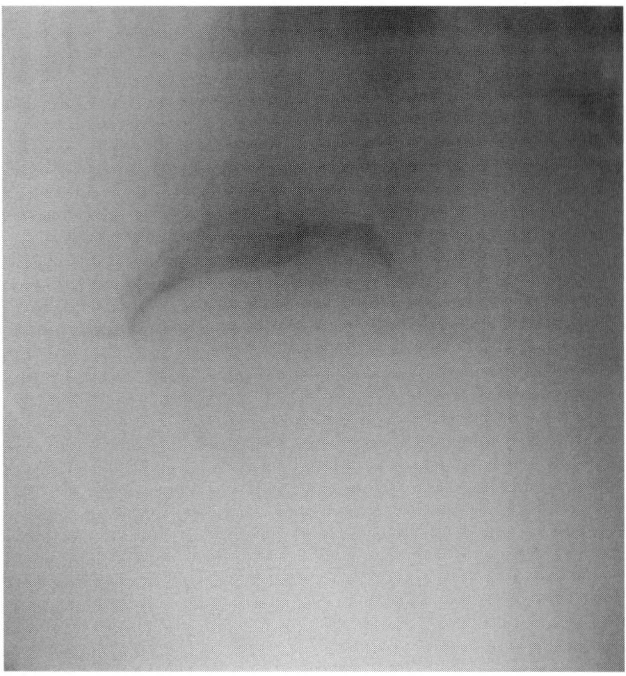

Fig. 35-30 Lateral radiograph of the cranial aspect of the thorax. A focal soft tissue mass is cranial to the heart. The dorsal aspect of this mass is convex. Opposite lateral radiographs of the cranial aspect of the thorax had a similar appearance, indicating the structure was on the midline. This mass was confirmed to be mediastinal lymphoma.

MEDIASTINAL DISEASE

Lymphadenopathy

The most common thoracic tumor in horses is lymphoma.[62] Lymphoma commonly results in a cranial mediastinal mass. Radiographically, this is seen as a soft tissue opacity cranial to the heart (Fig. 35-30).[75] With moderate cranial mediastinal lymphadenopathy the mediastinum is wide and the ventral

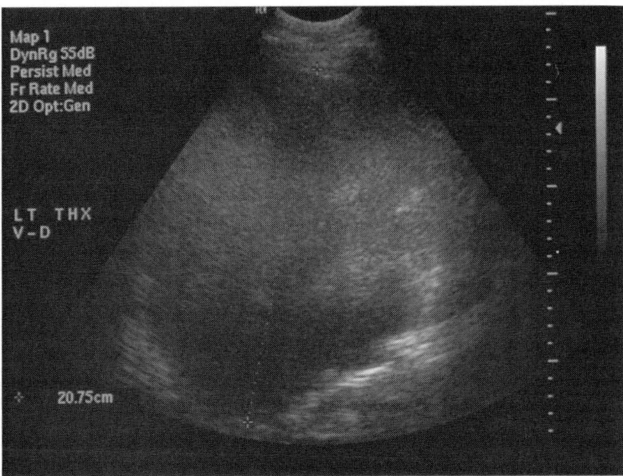

Fig. 35-31 A uniformly echoic mass can be seen in a transverse ultrasound image of the cranial aspect of the thorax of the horse in Figure 35-30.

border is irregular. More severe involvement causes loss of visualization of the normal aerated lung cranial to the heart as a result of atelectasis. Pleural fluid is also a common finding in lymphoma, which inhibits the radiographic detection of mediastinal masses.[76,77] Ultrasound is useful in these instances to characterize the quantity and quality of the fluid as well as the presence of a mass. Most masses are multilobular and uniformly hypoechoic and frequently displace the heart caudally (Fig. 35-31).[76]

A poorly defined soft tissue opacity dorsal to the carina that displaces the trachea dorsally or ventrally and silhouettes the ventral border of the aorta is indicative of tracheobronchial lymphadenopathy.[19,75] Tracheobronchial lymphadenopathy may be difficult to differentiate from a pulmonary mass. Opposite lateral radiographs are helpful because the lymph nodes are a midline structure and therefore should have the same appearance on both lateral radiographs. Computed tomography can also be used in foals to differentiate tracheobronchial lymphadenopathy from a pulmonary mass.[19]

Pneumomediastinum

Pneumomediastinum can occur as a result of punctures to the neck, rupture of the trachea, rupture of the esophagus, or a transtracheal wash. Linear gas opacities are seen tracking along the facial planes of the neck and mediastinum. This results in gas contrasting the trachea, esophagus, cranial vena cava, and aorta (Fig. 35-32). Pneumomediastinum can lead to pneumothorax.

TRACHEAL DISEASE

Tracheal collapse has been rarely reported in horses.[78] Dorsoventral flattening of the trachea is seen on the thoracic radiographs. Comparing radiographs obtained during inspiration and expiration may demonstrate a change in tracheal diameter associated with collapse.

Fluid can be seen pooled in the ventral aspect of the trachea at the thoracic inlet in horses that have aspirated. In severe tracheitis the tracheal wall may appear thick and irregular (Fig. 35-33).

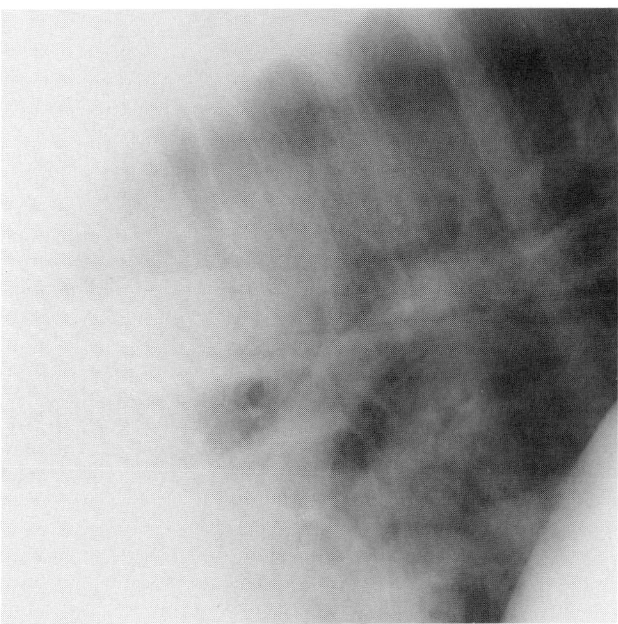

Fig. 35-32 Lateral radiograph of the craniodorsal aspect of the thorax. Gas is present in the cranial mediastinum. The gas contrasts with the esophagus, making it visible as a tubular soft tissue opacity dorsal to the trachea.

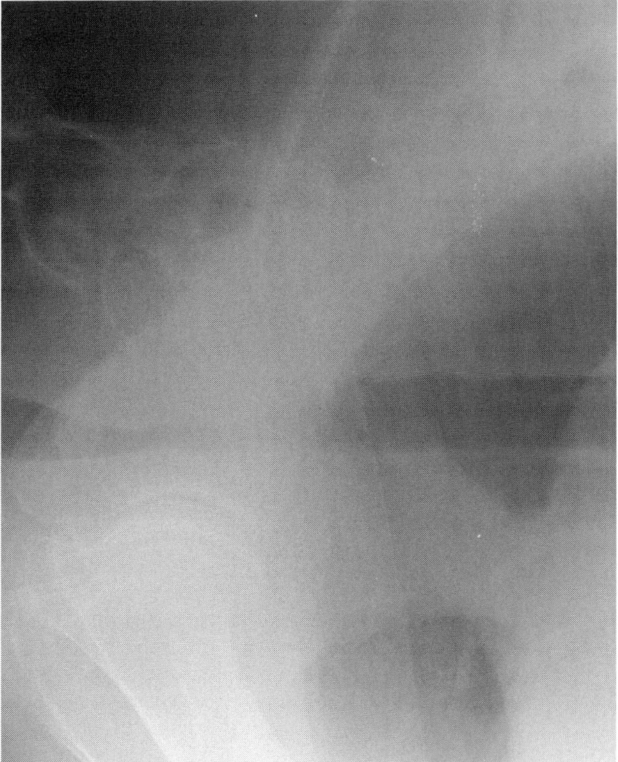

Fig. 35-33 Lateral radiograph of the cranial aspect of the thorax. The trachea is focally narrowed at the thoracic inlet, and the dorsal aspect of the lumen of the trachea has an irregular contour. This lesion was attributable to tracheal thickening from chronic tracheitis.

ESOPHAGEAL DISEASE

The most common esophageal disease of horses is idiopathic obstruction caused by impaction of ingesta (choke).[79] Reported esophageal disease in horses includes congenital or acquired strictures, esophageal duplication cyst, esophageal atresia, vascular ring anomalies, space-occupying lesions (abscess, tumor), megaesophagus, and esophagitis.[79-83] Regardless of the cause most esophageal disease results in impaction of food within the esophagus.[79]

The normal esophagus is not visible in survey radiographs. Contrast radiographs (esophography) are useful to evaluate the esophagus. Esophography can be performed with liquid or paste forms of barium as well as with barium-coated food administered orally. Barium paste coats the esophagus better, allowing the detection of mucosal abnormalities.[84] If the oropharyngeal phase of swallowing is not of interest, then the contrast medium can be administered directly into the cranial aspect of the esophagus with an esophageal tube. The use of certain sedatives and the placement of an esophageal tube, however, can result in dilation of the esophagus in normal horses.[85] The use of fluoroscopy to observe swallowing is best because it allows a dynamic assessment of the esophagus, but obtaining static radiographs after the administration of contrast medium can be diagnostic because most esophageal diseases result in delayed transit time.[85] Minimal contrast medium should be retained in the esophagus, outlining the esophageal folds after normal swallowing.[85,86]

With the exception of esophageal impactions in which focal enlargement of the esophagus with a granular radiopacity is seen, most esophageal diseases are not evident on survey radiographs.[86] In recurrent choke, esophography is indicated to evaluate for underlying primary esophageal disease.[79] Focal narrowing of the esophagus is indicative of a stricture or extraluminal mass causing compression of the esophagus. Filling the esophagus with a large amount of contrast medium (up to 500 mL) through a cuffed nasoesophageal tube may be necessary to distend the esophagus adequately enough to detect some strictures.[84] Esophagitis results in thickening of the esophageal wall, and accumulation of contrast medium may occur as a result of hypomotility. Focal esophageal ulcerations may be noted as the contrast medium adheres to the mucosa and creates irregular filling defects. In most horses, esophoscopy has replaced the need for contrast studies of the esophagus because of its ease and availability. However, for adequate assessment of esophageal motility and swallowing, esophography is still required.

CARDIAC DISEASE

Radiographic assessment of heart size is difficult in adult horses because of a lack of objective criteria and the inability to obtain orthogonal radiographs.[9] The entire heart should be imaged on one 14-inch × 17-inch radiographic cassette if possible but is often possible only in foals. Therefore echocardiography is the most common diagnostic test for cardiac disease in horses. The radiographic signs of cardiomegaly are the same as in small animals. Straightening of the caudal aspect of the heart, increased sternal and diaphragmatic contact, and dorsal displacement of the trachea are indications of left heart enlargement (Fig. 35-34).[9]

The radiographic signs of congestive heart failure are also the same as those seen in small animals. Pulmonary edema results in a diffuse to caudodorsal interstitial to alveolar lung pattern.[9,61] Pulmonary venous congestion may also be seen.[61] Pleural fluid may be evident if biventricular heart failure is present.[9,61] For the diagnosis of pericardial fluid and pericarditis, ultrasound is the best imaging modality.[87]

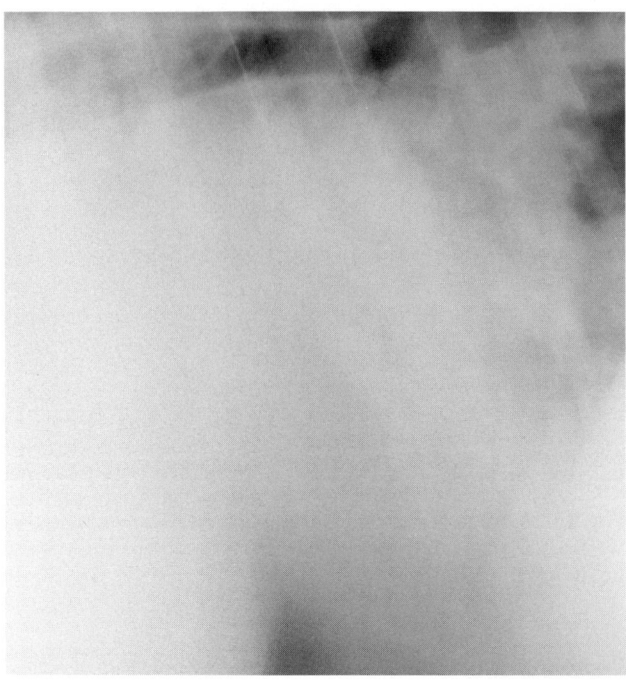

Fig. 35-34 Lateral radiograph of the thorax centered over the heart demonstrates loss of the caudal cardiac waist and dorsal displacement of the trachea, indicative of left-sided cardiomegaly. In the caudoventral lung field there is a mild soft tissue opacity. In the pattern recognition scheme this is an interstitial lung pattern. This change is attributed to pulmonary edema. (Courtesy Dr. Robert Bahr, Oklahoma State University, Stillwater, Okla.)

REFERENCES

1. Feeney D, Gordon B, Johnston G et al: A 200 centimeter focal spot-film distance (FFD) technique for equine radiography, *Vet Radiol* 23:13, 1982.
2. Wisner ER, O'Brien TR, Lakritz J et al: Radiographic and microscopic correlation of diffuse interstitial and bronchointerstitial pulmonary patterns in the caudodorsal lung of adult thoroughbred horses in race training, *Equine Vet J* 25:293, 1993.
3. Dyce KM, Sack WO, Wensing CJG: *Textbook of veterinary anatomy*, Philadelphia, 2002, WB Saunders.
4. Lamb C, O'Callaghan M, Paradis M: Thoracic radiography in the neonatal foal: a preliminary report, *Vet Radiol* 31:11, 1990.
5. Lester GD, Lester NV: Abdominal and thoracic radiography in the neonate, *Vet Clin North Am Equine Pract* 17:19, 2001.
6. Sanderson GN, O'Callaghan MW: Radiographic anatomy of the equine thorax as a basis for radiological interpretation, *N Z Vet J* 31:127, 1983.
7. Ainsworth DM, Beck KA, Boatwright CE et al: Lack of residual lung damage in horses in which *Rhodococcus equi*-induced pneumonia had been diagnosed, *Am J Vet Res* 54:2115, 1993.
8. Perron Lepage MF, Gerber V, Suter MM: A case of interstitial pneumonia associated with *Pneumocystis carinii* in a foal, *Vet Pathol* 36:621, 1999.
9. Koblik PD, Hornof WJ: Diagnostic radiology and nuclear cardiology. Their use in assessment of equine cardiovascular disease, *Vet Clin North Am Equine Pract* 1:289, 1985.

10. Hoskinson JJ, Tucker RL, Lillich J et al: Advanced diagnostic imaging modalities available at the referral center, *Vet Clin North Am Equine Pract* 13:601, 1997.
11. Rantanen N: Ultrasound appearance of normal lung borders and adjacent viscera in the horse, *Vet Radiol* 22:217, 1981.
12. Reef VB, Boy MG, Reid CF et al: Comparison between diagnostic ultrasonography and radiography in the evaluation of horses and cattle with thoracic disease: 56 cases (1984-1985), *J Am Vet Med Assoc* 198:2112, 1991.
13. Hinchcliff KW, Byrne BA: Clinical examination of the respiratory system, *Vet Clin North Am Equine Pract* 7:1, 1991.
14. Gross DK, Morley PS, Hinchcliff KW et al: Pulmonary ultrasonographic abnormalities associated with naturally occurring equine influenza virus infection in Standardbred racehorses, *J Vet Intern Med* 18:718, 2004.
15. Rantanen N: The diagnosis of lung consolidation in horses using linear array diagnostic ultrasound, *J Equine Vet Sci* 14:79, 1994.
16. Rush BR, Hoskinson JJ, Davis EG et al: Pulmonary distribution of aerosolized technetium Tc 99m pentetate after administration of a single dose of aerosolized albuterol sulfate in horses with recurrent airway obstruction, *Am J Vet Res* 60:764, 1999.
17. O'Callaghan MW, Hornof WJ, Fisher PE et al: Exercise-induced pulmonary haemorrhage in the horses: results of a detailed clinical, post mortem and imaging study. VII. Ventilation/perfusion scintigraphy in horses with EIPH, *Equine Vet J* 19:423, 1987.
18. Votion DM, Vandenput SN, Duvivier DH et al: Alveolar clearance in horses with chronic obstructive pulmonary disease, *Am J Vet Res* 60:495, 1999.
19. Wion L, Perkins G, Ainsworth DM et al: Use of computerised tomography to diagnose a Rhodococcus equi mediastinal abscess causing severe respiratory distress in a foal, *Equine Vet J* 33:523, 2001.
20. Bedenice D, Heuwieser W, Brawer R et al: Clinical and prognostic significance of radiographic pattern, distribution, and severity of thoracic radiographic changes in neonatal foals, *J Vet Intern Med* 17:876, 2003.
21. Farrow C: Radiographic aspects of inflammatory lung disease in the horse, *Vet Radiol* 22:107, 1981.
22. Nykamp S, Scrivani P, Dykes N: Radiographic signs of pulmonary disease: an alternative approach, *Compend Contin Ed Pract Vet* 24:25, 2002.
23. Wilkins PA: Lower respiratory problems of the neonate, *Vet Clin North Am Equine Pract* 19:19, 2003.
24. Wilkins PA: Lower airway diseases of the adult horse, *Vet Clin North Am Equine Pract* 19:101, 2003.
25. Kangstrom L: The radiological diagnosis of equine pneumonia, *J Am Vet Radiol Soc* 9:80, 1968.
26. Buergelt CD: Interstitial pneumonia in the horse: a fledgling morphological entity with mysterious causes, *Equine Vet J* 27:4, 1995.
27. Nout YS, Hinchcliff KW, Samii VF et al: Chronic pulmonary disease with radiographic interstitial opacity (interstitial pneumonia) in foals, 34:542, 2002.
28. Buergelt CD, Hines SA, Cantor G et al: A retrospective study of proliferative interstitial lung disease of horses in Florida, *Vet Pathol* 23:750, 1986.
29. Peek SF, Landolt G, Karasin AI et al: Acute respiratory distress syndrome and fatal interstitial pneumonia associated with equine influenza in a neonatal foal, *J Vet Intern Med* 18:132, 2004.
30. Lakritz J, Wilson WD, Berry CR et al: Bronchointerstitial pneumonia and respiratory distress in young horses: clinical, clinicopathologic, radiographic, and pathological findings in 23 cases (1984-1989), *J Vet Intern Med* 7:277, 1993.
31. Donaldson MT, Beech J, Ennulat D et al: Interstitial pneumonia and pulmonary fibrosis in a horse, *Equine Vet J* 30:173, 1998.
32. Hillidge CJ: Review of Corynebacterium (*Rhodococcus*) equi lung abscesses in foals: pathogenesis, diagnosis and treatment, *Vet Rec* 119:261, 1986.
33. Falcon J, Smith BP, O'Brien TR et al: Clinical and radiographic findings in *Corynebacterium equi* pneumonia of foals, *J Am Vet Med Assoc* 186:593, 1985.
34. Martens RJ, Martens JG, Fiske RA et al: *Rhodococcus equi* foal pneumonia: protective effects of immune plasma in experimentally infected foals, *Equine Vet J* 21:249, 1989.
35. Ainsworth DM, Eicker SW, Yeagar AE et al: Associations between physical examination, laboratory, and radiographic findings and outcome and subsequent racing performance of foals with *Rhodococcus equi* infection: 115 cases (1984-1992), *J Am Vet Med Assoc* 213:510, 1998.
36. Ramirez S, Lester GD, Roberts GR: Diagnostic contribution of thoracic ultrasonography in 17 foals with *Rhodococcus equi* pneumonia, *Vet Radiol Ultrasound* 45:172, 2004.
37. Green S, Hager D, Calderwood M et al: Acute diffuse mycotic pneumonia in a 7-month-old colt, *Vet Radiol* 28:216, 1987.
38. Maleski K, Magdesian KG, LaFranco-Scheuch L et al: Pulmonary coccidioidomycosis in a neonatal foal, *Vet Rec* 151:505, 2002.
39. Ziemer EL, Pappagianis D, Madigan JE et al: Coccidioidomycosis in horses: 15 cases (1975-1984), *J Am Vet Med Assoc* 201:910, 1992.
40. Toribio RE, Kohn CW, Lawrence AE et al: Thoracic and abdominal blastomycosis in a horse, *J Am Vet Med Assoc* 214:1357, 1999.
41. Mair TS, Lane JG: Pneumonia, lung abscesses and pleuritis in adult horses: a review of 51 cases, *Equine Vet J* 21:175, 1989.
42. Raphel CF, Beech J: Pleuritis secondary to pneumonia or lung abscessation in 90 horses, *J Am Vet Med Assoc* 181:808, 1982.
43. Lavoie JP, Fiset L, Laverty S: Review of 40 cases of lung abscesses in foals and adult horses, *Equine Vet J* 26:348, 1994.
44. Ainsworth DM, Erb HN, Eicker SW et al: Effects of pulmonary abscesses on racing performance of horses treated at referral veterinary medical teaching hospitals: 45 cases (1985-1997), *J Am Vet Med Assoc* 216:1282, 2000.
45. Reef VB: *Equine diagnostic ultrasound*, Philadelphia, 1998, WB Saunders.
46. Lavoie JP, Dalle S, Breton L et al: Bronchiectasis in three adult horses with heaves, *J Vet Intern Med* 18:757, 2004.
47. Koterba AM, Brewer BD, Tarplee FA: Clinical and clinicopathological characteristics of the septicaemic neonatal foal: review of 38 cases, *Equine Vet J* 16:376, 1984.
48. Jean D, Lavoie JP, Nunez L et al: Cutaneous hemangiosarcoma with pulmonary metastasis in a horse, *J Am Vet Med Assoc* 204:776, 1994.
49. Leguillette R: Recurrent airway obstruction—heaves, *Vet Clin North Am Equine Pract* 19:63, 2003.
50. Seahorn TL, Beadle RE: Summer pasture-associated obstructive pulmonary disease in horses: 21 cases (1983-1991), *J Am Vet Med Assoc* 202:779, 1993.
51. West JB, Mathieu-Costello O: Stress failure of pulmonary capillaries as a mechanism for exercise induced pulmonary haemorrhage in the horse, *Equine Vet J* 26:441, 1994.

52. Clarke AF: Review of exercise induced pulmonary haemorrhage and its possible relationship with mechanical stress, *Equine Vet J* 17:166, 1985.
53. O'Callaghan MW, Pascoe JR, O'Brien TR et al: Exercise-induced pulmonary haemorrhage in the horse: results of a detailed clinical, post mortem and imaging study. VI. Radiological/pathological correlations, *Equine Vet J* 19:419, 1987.
54. Doucet MY, Viel L: Clinical, radiographic, endoscopic, bronchoalveolar lavage and lung biopsy findings in horses with exercise-induced pulmonary hemorrhage, *Can Vet J* 43:195, 2002.
55. O'Callaghan MW, Sanderson GN: Clinical bronchography in the horse: development of a method using barium sulphate powder, *Equine Vet J* 14:282, 1982.
56. Sweeney CR: Exercise-induced pulmonary hemorrhage, *Vet Clin North Am Equine Pract* 7:93, 1991.
57. Birks EK, Durando MM, McBride S: Exercise-induced pulmonary hemorrhage, *Vet Clin North Am Equine Pract* 19:87, 2003.
58. Pascoe J, O'Brien T, Wheat J et al: Radiographic aspects of exercise-induced pulmonary hemorrhage in racing horses, *Vet Radiol* 24:85, 1983.
59. Riley CB, Bolton JR, Mills JN et al: Cryptococcosis in seven horses, *Aust Vet J* 69:135, 1992.
60. Kollias-Baker CA, Pipers FS, Heard D et al: Pulmonary edema associated with transient airway obstruction in three horses, *J Am Vet Med Assoc* 202:1116, 1993.
61. Davis JL, Gardner SY, Schwabenton B et al: Congestive heart failure in horses: 14 cases (1984-2001), *J Am Vet Med Assoc* 220:1512, 2002.
62. Sweeney CR, Gillette DM: Thoracic neoplasia in equids: 35 cases (1967-1987), *J Am Vet Med Assoc* 195:374, 1989.
63. Jorgensen JS, Geoly FJ, Berry CR et al: Lameness and pleural effusion associated with an aggressive fibrosarcoma in a horse, *J Am Vet Med Assoc* 210:1328, 1997.
64. Cook G, Divers TJ, Rowland PH: Hypercalcaemia and erythrocytosis in a mare associated with a metastatic carcinoma, *Equine Vet J* 27:316, 1995.
65. Facemire PR, Chilcoat CD, Sojka JE et al: Treatment of granular cell tumor via complete right lung resection in a horse, *J Am Vet Med Assoc* 217:1522, 2000.
66. Danton CA, Peacock PJ, May SA et al: Anaplastic sarcoma in the caudal thigh of a horse, *Vet Rec* 131:188, 1992.
67. Anderson JD, Leonard JM, Zeliff JA et al: Primary pulmonary neoplasm in a horse, *J Am Vet Med Assoc* 201:1399, 1992.
68. Prater PE, Patton CS, Held JP: Pleural effusion resulting from malignant hepatoblastoma in a horse, *J Am Vet Med Assoc* 194:383, 1989.
69. Rantanen N, Gage L, Paradis M: Ultrasonography as a diagnostic aid in pleural effusion of horses, *Vet Radiol* 22:211, 1981.
70. Boy MG, Sweeney CR: Pneumothorax in horses: 40 cases (1980-1997), *J Am Vet Med Assoc* 216:1955, 2000.
71. Perdrizet JA, Dill SG, Hackett RP: Diaphragmatic hernia as a cause of dyspnoea in a draft horse, *Equine Vet J* 21:302, 1989.
72. Verschooten F, Oyaert W, Muylle E et al: Diaphragmatic hernia in the horse: four case reports, *Vet Radiol Ultrasound* 18:45-50, 1977.
73. Everett KA, Chaffin MK, Brinsko SP: Diaphragmatic herniation as a cause of lethargy and exercise intolerance in a mare, *Cornell Vet* 82:217, 1992.
74. Hartzband L, Kerr D, Morris E: Ultrasonographic diagnosis of diaphragmatic rupture in a horse, *Vet Radiol Ultrasound* 31:42, 1990.
75. Berry CR, O'Brien TR, Madigan JE, et al: Thoracic radiographic features of silicosis in 19 horses, *J Vet Intern Med* 5:248, 1991.
76. Garber JL, Reef VB, Reimer JM: Sonographic findings in horses with mediastinal lymphosarcoma: 13 cases (1985-1992), *J Am Vet Med Assoc* 205:1432, 1994.
77. Mair TS, Lane JG, Lucke VM: Clinicopathological features of lymphosarcoma involving the thoracic cavity in the horse, *Equine Vet J* 17:428, 1985.
78. Carrig C, Groenendyk S, Seawright A: Dorsoventral flattening of the trachea in a horse and its attempted surgical correction: a case report, *J Am Vet Radiol Soc* 14:32, 1973.
79. Feige K, Schwarzwald C, Furst A et al: Esophageal obstruction in horses: a retrospective study of 34 cases, *Can Vet J* 41:207, 2000.
80. Clabough DL, Roberts MC, Robertson I: Probable congenital esophageal stenosis in a thoroughbred foal, *J Am Vet Med Assoc* 199:483, 1991.
81. Orsini JA, Sepesy L, Donawick WJ et al: Esophageal duplication cyst as a cause of choke in the horse, *J Am Vet Med Assoc* 193:474, 1988.
82. Murray MJ, Ball MM, Parker GA: Megaesophagus and aspiration pneumonia secondary to gastric ulceration in a foal, *J Am Vet Med Assoc* 192:381, 1988.
83. Baker SJ, Johnson PJ, David A et al: Idiopathic gastroesophageal reflux disease in an adult horse, *J Am Vet Med Assoc* 224:1967, 2004.
84. Green E: Esophageal obstruction. In Robinson N, editor: *Current therapy in equine medicine*, ed 3, Philadelphia, 1992, WB Saunders, pp 175-184.
85. King JN, Davies JV, Gerring EL: Contrast radiography of the equine oesophagus: effect of spasmolytic agents and passage of a nasogastric tube, *Equine Vet J* 22:133, 1990.
86. Greet TR: Observations on the potential role of oesophageal radiography in the horse, *Equine Vet J* 14:73, 1982.
87. Worth L, Reef V: Pericarditis in horses: 18 cases (1986-1995), *J Am Vet Med Assoc* 212:248, 1998.

ELECTRONIC RESOURCES evolve

Additional information related to the content in Chapter 35 can be found on the companion Web site at evolve http://evolve.elsevier.com/Thrall/vetrad/.

- Key Points
- Chapter Quiz
- Case Study 35-1
- Case Study 35-2

SECTION V

Canine and Feline Abdomen

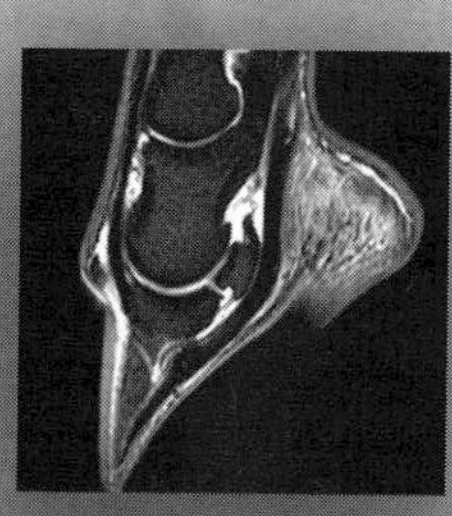
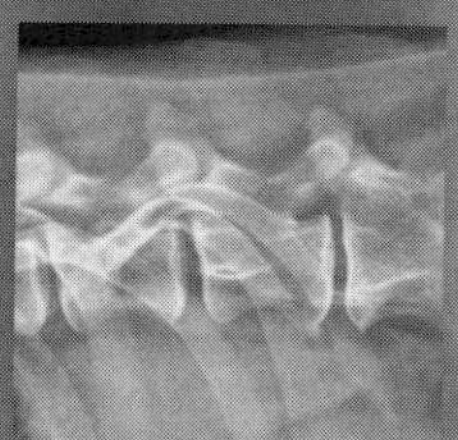
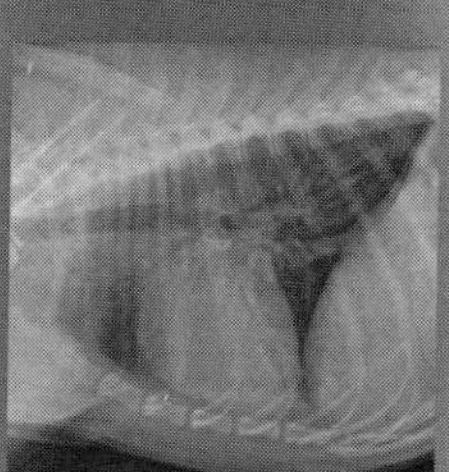
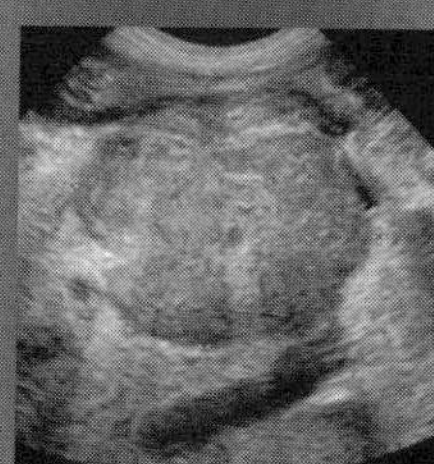
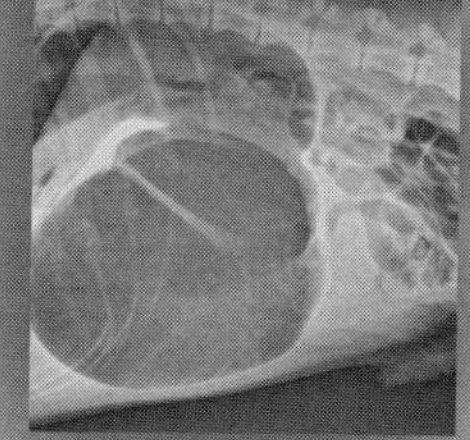

CHAPTER 36
Technical Issues and Interpretation Principles Relating to the Canine and Feline Abdomen

John P. Graham
Clifford R. Berry
Donald E. Thrall

This chapter provides a framework for beginning interpreters of abdominal radiographs. Basic information on how to produce a diagnostic abdominal radiograph, recommend views, and a structure for interpretation are presented. This chapter is not intended to be a standalone resource for abdominal image interpretation. Rather, it is an overview of some important principles to assist the reader in the evaluation of the more detailed chapters that focus on individual organs or abdominal regions.

Like the thorax, the abdomen contains multiple organ systems and is a complex, three-dimensional structure. Hence radiographic interpretation of the abdomen is challenging. The abdomen is not ideally suited to radiographic examination. Rather than having a natural radiographic contrast of air within the lungs, the abdomen depends on gas within the gastrointestinal tract and fat in the peritoneal and retroperitoneal space for radiographic contrast. Careful attention to technical detail is essential to get the best-quality abdominal radiographs.

TECHNICAL ASPECTS AND POSITIONING OF ABDOMINAL RADIOGRAPHY

The greatest technical problem in abdominal radiology is the relatively little contrast between intraabdominal organs and fat. To maximize the inherent contrast of the abdomen when using film-screen systems, a low kVp and high mAs technique should be used.[1] This includes a starting kVp of approximately 70 to 75 and an mAs setting of 6 to 8 for an average 13- to 15-cm dog abdomen. The best place to measure the abdomen is at its widest point, which typically is the cranial abdomen at the level of the liver. In very large dogs separate radiographs of the cranial and caudal aspects of the abdomen will need to be acquired, with specific measurements and radiographic technique for each section. If using primary digital acquisition, imaging the entire abdomen of a large dog may be possible with the same radiographic technique.

If the abdominal measurement exceeds 10 cm, a grid must be use to prevent scattered radiation from fogging the film and further degrading contrast in the image. Motion blurring can be avoided by making the exposure at end-expiration, when a brief pause usually occurs. Motion can also be diminished by selecting the highest milliamperage station allowable while maintaining the original mAs value. This will allow for the shortest exposure time setting.

The usual radiographic views of the abdomen include a right lateral and ventrodorsal radiograph (Fig. 36-1). A dorsoventral radiograph does not provide an adequate view of the entire abdomen; a dorsoventral view may be useful for evaluating a patient that cannot be positioned in dorsal recumbency but should never become routine for abdominal radiography. For the lateral view, the patient is positioned in right recumbency and the cranial margin of the radiograph should include the cranial most extent of the diaphragm. The caudal margin of the radiograph should include the coxofemoral joints. As noted above, in very large dogs this may require a cranial 14-inch × 17-inch radiograph and caudal 14-inch × 17-inch radiograph for both the lateral and ventrodorsal views (a total of four radiographs). The radiograph is exposed on end-expiration. If the patient is panting, blowing on the nose or cupping the nose with a hand may help momentarily suspend breathing and allow the exposure to be made without motion. The rotor should be running so that an exposure can be made when breathing stops.

Left lateral radiographs are helpful for repositioning gas within the stomach, small intestine, and large intestine (Fig. 36-2). Additional radiographic views that may be helpful in specific circumstances include a horizontal-beam radiograph, focal radiographs using a compression paddle to isolate a particular organ,[2] lateral radiographs in males made with the pelvic limbs pulled cranially for evaluation of the membranous and penile urethra, radiographs centered on the pelvis to evaluate the rectum, and radiographs obtained after the administration of a variety of contrast media. Details regarding special radiographic views that might be obtained with any abdominal special procedure are reviewed in other chapters.

A horizontal-beam ventrodorsal radiograph can be used to rule out free peritoneal air. This is described in detail in Chapter 38.

If a particular area of the abdomen cannot be assessed because of superimposed structures or a focal lesion (e.g., mass, mineralization, foreign body) is suspected, then the radiograph can be repeated with focal compression; such compression can be used in lateral or ventrodorsal views.[2] A nonradiopaque wooden cooking spoon or a plastic spoon can be used. The spoon is positioned on the area in question and gentle pressure is applied as the spoon is moved slightly cranially and caudally and then held stationery while making the exposure. The goal is to displace superimposed structures or move the area in question out from underneath these superimposed structures. The kVp is reduced by 15% because the thickness in that area is decreased as a result of the compression. This technique will not be successful in dogs or cats that have a tense abdomen, severe ascites, or a painful abdomen. This is a technique that can be used on the ventrodorsal radiograph to better evaluate the renal region.

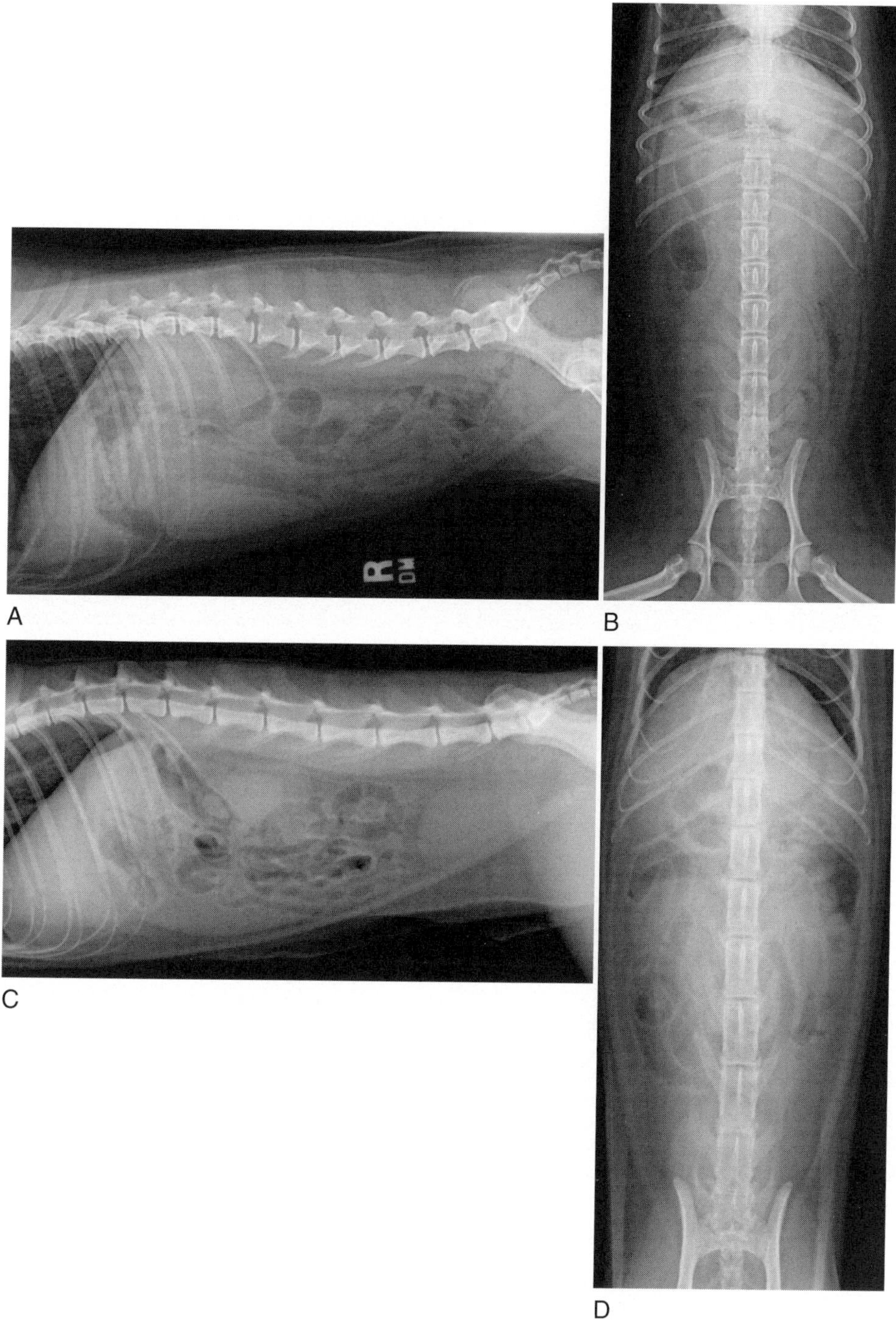

Fig. 36-1 Right lateral (A) and ventrodorsal (B) radiographs of the abdomen of a normal adult dog. Note the normal size and shape of the canine cecum. A gas-filled cecum will not be seen on feline abdominal radiographs. Right lateral (C) and ventrodorsal (D) abdominal radiographs of a normal cat.

The entire length of the penile urethra (from the prostatic urethra through the membranous urethra and the penile urethra) should be evaluated in male dogs that have a history of pollakiuria or stranguria. The dog is placed in right lateral recumbency and the pelvic limbs are pulled cranially so that they are not superimposed over the caudal aspect of the os penis on the lateral radiograph.

Because of the large number of organs and vascular and other structures in the abdomen, interpretation is better suited to a systematic structure-by-structure or organ-by-organ approach. By working through a checklist, the temptation to focus on an obvious lesion or the organ suspected to be abnormal based on clinical and historic data can be avoided.

A checklist for abdominal radiographic interpretation is provided on the Evolve Web site at http://evolve.elsevier.com/Thrall/vetrad/. Readers are encouraged to download this PDF file checklist, print it, and post it next to the viewing station so that radiographs can be reviewed in a systematic fashion.

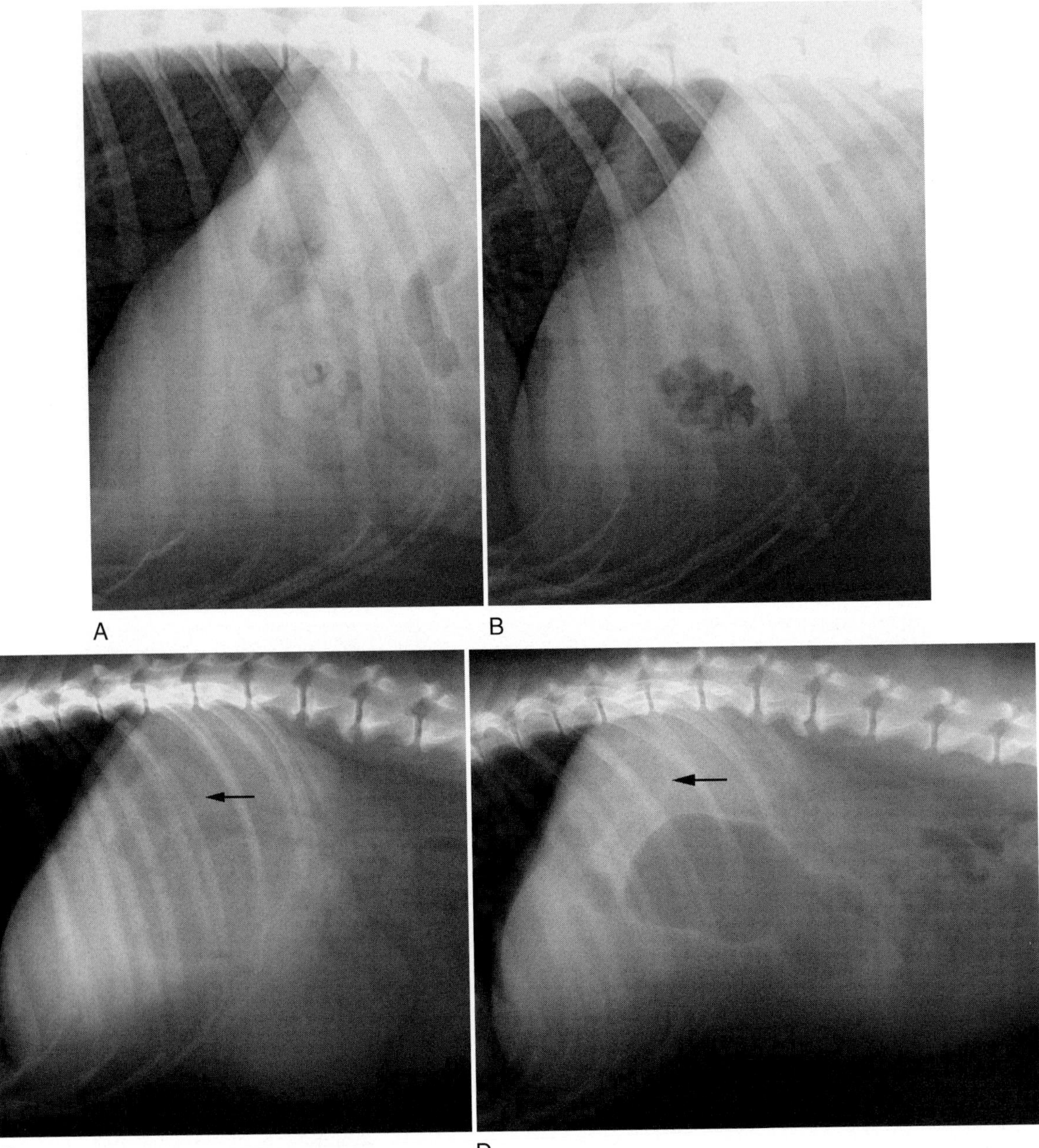

Fig. 36-2 Right lateral (A) and left lateral (B) radiographs of the cranial abdomen from a normal adult dog. Gas redistributes from the fundic portion of the stomach on the right lateral radiograph to the pylorus on the left lateral. Right lateral (C) and left lateral (D) radiographs from a dog with an obstruction of the cranial aspect of the duodenum (ball foreign body). On the right lateral view the ball (arrow) is harder to see, but on the left lateral view, when gas redistributes to the pylorus and proximal duodenum, the ball (arrow) is more clearly seen.

The basis for the interpretation paradigm is to divide the abdomen into four different compartments and evaluate each of these compartments, noting the roentgen abnormalities associated with each compartment. Remember that all interpretations are summaries, and as such the interpreter should always consider the possibility of missed lesions or inaccurate interpretations when bringing together all the findings as a specific disease process. Each roentgen abnormality can be thought of in terms of a window (past events), mirror (current problems), or a picture (predictor of future events) (see Chapter 5). For each of the four basic areas, a series of questions should be considered, and based on the answers to these questions appropriate differential lists can be formulated. The abdomen should be divided into the following four areas: (1) the extraabdominal structures—pelvis and pelvic limbs, lumbar and caudal thoracic vertebrae, ribs, diaphragm, caudal thorax, abdominal musculature and wall, and the soft tissues dorsal to the thoracic and lumbar spine; (2) the peritoneal and retroperitoneal space—predominantly a first-time overview of these areas, with emphasis on the serosal margin detail present within these spaces; (3) the gastrointestinal system, including the stomach, small intestine, large intestine, liver, spleen,

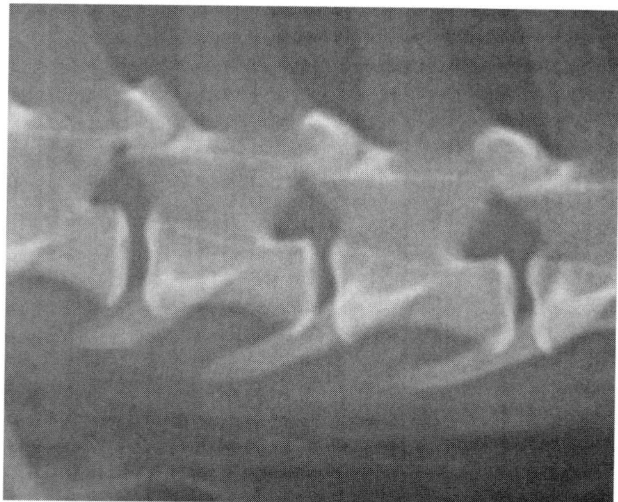

Fig. 36-3 Close-up of Figure 36-1, A. Note the transverse processes are superimposed at their origin from the vertebral bodies, thereby forming a single Nike brand "Swoosh." This can be used to determine whether the lateral radiograph is correctly positioned.

pancreas, and mid-abdomen; and (4) the urogenital system, including the region of the adrenal glands, medial iliac lymph nodes, kidneys, ureters, urinary bladder, and urethra as well as the reproductive tract. An overview of these four areas is presented in this chapter. As each area is presented, the first determination should be whether that specific area or structure is normal. By the end of the chapter, the reader should have a feel for what "normal" looks like. A picture of normal is easier to define for the abdomen than for the thorax because the abdomen presents a more constant picture, particularly in cats. Whenever considering the term *normal,* however, remember that every organ or structure has specific normal findings regarding the size, shape, position, margin (contours), location, number, and opacity. So the term *normal* is not as simple as it seems on first glance. Additionally, because overlap occurs between the four compartments of the abdomen, the interpreter will have a number of opportunities to evaluate a given organ, structure, or region. Follow-up questions to consider of a given area are presented to ensure that review of that particular area, organ, or structure has been completed. These follow-up questions also help identify the common radiographic abnormalities that may be associated with a given organ, structure, or area so that common disease entities are ruled in or out.

INTERPRETATION PARADIGM

Abdominal Wall and Extraabdominal Soft Tissue and Bone Structures

Before assessing extraabdominal structures, the radiographs should be assessed for appropriate technique and positioning. On the lateral radiograph, the transverse processes form a Nike-brand "Swoosh" sign at their junction with the vertebral body if the patient is straight (Fig. 36-3).[3] In addition, the overall body condition and age of the patient should be assessed. If the patient is cachectic, the abdomen should have a "tucked up" (concave ventral margin) appearance and poor serosal margin detail from the lack of peritoneal and retroperitoneal fat. If the dog or cat is less than 6 months of age, the intraabdominal detail is poor because of the presence of small amounts of peritoneal effusion, enlarged mesenteric lymph nodes, and the presence of immature fat that seems to have a different physical density than the final fat seen in adult dogs and cats. If the dog or cat is fat or in moderate body condition, then normal peritoneal and retroperitoneal detail with a rounded (convex) ventral body wall margin should be seen. If the patient is markedly obese, then a large amount of retroperitoneal fat and fat within the falciform ligament ventral to the liver should be seen. In cats that are fat, the small intestines tend to bunch in a right central abdominal position; this should not be mistaken for a mass or plication (Fig. 36-4).

The Abdominal Wall

Is the abdominal wall normal and visible along the entire length (ventral abdomen on the lateral radiograph and right and left sides on the ventrodorsal radiograph)?
Are any focal swellings or masses present?
Are any abnormal opacities present?
Is evidence of a body wall or diaphragmatic rupture present?
Are bone structures normal in radiographic appearance, including the ribs, vertebrae, pelvis, and pelvic limbs? In addition, appropriate positioning of the lateral radiograph should be verified.
Is the ventral abdominal wall pendulous or rounded? If yes, then ascites, obesity, hepatomegaly, and Cushing's disease should be considered. (These reasons will become more apparent as all the questions are answered regarding the other three areas of the abdominal interpretation paradigm.)

In a normal cat or dog the caudal surface of the diaphragm blends with the liver. In animals in good body condition, the inner margin of the abdominal wall is outlined by fat (see Fig. 36-1). Swellings or masses are usually evident clinically and should prompt the observer to evaluate the underlying body wall for evidence of disruption.

Diagnosing a diaphragmatic rupture is facilitated by detecting abdominal viscera in the thorax. Displaced organs may be obscured by pleural fluid, making the diagnosis of a hernia difficult. Secondary radiographic changes that suggest a ruptured diaphragm include absence of the normal falciform fat, absence of or cranial displacement of the liver and other viscera, and other signs of trauma, such as rib fractures.

Evaluation of the lumbar spine should include the ventral surfaces of the lumbar vertebrae. Ventral spondylosis deformans is commonly seen in older dogs and cats. The ventral cortex of the L3 and L4 vertebral bodies is normally thinner than the adjacent lumbar vertebrae because this is the site of the diaphragmatic attachment. Also, neoplasia (particularly prostatic, urinary bladder, or urethral carcinomas) may metastasize to the ventral aspects of the lumbar spine at L5-L7, with occasional involvement of the ventral aspect of the sacrum.[4,5] Other bone changes to evaluate for include degenerative changes of the intervertebral disc spaces; radiographic features of discospondylitis; osteolytic or osteoproliferative lesions of the vertebral bodies, ribs, pelvis, or pelvic limbs; and congenital abnormalities of the vertebral column.

The Peritoneum and Retroperitoneal Space

What is the patient's age and body condition?
Is the dog or cat thin, young, obese, or emaciated?
Are the retroperitoneal space and retroperitoneal detail and contrast normal?
Are the peritoneal space and peritoneal detail and contrast normal?

The conclusions drawn from the answers to these last two questions depend on the answer to the first question: the patient's age and body condition.

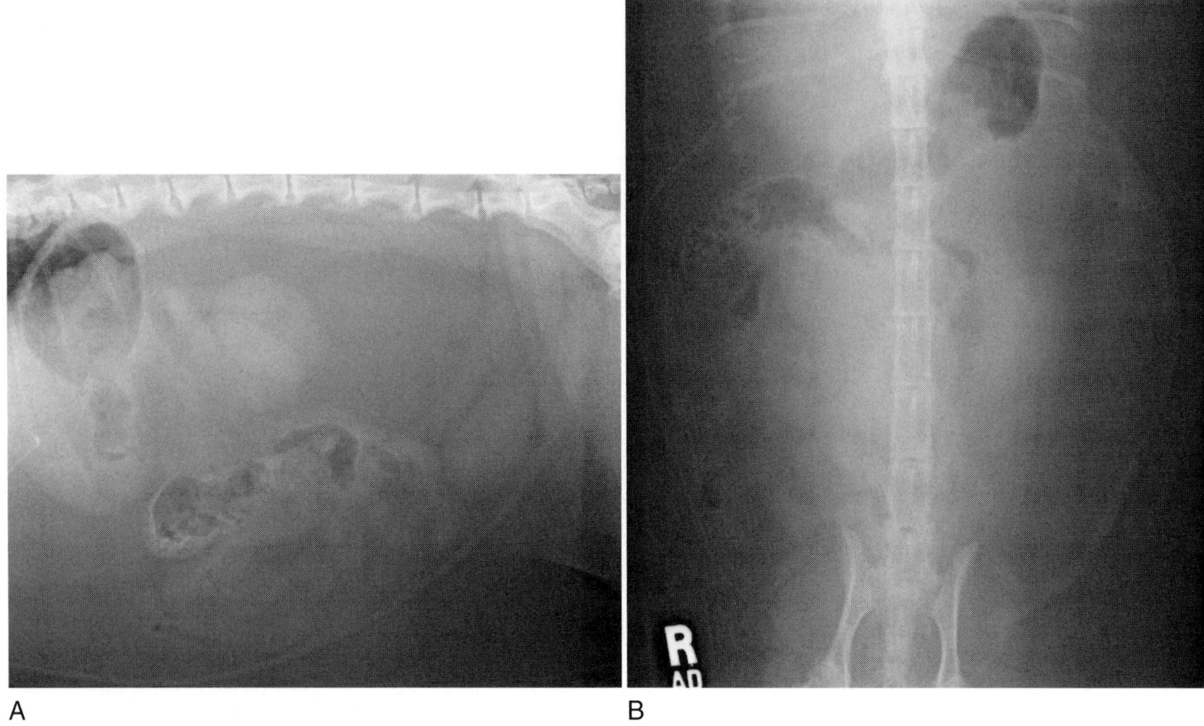

Fig. 36-4 Right lateral (A) and ventrodorsal (B) abdominal radiographs from an obese cat. A large amount of fat is within the falciform ligament, ventral to the liver, and the retroperitoneal space on the lateral radiograph. On the ventrodorsal radiograph, the spleen is seen along the left cranial abdominal wall, and the small and large intestines are displaced toward the right. In obese cats the small intestine is often displaced toward the right and may have a bunched appearance.

If the retroperitoneum is abnormal, is abnormal accumulation of fluid, gas, or mineral present?
If the peritoneum is abnormal, is abnormal accumulation fluid, gas, or mineral present?

Detail and contrast within the peritoneal and retroperitoneal spaces are essential for evaluating abdominal organs. The quality of contrast is determined by how much fat and the type of fat present. This is assessed by looking for subcutaneous fat, retroperitoneal fat, and fat within the falciform ligament ventral to the liver. In normal body condition, the complete outline of the left kidney and the caudal pole of the right kidney are visible in the adult dog. In healthy adult cats both kidneys should be clearly visible. The serosal edges of the abdominal organs and the inner margin of the muscle of the abdominal wall should be clearly visible in an animal in normal body condition. In animals with no body fat, neither peritoneal nor retroperitoneal organs can be discerned. This is normal in immature patients and is also seen in dogs or cats with cachexia as a result of severe, chronic illness. In patients in which detail is absent because of cachexia, the abdomen will have a tucked appearance.

Retroperitoneal fluid obliterates the outline of the kidneys (Fig. 36-5).[5] The degree to which the kidneys are obscured depends on the relative quantity of fluid versus fat. If a moderate or large volume of fluid is present, the retroperitoneal space is expanded, causing ventral displacement of the gastrointestinal tract. Retroperitoneal gas enhances detail in the dorsal abdomen, and structures such as the abdominal aorta and right kidney become clearly visible. Pneumoretroperitoneum is usually the result of extension of pneumomedi-

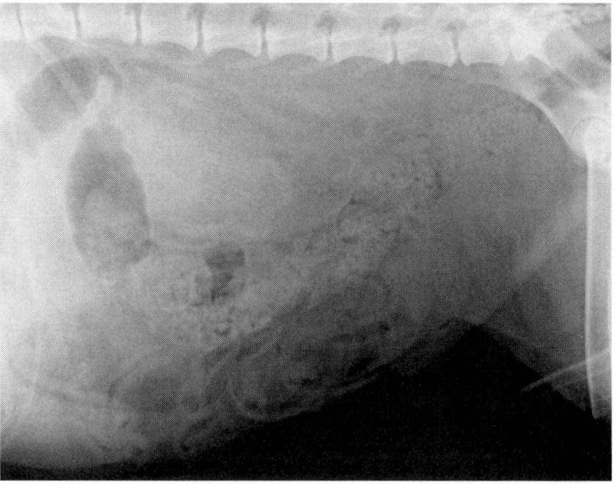

Fig. 36-5 Right lateral abdominal radiograph from a dog that had been hit by a car. The renal margins are indistinct, consistent with retroperitoneal effusion. Note the difference in clarity of visualization of organ edges in the retroperitoneal versus intraperitoneal spaces. This comparison is helpful in localizing fluid to one or both of these spaces. The effusion in this dog could be caused by hemorrhage, renal trauma with extravasation of urine, or both. An excretory urogram will help determine the vascular and ureteral integrity of the proximal urinary system. A positive contrast urethrogram would be needed to determine the integrity of the lower urinary tract (urinary bladder and urethra).

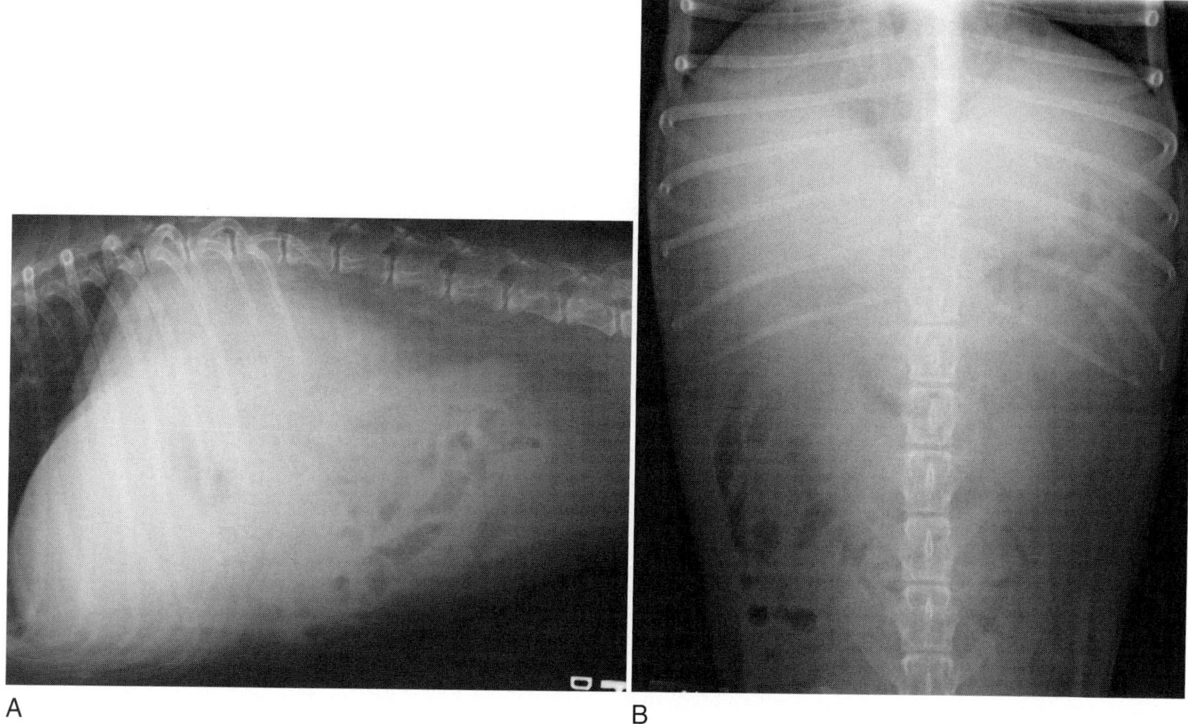

Fig. 36-6 Right lateral (A) and ventrodorsal (B) abdominal radiographs from a dog with severe pancreatitis. A focal mass effect is present in the region of the pancreas just caudal to the stomach. A decrease in the peritoneal detail is noted in the cranial abdomen. An enlarged pancreas, hyper-attenuating fat, and focal effusion were seen on abdominal ultrasound.

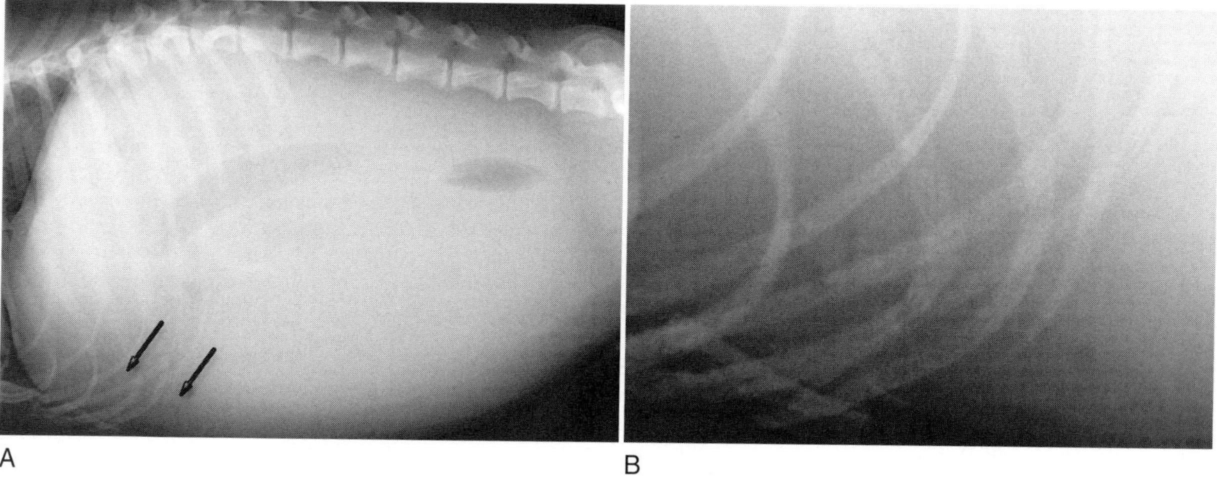

Fig. 36-7 Right lateral abdominal radiograph from a dog with generalized abdominal effusion caused by chronic hepatic cirrhosis. The small intestine is floating in the large amount of peritoneal fluid. Several small intestinal loops are abnormally gas dilated. In addition, multiple small areas of free air are noted in the cranioventral abdomen *(arrows)*. (**B**) A close-up view of the region indicated by *arrows* in **A.** This free gas was caused by perforation from a small intestinal tumor.

astinum as gas collects in the retroperitoneal space from the esophageal or aortic hiatus.

Peritoneal fluid results in a reduction in serosal margin detail and contrast. This may be confined to a specific part of the abdomen, as in pancreatitis, or the fluid may be generalized as in ascites. The degree of loss of detail depends on the relative quantities of fluid versus fat. A small quantity of fluid in a normal or obese animal produces a mottled, wispy, or streaky appearance and blurred serosal edges (Fig. 36-6). A large volume of fluid produces a more generalized increase in opacity with no serosal detail and usually a few gas-filled loops of intestine floating in the mid-abdomen (Fig. 36-7). This may be distinguished from cachexia by the shape of the abdomen and evaluation of retroperitoneal detail.

Peritoneal gas is a serious finding unless due to recent abdominal surgery. Large or moderate volumes of gas enhance

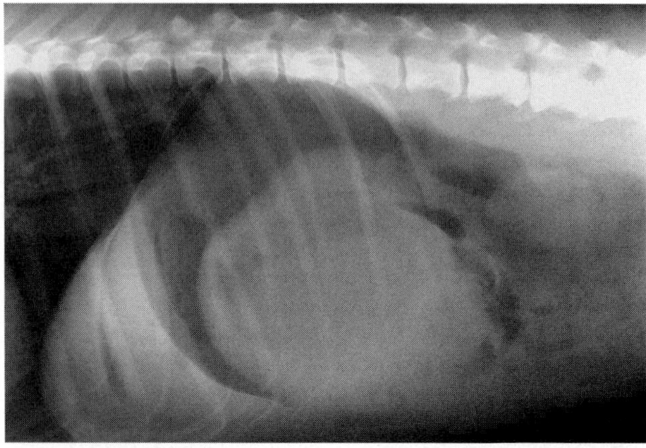

A

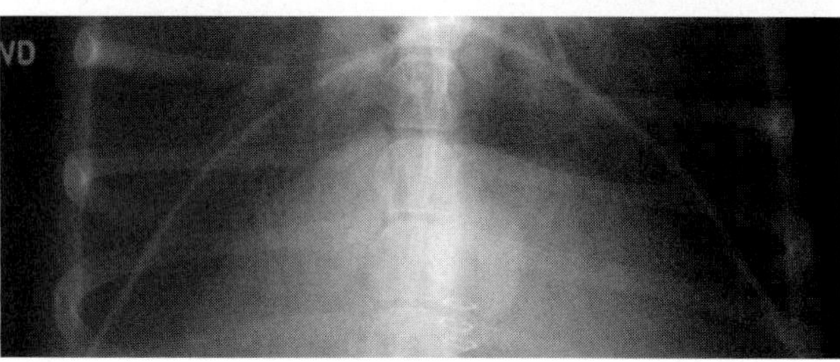

B

Fig. 36-8 Right lateral (A) abdominal radiograph from a dog with a gastrointestinal rupture and subsequent pneumoperitoneum. Air is noted caudal to the diaphragm and cranial to the liver margins. Peritoneal air is also present surrounding gastrointestinal structures. Follow-up close-up ventrodorsal radiograph of the same dog after surgery (B). Air is seen between the diaphragm and the cranial aspect of the liver. Several metallic staples are noted over the vertebral column.

the normal serosal detail and increase contrast (Fig. 36-8). Structures not normally seen, such as the caudal surface of the diaphragm and the caudate lobe of the liver, may be visible. Smaller bubbles are more difficult to detect but can be distinguished by a number of features. These bubbles may be seen at the periphery of the abdomen, away from the intestine. They may have distinct round shapes, especially if peritoneal fluid is present, or appear triangular as they outline the serosal edges of adjacent intestinal loops. Free peritoneal air may be confirmed by horizontal-beam radiography as previously described (see Chapter 38).

Peritoneal and retroperitoneal space mineralization is uncommon. A small, ovoid, mineralized intraperitoneal structure with an outer thicker wall occasionally will be seen as an incidental finding in older cats. This is a result of dystrophic mineralization of a cholesterol inclusion cyst. Additionally, in older cats the adrenal glands can become mineralized. Other retroperitoneal mineralization found in dogs and cats includes vascular mineralization that most often involves the abdominal aorta and arterial tree (Fig. 36-9). Another cause of focal retroperitoneal mineralizations are radiopaque ureteral calculi.

The Gastrointestinal Tract, Including the Liver, Spleen, Pancreas, and Mid-abdomen

The Stomach

Is the stomach normal for size, shape, margin, location, and opacity?

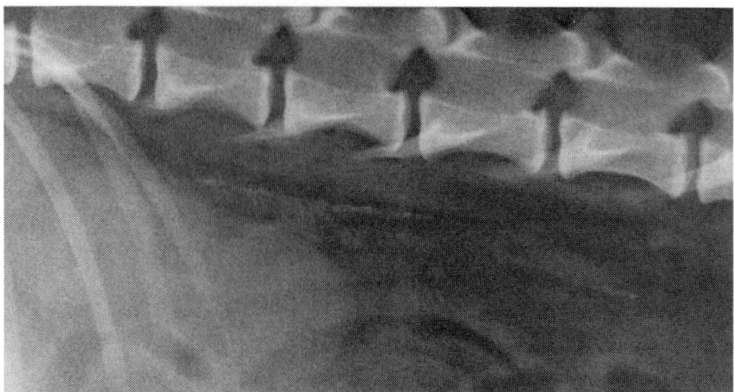

Fig. 36-9 Right lateral abdominal radiograph of a dog with chronic renal failure and metastatic mineralization of the abdominal aorta.

Is evidence of pyloric outflow obstruction present?
Is evidence of gastric dilation with or without volvulus present?
Is evidence of a gastric foreign body present?
Is evidence of a gastric wall mass present?
Is an abnormal accumulation of radiopaque or mineral material (gravel sign) present in the pyloric region of the stomach?

The normal canine stomach lies transversely across the abdomen with the fundus left and dorsal, the body noted just to the left of midline on the ventrodorsal radiograph and in a mid-abdominal position on the lateral radiograph.[6-16] The pyloric antrum is located to the right of midline and the pylorus on the right lateral radiograph, midway between dorsal and ventral (Fig. 36-10). In neonates and young patients, the stomach has a different anatomic location. On the ventrodorsal radiograph, the stomach resembles the letter J, with the body and fundus on the left and pyloric antrum and pylorus just to the right or on midline. In cats the stomach has a similar J shape and the pyloric antrum can have a midline position. Also in cats a radiolucent submucosal layer (fat) can be seen contrasting with the mucosal and muscularis layers in some adults, particularly on the ventrodorsal radiograph (Fig. 36-11). Obtaining ventrodorsal and left and right lateral radiographs and occasionally a dorsoventral radiograph is recommended in dogs or cats suspected to have gastric wall disease, especially masses. These four different radiographic projections allow for repositioning of gas and fluid within the lumen as well as evaluation of a larger majority of the inner mucosal margin than simply two orthogonal radiographs of the abdomen. However, stomach and intestinal wall thickness cannot be reliably assessed on survey radiographs; this is best done by using a contrast procedure or ultrasound. However, on the rare occasion of a dog or cat with a large gastric wall mass, the gas outlining the mass can document the true mucosal margin. This should be confirmed on multiple radiographs before making a specific diagnosis of a gastric wall mass (Fig. 36-12).

Chronic partial obstruction of the gastric outflow caused by hyperplasia of the mucosa and muscularis of the pylorus is a disease of small-breed dogs. The lesion causes progressively slower gastric emptying and results in gastric dilation. A severely dilated stomach may extend beyond the umbilicus (Fig. 36-13). The stomach is usually filled with fluid and a smaller quantity of gas. An accumulation of small mineral fragments (the gravel sign) may be seen in the pyloric antrum in patients with outflow obstruction caused by sedimentation of

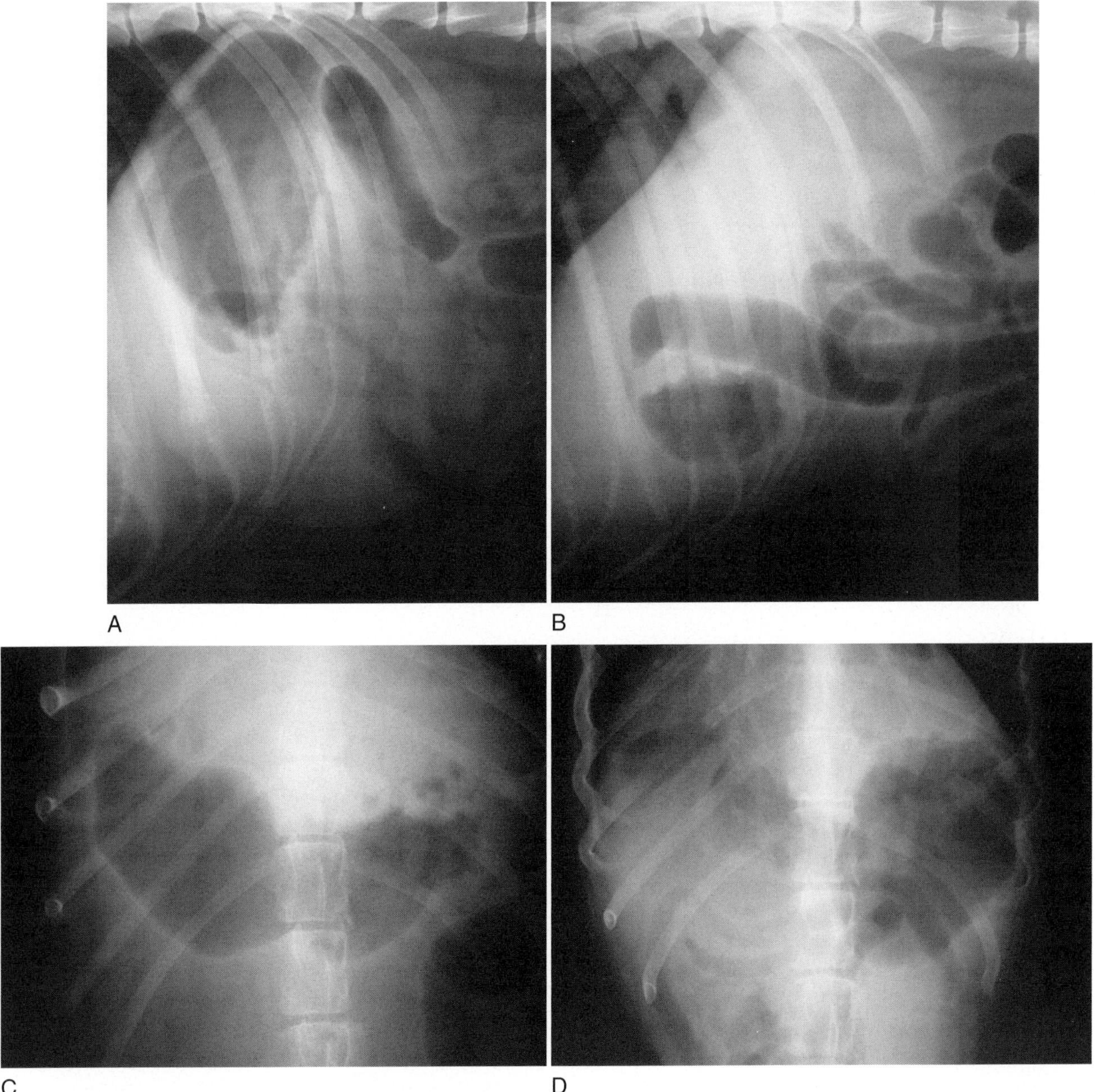

Fig. 36-10 Right lateral (A), left lateral (B), ventrodorsal (C), and dorsoventral (D) abdominal radiographs of a normal dog. Note the change in gas position in the stomach depending on the recumbent portion of the dog. Importantly, on the right lateral radiograph gas is located in the fundus and body of the stomach, whereas on the left lateral radiograph air is located in the pyloric antrum and pylorus.

heavier, indigestible food particles. The diagnosis may be confirmed by ultrasound examination.

Gastric dilation and volvulus is a life-threatening condition of large- and giant-breed dogs. A single right lateral recumbent radiograph may be sufficient to establish a diagnosis (Fig. 36-14). Alternatively, if the animal will not tolerate lateral recumbency, a dorsoventral radiograph should be made. The parts of the stomach must be identified, and whether they contain fluid or gas determines if they lie left or right of midline. If the stomach is in its normal position, a gas-filled fundus and body will be present in their normal positions. If the stomach has undergone a half turn (180 degrees) volvulus, the pylorus will be gas filled and located in the dorsal abdomen on the right or left lateral radiograph, indicating it is left of midline and in a dorsal location within the abdomen. If additional radiographs are required a dorsoventral and/or a left lateral recumbent radiograph may be helpful. Parts of the stomach are often easier to recognize if radiographs are obtained after initial decompression. If gastric wall necrosis has occurred, pneumoperitoneum, or gas within the portal venous system, can be seen.

The possibility of a gastric foreign body should be considered in animals with unresponsive vomiting and no radiographic evidence of small intestinal obstruction. If a foreign body is suspected, the radiographic examination consists of a four-view examination of the stomach (see Fig. 36-2). A

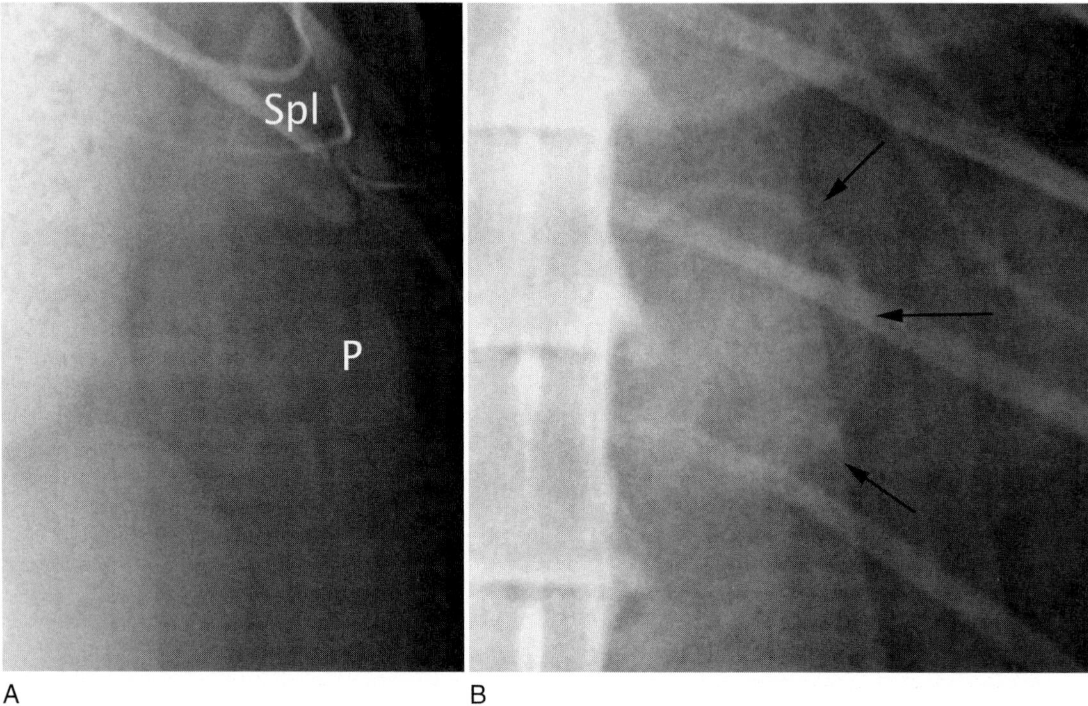

Fig. 36-11 Close-up ventrodorsal radiographs from two separate cats. In **A,** there is a soft tissue linear structure noted between the stomach and the spleen *(Spl)*. This is the left limb of the pancreas *(P)*. In **B** the stomach *(arrows)* is contracted and differential opacities are present within the gastric wall. This is as result of fat deposition within the gastric wall in normal cats. This is not normally seen in dogs.

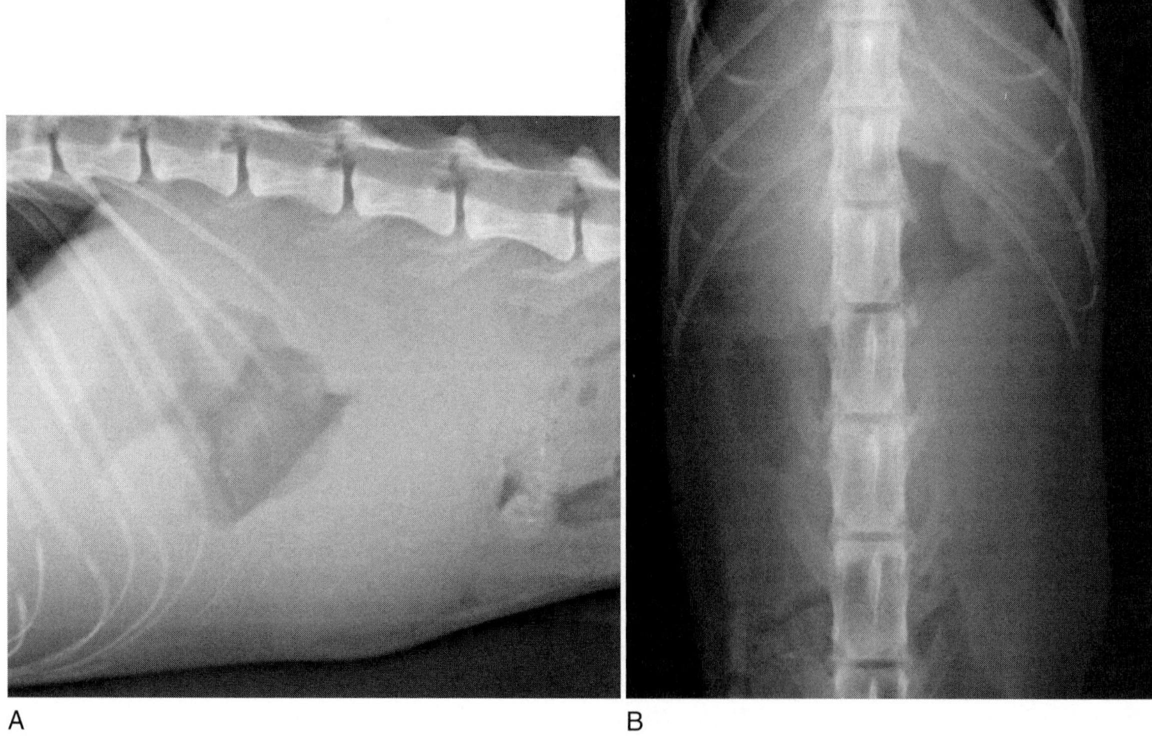

Fig. 36-12 Right lateral (**A**) and ventrodorsal (**B**) radiographs from a cat that was vomiting. The gastric wall is severely thickened on both the lateral and ventrodorsal radiographs. Intraluminal gas is present and outlines the true mucosal border. Serosal margin detail is decreased.

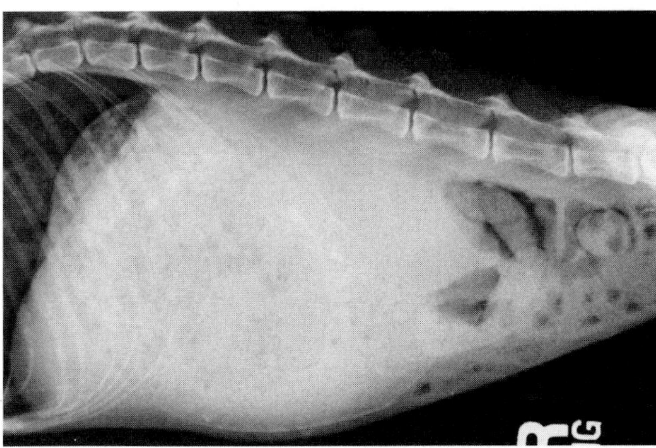

Fig. 36-13 Right lateral radiograph from a cat with chronic renal failure, gastric mucosal mineralization, and chronic pyloric outflow tract obstruction. The stomach is distended with a large amount of food material.

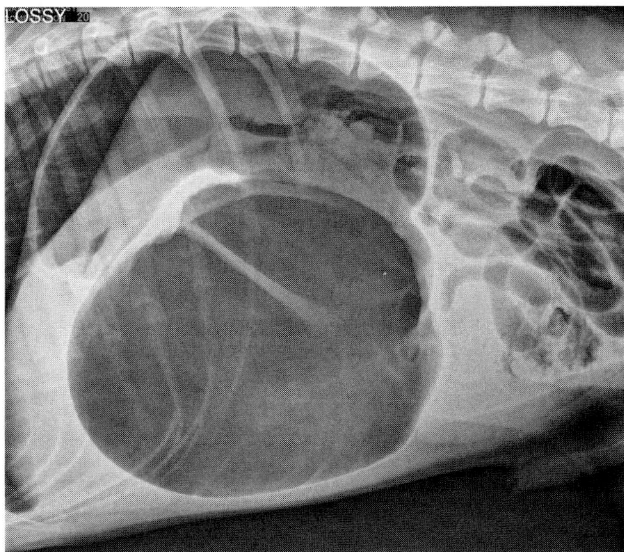

Fig. 36-14 Right lateral cranial abdominal radiograph from a dog with gastric dilation/volvulus. The stomach is severely gas distended and malpositioned. The pylorus is dorsally displaced on the lateral radiograph. Partial compartmentalization is also noted.

fluid-filled pylorus on the right lateral view should not be mistaken for a ball foreign body or mass because the pylorus will often have an almost perfectly round shape and uniform soft tissue opacity (Fig. 36-15). This is an easy trap for the novice radiologist but is easily avoided by making a left lateral radiograph, which will then show the pylorus filled with gas.

If a mass is suspected, the animal should be fasted for at least 12, and preferably 24, hours before radiography if possible. Radiographs are insensitive for the detection of gastric masses because most are located along the lesser curvature or are border effaced with the rest of the gastric soft tissue wall or contents. The presence of ingesta and fluid within the stomach may mimic wall thickening or obscure a mass. Suspected gastric tumors are best imaged by ultrasound, which allows for the assessment of the liver and regional lymph nodes for metastasis.

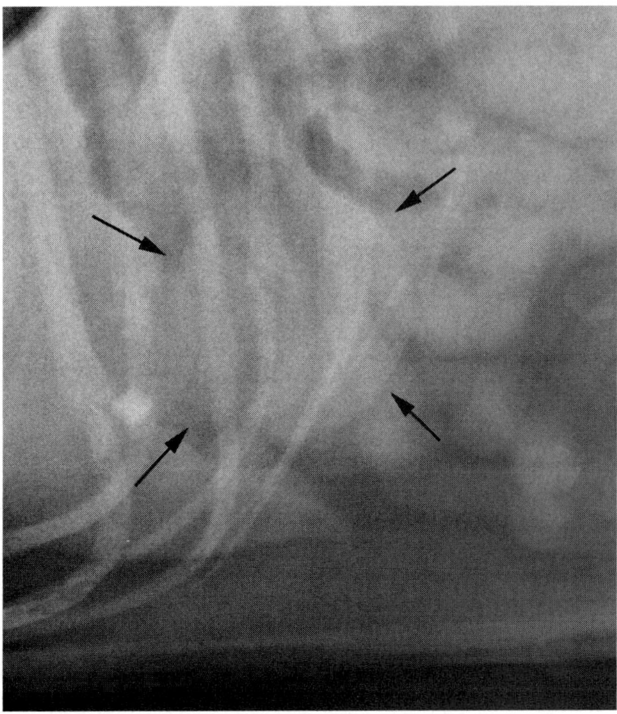

Fig. 36-15 Close-up right lateral radiograph. Fluid has gravitated to the pyloric antrum, creating a round opacity *(arrows)* that is often misinterpreted as a gastric foreign body.

Small Intestine

Is the small intestine normal for size, shape, position, number, contour, and opacity?

Is abnormal intestinal dilation present, with gas, fluid, or foreign material?

Is evidence of a linear foreign body present?

Is evidence of a gravel sign located in the mid-abdomen?

The normal small intestine fills the mid-abdomen and forms multiple smoothly margined, flowing loops. The normal feline small intestine contains little or no gas and should measure no more than 12 mm in diameter from serosal surface to serosal surface. In obese cats, the small intestine can be asymmetrically positioned in the right mid-abdomen in a ventrodorsal radiograph (see Fig. 36-4). This should not be mistaken for small intestinal plication, as seen with linear foreign bodies. Normal canine intestine contains a variable quantity of gas but should not be uniformly gas filled throughout the duodenum or jejunum. One rule of thumb is that the serosa-to-serosa width of a small intestinal segment in the dog should not exceed 1.6 times the height of the center of the fifth lumbar vertebral body.[11] The most common cause for an increased volume of intestinal gas is aerophagia either from dyspnea or stress, but this typically does not cause abnormal intestinal dilation. When evaluating abdominal radiographs, fluid-filled dilated loops should not be overlooked because they are much less conspicuous than gas-dilated segments.[12,16] After determining that the small intestine is abnormally dilated, the severity of the dilation and how much of the intestine is affected should be decided. Small intestinal obstruction will cause abnormal dilation of the small intestine proximal to the lesion. This is usually characterized by moderate to severe dilation of two to three loops proximal to the lesion (Fig. 36-16). If the obstruction is chronic and distal, the abnormally dilated small intestine may be extensive and involve most of the small intestine. If the obstruction is partial, then

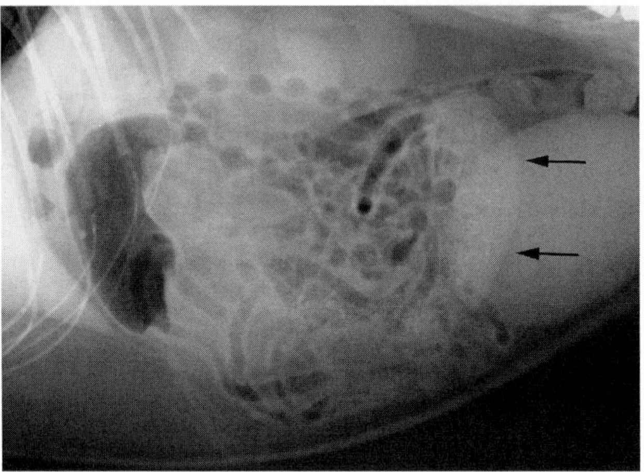

Fig. 36-16 A right lateral radiograph from a cat with long-term weight loss. A small intestinal segment is severely dilated and contains irregular radiopaque debris, sometimes called the gravel sign *(arrows)*. Fecal material is noted in the colon. The position of the dilated loop indicates it cannot be colon, even though its contents appear similar to feces. These changes are typical of a chronic partial obstruction, which is usually caused by a constricting annular lesion such as an ileal adenocarcinoma.

accumulation of larger radiopaque material (gravel sign) may be present just proximal to the site of obstruction (see Fig. 36-16). Recent or partial obstructions may have only limited dilation of one or several small intestinal loops.

A single dilated small intestinal loop is called a sentinel loop because it should alert the interpreter to the possibility of obstruction, which should be ruled out in these patients. The sentinel loop sign does not equal a mechanical obstruction, however, because it can also be caused by regional or generalized paralytic ileus.[12,16]

Obstruction of the duodenum may be difficult to confirm because accumulated secretions and gas proximal to the lesion are usually vomited, which prevents the development of gastric or duodenal dilation. Fabric foreign bodies may act as wicks, allowing the passage of intestinal fluid and minimizing the degree of dilation that may develop. In older animals chronic partial obstructions are often the result of intestinal tumors.

Neonates and very young patients can be a diagnostic challenge because they have little or no body fat. This lack of fat hampers the identification of any abnormally dilated fluid-filled stomach or small intestine. the presence of a normal gas shadow of the cecum in dogs and the colon in dogs and cats should be evaluated. Absence of these gas shadows may be a clue to the presence of an ileocolic or cecocolic intussusception. If the exact position of the colon is not known, a pneumocolon is a quick, inexpensive, and relatively noninvasive procedure that can be performed (Fig. 36-17).[17]

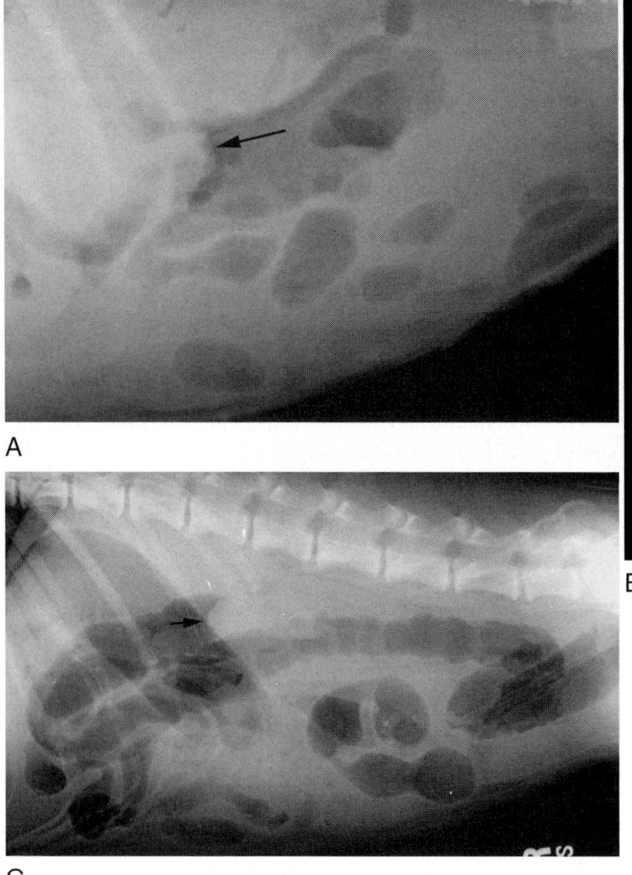

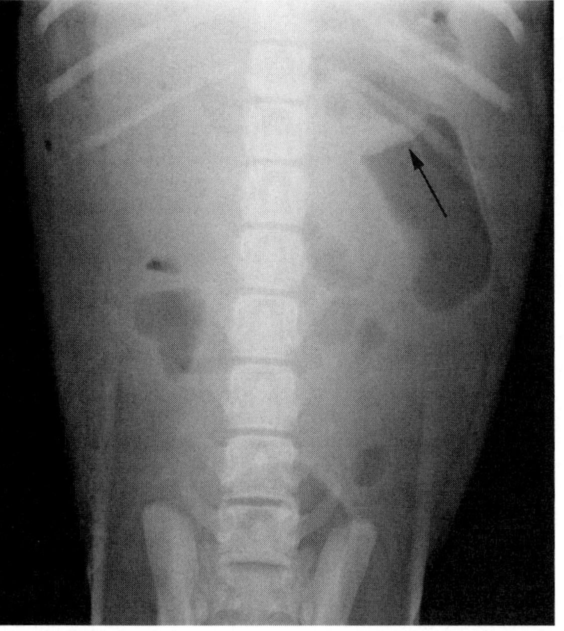

Fig. 36-17 Right lateral (A) and ventrodorsal (B) radiographs from a dog with an ileocolic intussusception. Gas is noted against the intussusceptum *(arrow)* within the colon. A right lateral (C) radiograph from another young dog with an intussusception. In this later dog, a pneumocolon was performed to provide contrast allowing the intussusceptum to be identified *(arrow)*.

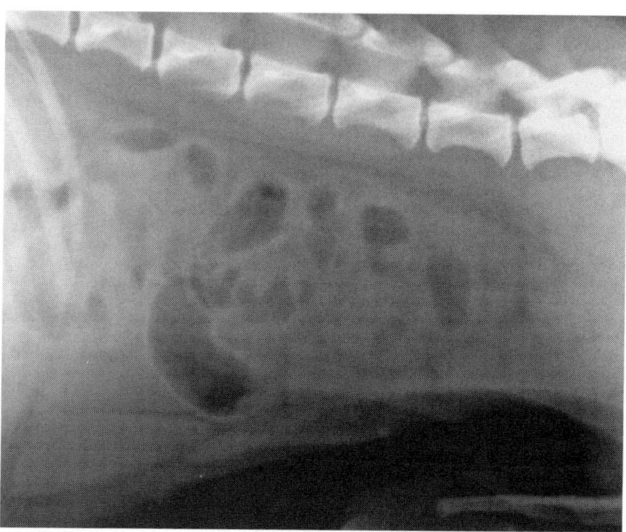

Fig. 36-18 Right lateral abdominal radiograph from an adult dog that has swallowed a linear foreign body. Abnormal plication of the small intestine is present along with abnormal, curved areas of small intestinal gas dilation.

Intestinal dilation may also be caused by a generalized paralytic ileus. Paralytic ileus commonly results in mild to moderate generalized gas or fluid distention of the small intestinal tract. Enteritis from acute inflammatory bowel disorders may also cause generalized bowel dilation. Severe enteritis, such as canine parvovirus infection or hemorrhagic gastroenteritis, may cause moderate to severe segmental or complete dilation of the intestinal tract and may be misdiagnosed as an obstructive small intestinal pattern. Most patients with gastroenteritis are radiographically normal or may have mild generalized gas dilation. Mild gas dilation is a nonspecific finding and should not be equated with a radiographic diagnosis of gastroenteritis.

Linear foreign bodies can be difficult to diagnose. If a linear foreign body becomes fixed at the base of the tongue, in the pylorus, or in the proximal duodenum, the intestine will become plicated as peristalsis tries to pull the object through. The small intestine may have a bunched appearance and look tightly stacked. The tight bunching of the small intestine produces abnormal gas bubbles that appear triangular or comma shaped, unlike the normal elongate ovoid gas bubbles routinely seen (Fig. 36-18). These abnormal gas bubble shapes are also located eccentrically, that is, toward the edge of the small intestinal loop rather than in the center. Linear foreign bodies are a challenging diagnosis and can quickly become life threatening. If a linear foreign body is suspected, an abdominal ultrasound or a positive-contrast upper gastrointestinal examination with water soluble contrast medium should be performed.

Large Intestine and Cecum

Is the cecum or large intestine normal for size, shape, position, contour, and opacity?

Is the cecum or large intestine abnormally dilated with gas, fluid, or foreign material?

Is the gas-filled cecal shadow in its expected location?

Is the colon or rectum abnormally displaced by other masses?

Is a pneumocolon needed to identify the exact location of the colon?

The cecum and colon are relatively fixed in their expected locations; however, they can contain variable amounts of gas and fecal material. The cecum is located to the right of midline at the level of L2 and L3 on the ventrodorsal radiograph, and in dogs has a characteristic gas distended letter C, spiral, or comma shape. The cecum is typically located just dorsal to a mid-abdominal position on the lateral radiographs (see Fig. 36-1). A gas-filled cecum is not found in the cat abdomen. The ileum connects with the colon at the ileocolic junction, which is located cranial and medial to the cecum on the ventrodorsal radiograph. The ascending colon extends cranially, curves to the left at the right colic flexure, extends across the abdomen as the transverse colon, and curves caudally at the left colic flexure. The colon continues as the descending colon, which is the longest segment of the colon. The descending colon empties into the rectum at the level of the pelvic inlet.

In dogs or cats with diarrhea, the colon may be fluid filled. In a young animal the exact position may not be known on survey radiographs. As previously stated, a pneumocolon is an easy technique to determine the exact position of the colon.[17] The colon is one of the abdominal structures that is easily displaced by abdominal masses, and if the only radiographic abnormality is a change in expected position, then the interpreter should look for a mass displacing the colon.

*The Liver**

Is the liver normal for size, shape, margin, position, location, and opacity?

Is the liver too small or enlarged?

Is the shape of the liver normal?

Is gas or mineralization present within the liver?

The liver is the largest solid organ in the abdomen.[18-20] The margins of the liver are best evaluated on the lateral radiograph and should have smooth surfaces with normal lobar edges that form acute angles. Liver size is usually assessed by using the position of adjacent organs and subjective criteria. The normal liver should lie beneath the ribs, extending almost to the arch of the ribs or just beyond the costal cartilages on a lateral radiograph. This depends on the degree of inspiration when the radiograph was made and also the breed of animal. A Doberman Pinscher liver may never extend beyond the costal cartilages on a lateral radiograph if made on inspiration, even if the liver is enlarged. If a line connecting the fundus and pylorus of the stomach is drawn, it should lie parallel to or angled slightly more caudal and dorsal than the caudal ribs in a normal dog or cat. A generalized reduction in liver size or cranial displacement of the liver (e.g., diaphragmatic hernia) results in cranial displacement of the gastric axis. Generalized hepatic enlargement causes caudal and dorsal displacement of the gastric axis and other abdominal viscera (Fig. 36-19). Hepatomegaly may be less dramatic in animals with hyperadrenocorticism because weakness of the abdominal muscles allows the liver to extend ventrally. Even severe hepatomegaly may have little effect on the position of the stomach. Extension beyond the ribs may indicate hepatomegaly, but this should be carefully interpreted because this appearance can be caused by other normal or abnormal conditions. This would include any disease that increases the intrathoracic volume, thereby displacing the diaphragm and the liver caudally. The liver often extends beyond the ribs in older animals as the ligaments that attach the liver to the diaphragm stretch. Conformational variations may also affect the relative position of the liver and adjacent viscera. Liver size is best assessed on the basis of a subjective assessment of whether the size is appropriate, too large, or too small for the patient. As a general guide, the liver size is more difficult to

*A review of the appearance of various abdominal masses, and their effect on other structures in the abdomen, can be found on the Evolve Web site at http://evolve.elsevier.com/Thrall/vetrad/.

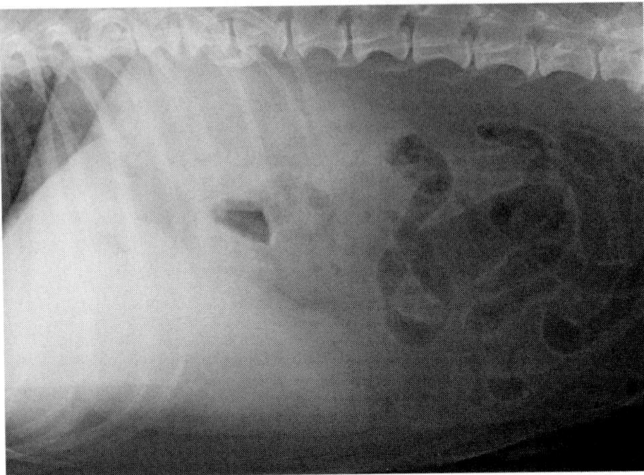

Fig. 36-19 Right lateral radiograph from a dog with pituitary-dependent Cushing disease. Generalized hepatomegaly with caudal and dorsal displacement of the gastric silhouette is present.

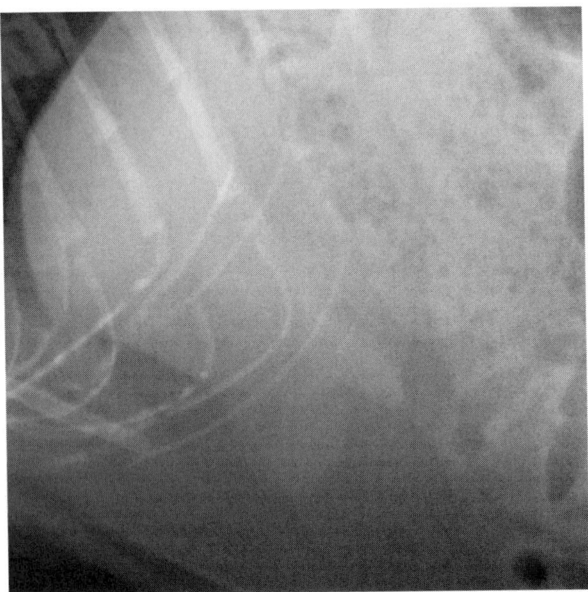

Fig. 36-20 Right lateral radiograph from a normal cat. The gallbladder margin is seen extending below the ventral aspect of the liver. This is a normal radiographic variant in cats and should not be mistaken for a mass.

assess on the ventrodorsal view. As such, hepatomegaly cannot definitively be identified unless focal enlargement of a specific region of the liver, such as a liver mass, is visualized. With microhepatia the cranial margin of the diaphragm is located less than two intercostal spaces from the main body of the stomach in a midline position. This later assessment is subjective and may help the interpreter feel more confident in the assessment of microhepatia on the basis of the lateral radiograph.

On the lateral radiograph, particularly in an obese animal, the renal fossa of the caudate lobe of the liver may be visualized. In these obese patients the right kidney is typically located caudal to and away from the renal fossa. Additionally, on the lateral radiograph of a cat, the gallbladder may normally extend below the ventral hepatic margin (Fig. 36-20).[20]

Intrahepatic lesions such as masses may alter the normal shape of the liver. Blunting or rounding of the normally

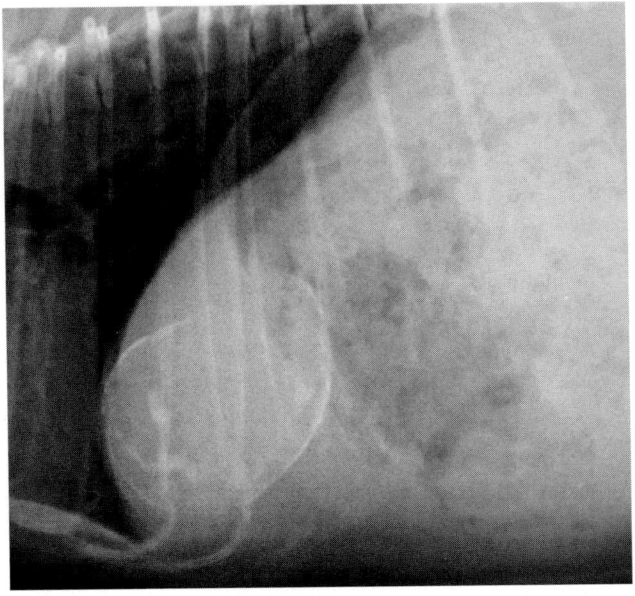

Fig. 36-21 Right lateral close-up radiograph from a dog with chronic cholecystitis. Mineralization is present in the wall of the gallbladder.

pointed lobar edges is the most reliable radiographic sign of hepatic disease. Nodules or masses may also protrude from the surface of the liver. The bulge of a full gallbladder on the ventral surface of the liver in cats should not be mistaken for a mass (see Fig. 36-20).

Intrahepatic mineralization is rare (Fig. 36-21). The presence of gas within the liver usually has grave prognostic implications. Linear gas shadows typically represent gas in the portal veins, hepatic veins, or intrahepatic bile ducts. A collection of small bubbles may be caused by emphysematous cholecystitis (right ventral liver) or abscess formation. Larger bubbles are usually within the gallbladder or an abscess cavity.

The Spleen

Is the spleen normal in size, shape, margin, position, and opacity?
Is generalized splenomegaly present?
Is a splenic mass (focal or the entire spleen) present?
Is the spleen malpositioned, or are abnormal accumulations of gas present within the spleen?

The spleen is an elongate, flattened, triangular organ with smooth surfaces and borders that form acute angles cranially and caudally. The proximal extremity of the spleen is relatively constant in position in the left craniodorsal abdomen because of the short gastrosplenic ligament that attaches the spleen to the body and fundus of the stomach.[21] The proximal extremity appears as a flattened triangular structure in the craniodorsal abdomen that may occasionally be seen on the lateral radiograph dorsal and caudal to the stomach. On the ventrodorsal radiograph, the spleen is typically seen lateral to the fundic portion of the stomach, medial to the body wall, and craniolateral to the cranial pole of the left kidney. The body and distal extremity are mobile and may be found almost anywhere in the abdomen depending on the size of the spleen. In cats, splenic size is relatively constant and only the proximal extremity of the spleen is seen on the ventrodorsal radiograph (see Figs. 36-1 and 36-11, *A*). If the distal extremity of the spleen is visible in the ventral abdomen on a lateral radiograph of a cat, it likely indicates an abnormally enlarged spleen. Splenic size in dogs is variable based on breed, age, and sedation. Factors such as stress also influence splenic size. Phenothiazine tranquilizers and barbiturate anesthetic agents cause splenic congestion and splenomegaly. The best radiographic indicator of pathologic splenic enlargement is rounding or blunting of the edges.

Splenic masses are the most commonly identified abdominal masses in older dogs (Fig. 36-22). If located in the body or tail of the spleen, the mass usually lies in the ventral midabdomen, causing caudal and dorsal displacement of the small intestine. The presence of peritoneal fluid may partly or completely obscure a mass, but a mass should be suspected if distribution of the small intestine is asymmetric. A pedunculated liver mass occasionally will be positioned caudal to the liver and be misinterpreted as a splenic mass (Fig. 36-23). A splenic torsion may appear as a large splenic mass or masses accompanied by peritoneal fluid. If little or no fluid is present, a characteristic folded, C-shaped spleen may be seen.

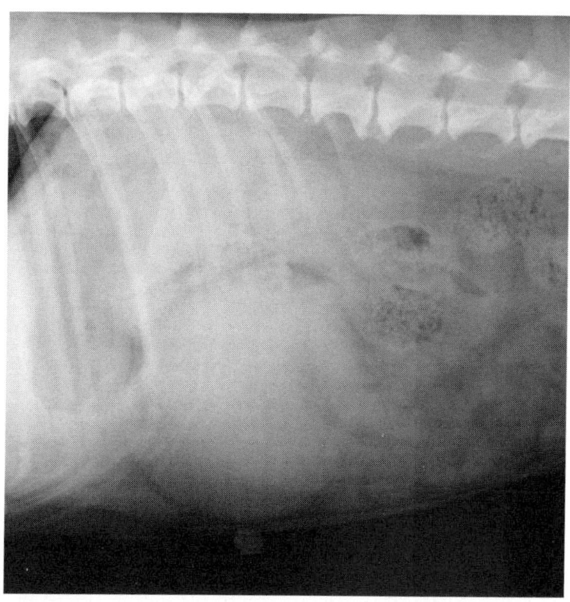

Fig. 36-22 Right lateral radiograph from a dog with a palpable mid-abdominal mass. A rounded, soft tissue, mid-abdominal mass has caused surrounding organ displacement. A splenic hemangiosarcoma was diagnosed following splenectomy.

The Pancreas

Is the pancreas visible on radiographs?
Is there evidence of pancreatitis?
Is there evidence of a pancreatic mass?

The normal pancreas is small and radiographically invisible. Pancreatitis may result in no radiographic abnormalities, so normal radiographs do not exclude pancreatitis. Moderate to severe pancreatitis triggers a severe inflammatory

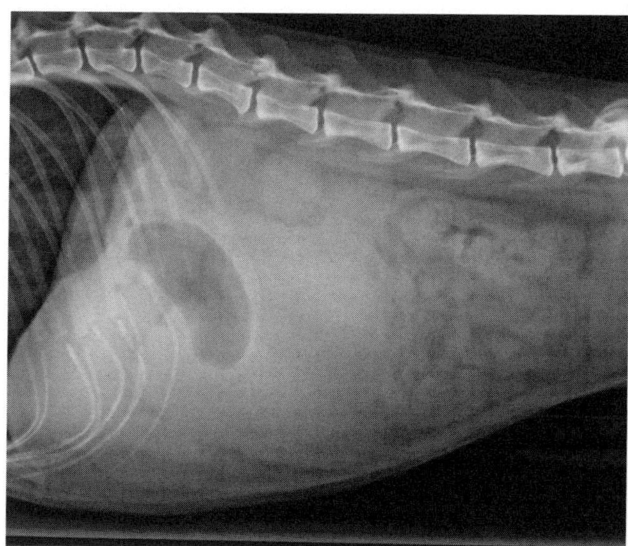

A

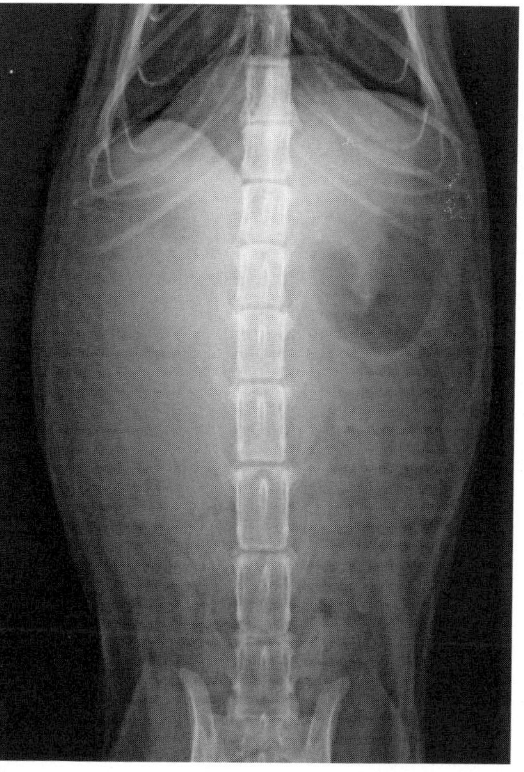

B

Fig. 36-23 Right lateral (A) and ventrodorsal (B) radiographs from a cat with a cranial abdominal mass. Even though this soft tissue mass appears caudal to the stomach on the lateral radiograph, this was a hepatic tumor (hepatocellular carcinoma). The stomach is displaced to the left by the right-sided tumor.

response in adjacent tissues.[13,14] This is seen as an ill-defined increase in soft tissue opacity and loss of detail within the cranial abdomen along the caudal border of the stomach and the descending duodenum (see Fig. 36-6). Caudal displacement of the transverse colon may be seen with pancreatitis affecting the left limb. If the right limb is affected, the descending duodenum may be displaced laterally and ventrally. Secondary peritonitis may cause a paralytic ileus of the descending duodenum that has a fixed, dilated appearance on sequential radiographs. Pancreatic masses cause similar organ displacements.

The Mid-abdomen

Is evidence of a mid-abdominal mass effect present?
Is evidence of inflammatory changes in the mid-abdomen present?
Are nodules within the mid-abdomen, and are margins of the serosal margins of mid-abdominal structures clearly visible?

The mid-abdomen is the most difficult part of the abdomen to evaluate.[15] Because a number of structures are superimposed and most of the small intestine is found in this region, a mass (5 to 8 cm in a large-breed dog) can be easily overlooked. The most common tissues of origin for a mass include the spleen, mesenteric lymph nodes, mesenteric cysts, or eccentric intestinal wall masses. Hints of a mid-abdominal abnormality may involve a mass effect, with displacement of the small or large intestinal tract. Focal peritoneal effusion may be present with multiple areas of decreased detail. Generalized peritoneal nodules as a result of tumor peritoneal seeding are called carcinomatosis. In dogs, multiple small soft tissue nodules within the peritoneum may be present. Cats with carcinomatosis typically have ascites and nodules cannot be seen.

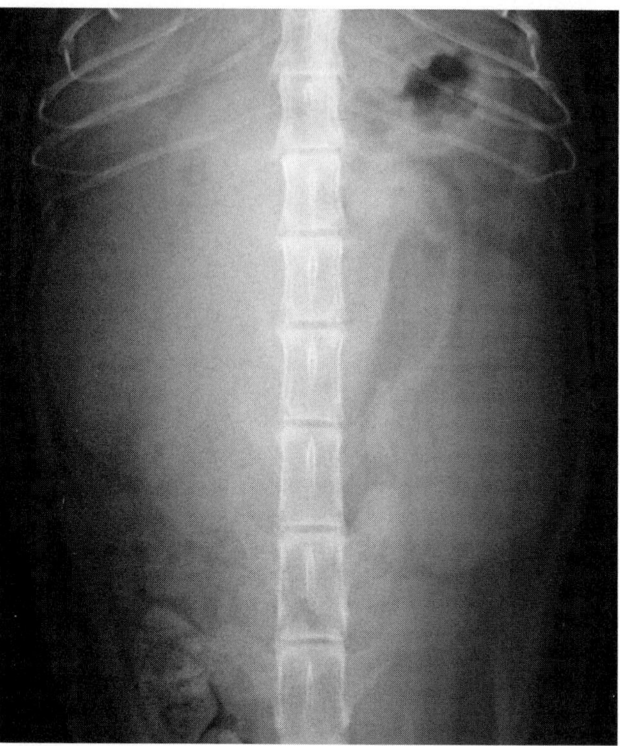

Fig. 36-24 Ventrodorsal abdominal radiograph from a cat with bilaterally enlarged kidneys. Differential diagnoses include lymphoma, bilateral hydronephrosis, polycystic kidney disease, and pseudocyst formation. In this cat, ultrasound confirmed pseudocyst formation.

Evaluation of the Urogenital System, the Adrenal Glands, and the Medial Iliac Lymph Nodes

Kidneys

Are the kidneys normal for size, shape, margin, number, location, and opacity?
Are the kidneys small?
Are the kidneys enlarged?
Do the kidneys have a normal shape, or are they irregular?
Is the renal radiographic opacity normal, or is mineralization present?

The left kidney is seen in most dogs with a normal body condition, but in many dogs only the caudal pole of the right kidney can be seen on the lateral radiograph and the entire right kidney may be difficult to see on the ventrodorsal radiograph.[22-26] Both kidneys should be clearly seen in any cat with a normal body condition. On the right lateral radiograph, the left kidney will be displaced from its dorsal position and may be in the mid-abdomen. Kidney size should be assessed on the ventrodorsal radiograph because renal positioning is more constant, thereby minimizing distortion. Normal canine kidneys measure 2.5 to 3.5 times the length of the second lumbar vertebra, whereas feline kidneys range from two to three times the length of the second lumbar vertebra. The kidneys should have smooth margins and be of homogeneous soft tissue opacity. Canine kidneys are somewhat elongated, whereas feline kidneys are shorter and rounder. In fact, when feline kidneys enlarge, they typically enlarge in a lateromedial versus craniocaudal direction. An obese cat will have some fat accumulation within the renal hilus, creating an apparent radiolucency that should not be mistaken for gas.

Small kidneys may be difficult to detect, especially if chronic renal insufficiency leads to cachexia. In young animals renal dysplasia or hypoplasia should be considered. In older animals most forms of chronic acquired renal disease will result in a reduction in size; these usually have an irregular shape and margin.

Renomegaly may affect one or both kidneys (Figs. 36-24 and 36-25). Left renal enlargement causes ventral, medial, and caudal displacement of the small intestine and descending colon. Right renal enlargement causes displacement of the descending duodenum and ascending and transverse colon ventrally, medially, and caudally. The small intestine is displaced toward midline ventrally and caudally. If the kidney is severely enlarged, identifying it as the organ of origin may be difficult. In such instances the absence of the normal renal silhouette suggests a renal origin for the mass. The shape and margin of the kidney are useful in refining a differential diagnosis list.

Urolithiasis and renal pelvic/diverticular mineralization is the most common cause of mineral opacity within the kidney. Renoliths may conform to the shape of the pelvis and diverticula and have a staghorn shape. Some renoliths are soft tissue rather than mineral opacity (cysteine and urate; recall the acronym "I can't C U") and can only be detected by a positive-contrast study (excretory urogram) or abdominal ultrasound. Small focal parenchymal mineralizations are common in chronic renal disease.

Urinary Bladder

Is the urinary bladder normal for shape, size, margins, location, and opacity?
Is the urinary bladder abnormally enlarged?
Is the urinary bladder shape normal or irregular?
Is the urinary bladder opacity uniformly soft tissue opaque, or are gas or areas of mineralization present?
Is the urinary bladder intact?

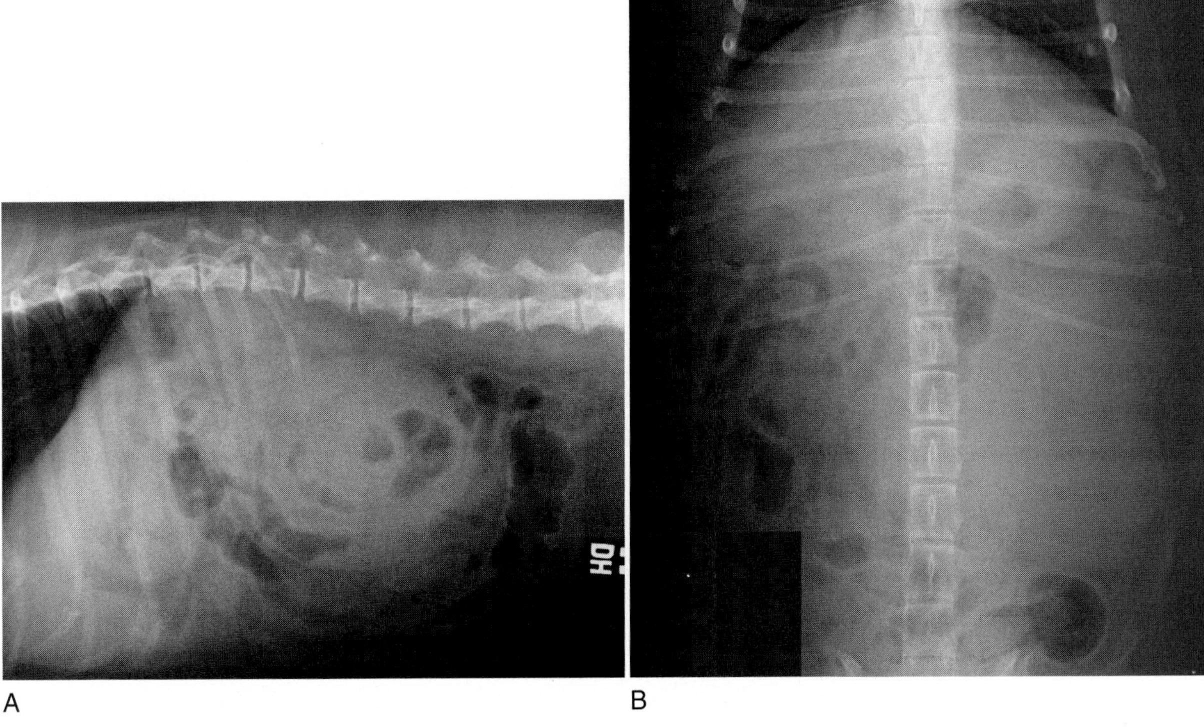

Fig. 36-25 Right lateral (A) and ventrodorsal (B) abdominal radiographs from a dog with a left renal mass. A renal cell carcinoma was diagnosed.

Do the urinary bladder and the cranioventral margin and the margin between the urinary bladder and the prostate in a male appear normal?

Are one or two teardrop-shaped margins noted in the caudal abdomen in a male dog?

The urinary bladder lies in the caudoventral abdomen. The normal canine bladder is pear shaped, with the neck located just cranial to the pubis. In the cat the bladder is more rounded and slightly more cranial. The normal urinary bladder size is difficult to define, but if the urinary bladder extends cranial to the umbilicus, diseases that can cause urine retention should be considered. Intramural tumors of the urinary bladder seldom alter the shape or opacity of the urinary bladder. In rare instances the contour of the bladder neck may be distorted or a poorly defined area of dystrophic mineralization may be present within the tumor. If a tumor is suspected, the presence of enlarged medial iliac lymph nodes should be investigated. Suspected tumors of the urinary bladder can be further investigated by contrast radiography and ultrasound. Uroliths may range from an accumulation of sandlike material to large stones. If uroliths are detected or suspected in male dogs, an additional radiograph of the penile urethra must be obtained (Fig. 36-26). Cysteine and urate uroliths are soft tissue opacity and cannot be detected on survey radiographs and require contrast radiography or ultrasound for diagnosis.

Urinary bladder rupture may occur as a result of blunt abdominal trauma or urethral obstruction. Rupture usually releases a moderate to large volume of fluid into the peritoneal cavity, with a consequent reduction in peritoneal detail and contrast. The absence of a normal urinary bladder outline with the presence of peritoneal fluid warrants a positive contrast cystogram to confirm or exclude a rupture. Entrapment of the urinary bladder in a perineal hernia is another consideration for a missing urinary bladder shadow in the caudal abdomen (Fig. 36-27).

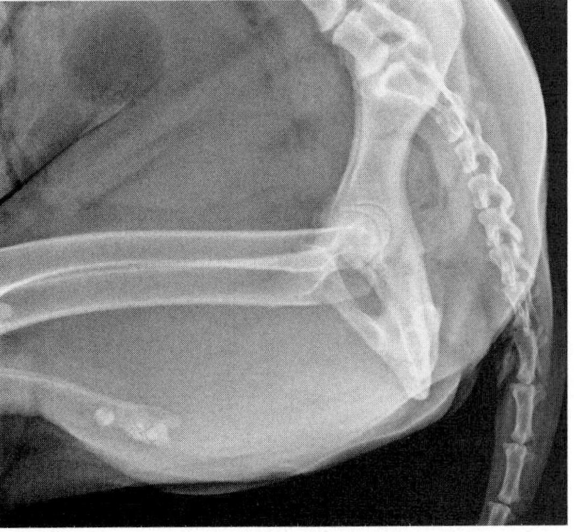

Fig. 36-26 Lateral radiograph of the perineal region of a dog made with the pelvic limbs pulled cranially. Note the calculi in the urethra at the base of the os penis. These calculi were less conspicuous in the conventional lateral view because they were superimposed over the femur.

Prostate

Is the prostate normal for size, shape, margin, location, and opacity?

Is the prostate enlarged?

Is the shape normal or irregular?

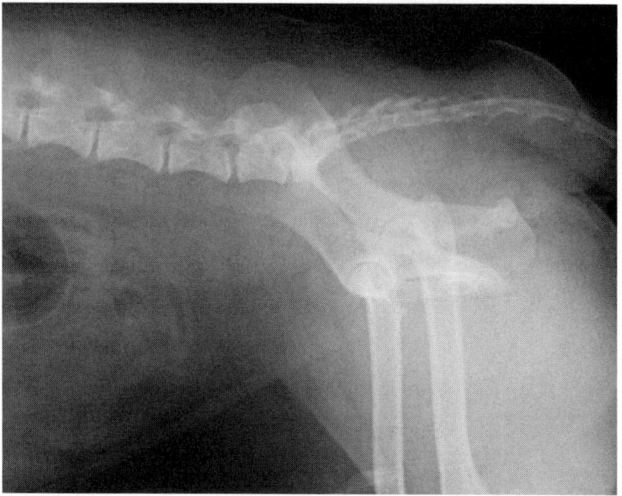

Fig. 36-27 Right lateral radiograph from a dog with a perineal hernia. The urinary bladder, which cannot be identified in this image, is caudally displaced into the hernia and is not visualized in the caudal abdomen.

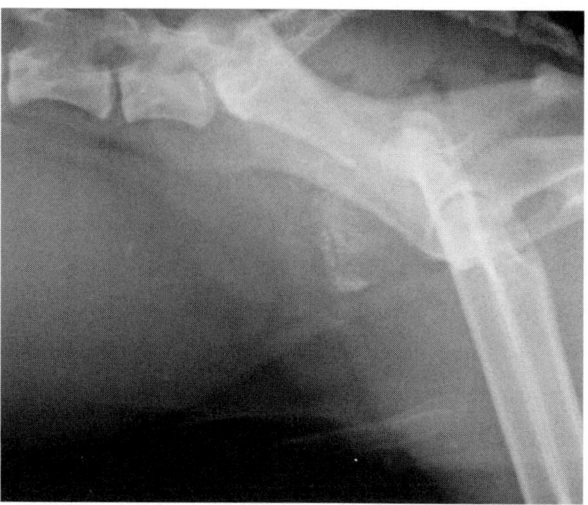

Fig. 36-28 Right lateral radiograph from a dog with an enlarged prostate with partial mineralization. The urinary bladder is distended. Carcinoma was diagnosed following fine-needle aspiration of the prostate.

Does evidence of a prostatic carcinoma exist, as evidenced by medial iliac lymph node enlargement, mineralization within the prostate, or irregular margination to the ventral vertebral bodies of the caudal lumbar and sacrum?

The normal prostate is usually contained within the pelvis. It may lie within the abdomen in young dogs when pulled cranially by a full urinary bladder and in normal older dogs. In a large-breed dog, the prostate is approximately the size of a walnut. Enlargement causes cranial displacement of the prostate and the bladder and dorsal displacement and compression of the colon (Fig. 36-28). Constipation may result from severe prostate enlargement. Irregularly marginated palisade-like new bone on the ventral cortex of the last two to three lumbar vertebrae, sacrum, and first few caudal vertebrae indicates metastatic tumor invasion of these structures.

Uterus and Ovaries

Is the uterus normal for size, shape, margin, location, number, and opacity?
Is the uterus enlarged?
Does evidence of a pregnancy exist?
Are signs of fetal death present?
Does a reason for dystocia exist?
Does evidence of an ovarian mass exist?

The normal uterus and ovaries are not radiographically visible, although the body of the uterus may sometimes be seen between the bladder neck and colon in obese animals.[27] Enlargement of both uterine horns produces a characteristic displacement of the small intestine toward midline and dorsally and cranially (Fig. 36-29). Pregnancy cannot be distinguished from pathologic causes of uteromegaly until fetal mineralization, which occurs after day 42 of pregnancy. Fetal death is more readily detected by ultrasound because radiographic changes take up to 24 hours to develop. Radiographically, the fetus may adopt a hyperextended or hyperflexed posture, or collapse and overlap of the skull bones may be visible. If putrefaction has begun, intrafetal and intrauterine gas may be present. In dystocia, fetal malposition or fetopelvic mismatch is sometimes apparent radiographically.

Ovarian masses tend to gravitate to the ventral midabdomen and cause displacement of the small intestine toward midline and away from the affected side. Ovarian teratomas often contain mineralization.

Adrenal Glands

Are the adrenal glands visible on the basis of a soft tissue mass or mineralization of an adrenal tumor?

The adrenal glands are normally not seen radiographically. They are located in the dorsal retroperitoneum dorsal to their corresponding phrenicoabdominal artery and vein. The right adrenal gland is located lateral to the caudal vena cava at the level of the right kidney in the dog and between the right kidney and the diaphragm in the cat. The left adrenal gland is located lateral to the abdominal aorta between the celiac and cranial mesenteric arteries and the left renal artery. The adrenal glands in older cats can be mineralized, and no significance is attached to this finding. Mineralized adrenal glands have also been reported in cats with muscular dystrophy. Adrenal tumors cause a mass in the mid- and cranial retroperitoneum (Fig. 36-30). Adrenal tumors can mineralize. Pheochromocytomas can also cause an adrenal mass with resultant retroperitoneal effusion.

Medial Iliac Lymphocenters (Lymph Nodes)

Are the medial iliac lymph nodes enlarged?
Is there any other evidence of urogenital tumors, lymphoma, pelvic masses, or tumors of the pelvic limbs?

The medial iliac lymph nodes are not normally visualized. They are located lateral to the caudal abdominal vessels at the level of the trifurcation of the caudal abdominal aorta (Fig. 36-31). A common radiographic mistake is misidentification of the iliolumbar blood vessels as the medial iliac lymph nodes (Fig. 36-32). The deep circumflex iliac arteries typically originate from the abdominal aorta at the level of L4, whereas the medial iliac lymph nodes are in a more caudal position, at the level of L6 and L7. Reactive lymphadenopathy from chronic cystitis or other focal inflammation usually will not result in lymph nodes that can be seen radiographically. Medial iliac lymph node enlargement is more common in dogs than in cats.

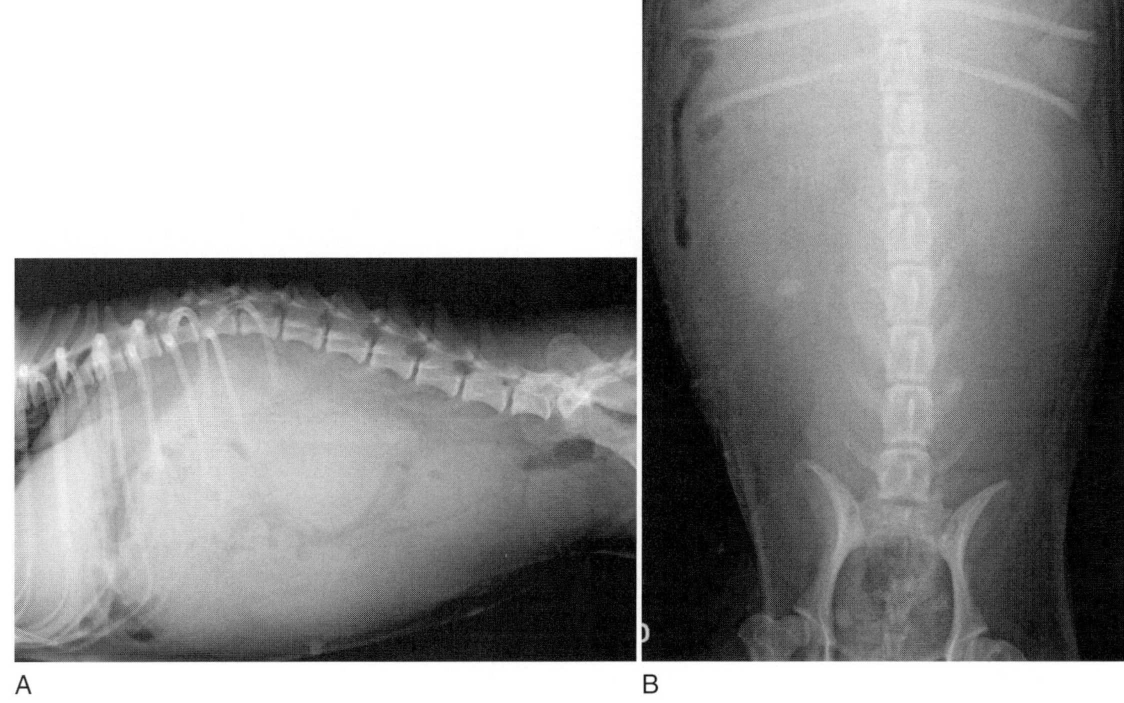

A B

Fig. 36-29 Right lateral (A) and ventrodorsal (B) radiographs from a dog. Multiple enlarged tubular soft tissue opacities are noted in the abdomen, displacing the small intestinal tract centrally and dorsally. These changes are consistent with uterine enlargement, and a pyometra was diagnosed at surgery.

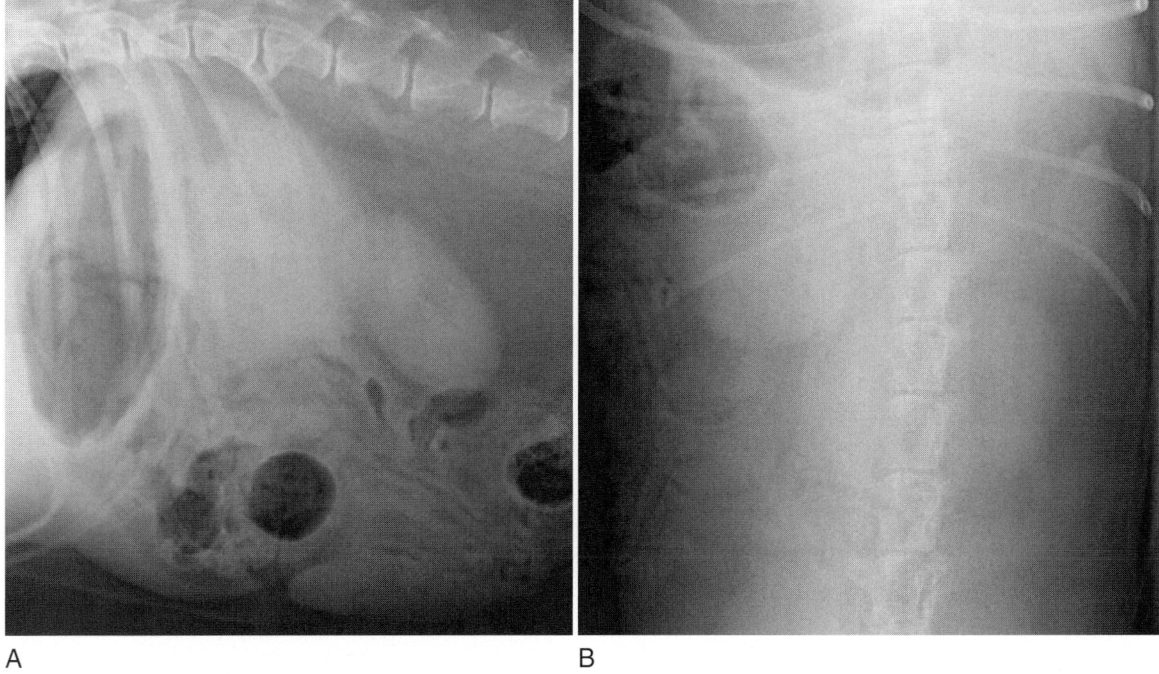

A B

Fig. 36-30 Right lateral (A) and ventrodorsal (B) radiographs from a dog with a dorsal, right-sided retroperitoneal mass. On the basis of the location, a mass originating from the right adrenal gland is a likely diagnosis. The right kidney is displaced caudally. An adrenal adenocarcinoma was diagnosed on histology.

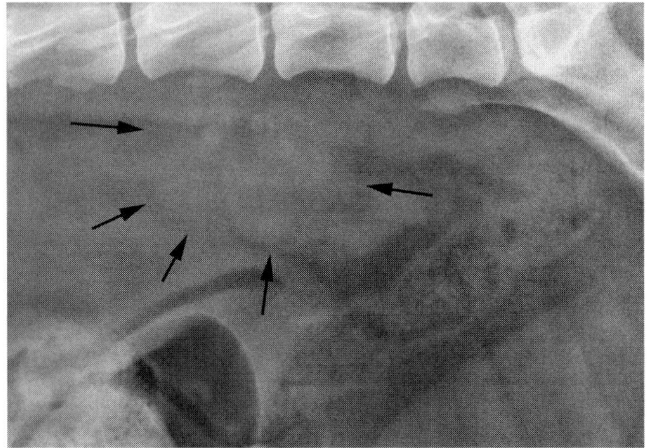

Fig. 36-31 Right lateral abdominal radiograph of a dog with lymphoma. The medial iliac lymph nodes are enlarged *(arrows)*.

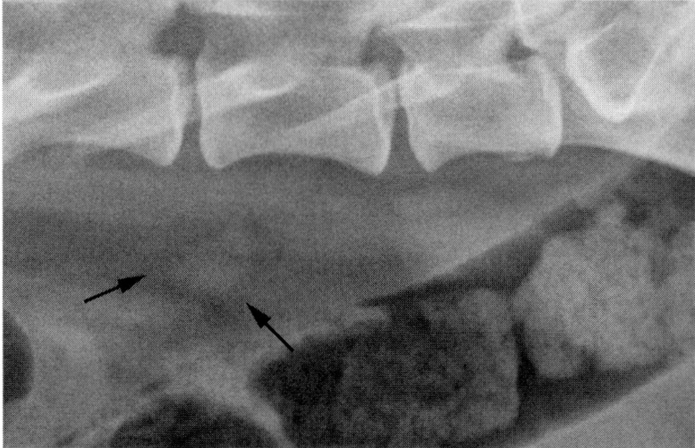

Fig. 36-32 Close-up view of the caudal retroperitoneal region of a normal dog. Sufficient retroperitoneal fat is present for the deep circumflex vessels to be seen. They are opaque because they are projected end on. These structures are sometimes misinterpreted as enlarged medial iliac lymph nodes.

REFERENCES

1. Lee R, Leowijuk C: Normal parameters in abnormal radiology of the dog and cat, *J Small Anim Pract* 23:251, 1982.
2. Carrig CB, Mostosky UV: The use of compression in abdominal radiography of the dog and cat, *J Am Vet Radiol Soc* 17:178, 1976.
3. Love NE, Berry CR: Interpretation paradigms for the abdomen—canine and feline. In Thrall DE, editor: *Textbook of veterinary radiology,* ed 4, Philadelphia, 2002, WB Saunders, p 483.
4. Feeney DA, Johnston GR, Klausner JS et al: Canine prostatic disease—comparison of radiographic appearance with morphologic and microbiologic findings; 30 cases (1981-1985), *J Am Vet Med Assoc* 190:1012, 1987.
5. Johnston DE, Christie BA: The retroperitoneum in the dog: retroperitoneal infections, *Comp Cont Educ Pract Vet* 12:1035, 1990.
6. Love NE: The appearance of the canine pyloric region in right versus left lateral recumbent radiographs, *Vet Radiol Ultrasound* 34:169, 1993.
7. Henley RK, Hager DA, Ackerman N: A comparison of two-dimensional ultrasonography and radiography for the detection of small amounts of free peritoneal fluid in the dog, *Vet Radiol* 30:121, 1989.
8. Kleine LJ, Lamb CR: Comparative organ imaging: the gastrointestinal tract, *Vet Radiol* 30:1123, 1989.
9. Jakovljevic S, Gibbs C: Radiographic assessment of gastric mucosal fold thickness in dogs, *Am J Vet Res* 54:1827, 1993.
10. Felts JF, Fox PR, Burk RL: Thread and sewing needles as gastrointestinal foreign bodies in the cat: a review of 64 cases, *J Am Vet Med Assoc* 184:56, 1984.
11. Graham JP, Lord PF, Harrison JM: Quantitative estimation of intestinal dilation as a predictor of obstruction, *J Small Anim Pract* 39:521, 1998.
12. Farrow CS: Radiographic appearance of canine parvovirus enteritis, *J Am Vet Med Assoc* 180:43, 1982.
13. Kleine LJ, Hornbuckle WE: Acute pancreatitis: the radiographic findings in 182 dogs, *J Am Vet Radiol Soc* 19:102, 1978.
14. Gibbs C, Denny HR, Minter HM et al: Radiological features of inflammatory conditions of the canine pancreas, *J Small Anim Pract* 13:531, 1972.
15. Root CR: Abdominal masses: the radiographic differential diagnosis, *J Am Vet Radiol Soc* 15:26, 1974.
16. Wise LA, Lappin MR: Canine dysautonomia, *Semin Vet Med Surg* 5:72, 1990.
17. Nyland TG, Ackerman N: Pneumocolon: a diagnostic aid in abdominal radiography, *J Am Vet Radiol Soc* 19:203, 1978.
18. Godshalk CP, Badertscher RR II, Rippy MK, et al: Quantitative ultrasonic assessment of liver size in the dog, *Vet Radiol* 29:162, 1988.
19. Barr F: Normal hepatic measurements in mature dogs, *J Small Anim Pract* 33:367, 1992.
20. Carlisle CH: Radiographic anatomy of the cat gallbladder, *Vet Radiol* 18:170, 1977.
21. Konde LJ, Wrigley RH, Lebel JL et al: Sonographic and radiographic changes associated with splenic torsion in the dog, *Vet Radiol* 30:41, 1989.
22. Shiroma JT, Gabriel JK, Carter TL et al: Effect of reproductive status on feline renal size, *Vet Radiol Ultrasound* 40:242, 1999.
23. McKenna SC, Carpenter JL: Polycystic disease of the kidney and liver in the Cairn Terrier, *Vet Pathol* 17:436, 1980.
24. Biller DS, Chew DJ, DiBartola SP: Polycystic kidney disease in a family of Persian cat, *J Am Vet Med Assoc* 196:1288, 1990.
25. Kirberger RM, Jacobson LS: Perinephric pseudocysts in a cat, *Aust Vet Pract* 22:160, 1992.
26. Finco Dr, Stiles NS, Kneler SK, et al: Radiologic estimation of kidney size in the dog, *J Am Vet Med Assoc* 159:995, 1971.
27. Ackerman N: Radiographic evaluation of the uterus: a review, *Vet Radiol* 22:252, 1981.

ELECTRONIC RESOURCES evolve

Additional information related to the content in Chapter 36 can be found on the companion Web site at evolve http://evolve.elsevier.com/Thrall/vetrad/.

- Key Points
- Chapter Quiz
- Systematic Checklist for Evaluating Abdominal Radiographs

CHAPTER • 37
Radiographic Anatomy of the Abdomen

James E. Smallwood
Kathy A. Spaulding

To use the roentgen sign method of recognizing abnormal radiographic findings effectively, an understanding of normal radiographic anatomy for the specific area of interest is required. This chapter provides a limited reference for the radiographic anatomy of the cardiopulmonary system. For more detailed information, readers are referred to a comprehensive text on radiographic anatomy.[1] The radiographic nomenclature used in this chapter was approved by the American College of Veterinary Radiology in 1983.[2]

REFERENCES

1. Schebitz H, Wilkens H: *Atlas of radiographic anatomy of the dog,* Stuttgart, Germany, 2005, Parey Verlag.
2. Smallwood JE, Shively MJ, Rendano VT et al: A standardized nomenclature for radiographic projections used in veterinary medicine, *Vet Radiol* 26:2, 1985.

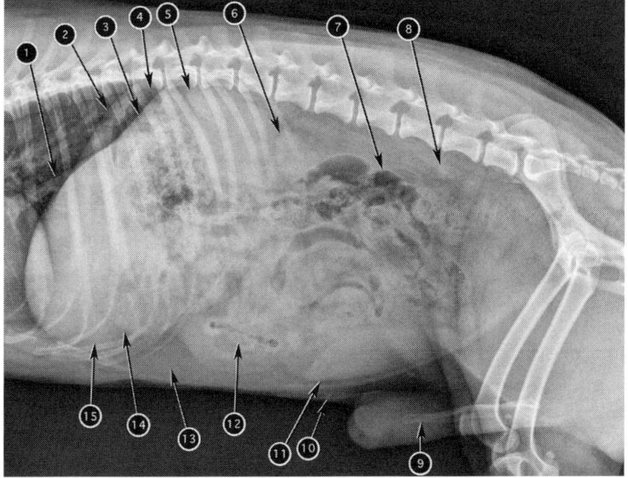

Fig. 37-1 Right-to-Left Lateral View of Canine Abdomen.
1. Caudal vena cava
2. Left crus of diaphragm
3. Right crus of diaphragm
4. Gas in fundus of stomach
5. Cranial extremity of right kidney
6. Cranial extremity of left kidney
7. Gas in descending colon
8. Deep circumflex iliac vessels
9. Os penis
10. Teat or nipple
11. Ventral region of spleen
12. Gas in small bowel
13. Fat in falciform ligament
14. Body of stomach
15. Liver

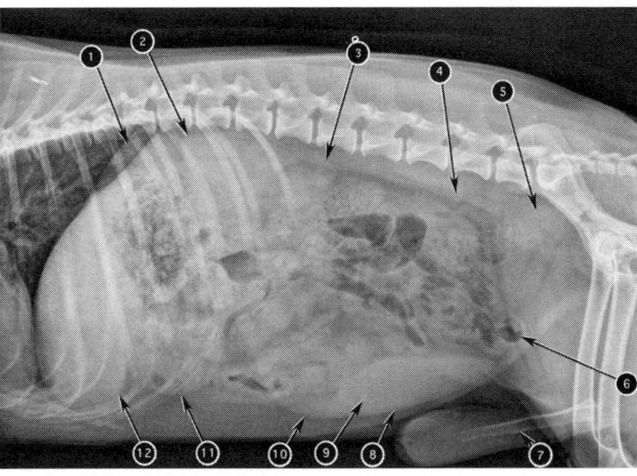

Fig. 37-2 Left-to-Right Lateral View of Canine Abdomen.
1. Gas and food in fundus of stomach
2. Cranial extremity of right kidney
3. Caudal extremity of left kidney
4. Deep circumflex iliac vessels
5. Feces in descending colon
6. Gas in small bowel
7. Os penis
8. Ventral region of spleen
9. Teat or nipple
10. Mid-ventral region of spleen
11. Body of stomach
12. Liver

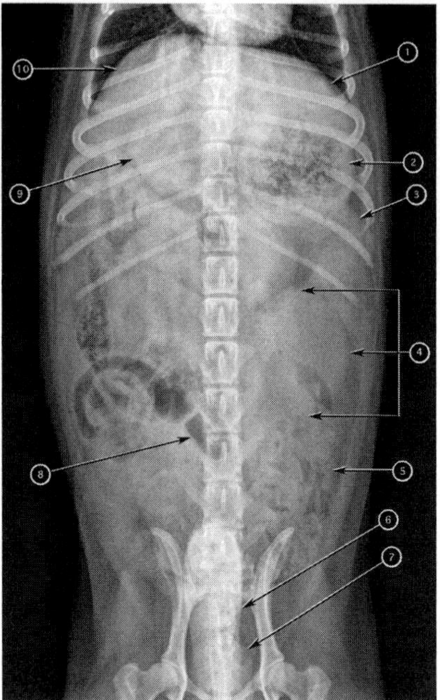

Fig. 37-3 Ventrodorsal Radiograph of Canine Abdomen.
1. Left lobe of liver
2. Gas and food in fundus of stomach
3. Mid-dorsal region of spleen
4. Left kidney
5. Feces in descending colon
6. Prepuce
7. Prostate
8. Gas in small bowel
9. Pyloric part of stomach
10. Right lobe of liver

ELECTRONIC RESOURCES evolve

Chapter 37 can also be found on the companion Web site at evolve http://evolve.elsevier.com/Thrall/vetrad/.

CHAPTER • 38
The Peritoneal Space

Paul M. Frank
Mary B. Mahaffey

The peritoneum, a thin, serous membrane, is divided into parietal, visceral, and connecting layers, which are all continuous.[1] The parietal peritoneum covers the inner surface of the abdominal cavity and is closely adhered to abdominal musculature; it separates extraperitoneal and intraperitoneal spaces. The visceral peritoneum covers the organs of the abdominal cavity either in whole or in part. The connecting peritoneum includes mesenteries, omenta, and intraabdominal ligaments. The peritoneal space, between the parietal and visceral peritoneal layers, normally contains only a small amount of fluid for lubrication.

The space between the dorsal margin of the parietal peritoneum and the abdominal wall is the retroperitoneal space. The retroperitoneal space is outside the peritoneal cavity and contains adrenal glands, kidneys, ureters, major blood vessels, and lymph nodes. The retroperitoneal space communicates with the mediastinum cranially and the pelvic canal caudally.[2]

Fat is usually deposited throughout the abdominal cavity, primarily in the falciform ligament, the greater omentum, the mesentery, and the retroperitoneal space. The presence of intraabdominal fat is important for visceral organ visualization because fat provides an interposed opacity between viscera (Fig. 38-1).

PERITONEAL SPACE

Increased Soft Tissue Opacity

Increased fluid within the peritoneal cavity causes a loss of the differential opacity interface between soft tissue and fat. Phrases commonly used to describe this loss of differential opacity are listed in Box 38-1.

Causes for loss of intraabdominal contrast include lack of fat, peritoneal effusion, peritonitis, and peritoneal neoplasia. A wet hair coat, or hair coated with ultrasound gel, may create the appearance of altered peritoneal space opacity.

Lack of intraabdominal fat may be the result of the age of the animal, or it may be caused by emaciation. Dogs and cats younger than a few months of age lack sufficient fat to provide intraabdominal contrast; thus the abdomen appears as relatively uniform and homogeneous, with soft tissue opacity. Another factor is that young patients have a relatively higher proportion of brown (multilocular) fat than adult dogs and cats. The major function of brown fat is heat production. As young animals mature, the relative weight of the brown fat decreases.[3] Brown fat has an opacity closer to that of soft tissue because of its higher water content. As this brown fat is replaced by white fat, the contrast between intraabdominal fat and soft tissues increases. The abdomen may also be somewhat pendulous in normal immature patients. Emaciation causes a similar homogeneous soft tissue opacity throughout the abdomen because of a lack of fat (see Fig. 38-1, C). In emaciated patients, the abdomen is often tucked up, which can be visualized on radiographs; however, the possibility of coexistent small-volume peritoneal effusion or peritonitis cannot be excluded.

Abdominal effusion refers to increased fluid within the peritoneal cavity. Fluid between abdominal viscera provides added overall opacity, and it causes border effacement of viscera and a loss of intraabdominal contrast. Classification of abdominal effusion is broad and includes transudates, exudates, blood, urine, bile, and chyle.[4] In practice, all abdominal fluids are of soft tissue opacity, comparable to the visceral organs. In many instances, the fluid is limited to the peritoneal space and contrast between the kidneys and adjacent retroperitoneal fat is preserved.

Peritonitis with edema and inflammation of serosal surfaces and adjacent fat may also cause loss of intraabdominal contrast. In addition, abdominal effusion is usually present with peritonitis. Peritoneal seeding of neoplastic foci can also cause a loss of intraabdominal contrast because of the soft tissue opacity of the nodules and possible coexistent effusion.

The radiographic appearance of the aforementioned conditions varies with the cause, the severity of the disease, and the relative amount of fluid versus fat present. The idea that accumulation of any amount of fluid results in complete obliteration of serosal margins is a common misconception. The degree to which serosal margin detail is obscured by fluid is determined by the relative amount of fat versus fluid; the more fat, the more fluid is needed to cause complete obliteration of serosal margins. Thus organ margins may still be visible when free fluid is present in the intraperitoneal space.

A large volume of abdominal fluid appears as a homogeneous fluid opacity uniformly distributed throughout the abdominal cavity (Fig. 38-2). The homogeneous appearance is caused by complete silhouetting of all soft tissue structures within the abdomen. A large volume of fluid often causes abdominal distention, with outward protrusion of the contour of the abdominal wall. Care must be taken because normal immature animals may have similar findings. A large volume of fluid may also displace the diaphragm cranially. If relatively mobile segments of bowel contain gas, they often float to the highest or uppermost area within the abdominal cavity. These segments will be located in the central portion of the abdomen on a lateral radiograph made in the routine fashion (i.e., with a vertical x-ray beam). The presence or absence of coexistent peritonitis cannot be ascertained radiographically in patients with a large intraperitoneal fluid volume.

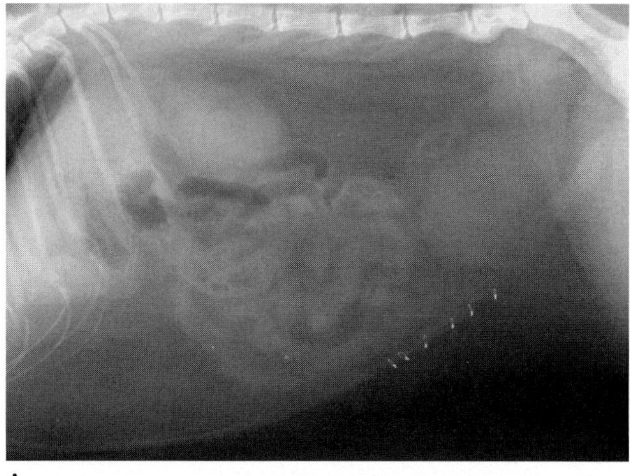
A

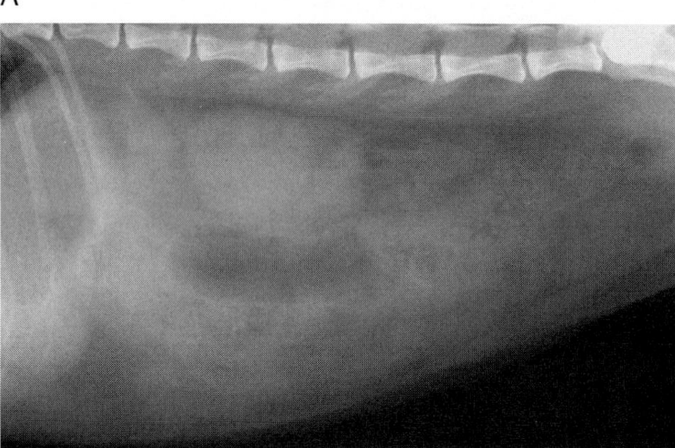
B

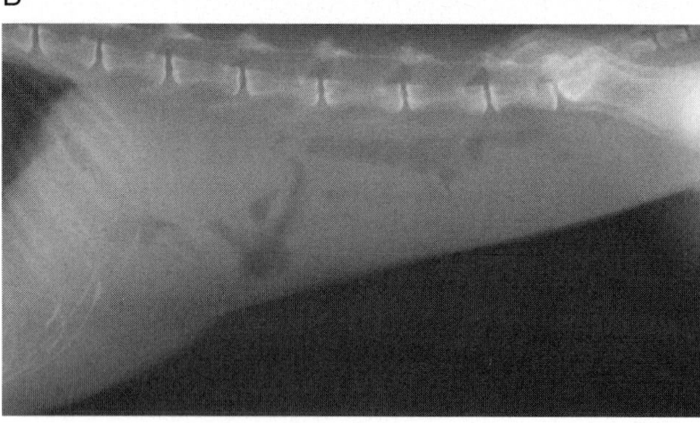
C

Fig. 38-1 Lateral views of the abdomen illustrating the effect of different amounts of abdominal fat. **A,** Obese cat. Extensive fat deposition in the falciform, omental, mesenteric, and retroperitoneal areas provides contrast between viscera of soft tissue opacity. (Metallic sutures in the ventral body wall are from prior surgery.) **B,** Normal cat. Fat deposition is less than that in **A** but is adequate to separate and allow visualization of viscera. **C,** Emaciated cat. Without interposed fat, border effacement of viscera is present, producing a uniform, homogeneous, soft tissue opacity throughout the abdomen except for gas in the bowel loops.

Smaller amounts of abdominal fluid or peritonitis may produce a mottled, hazy, or irregular fluid opacity on survey radiographs (Fig. 38-3). Individual viscera may be visualized, but the margins of soft tissue structures are indistinct or blurred. With small amounts of fluid, this appearance may be the result of interdigitation of fluid with folds in the greater omentum and small bowel but without a total silhouette effect.[5] Inflammation of the peritoneum or fat may produce a similar effect. Smaller amounts of effusion may be caused by early fluid accumulation of a generalized process or by more localized disease. Localized disease may lead to abnormal serosal margin detail in the area of the disease, with normal serosal margins visible elsewhere in the peritoneal space.

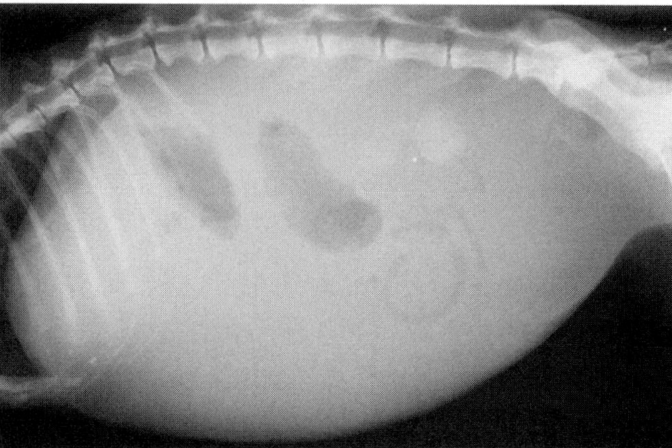

Fig. 38-2 Lateral view of the abdomen of a cat with a large volume of intraperitoneal fluid. Homogeneous fluid opacity is uniformly distributed throughout a distended abdomen. No fluid is in the retroperitoneal space, but fascial planes and organs in the retroperitoneal space are not visible because of superimposition of the distended abdomen.

Box • 38-1

Phrases Used To Describe Loss of Differential Opacity in the Abdomen

Loss of intraabdominal contrast
Decreased serosal surface visualization
Decreased serosal margin visualization
Decreased visualization of serosal surfaces
Increased intraabdominal soft tissue opacity
Increased intraabdominal fluid opacity
Decreased peritoneal detail

Manipulation of viscera during laparotomy produces changes that may appear comparable to peritonitis, and these changes may be modified by the amount of tissue trauma.[5] Solutions containing water, electrolytes, and relatively low molecular weight components are absorbed by the peritoneal membrane within 24 hours.[6] Proteinaceous fluids such as serum, blood, and lymph are absorbed more slowly and may be present for 1 to 2 weeks. These changes can be visualized after laparotomy, and they should not be mistaken for more significant complications. Static or increasing fluid accumulation during this period is abnormal.

One convenient method of assessing the intraperitoneal space for fluid accumulation is to compare the detail and contrast of the intraperitoneal space with the retroperitoneal space. Because many diseases resulting in intraperitoneal fluid accumulation do not affect the retroperitoneal space, retroperitoneal detail is often preserved when intraperitoneal fluid has altered the serosal margin of bowel and other

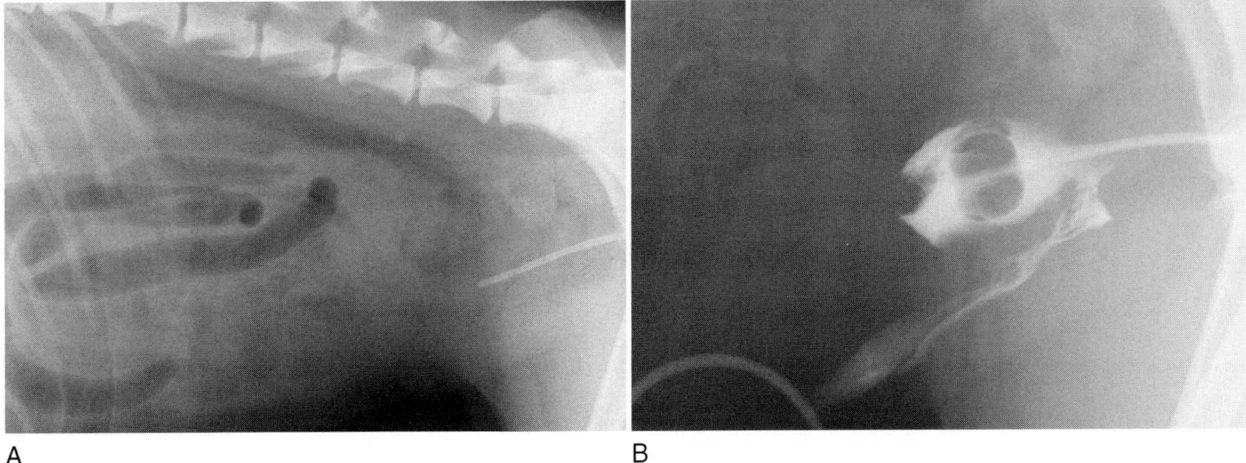

Fig. 38-3 A, Lateral survey radiograph of the abdomen of a dog who had been hit by a car. Mottled, hazy, irregular fluid opacity within the ventral half of the abdomen produces indistinctness or blurring of the margins of soft tissue structures. Note that the retroperitoneal space is normal. A urinary catheter is in place. **B,** Lateral cystogram of the same dog; the urinary bladder is ruptured.

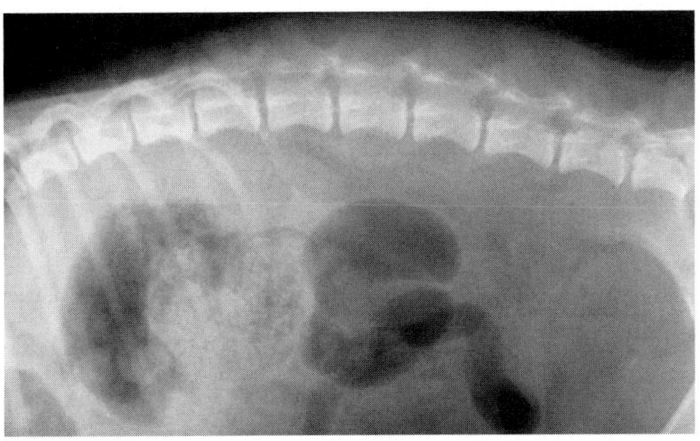

Fig. 38-4 Lateral view of the abdomen of a dog who had been hit by a car. Fluid opacity is in the retroperitoneal space with blurring of the margin of the lumbar musculature. The diagnosis was ruptured ureter.

intraperitoneal organs (see Fig. 38-3). Normally, detail and contrast in the intraperitoneal and retroperitoneal spaces should be identical. However, large volumes of intraabdominal fluid obscure the retroperitoneal space, even if the fluid is confined to the intraperitoneal space. This phenomenon is caused by superimposition by the large fluid volume. Loss of contrast and detail in the retroperitoneal space is an indication of fluid accumulation or, less commonly, inflammation. Fluid accumulation may be confined to the retroperitoneal space, with a normal appearance of the intraperitoneal space (Fig. 38-4). Often fluid within the retroperitoneal space leads to alternating fat and soft tissue opacities as the fluid dissects between fascial planes ("streaking"). The most common causes of isolated retroperitoneal fluid are hemorrhage and urine leakage. Inflammation and abscessation of the retroperitoneal space may be caused by migrating grass awns, penetrating wounds, foreign bodies, ligatures from ovariohysterectomy, and perforation of the urethra during catheterization.[7,8]

An ill-defined nodular or granular pattern to the abdomen (Fig. 38-5) may be caused by seeding of the peritoneum with multiple, metastatic neoplastic foci, or it may result from proteolytic enzymes escaping from an inflamed pancreas, causing saponification of omental and mesenteric fat. Examples of tumors associated with such spread include hemangiosarcoma of the spleen and carcinoma of various abdominal organs. The term *carcinomatosis* may be used to describe any cancer disseminated throughout the abdomen; it may be limited to carcinomas with this distribution or it can be used as a general term to describe loss of serosal detail with nodularity.[9]

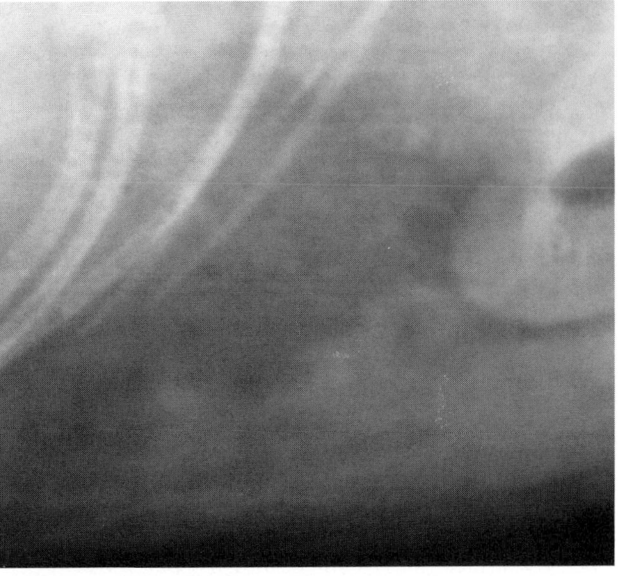

Fig. 38-5 Close-up of the cranioventral aspect of the abdomen of a dog with a colonic adenocarcinoma that had perforated the colon, leading to peritoneal carcinomatosis. The mottled appearance of the falciform fat is typical of carcinomatosis.

Localized radiographic changes of peritoneal disease are most often caused by a small amount of fluid or localized peritonitis (Fig. 38-6). Differential diagnoses for focal, ill-defined areas of increased opacity include pancreatitis, neoplasia, perforated gastrointestinal tract, compromised urinary tract, or trauma. The shape or contour of the abdomen should also be

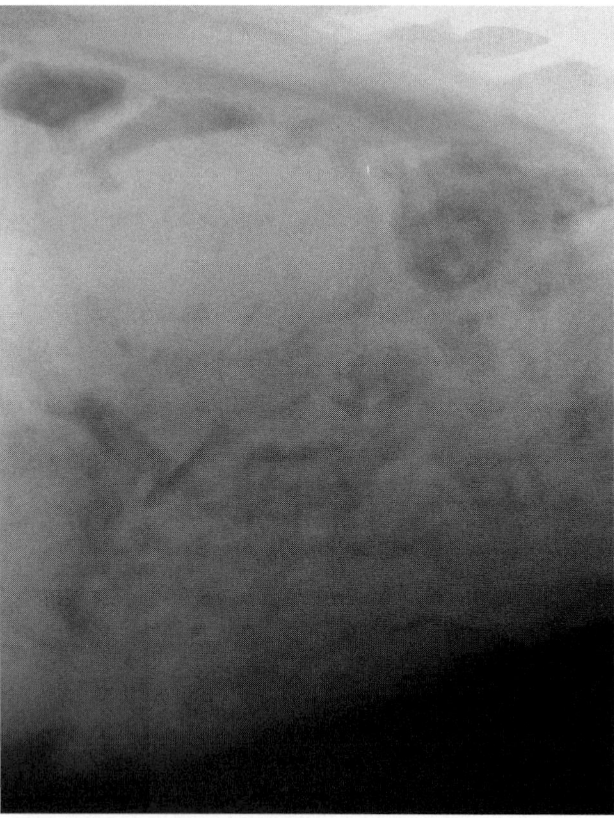

Fig. 38-6 Lateral view of a dog with poor serosal detail of the mid-ventral abdomen. The small intestines are bunched in this area. Note the greater detail in the retroperitoneal space compared with the intraperitoneal space. The diagnosis was adhesion formation as a result of prior enterotomy (foreign body removal).

Box • 38-2

Differential Diagnoses for Decreased Serosal Surface Visualization

- Lack of intraabdominal fat
- Young patient (brown fat)
- Peritoneal effusion (transudate, exudate, blood, urine, bile, chyle)
- Peritonitis
- Peritoneal neoplasia (primary or metastatic)
- Mass effect caused by crowding
- Superimposed external material (wet hair, ultrasound gel, etc.)
- Underexposure

evaluated. Large amounts of abdominal effusion result in a pendulous abdomen. However, the abdomen may also be pendulous from other causes, such as obesity and the muscle weakness of Cushing syndrome. Emaciation usually causes the abdomen to appear tucked up. Trauma to the abdominal wall or localized abdominal pain may produce asymmetrical contraction of abdominal muscles.[5] See Box 38-2 for causes of decreased serosal surface visualization.

Increased Gas Opacity

The two most common causes of free intraperitoneal gas are penetration of the abdominal wall, either by surgery or by penetrating wounds, and perforation of the bowel. However, not all bowel perforations lead to free abdominal gas.[10] Laparotomy is the most common cause of free abdominal gas, and the history is usually known in this instance. After laparotomy, a moderate amount of gas may persist for days to weeks.[11] Penetrating abdominal wounds are usually diagnosed by physical findings. In patients with a penetrating wound, differentiating whether free abdominal gas is caused solely by penetration of the abdomen or is the result of concurrent organ rupture is impossible to tell from radiographs.

A small volume of free abdominal gas is difficult to recognize on conventional radiographs made with a vertically directed x-ray beam because resulting bubbles are small and irregular in shape.[5] Larger gas volumes may coalesce into a larger bubble. This larger bubble may still be difficult to recognize on a radiograph made with a vertical x-ray beam because it is superimposed over other viscera. In addition, this larger bubble may simulate a gas-containing organ, such as the stomach. Such free abdominal gas usually floats to the highest point within the abdomen. In lateral recumbency, this point is usually under the caudal aspect of the ribs or in the mid-abdomen. The concurrent presence of abdominal effusion may make recognition of the gas bubble easier because the fluid provides a more uniform, homogeneous soft tissue background opacity (Fig. 38-7, *A*). A large volume of free abdominal gas is readily detected on survey radiographs because the gas provides contrast to outline serosal surfaces of viscera, such as bowel loops, the stomach, and the diaphragm (see Fig. 38-7, *B*).

Because free gas rises to the highest portion within the abdominal cavity, free gas may be visually isolated from superimposed structures by a horizontally directed x-ray beam. With a small volume of gas, putting the patient in position for 10 minutes before exposure may be helpful to allow most of the gas to migrate and coalesce at the uppermost portion of the abdomen. The most sensitive projection for detecting small volumes of gas is a lateral view, made with a horizontally directed x-ray beam, with the patient in dorsal recumbency and with the cranial portion of the abdomen slightly elevated so small amounts of gas will accumulate between the liver, diaphragm, and ventral aspect of the abdominal wall (Fig. 38-8, *A*).[12] Another projection used for documenting free gas is a ventrodorsal view obtained with the patient in left recumbency with the use of a horizontally directed x-ray beam. Gas usually localizes under the highest portion of the right abdominal wall (see Fig. 38-8, *B*), which is usually under the caudal aspect of the ribs. With larger volumes of gas, the bubble may extend under the diaphragm or along the abdominal wall caudally. Raising or lowering either end of the animal shifts the point of gas accumulation. Exposure factors should be lowered to underexpose the abdomen, and the right abdominal wall should be centered in the x-ray beam to avoid superimposition of abdominal organs created by divergence of the beam at its periphery. A view with the animal in right recumbency is not recommended because the gas bubble rises to the left side and may be confused with gas within the fundus of the stomach.

Gas may also accumulate in the retroperitoneal space.[8] Retroperitoneal gas is most often the result of extension of pneumomediastinum (see Chapter 31) or penetration of the abdominal wall. Retroperitoneal gas is confined to the retroperitoneal space in the dorsal abdomen and is best seen on a lateral radiograph (Fig. 38-9).

Intraabdominal Mineral Opacity

Increased mineral opacity not associated with the gastrointestinal tract can be seen in various sites within the abdomen. Focal calcified bodies (usually with a more opaque periphery) may be found in the peritoneal space (Fig. 38-10). These are

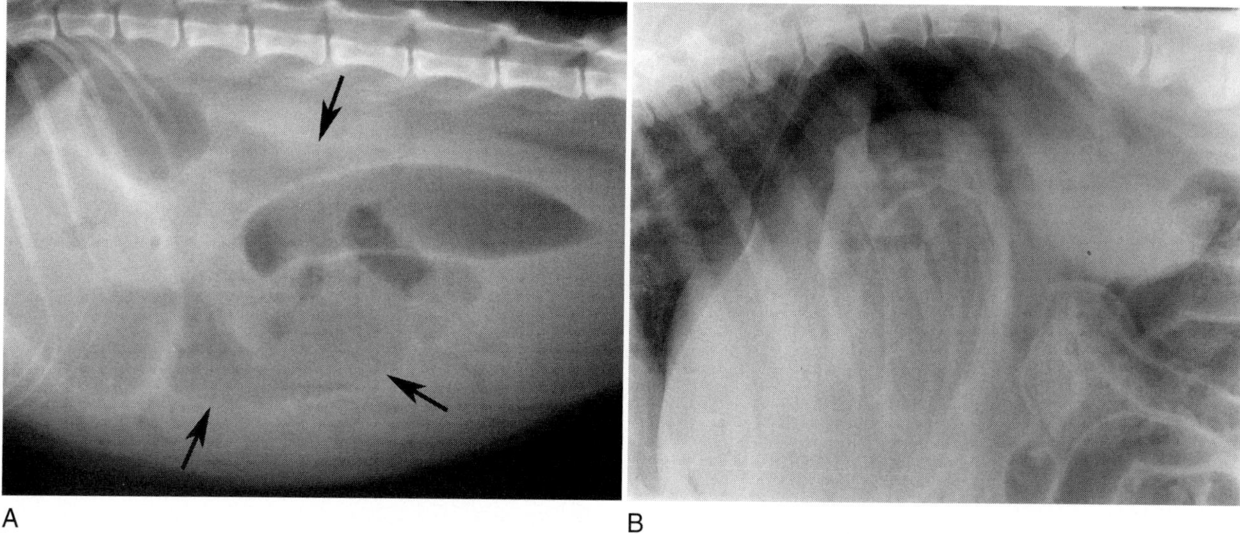

Fig. 38-7 A, Lateral survey radiograph of a cat with abdominal effusion and a moderate amount of free intraabdominal gas. *Arrows*, margins of the gas pocket. B, Lateral survey radiograph of the abdomen of a dog immediately after laparotomy. A large volume of free abdominal gas outlines the caudal surface of the right crus of the diaphragm, the cranial pole of the right kidney, the caudal surface of part of the liver, and the serosal surfaces of some bowel loops.

thought to be the result of dystrophic calcification of necrotic mesenteric fat and are not considered clinically significant.[13,14] Although not common, they are seen more often in cats than dogs. These have been referred to as Bates bodies.[14] Metastatic calcification of the abdominal vasculature is rare (Fig. 38-11) and is associated with abnormal calcium metabolism, primarily in animals with chronic uremia,[13,15] or in those with hypothyroidism. A mineralized fetus may be seen in the peritoneal space with ectopic pregnancy. Clinical signs may be caused by necrosis or mechanical interference, or the condition may be an incidental finding.[16]

Abdominal Wall Abnormalities

Mineralization may occasionally be visualized in the soft tissues surrounding the abdomen. For example, calcinosis associated with Cushing syndrome may produce nodular or linear calcification of soft tissues that may be visualized radiographically, most often dorsally and in the ventral abdominal wall.[17] Gas from a variety of causes may be seen in the soft tissues surrounding the abdomen. Abrasions with lacerations often produce a mottled, irregular gas pattern. Tubular or round gas pockets may be contained within herniated bowel loops (Fig. 38-12). Gas that dissects along fascial planes is most often caused by large open wounds, upper airway perforation, or pneumomediastinum. These patterns, however, are not pathognomonic for the cause of the gas accumulation. To assess accurately the location of extraabdominal lesions superimposed over the abdomen, two orthogonal views of the area must be made. In some instances, more than two views (i.e., oblique views) may be needed.

Sonography of the Peritoneal Space

Ultrasound is extremely useful for evaluating the peritoneal space, especially when increased fluid is suspected radiographically. Small volumes of fluid can be readily detected and samples collected by needle aspiration facilitated by ultrasound guidance. Fluid can be characterized by its echogenicity. Fluid with low cellular content such as urine or a transudate is anechoic (Fig. 38-13); fluid with moderate to high cellular content, such as exudate, blood, or chyle, is more echoic (Fig. 38-14). Peritoneal masses can be characterized as solid or cavitary (see Fig. 38-14, *B*), and samples can be obtained by needle aspiration for cytologic evaluation. Differentials are similar to those for any mass (cyst, hematoma, abscess, neoplasia, granuloma). Although uncommon, peritoneal metastases can be detected and appear as fingerlike projections of hypoechoic material scattered throughout the mesentery (Fig. 38-15). In the northwestern portion of the United States and Canada, as well as portions of Europe, peritoneal infection by *Mesocestoides* spp. tapeworms may manifest as varying sized, cavitary, septated structures with echogenic particles within the fluid.[18,19]

Small volumes of free peritoneal gas may appear as focal artifacts adjacent to the nondependent portion of the peritoneum. Small amounts of free peritoneal gas may not interfere with sonographic evaluation, but large volumes of gas may hinder complete evaluation of the peritoneal space and its contents. Survey and positional radiographs are the primary method of diagnosing pneumoperitoneum, but ultrasound may have a complementary role. In one study free peritoneal gas was found sonographically in patients in which it was not diagnosed radiographically, and sonography identified the specific location and cause of the pneumoperitoneum more frequently than radiographs. The findings of hyperechoic fat, free peritoneal fluid, and a dilated fluid-filled stomach or intestine were considered indirect evidence of gastrointestinal perforation.[20] As would be expected, pneumoperitoneum in conjunction with gastric dilatation or volvulus has been shown to be predictive for gastric necrosis. Prior percutaneous trocharization can confound the situation by leading to pneumoperitoneum and/or pneumatosis mimicking gastric necrosis.[21]

Abdominal Lymph Nodes

Abdominal lymph nodes can be divided into two groups: parietal and visceral. Parietal lymph nodes lie in the retroperitoneal space. These lymph nodes receive afferent lymphatics from the spine, adrenal glands, kidneys, caudodorsal abdomen, pelvis, and pelvic limbs. Efferent vessels from these lymph nodes drain into the lumbar trunk, which in turn empties into

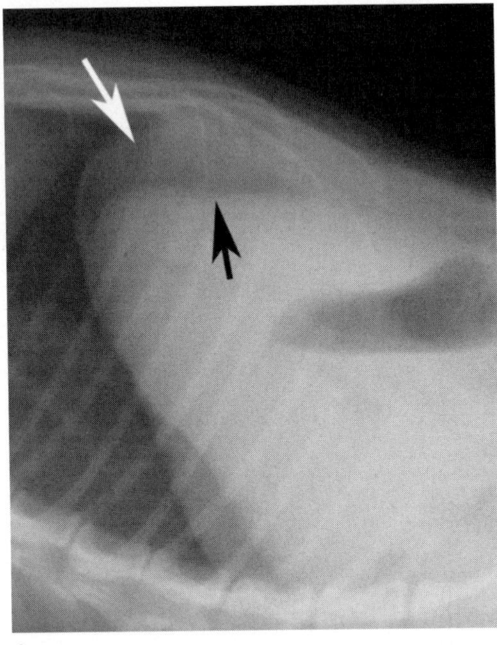
A

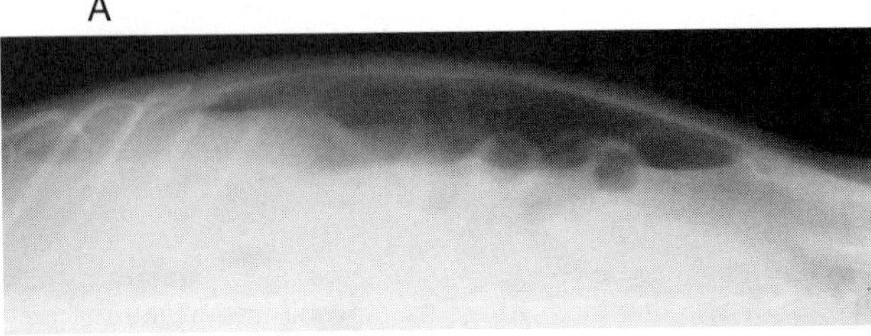
B

Fig. 38-8 A, Lateral view of the abdomen with the patient in dorsal recumbency, with the cranial abdomen slightly elevated and the use of a horizontally directed x-ray beam. Free abdominal gas has accumulated between the diaphragm *(white arrow)*, the liver *(black arrow)*, and the ventral abdominal wall. The diagnosis was ruptured stomach. **B,** Ventrodorsal view of the abdomen with the same patient in left recumbency and the use of a horizontally directed x-ray beam. The free abdominal gas pocket is located under the right abdominal wall and is projected separately from, rather than superimposed over, the abdominal fluid. Note the gas-filled intestines floating in the free peritoneal fluid.

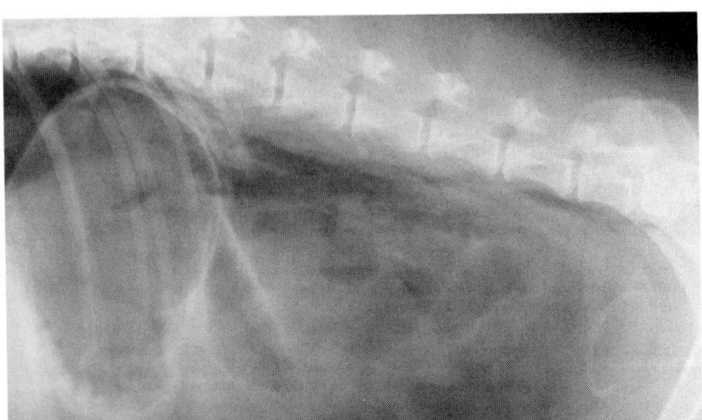

Fig. 38-9 Lateral view of a dog with pneumomediastinum. Some of this gas dissected along the fascial planes of the aorta and is located within the retroperitoneal space. Gas can be seen along the aorta (ventral to T12 and T13) and a urinary catheter is in place.

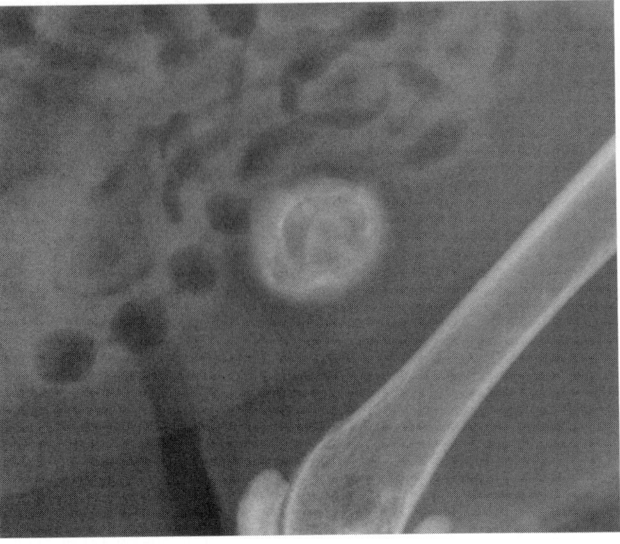

Fig. 38-10 Close-up lateral abdominal radiograph of a cat with a focal calcified body in the peritoneal space. The calcified body was an incidental finding and thought to be a result of dystrophic calcification of necrotic fat.

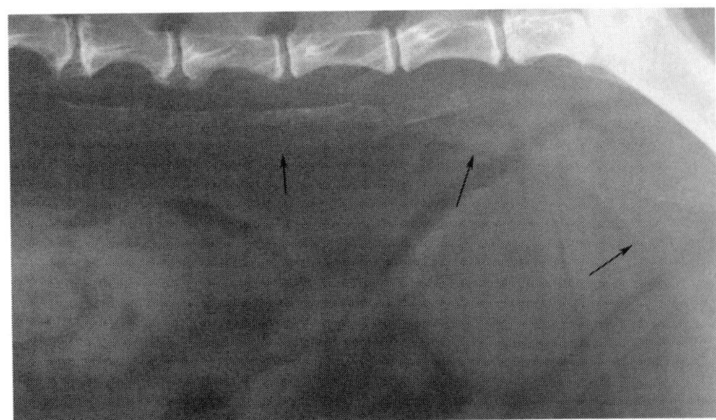

Fig. 38-11 Close-up lateral view of the caudal abdomen of a 13-year-old Shetland Sheepdog in chronic renal failure. The aorta, external iliac arteries, and femoral arteries *(arrows)* are visible because of metastatic calcification.

the cisterna chyli. The more cranially located of these lymph nodes may bypass the lumbar trunk and drain directly into the cisterna chyli. Many of the lymph nodes are inconsistently developed and may be absent; however, the medial iliac lymph nodes, the largest lymph nodes of the sublumbar group, are constant. The medial iliac lymph nodes, previously known as the external iliac lymph nodes,[1] are located ventral to the vertebra and between the deep circumflex iliac and external iliac arteries. Although some authors state that the medial iliac lymph nodes lie ventral to L5 and L6,[1] these lymph nodes often are located ventral to the bodies of L6 and L7.[5] One lymph node is usually present on each side, but occasionally two lymph nodes are on one or both sides. The medial iliac lymph nodes receive afferent lymphatics from the urogenital tract as well as from other structures in the caudal abdomen, pelvis, and pelvic limbs.

The visceral group of abdominal lymph nodes drains the liver, spleen, pancreas, stomach, and intestine. The largest of this group are the cranial mesenteric lymph nodes, which receive afferent lymphatics from the jejunum, ileum, and

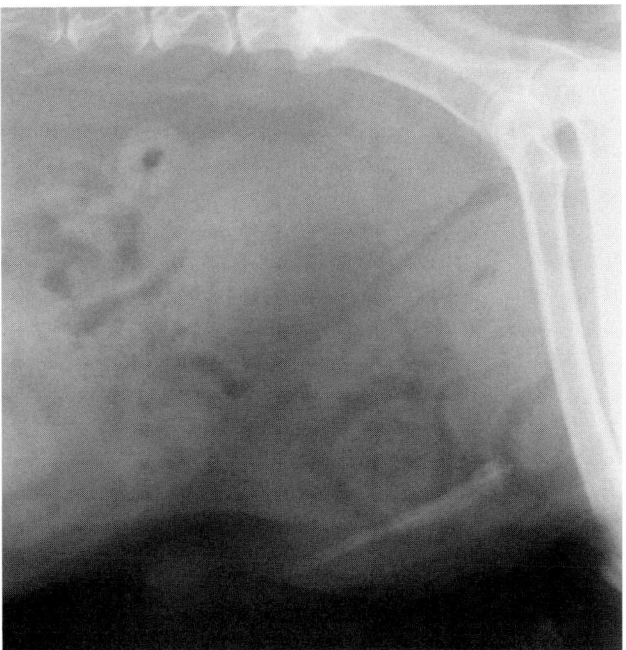

Fig. 38-12 Lateral view of the abdomen of a dog with a sharply marginated, tubular gas pocket ventral to the abdominal wall from an inguinal hernia with entrapped small intestine within the hernia.

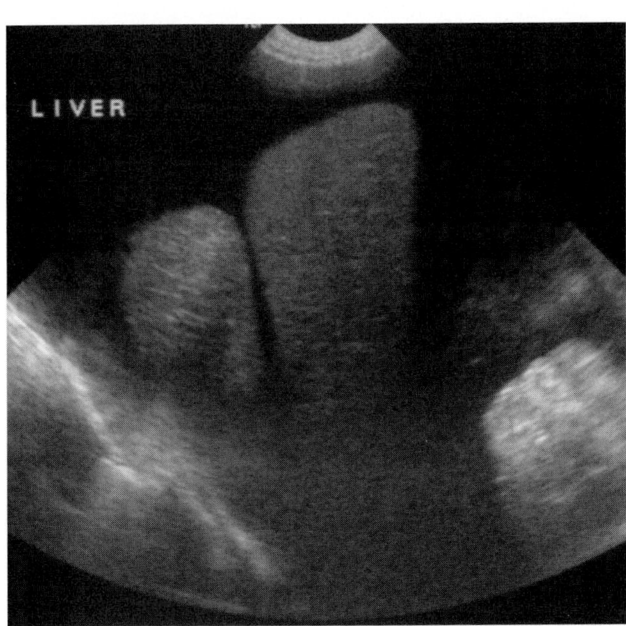

Fig. 38-13 Sagittal sonogram of a dog with ascites. Anechoic fluid is seen between and surrounding liver lobes. The lack of echoes in the fluid is consistent with the fluid being of low cellular content.

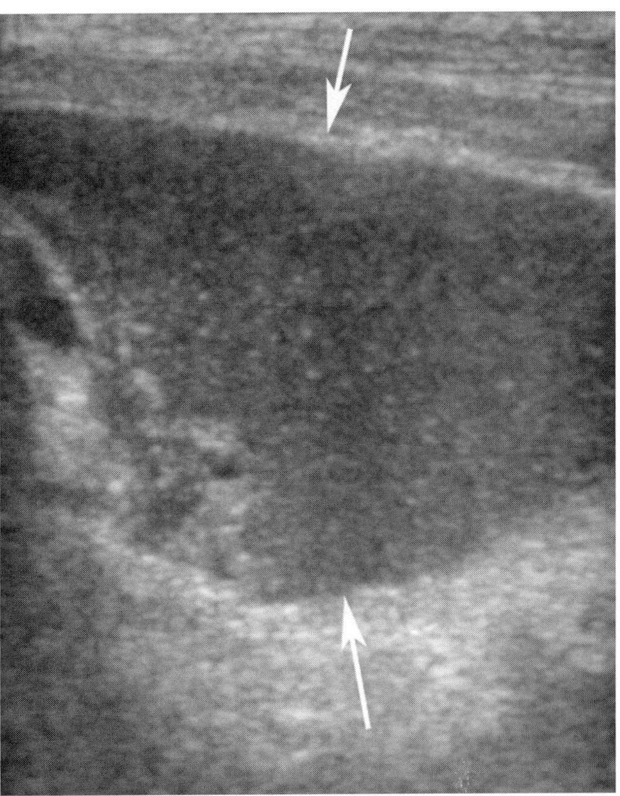

Fig. 38-14 Sagittal sonograms of a 6-year-old dog with an abdominal mass and peritoneal effusion. Free peritoneal fluid *(arrows)* with low-level echoes is compatible with highly cellular fluid.

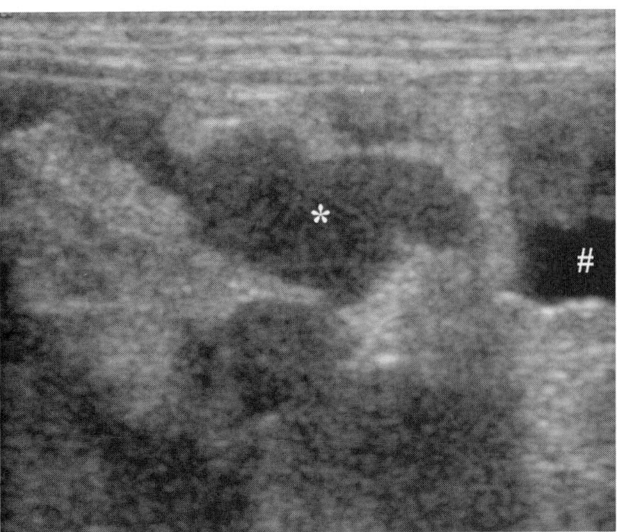

Fig. 38-15 Sagittal sonogram of a 9-year-old dog with peritoneal metastasis, which is seen as hypoechoic, irregularly shaped material *(asterisk)* interspersed through the more echogenic mesenteric fat. A small amount of anechoic peritoneal fluid can be seen on the right edge of the image *(#)*.

pancreas. The efferent vessels of the visceral lymph nodes drain into the intestinal trunk, which then empties into the cisterna chyli. Normal abdominal lymph nodes are not seen on survey radiographs because they are not of sufficient size or opacity to be seen as separate structures (Fig. 38-16).

Abnormalities of Lymph Nodes

Abdominal lymph nodes may be seen radiographically only if they are enlarged or mineralized. Abundant retroperitoneal fat present in most dogs also helps provide contrast between enlarged lymph nodes and surrounding soft tissue structures.

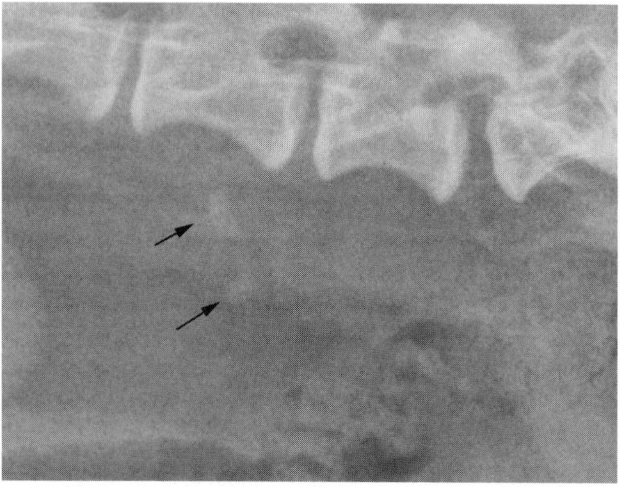

Fig. 38-16 Lateral view of the abdomen of a normal dog. Note the fat opacity within the retroperitoneal space. Ill-defined nodular soft tissue opacities in the caudal retroperitoneal space seen ventral to L6 (*arrows*) represent end-on projections of the deep circumflex iliac arteries and veins, not lymph nodes.

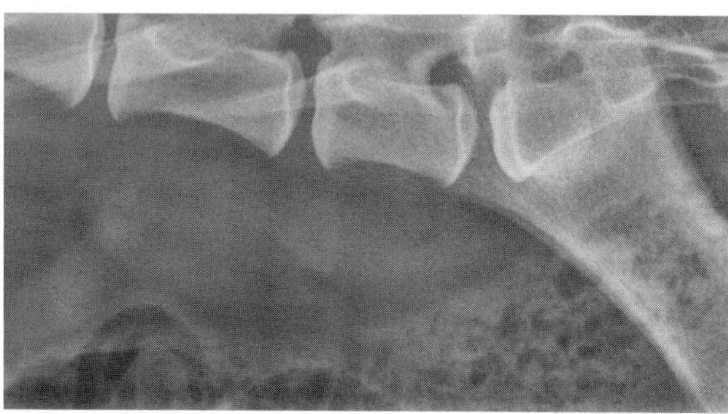

Fig. 38-17 Lateral view of the abdomen of a dog with anal gland adenocarcinoma. The medial iliac lymph nodes are enlarged and appear as a soft tissue mass with indistinct margins in the retroperitoneal space ventral to L6 and L7. The colon is displaced ventrally.

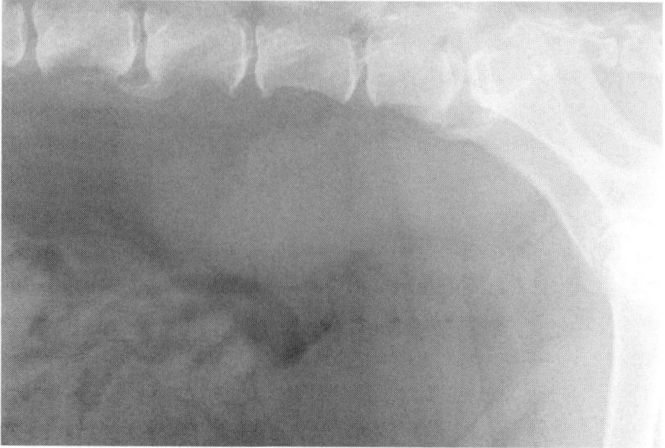

Fig. 38-18 Lateral view of the abdomen of a dog with lymphosarcoma. Medial iliac lymph node enlargement is severe and appears as a soft tissue mass in the retroperitoneal space extending caudally from L4-L5 into the pelvic canal.

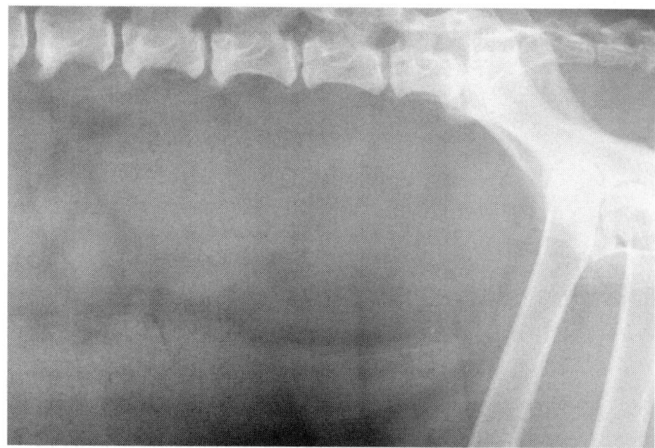

Fig. 38-19 Lateral view of the abdomen of a dog with metastatic mast cell tumor. A large soft tissue mass (lymph nodes) in the retroperitoneal space extends from L3-L4 into the pelvic canal, displacing the colon and rectum ventrally.

Of the parietal lymph nodes, the medial iliac nodes are usually the only nodes that enlarge to such a degree that they may be seen radiographically. Enlarged medial iliac lymph nodes appear as soft tissue masses in the retroperitoneal space ventral to L6 and L7 (Fig. 38-17). If node enlargement is severe, the lymph nodes may extend more cranially (Fig. 38-18). Enlarged lymph nodes frequently displace the descending colon and rectum ventrally (Fig. 38-19). However, a ventral course of the colon is not an indication of medial iliac lymph node enlargement unless a soft tissue mass is present where the lymph nodes are located. The colon may be normally positioned more ventral than usual without being displaced by a mass. The most common cause of medial iliac lymphadenopathy is neoplasia. Neoplastic lymph node involvement may be primary (e.g., lymphosarcoma) or metastatic (e.g., from caudal abdominal or pelvic neoplasms).[22] Inflammatory diseases may also cause node enlargement.

Visceral abdominal lymph nodes are not usually seen on radiographs. They rarely enlarge enough to be seen radiographically, tending to silhouette surrounding organs, and they are infrequently specifically recognized. However, cranial mesenteric lymph nodes may occasionally enlarge sufficiently so as to be seen as an ill-defined central abdominal mass displacing the intestine peripherally.

Sonography of Parietal and Visceral Lymph Nodes

Ultrasound is more sensitive than radiography for imaging lymph nodes. Because the medial iliac and jejunal lymph nodes are the largest and most consistent in the abdominal cavity, they can be found more often than other nodes when normal.[23] Normal lymph nodes tend to be similar in echogenicity to surrounding mesentery and adjacent musculature,[23] but knowledge of their location and careful identification of elongated structures of uniform echotexture and thin echogenic capsules can permit detection (Fig. 38-20). High-frequency transducers are necessary for obtaining resolution adequate for imaging normal lymph nodes. Lymph nodes are generally more easily identified in young or thin animals.[23] When abnormal, lymph nodes tend to enlarge and become more rounded and hypoechoic (Fig. 38-21).[23-25] When comparing reactive to neoplastic lymph nodes, neoplastic

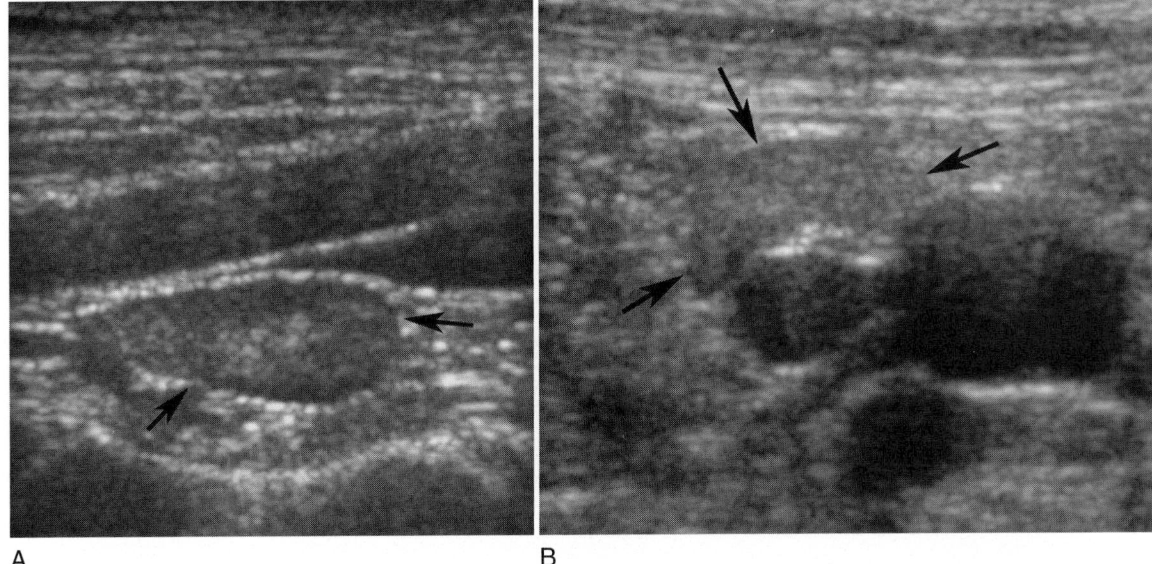

Fig. 38-20 Sagittal (A) and transverse (B) sonograms of a normal medial iliac lymph node. On the sagittal view, the lymph node *(arrows)* is seen as an elongated structure just ventral to the aorta near the aortic bifurcation. The lymph node is nearly isoechoic to surrounding structures and has a thin echogenic capsule. On the transverse image, the lymph node *(arrows)* is seen as a curved structure just ventrolateral to the aorta. Ventral is to the *top* (A and B), and the head is to the left (A).

lymph nodes tend to have a short-to-long axis ratio of more than 0.5, narrow or absent hilus, hypoechogenicity, sharp borders, a resistive index more than 0.65, a pulsatility index greater than 1.45, and often distal acoustic enhancement. These findings tend to not be present in reactive lymph nodes.[25] Fine-needle aspirates obtained with ultrasound guidance are helpful for determining the cause of lymph node enlargement, whether from metastasis or inflammation. The medial iliac lymph nodes can be found by scanning the caudal abdominal region and carefully searching the area around the terminal portions of the aorta and caudal vena cava. In some instances finding the lymph nodes by scanning in a transverse plane and looking for subtle rounded structures with thin echogenic borders (see Fig. 38-20, *B*) on either side of the aorta is easier. Alternatively, the medial iliac lymph nodes may be easier to find in the dorsal plane.[26] In the sagittal plane, the lymph nodes appear fusiform (see Fig. 38-20, *A*). The visceral lymph nodes are more often seen when abnormal and are encountered as hypoechoic nodules detected during routine scanning. They are identified as lymph nodes on the basis of their location.[23]

PANCREAS

The normal pancreas is not visualized on survey radiographs because of silhouetting with the adjacent tissues. The body (central portion) of the pancreas lies between the pylorus and the proximal descending duodenum. The right limb of the pancreas extends caudally from the body and lies adjacent to the descending duodenum. The left limb of the pancreas lies between the stomach and transverse colon, extending from the body towards the left kidney. Occasionally a poorly defined area of soft tissue opacity is seen in obese cats between the fundus of the stomach, the spleen, and the left kidney on ventrodorsal views. This may represent the left limb of the pancreas.

Abnormalities of the Pancreas

One of the more common causes of localized peritonitis is acute pancreatitis. The frequency and appearance of radiographic changes caused by acute pancreatitis are variable.[27-29] Changes can usually be localized to the right cranial abdomen, where the right lobe of the pancreas is closely associated with the proximal duodenum and pyloric antrum, or to the midline just caudal to the stomach, where the left lobe of the pancreas is located. The major radiographic abnormality is usually an increased, irregular soft tissue opacity in the right mid- to cranial abdomen, indicating localized peritonitis (Fig. 38-22, *A*). On the ventrodorsal view, the cranial right abdomen is normally more opaque than the left side, and care should be taken not to misdiagnose this normal opacity as pancreatitis.[5]

The proximal descending duodenum may be displaced ventrally or toward the right to produce a broad curvature, and the pylorus of the stomach may be displaced toward the left. Less frequently, the transverse colon may be displaced caudally. Bowel loops adjacent to the pancreas, such as the proximal descending duodenum, may contain gas; they may also have loss of tone and be dilated. This gas dilation of the duodenum may be referred to as the sentinel loop sign,[30] but this finding is not definitive evidence for pancreatitis. Spasticity of the duodenum has also been described. Foci of mineralization may occur in areas of fat necrosis.[28] Abscesses, inflammatory masses, and pseudocysts may be sequelae to pancreatitis (Box 38-3).[31-33]

Sonography of the Pancreas

Sonographic evaluation of the pancreas has become standard practice for evaluating patients suspected of having pancreatitis or pancreatic masses because the pancreas is better evaluated sonographically than radiographically. The normal pancreas is difficult to identify because of its small size, echogenicity similar to that of surrounding fat, and lack of a well-defined capsule.[34,35] In addition, gas in adjacent bowel

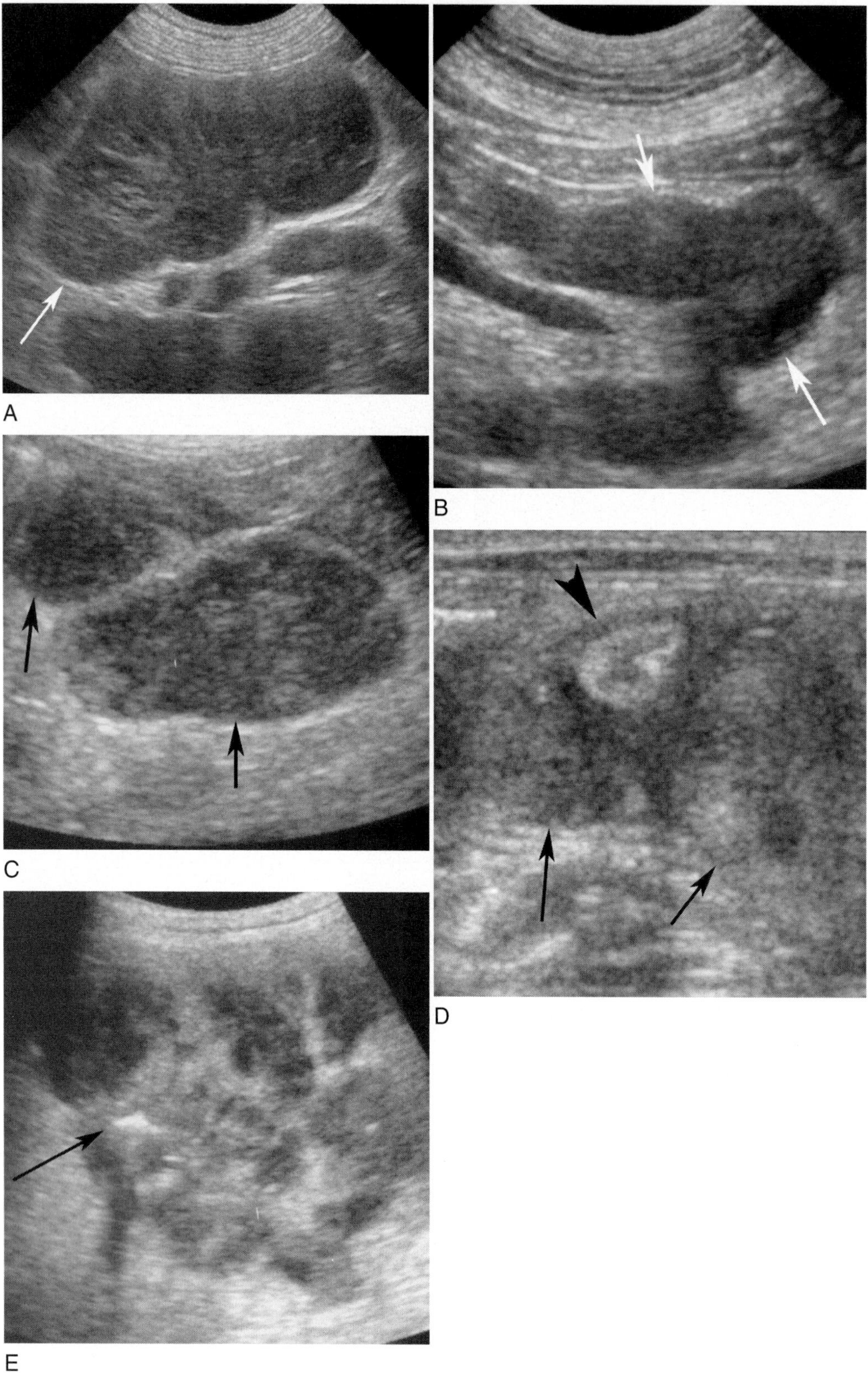

Fig. 38-21 Sonographic appearance of abnormal lymph nodes. **A,** Enlarged, hypoechoic medial iliac lymph node *(arrow)* surrounding the aorta in a dog with lymphosarcoma. **B,** Enlarged jejunal lymph node *(arrows)* in a dog with lymphosarcoma. This lymph node is hypoechoic to surrounding tissues and is irregular in shape. **C,** Enlarged jejunal lymph nodes *(arrows)* in a dog with inflammatory bowel disease. Lymphoid hyperplasia was found on evaluation of lymph node aspirates. Both nodes are hypoechoic and appear similar to those seen in the dog with lymphosarcoma (B). **D,** Enlarged ileocolic lymph nodes in a cat with lymphosarcoma. The ileum *(arrowhead)* is seen in cross section surrounded by enlarged hypoechoic lymph nodes *(arrows)*. **E,** Sonogram of a large (6 cm) mixed echogenic mass in the mid-abdomen of a dog. The mass incorporated intestinal segments. Gas *(arrow)* within one bowel segment is seen as an echogenic focus producing acoustic shadowing. The hypoechoic to nearly anechoic areas were presumed to be enlarged mesenteric lymph nodes because lymphosarcoma was diagnosed from aspirates of these structures.

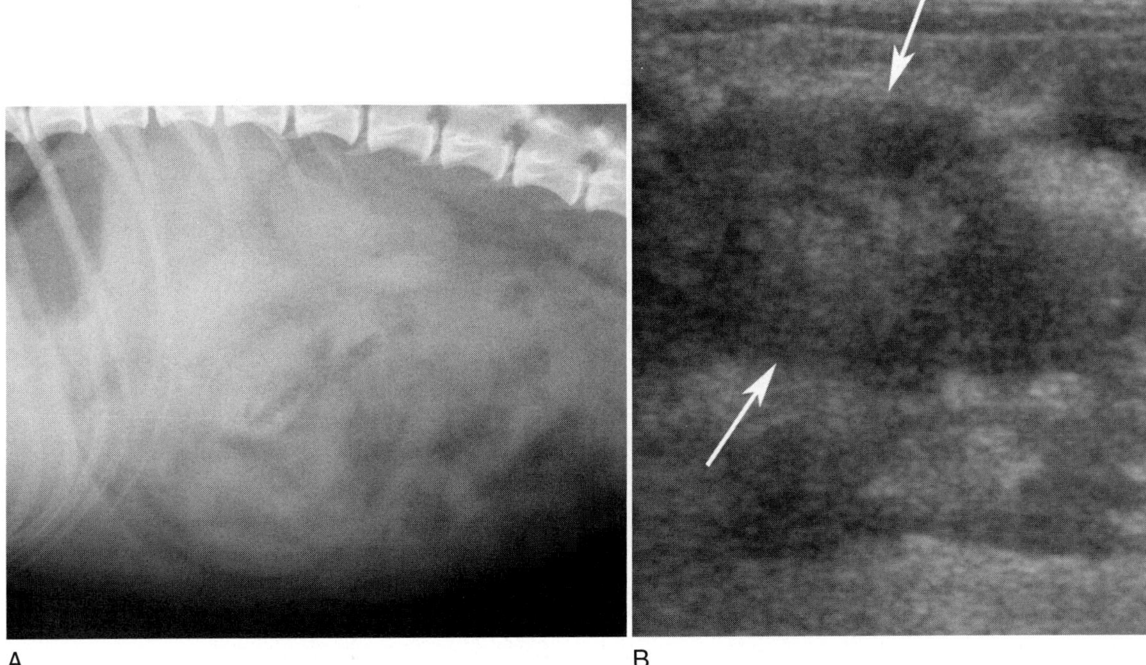

Fig. 38-22 A, Lateral survey radiograph of a dog with increased irregular soft tissue opacity in the mid-cranial to cranial abdomen as a result of localized peritonitis. This is a difficult assessment to make; recognizing this change requires high-contrast radiographs and a patient with adequate abdominal fat. B, Transverse ultrasonographic view of the right limb of the pancreas in the same dog. Note the pancreas *(arrows)* is enlarged, hypoechoic, and irregular in shape and the surrounding mesentery is hyperechoic. The diagnosis was pancreatitis.

Box • 38-3

Radiographic Signs of Pancreatitis

Increased soft tissue opacity, cranial right abdomen
Focal decrease in serosal detail, cranial right abdomen
Gas-distended descending duodenum (sentinel loop sign)
Displacement of adjacent intestinal structures
Radiographs may be normal

segments often obscures the pancreatic region. Therefore identifiable adjacent landmarks are used to scan the pancreatic area. Patients can be scanned in dorsal[36-39] or lateral recumbency[35] with the highest frequency transducer that will provide sufficient depth penetration. The body and right limb of the pancreas can be found by scanning the stomach in a sagittal (longitudinal) plane and sliding the transducer to the right until the duodenum can be identified. The right limb lies just dorsal and medial to the duodenum, medial to the right kidney, and lateral to the portal vein. Another approach is to scan the cranial pole of the right kidney in a sagittal plane and move the transducer medially or laterally until the descending duodenum is found. The left limb of the pancreas lies between the greater curvature of the stomach and the transverse colon and extends to the level of the spleen. The pancreatic area should be examined in both sagittal and transverse planes.

As mentioned, the normal pancreas is routinely difficult to identify; when seen, it has indistinct margins (Fig. 38-23).

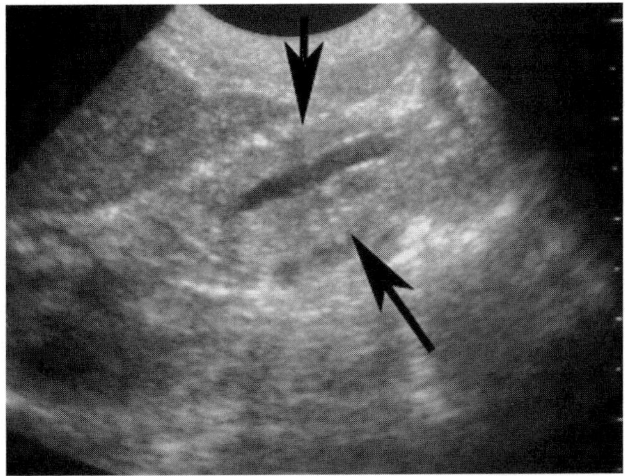

Fig. 38-23 Sagittal sonogram of the pancreatic region of a normal dog. The pancreas *(arrows)* is seen as a poorly defined structure adjacent to the liver. The pancreas is approximately the same echogenicity as the mesentery, and the hypoechoic structure in the middle of the pancreas is the pancreaticoduodenal vein.

The normal pancreas is somewhat hypoechoic, being less echogenic than the spleen[35] but more echogenic than the liver.[35,36] Occasionally, the pancreaticoduodenal vein, which lies within the pancreas and runs parallel to the duodenum, can be identified (see Fig. 38-23).[35-40] The pancreas is more likely to be identified in puppies, thin dogs, and dogs with

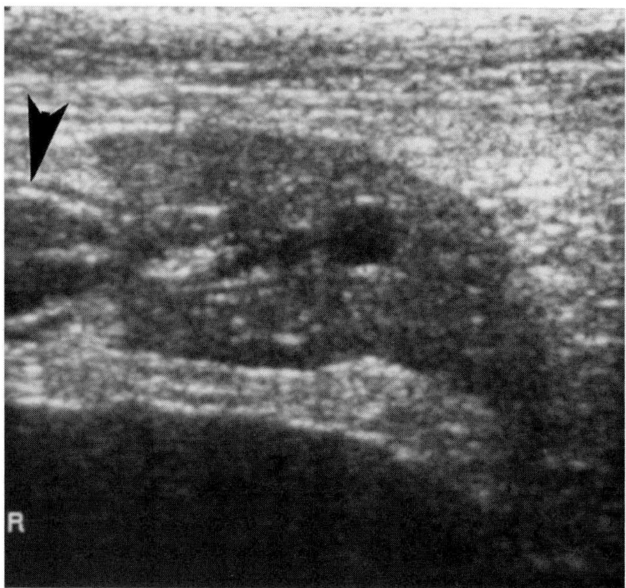

Fig. 38-24 Transverse sonogram of the right lobe of the pancreas of a dog with mild pancreatitis. The pancreas is less echogenic than normal and is seen as a triangular structure, hypoechoic to surrounding fat, just ventral to the liver and medial to the duodenum *(arrowhead)*. The pancreaticoduodenal vein is seen in cross section as a round anechoic structure within the pancreas.

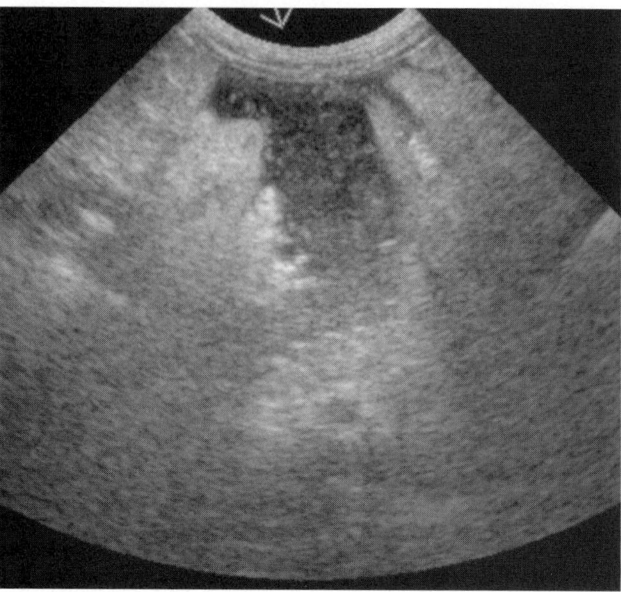

Fig. 38-25 Sagittal sonogram of the right lobe of the pancreas in a dog with pancreatitis. The pancreas is enlarged and hypoechoic, and the surrounding mesentery is hyperechoic. This is a common appearance in dogs with moderate to severe pancreatitis.

peritoneal fluid.[35] In human beings, fatty infiltration of the pancreas is associated with obesity and increased pancreatic echogenicity is associated with age, making the pancreas similar in echogenicity to surrounding fat and therefore difficult to identify.[41] In cats the normal pancreas is isoechoic to the liver and hypoechoic to the surrounding mesentery, findings that do not appear to change with age, gender, body weight, or body condition.[42,43] Normal feline pancreatic width (ventral to dorsal dimension) at the body was reported to be between 0.35 and 0.85 cm; the left limb was found to be between 0.26 to 0.95 cm. The width of the pancreatic duct was measured at 0.065 to 0.25 cm (95% confidence intervals).[42] Another study of cat pancreata found the thicknesses (in centimeters) to be 0.45 ± 0.087 for the right lobe, 0.66 ± 0.132 for the body, 0.54 ± 0.146 for the left lobe, and 0.08 ± 0.025 for the duct.[43]

Combined with history and clinical findings, ultrasound has become a useful diagnostic aid for patients with pancreatitis.[35,40,44-47] In patients with mild pancreatitis, the pancreas may be uniformly hypoechoic surrounded by more echogenic fat (Fig. 38-24).[35,45] Some believe that dilation of the pancreatic duct is more sensitive as an initial sign of pancreatitis in cats,[48] similar to children.[49] In more severe inflammation, the pancreas may be enlarged and contain irregularly shaped hypoechoic and hyperechoic areas (Fig. 38-25).[31,36,38] Other findings may include cavitary lesions, thickened duodenum, biliary obstruction, localized peritoneal fluid, and dilation of the pancreatic duct.[35,44-47,50] Hypoechoic areas within the pancreas are likely caused by inflammation, hemorrhage, necrosis, and edema.[36,46,51] Hyperechoic areas may be from fibrosis.[51] The surrounding tissue may be increased in echogenicity as a result of acoustic enhancement through hypoechoic areas or saponification of mesenteric fat.[31,35,46] In spite of these criteria, pancreatitis remains difficult to diagnose, especially in cats.[52] Differentiation of acute versus chronic pancreatitis also remains elusive.[53] However, ultrasound appears to be more sensitive than helical computed tomography in detecting pancreatitis in cats (Box 38-4).[54]

Box • 38-4

Ultrasonographic Signs of Pancreatitis

- Enlarged pancreas
- Hypoechoic pancreas
- Hyperechogenicity of the surrounding mesentery
- Possible cavitary lesions
- Possible dilation of biliary or pancreatic ducts
- May be normal

Pancreatic pseudocysts and abscesses may occur as a result of pancreatitis[4,6,33,55-59]; they appear as large, mostly anechoic masses in the pancreatic area with distal acoustic enhancement and low-level internal echoes (Fig. 38-26, *A*). They may be difficult to differentiate ultrasonographically; ultrasound-guided aspirates are helpful in differentiating the two.[6] If the location of a pancreatic mass lesion is near the opening of the common bile duct, biliary obstruction may result.[59] True pancreatic cysts are quite rare, but one has been reported in a cat. Clinical signs (vomiting) resolved after surgical removal of the cyst.[60] Another rare finding is a calculus within the pancreatic duct. A pancreatolith has been reported in a cat.[61]

Pancreatic neoplasms are uncommon but may be detected sonographically. Exocrine pancreatic carcinomas tend to invade the duodenum and often metastasize to regional lymph nodes, liver, and the peritoneum.[62] Functional islet cell tumors may be benign or malignant and should be suspected in dogs with persistent hypoglycemia. Both types of tumors may appear as discrete hypoechoic nodules or masses in the pancreatic region.[34,35,44,63] A potential source of error is misinterpretation of enlarged hypoechoic lymph nodes as pancreatic masses.[63] Islet cell tumors can be small and difficult to detect

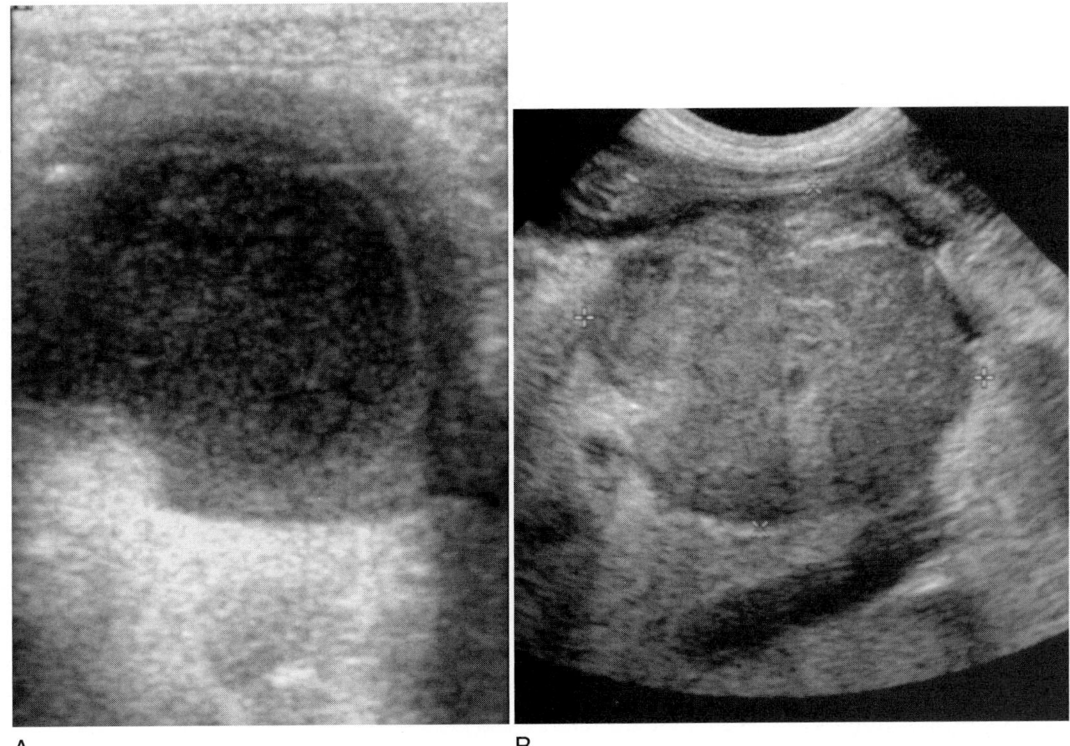

Fig. 38-26 A, Sagittal sonogram of the right limb of the pancreas in a dog. A large spherical mass is seen, with a thick hyperechoic capsule and less echogenic internal contents. This mass was confirmed to be a pancreatic abscess at surgery. **B,** Sagittal sonogram of the right limb of the pancreas in a dog. A solid, mid-level echogenic structure is seen *(cursors)* adjacent to the duodenum *(top right)*. This pancreatic mass is most consistent with the diagnosis of pancreatic neoplasia.

sonographically; therefore a normal examination does not rule out neoplasia.[35] Only approximately 30% of insulinomas can be detected with ultrasound.[64] Both pancreatitis and pancreatic neoplasms may cause biliary dilation, lymphadenopathy, and peritoneal fluid. Hyperechoic or heterogeneous masses are more often found in pancreatitis, and discrete hypoechoic nodules are more characteristic of neoplasia. Some suggest that the main sonographic features that may help distinguish between inflammation and neoplasia are findings of a diffusely hypoechoic pancreas in dogs with pancreatitis and hypoechoic nodules in dogs with neoplasms.[44] Others suggest that abnormalities of the liver and pancreas, combined with a lack of pain, are suggestive of neoplasia (see Fig. 38-26, *B*).[65]

Correlation with history, clinical signs, and other diagnostic findings may help increase suspicion of one condition versus another. In many patients, tissue sampling (e.g., fine-needle aspiration, biopsy, or surgical biopsy) is not required for adequate management. However, if a definitive diagnosis is needed, tissue sampling is necessary.[65] A single biopsy may not be sufficient because pancreatic diseases tend to be focal and randomly distributed in dogs.[66] Again, a normal sonographic examination of the pancreas does not rule out pancreatic disease, especially infiltrative or inflammatory disease. This is particularly true for cats.

ADRENAL GLANDS

The adrenal glands are located in the retroperitoneal space. The left adrenal gland is located more cranially with respect to its corresponding kidney than the right adrenal gland, which is located near the hilus of the right kidney. The right adrenal gland is bordered dorsally by the psoas minor muscle and the crus of the diaphragm, medially by the caudal vena cava, ventrolaterally by the right kidney, and cranioventrally by the right lateral liver lobe. The left adrenal gland is bordered dorsally by the psoas minor muscle, ventrally by the spleen, laterally by the left kidney, and medially by the aorta.[1] Because of their small size and soft tissue opacity, the adrenal glands are not usually seen radiographically.

Abnormalities of the Adrenal Glands

Adrenal glands may be seen radiographically only when they are enlarged or mineralized. Radiographically detectable adrenal gland enlargement may be caused by pheochromocytoma,[67] cortical carcinoma, or adenoma.[68,69] An adrenal mass should be suspected when a soft tissue or partially mineralized mass is present craniomedial to a kidney; the kidney may be displaced caudolaterally by the mass. Large left adrenal masses may displace the fundus of the stomach cranially, the transverse colon caudoventrally, and the left kidney caudally. Masses of the right adrenal gland may be more difficult to detect than those of the left because the right adrenal gland is in close proximity to the liver. Functional adrenal tumors (carcinomas and adenomas) occur with equal frequency in the right and left sides of the gland; adrenal tumors occasionally may occur bilaterally.[69,70] Functional adrenocortical neoplasms (carcinomas or adenomas) are found in 10% to 20% of dogs with Cushing syndrome.[71,72]

Dystrophic mineralization of adrenal tumors may occur and may be seen radiographically (Fig. 38-27).[68,69,73-75] Radiographically visible adrenal calcification in dogs with Cushing

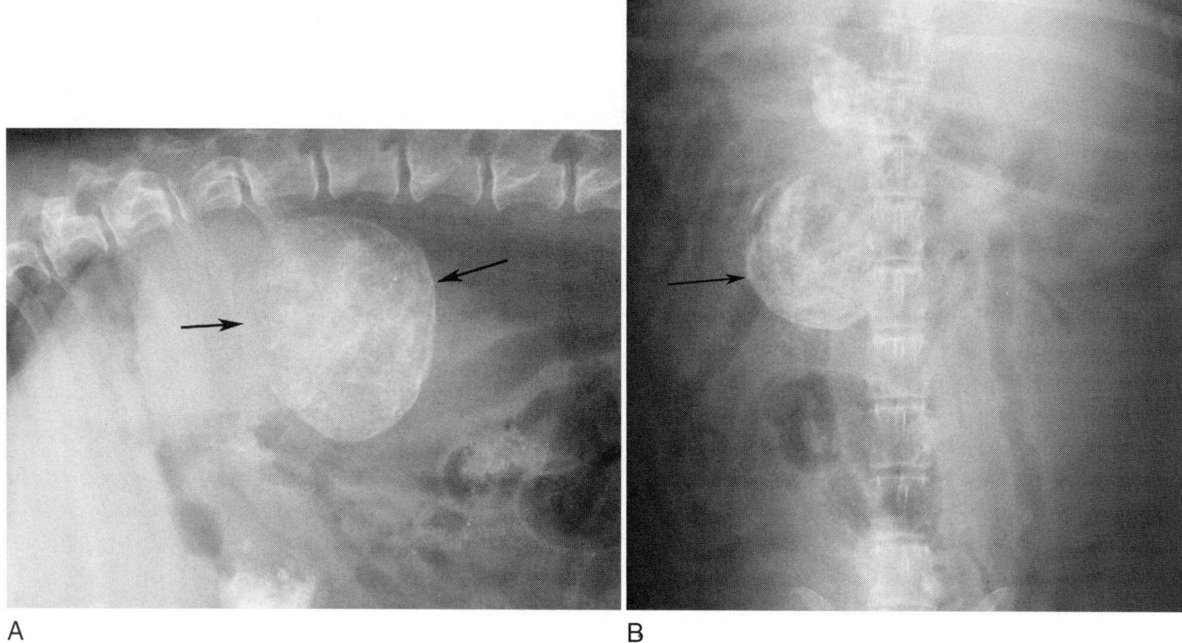

Fig. 38-27 Lateral (A) and ventrodorsal (B) abdominal radiographs of a 14-year-old dog. A large mineralized mass is located caudal to the stomach and just to the right of midline *(arrows)*. The liver is enlarged and the abdomen is pendulous. The mass is a malignant functional adrenocortical tumor causing hyperadrenocorticism. A small amount of mineralized ingesta is present within the pyloric region of the stomach.

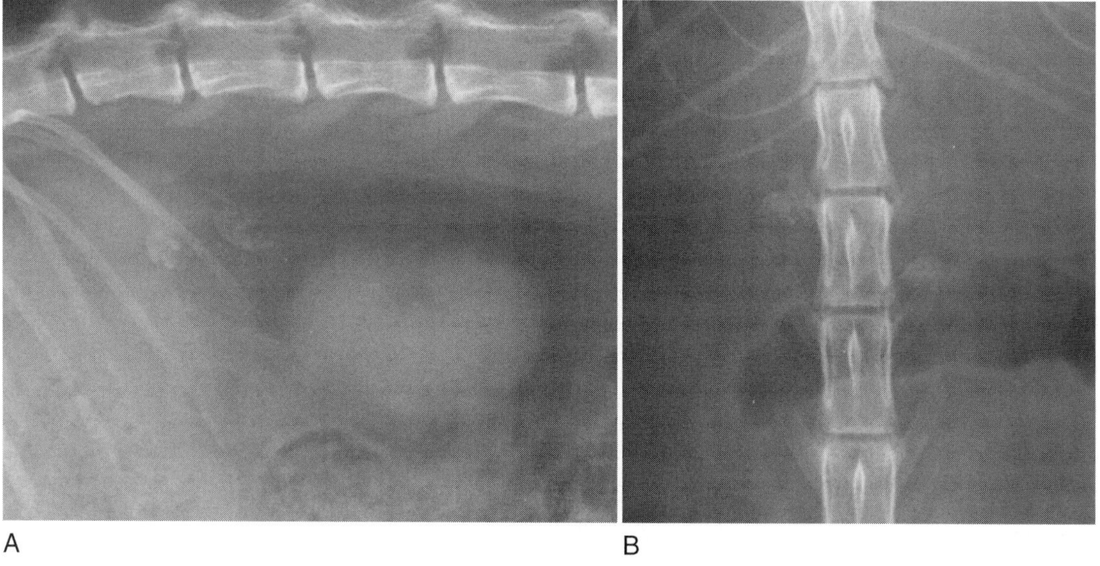

Fig. 38-28 Lateral (A) and ventrodorsal (B) radiographs (close-up views) of the abdomen of a 3-year-old Persian cat. Mineral opacities cranial to each kidney are adrenal glands with calcification of the zona reticularis. This finding is clinically insignificant.

syndrome is highly suggestive of neoplasia. In dogs with functional adrenal tumors, 92% and 54% of radiographically visible carcinomas and adenomas, respectively, were calcified.[69] In another study, adrenal calcification was found in 54% and 60% of carcinomas and adenomas, respectively.[68] Carcinomas may invade local tissues, including the caudal vena cava, and metastasize to the liver, lymph nodes, lungs, and kidneys.[69,76-78] When adrenal carcinomas are advanced, it may not be possible to determine the origin of the primary mass lesion radiographically. In such an instance, the metastases may be the major radiographic finding, although an ill-defined soft-tissue mass may be present in the craniodorsal abdomen.

Mineralization may occur in nonneoplastic adrenal glands (Fig. 38-28). Radiographically visible adrenal mineralization of unknown etiology has been reported in cats.[74,75] Histologic detection of adrenal calcification was reported in 3.5% of dogs,

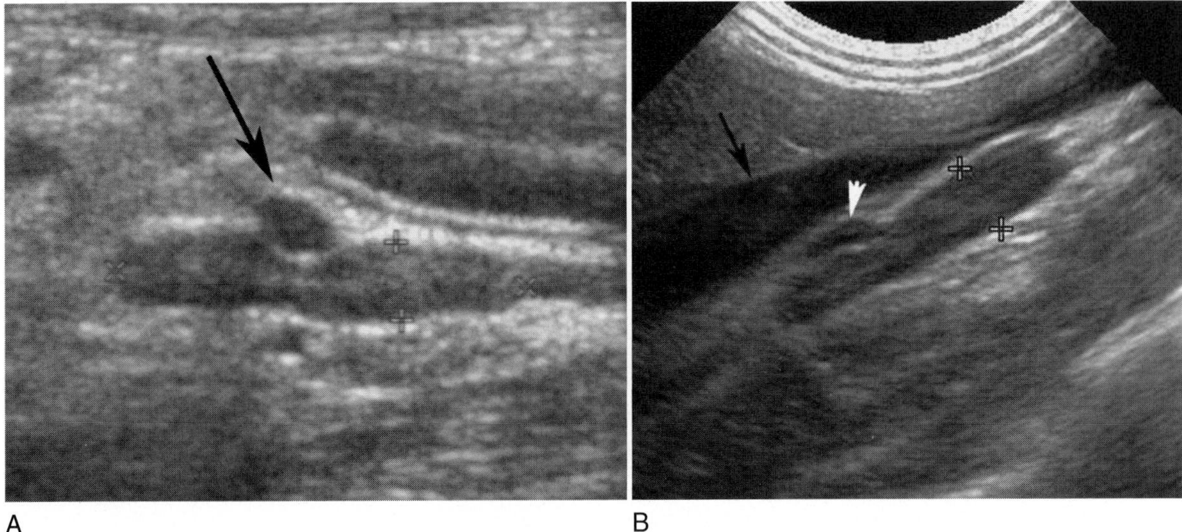

Fig. 38-29 Sagittal sonograms of the left (A) and right (B) adrenal gland of normal dogs. **A,** The left adrenal gland has a dumbbell shape and is seen just ventral to the phrenicoabdominal vein *(arrow)*. It is less echogenic than the surrounding fat. **B,** The right adrenal gland is seen as an elongated hypoechoic structure just dorsal to the caudal vena cava *(black arrow)*. The adrenal gland is surrounded by a hyperechoic capsule. The phrenicoabdominal vein *(white arrow)* is less often visualized on the right side. The head is to the left and ventral to the top.

30% of cats, and 50% of monkeys in one study[79] and in 25% of cats[80] and 1% of dogs[81] in two other studies. Calcification occurred in the zona reticularis of the adrenal cortex in the dogs, monkeys, and cats; however, in some cats, calcification affected the entire adrenal cortex and extended into the medulla.[82] Adrenal calcification was not associated with clinical findings. The cause and pathogenesis of adrenal calcification are unknown. In human beings, adrenal calcification has been associated with intraadrenal hemorrhage, tuberculosis, Addison's disease, tumors (benign and malignant), cysts, Niemann-Pick disease,[82] and Wolman's disease.[83]

Calcification of the adrenal glands appears to be relatively common in cats, but calcification in most animals is not sufficient to be seen radiographically. A mineralized adrenal gland of normal size and shape in cats and dogs is likely to have no clinical significance.

Adrenal gland dysfunction usually causes secondary changes that are visible radiographically. Radiographic findings that may be seen in patients with Cushing syndrome include hepatomegaly, bronchopulmonary mineralization, dystrophic mineralization of the skin and other soft tissues, and adrenal gland enlargement with mineralization when functional tumors are present.[68,74,75] Pulmonary arterial thrombosis has also been reported in dogs with Cushing syndrome.[84] Decreased size of the heart,[85-87] peripheral pulmonary arteries, caudal vena cava, and liver[87] has been associated with Addison's disease. Although esophageal dilation has been thought to be a feature of Addison's disease,[74] it is probably a rare finding because no evidence of esophageal dilation was found in a recent study of 22 affected dogs.[87]

Sonography of Adrenal Glands

Ultrasound is a useful imaging modality for evaluating the adrenal glands. It has been used to evaluate normal dog adrenal glands,[88-92] normal cat adrenal glands,[93,94] and dogs with hyperadrenocorticism,[69,88,90,91] hypoadrenocorticism,[95] and adrenal masses.[96,97] However, the ability to image the glands accurately depends highly on the quality of the equipment, operator experience, and size of the patient. The highest frequency transducer that produces adequate penetration is recommended. If possible, 7.5 MHz or higher transducers should be used, but lower frequency transducers may be necessary to obtain adequate penetration in larger dogs. The adrenal glands are more easily imaged in smaller patients in which higher resolution probes can be used to obtain quality images with adequate penetration. Overlying bowel gas often obscures the adrenal glands.

Most patients are scanned in dorsal recumbency. To find the left adrenal gland, scan the cranial pole of the left kidney in a sagittal plane, then slide the transducer medially to the aorta. The left adrenal gland lies just ventrolateral to the aorta between the cranial mesenteric and renal arteries. Occasionally the adrenal gland may be located slightly cranial to the celiac and cranial mesenteric arteries. To obtain a full longitudinal view of the adrenal gland, the probe may need to be rotated so the aorta is imaged obliquely. The left adrenal gland of the normal dog is usually described as shaped like a peanut shell[98] or dumbbell (Fig. 38-29, *A*).[99] Care should be taken to not confuse the adrenal gland with a lymph node. Both adrenal glands of dogs and cats are hypoechoic to the surrounding fat and hypoechoic or isoechoic when compared with the renal cortex. Occasionally the adrenal gland has a layered appearance, with the medulla being more echogenic than the cortex. This layered appearance has been ascribed to both normal[94,100] and hyperplastic glands.[101] A hyperechoic capsule can often be identified (see Fig. 38-29, *B*).[94,102] The right adrenal gland is more difficult to image, especially in larger dogs.[103] After the cranial pole of the right kidney is scanned in a sagittal plane, the transducer is moved medially to find the caudal vena cava. The right adrenal gland lies dorsolateral to the caudal vena cava and cranial to the renal vein. The phrenicoabdominal veins cross the ventral surfaces of both adrenal glands and can occasionally be identified with high-resolution transducers. The shape of the right adrenal gland of the dog is different from that of the left. The right has been described as having a comma-shaped[45] or bent arrow conformation.[99] In the authors' experience, many large-breed dogs have adrenal glands with an elongated, thin shape. This is suspected to be a normal variant. In cats, both adrenal glands are oblong and oval to bean shaped (see Fig. 38-29, *B*).[93,94] Overlying bowel gas obscuring the adrenal glands is a major problem, especially on the right side. If this happens, the patient or transducer can be repositioned in an attempt to move the overlying bowel. Sedation may be helpful in some patients who resist abdominal compression by the transducer. Imaging the adrenal glands in the dorsal plane is an alternate method of avoiding the overlying bowel gas problem and is preferred by some sonographers.[102] An intercostal approach may be necessary to image the right gland. Both adrenal glands can be imaged in a dorsal plane with the patient in lateral recumbency. Imaging the dependent adrenal gland is often made easier by placing the transducer under the patient and directing the sound beam upwards.

Ultrasonographic determination of adrenal size has been used as an aid for evaluating dogs suspected of having hyperadrenocorticism and hypoadrenocorticism. Adrenal size may depend on the age of the dog,[90] with middle-aged and older dogs having larger glands. The thickness (ventrodorsal dimension) of the gland is more accurate than adrenal length (craniocaudal dimension) or adrenal width (mediolateral dimension) in estimating gross adrenal size.[89] Adrenal gland length is proportional to body weight, but the diameter (thickness or width) is not.[88] Therefore cross-sectional measurements are more valuable than length in the assessment of adrenal gland size. Adrenal gland thickness greater than 0.6 cm in small-breed and 0.7 cm in middle-aged to older large-breed dogs has been used as the criterion for maximum normal adrenal gland size.[90] However, adrenal gland measurements alone should not be used to diagnose abnormalities because considerable overlap of adrenal size exists in normal and abnormal dogs. The shape of the glands, the response of the patient to pituitary-adrenal axis testing, and the patient's clinical signs must be correlated with the size of the adrenal glands when making a diagnosis.

The use of ultrasound as a screening test for hyperadrenocorticism is not recommended,[104] although ultrasound is considered useful in differentiating pituitary-dependent hyperadrenocorticism (PDH) and functional adrenocortical neoplasia.[88,89,105] In dogs with PDH, the adrenal glands have a plump appearance; they are bilaterally enlarged, uniformly hypoechoic, and normally shaped (Fig. 38-30).[88,90,91,105] Normal adrenal gland size does not rule out PDH.[90] Adrenal gland tumors cause gland enlargement with loss of normal shape and a change in echotexture (Figs. 38-31, 38-32, and 38-33). Tumors may occur bilaterally but are most often unilateral.[96,97] In dogs with functional adrenocortical tumors, the contralateral adrenal gland is often of normal size and can be imaged with ultrasound.[96,97,105] This is contrary to previous suggestions that the contralateral adrenal gland would atrophy.[45] Ultrasound is not useful in differentiating benign and malignant lesions because no consistent appearance for a tumor type exists.[96] Mineralization may be seen in both benign and malignant neoplasms as well as in adrenocortical hyperplasia.[90,96] In one report, pheochromocytomas and adenocarcinomas tended to be rounded masses; adenomas, hyperplasia, and adrenal metastasis tended to appear as nodules.[96] Because PDH-induced nodular cortical hyperplasia may appear similar to small functional adrenocortical tumors, ultrasound is not useful in differentiating the two.[90] Screening for hyperadrenocorticism by imaging of the adrenal glands with computed tomography or magnetic resonance imaging is also not recommended, although these modalities may be useful for imaging the pituitary gland.[104]

Ultrasound is helpful in evaluating extension of tumors into surrounding tissues, especially the caudal vena cava. The extension of the mass into the caudal vena cava may extend to the right atrium.[106] Lymphoma of the adrenal glands was

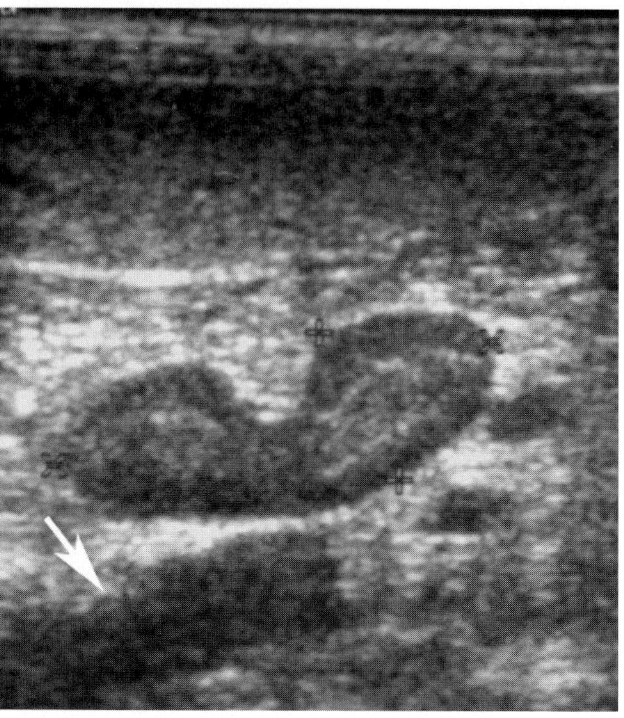

Fig. 38-30 Sagittal sonogram of the left adrenal gland *(cursors)* of a Dachshund with pituitary-dependent hyperadrenocorticism. The adrenal gland has a plump appearance but is normally shaped. The gland is enlarged measuring 2.59 cm in length and 0.97 cm in thickness. The hypoechoic cortex can be differentiated from the more echogenic medulla. This layered appearance has been described in normal dogs and in dogs with hyperadrenocorticism. The *arrow* points to the aorta.

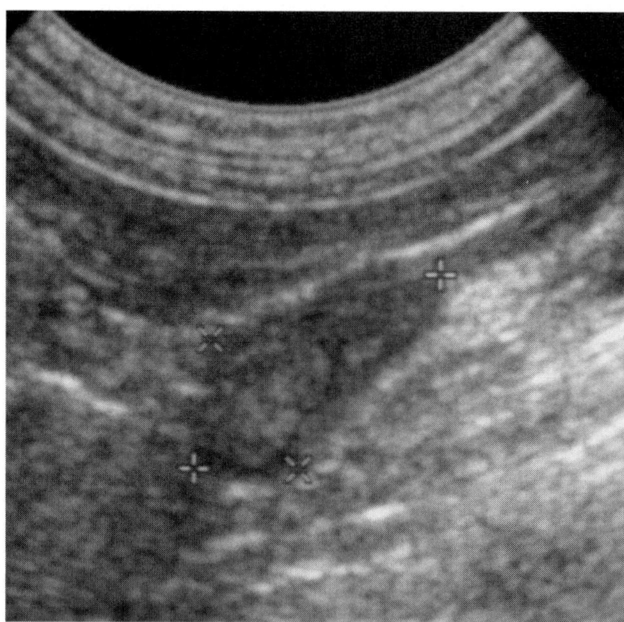

Fig. 38-31 Sagittal sonogram of the left adrenal gland *(cursors)* of a 12-year-old mixed-breed dog. A hyperechoic nodule is seen in the cranial pole of the adrenal gland. The ultrasonographic appearance of this nodule is not specific and could be caused by neoplasia (varying types), granuloma, or nodular hyperplasia.

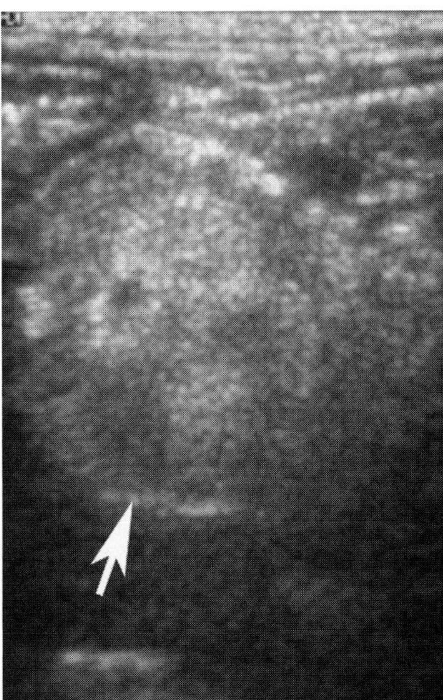

Fig. 38-32 Transverse sonogram of the right adrenal gland *(arrow)* of a 13-year-old Shih Tzu with hyperadrenocorticism. The adrenal gland is enlarged, rounded, and of mixed echogenicity, containing hyperechoic nodules. Histopathologically, the adrenal gland contained myelolipomas and adenomas.

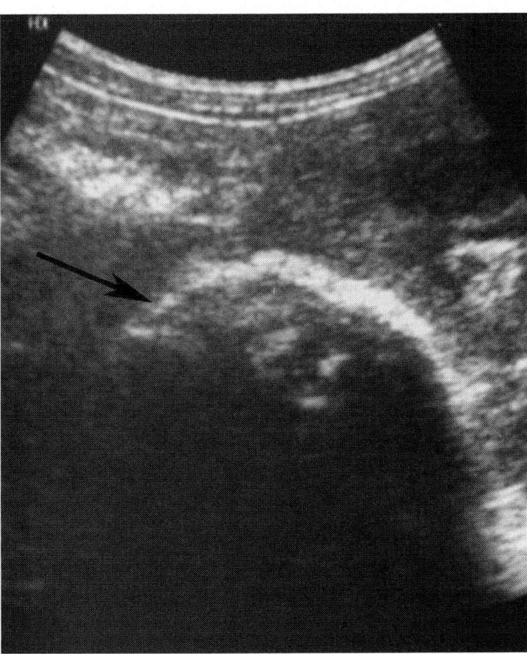

Fig. 38-33 Sagittal sonogram of the left adrenal gland of the same dog as that in Figure 38-27. The adrenal gland is seen as a large, curvilinear hyperechoic line with distal acoustic shadowing, consistent with the appearance of mineral. The diagnosis is adrenocortical tumor.

reported to appear as hypoechoic adrenal glands in one cat and a mass involving the adrenal glands and midline structures in another patient.[107] Another cat with a hypoechoic adrenal mass was demonstrated to have primary hyperaldosteronism.[108] Ultrasound-guided biopsy and fine-needle aspiration of the adrenal gland are not commonly performed in veterinary medicine, but they have been reported without complication in a small number of patients.[96,109-111] Many clinicians are wary of aspiration of adrenal masses because if the mass is a pheochromocytoma, the possibility exists of stimulating a hypertensive crisis from a massive release of catecholamines. Adrenal gland tumors have also been reported to hemorrhage spontaneously, leading to retroperitoneal hemorrhage[112] or complex masses of the adrenal glands (Box 38-5).[96]

Box • 38-5

Differential Diagnosis for Adrenal Masses

Adenoma
Nodular hyperplasia
Adrenocortical carcinoma
May be:
- Metabolically inactive
- Cortisol secreting
- Aldosterone secreting

Granuloma
Metastatic neoplasia
Pheochromocytoma

Treatment of patients with hyperadrenocorticism with either mitotane or the newer drug trilostane is common. Trilostane causes an increase in adrenal gland size,[113,114] with the maximum size seen at 6 weeks after initiation of therapy.[113] The differentiation of the layers within the adrenal glands is increased with the outer hypoechoic zone being increased in echogenicity and the inner hyperechoic zone being decreased in echogenicity. After 6 months to 1 year of treatment, the size of the adrenal glands is unchanged but the shape may become irregular and the parenchyma may become inhomogeneous with an inability to discern the layers of the glands.[113,114] These changes may be caused by coagulative necrosis.[115] Mitotane causes adrenal gland heterogeneity, presumably from necrosis.[100] Mitotane may also cause the adrenal glands to become smaller, in contrast to the effects of trilostane.[116]

In a study to determine the sensitivity and specificity of endogenous adrenocorticotropic hormone (ACTH) concentration and ultrasonography to determine the cause of hyperadrenocorticism (pituitary dependent [PDH] vs. adrenal dependent [ADH]), the size of the adrenal glands in dogs with PDH was right length, 1.05 to 4.0 cm (median, 2.22 cm); right width, 0.52 to 1.43 cm (median, 0.85 cm); left length, 1.1 to 3.81 cm (median, 2.08 cm); left width, 0.35 to 1.43 cm (median, 0.85 cm). The adrenal glands were hypoechoic to the renal cortex and of subjectively normal shape. In dogs with ADH the unaffected gland had a mean length of 2.19 cm and a mean width of 0.78 cm. This was only slightly smaller than the glands of PDH patients. PDH was diagnosed by ultrasound if both adrenal glands were of similar size and normal shape. If one was normal and the other was abnormally enlarged and rounded, a diagnosis of ADH was made. Both tests (ACTH and ultrasound) were found to have a sensitivity of 100% and a specificity of 95% in differentiating PDH from ADH in dogs with a previous diagnosis of hyperadrenocorticism.[105] Although uncommonly reported, enlarged adrenal glands can be found in patients with oversecretion of sex hormones.[117]

In six dogs with hypoadrenocorticism, the adrenal glands were measurably smaller than the adrenal glands of normal dogs.[95] This was a significant change in the left adrenal gland in which the median thickness was 0.24 cm in abnormal dogs and 0.41 cm in normal dogs. Cats with interstitial cystitis have been suggested to have primary adrenal insufficiency because these animals have small adrenal glands at necropsy. Antemortem imaging findings in these animals were not reported.[118]

REFERENCES

1. Evans HE, Christensen GC: *Miller's anatomy of the dog,* ed 3, Philadelphia, 1993, WB Saunders.
2. Johnson DE, Christie BA: The retroperitoneum in dogs: anatomy and clinical significance, *Comp Contin Educ Prac Vet* 12:1027, 1990.
3. Johnson PR, Greenwood MRC: The adipose tissue. In Weiss L editor: *Cell and tissue biology: a textbook of histology,* ed 6, Baltimore, 1988, Urban and Schwarzenberg.
4. Ettinger SJ, Barrett KA: Ascites, peritonitis, and other causes of abdominal distention. In Ettinger SJ, Feldman EC, editors: *Textbook of veterinary internal medicine,* ed 4, Philadelphia, 1995, WB Saunders.
5. O'Brien TR: *The radiographic diagnosis of abdominal disorders of the dog and cat,* Philadelphia, 1978, WB Saunders.
6. Boen ST: *Peritoneal dialysis in clinical practice,* Springfield, IL, 1964, Charles C. Thomas.
7. Johnston DE, Christie BA: The retroperitoneum in dogs: retroperitoneal infections, *Comp Contin Educ Prac Vet* 12:1035, 1990.
8. Roush JK, Bjorling DE, Lord P: Diseases of the retroperitoneal space in the dog and cat, *J Am Anim Hosp Assoc* 26:47, 1990.
9. Root CR, Lord PF: Peritoneal carcinomatosis in the dog and cat: its radiographic appearance, *J Am Vet Radiol Soc* 12:54, 1971.
10. Suter PF, Olsson SE: The diagnosis of injuries to the intestines, gall bladder and bile ducts in the dog, *J Small Anim Pract* 11:575, 1970.
11. Probst CW, Stickle RL, Bartlett PC: Duration of pneumoperitoneum in the dog, *Am J Vet Res* 47:176, 1986.
12. Guffy M: *A radiological study of hydroperitoneum and pneumoperitoneum in the dog [thesis],* Fort Collins, CO, 1966, Colorado State University.
13. Lamb CR, Kleine LJ, McMillan MC: Diagnosis of calcification on abdominal radiographs, *Vet Radiol* 32:211, 1991.
14. Schwarz T, Morandi F, Gnudi G et al: Nodular fat necrosis in the feline and canine abdomen, *Vet Radiol Ultrasound* 41:335, 2000.
15. Yaphe W, Forrester SD: Renal secondary hyperparathyroidism, pathophysiology, diagnosis, and treatment, *Comp Contin Educ Prac Vet* 16:73, 1994.
16. Johnson CA: Disorders of pregnancy, *Vet Clin N Am Small Anim Pract* 18;477, 1986.
17. Huntley K, Fraser J, Gibbs C et al: The radiological features of canine Cushing's syndrome: a review of forty-eight small cases, *J Small Anim Pract* 23:369, 1982.
18. Crosbie PR, Boyce WM, Platzer ED et al: Diagnostic procedures and treatment of eleven dogs with peritoneal infections caused by *Mesocestoides* spp, *J Am Vet Med Assoc* 213;1578, 1998.
19. Caruso KJ, James MP, Fisher D et al: Cytologic diagnosis of peritoneal cestodiasis in dogs caused by *Mesocestoides* sp, *Vet Clin Pathol* 32:50, 2003.
20. Boysen SR, Tidwell AS, Pennick DG: Ultrasonographic findings in dogs and cats with gastrointestinal perforation, *Vet Radiol Ultrasound* 44:556, 2003.
21. Fischetti AJ, Saunders HM, Drobatz KJ: Pneumatosis in canine gastric dilatation-volvulus syndrome, *Vet Radiol Ultrasound* 45:279, 2004.
22. Leav I, Ling GV: Adenocarcinoma of the canine prostate, *Cancer* 22:1329, 1968.
23. Pugh CR: Ultrasonographic examination of abdominal lymph nodes in the dog, *Vet Radiol Ultrasound* 35:110, 1994.
24. Homco LD: Lymph nodes. In Green RW, editor: *Small animal ultrasound,* Philadelphia, 1996, Lippincott-Raven.
25. Nyman HT, Kristensen AT, Flagstad A et al: A review of the sonographic assessment of tumor metastasis in liver and superficial lymph nodes, *Vet Radiol Ultrasound* 45:438, 2004.
26. Llabres-Diaz FJ: Ultrasonography of the medial iliac lymph nodes in the dog, *Vet Radiol Ultrasound* 45:156, 2004.
27. Gibbs C, Denny HR, Minter HM et al: Radiological features of inflammatory conditions of the canine pancreas, *J Small Anim Pract* 13:531, 1972.
28. Kleine LJ, Hornbuckle WE: Acute pancreatitis: The radiographic findings in 182 dogs, *J Am Vet Radiol Soc* 19:102, 1978.
29. Suter PF, Lowe R: Acute pancreatitis in the dog: a clinical study with emphasis on radiographic diagnosis, *Acta Radiol (Stockh)* 319(suppl):195, 1970.
30. Davis S, Parbhoo SP, Gibson MJ: The plain abdominal radiograph in acute pancreatitis, *Clin Radiol* 31:87, 1980.
31. Edwards DF, Bauer MS, Walker MA et al: Pancreatic masses in seven dogs following acute pancreatitis, *J Am Anim Hosp Assoc* 26:189, 1990.
32. Salisbury SK, Lantz GC, Nelson RW et al: Pancreatic abscesses in dogs: six cases (1978-1986), *J Am Vet Med Assoc* 193:1004, 1988.
33. Wolfsheimer KJ, Hedlund CS, Pechman RD: Pancreatic pseudocyst in a dog with chronic pancreatitis, *Canine Pract* 16:6, 1991.
34. Lamb CR: Abdominal ultrasonography in small animals: examination of the liver, spleen, and pancreas, *J Small Anim Pract* 31:6, 1990.
35. Saunders HM: Ultrasonography of the pancreas, *Probl Vet Med* 3:583, 1991.
36. Nyland TG, Mulvany MH, Strombeck DR: Ultrasonic features of experimentally induced, acute pancreatitis in the dog, *Vet Radiol* 24:260, 1983.
37. Nyland TG, Mattoon JS, Herrgesell EJ et al: Pancreas. In Nyland TG, Mattoon JS, editors: *Small animal diagnostic ultrasound,* Philadelphia, 2002, WB Saunders.
38. Murtaugh RJ, Herring DS, Jacobs RM et al: Pancreatic ultrasonography in dogs with experimentally induced acute pancreatitis, *Vet Radiol* 26:27, 1985.
39. Mahaffey MB: The pancreas. In Cartee RE, editor: *Practical veterinary ultrasound,* Philadelphia, 1995, Williams & Wilkins, p 52.
40. Lamb CR: Recent developments in diagnostic imaging of the gastrointestinal tract of the dog and cat, *Vet Clin North Am Small Anim Pract* 29:307, 1999.
41. Worthen NJ, Beabeau D: Normal pancreatic echogenicity: relation to age and body fat, *Am J Radiol* 139:1095, 1982.
42. Larson MM, Panciera DL, Ward DL et al: Age-related changes in the ultrasound appearance of the normal feline pancreas, *Vet Radiol Ultrasound* 46:238, 2005.
43. Etue SM, Penninck DG, Labato MA et al: Ultrasonography of the normal feline pancreas and associated anatomic landmarks: a prospective study of 20 cats, *Vet Radiol Ultrasound* 42:330, 2001.

44. Lamb CR, McEvoy FJ: Comparison of ultrasonographic findings in canine pancreatitis and pancreatic neoplasia [abstract], *Vet Radiol Ultrasound* 36:434, 1995.
45. Saunders HM, Pugh CR, Rhodes WH: Expanding applications of abdominal ultrasonography, *J Am Anim Hosp Assoc* 28:369, 1992.
46. Homco LD: Pancreas. In Green RW, editor: *Small animal ultrasound*, Philadelphia, 1996, Lippincott-Raven, p 177.
47. Simpson KW, Shiroma JT, Biller DS et al: Antemortem diagnosis of pancreatitis in four cats, *J Small Anim Pract* 35:93, 1994.
48. Wall M, Biller DS, Schoning P et al. Pancreatitis in a cat demonstrating pancreatic duct dilatation ultrasonographically, *J Am Anim Hosp Assoc* 37:49, 2001.
49. Siegel MJ, Martin KW, Worthington JL: Normal and abnormal pancreas in children: US studies, *Radiology* 165:15, 1987.
50. Lamb CR: Dilation of the pancreatic duct: an ultrasonographic finding in acute pancreatitis, *J Small Anim Pract* 30:410, 1989.
51. Saunders HM: *Ultrasonographic detection and characterization of pancreatitis in dogs*, Proceedings of the American College of Veterinary Radiology Annual Meeting, Nov 29-Dec 1, 1990, Chicago, IL, p 66.
52. Saunders HM, VanWinkle TJ, Drobatz K et al: Ultrasonographic findings in cats with clinical, gross pathologic, and histologic evidence of acute pancreatic necrosis: 20 cases (1994-2001), *J Am Vet Med Assoc* 221:1724, 2002.
53. Ferreri JA, Hardam E, Kimmel SE et al: Clinical differentiation of acute necrotizing from chronic nonsuppurative pancreatitis in cats: 63 cases (1996-2001), *J Am Vet Med Assoc* 223:469, 2003.
54. Forman MA, Marks SL, DeCock HEV et al: Evaluation of serum feline pancreatic lipase immunoreactivity and helical computed tomography versus conventional testing for the diagnosis of feline pancreatitis, *J Vet Intern Med* 18:807, 2004.
55. VanEnkevort BA, O'Brien RT, Young KM: Pancreatic pseudocysts in 4 dogs and 2 cats: ultrasonographic and clinicopathologic findings, *J Vet Intern Med* 13:309, 1999.
56. Rutgers C, Herring DS, Orton C: Pancreatic pseudocyst associated with acute pancreatitis in a dog: ultrasonographic diagnosis, *J Am Anim Hosp Assoc* 21:411, 1985.
57. Hines BL, Salisbury SK, Jakovljevic S et al: Pancreatic pseudocyst associated with chronic-active necrotizing pancreatitis in a cat, *J Am Anim Hosp Assoc* 32:147, 1996.
58. Barnhart MD, Smeak D: Pericolonic mass containing chyle as a presumed sequela to chronic pancreatitis in a dog, *J Am Vet Med Assoc* 212:70, 1998.
59. Marchevsky AM, Yovich JC, Wyatt KM: Pancreatic pseudocyst causing extrahepatic biliary obstruction in a dog, *Aust Vet J* 78:99, 2000.
60. Coleman MG, Robson MC, Harvey C: Pancreatic cyst in a cat, *N Zealand Vet J* 53:157, 2005.
61. Bailiff NL, Norris CR, Seguin B et al: Pancreatolithiasis and pancreatic pseudobladder associated with pancreatitis in a cat, *J Am Anim Hosp Assoc* 40:69, 2004.
62. Jubb KVF, Kennedy PC, Palmer N: The pancreas. In Jubb KVF, Kennedy PC, Palmer N, editors: *Pathology of domestic animals, vol 2*, ed 3, Orlando, FL, 1985, Academic Press.
63. Lamb CR, Simpson KW, Boswood A et al: Ultrasonography of pancreatic neoplasia in the dog: a retrospective review of 16 cases, *Vet Rec* 137:65, 1995.
64. Feldman EC, Nelson RW: *Canine and feline endocrinology and reproduction*, Philadelphia, 2004, WB Saunders.
65. Bennett PF, Hahn KA, Toal RL et al: Ultrasonographic and cytopathological diagnosis of exocrine pancreatic carcinoma in the dog and cat, *J Am Anim Hosp Assoc* 37:466, 2001.
66. Newman S, Steiner J, Woosley K et al. Localization of pancreatic inflammation and necrosis in dogs, *J Vet Intern Med* 18:488, 2004.
67. Schaer M: Pheochromocytoma in a dog: a case report, *J Am Anim Hosp Assoc* 16:583, 1980.
68. Pennick DG, Feldman EC, Nyland TG: Radiographic features of canine hyper-adrenocorticism caused by autonomously functioning adrenocortical tumors: 23 cases (1978-1986), *J Am Vet Med Assoc* 192:1604, 1988.
69. Reusch CE, Feldman EC: Canine hyperadrenocorticism due to adrenocortical neoplasia, *J Vet Intern Med* 5:3, 1991.
70. Ford SL, Feldman EC, Nelson RW: Hyperadrenocorticism caused by bilateral adrenocortical neoplasia in dogs: four cases (1983-1988), *J Am Vet Med Assoc* 202:789, 1993.
71. Meijer JC: Canine hyperadrenocorticism. In Kirk RW, editor: *Current veterinary therapy*, Philadelphia, 1980, WB Saunders.
72. Owens JM, Drucker WD: Hyperadrenocorticism in the dog: canine Cushing's syndrome, *Vet Clin North Am Small Anim Pract* 7:583, 1977.
73. Huntley K, Frazer J, Gibbs C et al: The radiological features of canine Cushing's syndrome: a review of forty-eight cases, *J Small Anim Pract* 23:369, 1982.
74. Ticer JW: Roentgen signs of endocrine disease, *Vet Clin North Am* 7:465, 1977.
75. Widmer WR, Guptill L: Imaging techniques for facilitating diagnosis of hyper-adrenocorticism in dogs and cats, *J Am Vet Med Assoc* 206:1857, 1995.
76. Jubb KVF, Kennedy PC: *Pathology of domestic animals*, ed 2, New York, 1970, Academic Press, p 427.
77. Kelly DF, Darke PGG: Cushing's syndrome in the dog, *Vet Rec* 98:28, 1976.
78. Siegel ET: *Endocrine disorders of the dog*, Philadelphia, 1977, Lea & Febiger, p 166.
79. Ross MA, Gainer JH, Innes JRM: Dystrophic calcification in the adrenal glands of monkeys, cats, and dogs, *Arch Pathol Lab Med* 60:655, 1955.
80. Marine D: Calcification of the suprarenal glands of cats, *J Exp Med* 43:495, 1926.
81. Rajan A, Mohiyuddeen S: Pathology of the adrenal gland in canines (*Canis familiaris*), *Indian J Anim Sci* 44:123, 1974.
82. Bergman SM, Scouras GC: Incidental bilateral adrenal calcification, *Urology* 22:665, 1983.
83. Raafat F, Hashemian MP, Abrishami MA: Wolman's disease: report of two new cases with a review of the literature, *Am J Clin Pathol* 59:490, 1973.
84. Burns MG, Kelly AB, Hornof WJ et al: Pulmonary artery thrombosis in three dogs with hyperadrenocorticism, *J Am Vet Med Assoc* 178:388, 1981.
85. Rendano VT, Alexander JE: Heart size changes in experimentally induced adrenal insufficiency in the dog: a radiographic study, *J Am Vet Radiol Soc* 17:57, 1976.
86. Scott DW: Hyperadrenocorticism (hyperadrenocorticoidism, hyperadrenocorticalism, Cushing's disease, Cushing's syndrome), *Vet Clin North Am* 9:3, 1979.
87. Melian C, Stefanacci J, Peterson ME et al: Radiographic findings in dogs with naturally-occurring primary hypoadrenocorticism. *J Am Anim Hosp Assoc* 35:208, 1999.
88. Barthez PY, Nyland TG, Feldman EC: Ultrasonographic evaluation of the adrenal glands in dogs, *J Am Vet Med Assoc* 207:1180, 1995.

89. Grooters AM, Biller DS, Miyabayashi T et al: Evaluation of routine abdominal ultrasonography as a technique for imaging the canine adrenal glands, *J Am Anim Hosp Assoc* 30:457, 1994.
90. Grooters AM, Biller DS, Theisen SK et al: Ultrasonographic characteristics of the adrenal glands in dogs with pituitary-dependent hyperadrenocorticism: comparison with normal dogs, *J Vet Intern Med* 10:110, 1996.
91. Hoerauf A, Reusch C: Ultrasonographic evaluation of the adrenal glands in healthy dogs, dogs with no evidence of endocrine disease, and dogs with Cushing's disease [abstract], *Vet Radiol Ultrasound* 36:434, 1995.
92. Douglass JP, Berry CR, James S: Ultrasonographic adrenal gland measurements in dogs without evidence of adrenal disease, *Vet Radiol Ultrasound* 38:124, 1997.
93. Cartee RE, Finn-Bodner ST, Gray BW: Ultrasound examination of the feline adrenal gland, *J Diagn Med Sonog* 9:327, 1993.
94. Zimmer C, Hoerauf A, Reusch C: Ultrasonographic examination of the adrenal gland and evaluation of the hypophyseal-adrenal axis in 20 cats, *J Small Anim Pract* 41:156, 2000.
95. Hoerauf A, Reusch C: Ultrasonographic evaluation of adrenal glands in six dogs with hypoadrenocorticism, *J Am Anim Hosp Assoc* 35:214, 1999.
96. Besso JG, Penninck DG, Gliatto JM: Retrospective ultrasonographic evaluation of adrenal lesions in 26 dogs, *Vet Radiol Ultrasound* 38:448, 1997.
97. Hoerauf A, Reusch C: Ultrasonographic characteristics of both adrenal glands in 15 dogs with functional adrenocortical tumors, *J Am Anim Hosp Assoc* 35:193, 1999.
98. Tidwell AS, Penninck DG, Besso JG: Imaging of adrenal gland disorders, *Vet Clin North Am Small Anim Pract* 27:237, 1997.
99. Schelling CG: Ultrasonography of the adrenal glands, *Probl Vet Med Ultrasound* 3:604, 1991.
100. Nyland TG, Mattoon JS, Herrgesell EJ et al: Adrenal glands. In Nyland TG, Mattoon JS, editors: *Small animal diagnostic ultrasound*, Philadelphia, 2002, WB Saunders.
101. Homco LD: Adrenal glands. In Green RW, editor: *Small animal ultrasound*, Philadelphia, 1996, Lippincott-Raven.
102. Barthez PY, Nyland TG, Feldman EC: Ultrasonography of the adrenal glands in the dog, cat, and ferret, *Vet Clin North Am Small Anim Pract* 28:869, 1998.
103. Grooters AM, Biller DS, Merryman J: Ultrasonographic parameters of normal canine adrenal glands: comparison to necropsy findings, *Vet Radiol Ultrasound* 36:126, 1995.
104. Behrend EN, Kemppainen, RJ: Diagnosis of canine hyperadrenocorticism, *Vet Clin N Am Small Anim Pract* 31:985, 2001.
105. Gould SM, Baines EA, Mannion PA et al: Use of endogenous ACTH concentration and adrenal ultrasonography to distinguish the cause of canine hyperadrenocorticism, *J Small Anim Prac* 42:113, 2001.
106. Pradelli D, Quintavalla C, Domenech O et al. Tumor thrombus: direct endoluminal 'caudal vena cava- right atrium' extension in a dog affected by adrenal neoplasia, *Vet Res Comm* 27:787, 2003.
107. Parnell NK, Powell LL, Hohenhaus AE et al: Hypoadrenocorticism as the primary manifestation of lymphoma in two cats, *J Am Vet Med Assoc* 214:1208, 1999.
108. Moore LE, Biller DS, Smith TA: Use of abdominal ultrasonography in the diagnosis of primary hyperaldosteronism in a cat, *J Am Vet Med Assoc* 217:213, 2000.
109. Moore LE, Biller DS, Smith TA: Use of abdominal ultrasonography in the diagnosis of primary hyperaldosteronism in a cat, *J Am Vet Med Assoc* 217:213, 2000.
110. Chun R, Jakovljevic S, Morrison WB et al: Apocrine gland adenocarcinoma and pheochromocytoma in a cat, *J Am Anim Hosp Assoc* 33:33, 1997.
111. Rosenstein DS: Diagnostic imaging in canine pheochromocytoma, *Vet Radiol Ultrasound* 41:499, 2000.
112. Whittemore JC, Preston CA, Kyles AE et al: Nontraumatic rupture of an adrenal gland tumor causing intra-abdominal or retroperitoneal hemorrhage in four dogs, *J Am Vet Med Assoc* 219:329, 2001.
113. Ruckstuhl NS, Nett CS, Reusch CE: Results of clinical examinations, laboratory tests, and ultrasonography in dogs with pituitary-dependent hyperadrenocorticism treated with trilostane, *Am J Vet Radiol* 63:506, 2002.
114. Mantis P, Lamb CR, Witt AL et al: Changes in ultrasonographic appearance of adrenal glands in dogs with pituitary-dependent hyperadrenocorticism treated with trilostane, *Vet Radiol Ultrasound* 44:682, 2003.
115. Chapman PS, Kelly DF, Archer J et al: Adrenal necrosis in a dog receiving trilostane for the treatment of hyperadrenocorticism, *J Small Anim Prac* 45:307, 2004.
116. Horauf A, Reusch C: Effects of mitotane therapy in dogs with pituitary dependent Cushing's syndrome on the adrenal gland size—an ultrasonographic study, *Schweiz Arch Tierheilkd* 141:239, 1999.
117. Boag AK, Neiger R, Church DB: Trilostane treatment of bilateral adrenal enlargement and excessive sex steroid hormone production in a cat, *J Small Anim Prac* 45:263, 2004.
118. Westropp JL, Welk KA, Buffington CA: Small adrenal glands in cats with feline interstitial cystitis, *J Urol* 170:2494, 2003.

ELECTRONIC RESOURCES evolve

Additional information related to the content in Chapter 38 can be found on the companion Web site at evolve http://evolve.elsevier.com/Thrall/vetrad/.

- Key Points
- Chapter Quiz
- Case Study 38-1

CHAPTER • 39
The Liver and Spleen

Martha Moon Larson

RADIOLOGY OF THE LIVER

The liver is the largest solid organ in the abdomen. Hepatic size, shape, location, and opacity can be determined radiographically in most patients.[1-7]

The liver is located in the cranial abdomen between the diaphragm, which delineates its cranial borders, and the stomach, right kidney, and cranial portion of the duodenum, which define the caudal extent. The liver is nearly entirely within the costal arch, with the caudal ventral border (composed of the left lateral liver lobe in the dog) extending just slightly beyond the costal arch (Fig. 39-1). In dogs with a deep thoracic cavity, the liver lies more completely within the costal arch, whereas greater caudal hepatic extension is seen in dogs with shallow, wide thoracic conformation. Abundant falciform fat, especially in cats, can result in dorsal displacement of the ventral liver margins on lateral views. This may give rise to a false impression of a small liver. On ventrodorsal views, the liver is fairly symmetrically distributed in dogs, but a larger portion of the liver is often right sided in cats (Fig. 39-2).

Hepatic shape may not be easily visualized without abundant surrounding omental and falciform fat. The caudoventral hepatic margin protruding slightly from the costal arch should be relatively sharply marginated. It may protrude farther caudally in right lateral recumbent views, where it may merge with the spleen, blurring exact definition. Obliqued lateral views can produce apparent rounding of the hepatic margins, which should not be confused with hepatic enlargement.

The gallbladder is located just to the right of midline, in the cranioventral portion of the liver, but is not normally visible because of silhouetting with the soft tissue of the liver (Fig. 39-3). In some cats, however, the gallbladder can be seen on lateral abdominal radiographs as a curved structure protruding from the ventral liver margin.[8]

Hepatomegaly

Hepatic enlargement can be detected radiographically, although mild changes in size cannot be accurately assessed. The classic radiographic signs of generalized hepatomegaly are rounding or blunting of the caudoventral liver margins, along with extension beyond the costal arch, and caudal, and perhaps medial, displacement of the gastric axis (Figs. 39-4 to 39-6).[9-11]

Several nonpathologic conditions can result in extension of hepatic margins beyond the costal arch, including overexpansion of the thorax or deep inspiration (Fig. 39-7). Geriatric dogs and cats can have stretching or elongation of the triangular ligaments attaching the liver to the diaphragm, resulting in "sagging" and caudal extension of the liver margin. The same phenomenon can also occur in obese dogs with a pendulous abdomen. In these dogs the liver does not extend as far dorsally. Some brachycephalic and chondrodystrophic breeds have caudal extension from a more horizontally aligned liver compared with deep-chested breeds. Because of the numerous normal variations that can cause hepatic lobe extension beyond the costal arch, rounding or blunting of these lobes should also be present before hepatomegaly is concluded. In addition, neonatal and young dogs and cats have a larger liver size compared with body size, creating the appearance of hepatomegaly without a true hepatic abnormality (Fig. 39-8).[1,12]

With generalized hepatomegaly, caudal displacement of the stomach, right kidney, and transverse colon as well as cranial duodenal flexure may occur, along with dorsal elevation of the pylorus. On ventrodorsal views, an increased opacity may be present in the right cranial abdominal quadrant along with displacement of the body and pyloric portion of the stomach caudally, dorsally, and to the left. Both lateral and ventrodorsal abdominal views should be examined to evaluate liver size because hepatomegaly is sometimes obvious only on one view. The position of the stomach is important in determining hepatomegaly, but the stomach may be poorly visualized if empty of gas or food. The addition of a small amount of barium (1 mL/kg) better defines the gastric position, helping evaluate hepatic size (Fig. 39-9).[7]

Considerations for generalized hepatomegaly are numerous, and radiology alone is insufficient in most instances to narrow the list. Hepatic congestion, steroid hepatopathy, hepatic lipidosis, inflammatory and infiltrative disease, and primary and metastatic neoplasia are all possibilities. Hepatic ultrasound can determine internal architecture and is better suited for more exact diagnoses.

Visualization of focal hepatomegaly depends on the degree of enlargement and the liver lobe affected. Focal hepatic masses usually result in distortion of the hepatic outline and are continuous with the liver in at least one projection.[9-11] Right-sided hepatic masses displace the stomach and duodenum to the left side and dorsally and the small bowel caudally (Fig. 39-10). The right kidney and distal extremity of the spleen may also be displaced caudally. Left hepatic masses result in displacement of the stomach and spleen dorsally and to the right. With few exceptions, masses located cranial to the ventral aspect of the stomach are hepatic in origin.[9] Although hepatic masses classically result in caudal displacement of the stomach, a focal mass can grow and extend caudal to the stomach (Fig. 39-11).[10,11] Differentiation of a caudally located hepatic mass from a splenic mass in these instances is difficult based on radiographs alone. Differentials for focal hepatic masses include primary and metastatic neoplasia, abscess, granuloma, and hepatic cyst.

As with subtle hepatomegaly, slight decreases in hepatic size are not accurately identified radiographically. Marked microhepatia will result in cranial displacement of the stomach and decreased distance between the diaphragm and gastric lumen (Fig. 39-12). Congenital portosystemic shunts and hepatic cirrhosis are the two most common causes of true microhepatia. Diaphragmatic hernia, with displacement of the

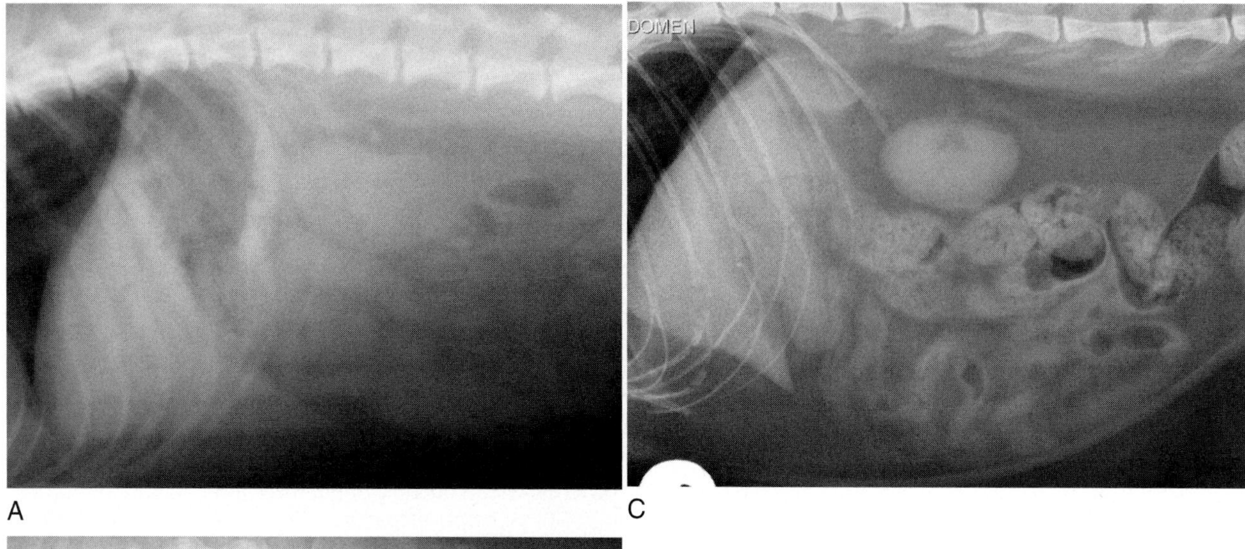

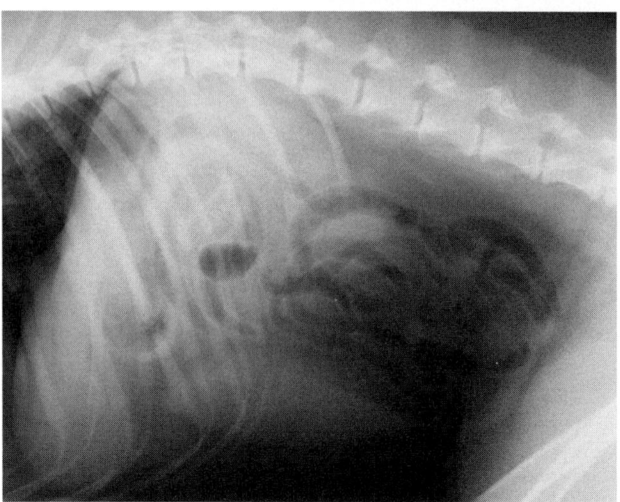

Fig. 39-1 A, Right lateral radiograph of the abdomen of a normal dog. The liver lies nearly entirely within the costal arch, with the sharply marginated caudoventral margin protruding slightly. B, Lateral radiograph of the abdomen of a dog with a deep thoracic cavity. The liver lies entirely within the costal arch, appearing small. The gastric axis is perpendicular to the spine, a normal variation for a dog with deep thoracic conformation. The distal extremity of the spleen lies immediately caudal to the liver. C, Lateral radiograph of the abdomen of a normal cat. The liver extends just slightly beyond the costal arch and has sharp margins. Abundant falciform fat results in dorsal displacement of the ventral liver margins. The proximal extremity of the spleen is noted craniodorsal to the kidney.

liver cranial to the diaphragm, gives the appearance of a small liver on abdominal radiographs.

Hepatic Opacity

The normal liver is of soft tissue opacity. Mineral opacities can occur within the hepatic parenchyma or biliary system.[13] Choleliths (gallbladder calculi) should be considered when focal mineral opacities are visible in the area of the gallbladder (Fig. 39-13). Linear "trails" of mineralized opacities extending peripherally are indicative of choledocholiths (bile duct calculi).[14] Biliary calculi are uncommon in dogs and cats but are visible radiographically if they contain sufficient calcium (Fig. 39-14).[15-22] These are usually incidental findings, but choledocholiths can cause biliary obstruction. Mineralization of the gallbladder wall (porcelain gallbladder) has been associated with gallbladder carcinoma as well as cholecystitis or cystic mucinous hyperplasia.[13,23]

Hepatic parenchymal mineralization may be localized or diffuse and have a variety of patterns.[13] Dystrophic calcification of hepatic granulomas, abscesses, hematomas, neoplastic masses, or areas of hepatic necrosis have been documented (see Fig. 39-10). Mineralization of the biliary tree occasionally is seen in dogs with bile duct carcinoma.[24] Alveolar echinococcosis infestation can result in large hepatic soft tissue masses with mineralization of varying patterns and should be considered in endemic areas.[25]

Radiolucent areas within the liver are indicative of intrahepatic gas, either in the biliary system, portal venous system, or hepatic parenchyma. Gas within portal vessels may occur as a result of severe necrotizing gastritis or enteritis, often associated with gastric dilation and volvulus complex. Gastrointestinal ulceration, distension, or trauma or interventional procedures may allow gas to ascend into the portovenous circulation.[1,26,27] A linear, branching radiolucent appearance, similar to air bronchograms, may be visible. Gas in or around the gallbladder occurs with emphysematous cholecystitis, reported in both diabetic and nondiabetic dogs.[28,29] Gas opacities are initially seen within the gallbladder wall, followed by more complete filling of the gallbladder lumen. The gas eventually extends to the pericholecystic tissues. Gas bubbles conforming to the shape of the distended gallbladder can be seen within 24 to 48 hours of onset of disease. Obstruction of the cystic duct may be a common predisposing factor in this disease. Gas lucencies within the biliary system can also be seen after surgery of the duodenum or biliary system.[1,4] Hepatic abscesses caused by gas-forming organisms may result in gas opacities within the hepatic parenchyma.[30-33] These abscesses appear as irregularly stippled or mottled gas patterns, usually in a localized area (Fig. 39-15). Hepatomegaly or hepatic mass is typically present with hepatic abscess, with or without gas formation.

Special Procedures of the Liver

Portosystemic shunts are congenital or acquired anomalies of the portal venous vasculature in which blood bypasses the liver and enters directly into the systemic circulation.[34]

Text continued on p. 674

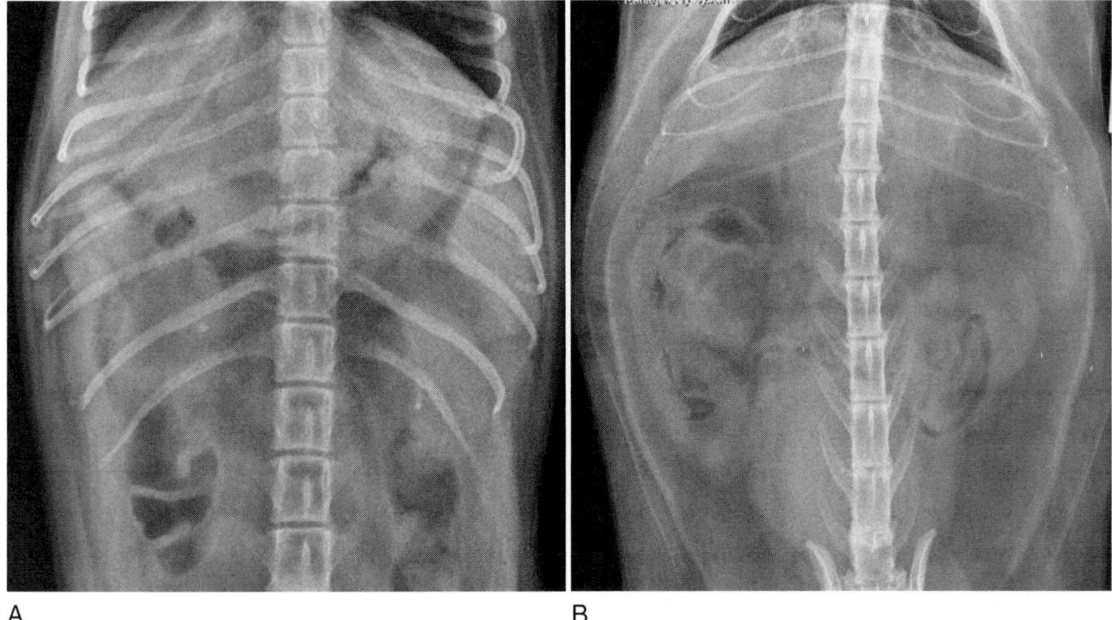

Fig. 39-2 **A,** Ventrodorsal radiograph of the cranial aspect of the abdomen of a normal dog. The liver lies cranial to and silhouettes the gastric shadow. Bilateral renal pelvic calculi are present. **B,** Ventrodorsal radiograph of the abdomen of a normal cat. The liver is more to the right side than in a dog and is better visualized in this cat because of surrounding abundant fat.

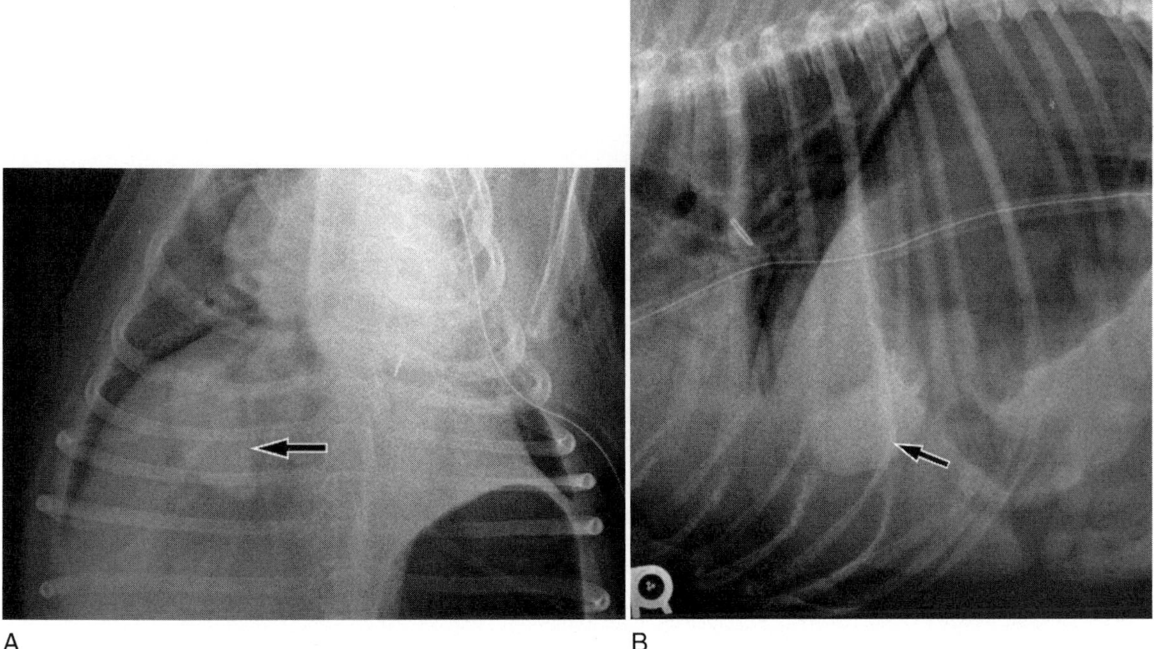

Fig. 39-3 Lateral and dorsoventral radiograph of the cranial abdomen in a dog made several hours after intravenous contrast medium administration for an excretory urogram. The gallbladder contains contrast medium because biliary excretion of iodinated contrast medium is a secondary route of excretion. The gallbladder is therefore conspicuous in the right cranial portion of the liver *(arrows)*. A chest tube extends across the cranial abdomen.

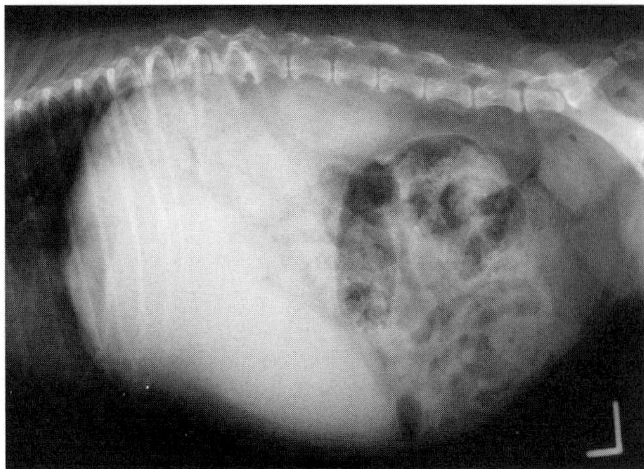

Fig. 39-4 Lateral radiograph of a dog with steroid hepatopathy and severe hepatomegaly. The liver has rounded, blunt margins and extends well beyond the costal arch.

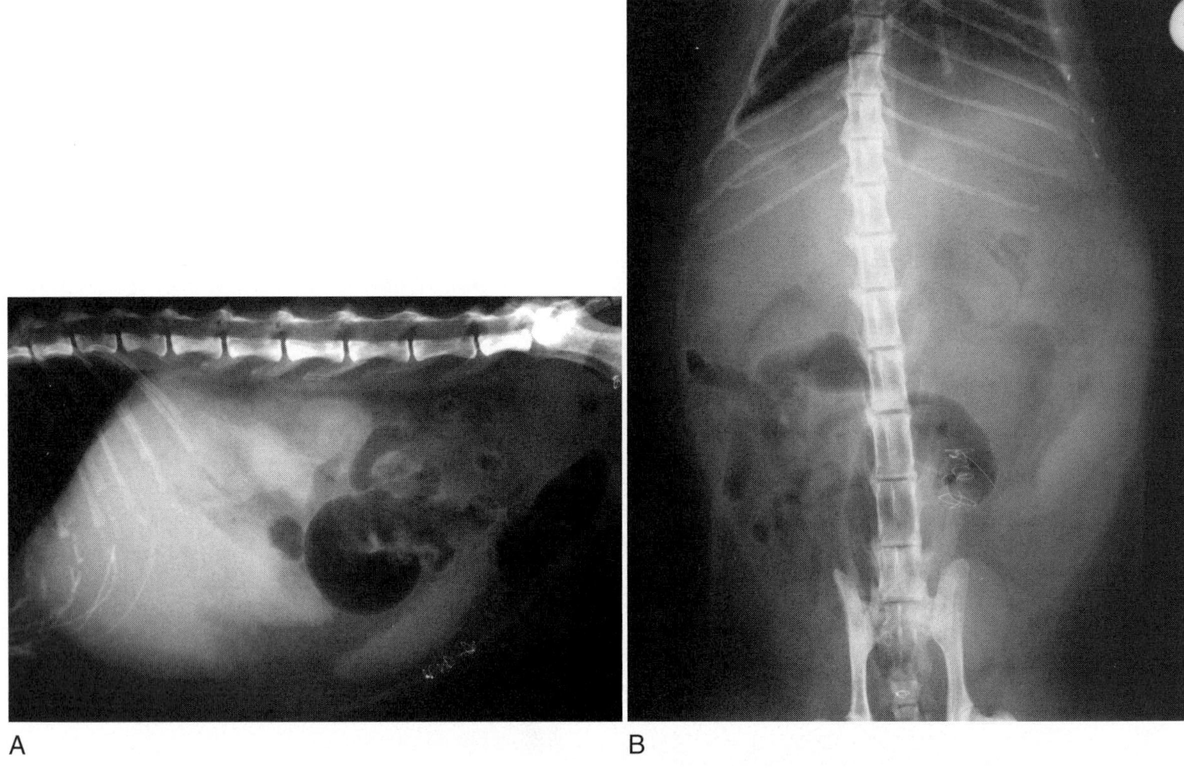

Fig. 39-5 Lateral (A) and ventrodorsal (B) radiographs of the abdomen of a cat with lymphosarcoma involving the liver and spleen. There is caudal, dorsal, and leftward displacement of the stomach as well as caudal extension of the liver margins. The spleen, which is also enlarged and has an irregular margin, is visualized extending along the ventral abdominal wall in **A**.

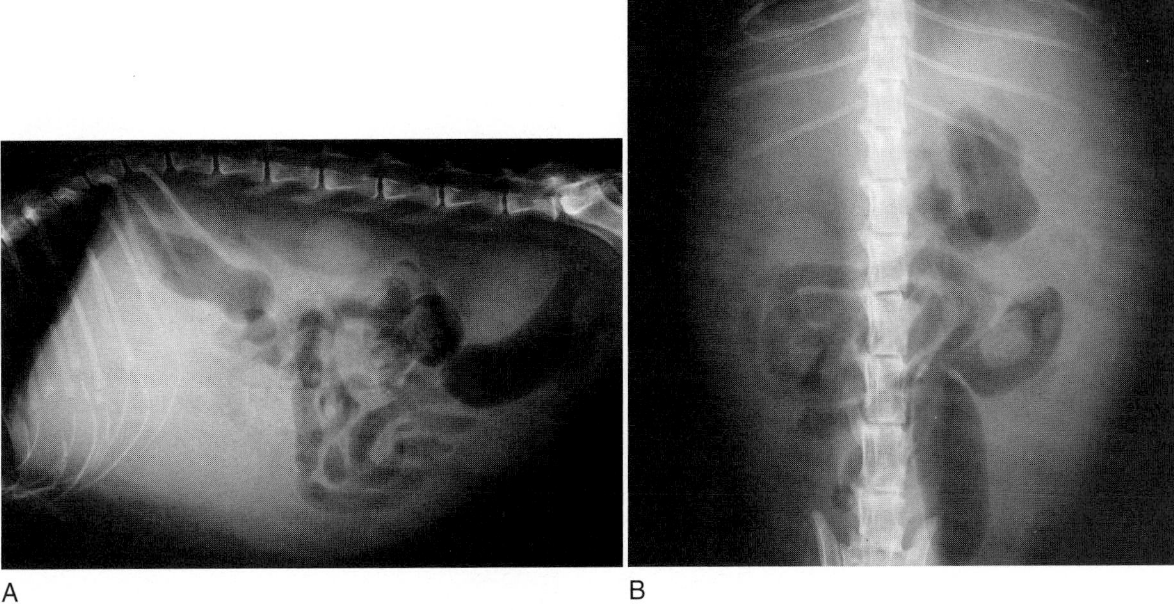

Fig. 39-6 Lateral (A) and ventrodorsal (B) radiographs of the abdomen of a cat with lymphosarcoma. Although peritoneal fluid obscures abdominal detail, the marked caudal, dorsal, and left-sided gastric displacement is consistent with severe hepatomegaly.

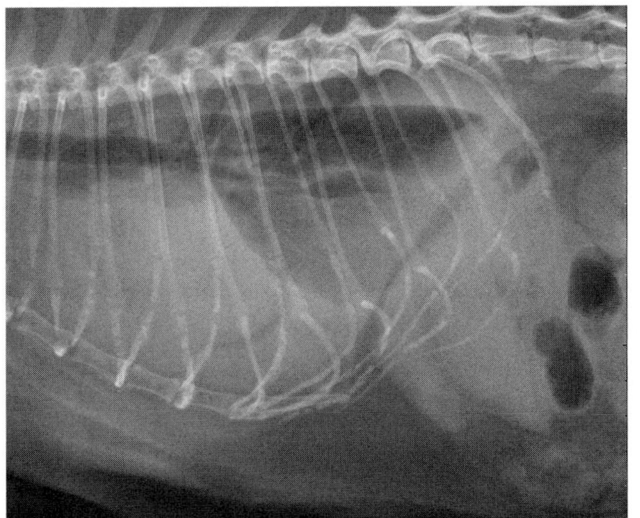

Fig. 39-7 Lateral radiograph of the thorax of a cat with pleural effusion. The overexpanded thorax results in caudal displacement of the diaphragm and liver margins, with subsequent apparent hepatomegaly. The liver margins remain relatively sharp.

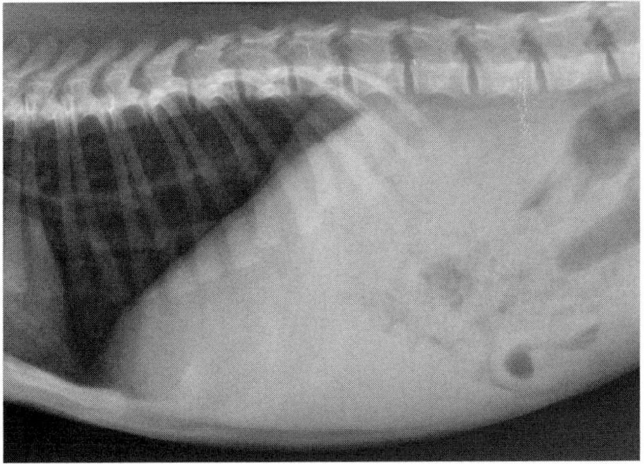

Fig. 39-8 Lateral radiograph of the abdomen of a normal puppy. The liver is large compared with overall abdominal size, a normal finding in young dogs and cats.

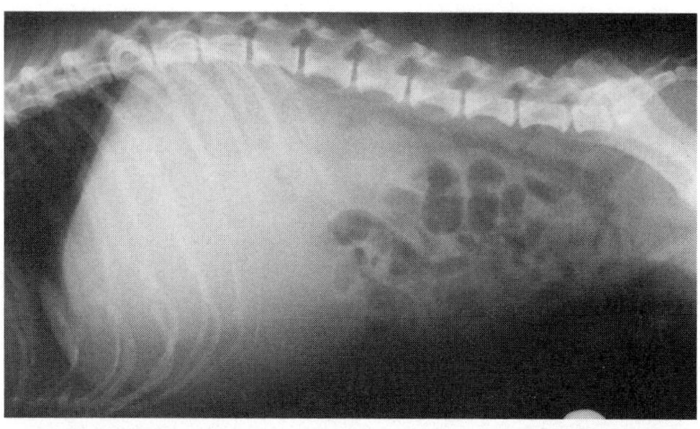

A

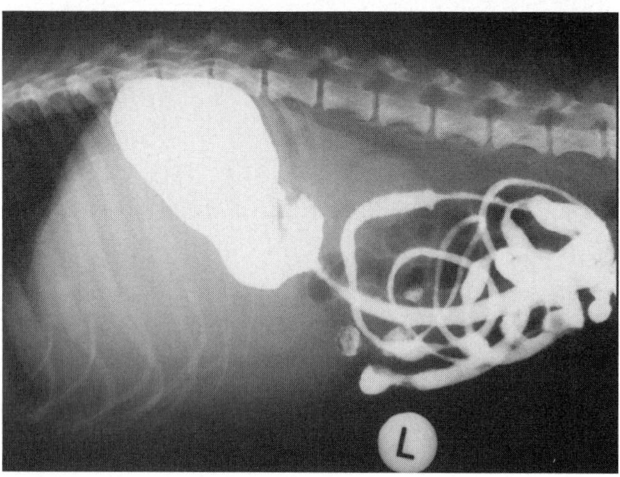

B

Fig. 39-9 Lateral radiographs of the abdomen of a dog taken before (A) and after (B) oral administration of barium. The enlarged liver is much better defined after the stomach is filled with barium and is more obviously displaced caudally and dorsally.

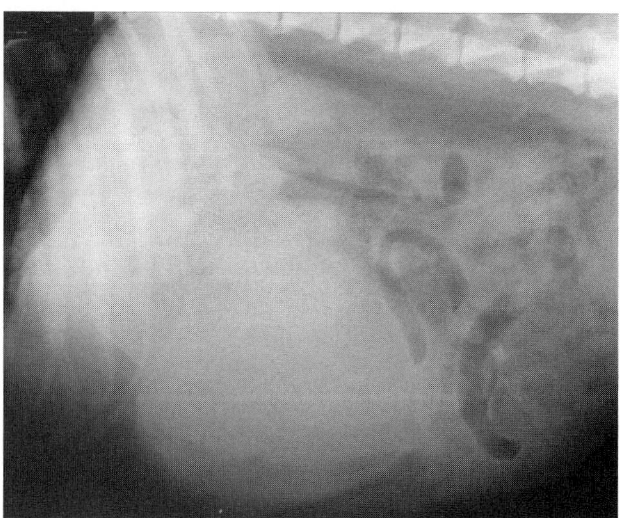

Fig. 39-11 Lateral radiograph of the abdomen of a dog with hepatic carcinoma. The hepatic mass extends caudal to the stomach, mimicking a splenic mass.

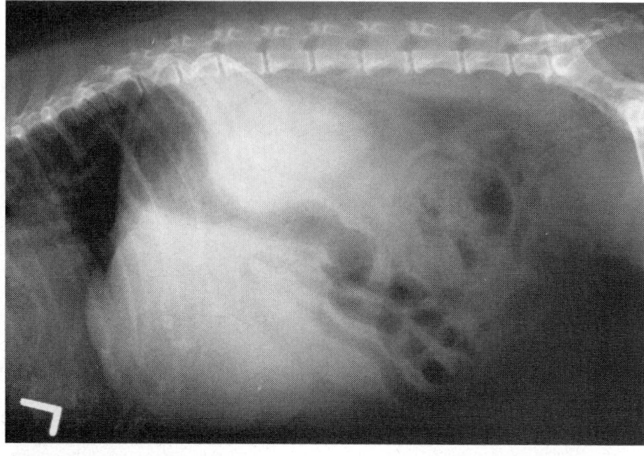

A

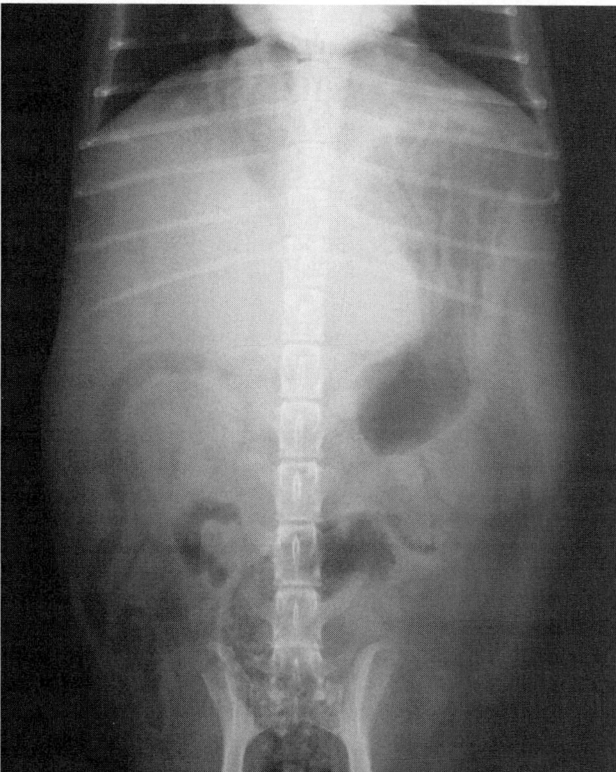

B

Fig. 39-10 Lateral (A) and ventrodorsal (B) radiographs of the abdomen of a dog with hepatic carcinoma. The right side of the liver is enlarged resulting in caudal, dorsal, and left-sided displacement of the stomach. The small bowel is displaced caudally. Faint mineralization is present in the ventral portion of the liver on the lateral view.

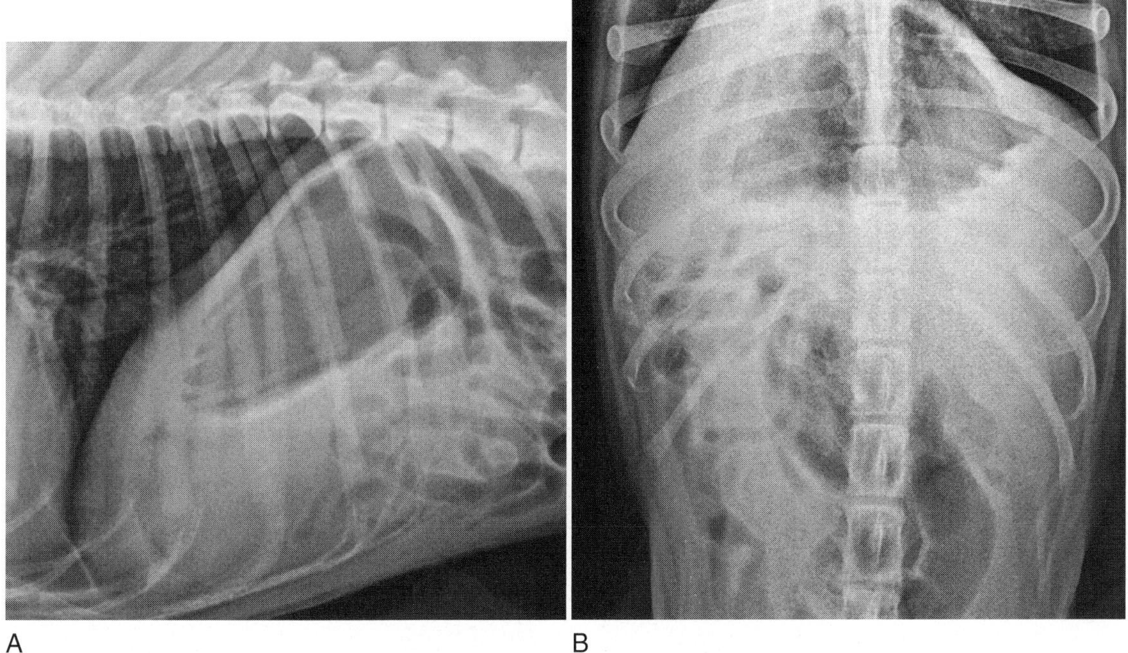

Fig. 39-12 Lateral (A) and ventrodorsal (B) radiograph of the abdomen of a dog with chronic hepatitis. Cranial displacement of the stomach is marked, consistent with microhepatia.

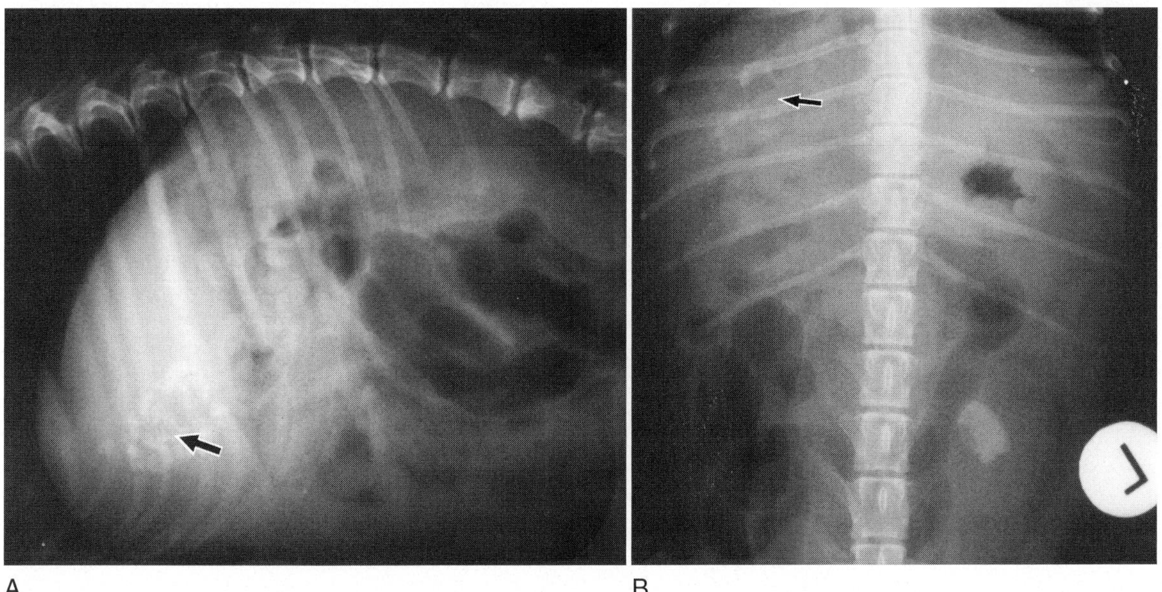

Fig. 39-13 Lateral (A) and ventrodorsal (B) radiographs of a dog with fever of unknown origin. Radiopaque choleliths are noted in the area of the gallbladder in the right cranial portion of the liver *(arrows)*. A left renal pelvic calculus is present.

Various imaging techniques have been used to demonstrate the anomalous vessels, including cranial mesenteric portography, percutaneous splenoportography, and operative mesenteric portography.[34-37] Angiography of the portal vein provides visualization of the anomalous vessel, any acquired collateral vessels, the direction of portal blood flow, and the patency of the portal vein and its branches. Intraoperative mesenteric portography is the most common angiographic procedure for assessing portosystemic shunts, involving intraoperative catheterization of a jejunal vein (or sometimes splenic vein) with subsequent injection of positive contrast medium to outline the portal system (Figs. 39-16 and 39-17). Ultrasound-guided splenic vein catheterization has been proposed as an alternative to laparoscopic catheter placement, but this technique may be somewhat challenging, especially in smaller patients.[38] Patient position during contrast medium injection may have an effect on the visualization of the opacified vessels as a result of gravity-dependent alterations in the distribution of portal blood flow. Contrast medium injection should be performed with the patient in left lateral and dorsal recumbent positions, followed by a repeat injection in right lateral recumbency if the results of the first two injections are negative or inconclusive.[39] The use of postshunt ligation intraoperative mesenteric portography provides confirmation that the

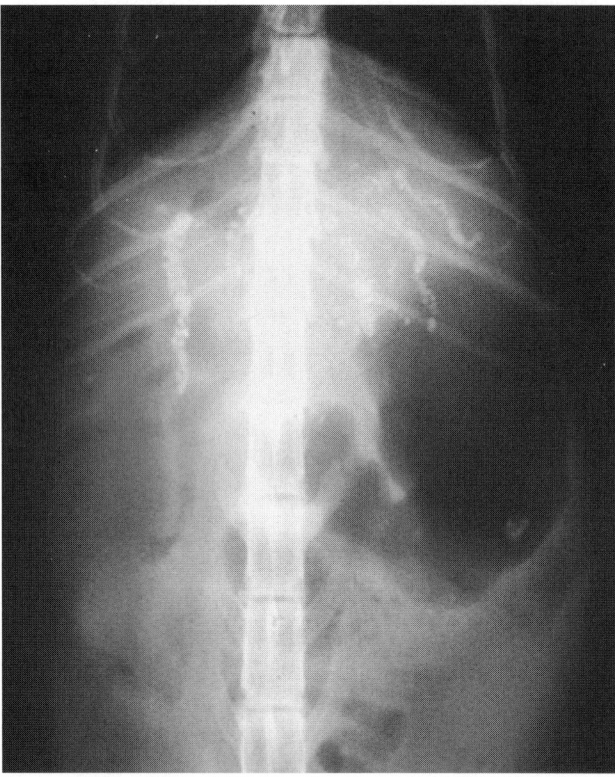

Fig. 39-14 Ventrodorsal radiograph of the abdomen of a clinically normal cat. Trails of mineralized choledocholiths are visible within the liver.

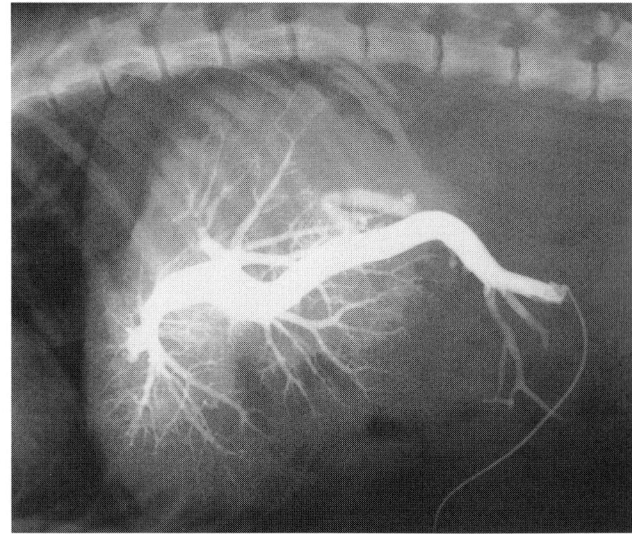

Fig. 39-16 Intraoperative mesenteric portogram (lateral view) of a normal dog outlining the normal portal vasculature.

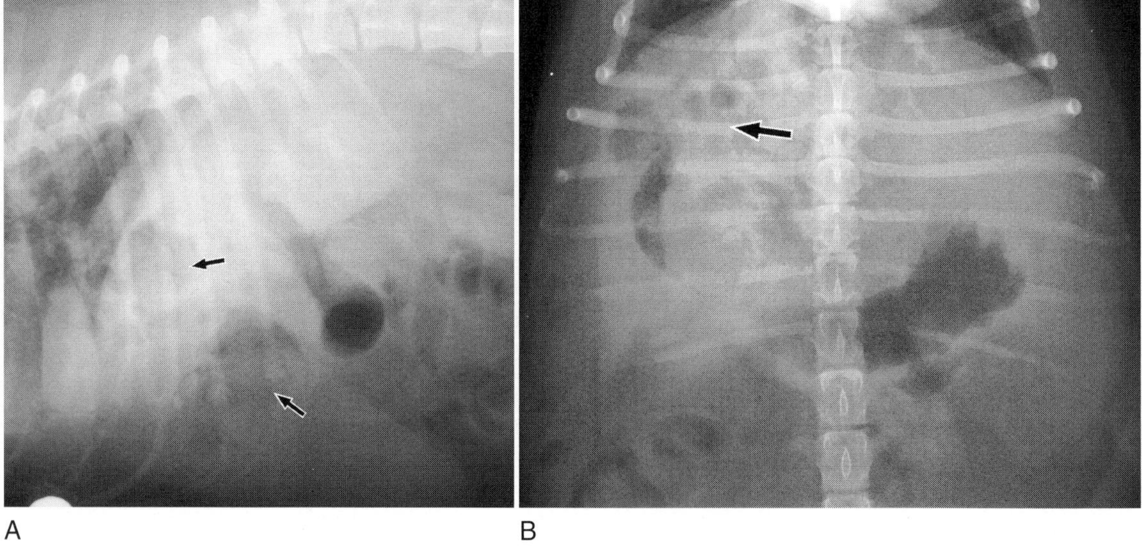

Fig. 39-15 Lateral (A) and ventrodorsal (B) radiographs of the abdomen of a dog with hepatic abscessation and emphysematous cholecystitis. Multiple poorly defined radiolucent gas shadows are visible in the area of the gallbladder and liver parenchyma *(arrows)*. Hepatomegaly is present.

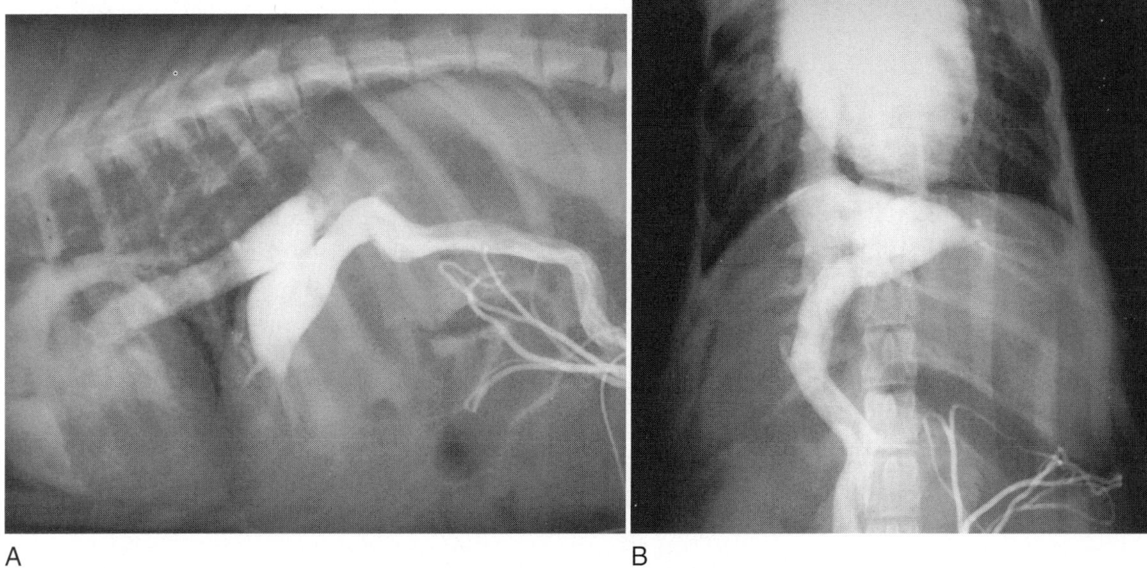

Fig. 39-17 Intraoperative mesenteric portogram (lateral [A] and ventrodorsal [B] views) outlining an intrahepatic portocaval shunt.

shunt has been correctly identified and ligated as well as information on the extent of hepatic portal vasculature.[40] Helical computed tomography combined with peripheral venous contrast injection has been used as a noninvasive imaging modality providing angiogram-like images of the normal and abnormal vasculature.[41,42]

Hepatic Ultrasound

Ultrasound examination of the liver allows more detailed evaluation of hepatic internal architecture, including the hepatic vasculature and biliary system. Ultrasound is also useful in guiding aspirates and biopsies for nonsurgical, less-invasive diagnoses.

The hepatic parenchyma has a medium-level echogenicity, with a homogeneous and uniform texture that is somewhat coarser than in the spleen.[43-45] The normal echogenicity of the liver is isoechoic to slightly hyperechoic to the renal cortex (caudate liver lobe and cranial pole of right kidney allow good comparisons) and hypoechoic to the spleen (Fig. 39-18). The liver margins should be smooth and sharp but are better visualized if adjacent peritoneal fluid is present (Fig. 39-19). The liver is bordered cranially and dorsally by an echogenic line representing the interface between the diaphragm and lung/pleura margins. A mirror-image artifact is frequently noted deep to the diaphragmatic interface, giving the false impression of liver on both sides of the diaphragm (see Chapter 3 for a detailed explanation of this artifact). The ultrasound assessment of hepatic size is subjective and based on operator experience.[46] A small liver is difficult to evaluate sonographically because of cranial displacement of the stomach, limiting the imaging window (Fig. 39-20). Liver size may appear decreased in dogs with a deep thoracic cavity in whom liver location is more completely within the costal arch. Intercostal ultrasound windows may be needed in these dogs as well as in patients with pathologically small livers. The enlarged liver can be examined relatively easily with ultrasound because it extends well beyond the xiphoid cartilage and more completely covers the right kidney (Fig. 39-21).

Hepatic and portal veins are routinely visualized within hepatic parenchyma. Portal veins are smoothly tapering vessels characterized by bright, echogenic borders.[43-45,47] The left and right branches originate from the main portal vein near the porta heptis, although they branch in different imaging planes.[47] Hepatic veins appear as anechoic linear structures extending through the parenchyma. Hepatic vein borders are not echogenic, with the exception of the veins near their confluence with the caudal vena cava, immediately adjacent to the diaphragm. A right lateral dorsal intercostal window provides an excellent window to the aorta, caudal vena cava, and main portal vein (Fig. 39-22). This window is also useful for more complete evaluation of the small liver. Normal hepatic arteries are not visualized without color Doppler examination. The caudal vena cava can be visualized coursing through the liver in the right lateral abdominal quadrant.

The gallbladder is well visualized as an oval, anechoic structure in the right cranioventral portion of the liver. Gallbladder size varies widely, and distension is normal in fasting or anorexic patients. Intraluminal contents are typically anechoic, although gallbladder sludge (dependent echogenic material without acoustic shadowing) is frequently seen and is considered an incidental finding (Fig. 39-23).[48] The normal gallbladder wall is thin and poorly visualized. In the cat, gallbladder wall thickness should be less than 1 mm or not visualized at all.[49] The normal canine gallbladder wall has been described as typically measuring 2 to 3 mm, but normal ranges have not been established.[50,51] A duplicate or septated gallbladder is occasionally seen as a normal variation in cats and is caused by a an abnormality in embryonic development.[52] The common bile duct is found immediately ventral to the portal vein but is more consistently visible in the cat, where it can frequently be followed to the duodenal papilla (Fig. 39-24). Normal diameter in the cat is 4 mm or less.[53] If visible, the canine bile duct should be 3 mm or less.[54] Intrahepatic bile ducts are not visible unless pathologically dilated.

Abnormal Appearance of the Liver

Ultrasound is helpful in differentiating between diffuse and focal hepatic disease. Diffuse hepatic disease can result in changes in shape, size, and echogenicity.[43-45,55-59] The hyperechoic liver parenchyma results in an abnormal echointensity of liver to adjacent organs (hyperechoic to renal cortex, isoechoic or hyperechoic to spleen), loss of visualization of the

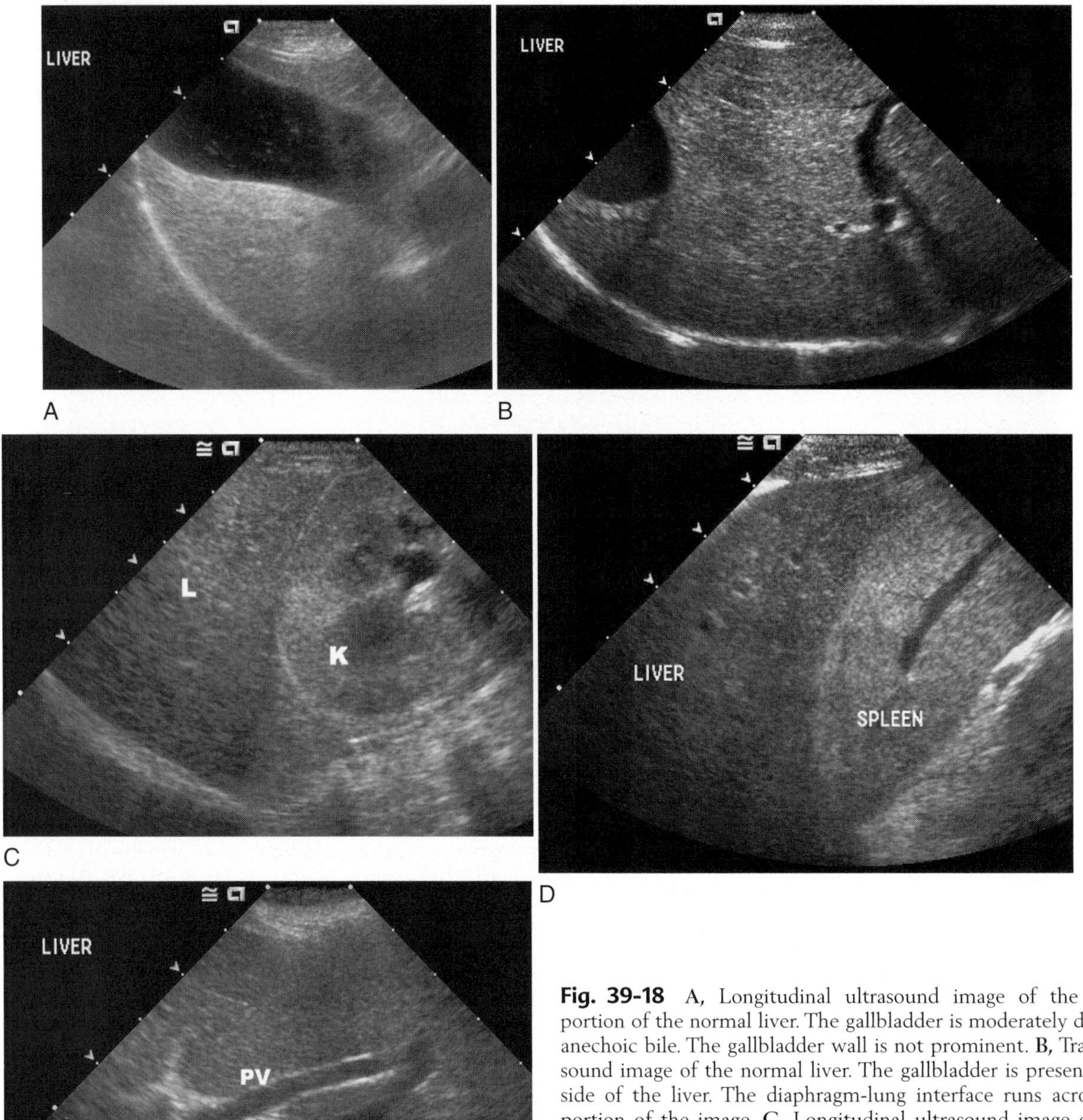

Fig. 39-18 **A,** Longitudinal ultrasound image of the right cranial portion of the normal liver. The gallbladder is moderately distended with anechoic bile. The gallbladder wall is not prominent. **B,** Transverse ultrasound image of the normal liver. The gallbladder is present on the right side of the liver. The diaphragm-lung interface runs across the dorsal portion of the image. **C,** Longitudinal ultrasound image of the normal caudate liver lobe and cranial pole of the right kidney. The liver is isoechoic to the renal cortex. *L,* Liver; *R,* right kidney. **D,** Longitudinal ultrasound image of the normal left liver and proximal portion of the spleen. The liver is hypoechoic to the spleen. **E,** Transverse ultrasound image of the normal canine liver. Portal veins *(P)* have a bright echogenic border, whereas hepatic veins *(H)* do not.

prominent periportal echoes, and increased attenuation of sound as it passes through the hyperechoic liver. Hepatic lipidosis and steroid hepatopathy commonly result in an enlarged, hyperechoic liver (see Fig. 39-21). In cats, liver parenchyma that is hyperechoic to adjacent falciform fat was considered highly suggestive of hepatic lipidosis.[57] Later reports state that this comparison may be normal in obese cats.[60] Chronic hepatitis with parenchymal fibrosis can also cause increased echogenicity, although liver size is variable and may be normal, increased, or decreased. Hepatic cirrhosis typically results in a small, irregular, hyperechoic liver (Fig. 39-25). Ascites often accompanies cirrhosis, enhancing visualization of irregular liver margins. Other hepatic diseases that may result in increased parenchymal echogenicity include lymphosarcoma, amyloidosis, and cholangiohepatitis. Mast cell infiltration in the liver results in a variable appearance, from normal to increased echogenicity and size. Hypoechoic nodules are occasionally noted as well.[61] A decrease in hepatic echogenicity results in prominence of the periportal echoes and abnormal comparison to the renal cortex (the liver becomes hypoechoic to the cortex). Decreased hepatic echogenicity is reported with hepatic congestion (along with dilated caudal vena cava and hepatic veins), lymphosarcoma, and cholangiohepatitis. Acute suppurative hepatitis is

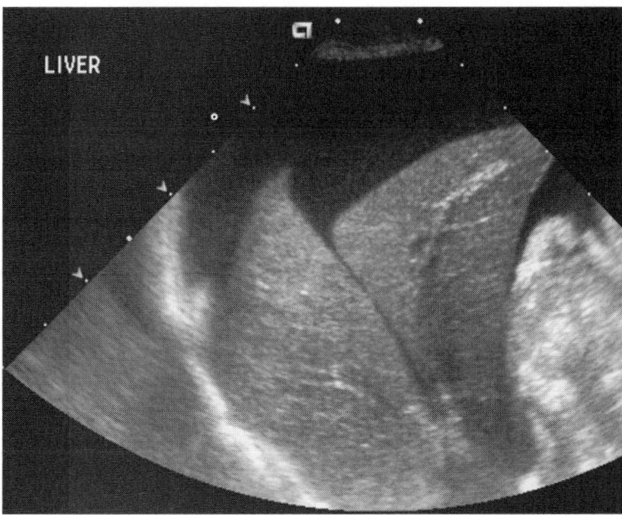

Fig. 39-19 Longitudinal ultrasound image of a dog with ascites. The normal liver lobes have a well-defined sharp, linear margin.

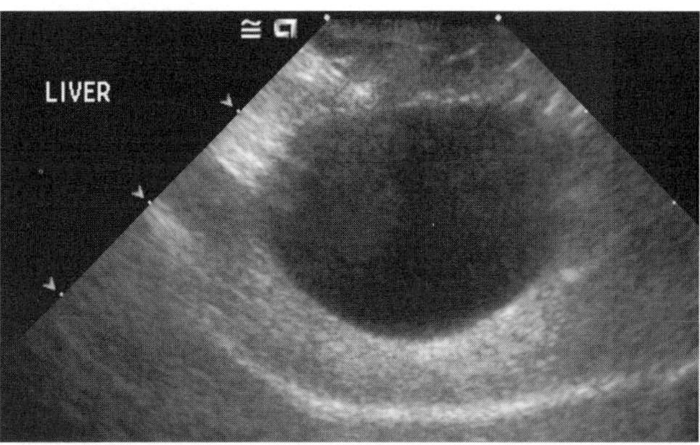

Fig. 39-20 Transverse ultrasound image of the liver in a dog with a portosystemic shunt. The liver is subjectively small, with the gallbladder occupying a large portion.

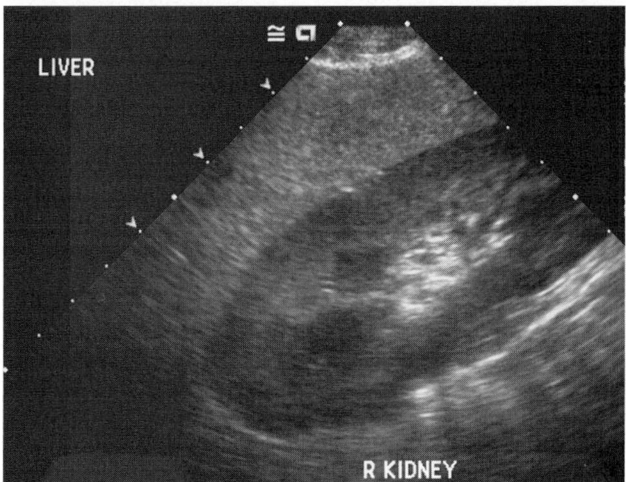

Fig. 39-21 Longitudinal ultrasound image of the caudate liver lobe and right kidney of a dog with hepatic lipidosis. The caudate liver lobe completely surrounds the right kidney, consistent with hepatomegaly. The liver is markedly hyperechoic to the renal cortex.

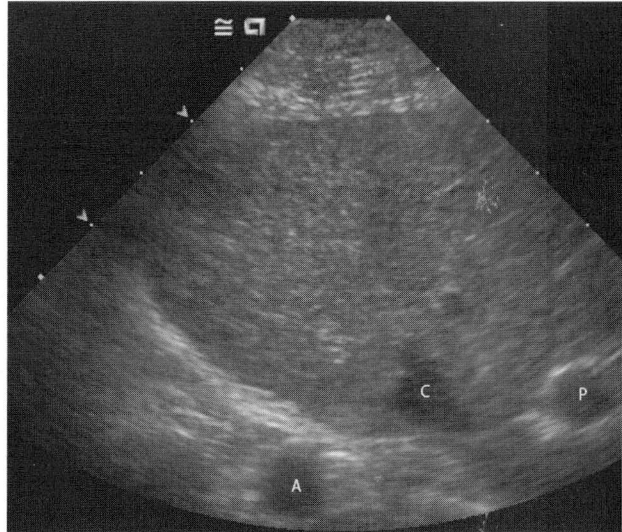

Fig. 39-22 Right lateral intercostal ultrasound image of a normal dog. Dorsal is at left and ventral is at right of the image. The top of the image represents the right abdominal wall with the left abdominal wall being at the bottom of the image. *A*, Aorta; *P*, portal vein; *C*, caudal vena cava.

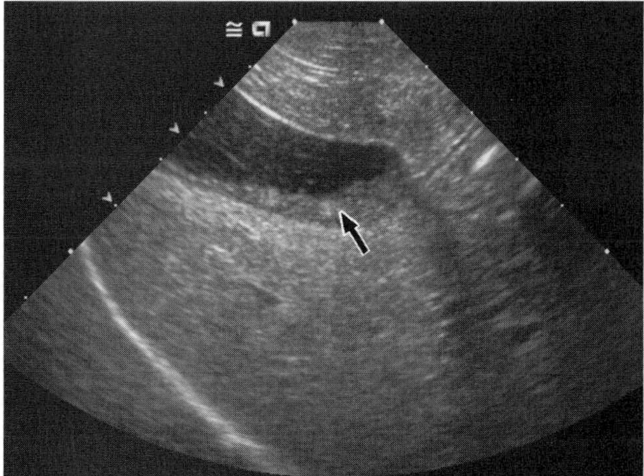

Fig. 39-23 Longitudinal ultrasound image of the liver and gallbladder of a normal dog. Echogenic biliary sludge is present on the dependent wall of the gallbladder.

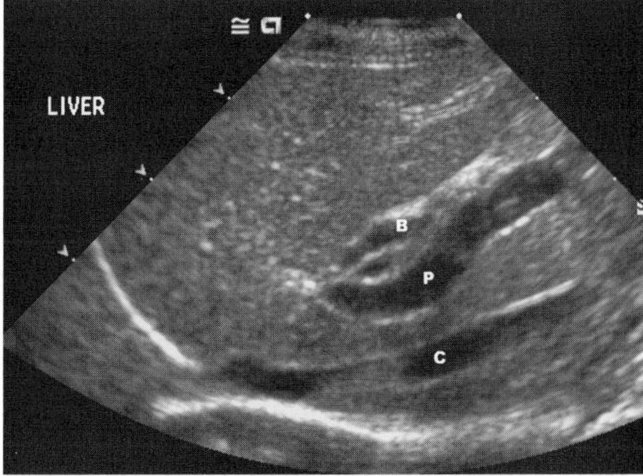

Fig. 39-24 Longitudinal ultrasound image of the liver in a normal cat. *C*, Caudal vena cava; *P*, portal vein; *B*, bile duct.

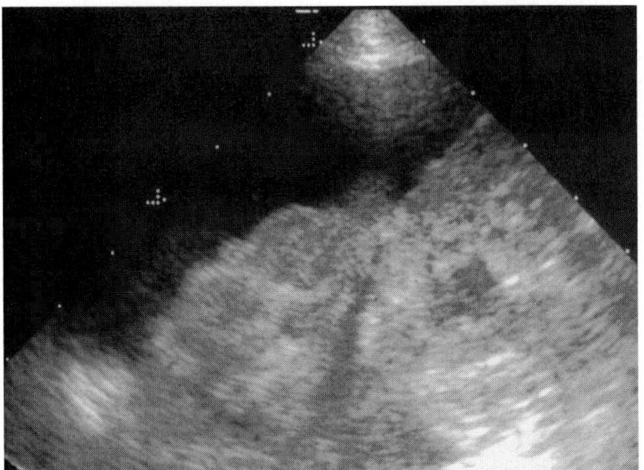

Fig. 39-25 Longitudinal ultrasound image of the liver in a dog with cirrhosis and ascites. The liver margins are irregular and rounded, and hypoechoic nodules are present within the liver parenchyma.

reported to cause hepatic hypoechogenicity from inflammation and edema. However, this finding may be uncommon, even with severe disease.[62] Of note, a normal hepatic ultrasound examination does not rule out diffuse disease because hepatic changes need to be severe before ultrasound changes are visible. Ultrasound appears to be relatively insensitive in detecting parenchymal changes of hepatic lymphosarcoma.[63,64] Subtle changes in hepatic echogenicity should be correlated with clinical signs and blood work, and a needle aspirate or biopsy is necessary for definitive diagnosis.[65,66] Prebiopsy coagulation screening is a useful precaution when liver disease is suspected.

Focal hepatic disease appears as a nodule or mass that differs in texture and echogenicity from surrounding normal liver parenchyma. Quite small nodules can be detected, especially when using high-frequency transducers. However, although ultrasound is sensitive in detecting hepatic nodules, it is not specific and numerous considerations are possible for focal disease. Cysts, abscesses, primary or metastatic neoplasia, hematomas, granulomas, nodular hyperplasia, and extramedullary hematopoiesis can all produce focal hepatic disease and may be difficult to differentiate on the basis of ultrasound appearance alone.[43-45,57] However, ultrasound is extremely useful in differentiating cystic versus solid masses; focal, multifocal, or diffuse distribution of masses; the relation of the mass to adjacent structures, such as large blood vessels or the gallbladder; and assessment of tumor vascularization patterns with Doppler imaging techniques.[11] Hepatic neoplasia has a variable appearance.[43-45,67] Primary hepatic neoplasia (carcinoma) may appear hypoechoic, hyperechoic, or of mixed echogenicity (Fig. 39-26). Primary neoplasia may be a solitary large mass confined to a single liver lobe; multifocal, involving several lobes; or multifocal or coalescing nodules in all liver lobes.[11,68] Hepatic lymphosarcoma, although sometimes seen as a change in size and echogenicity, can also result in focal nodules, usually hypoechoic.[63,64] Tumor type cannot be determined from the ultrasound appearance alone because varying amounts of hemorrhage, necrosis, and fatty infiltration within the tumor mass create an inconsistent appearance that varies even from liver lobe to liver lobe.[56,57] Likewise, hepatic metastatic disease is extremely variable in appearance but more often has a nodular or focal masslike appearance and is usually multifocal. Primary and metastatic neoplasia cannot be differentiated solely on ultrasound appearance. Target lesions (focal masses with a hyperechoic center and hypo-

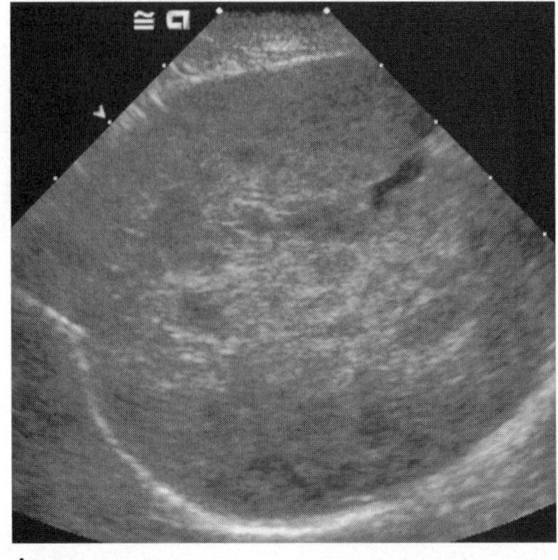

A

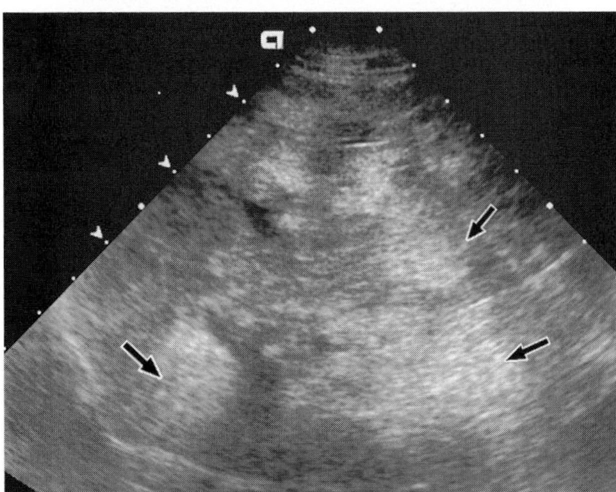

B

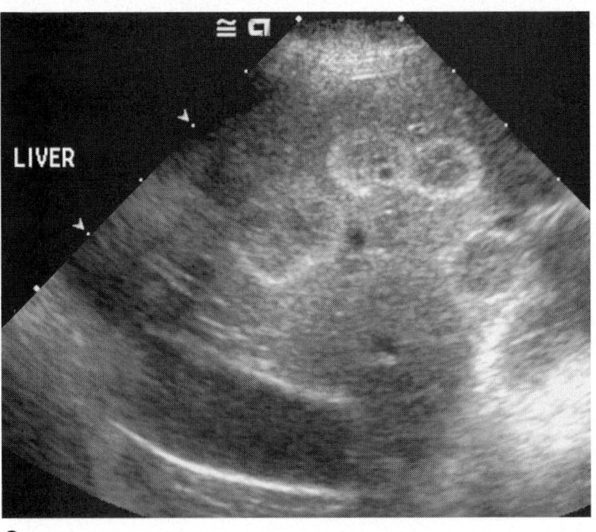

C

Fig. 39-26 A, Longitudinal ultrasound image of the liver from the cat in Figure 39-5. Multiple hypoechoic nodules are present in the enlarged liver (lymphosarcoma). B, Longitudinal ultrasound image of the liver from a dog with hepatic carcinoma. Multiple poorly defined hyperechoic nodules are distributed throughout the liver parenchyma *(arrows)*. C, Longitudinal ultrasound image of a liver from a dog with primary hepatic hemangiosarcoma. Multiple lesions (hyperechoic rim, hypoechoic center) are present.

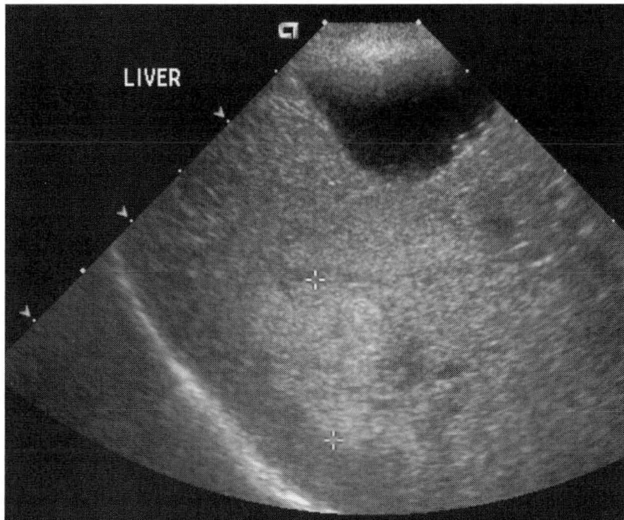

Fig. 39-27 Longitudinal ultrasound image of the liver from a dog with neurologic disease. A hyperechoic nodule is noted dorsal to the gallbladder (between calipers). The dog was euthanized for the neurologic disease, and nodular hyperplasia was diagnosed histopathologically.

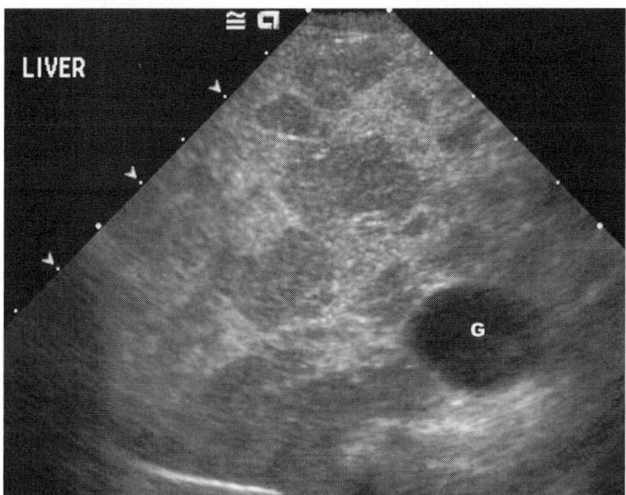

Fig. 39-28 Transverse ultrasound image of the liver from a dog with chronic hepatitis. Multiple hypoechoic nodules are present within a hyperechoic liver parenchyma. G, Gallbladder.

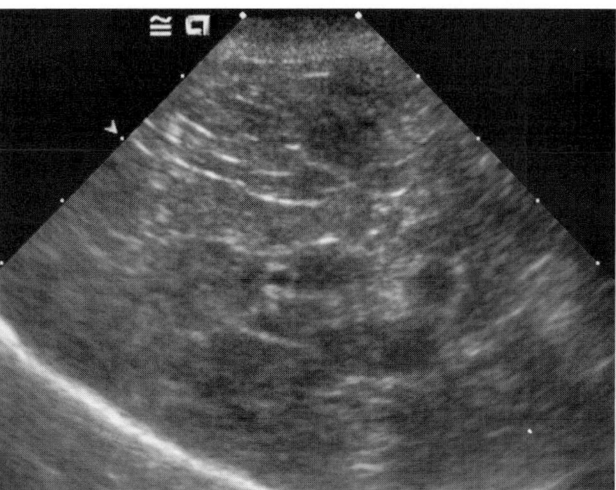

Fig. 39-29 Longitudinal ultrasound image of the liver from a dog with hepatocutaneous syndrome. Multiple hypoechoic nodules within the liver parenchyma result in a honeycomb appearance.

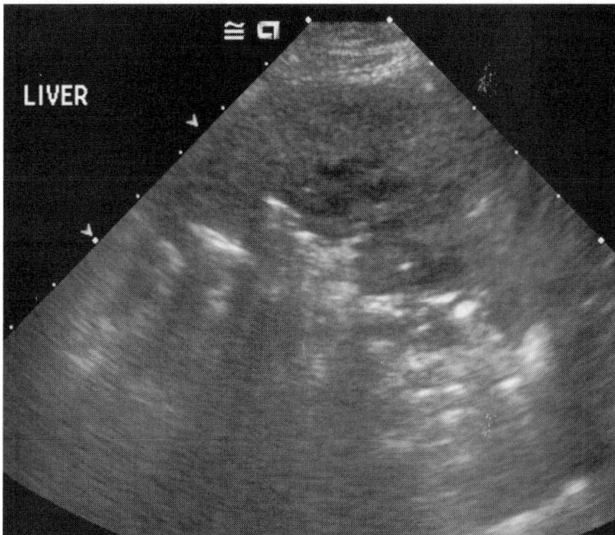

Fig. 39-30 Longitudinal ultrasound image of the liver from the dog in Figure 39-15. Echogenic shadows and reverberation artifacts are noted deep to gas pockets within the liver. This dog had emphysematous cholecystitis and hepatic abscessation.

echoic periphery) have been reported with both neoplastic and benign disease processes.[45,69] Contrast harmonic ultrasound is being used with some success in improving visualization of nodules and differentiating benign and malignant disease.[70,71] Hepatic nodular hyperplasia, a common benign lesion seen in the liver of older dogs, is usually clinically silent but may result in elevations in serum alkaline phosphatase.[72] It has a variety of appearances and cannot be differentiated from neoplasia without biopsy (Fig. 39-27). Hyperechoic, hypoechoic, isoechoic, and mixed echogenicity nodules, some with cavitation, are all possible.[73] Chronic hepatitis may also result in a diffuse nodular appearance (Fig. 39-28). Hyperechoic hepatic parenchyma surrounds multifocal hypoechoic nodules (nodular hyperplasia).[43,45,57] Liver size may be normal or decreased. Hepatocutaneous syndrome (superficial necrolytic dermatitis) results in a similar appearance. Hepatocutaneous syndrome should be suspected when the liver parenchyma has a "honeycomb" appearance, with hyperechoic hepatic parenchyma surrounding hypoechoic focal nodular areas (Fig. 39-29).[74-77] These patients have concurrent dermal lesions in the footpads and mucocutaneous junctions. An aspirate or biopsy is critical in making the diagnosis. Abscesses and hematomas have a variable appearance depending on duration. Abscesses often have an echogenic rim with a central anechoic or hypoechoic area.[31,33,78,79] They may contain gas, resulting in an echogenic interface with deep acoustic shadowing (Fig. 39-30). Hepatic abscesses commonly appear as a simple hypoechoic mass resembling nodular hyperplasia or neoplasia. Hematomas initially may be hyperechoic because of gas or red blood cell aggregates and then progress to hypoechoic or anechoic and finally back to hyperechoic because of reorganization or possible mineralization.[43,80,81] Hepatic cysts have a more consistent appearance, as a fluid-filled, anechoic structure with well-defined, thin walls and acoustic enhancement. Usually an incidental finding, hepatic cysts have the potential to produce clinical signs if large enough or numerous enough to replace liver parenchyma. They can be associated with polycystic kidney disease, so the kidneys should be carefully evaluated for cystic structures if hepatic cysts are noted. Biliary cystadenomas are benign cystic hepatic tumors seen mainly in older cats and may be focal or multifocal.[82] Although variable in appearance, the presence of a cystic component somewhere in the mass is a consistent finding (Fig. 39-31). Biliary cystadenomas may appear multilocular, containing thin-walled cysts, or as hyperechoic masses with a cystic component. Most cystic portions of these masses will be characterized by acoustic enhancement.

Disease of the Biliary System

Ultrasound is advantageous in the diagnosis of disease of the gallbladder and bile duct. Thickening of the gallbladder wall is a nonspecific sign reported with inflammatory conditions such as cholecystitis, cholangiohepatitis, and both acute and chronic hepatitis.[43,44] A double-layered (onion skin) appearance frequently is seen (Fig. 39-32). Wall edema results in a thickened hypoechoic wall with echogenic inner and outer rims, creating a layered appearance. Gallbladder wall thickening is also seen with right-sided congestive heart failure, hypoalbuminemia, sepsis, and neoplasia.[43,44,51,80] Peritoneal fluid surrounding the gallbladder can result in a false impression of wall prominence or thickening. Percutaneous cholecentesis for culture and cytology of the intraluminal bile should be performed with care.[51] Gallbladder thickening may be permanent as a result of inflammation and fibrosis despite resolution of the underlying disease process.[43] Choleliths are well visualized as echogenic focal structures, usually with acoustic shadowing, within the gallbladder lumen.[17,22,43] They may be single or multiple and are typically mobile, falling to the dependent gallbladder wall (Fig. 39-33). Although choleliths are usually incidental findings, they have the potential to obstruct the bile duct. Intraluminal biliary sludge is

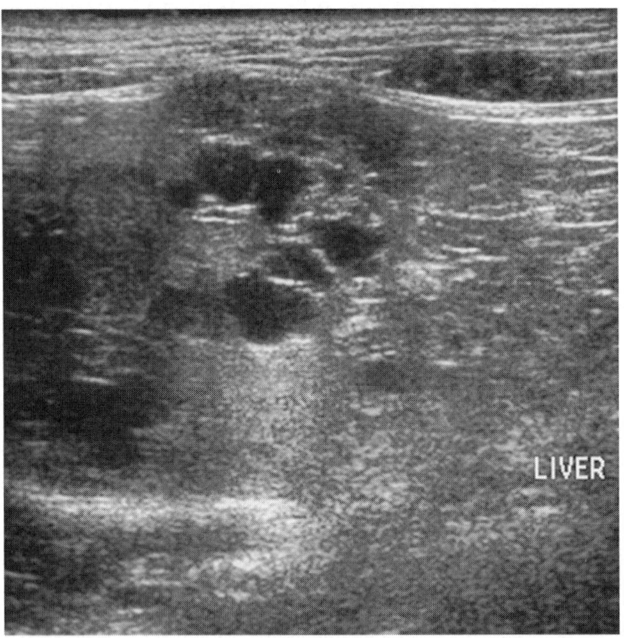

Fig. 39-31 Longitudinal ultrasound image of the liver from a cat with cystadenoma. A mass with anechoic cystic components, some with acoustic enhancement, is present.

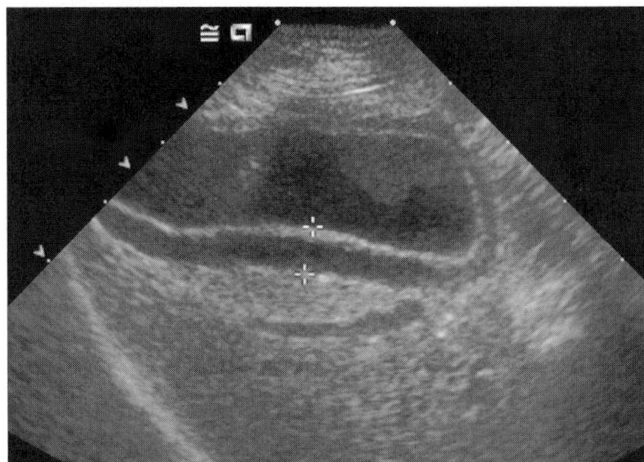

Fig. 39-32 Longitudinal ultrasound image of the liver and gallbladder from a dog with right-sided congestive heart failure. The gallbladder wall (between calipers) is thickened and has a layered appearance.

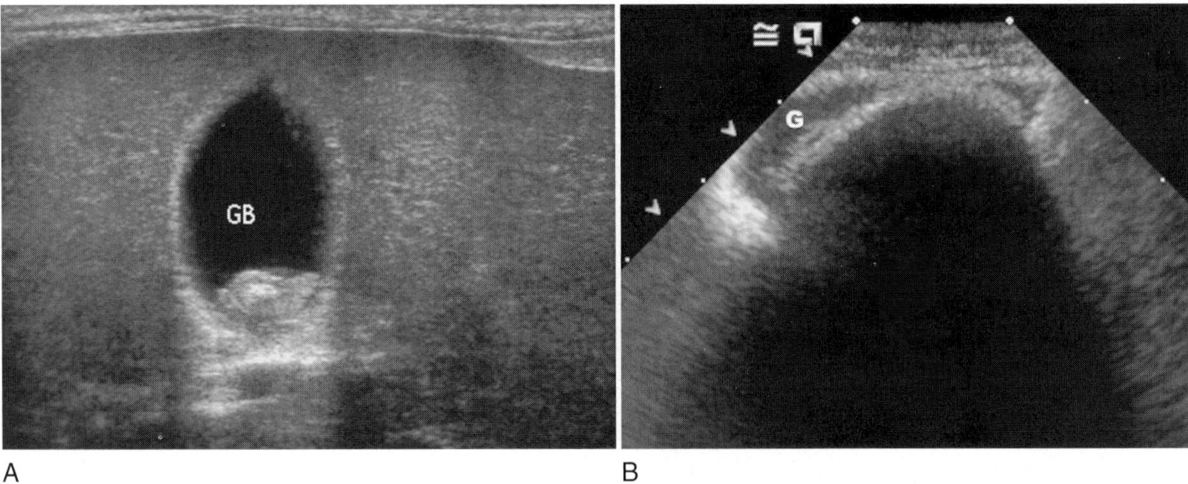

Fig. 39-33 Transverse ultrasound images of the gallbladder from two dogs. **A,** A small, dependent cholelith is present within the gallbladder lumen. Minimal shadowing is visible. *GB,* Gallbladder. **B,** A large, mineralized cholelith fills up most of the lumen of the gallbladder *(G)*. Only the echogenic rim of the cholelith and large acoustic shadow deep to the cholelith are visible.

usually of no clinical significance. However, a more organized form of nondependent sludge (semisolid mass of mucus), creating either a stellate or striated appearance within the gallbladder lumen, is termed biliary mucocele and may indicate gallbladder infection and necrosis (Fig. 39-34).[83-85] Hyperplasia of mucus-secreting glands within the gallbladder mucosa and abnormal accumulation of mucus within the gallbladder lumen occurs, with subsequent biliary obstruction by mucinous plugs within the cystic and bile duct. Distension of the intrahepatic and/or extrahepatic biliary system may be present. Ischemic necrosis of the gallbladder wall can lead to rupture. In one study, gallbladder mucoceles were associated with a 50% incidence of loss of gallbladder wall integrity and/or acute rupture.[83] The presence of discontinuity of gallbladder wall, pericholecystic hyperechoic fat, and/or pericholecystic fluid was strongly suggestive of gallbladder rupture in patients with biliary mucocele.[83,84] Cholecystocentesis should be discouraged in these patients because gallbladder wall rupture may be imminent.

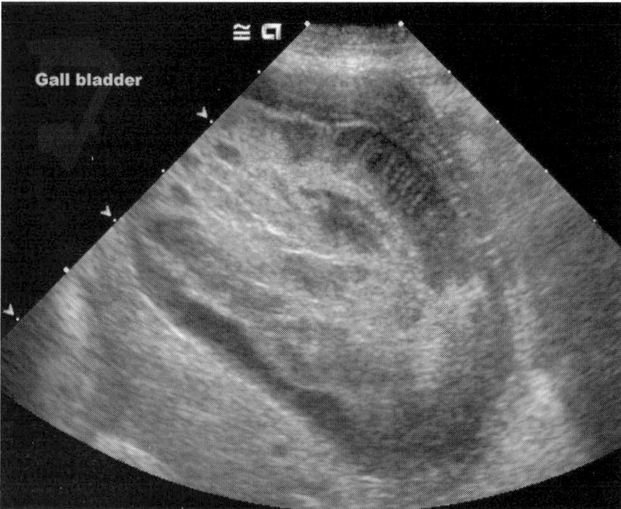

Fig. 39-34 Longitudinal ultrasound image of a gallbladder mucocele. Echogenic biliary sludge fills the gallbladder lumen, creating a striated appearance along the periphery.

Extrahepatic biliary obstruction results in a retrograde dilation of the biliary system.[86] With complete obstruction, the gallbladder and cystic duct distend within 24 hours, with progressive dilation of the common bile duct within 48 hours (Fig. 39-35). Gallbladder distension may be minimal in the face of chronic inflammation and fibrosis. Progressive dilation of the common bile duct and hepatic ducts occur during the next 3 to 4 days, with dilation of lobar and interlobar ducts seen by 7 days. This results in multiple tortuous, irregularly branching anechoic linear tracks within the liver. Although calculi in the bile duct can result in obstruction, more common causes include pancreatitis and neoplasia in the adjacent pancreas, duodenum, or liver.[87] Sludge accumulation within the bile duct associated with cholangiohepatitis can also result in extrahepatic biliary obstruction. Incomplete or early obstruction may not cause visible biliary dilation. Bile duct dilation may be prolonged, persisting after resolution of the obstruction.[43]

Vascular Disease

Venous congestion occurs with right-sided congestive heart failure or obstructive lesions in the caudal vena cava cranial to the diaphragm. Both hepatic caudal vena cava and hepatic veins dilate in response to the elevated pressures (Fig. 39-36). The liver may also enlarge and become hypoechoic, although echogenicity changes may not be consistent. Dilated caudal vena cava and hepatic veins, along with ascites, is suspicious of disease cranial to the diaphragm.

Ultrasonography can be used to identify most portosystemic shunts reliably, although detection of these vascular anomalies is operator dependent and requires a high skill level.[88] An abnormal shunting vessel is the most reliable indication of portosystemic shunt, but other changes, including a small liver, decreased or absent intrahepatic portal vasculature, increased vena cava size, enlarged kidneys, and renal and/or cystic calculi (urate calculi), are often present and are helpful in the diagnosis (Fig. 39-37).[43,88,89] With extrahepatic shunts (primarily affecting cats and small-breed dogs), the most common finding is a single shunt vessel connecting the portal vein, or a major tributary of the portal vein, to the left lateral aspect of the caudal vena cava between the right renal vein

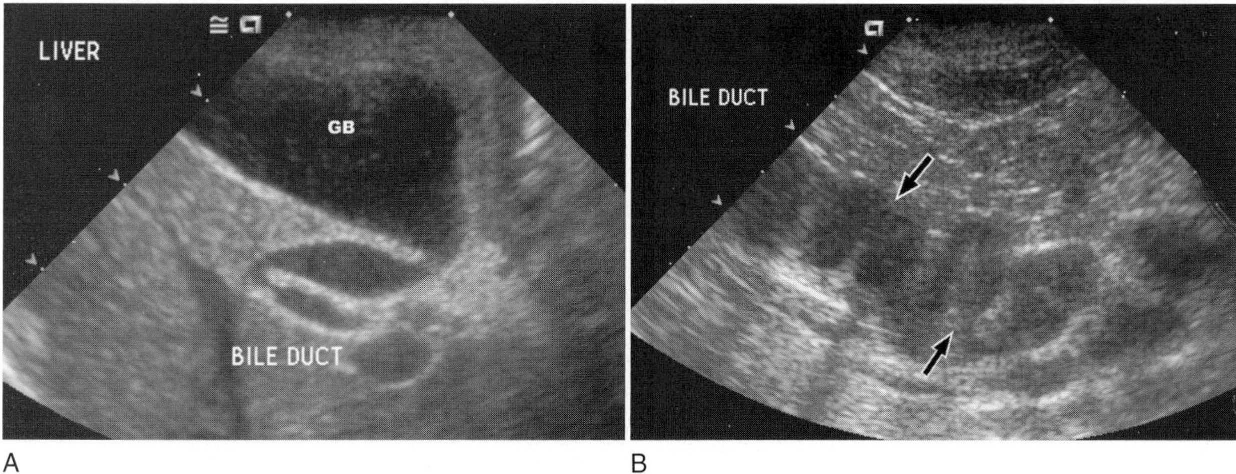

Fig. 39-35 Extrahepatic biliary obstruction. **A,** Longitudinal ultrasound image of a dog with extrahepatic biliary obstruction as a result of pancreatitis. The gallbladder *(GB)* and bile duct are moderately distended. **B,** Longitudinal ultrasound image of a cat with extrahepatic biliary obstruction caused by a pancreatic mass. The bile duct is dilated and tortuous *(arrows)*.

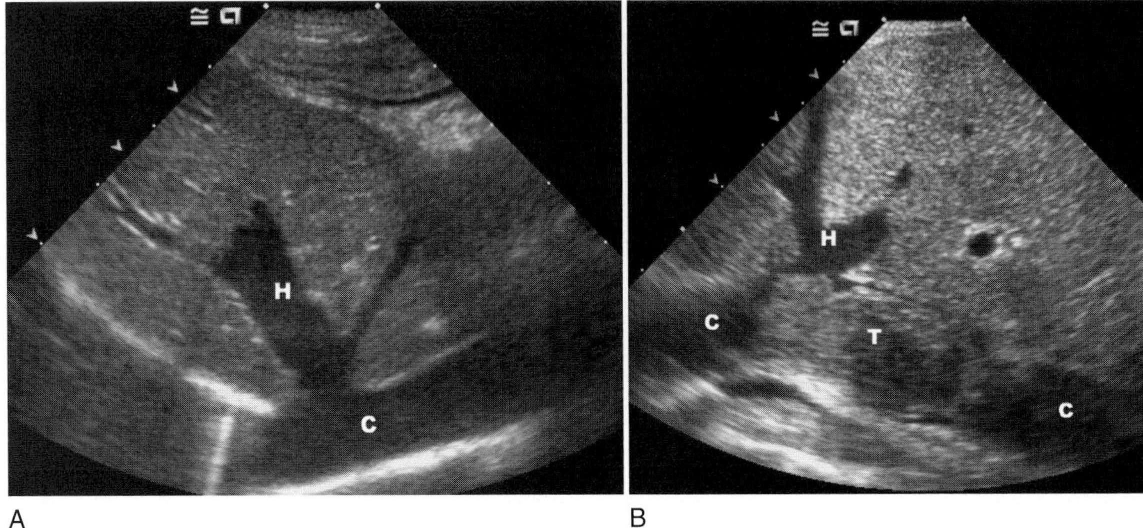

Fig. 39-36 Venous congestion. **A,** Right lateral oblique ultrasound image of the liver. The caudal vena cava and hepatic veins are distended as a result of right-sided congestive heart failure. C, Caudal vena cava; *H,* hepatic vein. **B,** Longitudinal ultrasound image of the liver in a dog with ascites. The lumen of the caudal vena cava *(C)* is filled with an echogenic thrombus *(T)*. The hepatic veins *(H)* are dilated as a result of the obstruction.

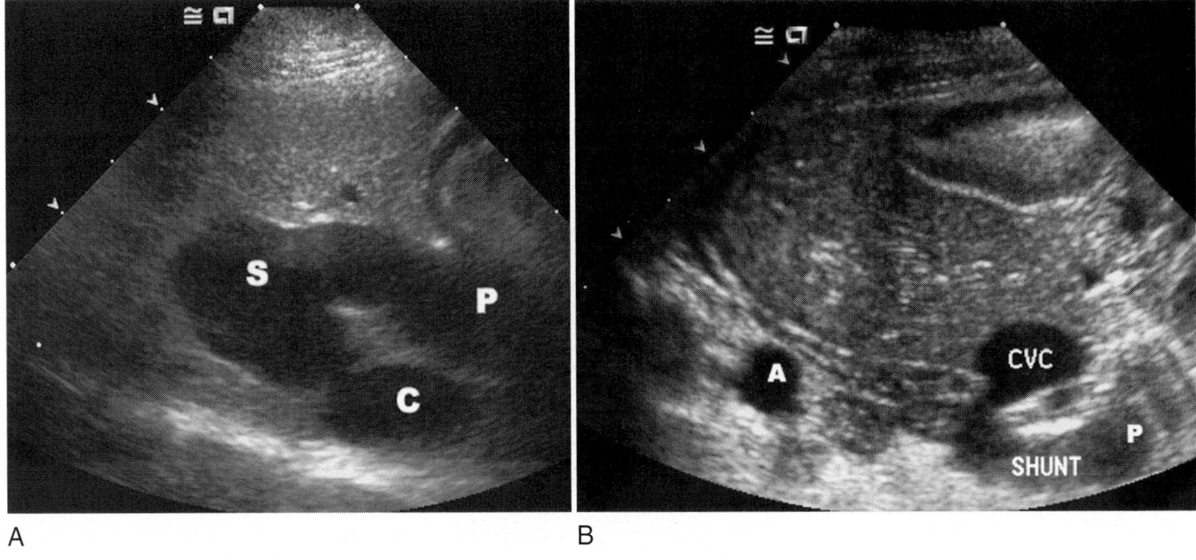

Fig. 39-37 Portosystemic shunts. **A,** Right lateral intercostal ultrasound image of a young dog with an intrahepatic portosystemic shunt. *P,* Portal vein; *S,* shunt; C, caudal vena cava. Dorsal is to the *left* of the image and right is at the *top* of the image. **B,** Right lateral intercostal ultrasound image of a young dog with an extrahepatic portosystemic shunt. *A,* Aorta; *CVC,* caudal vena cava; *P,* portal vein. Dorsal is to the *left* of the image, and right is at the *top* of the image.

and the hepatic veins.[89-92] Extrahepatic shunt vessels are more difficult to visualize because of poor acoustic windows (small liver) or the presence of bowel gas. A right dorsal intercostal window, in addition to routine views, is helpful in detecting the anomalous shunt vessel. In this window the portal vein and caudal vena cava are visible as they enter the porta hepatis, and abnormal shunting vessels may be more easily visualized. Pulsed-wave or color Doppler interrogation of the caudal vena cava is helpful in assessing for abnormal flow turbulence where a shunting vessel enters the vena cava.[88] Portoazygous shunts represent a less-common type of extrahepatic shunt. The presence of a large vessel in the craniodorsal abdomen coursing along the aorta, with flow directed cranially, is indicative of an abnormally enlarged azygous vein or the shunt vessel itself and is considered diagnostic for a portoazygous shunt.[88] Extrahepatic acquired shunt vessels attributable to hepatic disease and portal hypertension may appear as a grouping of multiple small, tortuous vessels, often medial to the spleen and left kidney. In some patients these abnormal vessels are not easily visualized without color flow Doppler imaging.[89] Intrahepatic shunts (primarily affecting small-breed dogs) may be somewhat easier to identify. A right lateral dorsal and left ventral intercostal window, in addition to the standard ventral abdominal approach, is helpful in visualizing intrahepatic anomalous vessels. These shunt vessels typically are large, with aberrant, tortuous courses connecting the intrahepatic portal vein and caudal vena cava and hepatic vein.[93] Measurement of portal flow velocity and the use of portal vein to aortic and portal vein to caudal vena cava ratios may also be valuable in the search for portosystemic shunts.[88] Contrast harmonic sonography has been used to detect increased hepatic arterial flow as an indicator of portosystemic shunting and may be useful as an additional diagnostic test.[94]

RADIOLOGY OF THE SPLEEN

The spleen is a dynamic organ whose normal size and location vary widely, especially in the dog. Subsequently, although usually visible, the radiographic appearance of the normal spleen can have numerous variations.[1-5] The spleen is typically divided into a proximal extremity (head of the spleen), a body, and a distal extremity (tail of the spleen). The proximal extremity is relatively fixed in the left craniodorsal aspect of the abdomen because of the gastrosplenic ligament. The distal extremity is not fixed and its position can vary considerably. On ventrodorsal views of the canine abdomen, the proximal extremity of the spleen is typically seen as a triangular soft tissue opacity caudolateral to the gastric fundus and craniolateral to the left kidney (Fig. 39-38). The remainder of the spleen may extend caudally, adjacent to the left lateral abdominal wall, or more medially across the midline. In this instance, the full length of the spleen is incompletely visualized. On lateral views, the triangular soft tissue opacity of the proximal extremity of the spleen is located dorsally, caudal to the stomach. The distal extremity is typically visualized as a triangular soft tissue opacity immediately caudal and slightly ventral to the pylorus or liver (Fig. 39-39). The distal extremity of the spleen is often more conspicuous on right lateral views of the abdomen but may silhouette the caudal margin of the liver and be poorly visualized as a separate structure.

The feline spleen is thinner and smaller compared with the dog and less variable in size and position (Fig 39-40; also see Fig. 39-1, C). Similar to the dog, the proximal extremity of the spleen can be visualized on ventrodorsal views in the left cranial abdomen, caudolateral to the stomach and craniolateral to the left kidney. The distal extremity usually extends caudally along the left lateral abdominal wall, allowing visualization of the entire spleen. On lateral abdominal views, the proximal extremity may be visualized caudal and dorsal to the gastric fundus. The distal extremity may occasionally be visible caudal to the stomach but is usually not seen in the normal cat.

Splenic Size

Radiographic assessment of splenic size is subjective, with the normal spleen size varying widely. Generalized splenomegaly results in rounded, blunted margins, with dorsal and caudal displacement of the small intestines on lateral views (Fig. 39-41). Organ displacement on ventrodorsal views depends on the portion of the spleen that is enlarged and the degree of enlargement. Small intestines may be displaced to the right or left, whereas an enlarged proximal extremity results in cranial displacement of the stomach. Considerations for diffuse splenomegaly are numerous and include inflammation (splenitis caused by infection with toxoplasmosis, fungal organisms, Haemobartonella, ehrlichiosis), hyperplasia (hemolytic disorders, systemic lupus erythematosus, chronic bacteremic disorders), congestion (impaired venous drainage, portal hypertension, splenic torsion/infarction, tranquilization and barbiturate administration), and infiltrative disease

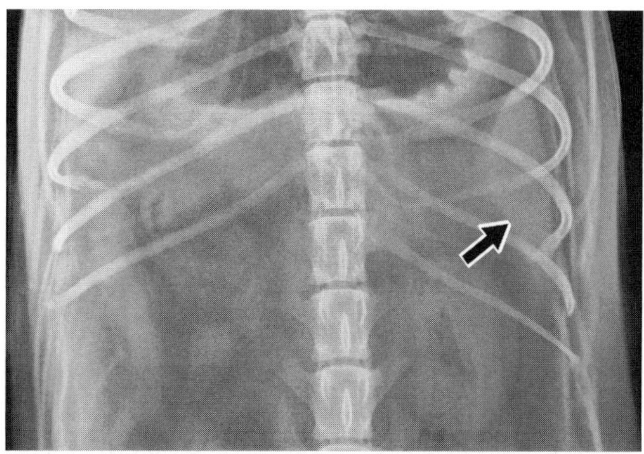

A

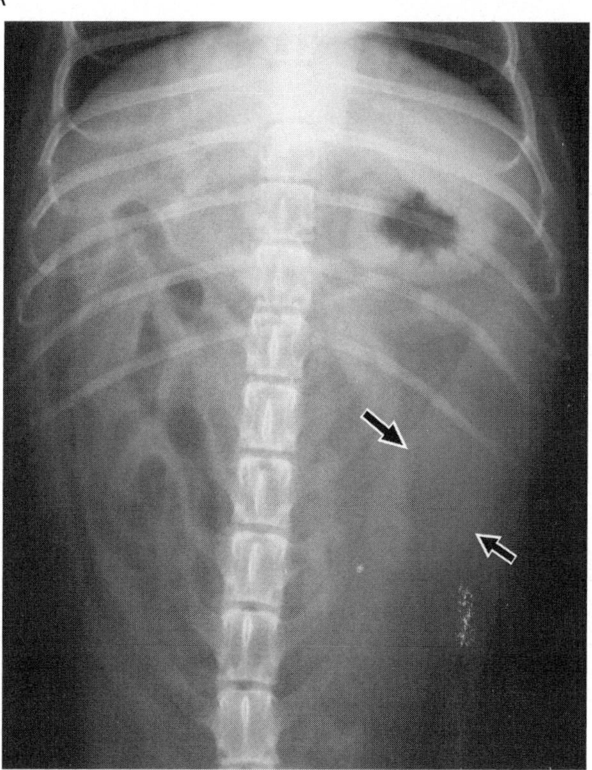

B

Fig. 39-38 Normal spleen. **A,** Ventrodorsal radiograph of the abdomen of a normal dog. The proximal portion of the spleen is visible in the left cranial abdomen, caudolateral to the gastric fundus and craniolateral to the left kidney *(arrow)*. **B,** Ventrodorsal radiograph of the abdomen of a normal dog. The entire spleen can be visualized extending down the left lateral abdomen *(arrows)*.

(neoplasia, both primary and metastatic; extramedullary hematopoiesis).[95] Lymphosarcoma, leukemia, systemic mastocytosis, multiple myeloma, and malignant histiocytosis can all result in diffuse neoplastic enlargement of the spleen. Compared with the dog, generalized splenomegaly in the cat is most commonly caused by neoplastic infiltration, primarily lymphosarcoma and mast cell tumor (Fig. 39-42; also see Fig. 39-5).[96,97]

Splenic torsion occurs when the spleen rotates around its mesenteric axis, resulting in complete occlusion of venous

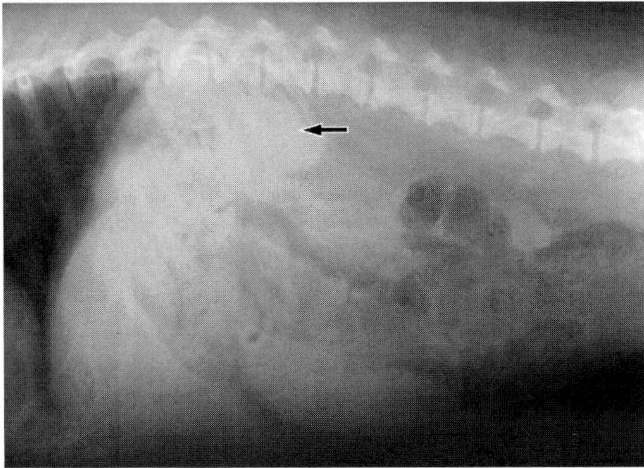

Fig. 39-39 Right lateral radiograph of the abdomen of a normal dog. The distal extremity of the spleen is visualized caudal to the liver. The proximal extremity is poorly visualized in the craniodorsal abdomen, caudal to the gastric fundus *(arrow)*.

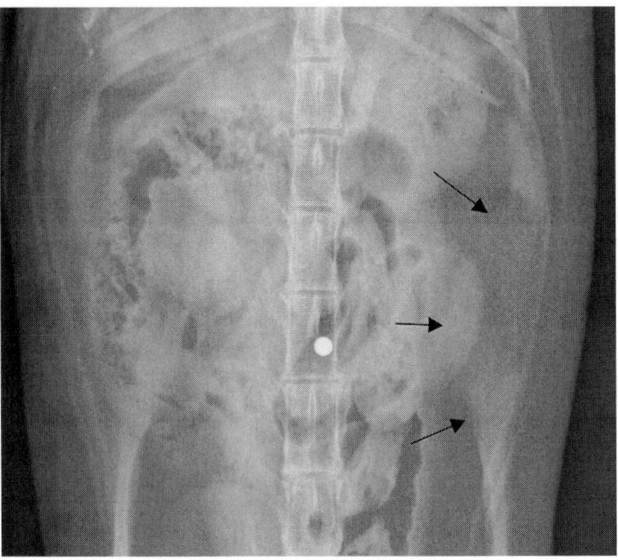

Fig. 39-40 Ventrodorsal radiograph of the abdomen of a normal cat. The entire spleen is visualized along the left lateral abdominal wall *(arrow)*.

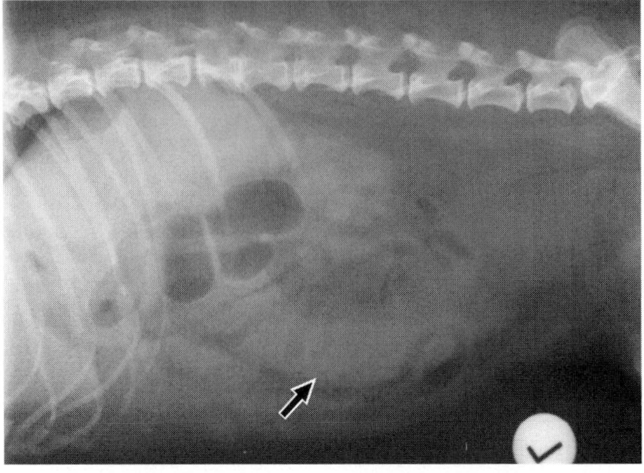

A

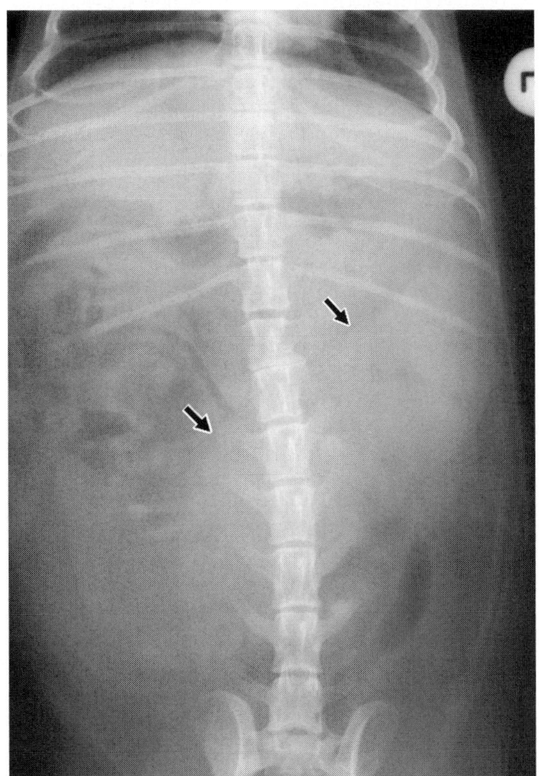

B

Fig. 39-41 Lateral (A) and ventrodorsal (B) radiographs of the abdomen of a dog with lymphosarcoma. The enlarged spleen is elongated, with rounded margins on both views *(arrows)*.

drainage and eventual arterial occlusion. This results in marked splenomegaly as well as atypical splenic location.* The spleen may acquire a C shape on the lateral view or may simply appear as a mass in the ventral abdomen (Fig. 39-43). Poor visualization of the spleen may be caused by accompanying peritoneal fluid. If gas-producing bacteria proliferate within the ischemic splenic parenchyma, emphysematous changes may occur, resulting in a mottled or foamy radiographic appearance.[26,99] Computed tomography has been used in the diagnosis of splenic torsion; findings include splenomegaly, a corkscrew-like soft tissue mass representing the rotated splenic pedicle, and lack of contrast enhancement.[100] The spleen may undergo torsion on its own or in association with gastric volvulus.

Focal splenic enlargement, as from a mass, results in local displacement of adjacent viscera depending on the location of the splenic mass (Figs. 39-44 and 39-45). Although often sharply marginated, the splenic mass may be obscured by peritoneal effusion associated with the mass (hemorrhage). A mass in the body or distal extremity of the spleen is probably the most common cause of a ventral abdominal mass, and on the lateral view results in dorsal and caudal displacement of the small intestines. On ventrodorsal views these masses may be midline in location or to the right or left of midline. Masses of the proximal extremity of the spleen are less common and may displace the stomach cranially, with caudal, medial, and ventral displacement of the small intestine and descending colon. The left kidney may be displaced caudally as well.

*References 1, 2, 5, 26, 98, 99.

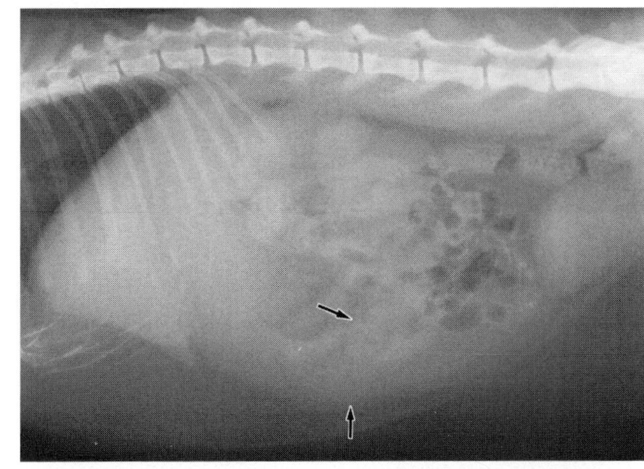

A

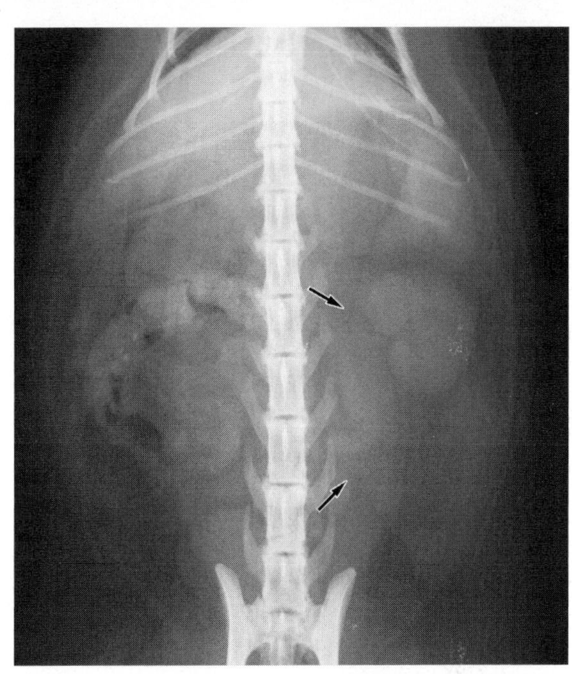

B

Fig. 39-42 Lateral (A) and ventrodorsal (B) radiographs of the abdomen of a cat with lymphosarcoma. The spleen is elongated and rounded and easily visualized on both views *(arrows)*.

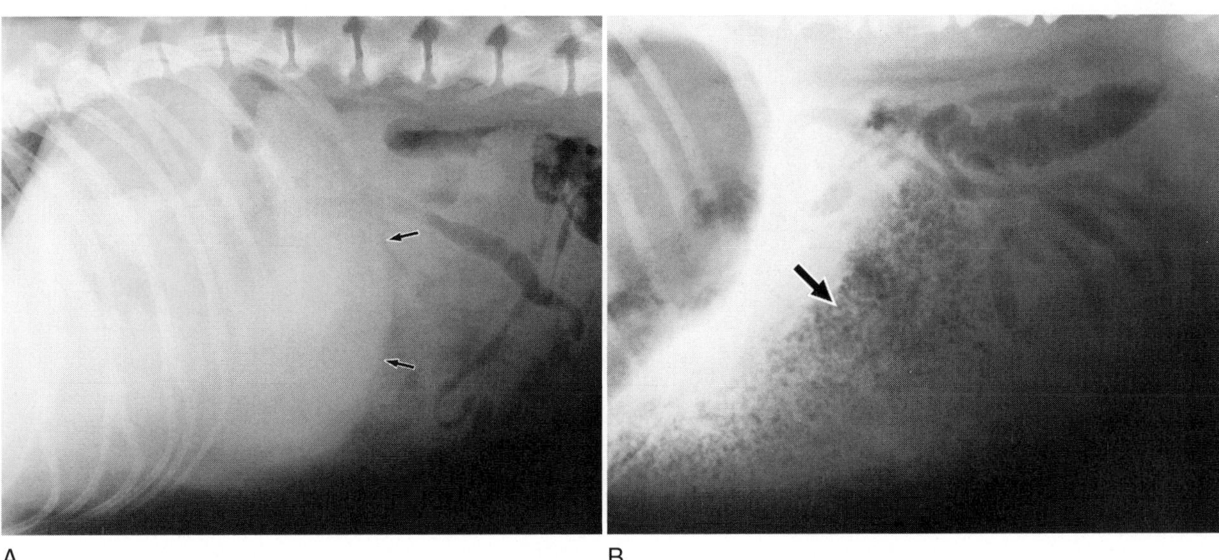

A B

Fig. 39-43 Splenic torsion. **A,** Lateral radiograph of the abdomen of a dog with splenic torsion. The spleen is enlarged and displaced caudally and dorsally *(arrows)*. **B,** Lateral radiograph of the abdomen of a dog with emphysematous splenic torsion. A mottled gas pattern is present within the enlarged and caudally displaced spleen *(arrows)*. Abdominal effusion obscures the splenic outline.

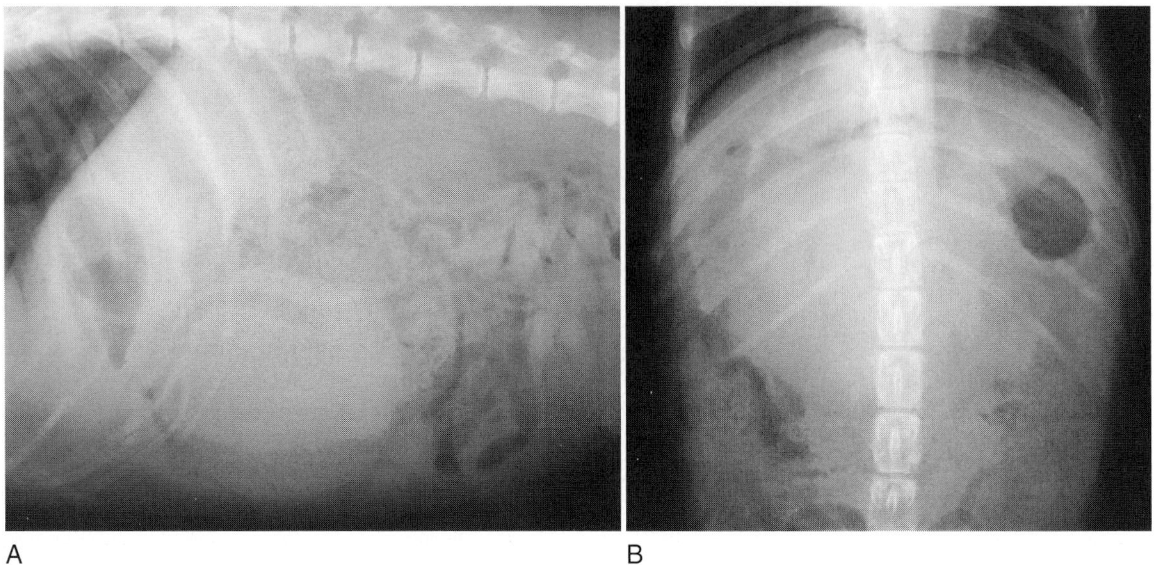

Fig. 39-44 Lateral (A) and ventrodorsal (B) radiographs of the abdomen of a dog with splenic hemangiosarcoma. A mass is present on the tail of the spleen, seen along the ventral abdomen on the lateral view, and on the cranial midline on the ventrodorsal view. The stomach is displaced cranially, with caudal displacement of the transverse colon on the ventrodorsal view.

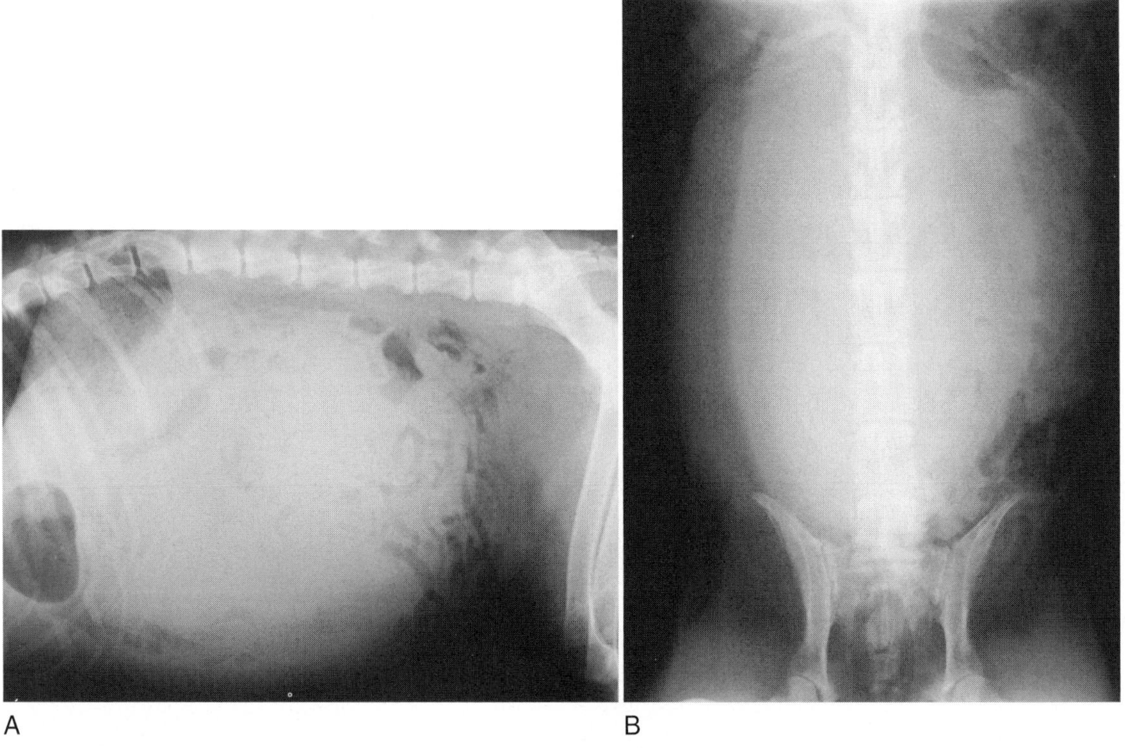

Fig. 39-45 Lateral (A) and ventrodorsal (B) radiographs of the abdomen of a dog with a splenic hematoma. The spleen is tremendously enlarged, with marked caudal and left-sided displacement of the small bowel.

Differentials for focal splenic enlargement include benign and neoplastic conditions. Primary and metastatic neoplasia, hematoma, nodular hyperplasia, extramedullary hematopoiesis, and abscess are all considerations.[97,101-103] Hemangiosarcoma is the most common neoplasm of the canine spleen, but splenic hematoma and hyperplastic nodules are the most common cause of splenic lesions.[103] Peritoneal effusion may accompany both benign and neoplastic diseases.

Normal splenic opacity is that of soft tissue. Mineralization of the spleen may be the result of dystrophic calcification of abscesses, hematomas, fungal granulomas, or neoplastic masses.[13] Gas within the spleen may be caused by splenic

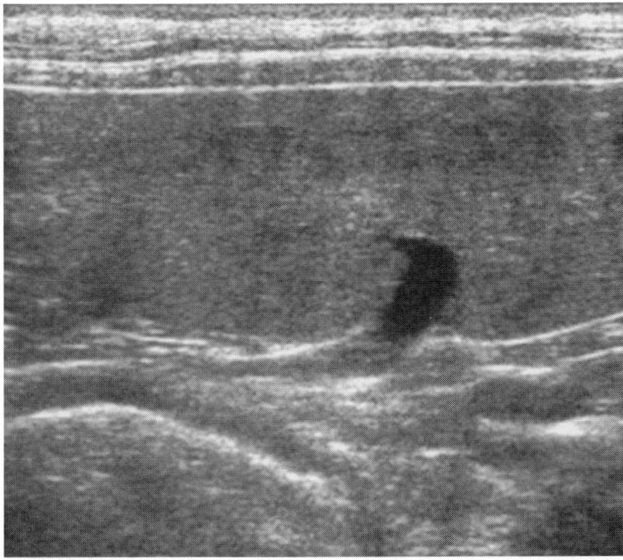

A

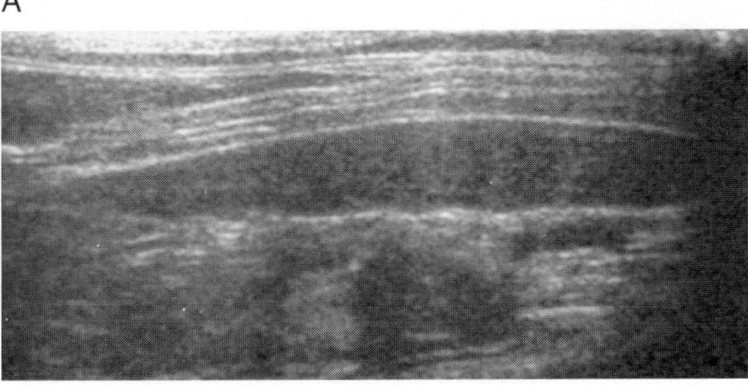

B

Fig. 39-46 Normal ultrasound appearance of the spleen. **A,** Longitudinal ultrasound image of the spleen in a normal dog. A splenic vein is seen leaving the splenic hilus. **B,** Longitudinal ultrasound image of the spleen in a normal cat. The feline spleen is typically a linear, thin structure, smaller in size compared with the dog.

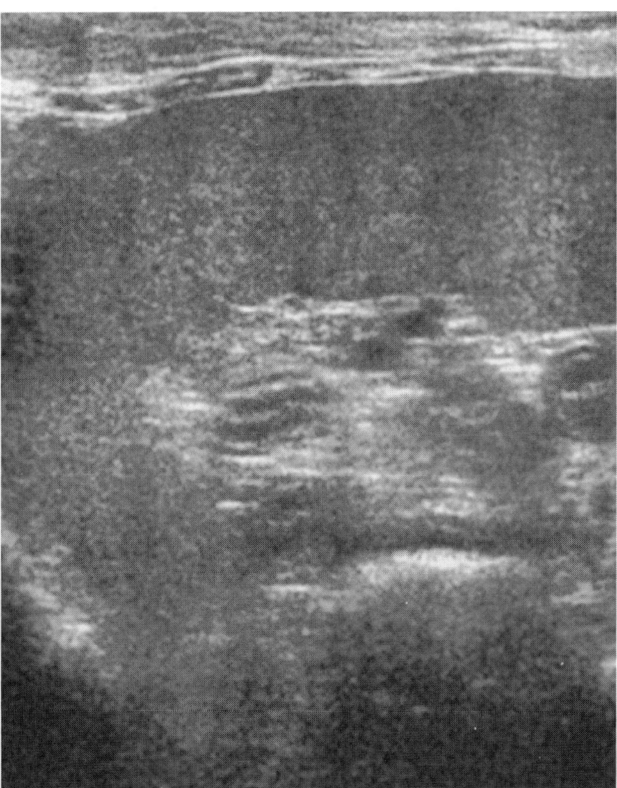

Fig. 39-47 Longitudinal ultrasound image of an enlarged spleen in a cat. The spleen is rounded and thickened, with folding of the cranial extremity (compare with Fig. 47, *B*). Mast cell tumor was diagnosed on fine-needle aspiration.

torsion (see Fig. 39-43, *B*). However, as in the liver, gas may ascend into the portovenous circulation and affect the spleen.[1,26,27] Infection with gas-forming organisms may involve the splenic or mesenteric vasculature.

Ultrasound of the Spleen

The canine spleen is well suited to ultrasound examination because of its superficial location and the lack of intervening gas-containing structures. The feline spleen may be difficult to image in some cats because of its smaller size.

Splenic location varies. The proximal extremity (head of the spleen) is located in the left craniolateral abdominal quadrant and may be beneath the costal arch. Intercostal windows may be necessary, especially in deep-chested dogs. The canine splenic body and distal extremity (tail of the spleen) may extend caudally along the left lateral abdomen or move medially across the ventral midline. It often appears folded on itself. The feline spleen is more consistent in location, along the left lateral abdominal wall, and rarely folds on itself unless enlarged.

The splenic parenchyma should be uniform, with a fine, dense pattern.[43] Echogenicity is slightly greater than the liver and renal cortex (Fig. 39-46). Splenic arteries are not usually seen without Doppler interrogation, but splenic veins are visualized as a Y-shaped confluence at the hilus. Tissue surrounding these vessels at the hilus may be highly echogenic because of capsular invagination and fat, considered a normal finding.[43] Splenic size is subjective and based on sonographer experience. When enlarged, the spleen may extend caudally or more completely cover the ventral abdomen. Splenic borders become rounded or blunted compared with the normal sharp, linear appearance. The spleen has no absolute size limits in the dog or cat (Fig. 39-47). Splenic size change suspected from sonography should be confirmed by palpation or abdominal radiographs.

Abnormal Splenic Sonographic Findings

Diffuse Disease

As in the liver, diffuse disease of the spleen potentially causes an increase in size or a change in echogenicity. However, these changes may be difficult to identify or characterize, especially with mild or early disease. Splenomegaly, with either normal or decreased echogenicity, is reported with numerous conditions, including congestion, neoplasia, infarction, inflammation, immune-mediated disease, chronic hemolytic anemia, parasitic infections, extramedullary hematopoiesis, and infection (bacterial or fungal).[43,61,96,98,104-110] Splenic congestion as a result of administration of phenothiazine and pentobarbital drug groups results in splenomegaly with no associated changes in echogenicity.[104] Congestion from portal hypertension appears similar, but dilated splenic veins may also be present. Splenic torsion, a form of splenic congestion, has a variety of appearances.[98,105] Splenomegaly may be the only finding. However, splenomegaly with a diffuse hypoechoic parenchyma, separated by linear echogenicities that represent dilated hyperechoic vessels, is highly suggestive of torsion

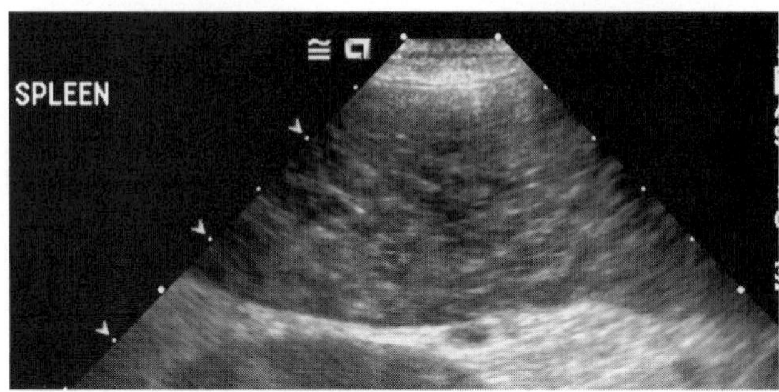

Fig. 39-48 Longitudinal ultrasound image of the spleen in a dog with splenic torsion. The spleen is enlarged and hypoechoic, with linear echogenicities representing dilated vessels.

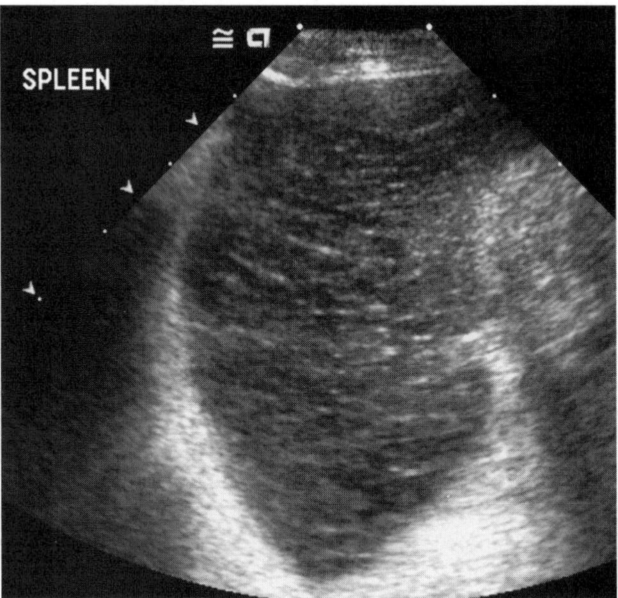

Fig. 39-49 Longitudinal ultrasound image of the spleen in a dog with complete splenic infarction. The spleen is enlarged and hypoechoic, with linear echogenicities throughout the parenchyma. The appearance is identical to splenic torsion (see Fig. 39-48).

(Fig. 39-48). Splenic veins may be dilated, with visible intravascular echogenicities representing formed thrombi or static echogenic blood. Complete absence of flow at the splenic hilus is also common, as is accompanying free peritoneal fluid. Gas shadows within the splenic parenchyma may indicate the presence of necrosis and gas-forming organisms. Diffuse splenic infarction as a result of other disease processes can have an identical appearance (Fig. 39-49).[106,107]

Diffuse neoplastic infiltration of the spleen has a variety of appearances, and tumor type cannot be determined from the ultrasound appearance (Fig. 39-50).[43,61,63,96,108-110] Lymphosarcoma, mast cell tumor, malignant histiocytosis, leukemic infiltration, and multiple myeloma can all result in splenomegaly with normal or decreased echogenicity. The parenchyma may appear uneven or coarse. Focal or multifocal nodules (usually hypoechoic) of varying sizes may also be present. A miliary nodular pattern of small hypoechoic nodules (moth eaten or Swiss cheese appearance) is suggestive of lymphosarcoma, but other neoplastic diseases, such as malignant histiocytosis, must also be considered.[110]

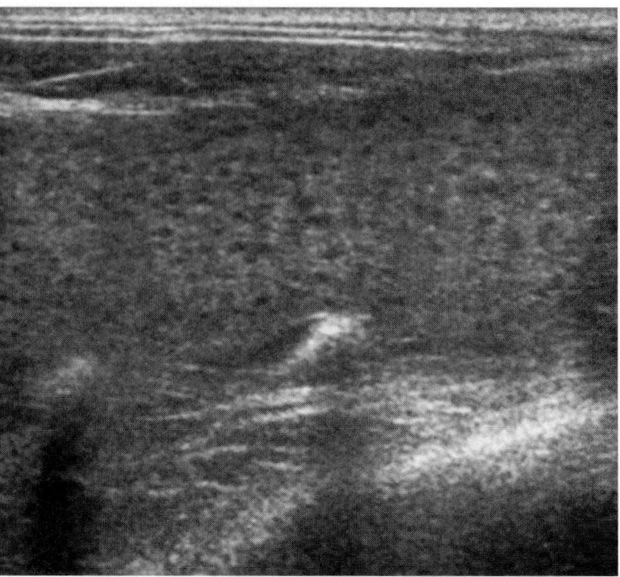

Fig. 39-50 Longitudinal ultrasound image of the spleen in a cat. The spleen is enlarged, with rounded margins. Multiple small hypoechoic nodules are present diffusely throughout the parenchyma. Lymphosarcoma was diagnosed on fine-needle aspiration.

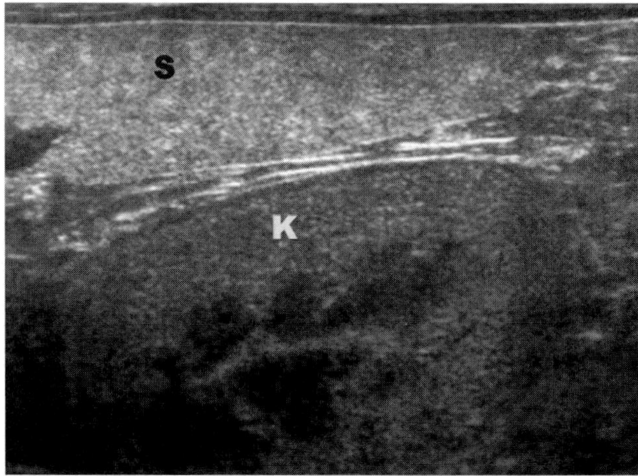

Fig. 39-51 Longitudinal ultrasound image of the spleen and left kidney in a dog. The spleen is markedly hyperechoic to the renal cortex, with poorly defined hyperechoic nodules. Extramedullary hematopoiesis was diagnosed by fine-needle aspiration. *S*, Spleen; *K*, kidney.

Diffuse increased echogenicity of the spleen is less common but may be seen with chronic vascular compromise, peritonitis, infection, or diffuse nonneoplastic infiltrative disease such as extramedullary hematopoiesis (Fig. 39-51).[43]

As in the liver, numerous considerations exist for focal disease, including primary and secondary neoplasia, nodular hyperplasia, hematoma, abscess, and infarction (Fig. 39-52). Lymphosarcoma, one of the most common splenic tumors, has a variety of appearances. In addition to the diffuse changes previously noted, lymphosarcoma may also produce focal hypoechoic or anechoic nodules or a single complex or cavitated mass.[63,96,110] Splenic masses attributable to hemangiosarcoma are typically complex, with hypoechoic,

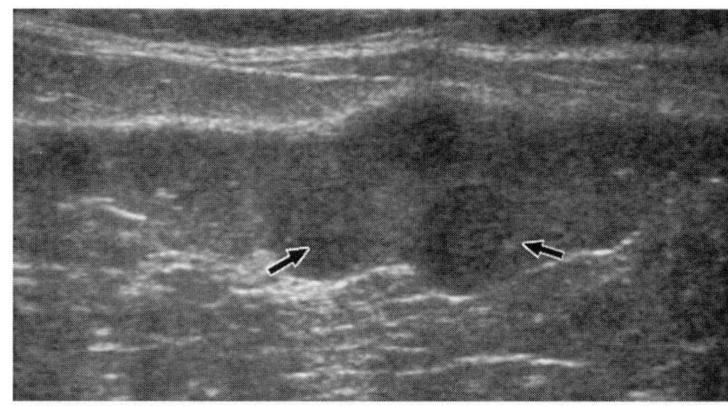

A

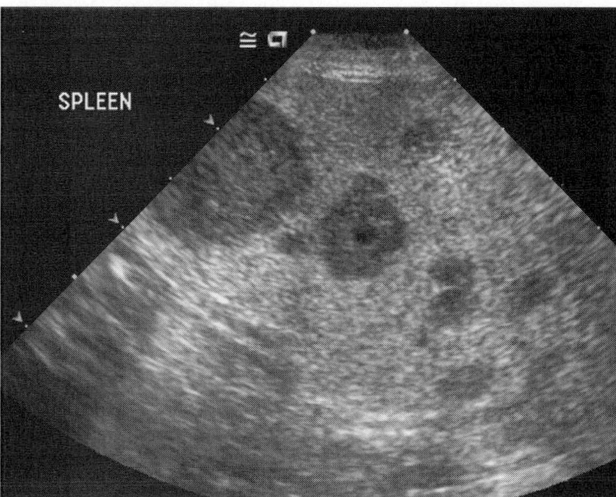

B

Fig. 39-52 Splenic nodules. **A,** Longitudinal ultrasound image of the spleen in a cat. Multiple hypoechoic nodules are present, causing focal bulging of the splenic margin *(arrows)*. Lymphosarcoma was diagnosed by fine-needle aspiration. **B,** Longitudinal ultrasound image of the spleen in a dog. Multiple irregular hypoechoic nodules are noted in the hyperechoic splenic parenchyma. Metastatic carcinoma was diagnosed at necropsy.

hyperechoic, and anechoic areas caused by hemorrhage, necrosis, and fibrotic or calcified tissue (Fig. 39-53).[43] Peritoneal fluid often accompanies hemangiosarcoma, and the liver should be carefully evaluated for accompanying metastasis. Splenic hematomas are similar in appearance to those described in the liver and may be associated with acute or previous trauma or develop from neoplastic disease (Fig. 39-54).[43,101,111] Hematomas are indistinguishable sonographically from hemangiosarcoma masses, and both may progress over time.[112] Splenic abscesses are relatively uncommon, but they can have a similar complex appearance.[43,113] Splenic abscesses can vary from a simple hypoechoic, poorly defined area to a complex, cavitated mass. Echogenic areas with shadowing within the mass may indicate gas formation. Myelolipomas are fatty, hyperechoic nodules occasionally seen in the normal spleen, especially along the peripheral margin or adjacent to vessels (Fig. 39-55).[114,115] Splenic myelolipomas are considered benign and incidental findings, but mast cell tumors have been reported to cause hyperechoic nodules in the spleen and should also be considered when hyperechoic foci are seen.[96] The echogenicity of focal splenic infarction changes over time. Initially infarcts are hypoechoic and may appear as a round or bulging mass or simple focal enlargement of the spleen (Fig. 39-56).[106,107] With age, infarcts become increasingly echogenic

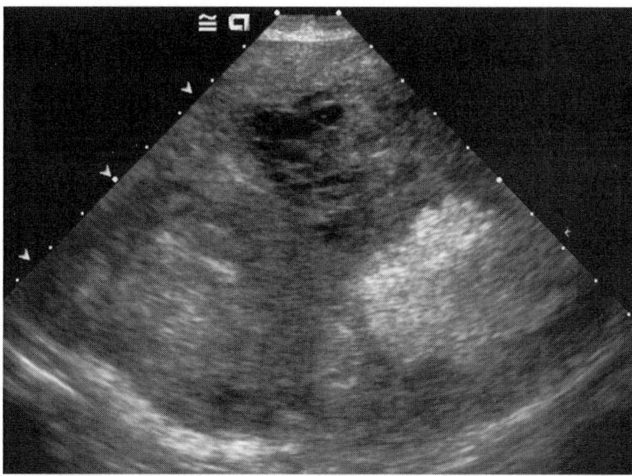

Fig. 39-53 Longitudinal ultrasound image of a splenic mass in a dog. Areas of hyperechogenicity, hypoechogenicity, and anechogenicity likely represent hemorrhage and necrosis. Hemangiosarcoma was diagnosed on histopathology.

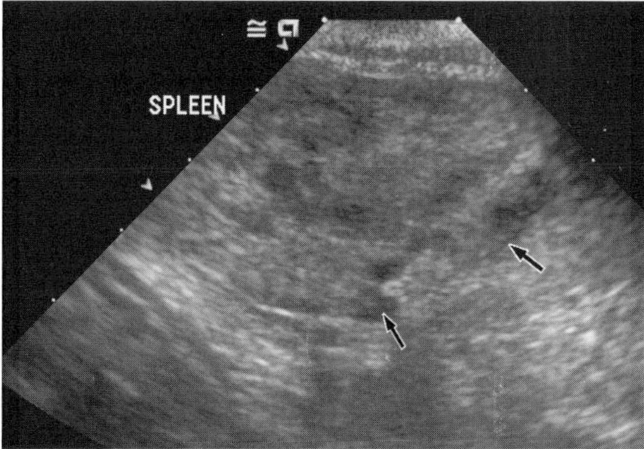

Fig. 39-54 Longitudinal ultrasound image of the distal extremity of the spleen in a dog presented for abdominal trauma (hit by car). Multiple poorly defined, coalescing hypoechoic nodules are present as a result of splenic hematoma formation. The spleen is outlined by *arrows.*

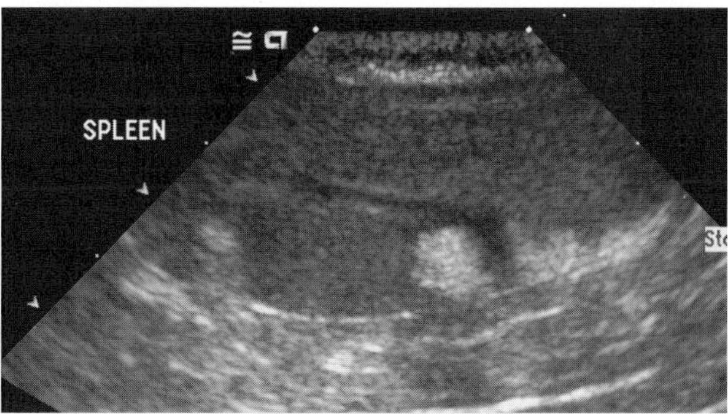

Fig. 39-55 Longitudinal ultrasound image of the spleen in a dog. Myelolipomas, seen as focal hyperechoic nodules, some with acoustic shadowing, are noted along the dorsal border.

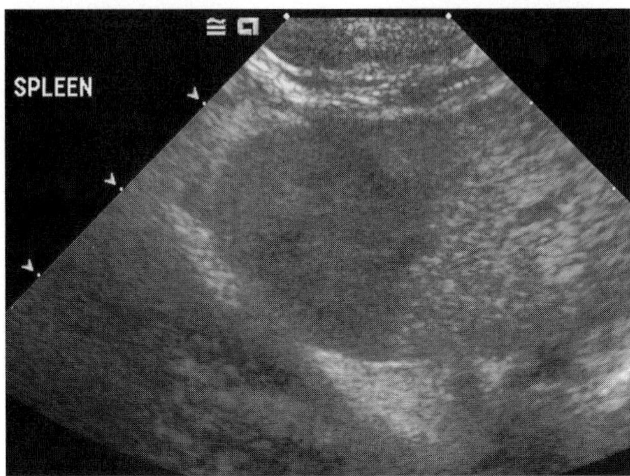

Fig. 39-56 Longitudinal ultrasound image of the spleen in a dog. The cranial extremity of the spleen is hypoechoic, with well-demarcated margins. No perfusion was present in the hypoechoic portion, consistent with an acute infarct.

and often are sharply demarcated from the normal splenic parenchyma. Nodular hyperplasia in the spleen has a similar appearance to that in the liver.[43] The splenic border may simply be smoothly irregular, or isoechoic, hypoechoic, or hyperechoic nodules may be present.

As in the liver, ultrasound is sensitive but not specific. Tissue samples are necessary for a more definitive diagnosis. Although diagnosis of diffuse splenic disease such as lymphosarcoma or extramedullary hematopoiesis may be achieved with needle aspiration, cavitated mass lesions such as hemangiosarcoma or hematoma may be more accurately diagnosed by splenectomy and histopathology of the mass.

REFERENCES

1. O'Brien T: The liver and spleen. In O'Brien T, editor: *Radiographic diagnosis of abdominal disorders in the dog and cat: radiographic interpretation, clinical signs, pathophysiology*, Philadelphia, 1979, WB Saunders.
2. Burt RL, Ackerman N: The abdomen. In Burt RL, Ackerman N, editors: *Small animal radiology and ultrasonography. a diagnostic atlas and text*, ed 2, Philadelphia, 1996, WB Saunders.
3. Farrow CF: The abdomen. In Farrow CF, editor: *Radiology of the cat*, St Louis, 1996, Mosby–Year Book.
4. Newell S, Graham JP: The liver and spleen. In Thrall DE, editor: *Textbook of veterinary diagnostic radiology*, ed 4, Philadelphia, 2002, WB Saunders.
5. Kealy JK: The liver and spleen. In Kealy JK, McCallister H, editors: *Diagnostic radiology & ultrasonography of the dog and cat*, ed 4, St Louis, 2005, Elsevier Saunders.
6. Suter PF: Radiographic diagnosis of liver disease in dogs and cats, *Vet Clin North Am* 12:153, 1982.
7. Biller DS, Partington BP: Hepatic imaging with radiology and ultrasound, *Vet Clin North Am Small Anim Pract* 25:305, 1995.
8. Carlisle CH: Radiographic anatomy of the cat gallbladder, *Vet Radiol* 18:170, 1977.
9. Root CR: Abdominal masses: the radiographic differential diagnosis, *Vet Radiol* 15:26, 1974.
10. Evans SM: The radiographic appearance of primary liver neoplasia in dogs, *Vet Radiol* 28:192, 1987.
11. Liptak JM, Cernell WS, Withrow SJ: Liver tumors in cats and dogs, *Compend Cont Educ Small Anim Pract* p. 50, January 2004.
12. Nickel R, Schummer A, Seiferle E et al: *The viscera of the domestic mammals*, Berlin, 1973, Verlag Paul Parey.
13. Lamb CR, Kleine LJ, McMillan MC: Diagnosis of calcification on abdominal radiographs, *Vet Radiol* 32:211, 1991.
14. Cantwell HD, Blevins WE, Hanika-Rebar C et al: Radiopaque hepatic and lobar duct choleliths in a dog, *Am Anim Hosp Assoc* 19:373, 1983.
15. Heidner GL, Campbell KL: Cholelithiasis in a cat, *J Am Vet Med Assoc* 186:176, 1985.
16. Jorgensen LS, Pentlarge VW, Flanders JA et al: Recurrent choleliths in a cat, *Compend Cont Educ Pract Vet* 9:265, 1987.
17. Kirpenstein J, Fingland RB, Ulrich T et al: Cholelithiasis in dogs: 29 cases (1980-1990), *J Am Vet Med Assoc* 202:1137, 1993.
18. Brömel C, Léveillé R, Scrivani PV, et al: Gallbladder perforation associated with cholelithiasis and cholecystitis in a dog, *J Small Anim Pract* 39:541, 1998.
19. Smith SA, Biller DS, Kraft SL et al: Diagnostic imaging of biliary obstruction, *Compend Cont Educ Pract Vet* 20:1225, 1998.
20. Rosenstein DS, Reif U, Stickle RL et al: Radiographic diagnosis: pericardioperitoneal diaphragm hernia and cholelithiasis in a dog, *Vet Radiol Ultrasound* 42:308-310, 2001.
21. Johnson SE: Cholelithiasis and cholangitis. In Kirk RW editors: *Current veterinary therapy X: small animal practice*, Philadelphia, 1989, WB Saunders.
22. Eich CS, Ludwig LL: The surgical treatment of cholelithiasis in cats: a study of nine cases, *J Am Anim Hosp Assoc* 38:290, 2002.
23. Brömel C, Smeak DD, Léveillé R: Porcelain gallbladder associated with primary biliary adenocarcinoma in a dog, *J Am Vet Med Assoc* 213:1137, 1998.
24. Thamm DH: Hepatobiliary tumors. In Withrow SJ, MacEwen EG editors: *Small animal clinical oncology*, Philadelphia, 2001, WB Saunders.
25. Scharf G, Deplazes P, Kaser-Hotz B et al: Radiographic, ultrasonographic, and computed tomographic appearance of alveolar echinococcosis in dogs, *Vet Radiol Ultrasound* 45:411, 2004.
26. Gaschen L, Kircher P, Venzin C et al: Imaging diagnosis: the abdominal air-vasculogram in a dog with splenic torsion and clostridial infection, *Vet Radiol Ultrasound* 44:553, 2003.
27. Sebastiá C, Quiroga S, Espin E et al: Portomesenteric vein gas: pathologic mechanisms, CT findings, and prognosis, *Radiographics* 20:1213, 2000.
28. Burk RL, Johnson GR: Emphysematous cholecystitis in the nondiabetic dog: three case histories, *Vet Radiol* 21:242, 1980.
29. Avgeris S, Hoskinson JJ: Emphysematous cholecystitis in a dog: a radiographic diagnosis, *J Am Anim Hosp Assoc* 28:344, 1992.
30. Lord PF, Carb A, Halliwell WH et al: Emphysematous hepatic abscess associated with trauma, necrotic hepatic nodular hyperplasia and adenoma in a dog: a case history report, *Vet Radiol* 23:46, 1982.
31. Grooters AM, Sherding RG, Biller DS et al: Hepatic abscess associated with diabetes mellitus in two dogs, *J Vet Intern Med* 8:203, 1994.
32. Grooters AM, Sherding RG, Johnson SE: Hepatic abscesses in dogs, *Compend Cont Educ* 17:833, 1995.
33. Farrar ET, Washabau RJ, Saunders HM: Hepatic abscesses in dogs: 14 cases (1982-1994), *J Am Vet Med Assoc* 208:243, 1996.
34. Suter P: Portal vein anomalies in the dog: their angiographic diagnosis, *J Am Vet Radiol Soc* 16:84, 1975.

35. Schmidt S, Suter PF: Angiography of the hepatic and portal venous system in the dog and cat: an investigative method, *Vet Radiol* 21:57, 1980.
36. Moon ML: Diagnostic imaging of portosystemic shunts, *Semin Vet Med Surg (SA)* 5: 120, 1990.
37. Lamb CR, Daniel GB: Diagnostic imaging of dogs with suspected portosystemic shunting, *Compend Cont Educ Small Anim Exotics* 24:626, 2002.
38. Hergessell EJ, Hornoff WJ, Koblik PD: Percutaneous ultrasound-guided trans-splenic catheterization of the portal vein in the dog, *Vet Radiol Ultrasound* 40:509, 1999.
39. Scrivani PV, Yeager AE, Dykes NL et al: Influence of patient positioning on sensitivity of mesenteric portography for detecting an anomalous portosystemic blood vessel in dogs: 34 cases (1997-2000), *J Am Vet Med Assoc* 219:1251, 2001.
40. White RN, Macdonald NJ, Burton CA: Use of intraoperative mesenteric portovenography in congenital portosystemic shunt surgery, *Vet Radiol Ultrasound* 44:514, 2003.
41. Thompson MS, Graham JP, Mariani CL: diagnosis of a porto-azygous shunt using helical computed tomography angiography, *Vet Radiol Ultrasound* 44:287, 2003.
42. Frank P, Mahaffey M, Egger C et al: Helical computed tomographic portography in ten normal dogs and ten dogs with a portosystemic shunt, *Vet Radiol Ultrasound* 44:392, 2003.
43. Nyland TG, Mattoon JS, Herrgesell EJ et al: Liver. In Nyland TG, Mattoon JS, editors: *Small animal diagnostic ultrasound,* ed 2, Philadelphia, 2002, WB Saunders.
44. Lamb CR: Ultrasonography of the liver and biliary tract, *Probl Vet Med* 3:555, 1991.
45. Nyland TG, Park RD: Hepatic ultrasonography in the dog, *Vet Radiol* 24:74, 1983.
46. Godshalk CP, Badertscher RR, Rippy MK et al: Quantitative ultrasonic assessment of live size in the dog, *Vet Radiol* 29:162, 1988.
47. Wu JX, Carlisle CH: Ultrasonographic examination of the canine liver based on recognition of hepatic and portal veins, *Vet Radiol Ultrasound* 36:234, 1995.
48. Brömel C, Barthez PY, Léveillé R et al: Prevalence of gallbladder sludge in dogs as assessed by ultrasonography, *Vet Radiol Ultrasound* 39:206, 1998.
49. Hittmair KM, Vielgrader HD, Loupal G: Ultrasonographic evaluation of gallbladder wall thickness in cats, *Vet Radiol Ultrasound* 42:149, 2001.
50. Spaulding KA: Ultrasound corner: gallbladder wall thickness, *Vet Radiol Ultrasound* 34:270, 1993.
51. Rivers BJ, Walther PA, Johnston GR et al: Acalculous cholecystitis in four canine cases: ultrasonographic findings and use of ultrasonographic-guided, percutaneous cholecystocentesis in diagnosis, *J Am Anim Hosp Assoc* 33:207, 1997.
52. Moentk J, Biller DS: Bilobed gallbladder in a cat: ultrasonographic appearance, *Vet Radiol Ultrasound* 34:354, 1993.
53. Léveillé R, Biller DS, Shiroma JJ: Sonographic evaluation of the common bile duct in cats, *J Vet Intern Med* 10:296, 1996.
54. Zeman RK, Taylor KJW, Rosenfield AT et al: Acute experimental biliary obstruction in the dog. Sonographic findings and clinical implications, *Am J Roentgenol* 136:965, 1981.
55. Biller DS, Kantrowitz B, Miyabayashi T: Ultrasonography of diffuse lever disease: a review, *J Vet Intern Med* 6:71, 1992.
56. Newell SM, Selcer BA, Girard E et al: Correlation between ultrasonographic findings and specific hepatic diseases in cats: 72 cases (1985-1997), *J Am Vet Med Assoc* 213:94, 1998.
57. Vörös K, Vrabély T, Papp et al: Correlation of ultrasonographic and patho-morphological findings in canine hepatic diseases, *J Small Anim Pract* 32:627, 1991.
58. Drost WT, Henry GA, Meinkoth JH et al: Quantification of hepatic and renal cortical echogenicity in clinically normal cats, *Am J Vet Res* 61:1016, 2000.
59. Yeager AE, Mohammed H, Accuracy of ultrasonography in the detection of severe hepatic lipidosis in cats, *Am J Vet Res* 53:597, 1992.
60. Nicoll RG, O'Brien RT, Jackson MW: Qualitative ultrasonography of the liver in obese cats, *Vet Radiol Ultrasound* 39:47-50, 1998.
61. Sato AF, Solano M: Ultrasonographic findings in abdominal mast cell disease: a retrospective study of 19 patients, *Vet Radiol Ultrasound* 45:51-57, 2004.
62. Tchelepi H, Ralls PW, Radin R et al: Sonography of diffuse liver disease, *J Ultrasound Med* 21:1023, 2002.
63. Lamb CR, Hartzband LE, Tidwell AS et al: Ultrasonographic findings in hepatic and splenic lymphosarcoma in dogs and cats, *Vet Radiol* 32:117, 1991.
64. Nyland TG: Ultrasonic patterns of canine hepatic lymphosarcoma, *Vet Radiol* 25:167, 1984.
65. Léveillé R, Partington BP, Biller DS et al: Complications after ultrasound–guided biopsy of abdominal structures in dogs and cats: 246 cases (1984-1991), *J Am Vet Med Assoc* 203:413-415, 1993.
66. De Rycke LM, Van Bree HJ, Simoens PJM: Ultrasound-guided soft tissue core biopsy of liver, spleen, and kidney in normal dogs, *Vet Radiol Ultrasound* 40:294, 1999.
67. Whiteley MB, Feeney DA, Whiteley LO et al: Ultrasonographic appearance of primary and metastatic canine hepatic tumors, *J Ultrasound Med* 8:621, 1989.
68. Liptak JM, Dernell, WS, Monnet E et al: Massive hepatocellular carcinoma in dogs: 48 cases (1992-2002), *J Am Vet Med Assoc* 225:1225, 2004.
69. Cuccouillo A, Lamb C: Cellular features of sonographic target lesions of the liver and spleen in 21 dogs and a cat, *Vet Radiol Ultrasound* 43:275, 2002.
70. Ziegler LE, O'Brien RT, Waller KR et al: Quantitative contrast harmonic ultrasound imaging of the normal canine liver, *Vet Radiol Ultrasound* 44:451, 2003.
71. O'Brien RT, Iani M, Matheson J et al: Contrast harmonic ultrasound of spontaneous liver nodules in 32 dogs, *Vet Radiol Ultrasound* 45:547, 2004.
72. Prause LC, Twedt DC: Hepatic nodular hyperplasia. In Bonagura JD, editor: *Current veterinary therapy XIII: small animal practice,* Philadelphia, 2000, WB Saunders.
73. Stowater JL, Lamb CR, Schelling SH: Ultrasonographic features of canine hepatic nodular hyperplasia, *Vet Radiol Ultrasound* 31:268, 1990.
74. Jacobson LS, Kirberger RM, Nesbit JW: Hepatic ultrasonography and pathological findings in dogs with hepatocutaneous syndrome: new concepts, *J Vet Intern Med* 9:399, 1995.
75. Nyland TG, Barthez PY, Ortega TM, et al: Hepatic ultrasonography and pathologic findings in dogs with canine superficial necrolytic dermatitis, *Vet Radiol Ultrasound* 37:200, 1996.
76. Kimmel SE, Christiansen W, Byrne KP: Clinicopathological, ultrasonographic, and histopathological findings of superficial necrolytic dermatitis with hepatopathy in a cat, *J Am Anim Hosp Assoc* 39:23, 2003.
77. March PA, Hiller A, Weisbrode SE et al: Superficial necrolytic dermatitis in 11 dogs with a history of phenobarbital administration (1995-2002), *J Vet Intern Med* 18:65, 2004.

78. Schwarz LA, Penninck DG, Léveillé-Webster C: Hepatic abscesses in 13 dogs: a review of the ultrasonographic findings, clinical data and therapeutic options, *Vet Radiol Ultrasound* 39:357, 1998.
79. Zatelli A, Bonfanti U, Zini E, et al: Percutaneous drainage and alcoholization of hepatic abscesses in five dogs and a cat, *J Am Anim Hosp Assoc* 41:34, 2005.
80. Nyland TG, Hager DA: Sonography of the liver, gallbladder, and spleen, *Vet Clin North Am Small Anim Pract* 15:1123, 1985.
81. Nyland TG, Hager DA, Herring DS: Sonography of the liver, gallbladder, and spleen, *Semin Vet Med Surg (Small Anim)* 4:13, 1989.
82. Nyland TG, Koblick PD, Tellyer SE: Ultrasonographic evaluation of biliary cystadenomas in cats, *Vet Radiol Ultrasound* 40:300, 1999.
83. Besso JG, Wrigley RH, Gliatto JM, et al: Ultrasonographic appearance and clinical findings in 14 dogs with gallbladder mucocele, *Vet Radiol Ultrasound* 41:261, 2000.
84. Pike FS, Berg J, King NW et al: Gallbladder mucocele in dogs: 30 cases (2000-2003), *J Am Vet Med Assoc* 224:1615, 2004.
85. Worley DR, Hottinger HA, Lawrence HJ: Surgical management of gallbladder mucoceles in dogs: 22 cases (1999-2003), *J Am Vet Med Assoc* 225:1418, 2004.
86. Nyland TG, Gillett NA: Sonographic evaluation of experimental bile duct ligation in the dog, *Vet Radiol* 23:252, 1982.
87. Fahie MA, Martin RA: Extrahepatic biliary tract obstruction: a retrospective study of 45 cases (1983-1993), *J Am Anim Hosp Assoc* 31:478, 1995.
88. D'Anjou MA, Penninck D, Cornejo L, et al: Ultrasonographic diagnosis of portosystemic shunting in dogs and cats, *Vet Radiol Ultrasound* 45:424, 2004.
89. Lamb CR: Ultrasonography of portosystemic shunts in dogs and cats, *Vet Clin North Am Small Anim Pract* 28:725, 1998.
90. Martin RA, Payne JT: Angiographic results of intrahepatic portocaval shunt attenuation in three dogs, *Semin Vet Med Surg (Small Animal Pract)* 5:134, 1990.
91. Lamb CR: Ultrasonographic diagnosis of congenital portosystemic shunts in dogs: results of a prospective study, *Vet Radiol Ultrasound* 37:281, 1996.
92. Lamb CR, White RN: Morphology of congenital intrahepatic portocaval shunts in dogs and cats, *Vet Rec* 142:55, 1998.
93. Holt DE, Schelling C, Saunders HM et al: Correlation of ultrasonographic findings with surgical, portographic, and necropsy findings in dogs and cats with portosystemic shunts: 63 cases (1987-1993), *J Am Vet Med Assoc* 207:1190, 1995.
94. Salwei RM, O'Brien RT, Mathieson JS: Use of contrast harmonic ultrasound for the diagnosis of congenital portosystemic shunts in three dogs, *Vet Radiol Ultrasound* 44:301, 2003.
95. Neer TM: Clinical approach to splenomegaly in dogs and cats, *Compend Small Anim* 18:35, 1996.
96. Hanson JA, Papageorges M, Girard E, at al: Ultrasonographic appearance of splenic disease in 101 cats, *Vet Radiol Ultrasound* 42:441, 2001.
97. Spangler WL, Culbertson MR: Prevalence and type of splenic disease in cats: 455 cases (1985-1991), *J Am Vet Med Assoc* 201:773, 1992.
98. Konde LJ, Wrigley RH, Lebel JL, et al: Sonographic and radiographic changes associated with splenic torsion in the dog, *Vet Radiol* 30:41, 1989.
99. Stickle RL: Radiographic signs of isolated splenic torsion in dogs: eight cases (1980-1987), *J Am Vet Med Assoc* 194:103, 1989.
100. Patsikas MN, Rallis T, Kladakis SE et al: Computed tomography diagnosis of isolated splenic torsion in a dog, *Vet Radiol Ultrasound* 42:235, 2001.
101. Wrigley RH, Konde LJ, Park RD et al: Clinical features and diagnosis of splenic hematomas in dogs: 10 cases (1980-1987), *J Am Anim Hosp Assoc* 25:371, 1989.
102. Weinstein MJ, Carpenter JL, Mehlaff Schunk CJ: Nonangiogenic and nonlymphomatous sarcomas of the canine spleen: 57 cases (1975-1987), *J Am Vet Med Assoc* 195:784, 1989.
103. Spangler WL, Culbertson MR: Prevalence, type, and importance of splenic diseases in dogs: 1,480 cases (1985-1989), *J Am Vet Med Assoc* 200:829, 1992.
104. O'Brien RT, Waller KR, Osgood TL: Sonographic features of drug-induced splenic congestion, *Vet Radiol Ultrasound* 45:225, 2004.
105. Saunders HM, Neath PJ, Brockman DJ: B-mode and Doppler ultrasound imaging of the spleen with canine splenic torsion: a retrospective evaluation, *Vet Radiol Ultrasound* 39:349, 1998.
106. Hardie EM, Vaden SL, Spaulding K et al: Splenic infarction in 16 dogs: a retrospective study, *J Vet Intern Med* 9:141, 1995.
107. Schelling CG, Wortman JA, Saunders MH: Ultrasonic detection of splenic necrosis in the dog. Three case reports of splenic necrosis secondary to infarction, *Vet Radiol* 29:227, 1988.
108. Cruz-Arámbulo R, Wrigley R, Powers B: Sonographic features of histiocytic neoplasms in the canine abdomen, *Vet Radiol Ultrasound* 45:554, 2004.
109. Ramirez S, Douglass JP, Robertson ID: Ultrasonographic features of canine abdominal malignant histiocytosis, *Vet Radiol Ultrasound* 43:167, 2002.
110. Wrigley RH, Konde LJ, Park RD, et al: Ultrasonographic features of splenic lymphosarcoma in dogs: 12 cases (1980-1986), *J Am Vet Med Assoc* 193:1565, 1988.
111. Hanson JA, Penninck DG: Ultrasonographic evaluation of a traumatic splenic hematoma and literature review, *Vet Radiol Ultrasound* 35:463, 1994.
112. Wrigley RH, Park RD, Konde LJ et al: Ultrasonographic features of splenic hemangiosarcoma in dogs: 18 cases (1980-1986), *J Am Vet Med Assoc* 192:1113, 1988.
113. Konde LJ, Lebel JL, Park RD et al: Sonographic application in the diagnosis of intraabdominal abscess in the dog, *Vet Radiol* 27:151, 1986.
114. Walzer C, Hittmair K, Walzer-Wagner C: Ultrasonographic identification and characterization of splenic nodular lipomatosis or myelolipomas in cheetahs (*Acinonyx jubatus*), *Vet Radiol Ultrasound* 37:289, 1996.
115. Schwarz LA, Penninck D, Gliatto J: Ultrasound corner: canine splenic myelolipomas, *Vet Radiol Ultrasound* 42:347, 2001.

ELECTRONIC RESOURCES evolve

Additional information related to the content in Chapter 39 can be found on the companion Web site at evolve http://evolve.elsevier.com/Thrall/vetrad/.

- Key Points
- Chapter Quiz
- Case Study 39-1
- Video 39-1 (in Case Study 39-1)
- Case Study 39-2
- Video 39-2 (in Case Study 39-2)
- Case Study 39-3
- Video 39-3 (in Case Study 39-3)
- Case Study 39-4
- Video 39-4 (in Case Study 39-4)

CHAPTER • 40
The Kidneys and Ureters

Daniel A. Feeney
Gary R. Johnston

THE KIDNEYS

Survey radiographs, procedures with contrast medium, and sonography can contribute much information toward the diagnosis of renal and ureteral diseases. The external boundaries of the kidneys can usually be identified on survey radiographs. This identification permits assessment of the size, shape, and radiographic opacity of the kidneys. However, when the kidneys cannot be assessed by survey radiographs, or when qualitative functional information is needed, ultrasonography or excretory urography may provide the clinician with important information.

The general goals of this chapter are to specify the radiographic and ultrasonographic imaging procedures applicable to the kidneys and ureters and place each of these procedures in perspective regarding indications, limitations, contraindications, and pitfalls when applicable. Subsequently, the normal radiographic and ultrasonographic findings based on geometric signs are described. In addition, the abnormal radiographic findings are described, and a partial list of conditions that should be considered in association with certain geometric signs is presented.

Imaging Procedures

Survey radiographs provide information on the external anatomy of the kidneys when radiographic contrast is adequate to permit their visualization. In addition, abnormal opacities near or within the kidneys can be assessed, such as air and mineral, that may be clues to the pathophysiologic mechanism for the clinical signs of renal disease.[1,2] Because the right lateral view permits greater longitudinal separation of the radiographic images of the right and left kidneys, it is the projection most applicable to radiography of the upper urinary tract.[3]

Survey radiographs may not provide adequate morphologic information when the patient is emaciated or has peritoneal or retroperitoneal fluid. Excretory urography is useful for defining anatomic structures and qualitatively assessing the function of the kidneys. It is a relatively simple means of verifying and localizing upper urinary tract disease, and it may be used to assess the reversibility of renal disease. Although excretory urography is not a quantitative measurement of renal function, it may be used to assess the relative function of the kidneys and may be loosely interpreted to assess the pathophysiologic mechanisms of renal failure.[4]

Excretory urography may be used in both azotemic and nonazotemic patients, provided hydration is adequate. As the degree of renal failure progresses, however, an increase in the dose of contrast medium may be necessary to provide adequate visualization of the kidneys. In any instance, patient hydration should be assessed and determined to be normal before any contrast medium is administered.[4] A temporary decrease in kidney function may occur after excretory urography; an in-depth discussion of this is beyond the scope of this text. The clinical significance of this decreased function is considered minimal in the presence of adequate urinary output and patient hydration.

Azotemia is not a contraindication in excretory urography, provided the patient is adequately hydrated. For information concerning the specific pathophysiologic characteristics and management of patients with the unlikely occurrence of contrast medium–induced renal disease or failure, readers are directed to texts on renal disease.[1,2]

The technique of excretory urography is described in detail in Box 40-1. The patient should be prepared as for survey radiographs; food is withheld and cleansing enemas are administered.[4-6] Generally, ionic iodinated contrast medium is used and given by bolus intravenous injection. However, if previous systemic reactions (e.g., shock) have occurred in the patient, or if the patient is severely compromised medically, nonionic contrast medium, such as iopamidol and iohexol, or an alternative procedure such as ultrasonography should be considered. The dose of contrast medium for excretory urography is 400 mg iodine per pound of body weight injected by a preplaced cephalic venous or jugular venous catheter.[4-7] Catheter placement should be maintained for at least 15 to 20 minutes after administration of the contrast medium because it provides a readily accessible route in the event of a hypotensive reaction to the contrast medium. Many filming sequences have been suggested; however, radiographs obtained immediately and 5, 20, and 40 minutes after injection of contrast medium generally yield the most information.[4,5,7]

The interpretative phases of the excretory urogram are the nephrographic and pyelographic phases. Opacification of the functional renal parenchyma is the nephrogram, and opacification of the renal pelvis, pelvic recesses, and ureters is the pyelogram. Each phase should be evaluated separately. Although procedures in which radiographic contrast medium is used provide considerable information relative to urinary tract disease, they may complicate some subsequent determinations for as long as 24 hours. For example, increased urine specific gravity from intravenously administered contrast medium may be erroneously interpreted as adequate renal concentrating ability.[8] In addition, although detailed in vivo studies are not available for all types of urinary pathogens, contrast medium inhibition of growth of some urinary tract organisms cannot be ignored.[9] Therefore samples for culture and renal concentrating ability studies, as well as for urine sediment cytologic analysis, should be performed before or at

Box • 40-1

Technique for Excretory Urography

Provide routine patient preparation
Allow 24 hours without food; water ad libitum
Perform cleansing enema at least 2 hours before radiography
Assess hydration status; proceed only if normal
Obtain survey radiographs
Infuse contrast medium intravenously by the cephalic or jugular vein as rapidly as possible (bolus injection)
Dose: 400 mg iodine/lb body weight
Use contrast medium: usually sodium iothalamate or sodium diatrizoate, but consider nonionic agents such as iopamidol or iohexol in high-risk patients
Obtain abdominal radiographs in the following sequence:

- Ventrodorsal views at 5 to 20 seconds, 5 minutes, 20 minutes, and 40 minutes after injection for general assessment
- Lateral view at 5 minutes after injection for general assessment
- Oblique views at 3 to 5 minutes after injection for ureteral termination in urinary bladder
- Lateral and ventrodorsal views at 30 to 40 minutes after injection to observe urinary bladder if retrograde cystography is contraindicated or impossible

Modified from Feeney DA, Barber DL, Johnston GR et al: The excretory urogram: techniques, normal radiographic appearance and misinterpretation, *Compend Contin Ed Vet Pract* 4:233, 1982.

Table • 40-1

Quantitative Appearance of Normal Canine and Feline Excretory Urograms

STRUCTURE	MEASUREMENT*	VALUE†
Kidney	Length	Dog 3.00 (0.25) (L2) 2.50 to 3.50 (L2) Cat 2.4 to 3.0 (L2) 4.0 to 4.5 cm
	Width	Dog 2.00 (0.20) (L2) Cat 3.0 to 3.5 cm
Renal pelvis	Width	Dog 0.03 (0.017) (L2) (generally 2.0 mm) Cat Not reported
Pelvic recesses	Width	Dog 0.02 (0.005) (L2) (generally 1.0 mm) Cat Not reported
Proximal ureter	Width	Dog 0.07 (0.018) (L2) (generally (2.5 mm) Cat Not reported
Distal ureter	Width	Not reported in dogs or cats

Modified from Feeney DA, Barber DL, Johnston GR et al: The excretory urogram: techniques, normal radiographic appearance and misinterpretation, *Compend Contin Ed Vet Pract* 4:233, 1982.
*Measurements apply only to the ventrodorsal view.
†The length of the body of the second lumbar vertebral body as visualized on the ventrodorsal view.

least 24 hours after (including several voidings) excretory urography.

Renal ultrasonography is a noninvasive technique in which sound is directed into the tissue and the reflected echoes are reconstructed into two-dimensional images.[10-15] With the use of sonography, information on renal architecture may be provided without the use of contrast medium.

Two-dimensional ultrasonography is based on the concept of tissue reflectivity (see Chapter 3). Sound exiting the transducer (handheld part of the instrument) traverses the tissues into which it is directed. Variances in tissue, fat, connective tissue content, and vascularity influence how much of the sound is reflected back to the transducer as it passes through tissues. The degree of sound reflection that occurs at a given tissue interface determines how echogenic (bright compared with the scan background) specific tissues or organs will be. Reflection dominates to the point of nothing visible (shadowing) beyond materials that are quite different from soft tissue (e.g., bone, air, metal). Simple fluids (e.g., transudates or normal urine) usually have no echoes and appear black. Of note, the image represents a "slice" of tissue, usually between 4 and 15 mm thick (depending on the ultrasound frequency and beam focusing used). The appearance of the kidney varies depending on the location (e.g., medial, cranial) of the slice, and the whole kidney should be scanned in a smooth, slow motion using standard imaging planes (e.g., sagittal, transverse, dorsal).

Normal Imaging Findings

The normal quantitative radiographic findings for the dog and cat kidney and ureter are listed in Table 40-1. The most widely used quantification of normal kidney size in the dog and cat is renal length assessed on survey radiographs.[1,3-5,7,16-18] In general, the dog kidney is approximately three times the length of the L2 vertebral body as visualized on the ventrodorsal view, with a normal range of 2.5 to 3.5 times the length of L2.[7,16] In the cat, the most accepted renal length is that of 2.4 to 3 times the length of the L2 vertebral body,[17] but other values have been suggested.[18] However, in the authors' experience, cats older than 10 years may have a renal length of approximately twice the length of L2. This suggestion has been supported by others.[19] No direct association exists between the apparent small kidney size and laboratory evidence of renal failure when the kidney length is between 2 and 2.4 times the length of L2. Therefore care must be taken not to overemphasize the significance of a renal size that is slightly outside the accepted normal range in cats, particularly if they are somewhat aged or neutered.

Other quantitative measurements visible only on excretory urograms that may be used to assess the kidneys include measurement of the pyelographic variables, including the width of the pelvic recesses, renal pelvis, and proximal ureter. In general, the renal pelvis and pelvic recesses (sometimes referred to as pelvic diverticula) in the dog do not exceed

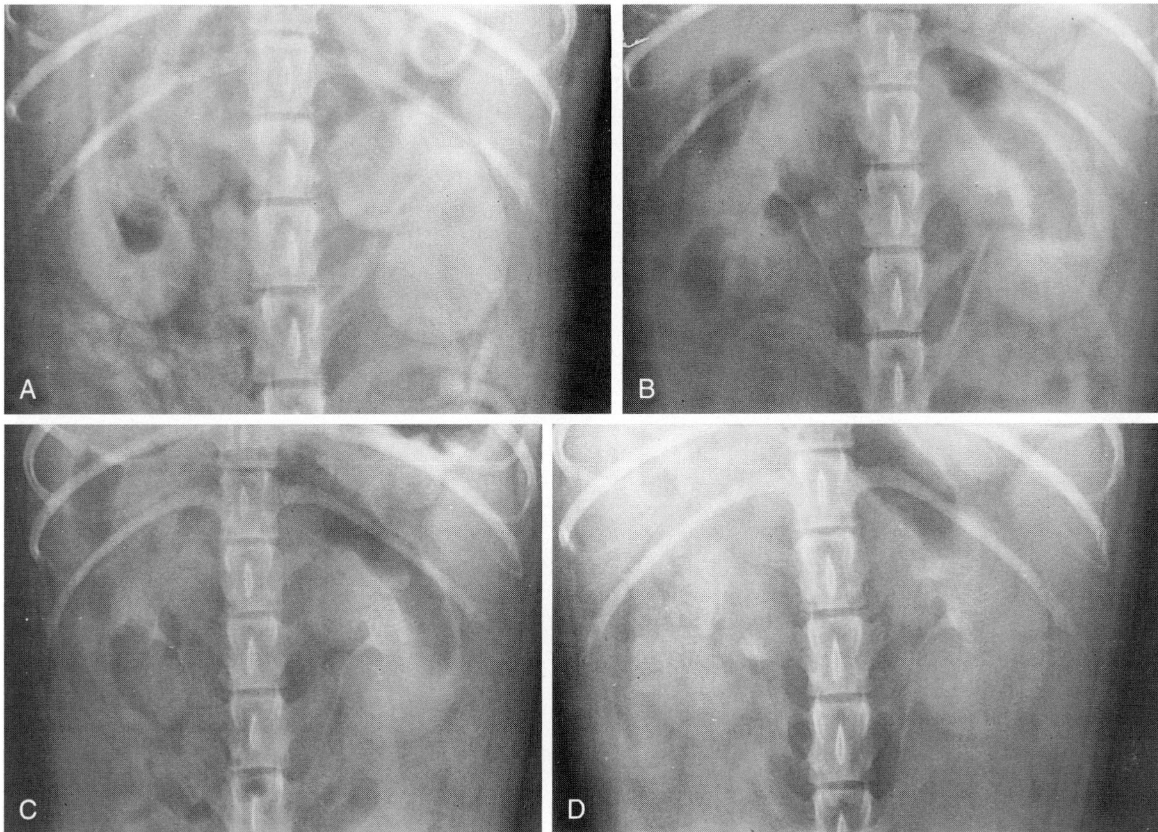

Fig. 40-1 Ventrodorsal views of a normal dog after intravenous administration of 400 mg iodine per pound of body weight in the form of sodium iothalamate. **A**, 10 seconds; **B**, 5 minutes; **C**, 20 minutes; and **D**, 40 minutes after injection.

1 or 2 mm in diameter, and the proximal ureter in the dog does not exceed 2 or 3 mm in diameter (see Table 40-1).[7]

The shape of the dog kidney is somewhat elongated, resembling that of a bean, whereas the ureter of the cat is somewhat more rounded although still somewhat elongated (Figs. 40-1 and 40-2).[1,4-6] The right kidney is usually more cranial than the left and, as previously mentioned, this separation can be enhanced on the right lateral view.

Renal opacity on survey radiographs is that of homogeneous soft tissue.[1,3] Visualization of the kidneys on survey radiographs relies on the presence of retroperitoneal fat surrounding the kidneys. During excretory urography the nephrogram is homogeneous, with the exception of the early combined vascular and tubular nephrograms, in which the cortex is more radiopaque than the medulla.[4,10] The pyelogram in the normally functioning kidney is more radiopaque than the nephrogram (see Figs. 40-1 and 40-2). On contrast-enhanced computed tomography, a nephrogram and pyelogram are also identified. The principles defined for these phases of the excretory urogram apply to computed tomography as well.

The dynamic aspects of excretory urography lie in the assessment of nephrographic opacification and fading sequences.[4,20] Visualization of renal opacification after intravenous injection of iodinated contrast medium depends on renal blood flow, glomerular filtration of the contrast medium, and tubular reabsorption of water, resulting in concentration of contrast medium in the tubules. The normal nephrogram should be most radiopaque within 10 to 30 seconds after bolus injection of contrast medium. With increasing delay after injection, the nephrographic opacity should progressively decrease; fewer than 25% of normal dogs have detectable nephrographic opacity 2 hours after injection. The pyelogram should be consistently opaque, and the diameter of the ureter should vary with time because of peristalsis (see Figs. 40-1 and 40-2). The degree of nephrographic and pyelographic opacification in combination with the opacification and fading patterns of the nephrogram can be used as a qualitative estimate of renal function.[6,21] In general, the poorer the renal function, the less opacified are the nephrographic and pyelographic phases of the excretory urogram.

Sonographically, the parts of the kidney that are routinely seen include the cortex, the medullary papillae, the arcuate vessels and pelvic recess interfaces, the renal vessels (in the hilus), and the fat in the renal hilus (Fig. 40-3). The renal pelvis is usually not seen. However, if high-resolution equipment (e.g., 7.5 to 10.0 MHz) is used, the pelvis may be visible as an anechoic (black) slit. Similarly, the ureter is usually not seen except where it enters the urinary bladder, where a jet of urine expelled from the ureter into the bladder can sometimes be seen. Aggressive fluid therapy may cause the renal pelvis and the pelvic recesses to dilate physiologically,[22] but the normal pelvis will still be less than 1 to 2 mm wide and the ureter less than 3 mm in diameter. The renal cortex in dogs typically appears either a little less or a little more bright than the liver background and should always be less bright than the spleen. Renal cortical echotexture in cats can be quite variable and is often equal to the liver and may approach that of the spleen.[23] The renal medulla in dogs and cats is less echogenic than the cortex. The echotexture consideration is important for assessing diseases that do not alter the kidney architecture (e.g., tubular necrosis, feline infectious peritoni-

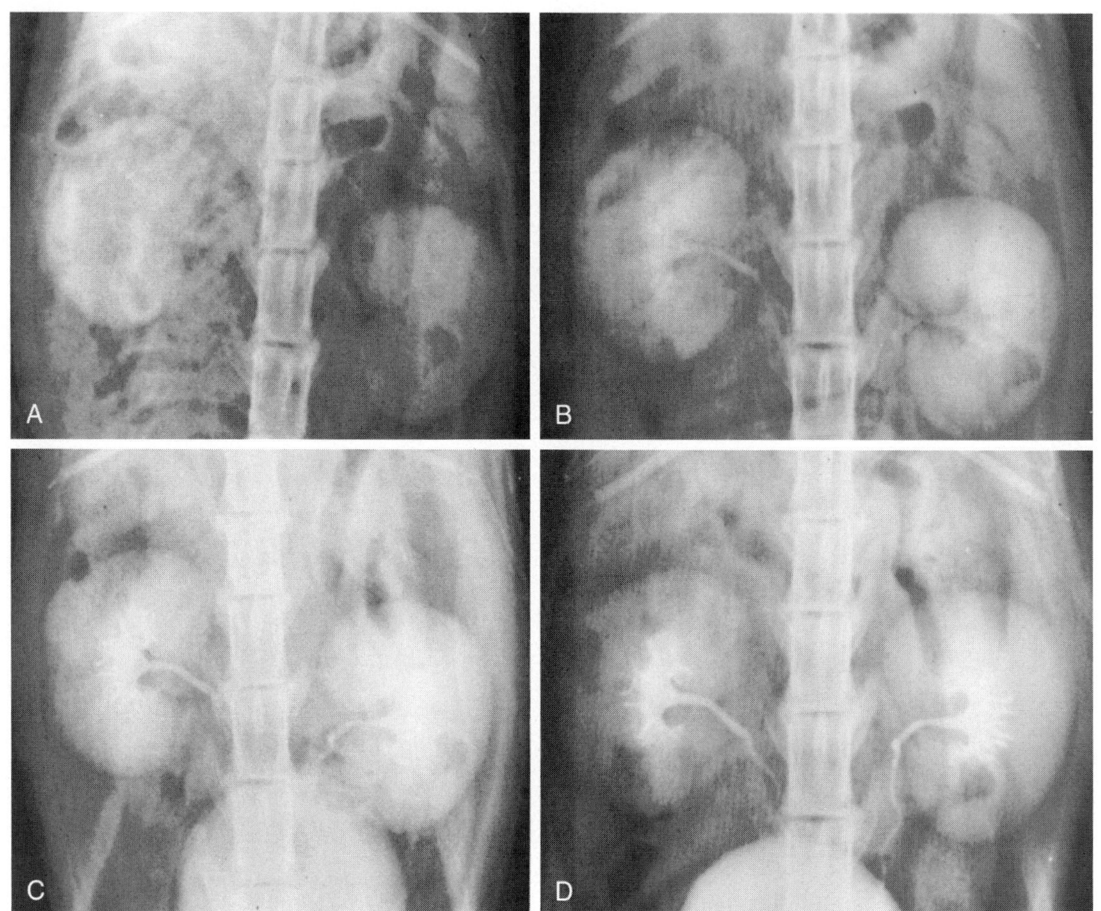

Fig. 40-2 Ventrodorsal views of a normal cat after intravenous administration of 400 mg iodine per pound of body weight in the form of sodium iothalamate. **A,** 10 seconds; **B,** 5 minutes; **C,** 20 minutes; and **D,** 40 minutes after injection.

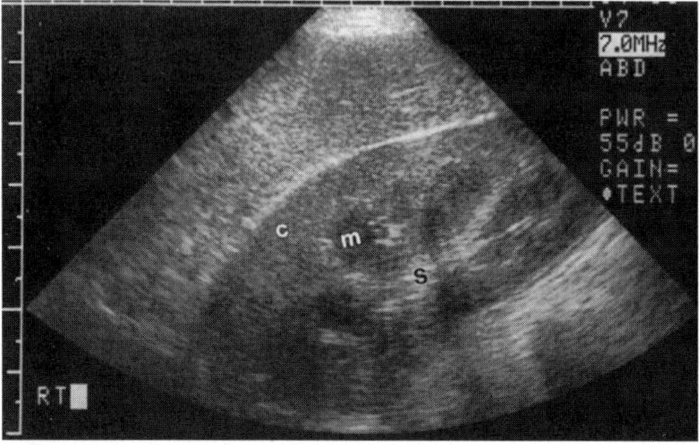

Fig. 40-3 Sagittal ultrasonogram of a normal right canine kidney as viewed through the liver. The renal cortex *(c)*, the renal medulla *(m)*, the renal sinus fat *(s)*, and the echogenic vascular structures at the corticomedullary junction can be identified.

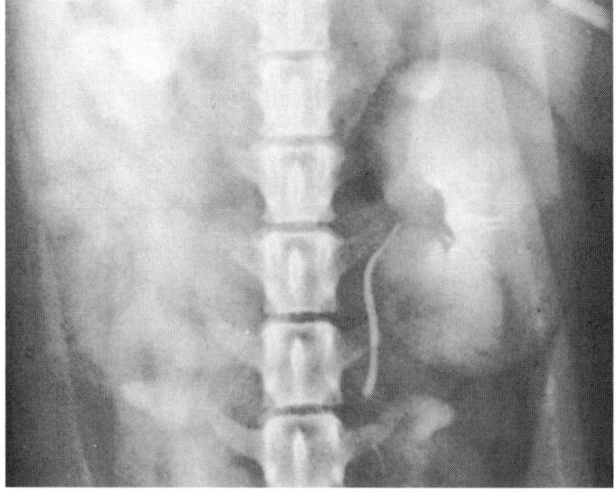

Fig. 40-4 Radiograph made as part of an excretory urogram. The left kidney is enlarged but is anatomically and functionally normal. The right kidney is not visualized. The left kidney has undergone functional and anatomic compensatory hypertrophy.

tis). Architectural disruptions of the kidney or ureter are interpreted similarly to the radiographic methods defined below.

Abnormal Imaging Findings

Number

Renal aplasia or agenesis may result in the inability to identify one of the kidneys.[1,2,24] Unilateral renal agenesis may result in compensatory hypertrophy of the unaffected kidney (Fig. 40-4). The possibility that more than the expected number of kidneys developed through renal duplication also exists.[25] The inability to visualize a kidney radiographically may be merely the result of extreme hypoplasia, the consequences of chronic disease, or both.

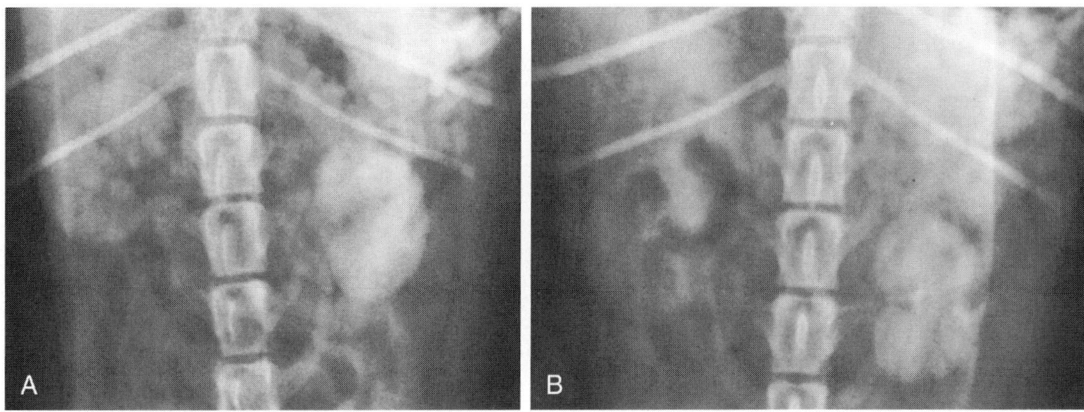

Fig. 40-5 Ventrodorsal views 10 seconds (A) and 5 minutes (B) after intravenous contrast medium injection for excretory urography in a 1-year-old Shih Tzu. The kidneys are small, nephrographic opacity is poor, and pyelographic opacity is minimal. Microscopic diagnosis was Shih Tzu familial renal disease.

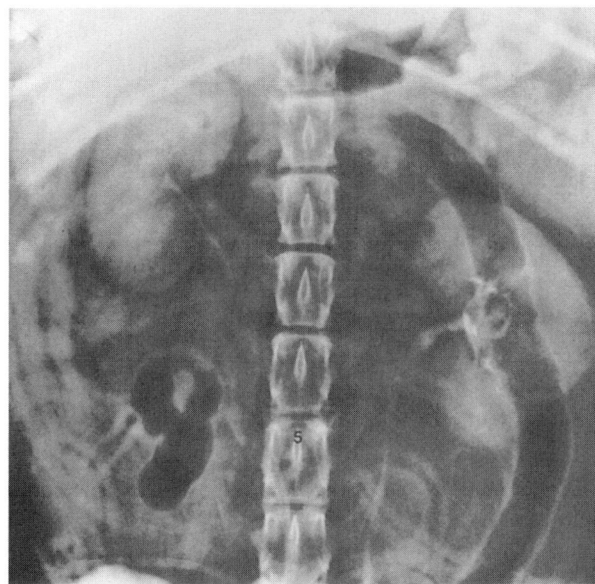

Fig. 40-6 Ventrodorsal view of a patient 5 minutes after intravenous contrast medium injection for excretory urography. In the mid-portion of the left kidney, there is a mass effect with compression and distortion of the renal pelvis and pelvic recesses in the adjacent area. Microscopic diagnosis was renal adenocarcinoma.

Size, Shape, and Margination

The combination of size, shape, and marginization, when applied to the abnormal appearance of the kidneys, may help the interpreter limit the possible considerations to a manageable number (listed below by size and shape variability)[1-3,6,10,18,20-40]:

- Normal size and shape
  - Amyloidosis
  - Glomerulonephritis
  - Acute pyelonephritis
  - Familial renal disease
- Normal size, irregular shape and margin
  - Focal
  - Infarct
  - Abscess
  - Diffuse
  - Chronic pyelonephritis
  - Polycystic renal disease
- Small size, regular shape and margin
  - Hypoplasia
  - Glomerulonephritis
  - Amyloidosis
  - Familial renal disease (Fig. 40-5)*
- Small size, irregular shape and margin
  - End-stage renal disease
  - Dysplasia
- Large size, regular shape and margin
  - Compensatory hypertrophy
  - Round cell neoplasia
  - Hydronephrosis
  - Dioctophyma renale
  - Amyloidosis
  - Glomerulonephritis
  - Perirenal pseudocyst
  - Perinephric abscess
  - Large solitary renal cyst
- Large size, irregular shape and margin
  - Focal
  - Primary tumor (Fig. 40-6)
  - Metastatic tumor
  - Hematoma

*Depending on the stage of juvenile or familial renal disease and the breed of dog involved, the kidneys may appear nearly normal, small, and smooth or small and irregular.[41-74] Familial or juvenile renal disease has been reported in the following breeds: Samoyed, Chow Chow, Newfoundland, Doberman Pinscher, Rottweiler, Standard Poodle, Chinese Shar Pei, soft-coated Wheaten Terrier, Cocker Spaniel, Norwegian Elkhound, Bull Terrier, Old English Sheepdog, Golden Retriever, Keesond, English Foxhound, Burmese Mountain Dog, Basenji, Lhasa Apso, Shih Tzu, German Shepherd, Dutch Kooiker, Beagle, Bedlington Terrier, Collie, Alaskan Malamute, Cairn Terrier, Pembroke Welsh Corgi, Airedale Terrier, Boxer, English Bulldog, Great Dane, Great Pyrenees, Pekingese, Shetland Sheepdog, Yorkshire Terrier, Miniature Schnauzer, and Cavalier King Charles Spaniel. Familial renal disease in cats has been recognized in two forms, including the multicavitary appearance of feline polycystic disease and the infiltrative appearance of feline amyloidosis.[33,54,60,75,76]

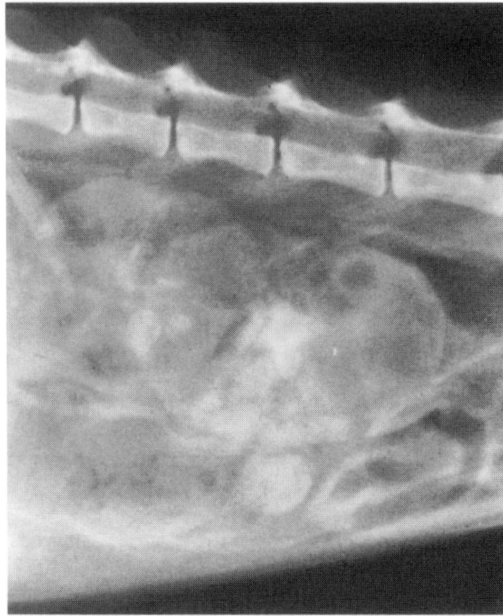

Fig. 40-7 Lateral view of a cat 5 minutes after intravenous contrast medium injection for excretory urography. Kidneys are enlarged and nephrographic opacification is variable in a random, patchy appearance. Microscopic diagnosis was feline polycystic kidney disease.

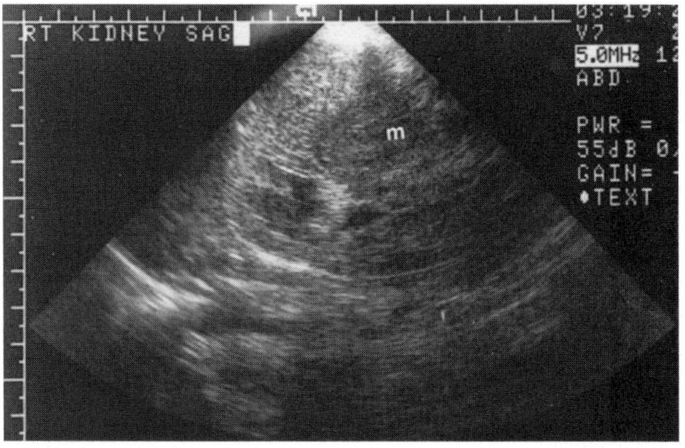

Fig. 40-8 Sagittal ultrasonogram of a canine kidney with a mass *(m)*.

- Perirenal pseudocyst
- Diffuse
- Polycystic renal disease (Fig. 40-7)
- Feline infectious peritonitis
- Round cell neoplasia

However, a number of plant, drug, and miscellaneous toxicities (e.g., snake bite) as well as specific infectious diseases (e.g., babesiosis, borreliosis, leptospirosis) can be the cause of or indirectly lead to acute renal failure that may not alter the architecture of the kidneys.[77]

The same principles of size, shape, margination, and number described for radiographic interpretation apply to ultrasonographic interpretation.[78,79] However, with ultrasonography the internal architecture can be visualized regardless of the renal functional status. The interpretation should still be based on focal or diffuse diseases of the parenchyma or diseases of the renal collecting system and ureter. The advantage of ultrasound is the ease with which the extent of the disease can be determined within the kidney for focal disease (Fig. 40-8) and the ease of assessment of renal pelvic

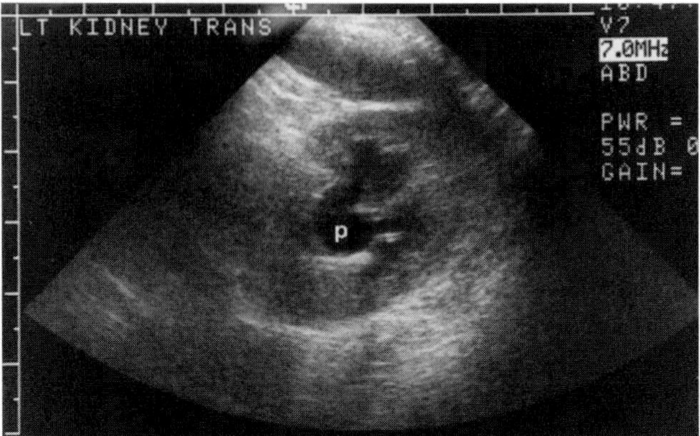

Fig. 40-9 Transverse ultrasonogram of a canine kidney at the level of the renal sinus. Note the dilated renal pelvis *(p)* typical of hydronephrosis.

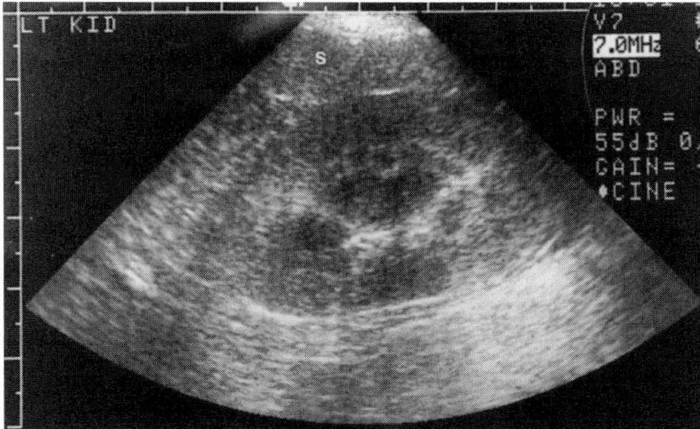

Fig. 40-10 Sagittal ultrasonogram of a canine kidney in which the renal cortices are as echogenic as the spleen *(s)*. Note how bright the renal cortex appears (compare with Fig. 40-3). Interpretation was infiltrative renal disease or acute tubular necrosis.

or ureteral dilation when fluid distended (Fig. 40-9). The location and relevance of renal mineralization can also be assessed. This is particularly relevant for survey radiographically identifiable focal renal pelvic or ureteral mineral opacities and the question of whether hydronephrosis is present.

A linear area of increased medullary echogenicity near and parallel to the corticomedullary junction has been referred to as the medullary rim sign.[80] The relevance of this nonspecific sign has been given perspective.[81] Histologically, it is an area of tubular mineralization that has no specific association with any given category of disease and is not a predictable indicator of renal dysfunction. It may, in fact, be an observation that indicates some degree of renal insult (e.g., hypercalcemia) or degeneration, but its relevance in the assessment of clinically relevant disease is questionable. Diffuse parenchymal disease presents more of an interpretive challenge. In these patients the renal architecture may not be disrupted, but the renal echotexture may be abnormal (e.g., greater than the spleen) (Fig. 40-10). This is particularly a problem in the pathophysiologic circumstances of acute tubular necrosis or acute renal failure. In dogs the renal cortical echointensity (brightness) typically is less than or equal to the liver.[82] In older dogs, the renal cortical echointensity may be equal to that of the liver, but it should always be less than the echointensity of the spleen. Biopsy or fine-needle aspiration can be expedited by ultrasonographic guidance, improving the margin of safety as well. This is particularly problematic in cats because of the normal benign fat infiltration that occurs, affecting the renal

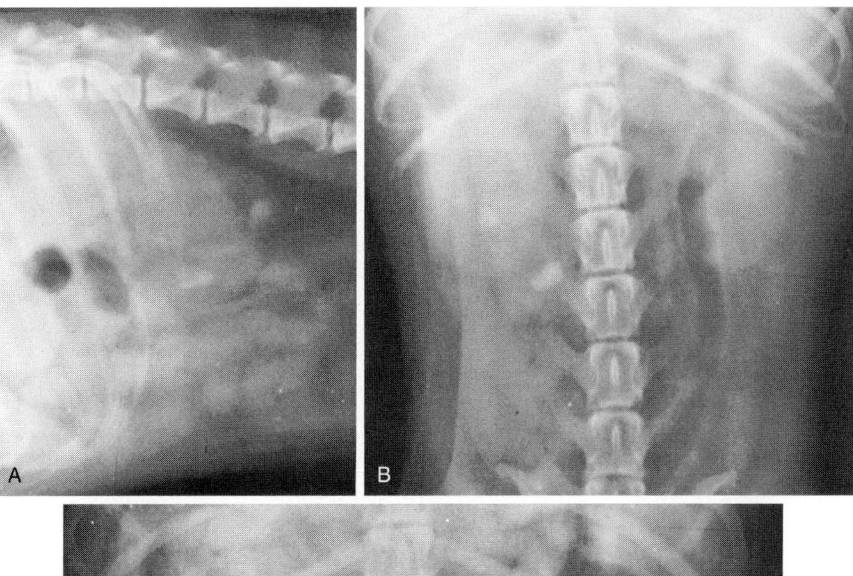

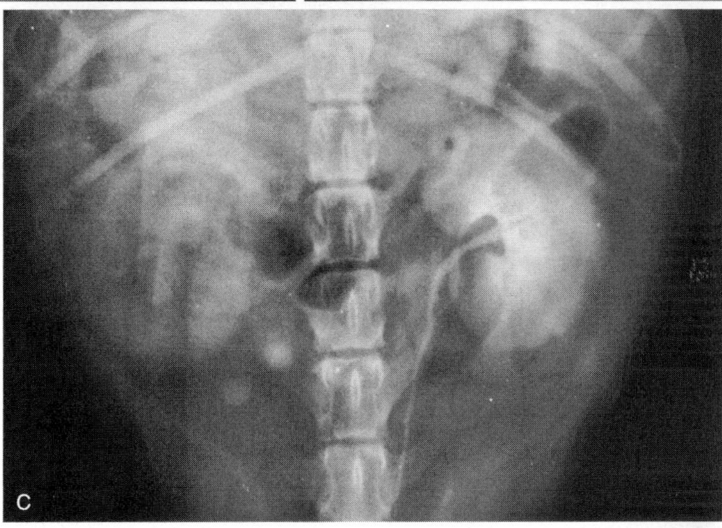

Fig. 40-11 Lateral (A) and ventrodorsal (B) radiographs in which there are smoothly marginated, oval, white calcific opacities in the area of the right kidney and ureter. **C,** Ventrodorsal view 5 minutes after intravenous injection of contrast medium for excretory urography. Peripheral opacification of the right nephrogram is identified without accompanying central or pyelographic opacification. Surgical diagnosis was right renal and ureteral calculi with ureteral obstruction and right renal hydronephrosis.

echogenicity.[15,23] Doppler ultrasound techniques have been applied to the kidney in an effort to measure resistance to renal parenchymal blood flow. Although not specific, increased renal blood flow resistance is associated with both parenchymal and collecting system disease.[83,84]

Location

Kidneys may maintain relatively normal function while being abnormally located. In animals and human beings, ectopic kidneys have been identified in the thorax, intraabdominal region (not the normal retroperitoneal space), and pelvic canal.[3,85-87] Excretory urography and ultrasonography are useful in confirming these unusually located masses as kidneys; excretory urography may help assess the functional potential.

In addition to an ectopic kidney, a kidney may be displaced by an adjacent mass.[3] In particular, adrenal masses may displace either kidney caudally; the right kidney may be displaced caudally by a liver mass, and the left kidney may be displaced caudally by a mass in the proximal extremity of the spleen. This indirect method of assessing abdominal masses by adjacent organ displacement may be used as an aid in establishing the differential diagnosis.

Radiopacity

On survey radiographs, variations in renal radiopacity (from the expected soft tissue appearance) are recognized. The most common opacities recognized include air or mineral. Air may result from vesicoureteral reflux from previous pneumocystography, but it may also be the result of trauma to the perirenal area with leakage of air from intraperitoneal or extraabdominal sources. Mineral radiopacity may be caused by the presence of renal calculi (Fig. 40-11), which are usually magnesium ammonium phosphate in both dogs and cats.[3,88,89] Other chemical types of calculi may be encountered with some frequency; however, the radiopacity may vary with the degree of mineralization and is not specific for chemical composition of the calculus. Other mineral opacities within the kidney that must be considered include mineralized cyst,[3] calcified tumors,[3] calcification of the renal parenchyma (nephrocalcinosis),[3,90] mineralized medullary areas from papillary necrosis, and osseous metaplasia of the renal pelvis in the presence of renal disease.[91,92] As previously mentioned, loss of retroperitoneal contrast because of emaciation, the presence of perirenal (retroperitoneal) fluids (blood or urine), or both may impede or preclude visualization of the kidneys. The determination of the need for immediate excretory urography or sonography must be made on the basis of the assessment of the remainder of the body fat stores as well as the clinical history.

Excretory urography causes an increase in the radiographic opacity of the renal parenchyma through the accumulation of contrast medium within the renal tubules and vasculature. The opacity of the renal outflow tract is also increased because

Box 40-2

Possible Structural Nephrographic Opacification Patterns Associated with Certain Renal Diseases*

Opacification Pattern	*Renal Disease*
Uniform	Normal Compensatory hypertrophy Acute glomerular or tubulointerstitial disease Perirenal pseudocysts Hypoplasia
Focal, nonuniform	Neoplasm Hematuria Cyst Single infarct Hydronephrosis Abscess
Multifocal, nonuniform	Polycystic disease Multiple infarcts Acute pyelonephritis Chronic generalized glomerular or tubulointerstitial disease Feline infectious peritonitis Infiltrative neoplasia
Nonopacification	Aplasia/agenesis† Renal artery obstruction† Nephrectomy or nonfunctional renal parenchyma† Insufficient or extravascular contrast medium injection

*Best identified on radiographs exposed 5 to 20 seconds or 5 minutes after contrast medium injection. Do not overinterpret corticomedullary separation on early postinjection radiographs.
†Only unilateral conditions compatible with life.

Box 40-3

Pyelographic Appearance of Some Common Diseases of the Kidney

Pyelonephritis
Acute

Pelvic dilation
Proximal ureteral dilation
Absent or incomplete filling of pelvic recesses

Chronic

With or without pelvic dilation with irregular borders
Proximal ureteral dilation
Short, blunt pelvic recesses

Hydronephrosis
Pelvic dilation
Dilation of pelvic recesses (recesses may not be distinguishable if pelvic dilation is severe)
Ureteral dilation

Neoplasia
Renal Parenchyma

Distortion or deviation of renal pelvis, with dilation
Distortion or deviation of pelvic recesses

Renal Pelvis

Distortion or dilation of renal pelvis
Filling defects in renal pelvis

Uroliths and Blood Clots
Filling defects in renal pelvis
Uroliths usually radiolucent compared with contrast medium; blood clots always are radiolucent compared with contrast medium

Reprinted from Feeney DA, Barber DL, Osborne CA: Advances in canine excretory urography. In *30th Gaines Veterinary Symposium,* White Plains, NY, 1981, Gaines Dog Research Center.

of urine that contains concentrated contrast medium. The identifiable structural alterations of both the nephrogram and the pyelogram are described in Boxes 40-2 and 40-3, respectively[4]; Figures 40-4 through 40-7 and Figure 40-11 provide examples of structural nephrographic alteration. Figures 40-12 and 40-13 are examples of two common causes that result in structural alteration of the pyelogram. Referring to Boxes 40-2 and 40-3 for the separate evaluation of the nephrographic and pyelographic architecture is suggested as a beginning; considerations occurring for each finding should then be pursued. The diagnostic considerations mentioned in these tables are applicable to ultrasonographic interpretation as well.

Function

The alterations in nephrographic opacification and fading sequences are described in detail in Box 40-4. In general, these changes are classified according to the degree of opacification encountered on the immediate postinjection radiograph as well as the relation of the subsequently encountered nephrographic opacity in the patient compared with the initial opacification.[4,20] Differential considerations for each of the nephrographic opacification sequences are listed, but they are not the only possibilities. Early first (10 to 30 seconds) nephrographic opacification may be delayed in animals with acute and subacute pyelonephritis.[93,94] Figure 40-14 is an example of an abnormal nephrographic opacity sequence (compare with Fig. 40-1).

A common alteration of the pyelographic phase of the excretory urogram is poor or undetectable opacification of the pyelogram. The opacity of the pyelogram depends on both the filtration of the contrast medium from the blood and the concentration of the contrast medium within the tubules. Loss of either of these capabilities within the kidneys (assuming adequate dosage and proper route of administration of contrast medium) may result in a less than optimal pyelogram. In patients with overt renal dysfunction identified on serum biochemical analyses, ultrasonography is a useful alternative to excretory urography.

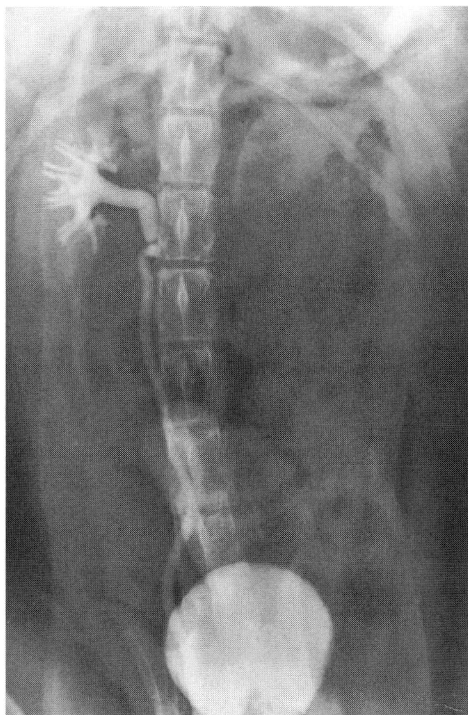

Fig. 40-12 Ventrodorsal view 40 minutes after intravenous contrast medium injection for excretory urography. The right ureter, renal pelvis, and pelvic recesses are symmetrically enlarged. The left kidney is dramatically enlarged, with only a rim of nephrographic opacification. The central portion of the left kidney is nonopacified, and no pyelogram is present. Necropsy confirmed moderate right and extreme left hydronephrosis caused by bilateral ureteral obstruction by a transitional cell carcinoma of the bladder.

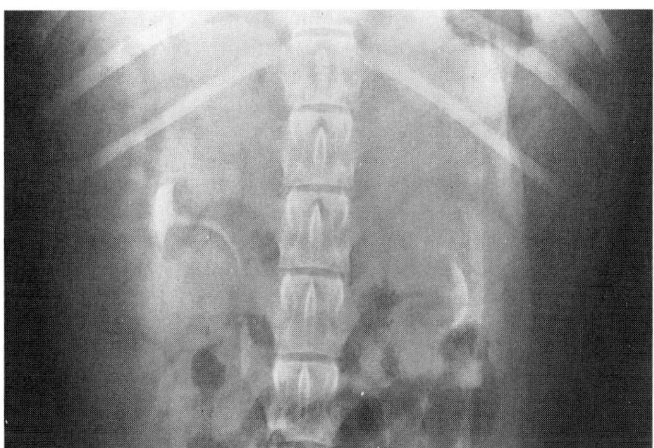

Fig. 40-13 Ventrodorsal view 20 minutes after intravenous injection of contrast medium for excretory urography. The right and left renal pelves are dilated, but the pelvic recesses cannot be identified. The ureters, particularly the right ureter, are mildly dilated. Radiologic diagnosis was bilateral chronic pyelonephritis.

Box • 40-4

Possible Nephrographic Opacification Sequences Associated with Certain Renal Disease Processes

Good initial opacification followed by progressively decreasing opacity:
- Normal

Fair to good initial opacification followed by progressively increasing opacity:
- Systemic hypotension from contrast agents
- Acute renal obstruction (including precipitated Tamm-Horsfall mucoprotein in renal tubules)
- Contrast medium–induced renal failure

Fair to good initial opacification followed by persistent opacity:
- Acute renal tubular necrosis (associated with toxicity)
- Contrast medium–induced renal failure
- Systemic hypotension from contrast agents

Poor initial opacification followed by progressively decreasing opacity:
- Primary polyuric renal failure
- Inadequate contrast medium dose

Poor initial opacification followed by progressively increasing opacity:
- Acute extrarenal obstruction
- Systemic hypotension existing before contrast medium administration
- Renal ischemia (arterial or venous)

Poor initial opacification followed by persistent opacity:
- Primary glomerular dysfunction (chronic)
- Severe generalized acute (toxic) or chronic (degenerative) renal disease

Reprinted from Feeney DA, Barber DL, Osborne CA: Functional aspects of the nephrogram in excretory urography: a review, *Vet Radiol* 23:42, 1982.

THE URETERS

Normal Radiographic Findings

The normal ureters are not visible on survey radiographs. As visualized at excretory urography, the diameter of each ureter is usually less than 2 or 3 mm at the hilus.[5,7] The shape of the ureters is tubular, with segmentation secondary to peristalsis.[4,5] The ureters are primarily retroperitoneal but become intraperitoneal as they approach their termination at the bladder trigone.[95-99] Care should be exercised in the interpretation of the end-on view of the deep circumflex iliac artery as a survey radiographic abnormality related to the ureter.[6] The normal findings for excretory urography relative to the ureter have been described (see Figs. 40-1 and 40-2).[4-7]

Abnormal Radiographic Findings

Number

As previously described, agenesis and aplasia of the kidneys and their associated ureters have been reported. Ureteral duplication in the presence of renal duplication in dogs has also been described.[26]

Size, Shape, and Margination

Information pertaining to the size of the ureter, its overall shape, and the mucosal margin characteristics may be combined to assist in the differential diagnosis of ureteral

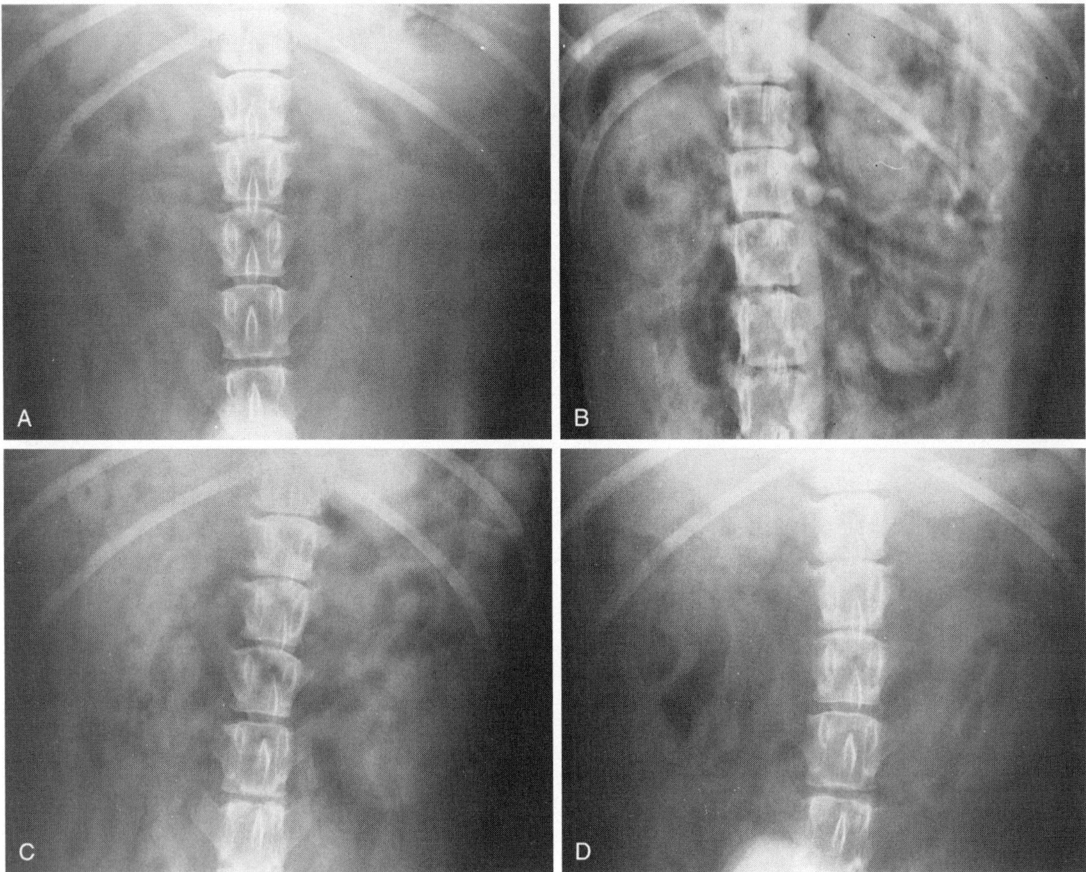

Fig. 40-14 Ventrodorsal views immediately before (A), 10 seconds after (B), 5 minutes after (C), and 40 minutes after (D) intravenous injection of contrast medium for excretory urography. The size of the kidneys is normal, but nephrographic opacification is poor. Microscopic diagnosis was glomerulonephritis caused by systemic lupus erythematosus.

disease.* In the following list, this triad of geometric signs is used and, if possible, differential considerations of disease processes are listed.

- Diffuse enlargement, regular shape, smooth mucosa
  - Obstruction at trigone
  - Ectopic ureter (Fig. 40-15)
  - Atony from infection or periureteral inflammation (rare)
  - Chronic vesicoureteral reflux (rare)
- Focal enlargement, smooth mucosa
  - Ureterocele (Fig. 40-16) including ectopic ureterocele
  - Diverticulum
- Diffuse enlargement, irregular mucosa
  - Fibrosis
- Focal enlargement, irregular mucosa
  - Neoplasia
  - Fibroepithelial polyps
- Focal enlargement, smooth mucosa
  - Focal obstruction distal to dilated segment
- Focal lumen narrowing, smooth mucosa
  - Extrinsic compression
  - Stricture
- Focal lumen narrowing, irregular mucosa
  - Stricture
  - Fibroepithelial polyps

Location

The abnormal location of the ureter most often encountered is ectopic ureter, in which the distal portion of the ureter terminates at a point other than the bladder trigone.[96-99] The most common site of abnormal ureteral termination is the vagina, followed in relative frequency by the urethra, bladder neck, and uterus. As previously mentioned, the affected ureter is usually dilated throughout its length (see Fig. 40-14). Another possible cause of abnormal location of the distal portion of the ureter is trauma, usually from avulsion of the ureter from the bladder neck. In ureteral avulsion, retroperitoneal effusion may also occur.

In addition to excretory urography (the authors' preference) for diagnosis of ectopic ureter, retrograde positive-contrast vaginography can be used.[112] In this technique, sterile, iodinated contrast medium is placed in the vestibule and vagina by a balloon catheter of suitable size to limit contrast medium extravasation around the balloon. The balloon is placed just inside the vulvar lips and contrast medium is infused until mild resistance is met. The goal of this procedure is to identify the ectopic ureters that enter the vagina. The advantage of this procedure is the definitive identification of ureters that terminate in the vagina (Fig. 40-17). The disadvantage of this procedure is that it requires general anesthesia and will not predictably allow identification of ureters that do not terminate in the vagina. The excretory urogram provides insight on ectopic ureters, regardless of where they terminate, and a physiologic means to fill the urinary bladder with positive-contrast medium to assess urethral sphincter continence. A more sophisticated approach to the diagnosis of ectopic ureters is spiral computed tomography.[113,114] This technique has been reported to be slightly more accurate than excretory urography.

*References 4-7, 10, 18, 26, 94, 96-111.

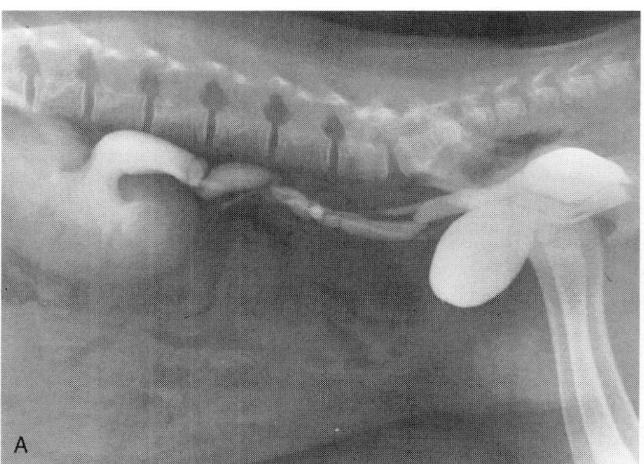

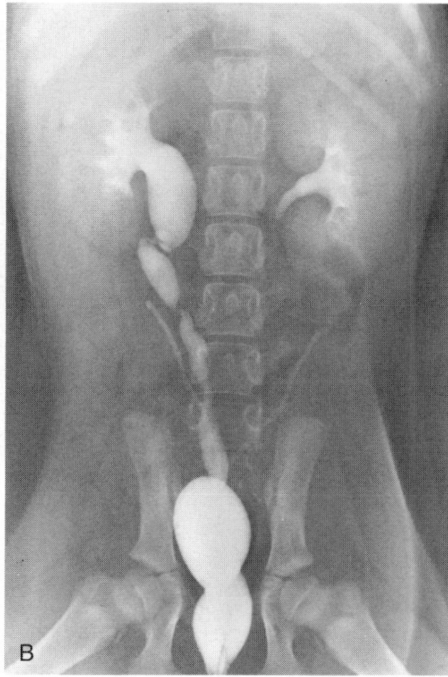

Fig. 40-15 Lateral (A) and ventrodorsal (B) views of a patient 40 minutes after intravenous injection of contrast medium for excretory urography. The right ureter is extremely dilated, as are the right renal pelvis and pelvic recesses. The right ureter extends dorsal to the bladder trigone and ventral to the vestibule and terminates in the urethra. A previous retrograde vaginogram outlined the termination of this ureter as well as the urethral orifice, the cervix, and the uterine horns. Radiologic diagnosis was ectopic ureter.

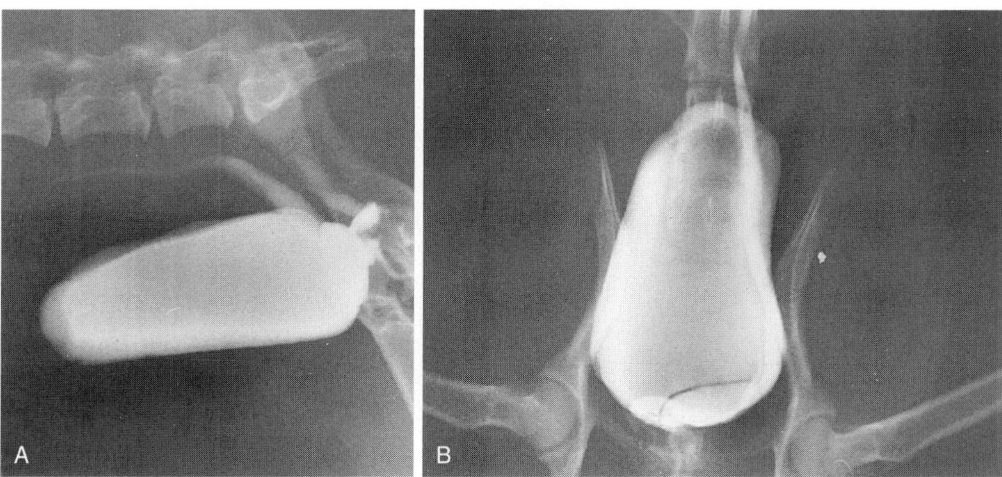

Fig. 40-16 Lateral (A) and ventrodorsal (B) views of a patient 40 minutes after intravenous injection of contrast medium for excretory urography. The terminal portion of the left ureter is dilated in its intramural and submucosal path in the urinary bladder and terminates in the proximal urethra. Radiologic diagnosis was ectopic ureter with ureterocele. The *radiolucent line* in the caudal aspect of the bladder in **B** is the wall of the ureterocele. It is visible because of adjacent contrast medium in the ureteral lumen and in the bladder lumen.

Radiopacity

Air in the ureters is most likely associated with vesicoureteral reflux caused by pneumocystography. Mineralization of the ureter is rare; most mineral opacities in the area of the ureter represent calculi (see Fig. 40-11).[4,6] Loss of retroperitoneal contrast in survey abdominal radiographs may be an indirect indication of the accumulation of blood or urine or both, including ureteral rupture (Fig. 40-18)[115] and urinoma.[116] This loss of retroperitoneal contrast must be interpreted in light of the body fat status in the remainder of the patient.

During excretory urography, a reproducible filling defect in the contrast medium column in the ureter may be caused by a calculus, a neoplasm, a polyp, infiltrative disease, or a stricture secondary to disease or external compression.[4,6,101-104] Assessment of the margination and opacity of these structures on survey radiographs in combination with the size, shape, and

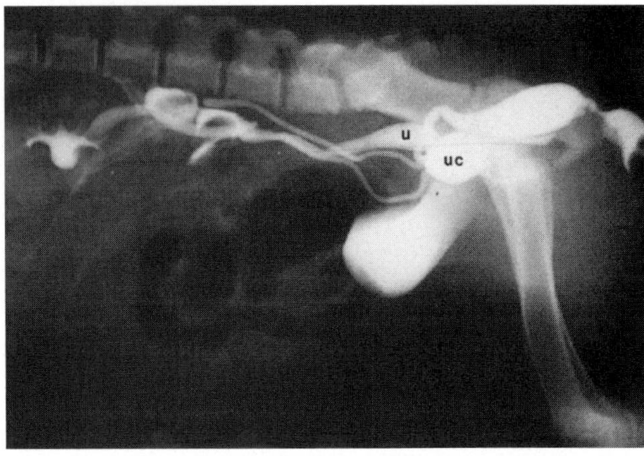

Fig. 40-17 Lateral view of a retrograde, positive-contrast vaginogram in a bitch with an ectopic ureter/ureterocele. The ectopic ureter *(u)* is dilated and ends in a ureterocele *(uc)*. (Reprinted from Johnston GR: *Contrast vaginography in the bitch: techniques and applications. Proceedings 319: reproduction and paediatrics*, Sydney, Australia, 1999, University of Sydney.)

margination of the ureter at excretory urographic examination may help differentiate these considerations. Nonvisualization of a ureteral segment is usually normal because of peristalsis.[4,5,7] However, this segment of the ureter should be visualized at some time in the sequence of radiographs. If the segment is not seen during the sequence, especially in the presence of contrast medium accumulation in the retroperitoneal space or loss of retroperitoneal contrast, ureteral rupture should be considered (see Fig. 40-18).[4,10,95] Another consideration in segmental nonvisualization of the ureter is stricture, but proximal dilation provides perspective on the nonvisualized segment.

A useful alternative to either ultrasonography or excretory urography alone is antegrade pyelography.[117] In this technique, sterile iodinated radiographic contrast medium is instilled into the usually somewhat dilated renal pelvis under ultrasonographic guidance with follow-up radiographs (often shortly after instillation and then 15 to 30 minutes later). The intent is to determine if a stonelike opacity along the suspected course of the ureter is actually in the ureter and the cause of the ureteropyelectasia.

Function

Ureteral atony or hypotonia may be induced as a result of intraluminal infection, periureteral inflammation, trauma, or

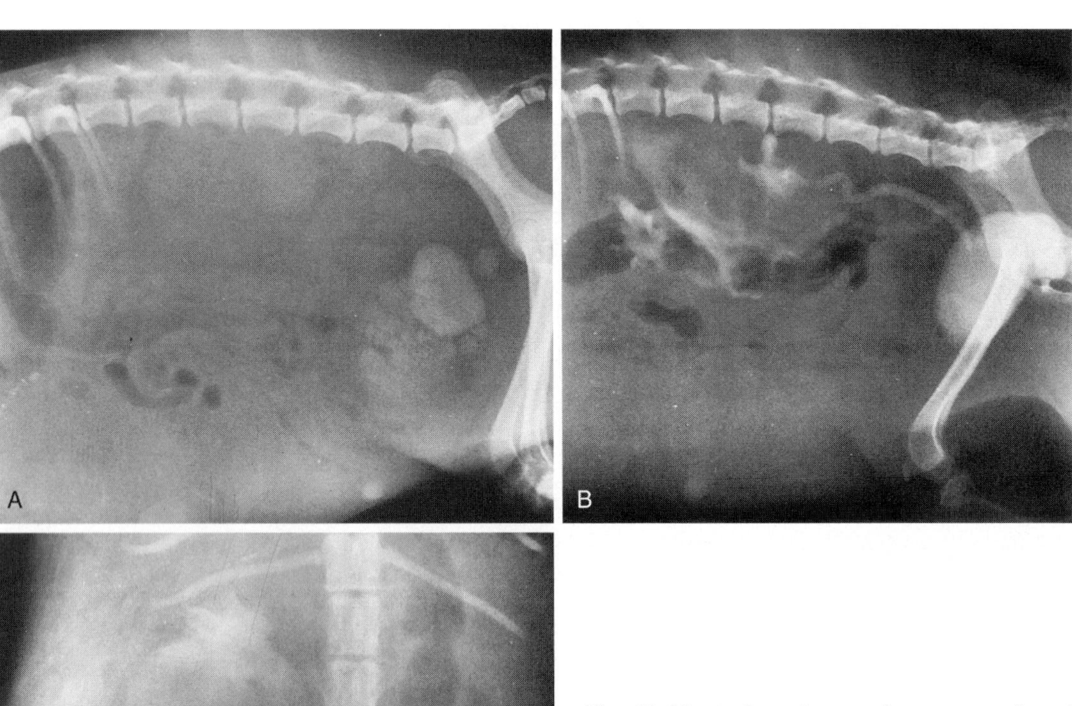

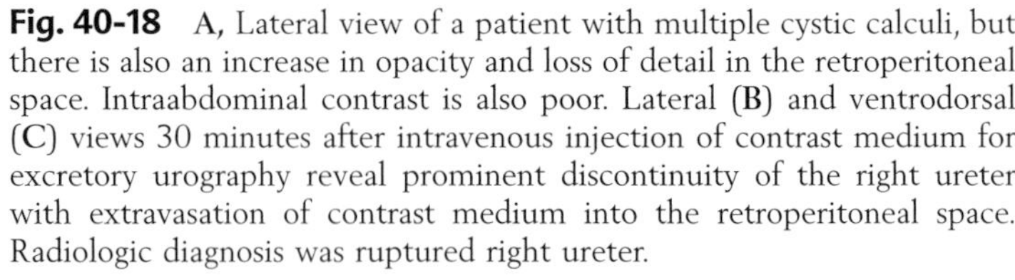

Fig. 40-18 A, Lateral view of a patient with multiple cystic calculi, but there is also an increase in opacity and loss of detail in the retroperitoneal space. Intraabdominal contrast is also poor. Lateral (B) and ventrodorsal (C) views 30 minutes after intravenous injection of contrast medium for excretory urography reveal prominent discontinuity of the right ureter with extravasation of contrast medium into the retroperitoneal space. Radiologic diagnosis was ruptured right ureter.

ureteral obstruction (see Figs. 40-12 and 40-15).[4,6,94,95,101,102] Differentiation among these possible causes requires complete assessment of the size, shape, and margination of the opacified ureter as well as observation of the site and character of ureteral termination. Comparison with the results of urine cytologic and culture studies is also of value.

Vesicoureteral reflux is the retrograde flow of urine from the bladder into the ureter either as a low-pressure phenomenon in the presence of incompletely filled bladder or as a high-pressure phenomenon in the presence of a filled bladder or during voiding.[106] Vesicoureteral reflux may be encountered in immature small animals and may be induced during retrograde radiographic procedures. Reflux may also be induced as a result of manual compression of the urinary bladder in an attempt to perform voiding urethrography. The major significance of vesicoureteral reflux lies in the potential of retrograde flow of urine contaminated with pathologic organisms from the urinary bladder toward the kidney.

The normal ureter is not visible sonographically as a tubular entity except as it enters the urinary bladder.[10,13,14,78,79] This is most easily recognized by the characteristic flow jet produced in the bladder lumen when the peristaltic ureter ejects urine. However, when the ureter is either focally or diffusely enlarged, it can be recognized as a fluid-containing tube that may or may not have evidence of peristalsis during real-time ultrasonography. As the ureter exits the kidney, it can create a circular black void in the otherwise uniformly bright renal sinus fat in the renal hilus when viewed in the sagittal plane. The dilated renal pelvis can be seen to make a funnel-shaped transition into a dilated ureter at the ureteropelvic junction when viewed on the transverse plane through the renal hilus. On occasion the dilated ureter can be traced along its retroperitoneal path by ultrasonography. However, the technique of excretory urography provides a better assessment of ipsilateral renal function and concentrating ability and the ureteral peristaltic capability than does ultrasonography.

REFERENCES

1. DiBartola SP: Clinical approach and laboratory evaluation of renal disease. In Ettinger SJ, editor: *Textbook of veterinary internal medicine,* ed 4, Philadelphia, 1995, WB Saunders.
2. Osborne CA, Polzin DJ, Feeney DA et al: The urinary system: pathophysiology, diagnosis, and therapy. In Gourley IA, Vasseur PB, editors: *General small animal surgery,* Philadelphia, 1985, J.B. Lippincott.
3. Allan G: Radiology in the diagnosis of kidney disease, *Aust Vet Pract* 12:97, 1982.
4. Feeney DA, Barber DL, Osborne CA: Advances in canine excretory urography. In *Proceedings of the 30th Gaines Veterinary Symposium,* White Plains, NY, 1981, Gaines Dog Research Center, p 8.
5. Feeney DA, Barber DL, Johnston GR et al: The excretory urogram: techniques, normal radiographic appearance, and misinterpretation, *Compend Contin Educ Pract Vet* 4:233, 1982.
6. Kneller SK: Role of excretory urography in the diagnosis of renal and ureteral disease, *Vet Clin North Am* 4:843, 1974.
7. Feeney DA, Thrall DE, Barber DL et al: Normal canine excretory urogram: effects of dose, time and individual dog variation, *Am J Vet Res* 40:1596, 1979.
8. Feeney DA, Osborne CA, Jessen CR: Effects of radiographic contrast media on the results of the urinalysis with emphasis on specific gravity, *J Am Vet Med Assoc* 176:1378, 1980.
9. Ruby AL, Ling GV, Ackerman N: Effects of sodium diatrizoate on the in vitro growth of 3 common canine urinary bacterial species, *Vet Radiol* 24:222, 1983.
10. Feeney DA, Johnston GR, Walter PA: Imaging the kidney and prostate gland in small animals: has gray-scale ultrasonography replaced contrast radiography? *Probl Vet Med* 3:619, 1991.
11. Konde LJ, Wrigley RH, Park RD et al: Ultrasound anatomy of the normal canine kidney, *Vet Radiol* 25:173, 1984.
12. Walter PA, Feeney DA, Johnston GR, Fletcher TF: The normal feline renal ultrasonogram: Quantitative analysis of imaged anatomy. Am J Vet Res 48:596, 1987.
13. Walter PA, Johnston GR, Feeney DA, O'Brien TD: Renal ultrasonography in healthy cats. Am J Vet Res 48:600, 1987.
14. Wood AKW, McCarthy PH: Ultrasonographic-anatomic correlation and an imaging protocol of the normal canine kidney, *Am J Vet Res* 51:103, 1990.
15. Yaeger AE, Anderson WI: Study of association between histologic features and echogenicity of architecturally normal cat kidneys, *Am J Vet Res* 50:860, 1989.
16. Finco DR, Stiles NS, Kneller SK et al: Radiologic estimation of kidney size in the dog, *J Am Vet Med Assoc* 159:995, 1971.
17. Barrett RB, Kneller SL: Feline kidney measuration, *Acta Radiol (Stockh)* 319(suppl):279, 1972.
18. Bartels JE: Feline intravenous urography, *J Am Anim Hosp Assoc* 9:349, 1973.
19. Shiroma JT, Gabriel JK, Carter TL et al: Effect of reproductive status on feline renal size, *Vet Radiol Ultrasound* 40:242, 1999.
20. Feeney DA, Barber DL, Osborne CA: Functional aspects of the nephrogram in excretory urography: a review, *Vet Radiol* 23:42, 1982.
21. Thrall DE, Finco DR: Canine excretory urography: is quality a function of BUN? *J Am Anim Hosp Assoc* 12:446, 1976.
22. Jakovljevic S, Rivers WJ, Chun R et al: Results of renal ultrasonography performed before and during administration of saline (0.9% NaCl) solution to induce diuresis in dogs, *Am J Vet Res* 60:405, 1999.
23. Drost WT, Henry GA, Meinkoth JH et al: Quantification of hepatic and renal cortical echogenicity in clinically normal cats, *Am J Vet Res* 61:1016, 2000.
24. Cuypers MD, Grooters AM, Williams J et al: Renomegaly in dogs and cats: differential diagnosis, *Compend Contin Educ Prac Vet* 19:1019, 1997.
25. Robinson GW: Uterus unicornus and unilateral renal agenesis, *J Am Vet Med Assoc* 147:516, 1965.
26. O'Handley P, Carrig CB, Walshaw R: Renal and ureteral duplication in a dog, *J Am Vet Med Assoc* 174:484, 1979.
27. Senior DF: Parasites of the urinary tract. In Kirk RW, editor: *Current veterinary therapy VII,* Philadelphia, 1980, WB Saunders.
28. Barsanti JA, Crowell R: Renal amyloidosis. In Kirk RW, editor: *Current veterinary therapy VII,* Philadelphia, 1980, WB Saunders.
29. Brace JJ: Perirenal cysts (pseudocysts) in the cat. In Kirk RW, editor: *Current veterinary therapy VII,* Philadelphia, 1980, WB Saunders.
30. Stowater JL: Congenital solitary renal cyst in a dog, *J Am Anim Hosp Assoc* 11:199, 1975.
31. Caywood DD, Osborne CA, Johnston GR: Neoplasms of the canine and feline urinary tracts, In Kirk RW, editor: *Current veterinary therapy VII,* Philadelphia, 1980, WB Saunders.

32. McKenna SC, Carpenter JL: Polycystic disease of the kidney and liver in the canine terrier, *Vet Pathol* 17:436, 1980.
33. Lulich JP, Osborne CA, Walter PA et al: Feline idiopathic polycystic kidney disease, *Compend Contin Educ Pract Vet Small Anim* 10:1030, 1988.
34. Rendano VT, Parker RB: Polycystic kidneys and peritoneal pericardial diaphragmatic hernia in a cat, *J Small Anim Pract* 17:479, 1976.
35. Crowell WA, Hubbell JJ, Riley JC: Polycystic renal disease in related cats, *J Am Vet Med Assoc* 175:286, 1979.
36. Osborne CA, Johnson KH, Kurtz HJ et al: Renal lymphoma in the dog and cat, *J Am Vet Med Assoc* 158:2058, 1971.
37. Barber DL: Radiographic evaluation of a focal inflammatory renal lesion, *J Am Anim Hosp Assoc* 12:451, 1976.
38. Chalifoux A, Phaneuf JB, Oliver N et al: Glomerular polycystic kidney disease in a dog, *Can Vet J* 23:365, 1982.
39. Essman SC, Drost WT, Hoover JP et al: Imaging of a cat with perirenal pseudocysts, *Vet Radiol Ultrasound* 41:329, 2000.
40. Churchill JA, Feeney DA, Fletcher TF et al: Effects of diet and aging on renal measurements in unnephrectomized geriatric bitches, *Vet Radiol Ultrasound* 40:233, 1999.
41. Bernard MA, Valli VE: Familial renal disease in Samoyed dogs, *Can Vet J* 18:181, 1977.
42. Brown CA, Crowell WA, Brown SA et al: Suspected familial renal disease in Chow Chows, *J Am Vet Med Assoc* 196:1279, 1990.
43. Casal ML, Giger Y, Bovee KC et al: Inheritance of cystinuria and renal defect in Newfoundlands, *J Am Vet Med Assoc* 207:1585, 1995.
44. Chew DJ, DiBartola SP, Boyce JT et al: Juvenile renal disease in Doberman Pinscher dogs, *J Am Vet Med Assoc* 182:481, 1983.
45. Cook SM, Dean DF, Golden DL et al: Renal failure attributable to atrophic glomerulopathy in four related Rottweilers, *J Am Vet Med Assoc* 202:107, 1993.
46. Davenport DJ, DiBartola SP, Chew DJ: Familial renal disease in the dog and cat, *Cont Issues Small Anim Pract* 4:137, 1986.
47. DiBartola SP, Chew DJ, Boyce JT: Juvenile renal disease in related standard poodles, *J Am Vet Med Assoc* 183:693, 1983.
48. DiBartola Sp, Tarr MJ, Webb DM et al: Familial renal amyloidosis in Chinese Shar Pei dogs, *J Am Vet Med Assoc* 197:483, 1990.
49. English PB, Winter H: Renal cortical hypoplasia in a dog, *Aust Vet J* 55:181, 1979.
50. Eriksen K, Grondalen J: Familial renal disease in soft-coated Wheaten Terriers, *J Small Anim Pract* 25:489, 1984.
51. Felkai C, Voros K, Vrabley T et al: Ultrasonographic findings of renal dysplasia in Cocker Spaniels: eight cases, *Acta Vet Hung* 45:397, 1997.
52. Finco DR: Congenital and inherited renal disease, *J Am Anim Hosp Assoc* 9:301, 1973.
53. Finco DR, Kurtz HJ, Low DG et al: Familial renal disease in Norwegian Elkhound dogs, *J Am Vet Med Assoc* 156:747, 1970.
54. Greco DS: Congenital and inherited renal disease of small animals, *Vet Clin North Am Small Anim Pract* 31:393, 2001.
55. Jones BR, Gething MA, Badcoe LM et al: Familial progressive nephropathy in young Bull Terriers, *N Z Vet J* 37:79, 1989.
56. Jones BR, Jones JM, Chen W et al: Chronic renal failure in young Old English Sheepdogs, *N Z Vet J* 38:118, 1990.
57. Kerlin RL, VanWinkle TJ: Renal dysplasia in Golden Retrievers, *Vet Pathol* 32:327, 1995.
58. Klopfer U, Neumann F, Trainin R: Renal cortical hypoplasia in a Keesond litter, *Vet Med Small Anim Clin* 70:1081, 1975.
59. Koeman JP, Biewenga WJ, Gruys E: Proteinuria associated with glomerulosclerosis and glomerular collagen formation in 3 Newfoundland dog littermates, *Vet Pathol* 31:188, 1984.
60. Lees G: Congenital renal diseases, *Vet Clin North Am Small Anim Pract* 26:1379, 1996.
61. Lees GE, Helman RG, Homco LD et al: Early diagnosis of familial nephropathy in English Cocker Spaniels, *J Am Anim Hosp Assoc* 34:189, 1998.
62. Lucke VM, Kelly DF, Darke PG et al: Chronic renal failure in young dogs: possible renal dysplasia, *J Small Anim Pract* 21:169, 1980.
63. Mason NJ, Dan MJ: Renal amyloidosis in related English Foxhounds, *J Small Anim Pract* 37:255, 1996.
64. Minkus G, Breuer W, Wanke R et al: Familial nephropathy in Burmese Mountain Dogs, *Vet Pathol* 31:421, 1994.
65. Morton LD: Familial nephropathy in Miniature Schnauzers, *Can Vet J* 32:389, 1991.
66. Noonan CHB, Kay JM: Prevalence and geographic distribution of Fanconi syndrome in Basenjis in the United States, *J Am Vet Med Assoc* 197:345, 1990.
67. O'Brien TD, Osborne CA, Yano BC et al: Clinicopathologic manifestations of progressive renal disease in Lhasa Apso and Shih Tzu dogs, *J Am Vet Med Assoc* 180:658, 1982.
68. Peeters D, Clerex C, Michiels L et al: Juvenile nephropathy in a Boxer, Rottweiler, a Collie and an Irish Wolfhound. *Aust Vet J* 78:162, 2000.
69. Perry W: Generalized nodular dermatofibrosis and renal cystadenoma in a series of 10 closely related German Shepherd dogs, *Aust Vet Pract* 25:90, 1995.
70. Reusch C, Hoerauf A, Lechner J et al: A new familial glomerulonephropathy in Burmese Mountain dogs, *Vet Rec* 134:411, 1994.
71. Robinson WF, Huxtable CR, Gooding JP: Familiar nephropathy in Cocker Spaniels, *Aust Vet J* 62:109, 1985.
72. Schulze C, Meyer HP, Blok Al et al: Renal dysplasia in 3 Dutch Kooiker dogs, *Vet Q* 20:146, 1998.
73. Witcock BP, Patterson JM: Familial glomerulosclerosis in Doberman Pinscher dogs, *Can Vet J* 20:244, 1979.
74. Zuilen CD, Nickel RF, VanDijk TH et al: Xanthinuria in a family of Cavalier King Charles Spaniels, *Vet Q* 19:172, 1997.
75. Chew DJ, DiBartola SP, Boyce JT et al: Renal amyloidosis in related Abyssinian cats, *J Am Vet Med Assoc* 181:139, 1982.
76. Tarr MJ, DiBartola SP: Familial amyloidosis in Abyssinian cats: a possible model for familial Mediterranean fever and pathogenesis of secondary amyloidosis, *Lab Invest* 52:67a, 1985.
77. Stokes JE and Forrester SD: New and unusual causes of acute renal failure in dogs and cats, *Vet Clin North Am Small Anim Pract* 34:909, 2004.
78. Konde LJ: Sonography of the kidney, *Vet Clin North Am* 15:1149, 1985.
79. Walter PA, Johnston GR, Feeney DA et al: Applications of ultrasonography in the diagnosis of parenchymal kidney disease in cats, *J Am Vet Med Assoc* 192:92, 1988.

80. Forrest LJ, O'Brien RT, Tremelling MS et al: Sonographic renal findings in 20 dogs with *Leptospirosis*, *Vet Radiol Ultrasound* 39:337, 1998.
81. Mantis P, Lamb CR: Most dogs with medullary rim sign on ultrasonography have no demonstrable renal dysfunction, *Vet Radiol Ultrasound* 41:164, 2000.
82. Churchill JA, Feeney DA, Fletcher TF et al: Age and diet effects on renal echogenicity in geriatric bitches, *Vet Radiol Ultrasound* 40:642, 1999.
83. Morrow KL, Salman MD, Lappin MR et al: Comparison of the resistive index to clinical parameters in dogs with renal disease, *Vet Radiol Ultrasound* 37:193, 1996.
84. Nyland TG, Fisher PE, Doverspike M et al: Diagnosis of urinary tract obstruction in dogs using duplex Doppler ultrasonography, *Vet Radiol Ultrasound* 34:348, 1993.
85. Allworth MS, Hoffman KL: Crossed renal ectopia with fusion in a cat, *Vet Radiol Ultrasound* 40:357, 1999.
86. Wells CA, Coyne JA, Prince JL: Ectopic kidney in a cat, *Mod Vet Pract* 61:693, 1980.
87. Johnson CA: Renal ectopia in a cat, *J Am Anim Hosp Assoc* 15:599, 1979.
88. Osborne CA, Klausner JS, Clinton CW: Analysis of canine and feline uroliths. In Kirk RW, editor: *Current veterinary therapy VIII*, Philadelphia, 1983, WB Saunders.
89. Ling GV, Ruby AL, Johnson DL et al: Renal calculi in dogs & cats: prevalence, mineral type, breed, age, and gender interrelationships, *J Vet Intern Med* 12:11, 1998.
90. Barber DL, Rowland GN: Radiographically detectable soft-tissue calcification in chronic renal failure, *Vet Radiol* 20:117, 1979.
91. Hall MA, Osborne CA, Stevens JB: Hydronephrosis with heteroplastic bone formation in a cat, *J Am Vet Med Assoc* 160:857, 1972.
92. Miller JB, Sande RD: Osseous metaplasia in the renal pelvis of a dog with hydronephrosis, *Vet Radiol* 21:146, 1980.
93. Fuller WJ: Subacute pyelonephritis with a unilaterally non-visualized pyelogram, *J Am Anim Hosp Assoc* 12:509, 1976.
94. Barber DL, Finco DR: Radiographic findings in induced bacterial pyelonephritis in dogs, *J Am Vet Med Assoc* 175:1183, 1979.
95. Selcer BA: Urinary tract trauma associated with pelvic trauma, *J Am Anim Hosp Assoc* 18:785, 1982.
96. Faulkner RT, Osborne CA, Feeney DA: Canine and feline ureteral ectopia. In Kirk RW, editor: *Current veterinary therapy VIII*, Philadelphia, 1983, WB Saunders.
97. Hagar DA, Blevins WE: Ectopic ureter in a dog: extension from the kidney to the urinary bladder and to the urethra, *J Am Vet Med Assoc* 189:309, 1986.
98. Hayes HM: Breed associations of canine ectopic ureter: a study of 217 female cases, *J Small Anim Pract* 25:501, 1984.
99. Owen RR: Canine ureteral ectopia, *J Small Anim Pract* 14:407, 1983.
100. Jakovljevic S, VanAlstine WG, Adams LG: Ureteral diverticula in two dogs, *Vet Radiol Ultrasound* 39:425, 1998.
101. Rose JG, Gillenwater JY: Effects of obstruction on ureteral function, *Invest Urol* 12:139, 1975.
102. Rose JG, Gillenwater JY: Effects of obstruction and infection upon ureteral function, *Invest Urol* 11:471, 1974.
103. Burton CA, Day MJ, Hotston-Moore A et al: Ureteric fibroepithelial polyps in 2 dogs, *J Small Animal Pract* 35:593, 1994.
104. Moroff SD, Brown BA, Matthiesen DT et al: Infiltrative ureteral disease in female dogs: 41 cases (1980-1987), *J Am Vet Med Assoc* 199:247, 1991.
105. Reichle JK, Peterson RA, Mahaffey MB: Ureteral fibroepithelial polyps in four dogs, *Vet Radiol Ultrasound* 44:433, 2003.
106. Klausner JS, Feeney DA: Vesicoureteral reflux. In Kirk RW, editor: *Current veterinary therapy VIII*, Philadelphia, 1983, WB Saunders.
107. Ross LA, Lamb CR: Reduction of hydronephrosis and hydroureter associated with ectopic ureters in two dogs after ureterovesical anastomosis, *J Am Vet Med Assoc* 196:1497, 1990.
108. Scott CW, Greene RW, Patnaik AK: Unilateral ureterocele associated with hydronephrosis in a dog, *J Am Anim Hosp Assoc* 10:126, 1974.
109. Takiguchi M, Uasuda J, Ochiari K et al: Ultrasonographic appearance of orthotopic ureterocele in a dog, *Vet Radiol Ultrasound* 38:398, 1997.
110. Smith CW, Park RD: Bilateral ectopic ureteroceles in a dog, *Canine Pract* 1:28, 1974.
111. Stowater JL, Springer AL: Ureterocele in a dog, *Vet Med Small Anim Pract* 74:1753, 1979.
112. Johnston GR, Osborne CA, Wilson JW et al: Familial ureteral ectopia in the dog, *J Am Anim Hosp Assoc* 13:168, 1977.
113. Rozear L, Tidwell AS: Evaluation of the ureter and ureterovesical junction using helical computed tomography excretory urography in healthy dogs, *Vet Radiol Ultrasound* 44:155, 2003.
114. Samii VF, McLoughlin MA, Mattoon JS et al: Digital fluoroscopic excretory urography, digital fluoroscopic urethrography, helical computed tomography and cystoscopy in 24 dogs with suspected ureteral ectopia, *J Vet Intern Med* 18:271, 2004.
115. Weisse C, Aronson LR, Drobatz K: Traumatic rupture of the ureters: 10 cases, *J Am Anim Hosp Assoc* 38:188, 2002.
116. Worth AJ, Tomlin SC: Post-traumatic paraureteral urinoma in a cat, *J Small Anim Pract* 45:413, 2004.
117. Adin CA, Herrgesell EJ, Nyland TG et al: Antegrade pyelography for suspected ureteral obstruction in cats 11 cases (1995-2001), *J Am Vet Med Assoc* 222:1576, 2003.

ELECTRONIC RESOURCES evolve

Additional information related to the content in Chapter 40 can be found on the companion Web site at evolve http://evolve.elsevier.com/Thrall/vetrad/.

- Key Points
- Chapter Quiz
- Case Study 40-1
- Case Study 40-2

CHAPTER • 41
The Urinary Bladder

Richard D. Park
Robert H. Wrigley

NORMAL ANATOMY

The urinary bladder is divided grossly into three parts: the vertex (apex vesicae) cranially, the body (corpus vesicae) in the middle, and the neck (cervix vesicae) caudally (Fig. 41-1).[1-3] Three ligaments formed from peritoneal reflections loosely hold the bladder in position.[3] The middle bladder ligament (ligamentum vesicae medianum) extends along the ventral bladder surface, and two lateral ligaments (ligamenta vesicae lateralia) extend along the lateral bladder surfaces. These ligaments often contain large fat deposits, facilitating radiographic visualization of the bladder neck and body. The cranial and dorsal surfaces of the bladder are radiographically visible because of adjacent fat within the omentum and mesentery (Fig. 41-2).

The urinary bladder wall is a musculomembranous structure consisting of mucosal, submucosal, and muscular layers; the peritoneum closely adheres to the serosal surface, providing a separate fourth layer. Bladder wall thickness and the mucosal surface of the bladder cannot be identified on survey radiographs because the adjacent urine has the same radiographic opacity, leading to border effacement.

Radiographic visualization of the urinary bladder is compromised by insufficient abdominal fat, inadequate distention, and superimposition opacities. Emaciated or young animals may not have sufficient abdominal fat to provide good tissue contrast adjacent to the urinary bladder. Ingested material in the small bowel, fecal material in the large bowel, pelvic limb muscle, and bone from the spine and pelvis cause superimposition opacities that may obscure all or part of the urinary bladder. Focal superimposition opacities may be created by fluid-filled small bowel, nipples, the prepuce, and cutaneous masses. Some of these superimposition opacities can be eliminated or minimized by withholding food for 24 hours preceding the study, giving cleansing enemas, and pulling the pelvic limbs caudally when the radiograph is made.

Bladder size varies with the amount of urine in the bladder. After the patient voids, the bladder is small and may not be visible radiographically. With extreme distention, the cranial bladder border may extend to the umbilicus. Severe distention may occur in a normal bladder if the animal has not had an opportunity to void or will not void because of a strange or unfamiliar environment. The urinary bladder in the dog is usually oval, but with distention it becomes more ellipsoid. The feline urinary bladder is almost always ellipsoid (Fig. 41-3).

The bladder is cranial to the pubis, dorsal to the rectus abdominis muscle, caudal to the small bowel and omentum, and ventral to the large bowel. In females the uterus lies between the bladder and the rectum. The normal urinary bladder may be partially within the pelvic canal or cranial to the pubis (external to the pelvic canal).[4,5] The distended urinary bladder is more often located cranial to the pubis but may be within the pelvic canal.[4,5] The normal urinary bladder in the cat is always intraabdominal and is located 2 to 3 cm cranial to the pubis. This positioning results from the long bladder neck in the cat, which is not always visible on survey radiographs.[6]

The urinary bladder is a soft tissue opaque structure. Any opacity greater or less than soft tissue detected within the bladder on survey radiographs is abnormal.

RADIOGRAPHIC SIGNS OF URINARY BLADDER DISEASE

Signs of urinary bladder disease on survey radiographs are limited. In many instances, the signs indicate disease in adjacent structures. Signs that indicate disease of the urinary bladder or adjacent structures are poor or nonexistent bladder visualization and abnormal bladder position, shape, size, and opacity (Table 41-1).

Poor radiographic visualization of the urinary bladder may occur if serosal detail in the caudal abdomen is good or decreased. If the serosal detail is good and the bladder is not seen, the bladder is empty or has been displaced caudally or ventrally. If serosal detail is decreased and the bladder surface is not distinctly seen, free peritoneal fluid or inadequate peritoneal fat may be the cause (Fig. 41-4).

The bladder may be abnormally displaced in various directions.[7] Sometimes the cause of bladder displacement may be determined by observation of surrounding structures (Fig. 41-5). With severe bladder displacement, as with hernias, the bladder may not be seen on survey radiographs but may be identified by cystography or ultrasonography. Bladder retroflexion was found in 12 (20%) of 61 dogs with a perineal hernia.[8] A urinary bladder partially within the pelvic canal (Fig. 41-6) may be associated with congenital urinary tract anomalies.[9] A minimally distended bladder may be pelvic in position and move more cranially when distended; pelvic bladders have been reported as a normal variation.[4,5] Incontinent female dogs with a pelvic bladder usually have shorter urethras than do continent dogs.[10] Because pelvic bladders do not always indicate a clinical problem, a pelvic bladder should be correlated with clinical signs to determine its clinical significance.

A change in shape of the urinary bladder is not commonly detected on survey radiographs. Abdominal masses adjacent to the serosal surface of the bladder may distort the bladder shape. Tumors originating from the bladder wall occasionally protrude from the serosal surface and produce a discernible bladder shape change (Fig. 41-7).[11] A pointed vertex with an

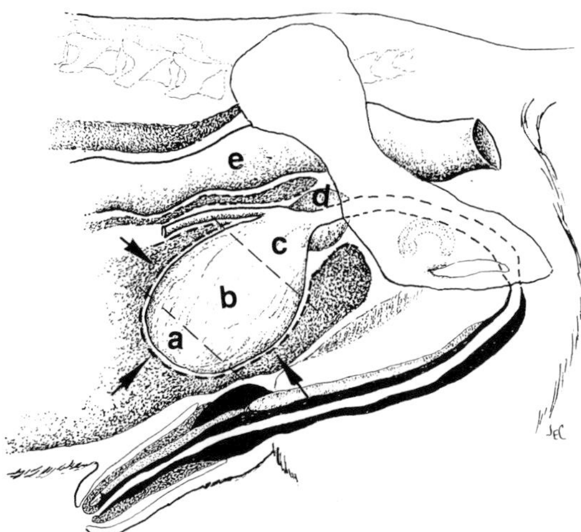

Fig. 41-1 Lateral view of the abdomen in a normal male dog. *a*, Vertex; *b*, body of the bladder; *c*, neck of the urinary bladder; *d*, prostate; *e*, large bowel. The *broken line* around the urinary bladder *(arrows)* represents the peritoneal reflection around and adherent to the serosal surface of the urinary bladder.

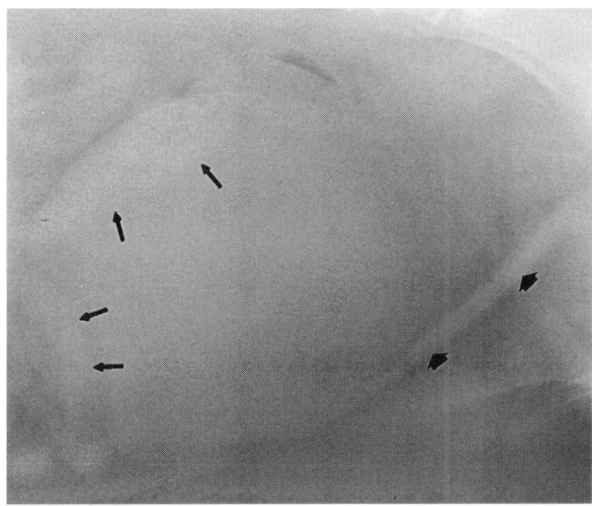

Fig. 41-2 Lateral radiograph of the caudal abdomen in a normal dog. The bladder neck is well visualized because of fat within the bladder ligaments. The rectus abdominis muscle *(short arrows)* is ventral to the bladder. Bowel is superimposed *(long arrows)* over the cranial and dorsal borders of the bladder.

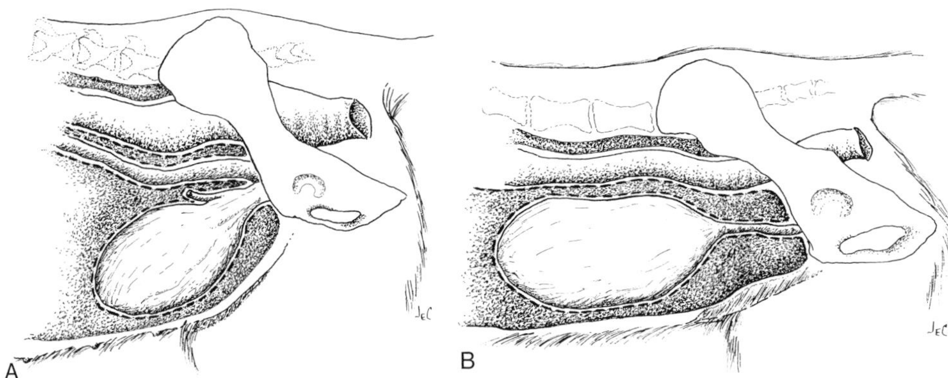

Fig. 41-3 A, Bladder in a normal female dog. The bladder is adjacent to the pubis and is oval. The broken line indicates the peritoneal reflection around the bladder. **B,** Bladder in a normal cat. The bladder is ellipsoid and has a long neck, which makes the bladder appear to be displaced cranially away from the pubis. The *broken line* denotes the peritoneal reflection around the bladder. (From Park RD: Radiology of the urinary bladder and urethra. In O'Brien TR, editor: *Radiographic diagnosis of abdominal disorders in the dog and cat,* Davis, CA, 1981, Covell Park Veterinary.)

elongated bladder may occur with a persistent urachal ligament in the cat.[12] An abnormally small or large urinary bladder is difficult to diagnose radiographically because of the wide normal variation in bladder size. In most instances a consistently small or large bladder with associated clinical signs is an indication that a contrast study or ultrasound examination should be performed to determine the cause of the small or large bladder.

Any change in radiographic opacity in the urinary bladder is abnormal and usually easy to detect. Gas in the bladder may be introduced iatrogenically from catheterization or cystocentesis. Small luminal gas bubbles are usually seen in the center of the bladder on the recumbent lateral view (Fig. 41-8). Gas in the bladder lumen, bladder wall, and occasionally the bladder ligaments occurs with emphysematous cystitis (Fig. 41-9). Emphysematous cystitis is produced by glucose-fermenting organisms and may be seen in association with diabetes mellitus.[13,14] Occurrence of emphysematous cystitis without diabetes mellitus also has been reported.[15,16]

Most radiopacities associated with the bladder are calculi. If cystic calculi are identified on radiographs, assessment of the remainder of the urinary tract is important as calculi are commonly present elsewhere (Fig. 41-10). Not all calculi are radiopaque, however; thus the absence of radiopacities within the bladder does not rule out the presence of cystic calculi (Table 41-2). A horizontal-beam radiograph can be made to diagnose sandlike material within the bladder. This is particularly helpful in cats with feline urologic syndrome.[17] Radiopacities in the urinary bladder can also be produced by mineralization of the bladder wall associated with neoplasia or chronic cystitis, but this is unusual.

CONTRAST CYSTOGRAPHY

Retrograde contrast cystography is a fast, simple, and inexpensive technique that may provide valuable diagnostic and prognostic information about bladder disease. Clinical

TABLE • 41-1

Urinary Bladder: Survey Radiographic Signs

RADIOGRAPHIC SIGN	GAMUT OF CONDITION(S) OR DISEASE(S)
Visualization	
Bladder not seen; abdominal serosal outlines are clear	Postvoiding
	Displaced bladder
	Perineal hernia
	Inguinal hernia
	Pelvic bladder
	Short urethra
	Ectopic ureter
	Congenital fistulas
	Normal pelvic bladder
Bladder not seen; abdominal serosal outlines are not clearly seen	Ruptured urinary bladder
	Peritoneal fluid
	Transudate
	Exudate
	Hemorrhage
	Emaciated animal
	Young animal (<4 months of age)
Abnormal Position	
Ventral displacement	Abdominal wall hernia
Cranial displacement	Inguinal hernia
	Prostatic disease
	Neoplasia
	Prostatitis
	Prostatic cyst
	Hypertrophy
Cranioventral displacement	Enlarged uterus
	Pyometra
	Pregnancy
	Sublumbar mass(es)
	Large bowel distention
	Uterine stump granuloma or abscess
	Persistent patent urachus or urachal ligament
Abnormal Position	
Caudal displacement	Perineal hernia
	Large abdominal mass(es)
	Congenital anomalies
	Short urethra
	Ectopic ureters
Dorsal displacement	Congenital fistulas
	Normal pelvic bladder
	Abdominal mass(es)
Abnormal Shape	Mesenchymal neoplasia
	Adjacent abdominal mass(es)
	Neoplasia
	Abscess or granuloma
	Persistent urachal ligament
Abnormal Size	
Increased size	Distal urinary obstruction
Decreased size	Urethral obstruction
	Bladder neck obstruction
	Neurologic deficiencies
	Congenital anomalies
	Ectopic ureters
	Fistulas
	Diffuse bladder wall disease
	Cystitis
	Neoplasia
	Hemorrhage
Opacity Changes	
Increased	Calculi
	Bladder wall mineralization
Decreased	Neoplasia
	Inflammation
	Gas
	Iatrogenic
	Emphysematous cystitis

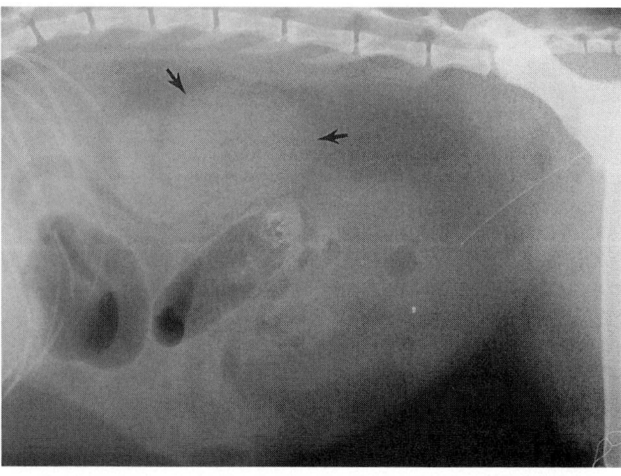

Fig. 41-4 Lateral radiograph of the abdomen of a cat. The kidneys are easily seen because they are surrounded retroperitoneal fat *(arrows)*. The serosal surfaces on the bowel and urinary bladder do not have distinct outlines because of free peritoneal fluid. A catheter is in the urinary bladder.

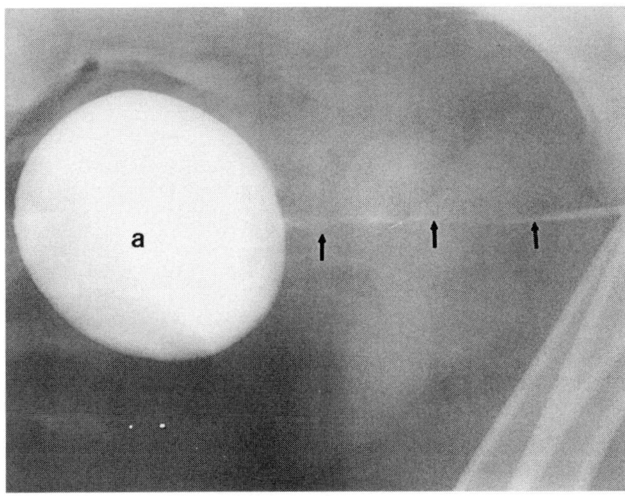

Fig. 41-5 Positive-contrast cystogram, lateral view, in a male dog. The urinary bladder *(a)* is displaced cranially from the pubis by a large prostatic mass. The urethra and bladder neck are filled with positive-contrast medium *(arrows)*. Diagnosis was prostatic carcinoma.

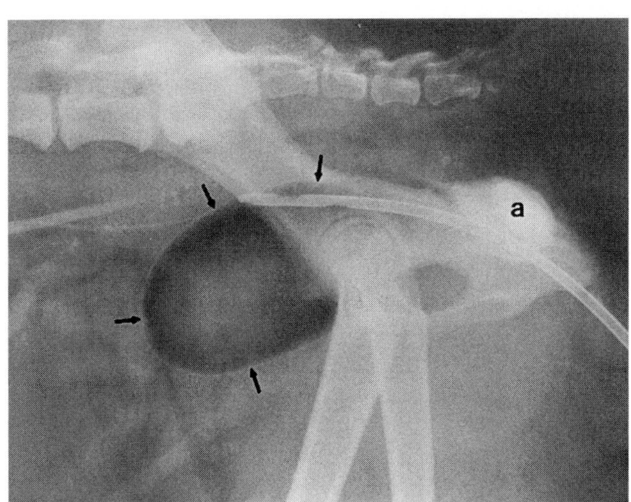

Fig. 41-6 Lateral radiograph of the caudal abdomen and pelvis after intravenous urography and double-contrast cystography. A radiopaque catheter is present within the bladder, and the bladder is partially within the pelvic canal *(arrows)*. Contrast medium has accumulated in the vagina *(a)* because of an ectopic ureter.

indications for cystography include dysuria, pollakiuria, and intermittent or persistent chronic hematuria. Radiographic signs that suggest a need for cystography include identification of increased or decreased opacity in the urinary bladder, evaluation of caudal abdominal masses that may be associated with the urinary bladder, nonvisualization of the bladder after abdominal trauma, and evaluation of the urinary bladder with an abnormal shape or location.

Voiding cystography is not discussed in this chapter. The reader is referred to other publications for more detailed information.[18-22] Voiding cystography, coupled with cystometry and urethral pressure profiles, is the technique of choice for investigating dynamic bladder diseases such as urinary incontinence and other voiding abnormalities.

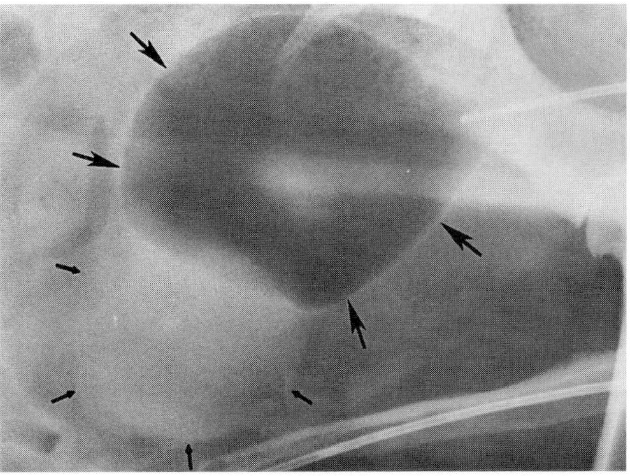

Fig. 41-7 Oblique view of the abdomen after double-contrast cystography. A mass *(small arrows)* is present on the cranioventral aspect of the gas-filled bladder *(large arrows)*. The mass is a leiomyosarcoma originating from the bladder; it gave the bladder a bilobed appearance on the survey radiograph.

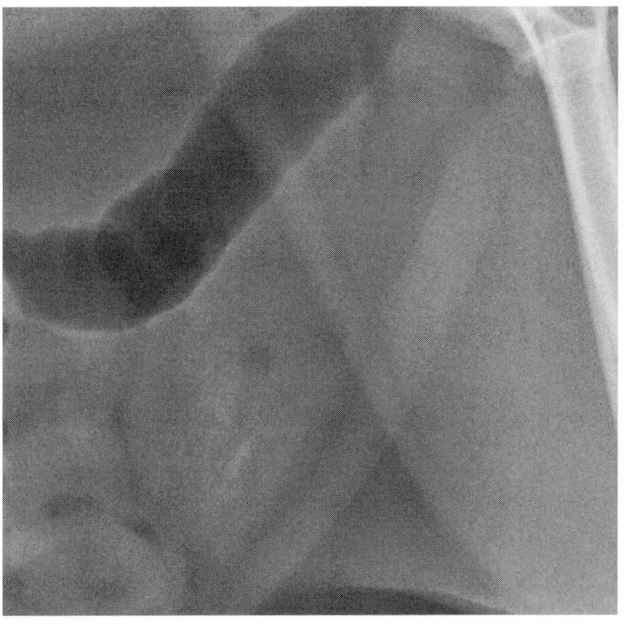

Fig. 41-8 Lateral view of the caudal abdomen of a cat with ill-defined regions of increased opacity in the cranioventral aspect of the bladder caused by mineralized concretions (sandlike material). A small central radiolucency is also present. This is an air bubble introduced inadvertently during cystocentesis. This radiolucency must not be misinterpreted as a calculus because no positive contrast medium has been administered. So-called radiolucent calculi are really of soft tissue opacity are not visible on survey radiographs. However, such calculi appear relatively radiolucent, creating a filling defect, when surrounded by a substance of an opacity greater than that of soft tissue, such as when contrast medium is in the bladder.

Cystography Technique

If possible, food should be withheld for 24 hours and an enema given preceding cystography. Fecal material superimposed over the urinary bladder may mask important radiographic information.

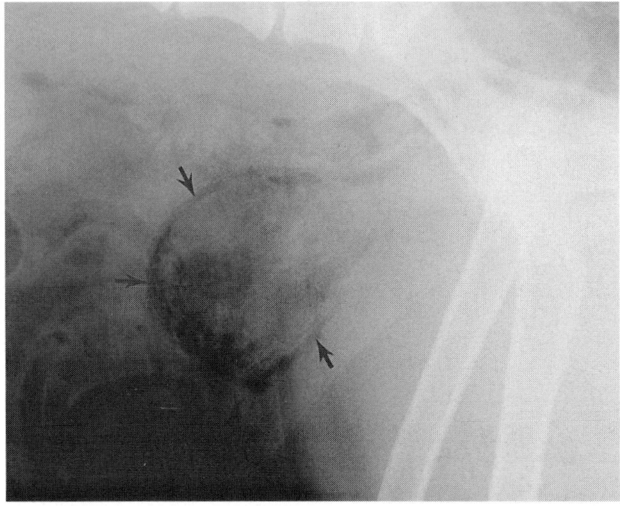

Fig. 41-9 Lateral view of the abdomen of a dog with gas within the bladder wall and lumen *(arrows)*. Gas in the surrounding bowel loops presents some difficulty in distinguishing gas within the bladder. The animal had cystitis caused by a gas-producing organism.

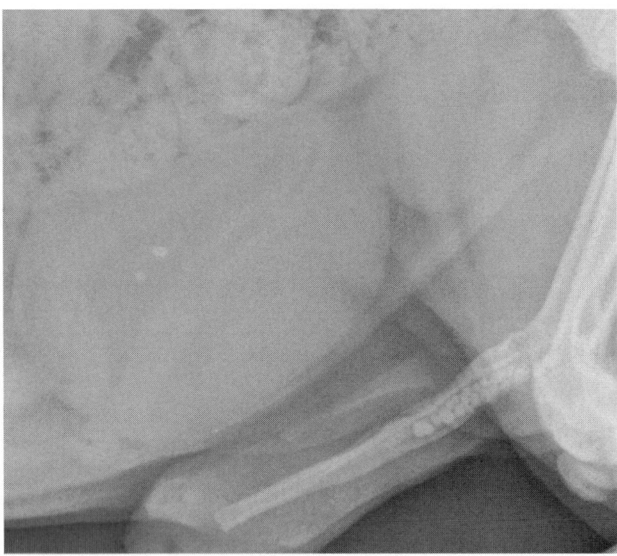

Fig. 41-10 Lateral radiograph of the caudal abdomen of a dog with two small cystic calculi. From this single view, whether these opacities are in the bladder cannot be determined with certainty. They appeared to be in the bladder on the ventrodorsal view, thereby establishing their position. If doubt exists regarding the presence, or existence, of calculi after examining orthogonal radiographs, sonography would be the most expeditious way to obtain further information. This dog also has multiple small calculi in the penile urethra. If cystic calculi are identified, the remainder of the urinary tract from the kidneys to the terminus of the urethra should be examined for additional calculi. Prostatomegaly is also present in this dog.

All catheters and equipment should be sterilized, and the genitalia should be cleaned before the bladder is catheterized. The equipment necessary for bladder catheterization is illustrated in Figure 41-11. To reduce bladder pain and spasm during cystography, 2 to 5 mL of 2% lidocaine (Xylocaine) without epinephrine may be injected into the bladder before cystography is performed.

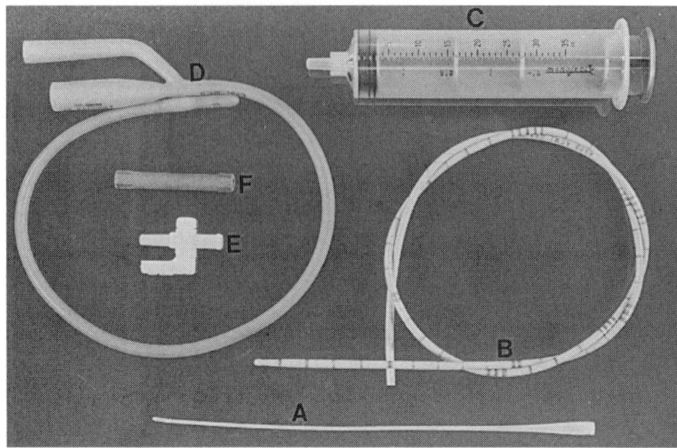

Fig. 41-11 Equipment for bladder catheterization and cystography. *A,* Tom Cat catheter; *B,* male urethral catheter; *C,* large syringe; *D,* Foley (balloon-type) catheter; *E,* three-way valve; *F,* catheter connector for use with the male urethral catheter. (From Park RD: Radiology of the urinary bladder and urethra. In O'Brien TR, editor: *Radiographic diagnosis of abdominal disorders in the dog and cat,* Davis, CA, 1981, Covell Park Veterinary.)

TABLE • 41-2

Radiopacity of Cystic Calculi on Survey Abdominal Radiographs

CALCULUS COMPOSITION	OPACITY
Calcium oxalate	Radiopaque
Silica	Radiopaque
Triple phosphate	Radiopaque; small calculi may be nonradiopaque
Cystine	Nonradiopaque but may have radiopaque stippling
Urate	Nonradiopaque

Complications resulting from catheterization and cystographic procedures occur infrequently and usually are not detrimental to the animal. Iatrogenic trauma, bacterial contamination,[23] or kinked[24] and knotted urethral catheters may occur from improper catheterization techniques. Intramural and subserosal accumulation of contrast medium in the bladder has been reported after maximal bladder distention with a Foley catheter (Fig. 41-12).[25-28] This complication occurs more frequently in cats, often with a nondistended bladder and minimal intravesicular pressure. It usually does not result in a clinical problem. Mucosal ulceration, inflammation, and granulomatous reactions may occur, but the changes are usually transitory and produce no serious clinical problems.[29] The most serious complication from negative-contrast cystography is gas embolization into the circulatory system, which may result in death (Fig. 41-13).[30-32] Fortunately such complications rarely occur. Death from gas embolism may be prevented by using nitrous oxide or carbon dioxide instead of room air.

Both negative- and positive-contrast media are used for cystography. Negative-contrast media include carbon dioxide and nitrous oxide. Positive-contrast media are water-soluble

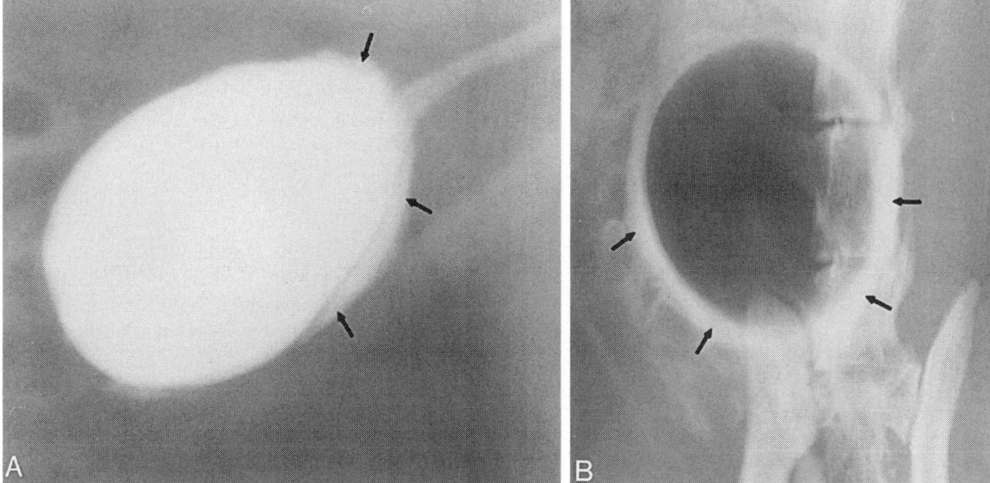

Fig. 41-12 Positive- (A) and double-contrast (B) cystograms in which subserosal accumulation of contrast medium may be seen *(arrows)*. This usually produces no severe or long-lasting complications. It is produced by a high intraluminal bladder pressure and is predisposed by bladder disease, particularly inflammation.

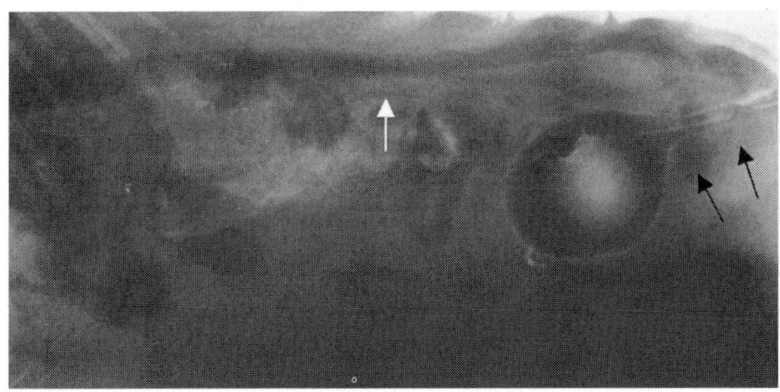

Fig. 41-13 Lateral abdominal radiograph of a cat after introduction of air into the bladder for a double-contrast cystogram. Gas is in the tissues immediately adjacent to the bladder *(black arrows)*, in a ureter *(white arrow)*, in the renal collecting system, in renal veins, and in the caudal vena cava. This was a fatal air embolic event. Air should not be used for negative- or double-contrast cystography, especially in patients with hematuria, because blood in the urine is evidence of communication between the bladder lumen and vascular system.

organic iodides that should be used in an approximate 20% iodine solution. Barium should never be used for cystography.[25,33] The volume of positive-contrast medium used for cystography varies with body weight, the species, and the pathologic process present in the bladder. An approximation of 10 mL, or a range of 3.5 to 13.1 mL of contrast medium per kilogram body weight, may be used.[33] The injection should be terminated before the estimated volume has been administered if the bladder feels adequately distended by external palpation, if reflux occurs around the catheter, or if back pressure is felt on the syringe plunger. Moderate bladder distention is recommended because complete distention may obliterate subtle mucosal and bladder wall changes.[34] Four radiographic views of the caudal abdomen (lateral; ventrodorsal; ventral left, dorsal right; ventral right, dorsal left) should be made to examine the contrast medium–filled bladder adequately.

Cystographic Procedures

Retrograde positive- and double-contrast procedures often are more useful to evaluate the bladder than is negative-contrast cystography. Positive-contrast cystography is performed by injecting a 20% solution of an organic iodide compound into an evacuated bladder by a urethral catheter. The procedure is the method of choice for identifying bladder location, demonstrating bladder tears or ruptures, and identifying abnormal communication with adjacent structures.

A double-contrast cystogram may be performed by injecting a small volume of undiluted positive-contrast medium into an empty bladder. The recommended dose of positive-contrast medium is 0.5 to 1 mL for a cat, 1 to 3 mL for a dog weighing less than 25 lb, and 3 to 6 mL for animals weighing more than 25 lb. Contrast medium injection is followed by bladder distention with negative-contrast medium (Fig. 41-14). Double-contrast cystography is superior for assessing bladder wall lesions and intraluminal filling defects. The selection of positive- or double-contrast cystography is based on clinical history, clinical signs, radiographic signs, and the character of aspirate obtained with bladder catheterization (Fig. 41-15).

Radiographic Signs with Contrast Cystography

Radiographic signs observed with urinary bladder disease include an irregular mucosal border, intramural thickening, filling defects, and extravasation patterns (Table 41-3).[35] These radiographic changes must be differentiated from artifacts such as air bubbles and inadequate bladder distention. By noting the number, severity, and distribution of radiographic signs, a specific diagnosis usually can be postulated or a differential diagnosis list can be developed. If nonspecific radiographic signs are present or further confirmation is necessary, further testing is necessary.

Mucosal Changes

The urinary bladder has a transitional epithelium, which appears smooth on a normal cystogram. The transitional bladder epithelium is capable of metaplastic, neoplastic, and nonneoplastic proliferation.[36] Mucosal proliferation appears as an irregular outline along the inside bladder surface and may be accentuated with inadequate bladder distention. The irregular mucosa is usually focally distributed but may be diffuse;

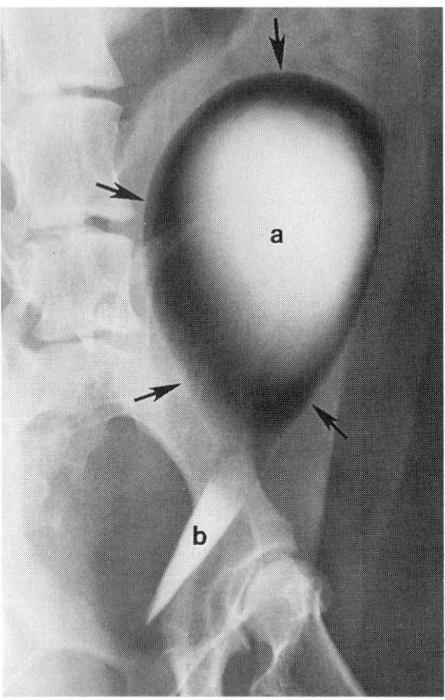

Fig. 41-14 Ventral left, dorsal right radiograph of a normal double-contrast cystogram. The urinary bladder wall *(arrows)* is clearly seen. The contrast "puddle" in the dependent portion of the bladder (**A**) and the contrast medium-filled urethra (**B**) are easily identified.

it may vary in severity from a slightly irregular brush-type surface to a severe "cobblestone" appearance (Fig. 41-16). Mild mucosal irregularity may be obliterated on a cystogram if the bladder is completely distended.[34] Ulcers may be present with mucosal proliferation. Ulcers can be identified with a double-contrast cystogram because contrast medium adheres to the ulcerated surface.

Intramural Changes (Bladder Wall Thickening)

The normal bladder wall is approximately 1 mm thick regardless of the degree of distention.[29] Intramural changes are demonstrated best with double-contrast cystography and include increased bladder wall thickness that is usually focal but may be diffuse (Fig. 41-17). Mild bladder wall thickening may be missed if the bladder is completely distended.[34] Bladder wall thickening may be caused by cellular infiltration or fibrous tissue proliferation. Cellular infiltration may result from inflammation, hemorrhage from trauma, or neoplasia. Intramural bladder thickening causes decreased bladder distensibility, which may be symmetric with diffuse intramural bladder disease or asymmetric with focal intramural bladder disease.

Filling Defects

A bladder filling defect is anything occupying space within the bladder lumen that alters normal filling; such a defect occupies space normally filled with contrast medium on a cystogram. All filling defects appear radiolucent when surrounded with positive-contrast medium even though they are not radiolucent in survey radiographs. The size, shape, number, border contour, position within the bladder, and attachment to the bladder wall should be examined with all bladder filling

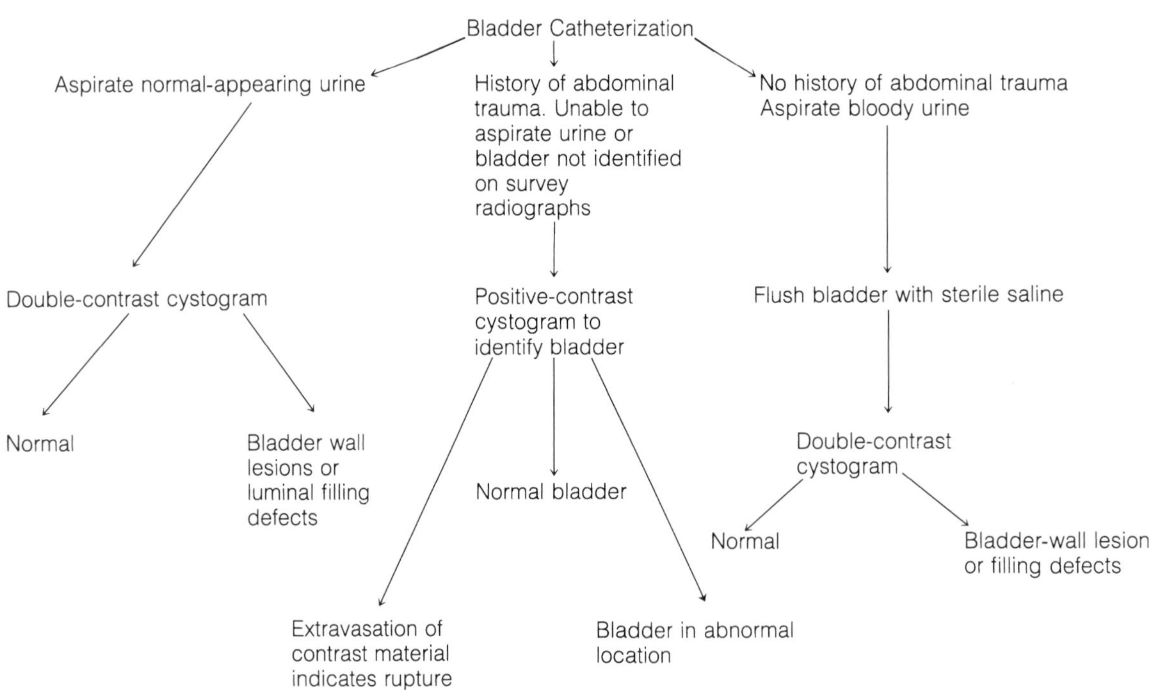

Fig. 41-15 Selection of cystographic procedure. (Modified from Park RD: Radiology of the urinary bladder and urethra. In O'Brien TR, editor: *Radiographic diagnosis of abdominal disorders in the dog and cat,* Davis, CA, 1981, Covell Park Veterinary.)

TABLE • 41-3

Radiographic Signs of Pathologic Processes of the Bladder

	MUCOSAL CHANGES		INTRAMURAL THICKENING		FILLING DEFECT		CONTRAST EXTRAVASATION	
DISEASE	**FOCAL**	**DIFFUSE**	**FOCAL**	**DIFFUSE**	**ATTACHED**	**FREE**	**SMOOTH**	**IRREGULAR**
Chronic cystitis	Cranioventral	Occasional	Cranioventral	Occasional (cytoxan-induced cystitis)	Blood clots	Blood clots, calculi	—	—
Polypoid cystitis	Cranioventral	—	Cranioventral	—	Cranioventral	Blood clots	—	—
Acute cystitis	—	—	—	—	—	Occasional blood clots	—	—
Cystic calculi	Cranioventral from cystitis	—	Cranioventral from cystitis	—	—	Calculi and occasional blood clots	—	—
Neoplasia	Any location within bladder	Occasional	Any location within bladder	Occasional	Sessile, occasionally pedunculated	Blood clots	—	—
Bladder contusion	Any location	Large areas of bladder often involved	Any location	Large areas of bladder often involved	Bladder wall hematoma	Blood clots	—	—
Bladder rupture or perforation	—	—	—	—	—	Blood clots	—	Most extravasate is into peritoneal cavity
Traumatic diverticula	—	—	—	—	—	Blood clots	Any location	—
Urachal diverticula	Cranioventral associated with cystitis	—	Cranioventral associated with cystitis	—	—	—	Cranioventral	—

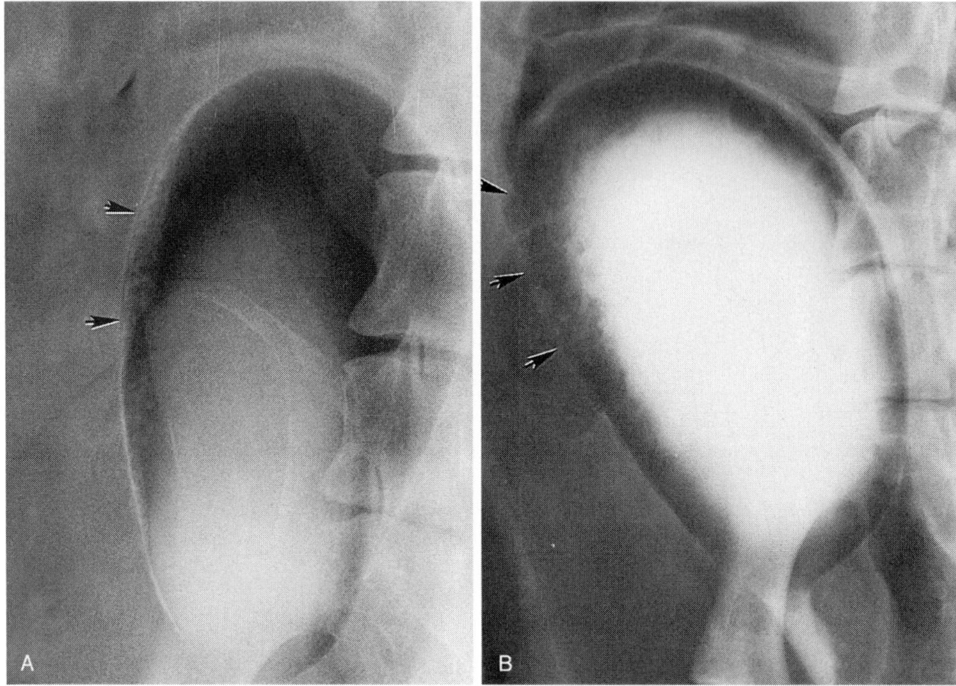

Fig. 41-16 A, Ventral right, dorsal left radiograph of the bladder during double-contrast cystography. Mild mucosal irregularity is present along the right ventral bladder *(arrows)* as a result of chronic bacterial cystitis. B, Ventral right, dorsal left radiograph of the bladder of another dog during double-contrast cystography. Severe mucosal irregularity and mild bladder wall thickening are present along the ventral right bladder *(arrows)*.

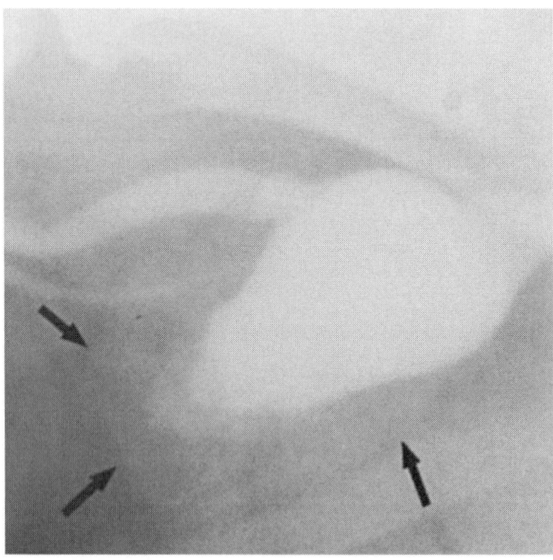

Fig. 41-17 Lateral radiograph of the urinary bladder filled with positive-contrast medium during intravenous urography. Diffuse bladder wall thickening is present as the result of cytoxan-induced cystitis. The serosal surface *(arrows)* is outlined by fat. Bladder distensibility is decreased by the severe intramural changes. One ureter is distended as a result of obstruction at the ureterovesical junction.

defects. Observing these filling defect characteristics helps determine the nature of the filling defect, which ultimately may prove helpful in reaching a diagnosis (Table 41-4).

Filling defects may be categorized as free or attached. Free luminal filling defects may be caused by air bubbles, calculi, sebaceous or mucous plugs,[35] or blood clots (Fig. 41-18). They are best demonstrated with double-contrast cystography and are seen within the dependent contrast puddle, which is in the center of the bladder on a recumbent lateral view. The concentration of the contrast medium and depth of the contrast puddle have an effect on visualization of cystic calculi of varying size and composition.[37,38] Attached filling defects may be caused by neoplasia (Fig. 41-19), inflammatory polyps, blood clots, iatrogenic hematomas, adherent calculi, and ureteroceles (Fig. 41-20).[39] With double-contrast cystography mural masses may be seen only on views in which the positive-contrast medium gravitates around the mass.[40] Mucosal irregularity and ulcers are frequently present on the surface of large attached filling defects. Bladder wall infiltration may be diagnosed as a thickened bladder wall adjacent to the filling defect.[41] Although a specific diagnosis cannot always be made from the cystogram when attached filling defects are present, the defects may be differentiated by surgical removal or ultrasound-guided biopsy.

Contrast Extravasation Patterns from the Urinary Bladder

Retrograde positive-contrast cystography is the best technique to assess urine malpositioning from the bladder. Urine malpositioning may occur within the urinary tract, into adjacent visceral soft tissue structures, or into the peritoneal cavity.

Urine malpositioning from the normal bladder confined within the urinary tract may be seen with vesicoureteral reflux, urachal anomalies (Fig. 41-21), and traumatic bladder diverticula (Fig. 41-22). Congenital urachal anomalies include diverticula,[42,43] cysts, and persistent patent urachus.[44-47] A urachal diverticulum can function as a cavity that may result in retention of urine (see Fig. 41-21).

The contrast medium borders produced by urine malpositioning within the urinary tract are usually smooth and may be identified as extensions from the urinary bladder.

TABLE • 41-4

Bladder Filling Defects

LESION	SHAPE	ATTACHMENT	BORDER/CONTOUR	BLADDER WALL INFILTRATION (THICKENING)
Calculi	Round to slightly irregular	Free in lumen; center of contrast puddle	Indistinct	Variable; usually cranioventral if associated with cystitis
Sebaceous or mucous plug	Round or irregular	Free in lumen; center of contrast puddle	Smooth or irregular, distinct or indistinct	Variable; associated with cystitis
Polyp	Pedunculated or convex	Stalk or sessile	Smooth or irregular, often with ulceration	Variable; bladder wall may be thick at attachment site
Epithelial neoplasia	Irregular or convex	Sessile	Irregular, often with ulceration	Bladder wall often thick or infiltrated at base of attachment
Mesenchymal neoplasia	Convex	Sessile	Usually smooth	Originates within the bladder wall
Blood clots	Irregular	Variable; may be free luminal	Irregular and indistinct	Thickened bladder wall from primary disease process
Bladder wall hematoma	Convex	Sessile	Smooth to slightly irregular	Originates within bladder wall
Ureterocele	Convex to round	Sessile	Smooth	Originates within trigone region of the bladder wall

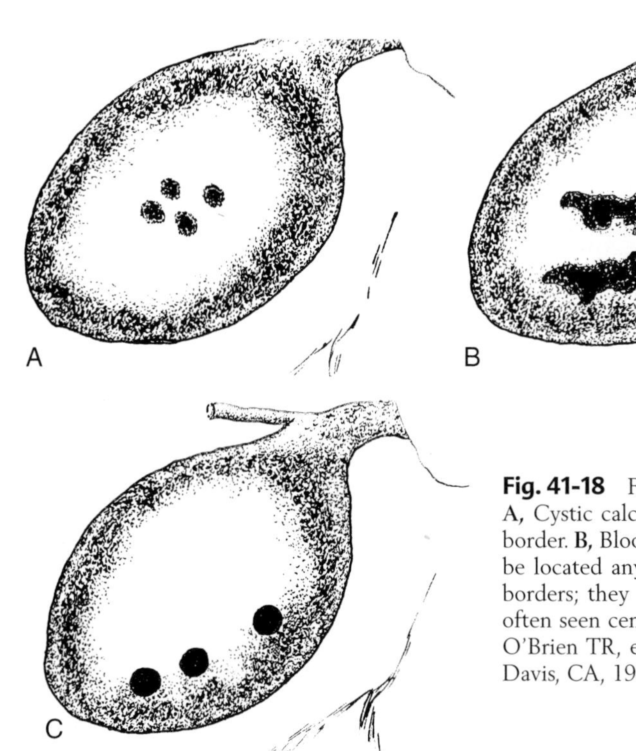
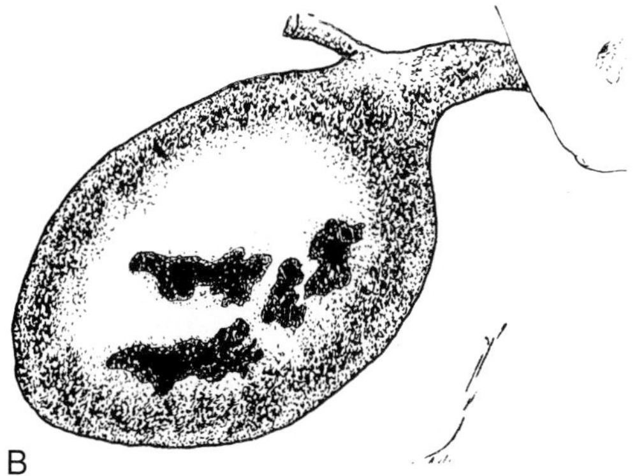

Fig. 41-18 Free luminal filling defects demonstrated by double-contrast cystography. **A,** Cystic calculi, in the center of the contrast "puddle," are round with an indistinct border. **B,** Blood clots are irregularly shaped with irregular, indistinct borders; they may be located anywhere in the bladder. **C,** Air bubbles are round with smooth, distinct borders; they are shown here at the periphery of the contrast puddle but are more often seen centrally. (From Park RD: Radiology of the urinary bladder and urethra. In O'Brien TR, editor: *Radiographic diagnosis of abdominal disorders in the dog and cat,* Davis, CA, 1981, Covell Park Veterinary.)

Contrast extravasation from the urinary bladder to adjacent visceral structures may be seen with either congenital or acquired fistulas. The organs most commonly involved are the rectum and the vagina. Such fistulas can usually be diagnosed with fluoroscopy or in an indirect fashion on contrast cystograms; that is, the structure that communicates with the bladder fills simultaneously or shortly after the bladder is filled with contrast medium.[48]

Contrast extravasation into the peritoneal cavity and surrounding soft tissues has an irregular outline and usually occurs simultaneously with injection of contrast medium into the bladder (Fig. 41-23). With small bladder neck tears, extravasation of contrast medium may be slow, with only a small volume extravasated.[6,43] In these instances, a second radiograph may be required 5 to 10 minutes after contrast medium injection to identify

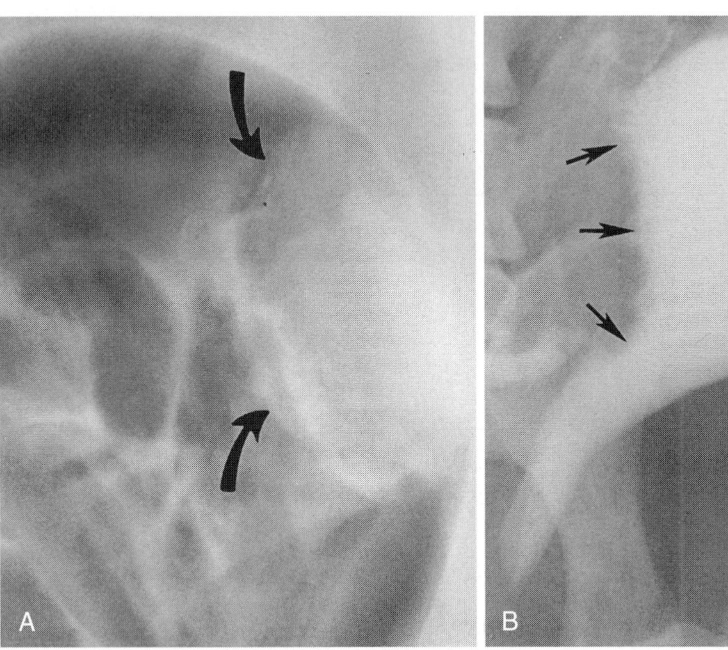

Fig. 41-19 A, Double-contrast cystogram. A large neoplastic mass *(arrows)* protrudes into the bladder lumen. Bladder wall infiltration is minimal. Contrast medium coats the ulcerated surface of the neoplasm. **B,** Positive-contrast cystogram. A large neoplastic lesion (transitional cell carcinoma) is present on the right side of the bladder *(arrows)*. The neoplasm causes a large filling defect with an irregular surface.

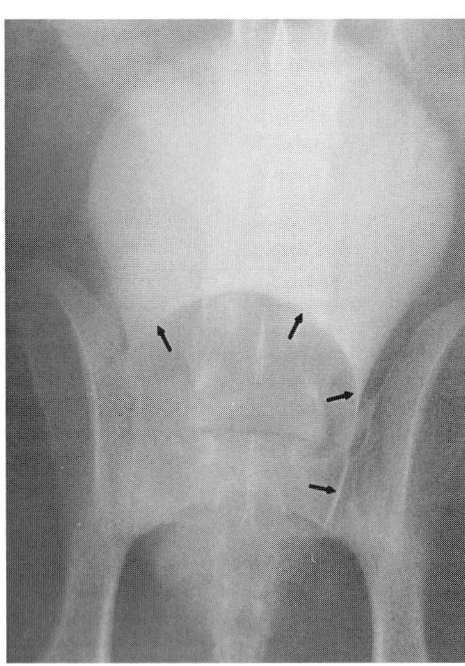

Fig. 41-20 Ventrodorsal radiograph of the bladder filled with contrast medium during intravenous urography. The smooth luminal filling defect *(arrows)* that projects into the bladder neck is a ureterocele.

delayed extravasation from the bladder into the peritoneal cavity.

Pitfalls with Cystographic Interpretation

Interpretation pitfalls are changes noted on the radiograph that mimic actual pathologic changes. These changes are artifacts that are created during the cystographic procedure. Pitfalls commonly seen with contrast cystography are air bubble artifacts and pseudofilling defects.

Three types of air bubble artifacts have been recognized: small air bubbles simulating calculi or other small luminal filling defects, a large air bubble simulating bladder wall thickening, and multiple air bubbles creating a honeycomb appearance (Fig. 41-24). Air bubbles are radiolucent and have smooth, distinct borders.

Pseudofilling defects may be mistaken for bladder neoplasia or other attached filling defects. These defects are created by inadequate bladder distention combined with external pressure from adjacent abdominal structures. Pseudofilling defects have a smooth surface and taper on both borders; they can be obliterated with further bladder distention (Fig. 41-25).

SONOGRAPHY

The fluid-filled urinary bladder is readily and easily evaluated by sonography. The superficial location enables high-resolution imaging, and the urine provides high sonographic contrast, which results in clear visualization of the bladder wall and intraluminal abnormalities. Urolithiasis and neoplasia from transitional cell carcinoma are readily and accurately identified by using sonography.[49,50]

High-resolution transducers (7 to 10 MHz) are best suited for examination of the bladder. A 5-MHz transducer may be necessary to penetrate to the far wall of a distended bladder in large-breed dogs. Linear and curved wide-aperture format transducers are particularly useful. A standoff pad should be used with a sector transducer to improve the image quality of the ventral bladder wall. Image contrast settings should be set to high-contrast display; acoustic power and near gain should be decreased to suppress reverberation echoes generated between the transducer, the skin, and abdominal wall structures.

The sonographic examination is best performed when the bladder is moderately full. A small bladder after recent urination is more difficult to locate; the wall is thicker and image contrast is reduced. Reexamination of the bladder should be done when the bladder is moderately distended after some hours of inside confinement, after administration of a diuretic, or after catheterization and saline injection. The wall of a flaccid bladder can be deviated inward by a distended colon, and the acoustic shadow artifacts generated by colonic

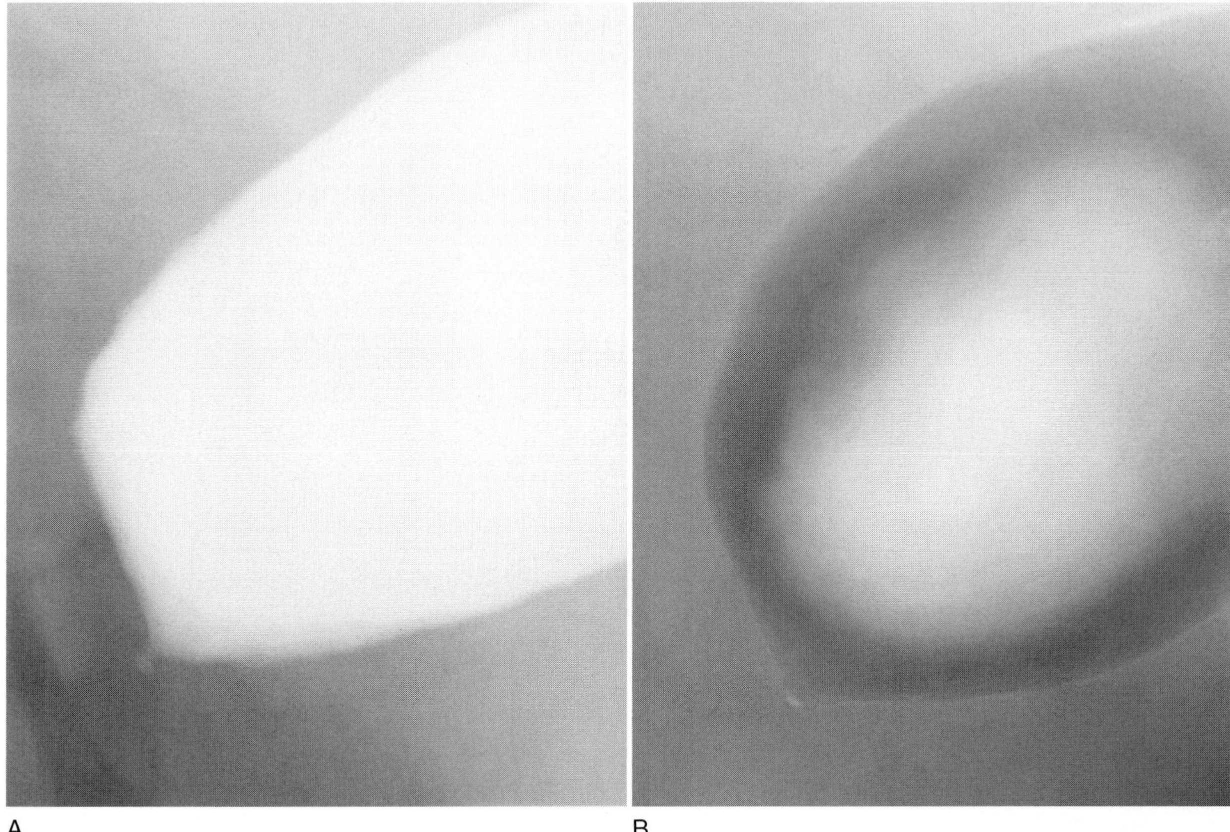

Fig. 41-21 Appearance of the cranioventral aspect of the bladder during positive-contrast (A) and double-contrast (B) cystography in a dog. A small urachal diverticulum fills with contrast medium in A. In B there is residual contrast medium in the diverticulum, suggesting urine retention that may predispose to urinary tract infections.

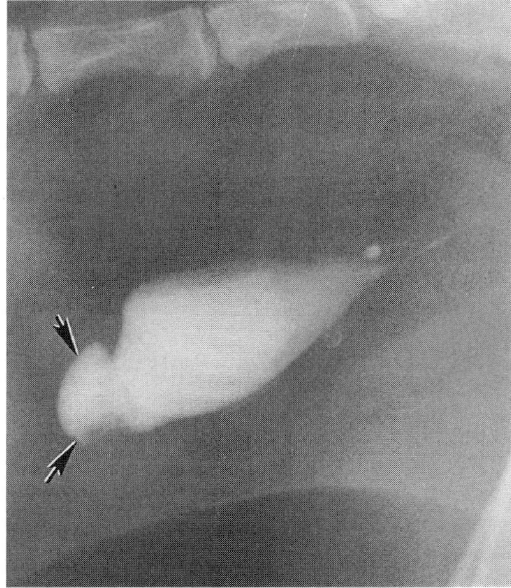

Fig. 41-22 A traumatic bladder diverticulum is identified *(arrows)*. Immediately after trauma, traumatic diverticula must be differentiated from a bladder contusion. Contusions usually heal within 48 hours and the bladder distends symmetrically.

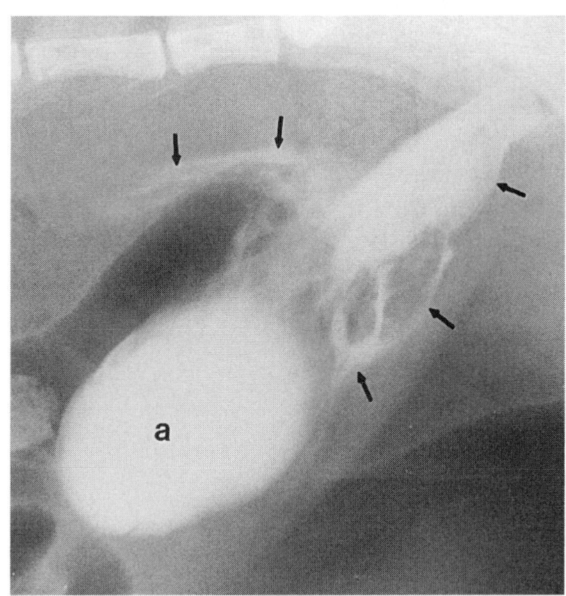

Fig. 41-23 Positive-contrast cystogram in a cat. Contrast medium fills the urinary bladder *(a)* but has also leaked into the peritoneal cavity *(arrows)*. The contrast medium leakage resulted from a bladder neck tear.

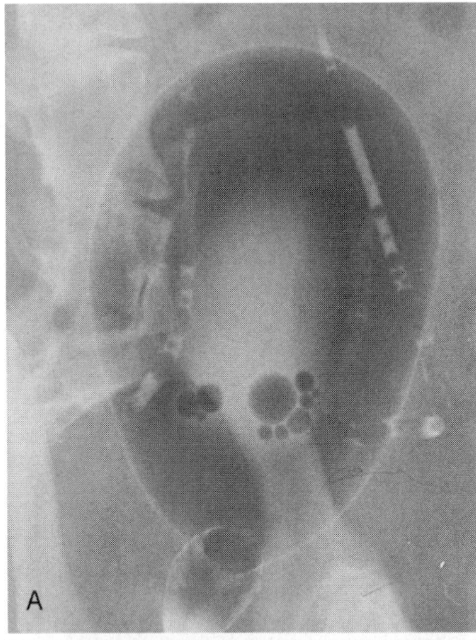

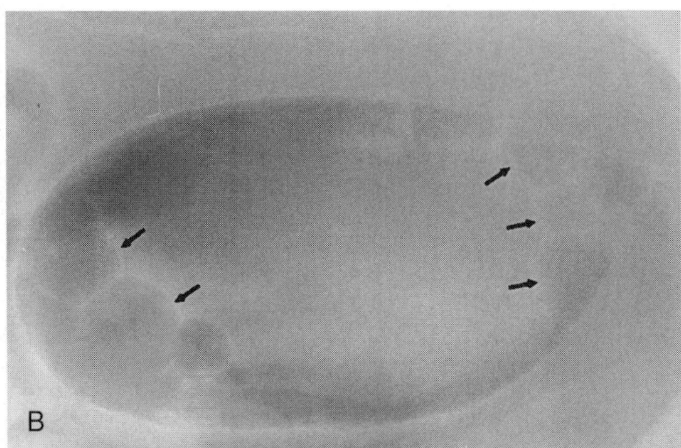

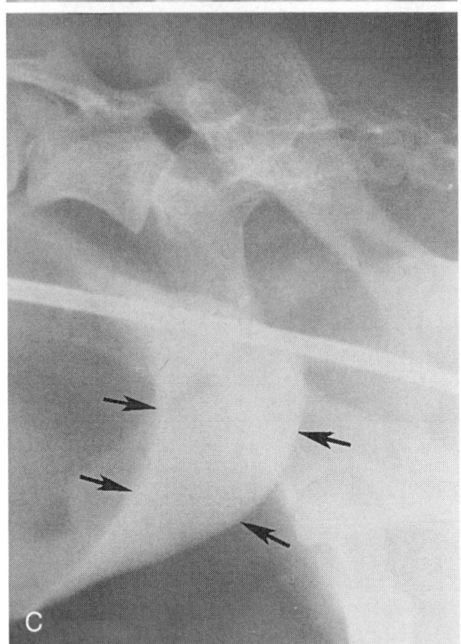

Fig. 41-24 Air bubble artifacts created by cystographic procedures. **A,** Small air bubbles that cause free luminal-type filling defects in the urinary bladder during double-contrast cystography. Bubbles are also present in both ureters. **B,** A honeycomb appearance created by several adjacent air bubbles *(arrows)*. A large air bubble in a mostly fluid-filled bladder may produce the appearance of a thick bladder wall. **C,** Positive-contrast medium and gas may produce a similar pattern *(arrows)*. The smooth borders of the pseudothick bladder wall are produced by the large air bubble border and the actual bladder wall or outer border of the contrast medium. The region between the *arrows* should be recognized as contrast medium because of its opacity.

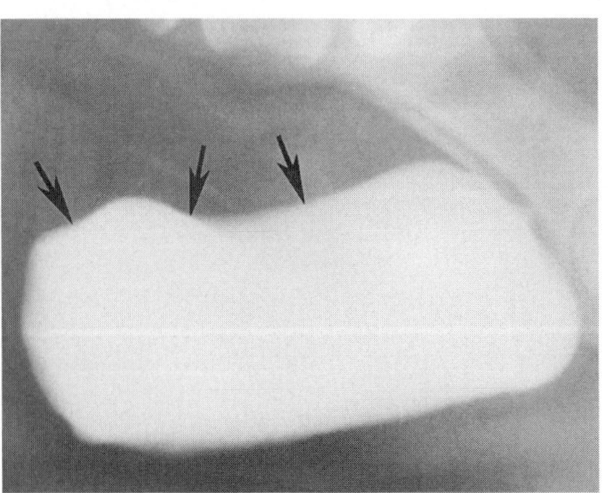

Fig. 41-25 Lateral radiograph of a contrast medium–filled bladder during intravenous urography. Pseudofilling defects *(arrows)* are created by pressure from adjacent abdominal structures on a partially distended bladder.

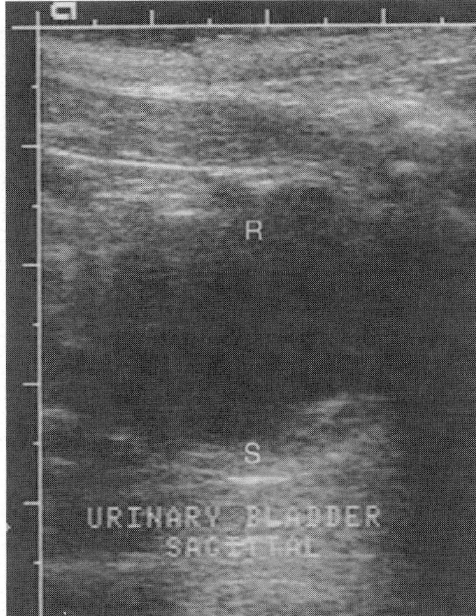

Fig. 41-26 Poor-quality sagittal sonogram of the urinary bladder. Excessive reverberation echoes *(R)* have been recorded, which prevents evaluation of the ventral bladder wall and nature of the urine. Also, spurious echoes *(S)* are present in the dorsal lumen of the bladder from side (grating) lobe artifact creating pseudoechogenic debris in the urine.[54]

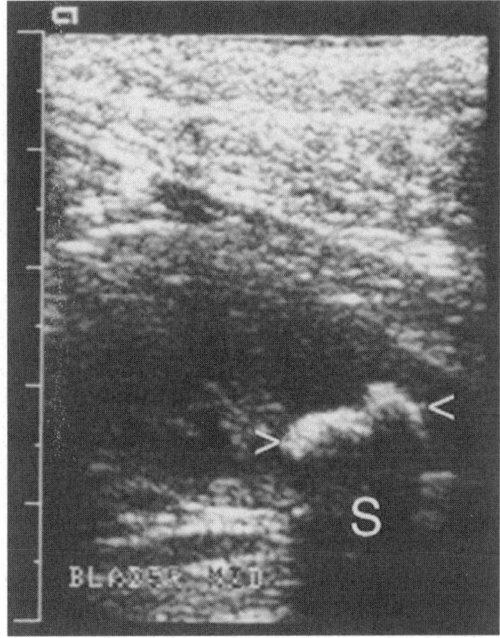

Fig. 41-27 Sagittal sonogram of the urinary bladder demonstrates calculi *(arrows)* creating characteristic acoustic shadows *(S)*.

contents often appear like the shadows generated by calculi.[51] In middle-sized to large-breed dogs, a fully distended bladder is also less desirable, but a lower frequency transducer that has lower resolution will be needed. Also, the thinner wall is more difficult to visualize and measure. Bladder wall thickness of normal dogs has been shown to vary depending on the degree of bladder distention.[52] The wall was reported to be 2.3 mm thick when the bladder was minimally distended and 1.4 mm with moderate distention (4 mL/kg).[52]

Bladder sonography can be performed with the dog in either dorsal or lateral recumbency. Thorough evaluation of the entire bladder should be done in a transverse plane and also orthogonally in either a sagittal or a dorsal plane. Accurate assessment of bladder wall thickness requires a perpendicular orientation of the ultrasound beam. Assessment of the cranial wall is challenging because of the suboptimal beam alignment and the adjacent gas-filled bowel.[53] Side and grating lobe artifacts generated by the adjacent colon can give rise to an erroneous display of echogenic material in the bladder lumen, and the curved bladder wall can create additional echoes adjacent to the dorsal bladder wall (Fig. 41-26).[54] Transducer rotation of 90 degrees over such suspicious areas is often helpful to enable recognition of the proximity of the colon and determination of the nature of the artifact. Free intraluminal abnormalities (e.g., calculi, sediment, and blood clots) gravitate to the most dependent side of the bladder. In lateral recumbency, careful examination of the most dependent area of the bladder is required so that small calculi are not overlooked. Ballottement is useful for initiating sediment swirling across the real-time display. Additional imaging after the animal has been positioned in the opposite lateral recumbent or standing position allows detection of gravitation of free intraluminal objects to a dependent position within the bladder.

The normal filled bladder is ovoid in shape, with a slight elongation caudally at the trigone. The ureters and urethra are not visualized unless they become distended with urine. With high-resolution transducers, the normal bladder wall can be seen to be divided into three distinct layers. The mucosa is a thin hyperechoic surface outlined against the urine, the middle muscle layer is hypoechoic, and the outer serosal layer is hyperechoic.[55] The cranioventral wall is slightly thinner than other regions. In normal adult cats, the mean bladder wall thickness did not exceed 1.7 mm ± 0.56 mm.[55] In normal adult dogs with mild bladder distention (2 mg/kg), the mean wall thickness was 1.6 mm, but this thickness does increase with body weight.[52] Normal urine is anechoic. The turbulence created by discharge of urine through the ureteral openings may generate transient echo jets in the bladder lumen adjacent to the trigone.[56]

Intraluminal Changes

Urinary calculi, cellular and crystalline debris, gas, and blood clots are readily detected by sonography. Consideration of the gravitational alignment is especially helpful in differentiating calculi and blood clots that fall downward from gas bubbles that rise upward. The location of cellular and crystalline debris and fresh hemorrhage is more variable. Sedimentation tends to occur, and vigorous ballottement will generate swirling echo patterns on real-time display.

Calculi

The urine/calculus interface is intensely hyperechoic and usually appears convex. Multiple calculi often aggregate together and give rise to an irregular, somewhat continuous surface, which makes distinguishing and measuring individual calculi difficult. Distinct acoustic shadows are observed deep to calculi that exceed the diameter of the sound beam (Fig. 41-27).[57] Smaller calculi may not generate the characteristic shadows until the beam focus is optimized at the depth of the calculi. Echogenicity and acoustic shadow generation are independent of chemical composition, so radiopaque and nonradiopaque calculi can be detected by sonography.[56] Ballottement usually does not cause calculi to move, but placing the animal in a standing position clearly allows detec-

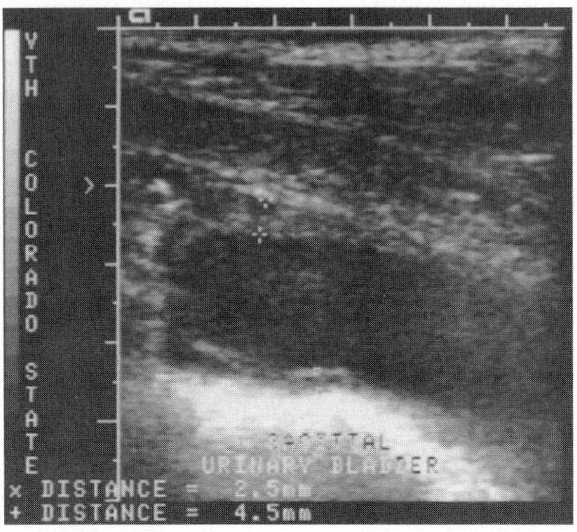

Fig. 41-28 Sagittal sonogram of the urinary bladder reveals an abnormal thickening of the cranioventral wall (4.5 mm) caused by cystitis. The urine is abnormally echogenic from hematuria.

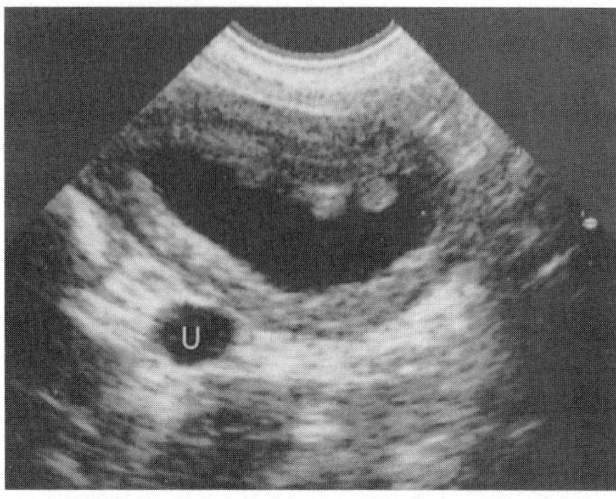

Fig. 41-29 Transverse sonogram of the urinary bladder reveals an abnormally thickened bladder wall. Sessile nodular masses protrude from the ventral bladder wall into the bladder lumen. Histology of the bladder wall revealed a transitional cell carcinoma that had obstructed the right ureter, causing hydroureter *(U)* and hydronephrosis.

tion of relocation of the calculi into the cranioventral aspect of the bladder. This action helps differentiate calculi from an adjacent colonic acoustic shadow and dystrophic mineralization in the bladder wall.

Gas bubbles accidentally introduced by bladder catheterization or cystocentesis appear echogenic and can generate acoustic shadows. Differentiation from calculi is easy because the bubble floats on top of the urine.

Crystalline and cellular sediments generate a variably echogenic pattern in more dependent urine. In cats, the crystalline deposits may become thick enough to form a hyperechoic layer confluent with the bladder wall that creates acoustic shadowing. Vigorous ballottement or placing the animal in a standing position allows visualization of the characteristic swirling pattern that helps differentiate thick sediment from calculi.

Blood clots tend to be associated with the clinical observation of severe hematuria. Relative to normal urine, a blood clot commonly appears as a hyperechoic, nonshadowing, mobile mass.[58,59] Sometimes the clot may be attached to the wall, covering or adjacent to a traumatic injury or a neoplastic mass. Alternately, severe acute hemorrhage can fill the bladder and give rise to a lacy hypoechoic pattern that changes little with ballottement or animal repositioning. A similar appearance can be observed with severe proteinuria and fat droplets.[60]

Mural Changes

Sonography is especially useful for detecting changes from chronic cystitis and neoplasia. Contrast radiographic techniques are superior to sonography in diagnosing congenital abnormalities of the urachus and ureters as well as ruptured bladders.

Cystitis

Chronic cystitis results in diffuse thickening of the bladder wall and is readily detected by sonography. The bladder wall becomes abnormally hypoechoic, and the normal layering becomes less parallel. Measurements reveal abnormal wall thickness (Fig. 41-28), and hypoechoic cellular debris frequently accumulates in the bladder lumen.[61] A normal sonographic appearance of the bladder does not rule out the presence of mild or acute cystitis or idiopathic lower urinary tract disease in cats. Small polypoid mucosal masses are also occasionally observed with chronic cystitis. Such masses are difficult to differentiate from bladder wall neoplasia. Follow-up sonographic evaluations should be made after treatment of the cystitis to reevaluate such masses. Persistence and especially enlargement of irregularly thickened or nodular masses indicate the need for biopsy because neoplasia may be present. Muscular hypertrophy resulting from chronic partial lower urinary tract obstruction can also cause bladder wall thickening and may simulate the sonographic appearance of cystitis. Emphysematous cystitis creates a confusing sonographic appearance because the gas artifacts may obscure all bladder anatomy. Radiography is more informed in these patients because the gas is more easily recognized within the bladder lining and wall.

Neoplasia

Sonography of transitional cell carcinoma of the bladder most frequently reveals irregularly shaped, broad-based, hypoechoic masses protruding into the bladder lumen.[50] Single or multiple masses may be present (Fig. 41-29). The echo pattern can vary if fibrosis, mineralization, and necrosis have developed. Adjacent blood clots are common and can falsely contribute to the size and echogenic texture of the mass. An abrupt transition is often observed between the neoplastic mass and the adjacent bladder wall.[50] Some highly aggressive carcinomas and mesenchymal tumors also tend to spread through the bladder wall. If a small intraluminal mass occurs, the bladder wall takes on the appearance of severe cystitis. Unfortunately, the sonographic appearance of polypoid cystitis, adherent blood clots, and mural hematomas is similar to that of bladder neoplasia. The observation of ureter dilation adjacent to the bladder wall mass (see Fig. 41-29) and focal medial iliac lymphadenopathy tends to support the diagnosis of neoplasia. An aspirate, biopsy, or both are necessary to confirm the presence of bladder neoplasia. The information gained from aspiration of a bladder mass percutaneously, however, must be weighed against the possibility of seeding the needle tract with tumor cells.[62]

REFERENCES

1. Fletcher TF: Anatomy of pelvic viscera, *Vet Clin North Am* 4:471, 1974.
2. International Committee on Veterinary Anatomical Nomenclature: *Nomina anatomica veterinaria,* Vienna, 1973, World Association of Veterinary Anatomists.
3. Evans HE: *Miller's anatomy of the dog,* ed 3, Philadelphia, 1993, W.B. Saunders.
4. Mahaffey MB, Barsanti JA, Barber DL et al: Pelvic bladders in dogs without urinary incontinence, *J Am Vet Med Assoc* 184:1477, 1984.
5. Johnston GR, Osborne CA, Jessen CR et al: Effects of urinary bladder distension on location of the urinary bladder and urethra of healthy dogs and cats, *Am J Vet Res* 47:404, 1986.
6. Nickel R, Schummer A, Seiferle E et al: *The viscera of the domestic mammals,* Berlin, 1973, Paul Parey.
7. Park RD: Radiology of the urinary bladder and urethra. In O'Brien TR, editor: *Radiographic diagnosis of abdominal disorders in the dog and cat,* Davis, CA, 1981, Covell Park Veterinary, p 543.
8. White RAS, Herrtage ME: Bladder retroflexion in the dog, *J Small Anim Pract* 27:735, 1986.
9. Adams WM, DiBartola SP: Radiographic and clinical features of pelvic bladder in the dog, *J Am Vet Med Assoc* 182:1212, 1983.
10. Holt PE: Urinary incontinence in the bitch due to sphincter mechanism incompetence: surgical treatment, *J Small Anim Pract* 26:237, 1985.
11. Patnaik AK, Greene RW: Intravenous leiomyoma of the bladder in a cat, *J Am Vet Med Assoc* 175:381, 1979.
12. Hansen JS: Persistent urachal ligament in the cat, *Vet Med Small Anim Clin* 67:1090, 1972.
13. Root CR, Scott RC: Emphysematous cystitis and other radiographic manifestations of diabetes mellitus in dogs and cats, *J Am Vet Med Assoc* 158:721, 1971.
14. Ellenbogen PH, Talner LB: Uroradiology of diabetes mellitus, *Urology* 8:413, 1967.
15. Middleton DJ, Lomas GR: Emphysematous cystitis due to *Clostridium perfringens* in a non-diabetic dog, *J Small Anim Pract* 20:433, 1979.
16. Sherding RG, Chew DJ: Nondiabetic emphysematous cystitis in two dogs, *J Am Vet Med Assoc* 174:1105, 1979.
17. Steyn PF, Lowry J: Positional radiography as an aid to diagnose sand-like uroliths in the urinary bladder of feline urologic syndrome cats, *Feline Pract* 19:21, 1991.
18. Moreau PM, Lees GE, Gross DR: Simultaneous cystometry and uroflowmetry (micturition study) for evaluation of the caudal part of the urinary tract in dogs: studies of the technique, *Am J Vet Res* 44:1769, 1983.
19. Moreau PM, Lees GE, Gross DR: Simultaneous cystometry and uroflowmetry (micturition study) for evaluation of the caudal part of the urinary tract function in dogs: reference values for healthy animals sedated with xylazine, *Am J Vet Res* 44:1774, 1983.
20. Moreau PM, Lees GE, Hobson HP: Simultaneous cystometry and uroflowmetry for evaluation of micturition in two dogs, *J Am Vet Med Assoc* 183:1083, 1983.
21. Rosin AE, Barsanti JA: Diagnosis of urinary incontinence in dogs: role of the urethral pressure profile, *J Am Vet Med Assoc* 178:814, 1981.
22. Oliver JE Jr, Young WO: Air cystometry in dogs under xylazine-induced restraint, *Am J Vet Res* 34:1433, 1973.
23. Mooney JK Jr, Cox EC, Heniman F: Vesical contamination from insertions of everting cot or catheter in inoculated canine urethra, *Invest Urol* 11:248, 1973.
24. Buchanan JW: Kinked catheter: a complication of pneumocystography, *J Am Vet Radiol Soc* 8:54, 1967.
25. Feeney DA, Johnston GR, Tomlinson MJ et al: Effects of sterilized micropulverized barium sulfate suspension and meglumine iothalamate solution on the genitourinary tract of healthy male dogs after retrograde urethrocystography, *Am J Vet Res* 45:730, 1984.
26. Johnston GR, Stevens JB, Jessen CR et al: Complications of retrograde contrast urethrography in dogs and cats, *Am J Vet Res* 44:1248, 1983.
27. Barsanti JA, Crowell W, Losonsky J et al: Complications of bladder distention during retrograde urethrography, *Am J Vet Res* 42:819, 1981.
28. Farrow CS: Exercises in diagnostic radiology, *Can Vet J* 22:260, 1981.
29. Mahaffey MB, Barber DL, Barsanti JA et al: Simultaneous double-contrast cystography and cystometry in dogs, *Vet Radiol* 25:254, 1984.
30. Ackerman N, Wingfield WE, Corley EA: Fatal air embolism associated with pneumourethrography and pneumocystography in a dog, *J Am Vet Med Assoc* 160:1616, 1972.
31. Zontine WJ, Andrews LK: Fatal air embolization as a complication of pneumocystography in two cats, *J Am Vet Radiol Soc* 19:8, 1978.
32. Thayer GW, Carrig CB, Evans AT: Fatal venous air embolism associated with pneumocystography in a cat, *J Am Vet Med Assoc* 176:643, 1980.
33. Brodeur AE, Goyer RA, Melick W: A potential hazard of barium cystography, *Radiology* 85:1080, 1965.
34. Mahaffey MB, Barsanti JA, Browell WA et al: Cystography: effect of technique on diagnosis of cystitis in dogs, *Vet Radiol* 30:261, 1989.
35. Johnston GR, Feeney DA: *Radiographic evaluation of the urinary tract in dogs and cats: contemporary issues in small animal practice. Vol 4: nephrology and urology,* New York, 1986, Churchill Livingstone, p 203.
36. Mostofi FK: Potentialities of bladder epithelium, *J Urol* 71:705, 1954.
37. Weichselbaum RC, Feeney DA, Jessen CR et al: In vitro evaluation of contrast medium concentration and depth effects on the radiographic appearance of specific canine urolith mineral types, *Vet Radiol Ultrasound* 39:396, 1998.
38. Weichselbaum RC, Feeney DA, Jessen CR et al: Urocystolith detection: comparison of survey, contrast radiographic and ultrasonographic techniques in an in vitro bladder phantom, *Vet Radiol Ultrasound* 40:386, 1999.
39. Stowater JL, Springer AL: Ureterocele in a dog: a case report, *Vet Med Small Anim Clin* 74:1753, 1979.
40. Scrivani PV, Leveille R, Collins RL: The effect of patient positioning on mural filling defects during double contrast cystography, *Vet Radiol Ultrasound* 38:355, 1997.
41. Archibald J: Urinary system. In Archibald J, editor: *Canine surgery,* Santa Barbara, CA, 1965, American Veterinary Publications.
42. Green RW, Bohning RH Jr: Patent persistent urachus associated with urolithiasis in a cat, *J Am Vet Med Assoc* 158:489, 1971.
43. Osborne CA, Johnston GR, Kruger JM et al: Etiopathogenesis and biological behavior of feline vesicourethral diverticula, *Vet Clin North Am Small Anim Pract* 3:697, 1987.

44. Hansen JS: Patent urachus in a cat, *Vet Med Small Anim Clin* 67:379, 1972.
45. Osborne CA, Rhoades JD, Hanlon GF: Patent urachus in the dog, *Anim Hosp* 2:245, 1966.
46. Scherzo CS: Cystic liver and persistent urachus in a cat, *J Am Vet Med Assoc* 151:1329, 1967.
47. Park RD: Radiographic contrast studies of the lower urinary tract, *Vet Clin North Am* 4:863, 1974.
48. Osuna DJ, Stone EA, Metcalf MR: A urethrorectal fistula with concurrent urolithiasis in a dog, *J Am Anim Hosp Assoc* 25:35, 1989.
49. Biller D, Kantrowitz B, Partinton R et al: Diagnostic ultrasound of the urinary bladder, *J Am Anim Hosp Assoc* 26:397, 1990.
50. Lévellé R, Biller D, Partington B et al: Sonographic investigation of transitional carcinoma of the urinary bladder in small animals, *Vet Radiol* 33:103, 1992.
51. Berry CR: Differentiating cystic calculi from colon, *Vet Radiol* 33:282, 1992.
52. Geisse AL, Lowry JE, Schaeffer DJ et al: Sonographic evaluation of urinary bladder wall thickness in normal dogs, *Vet Radiol Ultrasound* 38:132, 1997.
53. Douglas JP, Kremkan FW: Ultrasound corner: the urinary bladder wall hypoechoic pseudolesion, *Vet Radiol Ultrasound* 34:45, 1993.
54. Barthez PY, Lévellé R, Scrivani PV: Side lobes and grating lobes artifacts in ultrasound imaging, *Vet Radiol Ultrasound* 38:387, 1997.
55. Finn-Bodner ST, Carter RE, Gray BW: Sonographic architecture and morphometric evaluation of the normal feline urinary bladder wall. In *Proceedings of the annual meeting of the American College of Veterinary Radiology,* Orlando, 1992, American College of Veterinary Radiology.
56. Spaulding KA, Stone E: Color Doppler evaluation of ureteral flow dynamics in the dog as influenced by relative specific gravity. In *Proceedings of the annual scientific meeting of the American College of Veterinary Radiology,* Chicago, 1993, American College of Veterinary Radiology.
57. Vörös K, Wladàr S: Ultrasound of urinary bladder calculi in dogs, *Canine Pract* 18:29, 1993.
58. Feeney DA, Walter PA: Ultrasonography of the kidneys, adrenal glands and urinary bladder. In *Proceedings of the American Institute of Ultrasound in Medicine animal ultrasound course,* Phoenix, 1989, American Institute of Ultrasound in Medicine.
59. Ackerman N: *Radiology and ultrasound of urogenital disease in dogs and cats,* Ames, IA, 1991, Iowa State University, p 1.
60. Finn-Bodner ST: The urinary bladder. In Cartee RE, editor: *Practical veterinary ultrasound,* Philadelphia, 1995, Lea & Febiger, p 219.
61. Finn-Bodner ST, Hudson JA, Brewer WG: Transabdominal sonographic evaluation of experimentally induced cystitis of the feline urinary bladder. In *Proceedings of the annual scientific meeting of the American College of Veterinary Radiology,* Chicago, 1993, American College of Veterinary Radiology.
62. Gilson SD, Stone EA: Surgically induced tumor seeding in eight dogs and two cats, *J Am Vet Med Assoc* 196:1811, 1990.

ELECTRONIC RESOURCES evolve

Additional information related to the content in Chapter 41 can be found on the companion Web site at evolve http://evolve.elsevier.com/Thrall/vetrad/.

- Key Points
- Chapter Quiz
- Case Study 41-1

CHAPTER • 42
The Urethra

Robert D. Pechman, Jr.

ANATOMY

The urethra is a sphincter and a conduit for urine from the bladder.[1] In females the urethra is shorter and wider than in males; it terminates at the external urethral orifice on the ventral floor of the vagina. An external urethral sphincter is present in female dogs.[2]

In males the urethra is long and thin and is subdivided into three parts in dogs and two parts in cats (Fig. 42-1). The prostatic urethra extends from the bladder to the caudal border of the prostate gland in dogs. The membranous urethra extends from the caudal margin of the prostate gland to the urethral bulb of the penis in dogs and from the bladder to the bulbourethral glands in cats. In both species the distal extent of the membranous urethra is approximately at the caudal margin of the ischium. The penile urethra extends from the caudal edge of the pelvis to the tip of the penis. The penile urethra is considerably smaller than the membranous urethra in cats (Fig. 42-2); in dogs it is partially surrounded dorsally by the os penis.[1,2]

SURVEY RADIOGRAPHY

Radiographic evaluation of the urethra is performed most often in male dogs.[1] Radiographic examination of the urethra in male cats may be of value in patients with feline urologic syndrome with or without urethral obstruction.[3] Radiographic examination of the urethra is not often performed in female dogs or cats.

Survey radiographs of the urethra are rarely helpful, but they should be carefully examined for signs of urethral disease. Radiopaque urethral calculi may be seen on survey radiographs. Abnormal cranial displacement of the urinary bladder may occur as a result of urethral rupture. Pelvic fractures, particularly in male dogs, may result in urethral injury. Contrast urethrography is indicated in all instances of suspected urethral disease.[3,4]

CONTRAST URETHROGRAPHY

Water-soluble organic iodide contrast media should be used. Oil-based contrast media, barium suspensions, and air should not be used because of the risk of urethrocavernous reflux and contrast medium embolization.[1,4-6] Positive-contrast medium should be diluted with sterile saline or sterile water to approximately 15% of the original concentration.[1,4]

A balloon-tipped catheter should be used.[4] The catheter is inserted into the urethra and the balloon inflated to prevent reflux of contrast medium. A 10- to 15-mL volume of contrast medium is typically used in dogs; 5 to 10 mL is adequate in cats. Radiographic exposures should be made during injection of the last 2 or 3 mL of contrast medium. A lateral view is usually adequate for diagnosis of urethral disease, but right and left ventrodorsal oblique projections are sometimes helpful. Ventrodorsal views are not usually of value. In the lateral view, positioning the patient with the pelvic limbs pulled cranially is important to avoid superimposition of the femurs over the urethra.[1,4] Distention of the urethra, particularly the prostatic urethra, and overall quality of the contrast urethrogram may be improved if the urinary bladder is fully distended with urine, contrast medium, or sterile saline during urethrography.[5] Retrograde positive-contrast urethrography should be performed with care because complications can result.[7,8] Fortunately, most of these potential complications are transient and reversible.

Urethrography can be more difficult in females. As in males, a balloon-tipped catheter must be inserted into the urethra, the balloon inflated, and positive-contrast medium injected. An exposure is made during the injection. The normal urethral mucosal surface is smooth and may be characterized by several linear folds (Fig. 42-3).[4]

Vaginocystourethrography is another method of evaluating the urethra in female dogs. A large balloon-tipped catheter is placed in the vestibule and the balloon inflated to occlude outflow. Clamping the vulvar lips tightly around the catheter may be necessary to prevent reflux. The tip of the catheter distal to the balloon should be cut as short as possible to prevent it from entering the vagina. Positive-contrast medium is injected (10 to 15 mL in dogs and 5 to 10 mL in cats) through the catheter. The vagina will fill preferentially. With subsequent filling, and what sometimes seems like firm resistance to injection, the contrast medium will reflux into the urethra and into the bladder, yielding an excellent retrograde contrast urethrogram (Fig. 42-4). Patients must be given general anesthesia for vaginocystourethrography, and extreme injection pressures must be avoided to prevent rupture.

Urethrography is often helpful in patients with abnormal urination or hematuria thought to be of urethral origin. Pelvic fractures, especially in male dogs, are an indication for contrast urethrography if urinary tract injury is suspected.[4,9-11]

URETHRAL ULTRASONOGRAPHY

Ultrasonographic examination of the urethra is a relatively easy and noninvasive way to evaluate patients for urethral abnormalities. Transabdominal ultrasonography can be used to examine the proximal aspect of the urethra in females and at least a portion of the prostatic urethra in males (Fig. 42-5). However, the pubic bones limit the caudal extent of the urethra that can be examined with sonography. Transrectal sonography allows evaluation of the caudal urethra in females and the caudal portion of the prostatic urethra and the membranous urethra in males. Ultrasonography permits evaluation

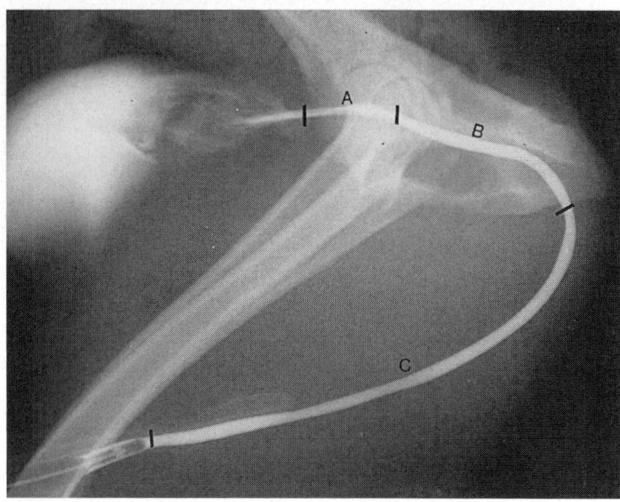

Fig. 42-1 Normal positive-contrast retrograde urethrogram in a dog. A balloon-tipped catheter is present within the penile urethra. The urethra is divided into three segments: *A*, the prostatic urethra; *B*, the membranous urethra; and C, the penile urethra. The urethral mucosa is smooth, and no filling defects are present in the contrast medium column.

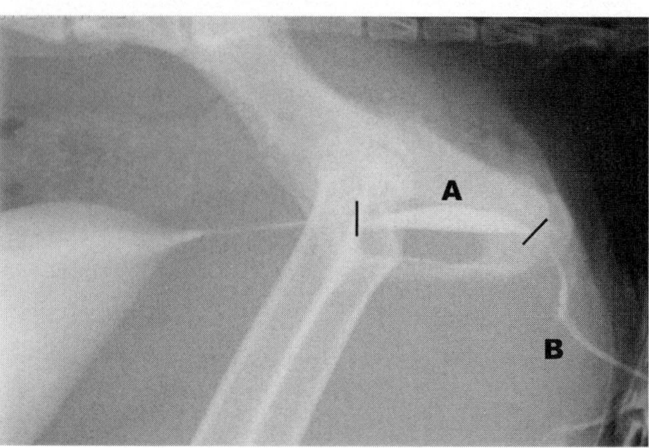

Fig. 42-2 A retrograde urethrogram in a male cat. The pelvic urethra (A) has a smooth mucosal surface and large diameter. The penile urethra (B) has a very small diameter and is nondistendable.

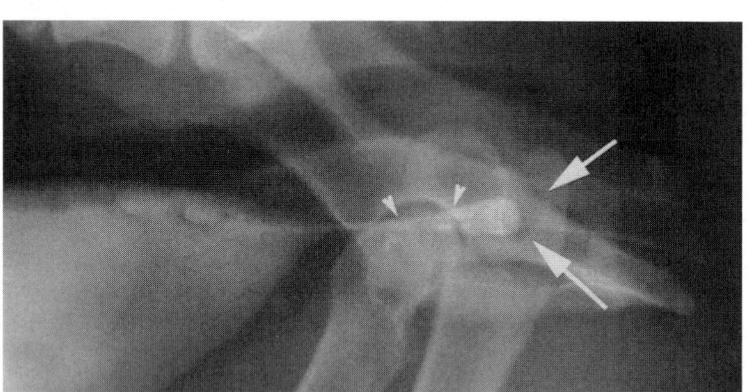

Fig. 42-3 A retrograde urethrogram in a female dog. The smooth, sharp mucosal surface *(arrowheads)* of the normal female is apparent. A balloon catheter was inserted into the urethral orifice *(arrows)* and inflated; positive-contrast medium was injected retrograde.

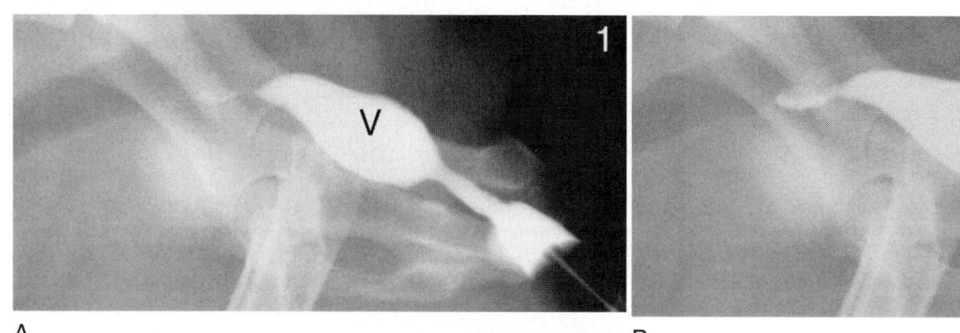

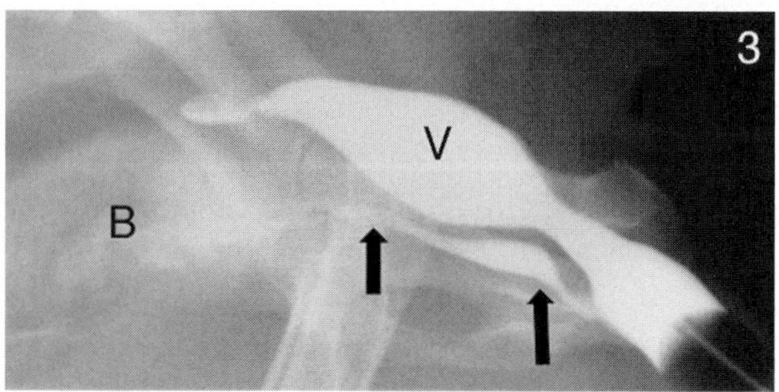

Fig. 42-4 A vaginocystourethrogram in a normal female dog. A, During injection of contrast medium the vagina *(V)* fills first. B, Contrast medium then begins to reflux into the urethra *(arrow)*. C, Contrast medium finally fills the urethra *(arrows)* and enters the urinary bladder (B). The urethral mucosal margins are smooth and sharp.

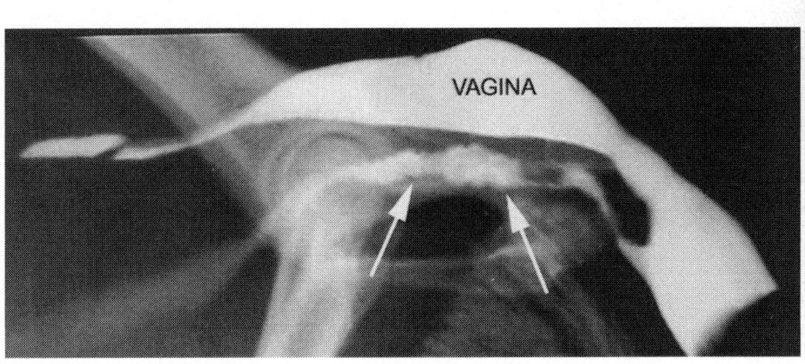

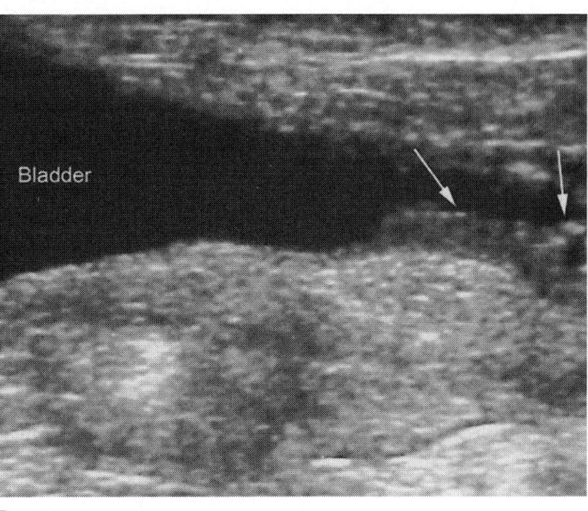

A B

Fig. 42-5 A, A vaginourethrogram in a female dog with stranguria. Reflux of contrast medium into the urethra and bladder is apparent. The urethral mucosa *(arrows)* in this dog is rough and irregular as a result of mural masses extending into the lumen. **B,** Transabdominal ultrasound image of the same female dog. A moderately echogenic tissue mass *(arrows)* has thickened the urethral wall and extends into the urethral lumen near the bladder neck. Diagnosis was transitional cell carcinoma. (Courtesy David Biller, DVM, Kansas State University, Manhattan, Kan.)

of the thickness of the wall of the urethra as well as the mucosal surface. The information acquired from ultrasonography is complementary to that gained from urethrography.[12]

RADIOGRAPHIC SIGNS OF URETHRAL DISEASE

Urethrographic signs of urethral disease may be classified as filling defects in the contrast medium column, extravasation of contrast medium from the urethral lumen,[1] or both.

Filling Defects

Filling defects may be intraluminal, intramural, or extramural. Intraluminal filling defects may be caused by air bubbles in the contrast medium column, mineralized or nonmineralized urethral calculi, or blood clots (Fig. 42-6). Air bubbles are round to oval and have smooth margins and a distinct, sharply defined border. Urethral calculi are variable in shape, have irregular margins, and usually are characterized by a poorly defined or blurred margin. If large enough, urethral calculi may produce widening of the urethral lumen. Blood clots are irregular in shape and have poorly defined margins.

Intramural filling defects may be attributable to neoplasia, inflammatory disease, or scar tissue from previous urethral surgery, or they may result from careless instrumentation. Intramural urethral lesions usually result in marked irregularity of the mucosal surface of the urethra (see Fig. 42-5) and may cause widening or narrowing of the urethral lumen. The transitional zone from normal to abnormal urethra is usually abrupt and sharply defined with intramural lesions.

Extramural filling defects result from compression by masses that surround the urethra. Prostatic hyperplasia or neoplasia may result in extramural filling defects. The mucosal surface remains smooth, and the margins of the extramural filling defect are smooth and tapered.[1]

Extravasation of Contrast Medium

Extravasation of contrast medium indicates a disruption in the integrity of the urethra (Fig. 42-7). Contrast medium may enter the peritoneal cavity if the urethral rent is near the bladder neck. Contrast medium may also enter the systemic venous circulation if urethrocavernous reflux of contrast medium occurs (Fig. 42-8).[1,11] Pelvic fractures or fractures of the os penis may produce urethral lacerations.[9-11] Abdominal trauma may be associated with urethral rupture at the vesicourethral junction.[10,11] Iatrogenic urethral disruptions may result from poor catheter manipulation or after urethral surgery.[1]

Extravasation of urethral contrast medium may also be seen when communication exists through fistulous tracts between the urethral lumen and the extraurinary organs.

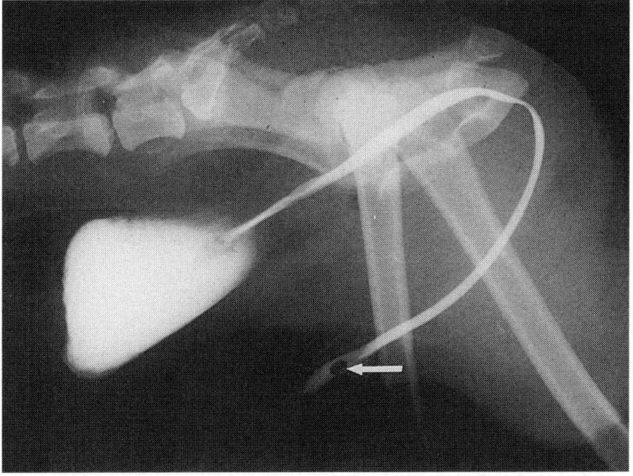

Fig. 42-6 Positive-contrast retrograde urethrogram in a male dog with a solitary urethral calculus. In survey radiographs a mineral opacity calculus was seen near the proximal os penis. With urethrography, the calculus appears as a radiolucent intraluminal filling defect in the contrast medium column *(arrow)*. The margins of the calculus are smooth and sharply defined. The remainder of the urethra is normal.

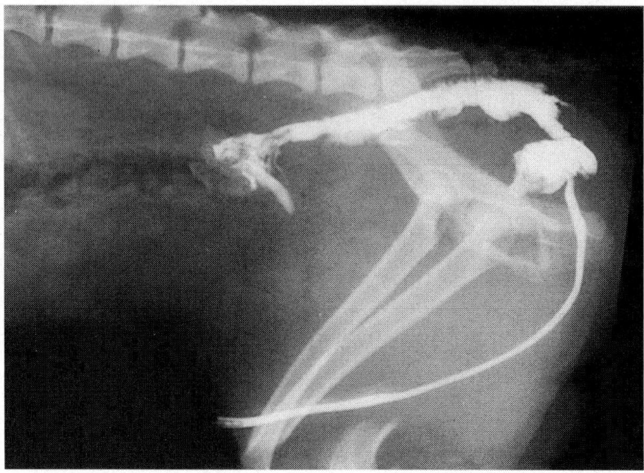

Fig. 42-7 Positive-contrast retrograde urethrogram in a male dog with fractures of the pelvis and femur. Extravasation of contrast medium into the perineal and pelvic soft tissues is visible. Complete transection of the membranous urethra was found at surgery.

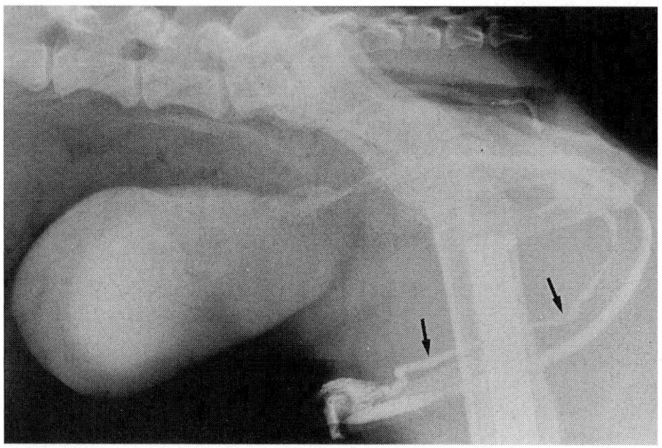

Fig. 42-8 Positive-contrast urethrogram in a male dog. Extravasation of contrast medium through a urethral laceration into the cavernous tissues of the penis is visible. The dorsal vein of the penis is opacified by contrast medium *(arrows)*. The patient was examined for stranguria. A fracture of the os penis at the site of the urethral laceration was apparent in survey radiographs. Note drainage of contrast medium into the caudal vena cava.

Urethrorectal and urethrovaginal fistulas have been reported[1,13]; these fistulas may be congenital or acquired.[1]

REFERENCES

1. Park RD: Radiology of the urinary bladder and urethra. In O'Brien TR, editor: *Radiographic diagnosis of abdominal disorders in the dog and cat,* Philadelphia, 1978, WB Saunders, p 605.
2. Osborne CA, Low DG, Finco DR: *Canine and feline urology,* Philadelphia, 1972, WB Saunders, p 7.
3. Johnston GR, Feeney DA, Osborne CA: Urethrography and cystography in cats: I. Techniques, normal radiographic anatomy, and artifacts. *Compend Contin Educ Pract Vet* 4:823, 1982.
4. Ticer JW, Spencer CP, Ackerman N: Positive contrast retrograde urethrography: a useful procedure for evaluating urethral disorders in the dog, *Vet Radiol* 21:2, 1980.
5. Johnston GR, Jessen CR, Osborne CA: Effects of bladder distention on canine and feline retrograde urethrography, *Vet Radiol* 24:271, 1983.
6. Ackerman N, Wingfield WE, Corley EA: Fatal air embolism associated with pneumourethrography and pneumocystography in a dog, *J Am Vet Med Assoc* 160:1616, 1972.
7. Johnston GR, Stevens JB, Jessen CR et al: Complications of retrograde contrast urethrography in dogs and cats, *Am J Vet Res* 44:1248, 1983.
8. Johnston GR, Feeney DA, Osborne CA: Urethrography and cystography in cats: II. Abnormal radiographic anatomy and complications, *Compend Contin Educ Pract Vet* 4:931, 1982.
9. Wingfield WE: Lower urinary tract injuries associated with pelvic trauma, *Canine Pract* 1:25, 1974.
10. Kleine LJ, Thornton GW: Radiographic diagnosis of urinary tract trauma, *J Am Anim Hosp Assoc* 7:318, 1971.
11. Pechman RD: Urinary trauma in dogs and cats: a review, *J Am Anim Hosp Assoc* 18:33, 1982.
12. Hanson JA, Tidwell AS: Ultrasonographic appearance of urethral transitional cell carcinoma in ten dogs, *Vet Radiol Ultrasound* 37:4, 1996.
13. Osborne CA, Engen MH, Yano BL et al: Congenital urethrorectal fistula in two dogs, *J Am Vet Med Assoc* 166:999, 1975.

ELECTRONIC RESOURCES evolve

Additional information related to the content in Chapter 42 can be found on the companion Web site at evolve http://evolve.elsevier.com/Thrall/vetrad/.

- Key Points
- Chapter Quiz
- Case Study 42-1
- Video 42-1

CHAPTER • 43
The Prostate Gland

Jimmy C. Lattimer
Stephanie C. Essman

NORMAL ANATOMY AND RADIOGRAPHIC APPEARANCE

The normal prostate gland surrounds the most proximal aspect of the urethra and lies ventral to the rectum and caudal to the urinary bladder, typically within the pelvic canal. The prostate gland is occasionally recognized radiographically in normal dogs by its round shape and soft tissue opacity and by the relation of the gland to the organs around it. More typically, the normal prostate gland is not seen radiographically in the dog; the normal prostate gland is not visible radiographically in the male cat. Lack of visualization of the normal prostate gland is influenced by the fact that the prostate gland is usually in direct contact with the rectum, resulting in the dorsal border of the prostate gland being effaced, especially if the rectum contains feces. A full rectum may also completely obscure the prostate gland on the ventrodorsal view. Also, if the shape or position of the prostate gland is altered, the gland may not be recognizable other than as a nondescript opacity between the bladder, rectum, and pelvis.[1]

DISEASES OF THE PROSTATE GLAND

Intrinsic disease of the prostate gland usually results in prostatic enlargement. Enlargement may also occur in response to extraprostatic diseases, such as an androgen-producing testicular tumor and orchitis.[2] Because of the close functional association of the prostate gland and testes, any animal with prostatic disease should also be examined (preferably ultrasonographically) for testicular disease.

The most common prostatic abnormality is benign prostatic hypertrophy, in which the prostate gland enlarges as a result of increased volume in the intercellular and ductal spaces rather than from increased intracellular volume or cell number. Thus once hypertrophy reaches a certain point, the development of dilated cystic spaces and ducts is inevitable. Solid and cystic hypertrophy are therefore different stages of the same disease, with the latter being the advanced form.[2,3] The size of the cystic spaces varies from microscopic to large; these spaces may become so large that they distort the shape of the entire prostate gland. A cystic prostate gland may have cysts of many different sizes. Large cystic spaces predispose the gland to infection.

Another common cause of prostatic enlargement is prostatitis, which is usually bacterial.[4] The infection may arise within the prostate gland or it may extend from other sources, such as the bladder or testicles.[5] Because many antibiotics do not readily penetrate the prostate gland, the gland may also be a reservoir for reinfection or for primary extension to other organs.[6,7] The degree of inflammation depends on the type of organism present and the condition of the prostate gland before infection. A normal prostate gland is more resistant to infection than is a hypertrophied gland with many secretion-filled cystic spaces. The inflammation may vary from a mild transient process that causes minimal or no clinical signs to a fulminating hemorrhagic process that rapidly destroys the entire gland.[8] The latter may result in rupture of the capsule with extension of infection to the peritoneal cavity, resulting in peritonitis.[7]

Chronic, recurrent prostatitis may result in a scarred, fibrotic prostate gland that is smaller than normal. Chronic scarring may result in stricture of the urethra.[9] Such a stricture is difficult to recognize radiographically unless a urethrogram is performed.

Prostatic abscesses may form as a result of prostatitis or primary cystic disease. As with cyst formation, abscesses may be small or large. Large abscesses distort the shape of the prostate gland and may eventually rupture, causing peritonitis. As previously mentioned, cysts form in advanced benign hypertrophy and are usually contained within the gland. However, cysts occasionally become so large that the shape of the gland is distorted and the predominant opacity seen on the radiograph is caused by the large cyst. Such large cysts are also referred to as *paraprostatic cysts* because they are no longer confined within the gland. These cysts are usually sterile but may become infected.[10]

Cysts occasionally result from neoplasia.[11] Formation of functional neoplastic secretory cells without an accompanying ductal system results in a cystic structure lined with neoplastic epithelium. Osteocollagenous retention cysts are rare and of unknown origin, but they do not appear to be the direct result of cystic hypertrophy.[12] A rare form of cyst, which is truly paraprostatic, is cystic enlargement of the mullerian ducts, called uterus masculinus.[13] Enlargement of the mullerian ducts results in a bilateral tubular mass that resembles uterine enlargement. The prostate gland itself may or may not be enlarged and usually is not distinguishable as a separate opacity.[9]

Prostatic adenocarcinoma is relatively uncommon; however, the incidence in intact and neutered males is similiar.[14,15] Prostatic adenocarcinoma is often advanced at presentation, with metastasis to regional lymph nodes, the pelvis, and distant sites such as the liver and lungs.[16-18] The prostate gland is massively enlarged by the tumor in some dogs, and in others the degree of enlargement is minimal. Small in situ prostatic carcinomas are unusual but do occur; they are usually discovered as a result of metastasis rather than from their local effects. Prostatic neoplasms are often secondarily infected or necrotic, and affected dogs may therefore have clinical signs

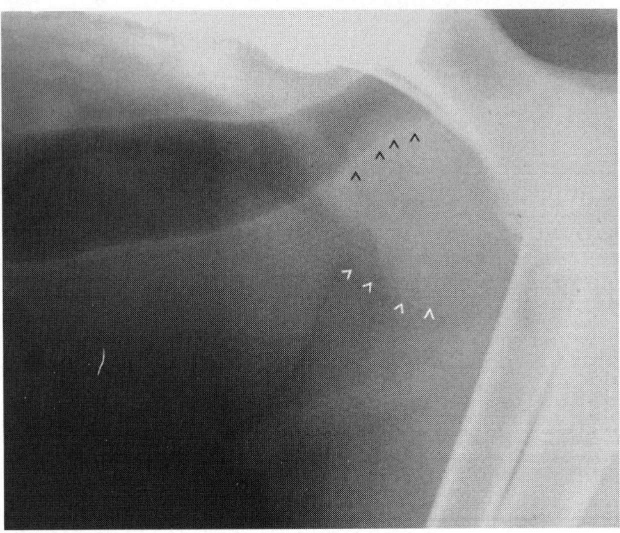

Fig. 43-1 Prostatic enlargement. The *white arrowheads* indicate the cranial margin of the prostate gland, which is displacing the bladder cranially. Notice the distinct triangular fat opacity region between the ventral caudal margin of the bladder and the cranial ventral margin of the prostate gland. The enlarged prostate gland is displacing the colon dorsally and indenting it *(black arrowheads)*. The enlargement seen here is relatively symmetric with relation to the neck of the bladder.

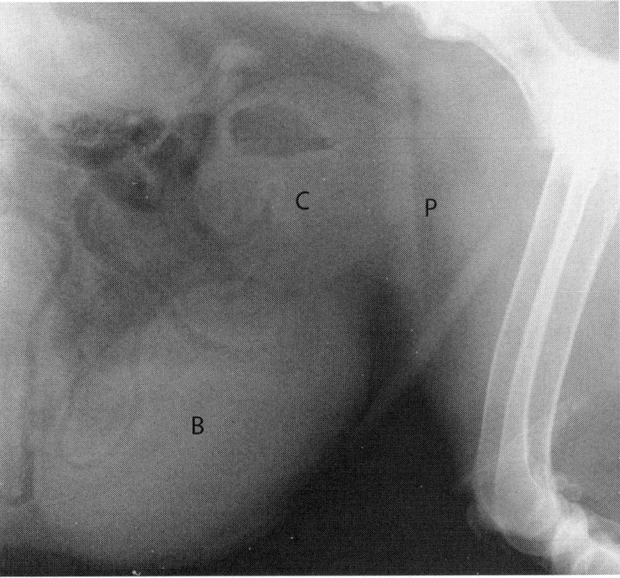

Fig. 43-2 A large, dorsally located paraprostatic cyst *(C)* arising from a prostate gland enlarged because of benign hypertrophy *(P)*. Note the cranial displacement of the urinary bladder *(B)* by the enlarged prostate gland and the asymmetric enlargement created by the cyst.

of prostatitis. These tumors are difficult to diagnose, unless signs of metastasis are present, because of the tendency of infection to overshadow neoplasia.[19-21]

Clinical Signs

The clinical signs of prostate gland disease are usually referable to either urinary or rectal problems. Stranguria, hematuria, and pyuria are commonly seen.[5,8,10,13] Complete urethral obstruction is unusual.[3,22] Another common symptom with prostatic disease is dyschezia, with small or ribbonlike stools.[8,22] As the enlarging prostate gland displaces the colon dorsally, it compresses it against the sacrum and pelvis, resulting in a decrease in rectal diameter (Fig. 43-1). Extreme straining to defecate may result in small amounts of fresh blood in the stool. Severe rectal compression by the prostate gland may cause clinical and radiographic signs of constipation or obstipation. The problem is then critical, and immediate treatment must be instituted. Another less common but important symptom is a pelvic limb gait abnormality. The animal may refuse to climb stairs and jump. Owners often believe the animal has developed osteoarthritis. Such animals may have severe, active septic prostatitis.[5,8] The pain caused by the prostatic infection is markedly exacerbated by walking, climbing, and jumping. Both pelvic limbs are usually affected uniformly because the pain is central. These animals are also usually sensitive to palpation of the caudal abdomen. Some erythema of the skin may be present from inflammation in this area. Gait abnormalities are seen rarely in uncomplicated benign prostatic hypertrophy.

Radiographic Changes

All common prostate gland diseases cause enlargement. The enlargement may be symmetric (diffuse in origin), asymmetric (focal in origin), or a combination of the two. Prostatic symmetry is usually judged by the shape of the prostate gland and the relative mass of the prostate gland with respect to the neck of the bladder. Hypertrophy and prostatitis are examples that usually cause symmetric enlargement (see Fig. 43-1), whereas neoplasia and cysts are examples that usually cause

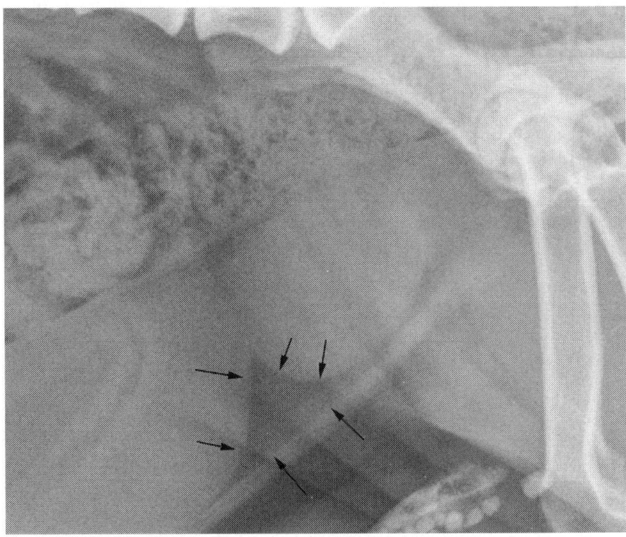

Fig. 43-3 Abdominal radiograph of a dog with prostatic hypertrophy. Note the cranial displacement of the bladder and the triangular region of fat between the caudoventral aspect of the bladder, the cranioventral aspect of the prostate gland, and the ventral abdominal wall *(arrows)*. This sign is a reliable indicator of a prostate-associated mass.

asymmetric enlargement (Fig. 43-2). Radiographic visualization of the prostate gland depends on the presence of surrounding fat; the gland may not be seen in very thin animals or those with fluid in the area of the neck of the bladder. A reliable sign of prostatomegaly is a triangular region of fat between the bladder, prostate gland, and ventral abdominal wall (Fig. 43-3).

Identification of prostatomegaly hinges on identification of a soft tissue mass in the caudal abdomen and on the relation of that mass to surrounding structures, principally the bladder and colon. Prostatomegaly typically displaces the bladder cranially because of the intimate relation between the prostate

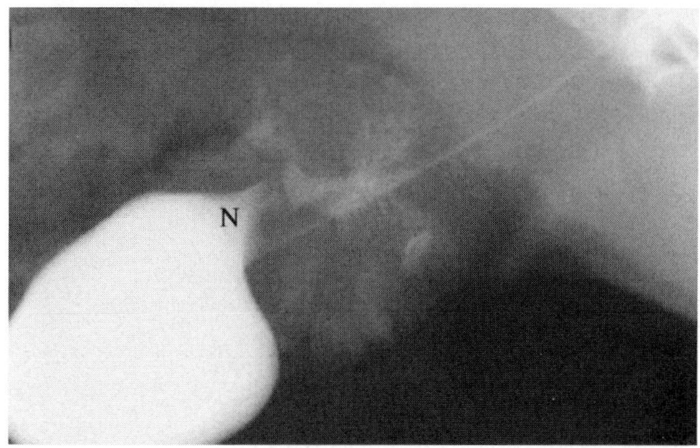

Fig. 43-4 Marked prostatic enlargement with dorsal elevation of the neck of the bladder *(N)*. In extreme instances the prostate gland may lift the bladder completely away from the floor of the abdominal wall. Note the reflux of contrast medium into the prostate gland and the way the enlarged prostate gland encompasses the neck of the bladder. A catheter is present in the urethra.

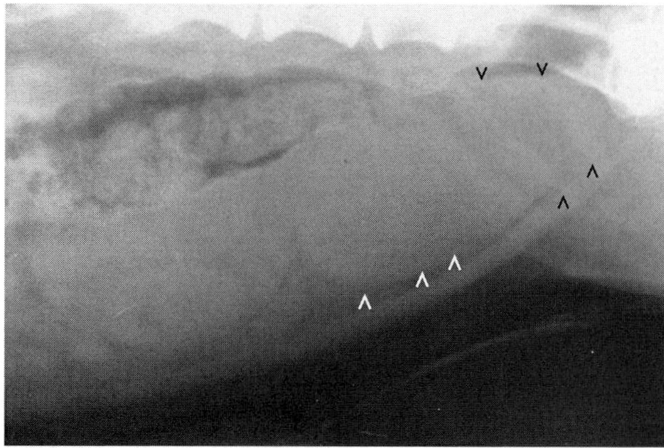

Fig. 43-5 An extremely enlarged prostate gland. The *black arrowheads* indicate the ventral and dorsal margins of the prostate gland. The *white arrowheads* indicate the ventral margin of a second lobular mass from the prostate gland. The urinary bladder is at the extreme left of the figure superimposed on the fluid-filled bowel loops. Subsequent studies indicated that multiple cysts arose from the prostate gland. Confusing the second cyst *(white arrowheads)* with the urinary bladder would be easy. Note the loss of the normal triangle of fat between the caudoventral aspect of the urinary bladder and the cranioventral aspect of the prostate gland.

gland and the urinary bladder (see Fig. 43-1). If prostatomegaly is uniform, bladder displacement is cranial along the floor of the abdomen. If prostatomegaly is eccentric, as often occurs with large cysts and abscesses, the direction of bladder displacement may be different. A cyst or abscess occasionally may extend dorsal to the bladder (see Fig. 43-2). Alternatively, with ventral prostatomegaly the bladder may be elevated (Fig. 43-4). Benign prostatic hyperplasia rarely results in asymmetric prostate enlargement; a large prostatic cyst or abscess extending ventral to the bladder is more common.

The more severe the enlargement of the prostate, the further cranially the bladder will be displaced (Fig. 43-5). Extreme enlargement is most commonly associated with a prostatic cyst, but other abnormalities may also be responsible. Extreme enlargement also frequently results in obliteration of the normal triangle of fat formed by the caudal ventral bladder and prostate gland (see Fig. 43-5).

The other major radiographic sign of prostatomegaly is dorsal displacement of the colon (see Figs. 43-1 and 43-5). Prostatic enlargement may also cause narrowing of the lumen of the colon or rectum. This compression may be visible radiographically, or the colon may simply become confluent with the prostate gland mass at the pelvic inlet (see Fig. 43-5). The latter appearance does not usually occur unless the prostate gland is quite enlarged.

The urethra, although not really displaced relative to the prostate gland, may be elevated from the pelvic floor or displaced laterally by an enlarged prostate gland. Urethral displacement is most often seen with asymmetric prostatic disease, such as tumors, cysts, and abscesses. The urethra is also often elongated by its passage through an enlarged prostate gland. The position of the urethra is impossible to ascertain radiographically unless contrast medium is used to outline it (see Fig. 43-8).

A tremendously enlarged prostate gland displaces other abdominal organs cranially. Huge prostatic lesions usually lie on the floor of the abdomen, so some dorsal displacement of the remainder of the abdominal contents occurs. Prostatic and paraprostatic cysts may become so large that they reach almost to the costal arch.[13] With masses of this magnitude, organ displacement is so severe that the actual source of the mass may be difficult to determine without the use of special radiographic procedures or sonography. Prostatic disease that results in urethral stricture may result in severe urinary bladder distention, which is then secondarily responsible for the displacement of the abdominal structures cranial and dorsal to it.

Prostatic size that exceeds 90% of the distance from the pubis to the sacral promontory is suggestive of a mass lesion (cyst, abscess, or neoplasm).[23] The actual degree of prostatic enlargement varies tremendously, however. For instance, prostatic size may vary from slight enlargement to 10 times normal size for benign prostatic hypertrophy, and the prostate gland may actually decrease in size in chronic prostatitis. Therefore if prostatic cysts or abscesses are present, the prostatic silhouette may be as great as 20 or more times normal size, or the degree of enlargement may be minimal. Acute prostatitis and neoplasia do not usually cause severe enlargement, as is seen with hypertrophy and cyst formation. Some small in situ prostatic tumors are not recognized until the animal is examined for another problem, such as cough and lameness caused by metastasis, or they may be discovered as an incidental finding at postmortem.

Paraprostatic cysts and abscesses usually have well-defined margins that are easily seen (see Fig. 43-2). An occasional abscess is poorly marginated, although this occurrence is the exception rather than the rule. A cyst or abscess occasionally may form in the pelvic canal; such lesions may not be readily visible on survey radiographs or produce the usual displacement of the bladder.[24] These lesions do, however, produce marked displacement and compression of the rectum and are therefore recognized as an intrapelvic mass. The lack of regional peritonitis associated with the large abscess may be caused in part to the thickness of the capsule and to the low virulence of the organism. Distinguishing a cyst from an abscess on the basis of radiographic examination alone is impossible.

When possible, evaluation of the margination of the prostate gland is important. The presence of adequate amounts of abdominal fat is essential to enable visualization of the prostatic margin. In the presence of emaciation, normally thin animals, pelvic trauma, or abdominal effusion, the prostatic margin and even the entire prostate gland itself may be indistinctly seen. If the prostate gland has a smooth margin that is easily seen, the disease involving the gland is likely to be benign or is slowly progressing (see Fig. 43-1), such as

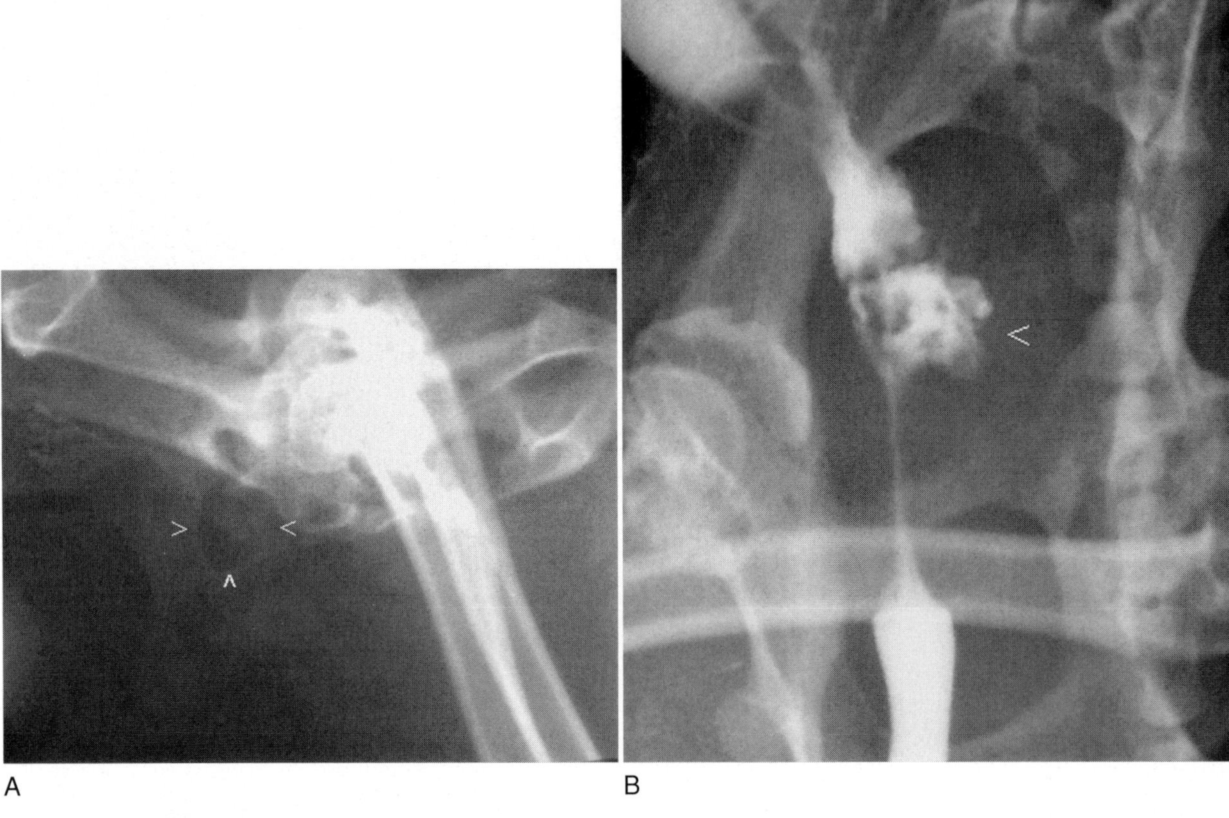

Fig. 43-6 Cavitation of the prostate gland. During a double-contrast cystogram an air-filled cavity was noted within the prostate gland (**A**). This cavity was irregular and thick walled. A urethrogram (**B**) clearly indicates the communication of the cavity with the urethra.

benign hypertrophy and low-grade or chronic prostatitis. A rough or indistinct margin in the presence of adequate abdominal fat is more likely to be caused by an acute or aggressive process such as neoplasia or prostatitis.[20,25,26] When the margin is indistinct or not discernible, the impression is that of a localized peritonitis in the caudal abdomen. Some secondary inflammation usually is in the surrounding tissues in most aggressive prostatic diseases.

Any change in the opacity of the prostate gland from its normal soft tissue opacity indicates severe or chronic disease. Areas of calcification within the gland are a sign either of long-standing prostatitis or of neoplasia.[13,21,23] Most prostate gland calcification is a result of neoplasia. Therefore, although calcification in the prostate gland is a serious finding that warrants biopsy,[24] prostate gland calcification is rarely observed radiographically. Prostate gland calcification is more commonly seen with sonography because that technique is more sensitive for its detection.

The presence of gas within the prostate gland is also an important sign. Because the prostate gland does not normally communicate with any air-containing organ, it should not contain gas. Such a finding is considered evidence of a gas-forming bacterial prostatitis unless the gas opacity can be attributed to an overlying gas-filled bowel loop. Coliform or clostridial prostatitis results in severe hemorrhagic necrosis of the gland, potentially causing a generalized peritonitis. Because of the rapidly fatal course of these infections, identification of noniatrogenic gas within the prostate gland should be viewed as an unfavorable prognostic sign. Even if the animal survives, severe permanent scarring of the prostate gland is likely. Sterility and urinary retention or incontinence may become long-term sequelae to such scarring.

The prostate gland may contain air because of reflux from the bladder during a negative- or double-contrast cystogram (Fig. 43-6). A small amount of reflux into prostatic ducts is a normal but not consistent occurrence. Simple filling of the ducts with air does not necessarily indicate prostatic disease. Filling of air in pockets within the prostate gland is abnormal, however, and is most often associated with cyst formation as a result of benign hypertrophy.

Palisade-type or smooth periosteal proliferation is sometimes seen on the ventral aspect of the caudal lumbar vertebrae and pelvis. Such proliferation is suggestive of regional metastasis from prostatic neoplasia.[20-23,27,28] Hyperostosis in this region from metastasis can also be caused by other urinary tumors or hematogenously metastasizing tumors of the pelvic canal or perineum.

SPECIAL RADIOGRAPHIC PROCEDURES FOR EVALUATING THE PROSTATE GLAND

Although ultrasonography has dramatically enhanced imaging of the prostatic parenchyma, retrograde urethrography is still an important and useful imaging procedure that should be considered in patients with suspected prostatic disease.

The only special radiographic procedure that has been found to be uniformly useful in evaluation of the prostate gland is the positive-contrast urethrogram. This procedure allows evaluation of the urethra itself and the position of the urethra in relation to suspected prostatic disease. Asymmetric positioning of the urethra indicates the enlargement is either extrinsic to the prostate gland or is occurring asymmetrically within the prostate gland (see Fig. 43-4), with the latter being more common.[23] Invasion or stricture of the urethra in association with a prostatic mass is a poor prognostic finding because of the danger that a urinary obstruction could occur and because it is a sign that aggressive disease is present.[23] Evidence of either prostatic asymmetrical enlargement or urethral abnormalities is a positive indication for prostatic biopsy.

Urethrography is easily performed in the male dog, and several methods may be used (see Chapter 42).[29,30] Urethrography provides only indirect evidence of prostatic disease. If the urethra is deviated around a large mass or does not pass directly through the center of the prostate gland, the disease within the prostate gland is asymmetric, such as a cyst. If the urethra passes directly through the middle of an enlarged prostate gland, the disease process is more likely to be diffuse throughout the gland, such as hypertrophy or prostatitis.

In addition, a urethrogram identifies the true location of the urinary bladder. In some instances, abdominal masses, such as an omental tumor, a paraprostatic cyst, or an enlarged retained testicle, lie just cranial to the bladder. This positioning closely mimics the appearance of an enlarged prostate gland displacing the bladder cranially, and verifying which opacity in the caudal abdomen is actually the bladder is important; urethrography is useful for this purpose. Survey radiographs and palpation do not always determine what is prostate gland and what is bladder (see Fig. 43-4). This identification is necessary if a blind percutaneous aspirate of the mass is to be attempted rather than a biopsy by laparotomy or with ultrasonographic guidance. When the positions of the bladder and urethra are identified with a urethrogram, the chances of injury to the urinary tract during biopsy procedures are lessened.

Direct signs of urethral disease of prostatic origin are urethral stricture, ulceration of the mucosa, and filling defects within the urethra. Ulceration or stricture of the prostatic urethra should be regarded as highly suggestive of neoplasia of the prostate gland.[6,23]

Extravasation of contrast medium into the prostate gland should not be interpreted as abnormal as long as only the prostatic ducts fill with contrast medium (Fig. 43-7). This appearance is often seen in animals with a normal prostate gland.[31] Only definite pooling of contrast medium within the prostate gland should be considered abnormal. Large, irregularly shaped cavities with rough walls that communicate with the urethra or cavitary smooth-walled lesions containing intraluminal masses are often associated with neoplasia; biopsy is indicated in these instances.[15,26] Conversely, if extravasation does not occur, the prostate gland is not necessarily normal or solid. Many times, large cavitary lesions, such as cysts and abscesses, attain their size because they do not communicate with the urethra.[10,13,22] If these cavities do fill with contrast medium, they are usually ovoid, with smooth walls.

The normal prostatic urethra as seen on the urethrogram has a smooth mucosal border. The urethra is usually slightly greater in diameter near the center of the prostate gland and tapers slightly at the cranial and caudal borders. The degree of the central dilation depends somewhat on the size of the prostate gland, the disease present, the degree of bladder distention, and the amount of pressure applied during injection.[32] A small filling defect in the dorsal wall of the urethra near the center of the prostate gland represents the colliculus seminalis and is a normal finding (Fig. 43-8). Some dogs may also have a normal groove in the colliculus.

The point at which the prostatic urethra joins the trigone of the bladder should be carefully evaluated. Small filling defects of mucosal ulcers that may be early lesions of transitional cell carcinoma may be detected. These small lesions may not be detected on a cystogram because they are obscured by the internal urethral sphincter, which is actually encircled by the prostate gland.[27]

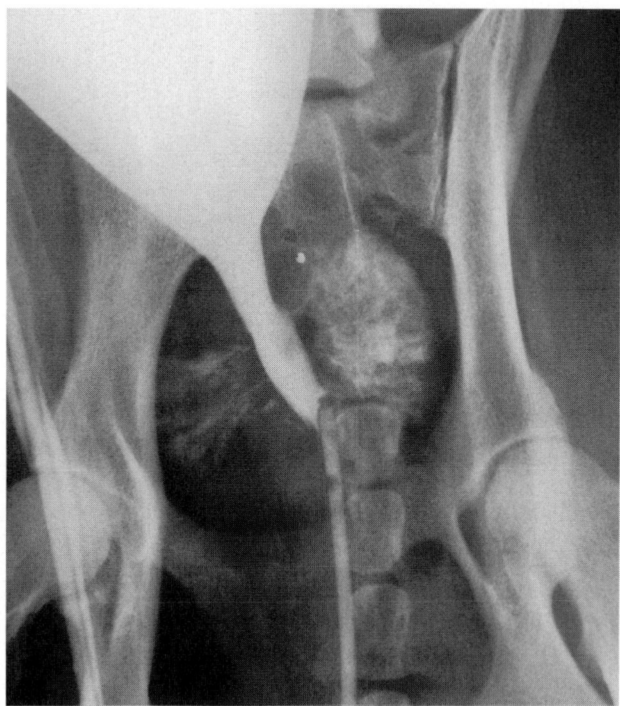

Fig. 43-7 Filling of the prostatic ducts with contrast medium. No cavities are present. Although the prostate gland in this dog is mildly enlarged, the filling of the prostatic ducts with contrast medium has no clinical significance.

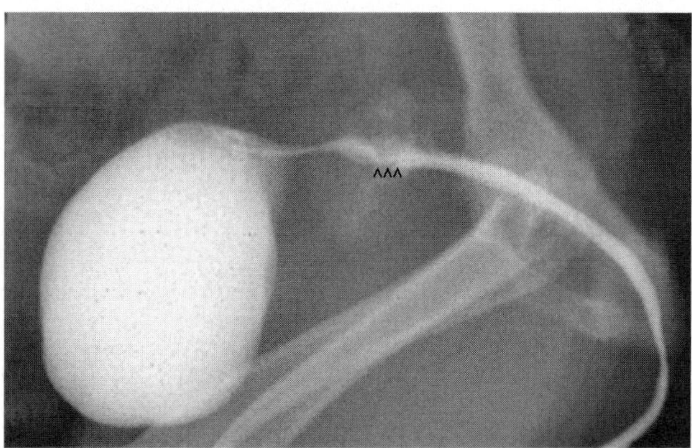

Fig. 43-8 The small filling defect (*black arrowheads* at the ventral aspect) in the dorsal wall of the prostatic urethra is a normal structure, the colliculus seminalis. It should not be mistaken for a lesion caused by prostatic or urethral disease.

SONOGRAPHY FOR EVALUATING THE PROSTATE GLAND

Diagnostic ultrasonography has largely supplanted radiography for the diagnosis of prostatic disease in practices in which it is available. Ultrasonography is easy, safe, and inexpensive to perform. The ultrasonographic examination can often be

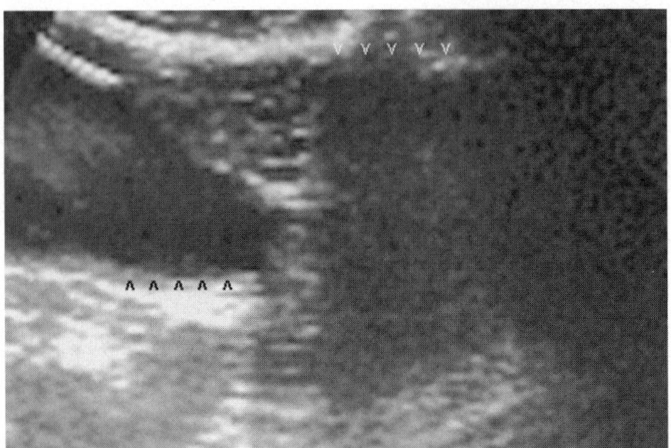

Fig. 43-9 This moderately enlarged prostate gland is difficult to image sonographically because of its intrapelvic location. The cranial aspect of the prostate gland is present between the bladder *(black arrowheads)* and the pubic brim shadow *(white arrowheads)*; the remainder of the gland cannot be seen. If the proper probe is available, this prostate gland could be imaged more completely with a transrectal approach.

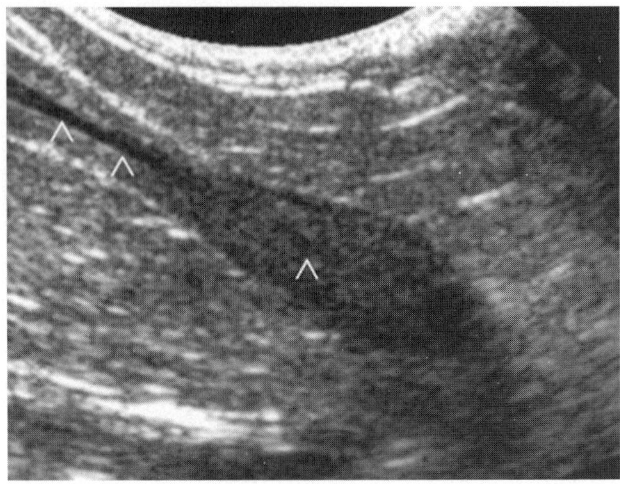

Fig. 43-10 Longitudinal sonographic image of normal prostate gland. The organ margins are distinct, and the echogenicity is close to that of the surrounding fat. The urethra is a small echolucency in the center of the gland *(white arrowheads)*.

performed in less time than a contrast examination, but the major advantage of ultrasonography is its ability to image the actual structure of the tissues within the prostate gland. This is important for delineating the differences between mass lesions such as cysts and tumors.

The sonographic examination of the prostate gland should include the bladder and testicles at a minimum. These associated structures may be secondarily affected in prostatic disease, or they may actually be the site of the primary disorder when the prostate gland is the secondary site of involvement. The ultrasonographic examination of the prostate gland should be performed from the prepubic position. The prostate gland in most dogs can be effectively examined with this approach. Very small normal glands such as those seen in neutered dogs may occasionally not be seen, but an abnormal prostate gland is rarely not seen cranial to the pubis (Fig. 43-9). The examination should consist of images of the prostate gland in the transverse, sagittal, and parasagittal planes. The prostate gland is most easily imaged from the right side of the os penis when the dog is on its back. In some dogs angling the probe caudally is necessary to see the caudal pole of the prostate gland where it lies just dorsal to the pubic brim. Measurement of the prostate gland and lesions within the prostate gland is easily performed with ultrasonography and has been found to be accurate.[33]

The normal prostate gland is uniformly echogenic with an echogenicity that is very similar to that of the surrounding fat. However, the echotexture of the prostate gland is different than that of fat because the prostate gland has a homogenous medium to fine texture and fat tends to be more coarsely echotextured. The urethra usually is seen as a small echolucency in the center of the gland with a narrow band of slightly hyperechoic tissue surrounding it (Fig. 43-10). Although the position of the urethra can usually be ascertained, involvement of the urethra by a disease process can only be inferred sonographically and must be confirmed by urethrography.

Benign prostatic hypertrophy usually appears sonographically as a uniformly enlarged gland that is mildly hyperechoic (bright) and has a smooth margin. The dorsal portion of the gland may be enlarged to a greater degree than the ventral, or vice versa, but the changes are symmetric from right to left (Fig. 43-11). This symmetry may be lost as the hypertrophy increases in severity and enters the cystic stage of the disorder. As cysts form, some invariably become larger than others and distort the shape of the prostate gland as they increase in size. Differentiating the solid and cystic forms of hypertrophy was generally not possible before the advent of ultrasound examination. A presumptive diagnosis of benign prostatic hypertrophy based on sonographic imaging characteristics must still be confirmed by biopsy.

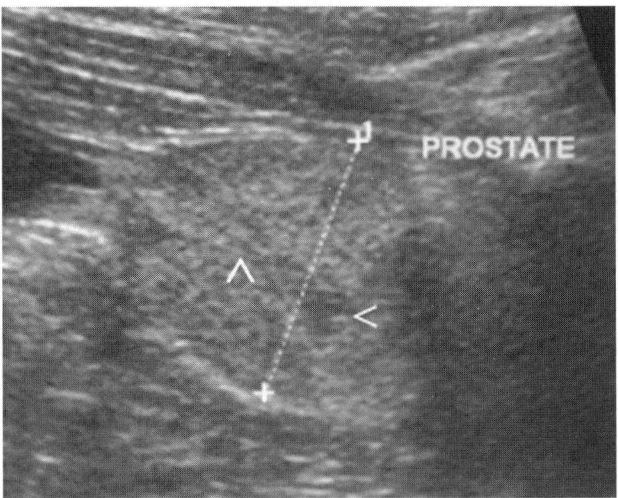

Fig. 43-11 Benign prostatic hypertrophy. The prostate gland is still relatively symmetric, as seen in this longitudinal section with only slight dorsal prominence, but is increased in echogenicity compared with the surrounding fat. The margins are not quite as distinct as normal. As the gland enlarges it will continue to lose its symmetry. The position of the urethra is indicated by *white arrowheads*.

The sonographic changes seen in prostatitis vary from mild hyperechogenicity and enlargement of the prostate gland to severe enlargement with a mottled hyperechoic to hypoechoic (dark) pattern (Fig. 43-12). The shape of the prostate gland is usually normal, but in severe prostatitis it may be somewhat distorted. This is especially true if abscess formation is present in the gland. Some dogs may have a hypoechoic band of edema in the joint capsule outlining the prostate gland. Other dogs, in which the inflammation has extended into the surrounding fat, may have hyperechoic fat surrounding

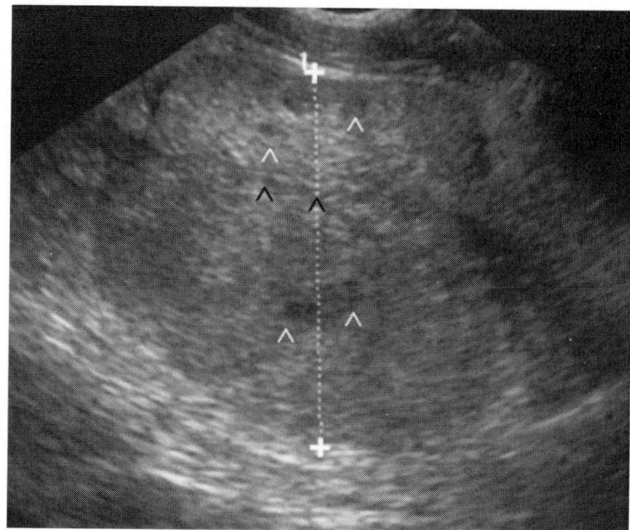

Fig. 43-12 Prostatitis. The prostate gland is slightly asymmetrically enlarged dorsally, and slightly sonolucent zones are suggestive of focal necrosis in the gland *(white arrowheads)*. Such a mottled appearance is typical of prostatitis but can be seen with neoplasia as well. *Black arrowheads* indicate the urethra.

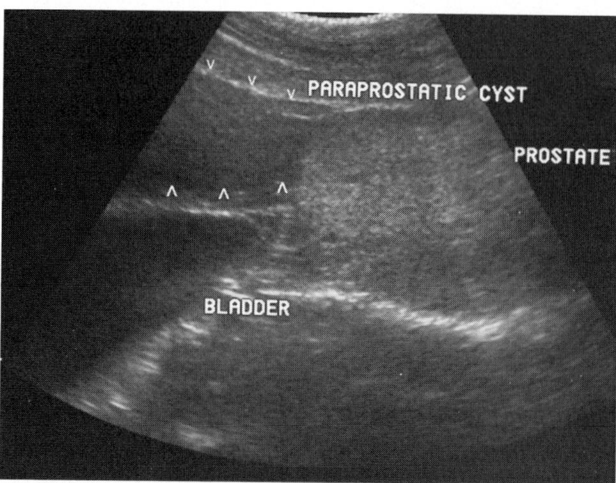

Fig. 43-13 A large paraprostatic cyst *(white arrowheads)* is present ventral and cranial to the prostate gland and ventral to the bladder. Notice the minimal evidence of cyst formation within the prostate gland itself, which is only mildly enlarged. The fluid in the cyst is more echogenic fluid than in the bladder.

the gland. In severe necrotizing prostatitis, the delineation of the gland from the surrounding fat may be lost and the prostate gland may appear as a dark structure with an irregular and indistinct margin along the surrounding hyperechoic fat.

Cysts and abscesses within and attached to the prostate gland appear as thin-walled structures with echolucent centers. They vary widely in size from a couple of millimeters to several centimeters. Their contents may be anechoic, or they may have varying amounts of cellular debris within the lumen.[34] As a general rule, the presence of septation or large amounts of debris within the lumen is more indicative of abscess, whereas anechoic contents are suggestive of a cyst; however, this is not a universally accurate distinction. The presence of through transmission deep to a highly echogenic structure is usually indicative of a fluid-filled rather than a solid cellular mass. Both cysts and abscesses occasionally may occur in conjunction with neoplasia. As with urethrography, cavitary lesions with rough or shaggy internal margins or solid tissue masses within them are highly suggestive of neoplasia, whereas smooth margins are more indicative of cysts (Fig. 43-13).

Calcification within the prostate gland, indicated sonographically by bright echoes that cast shadows, is generally considered a sign of malignancy, particularly if it is linear and irregular (Fig. 43-14). However, in some instances chronic inflammation can cause slight calcification of the prostate gland, which is detectable with ultrasonography. Thus a diagnosis of malignancy on the basis of calcification alone should not be made, but such a finding is strong justification for prostatic aspirate or biopsy.

Malignant neoplasia of the prostate gland in the dog is usually advanced at the time of presentation. These are highly aggressive disease processes that destroy the architecture of the gland, resulting in a mixed echogenic pattern that causes asymmetrical enlargement of the prostate gland (Fig. 43-15). When seen early, prostatic neoplasia may cause a single bright focus within one area of the gland, and the gland may or may not be distorted (Fig. 43-16).

A definitive diagnosis of any given prostatic disease should not be made on the basis of sonographic findings alone.[35] An ultrasonographically guided biopsy should be performed to support the sonographic diagnosis. In dogs with suspected

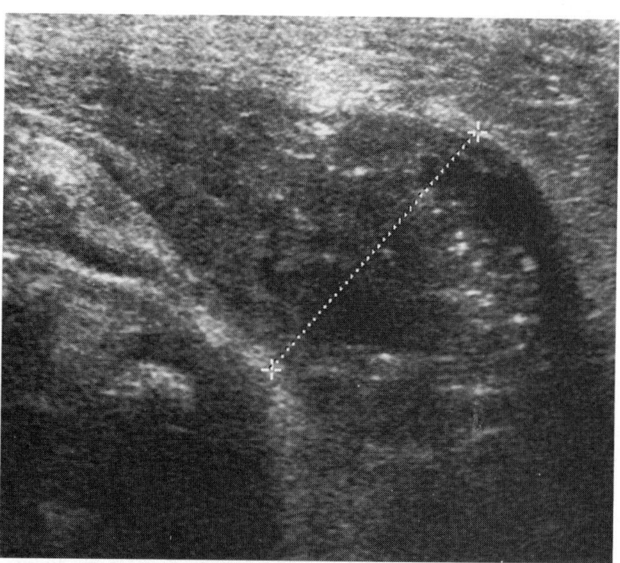

Fig. 43-14 Sonographic image of the prostate gland of a dog with a prostatic adenocarcinoma. The scattered focal hyperechoic regions represent mineralizations within the gland. These mineralizations, which are highly suggestive of prostatic neoplasia, were not visible radiographically. The *dotted line* indicates the location of a prostate gland measurement.

neoplasia, biopsies should be taken of the primary lesion of interest and the other quadrants of the gland.

COMPUTED TOMOGRAPHY AND MAGNETIC RESONANCE IMAGING

Few reports exist of computed tomography (CT) or magnetic resonance (MR) imaging being used for the evaluation of prostatic disease in dogs despite widespread use for this purpose in human beings. Both CT and MR imaging may be used to evaluate the prostate gland and surrounding tissues. These imaging systems result in tomographic or slicelike images through the prostate gland, removing superimposition of

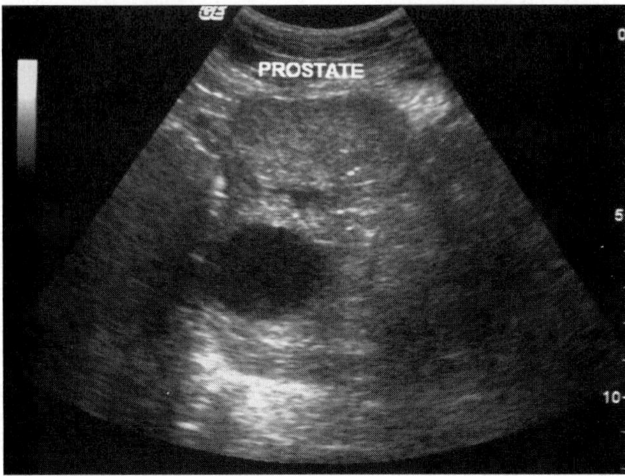

Fig. 43-15 This rough irregular cavity within the prostate gland is easily detected sonographically. Such cavities may represent small cysts or abscesses, but they are also seen with neoplasia. Such a finding warrants an ultrasound-guided biopsy or aspiration of the gland.

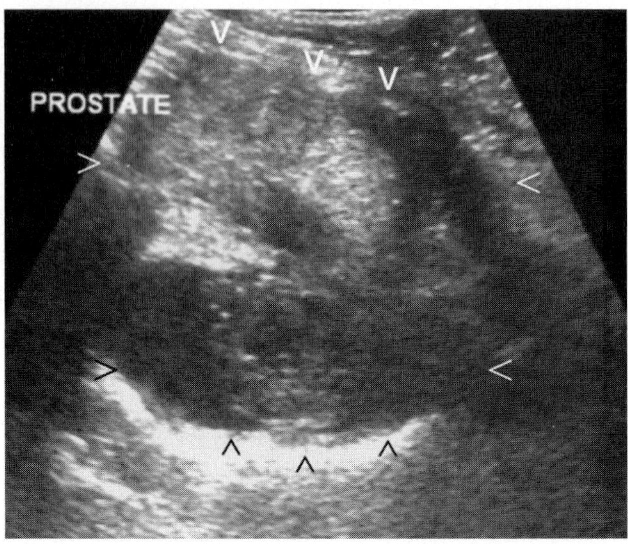

Fig. 43-16 Transverse sonographic image of the prostate gland. The margins of the gland *(black and white arrowheads)* are difficult to define. The prostate gland has a markedly mottled appearance. Some areas are quite hyperechoic and others almost sonolucent. Such a pattern is characteristic of neoplasia but may be seen in severe prostatitis.

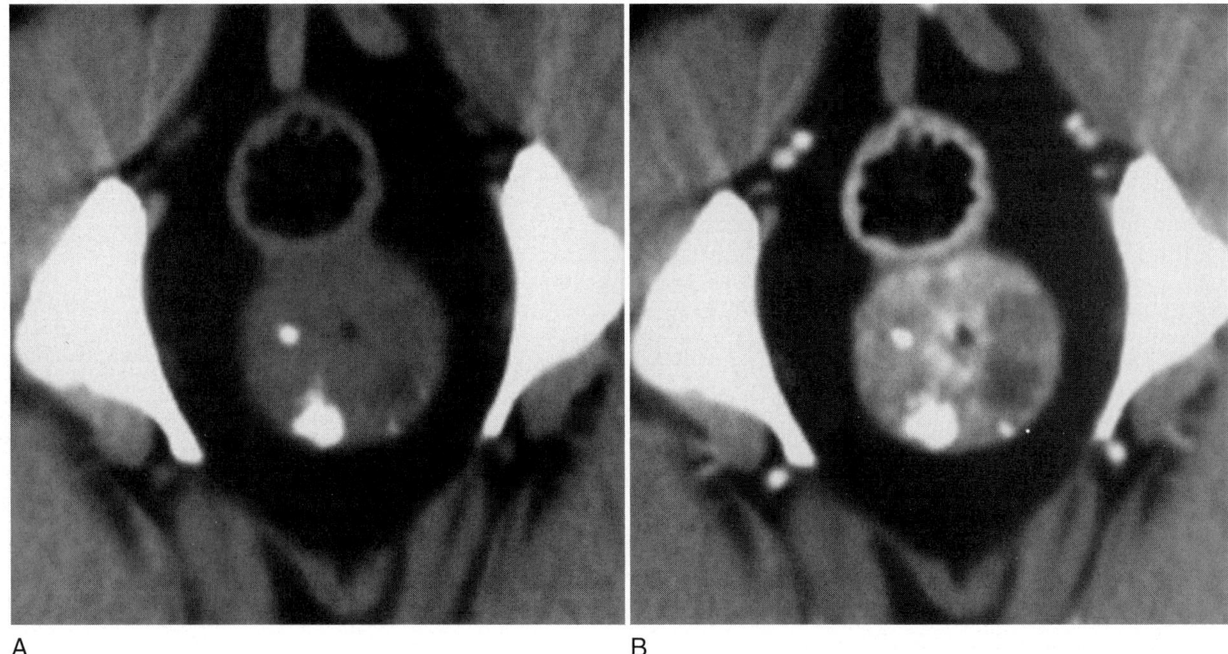

Fig. 43-17 CT examination of the prostate gland. **A,** This image indicates what appears to be symmetric enlargement of the prostate gland with irregular foci of calcification within it. **B,** This image acquired after the administration of intravenous contrast medium is at the same location as image **A**. Irregular contrast enhancement of the right side of the prostate gland and the area around the mineralization can be seen; this is consistent with the vascular lakes of neoplasia. The diagnosis of prostatic carcinoma was confirmed by ultrasound-guided biopsy.

tissue and the confusing shadows inherent in radiographs. Lesion conspicuity is less in CT images than in MR images. CT is more sensitive to changes in shape and opacity of the prostate gland than is standard radiography. For example, even without contrast medium administration, differentiation of cystic and solid cellular regions may be possible.

Contrast medium administered intravenously at the proper dose and time relative to scanning can markedly improve the diagnostic utility of CT. Contrast medium is conspicuous in the wall of cystic structures and the vascular lakes of most neoplastic lesions (Fig. 43-17). Hypertrophy of the gland and prostatitis are indicated by a uniform enlargement and change in attenuation with contrast. Minor changes in size and shape of the draining lymph nodes are also more easily detected with CT than with ultrasound. CT may also be used to guide biopsies of small intraglandular sites of suspicion with minimal special equipment needed.

MR imaging may also be used to assess the prostate gland; greater contrast generally exists between the prostate gland and the surrounding tissues and between normal and diseased prostate gland. In addition, cystic lesions can easily be detected without the use of contrast media, but small neoplastic lesions may not be. The greatest advantage of MR imaging is the excellent tissue contrast rendering afforded by the use of multiple different echo sequences, which allows better lesion characterization and and localization. The biggest drawback is the cost and availability of the procedure combined with availability of individuals experienced in the interpretation of the studies.

Within the next few years both CT and MR imaging will likely be increasingly used to characterize prostatic lesions and assess response to treatment as the availability of these modalities increases.

REFERENCES

1. Finco DR: Diseases of the prostate gland of the dog. In Morrow DA, editor: *Current therapy in theriogenology,* Philadelphia, 1980, WB Saunders.
2. O'Shea JD: Studies on the canine prostate gland: 1. Factors influencing its size and weight, *J Compend Pathol* 73:321, 1962.
3. Metten S: *A morphologic study of benign prostatic hypertrophy in the dog* [dissertation], Fort Collins, CO, 1978, Colorado State University.
4. Barsanti JA, Shotts EB Jr, Prasse K et al: Evaluation of diagnostic techniques for canine prostate disease, *J Am Vet Med Assoc* 177:160, 1980.
5. Gricne TP, Johnson RG: Diseases of the prostate gland. In Ettinger SI, editor: *Textbook of veterinary internal medicine: diseases of the dog and cat,* ed 2, Philadelphia, 1983, WB Saunders.
6. Rogers KS, Wanrschek L, Lees GE: Diagnostic evaluation of the canine prostate, *Compend Small Anim* 8:799, 1986.
7. Zolton GM, Gricner TP: Prostatic abscess: surgical approach, *J Am Anim Hosp Assoc* 14:698, 1978.
8. Barsanti JA, Finco DR: Canine bacterial prostatitis, *Vet Clin North Am* 9:679, 1979.
9. Kornegay J: Canine prostatic disease, *SW Vet* 26:257, 1973.
10. Zolton GM: Surgical techniques for the prostate, *Vet Clin North Am Small Anim Pract* 91:349, 1979.
11. Price D: Comparative aspects of development and structure in the prostate, *Natl Cancer Inst* 12:1, 1962.
12. Rife J, Thornburg LP: Osteocollagenous prostatic retention cyst in the canine, *Canine Pract* 7:44, 1980.
13. Weaver AD: Discrete prostatic (paraprostatic) cysts in the dog, *Vet Rec* 102:435, 1978.
14. O'Shea JD: Studies on the canine prostate gland: 11. Prostatic neoplasms, *J Comp Pathol* 73:244, 1963.
15. Weaver AD: Fifteen cases of prostatic carcinoma in the dog, *Vet Rec* 109:71, 1991.
16. Gill CW: Prostatic adenocarcinoma with concurrent Sertoli tumor in a dog, *Can Vet J* 22:230, 1981.
17. Grant CA: Carcinoma of the canine prostate, *Acta Pathol Scand* 40:197, 1957.
18. Rabaut SM, Kelch WJ: Undifferentiated carcinoma in the canine prostate, *Mod Vet Pract* 60:401, 1979.
19. Jameson RM: Prostatic abscess and carcinoma of the prostate, *Br J Urol* 40:288, 1968.
20. Leav E, Ling GV: Adenocarcinoma of the canine prostate, *Cancer* 22:1329, 1968.
21. Rendano VT Jr, Slauson DO: Hypertrophic osteopathy in a dog with prostate adenocarcinoma and without thoracic metastasis, *J Am Anim Hosp Assoc* 18:905, 1982.
22. Bortwiek R, Mackenzie CP: The signs and results of treatment of prostatic disease in dogs, *Vet Rec* 89:374, 1971.
23. Feeney DA, Johnston GR, Klausner JS et al: Canine prostatic disease—comparison of radiographic appearance with morphologic and microbiologic findings: 30 cases (1981-1985), *J Am Vet Med Assoc* 190:1018, 1987.
24. McClain DL: Surgical treatment of perineal prostatic abscesses, *J Am Anim Hosp Assoc* 18:794, 1982.
25. Zontine WJ: Radiographic interpretation: the prostate gland, *Mod Vet Pract* 56:341, 1975.
26. O'Brien T: Abdominal masses. In O'Brien T, Biery DN, editors: *Radiographic diagnosis of abdominal disorders in the dog and cat: radiographic interpretation, clinical signs, pathophysiology,* Philadelphia, 1978, WB Saunders, p 85.
27. Christensen GC: The urogenital apparatus. In Evans HE, Christensen GC, Miller ME, editors: *Miller's anatomy of the dog,* ed 2, Philadelphia, 1979, WB Saunders, p 565.
28. Franks LM: The spread of prostatic carcinoma to the bones, *J Pathol* 66:91, 1953.
29. Root CA: Urethrography. In Ticer JW, editor: *Radiographic techniques in veterinary practice,* ed 2, Philadelphia, 1984, WB Saunders, p 387.
30. Johnston GR, Feeney DA, Osborne CA, et al: Effects of intravesical hydrostatic pressure and volume on the distensibility of the canine prostatic portion of the urethra, *Am J Vet Res* 46:748, 1985.
31. Ackerman N: Prostatic reflux during positive contrast retrograde urethrography in the dog, *Vet Radiol* 24:251, 1983.
32. O'Brien T: Normal radiographic anatomy of the abdomen. In O'Brien T, Biery DN, editors: *Radiographic diagnosis of abdominal disorders in the dog and cat: radiographic interpretation, clinical signs, pathophysiology,* Philadelphia, 1978, WB Saunders, p 9.
33. Cartee RE, Rowles T: Transabdominal sonographic evaluation of the canine prostate, *Vet Radiol* 24:156, 1983.
34. Stowater JL, Lamb CR: Ultrasonographic features of paraprostatic cysts in 9 dogs, *Vet Radiol* 30:232, 1989.
35. Hager DA, Nyland TG, Fisher P: Ultrasound-guided biopsy of the canine liver, kidney and prostate, *Vet Radiol* 26:82, 1985.

ELECTRONIC RESOURCES evolve

Additional information related to the content in Chapter 43 can be found on the companion Web site at evolve http://evolve.elsevier.com/Thrall/vetrad/.

- Key Points
- Chapter Quiz
- Case Study 43-1

CHAPTER • 44
The Uterus, Ovaries, and Testes

Daniel A. Feeney
Gary R. Johnston

UTERUS

Imaging Procedures

The major applications of survey radiographs to diseases of the uterus lie in confirming that a palpable abdominal mass is consistent with an enlarged uterus or in identifying an enlarged uterus in a bitch that is difficult to palpate. Other uses for survey radiographs include assessment for the purposes of determining (1) fetal skeletons (i.e., number and degree of mineralization), (2) progress in variations of uterine size both during pregnancy and in disease states such as pyometra, and (3) to a limited degree, fetal viability, based principally on the absence of findings consistent with fetal demise. An understanding of possible conditions affecting the female genital tract is essential to the interpretation of the radiographic findings.[1-7]

Adequate attention must be paid to technical procedures to ensure maximal radiographic contrast because the uterus in disease states and without the presence of skeletal structures must be differentiated from the bladder, bowel, and other nonspecific abdominal masses. Unless the patient is critically ill, ideal preparation includes withholding food for 24 hours and administering enemas to evacuate the colon at least 2 hours before radiography.[8] Radiographic technique is also important when the early mineralization of fetal skeletons is assessed because, in the presence of a large uterus, early fetal mineralization may be masked by poor technique.

Abdominal compression has been suggested as a possible means by which the colon, uterus, and bladder may be differentiated radiographically.[8,9] The usefulness of this technique is basically limited to patients in which the uterus is not massively enlarged and can be aligned between the colon and urinary bladder by using a compression device—either a plastic paddle or a wooden kitchen spoon. An example of the type of separation that can be achieved is shown in Figure 44-1.

Ultrasonography is useful for the diagnosis of pregnancy in the bitch and the queen, for confirmation of fetal viability, and for development and use of tables to predict parturition date on the basis of fetal ultrasonographic characteristics.[1,7,10] It is also valuable in assessing a mildly enlarged uterus to determine whether the contents are fluid, as in pyometra; gestational sacs, indicative of pregnancy; a mixture of wall thickening and fluid suggestive of subinvolution[11]; or a mass, suggestive of neoplasia.[7,12-18]

In the normal anestrous bitch, the uterus is a tubular structure approximately the size of a collapsed small intestine. However, it lacks the central echogenic stripe seen in the submucosal and mucosal layers of the intestine. In a bitch in estrus, a limited echogenic stripe is seen in the area around the collapsed uterine lumen. Any fluid seen in the uterus is considered abnormal. This mildly echogenic stripe represents the development of the endometrium in response to hormonal stimulation. The normal uterus can be difficult to find, particularly in a bitch with gas accumulation in regional bowel structures. The normal uterus is easiest to locate between the urinary bladder and the colorectal junction. An example of normal uterus in an anestrous bitch is shown in Figure 44-2. Doppler ultrasound techniques have been applied to fetal and maternal assessments in the pregnant bitch but are not considered a routine part of a general work-up of either the pregnant or the nonpregnant bitch or queen.

Normal Imaging Findings

Nonpregnant Animal

The uterine body and horns cannot be seen in survey radiographs in the normal dog or cat unless the animal is pregnant.[3] The normal uterus is tubular, approximately 1 cm in diameter, and located in the mid- and caudal abdomen, with the uterine body between the colon and the bladder.[3] The radiopacity of the normal nongravid uterus is that of soft tissue, and it usually cannot be differentiated from small intestine on survey radiographs.

Pregnant Animal

The size, shape, and opacity of the canine uterus during pregnancy vary with the breed, the number of fetuses, and the stage of gestation. The fetal development and radiographic appearance of the uterus during gestation have been described in detail elsewhere,[6,8,19-23] but a brief summary follows. In general, uterine enlargement is detectable radiographically at approximately 30 days after ovulation.[6] The circumference of the uterine horns is then reported to be approximately 10 to 11 cm.[21] Spherical enlargements at the location of the gestational sacs are identifiable in the uterus between 30 and 40 days after ovulation.[6] The circumference at the spherical enlargement is then approximately 10 to 15 cm.[21] The uterus subsequently becomes smoothly tubular and has been described as sausage shaped at approximately 38 to 45 days after ovulation[6]; the circumference of the uterine horns is then approximately 12 to 17 cm.[21] Early fetal mineralization is identifiable by survey radiographs at or beyond 45 days after ovulation.[6] A near-term pregnancy in a normal bitch is shown radiographically in Figure 44-3.

The size, shape, and opacity of the feline uterus are similar to those of the dog. The feline uterus during gestation is described in considerable detail elsewhere,[23] but a brief summary follows. In the pregnant cat, radiographically detectable uterine enlargement occurs at approximately 25 to 35 days of gestation.

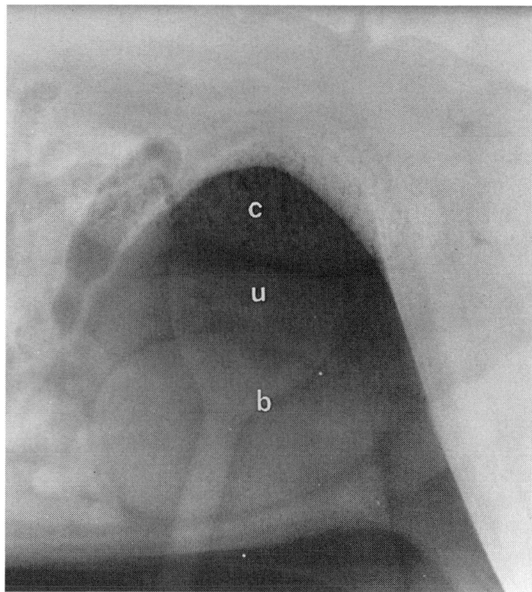

Fig. 44-1 Lateral view of the caudal abdomen. Local compression was applied during radiography with a wooden spoon. Note the separation of the colon *(c)*, uterus *(u)*, and urinary bladder *(b)*.

Fetal mineralization is identified at approximately 36 to 45 days of gestation and progresses beyond this time.

The location of the pregnant uterus in both the dog and the cat is in the mid- to caudal ventral abdomen at mid- to late gestation. The enlargement of the uterus at this site causes cranial and somewhat dorsal displacement of the small intestine, with dorsal and lateral displacement of the descending colon and some degree of ventral compression of the urinary bladder.[8]

Although details are available elsewhere,[13,14,16,17] the following is a working assessment of pregnancy focused on the dog. The earliest suggested time for ultrasonographic assessment of pregnancy is between 25 and 30 days' gestational age. The closer to 30 days' gestational age, the more likely a clearly defined heartbeat will be detected. A common problem is assessment too early in the gestation (particularly when the breeding dates are uncertain), which usually yields equivocal results. Although small cystlike gestational sacs can be found at approximately 20 days' gestational age, a true gestational sac is easily identified in the 25- to 30-day range (Fig. 44-4). In the 30- to 40-day range of gestational age, the conceptus begins to take shape (e.g., not just a disc or a rounded aggregate). After approximately 40 days, evidence of mineralization can be found and identification of the stomach, urinary bladder, heart, and great vessels becomes progressively easier with time (Fig. 44-5). In the authors' experience, the radiographic assessment of distal limb bone development is still the best predictor of late-term gestational age.[6,20] Similar

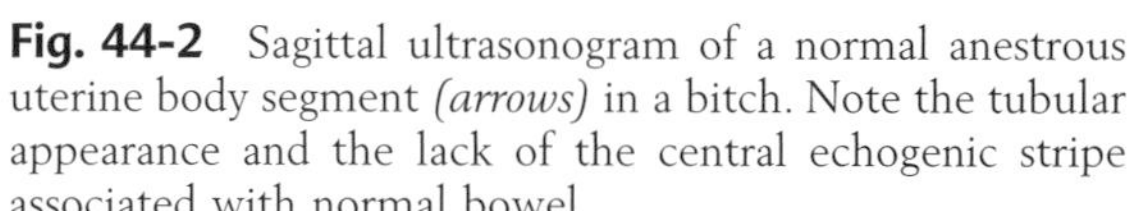

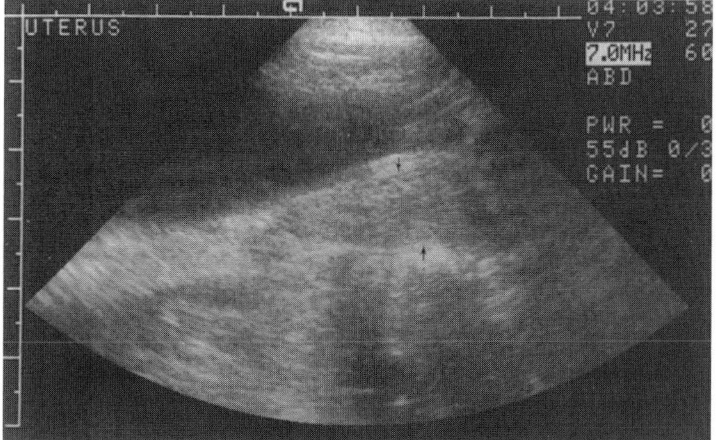

Fig. 44-2 Sagittal ultrasonogram of a normal anestrous uterine body segment *(arrows)* in a bitch. Note the tubular appearance and the lack of the central echogenic stripe associated with normal bowel.

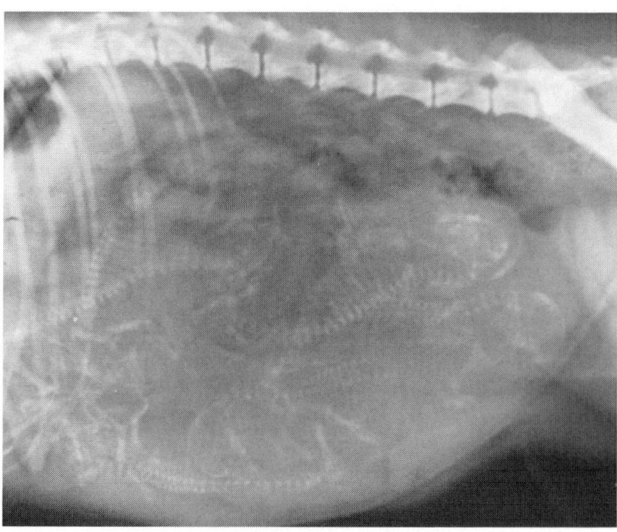

Fig. 44-3 A normal pregnancy, near term, in a bitch (lateral view). In the fetuses, note the mineralization and alignment of the skull bones as well as the arrangement of the cervical through lumbar vertebrae and the pelvis with the appendages.

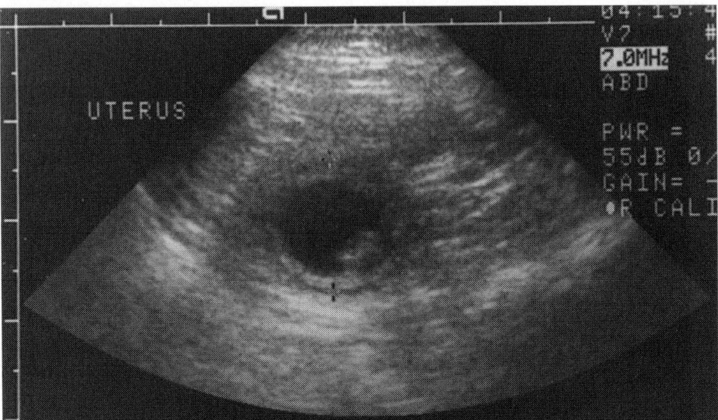

Fig. 44-4 Ultrasonogram of an early pregnancy (approximately 25 days' gestational age) in a dog. The fetal vesicle is within the *cursors.*

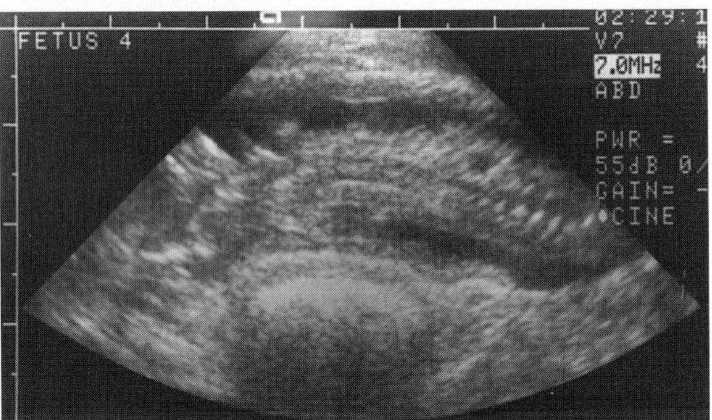

Fig. 44-5 Ultrasonogram of a late second- and early third-trimester pregnancy (±40 days' gestational age) in a bitch. The spine is clearly visible, but almost no shadowing is present because of limited mineralization.

information is available for the queen.[24] However, ultrasonographic assessment is best for assessing fetal viability and well-being.[17] As a rule of thumb, the fetal heart rate should be 1.5 to 2.0 times that of the bitch or queen. A slow heart rate raises concern about fetal distress. A search for a fetus must be made in an organized fashion by checking both horns and the body. As for late-term gestational aging, survey radiographs have been more accurate for counting fetuses than has ultrasound. Ultrasound is, however, a useful tool for assessment of the postpartum uterine status.[25]

Abnormal Imaging Findings

Number

Absence of one of the horns in a normally bicornuate uterus has been reported,[26] but this is rare.

Size

Generalized uterine enlargement seen radiographically in the absence of fetal mineralization is suggestive of a number of diseases in addition to the early phases of normal pregnancy before fetal mineralization. Differential diagnoses that should be considered under these circumstances include early pregnancy and possibly pseudopregnancy[6-8,27]; pyometra, hydrometra, and mucometra[3-8,27,28]; uterine torsion[3-8,29-31]; uterine entrapment[32]; hydrocolpos[33]; cystic endometrial hyperplasia[34]; and uterine adenomyosis.[35-37] Representative examples of diffuse uterine enlargement are shown in Figures 44-6 and 44-7.

Generalized uterine enlargement in the presence of fetal mineralization is suggestive of pregnancy, but the possibility of torsion of the pregnant uterus should not be excluded. Clinical signs and history must then be used to differentiate these possibilities.

Localized uterine enlargement is suggestive of a number of diseases, including neoplasia[3,38]; cystic endometrial hyperplasia[2,38]; localized or loculated pyometra, hydrometra, or mucometra[28]; uterine stump granuloma or abscess[7,8,39]; cystic uterine remnant[40]; and uterine adenomyosis.[35-37] Focal uterine body enlargement confirmed as a uterine stump granuloma with urinary bladder invasion and a fistulous tract draining into the flank are shown in Figure 44-8.

Location

The normal location of the uterus in the caudal ventral mid-abdomen has been discussed, and its detection, location, and effect on adjacent organs are highly dependent on its size.[3,8] Herniation of the uterus through discontinuities in the abdominal wall, including the inguinal ring, may occur and be congenital or acquired.[3,32] These herniations may also occur during pregnancy. An example of uterine herniation into the subcutaneous tissues by way of the inguinal canal is shown in Figure 44-9. This uterus was in the stages of gestation before fetal mineralization.

Radiopacity

The normal nonpregnant and early pregnant uterus is of soft tissue or fluid radiopacity.[3-8] Other uterine conditions that also have soft tissue radiographic characteristics are pyometra, hydrometra, mucometra, hydrocolpos, and uterine torsion.[3-8,29,31,33] As previously mentioned, history and clinical signs are necessary to differentiate these possibilities. Gas within the uterus is generally indicative of fetal death[3,5,6] or ischemia from uterine torsion,[2] but emphysematous pyometra has been reported.[41] In both instances the gas is caused by devitalization and breakdown of the tissues. An example of an emphysematous fetus is shown in Figure 44-10. Traumatic attempts at catheterization of the cervix can artifactually introduce gas and be overinterpreted as evidence of intrauterine disease. The other possibility is that a gas-forming organism within an abscess of the uterine stump in the neutered patient may cause focal accumulation of air, but this is highly unlikely.[8]

Mineralization within the uterus is usually indicative of fetal skeletons, but the alignment of the structures, such as vertebrae, ribs, and limbs, and the shape and alignment of skull bones must be assessed to differentiate a radiographically viable fetus, a dead fetus, and a mummified fetus.[5,6] In general, radiographic evidence of axial or appendicular skeletal malalignment or collapse of the skull bones is suggestive of fetal death. Overlap and apparent compression of the structures into a smaller than expected space is more suggestive of mummification than of a recent history of fetal death. An example of a mummified fetus is shown in Figure 44-11.

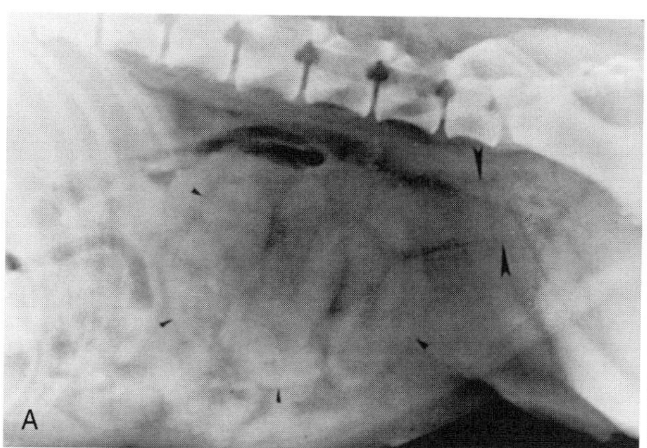

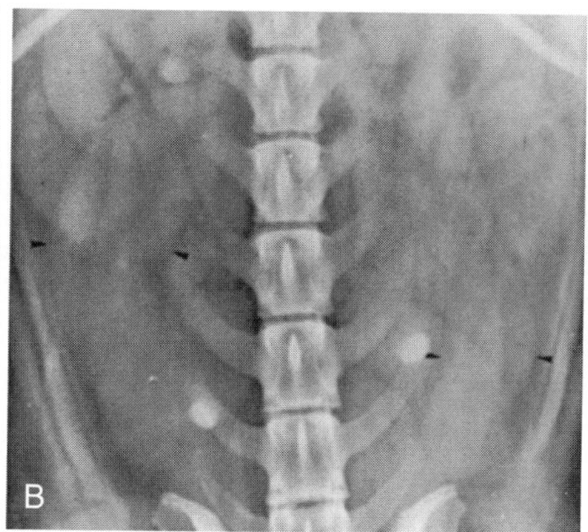

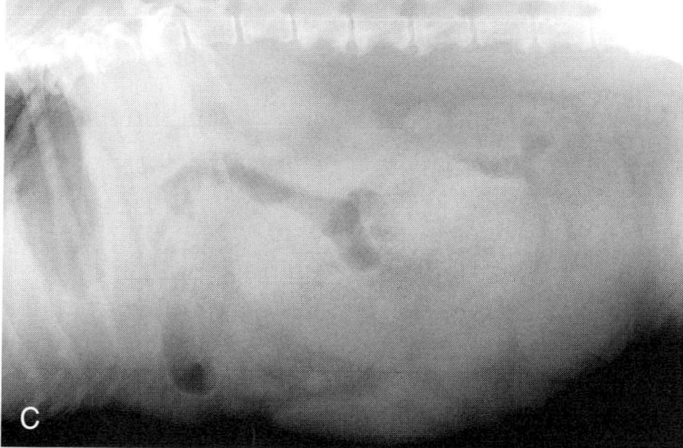

Fig. 44-6 Lateral (A) and ventrodorsal (B) radiographs of a patient with a tubular, coiled, soft tissue structure in the caudal abdomen that extends into the pelvis *(arrowheads)*. This is a moderately distended uterus, as found in pyometra. **C,** Lateral view of a patient with a caudoventral abdominal mass that occupies approximately 50% of the abdominal cavity. Displacement of the viscera is consistent with uterine enlargement.

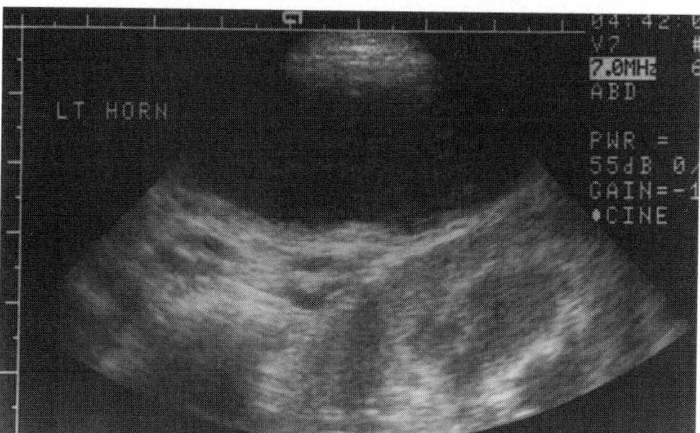

Fig. 44-7 Transverse ultrasonogram of the left uterine horn in a bitch that is filled with complex fluid. This is typical of what is seen in canine pyometra.

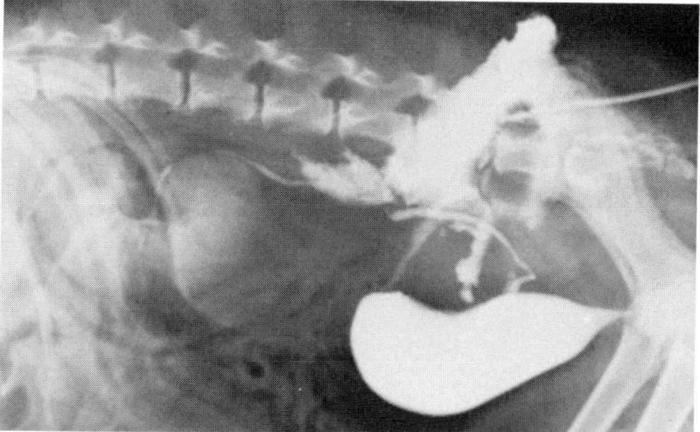

Fig. 44-8 Lateral view after excretory urography and left-flank fistulography. A draining tract in the left flank injected with contrast medium leads to a soft tissue mass, which displaces the urinary bladder ventrally and indents it dorsally. Only the right kidney and ureter are identified. Radiologic diagnosis was probable uterine stump granuloma with chronic obstruction of the left ureter. The diagnosis was confirmed at laparotomy.

If the fetal skeleton appears to be tightly curled, is more obvious than expected when surrounded by uterus, or is not associated with a tubular uterine radiopacity or its expected location, the possibility of ectopic pregnancy should be considered.[42-44] Peritoneal effusion may complicate the assessment of the uterine boundaries in these patients and may further confuse the diagnosis with the possibility of acute uterine rupture[45] rather than ectopic pregnancy.[42,43] Ultrasonography is of value in this situation.[7,18]

Function

Dystocia may be caused by both maternal and fetal factors.[46] Radiographs are of minimal value in determining the maternal factors, such as uterine contractility, other than for assessment of the size relation between the fetus and the maternal pelvic canal. Radiography may be helpful in assessing one of the fetal factors—positioning relative to the maternal pelvic canal—thus providing additional evidence for the necessity of cesarean section (Fig. 44-12). If no fetus is lodged in the birth canal, another consideration is uterine inertia. Survey radiographs may also be of value in the postpartum bitch to determine the possibility of a retained fetus, but routine follow-up radiography of every pregnancy is not indicated.

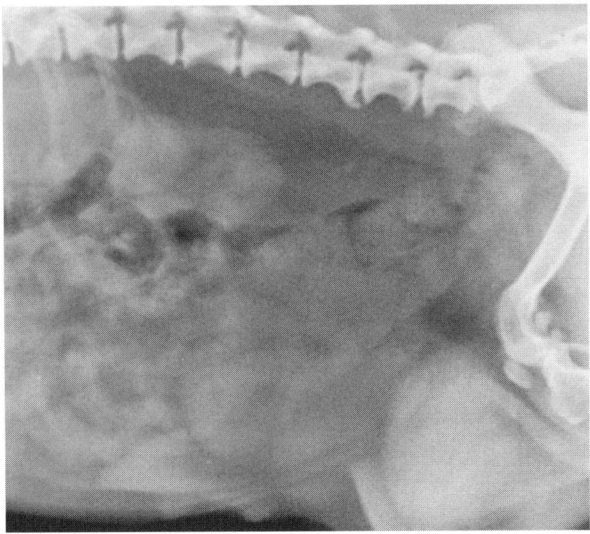

Fig. 44-9 Lateral view of a bitch in mid-term pregnancy with an inguinal mass. The tubular soft tissue opacity representing the uterus extends into the subcutaneous periinguinal tissues. Radiologic diagnosis was inguinal hernia containing a portion of dilated uterus, probably as a result of pregnancy.

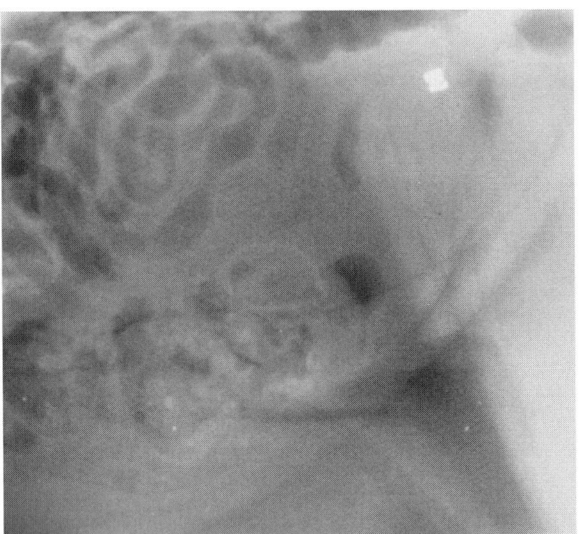

Fig. 44-10 Close-up lateral view of the ventral abdomen. A moderately mineralized fetus is within the uterus. Gas is surrounding the fetus, however. Radiologic diagnosis was emphysematous fetus.

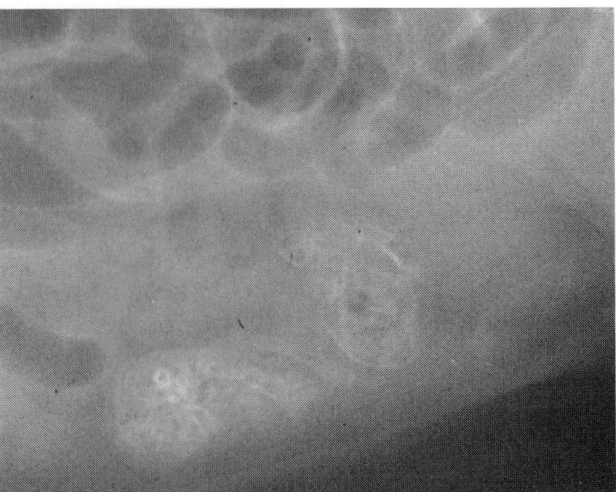

Fig. 44-11 Lateral view of a previously pregnant bitch. An irregularly mineralized mass with some evidence of skull and tubular bones is visible and located outside the intestinal tract and in a region consistent with that of the uterus. Radiologic diagnosis was mummified fetus. The diagnosis was confirmed at surgery.

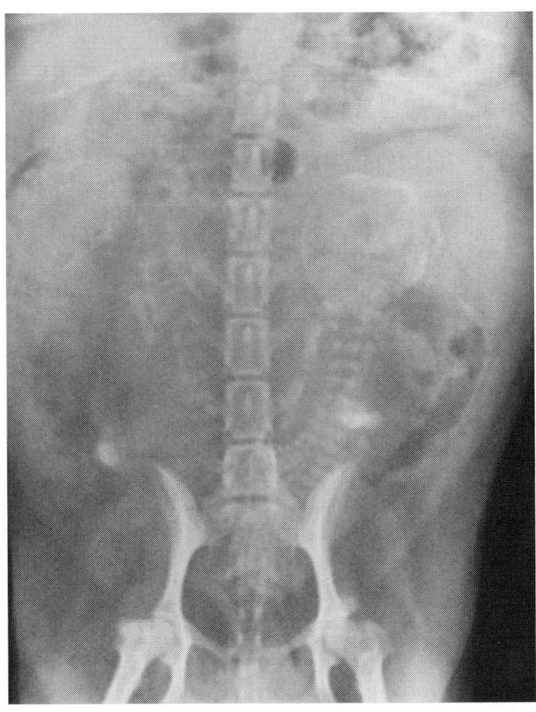

Fig. 44-12 Ventrodorsal view of a small-breed bitch in dystocia. Note the transverse presentation of the enlarged, but as determined radiographically, viable fetus. Surgical diagnosis was viable single fetus.

OVARIES

Imaging Procedures

Survey radiographs have limited applicability to the ovaries. Because ovaries are the basis of reproduction, exposure to ionizing radiation should be minimized. The major application of survey radiographs to the ovary is that of identifying a mass not palpable at physical examination or further localizing an abdominal mass to the ovary. On the basis of location, displacement of adjacent organs, and radiographic opacity, the organ of origin of the mass may be determined.[8] Survey radiographs are of considerable value in differentiating ovarian, splenic, and renal masses. The limitations are that normal ovaries cannot be visualized and the internal architecture of ovarian masses cannot be assessed by radiography unless mineralization is present; such mineralization is uncommon.

Excretory urography may be of assistance in assessing ovarian masses by assisting in the identification of and distinction from the ipsilateral kidney. Excretory urography may also be helpful to determine the degree of renal displacement and separate renal parenchyma from that of the ovary if the mass has not resulted in ventral migration of the ovary ventrally into the abdomen away from the kidney.

Another technique that is extremely valuable in assessing intraabdominal masses, including ovarian masses, is that of ultrasonography.[7,12-18] Ultrasonographic techniques are useful

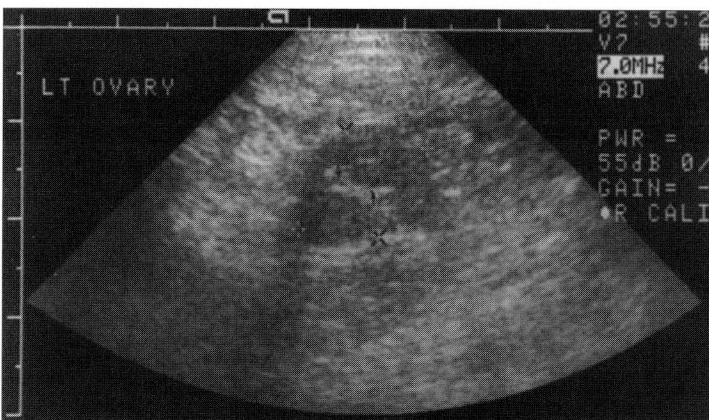

Fig. 44-13 Sagittal ultrasonogram of a normal anestrous ovary (within the *cursors*) in a bitch. Note the subtle follicles of fairly uniform size *(arrows)*.

in assessing general and follicular ovarian architecture, which facilitates determination of ovarian activity and staging of ovarian masses. The anestrous ovary in the bitch and the queen has follicles in the early stages of development (Fig. 44-13). It may also contain complex or echogenic areas indicative of corpora hemorrhagica or corpora lutea. As estrus approaches, selected follicles become disproportionately larger. The use of ultrasound to determine prime breeding time has not become a routine procedure in the bitch and queen as it has in the large domestic species, however. However, Doppler ultrasonographic techniques may provide some insight on ovarian circulatory status during the various phases of the estrus cycle.[47] Further details are available in the literature.[12,13]

Normal Imaging Findings

The normal ovaries, located just caudal to the kidneys, are not seen radiographically.[2,6] The ovaries are not, however, functionally retroperitoneal as are the kidneys, and ovarian masses gravitate ventrally without extensive ventral displacement of other abdominal viscera, such as that caused by a renal mass.[48]

Sonographically the normal ovary can be difficult to find unless the bitch or queen is cooperative or sedated. At sonography the ovary is often slightly ventral and slightly lateral to the caudal pole of the ipsilateral kidney. Visualization of the multiple anechoic follicles facilitates identification of the ovary and differentiation of it from other intraperitoneal structures.

Abnormal Imaging Findings

Number

Usually only one ovary, but occasionally both, may be radiographically abnormal. In the authors' opinion, the ovary must increase in size to at least the diameter of two bowel loops to be identifiable on survey radiographs. The shape of the abnormal ovary may be variable, but ovarian masses are usually well circumscribed.[8] If the ovarian mass is neoplastic, peritoneal fluid may also be present.

Size

A radiographically detectable mass in the appropriate anatomic region for the ovary, which is usually caudal to the respective kidney and originating from the dorsal abdominal wall, should have certain differential considerations: follicular cyst, [49,50] luteal cyst,[49,50] tumors of gonadostromal origin,[49,51] tumors of epithelial origin,[49,51] germ cell tumors,[49,52] tumors of mesodermal origin,[49,52] and hydrovarium.[28] An example of a well-circumscribed ovarian mass is shown in Figure 44-14.

Location

The normal ovaries lie caudal to their respective kidneys. As ovaries enlarge, they may displace the ipsilateral kidney cranially or laterally and may pull it ventrally. The degree and direction of adjacent organ displacement and the extent of ovarian mass migration depend on ovarian size and the position of the patient during radiography. Abdominal viscera other than those specifically described above may be displaced.

The role of ultrasonography in detecting ovarian mass lesions is fourfold. The first role is identification of the mass, particularly if it is not visible (but clinically suspected) on survey radiographs. Second, the determination must be made that the mass is an ovary, often by exclusion of association with other regional structures. Locating some small follicular structures on the perimeter is useful because the anestrous ovary can be difficult to locate (see Fig. 44-13). In that circumstance, what the mass is not attached to or an extension of must be determined, with ovarian mass being ruled out on the basis of location, including the controversial possibility of ovarian remnant.[53] Third, because many ovarian masses are malignant,[51,52,54-57] the concern is whether local or regional spread has occurred. The search for peritoneal seeding, abdominal fluid collections, and nodules in any other abdominal organs is the goal to stage the potential malignancy appropriately. Fourth, because malignant versus benign ovarian masses have no specific sonographic architecture to differentiate them, nearly the only architectural characteristic that can be comfortably assessed are follicular cysts. A fluid-filled cavity with no internal echoes; smooth, thin walls; and good echo enhancement beyond it is most likely to be a benign follicular cyst if the clinical signs are consistent.

Radiopacity

Ovarian cysts and most ovarian neoplasms are of soft tissue opacity.[49,51] Ovarian neoplasms may occasionally contain mineralized areas, including those with the opacity of bone or tooth enamel. Such masses are usually benign teratomas (dermoid cysts),[49,51] but malignant teratocarcinomas have also been reported to contain mineralization.[42] On the basis of this assessment and the vast difference in prognosis for these two types of tumors, basing prognosis on the presence of mineralization is ill advised.

Consideration

The possibility of intersex conditions should be considered, including the true and pseudohermaphrodite.[58,59] Complex anomalies encompassing the entire genital tract and involving the urinary tract should be considered in patients with other intraabdominal abnormalities or combined urinary and reproductive signs. Although contrast radiographic procedures and ultrasonographic evaluation may be of assistance in analyzing the anomaly, the anomalous tissue often needs to be removed and then evaluated by dissection and histologic examina-

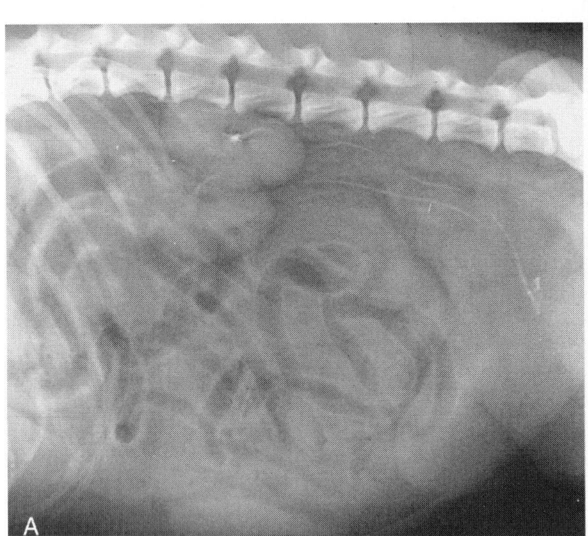

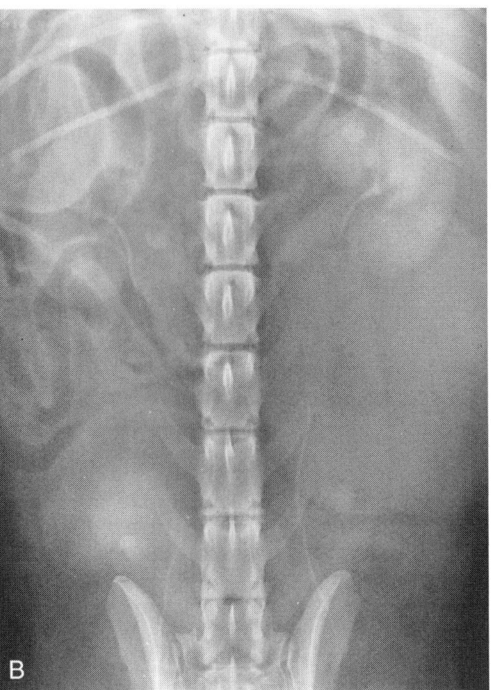

Fig. 44-14 Lateral (A) and ventrodorsal (B) views of a patient with a soft tissue abdominal mass approximately four times the size of the left kidney and located caudal and ventral to it. The mass is not clearly seen in the lateral view but is causing deformation of the dorsal and cranial aspects of the bladder by compression. Kidneys are opacified as a result of the injection of contrast medium. The location of the soft tissue mass is consistent with a mass arising from the ovary. Diagnosis was ovarian cyst (made at surgery).

tion.[7,18] Testosterone-producing female genital structures may also cause a complex clinical presentation and should be considered.[54]

TESTES

Imaging Procedures

Survey radiographs have limited applicability to the intrascrotal testes. Radiographs are, however, of value in the assessment of abdominal masses, which include neoplastic transformation of an intraabdominal testicle. In addition, testicular exposure to the mutagenic effects of ionizing radiation should be limited. An additional method that does provide information on the intrascrotal and intraabdominal testicular architecture is ultrasonography.[60-65] The testicle, particularly in the dog, is relatively easily scanned as long as it is in the scrotal sac. However, retained but normal testicles are at best difficult and often impossible to find if they are intraabdominal because of masking by bowel gas. Testicles between the inguinal ring and the scrotal sac can be identified if an organized and tedious search is implemented. For perspective, one study suggested that cryptorchidism is identified at the time of castration in approximately 6.8% of male dogs and approximately 1.3% of male cats.[66] The normal testicle has an echogenic capsule (tunica albuginea) and a uniform parenchymal echotexture similar to that of the spleen (Fig. 44-15). In the longitudinal center of the testicle, the mediastinal testes (rete testes) can be found. This is a useful architectural structure to help determine if parenchymal disruptions have changed the regional echotexture (e.g., an isoechoic mass). The epididymis is usually hypoechoic to the testicle and lies approximately dorsomedial to the testicle. It has a more coarse echotexture than

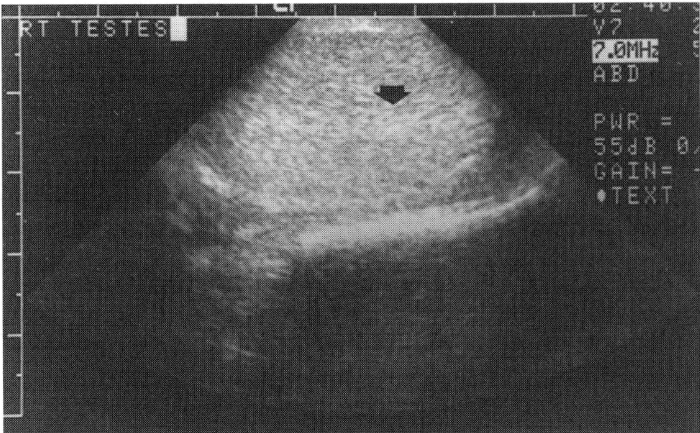

Fig. 44-15 Sagittal ultrasonogram of a normal canine testicle. Note the mediastinum testes *(arrow)*.

the testicle, but this is a subjective assessment. Any fluid seen in the scrotal sac is considered abnormal, and a search for its cause should be undertaken. Doppler techniques allow visualization of the arterial and venous flow in the testicle and the regional vascular structures.[67,68] If available, this is a useful tool in the noninvasive assessment of testicular torsion.

Normal Imaging Findings

Because the testicles, epididymis, and scrotum are all soft tissue structures, radiography is of minimal value in the evaluation of these organs in small animals. The accessibility of the scrotum to visual and digital inspection further minimizes the usefulness of radiography. Radiography may occasionally provide some information on the opacity (such as mineral and air) of an abnormality detected by palpation. Ultrasonography is of assistance in noninvasively assessing the internal architecture of the testicle and epididymis, accurately assessing testicular size[69] as well as clarifying the nature of scrotal enlargement.[60,62-65]

Abnormal Imaging Findings

Detailed discussion of the embryogenesis of the testes, gubernaculum, and scrotum is beyond the scope of this text, but further details can be found in the literature.[70,71] As with ovarian diseases, intersex anomalies must be considered. These anomalies may be evaluated by of contrast procedures of the lower and upper urinary tract as well as by ultrasonography, although the final diagnosis is usually determined surgically and microscopically.[58,70] Most of the following discussion deals with sequelae of cryptorchidism amenable to radiographic assessment.

Intraabdominal testicles of normal dimension usually cannot be identified radiographically. If the intraabdominal testicle enlarges, however, the following considerations may apply.

Size and Shape

To be detected radiographically, the enlarged intraabdominal testicle must be two or more times the diameter of the normal small intestine. When such a structure is identified, it must also be differentiated from other soft tissue structures in the abdomen, such as fluid-filled bowel, bladder, spleen, and possibly the prostate gland. In general, the radiologic consideration of the mass as an intraabdominal testicle results either from the knowledge that only one testicle was descended or identified at castration or by the fact that the mass cannot be associated with any other organ in a male patient. The shape of the enlarged, and probably neoplastically transformed, intraabdominal testicle is usually fairly symmetrical, with varying degrees of surface irregularity.

Number and Radiopacity

Usually only one of the testicles is responsible for the abdominal abnormalities in a given patient, even if both testicles are intraabdominal. The radiographic opacity of intraabdominal testicles is usually that of soft tissue, and no specificity may be assigned to the identification of calcific opacity within these masses; such an opacity is most likely to be dystrophic calcification rather than suggestive of teratoma and teratocarcinoma, as in the bitch.

Location

Intraabdominal testicles, when identified radiographically as an abdominal mass, usually lie somewhere in a parasagittal plane between the caudal pole of the ipsilateral kidney and the inguinal canal. The authors' experience suggests that these testicles usually gravitate to the ventral abdomen as they enlarge, causing dorsal and lateral displacement of the small intestine and possible indentation or caudal displacement of the urinary bladder. An example of a neoplastically transformed intraabdominal testicle is shown in Figure 44-16. Testicles may be identified in the inguinal canal or subcutaneous structures of the inguinal region. Subcutaneous soft tissue masses in this region in a male dog may be identified radiographically, but differentiation from lymph node, subcutaneous tumor, or another nonspecific mass requires ultrasonographic assessment (Fig. 44-17) and probable microscopic examination of a fine-needle aspirate.

Consideration

An intraabdominal mass identified in a male dog fitting the size, shape, and location criteria previously described must be differentiated from other intraabdominal organs, including

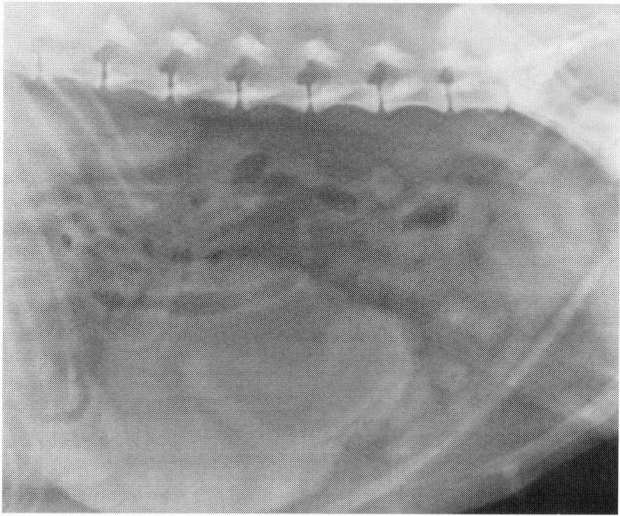

Fig. 44-16 Lateral radiograph of a male dog with an abdominal mass and only one palpable, descended testicle. The abdominal mass in the caudal midventral abdomen is approximately four to six times the size of the kidneys. Radiographic diagnosis was well-circumscribed intraabdominal mass, probably a retained intraabdominal testicle. The diagnosis was confirmed at laparotomy.

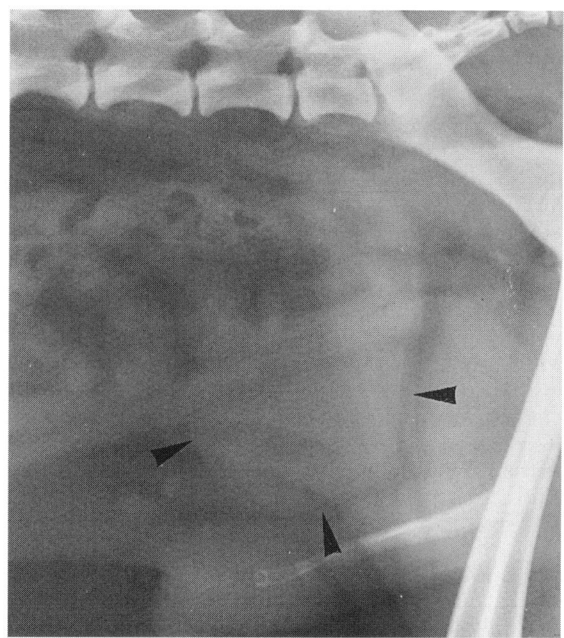

Fig. 44-17 Lateral view of a male dog in which only one testicle was intrascrotal. An ovoid soft tissue mass *(arrowheads)* is in the periinguinal soft tissues in the region of the os penis. Surgical diagnosis was malignant transformation of an incompletely descended testicle.

the spleen, bladder, cecum, and prostate gland; a nonspecific mesenteric mass; and a mass originating within the intestinal tract. Ultrasonographic examination can be valuable in this differentiation.[63] Fine-needle aspiration biopsy and laparotomy are alternatives worthy of consideration.

The mass, which is possibly testicle, may represent a neoplastically transformed, retained testicle[51] or torsion of an intraabdominal testicle without neoplastic transforma-

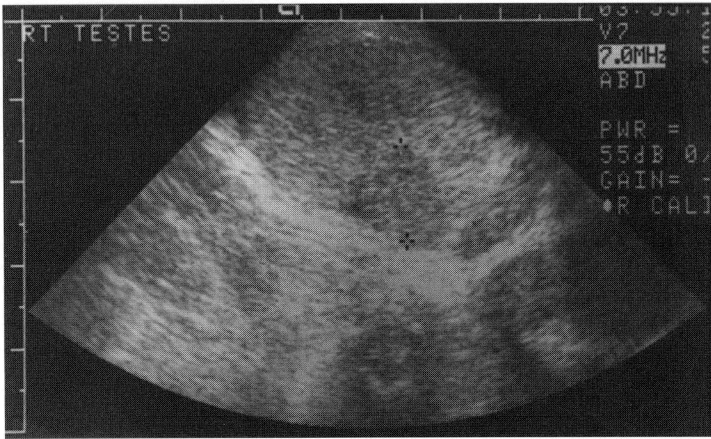

Fig. 44-18 Sagittal ultrasonogram of a testicle in which a hypoechoic mass (within the *cursors*) can be seen. Sonographic appearance is not specific for tumor cell type or differentiation of malignant versus benign lesions.

tion.[64,72,73] Differentiation of these processes is based on the history, abdominal palpation, and reproductive and cutaneous manifestations of endocrine abnormalities—that is, feminization—associated with neoplastic testicular tissue. Of note, some testicular tumors may invade locally or regionally and be locally invasive and metastasize to some unexpected distant organs.[74,75]

Intrascrotal Testicle

Size and shape are the major features used to assess the intrascrotal testicle for potential abnormalities. Symmetric enlargement of the testicle or hemiscrotum is suggestive of hydrocele,[63,75] orchitis,[77,78] intrascrotal testicular torsion,[63,72,79] parasitic migration,[80] feline infectious peritonitis in cats,[81] and nonspecific vascular abnormalities.[76] Observation of the testicular mass and spermatic cord at scrotal exploratory surgery is the most definitive means of differentiation among the scrotal contents and is not associated with the known genetic result of ionizing radiation to the opposite testicle. Asymmetric enlargement of the intrascrotal testicle is suggestive of neoplasia,[51] varicocele,[63] hematoma, abscess, epididymitis,[76] and epididymal sperm granulomas[82]; differentiation of these possibilities may be facilitated by information from the history and fine-needle aspiration biopsy.

As previously mentioned, an additional means of assessing the internal contents of the scrotum, including the testicle, is ultrasonography.[60-65] This method permits identification of the source of scrotal enlargement as to testicle, fluid retention, associated mass and, if the testicle is the site of enlargement, the internal architecture of the mass. An example of a focal testicular mass is shown in Figure 44-18.

ABNORMAL INTRAABDOMINAL FINDINGS RELATED TO THE UTERUS, OVARIES, AND TESTES

Unexplained intraabdominal calcific opacities may be related to previous uterine rupture or ectopic pregnancy and subsequent mummification of the involved fetuses. Careful radiographic scrutiny of the character of the calcified intraabdominal masses and the possible use of serial radiographs to assess reproducibility of the location are indicated. Occasionally, ingestion of an intact body of a puppy or other small mammal by the patient may complicate the diagnosis of intrauterine fetal calcification, intraabdominal ectopic pregnancy, or fetal mummification.

Variations in abdominal contrast may be somewhat nonspecific in that accumulation of abdominal fluid and free intraperitoneal air has numerous causes. The presence of abdominal fluid, however, especially if the patient has intestinal displacement (based on the intestine containing gas, so it can be recognized) consistent with an enlarged uterus, may be suggestive of uterine rupture with subsequent hemorrhage, ruptured pyometra, or hemorrhage from uterine torsion. Free intraperitoneal air in such patients, especially in the presence of intrauterine (perifetal) or intrafetal air, is highly suggestive of uterine rupture and fetal death.

Peritoneal effusion, which may occur from a wide variety of causes, may result from peritoneal seeding and diffuse metastasis of malignant ovarian tumors or hemorrhage from rupture of an ovarian tumor.[56] Although ovarian tumors are less often the cause of malignant effusion, abdominal hemorrhage, or both, these lesions should at least be considered as differential possibilities in an intact bitch.

Medial iliac lymphadenopathy may be identified in patients with testicular disease and is most suggestive of metastasis[78,83] or extension of an inflammatory process. Lumbar vertebral osteomyelitis and discospondylitis have been reported in patients with inflammatory diseases of the testicle, specifically including infection with *Brucella canis.*[84]

One final consideration of genital imaging is the vagina. Although this organ usually is accessible by direct visualization facilitated by various endoscopic devices, at times contrast radiographic imaging is the only method of viewing the area cranial to the vestibule. Positive-contrast vaginography is the retrograde filling of the vestibule and vagina.[85] Vaginography is performed with sterile, iodinated contrast medium diluted to approximately 150 to 200 mg of iodine/mL. The contrast medium is injected through a balloon catheter that has been placed just inside of the vulvar lips with appropriate sedation. Retrograde injection is performed until mild resistance to injection is met. A lateral view is made to determine the degree of filling. Retrograde injection is continued if the vagina is not well distended. Overdistention may result in expulsion of the contrast medium as a result of an abdominal press. Vaginography may be used to localize vaginal or vestibular masses, clefts, and stenoses or strictures.[7,86-88] An example of a vaginal stricture is shown in Figure 44-19. Vaginography may also be useful in the clarification of morphology in the incontinent bitch.[89] Vaginal pooling of urine mimicking incontinence caused by ectopic ureter or sphincter-related incontinence can be assessed by the combination of postvoiding radiographs after an excretory urogram (looking for vaginal staining/pooling) and a retrograde positive-contrast vaginogram (looking for strictures, masses, etc.) that could alter the normal relation among the external urethral orifice, the vagina, and the vestibule. When ectopic ureters connect to the vagina, vaginography can also further clarify this in addition to what is possible by excretory urography.[89]

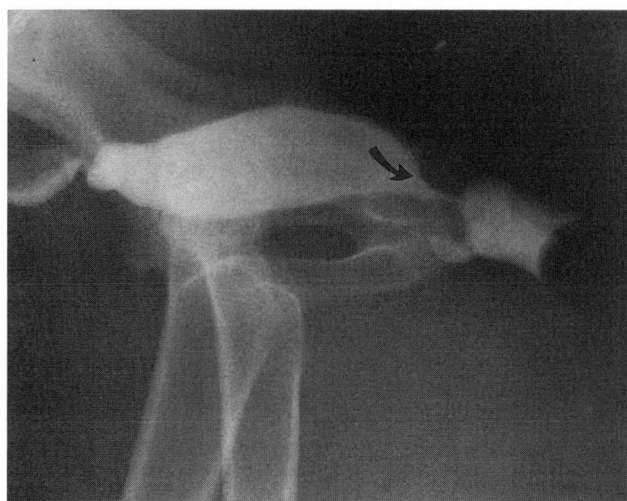

Fig. 44-19 Lateral view of a bitch during retrograde positive-contrast vaginography. Note the narrowing at the interface of the vestibule and the vagina *(arrow)*. Radiographic diagnosis was vaginal stricture.

REFERENCES

1. England G: Infertility in the bitch and queen. In Arthur GH, Noakes DE, Pearson H et al, editors: *Veterinary reproduction and obstetrics,* ed 7, Philadelphia, 1996, WB Saunders, p 516.
2. Morrow DA: *Current therapy in theriogenology,* Philadelphia, 1986, WB Saunders.
3. Ackerman N: Radiographic evaluation of the uterus: a review, *Vet Radiol* 22:252, 1981.
4. Kenney KJ, Matthiesen DT, Brown NO et al: Pyometra in cats: 183 cases (1979-1984), *J Am Vet Med Assoc* 191:1130, 1987.
5. Farrow CS, Morgan JP, Story EC: Late term fetal death in the dog: early radiographic diagnosis, *J Am Vet Radiol Soc* 17:11, 1976.
6. Rendano VJ: Radiographic evaluation of fetal development in the bitch and fetal death in the bitch and queen. In Kirk RW, editor: *Current veterinary therapy VIII,* Philadelphia, 1983, WB Saunders, p 947.
7. Rivers B, Johnston GR: Imaging of the reproductive organs of the bitch: methods and limitations, *Vet Clin North Am Small Anim Pract* 21:437, 1991.
8. Root CN: Interpretation of abdominal survey radiographs, *Vet Clin North Am* 4:763, 1974.
9. Ambrust LJ, Biller DS, Hoskinson JJ: Compression radiography: and old technique revisited, *J Am Anim Hosp Assoc* 36:537, 2000.
10. Son CH, Jeong KA, Kim JH et al: Establishment of the prediction table of parturition day with ultrasonography in small pet dogs, *J Vet Med Sci* 63:715, 2001.
11. Reberg SR, Peter AT, Blevins WE: Subinvolution of placental sites in dogs, *Compend Contin Educ Pract Vet* 14:789, 1992.
12. Allen WE, England GCW, White KB: Hydrops fetalis diagnosed by real-time ultrasonography in a Bichon frise bitch, *J Small Anim Pract* 30:465, 1989.
13. England GCW, Allen WE: Studies of canine pregnancy using B-mode ultrasound: diagnosis of early pregnancy and the number of conceptuses, *J Small Anim Pract* 31:321, 1990.
14. England GCW, Allen WE: Studies of canine pregnancy using B-mode ultrasound: development of the conceptus and determination of gestational age, *J Small Anim Pract* 31:324, 1990.
15. England GCW, Allen WE: Real-time ultrasonic imaging of the ovary and uterus of the dog, *J Reprod Fertil* 39:91, 1989.
16. England GCW, Yeager AW: Ultrasonographic appearance of the ovary and uterus of the bitch during oestrus, ovulation and early pregnancy, *J Reprod Fertil* 47(suppl):107, 1993.
17. Johnston SD, Smith FO, Bailie NC et al: Prenatal indicators of puppy viability at term, *Compend Contin Educ Pract Vet* 5:1013, 1983.
18. Poffenbarger EM, Feeney DA: Use of gray-scale ultrasonography in the diagnosis of reproductive disease in the bitch: 18 cases (1981-1984), *J Am Vet Med Assoc* 189:90, 1986.
19. Noakes DE: Pregnancy and its diagnosis. In Arthur GH, Noakes DE, Pearson H et al, editors: *Veterinary reproduction and obstetrics,* ed 7, Philadelphia, 1996, WB Saunders, p 63.
20. Rendano VT, Lein DH, Concannon PW: Radiographic evaluation of prenatal development in the Beagle: correlation with the time of breeding, LH release, and parturition, *Vet Radiol* 25:132, 1984.
21. Tsutsui T: Process of development of uterus, fetus, and fetal appendices during pregnancy in the dog, *Bull Nippon Vet Zootech Coll* 30:175, 1981.
22. Pharr JW, Post K: Ultrasonography and radiography of the canine post partum uterus, *Vet Radiol Ultrasound* 33:35, 1992.
23. Boyd JS: Radiographic identification of the various stages of pregnancy in the domestic cat, *J Small Anim Pract* 12:501, 1971.
24. Zambelli D, Canappele B, Bassi S, et al: Ultrasound aspects of fetal and extrafetal structures in pregnant cats, *J Feline Med Surg* 4:95, 2002.
25. Feretti, LM, Newell SM, Graham JP et al: Radiographic and ultrasonographic evaluation of the normal feline postpartum uterus, *Vet Radiol Ultrasound* 41:287, 2000.
26. Robinson GW: Uterus unicornis and unilateral renal agenesis in a cat, *J Am Vet Med Assoc* 147:516, 1965.
27. Stein BS: Obstetrics, surgical procedures and anesthesia. In Morrow DA, editor: *Current therapy in theriogenology,* Philadelphia, 1986, WB Saunders, p 865.
28. McAfee CT: Hydrouterus and hydrovarium in a Beagle bitch, *Canine Pract* 4:48, 1977.
29. Freeman LJ: Feline uterine torsion, *Compend Contin Educ Pract Vet* 10:1078, 1988.
30. Misumi K, Fujiki M, Miura N et al: Uterine horn torsion in two non-gravid bitches, *J Small Anim Pract* 41:468, 2000.
31. Shull RM, Johnston SD, Johnston GR et al: Bilateral torsion of the uterine horns in a nongravid bitch, *J Am Vet Med Assoc* 172:601, 1978.
32. Munro E, Stead C: Ultrasonographic diagnosis of uterine entrapment in an inguinal hernia, *J Small Anim Pract* 34:139, 1993.
33. Tsumagari S, Takagi K, Takeishi M et al: A case of a bitch with imperforate hymen and hydrocolpos, *J Vet Med Sci* 63:475, 2001.
34. Bigliardi E, Parmigiani E, Cavirani S et al: Ultrasonography and cystic hyperplasia-pyometra complex in the bitch, *Repro Domest Anim* 39:136, 2004.
35. Pack FD: Feline uterine adenomyosis, *Feline Pract* 10:45, 1980.
36. Potter K, Hancock DH, Gallina AM: Clinical and pathologic features of endometrial hyperplasia, pyometra and endometritis in cats: 79 cases (1980-1985), *J Am Vet Med Assoc* 198:1427, 1991.

37. Stocklin-Gautschi NM, Guscetti F, Reichler IM et al: Identification of focal adenomyosis as a uterine lesion in two dogs, *J Small Anim Pract* 42:413, 2001.
38. Brodey RS, Roszel JF: Neoplasms of the canine uterus, vagina and vulva: a clinicopathologic survey, *J Am Vet Med Assoc* 151:1294, 1967.
39. Spackman CJA, Caywood DD, Johnston GR, et al: Granulomas of the uterine and ovarian stumps: a case report, *J Am Anim Hosp Assoc* 20:449, 1984.
40. Franklin RT, Prescott JVB: Tenesmus and stranguria from a cystic uterine remnant, *Vet Radiol* 24:139, 1983.
41. Hernendez JL, Besso JG, Rault DN et al: Emphysematous pyometra in a dog, *Vet Radiol Ultrasound* 42:196, 2003.
42. Carrig CB, Gourley IM, Philbrick AL: Primary abdominal pregnancy in a cat subsequent to OHE, *J Am Vet Med Assoc* 160:308, 1972.
43. Tomlinson J, Jackson ML, Pharr JW: Extrauterine pregnancy in a cat, *Feline Pract* 10:18, 1980.
44. DeNooy PP: Extrauterine pregnancy and severe ascites in a cat, *Vet Med Small Anim Clin* 74:349, 1979.
45. Hayes G: Asymptomatic uterine rupture in a bitch, *Vet Rec* 154:438, 2004.
46. Bennett D: Canine dystocia—a review of the literature, *J Small Anim Pract* 15:101, 1974.
47. Koster K, Poulsen Nautrup C, Gunzel-Apel AR: A Doppler ultrasonographic study of cyclic changes of ovarian perfusion in the Beagle bitch, *Reproduction* 122:453, 2001.
48. Root CN: Abdominal masses: the radiographic differential diagnosis, *J Am Vet Radiol Soc* 15:26, 1974.
49. Dow C: Ovarian abnormalities in the bitch, *J Comp Pathol* 70:59, 1960.
50. Silva LDM, Onclin K, Verstegen JP: Assessment of ovarian changes around ovulation in bitches by ultrasonography, laparoscopy and hormonal changes, *Vet Radiol Ultrasound* 37:313, 1996.
51. Barrett RE, Theiler LH: Neoplasms of the canine and feline reproductive tracts. In Kirk RW, editor: *Current veterinary therapy VI*, Philadelphia, 1977, WB Saunders, p 1263.
52. Riser WH, Marcus JF, Gaibor EC et al: Dermoid cyst of the canine ovary, *J Am Vet Med Assoc* 134:27, 1959.
53. De Nardo GA, Becker K, Broan NO et al: Ovarian remnant syndrome: revascularization of free-floating ovarian tissue in the feline abdominal cavity, *J Am Anim Hosp Assoc* 37:290, 2001.
54. Cellio LM, Degner DA: Testosterone-producing thecoma in a female cat, *J Am Anim Hosp Assoc* 36:323, 2000.
55. Fernandez T, Diez-Bru N, Rios A et al: Intracranial metastases from an ovarian dysgerminoma in a 2-year old dog, *J Am Anim Hosp Assoc* 37:553, 2001.
56. Greene JA, Richardson RP, Thornhill JA et al: Ovarian papillary cystadenoma in a bitch, *J Am Anim Hosp Assoc* 15:351, 1979.
57. Patnaik AK, Shaer M, Parks JL et al: Metastasizing ovarian teratocarcinoma in dogs, *J Small Anim Pract* 17:235, 1976.
58. Murti GS, Gilbert DL, Bougmann AP: Canine intersex states, *J Am Vet Med Assoc* 149:1183, 1966.
59. Todoroff RJ: Canine urogenital anomalies, *Compend Contin Educ Pract Vet* 1:780, 1979.
60. Pugh CR, Konde LJ, Park RD: Testicular ultrasound in the normal dog, *Vet Radiol* 31:195, 1990.
61. Parkinson TJ: Fertility and infertility in male animals. In Arthur GH, Noakes DE, Pearson H et al, editors: *Veterinary reproduction and obstetrics*, ed 7, Philadelphia, 1996, WB Saunders, p 572.
62. Johnston GR, Feeney DA, Johnston SD et al: Ultrasonographic features of testicular neoplasms in dogs: 16 cases (1980-1988), *J Am Vet Med Assoc* 198:1770, 1991.
63. Johnston GR, Feeney DA, Rivers B et al: Diagnostic imaging of the male canine reproductive organs: methods and limitations, *Vet Clin North Am Small Anim Pract* 21:553, 1991.
64. Pearson H, Kelly DF: Testicular torsion in the dog: a review of 13 cases, *Vet Rec* 97:200, 1975.
65. Pugh CR, Konde LJ: Sonographic evaluation of canine testicular and scrotal abnormalities: a review of 26 case histories, *Vet Radiol Ultrasound* 32:243, 1991.
66. Yates D, Hayes G, Heffernan, M et al: Incidence of cryptorchidism in dogs and cats, *Vet Rec* 152:502, 2003.
67. Gumbsch, P, Gabler C, Holzmann A: Colour-coded duplex sonography of the testes of dogs, *Vet Rec* 151:140, 2002.
68. Gunzel-Apel AR, Mohrke C, Poulsen Nautrup C: Colour-coded and pulsed Doppler sonography of the canine testes, epididymis and prostate gland: physiological and pathological findings, *Reprod Domest Anim* 36:236, 2001.
69. Paltiel HJ, Diamond DA, Di Canzio J et al: Testicular volume: comparison of orchidometer and US measurements in dogs, *Radiology* 222:114, 2002.
70. Wensing CJ: Developmental anomalies including cryptorchidism. In Morrow DA, editor: *Current therapy in theriogenology*, Philadelphia, 1980, WB Saunders, p 583.
71. Bauran V, Dijkstra F, Wensing CJ: Testicular descent in the dog, *Acta Histol Embryol* 10:97, 1981.
72. Naylor RW, Thompson SMA: Intra-abdominal testicular torsion—a report of 2 cases, *J Am Anim Hosp Assoc* 15:763, 1979.
73. Hecht S, King R, Tidwell AS, et al: Ultrasound diagnosis: intra-abdominal torsion of a non-neoplastic testicle in a cryptorchid dog, *Vet Radiol Ultrasound* 45:58, 2004.
74. Wang FI, Laing SL, Chin SC: A primary retroperitoneal seminoma invading the kidneys of a cryptorchid dog, *Exp Anim* 50:341, 2001.
75. Rakiguchi M, Ida T, Kudo T, et al: Malignant seminoma with systemic metastases in the dog, *J Small Anim Pract* 42:360, 2001.
76. Leio DH: Canine orchitis. In Kirk RA, editor: *Current veterinary therapy VI*, Philadelphia, 1977, W.B. Saunders, p 1255.
77. Ober CP, Spaulding K, Breitschwerdt, EB et al: Orchitis in two dogs with Rocky Mountain spotted fever, *Vet Radiol Ultrasound* 45:458, 2004.
78. McNeil PE, Weaver AD: Massive scrotal swelling in two unusual cases of canine Sertoli cell tumor, *Vet Rec* 106:144, 1980.
79. Bartlett GR: What is your diagnosis? Testicular torsion, *J Small Anim Pract* 43:521, 2002.
80. Rodriguez F, Herraez P, Espinosa de los Monteros A et al: Testicular necrosis caused by Mesocestoides species in a dog, *Vet Rec* 153:275, 2003.
81. Sigurdardottir OG, Kolbjornsen O, Lutz H: Orchitis in a cat associated with coronavirus infection, *J Compend Pathol* 124:219, 2001.
82. Kawakami E, Koga H, Hori T et al: Sperm granuloma and sperm agglutination in a dog with asthenozoospermia, *J Vet Med Sci* 65:409, 2003.
83. Simon J, Rubin SB: Metastatic seminoma in a dog, *Vet Med Small Anim Clin* 74:941, 1979.
84. Henderson RA, Hoerline BF, Kramer TT et al: Discospondylitis in three dogs infected with *Brucella canis*, *J Am Vet Med Assoc* 165:451, 1974.
85. Allen WE, France C: A contrast radiographic study of the vagina and uterus of the normal bitch, *J Small Anim Pract* 26:153, 1985.
86. Gibbs PEC, Latham J: An evaluation of positive contrast vaginography as a diagnostic aid in the bitch, *J Small Anim Pract* 24:531, 1984.

87. Kyles AE, Vaden S, Hardie EM et al: Vestibulovaginal stenosis in dogs: 18 cases (1987-1995), *J Am Vet Med Assoc* 209:1189, 1996.
88. Root MV, Johnston SD, Johnston GR: Vaginal septa in dogs: 15 cases (1983-1992), *J Am Vet Med Assoc* 206:56, 1995.
89. Johnston GR, Osborne CA, Wilson JW et al: Familial ureteral ectopia in the dog, *J Am Anim Hosp Assoc* 13:168, 1977.

ELECTRONIC RESOURCES evolve

Additional information related to the content in Chapter 44 can be found on the companion Web site at evolve http://evolve.elsevier.com/Thrall/vetrad/.

- Key Points
- Chapter Quiz
- Case Study 44-1
- Case Study 44-2

CHAPTER • 45
The Stomach

Paul M. Frank
Mary B. Mahaffey

ANATOMY

The cranial surface of the stomach is in close apposition to the caudal surface of the liver. In the normal dog and cat, the empty stomach usually lies cranial to the last pair of ribs,[1,2] but it may extend slightly caudal to the costal arch. The stomach lies in a transverse plane, primarily to the left of the median plane.

The stomach is subdivided into the cardia, fundus, body, and pyloric portions (Fig. 45-1).[1] The cardia is a small area at the esophagogastric junction. The fundus is the dome or outpouching from the left dorsal aspect of the stomach. The body is the middle portion from the fundus to the pyloric portion and is the largest portion of the stomach. The distal third of the stomach is the pyloric portion, which is further subdivided into the pyloric antrum and the pyloric canal. The pyloric antrum is the proximal two thirds of the pyloric portion and is relatively thin walled and slightly expanded. The pyloric canal, the distal third of the pyloric portion, is more muscular and contains a double sphincter.

Additional landmarks of the stomach include the greater and lesser curvatures and the angular incisure (notch).[1] The greater curvature is the convex surface of the stomach that originates at the cardia and extends caudoventrally around to the pylorus. The lesser curvature is the concave surface that originates to the right of the cardia and extends cranioventrally to the pylorus. It is the shortest distance between the cardia and the pylorus. The angular notch is the point of acute angulation of the lesser curvature, located approximately at the junction of the body and the pyloric antrum. The mucosal surface of the stomach is characterized by numerous folds or ridges called rugal folds or rugae.

RADIOGRAPHIC EXAMINATION

Preparation

Ingesta within the stomach may obscure some lesions or simulate other lesions and thus create false-negative or false-positive results. Therefore, under ideal conditions, routine radiographic examination of the stomach should be performed on an animal that has fasted for 12 to 24 hours.[3-5] Nonirritating cleansing enemas may also be useful if a subsequent contrast study is contemplated. However, fasting is not feasible in many situations, and the inability to fast the patient is not a contraindication for abdominal radiography. Additionally, exceptions to fasting are possible because patients with emesis or anorexia may not require fasting. Also, fasting and enemas should be avoided in patients with acute abdominal disorders for which time delays are medically contraindicated or when fluid and gas patterns in the bowel may be of diagnostic importance.

Consideration of medications is also important. Many drugs used for treatment of gastrointestinal disorders or for chemical restraint affect gastric motility and may cause gaseous distention of the stomach and decreased motility. These preparations should be avoided or discontinued for an appropriate interval before any contrast study is undertaken.[6-10]

Radiographic Technique

Survey radiographs may be sufficient for diagnosing some gastric abnormalities. If contrast studies are deemed necessary, survey radiography of the stomach should always precede them. Various radiographic techniques are available and include conventional barium sulfate gastrography, low-volume gastrography, double-contrast gastrography, pneumogastrography, gastrography with iodinated contrast media, and gastric emptying studies with barium/food or radiopaque marker/food mixtures.[2,3,6,11-23] For one method of performing a positive contrast gastrogram, see Box 45-1.

For complete evaluation of the stomach, four conventional views are necessary: the ventrodorsal, the dorsoventral, the right recumbent lateral, and the left recumbent lateral. Oblique views may occasionally be of value to isolate or project certain areas of the stomach, such as the pylorus.

NORMAL RADIOGRAPHIC FINDINGS

The radiographic appearance of the normal stomach varies and depends on many factors, such as the species, breed, degree of gastric distention, volume and type of gastric content, position of the patient during radiography, and whether contrast medium was used.

The stomach usually is easy to recognize by its location and shape and the content of gas, ingesta, or both. The entire stomach may not be discernible on survey radiographs if it is empty or if the gastric fluid content silhouettes the liver or other abdominal structures. As a general guide, on the lateral view the axis of the stomach from the fundus through the body and pylorus is either perpendicular to the spine, parallel to the ribs, or somewhere between these angles (Fig. 45-2, *A*). On the lateral view, the pylorus may be superimposed over the body or located slightly cranial to the body. On the ventrodorsal view of the dog the cardia, fundus, and body of the stomach are located to the left of midline, and the pyloric portions are located to the right of midline. The pyloric

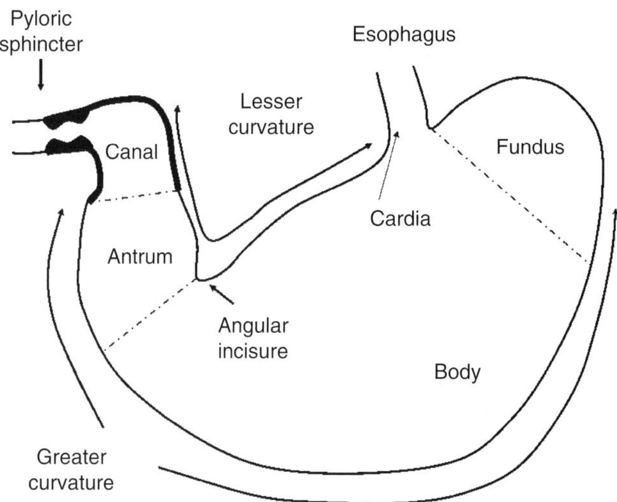

Fig. 45-1 The divisions of the stomach.

sphincter usually is located in the right cranial abdominal quadrant at approximately the level of the tenth or eleventh ribs and is usually cranial to the pyloric canal.[2] In immature dogs the pylorus may be located closer to midline than in adults.[11]

The long axis of the stomach may be perpendicular to the spine, with the stomach appearing to run transversely across the abdomen, making the angular notch difficult to identify (see Fig. 45-2, *B*). The stomach may also have a U-shaped appearance with a more obvious angular notch and still be within its normal location. On the ventrodorsal view of the cat, the stomach is more acutely angled with the pylorus located at or near the midline (see Fig. 45-2, C). Variations in the appearance of the stomach in the dog based on the shape of the thorax and cranial abdomen (i.e., breed conformation) have been described.[2] The actual shape of the stomach also varies with the degree of gastric distention because different portions of the stomach vary in their distensibility.

One of the most important factors in the appearance of the stomach is the position of the patient during radiography.[24] The relation between the position of the patient and the radiographic appearance of the stomach is an important concept that must be understood for accurate interpretation of radiographs and for demonstration of some gastric lesions. Variation in appearance of the stomach with different patient positions is caused by shifts in fluid and gas distribution within the lumen of the stomach. The stomach usually contains both fluid and gas, with the fluid being either of soft tissue (fluid) or mineral opacity. This fluid and gas distribution varies with the position of the patient because fluid settles dependently because of gravity, and gas rises to the highest part of the lumen. Gas and positive-contrast medium are relatively easy to visualize on radiographs, whereas fluid within the stomach may be more difficult to see because it may cause border effacement with other structures of similar opacity. Although the routine recommendation for radiography of suspected gastric disease is a single lateral radiographic projection and a ventrodorsal view, routine right and left lateral radiographic projections may be useful, along with a ventrodorsal radiograph when gastric disease is suspected.[25]

To explain the radiographic appearance of the stomach, the organ can be described as J shaped and positioned in a transverse plane in the cranial abdomen. Thus for example, with a patient positioned in dorsal recumbency for a ventrodorsal view, fluid within the lumen settles dependently to the fundus and body of the stomach. If enough fluid is present, the pyloric portion of the stomach also fills. Gas rises to the uppermost

Box 45-1

Positive-Contrast Gastrogram with Barium Sulfate

- Fast for 12 to 24 hours with or without cleansing enemas.
  - Food in the stomach will interfere with interpretation of gastric emptying time.
  - Ingesta may also obscure foreign bodies or small gastric lesions.
  - Gastrograms performed with food in the stomach are difficult to interpret.
- If possible, perform radiography without the use of sedatives.
  - Motility-altering drugs such as antiemetics may interfere with interpretation.
  - If sedatives are required because of the fractious nature of the patient, use the lowest dose possible and interpret gastric emptying times with caution.
- Perform survey radiographs to assess patient preparation, establish radiographic technique, and possibly identify the problem without gastrography.
- Administer barium sulphate suspension by an orogastric tube, with the patient on the x-ray table ready for radiography (cassette in position, technique set, etc.).
  - Barium USP powder mixed with water is not recommended.
- The dosage is 2.3 to 3.6 mL barium/kg body weight (5 to 8 mL/lb).
  - Feeding barium orally (i.e., without an orogastric tube) results in suboptimal distension of the stomach from emptying of the initial portions of barium before administration of the last portion.
  - Not administering enough barium is a common mistake. Small dogs typically need the high end of the dosage range and large dogs may only need the low end. This means a 100-lb dog gets at least 500 mL of barium.
  - Use caution to ensure that the orogastric tube is located in the esophagus, not the trachea.
    - Verify tube position by using fluoroscopy, survey radiograph, or palpation.
  - Before removing the tube, instill a small volume of air to clear the tube, then kink the tube before removal to prevent leakage of barium into the trachea.
- After removing the tube, immediately make radiographs centered over the stomach. All four views are recommended (right lateral, left lateral, dorsoventral, and ventrodorsal) and should be made as rapidly as possible.
- Additional radiographs (with or without obliques) should be made pending the results of the initial radiographs. If available, fluoroscopy is extremely helpful in the evaluation of gastrograms.
- Continue making radiographs (usually right lateral and ventrodorsal) until the majority of the barium is no longer seen within the stomach.
  - A small amount of residual barium coating the mucosa diffusely for several hours may be normal. Focal barium retention is suggestive of ulceration.
- The gastrogram may be combined with contrast evaluation of the small intestine.

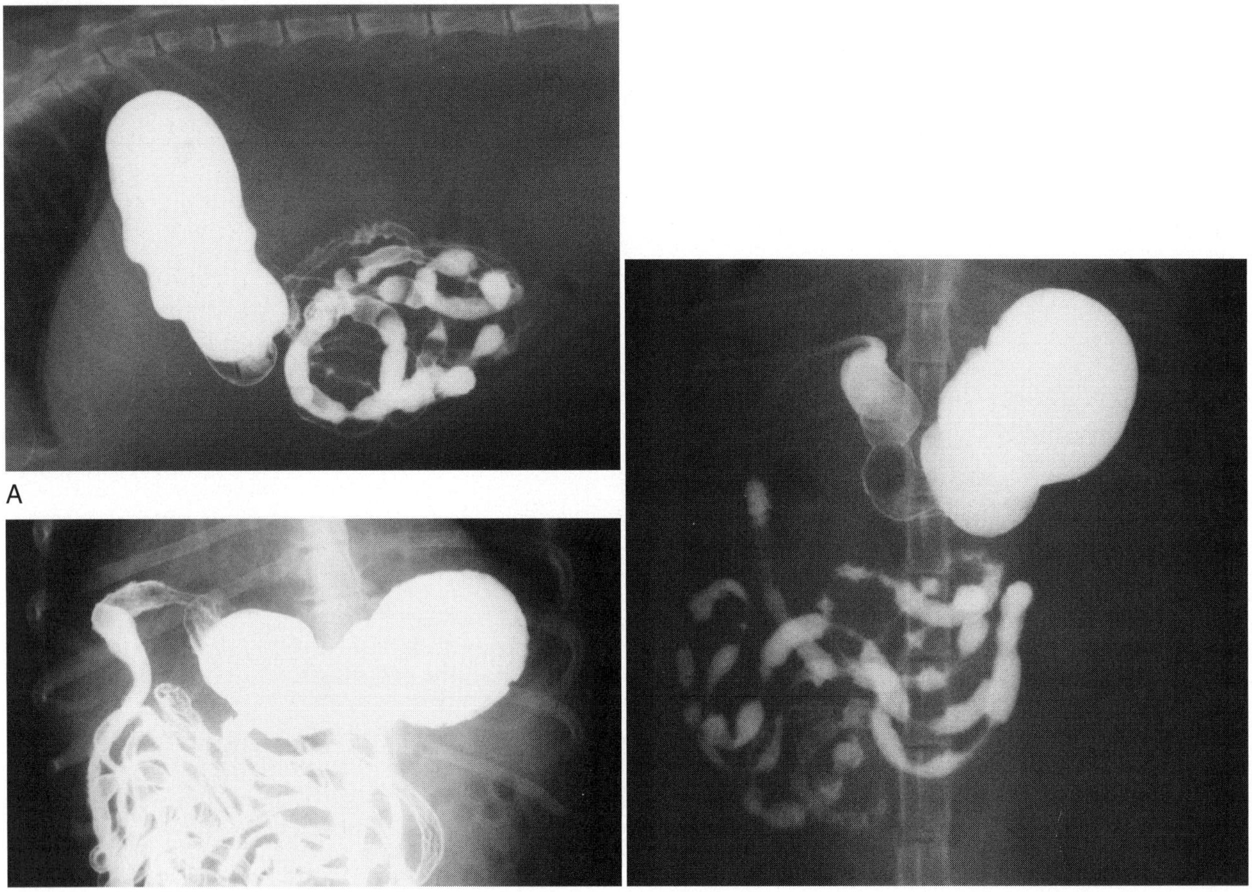

A

B

C

Fig. 45-2 Gastrograms illustrating normal positions of the stomach. **A,** Lateral view of a cat. The gastric axis is parallel with the ribs. **B,** Ventrodorsal view of a dog. The gastric axis of this dog is approximately perpendicular to the spine. Note that in some patients the stomach is U shaped. **C,** Ventrodorsal view of a cat. The stomach is acutely angled, with the pylorus located closer to midline.

portion, which is in the pyloric antrum and the body near midline. Figure 45-3 is a computed tomographic cross-sectional view of the cranial abdomen at the level of the stomach acquired with the dog in dorsal recumbency. Note the fluid opacity filling most of the stomach, with the gas bubble floating near midline. With this image as an example, predictions are possible for how the fluid and gas would be distributed if the animal were rotated in 90-degree increments for a left recumbent lateral view, a dorsoventral view in sternal recumbency, a right recumbent lateral view, and back to a ventrodorsal view in dorsal recumbency. These variations in appearance of the stomach are further altered by the volume and ratio of fluid to gas within the stomach. Examples of the appearance of the stomach with various views are illustrated in Figures 45-4 and 45-5; these views were made with a vertically directed x-ray beam.

On the ventrodorsal view (see Fig. 45-4, *A*), gas is located in the pyloric antrum and the body near midline. Fluid settles to fill the fundus, body, and pyloric portions of the stomach. Less fluid with a larger volume of gas would fill additional areas of the stomach with gas. If completely empty, the fundus and body may appear as a soft tissue mass on the ventrodorsal view. On a dorsoventral view (see Fig. 45-4, *B*) gas rises to the cardia and fundus, and fluid settles dependently to fill the pyloric portions and part of the body. On the left recumbent

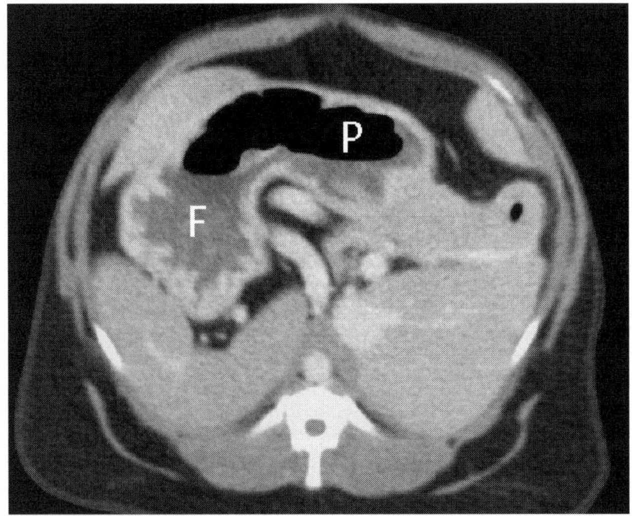

Fig. 45-3 Computed tomographic image of a normal dog in dorsal recumbency at the level of the stomach. Fluid fills most of the fundus *(F)* and part of the pylorus *(P)*, and the gas bubble floats near the midline.

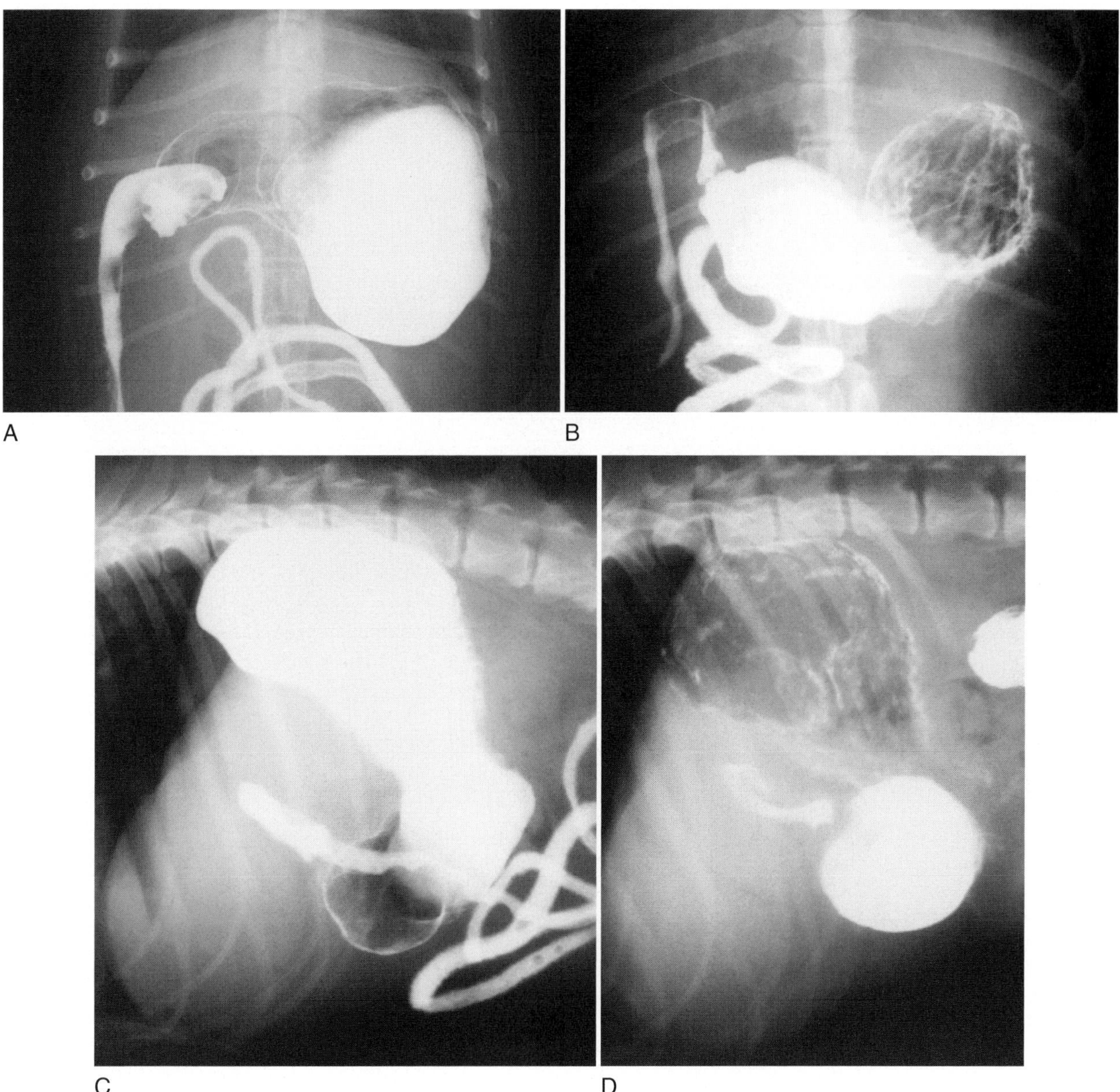

Fig. 45-4 Normal variations in fluid (barium) and gas distribution within the stomach with different patient positions. **A,** Ventrodorsal view, in dorsal recumbency. Gas is located in the body and pyloric antrum. Fluid settles dependently to fill the fundus, body, and pyloric portions (compare with Fig. 45-3). **B,** Dorsoventral view, in ventral recumbency. Gas rises to the cardia and fundus and fluid settles dependently to fill pyloric portions and part of the body. **C,** Left recumbent lateral view. Gas rises to the pyloric portion and fluid settles dependently to fill the fundus and body. **D,** Right recumbent lateral view. Gas rises to the fundus and body, which are coated with barium. Fluid settles dependently to fill the pyloric portion and part of the body.

lateral view (see Fig. 45-4, C) gas rises to the pyloric portion of the stomach, which is on the patient's right side and is thus the uppermost point of the stomach. Fluid settles dependently to the fundus and body. A gas pocket occasionally may be trapped in the fundic region. In this position the fundus and body are well visualized with positive-contrast medium but are more difficult to visualize if filled with fluid (Fig. 45-5, *A*). On the right recumbent lateral view (see Fig. 45-4, *D*), gas rises to the fundus and body, which are on the patient's left side and thus are uppermost. In the right lateral, the gas is often more spread out to fill the fundus and body (see Fig. 45-5, *B*) and may not stand out as discretely as on the left recumbent lateral view. In addition, fluid settles dependently to fill the pyloric portions and part of the body of the stomach. In this position the pyloric portion is well visualized with positive-contrast medium. The pyloric antrum and distal part of the body occasionally may appear in survey radiographs as a soft tissue mass in the right recumbent lateral view (see Fig. 45-5, *B*). If a mass or foreign body is suspected on a right recumbent lateral view in the pylorus, a left recumbent lateral view should be made to better visualize this area.

Recognizing that variations exist in the appearance of the normal stomach from factors such as the position of the patient and the volume and ratio of fluid to gas within

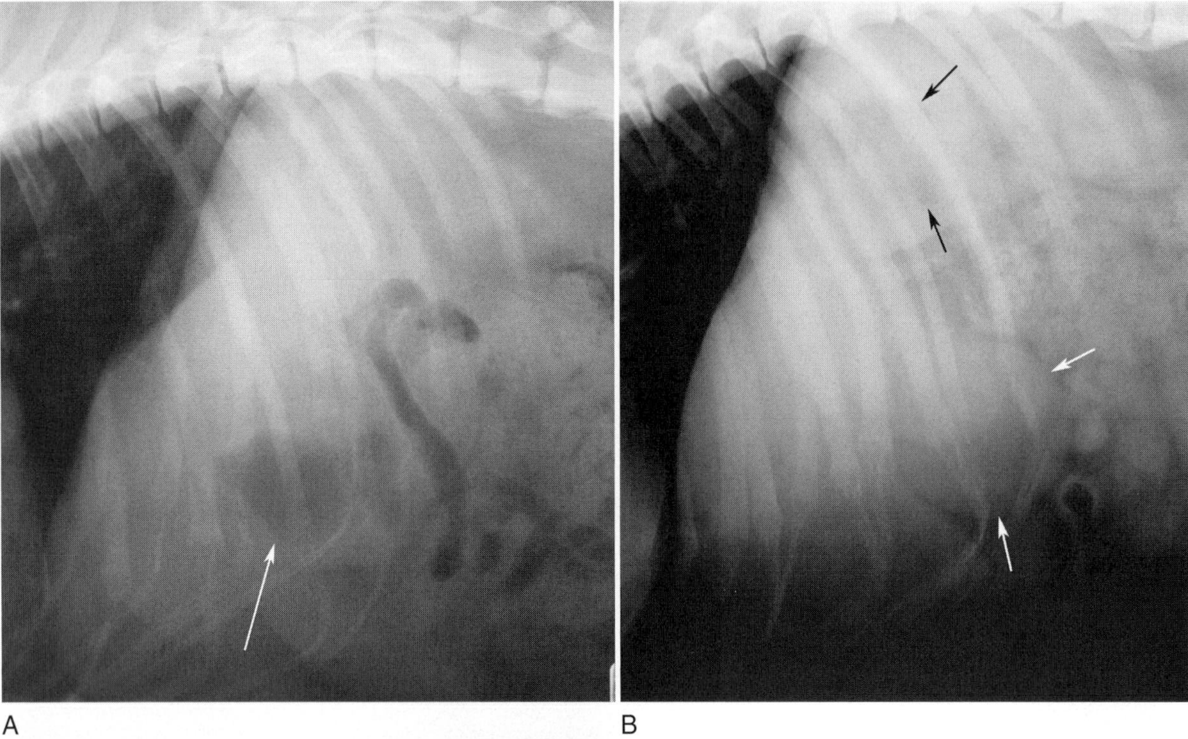

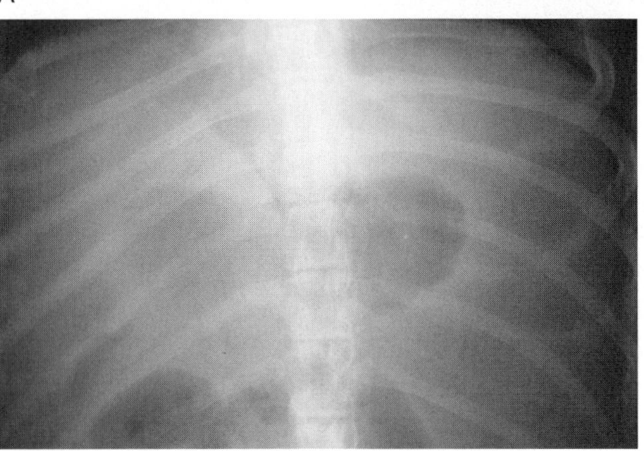

Fig. 45-5 Normal variations in fluid and gas distribution within the stomach on survey radiographs. **A,** Left recumbent lateral view. Gas rises to the pyloric portion *(arrow)* and part of the body, and a gas pocket remains near the cardia. Fluid settles dependently to the fundus and body, which are difficult to visualize when filled with fluid (compare with Fig. 45-4, C). **B,** Right recumbent lateral view. Gas rises to fill the fundus *(black arrows)* and the body. Fluid settles dependently to the pyloric portion, which appears as a soft tissue mass (*white arrows;* compare with Fig. 45-4, *D*). **C,** Ventrodorsal view made in dorsal recumbency. Gas rises across much of the stomach to outline the pylorus and body.

the stomach is important. The ability to take advantage of fluid and gas shifts within the stomach to visualize certain portions of the stomach more clearly is also important. Table 45-1 is a simplified summary of the expected changes in gas and fluid within the stomach on change in patient position.

Rugal folds are not seen well on survey radiographs. With positive-contrast gastrography, rugal folds are best seen at the peripheral portions of the stomach, where they may be visualized end on as regular small filling defects at the mucosal surface. If projected en face, rugal folds are not visible with positive-contrast gastrography unless the barium is well penetrated by the x-ray beam or the stomach has emptied much of the original dose. Rugal folds then appear as relatively radiolucent, linear filling defects separated by barium in the interrugal spaces (Fig. 45-6). Double-contrast gastrography provides the most detailed evaluation of the gastric mucosa and rugal folds.

Radiographic assessment of rugal folds is subjective because they vary in size and number[5,26] and their appearance depends on the degree of gastric distention. Rugal folds are more tortuous in the nondistended stomach and become more uniform and parallel to the gastric curvature with increasing distention.[5,12] Rugal folds are smaller and more spiral in the pyloric antrum.[27] Rugal folds may not be visible if the stomach is overdistended.[13] Rugal folds are smaller and fewer in number in cats than in dogs.[2] A reference range for normal

TABLE • 45-1

Distribution of Stomach Gas and Fluid as a Function of Radiographic Projection Using a Vertical X-ray Beam

RADIOGRAPHIC VIEW	LOCATION OF GAS	LOCATION OF FLUID
Dorsoventral	Fundus	Body/ pylorus
Ventrodorsal	Body (±pylorus)	Fundus
Left recumbent lateral	Pylorus (±body)	Fundus
Right recumbent lateral	Fundus	Pylorus

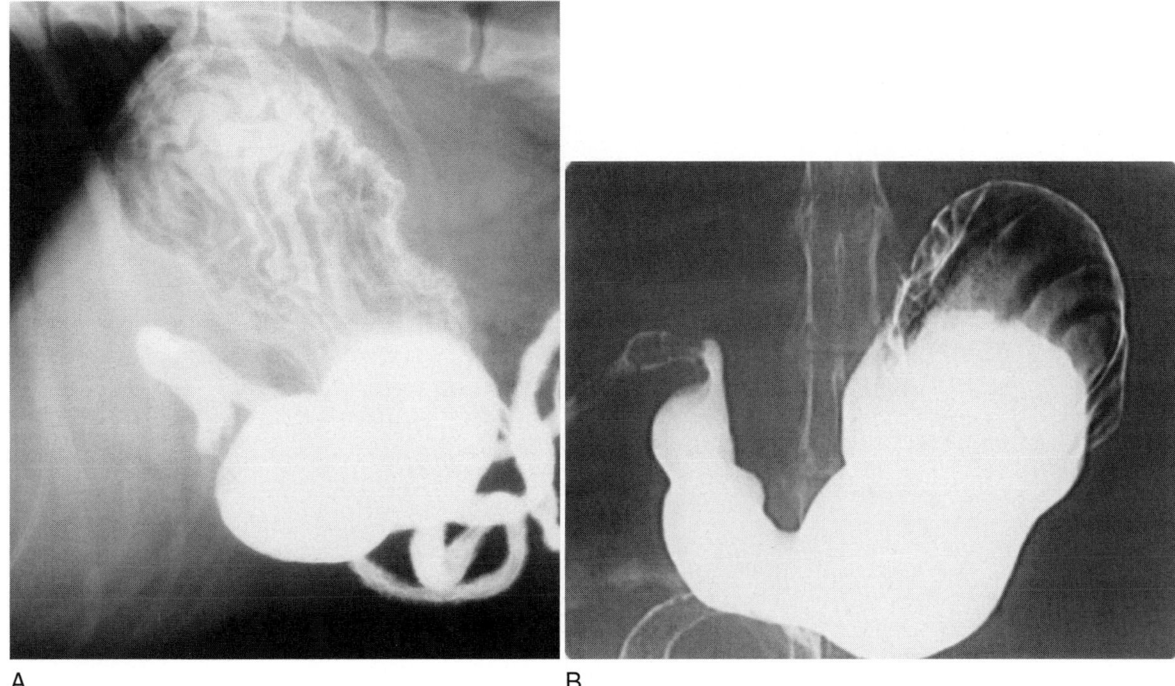

Fig. 45-6 A, Right recumbent lateral gastrogram. Note the multiple curvilinear filling defects in the fundic region of the stomach. These filling defects are the rugae. **B,** Dorsoventral gastrogram. Radiolucent linear filling defects are from rugal folds projected en face.

rugal fold thickness in dogs weighing 2 to 50 kg has been reported to be 1 to 8 mm.[26]

Gastric peristalsis and gastric emptying may be directly observed during fluoroscopy with the use of positive-contrast medium. Ultrasound can also be used to assess gastric motility. Although a peristaltic contraction may be seen on a conventional radiograph during gastrography, this is a chance event depending on when the radiograph was made. A peristaltic contraction appears as an indentation of the wall of the stomach with slight dilation of the lumen immediately preceding the contraction. Peristaltic contractions are stronger and most obvious in the pyloric portion of the stomach.

After administration of barium, gastric emptying should start within 15 minutes in most normal patients.[2,28,29] During gastrography with barium sulfate, the stomach generally empties within 1 to 4 hours in dogs.[6,28] Rapid emptying of the stomach has no clinical significance, whereas delayed emptying is more significant.

The rate of gastric emptying is a complex phenomenon that is altered by a variety of factors such as volume of contents, chemical and physical properties of chyme entering the duodenum, various reflex mechanisms, certain medications, and the type of contrast medium used. Thus a standard approach must be used to evaluate the rate of gastric emptying radiographically. Because the stomach starts to empty faster with an increased intraluminal volume,[14] the dosage of contrast medium should be standardized. Low dosages may result in delayed gastric emptying, which in turn may lead to a false impression of pyloric obstruction. The type of contrast medium used, the volume administered, and the presence or absence of medications that affect gastric emptying are all factors that must be considered and standardized. If these factors can be excluded as a cause of delayed gastric emptying, then delays in gastric emptying are most often related to psychological influences or actual disease at the pylorus. Emotional stress and noise may inhibit gastric movement.[30] Anxiety, fear, rage, or pain induced by physical manipulation of the patient, gastric intubation, and physical restraint may contribute to delayed gastric emptying. Thus patients with delayed gastric emptying must be allowed to calm down in a quiet environment before diagnostic significance is placed on this finding. Also for these reasons, minimal significance is usually placed on slight or minor delays in gastric emptying if the stomach proceeds to empty in a normal manner after an initial delay.

Studies that use barium-food mixtures have been performed in an attempt to further evaluate gastric function.[15,16] Emptying times for individual dogs were repeatable; however, the range of normal gastric emptying times was so wide (7 to 15 hours) that this procedure is not useful for evaluation of gastric emptying unless gross abnormalities are present.[15] In another study gastric emptying times for dogs and cats varied from 4 hours for high-moisture food to 16 hours for dry food.[5] An alternative technique for evaluating gastric emptying of solids in dogs and cats has been developed by using barium-impregnated polyethylene radiopaque spheres (BIPS, Chemstock Animal Health Ltd., Christchurch, New Zealand) mixed with food.[20-23] The number and size of radiopaque spheres, type and amount of food, and fasting period must be standardized. An advantage of the BIPS technique is that it can be performed in most veterinary practices; however, study times may be long (up to 10 hours). Some controversy exists about the usefulness of BIPS for gastric emptying analysis. Scintigraphic evaluation of gastric emptying of food may be considered the gold standard technique. Scintigraphy can be completed in 4 to 5 hours, but availability is limited.[9,31,32] Gastric emptying times are significantly different in both cats and dogs as measured by BIPS compared with scintigraphy. Emptying times measured by BIPS were significantly delayed relative to scintigraphy.[33,34]

A radiolucent line occasionally can be seen within the stomach wall of the cat. This has been determined to be composed of accumulated fat.[35] Distinguishing this finding from gas within the stomach wall may not always be possible.

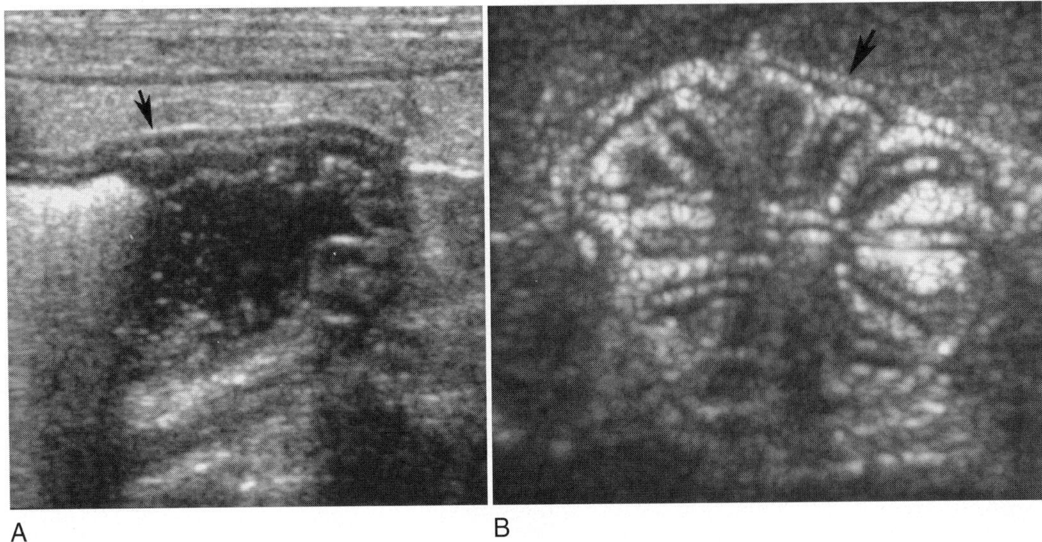

Fig. 45-7 Longitudinal ultrasonogram of the stomach in a normal dog (A) and a normal cat (B). **A,** The stomach is partially distended with gas and fluid. Gas within the lumen appears as a bright echo against the mucosal surface, producing reverberation artifact that prevents visualization of the far wall. Fluid within the caudal half of the stomach provides a window for identification of the far wall. The five normal layers of the stomach wall can be identified as well as several rugal folds. The *black arrowhead* identifies the bright serosal layer. **B,** The stomach is empty and contracted, giving it a "wagon wheel" appearance. The normal layered appearance of the stomach can be seen. The *black arrowhead* identifies the bright serosal surface. Caudal is to the *right,* and ventral is to the *top.*

ULTRASONOGRAPHIC EXAMINATION

Ultrasound examination is a useful addition to abdominal radiography for evaluation of the gastrointestinal tract. It may eliminate the need for contrast studies in many patients because gastric motility, wall thickness and architecture and, to a lesser extent, luminal contents may be evaluated. In addition, ultrasound examination is less expensive and quicker to perform than an upper gastrointestinal series and may be equally sensitive and specific for detection of gastric disease.[36] Gas and ingesta within the stomach may obscure the far wall and thus limit evaluation of the entire organ, but the lumen and far wall can be evaluated in those patients in which the stomach contains fluid and little gas (Fig. 45-7, *A*). Scanning ideally should be performed after a 12-hour fast and before barium contrast studies. If needed, intraluminal gas can be removed by an orogastric tube and the stomach distended with fluid to act as an acoustic window.[37,38] The stomach should be scanned in longitudinal and transverse planes. For evaluating stomach wall layers, 7.5-MHz (or higher) transducers are preferred, but 5-MHz transducers may be needed to evaluate deeper portions of the stomach. Ultrasound has been used to help diagnose gastric neoplasms,[39-46] inflammation or infection,[47] ulcers,[48] foreign bodies,[45,49] pyloric hypertrophy,[50] gastric mineralization,[51] gastroduodenal and gastrogastric and intussusceptions[52,53] and to evaluate gastropexy sites.[54,55]

NORMAL ULTRASONOGRAPHIC FINDINGS

The appearance of the stomach varies with the amount of distention and the extent of luminal contents. When empty, the stomach may have a "wagon wheel" appearance because of infolding of rugal folds (see Fig. 45-7, *B*). This is especially noticeable in the cat. With increasing distention, rugal folds become less conspicuous. Stomach wall thickness in dogs has been reported to be 3 to 5 mm depending on the location measured and the size of the dog, with larger dogs having larger measurements.[37,56] In cats the rugal fold thickness has been reported as 4.4 mm,[57] 2.6 mm,[57] or 2.0 mm[58] for the interrugal area and 2.1 mm for the pylorus.[58] Five wall layers corresponding to the mucosal surface, mucosa, submucosa, muscularis propria, and subserosa/serosa can be identified.[37] These layers have alternating hyperechoic and hypoechoic layers with mucosal surface, submucosa, and subserosa/serosa being hyperechoic and the mucosa and muscularis layers being hypoechoic (see Fig. 45-7). The mean number of peristaltic contractions observed ultrasonographically in dogs has been reported to be four to five contractions per minute.[37]

ABNORMAL RADIOGRAPHIC AND ULTRASONOGRAPHIC FINDINGS

Displacement

The position of the stomach may be a useful indicator for recognition or localization of some extragastric abnormalities in the cranial abdomen. Some diseases of the liver, spleen, pancreas, and diaphragm may affect the stomach. The relation between the stomach and a particular extragastric abnormality may help define the primary organ involved or the nature of the primary lesion.

The cranial surface of the stomach is in close apposition with the caudal surface of the liver. Thus changes in size or position of the liver may cause a change in position of the stomach. Generalized hepatomegaly often produces caudal and dorsal displacement of the stomach.[59] This displacement may be asymmetric if caused by a mass lesion.[2] However, because the cardia of the stomach is relatively fixed in

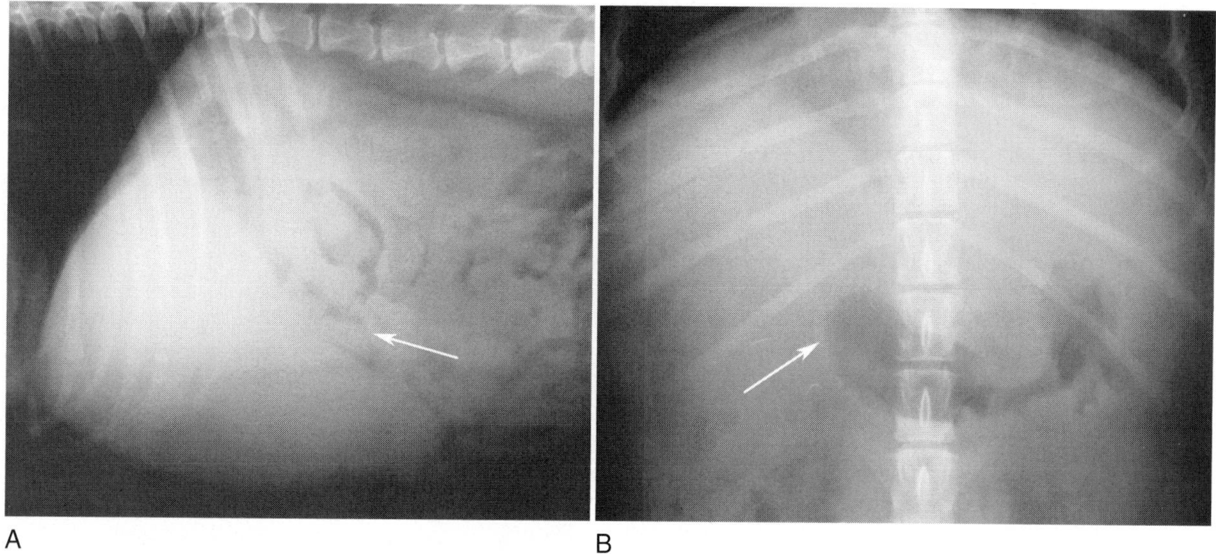

Fig. 45-8 Gastric displacement due to hepatomegaly. **A,** Lateral view. The pylorus *(arrow)* and body are displaced caudally. **B,** Ventrodorsal view. The pylorus *(arrow)* and body are displaced caudally and to the left.

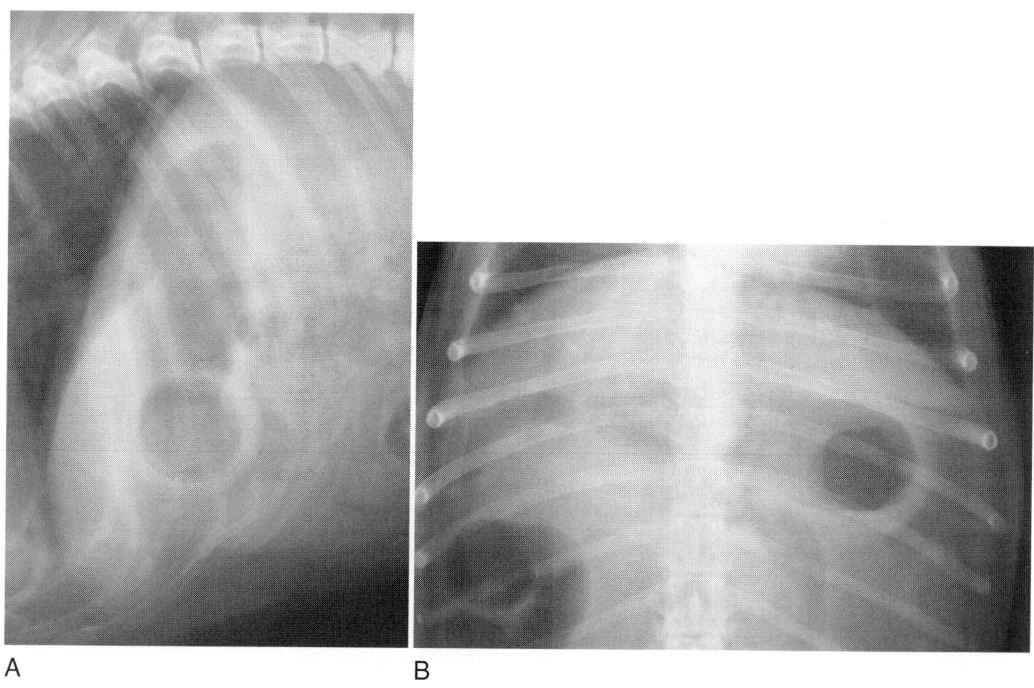

Fig. 45-9 Gastric displacement from a small liver. The pylorus and body are displaced cranially on lateral (A) and ventrodorsal (B) views. Final diagnosis was portosystemic shunt.

position, even generalized hepatomegaly produces a nonuniform displacement of the stomach. Thus on the lateral view generalized hepatomegaly often produces caudal and dorsal displacement of the pylorus and body of the stomach. This displacement changes the axis of the stomach so that the axis is no longer parallel with the ribs (Fig. 45-8, *A*). On the ventrodorsal or dorsoventral view, generalized hepatomegaly often causes displacement of the body and pylorus of the stomach caudally and toward the left from normal (see Fig. 45-8, *B*). This displacement changes the axis of the stomach so that it is no longer transverse.

Because a minimal number of objective radiographic criteria exist for liver size, displacement of the stomach helps in the recognition of hepatomegaly. Gastric displacement becomes especially valuable when the liver is not visible per se because of emaciation or abdominal effusion. In such patients air within the stomach may often be used to define the axis of the stomach. A small volume of room air or barium may also be given to confirm the axis of the stomach.

If the diaphragm is intact, cranial displacement of the stomach relative to the diaphragm can only occur with a decrease in the size of the liver (Fig. 45-9). Contrast studies are often of value to confirm cranial displacement of the stomach because a patient with a small liver may also be emaciated or have abdominal effusion, making the stomach difficult to see. Cranial displacement of the stomach may also occur with rupture of the diaphragm and herniation of the liver, part of the liver, or the stomach. Thus even though the stomach may not pass through a diaphragmatic hernia, the position of the stomach is an important consideration in patients suspected of having a diaphragmatic hernia. A cranial shift of the axis of the stomach may help define whether the liver has herniated cranially through the diaphragm. However, a normal axis of the stomach in such instances may still not completely exclude the possibility of herniation of part of the liver.

Abdominal masses that originate caudal to the stomach do not displace the stomach cranially because of the presence of the liver. Instead, such masses may distort the shape of the stomach as they press against and indent the stomach, or they may displace the stomach to the right or left. The relation of an abdominal mass to the stomach is often of value in helping define whether the mass originates in the liver, spleen, or pancreas (Fig. 45-10).

Gastric Foreign Bodies

Radiopaque material within the stomach is easily visualized and is commonly present on survey radiographs. These opacities are most often the result of ingested bone fragments and usually have no clinical significance. More clinically significant foreign bodies, such as fishhooks and needles, are also readily visualized and present no diagnostic problem. The stomach occasionally may contain nondescript radiopaque material of questionable significance. Close correlation with clinical signs is important (Fig. 45-11). Another important factor is persistence of the abnormality. If the patient is stable, repeat radiographs made 1 to 3 days later may provide valuable information. Judicious use of fasting or cleansing enemas may make these repeat radiographs more valuable.

A greater problem exists with radiographic diagnosis of nonopaque gastric foreign bodies. Such objects are usually difficult to see on survey radiographs. Gastric endoscopic examination is valuable and should be performed if the equipment is available. Contrast studies may be necessary for diagnosis. Several approaches exist to help in the radiographic identification of nonopaque gastric foreign bodies. The simplest is to

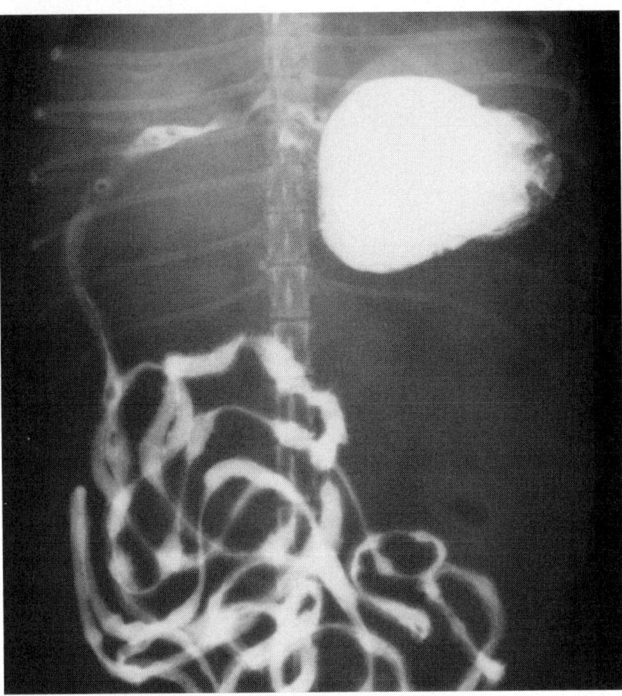

Fig. 45-10 Ventrodorsal radiograph of a dog with an abdominal mass; barium has been administered. The pylorus is displaced to the left; in addition, the cranial duodenal flexure and proximal part of the descending duodenum have a broad arc around the cranial surface of the mass, which itself is not visible. Final diagnosis was pancreatic abscess.

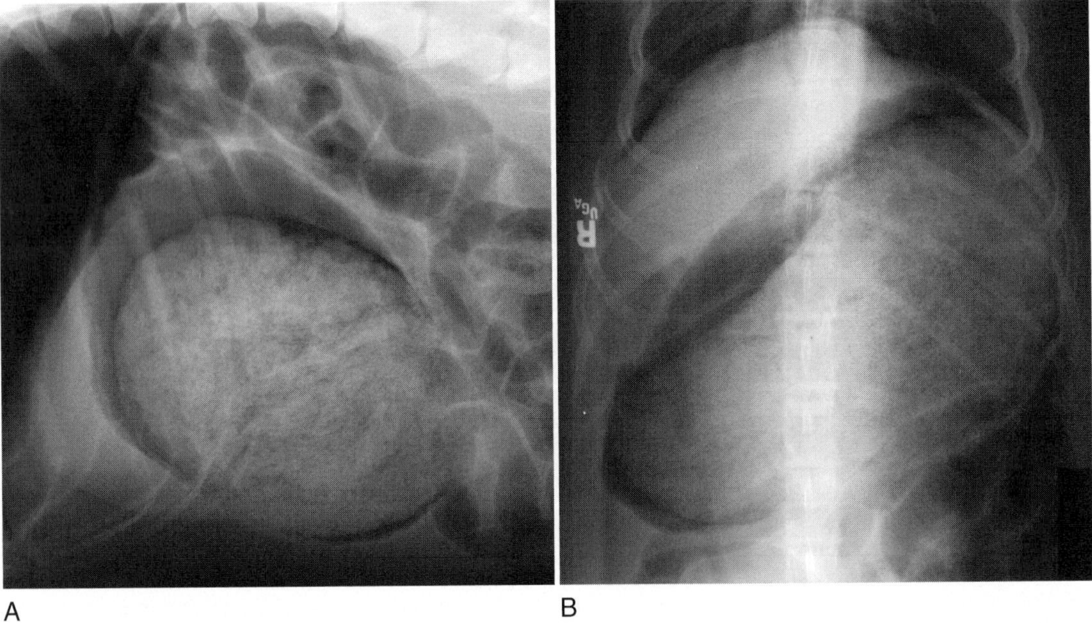

Fig. 45-11 Lateral (A) and ventrodorsal (B) radiographs of a gastric foreign body. This radiopaque material was easier to visualize because of the large amount of gas present surrounding the aggregated leaves and plant material.

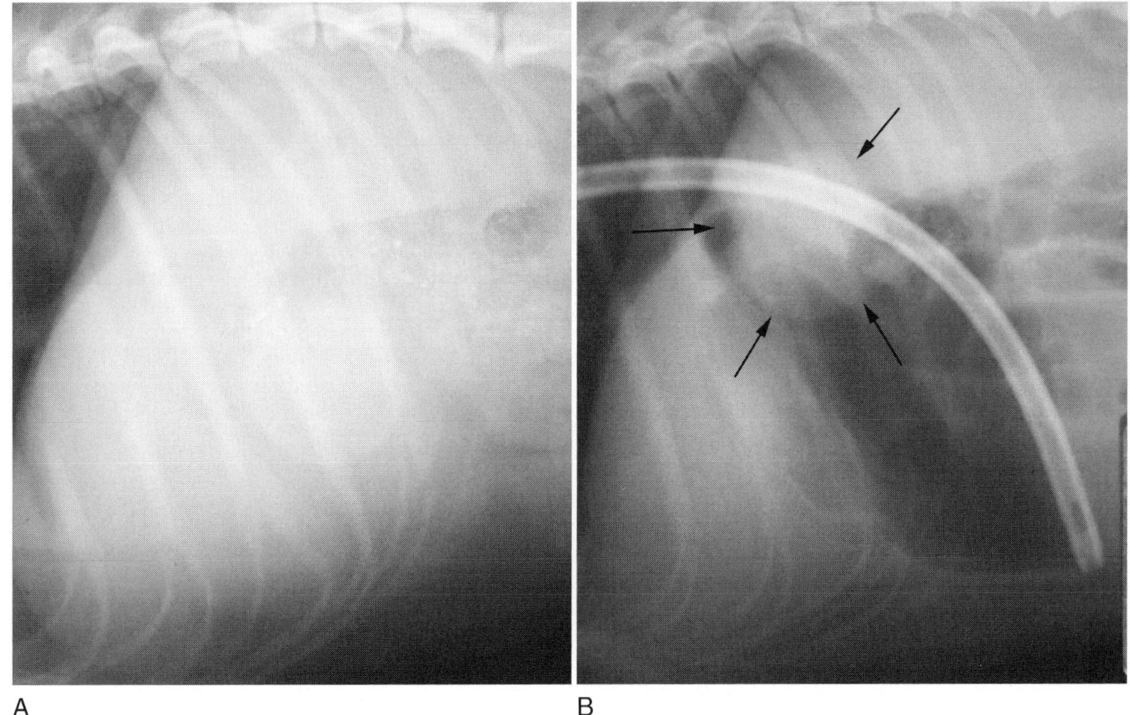

A B

Fig. 45-12 Gastric foreign body (ball) in the pyloric portion that is difficult to see well on the right recumbent lateral view (**A**) because of fluid in the pylorus. Gas has been administered by a gastric tube on the subsequent view (**B**), making the ball *(arrows)* easier to see. Note the ball has moved to the fundic region of the stomach.

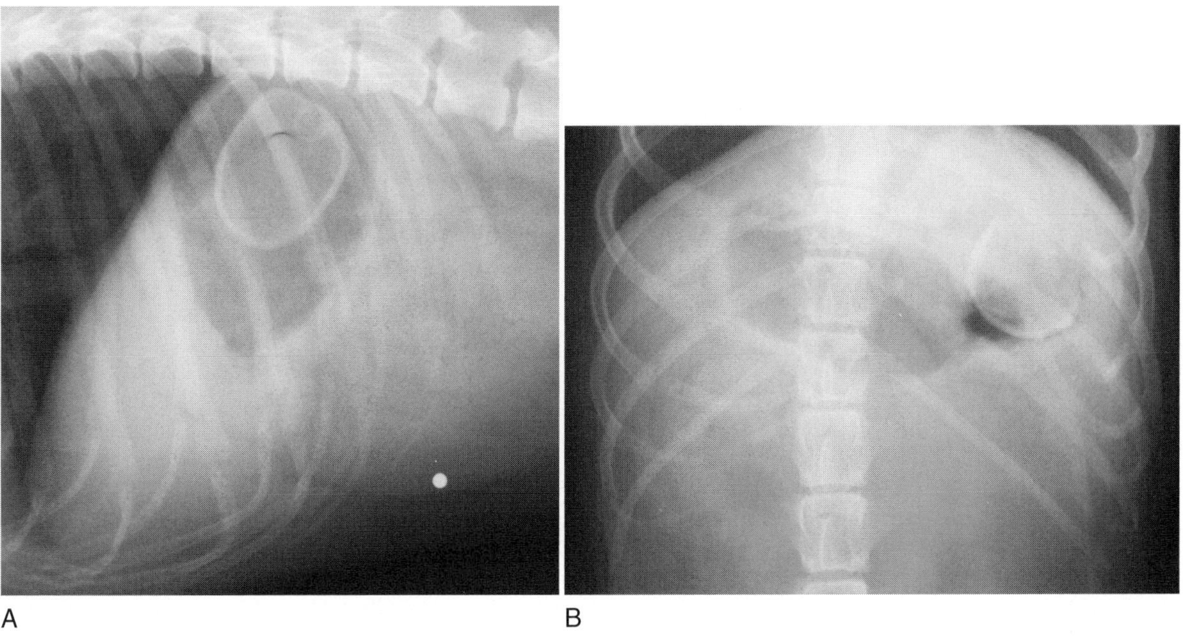

A B

Fig. 45-13 Gastric foreign body (ball) is seen on both views within the fundus.

use different patient positions. If the foreign body does not shift dependently with gastric fluid, then a different view may help outline the foreign body with gas. This approach is most valuable if the foreign body remains in the pyloric portion of the stomach and can be outlined with gas in a left recumbent lateral view. Giving a small amount of barium or gas (Fig. 45-12) or performing a double-contrast gastrogram may make such foreign bodies easier to visualize than with a standard gastrogram using a large volume of barium because a large volume of barium may completely obscure the foreign body and thus lead to a false-negative result. Knowledge of patient positioning is again important because gas within the stomach during a contrast study may simulate a filling defect comparable with that associated with a foreign body.

The appearance of a foreign body on a gastrogram varies depending on the type of foreign body present (Fig. 45-13).

An object such as a solid ball creates a round, discrete filling defect within the barium. If the object has a nonabsorbent surface it may not be visible after the stomach has emptied. Conversely, a rag or sock may not create an initial filling defect because the contrast medium may permeate the object. Because of absorption and retention of contrast medium, however, the foreign body may be better visualized after the stomach has emptied.

Gastric foreign bodies may be identified ultrasonographically.[45,49] The ability to detect these objects depends on the presence of other gastric contents (e.g., gas, fluid, and food), the position of the object relative to the sound beam, and the object composition. Strong acoustic shadows with or without an echogenic acoustic interface are strongly suggestive of foreign bodies. A semicircular border is suggestive of a ball. Intraluminal fluid surrounding foreign objects facilitates their detection and the ability to distinguish rounded reflective foreign body surfaces from intraluminal gas; therefore adding water to the stomach may be beneficial in some patients. Objects that transmit sound may be visualized more completely than those producing strong acoustic shadows.

Acute Gastric Dilation and Volvulus

Acute gastric dilation and gastric volvulus produce gaseous distention of the stomach. Although both fluid and gas are present in the stomach, gaseous distention is the predominant abnormality in these conditions. Gastric dilation and volvulus have been reported in a dog as young as 5 weeks old.[60] Although rare, a similar condition has been reported in the cat.[61]

Acute gaseous distention of the stomach may be attributable to a complex variety of causes. Gaseous distention of the stomach may also be caused by aerophagia as a result of severe dyspnea or pain. In such instances the gastric distention is usually less severe, and other correlative findings may be present to help in the differential diagnosis. With acute gastric dilation the stomach is enlarged and is filled primarily with gas but retains its normal position and anatomic relations. Thus the pylorus is still located on the right and the fundus on the left. The normal position of the stomach usually can be determined on survey radiographs by using and comparing the right recumbent and left recumbent lateral views or the ventrodorsal and dorsoventral views. Recognition of the pylorus of a distended stomach is usually easier on lateral views than on the ventrodorsal or dorsoventral view. Contrast gastrography may help in this localization but is usually not necessary.

Gastric volvulus is also associated with acute gaseous distention of the stomach. Gastric volvulus is differentiated from acute gaseous dilation by the presence of gastric malpositioning. Different directions and degrees of rotation of the stomach may be present at the time of radiography, and the radiographic appearance of the stomach varies depending on the type and degree of rotation and the amount of distention.[62,63] As the stomach dilates the fundus and greater curvature rotate (clockwise when viewed from caudal to cranial) to lie along the ventral abdominal wall. The pylorus therefore shifts dorsally, cranially, and to the left, and the body of the stomach shifts toward the right.[27] Because of the gastrosplenic ligament, the spleen follows the greater curvature toward the right.

The major radiographic feature of gastric volvulus is gas and fluid distention of the stomach (more gas than fluid). Additionally, the pylorus is usually displaced dorsally and to the left. Thus radiographic determination of the location of the pylorus is the key differentiating feature between gastric dilation and gastric volvulus. Radiographic localization of the pylorus is best accomplished by making left and right recumbent lateral views or ventrodorsal and dorsoventral views. Lateral views are usually of most value. When filled with gas, the pyloric portion of the stomach appears more tubular and narrower than the rest of the stomach. Although the stomach is filled primarily with gas, it usually contains enough fluid so that the pyloric portion may fill with fluid and thus not be seen. Both lateral views may be needed to ensure that the pylorus fills with gas and can thus be recognized. In the unstable, acutely ill patient in which gastric dilatation and volvulus are suspected, a right lateral radiograph should be made first. In many instances the diagnosis may be obvious on this one radiograph, and the unstable patient will not have to undergo manipulation to perform other positional radiographs. If the diagnosis is not obvious on this first radiograph, other radiographic views are necessary.

With the pylorus shifted to the left and with the patient in left recumbency, fluid in the stomach fills the pylorus and gas fills the rest of the stomach. With the patient in right recumbency, gas fills the pyloric portion and fluid shifts to the fundus or body of the stomach. This gas distribution is opposite to what is normally expected. Thus the radiographic finding that the pyloric portion fills with fluid on the left recumbent lateral view and fills with gas on the right recumbent lateral view indicates that the pylorus is on the left side and that the stomach has rotated (Figs. 45-14 and 45-15). Recognition of this shift is usually more difficult on the ventrodorsal and dorsoventral views because specific recognition of the pyloric portion may be more difficult. Positive-contrast gastrography may be performed but usually is not needed. An additional variation is a volvulus of 360 degrees in which the pylorus and fundus are in their normal positions (Fig. 45-16) and diagnosis depends on findings at physical examination or surgery.

Gastric volvulus may also be present without severe gastric distention. This situation may often exist for days or weeks after previous gastric decompression[64] or may be present at the time of initial presentation.[28] The aforementioned radiographic principles still apply as a means to recognize rotation of the stomach (see Fig. 45-14).

Compartmentalization is a term that refers to the radiographic appearance of soft tissue bands that project into or across the gas-filled lumen of the rotated stomach. These soft tissue bands result from folding of the stomach on itself as the folded wall projects into the lumen and is outlined by gas within the lumen.[2] These bands may become more obvious with greater degrees of distention (see Fig. 45-15). With progressive distention of the stomach, the stomach wall becomes thinner. Gas within the gastric wall, termed pneumatosis, has also been described but is infrequent.[2] Gastric pneumatosis or pneumoperitoneum should alert the clinician to the increased possibility of gastric necrosis. Prior trocharization of the stomach will obviously complicate assessing the significance of pneumatosis or pneumoperitoneum, and the lack of pneumatosis does not rule out the possibility of gastric necrosis.[65]

As the stomach enlarges other mobile structures within the abdomen are displaced caudally. With severe gastric distention, visualization of other abdominal organs is often difficult because of crowding. The spleen usually is also involved in gastric volvulus and may shift with the stomach. The spleen is usually enlarged because of impaired circulation, but its location may vary. Outright torsion of the malpositioned spleen may also occur; this further compromises the patient. The greater the gastric distention, the less likely the spleen is to be visualized radiographically because of crowding of abdominal viscera. Thus splenomegaly and splenic displacement may be more easily visualized with less-severe gastric volvulus. Other changes that may be seen with volvulus include reflex paralytic ileus of the small intestine, esophageal dilation, and microcardia and pulmonary hypovolemia (small vessels) associated with shock.

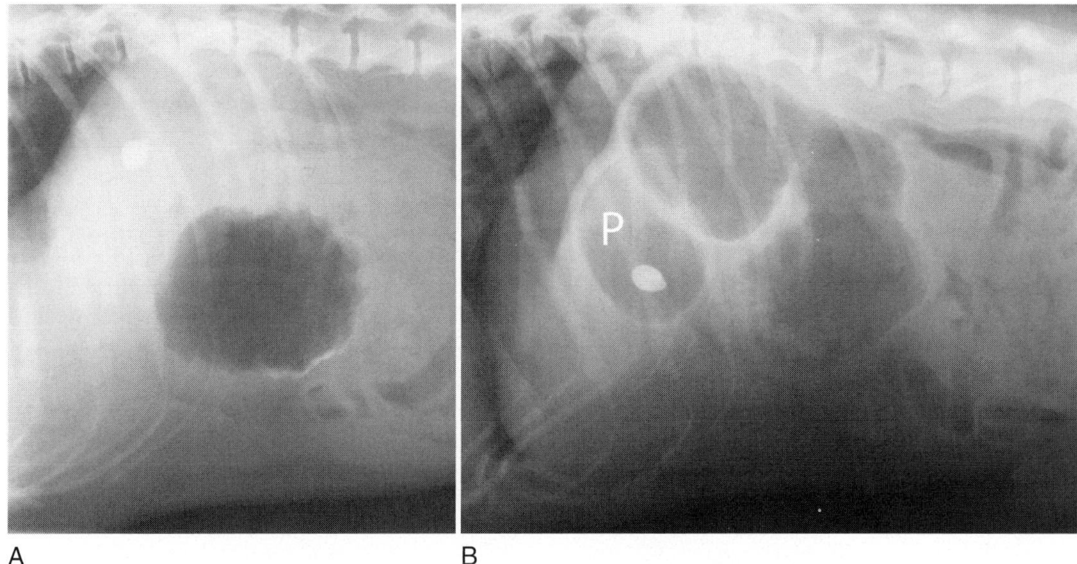

Fig. 45-14 Gastric volvulus. **A,** Left recumbent lateral view. The stomach is mildly distended with gas in the fundus and the body. Fluid fills the pyloric portion, which is not well visualized. An incidental mineral foreign body is seen within the pylorus. **B,** Right recumbent lateral view. The fluid shifts into the fundic portion, and gas outlines the pyloric portion *(P)* as well as the body and fundus. These changes indicate that the pylorus is on the left and the fundus is on the right and that there is a gastric volvulus. This patient has minimal dilation because of recent decompression by passage of an orogastric tube.

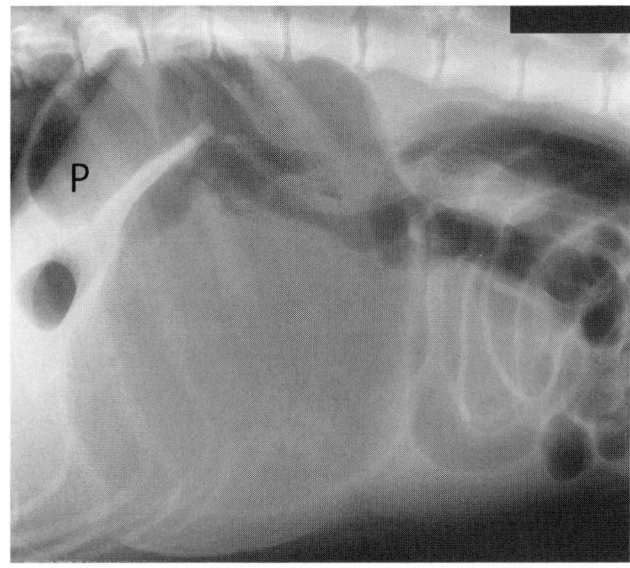

Fig. 45-15 Gastric volvulus, right recumbent lateral view. The pylorus *(P)* is directed cranioventrally. Compartmentalization of the stomach is evident. The majority of the small intestine is moderately distended, suggesting paralytic ileus.

Chronic Pyloric Obstruction

Obstruction of gastric emptying at the pylorus may be acute or chronic. Causes of acute obstruction include gastric volvulus and foreign bodies. Chronic pyloric obstruction is usually the result of narrowing of the pyloric orifice caused by diseases affecting the wall or blocking the orifice, such as hypertrophic pyloric stenosis, pylorospasm, inflammation or fibrosis, neoplasia, and mucosal antral hypertrophy. These conditions usually cause a chronic partial obstruction at the pylorus, leading to chronic retention of gastric content.

Chronic partial obstruction of the pylorus often manifests on survey radiographs as fluid-filled gastric distention as opposed to the acute gaseous distention of gastric volvulus (Fig. 45-17). The stomach may be quite large with chronic partial obstruction of the pylorus. However, the enlarged stomach may be more difficult to identify on survey radiographs when it is filled with fluid than when it is filled with gas. Even when distended with fluid, the stomach still contains some gas. In these instances, however, the gas does not totally outline or fill the entire stomach. Instead, the smaller amount of gas floats as a bubble on top of the fluid and should not be mistaken as the limits of the stomach or wall thickening (see Fig. 45-17, *B*).

The major effect of pyloric obstructive diseases is to restrict gastric emptying. Survey radiographic findings may vary from normal gastric size to enlargement depending on the severity and duration of the obstruction. With contrast studies, the major radiographic abnormality is delayed gastric emptying. However, an initial delay in gastric emptying may be of no clinical significance because of the influence of various psychologic or pharmacologic factors previously discussed. This point is especially important to remember if the stomach starts to empty normally after an initial delay or after the animal is allowed to calm down. Of more significance is a pronounced delay in gastric emptying when only a small amount of contrast medium passes from the stomach in a few hours. Because the normal stomach should be empty 1 to 4 hours after administration of contrast medium, retention of most of the barium within the stomach 3 or 4 hours after administration usually indicates pyloric obstructive disease (Fig. 45-18).

Differentiation of the pyloric obstructive diseases is difficult radiographically, especially without fluoroscopy. The stomach is a dynamic organ that rapidly changes appearance

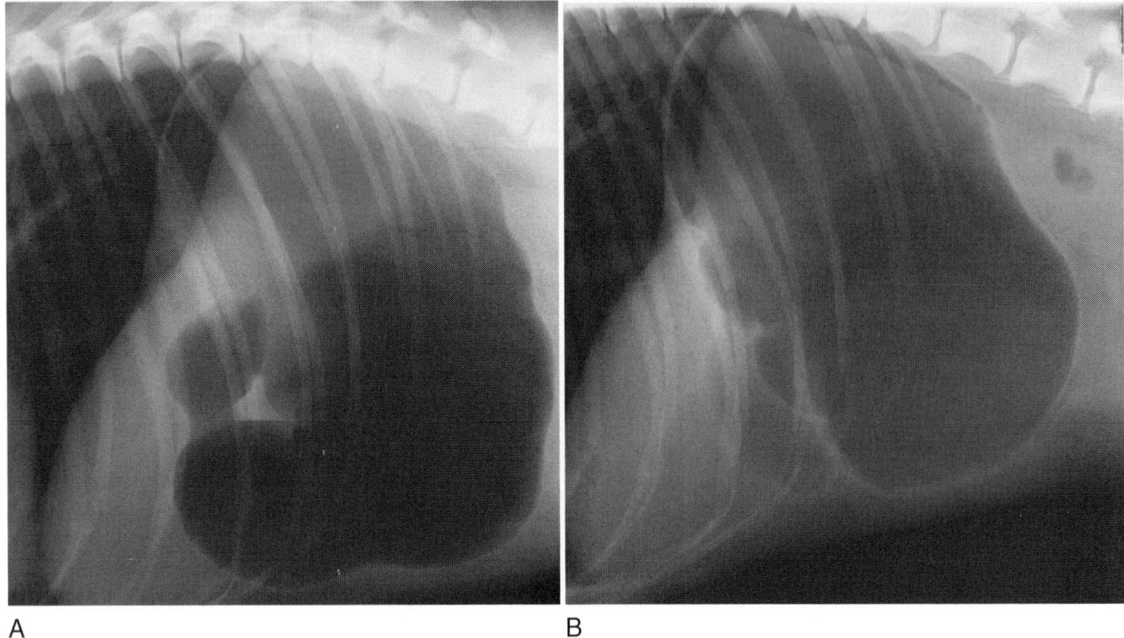

Fig. 45-16 Left recumbent (A) and right recumbent (B) lateral views of a dog with acute gastric dilatation. On the basis of these radiographic findings, the pylorus and the fundus are normally positioned. A gastric tube could not be passed into the stomach. Final diagnosis was 360-degree gastric volvulus.

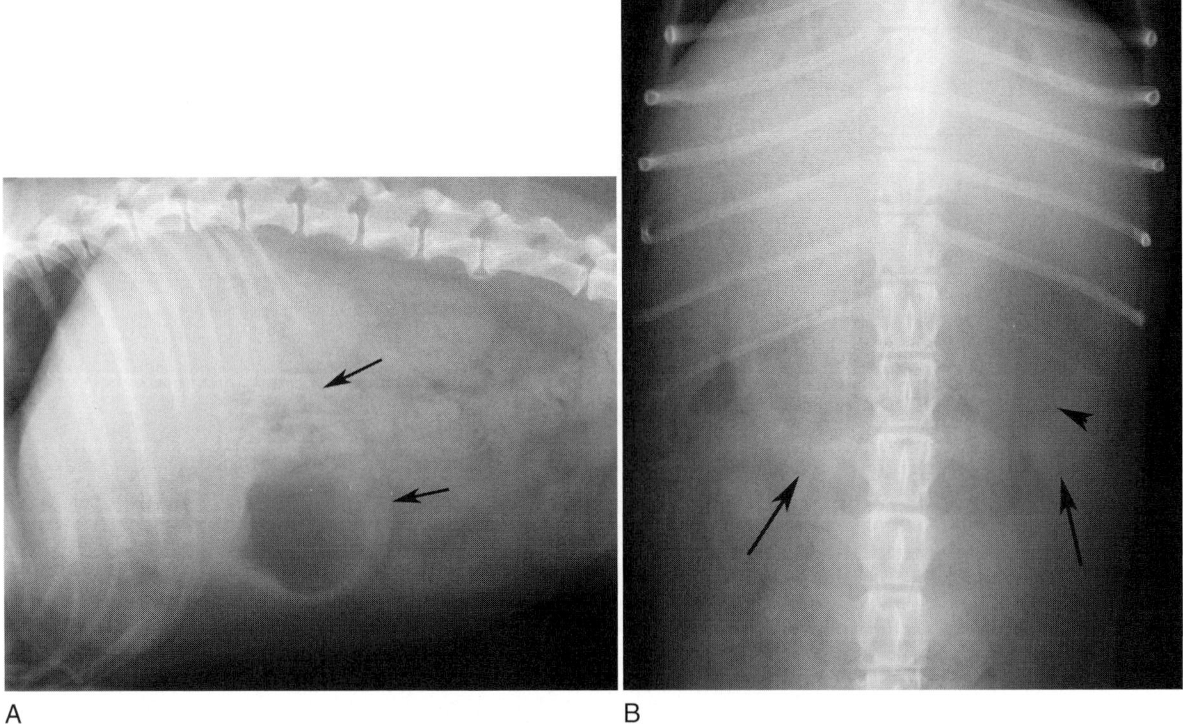

Fig. 45-17 Lateral (A) and ventrodorsal (B) radiographs of a dog with fluid-filled gastric distention caused by chronic pyloric obstruction. The stomach is more difficult to identify when filled with fluid instead of gas. The *long arrows* indicate the caudal margin of the stomach. The smaller gastric gas pocket (*short arrows* in B) should not be mistaken for gastric wall thickening.

because of peristaltic waves, and a radiograph is simply a snapshot of the morphologic features of the stomach. Thus the appearance of the stomach on a radiograph depends on when the exposure was made. Although some diseases may produce characteristic radiographic abnormalities, such abnormalities may be visible only during certain moments within the gastric cycle and thus are not likely to be seen on a randomly exposed radiograph. The advantage of fluoroscopy is that sequential changes of the shape of the stomach can be visualized; thus those momentary changes that may best demonstrate certain lesions of the stomach may be documented. Even with fluoroscopy, however, differentiating some pyloric obstructive diseases is not possible. For example, hypertrophic pyloric stenosis, neoplasia, and mural scarring all may produce an annular type of stricture of the pylorus that prevents the pylorus from opening adequately. Thus dividing obstructive pyloric diseases into those that encircle the pylorus, and are thus restrictive, and those that obstruct the pylorus by blocking its orifice may be a more practical choice.

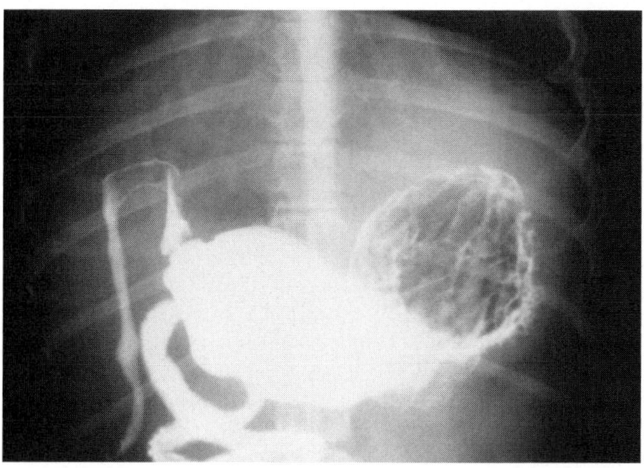

Fig. 45-18 Dorsoventral radiograph 5 hours after barium was given. A pronounced delay in gastric emptying is visible, with most of the contrast medium retained within the stomach.

Restrictive diseases of the pylorus include hypertrophic pyloric stenosis, pylorospasm, inflammation or scarring, and neoplasia. If characteristic abnormalities are present on radiographs, they are usually those of an annular type of stricture narrowing the pyloric sphincter. If barium fills only the entrance of the lumen at the pyloric sphincter, the resultant radiographic appearance is referred to as the beak sign.[66] If barium fills the length of the narrowed lumen through the pyloric sphincter, the resultant radiographic appearance is referred to as the string sign.[66] A tit sign has been described as a relatively sharp, pointed outpouching of the pyloric antrum along the lesser curvature as a peristaltic wave pushes contrast medium in a peristaltic pouch up against the mass-type lesion around the pylorus.[66] Variations in severity, symmetry, and radiographic projection all contribute to create variations in the radiographic appearance of pyloric restrictive lesions (Fig. 45-19). In dogs with chronic pyloric hypertrophy, the hypertrophic muscularis may be detected ultrasonographically. It is seen as a thick hypoechoic layer. The thickness of the muscularis has been reported to be greater than 3 mm in mild to moderate hypertrophy and greater than 8 mm in severely affected dogs. Vigorous, but ineffective, peristaltic contractions that fail to propel contents into the duodenum are seen in some patients.[50]

The second group of pyloric obstructive diseases includes gastric foreign bodies, mucosal inflammation or hypertrophy, and some mural lesions of the pyloric antrum. These types of lesions are more likely to produce filling defects within the lumen that occlude the orifice of the pyloric sphincter (Fig. 45-20). Again, radiographic recognition of such a lesion is usually diagnostically adequate, and specific differentiation of the underlying cause may not be possible on radiographs.

Gastric Ulcers

Gastric ulcers are difficult to identify on conventional radiographs. Gastric ulcers are more conspicuous in barium

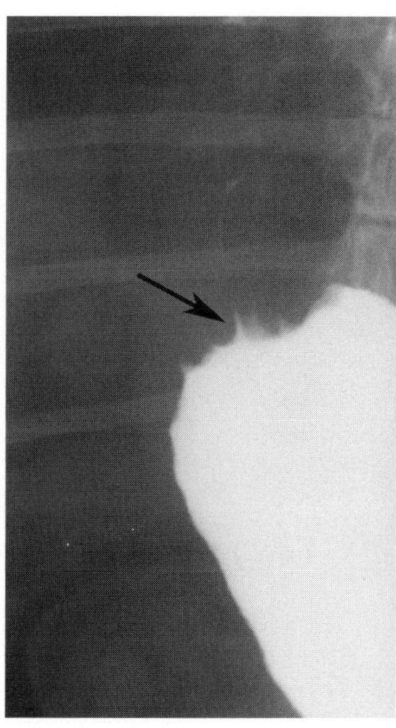

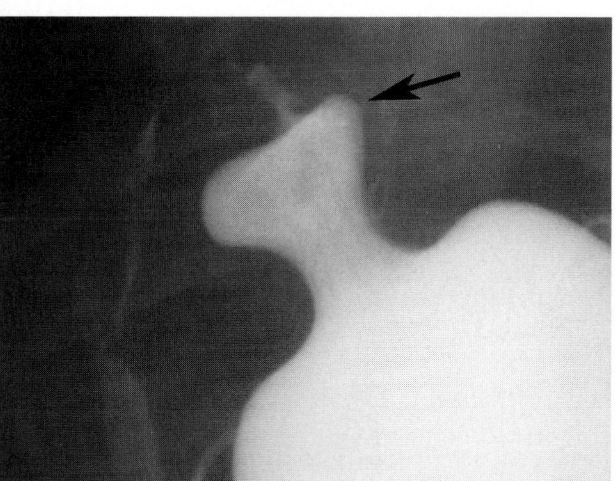

Fig. 45-19 A, Ventrodorsal radiograph of the pyloric region of a dog with restrictive disease of the pylorus. The "string" sign *(arrow)* is caused by barium that fills the length of the lumen of the narrowed pyloric sphincter because of an annular type of stricture. B, Ventrodorsal radiograph of the pyloric region of another dog with restrictive disease of the pylorus. The peristaltic pouch *(arrow)* is the outpouching of the pyloric antrum along the lesser curvature as a peristaltic wave pushes contrast medium up against the mass-type lesion encircling the pylorus. A pronounced delay in gastric emptying was also present.

studies, in which they produce craters in the wall of the stomach that appear as outpouchings from the lumen (Fig. 45-21). The radiographic appearance of a gastric ulcer may vary depending on whether the ulcer is projected in profile, en face, or obliquely.[67] The appearance of the ulcer may be further altered by gastric peristalsis. Manipulation of the patient during fluoroscopy allows a more complete and continuous evaluation of the margin and contour of the stomach. Double-contrast gastrography may also be of value because ulcers that are projected en face may be visualized with double-contrast studies but are obscured with positive-contrast gastrography.

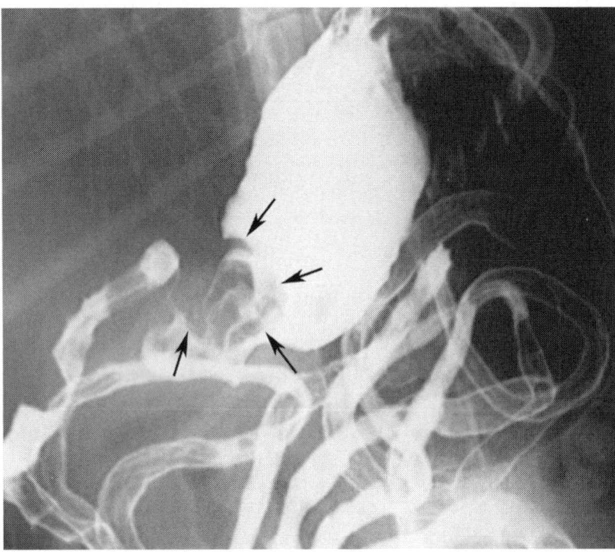

Fig. 45-20 Ventrodorsal oblique radiograph of the pylorus of a dog with obstructive disease of the pylorus. A hemispheric filling defect is at the pylorus that projects into the lumen. Pronounced delay in gastric emptying was present.

Gastric ulcers may be benign or malignant. Benign gastric ulcers may result from a variety of causes.[27,68,69] Use of nonsteroidal antiinflammatory drugs has become a common cause of benign gastric ulcers.[70-72] Dachshunds with disc prolapse were found to have a 76% prevalence of gastroduodenal ulceration.[73] This is thought to be from ulcerogenic drug administration as well as autonomic disturbances, stress, hypovolemia, and other factors.[73]

Malignant gastric ulcers occur in association with gastric neoplasia and may be caused by tumor necrosis.[69] Criteria have been established for the radiographic differentiation of benign and malignant gastric ulcers in human beings.[67,74,75] Thus although radiography may provide an excellent method for the recognition of gastric ulcers, infrequent use of single- and double-contrast gastrography, lack of fluoroscopy, and insufficient views all combine to limit the recognition of gastric ulcers in dogs and cats. In addition, experience is limited in radiographically differentiating benign and malignant gastric ulcers in dogs and cats. Ulceration is often associated with gastric carcinoma,[76,77] and gastric ulcers in dogs that are recognized on radiographs are often the result of neoplasia.[78] Thus the radiographic recognition of a gastric ulcer should lead to strong consideration of neoplasia and further evaluation of the stomach with endoscopic and biopsy studies or by surgical exploration.

Gastric ulcers may be detected on ultrasound examination (see Fig. 45-21, *B*) but are not always found even if present.[48,79] Features include the presence of a wall defect (crater) usually within the center of a locally thickened area of stomach wall. The thickened area may have loss of the normal layered appearance. Gastric fluid accumulation and decreased motility may also be noted. Ulcers from nonneoplastic causes do not appear distinctly different from those seen with neoplasms.

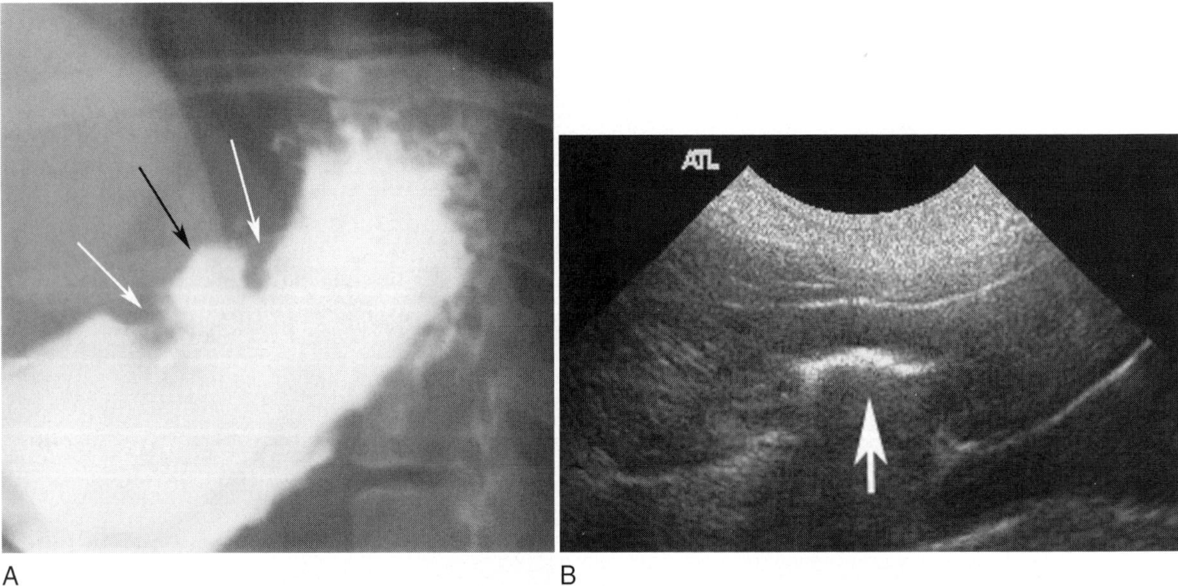

Fig. 45-21 **A,** Ventrodorsal oblique radiograph of the stomach of a dog with a gastric ulcer *(black arrow)*. Note the filling defects protruding into the stomach *(white arrows)* representing the "collar" of the ulcer. **B,** Sagittal sonograph of the stomach of another dog. The pyloric region of the stomach is diffusely thickened and layers are not identifiable. The *white arrow* indicates a portion of the stomach wall that is focally thinner than the remainder. The mucosal surface of this area is hyperechoic. A large ulcer was found in this area at necropsy; the diagnosis was adenocarcinoma.

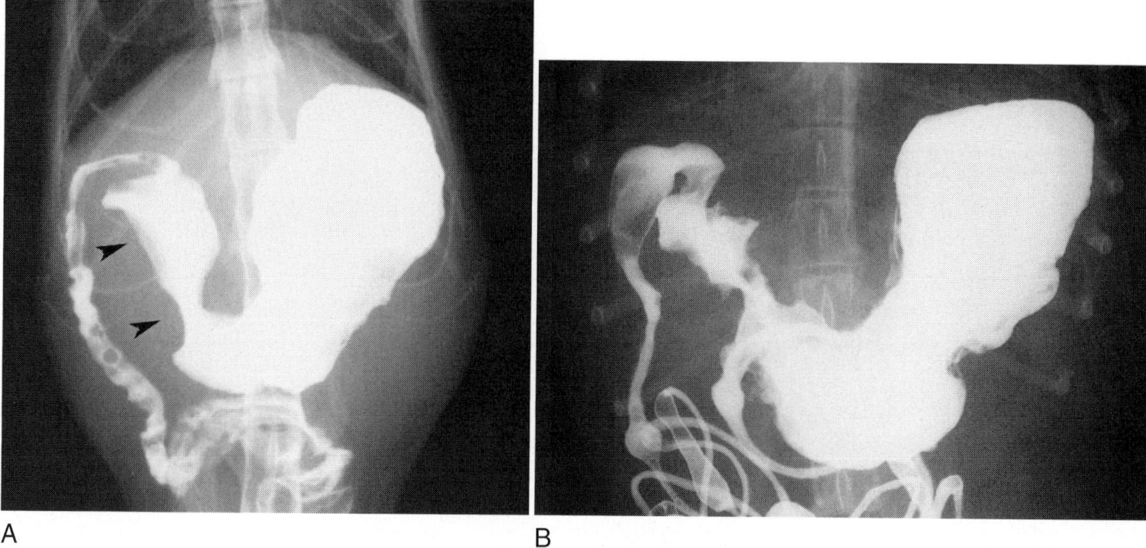

Fig. 45-22 A, Ventrodorsal gastrogram of a cat. A smooth filling defect is present from a mass lesion along the greater curvature *(arrows)*. B, Ventrodorsal gastrogram of a dog. An annular mass encircles the pyloric portion and part of the body. This area failed to distend even in sternal recumbency, and the abnormality persisted throughout the study. Final diagnosis was gastric adenocarcinoma.

Gastric Neoplasia

Several types of gastric neoplasms occur in the stomach, and any region of the stomach may be involved. Polyps may often be clinically silent and are most often found incidentally.[80] Adenocarcinoma is the most common malignant gastric tumor in dogs.[77,81] This tumor may occur in any region of the stomach but appears to be found most often in the pyloric portion.[76,82] Gastric neoplasia occurs less frequently in the cat than in the dog,[83] and lymphosarcoma is the most common type of feline gastric neoplasm.[84]

The radiographic appearance of gastric neoplasia varies and primarily depends on the size, shape, and location of the tumor. The major radiographic feature is that of a mass lesion that projects into the gastric lumen, creating a filling defect within the contrast medium. The more nodular and pedunculated the lesion, the easier to recognize it as a distinct mass (Fig. 45-22). Smaller mass lesions may be completely obscured by a relatively large volume of barium. Oblique projections, conformation of the stomach, and peristaltic contractions all may contribute to obscure some mass lesions of the stomach.

Tumors that are diffuse and less discrete are more difficult to identify. Diffuse infiltrative lesions of the stomach wall may not produce distinct filling defects. Instead, they may alter the shape of the stomach and produce decreased motility of the involved area. If such diffuse lesions encircle a portion of the stomach, the radiographic appearance may be that of an annular narrowing or one in which the stomach has decreased distensibility in the affected area (see Fig. 45-22, *B*). Because of variations in appearance of the stomach created by peristalsis, persistence of a suspected abnormality on sequential radiographs is important. The radiographic recognition of a gastric ulcer should also suggest the possibility of gastric neoplasia.

Gastric masses can be found on ultrasound examination of the stomach, thus eliminating the need for radiographic contrast studies. Common features include thickening of the stomach wall, distortion of the normal layered appearance of the wall, and decreased echogenicity and motility in the affected area (Fig. 45-23).[39-46] Although such lesions are most often associated with gastric neoplasia, similar changes have been reported in dogs with pythiosis[47] and zygomycosis.[85] Extension of the lesion through the serosal surface of the stomach has been reported in dogs with gastric carcinoma.[46] Another reported sonographic feature of gastric carcinoma is "pseudolayering" of the stomach wall, which is thought to be associated with uneven distribution of tumor in the layers of the stomach wall.[39,41] Instead of the five layers normally seen, a central, moderately echogenic zone between two lesser echogenic lines is seen. Loss of wall layering in the intestines has also been associated with neoplasia as opposed to inflammatory disease. Dogs with loss of layers were 50.9 times more likely to have neoplasia than inflammatory bowel disease.[86] Although the stomach was not included in this study, the same trend may exist for the stomach, with loss of layers being suggestive of neoplasia.

Concurrent regional lymph node enlargement and ulceration of the affected area have been reported in both gastric carcinoma and lymphosarcoma.[46] Reports of maximal gastric wall thickness range from 10 to 27 mm in dogs[41,42,46] and 8 to 25 mm in cats[40,43] with gastric neoplasia, measurements clearly greater than the reported normal gastric wall thickness of 3 to 5 mm (dogs) and 2 mm (cats). Gastric wall measurements greater than 6 to 7 mm have been proposed as being abnormal.[37] Although gastric wall thickening is an important abnormal finding, caution must be exercised when assessing wall thickness in a contracted, empty stomach because the stomach wall is normally thickened when empty and a false-positive diagnosis of gastric mass can be made.[87] Distending the stomach with water may help distinguish true- and false-positive lesions, but real-time observation of gastric motility may be an easier way to distinguish the two because a lack of motility usually is seen in an abnormal wall segment. Cytologic or histopathologic evaluation is necessary for a definitive diagnosis. Specimens can be obtained by ultrasound-guided fine-needle aspiration or tissue core biopsy.[88,89]

Diffuse Diseases of the Stomach

The stomach may be diffusely involved in a variety of diseases that produce inflammation, hypertrophy, atrophy, or mineral-

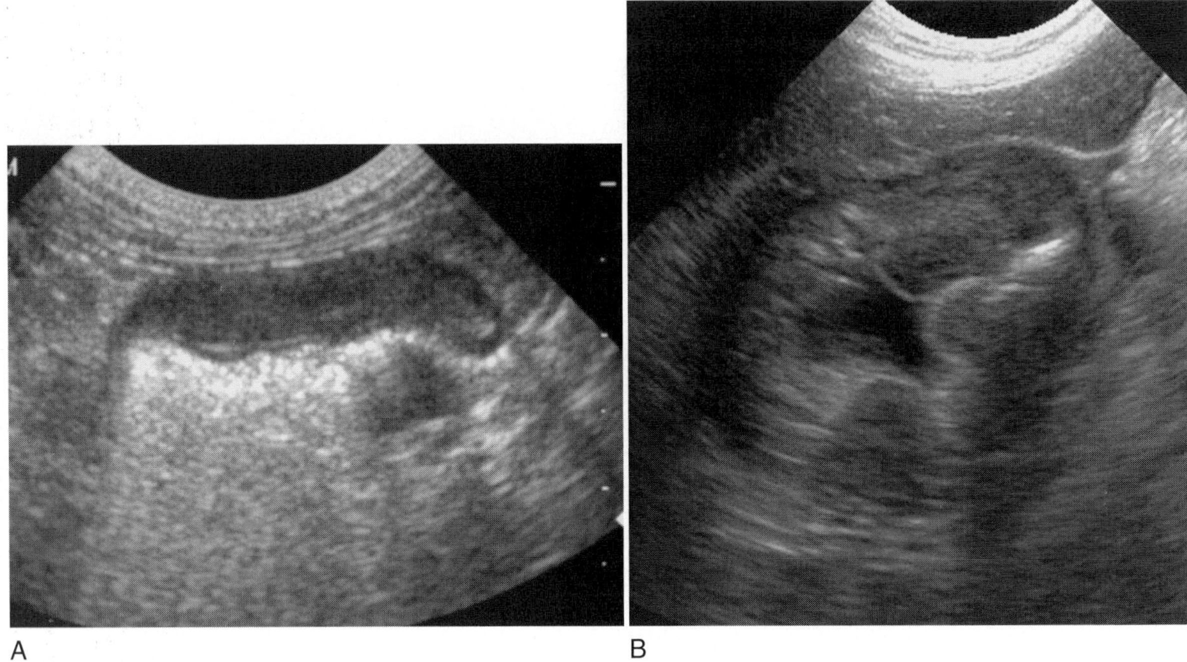

Fig. 45-23 Longitudinal ultrasonograms of gastric neoplasia. **A,** Lymphosarcoma in the stomach wall of a cat. The stomach wall is thickened, hypoechoic, and has lost the normal layered appearance. **B,** Suspected adenocarcinoma in the stomach wall of a dog. The wall is uniformly thickened and decreased in echogenicity. The normal layered appearance is disrupted. Caudal is to the *right*, and ventral is to the *top*.

ization. Acute gastritis may result from a variety of causes and is rarely associated with radiographic abnormalities. Chronic gastritis is infrequently diagnosed clinically and may also result from a variety of causes. Examples include diseases such as chronic atrophic gastritis, chronic hypertrophic gastritis, eosinophilic gastritis, and pythiosis and zygomycosis.[90,91] Paucity of rugal folds, large rugal folds, nodules, or a thickened gastric wall may be seen with these diseases (Fig. 45-24).[90] Care must be taken when evaluating stomach wall thickness on survey radiographs. Fluid within the stomach may cause border effacement with the stomach wall, creating the illusion of increased thickness.

Ultrasonographic findings of gastric pythiosis and zygomycosis are similar to those reported for gastric neoplasms.[47,85] Nonfungal inflammation may cause diffuse stomach wall thickening with maintenance of wall layers.[45,92] Although loss of the normal layered appearance of the intestines is generally associated with neoplasia,[86] some cases of inflammatory bowel disease or infectious gastritis (pythiosis) also demonstrate loss of the normal layered appearance.[47,93]

Soft tissue calcification may occur in association with chronic renal failure.[51,94,95] In such patients mineralization of the gastric wall may be visible radiographically as thin, linear, mineralized opacities (Fig. 45-25).[94] Rugal mineralization is often more easily visualized when the stomach is empty and the mineralized mucosal fold pattern is more tightly grouped. Ultrasonographic findings of dogs with uremic gastropathy include thickened gastric wall and rugal folds and a hyperechoic zone at the mucosal/luminal interface caused by mucosal mineralization.[51,92] Ultrasound was thought to be more sensitive than radiography for detection of gastric lesions associated with uremia.

Although in many patients endoscopy is the gold standard for the diagnosis of gastric diseases, in some patients the mucosal surface of the stomach may be normal, leading to

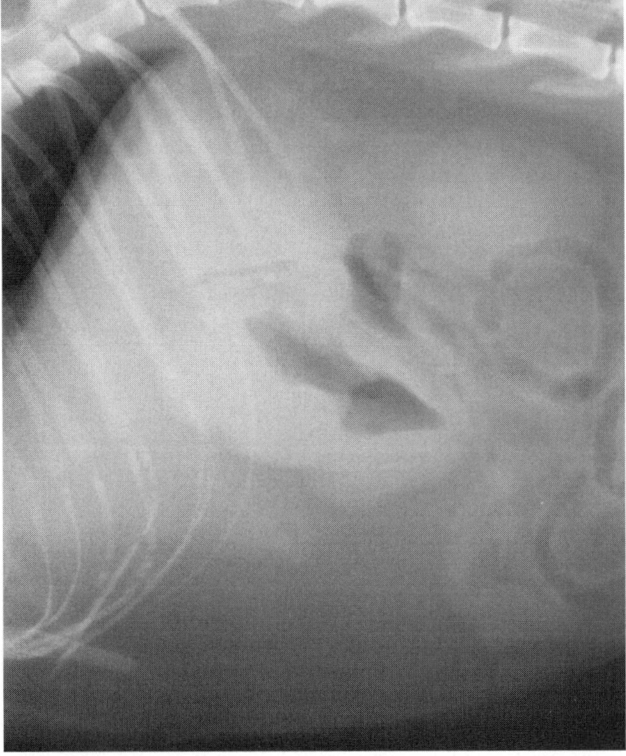

Fig. 45-24 Lateral survey radiograph of the abdomen of a cat with a thick gastric wall. The thickened wall is best visualized in the ventral mid-abdomen and is associated with a narrow, tubular, gas-filled lumen. Care should be taken when evaluating the stomach wall on survey radiographs.

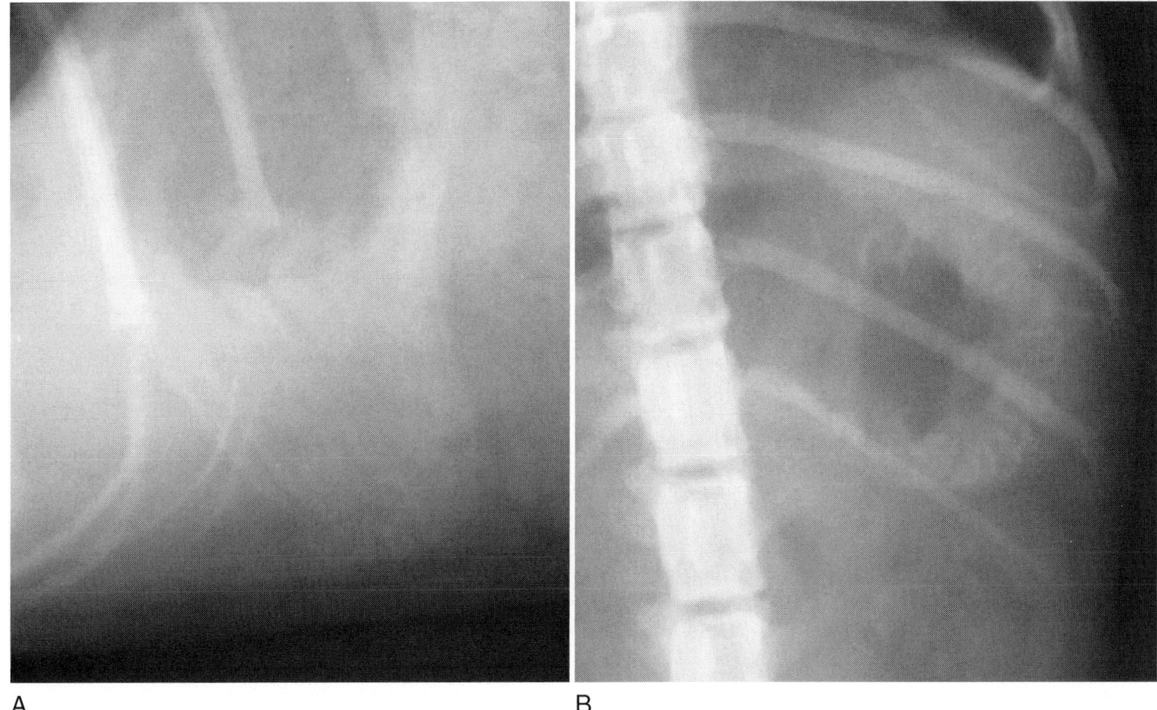

Fig. 45-25 Close-up right recumbent lateral (A) and ventrodorsal (B) survey radiographs of a dog with chronic renal failure. Thin, curvilinear, mineralized opacities that parallel the rugal folds of the stomach are caused by gastric calcification.

false-negative results by endoscopy. Ultrasound demonstrates the morphologic features of the entire gastric wall unless the wall is hidden by gas or echogenic ingesta. In some patients ultrasound may be more informative than endoscopy.[96]

REFERENCES

1. Evans HE: *Miller's anatomy of the dog,* ed 3, Philadelphia, 1993, WB Saunders.
2. O'Brien TR: *Radiographic diagnosis of abdominal disorders in the dog and cat,* Philadelphia, 1978, WB Saunders.
3. Brawner WR, Bartels JE: Contrast radiography of the digestive tract: indications, techniques, and complications, *Vet Clin North Am* 13:599, 1983.
4. Root CR: Interpretation of abdominal survey radiographs, *Vet Clin North Am* 4:763, 1974.
5. Arnbjerg J: Gastric emptying time in the dog and cat, *J Am Anim Hosp Assoc* 28:77, 1992.
6. Gomez JA: The gastrointestinal contrast study: methods and interpretation, *Vet Clin North Am* 4:805, 1974.
7. Bargai U: The effect of xylazine hydrochloride on the radiographic appearance of the stomach and intestine in the dog, *Vet Radiol* 23:60, 1982.
8. Hogan PM, Aronson E: Effect of sedation on transit time of feline gastrointestinal contrast studies, *Vet Radiol* 29:85, 1994.
9. Steyn PF, Twedt D, Toombs W: The effect of intravenous diazepam on solid phase gastric emptying in normal cats, *Vet Radiol Ultrasound* 38:469, 1997.
10. Scrivani PV, Bednarski RM, Meyer CW: Effects of acepromazine and butorphanol on positive-contrast upper gastrointestinal tract examination in dogs, *Am J Vet Res* 59:1227, 1998.
11. Miyabayashi T, Morgan JP: Upper gastrointestinal examinations: a radiographic study of clinically normal Beagle puppies, *J Small Anim Pract* 32:83, 1991.
12. Evans SM, Lauffer I: Double-contrast gastrography in the normal dog, *Vet Radiol* 22:2, 1981.
13. Evans SM, Biery DN: Double-contrast gastrography in the cat: technique and normal radiographic appearance, *Vet Radiol* 24:3, 1983.
14. Root CR, Morgan JP: Contrast radiography of the upper gastrointestinal tract in the dog, *J Small Anim Pract* 10:279, 1969.
15. Burns J, Fox SM: The use of a barium meal to evaluate total gastric emptying time in the dog, *Vet Radiol* 27:169, 1986.
16. Miybayashi T, Morgan JP: Gastric emptying in the normal dog: a contrast radiograph technique, *Vet Radiol* 25:187, 1984.
17. Allan GS, Rendano VT, Quick CB et al: Gastrografin as a gastrointestinal contrast medium in the cat, *Vet Radiol* 20:110, 1979.
18. Agut A, Sanchezvalverde MA, Torrecillas FE et al: Iohexol as a gastrointestinal contrast medium in the cat, *Vet Radiol Ultrasound* 35:164, 1994.
19. Williams J, Biller DS, Miyabayashi T et al: Evaluation of iohexol as a gastrointestinal contrast medium in normal cats, *Vet Radiol Ultrasound* 34:310, 1993.
20. Allan FJ, Guilford WG, Robertson ID et al: Gastric emptying of solid radiopaque markers in healthy dogs, *Vet Radiol Ultrasound* 37:336, 1996.
21. Guilford GW, Lawoko CRO, Allan FJ: Accuracy of localizing radiopaque markers by abdominal radiography and correlation between their gastric emptying rate and that of a canned food in dogs, *Am J Vet Res* 58:1359, 1997.
22. Chandler ML, Guilford G, Lawoko CRO: Radiopaque markers to evaluate gastric emptying and small intestinal transit time in healthy cats, *J Vet Intern Med* 11:361, 1997.
23. Hall JA, Willer RL, Seim HB et al: Gastric emptying of nondigestible radiopaque markers after circumcostal

gastropexy in clinically normal dogs and dogs with gastric dilatation-volvulus, *Am J Vet Res* 53:1961, 1992.
24. Grandage J: The radiologic appearance of stomach gas in the dog, *Aust Vet J* 50:529, 1974.
25. Armbrust LJ, Biller DS, Hoskinson JJ: Case examples demonstrating the clinical utility of obtaining both right and left lateral abdominal radiographs in small animals, *J Am Anim Hosp Assoc* 36:531, 2000.
26. Jakovljevic S, Gibbs C: Radiographic assessment of gastric mucosal fold thickness in dogs. *Am J Vet Res* 54:1827, 1993.
27. Twedt DC, Wingfield WE: Diseases of the stomach. In Ettinger SJ, editor: *Textbook of veterinary internal medicine, vol 2*, ed 2, Philadelphia, 1983, WB Saunders, p 1233.
28. Funkquist B, Garmer L: Pathogenetic and therapeutic aspects of torsion of the canine stomach, *J Small Anim Pract* 8:523, 1967.
29. Gibbs C, Pearson H: The radiological diagnosis of gastrointestinal obstruction in the dog, *J Small Anim Pract* 14:61, 1973.
30. Gue M, Fioramonti J, Frexinos J et al: Influence of acoustic stress by noise on gastrointestinal motility in dogs, *Dig Dis Sci* 32:1411, 1987.
31. Hornof WJ, Koblik PD, Strombeck DR et al: Scintigraphic evaluation of solid-phase gastric emptying in the dog, *Vet Radiol* 30:242, 1989.
32. Kunze CP, Hoskinson JJ, Butine MD et al: Evaluation of solid phase radiolabels of dog food for gastric emptying, *Vet Radiol Ultrasound* 40:169, 1999.
33. Lester NV, Roberts GD, Newell SM et al: Assessment of barium impregnated polyethylene spheres (BIPS) as a measure of solid-phase gastric emptying in normal dogs: comparison to scintigraphy, *Vet Radiol Ultrasound* 40;465, 1999.
34. Goggin JM, Hoskinson JJ, Kirk CA et al: Comparison of gastric emptying times in healthy cats simultaneously evaluated with radiopaque markers and nuclear scintigraphy, *Vet Radiol Ultrasound* 40;89, 1999.
35. Heng HG, Wrigley RH, Kraft SL, et al: Fat is responsible for an intramural radiolucent band in the feline stomach wall, *Vet Radiol Ultrasound* 46:54, 2005.
36. Keith DG, Wortman JA, Saunders HM et al: A comparison of the sensitivity and specificity of barium gastrography and ultrasonography for gastric and duodenal disease [abstract], *Vet Radiol Ultrasound* 40:657, 1999.
37. Penninck DG, Nyland TG, Fisher PE et al: Ultrasonography of the normal canine gastrointestinal tract, *Vet Radiol* 30:272, 1989.
38. Lamb CR: Abdominal ultrasonography in small animals: intestinal tract and mesentery, kidneys, adrenal glands, uterus, and prostate, *J Small Anim Pract* 31:295, 1990.
39. Penninck DG: Characteristics of gastrointestinal tumors, *Vet Clin North Am Small Anim Pract* 28:777, 1998.
40. Penninck DG, Moore AS, Tidwell AS et al: Ultrasonography of alimentary lymphosarcoma in the cat, *Vet Radiol Ultrasound* 35:299, 1994.
41. Penninck DG, Moore AS, Gliatto J: Ultrasonography of canine gastric epithelial neoplasia, *Vet Radiol Ultrasound* 39:342, 1998.
42. Kaser-Hotz B, Hauser B, Arnold P: Ultrasonographic findings in canine gastric neoplasia in 13 patients, *Vet Radiol Ultrasound* 37:51, 1996.
43. Grooters AM, Biller DS, Ward H et al: Ultrasonographic appearance of feline alimentary lymphoma, *Vet Radiol Ultrasound* 35:468, 1994.
44. Rivers BJ, Walter PA, Johnston GR et al: Canine gastric neoplasia: utility of ultrasonography in diagnosis, *J Am Anim Hosp Assoc* 33:144, 1997.
45. Penninck DG, Nyland TG, Kerr LY et al: Ultrasonographic evaluation of gastrointestinal diseases in small animals, *Vet Radiol Ultrasound* 31:134, 1990.
46. Lamb CR, Grierson J: Ultrasonographic appearance of primary gastric neoplasia in 21 dogs, *J Small Anim Pract* 40:211, 1999.
47. Graham JP, Newell SM, Roberts GD et al: Ultrasonographic features of canine gastrointestinal pythiosis, *Vet Radiol Ultrasound* 41:273, 2000.
48. Penninck DG, Matz M, Tidwell AS: Ultrasonography of gastric ulceration in the dog, *Vet Radiol Ultrasound* 38:308, 1997.
49. Tidwell AS, Penninck DG: Ultrasonography of gastrointestinal foreign bodies, *Vet Radiol Ultrasound* 33:160, 1992.
50. Biller DS, Partington BP, Miyabayashi T et al: Ultrasonographic appearance of chronic hypertrophic pyloric gastropathy in the dog, *Vet Radiol Ultrasound* 35:30, 1994.
51. Grooters AM, Miyabayashi T, Biller DS et al: Sonographic appearance of uremic gastropathy in four dogs, *Vet Radiol Ultrasound* 35:35, 1994.
52. Huml RA, Konde LJ, Sellon RK et al: Gastrogastric intussusception in a dog, *Vet Radiol Ultrasound* 33:150, 1992.
53. Watson PJ: Gastroduodenal intussusception in a young dog, *J Small Anim Pract* 38:163, 1997.
54. Tanno F, Weber U, Wacker CH et al: Ultrasonographic comparison of adhesions induced by two different methods of gastropexy in the dog, *J Small Anim Pract* 39:432, 1998.
55. Wacker CA, Weber UT, Tanno F et al: Ultrasonographic evaluation of adhesions induced by incisional gastropexy in 16 dogs., *J Small Anim Pract* 39:379, 1998.
56. Agut A, Wood AKW, Martin ICA: Sonographic observations of the gastroduodenal junction of dogs, *Am J Vet Res* 57:1266, 1996.
57. Newell SM, Graham JP, Roberts GD et al: Sonography of the normal feline gastrointestinal tract, *Vet Radiol Ultrasound* 40:40, 1999.
58. Goggin JM, Biller DS, Debey BM et al: Ultrasonographic measurement of gastrointestinal wall thickness and the ultrasonographic appearance of the ileocolic region in healthy cats, *J Am Anim Hosp Assoc* 36:224, 2000.
59. Suter PF: Radiographic diagnosis of liver disease in dogs and cats, *Vet Clin North Am Small Anim Pract* 12:153, 1982.
60. Mazin RM, Christman A, Pasek A: What is your diagnosis? GDV in a 5-week-old puppy, *J Am Vet Med Assoc* 221:489, 2002.
61. Bredal WP, Eggertsdottir AV, Austefjord O: Acute gastric dilatation in cats: a case series, *Acta Vet Scand* 37:445, 1996.
62. Funkquist B: Gastric torsion in the dog: I. Radiological picture during nonsurgical treatment related to the pathological anatomy and to the future clinical course, *J Small Anim Pract* 20:73, 1979.
63. Kneller SK: Radiographic interpretation of the gastric dilatation-volvulus complex in the dog, *J Am Anim Hosp Assoc* 12:154, 1976.
64. Frendin J, Funquist B, Stavenborn M et al: Gastric displacement in dogs without clinical signs of acute dilatation, *J Small Anim Pract* 29:775, 1988.
65. Fischetti AJ, Saunders HM, Drobatz KJ: Pneumatosis in canine gastric dilatation-volvulus syndrome, *Vet Radiol Ultrasound* 45:279, 2004.
66. Rhodes WH, Brodey RS: The differential diagnosis of pyloric obstructions in the dog, *J Am Vet Radiol Soc* 6:65, 1965.
67. Zboralske FF: Gastric ulcer. In Margulis AR, Burhenne HJ, editors: *Alimentary tract roentgenology*, St Louis, 1967, CV Mosby.

68. Howard EB, Sawa TR, Nielson SW et al: Mastocytoma and gastroduodenal ulceration. Vet Pathol 6:146, 1969.
69. Robbins SL: *Pathologic basis of disease*, Philadelphia, 1974, WB Saunders.
70. Jones RD, Baynes RE, Nimitz CT: Nonsteroidal anti-inflammatory drug toxicosis in dogs and cats: 240 cases (1989-1990), *J Am Vet Med Assoc* 201:475, 1992.
71. Stanton ME, Bright RM: Gastroduodenal ulceration in dogs, *J Vet Intern Med* 3:238, 1989.
72. Wallace MS, Zawie DA, Garvey MS et al: Gastric ulceration in the dog secondary to the use on nonsteroidal anti-inflammatory drugs, *J Am Anim Hosp Assoc* 26:467, 1990.
73. Dowdle SM, Joubert KE, Lambrechts NE et al: The prevalence of subclinical gastroduodenal ulceration in Dachshunds with intervertebral disc prolapse, *J S Afr Vet Assoc* 74:77, 2003.
74. Nelson SW: The discovery of gastric ulcers and the differential diagnosis between benignancy and malignancy, *Radiol Clin North Am* 7:5, 1969.
75. Porcher P, Buffard P: Malignancy of the stomach. In Margulis AR, Burhenne HJ, editors: *Alimentary tract roentgenology*, St Louis, 1967, C.V. Mosby.
76. Hayden DW, Nelson SW: Canine alimentary neoplasia, *Zentralbl Veterinarmed [A]* 20:1, 1973.
77. Sautter JH, Hanlon GF: Gastric neoplasms in the dog: a report of 20 cases, *J Am Vet Med Assoc* 166:691, 1975.
78. Barber DL: Radiographic aspects of gastric ulcers in dogs: a comparative review and report of 5 case histories, *Vet Radiol* 23:109, 1982.
79. Liptak JM, Hunt GB, Barrs VRD et al: Gastroduodenal ulceration in cats: eight cases and a review of the literature, *J Feline Med Surg* 4:27, 2002.
80. Willard MD: Diseases of the stomach. In Ettinger SJ, Feldman EC, editors: *Textbook of veterinary internal medicine, vol 2*, ed 4, Philadelphia, 1995, WB Saunders, p 1143.
81. Murray M, Robinson PB, McKeating FJ et al: Primary gastric neoplasia in the dog: a clinico-pathological study, *Vet Rec* 91:474, 1972.
82. Patnaik AK, Hurvitz AI, Johnson GE: Canine gastric adenocarcinoma, *Vet Pathol* 15:600, 1978.
83. Brodey RS: Alimentary tract neoplasms in the cat: a clinicopathologic survey of 46 cases, *Am J Vet Res* 27:74, 1966.
84. Tyler DE: Gastric neoplasia in the dog and cat [abstract], *Arch Am Coll Vet Surg* 6:47, 1977.
85. Burke RL, Ackerman N: The abdomen. In Burk RL, Ackerman N, editors: *Small animal radiology and ultrasonography: a diagnostic atlas and text*, ed 2, Philadelphia, 1996, WB Saunders.
86. Penninck D, Smyers B, Webster CR et al: Diagnostic value of ultrasonography in differentiating enteritis from intestinal neoplasia in dogs, *Vet Radiol Ultrasound* 44:570, 2003.
87. Lamb CR, Forster-van Hijfte M: Beware of the gastric pseudomass, *Vet Radiol Ultrasound* 35:398, 1994.
88. Penninck DG, Crystal MA, Matz ME et al: The technique of percutaneous ultrasound guided fine-needle aspiration biopsy and automated microcore biopsy in small animal gastrointestinal diseases, *Vet Radiol Ultrasound* 34:433, 1993.
89. Crystal MA, Penninck DG, Matz ME et al: Use of ultrasound-guided fine-needle aspiration biopsy and automated core biopsy for the diagnosis of gastrointestinal diseases in small animals, *Vet Radiol Ultrasound* 34:438, 1993.
90. Twedt DC, Magne ML: Diseases of the stomach. In Ettinger SJ, editor: *Textbook of veterinary internal medicine, vol 2*, ed 3, Philadelphia, 1989, WB Saunders, p 1289.
91. Miller RI: Gastrointestinal phycomycosis in 63 dogs, *J Am Vet Med Assoc* 165:473, 1985.
92. Homco LD: Gastrointestinal tract. In Green RW, editor: *Small animal ultrasound*, Philadelphia, 1996, Lippincott-Raven, p 149.
93. Baez JL, Hendrick MJ, Walker LM et al: Radiographic, ultrasonographic, and endoscopic findings in cats with inflammatory bowel disease of the stomach and small intestine: 33 cases (1990-1997), *J Am Vet Med Assoc* 215:349, 1999.
94. Barber DL, Rowland GN: Radiographically detectable soft tissue calcification in chronic renal failure, *Vet Radiol* 20:117, 1979.
95. Parfitt AM: Soft tissue calcification in uremia, *Arch Intern Med* 124:544, 1969.
96. Beck C, Slocombe RF, O'Neill T et al: The use of ultrasound in the investigation of gastric carcinoma in a dog, *Aust Vet J* 79:332, 2001.

ELECTRONIC RESOURCES evolve

Additional information related to the content in Chapter 45 can be found on the companion Web site at evolve http://evolve.elsevier.com/Thrall/vetrad/.

- Key Points
- Chapter Quiz
- Case Study 45-1

CHAPTER • 46
The Small Bowel

Elizabeth A. Riedesel

Abdominal radiographs can help the clinician make a definitive diagnosis or decide between medical or surgical treatment. However, radiographs should not take precedence over a complete history, a thorough physical examination, and pertinent laboratory tests. Survey radiographs, ultrasonography, and intestinal contrast examinations may be useful aids in the diagnosis of both acute and chronic intestinal disorders. The patient that does not respond to symptomatic therapy for vomiting or diarrhea should be given a more extensive evaluation, including radiographic and sonographic studies. Although radiographic and sonographic abnormalities are not present in every intestinal disorder, one or more of the roentgen signs and sonographic patterns discussed in this chapter characterize many lesions.

THE NORMAL SMALL BOWEL

Radiography

The standard views used to evaluate the small bowel are the recumbent left-to-right lateral and ventrodorsal views. Supplemental views can also be useful. The general intent of the supplemental views is to take advantage of the natural contrast of gas in the bowel in association with specific disease processes.[1,2] For elective abdominal radiographs of patients with chronic signs, food should be withheld for 24 hours and a cleansing enema administered 2 to 4 hours before the radiographic examination. This preparation produces the desired empty intestinal tract that facilitates assessment of the radiographs. However, for the patient with acute abdominal pain, acute persistent vomiting, or palpable, enlarged fluid- or gas-filled bowel, no specific preparation is necessary. In fact, in these patients, the pattern of gas and fluid can be helpful diagnostically, and this valuable information may be altered by an enema. The roentgen sign assessment for the small intestine is summarized in Box 46-1. Margination, size, position, shape, and radiopacity can be assessed by survey radiographs, but mucosal irregularities and abnormal peristalsis or transit time must be determined from contrast studies or ultrasound.

A moderate amount of intraperitoneal fat provides good contrast for definition of the intestinal serosal surfaces (Fig. 46-1). Animals younger than 6 months or emaciated animals have poor serosal definition because of a lack of intraabdominal fat for contrast.[3] Serosal surfaces should be smooth and are most easily seen in regions where superimposition of bowel is minimal. A false interpretation of decreased serosal definition often results when the small bowel loops are overlapping in the central abdomen, when loops are crowded together by an abdominal mass effect, or when little or no gas is present in the bowel lumen. These effects should not be misinterpreted as abdominal effusion.

Because of the variation in canine body size and the magnification effects of radiography, no accurate, specific measurement for normal diameter of the small bowel exists. Two schemes for relative bowel diameter have been developed that use nearby bones as reference structures. The maximal normal diameter (serosa to serosa) for the dog has been reported to be less than twice the width of a rib,[4] or less than 1.6 times the height of the body of L5 at its narrowest point.[5] Because most cats tend to have a similar body size, a more specific definition of normal bowel diameter has been defined as not exceeding 12 mm,[6] or twice the height of the central portion of the L4 vertebral body.[7] Although the duodenum may be slightly wider, the jejunum and ileum should have approximately the same diameter.[8] However, as a clinician gains experience in evaluating abdominal radiographs, qualitative assessment of bowel size may become just as accurate as measurement techniques.

Attempts to judge the thickness of the intestinal wall on survey radiographs are unreliable. An empty bowel loop with a small volume of intraluminal air should not be mistaken for a pathologically thickened segment. True thickening of the intestinal wall is better judged by ultrasound, contrast study, or palpation.[9]

The small bowel has fixed and movable segments. In the dog the cranial duodenal flexure is fixed along the caudal surface of the right side of the liver by the hepatoduodenal ligament. The descending duodenum lies along the right abdominal wall. The caudal duodenal flexure is located at a transverse plane through the tuber coxae, with the ascending duodenum continuing from this point on the left side of the root of the mesentery directly cranial to the stomach. The jejunoileum should be uniformly distributed throughout the peritoneal cavity, occupying space not taken up by distensible organs (stomach or urinary bladder), solid organs (liver, spleen, or kidneys), or fat. The ileum crosses from the left to the right mid-abdomen to terminate at the ileocolic junction.

The cat differs from the dog in the position of the cranial duodenal flexure. In the cat the cranial flexure usually creates a sharper angle with the pylorus and is located closer to the midline. The descending duodenum courses in a gently curved loop, positioning the caudal duodenal flexure at approximately mid-abdomen. As in the dog, the ascending duodenum courses in a cranial direction until it reaches the stomach; the jejunum is then located throughout the rest of the mesogastric area.

Common positional variations of small bowel seen in normal dogs and cats include (1) a full stomach displacing the bowel caudally, (2) a distended urinary bladder displacing the bowel cranially, (3) intraperitoneal fat in obese cats causing the small bowel to be located centrally and/or on the right side, (4) in very obese cats, fat displacing the bowel into the central region of the abdominal cavity and (5) in obese dogs, the bowel occupying the ventral portion of the pendulous abdominal cavity. Positional changes in the small intestine may also be indicative of disease in adjacent organs.

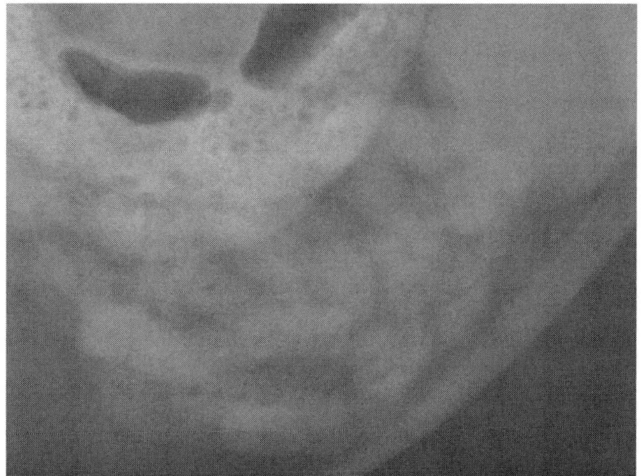

Fig. 46-1 Serosal edges of small intestine are easily seen in this cat with abundant intraperitoneal fat. Bowel segments seen end on appear as rings if the lumen contains air or as round nodules if the lumen is empty or contains fluid.

Box 46-1

Roentgen Signs in the Small Intestine

Margination: serosal surface definition
Size: diameter of lumen
Position: location within abdominal cavity
Shape: contour of bowel loops
Radiopacity: lumen contents and bowel wall
Architecture: mucosa/bowel wall smoothness
Motility: contrast medium transit time

The normal small bowel is recognized in survey radiographs as smooth, continuously curving tubes, or as solid circles or rings (see Fig. 46-1). These shapes are produced by the contractile activity of the smooth muscle. Segmental contractions give rise to spherical shapes, whereas peristaltic contractions cause long tubular shapes.

The radiopacity of the normal small intestine is variable because of differing opacities of material within the lumen. In a nonfasted animal, any of the following may be seen in the lumen: air; grainy-appearing mottled ingesta, which may include mineral or metal; or fluid of homogeneous soft tissue opacity. The nondiscretionary eating habits of some dogs and cats may result in mineral or metallic opacities of small size in the small bowel. Clay-based cat litter and small gravel from dog runs are common examples. Gastrointestinal medications that contain calcium, magnesium, aluminum, bismuth, or silicate can impart significant radiopacity to the intestinal content.[10] Some pet vitamin and mineral supplements contain sufficient mineral to be visible. In general, tablets or capsules containing minerals, either as active ingredients or in the coating, are more likely to be visible than liquids containing these minerals.[10] In a fasted animal, the lumen may contain a small amount of ingested air, or it may be of homogeneous fluid or soft tissue opacity.

Normal bowel gas is less common in the cat than in the dog. In the fasted cat, gas is rarely present in the small intestine, but in fasted dogs 30% to 60% of the small bowel content may be gas.[6,11] Animals stressed by handling or dyspneic animals frequently are aerophagic, with more air-containing small bowel. The bowel wall should be of uniform soft tissue opacity. This uniformity is most easily assessed in loops that contain air.

Positive-Contrast Examination

Indications

Contrast media used to increase the opacity of the bowel can be helpful. However, contrast studies of the bowel are inherently low-yield procedures and must, therefore be reserved for select patients and conducted appropriately. The complete upper gastrointestinal positive-contrast radiographic evaluation of the stomach and small bowel is time consuming for the veterinarian and can be expensive for the animal's owner. Because of the potential for a low yield of diagnostic information, a contrast study should be reserved for the patient in which a diagnosis or approach to treatment cannot be made from the combined clinical information and survey radiographs. In many patients ultrasound evaluation is capable of providing diagnostic information about the small bowel; this information often negates the need for a contrast radiographic study. However, accurate gastrointestinal sonography requires considerable skill and training.

The clinical signs that most frequently warrant an intestinal contrast study (or ultrasound imaging) include the following:

- Acute, persistent vomiting with negative findings on survey radiographs
- Recurrent vomiting, especially in animals refractory to symptomatic therapy and without other organ disease to explain the vomiting
- Palpable abdominal mass without obstructive bowel signs on survey radiographs
- Acute abdominal pain with an unusual or unexplained abnormality seen in the survey radiographs
- Weight loss with intermittent or recurrent diarrhea[8,12-15]
- Melena
- Hematemesis

Gastrointestinal tract contrast studies are frequently not informative in patients that have chronic diarrhea without vomiting. However, information that can be gained from a contrast study (or ultrasound imaging) in these patients includes the following:

- A more thorough evaluation of mucosal abnormalities
- Length of intestine affected (focal, regional, or generalized)
- Thickness of bowel wall
- Abnormalities in peristaltic activity and intestinal transit time
- Improved determination of luminal size
- A more complete evaluation of luminal contents
- Determination of patency of the lumen

Contraindications

Contrast evaluation is not warranted in the patient with survey radiographic evidence of bowel obstruction.[13] Minimal additional information will be gained because contrast medium may pass slowly through atonic bowel proximal to the obstruction, especially in the weakened or debilitated animal. If the clinical and survey radiographic findings are strongly suggestive of mechanical obstruction, surgery is indicated. Further attempts to define the specific site and type of obstructing lesion with contrast medium only delay and possibly complicate surgery and causes additional patient stress. The use of iodinated contrast medium and barium-impregnated markers is also not indicated in such patients.

Patients with survey radiographic evidence of free peritoneal gas that is not residual from recent celiotomy, from penetrating trauma, or abdominocentesis are also not appropriate patients for contrast intestinal studies. In these patients, the peritoneal gas is most likely from gastrointestinal perforation.[16] If perforation of the intestinal tract is suspected, use of barium sulfate is not recommended because the combination of barium and ingesta within the peritoneal cavity may cause more severe peritonitis, foreign body granulomas, or serosal adhesions.[13,17-19] Attempting to identify the location of the perforation is not as important as providing aggressive medical and surgical intervention. Ultrasound evaluation is probably an overall safer means for evaluating patients with suspected gastrointestinal perforation.

Water-soluble organic iodine contrast media are either ionic or nonionic. Most ionic contrast media are hypertonic and cause an influx of fluid into the gastrointestinal tract. Ionic iodinated contrast media are not recommended for oral administration in young and debilitated patients, and especially dehydrated patients, because the resultant fluid shift can worsen any hypovolemic state.[20]

Technique and General Interpretation

An empty gastrointestinal tract is preferred if optimal information is to be obtained from the contrast study. For the elective upper gastrointestinal tract examination, a 24-hour fast is recommended before contrast medium administration. An enema should be given 2 to 4 hours before the contrast study to allow emptying of residual fluid and air. However, for patients with acute severe abdominal distress, no preparation is usually possible. Additionally, the patient with an acute abdominal crisis may suffer additional injury from administration of laxatives or enemas.

Many pharmaceuticals affect gastrointestinal motility. General anesthetics (such as isoflurane), sedatives (such as xylazine hydrochloride), neuroleptanalgesics (such as fentanyl and droperidol), and tranquilizers (such as promazine hydrochloride) slow the passage of barium through the intestine.[21,22] The alpha$_2$ agonist metetomidine causes decreased gastrointestinal motility in dogs and cats. These drugs should be avoided when performing contrast studies. When tranquilization of a cat is necessary, a ketamine/diazepam combination (2.7 mg/kg ketamine hydrochloride and 0.09 mg/kg diazepam in separate syringes, given intramuscularly 20 minutes before administration of barium) has been shown to have minimal effect on motility.[23] Low-dose (0.05 mg/kg) intravenous acepromazine maleate has been recommended for tranquilization of fractious dogs.[24] Medications that contain anticholinergic drugs should also be discontinued at least 24 hours (preferably 48 to 72 hours) before the contrast study.[12] The influence of medications on the motility of the intestinal tract should be kept in mind when evaluating both survey radiographs and contrast radiographic studies.

The effect of various pharmaceuticals on the gastrointestinal tract should be considered relative to the interpretation of disease- versus drug-induced radiographic changes.[10] Among those noted to affect the small intestine are xylazine, which induces generalized bowel distention consistent with gastric dilation, as well as functional, or adynamic, ileus, which lasts for several hours. Opioid peptides (such as butorphanol) can have either a stimulatory or an inhibitory effect on gastrointestinal motility depending on the animal species and the region of the gastrointestinal tract affected. Several drugs, such as cisapride, are now commonly used for their gastroprokinetic effects. Although the major site of action of these drugs is the stomach, cisapride has a stimulatory effect in both the duodenum and the jejunum. Thus when a contrast study is used for assessment, these drugs may mask a small intestinal motility disorder pattern.[10]

Standard views are routinely used. Oblique views to project the pyloric sphincter or a particular abnormality may be added as needed.[25,26] Right-to-left lateral and dorsoventral views may add information to the evaluation of the pyloric antrum and duodenum at early times after contrast medium administration.

Three radiopaque liquid contrast media can be used to evaluate the small intestine: barium sulfate, ionic organic iodine, and nonionic organic iodine. Barium sulfate is available in a dry powder form or as a liquid suspension. The oral ionic organic iodine preparations are meglumine diatrizoate and sodium diatrizoate. The nonionic organic iodine product is iohexol. The advantages, disadvantages, and suggested uses of these products are summarized in Table 46-1.[12,15,20,27-31]

Commercially prepared barium sulfate suspension is the contrast medium of choice in most instances. If perforation of the intestinal tract is suspected, use of barium sulfate is not recommended, as previously mentioned. An organic iodine preparation designed for the gastrointestinal tract should be used when perforation is suspected. A small tear occasionally is missed because the iodine is reabsorbed rapidly by the serosa. If a tear is still suspected after an iodine study has been completed, barium may demonstrate the leak more obviously. Because of the more rapid passage of iodine preparations through the gastrointestinal tract, these agents may also be used to determine the patency of the lumen quickly. As previously noted, the nonionic organic iodine contrast media are typically hypertonic. These agents draw fluid into the bowel, causing dilution of contrast medium opacity, and may potentiate a hypovolemic state. The nonionic, water-soluble, iodinated contrast media are of low osmolality, and thus isotonic, and provoke less fluid movement into the bowel lumen but are relatively costly. Because they are clear liquids, the iodinated agents allow for endoscopic evaluation and sonography to be performed immediately after completion of the contrast study.

The volume of contrast medium present within the intestinal lumen is a critical factor in interpretation. The intestine should be distended to its reasonable physiologic maximum. Failure to administer an adequate volume of contrast medium is one of the most frequent causes for nondiagnostic barium studies. Some recommended dosages for contrast medium are given in Table 46-2.

Complete descriptions of the method for performing a barium upper gastrointestinal tract study and excellent examples of the normal appearance of the contrast-filled small bowel are available elsewhere.[6,12,14,15,25] Examples of the appearance of barium and iodine in normal small bowel are presented in Figures 46-2 and 46-3. A summary of the portions of the gastrointestinal tract seen at specific intervals after contrast medium administration is presented in Table 46-3.

Dogs often have multiple square-shaped outpocketings on the antimesenteric side of the descending duodenum. Only one may be present, or several may be visible. These are termed pseudoulcers and are normal and caused by mucosal depressions over submucosal lymphoid accumulations (Fig. 46-4). Pseudoulcers are not found in the cat. Approximately 30% of normal cats have strong segmental contractions throughout the length of the duodenum that produce a "string of pearls" effect during the contrast study (Fig. 46-5).[6] Pseudoulcers and the string of pearls appearance are seen only in barium contrast studies, not in survey radiographs.

In both the normal dog and the normal cat, the remaining small bowel should appear to have a smooth contrast/mucosa interface. A fine brush pattern, also called fimbriation, may occur in the dog. This is a normal pattern and is caused by barium between the intestinal villi (Fig. 46-6).[32] Concentric narrowing of short lengths of bowel is caused by peristalsis (Fig. 46-7). The location of such narrowings should vary during the time of study in the normal animal.

In a normal upper gastrointestinal study, barium and gas may be present simultaneously in loops (Fig. 46-8). A double-

TABLE • 46-1

Intestinal Contrast Agents

CONTRAST AGENT	ADVANTAGES	DISADVANTAGES	USES
Barium sulfate suspensions	Very radiopaque Excellent mucosal detail Remain in suspension Resist dilution Physiologically inert Low cost	May induce granulomas or adhesions if leaked into peritoneal cavity	Routine gastrointestinal tract contrast studies
Barium sulfate, USP	Inexpensive	Inadequate mucosal detail Tends to flocculate	Not recommended
Organic iodine (ionic) solutions	Rapid transit time Nonirritating to serosal surfaces Rapidly resorbed after extraluminal leakage	May form precipitates May be absorbed across mucosa and excreted by urinary tract Hypertonicity causes: Fluid flux into lumen Dilution of contrast medium Electrolyte imbalance Dehydration	Suspected intestinal perforation
Organic iodine (nonionic) solutions	Rapid transit time Nonirritating Resorbed after extraluminal leakage Low osmolality Does not become progressively dilute	Expensive	Suspected perforation before endoscopy Young or debilitated patient
Radiopaque markers (BIPS)	Ease of administration Not liquid Orogastric tubing not needed Can be given with food	No mucosal information	Assess orocolic transit rate Assess presence of absence of obstructive disease

TABLE • 46-2

Recommended Dose Rate for Contrast Medium

CONTRAST MEDIUM	DOG	CAT
Barium sulfate suspension*	6-12 mL/kg 20% (w/w)[14] or 6-10 mL/kg 60% (w/w)	12-16 mL/kg[6]
Organic iodine preparation (full strength)	2-3 mL/kg[8,14,15]	2 mL/kg[15]
Organic iodine, nonionic (240-300 mg I/mL)	10 mL/kg (1 : 2 dilution)[28]	10 mL/kg (1 : 2 dilution)[28,31]
Radiopaque markers (BIPS)†	10 5-mm and 30 1.5-mm spheres	10 5-mm and 30 1.5-mm spheres

*A large volume of relatively dilute contrast medium is preferred by some to distend the intestinal lumen but not to obscure radiolucent luminal filling defects. The author prefers a full-strength barium suspension for its superior mucosal pattern definition.
†Follow manufacturers' specific directions for administration with or without food.

contrast effect is present when the distention by gas is greater than that caused by the barium. The barium/mucosa interface typically appears in such loops as a thin opaque line. In other loops, gas may be present only as small bubbles. Findings on the barium contrast images that most strongly correlate with abnormalities are changes in the diameter of the bowel, changes in the barium/mucosa interface, and changes in the rate of passage of barium. The intestinal tract is normally characterized by dynamic changes; thus documenting a suspicious finding on multiple radiographs over time increases the significance of the finding.

Barium-impregnated polyethylene spheres (BIPS) (Chemstock Animal Health, Christchurch, New Zealand) have been designed for evaluation of gastric dysmotility and intestinal transit time in the dog and cat. Advantages and disadvantages of the use of these markers in the assessment of the small bowel are summarized in Table 46-1. The spheres are made in two sizes: 1.5-mm diameter and 5-mm diameter. The larger spheres are designed to become trapped at the oral aspect of an obstructing lesion, making them suitable for evaluation of partial and complete obstruction (Fig. 46-9).[33] BIPS are typically administered with a meal. The type of meal influences the rate of gastric emptying; thus strict adherence to the manufacturer's recommendations must be maintained when the product is used for calculation of gastric emptying times and assessment of orocolic transit.

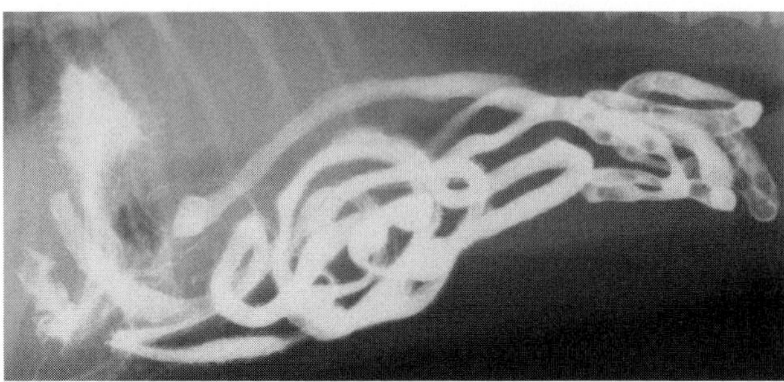

Fig. 46-2 Normal canine barium upper gastrointestinal tract study. Note the excellent radiopacity of the contrast medium and the sharp definition of the mucosal surface 15 minutes after contrast medium administration.

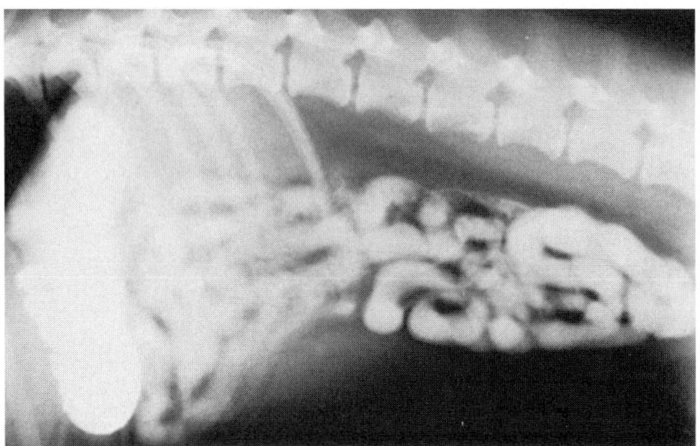

Fig. 46-3 Normal canine upper gastrointestinal tract study using water-soluble iodinated contrast medium. Whereas contrast medium opacity 30 minutes after administration is good in the bowel located in the caudal abdomen, the contrast medium is diluted (decreased opacity and poor definition of mucosa) in the cranial abdomen because of fluid entering the bowel in response to the hyperosmolar nature of the contrast medium.

TABLE • 46-3

Upper Gastrointestinal Tract Film Sequence

	BARIUM	IONIC AND NONIONIC ORGANIC IODINE	STRUCTURES USUALLY OPACIFIED IN NORMAL ANIMALS*
Dog	Immediate	Immediate	Stomach
	15 minutes		Stomach, duodenum
	30 minutes	15 minutes	Stomach, duodenum, jejunum
	1 hour		Stomach, duodenum, jejunum
	2 hours	30 minutes	Stomach, all parts of small bowel
	4 hours	1 hour	Small bowel, colon
Cat	Immediate	Immediate	Stomach
	5 minutes	5 minutes	Stomach, duodenum
	30 minutes	30 minutes	All parts of small bowel
	1 hour	1 hour	Small bowel, colon

*Because of the extreme variability of individual transit times, this list is only an approximation of the parts of the gastrointestinal tract seen at these times.

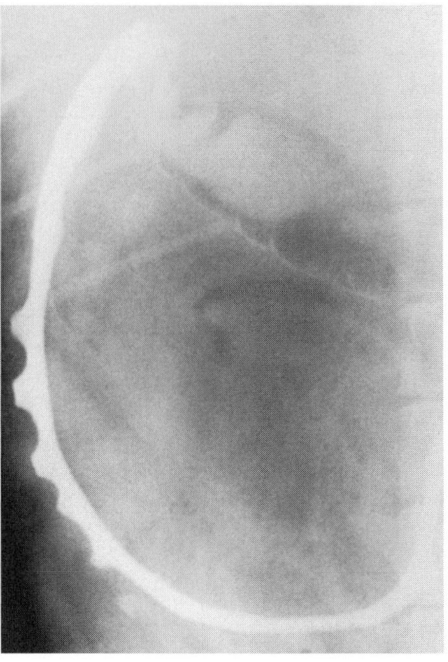

Fig. 46-4 Normal canine barium upper gastrointestinal tract study. Multiple pseudoulcers are present along the antimesenteric surface of the descending duodenum. These indentations are normal variations in the appearance of the duodenum of dogs and are caused by depression in the mucosa at sites of lymphoid follicles. Only one pseudoulcer may be present, or multiple, as in this dog.

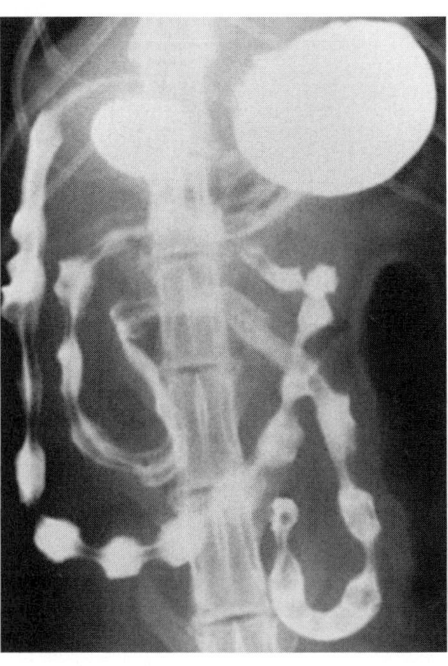

Fig. 46-5 Normal feline barium upper gastrointestinal tract study. Prominent circular muscle contractions cause almost complete obliteration of the duodenal lumen during segmental peristalsis. This string of pearls appearance is commonly seen in feline barium studies of the small bowel. The linear filling defect is a normal variant attributed to a longitudinal fold of mucosa in the incompletely distended intestine. This has been called the pseudostring sign and should not be misinterpreted as linear foreign material.

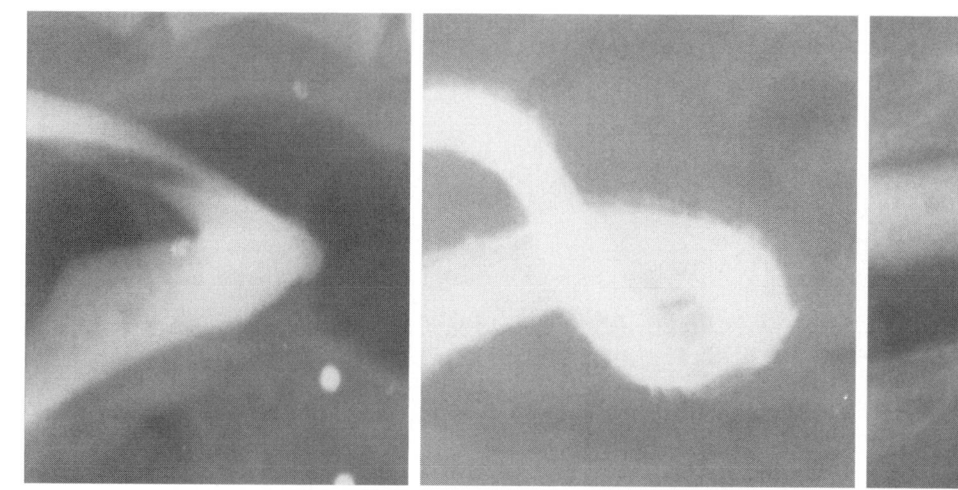
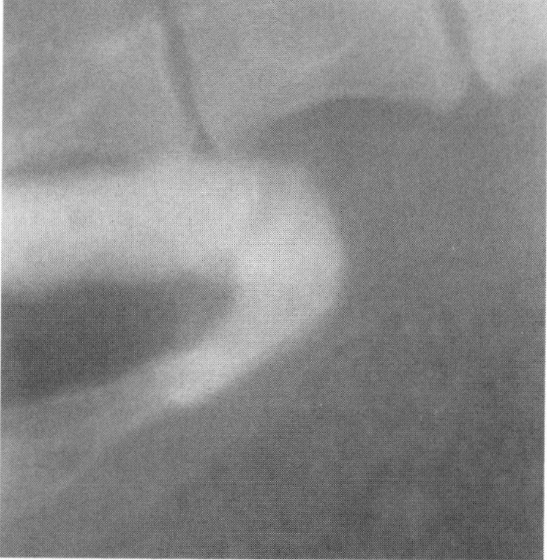

Fig. 46-6 Close-up views of the caudal duodenal flexure of three dogs demonstrate the variation in normal mucosal pattern seen during an upper gastrointestinal examination. The mucosal pattern can range from very smooth as in the *left panel,* to highly fimbriated, as in the *middle panel,* to a halo appearance, as in the *right panel.*

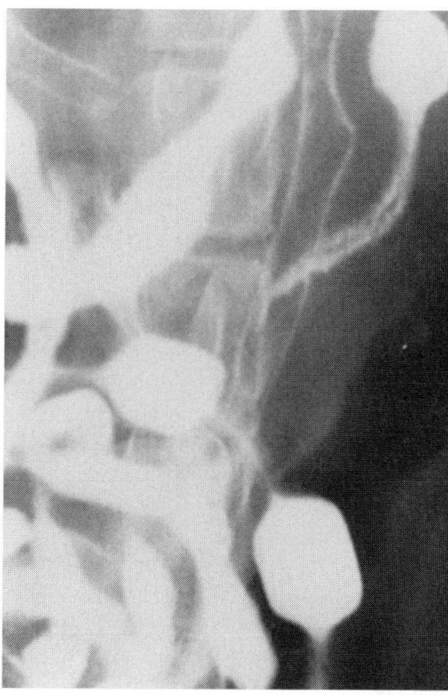

Fig. 46-7 Normal segmental intestinal contractions during a canine upper gastrointestinal tract study are indicated by symmetric indentations of the bowel wall on each side proximal and distal to the formed bolus of contrast medium.

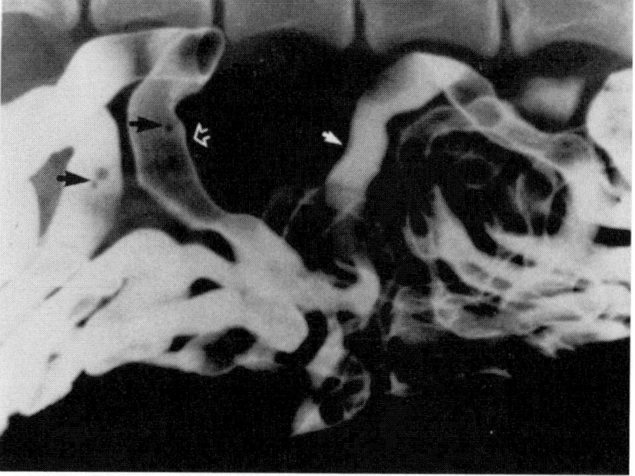

Fig. 46-8 Normal canine barium upper gastrointestinal tract study. The bowel segments filled with barium are uniformly opaque *(solid white arrow).* The mucosal surface/barium interface is flat and smooth. Bowel loops containing air have a double-contrast effect; barium coating the mucosa is seen as a *thin opaque line,* whereas intraluminal air is radiolucent *(open white arrow).* Small intraluminal gas bubbles are seen as sharply defined focal radiolucencies in two bowel segments *(black arrows).*

Ultrasound

Observations that can be made from intestinal sonography include assessment of wall thickness, wall layer pattern, and motility. Transducers frequencies of 7.5 MHz and higher enable the best identification of individual layers of the intestinal wall. Ultrasound imaging also allows assessment of structures adjacent to the intestine, such as the pancreas and lymph nodes, thus disclosing a nonintestinal primary cause for vomiting, anorexia, or weight loss that has not responded to symptomatic therapy. Ultrasound-guided fine-needle aspiration sampling for cytology and culture evaluation can be done in many patients.

The major obstacle for optimal ultrasound imaging is the presence of gas in the bowel. When gas is present, the far wall cannot be assessed. Repositioning the patient, using gravity-based transducer placement, administering fluid by orogastric intubation, or repeating the examination at a later time may overcome the artifacts induced by gas.

Wall thickness variations for the dog and cat are summarized in Table 46-4. Higher frequency transducers and measures of wall thickness in a longitudinal axis segment provide a correlation between the thickness of the duodenum and jejunum relative to the weight of dogs.[34] When a 10-MHz linear transducer is used in the normal cat, a subtle difference in thickness is found from the duodenum through the ileum.[35]

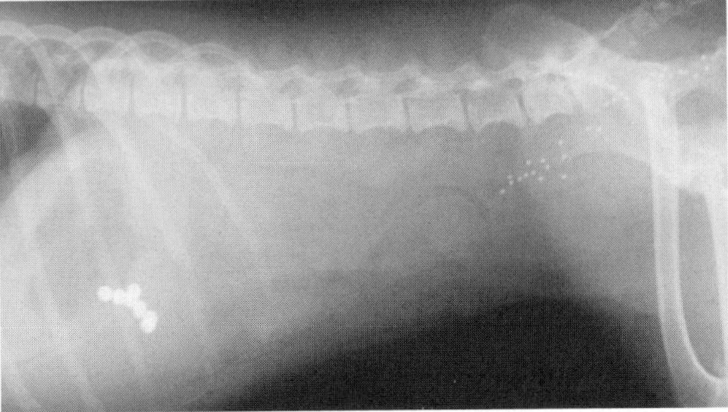

Fig. 46-9 Lateral abdominal radiograph made 18 hours after administration of large and small BIPS. The small spheres are in the colon, whereas the large spheres remain in the stomach. This pattern of sphere distribution is consistent with partial pyloric outflow obstruction.

TABLE • 46-4

Small Bowel Normal Measurements

	DOG	CAT
Radiographic*	≤2 times width of rib Ratio of maximal small bowel diameter to narrowest height of L5 body <1.6	≤12 mm ≤2 times the central height of L2
Ultrasound wall thickness† Duodenum	Up to 20 kg, ≤5.1 mm 20-29.9 kg, ≤5.3 mm >30 kg, ≤6.0 mm	2.0-2.4 mm
Ultrasound wall thickness† Jejunum	Up to 20 kg, ≤4.1 mm 20-29.9 kg, ≤4.4 mm >30 kg, ≤4.7 mm	2.1-2.5 mm
Ultrasound wall thickness† Ileum	Not specifically defined	2.5-3.2 mm

*Serosa to serosa.
†Mucosa to serosa.

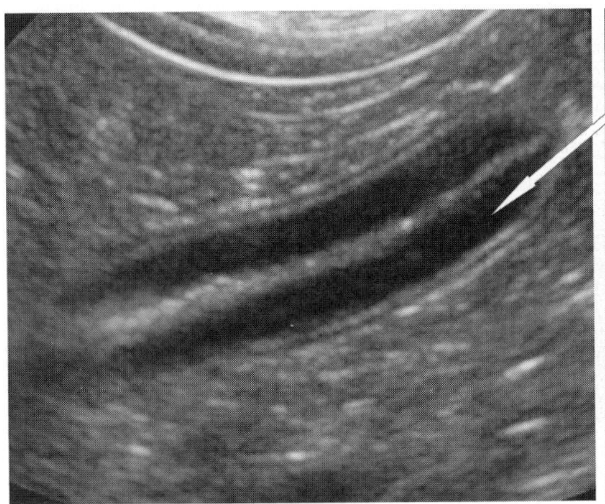

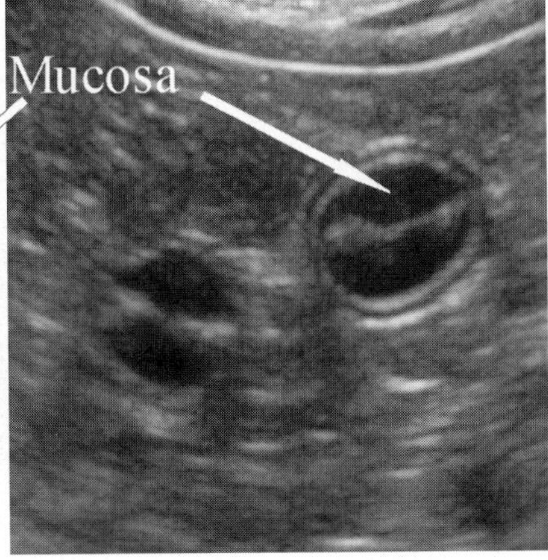

Fig. 46-10 Ultrasound images of a normal canine jejunum. The long axis is depicted on the *left* and transverse on the *right*. The five-layer alternating echogenicity pattern can be identified. The mucosal layer is indicated by *arrows*. The central hyperechoic *line* represents the empty lumen.

The normal small intestinal wall pattern consists of alternating hyperechoic and hypoechoic layers. When no fluid or gas is present, a thin, hyperechoic line represents the lumen. From the lumen to the serosa, the layers and echogenicities are as follows: mucosa and hypoechoic, submucosa and hyperechoic, muscularis and hypoechoic, and serosa and hyperechoic (Fig. 46-10). The hypoechoic mucosal layer is the thickest of the individual layers and thus is visually dominant.[36] When fluid is within the lumen, the mucosal surface is normally hyperechoic. If gas is present within the lumen, a prominent reverberation artifact occurs in a relatively long length of bowel and a "comet tail" reverberation artifact is present during peristaltic contraction. Acoustic shadowing artifact frequently occurs either with focal luminal gas or with dense particles of ingesta in transit. A short linear or focal hyperechogenicity frequently occurs at the equatorial tangents of transverse sections of empty bowel. This occurs as a result of widening of the intervillous space when the bowel folds.[37]

The normal duodenum can be distinctly identified by its superficial right-side location and can be traced cranially into the stomach and caudally to the descending loop, which courses to the left. With high-resolution transducers, the duodenal papilla can be seen in many cats and dogs. The feline duodenal papilla ranges from 2.9 to 5.5 mm wide and averages 4.0 mm in height when imaged in the transverse plane.[38] Pseudoulcers occasionally can be seen in the canine duodenum, and the strong segmental contractions described as the string of pearls in a barium series can be seen in the feline duodenum.

The jejunum and most of the ileum are seen as nondescript loops. The terminal 1- to 2-cm portion of the ileum, or the ileocolic junction, in the cat has the appearance of a wagon wheel because of projection of the mucosa into the lumen.[35] Peristaltic contractions are seen and vary from less than 1 to 3 per minute in the small intestine depending on the fasted state or amount of time after being fed.[10,39]

Normal mesenteric lymph nodes are unlikely to be seen with 5- to 7.5-MHz transducers; however, when 10-MHz or greater frequencies are used, these lymph nodes can be found in the relaxed patient.[35] Normal lymph nodes are typically isoechoic to adjacent fat and may not be readily apparent.

TABLE • 46-5

Pathologic Conditions by Length and Relative Distention of Affected Bowel

FOCAL/MILD	FOCAL/SEVERE	GENERALIZED/MILD	GENERALIZED/SEVERE
Regional enteritis	Mechanical ileus	Functional ileus	Mechanical ileus
Regional peritonitis	Foreign object	Enteritis	Complete obstruction, distal bowel
Mechanical ileus, partial obstruction	Intussusception	Anticholinergic drugs	Intussusception
Early functional ileus	Bowel wall neoplasia	Electrolyte imbalance	Foreign object
Vascular compromise	Granulomatous wall infiltrate	Malabsorption	Bowel wall neoplasia
	Bowel stricture	Abdominal pain	Functional ileus
	Stenosis/atresia	Mechanical	Recent abdominal surgery
	Postsurgical adhesion	Partial obstructions at ileocolic junction (usually cats)	Spinal trauma (neurologic injury)
	Herniation		Intestinal volvulus (rare)
	Functional ileus		
	Parvovirus enteritis		
	Dysautonomia		

However, the region of the jejunal lymph nodes should be assessed in any patient suspected of having small intestinal disease.[40]

ABNORMAL SMALL BOWEL

Disease Resulting in Bowel Dilation

Numerous diseases result in dilation of the small intestine. Failure of intestinal contents to pass through the tract is called ileus. Ileus can be mechanical, caused by physical obstruction of the bowel, or functional (paralysis), in which peristaltic contractions of the bowel cease as a result of vascular or neuromuscular abnormalities within the bowel wall. In functional ileus the bowel remains patent.

In general, the appearance of mechanically obstructed bowel differs from functionally obstructed bowel by the following parameters: (1) mechanically obstructed bowel is usually of larger diameter than functionally obstructed bowel; (2) both gas and fluid typically are in the lumen of mechanically obstructed bowel, whereas functionally obstructed bowel tends to contain more gas or may be completely gas filled; (3) patients with mechanical obstruction usually have some bowel segments of normal size, whereas patients with functional obstruction may have generalized involvement of the bowel. These parameters, however, are only guidelines and some overlap exists between mechanical and functional ileus, making the radiographic distinction impossible in some patients.

Table 46-5 lists diagnostic considerations for the more common patterns of bowel dilation. Patterns of dilation include (1) focal/mild: one to three loops are involved, and luminal distentions are 1.5 to 2 times normal; (2) focal/severe: one to three loops are involved, and luminal distention is greater than twice normal (Fig. 46-11); (3) generalized/mild: all loops are involved, and luminal distention is 1.5 to 2 times normal; and (4) generalized/severe: all loops are involved, and luminal distention is greater than twice normal.

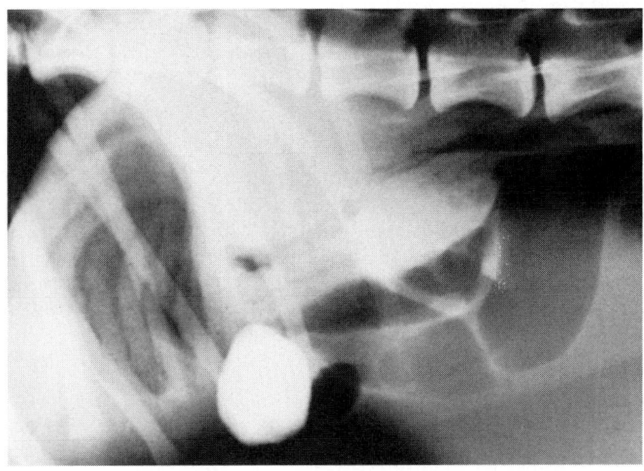

Fig. 46-11 Mechanical ileus, caused by a radiopaque foreign object (rock). Note the focal, extensively dilated small bowel loops.

Mechanical Ileus

The small intestinal lumen can be occluded by foreign objects, intussusception, masses from the wall of the bowel, or extrinsic lesions that compress the bowel. Mechanical obstruction can be complete or partial and can occur at any location through the tract. The most consistent radiographic sign of mechanical obstruction is a variable degree of dilation of bowel loops oral to the site of obstruction (Fig. 46-12). More complete and longer duration obstruction results in greater bowel distention. As more bowel becomes progressively distended, the segments often assume a "stacked" appearance as they become crowded into a relatively smaller space (Fig. 46-13).

A more distal (along the length of the small intestine) or more complete obstruction leads to a greater number of

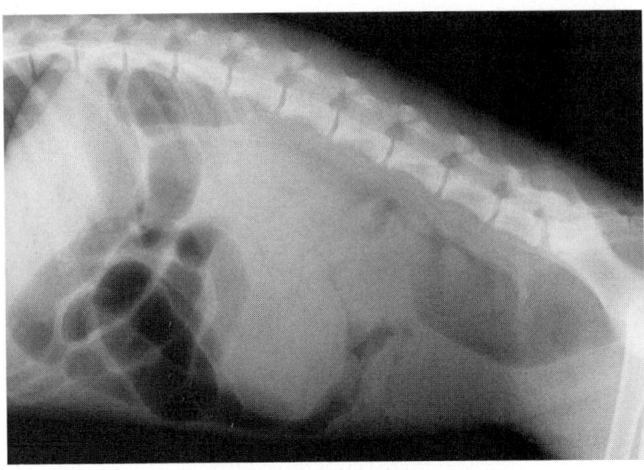

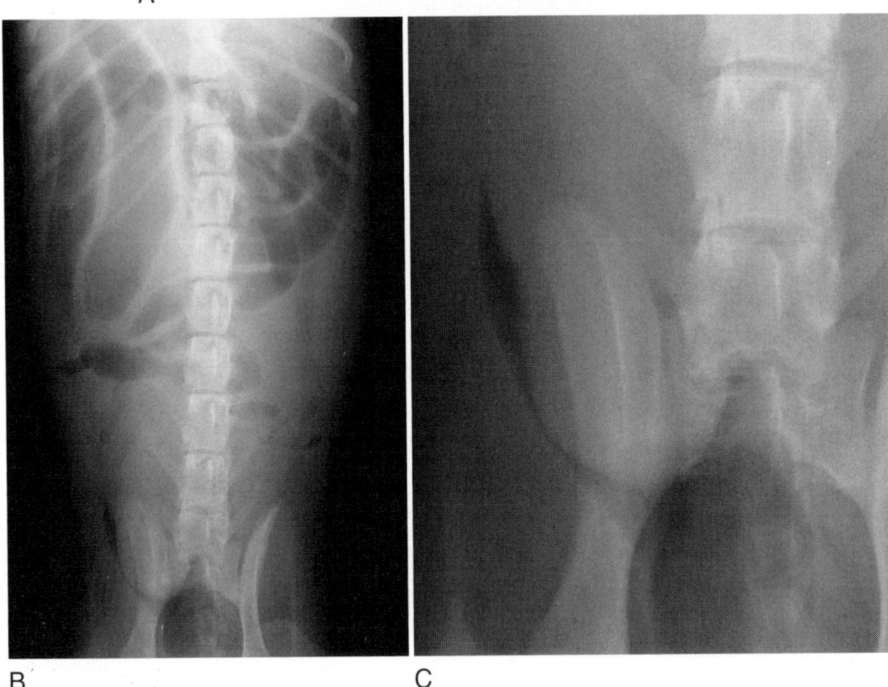

Fig. 46-12 Lateral (A) and ventrodorsal (B) radiographs of a dog with mechanical bowel obstruction caused by an ileocolic intussusception. Severely dilated bowel segments are present, but some segments are normal in size; this is much more consistent with a mechanical bowel obstruction than functional obstruction. Many times the cause of a mechanical bowel obstruction cannot be determined by survey radiographs, but in this dog the ileal intussusceptum can be seen within the descending colon. **C,** Close-up ventrodorsal view. A sharp interface is visible between the intussusceptum and the gas more distal in the colon. This finding is highly specific for ileocolic intussusception.

distended loops. Obstructed bowel typically contains both fluid and gas unless the obstruction is quite proximal, allowing gas and fluid to reflux into the stomach.

Acute obstructions of the duodenum are difficult to detect in survey radiographs because the stomach acts as a reservoir for gas and fluid that might collect. Also, if vomiting is frequent the accumulated fluid and gas are removed from the stomach and duodenum. With chronic duodenal obstruction, however, gastric distension becomes apparent (Fig. 46-14).

Partial obstructions may be difficult to detect. This is particularly true when the partial obstruction is of short duration and in the proximal duodenum. Dilation of such a relatively short length of duodenum may be easily overlooked. Longstanding partial obstructions that are distal in the bowel result in accumulation of opaque granular material proximal to the site of obstruction. This is caused by desiccation of ingesta that becomes trapped proximal to the obstruction. The desiccated material often has the appearance of feces, and the identification of this fecal-like material in small rather than large bowel is a reliable sign of partial distal small bowel obstruction. One scenario in which this type of obstruction occurs is elderly cats that develop ileal adenocarcinomas causing partial bowel obstruction (Fig. 46-15).

If a bowel obstruction is complete, the small intestine distal to the obstruction is likely to be empty. As a prediction for the presence of obstruction in the dog, a measured ratio less than 1.6 for the small intestine diameter relative to the L5 vertebral body height indicates that small intestinal obstruction is not likely.[5] Values greater than 1.6 are suggestive of obstruction. Alternatively, qualitative assessment of bowel size may be as accurate once a clinician has gained experience.

Foreign objects composed of mineral or metal are easily recognized (see Fig. 46-11). Disk-shaped metallic foreign objects consistent with a penny should be closely checked for erosion. Pennies minted since 1983 have a major zinc composition and can cause anemia from acute zinc toxicity.[41] Conversely, a patient with malaise and Heinz body anemia should be radiographed to assess for ingested zinc-containing coins or other objects (such as nuts or bolts).

Many small to moderately sized rocks are ingested by dogs and clay litter or hard-shelled seeds by cats and are identified incidentally as they pass without causing obstruction. However, small particles of radiopaque ingesta and debris can also accumulate proximal to a chronic partial obstruction (see Fig. 46-15). Nonmineralized, nonmetallic foreign objects are much more difficult to identify. Fruit pits, corncobs, and other nonopaque objects may be recognized by their geometrically shaped radiolucencies on survey radiographs (Fig. 46-16).[42] The nonopaque foreign object with irregular surfaces, especially with grooves, can entrap small, mineralized ingested debris and gas and may become more visible. Careful application of abdominal compression may enhance the conspicuity of these foreign objects.

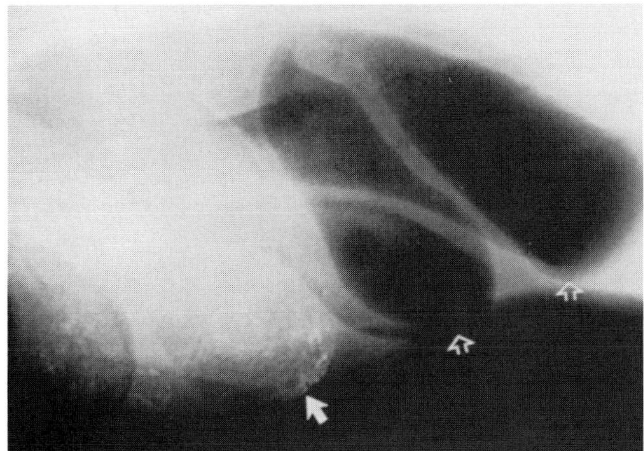

Fig. 46-13 Mechanical obstruction in a dog with an ileocolic intussusception. Although intussusception cannot be diagnosed from this image, the radiographic findings are strongly suggestive of mechanical obstruction because of the degree of dilation and the presence of both fluid and gas in the bowel. The distended loops are "stacked" as a result of their confinement in a relatively smaller space. Stacking of distended loops is highly suggestive of mechanical obstruction.

A pneumocolon can be used to differentiate questionably dilated small intestine from colon and define the location of mottled mineralized material to be in the small versus large bowel. On the basis of clinical signs, the use of 24-hour serial survey radiographs, a contrast study, or an ultrasound evaluation may be necessary to confirm the diagnosis of partial obstruction suggested by abnormal luminal contents. Persistence of small opaque foreign objects in the same intestinal location in serial radiographs over a 24- to 48-hour period should increase the suspicion of partial obstruction.

If obstruction is complete, the markedly reduced intestinal motility may significantly prolong barium transit to the site of obstruction. Dilated loops typically have a smooth barium/mucosa interface.[43] However, at the region of obstruction barium should outline the foreign object, with the object itself creating a filling defect in the barium column (Fig. 46-17). Figure 46-18 schematically depicts variations in the contrast/intraluminal object interface. Fenestrated foreign objects that cause only partial obstruction allow barium to pass around or through them. If only a small volume of barium passes through or around such an object, the volume may be insufficient to achieve physiologic distention of the remainder of the bowel. In Figure 46-19 barium accumulation can be seen in dilated bowel orad to a foreign object (baby bottle nipple) as can a thin stream of barium in the bowel distal to the partial obstruction. This reduced contrast volume may lead to a false impression of narrowed bowel diameter distal to the obstruction.

The ultrasonographic appearance of ingested foreign material varies according to the composition of the material.[44] The acoustic pattern caused by the rigid foreign object may have a shape that can be specifically recognized. Objects that transmit the beam, such as some types of rubber balls, are more readily identified. Those that create a strong reflection with marked acoustic shadowing may be more difficult to define

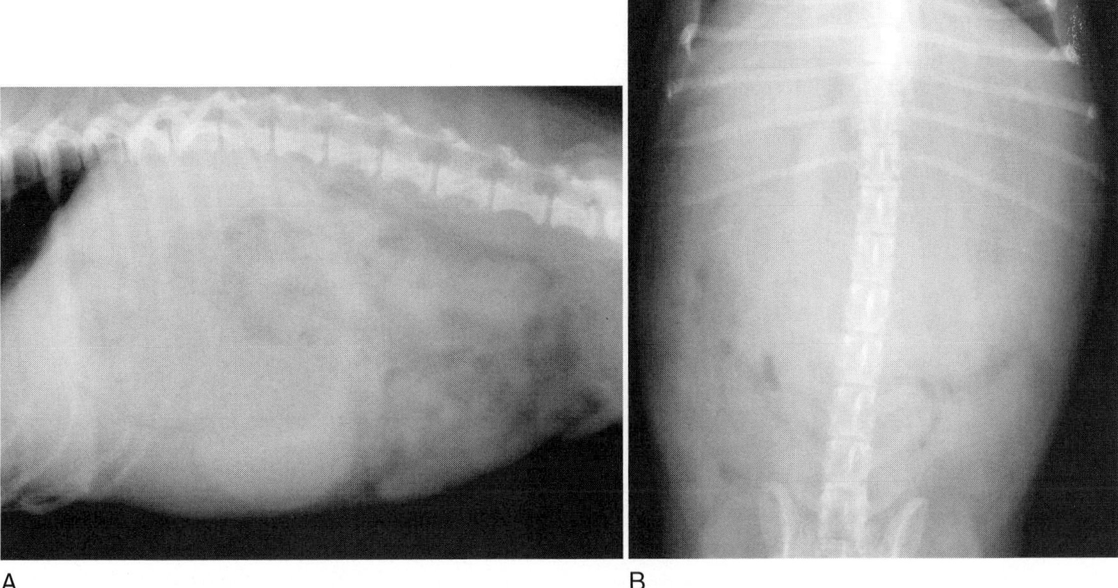

Fig. 46-14 Lateral (A) and ventrodorsal (B) radiographs of a dog with a chronic proximal small bowel obstruction. Proximal obstructions may not be apparent early, but later the stomach distends, as seen here. The stomach in this dog is quite large and contains both fluid and gas. The lateral is a left-to-right lateral and the round opacity in the cranioventral abdomen is the fluid-filled pylorus; this should not be confused with a foreign body or soft tissue mass. In both views the stomach wall appears thickened, but this is an illusion created by the combination of the gas and fluid in the lumen with the wall.

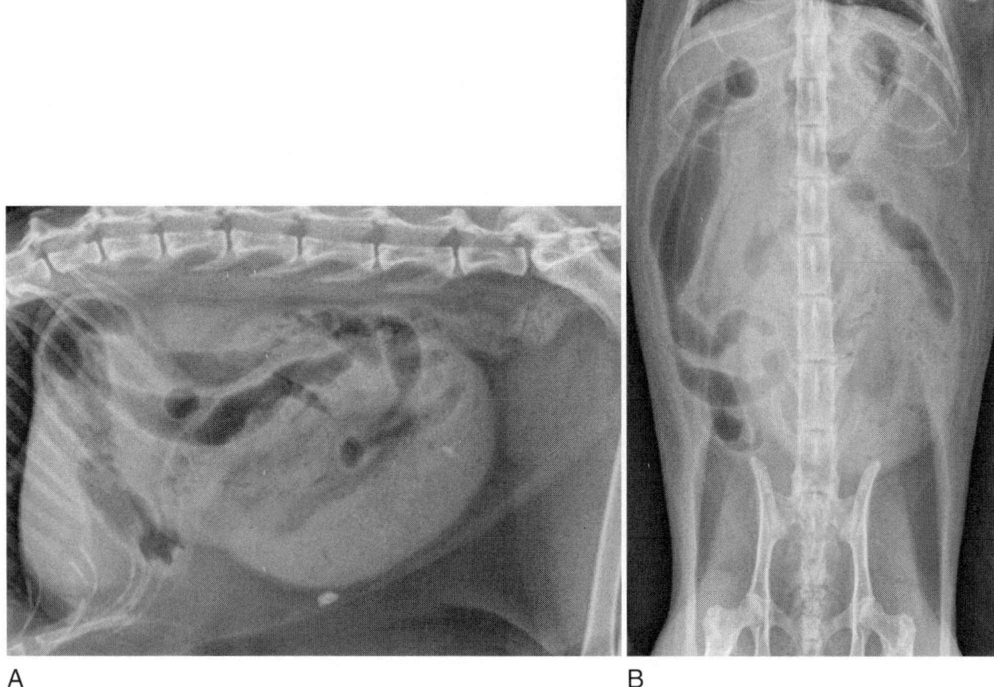

Fig. 46-15 Lateral (A) and ventrodorsal (B) radiographs of a cat with chronic partial ileal obstruction from an adenocarcinoma. The ileum is markedly distended with fecal-like material. This loop is differentiated from large bowel by its position ventral to the colon in **A** and its caudal turn in **B**; the colon does not have a caudal flexure as seen in **B**. The opacity of the material in the bowel is caused by continued desiccation because of its inability to pass the obstruction. More proximal bowel segments may continue to remain normal.

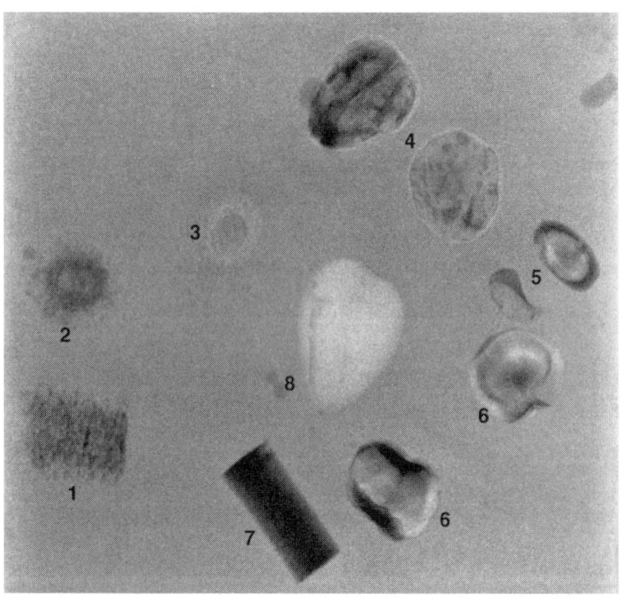

Fig. 46-16 Various nonopaque foreign bodies radiographed in a water bath. *1*, Section of corncob viewed side on; *2*, section of corncob viewed end on; *3*, peach pit; *4*, walnuts; *5*, acorns; *6*, chestnuts; *7*, wine cork; *8*, avocado pit. (From Lamb CR, Hanson K: Radiological identification of nonopaque intestinal foreign bodies, *Vet Radiol Ultrasound* 35:87, 1994.)

initially. When these objects cause incomplete obstruction, they are frequently associated with increased intestinal motility resulting from irritation. With more complete obstruction, the foreign object may be associated with accumulation of fluid in the associated bowel.

Linear foreign material (e.g., string, nylon hosiery) that becomes trapped in the intestine usually causes both an abnormal shape and contour of the loops and an abnormal luminal content pattern.[8] Some portion of the linear material typically becomes fixed at an orad location—most commonly in the stomach in dogs and under the tongue in cats.[45] The remainder of the length passes into the small intestine. The peristaltic action of the bowel causes it to "climb" up the linear foreign body, which results in a pleated, or plicated, appearance of the affected loops. These loops may not become particularly distended, but gas commonly becomes trapped in pockets formed by the pleats. The result is an abnormal pattern of round, tapered, short-tubular, and sometimes crescent-shaped, gas shapes (Fig. 46-20). If the linear material is absorptive in nature, such as fabric, it can absorb fluid incompletely and have a mottled to linear, streaked gas pattern.

A serious complication of chronic linear foreign body is laceration of the intestinal wall. If the laceration is small, serosal adhesion to an adjacent loop can occur, resulting in a fixed position of two or more loops. If the laceration is large, septic peritonitis and potential gas leakage occur. A comparative study between dogs and cats with linear foreign objects noted several significant differences: affected dogs tended to be older and had less irregularity in the gas pattern; one quarter of dogs had concurrent intussusception; on both radiographic and

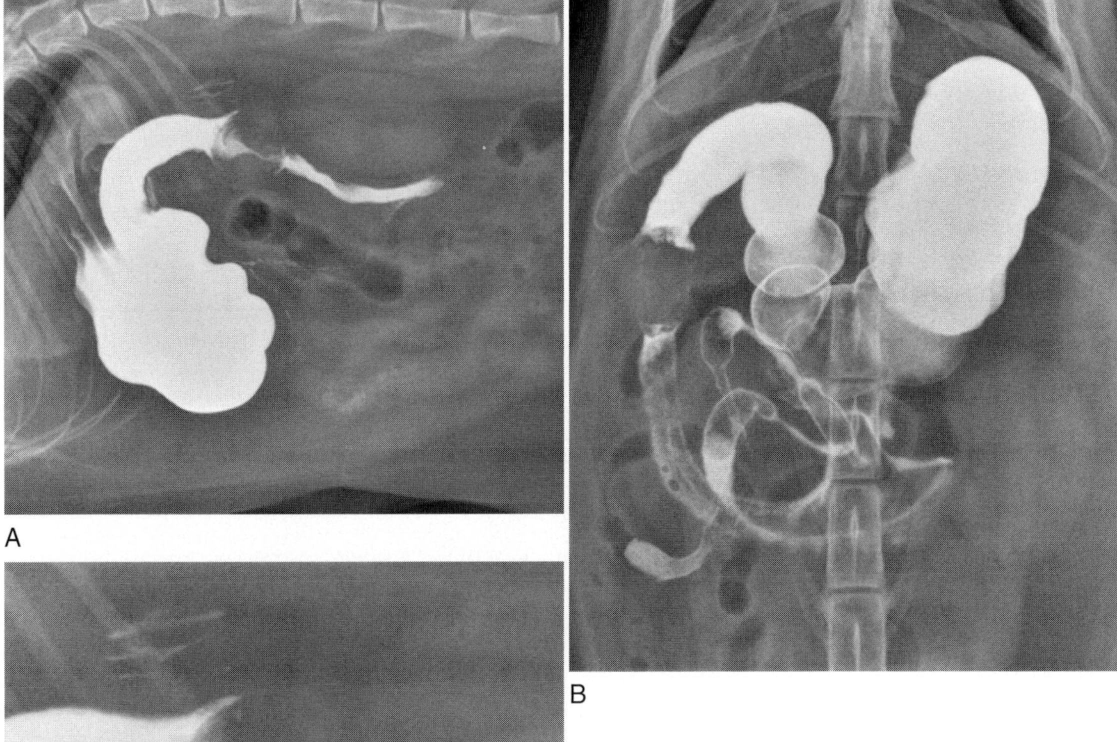

Fig. 46-17 Lateral (B), ventrodorsal (B), and close-up lateral (C) radiographs of the cranial abdomen of a cat with a duodenal foreign body that had been given barium. Radiographs were made 15 minutes after barium administration. The filling defect created by the foreign object is apparent. The lumen is not completely occluded because some barium is able to be propelled around the periphery of the foreign object. This is not the type of appearance that would result from a mural mass. The stomach is distended and hypercontractile; numerous peristaltic contractions are apparent.

surgical assessment, dogs revealed greater evidence of bowel trauma or bowel laceration and peritonitis; and the probability of death as a result of linear foreign body in dogs was nearly double that in cats.[45-47]

Barium contrast studies improve detection of the abnormal shape and contour of the loops containing the linear foreign material (Fig. 46-21). Thin linear material such as string or cord may not be visible as a filling defect. However, if the fixed component of the string is in a wad, this should be seen as a filling defect in the barium, such as in the pyloric region of the stomach. Such a mass of string in the stomach may not be seen in the initial views when a large volume of barium masks the material. However, in later images, when all barium should have exited the stomach, a barium-soaked or coated mass remains in the stomach, indicating the retained foreign material. For this reason, 12- to 24-hour postbarium films are suggested in suspect patients if standard postbarium radiographs are nondiagnostic. Patients suspected to have linear foreign bodies that also have reduced serosal detail have a reasonable likelihood of laceration of the bowel wall with secondary peritonitis. Contrast medium may leak from these lacerations (Fig. 46-22).

Enteric parasites occasionally are discovered by positive-contrast examinations. The linearity of an ascarid looks strikingly similar to that of a linear foreign body. However, with parasites, the bowel is not likely to be plicated.

The ultrasound appearance of linear material depends on the amount of gas and fluid accumulated around the foreign material. Plication (undulating mucosa) of the bowel around an echogenic line has been described most frequently.[44] This differs from the smooth, straight mucosa normally seen on either side of the bright linear stripe of an empty normal bowel lumen. If within the duodenum, the linear foreign material may be traceable into the stomach.[48] Thickening of the wall or obliteration of the wall layer pattern has not been described. Intestinal perforation caused by linear foreign material or other diseases (nonlinear penetrating foreign bodies, neoplasia, or drug-induced perforating ulcers) should be suspected when the ultrasound examination identifies a combination of focal hyperechoic mesenteric fat, echogenic peritoneal effusion, and fluid in the bowel.

Intussusception, the invagination of one portion (intussusceptum) of the gastrointestinal tract into the lumen (intussuscipiens) of an adjacent segment, can be initiated by many events, including motility disorders, inflammatory wall lesions, neoplasia, or idiopathic causes.[49] Although intussusceptions can occur anywhere along the digestive tract, the majority occur in the small intestinal tract and at the ileocolic or cecocolic junction. The radiographic appearance of intussusception is considerably influenced by the completeness of the occlusion of the lumen of the intussusceptum.[8] Many distal intussusceptions result in generalized severe distention of the small

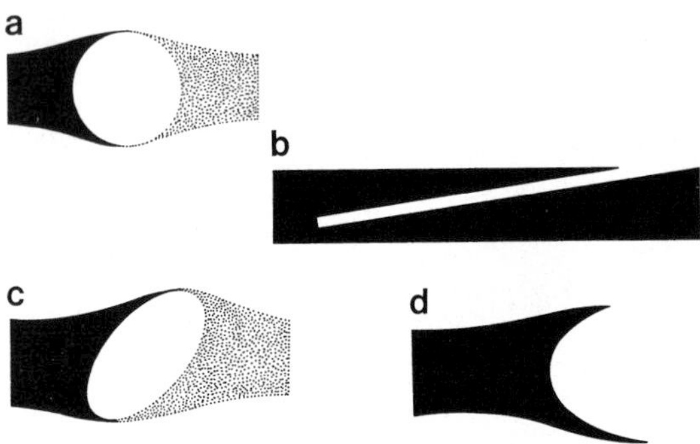

Fig. 46-18 Shapes of contrast interface with an intraluminal object. The barium column *(black)* fills the intestine and outlines one or several surfaces of the object. Partial obstruction of the lumen allows a smaller quantity of barium *(stippling)* to pass. With complete obstruction, no barium is in the bowel distal to it and therefore no definition is visible of the caudal surface of the object. *a*, A spherical mass (rubber ball) arising from the bowel mucosa (leiomyoma; rare). *b*, A flat, straight foreign object, such as hard plastic, leather, or wood splinter. *c*, Fruit pit or nut. *d*, Retrograde intussusception (invagination of bowel in the opposite direction of normal ingesta passage).

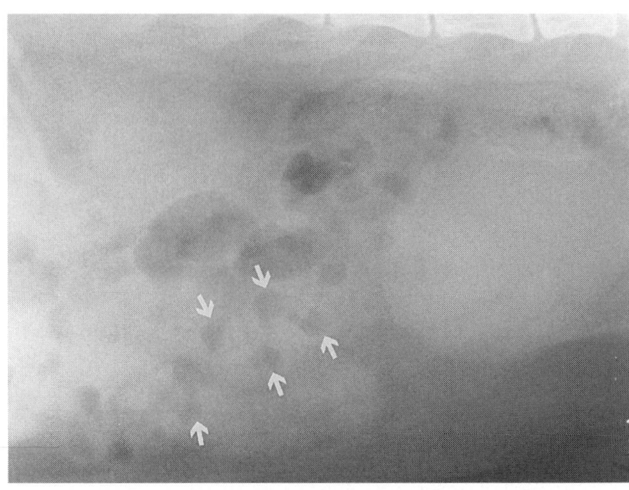

Fig. 46-20 Noncontinuous gas typical of plicated, zigzag, accordion-like contour of the small intestine *(arrows)* in a cat with a linear intestinal foreign object. A string was removed at surgery.

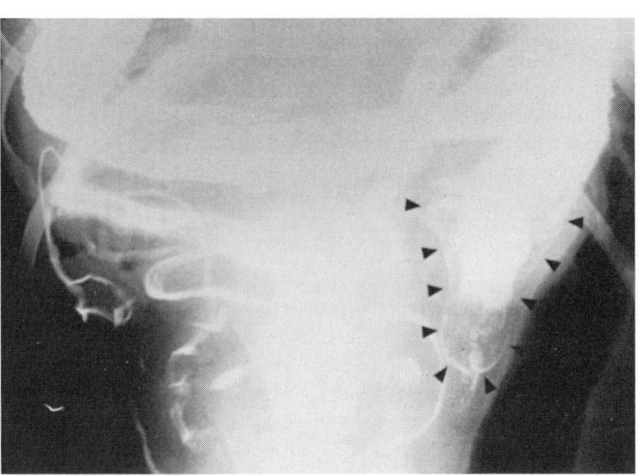

Fig. 46-19 Mechanical obstruction of the jejunum by a foreign object (baby bottle nipple *[arrows]*).

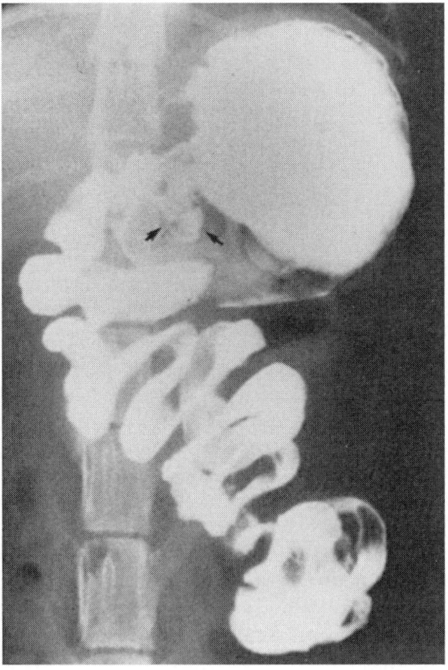

Fig. 46-21 Feline upper gastrointestinal tract study 20 minutes after administration of barium. The tightly pleated or "ribbon candy" appearance indicates the presence of linear foreign material. The proximal end of the foreign material is often wrapped around the base of the tongue or is caught in the pyloric antrum of the stomach *(arrows)*.

bowel; the intussusceptum occasionally can be seen in the colon if sufficient colon gas is present (see Fig. 46-12). In most patients, however, differentiating intussusception from other causes of mechanical obstruction solely on the basis of survey radiographs is not possible.

Left lateral survey radiographs and barium oral or barium enema contrast studies can be used to differentiate intussusception from other causes of bowel obstruction. A barium enema has a high probability of defining ileo-ceco-colic level intussusceptions, especially when the bowel is considerably dilated. Oral barium takes a long time to reach this distal level when motility is reduced. The pattern of barium at the lesion can vary depending on the degree of patency of the lumen through the length of the intussusceptum and the space remaining between the intussusceptum and the intussuscipiens. The longer the duration of the intussusception, the greater the edema in the affected bowel walls and the more complete the obstruction. In some patients a thin column of barium can be seen passing through the narrowed lumen of the intus-

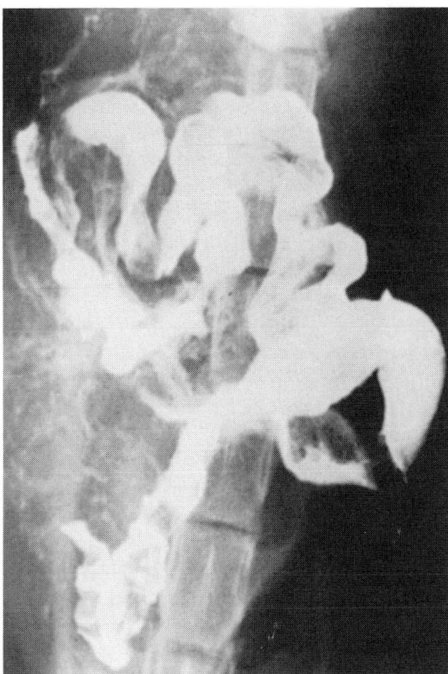

Fig. 46-22 Leakage of contrast medium into the peritoneal cavity occurred as a result of bowel necrosis at multiple sites. Iodine-containing, water-soluble contrast media are the agents of choice when bowel perforation is suspected. After this cat vomited iodine several times, barium was used to achieve a diagnostic study.

susceptum. If barium can seep between the invaginated and outer segments, a filling defect is demonstrated and a tube within a tube effect, or "coil-spring" effect, is seen.[8] With complete obstruction an abrupt end to the barium column is usually present with dilation orally.

Intussusceptions have a characteristic ultrasound pattern (Fig. 46-23). The telescoping effect results in a bull's-eye target, or concentric ring, appearance when viewed in the transverse plane of the lesion and a multilinear pattern when viewed in the longitudinal plane of the lesion.[50-52] A hyperechoic or anechoic region typically is noted in the center of or mildly eccentrically positioned within the concentric or linear pattern. The shape of this hyperechoic material may be round or semilunar and is caused by mesenteric fat pulled into the intussuscipiens. If anechoic, it most likely represents a small volume of fluid within the lumen of the inner loop or between the inner and outer loops. When viewed in the long axis, fluid distention is often seen in the bowel proximal to the lesion.

Proliferating tissue masses originating within the intestinal wall include tumors, polyps, and granulomatous infiltrates. The development of an obstructive bowel pattern from these lesions depends on the size of the lesion and whether growth of the lesion is directed toward or away from the lumen. Over time most could progress from no effect to partial obstruction to complete obstruction. Most present clinically during the phase of partial obstruction, with focal mild to severe distention. Additional features of these masses are discussed below.

Lesions originating outside the intestinal wall can cause compression on a loop and result in partial or complete obstruction. Lesions in this category include adhesions from prior surgery, abdominal boundary hernias (congenital or traumatic), and occasionally masses originating from other abdominal organs.

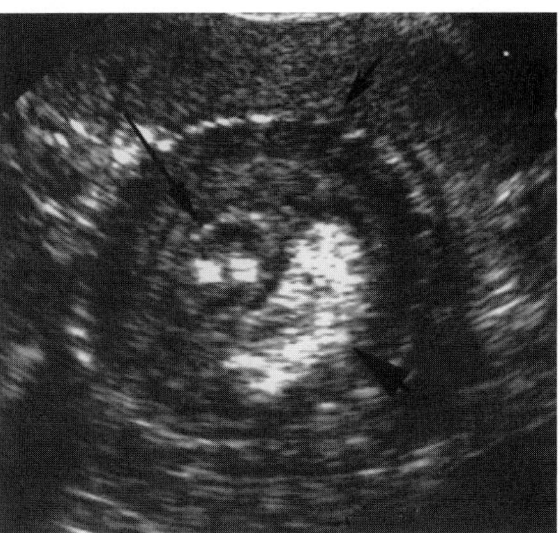

Fig. 46-23 Transverse ultrasound image showing a concentric ring pattern with an eccentric ovoid hyperechoic region. The central ring *(long arrow)* represents the intussusceptum. The eccentric hyperechoic material *(short arrows)* is most likely intussuscepted mesenteric fat.

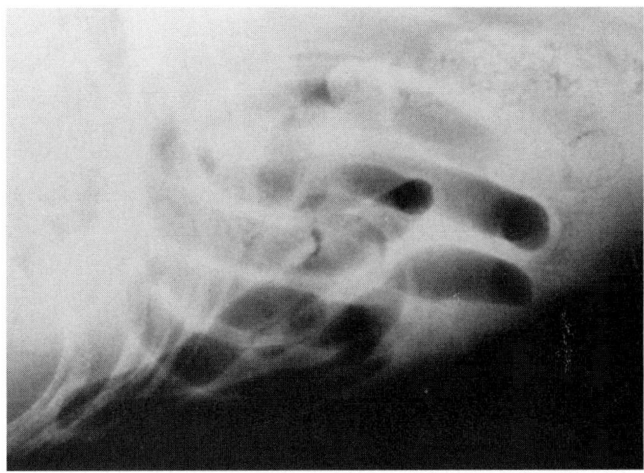

Fig. 46-24 Mild, generalized enlargement of small bowel lumen (approximately four times the width of the adjacent rib). This dog had a recently ruptured splenic hemangiosarcoma (not visible on this image) leading to abdominal pain and subsequent functional ileus.

Functional Ileus

When the peristaltic contractions of the bowel cease because of vascular or neuromuscular abnormalities within the bowel wall, the lumen dilates (Fig. 46-24). In functional ileus the bowel lumen remains patent. Many patients have no specific survey radiographic changes to differentiate the bowel dilation caused by functional ileus from that of mechanical ileus. As previously noted, the length of bowel affected may provide some differentiation, with localized dilation more likely from a mechanical cause and diffuse dilation more likely from functional ileus. However, obvious overlap between these two occurs. Furthermore, chronic moderate to severe mechanical obstruction can eventually lead to functional ileus.

A barium contrast study of patients with functional ileus should show uniformly distended bowel segments, delayed transit, and normal to nonspecific changes in the barium

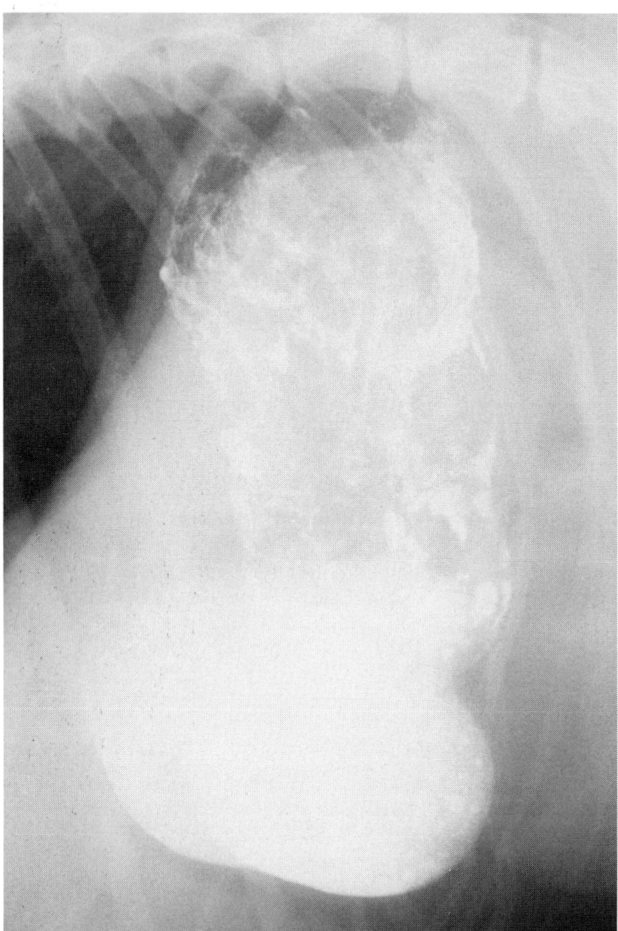

Fig. 46-25 Right lateral radiograph of a dog recently given barium. The barium is clumping or flocculating in the fundus. Flocculation is relatively nonspecific. However, when a commercially prepared barium suspension is used and flocculation is seen, altered pH or the presence of luminal hemorrhage, as might occur with functional ileus, should be considered. Conversely, flocculation with suspensions made from barium powder is so common that it has no significance.

texture and mucosal border. No barium contrast findings are specifically diagnostic of the diseases causing functional ileus. Flocculation of the barium (Fig. 46-25), a cobblestone appearance of the barium/mucosa interface, and an irregular undulation of the mucosal border can be seen throughout the progression of parvovirus enteritis.[53] Because these diseases mimic complete mechanical obstruction, the role of the barium contrast study is to exclude mechanical obstruction. However barium transit may be so severely prolonged that a conclusion of obstruction is reached in error.

No specific ultrasound features have been described to differentiate functional ileus from chronic complete mechanical obstruction. The finding of peristalsis suggests exclusion of functional ileus. A thorough search of the bowel should be done to look for obvious obstructive causes such as intussusception, intraluminal foreign material, or extrinsic masses. The finding of echogenic peritoneal effusion supports a diagnosis of peritonitis that can be confirmed by fluid sampling and analysis.

The more common diseases that cause functional ileus include viral enteritis (canine parvovirus-2 in particular), chronic mechanical obstruction, and peritonitis.[53] Other less-common diseases with a primary radiographic change of dilated intestinal loops include strangulation of the intestine through a hernia (vascular compromise), mesenteric volvulus (vascular compromise), spinal trauma (neurologic injury), segmental jejunal arterial thrombosis (vascular compromise), dysautonomia (autonomic nervous system disease), and intestinal pseudoobstruction (tunica muscularis fibrosis and atrophy). Small intestinal loops can slip through traumatic tears or developmental hernias of the peritoneal cavity boundaries. The identification of such loops in an extraabdominal location is often quite easy because of gas within their lumen. Bowel dilation occurs if the rent becomes constrictive or if the loop twists, effectively occluding its outflow.

Mesenteric volvulus results in occlusion of the cranial mesenteric artery. The reduced blood supply leads to ischemic necrosis, gastrointestinal toxin release, and shock.[54,55] The initiating event for volvulus typically is not known. The majority of dogs reported have been of larger breed size. Many dogs have no distant or immediate prior history of gastrointestinal signs and are presented for peracute or acute abdominal distension, abdominal pain, and shock. However, mesenteric volvulus has occurred subsequent to prior treatment for acute gastric dilatation with volvulus and for intussusception. A series of dogs with mesenteric volvulus had a previous clinical diagnosis of pancreatic insufficiency and clinical signs of vomiting.[56] The radiographic signs are moderate to severe dilation of the small intestine with fluid and gas. Peritoneal effusion may be concurrent. A cat with jejunal thrombosis resulting in segmental bowel infarction had radiographic evidence of segmental bowel dilation and delayed gastric emptying and intestinal transit times. Sonographically over the course of 72 hours this bowel segment underwent progressive wall thickening, conversion to loss of wall layers, and finally a generalized hypoechoic wall. Perienteric hyperechoic mesenteric fat also developed.[57]

A syndrome of intestinal pseudoobstruction, with histopathologic changes restricted to the tunica muscularis but apparently not involving the myenteric plexuses, has been reported in 8 dogs.[58-60] Diagnosis was based on full-thickness intestinal biopsy, which in the majority had tunica muscularis fibrosis, atrophy, and cellular infiltrate. One dog was suspected to have an immune-mediated etiology based on immunohistochemical staining features.[61] All dogs had progressive deterioration caused by emaciation from malabsorption.

Dysautonomia is an autonomic nervous system disease that among other clinical signs can include vomiting, diarrhea, and inappetence. Radiographs of the abdomen are often characterized by focal or diffuse gastrointestinal dilation. Barium transit is markedly delayed. The most unique feature of these patients is their geographic origin, the first being reported from the United Kingdom. Additional patients have been reported in Europe and predominately in Missouri and Kansas in the United States.[62-64]

The vaccination history (parvovirus), geographic region of origin (Missouri, Kansas, United Kingdom, and Europe) of a patient with concomitant signs of other autonomic nervous system dysfunction (dysautonomia), history of thromboembolic disease, and a thorough current history and physical examination are the most useful factors in ranking these causes of functional ileus as having a higher likelihood than the causes of mechanical obstruction.

Infiltrative Bowel Disease

Infiltrative bowel disease infers generalized or segmental infiltration of the bowel wall as a result of nonseptic inflammation, infection, or neoplasia. Some infiltrative bowel diseases, such as lymphocytic-plasmocytic enteritis, do not have a specific etiology and are characterized by inflammatory cell infiltration of the intestinal wall.[65] Bowel ischemia may also result in a bowel appearance in a barium contrast study similar to that produced from infiltrative disease.

With cellular infiltration into the layers of the bowel wall, the most anticipated change is an increase in bowel wall thickness. However, some infiltrations do not cause a radiographically detectable thickness change but alter the physiology of the bowel such that it appears abnormal radiographically, especially when barium has been given. Bowel wall thickness cannot be reliably detected from survey radiographs but can be evaluated in barium and ultrasound studies, the latter providing the most sensitive detection of thickening. Ultrasound is the only readily available imaging modality that can differentiate bowel wall layers. However, survey radiographic findings that should heighten the suspicion of infiltrative small bowel disease in a patient with appropriate clinical signs include increased small bowel gas in cats and decreased gas/fluid ratio in dogs.[11]

No radiographic or sonographic features are specific to infiltrative bowel disease. Survey radiographs are usually within normal limits. Because infiltrative bowel disease can be a diagnosis made by exclusion, the negative survey radiographic findings help exclude other diseases. Inflammatory infiltrates are suspected to increase bowel wall thickness. However, on the basis of wall thickness, one study could not differentiate healthy from abnormal dogs.[66] The finding of normal wall thickness may lead to a significant rate of false-negative diagnoses. Intestinal biopsy remains the definitive diagnostic test for infiltrative bowel disease.

Infectious enteritides may be caused by viruses, bacterial, rickettsial, or fungal organisms. Parvovirus (canine parvovirus-2)-induced radiographic changes have been discussed in a previous section with reference to a differential diagnosis for abnormal bowel dilation. When there is reasonable suspicion of parvoviral enteritis an enzyme-linked immunosorbent assay (ELISA) test for canine parvovirus-2 in the feces should be done before barium contrast or ultrasound is used. Other viral diseases that infect the small intestinal tract have not been shown to cause any specific radiographic or sonographic changes, and thus are not discussed here. Bacterial overgrowth in the small intestine has also not been related to specific radiographic or sonographic changes.

In infiltrative bowel disease, survey radiographs are usually normal or luminal fluid may be increased. In severe infiltrations an abnormal mucosal margin may be seen or the wall may appear thickened (Fig. 46-26). Although radiographic assessment of wall thickness is complicated by silhouetting of intraluminal fluid within the wall, it is hard to imagine how silhouetting could lead to the appearance seen in Figure 46-26.

In barium contrast studies of patients with infiltrative bowel disease, a lumen contour change, irregular mucosal interface, wall thickness change, or luminal size change may be present. Survey radiographic findings that warrant positive-contrast evaluation when infiltrative small bowel disease is strongly suspected include increased small bowel gas in cats and decreased gas/fluid ratio in dogs.[11] Unfortunately, no positive-contrast findings, either single or in combination, have been discovered to differentiate nonneoplastic from neoplastic infiltrative disease.[11] However, the positive-contrast study may be used to corroborate a suspicion of abnormality from the survey radiographs and better define the location of a lesion in regard to whether endoscopic versus surgical biopsy would be most effective. This is especially valid if ultrasound is not available.

Barium studies in patients with infiltrative bowel disease are often characterized by an appearance termed thumbprinting. Thumbprinting is characterized by irregularly arranged mural-based indentations into the adjacent barium column. Thumbprinting should not be confused with normal bowel peristalsis, which is common immediately after administration of barium. Peristalsis typically causes smooth symmetric mural indentations into the barium (Fig. 46-27). Thumbprinting, which may be localized or generalized, usually results in less-structured indentations into the barium column and barium collections that are less oval in shape (Figs. 46-28 to 46-30).

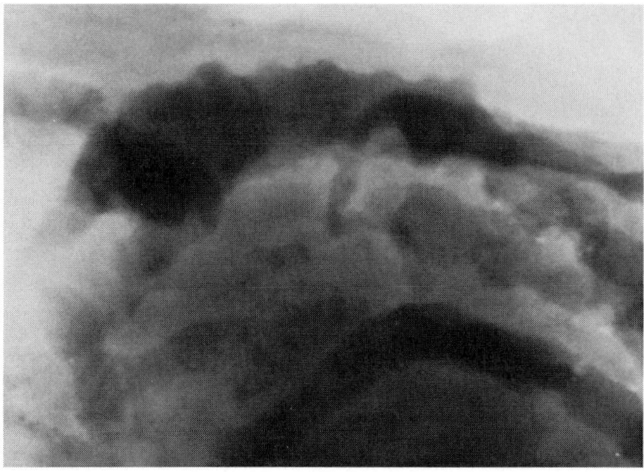

Fig. 46-26 Survey radiograph in which focal dilation and an irregular, scalloped mucosal surface of a small bowel segment are seen. Evaluation of the length of intestine affected and the severity of changes in the mucosa require a barium study or ultrasound evaluation. Most infiltrative bowel diseases will not produce this marked change in survey radiographs.

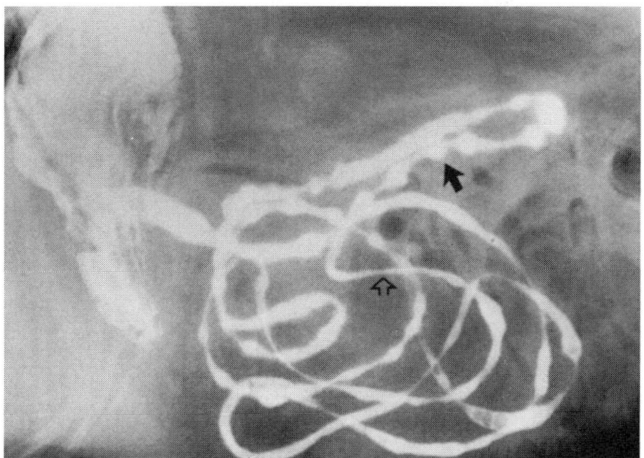

Fig. 46-27 Hyperperistalsis, which is clinically insignificant, is seen in this barium upper gastrointestinal tract study 5 minutes after contrast medium administration. Hypersegmentation causes numerous beadlike accumulations of contrast medium *(solid arrow)*. Thin strands of barium that extend for several centimeters *(open arrow)* can be seen when transit time through the small bowel is faster than normal, as in this patient. This appearance differs from thumbprinting; the indentations into the barium column are symmetric in the wall and quite smooth, and the "beads" are distinct, with round margins.

Bowel-Associated Masses

Bacterial abscesses can occur as focal lesions associated with the intestinal wall. A bowel-associated abscess can be a consequence of partial or complete intestinal perforation by

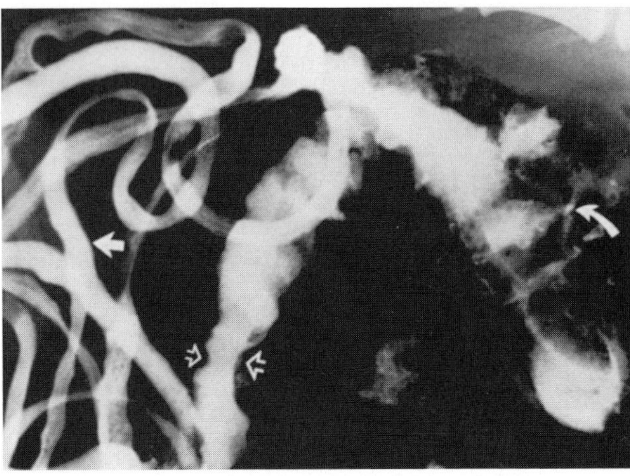

Fig. 46-28 Barium upper gastrointestinal tract study (same patient as in Fig. 46-26). Normal bowel is seen in the cranial abdomen *(solid arrow)*. Abnormal mucosal architecture is indicated by thumbprinting *(open arrows)* and a spiculated, ragged interface between the barium and the mucosa *(curved arrow)*. The affected section of bowel is also moderately dilated. This pattern is typical of infiltrative bowel disease and is nonspecific. Considerations include lymphocytic plasmocytic enteritis, eosinophilic enteritis, parvoviral infection, lymphoma, and ischemia. Histopathologic diagnosis was lymphosarcoma.

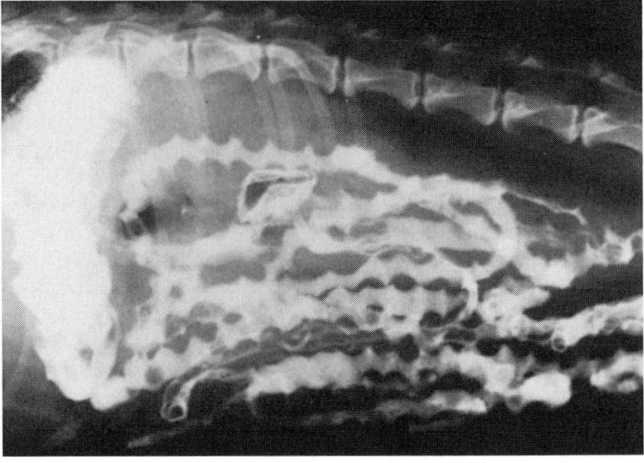

Fig. 46-30 Generalized asymmetric thumbprinting throughout the small bowel. This pattern suggests extensive infiltrative bowel disease such as lymphosarcoma, parvoviral enteritis, or lymphocytic-plasmacytic enteritis. Interestingly, the severity and distribution of this thumbprinting pattern may change with time during the barium study, sometimes becoming less extensive and more localized. This suggests that some of the thumbprinting seen in barium studies of patients with infiltrative bowel disease is caused by wall spasm rather than cellular infiltration. Histopathologic diagnosis was lymphocytic-plasmacytic enteritis.

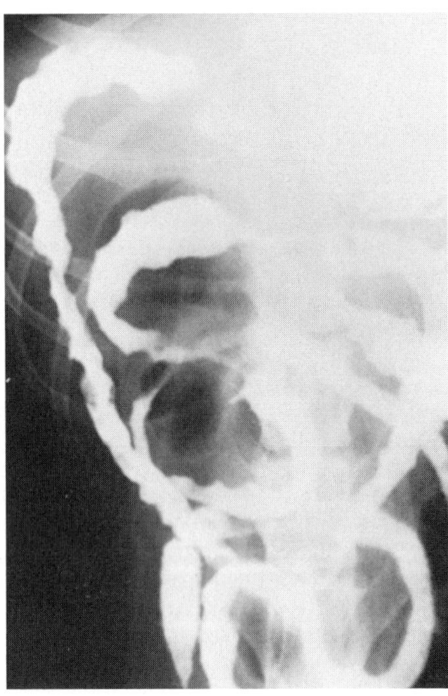

Fig. 46-29 Numerous mural indentations resulting in filling defects are seen in the duodenum and less prominently in the jejunum. These defects appear as thumbprintlike indentations of the barium column. The lumen diameter of the descending duodenum is narrowed. This pattern is typical of infiltrative bowel disease and is nonspecific. Considerations include lymphocytic plasmocytic enteritis, eosinophilic enteritis, parvoviral infection, lymphoma, and ischemia. Histopathologic diagnosis was lymphocytic plasmacytic enteritis.

foreign material, with subsequent adhesions and abscess formation. The mass may result in regional loss of serosal detail or may displace adjacent bowel (Fig. 48-31). A mottled appearance may be seen in bowel-associated abscesses when exudate from the abscess drains into the lumen and is replaced by gas. Abscesses associated with the small intestine may originate from a source extrinsic to the wall. This may occur as a result of retained surgical sponges or be caused by a pancreatic abscess. For example, inflammation of the proximal duodenum as a result of pancreatitis can cause the duodenum to take on a fixed or rigid appearance demonstrated radiographically by mild gas dilation.[67] A left lateral view may help show this mild dilation. Sonographically a corrugated mucosal and submucosal contour pattern has been observed to be associated with pancreatitis.[68] This corrugation may also be apparent in a barium study (see Fig. 46-30). However, this corrugated pattern is not specific to pancreatitis and can be seen with other causes of peritonitis as well as enteritis, neoplasia, and bowel wall ischemia.[68,69]

Although uncommon, mycotic infections of the intestinal tract include histoplasmosis, cryptococcosis,[70] and pythiosis. Pythiosis, an opportunistic water-borne fungus, has been diagnosed in dogs in Oklahoma (including the northern region) in addition to its more common endemic locale in the states along the Gulf Coast.[71,72] Pathologic changes are often advanced by the time of clinical presentation. Pyogranulomatous lesions cause localized thickening of the intestinal wall that frequently extends through the serosa, along the mesentery, and into the mesenteric lymph nodes. This combination results in a palpable abdominal mass. The ultrasound features of a series of dogs having pythiosis included thickening of the intestinal wall associated with loss of the layer pattern.[73] The sonographic features are similar to those of intestinal neoplasia. Histologic examination of tissue is required for diagnosis.

Common neoplasms of the small intestine include the malignant tumors: adenocarcinoma, lymphosarcoma, mastocytoma, and leiomyosarcoma. Atypical tumors reported are extraskeletal tumors, osteosarcoma, fibrosarcoma, carcinoid,

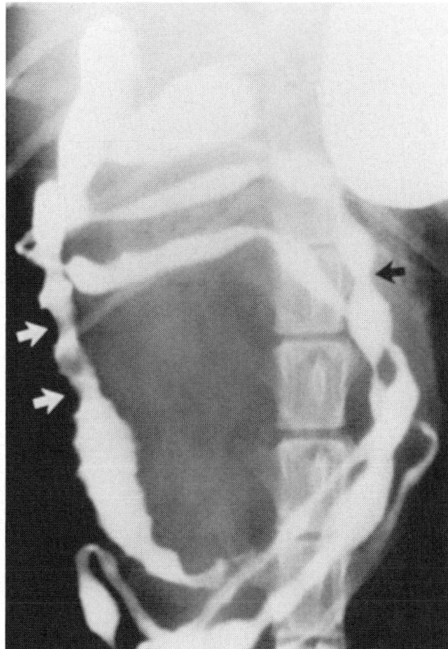

Fig. 46-31 Irritation of duodenum and jejunum is indicated by irregular, serrated mucosal surface *(white arrows)* of duodenum and hypersegmentation *(black arrow)*. The duodenum also appears displaced slightly to the right. The mid-central area, which is devoid of bowel loops, was caused by necrotic, hemorrhagic pancreatitis and abscess formation that resulted 10 days after a penetrating wound.

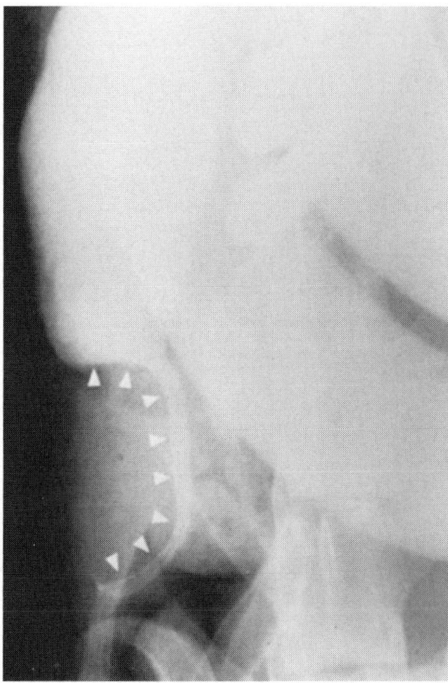

Fig. 46-32 Eccentrically narrowed bowel lumen, smooth mucosal surface, and dilation of bowel proximal to the narrowing characterize this focal intramural obstruction *(arrowheads)*. Histopathologic diagnosis was adenocarcinoma of bowel wall. Eccentric narrowing usually occurs with a mass lesion; a posttraumatic or postinflammatory stricture usually causes more symmetric narrowing.

neurilemmoma, and hemangiosarcoma.[74-87] Benign adenomatous polyps of the duodenum have also been reported in cats, with an increased frequency noted among Asian breeds.[88] In survey radiographs no signs unique to any of these tumors are noted. They may create no changes, be seen as soft tissue masses of variable size, or cause partial to complete obstruction resulting in bowel dilation signs. Accumulation of radiopaque foreign material may be seen as a consequence of partial obstruction. Identification of these bowel tumors is improved with either positive-contrast or ultrasound evaluation.

Masses associated with intestinal wall tumors typically cause smoothly rounded protrusions toward the lumen (Fig. 46-32). If the mural mass surrounds the lumen, the lumen often becomes enlarged and irregularly shaped (Fig. 46-33). Distinguishing between a large emphysematous mural tumor and a bowel-associated abscess may not be possible in most patients. The use of barium usually is unnecessary in such patients, but it can be administered to distinguish a bowel tumor from an adjacent abscess (Fig. 46-34). This distinction can also be made sonographically.

A pattern seen in barium studies of annular infiltration by adenocarcinoma is narrowing of the lumen by irregular indentations without a marked mural mass effect. This has been called an "apple core" appearance (Fig. 46-35).[13,79] It is not, however, specific for a diagnosis of neoplasia, and biopsy must be performed for diagnosis.[89-93]

When evaluated sonographically, intestinal neoplasia usually results in more extensive obliteration of the intestinal wall layering and greater wall thickness and is more likely to be focal than are inflammatory infiltrates.[11,94-98] In a study of 150 dogs, loss of wall layer pattern was the most predictive feature for differentiating between enteritis and neoplasia.[99] No ultrasonographic pattern is entirely specific for differentiating the types of small intestinal neoplasia. However, most (75%) cats with alimentary lymphosarcoma have transmural circumferential (as is seen in the transverse plane) thickening (4 to 22 mm), with the wall layers replaced by hypoechoic tissue. Half of these cats have associated enlargement of the mesenteric lymph nodes.[100,101] Intestinal adenocarcinoma of cats tends to cause transmural asymmetrical thickening, with the wall layer pattern lost and replaced by tissue of mixed echogenicity.[102]

Fewer sonographic characteristics have been described for specific intestinal neoplasms in the dog, with the exception of the smooth-muscle tumors, leiomyosarcoma and leiomyoma.[103] Leiomyosarcoma tends to be found as a large (2 to 8 cm thick), eccentrically positioned mass with mixed echogenicity. The larger the mass, the more likely that areas of necrosis will appear as hypoechoic foci. The large size of many leiomyosarcomas can cause difficulty determining that they are of bowel origin. Other tumors of the canine small intestine are insufficiently reported to enable any conclusions about trends in their sonographic appearance.[104] Ultrasound evaluation of the intestine combined with ultrasound-guided fine-needle aspiration and microcore biopsy is an accurate method of minimally invasive diagnosis.[105]

Miscellaneous Small Intestinal Diseases

Opacity changes in the intestinal wall are rare. Diffuse mineralization of the wall can occur by metastatic calcification as a result of hypercalcemia. Reports of dogs and cats poisoned by cholecalciferol-based rodenticides and having ingested human antipsoriasis ointment containing calcitriol analogues have noted clinical signs of vomiting, which may prompt radiography and/or ultrasonography of the abdomen.[106-109] Diffuse calcification of the gastrointestinal tract may be found in these patients. Radiographically the degree of calcification typically

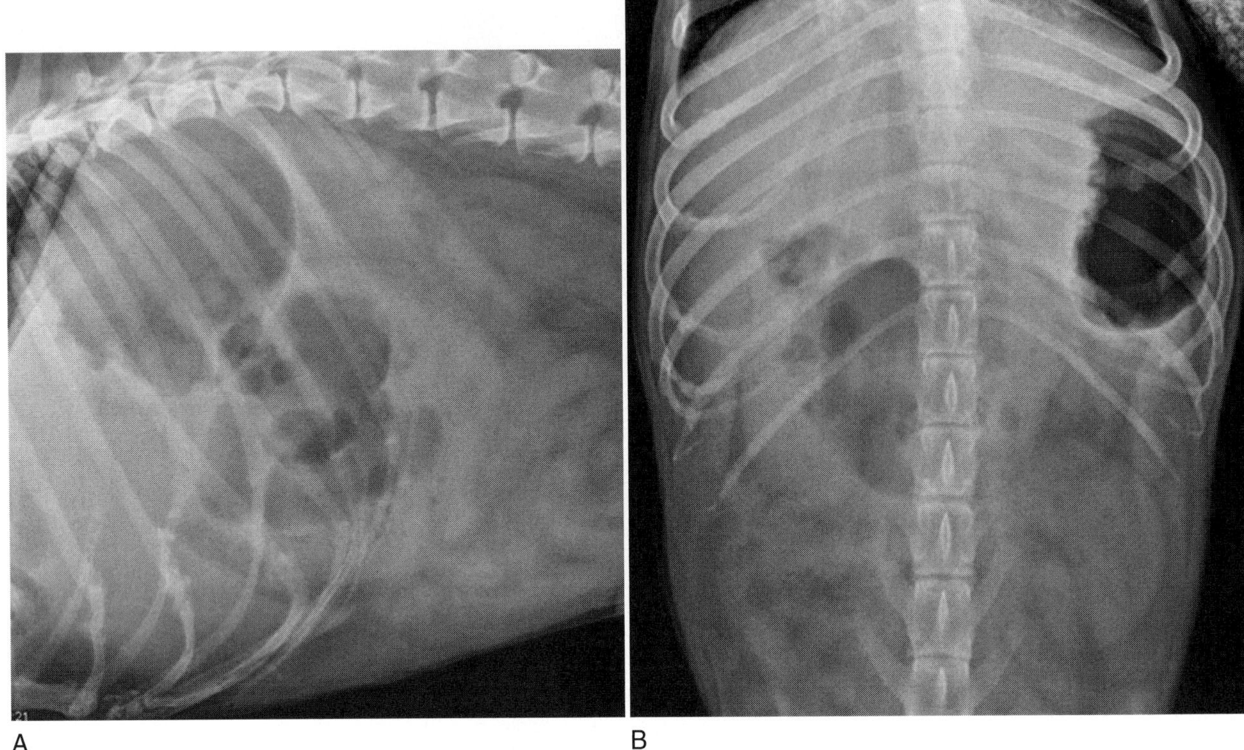

Fig. 46-33 Lateral (A) and ventrodorsal (B) radiographs of a dog with a large mural neoplasm of the jejunum located just caudal to the pylorus. The tumor has altered the shape of the lumen, which is now dilated and quite irregular. An intraabdominal abscess could have a similar appearance.

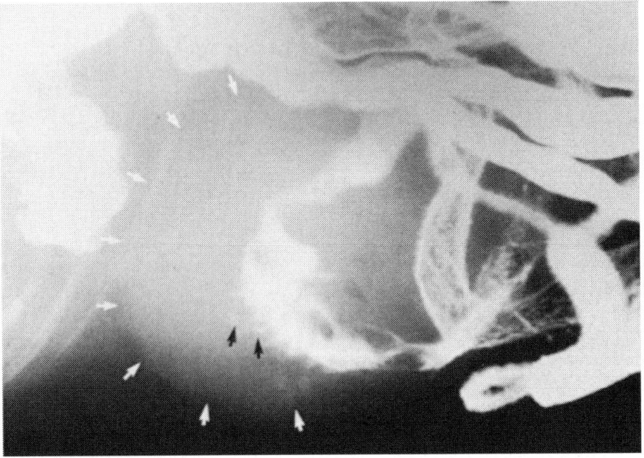

Fig. 46-34 Adenocarcinoma of the jejunum during a barium upper gastrointestinal tract study. Radiographic signs include soft tissue mass *(white arrows)*, mild focal enlargement of bowel lumen, irregular contour of mucosa, and extravasation of a small amount of contrast into the mass *(black arrows)*.

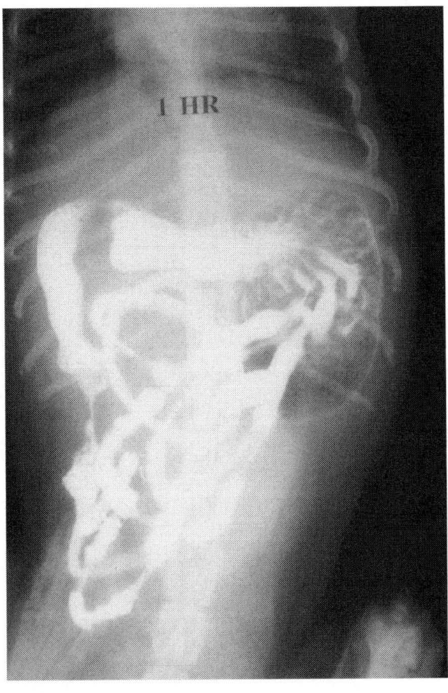

Fig. 46-35 Ventrodorsal view at 1 hour after barium administration in a dog with hematochezia and melena. Concentric luminal narrowing and an irregular mucosal pattern are present in the descending duodenum. This has been termed the "apple core" sign and is highly suggestive of a malignant mural mass.

creates a thin line of opacity, imparting an enhanced contrast effect. Differential diagnosis for this type of diffuse mineralization should include other causes of hypercalcemia, including severe primary renal disease.

Pneumatosis intestinalis and pneumatosis coli both refer to the presence of air in the intestinal wall.[110] Numerous underlying causes can lead to this gas accumulation, including necrotizing enterocolitis, ischemic necrosis caused by volvulus, trauma, and bacterial origin in immunocompromised patients. Pneumatosis intestinalis in small animals has not been reported; however, two patients with pneumatosis coli have been described, and the author has seen a dog with pneumatosis coli that occurred after numerous enemas.[111,112]

REFERENCES

1. Armbrust LJ, Biller DS, Hoskinson JJ: Case examples demonstrating the clinical utility of obtaining both right and left lateral abdominal radiographs in small animals, *J Am Anim Hosp Assoc* 36:531, 2000.
2. Armbrust LJ, Biller DS, Hoskinson JJ: Compression radiography: an old technique revisited, *J Am Anim Hosp Assoc* 36:537, 2000.
3. Root CR: Interpretation of abdominal survey radiographs, *Vet Clin North Am* 4:763, 1974.
4. Owens JM, Biery DN: *Radiographic interpretation for the small animal clinician,* ed 2, Baltimore, 1999, Williams & Wilkins.
5. Graham JP, Lord PF, Harrison JM: Quantitative estimation of intestinal dilation as a predictor of obstruction in the dog, *J Small Anim Pract* 39:521, 1998.
6. Morgan JP: The upper gastrointestinal examination in the cat: normal radiographic appearance using positive-contrast medium, *Vet Radiol* 22:159, 1981.
7. Riedesel EA: Unpublished data, 1996.
8. O'Brien TR: Small intestine. In O'Brien TR, editor: *Radiographic diagnosis of abdominal disorders in the dog and cat,* Philadelphia, 1978, WB Saunders.
9. Penninck DG, Nyland T, Fisher P et al: Ultrasonography of normal canine gastrointestinal tract, *Vet Radiol* 30:272, 1989.
10. Hall JA, Watrous BA: Effect of pharmaceuticals on radiographic appearance of selected examinations of the abdomen and thorax, *Vet Clin North Am Small Anim Pract* 30:349, 2000.
11. Weichselbaum RC, Feeney DA, Hayden DW: Comparison of upper gastrointestinal radiographic findings to histopathologic observations: a retrospective study of 41 dogs and cats with suspected small bowel infiltrative disease, *Vet Radiol Ultrasound* 35:418, 1994.
12. Brawner WR, Bartels JE: Contrast radiography of the digestive tract: indications, techniques and complications, *Vet Clin North Am Small Anim Pract* 13:599, 1983.
13. Gomez JA: The gastrointestinal contrast study, *Vet Clin North Am* 4:805, 1974.
14. Morgan JP, Silverman S: Radiographic evaluation of the digestive tract. In *Techniques of veterinary radiography,* ed 3, Davis, CA, 1982, Veterinary Radiology Associates.
15. Root CR: Contrast radiography of the alimentary tract. In Ticer JW, editor: *Radiographic technique in veterinary practice,* Philadelphia, 1984, WB Saunders.
16. Smelstoys JA, Davis GJ, Learn AE et al: Outcome of and prognostic indicators for dogs and cats with pneumoperitoneum and no history of penetration trauma: 54 cases (1988-2002), *J Am Vet Med Assoc* 225:251, 2004.
17. Foley MJ, Ghahremani GG, Rogers LF: Reappraisal of contrast media used to detect upper gastrointestinal perforations, *Radiology* 144:231, 1982.
18. Ott DJ, Gelfand DW: Gastrointestinal contrast agents: indications, uses, and risks, *JAMA* 249:2380, 1983.
19. Seltzer SE, Jones B, McLaughlin GC: Proper choice of contrast agents in emergency gastrointestinal radiology, *Crit Rev Diagn Imaging* 12:79, 1979.
20. Allan GS, Rendano VT, Quick CB et al: Gastrografin as a gastrointestinal contrast medium in the cat, *Vet Radiol* 20:3, 1979.
21. Hsu WH, McNeel SV: Effect of yohimbine on xylazine-induced prolongation of gastrointestinal transit in dogs, *J Am Vet Med Assoc* 183:297, 1983.
22. Zontine WJ: Effect of chemical restraint drugs on the passage of barium sulfate through the stomach and duodenum of dogs, *J Am Vet Med Assoc* 162:878, 1973.
23. Hogan PM, Aronson E: Effect of sedation on transit time of feline gastrointestinal contrast studies, *Vet Radiol* 29:85, 1988.
24. Kerr LV, Koblik PD: Contrast radiography. In Morgan R, editor: *Handbook of small animal practice,* New York, 1988, Churchill Livingstone.
25. Farrow CS, Green R, Shively M: *Radiology of the cat,* St Louis, 1994, Mosby–Year Book.
26. Ticer JW: The abdomen. In Ticer JW, editor: *Radiographic technique in veterinary practice,* Philadelphia, 1984, WB Saunders.
27. Root CR, Morgan JP: Contrast radiography of the upper gastrointestinal tract in the dog: a comparison of micropulverized barium, *J Small Anim Pract* 10:279, 1969.
28. Agut A, Sanchez-Valverde MA, Lasaosa JM et al: Use of Iohexol as a gastrointestinal contrast medium in the dog, *Vet Radiol Ultrasound* 34:71, 1993.
29. Agut A, Sanchez-Valverde ME, Torrecillas FE et al: Iohexol as a gastrointestinal contrast medium in the cat, *Vet Radiol Ultrasound* 35:164, 1993.
30. Williams J, Biller DS, Myer CW et al: Use of iohexol as a gastrointestinal contrast agent in three dogs, five cats and one bird, *J Am Vet Med Assoc* 202:624, 1993.
31. Williams J, Biller DS, Miyabayashi T et al: Evaluation of Iohexol as a gastrointestinal contrast medium in normal cats, *Vet Radiol Ultrasound* 34:310, 1993.
32. Thrall DE, Leininger JR: Irregular intestinal mucosal margination in the dog: normal or abnormal? *J Small Anim Pract* 17:305, 1976.
33. Robertson ID, Burbridge HM: Pros and cons of barium-impregnated polyethylene spheres in gastrointestinal disease, *Vet Clin North Am Small Anim Pract* 30:449, 2000.
34. Delaney F, O'Brien RT, Waller K: Ultrasound evaluation of small bowel thickness compared to weight in normal dogs, *Vet Radiol Ultrasound* 44:577, 2003.
35. Goggin JM, Biller DS, Debey BM et al: Ultrasonographic measurement of gastrointestinal wall thickness and the ultrasonographic appearance of the ileocolic region in healthy cats, *J Am Anim Hosp Assoc* 36:224, 2000.
36. Lamb CR: Recent developments in diagnostic imaging of the gastrointestinal tract of the dog and cat, *Vet Clin North Am Small Anim Pract* 29:307, 1999.
37. Rault DN, Besso JG, Boulouha L et al: Significance of a common extended mucosal interface observed in transverse small intestine sonograms, *Vet Radiol Ultrasound* 45:177, 2004.
38. Etue SM, Pennick DG, Labatto MA et al: Ultrasonography of the normal feline pancreas and associated anatomic landmarks: a prospective study of 20 cats, *Vet Radiol Ultrasound* 42:330, 2001.
39. An Y, Lee H, Chang D et al: Application of pulsed Doppler ultrasound for the evaluation of small intestinal motility in dogs, *J Vet Sci* 1:71, 2001.

40. Pugh CR: Ultrasonographic examination of the abdominal lymph nodes in the dog, *Vet Radiol Ultrasound* 35:110, 1994.
41. Luttgen PJ, Whitney MS, Wolf AM et al: Heinz body hemolytic anemia associated with high plasma zinc concentration in a dog, *J Am Vet Med Assoc* 197:1347, 1990.
42. Lamb DR, Hansson K: Radiological identification on nonopaque intestinal foreign bodies, *Vet Radiol Ultrasound* 35:87, 1994.
43. Kleine LJ: The role of radiography in the diagnosis of intestinal obstruction in dogs and cats, *Compend Contin Educ Vet Pract* 1:44, 1979.
44. Tidwell AS, Penninck DG: Ultrasonography of gastrointestinal foreign bodies, *Vet Radiol Ultrasound* 33:160, 1992.
45. Evans KL, Smeak DD, Biller DS: Gastrointestinal linear foreign bodies in 32 dogs: a retrospective evaluation and feline comparison, *J Am Anim Hosp Assoc* 30:445, 1994.
46. Felts JF, Fox PR, Burk RL: Thread and sewing needles as gastrointestinal foreign bodies in the cat: a review of 64 cases, *J Am Vet Med Assoc* 184:56, 1984.
47. Basher AW, Fowler JD: Conservative versus surgical management of gastrointestinal linear foreign bodies in the cat, *Vet Surg* 16:135, 1987.
48. Hoffmann, KL: Sonographic signs of gastroduodenal linear foreign body in 3 dogs, *Vet Radiol Ultrasound* 44:466, 2003.
49. Lewis DD, Ellison GW: Intussusception in dogs and cats, *Compend Contin Educ* 9:523, 1987.
50. Penninck DG, Nyland TG, Kerr LY et al: Ultrasonographic evaluation of gastrointestinal diseases in small animals, *Vet Radiol* 31:134, 1990.
51. Lamb CR, Mantis P: Ultrasonographic features of intestinal intussusception in 10 dogs, *J Small Anim Pract* 39:437, 1998.
52. Patsikas MN, Jakovljevic S, Moustardas et al: Ultrasonographic signs of intestinal intussusception associated with acute enteritis or gastroenteritis in 19 young dogs, *J Am Anim Hosp Assoc* 39:57, 2003.
53. Farrow CS: Radiographic appearance of canine parvovirus enteritis, *J Am Vet Med Assoc* 180:43, 1982.
54. Nemzek JA, Walshaw R, Hauptman JG: Mesenteric volvulus in the dog: a retrospective study, *J Am Anim Hosp Assoc* 29:357, 1993.
55. Junius G, Appeldoorn AM, Schrauwen E: Mesenteric volvulus in the dog: a retrospective study of 12 cases, *J Small Anim Pract* 45:104, 2004.
56. Westermarck E, Rinaila-Parnanen E: Mesenteric torsion in dogs with chronic pancreatic insufficiency: 21 cases (1978-1987), *J Am Vet Med Assoc* 195:1404, 1989.
57. Wallack ST, Hornof WJ, Herrgesell EJ: Ultrasonographic diagnosis-small bowel infarction in a cat, *Vet Radiol Ultrasound* 44:81, 2003.
58. Arrick RH, Kleine LJ: Intestinal pseudoobstruction in a dog, *J Am Vet Med Assoc* 172:1201, 1978.
59. Moore R, Carpenter J: Intestinal sclerosis with pseudo-obstruction in three dogs, *J Am Vet Med Assoc* 184:830, 1984.
60. Lamb WA, France MP: Chronic intestinal pseudo-obstruction in a dog, *Aust Vet J* 71:84, 1994.
61. Eastwood JM, McInnes EF, White RN et al: Cecal impaction and chronic intestinal pseudo-obstruction in dog, *J Am Vet Med Assoc* 52:43, 2005.
62. Longshore RC, O'Brien DP, Johnson GC et al: Dysautonomia in dogs: a retrospective study, *J Vet Intern Med* 10:103, 1996.
63. Detweiler DA, Biller DS, Hoskinson JJ et al: Radiographic findings of canine dysautonomia in twenty-four dogs, *Vet Radiol Ultrasound* 42:108, 2001.
64. O'Brien DP, Johnson GC: Dysautonomia and autonomic neuropathies, *Vet Clin North Am Small Anim Pract* 32:251, 2002.
65. Jergens AE: Inflammatory bowel disease: current perspectives, *Vet Clin North Am Small Anim Pract* 29:501, 1999.
66. Rudorf H, van Schaik G, O'Brien RT et al: Ultrasonographic evaluation of the thickness of the small intestinal wall in dogs with inflammatory bowel disease, *J Small Anim Pract* 46:322, 2005.
67. O'Brien TR: Liver, spleen and pancreas. In O'Brien TR, editor: *Radiographic diagnosis of abdominal disorders in the dog and cat,* Philadelphia, 1978, WB Saunders.
68. Moon ML, Billar DS, Armbrust LJ: Ultrasonographic appearance and etiology of corrugated small intestine, *Vet Radiol Ultrasound* 44:199, 2003.
69. Boysen SF, Tidwell AS, Pennick DG: Ultrasonographic findings in dogs and cats with gastrointestinal perforation, *Vet Radiol Ultrasound* 44:556, 2003.
70. Malik R, Hunt GB, Bellenger CR et al: Intra-abdominal cryptococcosis in two dogs, *J Small Anim Pract* 40:387, 1999.
71. Helman RG, Oliver J III: Pythiosis of the digestive tract in dogs from Oklahoma, *J Am Anim Hosp Assoc* 35:111, 1999.
72. Miller RI: Gastrointestinal phycomycosis, *J Am Vet Med Assoc* 186:473, 1985.
73. Graham JP, Newell SM, Roberts GD et al: Ultrasonographic features of canine gastrointestinal pythiosis, *Vet Radiol Ultrasound* 41:273, 2000.
74. Brodey RS: Alimentary tract neoplasms in the cat: a clinicopathologic survey of 46 cases, *Am J Vet Res* 27:74, 1966.
75. Patniak AK, Liu S-K, Jonhson GF: Feline intestinal adenocarcinoma, *Vet Pathol* 13:1, 1976.
76. Patniak AK, Hurvitz AI, Johnson GF: Canine gastrointestinal neoplasms, *Vet Pathol* 14:547, 1977.
77. Patniak AK, Hurvitz AI, Johnson GF: Canine intestinal adenocarcinoma and carcinoid, *Vet Pathol* 17:149, 1980.
78. Feeney DA, Klausner JS, Johnston GR: Chronic bowel obstruction caused by primary intestinal neoplasia: a report of five cases, *J Am Anim Hosp Assoc* 18:67, 1982.
79. Gibbs C, Pearson H: Localized tumors of the canine small intestine: a report of twenty cases, *J Small Anim Pract* 27:506, 1986.
80. Bruecker KA, Withrow SJ: Intestinal leiomyosarcomas in six dogs, *J Am Anim Hosp Assoc* 24:281, 1988.
81. Kosovsky JE, Matthiesen DT, Patnaik AK: Small intestinal adenocarcinoma in cats: 32 cases (1978-1985), *J Am Vet Med Assoc* 192:233, 1988.
82. Couto CG, Rutgers HC, Sherding RG et al: Gastrointestinal lymphoma in 20 dogs, *J Vet Intern Med* 3:73, 1989.
83. Pardo AD, Adams WH, McCracken MD et al: Primary jejunal osteosarcoma associated with a surgical sponge in a dog, *J Am Vet Med Assoc* 196:935, 1990.
84. Bortnowski HB, Rosenthal RC: Gastrointestinal mast cell tumors and eosinophilia in two cats, *J Am Anim Hosp Assoc* 28:271, 1992.
85. Crawshaw J, Berg J, Sardinas JC et al: Prognosis for dogs with nonlymphomatous, small intestinal tumors treated by surgical excision, *J Am Anim Hosp Assoc* 34:451, 1998.
86. Takahashi T, Kadosawa T, Nagase M et al: Visceral mast cell tumors in dogs: 10 cases (1982-1997), *J Am Vet Med Assoc* 216:222, 2000.
87. Theilen GH, Madewell BR: Tumors of the digestive tract. In Theilen GH, Madewell BR, editors: *Veterinary cancer medicine,* Philadelphia, 1979, Lea & Febiger.

88. MacDonald JM, Mullen HS, Moroff SD: Adenomatous polyps of the duodenum in cats: 18 cases (1985-1990), *J Am Vet Med Assoc* 202:647, 1993.
89. Happe RP, van der Gaag I, Lamers CBHW et al: Zollinger-Ellison syndrome in three dogs, *Vet Pathol* 17:177, 1980.
90. Moreland KJ: Ulcer disease of the upper gastrointestinal tract in small animals: pathophysiology, diagnosis, and management, *Compend Contin Educ Vet Pract* 10:1265, 1988.
91. Murray M, McKeating FJ, Baker GJ et al: Peptic ulceration in the dog: a clinico-pathological study, *Vet Rec* 91:441, 1971.
92. Zontine WJ, Meierhenry ER, Hicks RF: Perforated duodenal ulcer associated with mastocytoma in a dog: a case report, *J Am Vet Radiol Soc* 18:162, 1977.
93. Middleton DJ, Watson ADJ, Culvenor JE: Duodenal ulceration associated with gastrin-secreting pancreatic tumor in a cat, *J Am Vet Med Assoc* 183:461, 1983.
94. Burrows CF: Canine hemorrhagic gastroenteritis, *J Am Anim Hosp Assoc* 13:451, 1977.
95. Hayden DW, Van Kruiningen HJ: Lymphocytic-plasmacytic enteritis in German shepherd dogs, *J Am Anim Hosp Assoc* 18:89, 1982.
96. Vest B, Margulis AR: Experimental infarction of small bowel in dogs, *AJR* 92:1080, 1964.
97. Hendirk M: A spectrum of hypereosinophilic syndromes exemplified by six cats with eosinophilic enteritis, *Vet Pathol* 18:1888, 1981.
98. Tams TR: Chronic feline inflammatory bowel disorders: II. Feline eosinophilic enteritis and lymphosarcoma, *Compend Contin Educ Vet Pract* 8:464, 1986.
99. Penninck D, Smyers B, Webster CRL et al: Diagnostic value of ultrasonography in differentiating enteritis from intestinal neoplasia in dogs, *Vet Radiol Ultrasound* 44:570, 2003.
100. Grooters AM, Biller DS, Ward H et al: Ultrasonographic appearance of feline alimentary lymphoma, *Vet Radiol* Ultrasound 35:468, 1994.
101. Penninck DG, Moore AS, Tidwell AS et al: Ultrasonography of alimentary lymphosarcoma in the cat, *Vet Radiol Ultrasound* 35:299, 1994.
102. Rivers BJ, Walter PA, Feeney DA et al: Ultrasonographic features of intestinal adenocarcinoma in five cats, *Vet Radiol Ultrasound* 38:300, 1997.
103. Myers NC, Penninck DG: Ultrasonographic diagnosis of gastrointestinal smooth muscle tumors in the dog, *Vet Radiol Ultrasound* 35:391, 1994.
104. Paoloni MC, Pennick DG, Moore AS: Ultrasonographic and clinicopathologic findings in 21 dogs with intestinal adenocarcinoma, *Vet Radiol Ultrasound* 43:562, 2002.
105. Crystal MA, Penninck DG, Matz ME et al: Use of ultrasound-guided fine-needle aspiration biopsy and automated core biopsy for the diagnosis for gastrointestinal disease in small animals, *Vet Radiol Ultrasound* 34:438, 1993.
106. Gunther R, Felice LJ, Nelson RK et al: Toxicity of a vitamin D_3 rodenticide to dogs, *J Am Vet Med Assoc* 193:211, 1988.
107. Morita T, Awakura T, Shimada A et al: Vitamin D toxicosis in cats: natural outbreak and experimental study, *J Vet Med Sci* 57:831, 1995.
108. Fan TM, Simpson KW, Trasti S et al: Calcipotriol toxicity in a dog, *J Small Anim Pract* 39:581, 1998.
109. Hare WR, Dobbs CE, Slaymen SA et al: Calcipotriene poisoning in dogs, *Vet Med* 95:770, 2000.
110. Pear BL: Pneumatosis intestinalis: a review, *Radiology* 207:13, 1998.
111. Anderson GR, Geary JC: Pneumatosis coli (interstitial emphysema of colon): a case report, *J Am Anim Hosp Assoc* 9:352, 1973.
112. Morris EL: Pneumatosis coli in a dog, *Vet Radiol Ultrasound* 33:154, 1992.

ELECTRONIC RESOURCES evolve

Additional information related to the content in Chapter 46 can be found on the companion Web site at evolve http://evolve.elsevier.com/Thrall/vetrad/.

- Key Points
- Chapter Quiz
- Case Study 46-1

CHAPTER • 47
Large Bowel

Tobias Schwarz
Darryl N. Biery

IMAGING OPTIONS FOR LARGE BOWEL DISEASE

Survey and contrast radiographic procedures have been used to assess many colonic conditions.[1-3] After a survey radiographic examination, however, endoscopy (colonoscopy) now has largely replaced radiographic contrast studies of the colon. Most colonic diseases are diagnosed by endoscopy, especially when a flexible endoscope enables visualization of the transverse colon, ascending colon, and cecum with the additional advantage of obtaining aspirates and biopsies if needed.[4]

Ultrasound has become a sensitive and practical imaging modality that is usually less time consuming than many radiographic contrast studies of the colon; it also provides additional and complementary information to the clinical, endoscopic, and survey radiographic findings.[5] Although air and feces in the bowel are limiting factors for ultrasound studies, ultrasound examination allows assessment of near-field bowel wall thickness and symmetry, mural and extramural bowel masses, the regional lymph nodes, intussusceptions, and other abdominal viscera. Transabdominal needle aspiration and biopsies of colonic masses can also be obtained with ultrasound-guided techniques.[6,7] In addition, new techniques of endoscopic sonography are now beginning to be used for detailed evaluation of mural and extramural colonic structures.

Less commonly used imaging techniques for colonic disease include rectocolonic lymphangiography, mesenteric angiography, and colonic transit scintigraphy. These techniques enable assessment of anatomic or functional abnormalities but require specialized equipment and expertise.[8-10]

NORMAL RADIOGRAPHIC ANATOMY

The large bowel of the dog and cat is composed of the cecum, colon, rectum, and anal canal (Fig. 47-1). The cecum, a diverticulum of the proximal colon, has different anatomic and radiographic appearances in the dog and the cat (Fig. 47-2).[1] The canine cecum is semicircular (corkscrew or C-shaped) and compartmentalized with a cecocolic junction and normally contains some intraluminal gas. The intraluminal gas and characteristic shape enable easy recognition of the cecum in the right mid-abdomen on most survey radiographs. The feline cecum, however, is usually not visible on survey radiographs. It is a short, cone-like diverticulum of the colon with no distinct cecocolic junction and no compartmentalization; it rarely contains gas.

The colon of the dog and the cat, the longest segment of the large bowel, is a thin-walled distensible tube that is divided into ascending, transverse, and descending parts. These divisions are easily recognized on survey abdominal radiographs based on their shape, size, and location. The distal ileum enters the ascending colon from a medial direction by way of the ileocecal sphincter. This circular sphincter is usually not visible on survey radiographs, but it is usually easy to identify as a filling defect when barium is present in the lumen of the colon adjacent to the sphincter. The colon has a shape similar to that of a question mark or a shepherd's crook (see Fig. 47-1). The junction between the ascending and transverse colon is the right colic flexure, and the junction between the transverse and descending colon is the left colic flexure. The ascending colon and right colic flexure are located to the right of midline. The transverse colon, which passes from right to left, lies cranial to the root of the mesentery. The left colic flexure and proximal descending colon are located to the left of midline. The distal descending colon courses to the midline and enters the pelvic canal to become the rectum. The rectum is the terminal portion of the colon, beginning at the pelvic inlet and ending at the anal canal.

An understanding of the anatomic relation of the large bowel to other viscera is extremely important for the radiographic recognition of diseases of the large bowel and adjacent organs (Fig. 47-3). The ascending colon lies adjacent to the descending duodenum, right lobe of the pancreas, right kidney, mesentery, and small bowel. The transverse colon lies adjacent to the greater curvature of the stomach, left lobe of the pancreas, liver, small intestine, and root of the mesentery. The proximal descending colon lies in close proximity to the left kidney and to the ureter, spleen, and small bowel. The mid-portion of the descending colon lies adjacent to the small bowel, urinary bladder, and uterus. Because it is less fixed, the mid-portion of the descending colon has a variety of normal positions in the caudal left abdomen. In some dogs the descending colon is positioned along or slightly right to the median axis of the body. Such normal variations are caused by various amounts of ingesta within the bowel, intraabdominal fat, and urinary bladder distention (see Fig. 47-1). Some dogs appear to have an excess of length of colon. This finding, called redundant colon, is considered a variant of normal and is not clinically significant.[1,3,11]

The distal portions of the descending colon and rectum are also closely associated with the urethra, the medial iliac and sacral lymph nodes, the prostate or uterus and vagina, and the pelvic diaphragm.

RADIOGRAPHIC TECHNIQUES OF LARGE BOWEL EVALUATION

Survey Radiography

Because feces and gas produce contrasting radiographic opacities and are usually present in the large bowel, a part or the

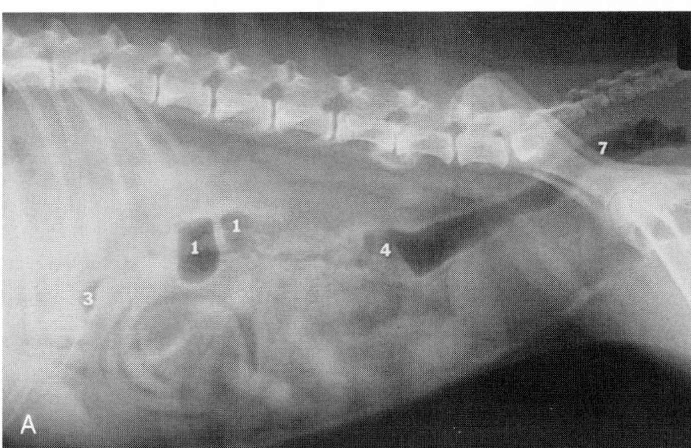

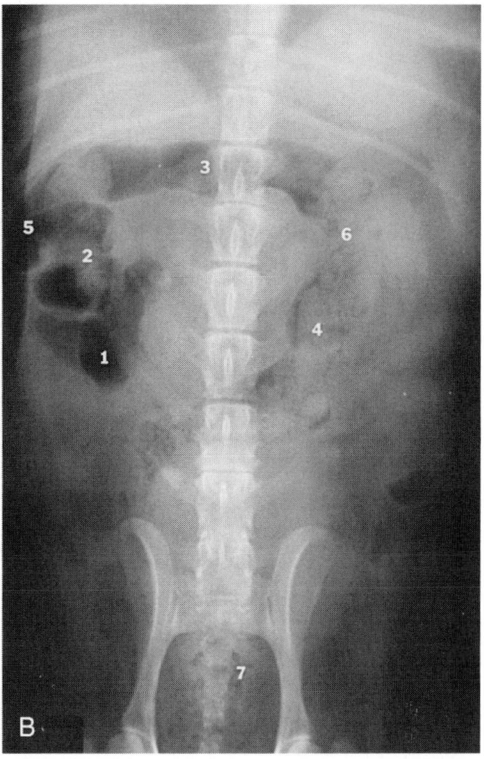

Fig. 47-1 Survey lateral (A) and ventrodorsal (B) radiographs of a normal canine abdomen. The large bowel is divided into the cecum *(1)*, ascending colon *(2)*, transverse colon *(3)*, descending colon *(4)*, right colic flexure *(5)*, left colic flexure *(6)*, rectum *(7)*, and anal canal. Note the admixture of gas and feces in the cecum, colon, and rectum. In **B,** the descending colon is displaced toward the right by a normally distended urinary bladder.

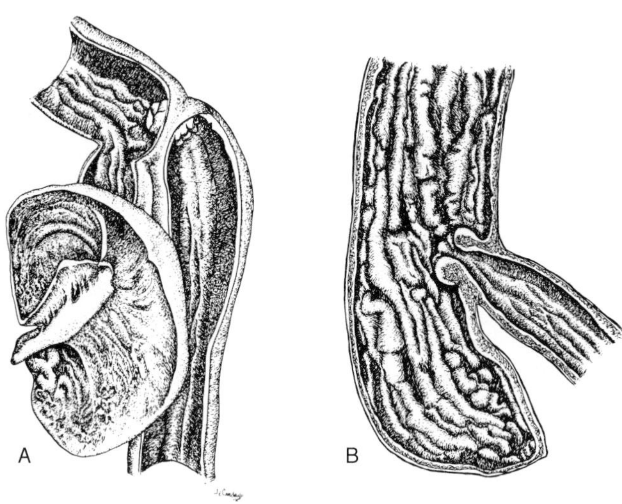

Fig. 47-2 The cecum of the dog (A) and of the cat (B) are anatomically and radiographically different. The canine cecum is semicircular and compartmentalized and normally contains some gas. The feline cecum, however, is a short, conelike structure with no compartmentalization; it rarely contains gas. (Reprinted from O'Brien TR: *Radiographic diagnosis of abdominal disorders in the dog and cat,* Davis, CA, 1981, Covell Park Veterinary, 1981.)

entire large bowel is identifiable on survey radiographs of the abdomen. The different body positions used for survey radiography distribute intraluminal gas to different parts of the large bowel, largely because of gravity. Thus, gas is usually present in the more nondependent portions of the colon. Normal large bowel content usually has a characteristic pattern of fine and evenly distributed gas bubbles, which is helpful in differentiating the colon from small intestinal loops and abnormal conditions of the large bowel. When present, mineral- or metal-opaque foreign bodies (e.g., pieces of bone, safety pin, wire) are easily recognized on survey radiographs. Neither the wall thickness nor the mucosal pattern of the large bowel can be evaluated from survey radiographs.

When the large bowel is evaluated radiographically, the entire abdomen and pelvic area must be included on two orthogonal radiographic views. The urinary bladder should be empty. Rectal examination, vigorous abdominal palpation, aerophagia from restraint and struggling, and enemas before survey radiography may increase the amount of gas or fluid present within the colon and in other parts of the gastrointestinal tract. Although an abnormality in position, size, or shape of the large bowel may be seen on survey radiographs, it may not be a significant finding, and a diagnosis may not be possible.

Compression Radiography

Compression radiography of the abdomen is a simple technique that may help further delineate the presence of a lesion.

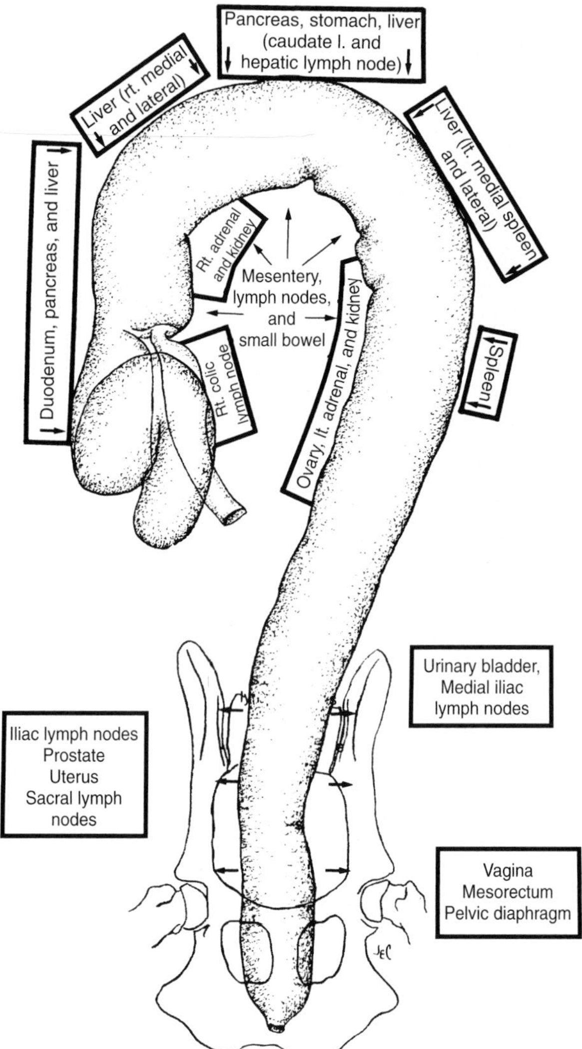

Fig. 47-3 Viscera adjacent to the large bowel, on a ventrodorsal radiographic view, may cause a change in position of a portion of the colon. This change in position may be indicative of disease or a variant of normal, depending on the cause of the deviation (e.g., enlarged bladder versus enlarged medial iliac lymph nodes). *Arrows,* Usual direction of large bowel position displacement when an organ enlarges (see Fig. 47-10). (Reprinted from O'Brien TR: *Radiographic diagnosis of abdominal disorders in the dog and cat,* Davis, CA, 1981, Covell Park Veterinary.)

When the abdomen is compressed with a wooden or plastic spoon or paddle, bowel or masses adjacent to the large intestine are displaced or compressed, which enhances radiographic detail (Fig. 47-4). More definitive radiographic evaluation of the large bowel usually requires a contrast study with barium sulfate suspension (barium enema), air (pneumocolon), or a combination of barium sulfate suspension and air (double-contrast study).

Barium Enema

After survey radiographs, the barium enema is the most common radiographic study for examination of the large bowel. The radiographic findings (barium enema or double-contrast study) in large bowel disease include (1) irregularity of the barium/–mucosa interface, (2) spasm of the bowel lumen, (3) partial or complete occlusion of the bowel lumen, (4) outpouching of the bowel wall from a hernia or diverticulum, (5) displacement of bowel, and (6) perforation with peritonitis. Similar to the alterations seen on survey radiographs, the contrast study findings are usually nonspecific. Although spasm and mucosal irregularity are commonly associated with severe local inflammation, other causes include toxicity, reflex mechanism, and idiopathic factors. Bowel inflammation (e.g., typhlitis and colitis) may occur with generalized or regional areas of bowel wall thickening from edema and small ulcerations. The acute stages of bowel inflammation frequently have no abnormal radiographic findings.

A barium enema currently is most indicated when (1) narrowing of the lumen prevents passage of an endoscope, (2) limitations of the endoscope prevent examination of all the colon and cecum, and (3) a mural or extramural lesion is suspected, and the mucosa is found to be normal on endoscopic examination.[4] Survey radiographs should be made as a first diagnostic step and also before the contrast study to determine correct radiographic exposure techniques and ascertain adequate patient preparation for the contrast study. For a high-quality diagnostic study, the colon should be thoroughly cleansed before the contrast study. This is best done by withholding food for 24 to 36 hours, and by cleansing the colon with both an orally administered cathartic and warm water enemas before the procedure. The colonic mucosa and lumen should be free of fecal material with a clear effluent visible on an enema immediately before the study. Generally, the radiographic technique should be increased by 6 to 8 kVp over the survey technique when barium is used. Although barium enema techniques may vary, barium at room temperature is administered through an inflatable cuffed catheter placed in the distal rectum to prevent the barium from leaking from the colon, and obtain adequate distention of the colon.[1,11-13] General anesthesia is almost always necessary. Micropulverized barium suspension is the contrast medium of choice for obtaining a smooth coating of the mucosal surface. The colon should be slowly filled with barium by a gravity system, preferably with fluoroscopic observation. Because fluoroscopic equipment may not be available and the volume of barium needed to fill the colon is extremely variable, the contrast medium should be given in several small increments until the desired effect is seen radiographically. Usually the barium dosage is 7 to 15 mL per kilogram of body weight. Multiple radiographic views—left lateral; ventrodorsal; right ventral, left dorsal oblique; and left ventral, right dorsal oblique—should be made when the colon is distended with barium and again after evacuation of the barium from the colon. The detection of subtle mucosal lesions may be enhanced by a double-contrast study. In most instances, this is done by removing as much of the barium as possible and inflating the colon with room air through the catheter.

When distended with barium, the normal colon has a smooth contrast medium/mucosa interface and a uniform diameter. After evacuation of the barium, longitudinal mucosal folds are visible. If air is then infused, a double-contrast study is obtained, which provides the most detailed visualization of the mucosal surface.

A variety of radiographic appearances result from adherence of barium to mucus, clumping and flocculation of barium, and filling defects of feces that are either within the lumen or attached to the wall. The colon of the dog and the cecum and colon of the cat have lymph follicles in the mucosa, which appear as spicules on a barium enema study, or as pinpoint radiopacities when visualized en face with a double-contrast study. These normal follicles must be differentiated from small ulcers.

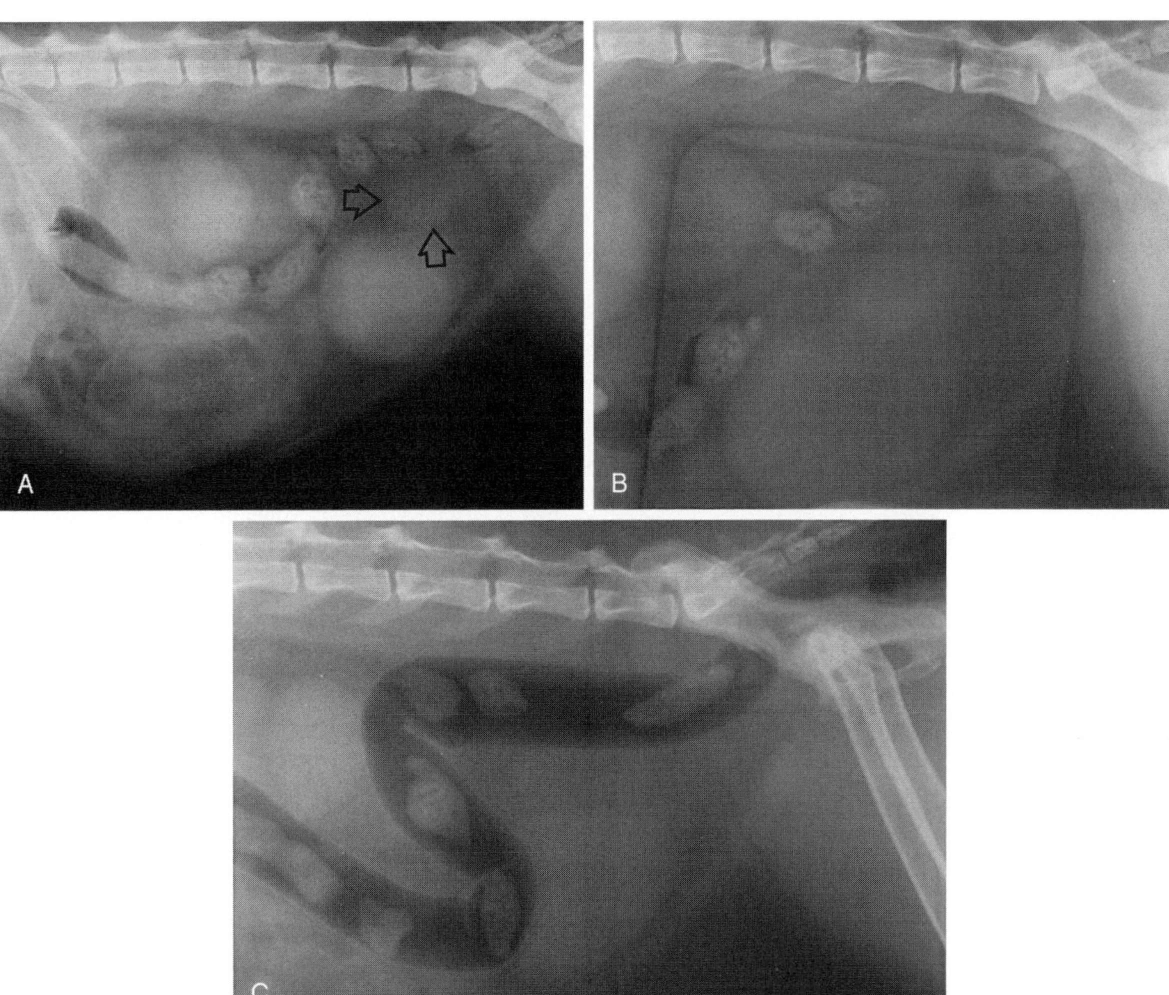

Fig. 47-4 A 5-year-old neutered domestic shorthaired female cat. **A,** Survey radiograph. A soft tissue mass *(arrows)* is interposed between the descending colon and the urinary bladder. At surgery, the mass was found to be a uterine stump pyometra. **B,** Survey lateral recumbent radiograph of the abdomen with a compression paddle applied. The mass appears fixed and separate from the descending colon and urinary bladder. **C,** Survey lateral radiograph of the abdomen after a partial pneumocolon study performed by retrograde introduction of gas. The soft tissue mass (uterine stump pyometra) is visualized as an extramural mass. Feces were not removed before the contrast study was conducted.

The large bowel cannot be properly evaluated after oral administration of contrast medium because large bowel luminal distention is usually inadequate; intraluminal filling defects from feces also occur frequently.

Complete large bowel contrast studies are time consuming and must be done meticulously performed to assess the mucosa, wall, lumen, and adjacent viscera as well as to avoid artifacts, complications, and technical failures, such as contrast medium on the veterinarian, equipment, and patient. Partial large bowel contrast studies, which are less thorough, quicker, and easier, may be performed with the introduction of small amounts of air or barium into the rectum through dose syringe. These studies do not allow visualization of the entire large bowel or of small lesions, such as mucosal irregularities; however, they may enable visualization of large intraluminal lesions and differentiation of the colon from adjacent organs and masses (see Fig. 47-4, C).

Complications Associated with Contrast Studies

Complications related to contrast studies of the colon may occur. The most serious complication is perforation and subsequent peritonitis (Fig. 47-5). Rupture can occur from a cleansing enema, improper selection or use of a barium enema catheter, and overdistention of weakened or diseased bowel, or after a biopsy.[14-16] If colonic perforation is suspected, a 15% to 20% concentration of nonionic aqueous iodine contrast medium can be substituted for the barium, but mucosal detail will be significantly diminished.[12]

A common inconsequential complication is retrograde filling of the distal small bowel; such reflux may obscure visualization of the colon. This complication has been reported in approximately one third of dogs and may occur without overdistention of the colon.[11] Spasm, which is usually transient, may also occur when the contrast medium is cold, when narcotic premedications are used, or when the wall is irritated by the catheter (Fig. 47-6).

RADIOGRAPHIC FINDINGS IN LARGE BOWEL DISEASE

Disease involving or adjacent to the large bowel may produce radiographic alterations in size, shape, location, and radiopacity.[1-4] Although function cannot be evaluated radiographically, the quantity or location of feces may suggest impaired motility. A colon filled with homogeneous soft tissue opaque material without the finely dispersed gas pattern typical for formed feces is suggestive of diarrhea. A soft tissue mass or an intussusception also appears as a homogeneous soft tissue radiopacity. A curved gas/soft tissue interface of a homogeneous luminal soft tissue opacity in the large bowel can sometimes be seen at the edge of an intussusception and is sometimes referred to as a meniscus sign (Fig. 47-7).[17] Most radiographic findings in large bowel disease are not pathognomonic. Many different diseases have similar radiographic findings, and any particular disease may have a spectrum of different appearances. In addition, parasitic, dietary, and other inflammatory causes of large bowel disease commonly have no detectable radiographic abnormality.

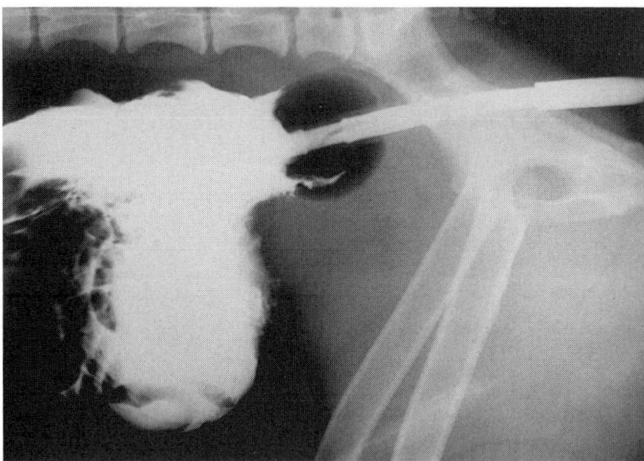

Fig. 47-5 Lateral radiograph of a 5-year-old male Irish Setter in which perforation of the colon occurred during a barium enema study. This complication may occur from improper catheter type, improper catheter use, or disease of the colon. The dog had a 4-month history of weight loss and straining to defecate. At necropsy, chronic prostatitis with adhesions to the colon and a localized peritonitis were evident.

In the normal large bowel, the colon contains most of the feces, with small amounts of or no feces in the rectum (see Fig. 47-1). The diameter of the normal colon varies with the amount of feces present and individual defecation habits. As a rule of thumb, the diameter of the normal colon should be less than the length of the body of L7.[1]

Colonic impaction is characterized radiographically by accumulation of the feces that are more radiopaque than normal as a consequence of constipation, obstipation, or megacolon. Chronic impaction can also result in generalized enlargement of the colon.

Localized dilatation of the colon is usually related to impaction or localized diseases such as mechanical obstruction (e.g., ileocolic and cecocolic intussusception, cecal and colic volvulus, strangulation by ruptured duodenocolic ligament), narrowed pelvic canal from fracture, intramural or extramural colonic tumor (Fig. 47-8), stricture, or foreign body.

Generalized enlargement of the colon is commonly referred to as megacolon, a condition caused by mechanical or functional obstruction and characterized by diffuse colonic dilation with ineffective motility. Megacolon may be idiopathic or associated with numerous underlying causes such as (1) chronic constipation and obstipation from nutritional, metabolic, or mechanical causes; (2) feline idiopathic megacolon; (3) spinal anomalies (e.g., cauda equina syndrome, sacrococcygeal agenesis in Manx cats); (4) neuromuscular disorders (e.g., feline dysautonomia, aganglionosis, or Hirschsprung's disease [Fig. 47-9]); (5) metabolic disorders (e.g., hypokalemia, hypothyroidism); (6) surgical ureterocolic diversion techniques; (7) perineal hernia; and (8) anorectal congenital anomalies.[1,3,18-22] Mechanical causes of colonic obstruction include narrowing of the pelvic canal from pelvic malunion fractures, prostatomegaly, lymphadenopathy, colonic masses, and foreign bodies.

Congenital anomalies of the large bowel are rare in the dog and the cat. Anomalies reported include imperforate anus, atresia recti, atresia coli, fistulation, diverticula, duplication of the large bowel and rectum, and a short, straight colon with the cecum in the left hemiabdomen.[1,3,23-29]

The size and shape of the colon may also be altered by numerous chronic inflammatory diseases of the large bowel and adjacent viscera. These inflammatory changes may result in localized or generalized irregularity and ulceration

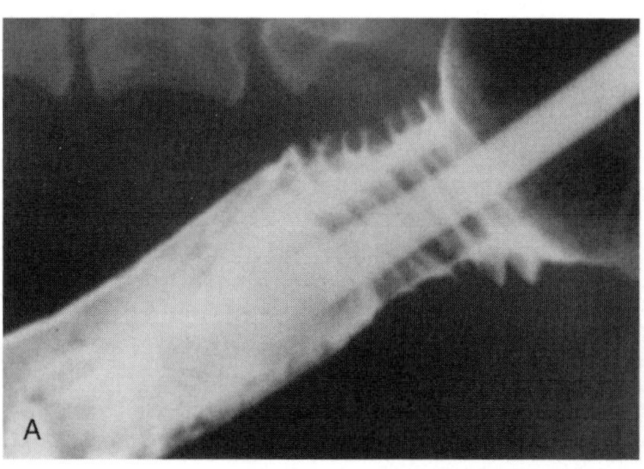

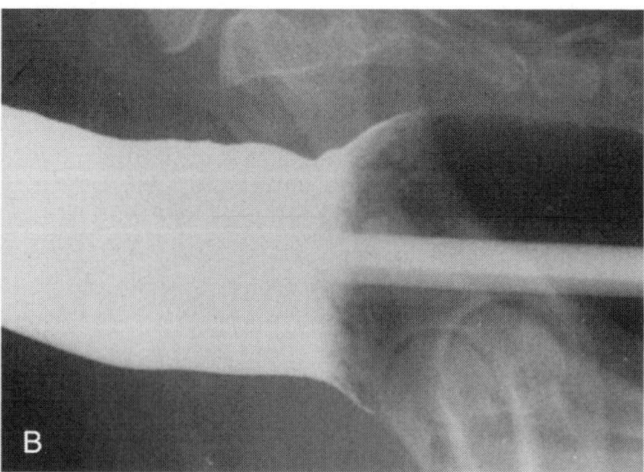

Fig. 47-6 Narrowing and irregularity of the descending colon are present immediately cranial to the air-inflated catheter cuff. This was a spasm **(A)** and was transient based on a subsequent radiograph **(B)** made several minutes later.

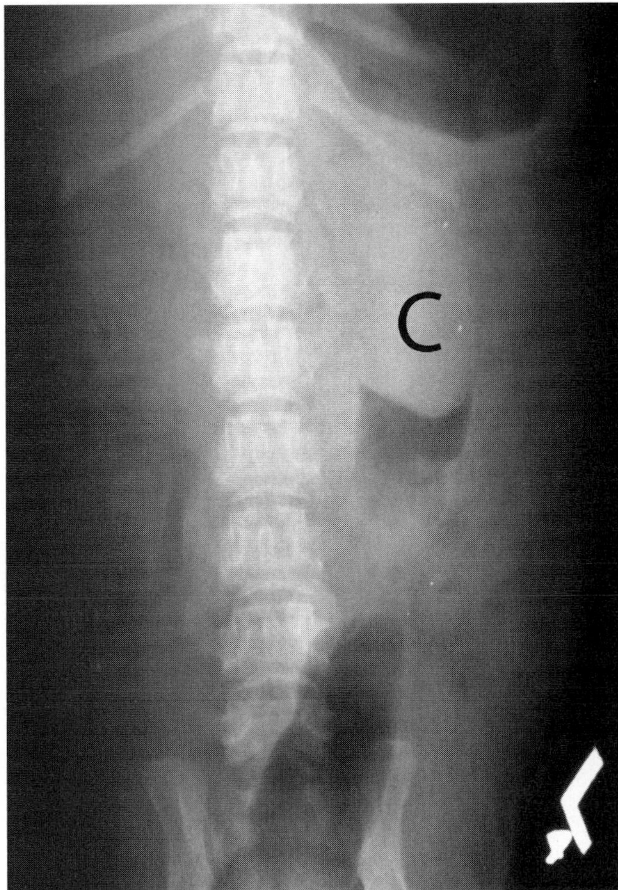

Fig. 47-7 Survey ventrodorsal abdominal radiograph of a 3-month-old Basset Hound with a 1-one day history of vomiting and diarrhea and a palpable abdominal mass. Abdominal detail is poor, but this is typical of a patient of this age. The proximal descending colon *(C)* is distended by homogeneously soft-tissue opaque material with a curved gas interface caudally, sometimes referred to as a meniscus sign. Final diagnosis was colocolic intussusception.

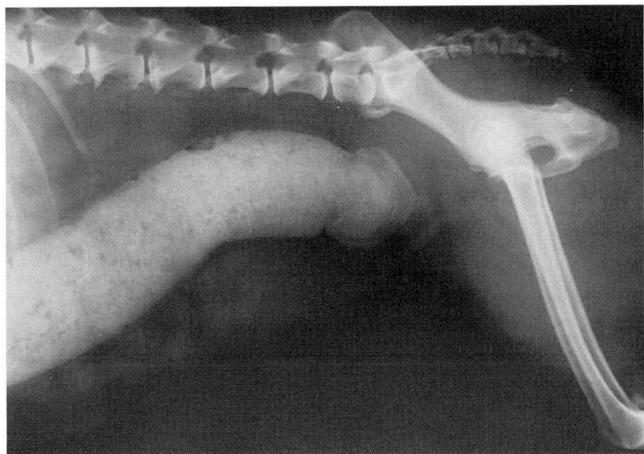

Fig. 47-8 Survey lateral recumbent radiograph of the abdomen of a 9-year-old neutered female, mixed-breed dog with 5 months of progressive difficulty urinating and straining to defecate. The stools were flattened, and a rectal mass was palpable. The mass within the pelvis was a fibroleiomyoma causing partial colonic obstruction and megacolon. Unrelated L7-S1 spondylosis deformans is also present.

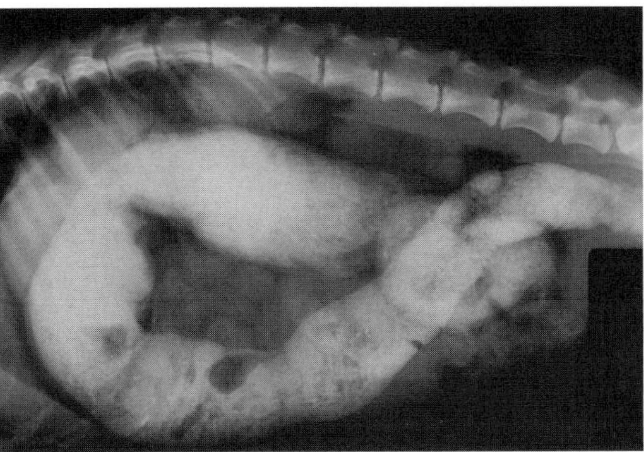

Fig. 47-9 Generalized megacolon is present. This 5-month-old female mixed-breed dog had functional ileus and histologic evidence of Hirschsprung's disease.

of the mucosa with diverticula, adhesions, or shortening of the colon.

Abnormal location of the large bowel is a common radiographic alteration seen with large bowel disease in the dog and cat. Although the normal location of the large bowel varies, mass lesions, particularly those of organs adjacent to the colon, cause displacement of the cecum, colon, or rectum (Fig. 47-10; see also Fig. 47-3). Masses or enlargement of the uterus, prostate, and lymph nodes (mesenteric, para-aortic, and iliac) commonly alter the position and shape of the large bowel.

Many large bowel diseases exhibit radiographic changes in the colon similar to those in other parts of the gastrointestinal tract. These conditions include (1) foreign bodies; (2) obstruction, including ileocolic (Fig. 47-11) and cecocolic intussusception (Fig. 47-12), volvulus, and strangulation; (3) inflammation (Fig. 47-13); (4) stricture (Fig. 47-14); (5) neoplasms (Fig. 47-15); (6) perforation; (7) adhesions; and (8) diverticula or hernia (Fig. 47-16).[30-41]

Differences in the appearance of intraluminal, intramural, and extramural lesions of the large bowel are important to recognize in a contrast study. These classifications regarding site of origin allow differentiation of conditions such as foreign bodies, intussusception, inflammation, and benign or malignant tumors. For example, a lesion that is plaquelike is intramural and arises from the mucosal or submucosal tissues. An extramural mass usually causes extrinsic narrowing of the lumen, displacement of the bowel and adjacent viscera, or both. In most diseases of the large bowel, particularly those that are not extramural, a contrast study is required for detection and for decision making regarding the most probable diagnosis (Fig. 47-17).

A severe form of inflammatory disease in the dog, known as ulcerative colitis, has a spectrum of radiographic findings that consists of mucosal and submucosal ulcers, spasticity, rigidity, and shortening of the colon (see Fig. 47-13).

Narrowing of the large bowel lumen results from spasm or constriction caused by neoplasia, scar tissue, or direct trauma to the bowel wall. Unlike constriction, spasm is transient and frequently is caused by the barium enema technique (see Fig. 47-6). When evaluating a constriction with a barium enema examination, the base and length of the defect, the mucosal surface, and the mural involvement should be assessed (see Fig. 47-14). Most constrictions of the large bowel are produced by neoplasms (usually carcinoma and lymphosarcoma),

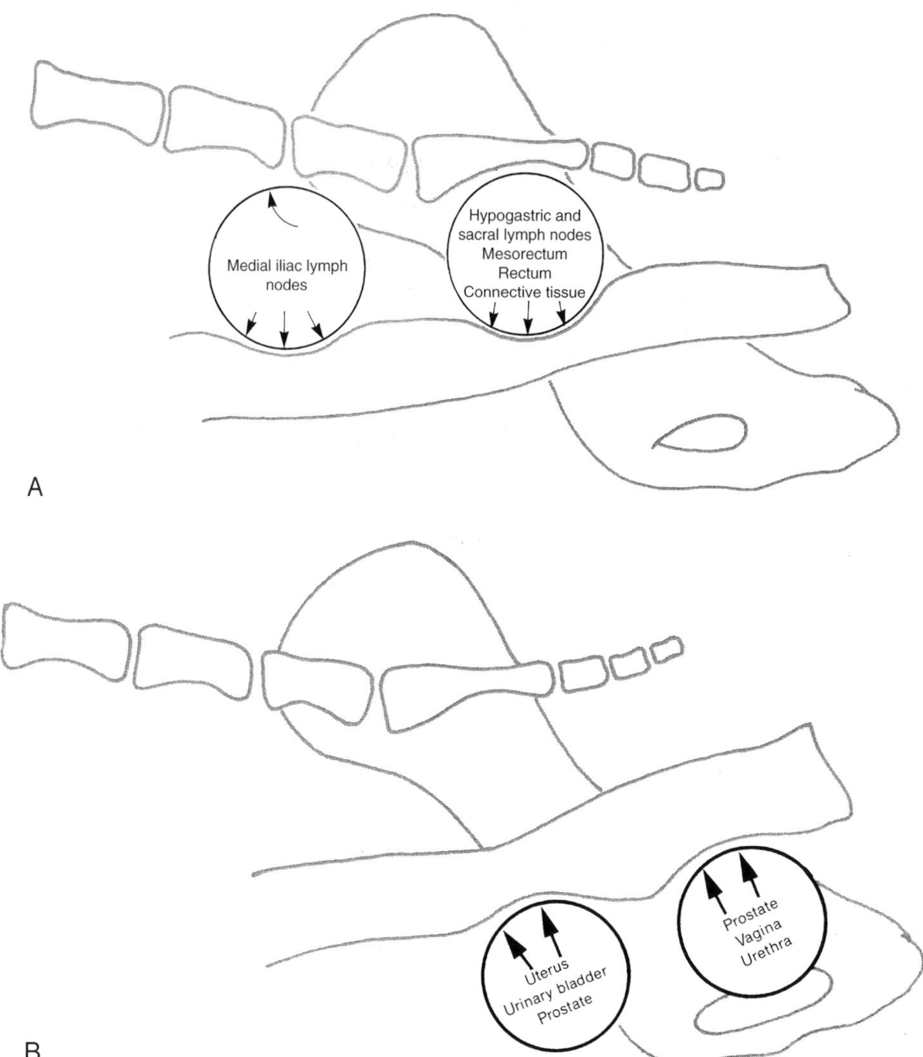

Fig. 47-10 Terminal colon and rectal displacement by adjacent organ enlargement. **A,** Ventral displacement of the terminal colon and rectum commonly results from medial iliac (previously called sublumbar or external iliac lymph nodes) and sacral lymph node enlargement. Although less common, a hematoma, abscess, or tumor may produce similar displacement alterations. **B,** Dorsal displacement of the rectum commonly results from enlargement of the prostate, the uterus, the vagina, or the intrapelvic urinary bladder. (Reprinted from O'Brien TR: *Radiographic diagnosis of abdominal disorders in the dog and cat,* Davis, CA, 1981, Covell Park Veterinary, 1981.)

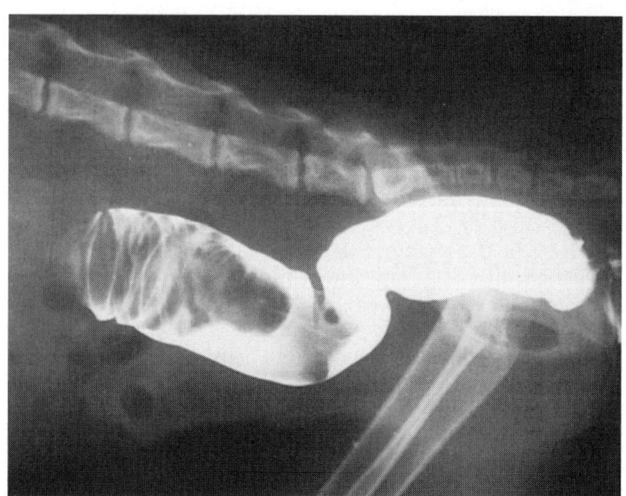

Fig. 47-11 A 4-month-old male Siamese cat with colocolic intussusception. Note the radiolucent filling defect and the coiled-spring appearance created by the intussusceptum being outlined by barium.

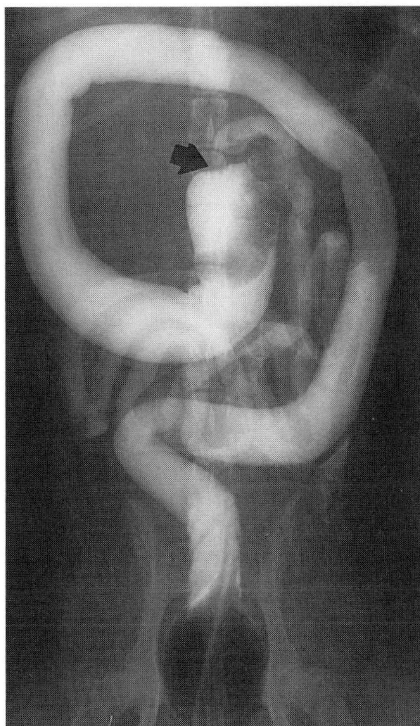

Fig. 47-12 A 14-month-old male Beagle had intermittent diarrhea with shreds of mucosa and blood in the stool for 5 months. On the ventrodorsal view during a barium enema examination, a cecocolic intussusception is visible as a radiolucent filling defect. Note that the remainder of the large bowel, ileocolic junction *(arrow)*, and distal ileum are normal. The cecocolic intussusception had not been visible on two previous barium upper gastrointestinal tract studies.

but benign disease such as adenoma, scar tissue, eosinophilic colitis, and ulcerative colitis may mimic the radiographic findings of a malignant lesion.

ULTRASONOGRAPHIC EVALUATION OF THE LARGE BOWEL

Ultrasonographic evaluation of the colon and cecum follows the same principles that apply to the small intestine but is somewhat limited because of the reflective nature of feces and gas and the thinner wall thickness of the large intestine. The parts of the intestinal wall that are distant to reflective content cannot be assessed. Despite these limitations an assessment of the colon should be part of a standard abdominal ultrasonographic examination. The colon can be identified in a transverse plane in the region of the urinary bladder neck as the only multilayered tubular structure and by the curved shadowing hyperechoic rim emanating from colonic gas or fecal material (Fig. 47-18). In female animals care should be taken to differentiate colon from the uterine body (or stump in neutered animals) which is smaller, lacks wall layering, bifurcates (in intact females), and normally does not contain reflective material. The colon can then be followed cranially, although not always along its entire course. The cecum and ascending colon are best located by first identifying the terminal ileum, which has a prominent muscularis layer and ileocolic junction in the right mid-abdomen, in proximity to the right kidney and caudal duodenal flexure (Fig. 47-19). Contrary to common belief, cats do have a cecum that is ultrasonographically visible. The cecum should not be confused with abnormally distended small bowel loops or other tubular structures. Under optimal conditions five wall layers can be distinguished in the large intestinal wall, similar to the small bowel (see Fig. 47-18). However, the large intestine has a very

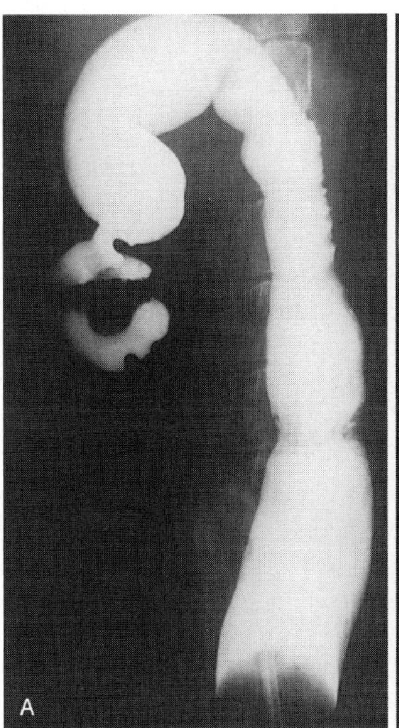

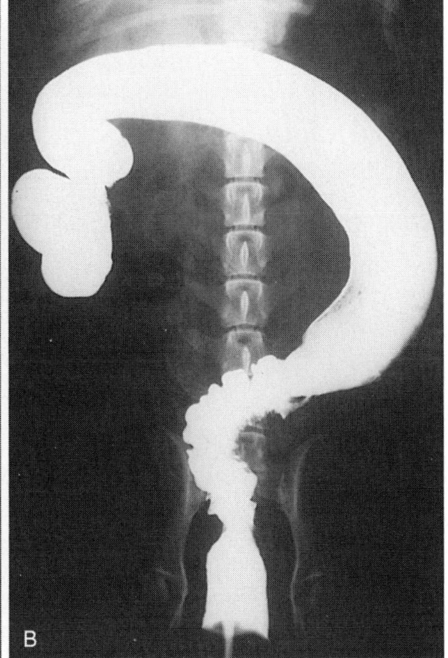

Fig. 47-13 Barium enema examination in two dogs, one with generalized colitis **(A)** and the other with localized colitis **(B)**. Note the nondistensible descending colon and cecum and shortening of the colon in the more advanced and generalized disease. The localized colitis is characterized by nondistensibility and mucosal irregularity of the distal portion of the descending colon.

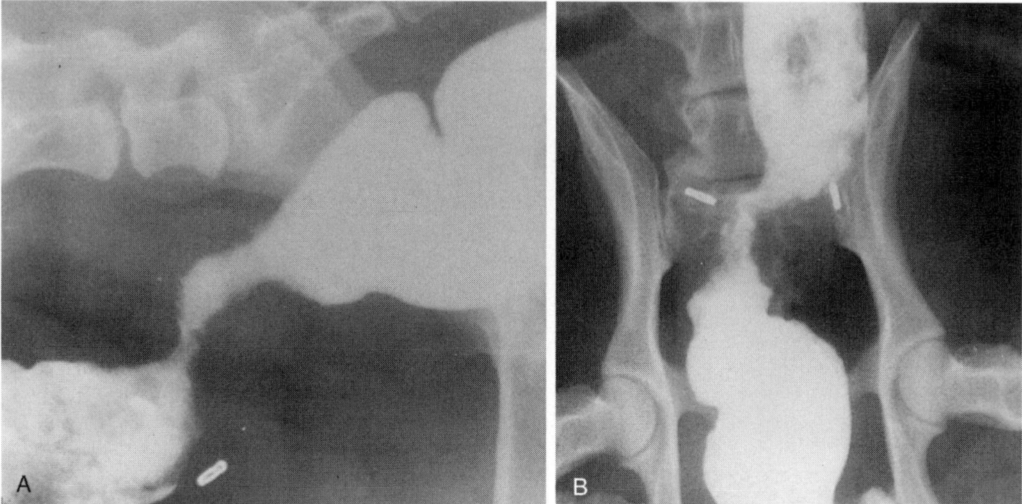

Fig. 47-14 An 11-year-old female, neutered miniature Schnauzer had a 3-year history of straining to defecate with occasional soft and bloody stools. In lateral (**A**) and ventrodorsal (**B**) views of the barium enemation there is an irregular and circumferential narrowing at the junction of the descending colon and rectum. At surgery and biopsy, this narrowing was a benign stricture, presumed to be caused by previous ovariohysterectomy (note surgical clips).

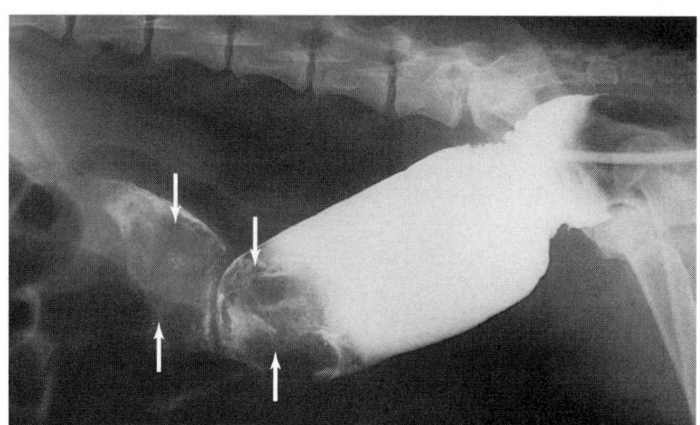

Fig. 47-15 A barium enema study in a 6-year-old female German Shepherd dog. An intraluminal mass *(arrows)* is seen as a polypoid filling defect in the mid-portion of the descending colon. The mass was lymphoma of the colon.

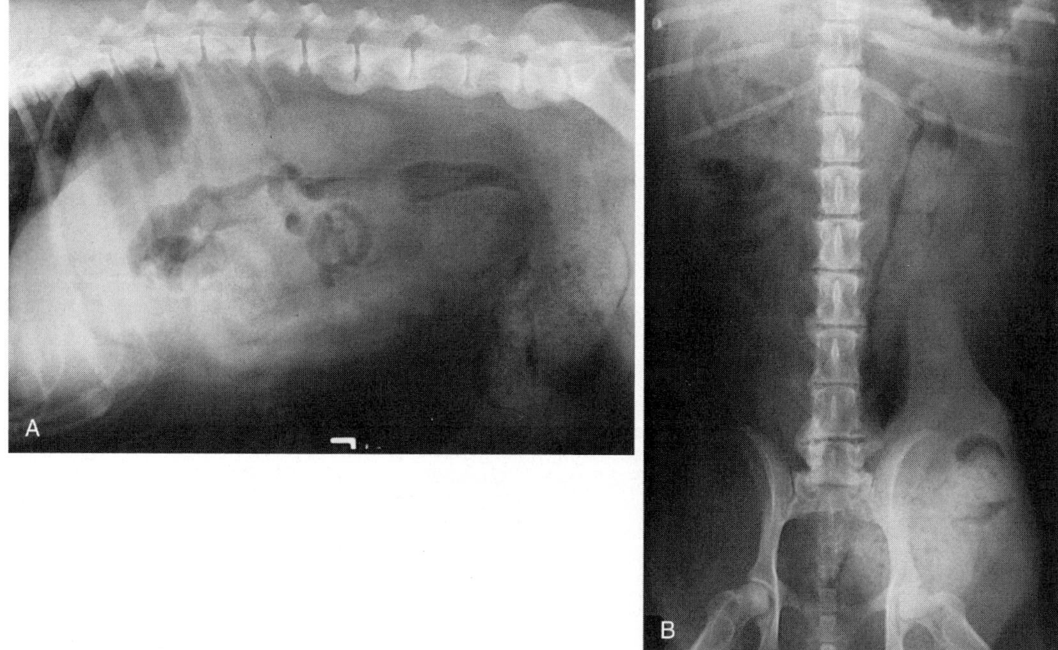

Fig. 47-16 A 17-month-old female, neutered mixed-breed dog had a painful abdomen and lethargy after fighting with a larger dog. In survey lateral (**A**) and ventrodorsal (**B**) radiographs, a localized and dilated feces-filled segment of the descending colon was seen. This represents a partial obstruction, within a left inguinal hernia.

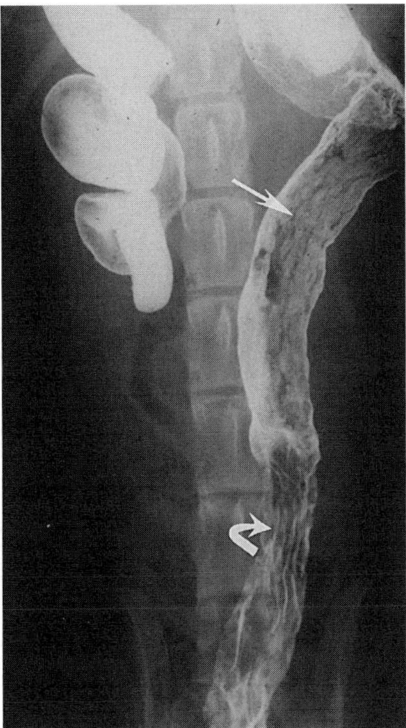

Fig. 47-17 Postevacuation ventrodorsal radiograph of a barium enema. Normal longitudinal mucosal folds of the colon *(curved arrow)* and an abnormal mucosal pattern *(straight arrow)* are visualized. The abnormal area was localized colitis and was not visible on other radiographs obtained with the colon distended with barium.

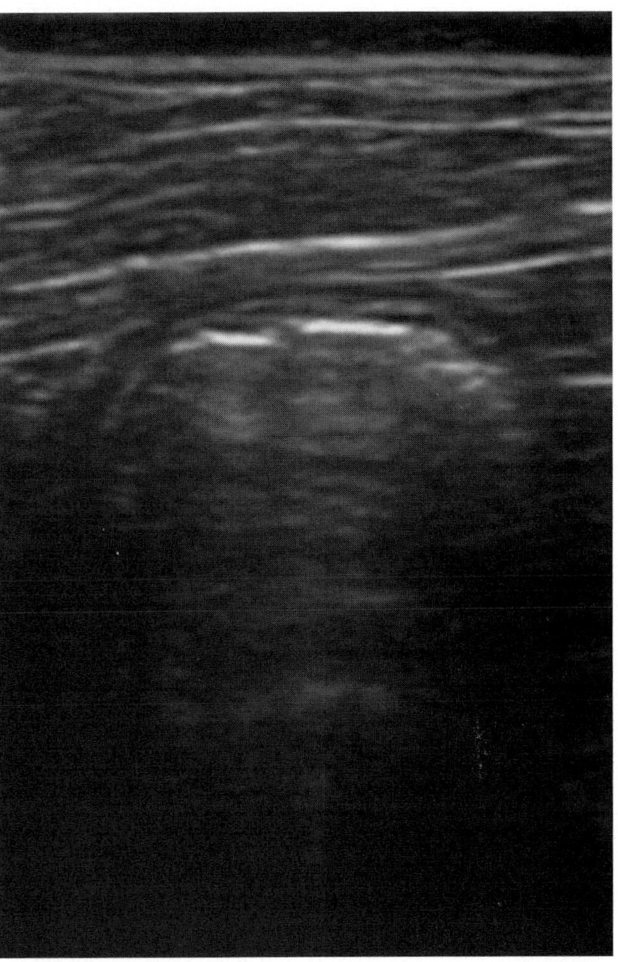

Fig. 47-18 Transverse ultrasonogram of a normal descending colon of a dog. Despite the fact that the wall is thinner (2.5 mm) than that of small bowel, five wall layers with alternating echogenicity can still be distinguished. The colonic content appears as a heterogeneously hyperechoic curved rim with dirty distal shadowing that prohibits assessment of the colon wall in the far field.

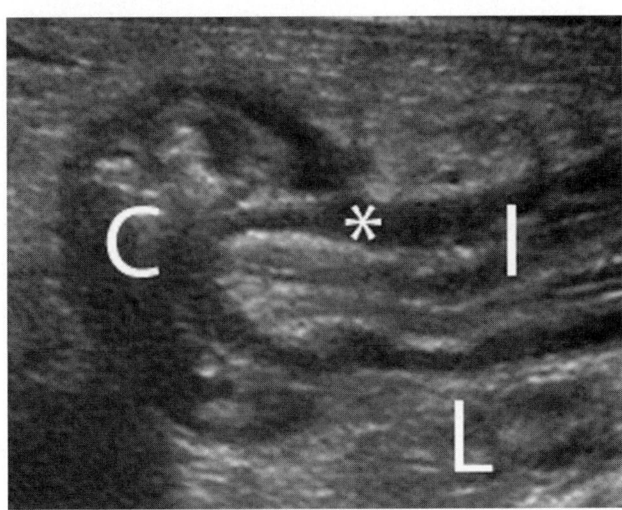

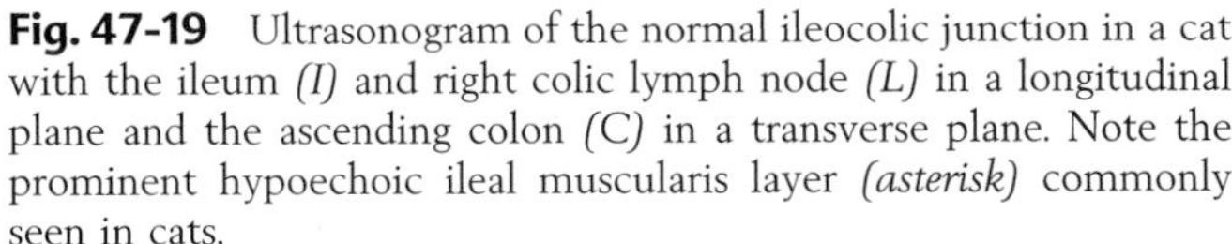

Fig. 47-19 Ultrasonogram of the normal ileocolic junction in a cat with the ileum *(I)* and right colic lymph node *(L)* in a longitudinal plane and the ascending colon *(C)* in a transverse plane. Note the prominent hypoechoic ileal muscularis layer *(asterisk)* commonly seen in cats.

thin wall (2 to 3 mm in dogs, 1.7 mm in cats), and layers are not always distinguishable.[42,43] The colon is accompanied by left, middle, and right colic lymphocenters in the adjacent mesocolon.[44,45] The right colic lymph node is located in the vicinity of the ileocolic junction and is normally visible as a small ovoid structure with a homogenous echogenicity similar to other abdominal lymph nodes (see Fig. 47-19). The middle and left colic lymph nodes, which are adjacent to the transverse and descending colon, respectively, usually are only visible if abnormal. Abnormal lymph nodes are enlarged, often abnormally shaped, hypoechoic, and are indicative of reactive or neoplastic (infiltrative, metastatic) disease (Fig. 47-20). The same differential diagnosis applies to abnormally thick large bowel walls with or without loss of wall layering and mucosal surface irregularities. A distinction between extramural and intramural masses usually can be made. Most ultrasonographic large bowel abnormalities are not specific and should be interpreted along with other imaging findings, lesion extent and, if possible, guided aspirates or biopsy. Intussusception, however, has a pathognomonic ultrasonographic appearance. Juxtaposition of the combined wall layers of the intussuscipiens and intussusceptum creates a concentric ring sign in transverse images and multiple parallel lines with alternating echogenicity in longitudinal views (Fig. 47-21).[17] The mesentery entrapped between the two intestinal segments appears as a hyperechoic region within the lesion. Reducibility of intestinal intussusception depends on tissue viability and intact blood supply and can be predicted with color Doppler studies.[46] Intestinal masses can be involved in intussusception and interrupt the layered appearance. Ulcerations and perforations of the large intestine are quite difficult to diagnose or rule out ultrasonographically with certainty, because colonic reflective material (gas, feces) prohibits evaluation the large bowel wall distant to the reflection. Ultrasonographic assessment of the rectum is best performed intrarectally, which requires an obstetric probe, general anesthesia, and previous bowel evacuation. However, an assessment of the anal and perianal region can be made with a standard small footprint probe with a perianal approach. This allows visualization of the anal gland sacs and evaluation of their possible involvement in perianal masses and fistulae.

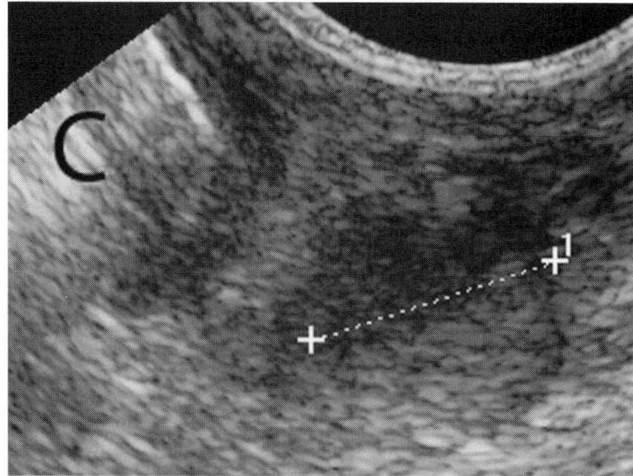

Fig. 47-20 Ultrasonogram of the ascending colon *(C)* in short axis and an adjacent, moderately enlarged (1 cm thick) normoechoic right colic lymph node (between calipers) of a 3-year-old cat with feline infectious peritonitis.

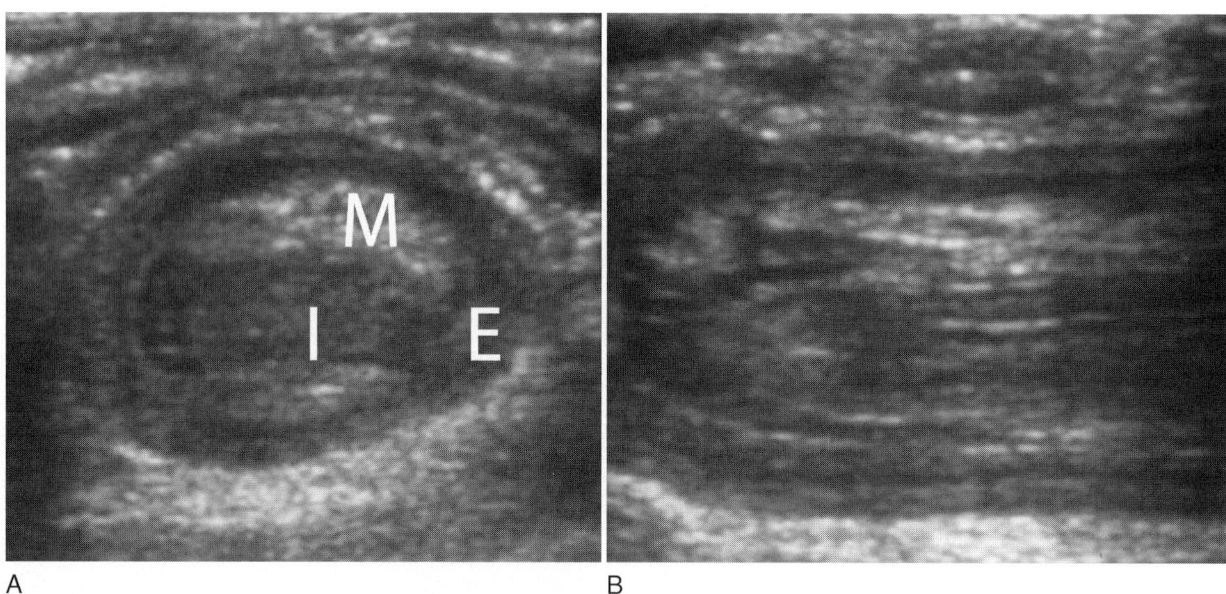

Fig. 47-21 Ultrasonogram in transverse (**A**) and longitudinal (**B**) planes of the descending colon of the same dog as in Figure 47-7. In **A**, note the ringlike juxtaposed wall layers with alternating echogenicity of the external intussuscipiens *(E)* and internal intussusceptum *(I)* (concentric ring sign) as well as the entrapped hyperechoic mesentery between the segments *(M)*. In (**B**) the same wall layers have a parallel orientation.

REFERENCES

1. O'Brien TR: *Radiographic diagnosis of abdominal disorders in the dog and cat,* Davis, CA, 1981, Covell Park Veterinary.
2. Farrow CS, Green R, Shiveley M: *Radiology of the cat,* St Louis, 1995, Mosby.
3. Kealy KJ, McAllister H: *Diagnostic radiology and ultrasonography of the dog and cat,* ed 3, Philadelphia, 2000, WB Saunders.
4. Jergens AE, Willard MD: Diseases of the large intestine. In Ettinger SJ, Feldman EC, editors: *Text book of veterinary internal medicine,* ed 5, Philadelphia, 2000, WB Saunders, p 1238.
5. Lamb CR: Recent developments in diagnostic imaging of the gastrointestinal tract of the dog and cat, *Vet Clin North Am Small Anim Pract* 29:307, 1999.
6. Homco LD: Gastrointestinal tract. In Green R, editor: *Small animal ultrasound,* Philadelphia, 1996, Lippincott Raven.
7. Penninck DG: Ultrasonography of the gastrointestinal tract. In Nyland T, Mattoon J, editors: *Veterinary diagnostic ultrasound,* ed 2, Philadelphia, 2002, WB Saunders.
8. Becker M, Adler L, Parish JF: Rectal lymphangiography in dogs, *Radiology* 91:1037, 1968.
9. Gomez JA, Korobkin M, Lawson TL et al: Selective abdominal angiography in the dog, *J Am Vet Radiol Soc* 14:72, 1973.
10. Krevsky B, Somers MB, Mauere AH et al: Quantitative measurement of feline colonic transit, *Am J Physiol* 255:G529, 1988.
11. Ticer JW: *Radiographic technique in veterinary practice,* ed 2, Philadelphia, 1984, WB Saunders.
12. Kleine LJ, Lamb CR: Comparative organ imaging: the gastrointestinal tract, *Vet Radiol* 30:133, 1989.
13. Brawner WB, Bartels JE: Contrast radiography of the digestive tract: indications, techniques, and complications, *Vet Clin North Am* 13:599, 1983.
14. Seaman WB, Walls J: Complications of the barium enema, *Gastroenterology* 48:728, 1965.
15. Toombs JP, Caywood DD, Lipowitz AJ et al: Colonic perforation following neurosurgical procedures and corticosteroid therapy in four dogs, *J Am Vet Med Assoc* 177:68, 1980.
16. Toombs JP, Collins LG, Graves GM et al: Colonic perforation in corticosteroid-treated dog, *J Am Vet Med Assoc* 188:145, 1986.
17. Lamb CR, Mantis P: Ultrasonographic features of intestinal intussusception in 10 dogs, *J Small Anim Pract* 39:437, 1998.
18. Washabau RJ, Hasler AH: Constipation, obstipation and megacolon. In August JR, editor: *Consultations in feline internal medicine,* ed 3, Philadelphia, 1997, WB Saunders.
19. Matthiesen DT, Scale TD, Whitney WO: Megacolon secondary to pelvic fractures, *Vet Surg* 20:113, 1991.
20. Sharp NJH, Nash AS, Griffiths IR: Feline dysautonomia (Key-Gaskell syndrome): a clinical and pathologic study of forty cases, *J Small Anim Pract* 25:599, 1984.
21. DeForest ME, Gasrur PK: Malformations and the Manx syndrome in cats, *Can Vet J* 2:304, 1979.
22. Jones BR, Gruffydd-Jones TJ, Sparkes AK: Preliminary studies on congenital hypothyroidism in a family of Abyssinian cats, *Vet Rec* 131:145, 1992.
23. Rawlings CA, Capps WF: Rectovaginal fistula and imperforate anus in a dog, *J Am Vet Med Assoc* 159:320, 1971.
24. Fluke MH, Hawkins EC, Elliott GS et al: Short colon in two cats and a dog, *J Am Vet Med Assoc* 195:87, 1989.
25. Jakowski RM: Duplication of colon in a Labrador retriever with abnormal spinal column, *Vet Pathol* 14:256, 1977.
26. Bredal WP, Thoresen SI, Kvellestad A: Atresia coli in a nine week old kitten, *J Small Anim Pract* 35:643, 1994.
27. Longhofer SL, Jackson RK, Cooley AJ: Hindgut and bladder duplication in a dog, *J Am Anim Hosp Assoc* 27:97, 1991.
28. Schlesinger DP, Philbert D, Breur GJ: Agenesis of the cecum and the ascending and transverse colon in a twelve year old cat, *Can Vet J* 33:544, 1992.
29. Shinozaki JK, Sellon RK, Tobias KM et al: Tubular colonic duplication in a dog, *J Am Anim Hosp Assoc* 36:209, 2000.
30. Guffy MM, Wallace L, Anderson NV: Inversion of the cecum into the colon of a dog, *J Am Vet Med Assoc* 156:183, 1970.
31. Kolata RJ, Wright JH: Inflammation and inversion of the cecum in a cat, *J Am Vet Med Assoc* 162:958, 1976.
32. Lansdown ABG, Fox EA: Colorectal intussusception in a young cat, *Vet Record* 19:429, 1991.
33. Carberry CA, Flanders JA: Cecal-colic volvulus in two dogs, *Vet Surg* 22:225, 1993.
34. Drobatz KJ, Hughes D, Hill C et al: Volvulus of the colon in a cat, *J Vet Emerg Crit Care* 6:99, 1996.
35. Hassinger KA: Intestinal entrapment and strangulation caused by rupture of the duodenocolic ligament in four dogs, *Vet Surg* 26:275, 1997.
36. Morris EL: Pneumatosis coli in a dog, *Vet Radiol Ultrasound* 33:154, 1992.
37. Bolton GR, Brown TT: Mycotic colitis in a cat, *Vet Med Small Anim Clin* 67:978, 1972.
38. Birchard SJ, Couto CG, Johnson S: Nonlymphoid intestinal neoplasia in 32 dogs and 14 cats, *J Am Anim Hosp Assoc* 22:533, 1986.
39. Slawienski MJ, Mauldin GE, Mauldin GN et al: Malignant colonic neoplasia in cats, *J Am Vet Med Assoc* 211:878, 1997.
40. Sealer RJ: Colorectal polyps of the dog: a clinicopathologic study of 17 cases, *J Am Vet Med Assoc* 174:72, 1979.
41. Welches CD, Scavelli TD, Aronsohn MG et al: Perineal hernia in the cat: a retrospective study of 40 cases, *J Am Anim Hosp Assoc* 28:431, 1992.
42. Penninck DG, Nyland TG, Fisher PE et al: Ultrasonography of the normal canine gastrointestinal tract, *Vet Radiol* 30:272, 1989.
43. Newell SM, Graham JP, Roberts GD et al: Sonography of the normal feline gastrointestinal tract, *Vet Radiol Ultrasound* 40:40, 1999.
44. Bezuidenhout AJ: The lymphatic system. In Evans HE, editor: *Miller's anatomy of the dog,* ed 3, Philadelphia, 1993, WB Saunders.
45. Pugh CR: Ultrasonographic examination of abdominal lymph nodes in the dog, *Vet Radiol Ultrasound* 35:110, 1994.
46. Patsikas MN, Papazoglou LG, Jakovljevic S et al: Color Doppler ultrasonography in prediction of the reducibility of intussuscepted bowel in 15 young dogs, *Vet Radiol Ultrasound* 46:313, 2005.

ELECTRONIC RESOURCES evolve

Additional information related to the content in Chapter 47 can be found on the companion Web site at evolve http://evolve.elsevier.com/Thrall/vetrad/

- Key Points
- Chapter Quiz
- Case Study 47-1

INDEX

Page numbers followed by f indicate figures; t, tables; b, boxes.

C

D

E

N

Q

R

S

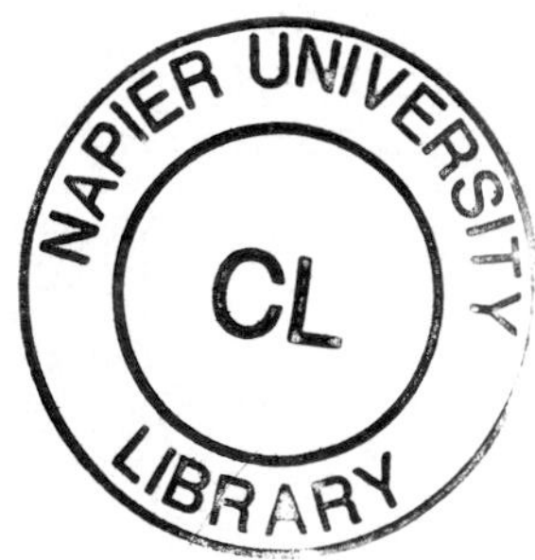